Oxford Textbook of
Palliative Medicine

Free personal online access for 12 months

Individual purchasers of this book are also entitled to free personal access to the online edition for 12 months on *Oxford Medicine Online* (www.oxfordmedicine.com). Please refer to the access token card for instructions on token redemption and access.

Online ancillary materials, where available, are noted at the end of the respective chapters in this book. Additionally, *Oxford Medicine Online* allows you to print, save, cite, email, and share content; download high-resolution figures as Microsoft PowerPoint slides; save often-used books, chapters, or searches; annotate; and quickly jump to other chapters or related material on a mobile-optimised platform.

We encourage you to take advantage of these features. If you are interested in ongoing access after the 12-month gift period, please consider an individual subscription or consult with your librarian.

Oxford Textbook of
Palliative Medicine

FIFTH EDITION

Edited by

Nathan I. Cherny

Marie T. Fallon

Stein Kaasa

Russell K. Portenoy

David C. Currow

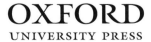

OXFORD
UNIVERSITY PRESS

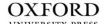
OXFORD
UNIVERSITY PRESS

Great Clarendon Street, Oxford, OX2 6DP,
United Kingdom

Oxford University Press is a department of the University of Oxford.
It furthers the University's objective of excellence in research, scholarship,
and education by publishing worldwide. Oxford is a registered trade mark of
Oxford University Press in the UK and in certain other countries

First Edition published in 1993
Second Edition published in 1998
Third Edition published in 2004
Fourth Edition published in 2010
Fifth Edition published in 2015

Impression: 1

Published in the United States of America by Oxford University Press
198 Madison Avenue, New York, NY 10016, United States of America

British Library Cataloguing in Publication Data
Data available

Library of Congress Control Number: 2014948994

ISBN 978–0–19–965609–7

Printed and bound in Great Britain by
Bell & Bain, Glasgow

Preface

Facing the challenges of continuity and change

This edition is dedicated to the memory of Professor Geoffrey Hanks, one of the three founding editors of the textbook and co-editor of the first four editions, who died in June 2013. The standing and quality of the textbook as a work of academic excellence reflects Geoffrey's legacy that spanned almost four decades as a clinician, researcher, teacher, and editor. He was a man of great compassion, wisdom, humour, personal charm, humility, and courage. He served as a teacher, friend, and colleague to all of us. While we are greatly saddened by his untimely death, we are inspired by his legacy. Professor Hanks did not participate in the editing of this edition, but he entrusted the development of this fifth edition to an international team including Nathan I. Cherny (Israel), Marie T. Fallon (Scotland), Russell K. Portenoy (United States), Stein Kaasa (Norway), and David Currow (Australia).

In developing the textbook, we are constantly listening to the feedback of the thousands of clinicians and researchers who use this text as a resource and as a benchmark of excellence. The new edition has been substantially revamped. It has many new chapters and new authors, and has new sections devoted to assessment tools, issues in patients with cancer, issues of the very young and very old, and research in palliative care. We also have improved the readability and utility of the textbook by producing a smaller and less cumbersome print version and an online version with expanded references, and in some cases, expanded text versions of the chapters. There is extraordinary talent and thoughtfulness in the world of palliative medicine and we invite the readers of this book to contribute to its continued evolution by providing feedback to the editors about the book, as a whole or its individual chapters. The information you provide will be used to develop subsequent editions. Comments can be sent to us at editors@OTPM5.org

The two decades since the first edition of this textbook was published have witnessed truly remarkable growth in palliative care—as a specialty practice for many disciplines, as diverse types of health-care delivery systems, and as an intellectual framework for the development of an evidence base, clinical guidelines, and professional education. Growth of their scale is challenging to master, and brings both uncertainties and optimism about the future. In this process we see the challenge in complex issues of continuity, development, and change.

Continuity: cardinal concepts underlying the philosophy of palliative medicine

Palliative medicine asserts, boldly and optimistically, that even in the face of overwhelming illness, suffering can and must be relieved. This assertion is derived from a rights ethos. There may be individual barriers that patients or families bring to the clinical setting, or larger pragmatic, economic, geopolitical, or social reasons that make it difficult to provide palliative care, but none of these concerns undermine the duty to prioritize the relief of suffering for people with incurable illnesses and the families that support them.

The factors that motivate palliative medicine practitioners to do what they do in the face of great challenges are the underlying axioms of our professional endeavours. These axioms should be clearly articulated because they underlie the personal, professional, and societal investments that address intense human suffering in the context of inexorably progressive illnesses and impending death.

Care, compassion, empathy, and justice

Care is the recognition that the well-being of others is a matter of consequence. As an integral part of the human experience, it is a motivating force that influences the nature and dynamic of interpersonal behaviours. Compassion is that aspect of care that recognizes the emotional dimension of the human experience and encompasses sympathy for another's loss.

Empathy, the ability to perceive and to understand the emotional experience of others and to relate to it in a meaningful and appropriate manner, predicates care and compassion. In the clinical context, an empathic connection occurs when the clinician understands what his or her patient is experiencing, and communicates it (verbally or non-verbally) such that the patient feels that he or she is understood. The empathic connection is often therapeutic in itself. Beyond that, it contributes to a bond which, in turn, facilitates the trust necessary to forge an effective and sustained therapeutic relationship.

Care and empathy interface with the perception of justice. The claim that access to the means to relieve suffering is a human right derives from the empathic experience; that is, that unnecessary suffering is a profound matter of consequence and that it demands a constructive response. Care, compassion, and empathy motivate sensitivity, respect, concern, charity, generosity, altruism, and, sometimes, self-sacrifice. The absence of care implies that the well-being of the other is inconsequential and, in its absence, human interaction is often characterized by insensitivity, neglect or negligence.

Resilience in professional caregiving

In taking on the task of palliative care, a professional caregiver willingly accepts the role as first-hand witness to physical, emotional, and existential distress. Caring for people at the end of life and their families in this context day after day (and, in many cases, for years on end), challenges us as professionals and as individuals. Each member of an interdisciplinary team brings personal needs and resources to the clinical experience, and the different stressors born by members of the team can strain even the best of collaborative relationships.

Resilience is the quality that enables professional caregivers to cope, adapt, and continue giving and growing, despite the tidal surge of suffering that we dare to confront. Resilience is buffered by the skills acquired through years of training, and by dedication and good intentions. As teams, resilience is the flexible, binding matrix that keeps us working constructively together despite stress, conflict, interpersonal frictions, and grievances that would potentially fragment or undermine our ability to deliver care.

Common experience suggests that resilience characterizes most clinicians who choose palliative care as a career. These clinicians are self-motivated and driven to develop the skills and relationships that support their ongoing ability to contextualize and manage the suffering they encounter. Not all who work in palliative care do so by choice, however. Interns, resident staff, nursing students, junior members of the allied health team, administrative and support staffs may find themselves addressing the problems of patients with advanced illness by consignment rather than by choice. For those without the resilience of the clinicians who seek to specialize in palliative care, and without good support systems, this can be a high-stress challenge that can only be endured in an understanding and supportive environment that helps foster coping and resilience.

The patients and families we seek to help have not chosen their fate. How they cope, or are helped to cope, hinges on both the provision of meticulous care and the fostering of resilience in the patient, individual family members, and the family unit as a whole. Some patients come with rich sources of personal and family resilience. Others are overwhelmed. Competent palliative care will always seek to support adaptive coping, and psychological and spiritual healing of both patients and families.

Courage

For the incurably ill, fear may be a part of life. There is just so much to fear: death, physical distress and debilitation, dependency, and so many losses: personal control over biological functioning, mental faculties, potency, beauty, future hopes, separation, and loss of life itself.

Courage takes many forms in the lives of our patients and the families who care for them. They need courage to seek meaning in a life that is now demonstrably finite and to savour the remaining life while grieving for the hopes and dreams that cannot and will not be fulfilled. They need courage to confront difficult decisions about treatment options that have both the potential to either improve quality of life or possibly undermine it. No one wants to live with a gastrostomy, to wear a diaper, to have an intercostal catheter, to have a limb amputated, or to undergo endoscopic stent insertion. For many patients, consenting to even simple interventions requires great courage, and the need to believe that the recommendation is born of both knowledge and compassion.

We often try to support our patients in a process that changes focus from 'everything to live longer' to 'everything to live better'. We must acknowledge that there is great courage in making decisions to desist from, to forgo, or to withdraw treatments or interventions, and sometimes even greater courage than the decision to undergo another gruelling intervention to try live a short time more.

Humility and audacity

The many issues our patients confront pose challenges to the limits of the art and science of palliative medicine. Understanding the limits of what can be reasonably expected from our care underscores the need to present treatment plans with both hope and humility. Often, there is more than one option that is, potentially, of equal benefit for a patient, and, in presenting therapeutic options, we need to explain not only what we know, but also the manifest uncertainties involved.

An excess of optimism or overconfidence about anticipated treatment outcomes poses the risk of undermining one's credibility. At some point, it becomes hubris. Experienced clinicians desist from saying a treatment 'will help', and rather invoke the contingency 'may help.' We must always commit to vigilant monitoring of outcomes and be ready to readdress the treatment with honesty and a commitment to care that encourages and fosters trust.

Honest and humble evaluation of what we can reasonably expect as outcomes of our care makes us aware of the limitations in treatment options, resources, and clinician knowledge that undermine our ability to provide optimal outcomes for all. It is this critical element of humility that provides the impetus for programme development, political activism to improve resource allocation, and research to improve the knowledge base for the delivery of the best patient-centred care that is possible.

Humility should not prevent us from audacious thought, however. The Serenity Prayer implores us to 'Accept the things we cannot change, to change the things we can and to have the wisdom to know the difference'. The issues that we confront in palliative medicine compel us to seek ways to shift the boundaries between the 'things that cannot be changed' and those that are amenable to intervention and change. This is the dimension of audacity and the imperative of research.

Sensitivity to differences

There is no one best way to deal with life-threatening illness and cultural, religious, and interpersonal factors strongly affect individual approaches. Individualized care is grounded in the recognition that human responses to the same event vary dramatically and that only part of this variation is predictable.

Cultural sensitivity also must recognize the heterogeneity of different cultural and religious communities. Indeed reductionist anthropological approaches that foster cultural stereotyping are best avoided in favour of an individualized approach that explores the values and goals of the individual patient and his or her family within his or her environment.

Trust

Through empathy, compassion, honesty, humility, sensitivity, and diligence we aim to develop a bond of trust. We aim to build a trust that is sufficiently robust such that patients and their families feel secure in effective care planning, and develop courage and resilience despite the profound difficulties of their circumstances.

Development: education, service delivery, availability, and therapeutics

Education

The maturing of palliative medicine as a profession has been accompanied by the ongoing development of palliative medicine education and educational resources all over the world.

Globally, the principles and precepts of palliative care are finding a new home in medical education. Palliative care is an excellent framework for teaching the biopsychosocial model of illness and the inter-professional approach to complex health-care problems. Curricula have been developed and published in many countries, universities, and individual faculties; moreover, there is a plethora of teaching models and aids that have been published and disseminated.

Undergraduate training raises consciousness and plants a seed that could germinate and grow during postgraduate education. Clinicians who do not choose to specialize in palliative medicine may or may not encounter a systematic effort to promote competency in generalist-level palliative care during the next phase of training. Much more needs to be done to introduce palliative care into the curriculum of training in every specialty that provides care to populations with serious or life-threatening illness. This is especially true for specialists in oncology, intensive care, geriatrics, neurology, nephrology, cardiology, and pulmonology. In all of these specialties, there have been important developments, such as changes in curriculum, training initiatives, publications, and research. Still, change around the world is inconsistent at best, and at worst, disappointing. Despite evidence of progress, the development of a high level of skill and understanding of palliative medicine remains a goal that has yet to be achieved.

Advanced training in palliative medicine has developed substantially but is still very limited around the world. Palliative medicine is now a recognized medical specialty or subspecialty in over 20 countries, and in others application for specialty or subspecialty accreditation are underway or pending.

There is no consensus as to how to best train palliative medicine specialists. The content and duration of advanced training programmes vary greatly around the globe; it is 1 year in the United States, 4 years in the United Kingdom, and 3 years in Australia. Some programmes insist on a research component and others make no such demand. Given that the level of training not only affects competence and service delivery, but also influences the role and well-being of specialist clinicians working in the field, the issue of adequate training is salient. How best to adequately equip specialist palliative care clinicians remains an open question worthy of further evaluation and research.

Research in palliative care

Preclinical, translational, and clinical research are all badly needed to expand the boundaries of knowledge and provide an evidence base for patient care. This truism is valid for the medical endeavour in general, and is particularly relevant to palliative medicine, in which evidence-based practice is still relatively underdeveloped. The proliferation of research relevant to the care of the incurably ill has been a critical part of the maturation of palliative medicine. Research findings have sharpened our understanding of the mechanisms of symptoms we seek to relieve, helped define the limits of old approaches, and have uncovered new approaches to the challenging problems that have hitherto been refractory to older treatments. Indeed, this edition of the textbook is replete with many new insights and evidence-based therapeutic approaches that have been derived from these research endeavours.

By its nature, research in palliative medicine is very broad in its scope. Palliative care needs research in communication, service delivery, quality, and ethics as much as it needs biomedical and psychological research. Rigorous observational studies and well-crafted clinical trials are both essential at this point. The care of the incurably ill and their families is a 'complex system' challenge requiring multiple inputs, resource allocation, pharmacotherapeutic and psychological skills, and social understanding. All of these factors are increasingly represented in the evolving research culture that we encourage and cultivate.

Some believe that palliative care is unlike other disciplines in that it is not possible to inform practice with rigorous trials. We do not believe this. We must learn from our colleagues in other disciplines and ensure that, whenever possible, we run multisite studies.

Given that access to palliative care around the world largely relies on the referral of people with life-limiting illnesses to specialist services, any research done will help to inform the clinical care of those who are *not* referred. Our colleagues in medicine and other specialties will value high-quality data to inform their care of people with life-limiting illnesses.

The research imperative in palliative medicine faces many challenges. Funding is problematic, despite the new funding initiatives discussed in Chapter 19.1. There are few experienced investigators and the populations under study are vulnerable and may be reluctant or unable to participate. These challenges must be met if the field is to progress.

Service delivery

The past two decades have seen a flourishing of palliative medicine services in different settings worldwide. This has been well documented and monitored by the International Observatory of End of Life Care Project. There is not a region in the world that has not observed growth in palliative medicine services in the past 20 years. While there are areas where penetration and integration are tremendous, there are others in which programme development is still evolving and, unfortunately, many in which services are scarce and rudimentary.

There are now a great many models of palliative medicine service delivery: inpatient and home-based hospices, hospital consultation services, acute palliative care wards and day hospitals, ambulatory clinics, and mobile clinics. Although the underlying principles and philosophy are consistent, the spectrum of observed problems may be profoundly different depending on the care settings.

This is particularly true with the increasing movement towards 'upstream palliative medicine' in which palliative medicine is being delivered at an earlier stage of the trajectory of illness. The issues confronted by clinicians working in early stage palliative medicine units, such as those in acute palliative medicine units, are often quite different from those confronted by clinicians who are providing immediate end-of-life care. The goals of care are different with a greater emphasis on optimizing function and, often, life prolongation (even in the face of progressive incurable disease). In such cases, the duration of care will be prolonged and the fluctuating status of illness (with treatment-induced remissions and relapses) may involve rapidly changing care needs, problem lists, and priorities.

The quality of care that is offered through these services must be measured and responses to variations in the quality of care or its outcomes actively addressed. As in all areas of clinical care, we must each be striving to improve the care offered. In palliative medicine, as in any area of clinical practice, we can and do cause morbidity and, at times, premature mortality. To ensure the ongoing development of the specialty, such outcomes must be acknowledged and critically addressed.

Journals

There are now more than 14 peer-reviewed journals dedicated to issues of palliative care. Additionally, the major journals of many other subspecialties have increasingly embraced palliative care issues. Dedicated palliative care sections in general journals, such as have appeared in *The BMJ, JAMA: The Journal of the American Medical Association*, and the *Journal of Clinical Oncology*, bring palliative care to a wider audience.

Evolution: change and challenges in palliative medicine

One of the early axioms of palliative care is that it sought to provide an alternative to 'aggressive' or 'highly technical' medical care. Indeed palliative care was often presented as 'strong' on care and 'low' on technology. In the 1960s and early 1970s, when these concepts were initially articulated, low technology options were often indeed the very best that could be offered to help relieve patient distress. At that time, there were very few truly effective palliative anti-tumour options beyond radiotherapy, and endoscopy and interventional radiology were in their absolute infancy.

The extraordinary development of non-curative, but potentially beneficial, interventions to address so many of the conditions, symptoms, and complications confronted by patients has created new opportunities, tensions, and dilemmas for palliative medicine clinicians.

New therapeutic opportunities

The last 20 years have seen dramatic changes in the non-curative treatment options for many of the conditions we encounter, particularly in cancer, HIV, and cardiology. These interventions have shifted the natural history of advanced illness. While these interventions cannot cure, they have created new opportunities to prolong life while better controlling the ravages of disease. Some interventions may add months, others, possibly years to survival.

Whereas previously it was often the role of the palliative medicine clinician to present a counterpoint to the high morbidity and low likely benefit of chemotherapy, these developments have necessitated a change. Palliative medicine clinicians now must possess a more sophisticated understanding of disease-modifying palliative approaches for a broad array of common diseases. They often must contribute to a discussion of the risks and burdens versus the potential benefits of these therapies, even as they encourage a broader understanding of the options for care.

New palliative interventions exist not only for specific disease states but also for specific disease complications and symptoms. For example, endoscopic interventions and interventional radiology have radically broadened the range of options in the cases of obstruction of luminal structures (gastrointestinal, genitourinary, vascular, and respiratory). These approaches have altered the management of intestinal, biliary, ureteric, and bronchial obstruction, venous compression syndromes, and, in select cases, pain management. Surgical approaches have made major contributions to the management of complications of cancer such as spinal cord compression, brain metastases, and impending fractures (see Section 12)

Development of a palliative plan of care, and education of the patient and family, requires an understanding of these interventions. Palliative medicine clinicians should be taking an increasing role in the development, evaluation, and advancement of these innovations and developments.

New tensions

Concern is often expressed that the increased availability of technical interventions to relieve distress somehow diminishes from the ability to care, or from the heart of palliative care. The worry is that palliative care is being excessively 'medicalized' or 'professionalized'.

However, just as there is a romantic image of the nineteenth-century physician at the bedside of his patient dying of tuberculosis, who offers perhaps a tincture of opium but primarily provides comfort through his mere presence, there is also a tendency to romanticize the early days of palliative care, which focused on simple symptomatic treatments.

Today, we and the patients we serve have more and better therapeutic options to promote the pursuit of our common goals. Increasingly, palliative care services are integrated with oncology, respiratory medicine, cardiology, and other medical specialties so that appropriate sophisticated treatments may be used with the intent of either palliation or life prolongation (provided that this is a legitimate and compassionate option). This integrated approach needs careful discussion with the patient and their family. This discussion must include clear information about the likelihood of benefits, risks, and alternative approaches.

Many dying patients are not in a rush to die and their desire for life-prolonging treatments is understandable, and often within the bounds of potentially appropriate medical care. Although the World Health Organization's definition of palliative care includes the statement that palliative care 'intends neither to hasten nor postpone death', one must recognize that there is a difference between prolonging dying and prolonging a life in the face of incurable illness. Unfortunately, this distinction is often confused, leading people to believe that non-curative disease-modifying drugs or other high-tech palliative interventions are not part of palliative care. The consequence of this confusion is substantial. Indeed, some patients are denied palliative care services because they are interested in these interventions or treatments, and others are denied access to treatments that would otherwise serve their goals of care because they are in a palliative care clinical pathway.

New challenges

In some countries, the service delivery models for palliative care were developed with the aim of offering a more cost-effective way of managing patients with incurable illness. Many programmes are budgeted based on assumptions of great savings for the health-care funders.

Cost savings is not a primary objective of palliative care, but it may be an unintended consequence of a focus on medically appropriate care guided in shared decision-making by an informed patient and family. It is essential that policymakers understand this principle and also accept that cost savings is an aggregate concept. For some patients, palliative care is not inexpensive. Specialist palliative care always requires intensive skilled human resources, with adequate staff to allow for the provision of individualized care, and it may require costly technology or pharmaceuticals.

When a system of palliative care is supported in a capitated model, financial sustainability requires careful management of the care and a large enough group to benefit from a risk pool. In the United States, many hospices are small and are forced to limit access or deny treatment with accepted palliative interventions because reimbursements are too low. Even large hospices with access to a substantial risk pool cannot accept patients receiving modern chemotherapy and targeted therapy for cancer, even if the treatment is clearly palliative and minimally life-prolonging. How systems like this one, and many others around the world predicated on payment models that have not yet adapted to the evolving nature of palliative care, will cope with an ever-increasing need for services, is unknown. The developed world has resources but re-distribution of funds to underwrite the development and dissemination of specialist palliative care is needed; the developing world lacks resources. Identifying the means to pay for this necessary care is among the greatest challenges we face.

Conclusion

Noting that we may be professional carers now and will be patients later, Professor Balfour Mount has said that 'We are all in the same boat'—we all need the care and the services that form the mission of palliative care. In our professional roles too, we are all in the same boat: despite our varying settings and circumstances, we struggle with a similar spectrum of problems, challenges, and questions.

In this text you will find some of the answers to many of the questions. Humility demands that we recognize that, with what we know, not all of the questions can yet be answered. Indeed, often the best that can be offered is a range of suboptimal options to be considered and possibly tried on a sequential basis. This underlies the imperative to work together to push forward the boundaries of what we know, and improve the way in which we apply it to the care of the incurably ill.

We hope that this fifth edition of the *Oxford Textbook of Palliative Medicine* will help in this endeavour.

Nathan I. Cherny, Jerusalem, Israel
Marie T. Fallon, Edinburgh, United Kingdom
Stein Kaasa, Trondheim, Norway
Russell K. Portenoy, New York, United States
David C. Currow, Adelaide, Australia

Contents

List of Abbreviations

5-FU	5-fluorouracil	BE	bronchial arterial embolization
5-HIAA	5-hydroxyindoleacetic acid	BMI	body mass index
5-HT	5-hydroxytryptamine (serotonin)	BNP	brain natriuretic peptide
5-HTP	5-hydroxytryptophan	BPH	benign prostatic hyperplasia
AAC	augmentative or alternative communication	BPI	Brief Pain Inventory
AAHPM	American Academy of Hospice and Palliative Medicine	BTP	breakthrough pain
		BTX	botulinum toxin
ACD	Anaemia of chronic disease	CAM	complementary and alternative medicine
ACEI	angiotensin-converting enzyme inhibitor	CAUTI	catheter-associated urinary tract infection
ACGME	Accreditation Council for Graduate Medical Education	CBC	complete blood cell
		CBO	carotid blow-out
ACP	advance care planning	CBT	cognitive behavioural therapy
ACPOPC	Association of Physiotherapists in Oncology and Palliative Care	CBT-I	cognitive behaviour therapy for insomnia
		CDS	continuous deep sedation
ACTH	adrenocorticotropic hormone	CEE	Central and Eastern Europe
AD	adjustment disorder	CESCR	Committee on Economic, Social and Cultural Rights
ADLs	activities of daily living		
ADT	androgen deprivation therapy	CES-D	Center for Epidemiologic Studies of Depression Scale
AECOPD	acute exacerbation of chronic obstructive pulmonary disease		
		CF	cystic fibrosis
AED	antiepileptic drug	CGRP	calcitonin gene-related peptide
AFO	ankle–foot orthosis	CHF	congestive heart failure
AIDS	acquired immunodeficiency syndrome	CHPCA	Canadian Hospice Palliative Care Association
ALP	alkaline phosphatase	CI	confidence interval
ALS	amyotrophic lateral sclerosis	CIBP	cancer-induced bone pain
AMPA	α-amino-3-hydroxy-5-methyl-4-isoxazole propionic acid	CIC	clean intermittent catheterization
		CID	clinically important difference
ANC	absolute neutrophil count	CINV	chemotherapy-induced nausea and vomiting
ANH	artificial nutrition and hydration	CIS	Commonwealth of Independent States
ANZSPM	Australian and New Zealand Society of Palliative Medicine	CKD	chronic kidney disease
		CMV	cytomegalovirus
APC	argon plasma coagulation	CNS	central nervous system *or* clinical nurse specialist
APM	Association for Palliative Medicine for the United Kingdom and Ireland	COPD	chronic obstructive pulmonary disease
		COX	cyclooxygenase
APN	advanced practice nurse	CPE	clinical pastoral education
ARB	angiotensin receptor blocker	CPR	cardiopulmonary resuscitation
ASA	acetylsalicylic acid	CPS	clinical prediction of survival
ASCO	American Society of Clinical Oncology	CRP	C-reactive protein
ASHA	American Speech-Language-Hearing Association	CRS-R	Coma Recovery Scale-Revised
ASIC	acid sensing ion channel;	CRQ	Chronic Respiratory Disease Questionnaire
ATF-3	activating transcription factor	CRT	cardiac resynchronization therapy
ATP	adenosine triphosphate	CSF	cerebrospinal fluid
AVP	arginine vasopressin	CSP	Chartered Society of Physiotherapy

CSPCP	Canadian Society of Palliative Care Physicians
CT	computed tomography
CTCAE	Common Terminology Criteria for Adverse Events
CTZ	chemoreceptor trigger zone
CYP	cytochrome P450
DBS	deep brain stimulation
ddC	dideoxycytidine
DIC	disseminated intravascular coagulopathy
DLB	dementia with Lewy bodies
DM	dermatomyositis
DME	durable medical equipment
DNI	do not intubate
DNR	do not resuscitate
DSM	*Diagnostic and Statistical Manual of Mental Disorders*
DVIU	direct vision internal urethrotomy
DVT	deep vein thrombosis
EACA	epsilon aminocaproic acid
EAPC	European Association for Palliative Care
EAS	euthanasia or physician-assisted suicide
EBM	evidence-based medicine
EBP	evidence-based practice
ECEPT	Eastern and Central Europe Palliative Task Force
ECMO	extracorporeal membrane oxygenation
ECOG	Eastern Cooperative Oncology Group
ECT	electrochemotherapy
EEG	electroencephalography
EFGR	epidermal growth factor receptor
EFNS	European Federation of Neurological Societies
EFPPEC	Educating Future Physicians in Palliative and End-of-Life Care
EHR	electronic health record
EP	endoprostinoid
EPA	eicosapentaenoic acid
EPEC	Education in Palliative and End of Life Care
EPEC-EM	Education in Palliative and End of Life Care for Emergency Medicine
ERCP	endoscopic retrograde cholangiopancreatography
ESA	erythropoietin-stimulating agent
ESAS	Edmonton Symptom Assessment System
ESMO	European Society of Medical Oncology
ESKD	end-stage kidney disease
ESS	Epworth Sleepiness Scale
EU	European Union
FACIT-F	Functional Assessment of Chronic Illness Therapy—Fatigue
FACIT-Sp	Functional Assessment of Chronic Illness Therapy—Spiritual
FDA	Food and Drug Administration
FDG	fluorodeoxyglucose
FEV_1	forced expiratory volume in 1 second
FFGT	family-focused grief therapy
FIM	Functional Independence Measure
fMRI	functional magnetic resonance imaging
FPZV	Federatie Palliatieve Zorg Vlaanderen vzw
FTC	Federal Trade Commission
GABA	gamma-aminobutyric acid
GBD	Global Burden of Disease
G-CSF	granulocyte colony-stimulating factor

GDP	gross domestic product
GGT	gamma-glutamyl transferase
GI	gastrointestinal
GnRH	gonadotropin-releasing hormone
GORD	gastro-oesophageal reflux disease
GP	general practitioner
GPCR	G protein-coupled receptor
GRK	G protein coupled receptor kinase
GVHD	graft-versus-host disease
HAART	highly active antiretroviral therapy
HADS	Hospital Anxiety and Depression Scale
HCC	hepatocellular carcinoma
HCV	hepatitis C virus
HF	heart failure
HFPEF	heart failure with preserved ejection fraction
HFREF	heart failure with reduced ejection fraction
HIPEC	hyperthermic intraperitoneal chemotherapy
HIT	health information technology
HIV	human immunodeficiency virus
HNC	head and neck cancer
HPA	hypothalamic–pituitary–adrenal
HPNA	Hospice and Palliative Nurses Association
HPV	human papilloma virus
HRO	high-reliability organization
HRQOL	health-related quality of life
HRW	Human Rights Watch
IAHPC	International Association of Hospice and Palliative Care
IASP	International Association for the Study of Pain
ICD	implantable cardioverter defibrillator
ICESCR	International Covenant of Economic, Social and Cultural Rights
ICP	integrated care pathway *or* intracranial pressure
ICPCN	International Children's Palliative Care Network
ICU	intensive care unit
IDT	interdisciplinary team
IGF	insulin-like growth factor
IL	interleukin
ILF	International Lymphoedema Framework
IM	intramuscular
IMCP	individual meaning-centered psychotherapy
IMRT	intensity-modulated radiotherapy
INCB	International Narcotics Control Board
INED	Institut national d'études démographiques
INR	international normalized ratio
INSTI	integrase strand transfer inhibitor
IOELC	International Observatory on End of Life Care
IOM	Institute of Medicine
IPT	interpersonal psychotherapy
IV	intravenous
KNMG	Koninklijke Nederlandsche Maatschappij tot bevordering der Geneeskunst
KPS	Karnofsky Performance Status
LHRH	Luteinizing Hormone-Releasing Hormone
LIS	locked-in state
LMWH	low-molecular-weight heparin
LP	lumbar puncture
LST	life-sustaining treatment
LVAD	left ventricular assist device

M3G	morphine-3-glucuronide	NS	nociceptive specific
M6G	morphine-6-glucuronide	NSAID	non-steroidal anti-inflammatory drug
MAC	*Mycobacterium avium* complex	NSCLC	non-small cell lung cancer
MAOI	monoamine oxidase inhibitor	NTS	nucleus tractus solitarius
MBO	malignant bowel obstruction	NV	nausea and vomiting
MBSR	mindfulness-based stress reduction	NYHA	New York Heart Association
MCC	mucociliary clearance	OIH	opioid-induced hypersensitivity
MCS	motor cortex stimulation	OOH	out of hours
MDASI	MD Anderson Symptom Inventory	ORN	osteoradionecrosis
MDT	multidisciplinary team	OSF	Open Society Foundations
MID	minimal important difference	OT	occupational therapist
MLD	manual lymphatic drainage	OTFC	oral transmucosal fentanyl citrate
MLT	melatonin	PAG	periaqueductal grey
MMSE	Mini-Mental Status Examination	PaP	Palliative Prognostic
MND	motor neurone disease	PAS	physician-assisted suicide
MoCA	Montreal Cognitive Assessment	PCU	palliative care unit
MP	megestrol acetate	PD	Parkinson's disease
MPA	medroxyprogesterone acetate	PDE	principle of double effect
MPAC	Memorial Pain Assessment Card	PDI	Patient Dignity Inventory
MPQ	McGill Pain Questionnaire	PE	pulmonary embolism
MRA	mineralocorticoid antagonist	PEG	percutaneous endoscopic gastrostomy
MRC	Medical Research Council	PEPFAR	President's Emergency Plan for AIDS Relief
MRCP	magnetic resonance cholangiopancreatography	PET	positron emission tomography
MRI	magnetic resonance imaging	PFR	pulsed radiofrequency
MSA	multiple system atrophy	PG	prostaglandin
MSAS	Memorial Symptom Assessment Scale	PHQ-4	Patient Health Questionnaire-4
MSM	men who have sex with men	PI	protease inhibitor
NASW	National Association of Social Workers	PICU	paediatric intensive care unit
NaV	sodium channel	PIL	patient information leaflet
NCC	National Consensus Conference	PiPS	Prognosis in Palliative care Study
NCCAM	National Center of Complementary and Alternative Medicine	PJP	*Pneumocystis jirovecii* pneumonia
		PM&R	Physical medicine and rehabilitation
NCCN	National Comprehensive Cancer Network	PML	progressive multifocal leucoencephalopathy
NCI	National Cancer Institute	PNS	paraneoplastic neurological syndrome
NCPB	neurolytic coeliac plexus block	PO	*per os* (orally)
NCTC	National Collection of Type Culture	POAH	preoptic and anterior hypothalamus
NEST	Needs at the End-of-Life Screening Tool	POS	Palliative care Outcomes Scale
NEWS	National Early Warning Score	PPCS	Pain and Palliative Care Society
NGF	nerve growth factor	PPI	Palliative Prognostic Index *or* proton pump inhibitor
NGO	non-governmental organization		
NGT	nasogastric tube	PPS	Palliative Performance Scale
NHPCO	National Hospice and Palliative Care Organization	PPV	positive predictive value
NHS	National Health Service	PRN	*pro re nata* (as needed)
NICE	National Institute for Health and Care Excellence	PRO	patient-reported outcome
NIH	National Institutes of Health	PROM	patient-reported outcome measure
NK1	neurokinin 1	PROMIS*	Patient-Reported Outcome Measurement Information System*
NIPPV	non-invasive positive pressure ventilation		
NIV	non-invasive ventilation	PSP	progressive supranuclear palsy
NLSB	neurolytic lumbar sympathetic block	PSQI	Pittsburgh Sleep Quality Index
NMDA	*N*-methyl-D-aspartate receptor	PT	physiotherapist *or* physical therapy
NMT	neurologic music therapy	PTC	percutaneous transhepatic cholangiography
NNH	number needed to harm	PTHrP	parathyroid hormone-related peptide
NNRTI	non-nucleoside reverse transcriptase inhibitor	PTSD	post-traumatic stress disorder
NNT	number needed to treat	PVS	persistent vegetative state
NRTI	nucleoside reverse transcriptase inhibitor	QI	quality improvement
NP	nurse practitioner	QOL	quality of life
NPV	negative predictive value	RANK	receptor activator of nuclear factor kappa B
NRS	numerical rating scale	RANKL	ligand for the receptor activator of nuclear factor kappa B
NRTI	nucleoside reverse transcriptase inhibitor		

RAVE	receptor activation versus endocytosis	TACO	transfusion-associated circulatory overload
RBF	renal blood flow	TAE	transcatheter arterial embolization
RBD	REM sleep behaviour disorder	TBI	traumatic brain injury
RCP	Royal College of Physicians	TCA	tricyclic antidepressant
RCSLT	Royal College of Speech and Language Therapists	tDCS	transcranial direct current stimulation
RCT	randomized controlled trial	TENS	transcutaneous electrical nerve stimulation
REM	rapid eye movement	THC	delta (9)-tetrahydrocannabinol
RF	radiofrequency	TMS	transcranial magnetic stimulation
RFA	radiofrequency ablation	TNF-α	tumour necrosis factor-alpha
RGS	regulators of G-protein signalling	TRP	transient receptor potential
RLS	restless legs syndrome	TRPM8	transient receptor potential menthol receptor
R/S	religious/spiritual	TRVP1	transient receptor potential cation channel
RSCL	Rotterdam Symptom Checklist		subfamily V member 1 (capsaicin receptor/
rTMS	repetitive transcranial magnetic stimulation		vanilloid receptor 1)
RVM	rostroventral medial medulla	TSH	thyroid stimulating hormone
SC	subcutaneous	TURP	transurethral resection of prostate
SCC	spinal cord compression	UACS	upper airway cough syndrome
SCI	problem solving	UFH	unfractionated heparin
SD	standard deviation	UN	United Nations
SDH	superficial dorsal horn	UV	ultraviolet
SDS	Symptom Distress Scale	USAID	United States Agency for International
SEMS	self-expandable metal stent		Development
SGD	salivary gland dysfunction	USRDS	United States Renal Data System
SIAD	syndrome of inappropriate diuresis	VAD	ventricular assist device
SLT	speech and language therapy/therapist	VAS	visual analogue scale
SNRI	serotonin-norepinephrine reuptake inhibitor	VC	vomiting centre
SPARC-45	Sheffield Profile for Assessment and Referral to Care	VDS	visual descriptive scale
		VEGF	vascular endothelial growth factor
SPEED	Screen for Palliative and End-of-life care needs in the Emergency Department	VGCC	voltage-gated calcium channels
		VIP	vasoactive intestinal peptide
SRH	self-rated health	VTE	venous thromboembolism
SSRI	selective serotonin reuptake inhibitor	WBP	wound bed preparation
SUPPORT	Study to Understand Prognosis and Preferences for the Outcomes and Risks of Treatment	WDR	wide dynamic range
		WHO	World Health Organization
SWS	slow-wave sleep	WHOQOL	World Health Organization Quality of Life
TA	tranexamic acid	WPCA	Worldwide Palliative Care Alliance

List of Contributors

Amy P. Abernethy, Center for Learning Health Care, Duke Clinical Research Institute, Duke University School of Medicine, Durham, NC, USA

Janet L. Abrahm, Department of Psychosocial Oncology and Palliative Care, Dana-Farber Cancer Institute, Boston, MA; Harvard Medical School, Boston, MN, USA

Andy Adam, Department of Physical Medicine and Rehabilitation, Mayo Clinic, MN, USA

Michael L. Adams, Anesthesiologist, Private Practice, Las Vegas, NV, USA

Meera Agar, Department of Palliative Care and Supportive Services, Flinders University, Braeside Hospital HammondCare, Sydney, NSW, Australia

Yesne Alici, Department of Psychiatry and Behavioral Sciences, Memorial Sloan Kettering Cancer Center, New York, NY, USA

Terry Altilio, Department of Pain Medicine and Palliative Care, Beth Israel Medical Center, New York, NY, USA

Limor Amit, Department of Medical Oncology, Davidoff Cancer Center, Beilinson Hospital, Petach Tikvah, Israel

Bethany M. Andrews, School of Nursing, Vanderbilt University, Nashville, TN, USA

Barry R. Ashpole, Guelph, ON, Canada

Thomas M. Atkinson, Department of Psychiatry and Behavioral Sciences, Memorial Sloan Kettering Cancer Center, New York, NY, USA

Brian Badgwell, Department of Surgery, MD, Anderson Cancer Center, Houston, TX, USA

Lea Baider, Psychological Services, Assuta Hospital, Tel Aviv; Hebrew University, Jerusalem, Israel

Vickie E. Baracos, Department of Oncology, University of Alberta, Edmonton, AB, Canada

Jane Ellen Barr, WOC Patient Care Services, Department of Nursing Administration, North Shore-LIJ Health System; Long Island Jewish Medical Center, New Hyde Park, NY, USA

Jeffrey R. Basford, Department of Physical Medicine and Rehabilitation, Mayo Clinic, MN, USA

Steven Bayles, Vanderbilt-Bill Wilkerson Center for Otolaryngology and Communication Sciences, Nashville, TN, USA

Michael I. Bennett, Academic Unit of Palliative Care, Leeds Institute of Health Sciences, School of Medicine, University of Leeds, Leeds, UK

Rachelle Bernacki, Department of Psychosocial Oncology and Palliative Care, Dana-Farber Cancer Institute, Boston, MA, USA

Cheryl R. Billante, Vanderbilt Voice Center, Nashville, TN, USA

Craig D. Blinderman, Adult Palliative Care Services, Center for Supportive Care & Clinical Ethics, Department of Medicine, Columbia University, New York, NY, USA

Stewart Bond, Research Assistant Professor, Vanderbilt University School of Nursing, Nashville, TN, USA

Georg Bosshard, Clinic for Geriatric Medicine, Zurich University Hospital; Center on Aging and Mobility, University of Zurich, Zurich, Switzerland

Mark Bower, National Centre for HIV Malignancy, Chelsea & Westminster Hospital, London, UK

Ruth Branford, Greenwich & Bexley Community Hospice, London, UK

William S. Breitbart, Chairman, Department of Psychiatry and Behavioral Sciences, Memorial Sloan Kettering Cancer Center, New York, NY, USA

Frank Brennan, Department of Palliative Care, Calvary and St George Hospitals, Kogarah, Sydney, Australia

Jennifer Brodeur, Palliative Care Unit, Division of Palliative Care, The Ottawa Hospital; Bruyère Continuing Care, University of Ottawa, Ottawa, ON, Canada

Eduardo Bruera, Department of Palliative Care & Rehabilitation Medicine, The University of Texas MD Anderson Cancer Center, Houston, TX, USA

Kirsty Campbell, Department of Pain Medicine and Palliative Care, The Children's Hospital at Westmead, Sydney, Australia

Augusto Caraceni, Fondazione IRCCS Istituto Tumori di Milano, Milan, Italy; European Palliative Care Research Centre, Norwegian University of Science and Technology, Trondheim, Norway

David Casarett, Professor of Medicine, Director of Hospice and Palliative Care, University of Pennsylvania, Philadelphia, PA, USA

J. Brian Cassel, Division of Hematology/Oncology & Palliative Care, Massey Cancer Center, Virginia Commonwealth University, Richmond, VA, USA

Barrie R. Cassileth, Memorial Sloan Kettering Cancer Center, New York, NY, USA

Kin-Sang Chan, Department of Medicine, Haven of Hope Hospital, Tseung Kwan O, Hong Kong

Victor T. Chang, Rutgers—New Jersey Medical School, Section Hematology Oncology; VA New Jersey Health Care System, East Orange, NJ, USA

Martin Chasen, Elisabeth Bruyere Hospital and University of Ottawa, Ottawa, ON, Canada

Nathan I. Cherny, Shaare Zedek Medical Center, Jerusalem, Israel

Andrea L. Cheville, Associate Professor, Department of Physical Medicine and Rehabilitation, Mayo Clinic, MN, USA

Harvey Max Chochinov, Department of Psychiatry, Faculty of Medicine, University of Manitoba; Manitoba Palliative Care Research Unit, CancerCare Manitoba, Winnipeg, MB, Canada

Katherine Clark, Calvary Mater Newcastle, The University of Newcastle, Newcastle, Australia

Josephine M. Clayton, HammondCare Palliative and Supportive Care Service, Greenwich Hospital, Sydney; Sydney Medical School, University of Sydney, Sydney, Australia

Anthony J. Cmelak, Associate Professor, Department of Radiation Oncology, Vanderbilt-Ingram Cancer Center, Nashville, TN, USA

John J. Collins, Department of Pain Medicine and Palliative Care, The Children's Hospital at Westmead, Sydney, Australia

Lesley A. Colvin, Department of Anaesthesia, Critical Care & Pain Medicine, Western General Hospital, Edinburgh, UK

Jill Cooper, The Royal Marsden NHS Foundation Trust, London, UK

Michael J. Cousins, Pain Management & Research Centre, University of Sydney, Royal North Shore Hospital, Sydney, NSW, Australia

Sarah Cox, Department of Palliative Care, Chelsea and Westminster NHS Foundation Trust and Trinity Hospice, London, UK

LaVera Crawley, Assistant Professor (Research), Department of Paediatrics, Stanford University Center for Biomedical Ethics, California, CA, USA

Ricardo A. Cruciani, Director, Center for Comprehensive Pain Medicine and Palliative Care, Institute for Neurosciences, Capital Health Medical Center, Hopewell, NJ, USA

David C. Currow, Discipline of Palliative and Supportive Services, Flinders University, Adelaide, SA, Australia

David Dahan, Department of Intensive Care, Shaare Zedek Medical Center, Jerusalem, Israel

Patricia M. Davidson, School of Nursing, Johns Hopkins University, Baltimore, MD, USA

Isobel Davidson, School of Health Sciences, Queen Margaret University, Edinburgh, UK

Andrew N. Davies, Supportive & Palliative Care Department, Royal Surrey County Hospital NHS Foundation Trust, Guildford, UK

Liliana De Lima, International Association for Hospice and Palliative Care, Houston, TX, USA

Luc Deliens, End-of-Life Care Research Group, Vrije Universiteit Brussel and Ghent University, Brussels, Belgium; Department of Public and Occupational Health, EMGO Institute for Health and Care Research, VU University Medical Centre, Amsterdam, The Netherlands

Jane deLima Thomas, Instructor in Medicine, Harvard Medical School; Attending Physician, Department of Psychosocial Oncology and Palliative Care, Dana-Farber Cancer Institute, Boston, MA, USA

Gary Deng, Integrative Medicine Service, Memorial Sloan Kettering Cancer Center, New York, NY, USA

Paul L. DeSandre, Emory Palliative Care Center and Department of Emergency Medicine, Emory University School of Medicine, Atlanta, GA, USA

Lara Dhingra, Director, Health Disparities and Outcomes Research, MJHS Institute for Innovation in Palliative Care, New York, NY, USA

Anthony H. Dickenson, Department of Neuroscience, Physiology and Pharmacology, University College London, London, UK

Matthew Doolittle, Department of Psychiatry and Behavioral Sciences, Memorial Sloan-Kettering Cancer Center, New York, NY, USA

Ellie Dowling, Vanderbilt-Bill Wilkerson Center for Otolaryngology and Communication Sciences, Nashville, TN, USA

Alexandra M. Easson, Attending Physician, Mount Sinai Hospital; Assistant Professor, Department of Surgery, University of Toronto, Toronto, ON, Canada

Wendy Edmonds, Department of Pain Medicine and Palliative Care, The Children's Hospital at Westmead, Sydney, Australia

Sharon Einav, Department of Intensive Care, Shaare Zedek Medical Center, Jerusalem, Israel

Jackie Ellis, Post Doctoral Research Fellow, Academic Palliative and Supportive Care Studies (APSCS), University of Liverpool, UK

Frank Elsner, Department of Palliative Medicine, RWTH Aachen University, Aachen, Germany

Linda L. Emanuel, Buehler Center on Aging, Health & Society, Feinberg School of Medicine, Northwestern University, Chicago, IL, USA

Anne M. English, Dove House Hospice/Humber NHS Foundation Trust, Hull, UK

Christopher P. Evans, Department of Urology, University of California, Davis School of Medicine and Comprehensive Cancer Center, Sacramento, CA, USA

Marie T. Fallon, Edinburgh Cancer Research Centre, Institute of Genetic and Molecular Medicine, Edinburgh, UK

John T. Farrar, Associate Professor of Epidemiology, University of Pennsylvania, Philadelphia, PA, USA

Kenneth C. H. Fearon, Professor of Surgical Oncology, Consultant Colorectal Surgeon, Edinburgh, Scotland

Nanna Brix Finnerup, Danish Pain Research Center, Department of Clinical Medicine, Aarhus University Hospital, Aarhus, Denmark

Joseph J. Fins, Weill Cornell Medical College, New York, NY, USA

Katie Fitzgerald Jones, Nurse Practitioner Palliative Care, Hebrew Senior Life, Beth Isreal Deconess Hospital and Harvard Medical School; Dana-Farber Cancer Institute, Boston, MA, USA

Kate Flemming, Department of Health Sciences, University of York, York, UK

David C. Free, National Palliative Care Coordinator, Seasons Hospice & Palliative Care, Baltimore, MD, USA

Anne Marie Flores, Assistant Professor of Orthopaedics and Rehabilitation, Vanderbilt University Medical Center, Nashville, TN, USA

Karen Forbes, Department of Palliative Medicine, Bristol Haematology and Oncology Centre, University of Bristol and University Hospitals Bristol NHS Trust, Bristol, UK

Nicos I. Fotiadis, Palliative Care & Rehabilitation Medicine, MD Anderson Cancer Center, Houston, TX, USA

Deborah Julie Franklin, Department of Rehabilitation Medicine, Thomas Jefferson University Health System, Philadelphia, PA, USA

Judith Frost, Department of Pain Medicine and Palliative Care, The Children's Hospital at Westmead, Sydney, Australia

Reena George, Christian Medical College, Vellore, India

Georgina Gethin, School of Nursing and Midwifery, National University of Ireland, Galway, Ireland

Hans Gerdes, Attending Physician, Director of GI Endoscopy, Memorial Sloan-Kettering Cancer Center; Professor of Clinical Medicine, Weill Medical College of Cornell University, New York, NY, USA

Margaret Gibbs, St Christopher's Hospice, Sydenham, London, UK

Jane Gibbins, Cornwall Hospice Care, Royal Cornwall Hospital Trust and Peninsula Medical School

Gordon Giddings, Elisabeth Bruyere Hospital and University of Ottawa, Ottawa, ON, Canada

Afaf Girgis, Psycho-Oncology Research Group, Ingham Institute for Applied Medical Research, University of New South Wales, Liverpool, NSW, Australia

Paul Glare, Palliative Medicine Service, Department of Medicine, Memorial Sloan Kettering Cancer Center, New York; Department of Medicine, Weill Cornell Medical College, New York, NY, USA

Richard M. Gordon-Williams, Medical doctor, Neuroscience, Physiology and Pharmacology, University College, London, UK

Patricia Grocott, Reader in Palliative Wound Care, Department of Postgraduate Research, Florence Nightingale School of Nursing and Midwifery, King's College London, London, UK

Liz Gwyther, School of Public Health and Family Medicine, University of Cape Town, Cape Town, South Africa

Richard D.W. Hain, Children's Hospital, Cardiff, UK

Kirsten Haman, Assistant Professor of Clinical Psychiatry, Department of Psychiatry, Vanderbilt University Medical Center, Nashville, TN, USA

George Handzo, HealthCare Chaplaincy Network, New York, NY, USA

Joy Hao, Assistant Professor in Clinical Health Sciences, Department of Family Medicine, Center for Behavioral and Addiction Medicine, University of California, Los Angeles, CA, USA

Janet R. Hardy, Department of Supportive and Palliative Care, Mater Health Services, Mater Research—University of Queensland, Brisbane, QLD, Australia

Dagny Faksvåg Haugen, Regional Centre of Excellence for Palliative Care, Western Norway, Haukeland University Hospital, Bergen; Department of Clinical Medicine K1, University of Bergen, Bergen, Norway

Alric D. Hawkins, Psychiatrist, Houston Methodist Hospital, Houston, TX, USA

John H. Healey, Memorial Sloan-Kettering Cancer Center, New York; Weill Medical College of Cornell University, New York, NY, USA

Irene J. Higginson, Cicely Saunders Institute, Faculty of Life Sciences and Medicine, King's College London, London, UK

Amanda Hordern, Bayside Healthy Living, Hampton, VIC, Australia

Robert Horton, Palliative Medicine Consultant, Department of Medicine, Dalhousie University, QEII Health Sciences Centre, Halifax, NS, Canada

Annmarie Hosie, The University of Notre Dame Australia, School of Nursing, Darlinghurst, NSW, Australia

Peter J. Hoskin, Consultant in Clinical Oncology, Mount Vernon Cancer Centre, Middlesex; Professor in Clinical Oncology, University College London, UK

Jane M. Ingham, UNSW Australia, Faculty of Medicine, St Vincent's Clinical School, Cunningham Centre for Palliative Care, Sacred Heart Health Service, Darlinghurst, NSW, Australia

Troels Staehelin Jensen, Danish Pain Research Center and Department of Neurology, Aarhus University Hospital, Aarhus, Denmark

Rebecca Johnson, Buehler Center on Aging, Health & Society, Northwestern University, Feinberg School of Medicine, Chicago, IL, USA

Stein Kaasa, European Palliative Care Research Centre (PRC), Department of Cancer Research and Molecular Medicine, Faculty of Medicine, Norwegian University of Science and Technology (NTNU); St. Olavs Hospital, Trondheim University Hospital, Trondheim, Norway; Cancer

Clinic, St. Olavs Hospital, Trondheim University Hospital, Trondheim, Norway

Menelaos Karanikolas, Department of Anesthesiology, Washington University School of Medicine, St. Louis, MO, USA

Michael Kearney, Medical Director of the Palliative Care Service, Santa Barbara Cottage Hospital, Santa Barbera, CA, USA

Vaughan Keeley, Consultant in Palliative Medicine, Derby, UK

Jeremy Keen, Highland Hospice, Inverness, UK

Jonathan Koffman, Cicely Saunders Institute, Department of Palliative Care, Policy and Rehabilitation, King's College London, London, UK

Helena Knotkova, Director of Clinical Studies and Analytics, MJHS Institute for Innovation in Palliative Care, New York, NY, USA

Rae Lynne Kinler, Department of Pain Medicine and Palliative Care, Beth Israel Medical Center, New York, NY, USA

Timothy W. Kirk, City University of New York, York College, New York, NY, USA

David W. Kissane, Department of Psychiatry, Monash University, Clayton, VIC, Australia; Department of Psychiatry, Weill Medical College of Cornell University; Department of Psychiatry and Behavioral Sciences, Memorial Sloan-Kettering Cancer Center, New York, NY, USA

Nina Kite, The Royal Marsden NHS Foundation Trust, London, UK

Danielle N. Ko, Department of Palliative and Supportive Care, Royal Melbourne Hospital, Victoria, Australia

Eric L. Krakauer, International Programs, Center for Palliative Care, Harvard Medical School; Division of Palliative Care, Massachusetts General Hospital, Boston, MA, USA

Maia S. Kredentser, Department of Psychology, Faculty of Graduate Studies, University of Manitoba; Manitoba Palliative Care Research Unit, CancerCare Manitoba, Winnipeg, MB, Canada

Robert S. Krouse, Department of Surgery, Southern Arizona Health Care System and University of Arizona, Tucson, AZ, USA

Judith Lacey, Palliative and Suportive Care Consultant Physician, St George Private Hospital, Sydney, NSW, Australia

Nina Laing, New York Department of Education, Brooklyn, NY, USA

Barry J.A. Laird, University of Edinburgh, Edinburgh, UK; European Palliative Care Research Centre, Trondheim, Norway

Thomas W. LeBlanc, Division of Hematologic Malignancies and Cellular Therapy, Department of Medicine, Duke University School of Medicine, Durham, NC, USA

Olivia T. Lee, Department of Urology, Davis School of Medicine, University of California, Sacramento, CA, USA

Carrie Lethborg, Department of Psychiatry, Monash University, Clayton, Psychosocial Cancer Research, Cancer Services, St Vincent's Hospital, Melbourne University, Clayton, VIC, Australia

Mari Lloyd-Williams, Director and Professor of Academic Palliative and Supportive Care Studies (APSCS), University of Liverpool, UK

Jon Håvard Loge, Department of Behavioural Sciences in Medicine, Institute of Basic Medical Sciences, University of Oslo, Oslo, Norway

Charles L. Loprinzi, Department of Oncology, Mayo Clinic, Rochester, MN, USA

Stefan Lorenzl, Department of Neurology, LMU University Hospital Agatharied, Agatharied, Germany; University of Salzburg, Salzburg, Austria; Clinic and Policlinic of Palliative Care, LMU University Hospital Grosshadern, Munich, Germany

Michal Lotem, Center for Melanoma and Cancer Immunotherapy, Sharett Institute of Oncology, Hadassah Hebrew University Medical Center, Jerusalem, Israel

Tim Luckett, Improving Palliative Care through Clinical Trials (ImPaCCT), University of Technology, Sydney; University of New South Wales, Sydney, NSW, Australia

David Lussier, Insitut universitaire de gériatrie de Montréal, University of Montreal; Division of Geriatric Medicine and Alan-Edwards Centre for Research on Pain, McGill University, Montreal, QC, Canada

Tom Lynch, Department of Anesthesiology and Critical Care Medicine & Palliative Care Program, Kimmel Cancer Center at Johns Hopkins Core Faculty, Armstrong Institute for Patient Safety and Quality, The Johns Hopkins School of Medicine, Baltimore, MD, USA

Kathryn A. Mannix, Consultant in Palliative Medicine, Palliative Care Lead, NUTH, Netherlands

Cinzia Martini, Fondazione IRCCS Istituto Nazionale dei Tumori, Milan, Italy

Lars Johan Materstvedt, Department of Philosophy and Religious Studies, Faculty of Humanities, Norwegian University of Science and Technology (NTNU), Trondheim, Norway

Karen May, Piedmont Atlanta Hospital, Atlanta, GA; Visiting Nurse Health System, Hospice Atlanta, Atlanta, GA, USA

Susan E. McClement, College of Nursing, Faculty of Health Sciences, University of Manitoba; Manitoba Palliative Care Research Unit, CancerCare Manitoba, Winnipeg, MB, Canada

Renée McCulloch, Great Ormond Street Hospital, London; Institute of Child Health, University College London, London, UK

David McKeown, Memorial Sloan-Kettering Cancer Center, New York, NY, USA

Anja Mehnert, Division of Psychosocial Oncology, Department of Medical Psychology and Medical Sociology, University Medical Centre Leipzig, Leipzig, Saxony, Germany

Sharon Merims, Sharett Institute of Oncology, Hadassah Hebrew University Medical Center, Jerusalem, Israel

Jessica S. Merlin, Division of Infectious Diseases, Division of Gerontology, Geriatrics, and Palliative Care, University of Alabama at Birmingham, Birmingham, AL, USA

Frederick J. Meyers, School of Medicine, University of California, Davis School of Medicine, Sacramento, CA, USA

Martha F. Mherekumombe, Department of Pain Medicine and Palliative Care, The Children's Hospital at Westmead, Sydney, Australia

Joanne Michaud-Young, Department of Health—Province of New Brunswick, Chronic Disease Prevention and Management Unit, Fredericton, NB, Canada

Kelly Nichole Michelson, Associate Professor of Pediatrics and Buehler Center on Aging, Health & Society, Northwestern University Feinberg School of Medicine; Attending Physician, Ann & Robert H. Lurie Children's Hospital, Chicago, IL, USA

Fliss E.M. Murtagh, Reader and Consultant in Palliative Medicine, King's College London, Cicely Saunders Institute, Department of Palliative Care, Policy and Rehabilitation, London, UK

Amanda Moment, Dana Farber/Brigham and Women's Cancer Center, Brigham and Women's Hospital, Boston, MA, USA

Helen M. Moore, Sacred Heart Health Service, St Vincent's Hospital, Sydney; UNSW Australia, St Vincent's Clinical School, Sydney, NSW, Australia

Anna C. Muriel, Harvard Medical School, Department of Psychosocial Oncology and Palliative Care, Dana-Farber Cancer Institute, Boston, MA, USA

Barbara A. Murphy, Associate Professor, Department of Medicine, Vanderbilt-Ingram Cancer Center, Nashville, TN, USA

Kyriaki Mystakidou, Pain Relief and Palliative Care Unit, University of Athens, School of Medicine, Department of Radiology, Aretaieion Hospital, Athens, Greece

Friedemann Nauck, Department of Palliative Medicine, University Medicine Göttingen, Georg August University, Göttingen, Germany

Georg S. Nübling, Departments of Neurology and Palliative Care, Klinikum der Universität München, Ludwig-Maximilians-University, Munich, Germany

Clare O'Callaghan, Caritas Christi Hospice, St Vincent's Hospital; Palliative Care Service, Cabrini Health, Melbourne, Australia

Dianne L. O'Connell, Cancer Research Division, Cancer Council NSW, Woolloomooloo NSW, Australia

Meera Pahuja, Division of Hematology/Oncology & Palliative Care, Division of Infectious Diseases, Virginia Commonwealth University, Richmond, VA, USA

Irene Panagiotou, Cicely Saunders Institute, Faculty of Life Sciences and Medicine, King's College London, London, UK

Wisawatapnimit Panarut, Doctoral Student School of Nursing, Vanderbilt University, Nashville, TN, USA

Steven Z. Pantilat, Palliative Care Program, Division of Hospital Medicine, Department of Medicine, University of California, San Francisco, CA, USA

Efi Parpa, Pain Relief & Palliative Care Unit, Areteion Hospital; Department of Radiology, School of Medicine, University of Athens, Athens, Greece

Steven D. Passik, Associate Attending Psychologist, Department of Psychiatry and Behavioral Sciences, Memorial Sloan-Kettering Cancer center, New York, NY, USA

Sheila Payne, International Observatory on End of Life Care, Lancaster University, Lancaster, UK

Jose Pereira, Professor and Head, Division of Palliative Care, Department of Medicine, University of Ottawa and Medical

Chief, Palliative Medicine, Bruyere Continuing Care and Ottawa Hospital, Ottawa, ON, Canada

Jane L. Phillips, Professor Nursing (Palliative Care), Director Centre for Cardiovascular and Chronic Care, Faculty of Health, University of Technology, Sydney, Australia; Adjunct Professor of Palliative Nursing, University of Notre Dame, and the School of Medicine, Sydney University, Australia

Thomas P. Pittelkow, Department of Physical Medicine & Rehabilitation, Mayo Clinic, College of Medicine, Rochester, MN, USA

Mark R. Pittelkow, Department of Dermatology, Mayo Clinic Arizona, Scottsdale, AZ, USA

Michael Piza, Clinical Governance Unit, South Eastern Sydney Local Health District; UNSW Australia, School of Public Health and Community Medicine, Sydney, NSW, Australia

Barbara Pohl, Division of Medical Ethics, Weill Cornell Medical College, New York, NY, USA

Russell K. Portenoy, MJHS Institute for Innovation in Palliative Care, Chief Medical Officer, MJHS Hospice and Palliative Care, New York, NY, USA; Professor of Neurology, Albert Einstein College of Medicine Bronx, New York, NY, USA

Richard A. Powell, Nairobi, Kenya

Julie R. Price, Assistant Professor of Clinical Psychiatry, Assistant Professor of Physical Medicine & Rehabilitation, Vanderbilt University School of Medicine, Nashville, TN, USA

Sebastian Probst, Zurich University of Applied Sciences, Institute of Nursing, Winterthur, Switzerland

Christina M. Puchalski, Professor, Medicine and Health Sciences Director, George Washington Institute for Spirituality and Health, The George Washington University School of Medicine and Health Sciences, WA, USA

Lukas Radbruch, Department of Palliative Medicine, University Hospital Bonn, Bonn, Germany

M. R. Rajagopal, WHO Collaborating Centre for Training and Policy on Access to Pain Relief, Trivandrum, Kerala, India

Lesley K. Rao, Department of Anesthsiology, Division of Pain Management, Washington University School of Medicine in St. Louis, St. Louis, MO, USA

Paula K. Rauch, Marjorie E. Korff Parenting At a Challenging Time Program, Department of Psychiatry, Massachusetts General Hospital, Boston, MA, USA

Clare Rayment, Marie Curie Hospice, Bradford, Bradford, UK

Katherine L.P. Reid, Speech Pathology Department, Calvary Health Care Sydney; Department of Linguistics, Macquarie University Hospital, Sydney, NSW, Australia

Rosemary Richardson, Macmillan Supporters Service, Vale of Leven Hospital, Alexandria, UK

Sheila Ridner, Associate Professor, Vanderbilt University School of Nursing, Nashville, TN, USA

Carla I. Ripamonti, Head, Supportive Care in Cancer Unit, Department of Hematology and Pediatric Onco-Hematology, Fondazione IRCCS; Istituto Nazionale Tumori, Milan, Italy

Louise Robinson, Chelsea and Westminster Hospital, London, UK

Graeme M. Rocker, Division of Respirology, Dalhousie University, Capital Health, Halifax, NS, Canada

Joy Ross, Royal Marsden and Royal Brompton Palliative Care Service, Royal Marsden NHS Foundation Trust, London, UK

Tarun Sabharwal, Consultant Interventional Radiologist, Department of Radiology, St Thomas's Hospital, London, UK

Natasha Samy, Department of Pain Medicine and Palliative Care, The Children's Hospital at Westmead, Sydney, Australia

Megan B. Sands, The Prince of Wales Hospital and Community Services, Sydney; University of New South Wales, Sydney, NSW, Australia

Dirk Schrijvers, Department of Medical Oncology, Ziekenhuisnetwerk Antwerpen-Middelheim, Antwerp, Belgium

Erin E. Schweers, Department of Psychiatry and Behavioral Sciences, Memorial Sloan-Kettering Cancer Center, New York, NY, USA

Peter A. Selwyn, Department of Family and Social Medicine, Montefiore Medical Center/Albert Einstein College of Medicine, Bronx, NY, USA

Michael M.K. Sham, Palliative Medical Unit, Grantham Hospital, Hong Kong

Deborah Witt Sherman, Associate Dean of Academic Affairs, College of Nursing and Health Sciences, Florida International University, Miami, FL, USA

Fabio Simonetti, Fondazione IRCCS Istituto Nazionale dei Tumori, Milan, Italy

Christian T. Sinclair, Assistant Professor, University of Kansas Medical Center, Kansas City, KS, USA

Per Sjøgren, Section of Palliative Medicine, Department of Oncology, Rigshospitalet, Denmark

Tinne Smets, End-of-Life Care Research Group VUB & Ghent University, Department of Family Medicine and Chronic Care, Vrije Universiteit Brussel, Brussels, Belgium

Thomas J. Smith, Professor of Oncology, Harry J. Duffey Family Professor of Palliative Medicine, Director of Palliative Medicine, JHMI, The Johns Hopkins Hospital, Baltimore, MD, USA

Eliezer Soto, Anesthesia Pain Care Consultants, Tamarac, FL, USA

Anthony E. Steimle, Department of Cardiology, Kaiser Permanente Santa Clara Medical Center, Santa Clara, CA, USA

Karen E. Steinhauser, Center for Health Services Research in Primary Care, VA Medical Center; Division of Internal Medicine, Department of Medicine, Duke University, Durham NC, USA

Patrick Stone, Marie Curie Chair of Palliative and End of Life Care, Palliative Care Research Department, Division of Psychiatry, University College London (UCL), London, UK

Annette F. Street, Palliative Care Unit, La Trobe University, Melbourne, VIC, Australia

Robert A. Swarm, Division of Pain Management, Washington University School of Medicine, St. Louis, MO, USA

Nigel P. Sykes, St Christopher's Hospice, London, UK

Jennifer J. Tieman, Discipline of Palliative and Supportive Services, Flinders University, Bedford Park, SA, Australia

Doris M.W. Tse, Caritas Medical Centre, Hong Kong

Eleni Tsilika, Pain Relief and Palliative Care Unit, University of Athens, School of Medicine, Department of Radiology, Aretaieion Hospital, Athens, Greece

James A. Tulsky, Duke Palliative Care, Duke University, Durham, NC, USA

Raymond Voltz, Department of Palliative Medicine, University Hospital, Cologne, Germany

Amy Waller, Health Behaviour Research Group, University of Newcastle, Callaghan, NSW, Australia

Sharon M. Watanabe, Division of Palliative Care Medicine, Department of Oncology, University of Alberta, Edmonton, AB, Canada

Simon Wein, Palliative Medicine, Davidoff Cancer Center, Beilinson Hospital, Petach Tikvah, Israel

Batsheva Werman, Senior physician and palliative care fellow, Department of Oncolgy and Palliative Care, Shaare Zedek Medical Center, Jerrusalem, Israel

Eric Widera, Division of Geriatrics, Department of Medicine, University of California, San Francisco, CA, USA

Emily Wighton, The Royal Marsden & Royal Brompton Palliative Care Service, The Royal Marsden NHS Foundation Trust, London, UK

Michèle J.M. Wood, Marie Curie Hospice, London; Department of Psychology, University of Roehampton, London, UK

Cynthia Wu, Department of Medicine, University of Alberta Hospital, Edmonton, AB, Canada

Jennifer N. Wu, Department of Urology and Cancer Center, University of California, Davis, Sacramento, CA, USA

Patsy Yates, Head of School of Nursing and Midwifery, Queensland University of Technology, Kelvin Grove, QLD, Australia

Sriram Yennurajalingam, Department of Urology and Cancer Center, University of California, Davis, Sacramento, CA, USA

Talia I. Zaider, Department of Psychiatry and Behavioral Sciences, Memorial Sloan-Kettering Cancer Center; Department of Psychiatry, Weill Medical College of Cornell University, New York, NY, USA

Lauren A. Zatarain, Hematology/Oncology Fellow, Vanderbilt-Ingram Cancer Center, Nashville, TN, USA

Nancy Y. Zhu, Division of Hematology, Department of Medicine, University of Alberta, University of Alberta Hospital, Edmonton, AB, Canada

SECTION 1

The worldwide status of palliative care

International progress in creating palliative medicine as a specialized discipline and the development of palliative care

Sheila Payne and Tom Lynch

Introduction to international progress in creating palliative medicine

Throughout the world approximately 56 million people die each year, with the majority dying with or from non-communicable diseases, often in older age. The populations of Europe, North America, Australasia, and parts of Asia are ageing; increasingly, older people live with chronic and advanced conditions before they die. In other parts of the world, such as sub-Saharan Africa, communicable diseases, including HIV/AIDS, tuberculosis, and malaria, place major demands on palliative care. Palliative medicine offers opportunities for clinicians and other disciplines to work in partnership, to forge innovative alliances to shape the compassionate care of persons facing the final stages of life. Palliative care refers to enhancing the physical, psychological, emotional, social, spiritual, and existential well-being of patients and their families (Sepulveda et al., 2002).

The main objective of this chapter is to review the development of palliative medicine as a specialized discipline, and to trace the development of international initiatives, highlighting achievements and limitations in current comparative methodologies. We offer evidence on the progress of educational initiatives, both within medicine and for other members of the multidisciplinary team, at undergraduate and post-qualification level. It is beyond the scope of this chapter to review the training needs of volunteers or family carers. Finally, we consider what areas of palliative medicine require further development.

The chapter will focus upon developments in palliative medicine that relate to the care of adults, rather than children. The expansion of palliative care into specialist areas, such as cardiology, stroke medicine, or neurology, may increase demands for dual qualifications. Likewise, there are new developments in oncology practice which call for a more explicit integration of palliative care throughout the trajectory of illness and into protracted periods of survivorship with advanced disease (Kaasa et al., 2011).

Progress in international development in palliative care

History of key developments

Prior to the beginning of the twenty-first century, there had only been sporadic progress in the development of palliative care internationally. The first hospices were opened over a century ago in Dublin (Our Lady's Hospice) and in the East End of London (St Joseph's Hospice, Hackney) by Catholic nuns as a charitable and religious mission caring for those dying of tuberculosis and living in poverty (Humphreys, 2001; Winslow and Clark, 2005). Considerably later, St Christopher's Hospice opened in South London in 1967, following the pioneering work of Dame Cicely Saunders, and this was soon followed by hospice and palliative care initiatives in Western European countries (Table 1.1.1).

The first hospital palliative care team was established in the Royal Victoria Hospital, Montreal, by Balfour Mount in 1976, followed by the St Thomas' Hospital, London, team in 1977.

In the United States, hospice programmes began in the 1970s and Medicare funding was secured in 1982 (providing reimbursement of costs through insurance but requiring relinquishment of curative treatments). In 1988, the European Association for Palliative Care (EAPC) was formed (Blumhuber et al., 2002), and in the mid 1990s the International Association of Hospice and Palliative Care (IAHPC) was established in the United States. In South America, the 1994 Declaration of Florianopolis raised awareness of barriers to the accessibility and availability of opioids in the region (Stjernswärd et al., 1995), and in 2000, the Latin American Association of Palliative Care was formed.

During communist rule in the countries of Central and Eastern Europe and Commonwealth of Independent States (CEE/CIS), there had been few significant palliative care developments. Following the political changes of the 1990s, there was a steady development of palliative care services in this region (Table 1.1.2). This was due in part to initiatives such as the Poznan Declaration ('The Poznan Declaration 1998', 1999) and the Eastern and Central Europe Palliative Task Force (ECEPT) which commenced

Table 1.1.1 Palliative care in Western Europe

Western European country	Year hospice services commenced
United Kingdom	1967
Sweden	1977
Italy	1980
Germany	1983
Spain	1984
Belgium	1985
Netherlands	1991

Table 1.1.2 Palliative care in Central and Eastern Europe/Former Soviet Union (CEE/FSU)

CEE/FSU country	Year hospice services commenced
Poland	1976
Russia	1990
Hungary	1991
Bulgaria	1992
Czech Republic	1992
Romania	1992
Slovenia	1992
Albania	1993
Kyrgyzstan	1993
Lithuania	1993
Belarus	1994
Croatia	1994
Ukraine	1996
Estonia	1997
Latvia	1997
Azerbaijan	1998
Bosnia Herzegovina	1998
Republic of Macedonia	1998
Republic of Moldova	1998
Armenia	1999
Kazakhstan	1999
Slovakia	1999
Serbia and Montenegro	2000
Georgia	2001

in 1999 (ECEPT, n.d.). Financial support to the palliative care programmes within CEE and CIS came from the Open Society Foundations (OSF) Public Health Program (OSF, 2014), one of very few donors at the start of the new millennium supporting palliative care in this geographical area.

The early part of the twenty-first century witnessed a number of significant international developments: the Asia Pacific Hospice Palliative Care Network was formed in 2001 (Goh, 2002); in 2002, the Hospice Information Service recommenced in the United Kingdom; the first conference focusing on international development of palliative care was held at the Hague in 2003, and in the same year the European Society for Medical Oncology officially recognized the discipline (Cherny et al., 2003). Also in 2003, palliative care development in the CEE/CIS region was stimulated by the Council of Europe (2003) report on palliative care which provided specific guidelines provision. In 2004, the African Palliative Care Association was formed and two World Health Organization (WHO) publications aimed to improve the quality of care provided at the end of life (Davies and Higginson, 2004a, 2000b). Also in 2004, the United States Agency for International Development (USAID) launched the President's Emergency Plan for AIDS Relief (PEPFAR), which allocated funds to the development of hospice and palliative care. The second conference on international palliative care development was held in Seoul in 2005, and the first World Hospice and Palliative Care Day was celebrated in the same year.

Regular congresses organized by the EAPC provided excellent platforms for increased collaboration in international development of palliative care and by 2012 these had become designated as world congresses. In 2006, a Declaration was compiled that stressed the need for increased palliative care research in resource-poor countries, leading to a pledge to improve palliative care across Europe in 2007 (Radbruch et al., 2007). In the same year, the IAHPC and WHO led in producing a list of 34 essential medicines for palliative care. The Worldwide Palliative Care Alliance (WPCA) was formally constituted in 2009.

Achievements in the mapping and measuring of global palliative care development

Relatively recently, studies which generate comparative analyses of palliative care development and attempt to map the development of palliative care across countries, regions, and continents have begun to occur. The first study focused on seven countries in Western Europe (Clark et al., 2000) and was followed by mapping of 28 countries in Eastern Europe and Central Asia (Clark and Wright 2003). As a result of the latter project, the International Observatory on End of Life Care (IOELC) was established in 2003. The IOELC used comparative methods based on a common template to present its research-based country reports. This resulted in reviews of palliative care development in Africa (26 countries) (Wright et al., 2008), the Middle East (six countries), and South East Asia (three countries) (Wright et al., 2010), as well as India (McDermott et al., 2008).

Two further comparative studies of European palliative care development were undertaken. The first study focused on 11 European countries (Jaspers and Schindler, 2004). The second study focused on 16 European countries (Project on Hospice and Palliative Care in Europe n.d.), including the Czech Republic, Estonia, Hungary, Latvia, Lithuania, Poland, Slovakia, and Ukraine.

The EAPC Task Force on the Development of Palliative Care in Europe was founded in 2003, and has contributed substantially to documenting the progress of palliative care, producing, for the first time, comparative data on the status of services across the whole of the WHO European Region (a geographic area of 53 countries and a population of 879 million people) (Centeno et al., 2004). The Task Force works closely with a number of international hospice and palliative care organizations; in particular, IOELC, IAHPC, and Help the Hospices (HTH). In 2006, the initial findings of the Task Force were presented in the form of a map of specific resources of palliative care in Europe. In 2007, the Task Force produced a set of country reports that documented the existence of palliative care services using a common template to facilitate cross-national and regional comparison, published as a European Atlas of Palliative Care (Centeno et al., 2007a), and disseminated via the web pages of the EAPC (EAPC, 2013). They function as benchmarks, to enable countries to ascertain their level of palliative care development compared with others in their region and to track developments over time.

The *EAPC Review of Palliative Care in Europe* (Rocafort and Centeno, 2008), and associated articles were published in peer-reviewed journals. One article examined data on palliative medicine as an area of certified specialization in 52 European countries (Centeno, et al., 2007b). Another compiled facts and indicators on the development of palliative care in those countries (Centeno et al., 2007c). Two further articles examined barriers to the development of palliative care in both CEE/CIS (Lynch et al., 2009) and Western Europe (Lynch et al., 2010).

Emerging from this series of studies was an ambitious attempt in 2006 to measure and classify global palliative care development. The IOELC built on a basic description that had been produced by the Hospice Information Service but attempted to build more depth into the analysis, by developing a four-part typology, depicting levels of hospice-palliative care development across the globe: no known hospice-palliative care activity (group 1 countries); capacity building activity (group 2 countries); localized hospice-palliative care provision (group 3 countries); and countries where hospice-palliative care services were reaching a measure of integration with the mainstream health-care system (group 4 countries). By presenting a 'world map', the study sought to contribute to debate about the growth and recognition of palliative care services and, in particular, whether or not the four-part typology reflected sequential levels of development (Wright et al., 2008).

Since 2006, there have been further comparative studies of palliative care development. For example, in 2008, the work of the EAPC Task Force was extended in a collaborative study which specifically focused on the 27 member states of the European Union (EU) (Martin-Moreno et al., 2008). This study moved beyond a descriptive comparison of the data, to sketch out the beginnings of a more detailed method for ranking the 27 countries by the level of their palliative care development. A study commissioned by the Lien Foundation in Singapore and carried out by the Economist Intelligence Unit was published in 2010. This produced a ranking of palliative care development; this time in 40 countries of the world, and with a more complex set of indicators (Economist Intelligence Unit 2010). In 2011, a report from Human Rights Watch also documented the state of pain and palliative care services in 40 countries (Human Rights Watch 2011).

Methods for measuring progress and mapping: challenges and limitations

There are a number of practical and methodological challenges inherent in the mapping and measuring of global palliative care

development. In 2011, the EAPC Task Force embarked upon a new programme of work to refine its original methods and to produce updated information on the status of palliative care in each European country. The work culminated in the production of a second edition of the *EAPC Atlas of Palliative Care in Europe* that was launched at the EAPC Congress in Prague, June 2013. The Atlas addresses limitations and difficulties associated with standardization of terminology relating to hospice and palliative care services. It also addresses some of the unintended negative effects that may occur when benchmarking studies are undertaken, such as the role of 'human emotions' within the process of collecting the data—the fact that data provided by 'key persons' and national associations could have been inflated by 'competitive tendencies'.

The 2006 study that mapped the global development of palliative care was revised by the Worldwide Palliative Care Alliance in 2011, to update the original findings and facilitate cross-national comparative analysis and stimulate advocacy, policymaking, and service development. The results of the mapping study are shown in Fig. 1.1.1 (Lynch et al 2011).

Although the 2006 study had been heavily cited and adopted as a tool for international palliative care advocacy, it became clear that the rankings might benefit from refinement and the method of categorization could also be made more robust. Consequently, within the revised typology, changes were made to the criteria for the levels of palliative care development in groups 3 and 4 and these were subdivided to produce two additional levels of categorization: 3a/3b (isolated palliative care provision/generalized palliative care provision) and 4a/4b (countries where hospice-palliative care services are at a stage of preliminary integration into mainstream service provision/countries where hospice-palliative care services are at a stage of advanced integration into mainstream service provision). In addition, the EAPC undertook an extensive, consultative, and consensus-building exercise to agree norms and standards for palliative care within Europe (Radbruch and Payne 2009, 2010).

It was acknowledged that the global mapping study had other limitations. As with the 2006 study, there remained an absence of data for some countries, and respondents often experienced difficulty in choosing between the newly divided categories. Some respondents suggested that their country 'did not fit into any category', that their country was 'somewhere on the border' between two categories, or that 'strengths and limitations' existed within each subcategory. Achieving comparability between settings and the way in which services are counted also proved problematic. Two systems operate in tandem. Services in five of the six continents tend to be counted by provider, irrespective of the number of services. In Europe, they are usually counted by type (e.g. home care, day care, inpatient units, or hospital teams). Although this allows a degree of comparability for services in the countries of Europe and within and across the other five continents, it also inhibits any comparable worldwide analysis. In addition, listing services by provider could be a source of bias as a country with fewer but larger-scale provider organizations would show a lower ratio of services per capita compared with a country having several small providers. Differences in the way in which services are counted may be an artefact of the procedures for 'counting' organizations. The authors attempted to address these issues by listing the number of providers and services in the same category of data under the heading 'services/providers', and attempting to glean clarification from 'key persons' and local palliative care experts.

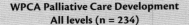

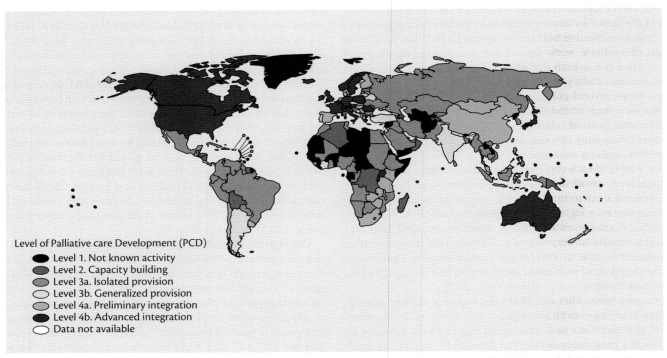

The boundaries and names shown and the designations used on this map do not imply the expression of any opinion whatsoever on the part of the WPCA concerning the legal status of any country, territory, city or areas of its authorities, or concerning the delimitation of its frontiers or boundaries. Dotted lines on maps represent approximate border lines for which there may not yet be full agreement.

Fig. 1.1.1 Mapping levels of palliative care development: a global update.
Reproduced with permission from Lynch, T., Clark, D., and Connor, S.R., *Mapping levels of palliative care development: A global update*, Worldwide Palliative Care Alliance, Copyright © 2011.

A major problem faced in this and other studies was that of standardization and definition in how services are characterized. Terms such as 'hospice', 'inpatient unit', or 'mobile team' do not have a universal currency and globally there were difficulties in comparing them. The authors also note the diversity of provision and the different 'histories' of palliative care in specific jurisdictions and acknowledge the absence of agreed standards and quality measures globally. In addition, the vast majority of data relating to palliative care development originated from palliative care activists and this was acknowledged as a potential source of bias or inaccuracy, with the inherent risk of data that either under-reported or over-reported the number of services.

From mapping, to research, to advocacy

The Access to Opioid Medication in Europe project

The 5-year Access to Opioid Medication in Europe (ATOME) project commenced in December 2009, funded by the European Commission's 7th Framework Programme. The aim of the project is to improve access to opioids in 12 European countries where there is statistical evidence of very low morphine per capita consumption: Estonia, Latvia, Lithuania, Poland, Slovakia, Hungary, Slovenia, Serbia, Bulgaria, Greece, Turkey, and Cyprus. The ten partners of the ATOME project work with country teams, including government officials and public health and medicine experts, to carry out legislative and policy reviews, leading to

recommendations that will facilitate access for all patients requiring treatment with medicines controlled under the international drug conventions. The integration of palliative care and harm reduction is a key aim of the project.

The project is undertaking a national situational analysis in each country with regard to the accessibility and availability of controlled medicines, including their use and causes for underuse. It is conducting an external review of relevant national legislation in each country and recommending appropriate amendments to governments. It is anticipated that the project will improve access to essential controlled medicines, including opioid analgesics and opioids used in substitution therapy for the treatment of opioid dependence, in the majority of the 12 European countries. Improved access will also contribute to the effective prevention of HIV/AIDS transmission among and from injecting drug user populations.

There are a number of research initiatives being undertaken within the ATOME project. For example, the principle of 'balance' in opioid control policy requires governments not only to prevent drug abuse, but also to ensure the availability of opioid analgesics for medical purposes. Efforts to prevent drug abuse and diversion must not interfere with the adequate availability of medication for patients' pain relief and drug substitution therapy. Within this context, the ATOME project has revised the WHO guidelines *Ensuring Balance in National Policies on Controlled Substances* (WHO 2011).

Two ATOME workshops (involving six countries each) drew together relevant stakeholders who formed a country team that analysed their country situation using a checklist developed by the WHO and the WHO Collaborating Centre for Communication and Policy in Cancer Care (University of Wisconsin, United States). The checklist was used by each country team to identify existing barriers for access to controlled medications at all levels of their respective health-care and legislative systems. As a follow-up to these workshops, 1-day national conferences are being organized in each of the 12 target countries (in collaboration with the country teams) in order to evaluate the implementation of the revised guidelines and to disseminate the project's findings and recommendations to relevant ministries, health-care professionals, and the general public, including patients and their families. Promoting the acceptance of rational use of opioids as medicines, both for pain management and substitution therapy, is also a priority of each conference.

In addition, a workshop was held to discuss the training of lawyers and national counterparts on how to review national controlled substance legislation from the perspective of balancing availability and prevention of abuse; lawyers from each country and 12 national counterparts identified from within the Ministry of Health were in attendance. Recommendations have been drafted to lift these barriers in such a way that prevention of drug abuse is warranted.

It is anticipated that collaboration between government officials and national health professionals in the project's 12 country teams will contribute to research in the area of pain management policy. A strong focus on the recommendations for policy and legislative change and their dissemination to key decision-makers at national and European level will help to ensure that causes of inappropriate prescribing and poor compliance will be identified and policy recommendations for safe, effective, and cost-effective use of medicines in Europe developed. The ATOME project draws on the successful lessons learned in Romania.

Open Society Foundations' International Palliative Care Initiative: the Romanian experience

The International Palliative Care Initiative (IPCI) was established in 2000 with an overall goal of integrating palliative care into national health-care systems. The IPCI promotes the WHO public health model, adopting a multi-pronged strategy that includes legal and policy reform, including drug availability and standards development, as well as education, training, and financing. The economic costs and benefits of palliative care are considered as key themes, as support for health budget monitoring activities may enable access to funding for palliative care treatment. In several countries, the IPCI, in collaboration with the OSF Public Health Program Health Budget Monitoring Advocacy project (HBMA), have managed to get members of the Ministry of Health and other key players (e.g. pharmaceutical and insurance companies) aligned to their way of thinking. This has been achieved through their support for policy analysis debate and for national and regional workshops.

Initially, Romania had a very restrictive controlled drugs legislation, dating back to 1963, which did not allow for adequate pain management or adequate treatment of opioid dependence. Terminally ill cancer patients could qualify for pain medication, but still had to overcome several serious barriers to access it. All other moderate and severe pain patients were excluded from adequate pain relief with opioid analgesics.

In 2002, the IPCI and the Pain and Policy Studies Group (PPSG) WHO Centre for Policy and Communications in Cancer Care, organized a regional workshop with representatives from Ministries of Health, narcotics control, and national HIV and cancer control programmes from six countries: Bulgaria, Croatia, Hungary, Lithuania, Poland, and Romania. Action plans were developed and technical assistance was provided by the Centre, leading to a significant change in legislation in Romania in 2005. This proved to be a watershed event for palliative care development not only in Romania, but more broadly both in the CEE/CIS region and throughout the world. Another activity developed in cooperation with the Romanian Ministry of Health was a workshop on controlled drugs legislation, held in Bucharest under the EU PHARE Programme in December 2003.

Following these initiatives, the Romanian government developed a new controlled drugs act, which was enforced in June 2006. To ensure proper implementation, the WHO Department of Medicines Policy and Standards, PPSG, Hospice Casa Sperantei, and the Romanian Ministry of Health, co-organized a workshop in 2006 where the implementation of the recent legislation was discussed. Policy was also developed for the training of physicians in prescribing opioid analgesics. Furthermore, the government established treatment facilities for opioid dependence in each province and in three prisons. Romania had laid the foundations for adequate access to essential controlled medicines.

Thanks to the IPCI and HBMA's support for budget monitoring activities, in April 2010 the Romanian Ministry of Health decided to finance palliative care and also to contribute to paying the costs of home-based care. Prior to this project, there was no government coverage of palliative care treatment. This project not only enabled access to funding for palliative care treatment, but also, unexpectedly, helped sharpen the national definition of palliative care.

Key initiatives in strengthening education and development of specialized disciplines

Future increases in the need for palliative care will place demands upon knowledge transfer across the whole workforce of those people who are involved. This section will review definitions of education and scholarship, and consider the extent to which early calls for integration between palliative care practice and education have been achieved (Sheldon and Smith, 1996). We draw upon the work of a number of task forces (time-limited expert working groups) convened by the EAPC, who, over the last decade, have made proposals for core educational curricula in medicine, nursing, and psychology. This leads on to discussion of the international growth of specialist palliative medicine as a discipline, highlighting potential advantages and disadvantages of this growth. Finally, we review the opportunities that innovations in communication and information technologies offer in terms of education and knowledge transfer.

Separating education and training as distinct elements of learning might be helpful at the outset. According to Wee and Hughes (2007, p. 2), 'Education is the process through which learning occurs. Training, on the other hand, is about the acquisition of knowledge or skills to deal with particular types of event'. Arguably education is a life-long endeavour, in which new knowledge is gained, embedded in the context of appropriate attitudes and values, which are used to inform high-quality practice. Palliative care draws upon pedagogical theories that are common to other health and social disciplines, which may be influenced by fashions, trends, and new developments. It is important to recognize that the content of education programmes—the curriculum—has three aspects: the formal curriculum as defined by educators, and often directed by statutory or disciplinary requirements; the informal curriculum which arises out of the interaction between learners and teachers; and the hidden curriculum which refers to the cultural learning environment (Wee and Hughes, 2007). Congruence between all three elements enhances the educational experience.

Multidisciplinary palliative care educational developments have progressed greatly in the United States (Weissman et al., 2007), including those in specific clinical contexts such as cancer care (Coyne et al., 2007) and intensive care (Ferrell et al., 2007). In Europe, the EAPC has coordinated a number of task forces focused on core professional disciplines within palliative care including nurse education (De Vlieger et al., 2004), undergraduate medical education within medicine (EAPC, 2007), postgraduate education for physicians (EAPC, 2009), and postgraduate education for psychologists (Junger and Payne, 2011). Further work is currently underway to identify a core educational curriculum for social workers and in the specialist area of paediatric palliative care. Ten core competences in interdisciplinary palliative care have been drawn together following a rigorous review and consensus process, to provide a framework for practitioners who work within the field (Gamondi et al., 2013a, 2013b). These core competences in palliative care, for all disciplines, provide a benchmark against which educational programme content and assessment can be matched, across institutions and internationally.

There is anecdotal evidence of considerable growth in the provision of post-qualification education in palliative care, but in the absence of collective databases of provision or any assessment of their level and quality, it is remarkably difficult to make accurate estimates of the number of programmes, the level of provision, and the quality of education offered. Moreover, programmes are currently offered by many organizations including hospices, hospitals, higher education and universities, with course lengths varying from a few hours to years. To address this gap in knowledge, a project undertaken by the IOELC has mapped educational provision at post-qualification level. We are aware of increasing numbers of certificated higher education awards being offered by universities; for example, in Asia, Masters in Palliative Care are available in Japan, and doctorate programmes are available for physicians, nurses, and allied health professionals in Singapore, Japan, and Korea (Payne et al., 2012). In Europe, there are exciting innovations with blended-learning programmes leading to a PhD in Palliative Care now being offered in the United Kingdom and Norway, and a large European Commission funded project designed to offer training to 12 PhD students and four post-doctoral fellows (End-of-Life Care 2011). The European Palliative Care Academy, funded by the Bosch Foundation, launched an international programme to enhance palliative care education and leadership training for clinicians across Europe in 2013.

An important drive to improve palliative care for all patients is the implementation of basic education in undergraduate curricula throughout all medical, nursing, and health professional courses globally, with an introduction to the principles of palliative care practice, including symptom control and communication skills. This should be supplemented by supervised clinical placements in palliative care so that students can engage in experiential learning. This is likely to raise awareness of what palliative care services can offer and means more appropriate and timely referrals of those with complex problems, and empowers professionals to manage better those with less need for specialist input.

Palliative medicine has been recognized as a specialty within the United Kingdom since 1987 and doctors wishing to achieve specialist registration must undergo post-registration specialist clinical training (Centeno et al., 2007b). The number of countries with specialist physician status for palliative medicine continues to grow including Ireland, Israel, and Germany. There remains some debate as to whether subspecialty status, for example, with registration in internal medicine or oncology, offers a better way to encourage high-quality physicians to enter this field and to prevent palliative medicine from becoming marginalized. Within nursing, similar development of specialist training and practice are evident, particularly in resource-rich regions, where clinical nurse specialists in palliative care have been shown to be effective (Larkin, 2008).

Conclusion

To sum up, given that this chapter has covered both a rapid overview of the development of palliative care and has highlighted key developments in palliative care education, it seems safe to conclude that, in some parts of the world, palliative care can be regarded as a success. There is evidence of increasing integration, with mainstream health-care provision, the inclusion of palliative care into national health-care planning process, and in a few places specific Palliative Care Strategic Plans have been adopted. This bodes well, even in times of financial constraint and uncertainty. However, countries with this level of development are very few, and even within these countries there may be inequity for particular patients, such as the very old, those with dementia, and who do not fit comfortably into mainstream society (Oliviere et al., 2011). In our view, one of the major challenges for the future is to improve equity of access to good quality care during the final phase of life, however long that may last. It is likely that advances in medicine and health technologies will mean that greater numbers of people will survive for longer with complex health and social care needs. This will mean a different type of workforce is required to provide basic palliative care wherever the patient and family are located and opportunities for advice, support, and referral to specialist palliative care providers. This will challenge specialist professionals to facilitate and coordinate care, rather than provide 'hands-on' care, which means that developing knowledge and skills in consultancy, advocacy, education, and leadership will form essential components alongside well-recognized knowledge in pain and symptom management, and psychosocial and existential support. A key component of specialist palliative care, however, must be the continued provision of care, otherwise the workforce deskills itself and loses credibility. In economically disadvantaged countries, it is essential that appropriate, sustainable models are developed.

Online materials

Complete references for this chapter are available online at <http://www.oxfordmedicine.com>.

References

Centeno, C., Clark, D., Lynch, T., *et al.* (2007a). *EAPC Atlas of Palliative Care in Europe*. Milan: European Association for Palliative Care.

Economist Intelligence Unit (2010). *The Quality of Death: Ranking End-Of-Life Care Across the World*. London: Economist Intelligence Unit. Available at: <http://www.eiu.com/sponsor/lienfoundation/qualityofdeath>.

Gamondi, C., Larkin, P., and Payne, S. (2013a). Core competencies in palliative care: an EAPC White Paper on palliative care education—Part 1. *European Journal of Palliative Care*, 20(2), 86–91.

Gamondi, C., Larkin, P., and Payne, S. (2013b). Core competencies in palliative care: an EAPC White Paper on palliative care education—Part 2. *European Journal of Palliative Care*, 20(3), 140–145.

Human Rights Watch (2011). *Global State of Pain Treatment: Access to Palliative Care as a Human Right*. [Online] Available at: <http://www.hrw.org/reports/2011/06/01/global-state-pain-treatment-0>.

Lynch, T., Clark, D., Centeno, C., *et al.* (2009). Barriers to the development of palliative care in CEE and CIS. *Journal of Pain and Symptom Management*, 37(3), 305–315.

Lynch, T., Clark, D., Centeno, C., *et al.* (2010). Barriers to the development of palliative care in Western Europe. *Palliative Medicine*, 24(8), 812–819.

Lynch, T., Clark, D., and Connor, S.R. (2011). *Mapping Levels of Palliative Care Development: A Global Update*. London: Worldwide Palliative Care Alliance.

Payne, S., Chan, N., Davies, A., Poon, E., Connor, S., and Goh, C. (2012). Supportive, palliative and end-of-life care for Asian patients with cancer. *The Lancet Oncology*, 13(11), 492–500.

Radbruch, L. and Payne, S. (2009). White Paper on standards and norms for hospice and palliative care in Europe: part 1. *European Journal of Palliative Care*, 16(6), 278–289.

Radbruch, L. and Payne, S. (2010). White Paper on standards and norms for hospice and palliative care in Europe: part 2. *European Journal of Palliative Care*, 17(1), 22–33.

Sepulveda, C., Marlin, A., Yoshida, T., and Ullrich, A. (2002). Palliative care: the World Health Organization's global perspective. *Journal of Pain and Symptom Management*, 24(2), 91–96.

World Health Organization (2011). *Ensuring Balance in National Policies on Controlled Substances*. Geneva: WHO.

Wright, M., Hamzah, E., Phungrassami, T., and Bausa-Claudio, A. (2010). *Hospice and Palliative Care in Southeast Asia. A Review of developments and Challenges in Malaysia, Thailand and the Philippines*. New York: Oxford University Press.

Wright, M., Wood, J., Lynch, T., and Clark, D. (2008). Mapping levels of palliative care development: a global view. *Journal of Pain and Symptom Management*, 35(5), 469–85.

Providing palliative care in economically disadvantaged countries

M.R. Rajagopal and Reena George

Introduction

A mother in Colombia advertises in a newspaper with a desperate plea to the government to make morphine available to her dying daughter. A man with cancer in India wants to end his life because his doctors would not relieve his pain (Human Rights Watch, 2010). Stories like this are commonplace all over the developing world. Eighty-three per cent of people who live in low- and middle-income countries get only 7% of the world's medical morphine (Pain and Policy Studies Group, 2009).

These inadequacies raise difficult questions for the worldwide palliative care community. How does one provide palliative care when there are so many other disparities in health and economic indices between the rich and poor nations of the world? Table 1.2.1 shows some figures from the reports of the World Health Organization (WHO). The life expectancy in the African Region of the WHO is 20 years less than in Europe. HIV mortality was 40-fold higher. Cardiovascular diseases, the leading cause of death worldwide, are three times as likely to be fatal in resource poor regions (WHO, 2012a).

Eighty per cent of the 17.3 million annual deaths due to cardiovascular diseases and 70% of the 7.6 million annual cancer deaths occurred in low- and middle-income countries. Twenty-five million people have died of HIV in the last three decades, the vast majority in economically disadvantaged countries (WHO, 2012b).

Given the fact that the total annual number of deaths in developing countries will soon reach 50 million, and that about two-thirds of dying patients would probably benefit from palliative care, the only way for universal access to be achieved in resource-poor countries will be by adopting a public health approach (Stjernswärd et al., 2007a, 2007b). The patterns which have evolved, for example, in the United Kingdom and the United States are just far too expensive and, if transplanted into low-income countries, would not reach more than a small percentage of those in need. Any initiatives will have to take into consideration the available resources and ground realities, economic and otherwise, within the developing world.

Important factors influencing the delivery of palliative care in low- and middle-income countries

Poverty and the economic impact of illness

In Africa and India, each with a population of over a billion, about 40% of people live on less than US$1 a day. Government spending on health is disproportionately low (WHO, 2012a). Out-of-pocket expenses for health care, combined with the lack of social security, can have a domino effect on poor families. Treatment-related debt and the loss of a livelihood push families below the poverty line, and children out of schools (Emanuel et al., 2010). Seventy per cent of HIV patients in Africa reported hunger as a symptom (Harding et al., 2012). Palliative care programmes have to find resources to provide free medicines, to support the education of children, and find an alternative source of livelihood for needy families. In Africa, the needs of hundreds of thousands of children orphaned by AIDS have severely stretched the timeline and boundaries of palliative care provision. Many programmes collaborate with other agencies to provide nutritional assistance, safe housing, and income-generation projects (Harding et al., 2003). Currently, only six of 54 African countries have anything approaching a country-wide network of palliative care services, namely South Africa, Kenya, Uganda, Zimbabwe, Zambia, and Malawi (Lynch et al., 2011).

The role of families

In traditional societies, it is rare to find a patient dying alone in a hospital or nursing home. Family members are actively involved in providing physical care and companionship. This is an invaluable resource to build on. Willing hands can be trained in wound management, subcutaneous drug administration, and other tasks. For this to work, palliative care services should develop simple drug and nursing protocols, and respond thoughtfully and sensitively to the caregivers' emotional and financial struggles and their concerns about contagion, addiction, and truth telling.

Table 1.2.1 Disparities in health and economic indices

	Global	High-income countries	Low-income countries	Africa	Europe
Non-communicable diseases age-standardized mortality	573	380	757	779	532
Cardiovascular diseases age-standardized mortality per 100,000, 30–70 years	245	105	375	382	238
Cancer age standardized mortality per 100,000, 30–70 years	150	141	154	147	166
HIV mortality per 100,000	27	2.6	85	160	9.6
HIV prevalence per 100,000	502	207	1445	2740	257
Per capita government expenditure on health in US$	549	2946	10	41	1677
Percentage of population living on less than US$1 per day	22.7	0	48.8	42.6	0
Life expectancy at birth (years)	64	76	52	51	71

Source: data from World Health Organization, *World Health Statistics*, Copyright © 2012 World Health Organization, available from <http://www.who.int/gho/publications/world_health_statistics/EN_WHS2012_Full.pdf>.

Family involvement has its negative aspect too. In societies where the family can override the autonomy of the patient, relatives may demand the continuation of futile treatments, regardless of the wishes of the patient. On the other hand, a fatalistic attitude towards suffering and death may limit care. The health-care team may have to negotiate with numerous relatives before they are allowed to discuss prognosis and options with the patient. Unsolicited advice from the extended family, differences of opinion with accusations about 'not doing enough', and a lack of respect for privacy can also create problems for the patient.

The disease spectrum and dichotomies in existing services

In developing countries, there is often confusion about which diseases fall within the remit of palliative care. In some African countries, more than 20% of the adult population is HIV positive. Twenty-five million people have died of HIV in the last three decades, the vast majority in economically disadvantaged countries. In countries, however, where antiretroviral therapy is provided, HIV is no longer the 'killer' it was (WHO, 2012a).

Financial support from the international donor community is often conditional, for example, limited to people who are HIV positive and with the stipulation that specialized palliative care units take on stable HIV patients just for support care. This impacts adversely on available time and resources and therefore disadvantages many dying patients. People with severe chronic obstructive pulmonary disease may not be eligible for care, even though the suffering may be no less. Cancer in Africa has doubled in incidence with the advent of HIV. Where oncology services and palliative radiotherapy are non-existent, there can be protracted suffering from pain and fungating wounds (Currow et al., 2011).

On the other hand, affluent people in the Middle East, India, and China can easily access state-of-the-art technology for anti-cancer treatment, but not facilities for palliative care. Many centres with the latest machines and anti-cancer treatments do not stock oral morphine for home-based care. The intensive care unit becomes the 'respectable' place to admit the dying patient.

The original WHO description of palliative care as applicable when 'the disease is no longer amenable to curative treatment' may have inadvertently caused suffering by sometimes denying symptom relief and psychosocial support when anti-cancer treatment was still in progress. Those trained in palliative care must be equipped to care for patients with life-limiting illness, whether or not they are at the end of life.

Foundation measures for a public health approach

Palliative care should be integrated with, and not separated from, the mainstream of health care. A public health approach means that the methods adopted must be valid scientifically as well as acceptable, sustainable, and affordable at the community level. The four components of the WHO Public Health Model are:

- appropriate policies
- adequate drug availability
- education of health-care workers and the public
- the implementation of palliative care services at all levels in society (Stjernswärd et al., 2007a).

Mongolia is a good example of a successful top-down implementation of the public health strategy. Initial collaboration between the government, local pioneers, and WHO experts led, within just a few years, to modified narcotic prescribing laws, availability of generic morphine, translation of clinical guidelines into the local language, training programmes, and budgetary support for palliative care. Within the first decade, beds were earmarked in government hospitals for patients needing palliative care, palliative care was included within undergraduate medical and nursing curricula, and courses for specialist training were started (Davaasuren et al., 2007).

In larger populations or where consistent government support is lacking, the process may be slower and more fragmented. Nevertheless it is possible to make a start.

Planting palliative care: international collaboration as a fulcrum

The WHO, through its collaborating centres, recognizes that policymaking bodies need individuals and beacon services as fulcra to initiate implementation. Local pioneers can be empowered with advocacy tools, teaching curricula, clinical guidelines, and policy documents developed by international organizations, associations, and academic centres without having to reinvent the wheel. International funding is vital at this stage (Callaway et al., 2007; Praill and Pahl, 2007; Stjernswärd et al., 2007b; Pantilat et al., 2012).

Propagating palliative care: adapting to the local context and multiplying

Pioneers who start with an existing palliative care 'recipe' should review it carefully to discriminate between the essentials to be retained and elements that need to be adapted to local ingredients (resources), cooking methods (health and family systems), and tastes (cultural appropriateness). The adapted recipe becomes a palatable and doable way to propagate palliative care; progressively reducing reliance on external resources and models, but striving to maintain essential standards (Ferris et al., 2007; Pallium India, 2010).

For example, the British inpatient hospice system cannot be replicated widely in developing countries. It is unjust to give superlative care at great cost to 250 inpatients per annum if 2500 others (or more) are denied any help. Furthermore, experience in Uganda and India has shown that care at home, supported by an outpatient clinic and occasional home visits, is cost-effective in terms of achieving population-wide coverage, with a 'back-up' inpatient facility for those with overwhelming problems, or no family and home.

It is likely that a palliative care service in a resource-poor country will, sooner or later, become swamped with patients, and that the service will have to expand indefinitely and/or reduce the quality of the care. So, given the likelihood of an increasing demand for care, it is essential for new services to have a policy which deals with this eventuality. If possible, such a policy should be based on a properly conducted needs assessment. In all this, it is important to keep the following points in mind:

◆ The palliative care delivery system should be realistic and sustainable.

◆ Patients' needs should come first. This is not automatically the case; the success of the organization or department may effectively become the team's main concern.

◆ A partnership in care needs to be established with the patient. Doctors have no right to force decisions on the patient. Formal education and wisdom are not synonymous.

◆ A partnership in care needs to be established with the family. Enough trained nurses will not be available to care for literally millions of patients. However, success is still possible by empowering the relatives to care for the patient.

◆ The family's finances need to be considered before advising on treatment.

◆ Existing resources should be utilized optimally. Constructing new palliative care centres is likely to exhaust available resources. Wherever possible, use should be made of existing facilities, that is, hospitals and primary health centres.

◆ Deficiencies in existing facilities need to be supplemented by non-governmental organizations (NGOs). Ways must be found to complement existing services, thereby 'plugging gaps' and evolving a seamless integrated service. Experience has shown that, with determination and diplomacy, it is generally possible for NGOs to work successfully alongside government health services.

◆ Volunteers can be the backbone of the palliative care service. There are numerous individuals who are kind-hearted and willing to help. However, this potential work force needs to be trained.

◆ Advocacy is essential. A strategy is necessary to influence policy and to improve funding and drug availability. There is a need both to approach health department decision-makers directly and to influence them indirectly through the public.

Prioritizing palliative care: integration into national health policies

Services may begin as a result of the efforts of local and national 'champions' but in order to achieve population-wide coverage, palliative care needs to be integrated into mainstream health care. This requires government policy for palliative care to be an essential or core element of the national health services. Ideally, there should be a comprehensive generic plan for the development of a palliative care programme for non-communicable diseases including cancer and other end-stage diseases, for HIV/AIDS, and for the care of older people with advanced chronic illnesses which can be implemented worldwide (Stjernswärd et al., 2007b). Inevitably, there will be some disease-specific measures; for example, antiretroviral drugs for those infected with HIV. Policies will not work without action plans, time lines, resources, and accountability for implementation. To achieve this amid all the other claims on very limited health budgets, there needs to be strong, well-reasoned advocacy from community groups, the health professions, and the wider public, such as has been the case in relation to AIDS.

Preserving the soul of palliative care: the need to keep the patient at the centre

A public health strategy is not incompatible with remembering the centrality of the patient, and the deep needs for meaning, connection, and peace at the end of life—concepts fundamental to palliative care, whatever the setting (Selman et al., 2011):

> A patient said 'Thank you. And not just for your pills but for your heart . . . '. (Saunders, 2003, p. 40)
>
> Here again comes a key phrase I have often quoted 'I look for someone to look as if they are trying to understand me.' These patients are not looking for pity and indulgence but that we should look at them with respect and an expectation of courage. (Saunders, 2003, p. 3)

Indeed, the remarkable courage and grace with which many desperately poor people face life and death, can evoke not just respect, but awe, in those privileged to be present with them (George, 2010).

Education

The caregivers, whether professional, volunteer, or family, all need training to enable them to acquire the necessary knowledge, attitude, and skills. Education about palliative care must also be extended to the public at large, policy-makers, and health service administrators.

Advocacy and public awareness

Experience has shown repeatedly that the general public is often more open to new ideas than health-care professionals or administrators. Some doctors may see palliative care as an admission of failure, or as a threat to their earnings. Others may assume they already have the necessary skills. Even when a specialist is reluctant to refer patients to a palliative care service, repeated demands by patients eventually can force a change in attitude.

Public understanding is also necessary to overcome the current problem of over-medicalization of death. It is a disturbing paradox that, in cities in economically backward countries, the dying are often subjected to inappropriate high-tech interventions. People with irreversible end-stage disease frequently die while still on ventilators, the family ruined by the high cost of treatment. Those who choose to withdraw life supports in a futile situation have to assume the guilt and the responsibility of being 'discharged against medical advice'. There is often public discussion about euthanasia but rarely about the possibilities of palliative care as an alternative to suffering or to inappropriate high-tech care.

Public demand can also lead to administrative reforms. Advocacy programmes have an important role to play, as shown by tobacco control programmes. It is up to the palliative care fraternity to bring these issues to public attention through a range of activities that could include:

- articles and real-life stories in newspapers, on television, and the Internet
- inviting key decision-makers and celebrities to Palliative Care Day celebrations
- public awareness programmes as part of community activities
- involving public figures who have encountered palliative care as 'mascots' for palliative care
- involving corporate organizations, clubs, and professional associations in supporting palliative care as a 'worthy cause'
- teaching palliative care and related matters in school and college education.

Training palliative care workers

Palliative care training must address not only knowledge acquisition (*head*) but also attitudes (*heart*) and skills (*hands*). Although it is effective in conveying book knowledge, didactic training seldom changes practice because it seldom changes attitudes and does not improve skills. The best way to learn any aspect of medicine is by the bedside, including 'hands-on' training. Unfortunately, this cannot always be arranged. When a short didactic course is all that can be offered, it helps if:

- one to two sessions include a clinical presentation with the patient in the classroom
- course participants can spend 1–2 hours observing a palliative clinic in action
- course participants can join in for a home visit.

Professional and volunteer education is essential at all levels of health care. The following examples from the grass-roots and the tertiary levels illustrate the range of possibilities in the developing world.

Educational initiatives from the grass roots

The Palliative Care Toolkit (Lavy et al., 2008) is a good example of an open-access, easy-to-use curriculum, developed within low-income countries and based on local case studies and available clinical resources.

The Toolkit was written to empower health workers to integrate symptom control and holistic support into the care they are already giving. It takes a 'can-do' approach, encouraging health workers at all levels that, with some basic training, they can make a difference to the lives of patients for whom cure is not possible (Coombes, 2008).

Advice on non-drug treatment runs alongside the medical guide to symptom control, equipping non-prescribers and lay volunteers to give good nursing care even where drugs are not available. Communication skills and psychological and spiritual support are addressed, with attention paid to the special needs of children. A set of tools to be used in the field includes forms for patient records and data collection, advocacy material, teaching aids, and a basic drug list.

The Toolkit training manual (Lavy, 2009) contains ready-made teaching material based on the Toolkit. It has been written for health workers doing palliative care who want to train others but have minimal experience in teaching and little time for preparation. Separate modules can be used as single sessions, or put together to create courses for different audiences and settings. Teaching materials, such as case studies, discussion topics, questions, and answers, are provided.

The Toolkit has been translated and is available at no cost on the Worldwide Palliative Care Alliance website in eight languages (Worldwide Palliative Care Alliance, 2009). Training grants have been awarded to organizations across India, sub-Saharan Africa, and Latin America (Help the Hospices, 2009).

Educational initiatives from national authorities

The notification of a higher speciality training programme, MD (Palliative Medicine), by the Medical Council of India and the Indian government is a significant milestone within the developing world towards developing a cadre of leaders and trainers for the future and integrating palliative medicine in medical education (Medical Council of India, 2010).

Drug availability

It is generally agreed that opioid analgesics are the mainstay of cancer pain management (WHO, 1986). Policies and recommendations for rational public health implementation are available (Joranson and Ryan, 2007), and essential drug policies have been established (De Lima, 2006)

Despite this, limited drug availability, specifically of morphine, continues to be a major obstacle to the development of palliative care. David Joranson, former Director of the Pain and Policy Studies Group, University of Wisconsin Comprehensive Cancer Center, and the team at the WHO Collaborating Center for Policy and Communications in Cancer Care, have helped local palliative care activists in many countries over the last 15 years (Mosoiu et al., 2006). However, it seems that one has to be Houdini to escape from the ensnarement of bureaucratic (and indifferent) red tape.

Widespread poverty in low- and middle-income countries means that, unless drugs are inexpensive, overcoming regulatory barriers alone does not translate into pain relief. Uganda has developed a simple protocol for local pharmacies to prepare inexpensive oral morphine solution from powder (Merriman and Harding, 2010). Through advocacy from Hospice Africa Uganda, with continued funding through Hospice Africa (UK), affordable oral morphine has been introduced to Tanzania, Malawi, Sierra Leone, Nigeria, Cameroon, and Ethiopia. A survey in 12 African countries identified an interplay of factors—regulatory barriers, fear of addiction and punitive regulations, a shortage of drug stocks, prescribers, and dispensers—affecting the availability of analgesics and other essential drugs (Harding et al., 2010).

Paradoxically, expensive drugs are frequently available in many countries. The power of drug companies to buy influence over every key group in health care—doctors, NGOs, charities, patient groups, journalists, politicians—is deeply disturbing (Ferner, 2005). In the absence of close monitoring, questionable practices go undocumented in developing countries.

Put at its simplest, the pharmaceutical industry tends to promote expensive new analgesics. As this is not balanced by medical education in the use of less expensive drugs, this leads to the unnecessary prescription of expensive drugs. It is shameful that many institutions have expensive sustained-release morphine, but not inexpensive ordinary morphine preparations. Many centres use transdermal fentanyl as the first-line strong opioid. Limited resources are thus spent unnecessarily, and thousands of other people are denied pain relief as a consequence. Pharmaco-economics are an important aspect of the implementation of palliative care services. The Morphine Manifesto, which was endorsed by 64 international organizations in 2012, warns governments and medical institutions against this danger (Pallium India et al., 2012).

Implementation

Possibilities and challenges at the national level: two examples of palliative care development in economically disadvantaged settings

Example 1: Uganda

Currently Uganda is the only low-income country in the world with a fully integrated palliative care service (Lynch et al., 2011). This development illustrates the steps of planting, propagation, and prioritization:

Hospice Africa (UK) supported the development of a cost-effective and culturally acceptable model in an African country, which could be adapted to the needs of other African countries. Hospice Africa Uganda started as a pilot project in 1993. A viable home care model was developed, oral morphine was formulated locally, and doctor and nurse training commenced. Sustained advocacy and partnership with the Ministry of Health led to a stakeholders workshop in 1998 supported by the WHO. Palliative care for people with AIDS and cancer was made a priority in the National Health Plan, where it is classed as 'essential clinical care for all Ugandans'. The government committed itself to putting resources and systems in place. Legislation was changed to allow nurses and clinical officers to prescribe oral morphine after they had completed a closely mentored 9-month training programme (Jagwe and Merriman, 2007; Merriman and Harding, 2010).

Uganda has thus established all the foundation measures as recommended by the WHO:

◆ a clear national policy has been agreed

◆ education in palliative care is incorporated into the undergraduate curricula of doctors and nurses

◆ courses and workshops in pain relief and palliative care, are available to health care professionals at all levels

◆ affordable morphine is produced generically within the country

◆ the Ministry of Health has published guidelines for handling morphine and other strong opioids

◆ nurses qualified in palliative care are able to prescribe morphine.

Uganda was a key demonstration country in the WHO's community health approach to palliative care for HIV/AIDS and cancer patients in Africa, a joint project between Botswana, Ethiopia, Tanzania, Uganda, and Zimbabwe (WHO, 2004). It has demonstrated the importance and success of a harmoniously integrated government approach with clear policies and a decentralized, community-based approach, linked to its HIV/AIDS programme.

The African Palliative Care Association was established in 2003. The Association works closely with existing palliative care services throughout Africa to promote advocacy, service development, education, research, and appropriate standards.

Example 2: India

In the early 1980s, there were only a few pain clinics in various parts of India. Modern palliative care was first introduced in 1986 in the form of Shanti Avedna Ashram, an inpatient hospice in Bombay. However, the more widespread development of palliative care was minimal until 1993 when the Indian Association of Palliative Care was launched and the Pain and Palliative Care Society (PPCS) in Kozhikode, Kerala was founded.

The PPCS succeeded in developing an effective, low-cost, home-care system based on an outpatient clinic functioning 6 days a week, supported by home visits when possible, and inpatient facility when essential (Ajithakumari et al., 1997; Rajagopal and Kumar, 1999). In 1995, the PPCS was designated a WHO demonstration project for a community-based approach. The PPCS trained and involved an increasing number of doctors and members of the public in providing palliative care. By working with lay volunteers, a network of 33 palliative care clinics developed in the surrounding part of Kerala over the next 7 years. Typically, these functioned on 1 or 2 days per week (Rajagopal and Venkateswaran, 2003).

Because there are no support systems for the chronically ill, palliative care services were not restricted to people with cancer and AIDS, but extended to:

◆ stable chronic disorders, such as post-traumatic paraplegia

◆ fluctuating chronic disorders, such as filarial lymphoedema and sickle-cell disease

◆ slowly progressive diseases, such as peripheral vascular disease

◆ all end-stage progressive diseases, such as renal failure and chronic obstructive pulmonary disease with respiratory failure.

Since the turn of the century, Neighbourhood Networks in Palliative Care have been established (Kumar, 2004). These are mainly volunteer driven and community owned. Questions have been raised about the quality of care that such teams can give (Gupta, 2004). While there is a need for the care system to be evaluated systematically, there is little doubt that these programmes have increased the community's awareness and participation in providing access to palliative care (Downing et al., 2005).

The Indian Association of Palliative Care has been a major force in bringing together palliative care workers in a large country and in sharing ideas. The association has been involved in advocacy, education, and research over 20 years. With support from many funding agencies, Pallium India, an NGO, has catalysed the development of eight palliative care centres in major teaching health-care institutions in North and North-East India and facilitated the initiation of two palliative care training centres in South India.

Although most palliative care delivery in India has been driven by NGOs, government involvement has also been important. For example:

◆ Palliative care centres have been exempted from the need for a 'drug licence', thereby enabling them to dispense morphine without an obligation to employ a qualified pharmacist, something which most centres could not afford (Joranson et al., 2002).

◆ Narcotic regulations have been simplified in 13 of 28 states and there are current efforts to change central legislation to improve access to opioids (Palat and Rajagopal, 2006).

◆ An uninterrupted supply of morphine sulphate powder has been guaranteed from government opium and alkaloid factories (Rajagopal et al., 2001).

◆ Palliative care is now part of the government's national programme for prevention and control of cancer, diabetes, cardiovascular diseases, and stroke (Government of India, 2010).

◆ The Government of Kerala declared a palliative care policy in 2008 integrating palliative care into the government's health-care system (Government of Kerala, 2008).

◆ The Medical Council of India has approved higher speciality training in palliative medicine.

Implementation at the grass roots: small beginnings matter too

Worldwide, only a minority of governments in economically disadvantaged countries have implemented palliative care policies effectively. For much of the world's population, comprehensive top-down approaches providing palliative care may not happen in the near future. The efforts, big and small, of individuals remain invaluable. Those who wish to help, but are uncertain as to how, can use the WHO framework as they plan service development at the grass roots.

'Start low, go slow, but do so' is a good motto when a worthwhile task seems daunting. Many beacon services began as small initiatives when someone was moved by an unmet need, and tried to make a small beginning by using what was available, and supplementing what was not.

But how does one begin? A few questions are helpful:

A. Needs assessment

1. Who needs palliative care where we are working?

2. What are their main problems?

3. What help are they getting at present? What is already available and what is not?

4. What could be added to improve their care and make it holistic (Lavy et al., 2008)?

These questions help think through the complex social and clinical needs to be met, to brainstorm the resources available, and to consider how the gaps could be filled using existing personnel. Allies can be found within and beyond the health-care system- individuals of goodwill in the community, groups involved in areas such as poverty alleviation and literacy, or the care of vulnerable people. As people come together to work for a common goal, new ideas are generated, resources are optimally used, change begins, others join, and the momentum grows.

The service in Kozhikode, India, for example, began with a doctor and a housewife from the community giving a few hours a week to provide pain management and counselling within a government hospital. In less than 5 years the service became a WHO demonstration centre for the developing world. A group of committed people in the United Kingdom provided the support that enabled Anne Merriman to pilot a palliative care programme that later became a model for Africa.

Fig. 1.2.1 from the Palliative Care Toolkit, shows palliative care as a tree. Its roots are the four elements of holistic care: physical, psychological, social and spiritual. Each of these roots can be made up from different components, e.g. existing clinics, faith communities, local NGOs. The branches and leaves which grow from these roots represent holistic palliative care in its different forms—different 'models of care' (Lavy et al., 2008, p. 6).

B. Strategy

What is already available and what is not?

What would be the most appropriate setting to begin in our context, home care? Outpatient clinic? Hospital support team?

Which locally appropriate models can we visit and learn from?

Can any part of the work be undertaken by existing organizations?

C. Education

Do we have a trained doctor and nurse?

Can we develop volunteers to act as the link between the patients and the health-care professionals?

How will we empower families to care for patients?

Are our colleagues sufficiently educated to refer appropriate patients to the new service?

Is the public aware of the benefits of a palliative care service?

D. Drug availability

Do we know how to procure strong opioids, particularly inexpensive preparations of morphine?

How much morphine should we stock?

How much free treatment will we be able to provide?

Do we have enough money for an uninterrupted supply of essential drugs?

E. Implementation

Have we made a practical action plan with short-term, medium-term, and long-term goals?

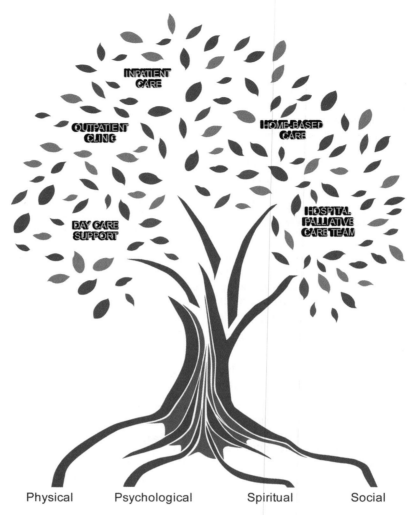

Fig. 1.2.1 Growing a model of care from available resources.

PHYSICAL	PSYCHOLOGICAL	SPIRITUAL	SOCIAL
Patient care:	Counselling:	Individuals:	NGOs:
Health centre	Social worker	Local religious leaders	FBOs
Local hospital	Trained volunteer	Volunteers from faith communities	Food supply work
Private clinics	HIV counselor	Social workers	OVC groups
Traditional healers	Patient advocates –	Family members	Income generation schemes
NGOs doing healthcare	Others with the same illness		Small loan schemes
ART clinic		Groups:	
	Support groups:	Faith community, e.g. church,	Individual professionals:
Drug supply:	PLHIV group	mosque, temple, synagogue	Social worker
Hospital pharmacy	Women's group	Women's groups	Legal advisor, for making wills
Local pharmacy shops	Youth organizations	Hospital visiting team	
		Children's groups	Involving others:
Advice and support:	Support at home:		Community leaders
Local doctor/nurse/clinician	HBC volunteers		Local schools and colleges
Local physiotherapist	Family members		Community groups
National palliative care association			

FBO: faith-based organization; HBC: home-based care; OVC: orphans and vulnerable care groups; PLHIV: people living with HIV.

Reproduced from Lavy V., Bond, C., and Woolridge, R., (2008) Palliative care toolkit: improving care from the roots up in resource-limited settings, Help the Hospices, London, with kind permission.

Do we have stated deadlines for drug availability and educational activities?

When do we schedule our reviews?

What performance indices should we monitor? Are they important and measurable (Downing et al., 2012)?

Implementation in the longer term

Building up without burning out

It is not easy to be a pioneer in palliative care in the developing world. The numbers unreached, intensity of suffering, and abject poverty create an urgent imperative. Juxtaposed with this, the lack of trained hands, essential drugs, acceptance within mainstream health care, and sustainable funding can be demoralizing. The gaps between needs and resources on the one hand, and idealism and personal limitations on the other, increase the risk of burnout.

Burnout happens in many professions and contexts (Maslach et al., 2001). It is touched upon in this chapter because both the risk of burnout and its impact on the provision of palliative care are likely to be significant, albeit unacknowledged in economically disadvantaged settings. To take an analogy from mountaineering, climbing an uncharted peak is more challenging and risky than when there are maps, systems, and resources in place.

Palliative care pioneers could base preventive measures on the same strategies that mountain climbers use in preparing for the long haul. The acronym '*TEAMS*' summarizes some important components: *training* that is multifaceted, *equipment* and resources that are appropriate, *awareness* of possible dangers, *mentors* to accompany, and *spaces* that are base camps to recuperate and recharge (see Box 1.2.1).

In many resource-poor settings, there may be not be occupational health services or human resource departments to deal with staff stress and burnout. Developing creative and accessible ways to address these issues should be a part of the strategy to provide sustainable palliative care in the developing world.

Charisma versus routinization

It has been said that history alternates between charisma and routinization. In this context, charisma refers to the ability of exceptional individuals to act as a catalyst for social change, and acknowledges the impact of personality in bringing about radical innovation in institutions and established beliefs. In relation to the evolution of palliative care in the United Kingdom, United States, and other English-speaking Western countries, Cicely Saunders was the initial charismatic influence. Now, in countries where palliative care is well established and fully integrated into the National Health Service, a major challenge is to prevent palliative care moving from the creative and disruptive influence of charisma to the cosy ambience of routinization (Twycross, 2002).

Conclusion

It is crucial to the continuing development of palliative care worldwide that palliative care remains *a movement with momentum*, manifesting an ongoing creative tension between charisma and routinization. Fortunately, so far, this often seems to be the case. It is heartening that in many countries palliative care is breaking out of its original cocoon, and is responding imaginatively and compassionately to neglected and unsupported suffering of many kinds in the community.

Box 1.2.1 'TEAMS': Strategies to reduce burnout in palliative care workers

Training: training in areas of management such as strategic planning, writing a business plan, assertiveness, working in teams, fundraising, setting boundaries, and conflict management.

Equipping: human resources and funds, even within resource-limited settings, need to be reasonably proportional to the expectations from the service. Training, empowering, involving the community, and developing a public health approach are long-term strategies for sustainability. However, during lean periods, when staffing and resources are low, it may be necessary to take difficult decisions about what to prioritize, what to cut out, and how to invest in obtaining more resources before the service itself 'burns out' trying to be all things to all people.

Awareness: pioneers need to be aware of the possibility of burnout, to develop the maturity to be self-aware, recognize danger signs, and accept constructive criticism (Maslach et al., 2014). Colleagues, patients, and family members may recognize withdrawal, cynicism, or emotional exhaustion long before the person affected acknowledges it.

Mentorship: mentorship can be provided by local colleagues as well as by advisors who are experienced in palliative care, administration, policymaking, and stress management. Resilient and balanced teams protect against burnout as they understand the strengths, interests, and weaknesses of team members, deploy this diversity in varied team roles (HumanMetrics, n.d.), and are willing to give and receive mutual support.

Safe spaces: pacing oneself, by interspersing activities that provide renewal and rest, is legitimate and not 'selfish' when so much remains to be done. Wisely investing off-duty hours in hobbies, holidays, family pursuits, sleep, physical fitness, and spirituality are good external ways to recharge from the demands of work. Within work itself, an analysis of one's motivations and talents (Assessment. com, 2014), can identify specific activities, for example, teaching, research, or networking that are invigorating. Making space to look back and be grateful for what has already been achieved can guard against a reduced sense of personal accomplishment.

Online materials

Complete references for this chapter are available online at <http://www.oxfordmedicine.com>.

References

Callaway, M., Foley, K.M., De Lima, L., *et al.* (2007). Funding for palliative care programs in developing countries. *Journal of Pain and Symptom Management*, 33, 509–513.

Currow, D.C., Wheeler, J.L., and Abernethy, A.P., (2011). International perspective: outcomes of palliative oncology. *Seminars in Oncology*, 38, 343–350.

Davaasuren, O., Stjernswärd, J., Callaway, M., *et al.* (2007). Mongolia: establishing a national palliative care program. *Journal of Pain and Symptom Management*, 33, 568–572.

De Lima, L. (2006). The international association for hospice and palliative care list of essential medicines for palliative care. *Palliative Medicine*, 20, 647–651.

Downing, J., Simon, S.T., Mwangi-Powell, F.N., *et al*. (2012). Outcomes 'out of Africa': the selection and implementation of outcome measures for palliative care in Africa. *BMC Palliative Care*, 11, 1.

Emanuel, N., Simon, M.A., Burt, M., *et al*. (2010). Economic impact of terminal illness and the willingness to change it. *Journal of Palliative Medicine*, 13, 941–944.

Ferris, F.D., Gómez-Batiste, X., Fürst, C.J., and Connor, S., (2007). Implementing quality palliative care. *Journal of Pain and Symptom Management*, 33, 533–541.

George, R. (2010). Life's lessons lost . . . and learned. *Journal of Clinical Oncology*, 28, 1806–1807.

Government of India (2010). *NPCDCS Guidelines*. [Online] Available at: <http://health.bih.nic.in/Docs/Guidelines-NPCDCS.pdf>.

Government of Kerala (2008). *Palliative Care Policy*. [Online] Available at: <http://www.kerala.gov.in/docs/policies/pain.pdf>.

Harding, R., Powell, R.A., Kiyange, F., Downing, J., and Mwangi-Powell, F., (2010). Provision of pain- and symptom-relieving drugs for HIV/AIDS in sub-Saharan Africa. *Journal of Pain and Symptom Management*, 40, 405–415.

Harding, R., Selman, L., Agupio, G., *et al*. (2012). Prevalence, burden, and correlates of physical and psychological symptoms among HIV palliative care patients in sub-Saharan Africa: an international multi-center study. *Journal of Pain and Symptom Management*, 44, 1–9.

Harding, R., Stewart, K., Marconi, K., O'Neill, J.F., and Higginson, I.J. (2003). Current HIV/AIDS end-of-life care in sub-Saharan Africa: a survey of models, services, challenges and priorities. *BMC Public Health*, 3, 33.

Help the Hospices (2009). *Palliative Care Toolkit Grants: Round One*. [Online] Available at: <http://www.helpthehospices.org.uk/our-services/grants/case-studies/palliative-care-toolkit-grants-round-one/>.

Jagwe, J. and Merriman, A. (2007). Uganda: delivering analgesia in rural Africa: opioid availability and nurse prescribing. *Journal of Pain and Symptom Management*, 33, 547–551.

Joranson, D.E., Rajagopal, M.R., and Gilson, A.M. (2002). Improving access to opioid analgesics for palliative care in India. *Journal of Pain and Symptom Management*, 24, 152–159.

Joranson, D.E. and Ryan, K.M. (2007). Ensuring opioid availability: methods and resources. *Journal of Pain and Symptom Management*, 33, 527–532.

Kumar, S. (2004). Learning from low income countries: what are the lessons? Palliative care can be delivered through neighbourhood networks. *BMJ*, 329, 1184.

Lavy, V. (2009). *Palliative Care Toolkit: Trainer's Manual*. London: Help the Hospices.

Lavy, V., Bond, C., and Woolridge, R. (2008). *Palliative Care Toolkit: Improving Care From the Roots Up in Resource-Limited Settings*. London: Help the Hospices.

Lynch T., Clark D., Connor R., *et al*. (2011). *Mapping Levels of Palliative Care Development: A Global Update 2011*. [Online] Worldwide Palliative Care Alliance. Available at: <http://www.thewpca.org/resources/>.

Maslach, C., Schaufeli, W.B., and Leiter, M.P. (2001). Job burnout. *Annual Review of Psychology*, 52, 397–422.

Merriman, A. and Harding, R., (2010). Pain control in the African context: the Ugandan introduction of affordable morphine to relieve suffering at the end of life. *Philosophy, Ethics, and Humanities in Medicine*, 5, 10.

Mosoiu, D., Ryan, K.M., Joranson, D.E., and Garthwaite, J.P. (2006). Reform of drug control policy for palliative care in Romania. *The Lancet*, 367, 2110–2117.

Pain and Policy Studies Group. (2009). *Opioid Consumption Data*. [Online] Available at: <http://painpolicy.wordpress.com/2011/10/18/2009-incb-opioid-consumption-data-now-available-on-ppsg-website/>.

Pallium India (2010). *Standards Audit Tools for Palliative Care Programs*. [Online] Available at: <http://palliumindia.org/cms/wp-content/uploads/2010/01/palliumindia-standardstool.pdf>.

Pallium India, International Association for Hospice and Palliative Care, and Pain & Policy Studies Group/WHO Collaborating Center (2012). *The Morphine Manifesto: A Call for Affordable Access to Immediate Release Oral Morphine*. [Online] Available at: <http://palliumindia.org/manifesto/>.

Praill, D. and Pahl, N., (2007). The worldwide palliative care alliance: networking national associations. *Journal of Pain and Symptom Management*, 33, 506–508.

Rajagopal, M.R., Joranson D.E., and Gilson A.M. (2001). Medical use, misuse, and diversion of opioids in India. *The Lancet*, 358, 139–143.

Rajagopal, M.R. and Kumar, S. (1999). A model for delivery of palliative care in India—the Calicut experiment. *Journal of Palliative Care*, 15, 44–49.

Rajagopal M.R. and Venkateswaran C. (2003). Palliative care in India: successes and limitations. *Journal of Pain & Palliative Care Pharmacotherapy*, 17, 121–128.

Saunders, C. (2003). *Watch with Me: Inspiration for a Life in Hospice Care*. Sheffield: Mortal Press.

Selman, L.E., Higginson, I.J., Agupio, G., *et al*. (2011). Quality of life among patients receiving palliative care in South Africa and Uganda: a multi-centred study. *Health and Quality of Life Outcomes*, 9, 21.

Stjernswärd, J., Foley, K.M., and Ferris, F.D. (2007a). The public health strategy for palliative care. *Journal of Pain and Symptom Management*, 33, 486–493.

Stjernswärd, J., Foley, K.M., and Ferris, F.D. (2007b). Integrating palliative care into national policies. *Journal of Pain and Symptom Management*, 33, 514–520.

Twycross, R.G. (2002). Palliative care: an international necessity. *Journal of Pain & Palliative Care Pharmacotherapy*, 16, 61–79.

World Health Organisation (2004). *A Community Health Approach to Palliative Care for HIV/AIDS and Cancer Patients in Sub-Saharan Africa*. Geneva: WHO.

World Health Organization (2012a). *World Health Statistics*. [Online] Available at: <http://www.who.int/gho/publications/world_health_statistics/EN_WHS2012_Full.pdf>.

World Health Organization (2012b). *Fact Sheets*. [Online] Available at: <http://www.who.int/mediacentre/factsheets/fs355/en/index.html>.

Worldwide Palliative Care Alliance (2009). *Resources*. Available at: <http://www.thewpca.org/resources/>.

1.3

Essential medicines for palliative care

Liliana De Lima, Lukas Radbruch, and Eduardo Bruera

Introduction to essential medicines for palliative care

The 'essential medicines' concept developed by the World Health Organization (WHO) states that there is a list of minimum medicines for a basic health-care system, including the most efficacious, safe, and cost-effective ones for priority conditions (WHO, 2012). According to the WHO, essential medicines are those that satisfy the primary health-care needs of the population (WHO, 2000). Thus, essential medicines should always be available, affordable, and used adequately.

Access to essential medicines as part of the right to the highest attainable standard of health ('the right to health') is well founded in international law. The right to health first emerged as a social right in the WHO Constitution (International Health Conference, 1946) and in the Universal Declaration of Human Rights (United Nations (UN), 1948). The binding International Covenant on Economic, Social, and Cultural Rights (ICESCR) of 1966 details the progressive realization of the right to health through four concrete steps, including access to health facilities, goods, and services. The General Comment 14 (UN, 2000a) further applies the principles of accessibility, availability, appropriateness, and assured quality to goods and services, which include essential medicines as defined by the WHO. In accordance with this, Target 8E of the eighth Millennium Development Goal (UN, 2000b) relates to access to essential medicines: 'In cooperation with pharmaceutical companies, provide access to affordable essential medicines in developing countries was measured using nine indicators for measuring access to medicines using data collected by WHO and its partners'. In addition, access to medical products and technologies as part of the right to health recognized in countries' constitutions or national legislation is the first country progress indicator for Strategic Objective 11 ('Ensure improved access, quality and use of medical products and technologies') of the WHO *Medium-Term Strategic Plan for 2008–2013* (WHO, 2008). In spite of all these efforts and commitments, the vast majority of the global population still does not have access to essential medicines. A UN report (UN, 2011) found that in the public sector, generic medicines are only available in 38.1% of facilities, and on average cost 250% more than the international reference price. In the private sector, those same medicines are available in 63.3% of facilities, but cost on average about 610% more than the international reference price. High prices limit access to medicines with common treatment regimens, costing a significant portion of the salary of workers in developing countries. The cost of treatment for chronic diseases is particularly unaffordable because of the need for long-term treatment protocols. Although there are no specific reports on access to essential medicines used in palliative care, many of these global reports include medications used in palliative care, such as potent analgesics, antidepressants, laxatives, and others. Of these, lack of access to opioids is a global problem which has been highlighted in many global and regional reports (African Palliative Care Association, 2006; International Narcotics Control Board, 2011; European School of Medical Oncology, 2012). The WHO estimates that 80% of the world's population, including tens of millions of people worldwide who suffer from moderate to severe pain, does not have adequate access to pain treatment. This includes 5.5 million terminal cancer and 1 million end-stage AIDS patients (WHO 2009). Many organizations, including UN bodies and non-governmental organizations, have called on governments to improve availability of these essential medicines and developed programmes and projects to increase awareness and knowledge. This chapter describes two such projects developed by the International Association for Hospice and Palliative Care (IAHPC), based on the 'essential medications' concept: they are the IAHPC List of Essential Medicines in Palliative Care and the Opioid Essential Prescription Package (OEPP). The main goal of these projects is to improve access to medicines and better patient care throughout the world.

The first section of this chapter describes the development of the IAHPC List of Essential Medicines followed by a description of the development of the OEPP. The final section describes the dissemination strategies and future developments for each.

IAHPC List of Essential Medicines in Palliative Care

In 2004, the WHO requested support from the IAHPC to develop a list of essential medicines for palliative care. At that time, the WHO Model List of Essential Medicines (WHO, 2005) had a section called 'Palliative Care', which did not list any medications, but contained a paragraph suggesting that all drugs mentioned in the WHO publication *Cancer Pain Relief with a Guide to Opioid Availability* (2nd ed.) (WHO, 1996) be considered essential. This publication has since been revised by WHO and replaced by other publications including *WHO Guidelines on the Pharmacological Treatment of Persisting Pain in Children with Medical Illnesses* (WHO, 2012) and two more currently in preparation: *WHO*

Guidelines on the Pharmacological Treatment of Persisting Pain in Adults with Medical Illnesses, and the *WHO Guidelines on the Pharmacological Treatment of Acute Pain.* The List of Essential Medicines in Palliative Care was completed in 2006.

The IAHPC convened a working group of international experts in the field. The Committee developed a plan of action, with the following steps:

Identification of the most prevalent symptoms in palliative care: it was agreed that the list would focus on medications to treat symptoms and not underlying conditions. As an example, disease-modifying treatments for cancers and HIV were excluded. An initial list of the 21 most common symptoms in palliative care was developed by the working group based on a review of the published literature at that time (Box 1.3.1) (Education for Physicians on End-of-Life Care, 1999; Lipman et al., 2000; Carr et al., 2002; Potter et al., 2003; Plan and Arnold, 2005; Solano et al., 2006).

Development of a baseline list: palliative care leaders from around the world were asked to propose appropriate medications for the 21 most frequently encountered symptoms. Of a total of 40 people who responded, 34 were physicians (85%) and 15 were from developing countries. In total, they recommended 147 products. This initial list was decreased to 120 by removing non-medications (e.g. oxygen and vitamins) and duplicates.

Delphi survey: an online survey with rating panels was sent to 112 physicians and pharmacists (77 from developing countries). Using a scale of 1–9, participants were asked to rate the safety and efficacy of each medication. Seventy-one participants (63% RR) responded.

Development of the final list: 28 global, regional, and professional representatives of pain and palliative care organizations were invited to a face-to-face-meeting in May 2006. Representatives from 26 of these organizations attended. Through a discussion and consensus process, each one of the medications resulting from the modified Delphi process was reviewed, based on the available evidence and the participants' own experience. Thirty-three medications for which there was consensus on efficacy and safety were included in the list. The resulting list was approved by all the participants as the IAHPC Essential Medicines List for Palliative Care (Table 1.3.1).

The group agreed that there was not enough evidence to recommend any medications as both safe and effective for five symptoms—bone pain, dry mouth, sweating, fatigue, and hiccups—and recognized that additional research was needed to identify safe and effective medications to treat these symptoms.

The resulting IAHPC List of Essential Medicines was published in several journals and widely disseminated (De Lima, 2006).

Opioid essential prescription package

The IAHPC List of Essential Medicines in Palliative Care does not specify dosages or combinations of treatment regimens such as those needed for chronic pain treatment, for example, the list does not recommend which opioid, laxative, and antiemetic may be most safe and effective in the treatment of chronic pain in patients who require initiation of strong opioids. In 2011, the IAHPC wanted to recommend an essential package of medications that could ensure that opioids are more available to patients and therefore lead to more sustained improvements in pain control.

Opioid medications are the mainstay of moderate to severe pain treatment (WHO, 2002). However, an estimated 80% of patients in need do not have adequate access to analgesics (WHO, 2007; Deandrea et al., 2008). Regulatory barriers and limited resources are among several causes of poor availability of medications. In addition, inadequate training of health-care professionals and poor communication between physicians and patients often lead to undertreated pain and the presence of adverse effects which are preventable or treatable.

Adverse effects of opioids, such as constipation and nausea, may limit the dosing of opioids and lead to early discontinuation and inadequate analgesia.

Constipation affects up to 87% of people with advanced conditions who are receiving opioids (Sykes, 1998). There are recommendations that laxative prophylaxis for prevention of constipation should be a priority when patients are starting opioid medication (Larkin et al., 2008). Laxatives can be separated into two types: those that act by softening faecal matter and those that act through direct stimulation of peristalsis. The evidence to favour one laxative over another in palliative care is scarce. Only a few trials show that oral lactulose, polyethylene glycol/electrolyte solutions, and senna are effective in people with opioid-induced constipation (Agra et al., 1998; Ramesh et al., 1998).

Nausea and vomiting occur in 15–40% of patients (Campora et al., 1991; Aparasu et al., 1999). Some health-care professionals suggest using antiemetics for the prevention of nausea and vomiting whenever opioids are prescribed, but there is limited evidence to support this recommendation (Nicholson, 2003). Metoclopramide is generally recommended as first-line therapy given that it has central effects as well as aids gastric emptying. Medications with

---

Box 1.3.1 Most common symptoms in palliative care

Anorexia–cachexia
Anxiety
Constipation
Delirium
Depression
Diarrhoea
Dry mouth
Dyspnoea
Fatigue
Hiccups
Insomnia
Nausea
Pain (intensity):
    mild to moderate
    moderate to severe
Pain (type):
    bone
    neuropathic
    visceral
Sweating
Terminal respiratory congestion
Terminal restlessness
Vomiting

Table 1.3.1 IAHPC List of Essential Medicines for Palliative Care©

Medication	Formulation	Indication for palliative care
*Amitriptyline**	50–150 mg tablets	Depression
		Neuropathic pain
Bisacodyl	10 mg tablets	Constipation
	10 mg rectal suppositories	
Carbamazepine**	100–200 mg tablet	Neuropathic pain
Citalopram (*or any other equivalent generic SSRI except paroxetine and fluvoxamine*)	20 mg tablets	Depression
	10 mg/5mL oral solution	
	20–40 mg injectable	
Codeine	30 mg tablets	Diarrhoea
		Pain—mild to moderate
Dexamethasone	0.5–4 mg tablets	Anorexia
	4 mg/mL injectable	Nausea
		Neuropathic pain
		Vomiting
Diazepam	2.5–10 mg tablets	Anxiety
	5 mg/mL injectable	
	10 mg rectal suppository	
Diclofenac	25–50 mg tablets	Pain—mild to moderate
	50 and 75 mg/3 mL injectable	
Diphenhydramine	25 mg tablets	Nausea
	50 mg/mL injectable	Vomiting
Fentanyl (*transdermal patch*)	25 micrograms/hour	Pain—moderate to severe
	50 micrograms/hour	
Gabapentin	300 mg or 400 mg tablets	Neuropathic pain
Haloperidol	0.5–5 mg tablets	Delirium
	0.5–5 mg drops	Nausea
	0.5–5 mg/mL injectable	Vomiting
		Terminal restlessness
Hyoscine butylbromide	20 mg/1 mL oral solution	Nausea
	10 mg tablets	Terminal respiratory congestion
	10 mg/mL injectable	Visceral pain
		Vomiting
Ibuprofen	200 mg tablets	Pain—mild to moderate
	400 mg tablets	
Levomepromazine	5–50 mg tablets	Delirium
	25 mg/mL injectable	Terminal restlessness
Loperamide	2 mg tablets	Diarrhoea
Lorazepam***	0.5–2 mg tablets	Anxiety
	2 mg/mL liquid/drops	Insomnia
	2–4 mg/mL injectable	
Megestrol acetate	160 mg tablets	Anorexia
	40 mg/mL solution	
Methadone (*immediate release*)	5 mg tablets	Pain—moderate to severe
	1 mg/mL oral solution	
Metoclopramide	10 mg tablets	Nausea
	5 mg/mL injectable	Vomiting

(*continued*)

Table 1.3.1 Continued

Medication	Formulation	Indication for palliative care
Midazolam	1–5 mg/mL injectable	Anxiety Terminal restlessness
Mineral oil enema		
Mirtazapine *(or any other generic dual action NassA or SNRI)*	15–30 mg tablets 7.5–15 mg injectable	Depression
Morphine	Immediate release: 10–60 mg tablets Immediate release: 10 mg/5 mL oral solution Immediate release: 10 mg/mL injectable Sustained release: 10 mg tablets Sustained release: 30 mg tablets	Dyspnoea Pain—moderate to severe
Octreotide	100 micrograms/mL injectable	Diarrhoea Vomiting
Oral rehydration salts		Diarrhoea
Oxycodone	5 mg tablet	Pain—moderate to severe
Paracetamol (Acetaminophen)	100–500 mg tablets 500 mg rectal suppositories	Pain—mild to moderate
Prednisolone *(as an alternative to dexamethasone)*	5 mg tablet	Anorexia
Senna	8.6 mg tablets	Constipation
Tramadol	50 mg immediate release tablets/capsules 100 mg/1 mL oral solution 50 mg/mL injectable	Pain—mild to moderate
Trazodone	25–75 mg tablets 50 mg injectable	Insomnia
Zolpidem *(still patented)*	5–10 mg tablets	Insomnia

Complementary: require special training and/or delivery method.
* Side effects limit dose.
** Alternatives to amitriptyline and tricyclic antidepressants (should have at least one drug other than dexamethasone).
*** For short-term use in insomnia.

Notes:
Non-benzodiazepines should be used in the elderly.
Non-steroidal anti-inflammatory medicines (NSAIMs) should be used for brief periods of time
No government should approve modified-release morphine, fentanyl, or oxycodone without also guaranteeing widely available immediate release oral morphine.

central nervous system effects, such as haloperidol (Vella-Brincat and Macleod, 2004), levomepromazine (Twycross et al., 1997), and cyclizine (Walder and Aitkenhead, 1995), have been shown to be effective but may cause sedation and other adverse effects. There are no studies to indicate the effectiveness of one antiemetic over another in the management of opioid-induced nausea.

The IAHPC convened a working group of international experts from academic and research institutions. The working group designed the study using the following steps.

A Delphi technique with two rounds was used to determine consensus. The survey contained medications listed in the IAHPC List of Essential Medicines for Palliative Care for the treatment of severe pain, nausea and vomiting, and constipation plus additional medications for which additional studies have been published since the development of the IAHPC list (Thomas and Cooney, 2008; Cherny et al., 2010; National Cancer Institute, 2010):

◆ *opioids*: morphine, oxycodone, methadone, and fentanyl (transdermal patch)

◆ *laxatives*: bisacodyl, sennosides, lactulose, polyethylene glycol, and magnesium hydroxide (oral liquid—Milk of Magnesia)

◆ *antiemetics*: metoclopramide, haloperidol, and levomepromazine.

Participants were asked to rank a list of medications in order of preference from 'most safe and effective' to 'least safe and effective' for the treatment of moderate to severe chronic pain due to cancer and other life-threatening conditions in adults initiating strong opioids. They were also given the opportunity to suggest other medications not included in the survey. In addition, participants were asked if their patients had difficulties accessing any of the medications listed in the study and if so, which medications.

Quantitative data were analysed using simple descriptive statistics. Open responses were coded, categorized, and used to inform the final OEPP. The components of the final OEPP were based on whether consensus was reached for drug and administration selection after both Delphi rounds.

Sixty pain and palliative care physicians agreed to participate in the study.

Preferred opioid: in the first round, morphine was selected by 89.4% (n = 51) of the participants, achieving consensus as the opioid of first choice to be included in OEPP. Hydromorphone was suggested as an alternative opioid and therefore included in the second round. In the second round, the vast majority agreed to oral morphine 5 mg every 4 hours as the first line of treatment. No consensus was reached regarding an alternative opioid of choice in case of lack of availability of morphine.

Preferred laxative: after both rounds, there was no clear consensus regarding a laxative of first choice with the combination of sennosides and docusate reaching the highest level of agreement, 59.2% (n = 29), followed by bisacodyl, 24.5% (n = 12). There was consensus that laxatives should always be given when opioid treatment is started, 93% (n = 53).

Preferred antiemetic: after both rounds metoclopramide reached a consensus of 75.5% (n = 37) as the antiemetic of first choice. No consensus was reached regarding frequency of antiemetic administration. After both rounds, 51.0% (n = 25) chose 'as needed' while 49.0% (n = 24) selected 'regularly'.

Availability and access to medications: a substantial proportion of participants had difficulty accessing opioids in their country, ranging from 33% (morphine) to 45% (methadone). Most laxatives are more readily available, although over one-third of participants (38.8%) would have difficulty accessing sennosides and docusate. Of the three antiemetics, the highest frequency in terms of problems with medication access was for levomepromazine (46.9%). Poor access to opioids, except fentanyl, was significantly higher in middle-low- and low-income countries (p < 0.05). No significant differences in accessibility for laxatives were found between high- and low-income countries. Access to levomepromazine was significantly more difficult in middle-low- and low-income countries. The number of participants in each geographical region was too small to determine significant differences among the responses from participants in each region.

OEPP: using the results from both rounds, members of the working group developed the OEPP and identified the appropriate dosage and route of administration for each medication in accordance with the Food and Drug Administration's approved manufacturer's recommendation. Box 1.3.2 shows the resulting OEPP.

The underlying aim of these two projects is to facilitate and improve care provision and effective symptom control.

Box 1.3.2 IAHPC Opioid Essential Prescription Package (OEPP)©

Opioid

Morphine, oral, 5 mg every 4 hours.

Laxative

Combination of senna and docusate, oral, 8.6 mg/50 mg every 12 hours.

OR:

Bisacodyl, oral, 5 mg every 12 hours.

Antiemetic

Metoclopramide, oral, 10 mg every 4 hours OR as needed.

Reproduced from Vignaroli E et al., Strategic Pain Management: The Identification and Development of the IAHPC Opioid Essential Prescription Package, *Journal of Palliative Medicine*, Volume 15, Number 2, Copyright © Mary Ann Liebert, Inc. 2012, with permission from Mary Ann Liebert, Inc.

The selection of the medications for the IAHPC List of Essential Medicines for Palliative Care and in the OEPP is consistent with different clinical guidelines and critical reviews in symptom management (Hanks et al., 2001; Davis et al., 2005).

A significant percentage of participants in both projects reported problems with availability and access of medications, especially opioids. Challenges in the provision of pain treatment in many developing countries are complex and include poverty; illiteracy; language barriers; limited health-care resources; lack of training; and unnecessarily restrictive laws and regulations which limit the distribution, prescription, dispensation, and use of controlled medications (Joranson and Ryan, 2007; Human Rights Watch, 2009). In some countries, more expensive medications and formulations become available before cheaper medications or formulations. In response to this situation, the IAHPC included a footnote in the List of Essential Medicines for Palliative care, stating that no government should approve modified-release morphine, fentanyl, or oxycodone without also guaranteeing the availability of immediate-release oral morphine.

The IAHPC List of Essential Medicines in Palliative Care and the OEPP are not directives, but rather are offered for guidance. In order for these resources to be useful, it is necessary that:

◆ physicians, nurses, pharmacists, and students in these disciplines are taught how to use these medicines in palliative care

◆ the medicines are available and accessible

◆ they are part of a broad palliative care strategy, both at the institutional and national levels.

Limitations of these studies

Both studies have several limitations:

◆ Participants were selected from convenience samples.

◆ The final results were based on consensus expert opinion. Additional research to evaluate the safety and efficacy of these medications needs to be carried out.

◆ These projects did not address cost and affordability issues—this is work that is needed.

◆ The list was developed for adult patients—a list for children with palliative care needs is urgent and should be developed.

Dissemination and future work

As the holder of the copyrights to the IAHPC List of Essential Medicines for Palliative Care and the OEPP, the IAHPC grants permission to all those interested in reproducing and using both resources as educational and advocacy tools to promote access to medicines and palliative care. It especially encourages use of the list and the OEPP as models for countries in which there currently is limited availability of drugs as well as those which are developing national palliative medication lists tailored to local needs and resources.

IAHPC distributed the List of Essential Medicines for Palliative Care and the OEPP to editors in different journals requesting them to announce and disseminate them.

The IAHPC will conduct a review and update of the List of Essential Medicines for Palliative Care in 2015 taking into account new evidence on safety and efficacy of medications, as well as new formulations which have since become available.

Further work is also needed to update the OEPP to establish a recommended type and dose of laxative, as well as a dosing schedule for metoclopramide and to compare the use of these medications on outcomes such as symptom prevalence and intensity, improvements in patient compliance, and reduction of adverse effects.

The IAHPC OEPP is designed for moderate to severe chronic pain in adult patients who require initiation of strong opioids. Further work is needed to examine the effectiveness of the OEPP compared to usual care in reducing adverse effects and improving tolerability of opioid treatment, leading to better pain management.

Recent Developments

Two important developments occurred recently which have global implications: In 2013, a section with medicines for pain and palliative care was included in both WHO Model Lists of Essential Medicines for adults (EML) and for children (EMLc) following an application of the IAHPC. (WHO EML 20013, WHO EMLc 2013). And in 2014 the World Health Assembly adopted a PC resolution which among other things, calls on governments to update national EM lists, in the light of the changes in the WHO EML (WHA 2014).

Online materials

Complete references for this chapter are available online at <http://www.oxfordmedicine.com>.

References

Carr, D., Goudas, L., Lawrence, D., *et al.* (2002). *Management of Cancer Symptoms: Pain, Depression, and Fatigue.* Evidence Report/Technology Assessment Number 61. Rockville, MD: Agency for Healthcare Research and Quality, US Department of Health and Human Services. Available at: http://archive.ahrq.gov/downloads/pub/evidence/pdf/cansymp/cansymp.pdf.

Cherny, N.I., Baselga, J., de Conno, F., and Radbruch, L. (2010). Formulary availability and regulatory barriers to accessibility of opioids for cancer pain in Europe: a report from the ESMO/EAPC Opioid Policy Initiative. *Annals of Oncology*, 21, 615–626.

Deandrea, S., Montanari, M., Moja, L., and Apolone, G. (2008). Prevalence of undertreatment in cancer pain. A review of published literature. *Annals of Oncology*, 19(12), 1985–1991.

De Lima, L. (2006). The International Association for Hospice and Palliative Care List of Essential Medicines for Palliative Care. *Palliative Medicine*, 20(7), 647–651.

Hanks, G.W., De Conno, F., Cherny, N., *et al.* (2001). Morphine and alternative opioids in cancer pain: the EAPC recommendations. *British Journal of Cancer*, 84(5), 587–593.

Human Rights Watch (2009). *'Please, Do Not Make Us Suffer Any More . . .': Access to Pain Treatment as a Human Right.* New York: Human Rights Watch. Available at: <http://www.hrw.org/en/reports/2009/03/02/please-do-not-make-us-suffer-any-more-0>.

Joranson, D.E. and Ryan, K.M. (2007). Ensuring opioid availability: methods and resources. *Journal of Pain and Symptom Management*, 33(5), 527–532.

Larkin, P.J., Sykes, N.P., Centeno, C., *et al.* (2008). The management of constipation in palliative care: clinical practice recommendations. *Palliative Medicine*, 22(7), 796–807.

Lipman, A.G. (2000). Evolving resources to support improvement of pain and symptom control at end of life. *Journal of Pharmaceutical Care in Pain & Symptom Control*, 8(3), 49–60.

Nicholson, B. (2003). Responsible prescribing of opioids for the management of chronic pain. *Drugs*, 63(1), 17–32.

Plan, W.M. and Arnold, R.M. (2005). Terminal care: the last weeks of life. *Journal of Palliative Medicine*, 8(5), 1042–1054.

Potter, J., Hami, F., Bryan, T., and Quigley, C. (2003). Symptoms in 400 patients referred to palliative care services: prevalence and patterns. *Palliative Medicine*, 17, 310–314.

Solano, J.P., Gomes, B., and Higginson, I. (2006). A comparison of symptom prevalence in far advanced cancer, AIDS, heart disease, chronic obstructive pulmonary disease and renal disease. *Journal of Pain and Symptom Management*, 13(1), 58–69.

Thomas, J.R. and Cooney, G.A. (2008). Palliative care and pain: new strategies for managing opioid bowel dysfunction. *Journal of Palliative Medicine*, 11(Suppl. 1), S1–S19.

National Cancer Institute (2010). University of Texas MD Anderson Cancer Center algorithm for the prevention of opioid-induced constipation. In *Gastrointestinal Complications*. [Online] National Cancer Institute. Available at: <http://www.cancer.gov/cancertopics/pdq/supportivecare/gastrointestinalcomplications/HealthProfessional/page3>.

United Nations (2011). *MDG Gap Task Force Report. The Global Partnership for Development: Time to Deliver.* New York: UN. Available at: <http://www.un.org/en/development/desa/policy/mdg_gap/mdg_gap2011/mdg8report2011_engw.pdf >

Vignaroli, E., Bennett, M.I., Nekolaichuk, C., *et al.* (2012). Strategic pain management: the identification and development of the IAHPC Opioid Essential Prescription Package. *Journal of Palliative Medicine*, 15(2), 186–191.

World Health Organization (1996). *Cancer Pain Relief with a Guide to Opioid Availability* (2nd ed). Geneva: WHO.

World Health Organization (2000). *Essential Drugs and Medicines Policy. The Essential Drug Strategy.* Geneva: WHO.

World Health Organization (2007). *Access to Controlled Medications Programme.* Geneva: WHO. Available at: <http://www.who.int/medicines/areas/quality_safety/access_to_controlled_medications_brnote_english.pdf>.

World Health Organization (2009). *Access to Controlled Medications Programme.* Briefing note. Geneva: WHO.

World Health Organization (2012). *WHO Guidelines on the Pharmacological Treatment of Persisting Pain in Children with Medical Illnesses.* WHO: Geneva. Available at: <http://whqlibdoc.who.int/publications/2012/9789241548120_Guidelines.pdf>.

1.4

Policy in palliative care

David C. Currow and Stein Kaasa

Hospice and palliative care

Hospice and palliative care services have developed in very different ways around the world due to local experts (and their networks of colleagues), differing health and social systems, differing sources of funding, and different perceptions of needs by the communities served by these services. In the 1950s, 1960s, and 1970s much of the developmental stage of hospice and palliative care around the world was as a counterculture, explicitly outside the normal health system policy and planning processes (Clark, 2000). It is doubtful that any country in the world has commenced hospice or palliative care services in response to well-formed national policies with an adequately funded planning and development phase. Instead, most settings have built hospice/palliative care on the momentum of visionary clinicians and funders who have responded to perceived needs from health-care providers, patients, families, and the communities in which they live. This background is important, because it places in context the work that is being done at pan-national, national, and sub-national levels to create effective policies that can further the key work of hospice/palliative care long after services have commenced and, often, after a large number of apparently unconnected local services have been well established.

Policy considerations—general

National policy initiatives reflect the breadth of service provision, the diversity of service delivery models (in response to local funding and broader health service provision models in health and social services), and the basic philosophies about life, death, and care in the communities in which the services have been built. In some specific cases, policy generation (and any accompanying legislation or regulation) may also reflect specific political imperatives at particular time points in a jurisdictional environment.

A fundamental aim of good government is to develop and implement policy that optimizes the well-being of its citizens. Given the universal nature of death, and the increasing prevalence of 'expected' death from chronic, progressive conditions, it should be expected that there are policies and even legislation that ensure good care is given to people at the end of life. Such policy must be informed by the best possible data, and seek to understand explicitly the needs of people at the end of life and their caregivers in order to generate the best possible frameworks for care delivery and support.

Policy in health and social services reflects the complex political processes that underpin priorities and the subsequent responses that may or may not include budgetary allocation and changes to legislation, regulations, or both. In most settings around the world, formulation of health policy is variously shared between politicians, professional organizations (such as medical and nursing societies), patient organizations, public servants, and the general society. In some cases, policy is driven by a political imperative and at other times by public servants or other bodies presenting key issues to their government, with proposals to prioritize a particular issue and on how best to prosecute the issue in public policy. In most settings, this makes for a dynamic process of tacit or overt negotiation between the political and operational arms of government.

Any policy is a series of compromises: there are always competing interests that will help shape the final results. The factors that influence policy are not always explicit and may relate, at times, to policy initiatives that are seemingly unrelated. Tracing such processes is almost impossible. Changes in health-care policy will often take time, and consistent work is often needed to generate and sustain any change in direction.

At times, there may also be differences in the approach between various levels of government and public administration within the same country. This may lead to differences in policies and documents that may be difficult to reconcile. Vested interests abound in bringing together the wide variety of opinions that help to inform any societal policy, given the increasing plurality seen in many communities around the world.

Policy that relates to health service delivery will have significant pressure exerted on it, depending on the funding models that are used to pay for health care. Private practitioners operating on a fee-for-service basis may bring very different pressures to negotiations than a health system where payment is primarily through capitation. Financial gains and losses are powerful factors in influencing policy and hence referral from one clinical service to another.

Health policy—palliative care

There are particular challenges in forming public policy on hospice/palliative care, and especially the end-of-life component. In so many ways, such conversations go to the very heart of existential beliefs and how these beliefs are manifest in the day-to-day lives of individuals and of whole communities. How individuals and groups within communities view death will have influence on the policies that are put in place for hospice/palliative care.

Accommodating widely varying and, at times, diametrically opposed views is a key challenge in the development of any relevant public policy that will actually have meaning in helping to shape the care provided in such communities. The spectrum of beliefs is wide: at one extreme there may be a belief that any life is sacred in and of itself, even in a vegetative state; the other extreme is that life can only be enjoyed if there is little or no compromise to physical and psychological well-being. The number of variations along this spectrum makes any public policy in this area incredibly difficult to generate in a way that all people are satisfied. First and foremost, good public policy is about ensuring that the well-being of all people, including the weak and voiceless, is respected and protected. This often does not, in itself, deliver policy that will necessarily please every lobby group, but it is a crucial tenet around which to build strong public policy. Depending upon the society, the basic values held by the community, the economic strength of that community, and the health-care system in which hospice/palliative care services are being built are among other intrinsic factors which influence priorities between treatments: cure, life prolongation, or relief of symptoms at the end-of-life care. Such priorities may be challenging for developing good end-of-life care. For example, in many health systems, the drivers to invest in marginal life prolongations seem to be many with economic, marketing, and professional pressures all influencing the ultimate policy decision.

'Patients' voices'

The voice of the community in democratic societies helps to inform health policies including end-of-life care. A key challenge in hospice/palliative care is the lack of an effective patient voice. People at the end of life can rarely find the sustained voice needed to truly influence public policy. Caregivers for people at the end of life are working tirelessly to provide care for the person with the life-limiting illness. After the care recipient dies, many caregivers are unable to devote significant time and energy to advocacy. Often this leaves professional bodies in the role of social advocates, with the inherent concern that there may be an element of self-interest in the requests being made by health professionals, seemingly on behalf of their patients.

The almost absent voice of consumers in service development means that in the public discourse of policy development, it is easy to drown out key views and values that are important to people with life-limiting illnesses and their caregivers. Simply asking the well population what they would like at the end of life is unlikely to be sufficient, and may lead to policy that is not congruent with the wishes of people actually facing an advanced, progressive, life-limiting illness. By definition, such a lack of advocacy is likely to continue to be there, and finding ways of respectfully but adequately consulting people at the end of life about such policy remains an ongoing challenge.

Policy documents

Several key initiatives are underway around the world to improve the quality of care and to provide stronger data to inform policy. Initiatives across the globe are each seeking to have a stronger framework to reflect the feedback of the actual experience of patients and caregivers (Barbera et al., 2010; Bausewein et al., 2010; Eagar et al., 2010; Payne and the EAPC Task Force on Family Carers, 2010a, 2010b; Kamal et al., 2011; Casarett et al., 2012; Centeno et al., 2013).

From evidence-based medicine to evidence-based practice

Evidence-based public policy is as important as evidence-based clinical practice, and where sufficient evidence is not available, it

Table 1.4.1 From evidence-based medicine to evidence-based practice

Step 1	Literature reviews ± Review of best practice
Step II	International/national guidelines
Step III	Clinical care pathway(s)
Step IV	Audit/assessment of outcomes(s)

is imperative that adequate research is done to understand the net effects (benefits and harms) not just with highly motivated clinicians who are willing to participate in such studies, but in 'greenfield' hospice/palliative care sites that are not particularly invested in the process. Further, after implementation, sufficient resources need to be invested in the ongoing evaluation of the training required, the uptake, and the outcomes using prospectively collected data with specific questions about the performance of the programme as well as seeking signals of any untoward or unintended consequences, as part of a learning health-care system (Basch and Abernethy, 2011).

Ideally good public policy is informed by the best available evidence, not simply political expediency (Loman, 2000; Alliance for Health Policy and Systems Research, 2007; Head, 2007; Banks, 2009; Brownson et al., 2009; Gluckman, 2011) A formal structure applied in several areas of medicine may also be applied in palliative care (Table 1.4.1). Step II and step III should ideally be endorsed by national or regional health-care authorities in order to assure the allocation of sufficient resources to implement the pathways and evaluate the pathways' impacts on health outcomes. This assessment must include the effectiveness of introducing these measures, levels of adherence to the pathways, and reasons for non-adherence or poor uptake. Ideally the effect/outcomes on patient care before and after the introduction of a pathway should be prospectively assessed. This assessment can be conducted at patient level but also through pre-defined quality indicators at institutional, regional, and/or national level.

For example, the wide uptake into health policy of the Liverpool Care Pathway (LCP) with all of its strengths and weaknesses deserves careful exploration (Currow and Abernethy, 2014). What was the level of evidence that was available to policymakers as they mandated uptake of the LCP across the health system in the United Kingdom? It could be argued that there was no level II or level I evidence, and the generalizability from the studies which had been reported by the time of the initial decision to mandate widespread uptake were not sufficient to ensure that the net effects of the LCP were known (Costantini et al., 2014). The UK government has subsequently taken the step not to recommend the use of the LCP in the United Kingdom at this time. This decision itself has sparked debate (The Lancet Oncology, 2013).

The World Health Organization and hospice/palliative care policy

Policy documents reveal the wide range of responsibilities and mandates of health and social services around the world. This section presents an overview of a sample of international and national policy documents that relate to hospice/palliative care. The list is not exhaustive, but serves to illustrate the issues frequently seen in health policy relating to end-of-life care.

The WHO most recently published its 'Knowledge into Action: WHO Guide for Effective Programmes' modules in which palliative care sits under 'Cancer Control' (WHO, 2007). The overarching aim of the document is to 'reduce unnecessary suffering of patients and their families'. In this, palliative care is embedded as one key aspect of cancer control although the palliative care aspects of the document are not limited to people with the diagnosis of cancer. The palliative care module contains three steps for planning strategically to improve hospice/palliative care:

◆ understanding the current context of palliative care

◆ determining where a programme wants to be within the next 5 years

◆ mapping out ways to achieve this outcome.

In policy terms, the WHO document frames hospice/palliative care in the context of the humanitarian needs that must be met. Internationally, this then defines the greatest needs as those of low- and medium-resource level countries where the highest proportion of patients present with advanced disease, and hence where little can be done to modify the course of the life-limiting illness. Emphasis is placed on the integration of hospice/palliative care into the existing health system whether in the public or private sector, rather than creating a parallel system of care, with an understandable focus on community and home-based care. Explicitly, the document outlines the need to adapt these three principles in ways that respect the cultural, social, and economic settings in which the care is being delivered. The document also reflects the need to cover all age groups including children. Interestingly, one key message from the document is that palliation should be linked to other aspects of the continuum of cancer control: prevention, early detection, and treatment services. The WHO document also clearly states that hospice/palliative care services should be able to work alongside therapies that may improve prognosis, such as chemotherapy or radiotherapy in the case of cancer.

Adopting a public health approach to palliative care was the framework deliberately chosen by the WHO as far back as 1996 (Stjernswärd et al., 1996). The three key elements outlined in a public health approach were:

◆ a government policy ensuring integration with other health services

◆ an education policy spanning health-care workers (including volunteers) and the public

◆ a medication policy that ensured the availability of essential medications (see Chapter 2.3).

These key elements are based on work defining the greatest perceived needs of people at the end of life from work done by the WHO: pain relief, accessible and affordable medications, and financial support. The WHO guide also outlines the aspirational goal of having 80% of all people who die from cancer seen by a palliative care service (and 60–80% of people dying from AIDS). Of note, the WHO guide includes an outline of the need for adequate information systems to complement physical, human, and financial resources for a comprehensive programme. The need for protocols, guidelines, and standards are also integral to successful programmes.

Accompanying the principles just outlined, the WHO guide provides a step-by-step process of planning, implementing, and evaluating a hospice/palliative care programme at a national level. This guidance encourages national policies explicitly to take into account the financial, cultural, and ethical context in which the programme is going to exist.

The WHO has in place an important framework that can influence policy at national and sub-national levels but there is no direct effector arm. The care of people at the end of life and the way that care is delivered through policy, associated funding models, and the other resources made available are beyond the jurisdiction of the WHO/United Nations. Although the WHO guide is a seminal document, it has no direct mandate in jurisdictions that choose to ignore it.

Country- state-, and topic-specific examples

The following subsections do not exhaustively outline every national policy document that has been published, but seek instead to reflect on aspects of several national policy documents or legislation in order to highlight key aspects that illustrate the breadth and complexity of public policy in any setting.

Most have themes that fit broadly with the year 2000 Australian *National Palliative Care Strategy: A National Framework for Palliative Care Service Development* which include:

◆ raising awareness and understanding about palliative care

◆ improving the quality and effectiveness services

◆ enhancing partnerships between service providers (Anonymous 2000).

By way of integration of policy, these principles are then reflected in other key national strategy documents: the *National Chronic Disease Strategy*; the *National Service Improvement Framework for Cancer*; and the *National Service Improvement Framework for Heart, Stroke and Vascular Disease* (Dowrick, 2006).

Country-specific example: the United States

Internationally, a watershed moment was in the early 1980s when the United States passed legislation to include an explicit payment provision for hospice care in the 1982 Tax Equity and Fiscal Responsibility Act. This allowed for a per diem payment for people who had limited prognosis and were eligible for Medicare payments. An act by any legislature is the mechanism that enshrines policy in the most overt way. As this Act had a sunset clause of 1986, the Congress replaced it permanently with a Medicare Hospice Benefit that year (Miller and Mike, 1995). This was a world-first legislation in recognizing the needs of people at the end of life and the care they required.

There were arguably two effects from this landmark legislation by the United States: it enshrined hospice/palliative care in law which was a positive outcome; but because it was a legislated per diem payment that was limited to the last 6 months of life, it may have limited referral to hospice services to later in the disease trajectory than intended (Christakis and Iwashyna, 2003). The legislation did not index the payment, thereby also potentially subsequently limiting the care that could be purchased in later years.

Country-specific example: Norway

The development of palliative care in Norway, as in many other countries has an evolutionary pattern. It started from the late

1970s with the establishment of informal palliative care groups in most health regions in the country. The primary goal of these groups was to inform, promote, and teach about palliative care at a local level. The needs were seen from the patients' and health-care pioneers' points of view. This first phase can be categorized as an 'information and policymaking phase'. Key politicians locally and nationally were approached with the aim to build a more formal platform for palliative care.

This process culminated in a national governmental report on care for dying patients in 1984 (Official Norwegian Reports, 1984). This report recommended establishing institutional sites. The governmental report from 1984 was used actively by the health-care providers in the field of palliative care to promote the need for establishing the combined academic and clinical units. It took almost 10 years (1993) to establish the first academic palliative care unit in Trondheim. It was established within the Department of Oncology at the Trondheim University Hospital with a full-time professor. Simultaneously, patient care was established in the Oslo region and in Bergen. In this process a non-governmental organization (NGO)—the Norwegian Cancer Society—was involved and, through a major grant to the Trondheim University Hospital, the professorial chair was funded for 5 years with an agreement that the university (the public health-care system) should continue to pay for this position after this time. The Norwegian Cancer Society also paid for the establishment of an inpatient unit at the Trondheim University Hospital at the same time.

This is an example of the use of a government report, involvement by an NGO and consistent policy work by health-care providers succeeding in developing palliative care in the country. Such an investment provided impetus for a second national government report in the form of a national cancer plan (Official Norwegian Reports, 1997) which included recommendations on the future development of palliative care and a report on care for the dying which was released in 1999 (Official Norwegian Reports, 1999).

Public health-care in Norway is fully paid for by the government. The financial system is based upon a basic payment of approximately 50% and a diagnosed-related group (DRG) by the remaining 50%. In order to further develop palliative care, a special DRG was established to make it economically feasible for health-care institutions to establish palliative care teams in hospitals and also community outreach teams. The DRG was followed by national standards on how to organize palliative care in teaching and local hospitals, as well as in community care. This combination of an official national policy on how to organize palliative care matched by DRG-based funding mechanisms had a catalytic effect on the development of clinical palliative care across Norway.

Country-specific example: Germany

In Germany, palliative care has developed rapidly since the establishment of the first palliative care unit in 1983 and the first inpatient hospice in 1986, using a two-pronged approach. Palliative care pioneers worked within the health-care system, while hospice care was established as a community-based citizens' movement, with a major focus on volunteers. Despite some conflicts between these two tiers (e.g. warning against a medicalization of palliative care), both approaches now collaborate and have succeeded in integrating palliative and hospice care in the health-care system. This is evident not only from the large and still increasing number

of specialist inpatient and outpatient services (195 inpatient hospices and 231 palliative care units in hospitals in 2011, 1500 home care services with volunteers), but also from the establishment of academic palliative care departments across the country (Aachen, Bonn, Cologne, Erlangen, Freiburg, Göttingen, Mainz, München, and Münster).

Recently, medical education in palliative medicine has been incorporated as an integral part of medical studies at German universities. As part of national policy, starting in 2014, physicians applying for a licence to practise medicine will have to provide a certificate of basic training in palliative medicine—a world first. A challenge in upcoming years will be establishing and enhancing comprehensive, standardized, and quality-controlled education within universities.

Only minimal requirements are legislatively specified for education of nurses in palliative care. However, standardized and quality-controlled advanced training courses are available. This training is more frequently being requested as a prerequisite for nurses working in palliative care.

Changes in the legislation have influenced the situation for home care enormously in the last 5 years, also making it more complex. With the Law for the Consolidation of the Competition in Compulsory Health Insurance (Gesetz zur Stärkung des Wettbewerbs in der gesetzlichen Krankenversicherung), a legal claim for palliative home care has been implemented in the fifth book of the social law in 2007. The ambitious goal of full coverage with comprehensive palliative home care has still not been achieved in most locations. However, after initial negotiation difficulties between palliative care providers and health insurance funds, an increasing number of contracts have been signed. As a consequence, more than 100 palliative care teams have begun work in the field of specialized palliative home care. Legal regulations for the supply of opioids and other medications for the treatment of patients at home have been adapted recently, thus, facilitating faster and more comprehensive medical treatment in emergency situations. Volunteer hospice services receive reimbursements for payment of the coordinators from the sickness funds. Overall, the legislation has been adapted significantly, contributing to improvements for patients requiring palliative care.

Even though hospice and palliative care is gaining increasing acknowledgement from political stakeholders, a national strategy on palliative and hospice care is still lacking. The German Association for Palliative Care in collaboration with the German Hospice Association and the German Medical Association has produced the 'Charter for the Care of Severely Ill and Dying Patients in Germany' as the German contribution to the Budapest Commitments, and is currently using this charter as the basis for the development of a national strategy. A research agenda for palliative care has also been commissioned by the Leopoldina German Academy of Science and will be published in 2014.

Country-specific example: Canada

Canada continues to be a leader in hospice/palliative care, in part because of a strong policy framework that has underpinned the development of services and the environment within which those services operate. Canada has not only set up a national strategy on palliative and end-of-life care, but has also publically evaluated it in a way that allows others to learn from it (Anonymous, 2007). In the life of that strategy, five working groups were established and each took forward a work programme which was coordinated with the other groups. They were:

- Best practices and quality care working group
- Education for formal caregivers working group
- Public information and awareness working group
- Research working group
- Surveillance working group.

These groups cover the full spectrum of hospice/palliative care public policy. Of particular note, the last group was charged with the role of developing a system for collecting and utilizing information about palliative and end-of-life care. The two key foci were *who used services* and *how the quality of those services could be systematically measured*. A whole-of-government approach utilizing existing organizations charged with understanding the measurement and reporting of the health system were engaged in the process. A key outcome of such far-reaching policy work was an inventory of performance measures in palliative and end-of-life care. The outputs also included a standard dataset to be collected on palliative care patients across participating services, complementing the work done by the *Best practices and quality care working group*.

The importance of a public awareness arm of any policy should not be overlooked. The programme of this working group encompassed the processes of both understanding what Canadians knew and thought about palliative and end-of-life care and, from that, what key messages needed to be more widely understood. This group also took explicit responsibility for the informational needs for family and friends as caregivers.

Country-specific example: New Zealand

New Zealand published a review of its government's policies regarding palliative and end-of-life care (Anonymous, 2010). It highlights many of the fundamental challenges of any policy: how was it implemented and how have outcomes been measured? Although there are no issues that are unique to any one jurisdiction, the challenges faced by New Zealand bring into sharp focus the issues of the social determinants of health and the impact that socioeconomic status still manifests at the end of life (Currow, 2009). In public policy, such recognition is crucial as, reproducibly across the globe, people from rural areas, the socioeconomically disadvantaged, people from first nations, and those whose birth place was not their country of residence, especially if the language is different, have poorer health outcomes, even at the end of life. Principles espoused in the policy include universal access to hospice/palliative care services irrespective of diagnosis and geography. Importantly, documents from New Zealand also do not limit access by prognosis.

The document highlights that, despite substantial investments by governments, measures have not been agreed universally for the evaluation of the impact of hospice/palliative care services. As such, data to evaluate the impact of a national approach are not available and become a key priority for the next iteration of a national approach to improving access and uptake of hospice/palliative care by moving towards 'an outcomes focused monitoring and evaluation framework'. The stated aim of 'a systematic and informed approach to the provision and funding of palliative care services' is challenging to achieve without measures being routinely collected and analysed. Without a specific investment in

measuring performance, it will continue to be difficult to understand fully the benefits of the national policy.

The first national strategy was put in place in 2001 in New Zealand (Anonymous, 2001). A long-term commitment by funders and policymakers is required if the benefits of a more systematic approach to the availability and uptake of hospice/palliative care is going to be taken. Such a lead time should ideally see greater uptake into policy documents in areas that interface with hospice/palliative care and, arguably, is a key measure for the evaluation of the success of policy at the level of policymakers.

Country-specific example: Romania

In Romania, hospice/palliative care services are potentially in a position not encountered in some more resource-advantaged countries—the ability to build hospice/palliative care services strategically as an integral part of a rapidly evolving health system. Such services are a mixture of public, charitable, and for-profit services arising where key opinion leaders and communities have sought and developed local solutions. Payment models include per diem payments for inpatients and fee-for-service for community-based care.

The national strategy is refreshingly honest—each service develops relationship with referring services according to the local service's own strategy (Mosoiu, 2009). Although this happens right around the world, few policy documents reflect the status quo with such accuracy. Given resource constraints, the national strategy has limited itself to people 'whose disease is not responsive to curative treatment' (WHO, 1990) thus temporarily rejecting the broader definition adopted by the international agency in 2002 which included a broader timeframe across the disease trajectory. The timeframe for review of this Romania stance is set for 2020.

The principles around which the Romanian National Strategy document has been built have universal application:

- the need for services to meet the 'specific and distinctive needs of the people they are intended for'
- availability (including availability at times convenient to service users not just providers)
- accessibility (financial, geographic, language, and culture-related issues, spanning all tiers of educational ability)
- quality care
- providing true continuity of care
- in an economically sustainable way.

The implementation of such principles in any national or state/provincial setting is likely to lead to significantly improved services.

The document also candidly addresses the challenge of the interface between specialist and generalist services as more health professional devote themselves full time to palliative care practice. This leads to the challenges in continuity of care especially at times of transition between physical locations of care. In any health system this creates difficulties, but at the end of life such fractured service delivery is arguably even more counter-productive. Given the small number of services for a large population, the other challenge is to ensure that additional services are created in geographic areas where currently there is no coverage.

State-specific example: Kerala

Kerala, in India's south west, is a populous state with excellent levels of education and infrastructure. Its palliative care services are examples of what can be achieved with high levels of commitment to local service delivery that is relevant, affordable, and patient centred. The programme of work, underpinned by a strong policy document, delivers a level of support that few would have thought possible three decades ago (Anonymous, 2008). The programme seeks to embrace both those who are dying and those with chronic conditions that would benefit from a palliative approach. Such population coverage requires the programme to be predominantly delivered by primary care. As such, palliative care was accorded 'priority status in public health and disease control programmes'. This enshrines the need to grow palliative care as an integral part of the health system and, unlike many countries with greater resources where palliative care will only be funded when everything else has been developed, it allows genuine integration of palliative care right across the spectrum of health service provision.

Ultimately the policies in Kerala set out a clear manifesto—good palliative care is everybody's business—from the most junior and least skilled health worker to the most highly trained specialist in any field of clinical endeavour. Care must be based around a person's home with their family and community providing care, supported by health professionals that are also locally based.

The policy also draws strongly on trained volunteers to achieve the immediate, medium-, and long-term aims of improving the well-being of people in the state by systematically decreasing suffering. Volunteers may not be paid, but their training and ongoing supervision requires explicit resources.

In policy, good palliative care delivery in the community also relies heavily on cross-sectoral support and cooperation. This requires governments, health services, professionals and their associated professional bodies, and community organizations to work closely together for a common goal. Each has a role not only in coordinating service delivery but also in building the capacity of the whole community, not just health professionals, to provide such care. This also requires close integration with other key policies in terms of cross-referencing and in prioritizing the available resources.

Topic-specific example: improving access to palliative care medications in Australia

There was a community imperative to improve community-based care in Australia. One key aspect of this was the availability of key symptom control medications in the community. At a policy level, such a process had to be completed within current legislative and regulatory frameworks (Rowett et al., 2009). A true whole-of-government, whole-of-community working party was established in 2002 to address this issue in the context of a national policy commitment to improve end-of-life care systematically.

The work was underpinned by a national survey to define medications essential to good palliation, the level of evidence underpinning such processes, and the current (subsidized) availability of the medication (Good et al., 2006). The survey identified many medications, most of which did not have sufficient evidence to support registration nor subsidy (comparative cost-effectiveness) applications. For those medications that were considered essential and did have sufficient evidence, a new section of the national subsidized formulary was created for palliative care patients. (In policy terms, this was the first patient-defined section of the formulary. Until that time it had always been defined in terms of the medications that different practitioners could prescribe. The

process has since been replicated in paediatrics and Aboriginal and Torres Strait Islander populations, demonstrating that good palliative care policy can positively influence policy in other parts of health.)

A work programme to improve systematically the evidence to inform prescribing has grown out of this work, with studies designed in consultation with regulatory and funding bodies to ensure the quality of the evidence will satisfy them if the studies are positive. Such national policy has collateral benefits around the world, given that phase III data are somewhat limited in their availability in hospice/palliative care. A national policy that community-based medications become more available has led to a number of benefits to patients including better evidence for how to use key medications in helping to relieve suffering in people with life-limiting illnesses.

Policy and hospice/palliative care

Ultimately, successfully developing hospice/palliative care services requires every level of government, funders, and the community to develop and support policies that can ensure the widest reach of services, and the most equitable distribution of limited resources. This requires the development and maintenance of close ties with existing health and social policymakers and funders. Building on international, national, and sub-national initiatives is delivering improved access to hospice/palliative care services around the globe.

References

Alliance for Health Policy and Systems Research (2007). *Sound Choices: Enhancing Capacity for Evidence-Informed Health Policy.* Geneva: WHO.

Anonymous (2000). *National Palliative Care Strategy: A National Framework for Palliative Care Service Development.* Canberra: Publications Production Unit (Public Affairs, Parliamentary and Access Branch).

Anonymous (2001). *The New Zealand Palliative Care Strategy.* Wellington: Ministry of Health.

Anonymous (2007). *Canadian Strategy on Palliative and End-of-Life Care—Final Report of the Coordinating Committee.* Ottawa: Health Canada.

Anonymous (2008). *Palliative Care Policy for Kerala.*

Anonymous (2010). *Positioning Palliative Care in New Zealand.* Wellington: Cancer Control New Zealand.

Banks, G. (2009). *Evidence-Based Policy Making: What is It? How Do We Get It?* ANZSOG/ANU Public Lecture Series, 4 February, Canberra. [Online] Productivity Commission. Available at: <http://www.pc.gov. au/__data/assets/pdf_file/0003/85836/cs20090204.pdf>.

Barbera, L., Seow, H., and Howell, D., *et al.* (2010). Symptom burden and performance status in a population-based cohort of ambulatory cancer patients. *Cancer*, 116(24), 5767–5776.

Basch, E. and Abernethy, A.P. (2011). Supporting clinical practice decisions with real-time patient-reported outcomes. *Journal of Clinical Oncology*, 29(8), 954–956.

Bausewein, C., Daveson, B., Benalia, H., Simon, S., and Higginson, I. (2010). *Outcome Measurement in Palliative Care: The Essentials.* [Online] PRISMA. Available at: <http://www.csi.kcl.ac.uk/files/ Guidance%20on%20Outcome%20Measurement%20in%20 Palliative%20Care.pdf>.

Brownson, R.C., Chriqui, J.F., and Stamatakis, K.A. (2009). Understanding evidence-based public health policy. *American Journal of Public Health*, 99(9), 1576–1583.

Casarett, D.J., Harrold, J., Oldanie, B., Prince-Paul, M., and Teno, J. (2012). Advancing the science of hospice care: Coalition of Hospices

Organized to Investigate Comparative Effectiveness. *Current Opiion inn Supportive Palliative Care*, 6(4), 459–464.

Centeno, C., Lynch, T., Donea, O., Rocafort, J., and Clark, D. (2013). *EAPC Atlas of Palliative Care in Europe* 2013—*Full Edition*. Milan: European Association for Palliative Care.

Christakis, N.A. and Iwashyna, T.J. (2003). The health impact of health care on families: a matched cohort study of hospice use by decedents and mortality outcomes in surviving, widowed spouses. *Social Science & Medicine*, 57(3), 465–475.

Clark, D. (2000). Palliative care history: a ritual process. *European Journal of Palliative Care*, 7(2), 50–55.

Costantini, M., Romoli, V., Leo, S.D., *et al.* (2014). Liverpool Care Pathway for patients with cancer in hospital: a cluster randomised trial. *The Lancet*, 383(9913), 226–237.

Currow, D.C. (2009). Even in death. *Journal of Palliative Medicine*, 12(11), 983–984.

Currow, D.C. and Abernethy, A.P. (2014). The Liverpool Care Pathway Randomised Controlled Trial. *The Lancet*, 383(9913), 192–193.

Dowrick, C. (2006). The chronic disease strategy for Australia. *Medical Journal of Australia*, 185(2), 61.

Eagar, K., Watters, P., Currow, D.C., Aoun, S.M., and Yates, P. (2010). The Australian Palliative Care Outcomes Collaboration (PCOC)—measuring the quality and outcomes of palliative care on a routine basis. *Australian Health Review*, 34(2), 186–192.

Gluckman, P. (2011). *Towards Better Use of Evidence in Policy Formation: A Discussion Paper*. Auckland: Office of the Prime Minister's Science Advisory Committee.

Good, P.D., Cavenagh, J.D., Currow, D.C., Woods, D.A., Tuffin, P.H., and Ravenscroft, P.J. (2006). What are the essential medications in palliative care?—a survey of Australian palliative care doctors. *Australian Family Physician*, 35(4), 261–264.

Head, B. (2007). Three lenses of evidence-based policy. *The Australian Journal of Public Administration*, 67(1), 1–11.

Kamal, A.H., Currow, D.C., Ritchie, C., Bull, J., Wheeler, J.L., and Abernethy, A.P. (2011). The value of data collection within a palliative care program. *Current Oncology Reports*, 13(4), 308–315.

Loman, J. (2000). Connecting research and policy. *Canadian Journal of Policy Research*, 1, 140–144.

Miller, P.J. and Mike, P.B. (1995). The Medicare hospice benefit: ten years of federal policy for the terminally ill. *Death studies*, 19(6), 531–542.

Mosoiu, D. (2009). *National Strategy for Palliative Care in Romania*. Worldwide Palliative Care Alliance Summit 2009.

Official Norwegian Reports (1984). *Care for the Sick and Dying People*. Oslo: Ministry of Health and Care Services.

Official Norwegian Reports (1997). *Care and Knowledge: 'Norwegian Cancer Plan'*. Oslo: Ministry of Health and Care Services.

Official Norwegian Reports (1999). *Treatment and Care for the Terminally Ill and Dying*. Oslo: Ministry of Health Care Services.

Payne, S. and the EAPC Task Force on Family Carers (2010). White paper on improving support for family carers in palliative care: part 1. *European Journal of Palliative Care*, 17(5), 238–245.

Payne, S. and the EAPC Task Force on Family Carers (2010). White paper on improving support for family carers in palliative care: part 2. *European Journal of Palliative Care*, 17(6), 286–290.

Rowett, D., Ravenscroft, P.J., Hardy, J., and Currow, D.C. (2009). Using national health policies to improve access to palliative care medications in the community. *Journal of Pain and Symptom Management*, 37(3), 395–402.

Stjernswärd, J., Colleau, S.M., and Ventafridda, V. (1996). The World Health Organization cancer pain and palliative care program past, present, and future. *Journal of Pain and Symptom Management*, 12(2), 65–72.

Tax Equity and Fiscal Responsibility Act of 1982, Pub. L. 97–248.

The Lancet Oncology (2013). Dignity in death: the triumph of politics over evidence. *The Lancet Oncology*, 14(13), 1243.

World Health Organization (1990). *Cancer Pain Relief and Palliative Care: A Report of a WHO Expert Committee*. WHO Technical Report Series, No. 804. Geneva: World Health Organization.

World Health Organization (2007). *Cancer Control: Knowledge into Action: WHO Guide for Effective Programmes*. Geneva: World Health Organization.

SECTION 2

The challenge of palliative medicine

The problem of suffering and the principles of assessment in palliative medicine

Nathan I. Cherny

Introduction to the problem of suffering and the principles of assessment in palliative medicine

Despite the advances of modern medicine, many illnesses continue to evade cure. Chronic, progressive, incurable illness is a major cause of disability, distress, suffering, and, ultimately, death. This is true for many causes of cancer, progressive neurological disorders, AIDS, and other disorders of vital organs. Progressive chronic diseases of this ilk are most common in late adulthood and old age, but they occur in all ages.

When cure is not possible, as often it is not, the relief of suffering is the cardinal goal of medicine. Recognition of this axiom is at the heart of the philosophy, science, and practice of palliative medicine.

Understanding suffering

For the patient with incurable illnesses such as cancer, the goals of care may be stated as the alleviation of suffering, the optimization of quality of life until death ensues, and the provision of comfort in death (Wanzer et al., 1989; Duggleby and Berry, 2005). Persistent suffering that is inadequately relieved (or the anticipation of this situation) undermines, for the sufferer, the value of life. Without hope that this situation will be relieved, patients, their families, and professional health-care providers may see elective death by suicide, euthanasia, or assisted suicide as their only alternatives. The truth of the perception that patients need to be killed or assisted to kill themselves to be adequately relieved of suffering depends upon the adequacy of the available measures to relieve suffering. The essence of the controversy is the problem of suffering.

The alleviation of suffering is universally acknowledged as a cardinal goal of medical care (Angell, 1982; President's Commission for the Study of Ethical Problems in Medical and Biomedical and Behavioral Research, 1983; Wanzer et al., 1989; Roy, 1991, 1993; American Nurses Association Center for Ethics and Human Rights Task Force on the Nurse's Role in End-of-Life Decisions, 1992; American Medical Association, 1996; Rich, 2001; Snyder and Leffler, 2005). The ability to formulate a response to the challenge of suffering requires a clinically relevant understanding of the nature of the problem.

A conceptual framework for suffering

Suffering can be defined as an aversive experience characterized by the perception of personal distress that is generated by adverse factors that undermine quality of life (Cassell, 1982, 1991; Saunders, 1984; Cherny et al., 1994a; Krikorian et al., 2012). The defining characteristics of suffering include (1) the presence of perceptual capacity (sentience), (2) that the factors undermining quality of life are appraised as distressing, and (3) that the experience is aversive. According to this definition, suffering is a phenomenon of conscious human existence, the intensity of which is determined by the number and severity of the factors reducing quality of life, the processes of appraisal, and perception. Each of these variables is amenable to therapeutic interventions.

The encounter with terminal illness is a potential cause of great distress to patients, their families, and the professional caregivers attending them. Among patients with incurable illness, significant pain and numerous other physical symptoms can diminish the patient's quality of life. Furthermore, many patients endure enormous psychological distress, and in some cases, form an existential perspective that, even without pain or other physical symptoms, continued life may be without meaning. For the families and loved ones of patients there is, likewise, great distress in this process: anticipated loss, standing witness to the physical and emotional distress of the patient, and bearing the burdens of care. Finally, professional caregivers may potentially be stressed by the suffering which they witness and which challenges their clinical and emotional resources. According to this model (Cherny et al., 1994a), the suffering of each of these three groups is inextricably interrelated such that the perceived distress of any one of these three groups may amplify the distress of the others (Fig. 2.1.1); this has been called reciprocal suffering (Wittenberg-Lyles et al., 2011).

Suffering, personal growth, and resilience

The potential for personal development and net positive gain in overcoming situations of adversity and suffering is widely recognized and it is often referred to as post-traumatic growth (Block,

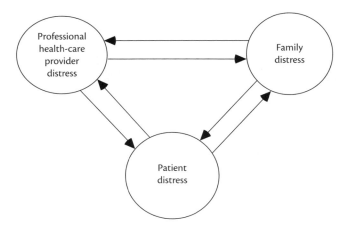

Fig. 2.1.1 The interrelationship between the distress of the patient, the family, and the health-care providers.

2001; Hefferon et al., 2009). This potential, however, is predicated on the ability to cope with the prevailing problems and challenges. It is the phenomenon of coping that generates the potential for growth and reward (Lazarus, 1985; Folkman et al., 1986; Block, 2001). Coping does not occur if the demands of the situation *are* overwhelming (as distinct from merely being appraised as overwhelming). For example, the patient with inadequately relieved pain, shortness of breath, or vomiting may be absolutely unable to address issues related to his offspring and spouse. The spouse and offspring who are overwhelmed by problems of daily care requirements may be absolutely unable to appreciate time with the patient.

Suffering in chronic debilitating illness cannot be eliminated, but if adequate relief is achieved then coping and growth can occur. By understanding and addressing the factors that may potentially overwhelm the patient, family, and health-care providers, the necessary preconditions for coping and growth are established. Intervention programmes focusing on mindfulness, healing arts, and spiritual care can facilitate post-traumatic growth of this sort (Block, 2001; Garland et al., 2007).

The potential for growth and adaptation are related to the quality and process of resilience (Hefferon et al., 2009). Resilience is the capacity of an individual person or a social system to grow and to develop in the face of very difficult circumstances (Vanistendael, 1996; Woodgate, 1999; Lloyd, 2006). The situational challenges may trigger the development of hitherto hidden or poorly developed resources and strengths in a person, triggering a process of personal development and growth.

Resilience is not limited to victims and patients, but also to their families and friends, and to the staff providing care. Resilience has several important attributes: resilience is not an absolute; rather it is a relative personal attribute which may vary over time. It consists of dimensions of resistance to adversity and the ability to make constructive adaptation. This latter characteristic implies the capacity to transform a negative event into an element of growth. It is important to emphasize that resilience does not ignore the need to deal with problems and negative situations: it involves processes of grieving and negative emotions such as sadness and fear but also involves looking for positive elements to (re) build life. Resilience does not invoke denial, but, rather, a realistic

appraisal that is not exclusively focused on problems and which recognizes and identifies positive opportunities (Woodgate, 1999; Lloyd, 2006).

Relieving suffering: a right

It is widely held that terminally ill patients have a right to adequate relief of uncontrolled suffering (Brennan, 2007; Gwyther et al., 2009). Indeed, the World Health Organization asserts that the relief of pain and other symptoms is a right of the patient with advanced and incurable cancer (World Health Organization, 1996) and the right to the adequate provision of palliative care for the terminally ill has been ratified by a host of medical societies and professional organizations. The right has legal status recognized by the Supreme Court of the United States (Burt, 1997) and an Israeli statute law defining the rights of the dying (Steinberg and Sprung, 2006).

The corollary of this right is the responsibility of caregivers to ensure that adequate provisions are made for relief. The formulation of a therapeutic response to suffering, however, requires an understanding of the phenomenon of suffering and of the factors that contribute to it. Indeed, the failure to appreciate, or to effectively address, the full diversity of contributing factors may confound effective therapeutic strategies (Krikorian et al., 2012).

Patient distress

Physical symptoms

Among patients with advanced incurable illness, physical symptoms are common—they are often multiple and they cause a variable degree of distress (Kirkova et al., 2010b; Seng Beng et al., 2013) (see Section 8).

Among patients with advanced cancer, 70–90% will have significant pain that requires the use of opioid drugs (van den Beuken-van Everdingen et al., 2007). Persistent pain interferes with the ability to eat (Feuz and Rapin, 1994), sleep (Hugel et al., 2004), think, interact with others (Ferrell, 1995), and is correlated with fatigue (Burrows et al., 1998), depression, and anxiety (Mystakidou et al., 2006). The prevalence of symptoms other than pain in the advanced cancer patient has been well documented in the hospice and palliative care literature (Teunissen et al., 2007). Symptoms often appear to cluster and indeed several common patterns of symptom clusters have been recognized including one cluster of nausea–vomiting, anxiety–depression, fatigue–drowsiness, and pain–constipation, and another of nausea–vomiting, anxiety–depression, and dyspnoea–cough (Kirkova et al., 2010a, 2011). Multiple, concurrent physical symptoms are common during the last weeks of life with a particularly high prevalence of fatigue and generalized weakness (Chang et al., 2000), and in the last few days of life dyspnoea, delirium, nausea and vomiting are most common (Reuben et al., 1988; Coyle, 1990; Lichter and Hunt, 1990; Ventafridda et al., 1990; Fainsinger et al., 1991; Henteleff, 1991; Johanson, 1991).

The data on the prevalence of physical symptoms among children with advanced and incurable cancer are similarly dramatic. In a Swedish survey of the parents of dying children, the symptoms which had a moderate or high impact on the child's well-being were physical fatigue (86%), reduced mobility (76%), pain (73%), and decreased appetite (71%) (Jalmsell et al., 2006). Findings from an English survey were similar: pain was observed in 71–92% of children and the other major symptoms were anorexia, weight loss, and weakness (Goldman et al., 2006).

The symptoms at the end of life in disease other than cancer are remarkably similar to those experienced by cancer patients (Janssen et al., 2008a, 2008b). In a study that evaluated the relative prevalence of 11 common symptoms (pain, depression, anxiety, confusion, fatigue, dyspnoea, insomnia, nausea, constipation, diarrhoea, and anorexia) among end-stage patients suffering from five common, chronic, and progressive diseases (cancer, AIDS, heart disease, chronic obstructive pulmonary disease (COPD), and renal disease), three symptoms—pain, breathlessness, and fatigue—were found among more than 50% of patients, for all five diseases. The great similarity in the spectrum of symptoms seen across all illness groups suggests that there are a number of common symptoms found as patients approach death in in both malignant and non-malignant chronic illnesses (Solano et al., 2006).

Psychological symptoms

Anxiety, depression, confusion, and insomnia are all common problems in cancer and non-cancer-related chronic terminal diseases including COPD, renal failure, and heart failure (Solano et al., 2006) (see Section 17).

Among cancer patients, the prevalence of psychiatric distress is variably estimated from 12% (Kadan-Lottick et al., 2005), 40% (Grabsch et al., 2006), to upwards of 60% of patients with far advanced cancer (Breitbart et al., 1995; Breitbart and Jacobsen, 1996). Whatever the prevalence, there is agreement that the most common problems are adjustment disorders, depression, anxiety, and delirium (Portenoy et al., 1994; Breitbart and Jacobsen, 1996; Grabsch et al., 2006; Strong et al., 2007; Annunziata et al., 2012). All four of these symptoms may contribute to the development of suicidal thoughts, and indeed, psychiatric disorders are present in the vast majority of cancer patients who are suicidal (Breitbart, 1988; Breitbart et al., 2010).

Factors that adversely influence the prevalence and severity of psychological distress are the presence of advanced disease; distressing physical symptoms (especially pain) (Derogatis et al., 1983; Mystakidou et al., 2006); disability; unresolved previous experiences of loss or separation (Nordin et al., 2001); feelings of frustration and hopelessness (Nordin et al., 2001); a lack of perceived support from at least one loved person (Stedeford, 1984); strained interpersonal relationships (Stedeford, 1984); controlling personality trait (Watson et al., 1990); difficulties in adapting to the illness and its implications (Farberow et al., 1963); economic concerns (Hanratty et al., 2007; Sharp et al., 2012); impaired cognitive abilities (Nordin et al., 2001); and unsatisfactory communication regarding illness or treatment (particularly where there has been the precipitous disclosure of poor prognosis without allowance for a process of adjustment and assimilation of information) (Mager and Andrykowski, 2002). Uncontrolled pain is an important precipitant of psychological distress and is a suicide risk factor (Laird et al., 2009; Breitbart et al., 2010). In a large prospective study of psychological symptoms in cancer patients (Derogatis et al., 1983), the prevalence of cancer-related pain was 39% in those who had a psychiatric diagnosis and only 19% in those without such a diagnosis. Indeed, it has been observed that psychiatric symptoms commonly resolve with adequate pain relief (Mystakidou et al., 2006).

Spiritual and existential distress

The importance of spirituality in care of the dying is increasingly acknowledged by clinicians, researchers, and educators in end-of-life care. The Institute of Medicine (Field and Cassel, 1997) lists spiritual well-being as one of six domains of quality supportive care of the dying. Consequentially, exploring this dimension of well-being is an important part of routine physician inquiry, especially among patients with advanced and incurable illness (Ambuel, 2003; Pearce et al., 2012; Seng Beng et al., 2013) (see Chapter 17.1).

Defining existential issues such as spirituality is challenging and definitions abound. One comprehensive review of the health literature documented 92 definitions of the term 'spirituality' (Unruh et al., 2002). This review identified seven definitional themes: relationship to God, a spiritual being, a higher power, or a reality greater than the self; not of the self; transcendence or connectedness to a bigger picture but unrelated to a belief in a higher being; a conviction that there is more to life than what we can observe materially; meaning and purpose in life; life force of the person, integrating aspects of the person; and summative definitions that combined multiple themes. In another interesting study that evaluated Buddhist and Christian terminally ill patients in Taiwan (Chao et al., 2002), ten themes in four broad categories emerged: communion with self (self-identity, wholeness, inner peace); communion with others (love, reconciliation); communion with nature (inspiration creativity); and communion with a higher being (faithfulness, hope, gratitude).

Positive connections to life around us inspire a conscious or unconscious perception that life has significance, purpose, and meaning. This is of practical consequence, particularly in the context of discovering or building connections. These connections may be with God, relations, projects, responsibilities, special objects, rituals, non-sectarian religion or philosophy, or even the shared appreciation of beauty, poetry, or music (Vanistendael, 2007). While the source of inspiration for such significance will vary from person to person, what they hold in common is their ability to imbue life with an overarching sense of purpose and meaning, including a sustained investment in life itself.

Within the religious world view, spirituality is usually associated with a sense of connectedness to a God, whereas within the secular realm, it often invokes a search for significance and meaning. According to Viktor Frankl, having a sense that one's life has meaning involves the conviction that one is fulfilling a unique role and purpose in life. He suggests that life is a gift that comes with a responsibility to live to one's full potential as a human being, and that through this process one can achieve a sense of peace, contentment, or even transcendence through connectedness with something greater than oneself. He describes central paths to fulfil one's potential as a human being through (1) involvement in creative or productive actions, (2) life experience, and (3) connectedness and love. Of these three paths he ascribes greatest importance to connectedness and love (Frankl, 1992).

Among patients with advanced cancer, unmnet spiritual needs are common (Moadel et al., 1999; Pearce et al., 2012). One study of 248 cancer outpatients found that spiritual or existential needs were commonly unmet; common among them were overcoming fears (51%), finding hope (42%) and meaning in life (40%), finding spiritual resources (39%), and having someone to talk with about the meaning of life and death (25%) (Moadel et al., 1999).

The common existential issues for patients with advanced cancer include hopelessness, futility, meaninglessness, disappointment, remorse, death anxiety, and disruption of personal identity. Existential distresses may be related to past, present, or future concerns. Current personal integrity, the sense of who one is as a person, can be disrupted by changes in body image; somatic, intellectual, social and professional function; and in perceived attractiveness as a person and as a sexual partner (Cassell, 1982; Bolmsjo, 2000). For some patients retrospection can trigger profound disappointment (from unfulfilled aspirations or a deprecation of the value of previous achievements), or remorse from unresolved guilt (Yalom, 1980; Cassell, 1982; Bolmsjo, 2000).

If life is perceived to offer, at best, comfort in the setting of fading potency or, at worst, ongoing physical and emotional distress as days pass slowly until death, anticipation of the future may be associated with feelings of hopelessness, futility, or meaninglessness such that the patient sees no value in continuing to live. Death anxiety is common among cancer patients; surveys have shown that 50–80% of terminally ill patients have concerns or troubling thoughts about death, and that only a minority achieve an untroubled acceptance of death (Bolmsjo, 2000). Together, these symptoms have been labelled a 'demoralization syndrome' (Kissane et al., 2001).

More recent studies indicate that the same spectrum of spiritual distress is observed in patients suffering from chronic life-threatening diseases other than cancer (Selman et al., 2007; Haynes and Watt, 2008; Bekelman et al., 2009; Steinhauser et al., 2011). Although these existential issues are sometimes referred to as 'spiritual', they appear to be universal, and independent of religion and religious practice (Yalom, 1980; Kissane, 2000).

Family/social distress

The perception by the patient of the distress of family, friends, and health-care providers can further amplify the patient's distress, and thus contribute to the nihilistic conclusion that ongoing existence only constitutes a perpetuation of the burden to self and to others.

Family distress

The development of a chronic life-limiting illness in a family member impacts upon the entire family (King and Quill, 2006; Janssen et al., 2011; Seng Beng et al., 2013). The challenges confronting the family—to acknowledge the ending of life as they have known it, and to define a new way of constructively living out their final days together as best possible—engender great stresses (Davies et al., 1990; King and Quill, 2006). Among the contributing factors to the ensuing distress are empathic suffering with the distress of the patient; grief and bereavement; role changes; and the physical, financial, and psychological sequelae of the burdens of care (Wittenberg-Lyles et al., 2011; Seng Beng et al., 2013) (see Chapter 17.6).

Furthermore, the family carers of adults with advanced chronic illness have been shown to constitute a vulnerable population (Janssen et al., 2011). In one study, almost a quarter of the family caregivers for the terminally ill had chronic health problems themselves (West et al., 1986), and others have highlighted the further detriment to health incurred by family carers (Schachter, 1992). A very high prevalence of anxiety and adjustment difficulties have also been identified among family members, the severity of which is often as great as that of the patients themselves (Grov et al., 2005, 2006).

Family needs

The needs of the families of patients with advanced cancer (Kristjanson, 1989; Ferrell et al., 1991a, 1991b; Kristjanson et al., 1995, 1997a; Milberg and Strang, 2000; Steinhauser et al., 2000; Soothill et al., 2001; Scott et al., 2001; Funk et al., 2010; Stajduhar et al., 2010, 2011) and other chronic illnesses (Scott et al., 2001; Goy et al., 2008; Ben Natan et al., 2010) have been surveyed by several researchers. The prompt and effective relief of patient symptoms is a major priority for family members, as are the needs for education in the comfort care of the patient, and for physician and nursing availability (Kristjanson et al., 1997a; Steinhauser et al., 2000; Fridriksdottir et al., 2006; Funk et al., 2010; Stajduhar et al., 2010, 2011;). Families often express the need for communication from health-care providers that is honest, direct, and compassionate, in which family concerns and opinions are heard and valued, and that conveys information that can help in patient care (Steinhauser et al., 2000; Scott et al., 2001; Goy et al., 2008; Adams et al., 2009; Funk et al., 2010; Stajduhar et al., 2010, 2011). Material supports such as a hospital bed, and professional supports in the framework of family meetings are similarly valued (Funk et al., 2010; Stajduhar et al., 2010, 2011). Besides lack of professional, financial, and home management supports which are endemic, other commonly unmet needs include the need to receive assurance of the patient's comfort; to be informed of the patient's condition; to ventilate emotions; to receive comfort and support from family members; and to receive acceptance, support, and comfort from health-care professionals (Sharpe et al., 2005).

Psychosocial distress among family members

Psychological distress among family caregivers is very common, occurring in 40–60% of family caregivers who care for a loved one during the end-of-life experience, especially as the patient's level of autonomy diminishes.

A review of the data on the impact of cancer on family members identified 11 major issues for family members: emotional strain, physical demands, uncertainty, fear that the patient will die, alteration in roles and lifestyles, financial concerns, ways to comfort the patient, perceived inadequacy of care services, existential concerns, sexuality, and non-convergent needs among family members (Lewis, 1986). These issues can be profoundly influenced by the trajectory of the illness. For example, a long illness characterized by a remitting and relapsing course may produce persistent anxiety and uncertainty which can produce severe emotional fatigue (Blood et al., 1994; Steele, 2000). To resolve those feelings, family members may, in some circumstances, hope for the patient's rapid demise. In contrast, when the time from diagnosis to impending death has been short, there may be little opportunity for family members to come to terms with the presence of life-threatening illness let alone impending death (Coolican, 1994; Casarett et al., 2001).

Psychological problems of anxiety, depression, and adjustment disorder are common among family members of patients with advanced cancer (Dumont et al., 2006; Gaudio et al., 2012; Seng Beng et al., 2013). Studies of family cohesiveness indicate that these problems are more prevalent in families with low levels of cohesiveness and high levels of conflict (Ozono et al., 2005). Good communication within the family mitigates against psychological distress in general (Ozono et al., 2005) and anxiety in particular (Edwards and Clarke, 2004).

Grief

In most cases, the pre-terminal phase of the chronic fatal illness experience is associated with a period of anticipatory grieving (Kissane et al., 1997; Simon, 2008; Johansson and Grimby, 2012, Johansson et al., 2012) in which the family undergoes a transition associated with the patient's 'fading away' (Davies et al., 1990). In one study (Davies et al., 1990), the onset of this transition was generally heralded by a deterioration in the patient's condition that challenged ongoing denial. The most heralding events were unrecoverable weakness, loss of independence in ambulation and personal care, and loss of mental clarity. These events are distressing in that they constitute losses, diminish hope for recovery, and focus attention on the inevitability of the patient's demise.

Caregiver burden

Although most patients die in the hospital setting, most of the care prior to dying is carried out at home by the family members with the support of health-care professionals. The care of a terminally ill family member greatly strains the physical, emotional, and psychological resources of the family unit and its individual members (Bialon and Coke, 2012; Seng Beng et al., 2013).

Home care often involves participation in personal hygiene needs, administration of medication by non-invasive or invasive routes, attention to nutritional needs, psychological support, and emergency management of such problems as pain, dyspnoea, or bleeding. The heavy physical work of transferring a weak or immobile patient, and attending to other needs (such as laundering or cleaning), is often further compounded by exhaustion as a result of sleep deprivation due to anxious thoughts or patient care needs (Aoun et al., 2010). For many this is a new experience and the uncertainties about the dying process, and the ability to cope with the problems that lie ahead, may become a focus for anxiety or ruminative thoughts. Family caregivers may be ill prepared to assume these tasks, requiring information on the disease and treatment, as well as instruction in technical and care skills. Moreover, caregiving must be balanced against already established roles and role responsibilities.

Financial distress

Financial distress has been underappreciated and is often neglected in routine care (Rabow et al., 2004; Longo et al., 2006; Hanratty et al., 2007). Studies comparing the relative costs of home- and hospital-based terminal care (Ventafridda et al., 1989; Beck-Friis et al., 1991) have generally neglected the financial and social costs to the family. In the National Hospice Study, 26% of primary care takers either left their work or lost their jobs, and 60% reported a significant reduction in income due to either absenteeism or a change in work arrangements (Muurinen, 1986). Permanent loss of employment occurred most frequently among those who could least afford it: older women and low-income families (Muurinen, 1986). The costs of caring for a family member can leave the surviving family with severely compromised resources (Grunfeld et al., 2004a). This distress is often exacerbated by inadequate insurance coverage.

Caregiver conflicts

The caregiver may experience profound conflict in this situation: conflict between the desire to provide adequate relief of distressing symptoms while, at the same time, wanting to preserve their loved one's alertness, and to avoid hastening death; and conflict between the duty to care for a loved one and to care for oneself, and one's other responsibilities. Additionally, there is often conflict between caregiving family members regarding goals of care, limits of care, and aggressiveness of care (Kramer et al., 2006; Kramer et al., 2010). Guilt, anger, denial, and other emotional influences sometimes compel family members into conflicted opinions whether to treat a devastating illness aggressively or discontinue life-sustaining measures (Bloche, 2005). These conflicts may reflect low levels of pre-existing cohesiveness, or they may threaten family closeness and collaboration in previously cohesive families.

Identifying families at risk

The endurability of the burdens of care is an important consideration in long-term care planning; the family members' current and future welfare is an important consideration when care demands are great and supportive resources for home care are limited (Callahan, 1988; Given et al., 2001, 2004). The ability and willingness of family members to participate in care is very variable (Abernethy et al., 2009) and in one retrospective survey, 22% of families of terminally ill patients were unable or unwilling to provide personal or medical care (Wellisch et al., 1989).

The identification of populations at particularly high risk for early intervention is facilitated by an assessment of stressors, particular family needs, and the resources available to the family. A survey of bereavement councillors highlighted several different risk factors: perceived lack of caregiver social support (70%), caregiver history of drug/alcohol abuse (68%), poor caregiver coping skills (68%), caregiver history of mental illness (67%), and patient is a child (63%) (Ellifritt et al., 2003).

Another approach has been to look at global family functioning as a predictor of coping. In a large longitudinal study, Kissane and colleagues identified characteristics of families with high prevalence of distress and poor coping (Kissane et al., 2003). Families classified as 'hostile' were characterized by low cohesiveness, low expressiveness, and high conflict. Family members typically described family life as fraught with frequent arguing, little teamwork or felt closeness among members, and minimal communication. Families classified as 'sullen' were also characterized by reduced cohesiveness and expressiveness, but only mild to moderate conflict. Reports of overt hostility were low in this group, suggesting that anger is muted, with depression gaining more prominence as the anger is directed inwards.

In contrast, the attributes identified to facilitate effective function include the ability to work cohesively, prior successful experience in handling stress, a substantial and flexible repertoire of coping strategies, family stability, financial security, the availability of outside supports to which the family is receptive, and a readiness to view this difficult period as potentially growth-producing (Quinn and Herndon, 1986). Kissane et al. identified two positive patterns of family function predictive of good coping. 'Supportive families' described family life as intimate and mutually supportive, with open and honest communication among its members, tolerance of emotional expression, and little to no escalation in conflict. Similarly 'conflict-resolving' families which had cohesiveness and above-average expressiveness, but also the presence of conflict but with good conflict management (characterized by the ability to both voice and resolve differences between family members) (Kissane et al., 2003).

Health-care professional distress

Stressors

Health-care professionals may experience distress due to the constant exposure to suffering, loss, and grief that they are expected to be able to ease or relieve. Among the stressors experienced by professionals working in this field are patients who experience high morbidity and mortality; high work pressure; frequent life and death decisions (which sometimes occur in ambiguous circumstances); high consumer expectations; interstaff conflict; severe patient dependency, debilitation, or disfigurement; severe emotional distress among patients and their families; and issues relating to suffering and distress caused by the treatments themselves (Kash et al., 2000). It is not unusual for clinicians to bond strongly with patients who remind them of someone special in their lives or identify with patients who are similar to themselves in age, appearance, or background (Meier et al., 2001; Ekedahl and Wengstrom, 2007). Identification with patients can revive personal pain and heighten feelings of guilt or a lack of control, resulting in burnout (Escot et al., 2001; Keidel, 2002; Ekedahl and Wengstrom, 2007) (see Chapter 4.16).

Physician distress

There is a paucity of data on physician burnout among palliative medicine specialists and much of the understanding regarding burnout is derived from studies of oncologists who deal with patients with advanced cancer (Martins Pereira et al., 2011). Stress and burnout are common phenomenon among clinicians managing patients with incurable cancer. Among oncologists, various studies have demonstrated prevalence rates of 25–56% (Whippen and Canellos, 1991; Ramirez et al., 1995; Akroyd et al., 2002; Elit et al., 2004; Grunfeld et al., 2004b; Asai et al., 2006). Multiple factors contribute to stress in oncology clinicians. There is an increasing awareness of the major contribution of workload and life balance issues (Grunfeld et al., 2004b; Shanafelt, 2005): volume overload, difficulty balancing personal and professional lives, inadequate staffing to do the job properly, the challenge of keeping current with medical literature, and pressures to obtain grants and to publish. Mounting administrative issues add to this. Interpersonal conflict and difficulties in relationships with colleagues, junior staff, nurses, administrative staff, and administration are common. To all of these are added the challenges of end-of-life care: dealing and being involved with the physical and emotional suffering of patients, delivering bad news, and having to deal with distressed, angry, or blaming relatives. Oncologists must deal daily with stressed patients and families, disproportionate hopes and expectations, emotionally laden dialogues with patients and families, and the limitations of treatments that are unable to deliver cures.

Regarding the contribution of end of life on oncologist burnout, a European Society for Medical Oncology survey of almost 900 medical oncologists regarding their attitudes to and involvement with the management of advanced cancer (Cherny and Catane, 2003) found that just over a third of respondents reported that they felt emotionally burned out by having to deal with too many deaths. This predilection to burnout was associated closely with negative attitudes to involvement in supportive and palliative care and low levels of actual involvement or referral to palliative care colleagues. This study suggests that burnout from end-of-life care was not so much associated to over-exposure rather to poor attitudinal preparedness and aberrant role definition. These finding suggest that positive attitudes and involvement in palliative care are all resilience factors that helps prevent burnout caused by exposure to advanced cancer.

In a survey of 81 French general practitioners (Schaerer, 1993), 86% endorsed the assertion that encounters with death were a cause of physician suffering. The major causes of physician suffering were the end of the doctor–patient relationship (58%), feelings of uselessness (55%) and failure (38%), increased awareness of their own mortality (49%), and the presence of 'questions without answers' (31%). The most commonly reported feelings that were experienced by these physicians at the bedside of the dying patient were sadness (94%), helplessness (89%), failure (61%), disappointment (59%), and loneliness (51%).

Nursing distress

Studies of nurses working in palliative care have yielded mixed results; an international study evaluating stress levels and coping mechanisms among professionals who work with illness and death found that palliative care and hospice workers had less stress and better coping than those in other fields (Vachon, 1995; Hackett et al., 2009; Martins Pereira et al., 2011). Despite this, the potential for exhaustion and burnout is well described (Vachon, 1995; Astudillo and Mendinueta, 1996a; Peterson et al., 2010). Major sources of stress include perceived deficiencies in symptom control, deep emotional involvement in work, dealing with young patients, dealing with the emotional needs of distressed relatives, and conflict with the participating physicians over the goals of care (Harris et al., 1990; Newton and Waters, 2001; Wilkes and Beale, 2001; Hackett et al., 2009; Peterson et al., 2010).

Research among nurses has demonstrated both vulnerability and resilience factors. Personality characteristics such as perfectionism and over-involvement with patients may contribute to compassion fatigue or burnout. Self-esteem, sense of mastery, purpose in life, and a clear philosophy of life are protective factors.

Younger nurses with fewer years of experience report higher levels of distress (van Staa et al., 2000). A qualitative study of palliative care professionals found that less experienced clinicians focused on the technical aspects of care. Clinicians with more than 10 years' experience focused on their commitment to patient and family and developing trusting and open therapeutic relationships. They were also likely to recognize the stressful nature of end-of-life care and to understand the experience from the perspective of the patient and family, as well as the meaning of the experience to themselves, both personally and professionally (Farber et al., 2003).

Assessment and planning

An effective approach to the alleviation of suffering for patients with incurable or terminal illness is predicated upon careful case assessment, identification of care needs, formulation of a multi-disciplinary therapeutic intervention to address those needs, and the provision of ongoing monitoring with readiness to re-evaluate the care plan as problems arise or needs change.

Assessment

An appreciation of the full diversity of factors that may contribute to suffering underscores the need for a methodical approach to the assessment of each individual case. The objectives of the assessment are to identify current problems that are a source of distress to each of the parties, to assess their care needs, and to evaluate the adequacy of the available resources. This evaluation must incorporate medical variables in the patient, family, and available community medical system; psychological variables in the patient, family, and psychosocial community supports; and social and financial variables in the patient and family. Since both the patient and the family are part of the unit of care, assessment requires discussion with both. The clinician must maintain a clinical posture that affirms relief of suffering as the central goal of therapy, and which encourages open and effective communication about perceived problems.

Patient assessment

The prevalence of poorly controlled pain and other physical symptoms, and the impact of these factors on the lives of all involved, emphasize the importance of addressing these issues at the earliest opportunity. The early establishment of good symptom control conveys concern, builds the trust of patients and their families, and facilitates the ability to address other important issues.

Patient variables that must be assessed include the disease status, expected disease progression, present functional level, symptoms, current therapies, and anticipated future problems. Of particular importance is the patient's level of function, reflecting his or her mobility (e.g. fully bedbound or fully mobile without aids), ability to communicate (from severe as with brain tumours to minimal impairment), ability to perform activities of daily living, bowel and bladder function (from incontinence to full self-care), and level of alertness (from coma to full alertness). The use of validated pain and symptom assessment instruments can provide a format for communication between the patient and health-care professionals and can also be used to monitor the adequacy of therapy.

It is important to ascertain the patient's and the family's understanding of the nature and extent of the illness and their expectations of treatment and outcome. As part of this process, the clinician must develop an understanding of the patient's prioritization of the sometimes conflicting goals of care: optimization of comfort, function (interactional function in particular), and duration of survival.

Family assessment

Family assessment should encompass medical variables, psychosocial concerns, and the adequacy and availability of supports. Evaluation of the willingness and ability of home carers to provide home care and the availability of supports are essential. Concurrent medical problems in a family member, particularly a primary caregiver, need to be evaluated since the viability of the home care plan may depend upon the family member's ability to participate in care. Since the ability of families to cope with home care is largely determined by the nature of the available home-care supports (Kristjanson et al., 1997b; Redinbaugh et al.,

2003; Limpanichkul and Magilvy, 2004), the family assessment must include an assessment of available health-care professional and community supports.

It is important to ascertain the family's understanding of the nature and extent of the patient's cancer and their expectations of treatment and outcome. Discrepancies between what is known and understood by the patient and the family should be identified, and the reasons for these discrepancies should be tactfully explored. Knowledge deficits may have been deliberately maintained: the family or patient not wanting information overload, the patient protecting the family from knowledge of poor prognosis, or the family protecting the patient from the impact of such information (Dalla-Vorgia et al., 1992; Mystakidou et al., 2005). This part of the assessment requires a non-judgemental posture, and sensitivity to psychological and cultural factors that may influence the transmission of information.

Health-care professional assessment

Evaluation of the professional caregiver supports usually requires greater detail than that which can be provided by the patient and family alone. To effectively plan for ongoing care, the clinical coordinator must understand the limitations of the involved health-care professionals (knowledge, experience, and availability for home care), their difficulties in coping with the situation, and their perceived needs to improve the care outcome. As previously described, the coping of professional caregivers may be severely strained by issues pertaining to communication; conflict with the patient, family, or colleagues; perceived therapeutic failure; excessive workload or emotional strain; and difficult therapeutic or ethical decisions.

Awareness of this interrelated construct enables the clinician to construct a series of critical questions regarding each of these domains, the answers to which constitute the basis of a patient assessment.

The patient

Several tools gave been developed to help evaluate patient suffering or distress (Krikorian et al., 2013) (see section 7).

Who is the patient and what is their social context? It is critically important to be aware of who the person is who is now needing care. This includes collection of information about basic demographics, family structure, other significant relationships, professional and education history, and place of dwelling. This phase should also incorporate past medical history and significant elements of family health and social history.

What is the patient's illness and where is the patient in the natural history of the condition? More often than not, this information will be available from the referring clinician and the patient's medical record. Specific information is required regarding the diagnosis, sites of disease, active medical problems, and anticipated prognosis. Anticipated prognosis relates not only to life expectancy, rather a broader concept that incorporates the projected course of illness and anticipated complications or problems.

Is the patient clear headed, if not why not? Cognitive impairment is very common among patients with advanced cancer and among other patients needing palliative care (Minagawa et al., 1996; Breitbart et al., 1997; Pereira et al., 1997). The presence of delirium impairs the ability to obtain direct information from the patient and will impair the ability to directly address many of the subsequent assessment issues without involvement of family and health-care providers. When cognitive impairment is identified, efforts should be made to identify reversible contributing factors. The chronology of the problem must be assessed, including pre-morbid level of function, the time course of the deterioration in cognitive function, precipitating or alleviating factors, and other features of co-morbidity that may help identify the underlying problem. In this setting, the clinician will need to obtain the greater part of the clinical information from the family members or other involved observers. Since iatrogenic cognitive impairment caused by centrally acting drugs is common, it is important to review the patient's drug chart and to ask about the ingestion of any other substances (such as 'medicinal' mushrooms) which may be implicated.

What does the patient understand of the illness? Care planning and further evaluations require that the clinician is aware of the extent of the patient's familiarity with his/her condition and what the patient's communication preferences are. Although there is extensive data indicating that most patients want accurate information regarding their medical status, this is not universal (Walsh et al., 1998). Some patients want only limited information and a few want no information (Walsh et al., 1998). Excessive candour in the setting of impaired coping or in a patient who expresses a desire not to receive information may constitute a maleficent assault (Campbell and Sanson-Fisher, 1998; Girgis and Sanson-Fisher, 1998; Walsh et al., 1998).

What are the current goals of care? The goals of care are often complex, but can generally be grouped into three broad categories: (1) prolonging survival, (2) optimizing comfort, and (3) optimizing function (Cherny et al., 1994b). The relative priority of these goals provides an essential context for therapeutic decision-making (Fins et al., 1999). The prioritization of these goals is a dynamic phenomenon which changes with the evolution of the disease. For some patients requiring palliative care the optimization of comfort, function, and survival may share equal priority whereas the provision of comfort usually assumes overriding priority as death approaches.

Awareness of goals has major implications for care and therapeutic decision-making and it influences the evaluation process. When patients equally prioritize optimal comfort and function, the therapeutic intent is to achieve an adequate degree of relief without compromising cognitive and physical function. In this setting, impairments to physical, psychological, or social function require careful evaluation in order to guide care needs. When, however, comfort is the overriding goal of care, and the overriding intent is to achieve relief of discomfort, there may be areas of function or of disease status that are no longer an essential part of the assessment.

What are the physical consequences of the illness? Is the patient coping? Are there physical problems that are not well controlled? Patients needing palliative care are typically polysymptomatic and often have severe limitations in activities of daily living. Data from a number of studies have demonstrated that patients commonly have six to ten active distressing symptoms (Teunissen et al., 2007). Symptom assessment aims to identify the active symptoms, their severity, and the degree of distress that they are engendering for the patient. Several well-validated tools have been developed to help screen patients for physical and psychological symptoms and to monitor their severity (Kirkova et al., 2009).

Pain in particular needs detailed evaluation; this is addressed in greater detail in Section 13.

Symptom evaluation must be accompanied an evaluation of function. This should incorporate activities of daily living such as ambulation, toileting, dressing, eating, sleeping and sexual function (if clinically appropriate).

The extent of the physical examination will be determined, in part, by the patient's prevailing condition and the goals of care. The physical examination often helps refine the differential diagnosis of problems indicated by the clinical history. Details of physical examination are beyond the scope of this introduction: suffice it to say that special attention must be paid to common problems associated with advanced illness including mouth care and skin integrity as well as to sites affected by the patient's symptoms or which may be commonly involved in the disease from which the patient suffers. When the patient suffers from pain or from neurological symptoms, the valuation should incorporate a neurological examination.

All relevant pre-existing diagnostic investigations should be reviewed. These often reveal important information that may explain current symptoms or help focus the need for any future diagnostic interventions.

Psychologically, how is the patient coping? What is he/she thinking? What are his/her active fears or concerns? Fear, anxiety, sadness, depression, and sleep disturbance are among the most common symptoms of advanced cancer. They are a substantial cause of distress, undermine coping, and are a major contributing factor for suicidal ideation and the desire for death. Patients should be asked how they are coping. This serves as a useful opening to explore more specific psychological and social issues. Inquiry about coping conveys concern. This, in turn, contributes to the development of trust and facilitates development of the therapeutic relationship. Specific enquiries should be made regarding feelings of sadness, anxiety, or persistent fears. If acknowledged, these symptoms should be further evaluated to identify the contributing factors, severity of the symptoms, and the impact of the psychological distress on patient function.

When patients express fears or anxiety, it is important to clarify the specific fears. Often fears are based either on misinformation or on anticipated problems that are very unlikely to occur. In other situations, patient fears are appropriate but are magnified either by poor communication or by a lack of communication. Patients with advanced cancer often harbour fears of uncontrolled pain, dyspnoea, or some other form of uncontrolled suffering at the end of life. These fears can be addressed through counselling, a commitment to continuity of care and to adequate palliation, and meticulous clinical follow-up with implementation of those commitments.

On a day-to-day basis, how is the patient coping and do they have adequate supports? Effective day-to-day coping requires an integration between physical, psychological, and disease-related factors in coordination with environmental factors related to family, friend, and health-care supports. This complex interaction must be evaluated. Asking patients about their day-to-day coping is a technique to open a dialogue regarding this complex interaction. Similarly, one can ask the patient if they have adequate supports. Support and coping are deliberately general queries that may evoke responses relating very diverse issues and concerns. Commonly expressed concerns include financial concerns, fears of family burnout, lack of availability of medical and nursing staff, difficulties in obtaining parking at the hospital, communication concerns with clinical staff, and inadequately controlled symptoms.

What are the deeper thoughts that the patient harbours? What sort of life have they had? Do they have unfulfilled dreams or aspirations? What have been the things that have made them sad or happy? How do they see the future? Existential and spiritual issues may relate to the past, present, or future. As people approach the end of life, they commonly have many thoughts relating to the life that they have lived, issues of legacy, the life that they are currently living, and concerns about the time that remains ahead of them. Additionally, many patients harbour transcendental thoughts relating to their place in the world, their relationship to God, and thoughts related to an afterlife. These concerns are universal, cross-cultural, and are probably intrinsic to mortal life. The relative weight of these issues is influenced by culture, past, cognitive function, and the place in the life cycle at which the patient is confronting their mortality.

Evaluating these deeply personal issues requires the prior development of a trusting relationship. Exploration and disclosure of these issues is usually undertaken over time. In many instances the patient may choose to disclose and discuss different issues with different staff members. This may reflect interpersonal dynamics, specific clinical skills, or perceived roles. Information sharing, with the patient's permission, with other members of the interdisciplinary team helps sensitize other participating caregivers to the specific cares, concerns, and sensitivities of the patient. When patients feel understood, they are more likely to feel trust in the care team and environment.

Life-review techniques can help identify points of meaning about important issues of legacy as well as unresolved issues related to the past such as remorse, unfulfilled ambitions, or guilt. Direct questioning can be used to evaluate the patient's coping in the family, at work, and in significant relationships.

Fear of death is commonplace. Specific death-related fears may include fears of pain, dyspnoea, loss of control, medical abandonment or overtreatment, oblivion, and concern for surviving family members. Frequently, specific goals or uncompleted tasks will be identified. This information may be critical for life planning in the time that remains for the patient.

What future problems are anticipated? What provisional steps can be taken to cover contingencies? Careful contingency planning can help avoid crises. Contingency planning should relate to specific anticipated physical problems (such as pain, dyspnoea, immobility, wound breakdown, or bleeding), psychological problems (such as anxiety, sleep disturbance, or delirium), and home-care problems (such as failing supports, family burnout, or access problems). By identifying probable contingencies one can implement and prepare a back-up plan. Examples of this sort of planning include provision of opioids and antipsychotics if pain or delirium is anticipated, oxygen if hypoxaemia is anticipated, and bathroom railing if immobility is anticipated. When home death is anticipated, it is helpful to have a prepared programme for the family of who needs to be called with all phone numbers prepared and any paperwork ready and available.

In some circumstances, the nature of the anticipated contingency may be such that it may impact on the immediate care plan. This is especially true when catastrophic bleeding from a carotid or femoral blow-out is anticipated. If the patient lives alone or

with a companion who may be significantly traumatized by this sort of horrid event, anticipatory admission to a hospital or palliative care unit may be appropriate. This is true for patients who may suffer asphyxiation from upper airway tumour.

Family

Screening tools to evaluate the distress and needs of family caregivers have been developed (Shim et al., 2010; Ewing and Grande, 2013). These tools address components of the following eight domains (see Chapter 7.4).

Who is the family and what is their social context? This is well achieved using a family map. Critical issues for assessment of each family member include age, place of residence, health status, occupation, nuclear family relationships, and geographic and emotional proximity to the patient. Some family members may have unresolved past issues with the patent and, as far as is possible, it is helpful to identify these.

How is the physical and psychological well-being of the family member? Since advanced and incurable illnesses are most commonly a problem of the elderly, often the caring family member may be in poor physical health. Similarly, significant illness in a family is a major emotional stress and indeed, family members often suffer from anxiety, depression, and adjustment disorder or difficulty. It is important that the members of the care team be aware of these factors as they will impact on the ability of the family member to participate in care and they indicate specific care needs of their own.

What do the family members understand of the patient's condition and the goals of care? Discrepancies between the patient's and the family members' understanding of the patient's diagnosis, treatments, anticipated outcomes of treatment, prognosis, and goals of care are commonplace (Purandare, 1997). It is only by asking family members what they understand of the illness that these discrepancies can be identified. When discrepancies are identified, the clinician must evaluate if there is a specific reason that they exist. Occasionally the patient may have specifically requested that information not be disclosed to family members or to a specific family member. When this has been the case, the reasons for concealment of this sort should be explored with the patient.

Emotionally, how are they coping with the prevailing situation? Are they adequately supported? Are they coping?

Life-threatening disease in a family member is a major life stress. Coping with this sort of stress is very variable and it has both psychological and physical dimensions. When emotional coping is difficult or when failure of coping occurs this impacts on everyone else involved in the care dynamic including the patient, other family members, and the professional health-care team (Vachon, 1998). Coping with physical care needs can be severely compromised when there is a failure of emotional coping. It is, therefore important to explore issues of emotional coping of the family members. Common issues include anticipatory grief, anxiety, and depression. Changes in the patient's condition commonly precipitate a transient adjustment disorder that may manifest as anxiety, panic, depression, psychomotor retardation, or acting-out.

Physically, how are they coping with the prevailing situation? Are they adequately supported? It is important to evaluate the family members' ability to cope with the patients care needs, to identify the role of pre-emptive or remedial assistance when available, and to identify impending breakdown in coping (which may require urgent intervention such as respite admission) (Bramwell et al., 1995; Astudillo and Mendinueta, 1996b; Karlsen and Addington-Hall, 1998). This process aims to evaluate the limits of the family's coping resources for home care. If the patient's care needs exceed these limits, other care plans will need to be activated. Coping with physical care needs can be supported by the provision of appropriate physical supports (such as a wheelchair, hospital bed, or toileting equipment), education in care provision, and professional or volunteer assistance.

What are the deeper thoughts that the family member harbours? What sort of life have they had? Do they have unfulfilled dreams or aspirations? What have been the things that have made them sad or happy? How do they see the future? Life-threatening illness in a spouse, sibling, or parent threatens a significant relationship, and it impacts on the way family members relate to their past, present, and future. Family members may suffer the same spectrum of existential issues as the patients themselves (Carson, 1997). As with the patient, life-review techniques may identify unfilled ambitions, regrets, and remorse related to relationship issues with the patient, as well as help highlight positive aspects of their shared experiences. The patient's illness may have altered the structure of the family relationships. Often, evaluation of future goals can identify specific targets that may not be achievable with the involvement of the patient unless they are brought forward. In many instances, discussion of these issues has brought forward major life events such as weddings, long-distance travel, or family reunions.

What are their concerns for the future? Family members often have specific fears regarding anticipated future events in relation to the patient. Common fears include fears of uncontrolled pain, confusion, incontinence, loss of ambulatory function, bleeding, addiction, abandonment, and lack of supports. Once identified, these fears are often amenable to intervention either through counselling, information transfer, family meetings, or the development of clear contingency plans and lines of communication.

Have they suffered other losses in the past? In what circumstances? How did they deal with them? How are these losses impacting on what is happening now? Previous grief experiences impact on the distress of impending bereavement (Janson and Sloan, 1991; Murphy et al., 1997). Knowing about the experiences of previous losses can help the professional caregiver address issues related to the current situation. Family members who have experienced multiple grief experiences may be suffering from cumulative losses. In other situations, family members have fears based on previous death experiences. Consequently it is important to ask family members about previous death experiences: what happened? How did they cope? Did the experience leave them with any specific fears or hopes regarding death and end-of-life care?

Health-care providers

Who is involved in the patient's care? Patients commonly have multiple professionals involved in their care. It is critical to identify them, their roles, the limits of their availability, the cost of their services, and the extent of their communication. Contact details should be made available and clear lines of communication and responsibility established. A clinician should be nominated as the coordinating clinician who is ultimately responsible for the coordination of professional caregiver activities.

What is the experience and expertise of the professional health-care providers with the prevailing problems? Health-care professionals constitute a heterogeneous group. Professionals vary greatly in their experience, training, and attitudes regarding palliative care and end-of-life care. Since knowledge deficits are endemic, it is important to understand the specific professional background of each of the participating clinicians. Where lack of experience or lack of knowledge in palliative care is identified in the care team, special provision for expert backup or remedial education may be required.

What do the professional health-care providers understand of the illness and of the goals of care? It is important to clarify the understanding of all participating caregivers regarding the goals of care and of their specific care goals. Miscommunication of the goals of care or lack of concordance between professional caregivers on this issue can contribute to conflict and confusion.

What are the limits of care that they can reasonably provide? Do they have adequate human resources to deal with the prevailing problems? Are they coping? Usually, there are limits to the professional services and personnel resources available for the care of patients. These limits need to be determined. Once determined, it is important to assess the likelihood that they will be adequate to meet the patient's and family's care needs. When the care needs are great and the professional caregiver resources are limited, it is important to assess professional caregiver coping. When there is mismatch between care needs and available services, particularly in the setting of home care, alternative care arrangements in hospital or a palliative care department or hospice may need to be considered.

How are they coping with the emotional impact of the situation? Caring for incurable patients and their families places a great stress on the emotional coping resources of health-care professionals and sometimes professionals feel inadequately prepared for the emotion-laden nature of this work. Consequently, it is important to assess the coping of the members of the care team with the emotional issues to which they are being exposed. As part of this assessment, it is important to check that the emotional care burden is being distributed between the professional carers and that there is provision for debriefing.

Do they have adequate physical resources? Home care of patients needing palliative care often requires equipment such as a hospital bed, ambulating assist devices (such as a walking frame or wheelchair), toileting equipment, oxygen, suction device, or specific medications. It is incumbent to evaluate what resources are needed and the evaluate availability and cost (if any).

What future problems are anticipated? What provisional steps can be taken to cover contingencies? The issue of contingency planning was addressed as part of the patient assessment. The evaluation of the care services must include an evaluation of the implementation of the contingency arrangements. Lines of communications should be clarified and the extent of available cover for emergencies checked. If the need for admission is foreseen, communication including a letter of introduction should be prepared in advance. When it is anticipated that the patient will die in the near future, there should be clear instructions for the family indicating who to contact, including the details of funeral company contacts.

Table 2.1.1 The dimensions of patient distress, management approaches, and potential therapeutic resources

Dimension	Distress	Intervention(s)	Therapist(s)
Physical	Pain	Comprehensive pain management	MD, Nur, Anaesth,
	Other physical symptoms	Comprehensive therapy	PCS, Physiat,
	Physical disability	Physiatric review and therapy	OT, PT.
Psychological	Anxiety	Careful assessment for reversible factors	Onc, Nur, SW,
	Depression	Psychotherapy ± pharmacotherapy	Psych, Neur, PCS
	Adjustment difficulties	Cognitive or behavioural interventions	
	Cognitive impairment		
	Unresolved previous loss or separation		
	Control		
Social	Strained family relationships	Family assessment, supportive intervention	MD, Nur, SW,
	Unsatisfactory communication regarding illness or treatment	Assessment and facilitation	Psych, PCS
	Economic	Assessment and support	
	Family related	Address issues of family distress	See Table 2.1.2
	Feeling an excessive care burden		
	Feeling an excessive emotional burden		
	Feeling an excessive economic burden		
	Doctor related	Evaluate limits of available medical supports	PCS, Psych, SW,
	Lack of MD attention to current problems	Expert consultation	Nurs
	Lack of empathic support from MD		
	MD excessively hopeful or pessimistic		
Existential	Current personal integrity	Attention to reversible factors	MD, Nur, SW, Phys,
	Changes in body image and function	Use of prosthetic, cosmetic, orthotic or functional supports	Psych, Chap, PCS,
	Changes in intellectual function	Cognitive, behavioural and supportive psychotherapies to enhance coping	Physiat, OT, PT, ST,
	Changes in social and professional function		Cosmet
	Changes in attractiveness as a sexual partner		
	Retrospective distress	Cognitive restructuring	SW, Psych, Chap, MD,
	Disappointment	Life-review techniques	Nurs, PCS, MT, RecT
	Remorse		
	Anticipation	Cognitive restructuring and goal reprioritization	Psych, SW, MD, Nur,
	Hopelessness	Identification of short-term achievable goals	Chap, PCS, ClinEth
	Futility	Abandonment of unachievable goals	
	Meaninglessness	Addressing fears associated with death	
	Death concerns		

Anaeth: Anaesthetist; Chap: Chaplain; ClinEth: Clinical ethicist; Cosmet: Cosmetician; MD: Doctor; MT: Music therapist; Nurs: Nurse; OT: Occupational therapist; PCS: Palliative care specialist; Physiat: Physiatrist; Psych: Psychiatrist; PT: Physical therapist; RecT: Recreation therapist; SW: Social worker.

Formulating a care plan

Based on this assessment one can formulate a care plan that addresses all aspects of the care trilogy: patient, family, and caregivers. The formulation can be summarized in a document or report that describes the following:

1. The medical condition of the patient and the goals of care.

2. Description of the involved family and professional carers.

3. Patient issues: physical, psychological, existential, social, communication, understanding.

4. Family issues: physical, psychological, existential, social, communication, understanding.

5. Professional carer issues: staffing, training, resources, resource/need match, emotional coping.

Table 2.1.2 The dimensions of family member distress, management approaches, and potential therapeutic resources

Dimension	Distress	Intervention	Therapist(s)
Patient related	Patient in physical distress.	Treat patient and support family	MD, Nurs, Psych,
	Patient in psychological distress.	Treat patient and support family	Chap, ClinEth
	Patient in existential distress.	Treat patient and support family	
Physical	Illness	Comprehensive therapy	MD, Nur,
	Physical disability	Physiatric review and therapy	
Psychological	Anxiety	Psychotherapy ± pharmacotherapy	MD, Nur, SW,
	Depression	Cognitive or behavioural interventions	Psych, Neur, PCS
	Adjustment difficulties		Chap
	Unresolved previous loss or separation		
	Uncertainty		
Social	Alteration in roles and lifestyles	Acknowledge difficulties	MD, Nur, SW,
	Unsatisfactory communication regarding illness or treatment	Explore specific problems of family and supports. Assess information needs and address them	Psych, PCS
	Lack of comfort and support from family members	Provide sensitive information and express readiness to provide appropriate supports	
	Lack of support and comfort from health-care professionals	Express readiness to deal with whatever difficulties may arise	
	Non-convergent needs among family members	Identify family members in need of psychological or psychiatric support	
	Economic/employment		
Personal resources	Excessive physical demands	Optimize home supports	SW, Nurs, MD
	Excessive complexity of care	Provide effective backup	
	Exhaustion	Consider alternative care arrangements	
		Consider respite care	

Chap: Chaplain; ClinEth: Clinical ethicist; Cosmet: Cosmetician; MD: Doctor; MT: Music therapist; Nurs: Nurse; OT: Occupational therapist; PCS: Palliative care specialist; Physiat: Physiatrist; Psych: Psychiatrist; PT: Physical therapist; RecT: Recreation therapist; SW: Social worker.

6. Coping assessment: patient, family, and professional staff.

7. Contingency planning: anticipated contingencies, planned interventions.

Tables 2.1.1 and 2.1.2 illustrate interdisciplinary care plans to address patient and family needs in each of the dimensions of care.

Implementation of ongoing assessment

Advanced incurable illness leading towards death is characterized by the potential for rapid and dramatic change and the overall tendency for change, increasing dependency, and an increasingly complex confluence of physical, psychological, existential, ethical, and social concerns. Just as care for the palliative care patient is a longitudinal commitment, so is assessment. Consequently, this assessment must be repeated at appropriate intervals which will be determined by the rate of change in the patient's clinical condition or at points of major change in goals, care plan, or the patient's condition.

Family meetings

A common source of distress for patient, family, and professional carers occurs when there is a lack of coordination in the desired goals of patient care. The goals of care are often complex, but can generally be grouped into three broad categories: (1) prolonging survival, (2) optimizing comfort, and (3) optimizing function. The relative priority of these goals provides an essential context for therapeutic decision-making. The prioritization of these goals is a dynamic phenomenon which changes with the evolution of the disease: whereas the optimization of comfort, function, and survival may share equal priority during the phase of ambulatory palliation, the provision of comfort usually assumes overriding priority as death approaches. When patients equally prioritize optimal comfort and function, the therapeutic intent is to achieve an adequate degree of relief without compromising cognitive and physical function. When comfort is the overriding goal of care, the overriding intent is to achieve relief. In the latter circumstance, there is a willingness to continue therapies that may impair function, or even foreshorten life expectancy.

Family meetings, with relevant members of the professional health-care team, provide a useful format for discussing the needs of all parties involved, clarifying care goals, sharing and exploring concerns, and developing a therapeutic plan that adequately addresses those needs (Rabow et al., 2004; Weissman, 2004; Fineberg, 2005; Lautrette et al., 2006). The participants should be determined on an individual case basis. Since the family is an appropriate unit of care, and its members have a right to confidentiality, it may be appropriate, on occasion, to meet without the participation of the patient to address their concerns and needs. Meetings with the participation of all people who are involved can open communication, improve coordination in the formulation of a care plan, and facilitate better personal coping for each of the individuals involved.

Formulation and implementation of a care plan

Coordination of the many participants in this sort of multidisciplinary care requires an identified leader for each case. This role is usually filled by either a physician or nurse, and the specific person may change in the course of an illness as the predominant care needs change. For example, with the progression of a cancer from a diagnostic stage to a palliative stage, the responsibility may shift sequentially from a surgeon, to a medical oncologist, and finally, to a palliative care nurse. The coordinator, or case manager, is responsible for monitoring the degree to which care needs are being met, and for facilitating change when necessary. Similarly the well-being and function of the health-care professionals must be monitored, ensuring the availability of appropriate manpower and expertise to effectively manage the prevailing problems. For security and safety in the event of a clinical crisis, it is essential that the patient and family have access to a contact person with 24-hour availability. This model represents a family-centred, multidisciplinary, collaborative approach between physicians, nurses, social workers, other therapists, and community supports.

Conclusion

An understanding of the nature of suffering and of the factors that contribute to it are essential to the task of palliative medicine. Suffering is a complex human experience which requires evaluation in order to construct an effective therapeutic response that is appropriate to presenting problems. An effective approach incorporates careful case assessment, identification of care needs, formulation of a multidisciplinary therapeutic intervention to address those needs, and the provision of ongoing monitoring with readiness to re-evaluate the care plan as problems arise or needs change.

References

Adams, E., Boulton, M., and Watson, E. (2009). The information needs of partners and family members of cancer patients: a systematic literature review. *Patient Education and Counseling*, 77, 179–186.

Angell, M. (1982). The quality of mercy. *The New England Journal of Medicine*, 306, 98–99.

Annunziata, M.A., Muzzatti, B., Bidoli, E., and Veronesi, A. (2012). Emotional distress and needs in Italian cancer patients: prevalence and associations with socio-demographic and clinical factors. *Tumori*, 98, 119–125.

Aoun, S., McConigley, R., Abernethy, A., and Currow, D.C. (2010). Caregivers of people with neurodegenerative diseases: profile and unmet needs from a population-based survey in South Australia. *Journal of Palliative Medicine*, 13, 653–661.

Ben Natan, M., Garfinkel, D., and Shachar, I. (2010). End-of-life needs as perceived by terminally ill older adult patients, family and staff. *European Journal of Oncology Nursing*, 14, 299–303.

Bloche, M.G. (2005). Managing conflict at the end of life. *The New England Journal of Medicine*, 352, 2371–2373.

Brennan, F. (2007). Palliative care as an international human right. *Journal of Pain and Symptom Management*, 33, 494–499.

Cassell, E.J. (1982). The nature of suffering and the goals of medicine. *The New England Journal of Medicine*, 306, 639–645.

Cassell, E.J. (1991). Recognizing suffering. *Hastings Center Report*, 21, 24–31.

Cherny, N.I., Coyle, N., and Foley, K.M. (1994b). The treatment of suffering when patients request elective death. *Journal of Palliative Care*, 10, 71–79.

Dumont, S., Turgeon, J., Allard, P., Gagnon, P., Charbonneau, C., and Vezina, L. (2006). Caring for a loved one with advanced cancer: determinants of psychological distress in family caregivers. *Journal of Palliative Medicine*, 9, 912–921.

Ewing, G. and Grande, G. (2013). Development of a Carer Support Needs Assessment Tool (CSNAT) for end-of-life care practice at home: a qualitative study. *Palliative Medicine*, 27(3), 244–256.

Fridriksdottir, N., Sigurdardottir, V., and Gunnarsdottir, S. (2006). Important needs of families in acute and palliative care settings assessed with the family inventory of needs. *Palliat Med*, 20, 425–432.

Funk, L., Stajduhar, K., Toye, C., Aoun, S., Grande, G., and Todd, C. (2010). Part 2: home-based family caregiving at the end of life: a comprehensive review of published qualitative research (1998–2008). *Palliative Medicine*, 24, 594–607.

Garland, S.N., Carlson, L.E., Cook, S., Lansdell, L., and Speca, M. (2007). A non-randomized comparison of mindfulness-based stress reduction and healing arts programs for facilitating post-traumatic growth and spirituality in cancer outpatients. *Supportive Care in Cancer*, 15, 949–961.

Gaudio, F.D., Zaider, T.I., Brier, M., and Kissane, D. (2012). Challenges in providing family-centered support to families in palliative care. *Palliative Medicine*, 26(8), 1025–1033.

Given, B.A., Given, C.W., and Kozachik, S. (2001). Family support in advanced cancer. *CA: A Cancer Journal for Clinicians*, 51, 213–231.

Gomes, B., Calazani, N., Curiale, V., McCrone, P., and Higginson, I. J. (2013). Effectiveness and cost-effectiveness of home palliative care services for adults with advanced illness and their caregivers. *Cochrane Database Syst Rev*, 6, CD007760.

Goy, E.R., Carter, J.H., and Ganzini, L. (2008). Needs and experiences of caregivers for family members dying with Parkinson disease. *J Palliat Care*, 24, 69–75.

Grov, E.K., Dahl, A.A., Moum, T., and Fossa, S.D. (2005). Anxiety, depression, and quality of life in caregivers of patients with cancer in late palliative phase. *Annals of Oncology*.

Grunfeld, E., Zitzelsberger, L., Coristine, M., Whelan, T.J., Aspelund, F., and Evans, W.K. (2004b). Job stress and job satisfaction of cancer care workers. *Psychooncology*.

Hanratty, B., Holland, P., Jacoby, A., and Whitehead, M. (2007). Financial stress and strain associated with terminal cancer a review of the evidence. *Palliative Medicine*, 21, 595–607.

Hefferon, K., Grealy, M., and Mutrie, N. (2009). Post-traumatic growth and life threatening physical illness: a systematic review of the qualitative literature. *British Journal of Health Psychology*, 14, 343–378.

Janssen, D.J., Spruit, M.A., Wouters, E.F., and Schols, J.M. (2008a). Daily symptom burden in end-stage chronic organ failure: a systematic review. *Palliative Medicine*, 22, 938–948.

Kadan-Lottick, N.S., Vanderwerker, L.C., Block, S.D., Zhang, B., and Prigerson, H.G. (2005). Psychiatric disorders and mental health service use in patients with advanced cancer: a report from the coping with cancer study. *Cancer*, 104, 2872–2881.

King, D.A. and Quill, T. (2006). Working with families in palliative care: one size does not fit all. *Journal of Palliative Medicine*, 9, 704–715.

Kirkova, J., Walsh, D., Rybicki, L., Davis, M.P., Aktas, A., Tao, J., and Homsi, J. (2010b). Symptom severity and distress in advanced cancer. *Palliative Medicine*, 24, 330–339.

Kissane, D.W., Clarke, D.M., and Street, A.F. (2001). Demoralization syndrome—a relevant psychiatric diagnosis for palliative care. *Journal of Palliative Care*, 17, 12–21.

Kramer, B., Kavanaugh, M., Trentham-Dietz, A., Walsh, M., and Yonke, R.J. (2010). Predictors of family conflict at the end of life: the experience of spouses and adult children of persons with lung cancer. *Gerontologist*, 50, 215–225.

Krikorian, A., Limonero, J.T., and Corey, M.T. (2013). Suffering assessment: a review of available instruments for use in palliative care. *Journal of Palliative Medicine*, 16, 130–142.

Krikorian, A., Limonero, J.T. and Mate, J. (2011). Suffering and distress at the end-of-life. *Psychooncology*.

Lautrette, A., Ciroldi, M., Ksibi, H., and Azoulay, E. (2006). End-of-life family conferences: rooted in the evidence. *Critical Care Medicine*, 34, S364–S372.

Mystakidou, K., Tsilika, E., Parpa, E., Katsouda, E., Galanos, A., and Vlahos, L. (2006). Psychological distress of patients with advanced cancer: influence and contribution of pain severity and pain interference. *Cancer Nursing*, 29, 400–405.

Pearce, M.J., Coan, A.D., Herndon, J.E., 2nd, Koenig, H.G., and Abernethy, A.P. 2011. Unmet spiritual care needs impact emotional and spiritual well-being in advanced cancer patients. *Support Care Cancer*.

Sharpe, L., Butow, P., Smith, C., Mcconnell, D., and Clarke, S. (2005). The relationship between available support, unmet needs and caregiver burden in patients with advanced cancer and their carers. *Psycho-Oncology*, 14, 102–114.

Shim, E.J., Lee, K.S., and Park, J.H. (2010). Comprehensive needs assessment tool in cancer (CNAT): the development and validation. *Supportive Care in Cancer*, 19, 1957–1968.

Simon, J.L. (2008). Anticipatory grief: recognition and coping. *Journal of Palliative Medicine*, 11, 1280–1281.

Stajduhar, K., Funk, L., Toye, C., Grande, G., Aoun, S., and Todd, C. (2010). Part 1: home-based family caregiving at the end of life: a comprehensive review of published quantitative research (1998–2008). *Palliative Medicine*, 24, 573–593.

Stajduhar, K.I., Funk, L., Cohen, S.R., *et al.* (2011). Bereaved family members' assessments of the quality of end-of-life care: what is important? *Journal of Palliative Care*, 27, 261–269.

Strong, V., Waters, R., and Hibberd, C. (2007). Emotional distress in cancer patients: the Edinburgh Cancer Centre symptom study. *British Journal of Cancer*, 96, 868–874.

Teunissen, S.C., Wesker, W., Kruitwagen, C., De Haes, H.C., Voest, E.E., and De Graeff, A. (2007). Symptom prevalence in patients with incurable cancer: a systematic review. *Journal of Pain and Symptom Management*, 34, 94–104.

The epidemiology of death and symptoms: planning for population-based palliative care

Megan B. Sands, Dianne L. O'Connell, Michael Piza, and Jane M. Ingham

Introduction to the epidemiology of death and symptoms

The epidemiology of the end-of-life experience

Epidemiology is defined as 'the study of the distribution and determinants of disease frequency' (Hennekins et al., 1987). Epidemiology is central to the development of strategies for the prevention and management of disease in populations and for the planning of health services. Epidemiological data can also provide information about the nature of the progression of specific diseases and treatment outcomes. For palliative care, epidemiology can provide important information about disease and symptom occurrence as well as health-care needs. In this chapter, we take a broad view of the epidemiology of 'disease' towards the end of life and discuss epidemiology as it relates to the 'human experience' with an emphasis on disease, symptoms, psychosocial experiences, and access to health services. Areas where information about a population is available and where it is needed, but lacking, are highlighted. Examples of the way in which epidemiological data have informed planning, policy, or patient care are highlighted throughout this chapter. Epidemiological studies on populations at the end of life are relatively few. Where data from large or whole population studies are unavailable, smaller studies such as those derived from service-based data, have been used to illustrate aspects of the human experience towards the end of life. The attainment of high-quality population-based data is essential to understanding the needs that inform service development and provision of care across settings.

Important definitions

The population base for palliative care

The World Health Organization (WHO) has defined palliative care. A definition of the palliative care population is important as it helps to articulate what palliative care is, who needs it, who should provide it (Rosenwax et al., 2006), and how well it is provided across health systems. A definition of the palliative care population is therefore a vital part of planning for palliative care service delivery. Notwithstanding this, defining the 'palliative care population' has been problematic. To date, among the approaches to defining the population have been the use of specific conditions, patient needs, and all deaths (Rosenwax et al., 2006). Definitions of the palliative care population may vary but it is essential to identifying who would benefit from palliative care and therefore remains a core challenge. The focus of research in this area has more recently centred on identifying markers of 'palliative care needs' as a basis for defining 'the palliative care population' (Boyd and Murray, 2010; Waller et al., 2010). Defining appropriate quality indicators is another important area of research. The type of diseases encountered as well as the socio-economic, cultural, home, and natural environments that patients inhabit are all important variables that influence the spectrum of a population's palliative care needs.

Incidence and prevalence

Incidence and prevalence are two important epidemiological measures. 'Incidence quantifies the number of new events or cases of disease that develop in a population of individuals at risk during a specified time interval' (Hennekins et al., 1987) and can be summarized as:

$$\frac{\text{Number of new cases}}{\text{Total population at risk}}$$

'Prevalence quantifies the proportion of individuals in a population who have the disease at a specific instant and provides an estimate of the probability (risk) that an individual will be ill at a point in time' (Hennekins et al., 1987) and can be summarized as:

$$\frac{\text{Number of cases}}{\text{Total population at a given point in time}}$$

Epidemiology of death worldwide

Limitations of mortality statistics

Mortality statistics provide information on death rates and causes of death in populations and therefore provide important epidemiological data for palliative care. In reviewing mortality data, it is important to have an understanding of the limitations of data which are derived from diverse sources, each with its own limitations. The Global Burden of Disease (GBD) study, which was initiated in 1993 to provide comprehensive mortality and morbidity data, has been a collaboration involving the WHO, the World Bank, and other organizations. This study is ongoing, and since its first publication in 1994 the GBD data has been updated (Lozano et al., 2012; Murray, 2012; WHO, 2013a). Estimates of mortality relating to deaths in 2011 were published in 2013 and were largely obtained using the same methods as those used to produce previously published mortality estimates but were derived from more recent information from vital registration data (WHO, 2013b) (see Box 2.2.1).

Mortality estimates from the GBD are obtained from four general sources (Lopez et al., 2006):

1. Death registration systems: these provide information, not always complete, on the causes of death for most high-income countries as well as many countries in Eastern Europe, Central Asia, Latin America, and the Caribbean (Maudsley et al., 1996).

2. Sample death registration systems: these register a sample of the population and establish death rates within the sample population which are then extrapolated to estimate data about the broader population. They are used to estimate mortality data in areas where deaths are not registered for a large proportion of the population, and are frequently necessary, for example, to estimate deaths in rural areas. Sample death registration systems contribute particularly to statistics regarding deaths in China and India, which together have more than one-third of the world's population (WHO, 2013a).

3. Epidemiological assessments: these provide estimates of deaths for major diseases, such as cancer, HIV/AIDS, malaria, and tuberculosis, for countries in the regions most affected by these conditions. Epidemiological assessments deduce case fatality rates (i.e. people who have a specified disease and who die as a result of that disease within a given period of time) from surveys on the incidence or prevalence of a specific disease over a specific period of time combined with knowledge of the usual mortality for that condition.

4. Cause of death models: these are used to estimate deaths according to broad cause groups in regions (including most of sub-Saharan Africa) with non-existent or incomplete mortality data.

Only a third of the world's population resides in regions where complete civil registration systems exist that provide adequate, cause-specific mortality data. In most of Africa, South East Asia, the Middle East, and parts of the Pacific, where over one-quarter of the world's population resides, there has until recently been little or no mortality monitoring (Rao et al., 2005; Lopez, 2006). Notable increases in the collection of data have been reported in Thailand and South Africa in publications from the WHO (2011).

It can be seen therefore, that reporting errors and inaccuracies relating to cause of death are a worldwide problem. Even in countries where deaths are reported with reasonable consistency, significant proportions of reports of death contain reporting errors (Maudsley et al., 1996; Rao et al., 2005; Mathers et al., 2006a). There are many reasons why death data may be unrepresentative. For example, in an effort to reduce complexity, mortality data are usually reported by single cause of death despite the fact that several co-morbidities and health risks may significantly contribute to death. This may introduce biases. These include, but are not limited to, economic constraints on various capacities for data collection and reporting, as well as political and other factors; these factors must be considered when assessing the limitations of global health data (Murray et al., 2004; Lopez et al., 2006; Mathers et al., 2006b; Wang et al. 2012).

Coding and reporting systems also influence the data available but increased adoption of standardized reporting systems such as the International Classification of Diseases (ICD; WHO a), by the majority of countries (from four countries in 1994 to more than one hundred in 2014) has resulted in improvements in 'real-time' availability of data relating to cause of death (WHO, b). Cumulative developments in information systems have potential for fostering further improvements in the comprehensiveness and accuracy of mortality statistics. Despite this, significant reporting delays exist in many regions in cause of death, location of death, and co-morbidities. The absence of these can impact on the service planning that is critical for optimizing the delivery of population-based care at the end of life (Wang et al., 2012).

Life expectancy

Life expectancies vary greatly worldwide (see Fig. 2.2.1) (Institut national d'études démographiques (INED), 2012). These variations are associated with demographic characteristics such as occupational, political, cultural, and lifestyle risks as well as ethnicity, gender, and genetics (Commission on Social Determinants of Health, 2008; WHO, 2009, Institute for Health Metrics and Evaluation, 2010; Lim et al., 2013). Populations from low-income countries have not experienced the increase in life expectancy observed in the rest of the world, and communicable diseases and conditions of the newborn continue to be a significant cause of death. For several countries of sub-Saharan Africa,

---

Box 2.2.1 Resource list

◆ Global burden of disease interactive cause and risk heat map <https://www.healthdata.org/data-visualization/gbd-heatmap>

◆ Data visualizations: <https://www.healthdata.org/results/data-visualizations>

◆ Estimates and analysis of mortality and burden of disease: WHO Global Health Observatory <http://www.who.int/gho/mortality_burden_disease/en/index.html>

◆ The ten leading causes of death by income group (2011): <http://www.who.int/mediacentre/factsheets/fs310/en/index1.html>

◆ Adult mortality rate, 1990–2011: <http://www.who.int/gho/mortality_burden_disease/mortality_adult/situation_trends/en/index.html>

◆ First ever global atlas identifies unmet need for palliative care: <http://www.thewpca.org/resources/global-atlas-of-palliative-care/>

◆ Gapminder, interactive visualizations of health and wealth of nations at www.gapminder.org <http://www.bit.ly/1c4x55x>

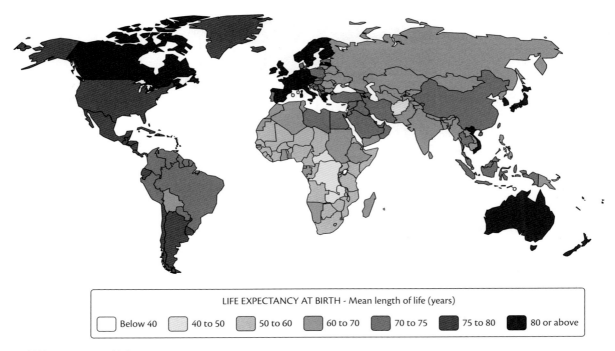

Fig. 2.2.1 World life expectancy at birth, 2013.
Reproduced from French National Institute for Demographic Studies (INED), *Interactive maps of the world population*, Copyright © 2014, with the permission of the French National Institute for Demographic Studies (INED), available at from http://www.ined.fr/en/everything_about_population/interactive_maps/

life expectancy in the 1990s had declined to 40 years or below (WHO, 2006). There have been some areas of notable improvement since that time; however, data demonstrate that countries in some regions have life expectancies less than or close to 50 years (INED, 2012).

Globally, life expectancy for 2012 has been estimated as 66 years for men and 71 years for women. In more developed regions the life expectancy at birth for both sexes is currently estimated to be 76.9 years and, in the least developed regions, 58.4 years (United Nations, 2013).

In addition to life expectancy, it is important to consider infant mortality. Within countries and across regions of the world, infant mortality varies. Across the world, the infant mortality rate has been projected to be 41.5 deaths per 1000 live births (INED, 2012). Two types of figures are reported for this very young age group—infant mortality per 1000 live births and infant deaths under the age of 1 year—and great variability exists for both. Afghanistan has, for example, had a very high infant mortality with projections of 123 deaths per 1000 live births in 2013 whereas projections for Iceland for the same year were for two deaths per 1000 live births (INED, 2012). In the contemporary era many countries have seen a decrease in child mortality. Others have been slower to achieve a decrease (Gapminder, 2010; INED, 2012).

Leading causes of death

In 2011, there were approximately 54.5 million deaths estimated throughout the world (WHO, 2013b). Fig. 2.2.2 presents the ten leading causes of death worldwide for 2011 (WHO, 2013c). As reports reflect individual cancers the general diagnosis of 'cancer' itself does not rank among the leading ten causes although lung cancers rank 6th with 1.5 million deaths (WHO, 2013d). The

leading reported causes of death vary among regions at different levels of economic development and illustrate some of the health disparities associated with economic issues. The World Bank now classifies countries into four income groups: low, lower-middle, upper-middle, and high. The most recent data on causes of death by income categories are for 2011 (see Box 2.2.1). Globally, adult mortality rate declined from 204 per 1000 population in 1990 to 160 per 1000 population in 2011 (WHO, 2013a).

Disparities in causes of death between countries reflect divergent levels of economic development. More specifically, communicable diseases and conditions of the newborn are the predominant causes of death in low-income countries. These causes of death also vary between demographic groups within countries defined, for example, by socioeconomic status, gender, age, and ethnicity. The disparity in global mortality is greatest for low-income countries which constitute 11.4% of the world's population but account for 16.3% of the world's deaths (WHO, 2008).

Another example of where differences in health status, life expectancy, and causes of death exist is between ethnic groups within some high-income countries in which some indigenous populations have comparatively higher rates of death and morbidity from diseases including cancer, respiratory disease, stroke, injury, and diabetes when compared to the non-indigenous population of the same country (see Box 2.2.1) (Stevenson et al., 1998; Horton, 2006; Australian Bureau of Statistics, 2011a, 2011b; WHO, 2011).

Differences in the ranking of causes of death between time periods have been demonstrated, most notably by the data presented in the GBD study which presented comparative data from 1990 and 2010. For instance, while many communicable diseases have decreased in frequency, death from HIV/AIDS has moved from

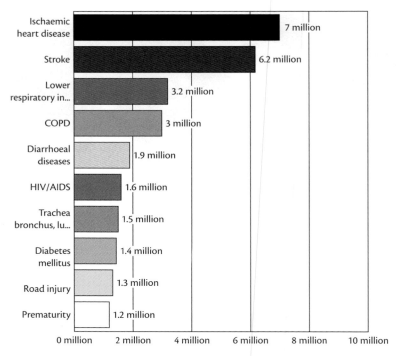

Fig. 2.2.2 Leading causes of death in the world in 2011.
Reproduced with permission from World Health Organization, *The Top 10 Causes of Death, Fact Sheet Number 310,* Copyright © World Health Organization 2013, available from http://www. who.int/mediacentre/factsheets/fs310/en/index.html.

33rd ranking to 6th, and road injury and self-harm have remained significant causes of death at 8th and 13th rank in 2010 (cf. 10th and 14th rank in 1990). Over those two decades, lung cancer has increased in frequency changing from 8th rank to 5th and diabetes has changed from 15th rank to 9th (Institute for Health Metrics and Evaluation, n.d.). WHO estimates comparing cause of death between the years 2000 and 2011 are available online (WHO, 2013d).

Projections for the future: leading causes of death

Mortality projections can assist in the planning of services that will be required to meet the needs of populations in the future and provide insight into requirements for the spectrum of knowledge and skills needed by palliative care clinicians (K. Strong et al., 2008).

Recently updated projections of mortality and cause of death have been released by the WHO and are summarized in Table 2.2.1. The death rates from various causes were estimated using data from 2011 (WHO, 2013d). An in-depth discussion of age-standardized mortality projections of cause of deaths for 2030 using 2002 data has been published by Mathers and colleagues. Among other estimates, they present data demonstrating expected increases by 2030 in deaths from HIV/AIDS, lung cancer, diabetes, chronic respiratory diseases, road traffic accidents, violence, and war (Mathers et al., 2006a). These 2002 projections for 2030 provide three kinds of estimates: baseline, pessimistic, and optimistic (Mathers et al., 2006a). Under the optimistic scenario, 64.9 million deaths worldwide were projected and under the pessimistic scenario 80.7 million. With respect to HIV/AIDS, a baseline projection estimates

deaths from this cause will increase from 2.8 million in 2002 to 6.5 million in 2030. Deaths from other infective conditions or perinatal conditions are projected to fall. Over the same time period baseline projections of deaths from cancer suggest an increase from 7.1 million to 11.5 million, and cardiovascular deaths from 16.7 to 23.3 million. Combined deaths from cancer and chronic non-infective and non-cancer illnesses are expected to account for 70% of deaths in 2030. The third major mortality grouping is related to deaths from injury and accidents and notable in this group was a 40% expected increase predominantly accounted for by road traffic accidents which were projected to increase from 1.2 in 2002 to 2.1 million in 2030 (Mathers et al., 2006a).

Projections are developed to reflect various contributing factors including the success of preventive action. Projections may vary if behaviours related to disease incidence or disease related-mortality change. Examples of important factors that may impact projections include tobacco use, the incidence of obesity, the incidence of infective causes of death, and whether prevention efforts have a greater or lesser impact than expected (Olshansky et al., 2005; Strong et al., 2008; Wang et al., 2012; WHO, 2012). For example, deaths attributed to tobacco use are estimated to be likely to account for 8 million deaths worldwide annually (WHO, 2013f); if preventive efforts are less or more successful than predicted, the death rates for tobacco-related diseases will change. Given the uncertainties that exist concerning influential variables including economic, environmental, social and, technological factors variations can be expected between actual and projected mortality (Mathers et al., 2006). Deviations from the projected mortality will affect palliative care services planning.

Table 2.2.1 Projected leading causes of death in 2030 (based on 2011 data)

Low-income countries			Lower-middle-income countries			Upper-middle-income countries			High-income countries		
Cause	Deaths (000s)	%	Cause	Deaths (000s)	%	Cause	Deaths (000s)	%	Cause	Deaths (000s)	%
Stroke	905	8.9	Ischaemic heart disease	3544	13.4	Stroke	3701	16.8	Ischaemic heart disease	1393	12.1
Lower respiratory infections	810	7.9	Stroke	3105	11.8	Ischaemic heart disease	3528	16.0	Stroke	867	7.6
Ischaemic heart disease	780	7.6	Chronic obstructive pulmonary disease	2213	8.4	Chronic obstructive pulmonary disease	1573	7.1	Alzheimer's disease and other dementias	728	6.4
HIV/AIDS	650	6.4	Lower respiratory infections	1509	5.7	Trachea, bronchus, lung cancers	1268	5.8	Trachea, bronchus, lung cancers	627	5.5
Diarrhoeal diseases	422	4.1	Diarrhoeal diseases	1064	4.0	Diabetes mellitus	782	3.6	Lower respiratory infections	525	4.6
Road injury	421	4.1	Diabetes mellitus	971	3.7	Liver cancer	717	3.3	Chronic obstructive pulmonary disease	446	3.9
Diabetes mellitus	369	3.6	Road injury	940	3.6	Stomach cancer	712	3.2	Colon and rectum cancers	403	3.5
Chronic obstructive pulmonary disease	336	3.3	HIV/AIDS	629	2.4	Lower respiratory infections	692	3.1	Diabetes mellitus	342	3.0
Preterm birth complications	327	3.2	Cirrhosis of the liver	557	2.1	Hypertensive heart disease	547	2.5	Hypertensive heart disease	252	2.2
Malaria	247	2.4	Falls	517	2.0	HIV/AIDS	463	2.1	Kidney diseases	249	2.2

Place of care: where are palliative care services and support needed and where do we die?

One aim of health-care service providers is to offer care, where possible, in a location that matches the patient's preference. Data reporting concordance between preferred place of death and actual place of death has been much less common than data that simply reports place of death (Pritchard et al., 1998; Gomes et al., 2012a).

Data reporting 'place of death' are for the most part collected only in high-income nations. In general, it is clear that for many individuals in low-income countries hospital care is not available, which would suggest that the vast majority of people in these regions die outside the hospital setting (English et al., 2006). The opposite is true in many high-income countries where death in hospital is common. The available data suggest that more than 50% of deaths in England, the United States, Germany, Switzerland, and France take place in the hospital (Gomes, 2013). Significant variations in place of death nonetheless exist among high-income countries, with lower rates of hospital death reported in the Netherlands (35%), Ireland (30%), and Italy (35%) (Klinkenberg et al., 2005; Beccaro et al., 2007).

Some studies have provided projections of where people in high-income populations are likely to die in the future, and suggest that the rate of death at home will decline over time (Gomes et al., 2008). Despite this, other data indicate that this trend may not necessarily continue and reports from several countries suggest there will be an increase in the proportion of patients who die at home, at least with respect to cancer deaths in populations which are served by specialist palliative care (Gomes et al., 2012a).

When asked about preferred place of death, the overwhelming majority of well people indicate a preference for care at home up until, and including, the time of death (Foreman et al., 2006; Beccaro et al., 2007; Gomes et al., 2012b; Gomes, 2013). This contrasts with actual place of death for the majority (McNamara et al., 2007; Gomes et al., 2012a; Gomes, 2013). The reasons for this disparity have been investigated, revealing that many factors, including access to care, influence this observation. For example, where inpatient beds are available, more inpatient care occurs (Pritchard et al., 1998; Higginson and Costantini, 2008). Recent research that has focused on 'preferred place of care' rather than only on 'place of death' takes into account the observation that the preferences of ill patients may change along the illness trajectory, and may be different to the preferences elicited from well people with or without life-threatening illness (Storey et al., 2003; Munday et al., 2007; Agar et al., 2008; Gomes et al., 2008; Gomes, 2013). These types of data illustrate some of the subtle, less acknowledged, reasons behind patients' changes in their preferred 'place of care' (see Fig. 2.2.3). When collected longitudinally, rather than at a single point in time, data that compares actual place of care to preferred place can also help to inform planning and support flexibility in service provision up until and including the time of death (Agar et al., 2008). Further research is required to explore factors associated with the disparities between desired place of death and actual place of death that have been identified (Gomes, 2013).

The availability of, and access to, palliative care expertise

Epidemiological data related to the provision of palliative care are important for understanding whether there is population-wide access to appropriate care. It also helps to identify populations in need of palliative care and, in relation to care towards the end of life, whether care is available in the patient's preferred place of care. These types of data allow for designing and refining models of palliative care delivery that aim to provide appropriate care and, where possible to provide it in patients' locations of choice. The WHO has endorsed palliative care as an essential component of health care (see Box 2.2.1) (WHO, 2014). To achieve this, it is vital that generalist and most specialist health practitioners have fundamental competencies in symptom management towards the end of life (Dudgeon et al., 2008; Shipman et al., 2008). It is generally accepted that there is also a need for patients to have access to specialist palliative care services when needed (Field and Cassel, 1997; National Institute for Clinical Excellence, 2004; WHO, 2007; Martin-Moreno et al., 2008; Temel et al., 2010; National Gold Standards Framework Centre, 2012).

It is evident that specialist palliative care services are becoming available for cancer and non-cancer diagnoses in most high-income countries through mainstream health services in community, inpatient, and acute hospital settings but availability is much more limited in middle-income and low-income countries (Fig. 2.2.4) (Morris, 2011). In high-income countries, many tertiary-referral centres accommodate integrated consultative, specialist palliative care services within acute and subacute settings (Glare et al., 2003; Mercadante et al., 2008). Studies have highlighted that palliative care specialist services in most middle-income countries are available but only for some of the patients in need, and are frequently unavailable for the poor and those living in rural and remote regions (Morris, 2011). Specifically, in low-income countries, the majority of those dying do not have any access to specialist services and those services that do exist reach only a very small proportion of the people in need (Kikule, 2003; Morris, 2011). The majority of dying people in these areas are cared for at home and in communities by family and/or neighbours. Regarding needs in these countries, one cross-sectional study identified three main areas of palliative care need in low-income areas —symptom management, counselling, and financial assistance (Kikule, 2003).

Despite the availability of services, for a significant proportion of patients with far advanced disease, even in high-income countries there are limits on access to symptom management and end-of-life care (Higginson, 1997; Pritchard et al., 1998; Rosenwax et al., 2006; Beccaro et al., 2007; Goldsmith et al., 2008). As an example of the impact of epidemiological data supporting this claim, a West Australian study showed that patients dying from illnesses other than cancer are less likely (8%) than those with cancer (68%) to receive specialist palliative care (Rosenwax et al., 2006). Studies elsewhere have raised similar access issues when considering palliative care (Solano et al., 2006; Murray et al., 2008).

Examples of the wealth of information that can be provided by generating epidemiological reports from carefully collected clinical data are reports such as those from Seow et al. (2012) and Laugsand et al. (2011) that describe components of multidisciplinary service provision, symptom management, prognosis, diagnoses, and co-morbidity. While not necessarily generalizable to other regions, these data provide information that could be highly useful in planning and tailoring regional services for the areas in which data was collected. Of note is that local needs assessments, using defined criteria, such as performance status, symptom prevalence, and prognosis, may also allow further comparison and

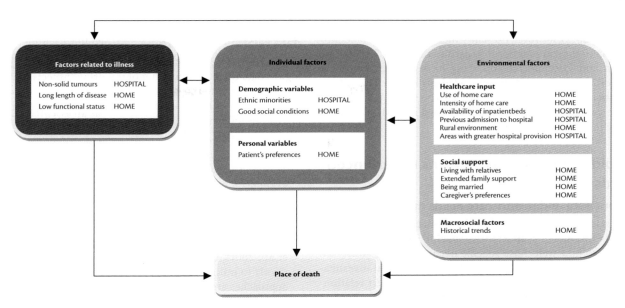

Fig. 2.2.3 Factors influencing place of death.

Reprinted from *The European Journal of Cancer*, Volume 44, Issue 10, Higginson, I.J. and Costantini, M., Dying with cancer, living well with advanced cancer, pp.1414–24, Copyright © 2008, with permission from Elsevier, http://www.sciencedirect.com/science/journal/09598049.

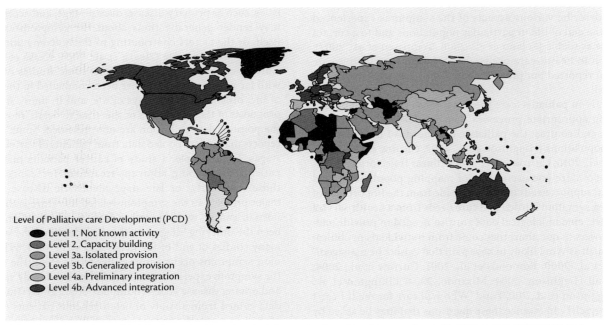

The boundaries and names shown and the designations used on this map do not imply the expression of any opinion whatsoever on the part of the WPCA concerning the legal status of any country, territory, city or areas of its authorities, or concerning the delimitation of its frontiers or boundaries. Dotted lines on maps represent approximate border lines for which there may not yet be full agreement.

Fig. 2.2.4 Palliative care development all levels.

Reproduced from Lynch, T. et al., *Mapping levels of palliative care development: a global update 2011*, Worldwide Palliative Care Alliance, Copyright © 2011, with permission from the Worldwide Palliative Care Alliance.

benchmarking in relation to palliative care access—an approach such as that recommended by Kaasa and colleagues and others (Kaasa et al., 2008; Boyd and Murray, 2010; Currow et al., 2012).

Studies such as those just mentioned can assist identifying the extent to which people and populations with palliative care needs are accessing services. Methodical enquiry into this matter is important especially where disparities exist and/or access is not clearly defined as needs based. An emphasis on needs-based care, rather than on diagnosis- or prognosis-based provision of care, has been advocated by many (Davies and Higginson, 2004;

Rosenwax et al., 2006; Young et al., 2008; Boyd and Murray, 2010; Waller et al., 2012); however, presently there are limited epidemiological data to inform practice in regard to this area. The routine collection and systematized reporting of data relating to care needs is crucial to this and the review, identification, and refinement of tools to help in identifying those who would benefit from palliative care will assist this process (Boyd and Murray, 2010; Waller et al., 2010; Weissman et al., 2011).

The epidemiology of symptoms experienced towards the end of life

Symptom data and health-care needs in palliative care

In the previous section, access to health services in relation to care needs was discussed. Importantly, specific research questions in relation to how well those specific needs are being addressed within populations generally warrant epidemiological investigation. Health-care needs at the end of life have a direct relationship with symptoms experienced during that time; in the context of palliative care (Franks et al., 2000; Mirando, 2004; Higginson et al., 2007), and in relation to many specific diseases at the end of life (Edmonds et al., 2001; Elkington et al., 2005), symptom management is also generally acknowledged as an important need, among many palliative care needs. Some data which quantify and describe various aspects of the symptoms experienced towards the end of life in particular populations and to a certain extent are available (Solano et al., 2006; Teunissen et al., 2007). In relation to health-care needs, data relevant to palliative care have been reported but prevalence has not necessarily been well quantified.

Currently in palliative care there is a focus on developing and describing appropriate processes that can be used to identify, compare, and contrast the palliative care needs of different people and populations (Higginson et al., 2007; Currow et al., 2008a; Waller et al., 2010; Currow et al., 2012). Illness trajectories, as discussed below, are one useful way of mapping population-based functional support needs over time. Aside from the importance of addressing symptom burden and care needs from a health-service perspective, epidemiological data are also needed to provide adequate answers to questions that come from individuals in clinical settings such as 'Am I likely to have pain that cannot be managed?' (Franks et al., 2000; Edmonds et al., 2001; Currow et al., 2004; Davies and Higginson, 2004; Mirando, 2004; Elkington et al., 2005; Higginson et al., 2007) and 'Who will care for me if I can't care for myself?'. In essence these questions that may be asked by patients and carers are the corollary of questions asked by palliative care providers, that is, 'What needs are best met by specialist palliative care providers?' and 'How can we ensure that people who may not require specialist palliative care have their needs at the end of life met?'

With respect to symptom management, biomedical ethics and contemporary liberal philosophy suggest that there is not only justification for symptom management at the end of life, but an ethical (Sen, 1993; Freeman, 2007) and legal (Brennan, 2007) imperative for it. Within health services and/or specific populations, it's important to develop benchmarks to assess outcomes and quality of care and to carefully describe study populations so as to facilitate comparisons across settings.

Methodological issues and limitations of data relating to symptoms

When reviewing and interpreting symptom-related epidemiological data there are a number of important aspects that must be considered. A summary of the key points to take into consideration in the interpretation of data reporting the epidemiology of symptoms follows:

1. *It is crucial to consider symptom-related epidemiological data in the context of the availability of effective symptom management.* This is especially important for patients and caregivers. For example, a prevalence estimate of 70% for severe pain can be alarming for patients and caregivers unless placed in context. While this figure may reflect the true point prevalence it does not convey the important information that the overwhelming majority of pain can be appropriately treated (Meuser et al., 2001), or that for the 10–15% of patients who respond poorly to initial pain management, standard multidisciplinary approaches are available to improve the refractory pain, suffering, and symptom burden (Hanks et al., 1992).

2. *Defining the population from which data are obtained is extremely important.* Care must be exercised when interpreting findings and, for the most part, extrapolation beyond the source population is best avoided. Heterogeneity in patient characteristics, such as primary disease, disease stage, and access to care, may render generalizations about the symptom-experience itself, or the factors contributing to the outcome under investigation, inappropriate (Hearn et al., 2003; Kaasa et al., 2006; Currow et al., 2008b). For example, some studies of patients with far-advanced disease have been conducted in the last year of life, others in the last days of life, and in many studies the prognosis of the population or the 'time to death' in relation to the point of data collection are not presented. Some symptom reports may reflect pooled data from patients at various disease stages. For example, a study of cancer patients may include patients undergoing adjuvant treatment for cancer, and/or those with early- or late-stage metastatic disease. Another major problem in the symptom-related literature is that a diagnosis of 'cancer' without further detail (e.g. lung, colon, etc.) has been the unifying 'diagnosis' that has identified the subjects in many studies of end-of-life needs and symptoms. While common symptoms occur across different diseases, the nature of the symptom experience and health-care needs may vary across and among disease states (Edmonds et al., 2001). Interpreting data gained from a study of heterogeneous patients even with respect to a specific primary malignancy (e.g. 'breast cancer') can present significant problems (Greenwald et al., 1987; Kaasa et al., 2006).

3. *The patient experience is personal and subjective*—attempts to characterize it may require a diverse spectrum of research methods and when a type of method is selected, it should be standardized and consistent to allow comparison with other studies using the same or similar methodology; this has not always been the case (Payne et al., 2008). With respect to symptom occurrence studies, for instance, although for each symptom a number of studies may be identified, heterogeneous target populations and/or poorly described characteristics of the populations, can mean that it is very difficult to compare

studies or to pool data in meta-analyses (van den Beuken-van Everdingen et al., 2007).

4. *The accuracy of data is dependent on the accuracy of information communicated between subject and researcher.* For example, the accuracy of the medical record as a source of data and the use of proxy symptom ratings will affect the data and limit interpretation (Addington-Hall, 2002; McPherson et al., 2003; Higginson, 2013). No matter which tool is used within a study, the validity of the tool in the context in which it has been used must be considered carefully (National Institutes of Health, 2004; Higginson, 2013).

   In addition, patient symptom reports are different to clinical diagnoses of syndromes. For example, with respect to delirium, if a study reports categories such as confusion, cognitive symptoms, and neurological symptoms separately rather than syndromal delirium, conclusions about the presence or absence of delirium become difficult to draw. Patients or proxies cannot be asked to rate the presence of 'delirium' which is a diagnosis not a symptom. Meta-analyses cannot reverse the impact of poorly defined symptoms or syndromes as the categories reported are determined by the methods used in the individual studies. The importance of study methods in terms of choosing the correct tools to address the hypothesis and carefully describing the population is again emphasized (Kaasa et al., 2008).

5. *An individual's symptom experience changes over time and the burden imposed by a particular symptom may change over time* (Hwang et al., 2003; Sharpe et al., 2005). The temporally isolated nature of point prevalence data does not reflect the dynamic changes of the symptom experience over time. Likewise, health-care needs at the end of life are dynamic and longitudinal studies are required to adequately describe them.

6. *The symptom experience is multidimensional, inter-relates with the bio-psychosocial, spiritual, and cultural domains, and may have characteristics linked with particular populations.* Some studies have addressed this by investigating symptom burden or distress in addition to symptom prevalence and/or incidence (Hwang et al., 2003; Potter et al., 2003; Strong et al., 2007; Blinderman et al., 2008). Other experts have reviewed and highlighted important priorities relating to care at the end of life and identified approaches and directions for future research that relate to measuring complex, and/or multicomponent interventions towards the end of life (National Institutes of Health, 2004; Higginson, 2013).

7. *Despite the limitations and challenges of study in this area, and considering the overall experience of symptom burden and distress towards the end of life, questions still exist as to which symptoms or health-care needs are the most common and/or most burdensome in the context of particular conditions or within particular health systems, and whether the common symptoms or needs are appropriately addressed* (Hearn et al., 1999). The management of uncommon but troubling symptoms is also of clinical importance; however, there is a paucity of epidemiological data for uncommon symptoms. Meta-analyses have been used to address the problem of small sample size, although as highlighted previously, the heterogeneity of studies included in meta-analyses is also problematic.

Collaborative, multi-centre studies with attention to inclusion criteria that carefully define the population reported can go a long way towards improving case recruitment as well as maximizing the homogeneity of the data (Currow et al., 2008a; Kaasa et al., 2008). Electronic record linkage has proven to be a powerful tool for palliative care health service research in areas such as estimating patients' needs, service utilization, cost, and place of care (Fassbender et al., 2005; Rosenwax et al., 2006; McNamara et al., 2007) but not in exploring the symptom experience as such.

The aim of this section has been to illustrate the relationship between empirical data and the symptom experience, and the uses, limitations, and challenges inherent in the interpretation of symptom-based epidemiological data. The following sections review existing epidemiological data related to symptoms and health-care needs at the end of life in the light of their incidence and prevalence, severity, frequency, associated distress, and in relation to impact on function and global burden for patients as well as caregivers.

Symptom occurrence by cause of death: what symptoms can be expected over time?

Until recently, symptom prevalence studies in the palliative care setting have focused predominantly on patients with cancer diagnoses. There are now a number of good quality studies that have explored the prevalence of symptoms in patients with life-threatening and far-advanced chronic lung disease (Elkington et al., 2005; Walke et al., 2007) and cardiovascular disease (Addington-Hall et al., 1998a; Solano et al., 2006; Young et al., 2008). Large population-based data sets describing symptom prevalence are lacking; however, two systematic reviews of studies reporting point estimates of the prevalence of different symptoms have provided excellent overviews of symptoms experienced near the end of life (Solano et al., 2006; Teunissen et al., 2007).

Although generalizing is problematic, the available evidence suggests that for people with advanced, progressive life-limiting illness, there is a core group of symptoms, including pain, depression, dyspnoea, and fatigue, experienced across disease states in the last days, and probably the last year of life. Table 2.2.2 presents the data from a meta-analysis which included 64 studies across progressive cancer and non-cancer illnesses (Solano et al., 2006). The authors defined the study time-frame in the included patients' end of life care and targeted 11 predicated symptoms. Studies restricted to the last hours of life were excluded. Notably this meta-analysis did not include cerebrovascular disease (stroke), now ranked the second most common cause of death worldwide, or Alzheimer's dementia which is now reported as the fourth most common cause of death in high-income countries according to 2011 data (WHO, 2013e).

Physical symptoms during the last year of life: what will it be like?

In a meta-analysis of 26 223 patients (Teunissen et al., 2007), studies relating to two time periods were analysed independently and data were presented in two groups relating to the time periods. The two groups were studies prior to the last 2 weeks of life (identified as 'group 1' in the original article) and studies

Table 2.2.2 Symptom prevalence in specific life-threatening diseases

Symptoms	Cancer	AIDS	HD	COPD	RD
Pain	35–96%[7,8,11,19,33–47]	63–80%[48–50]	41–77%[22,34,51,52]	34–77%[4,22,53]	47–50%[54,55]
	N = 10 379[a]	N = 942	N = 882[a]	N = 372	N = 370
Depression	3–77%[7,11,19,20,33,36,41,43,45,47,56–63]	10–82%[50,61,64,65]	9–36%[52,66]	37–71%[4,53]	5–60%[67–72]
	N = 4378[a]	N = 616[a]	N = 80[a]	N = 150	N = 956[a]
Anxiety	13–79%[19,33,36,41,45,47,58,62,63]	8–34%[12,64,73]	49%[52]	51–75%[74]	39–70%[67,68]
	N = 3274	N = 346[a]	N = 80	N = 1008	N = 72[a]
Confusion	6–93%[7,19,20,34,36,39,42–47,60,75–81]	30–65%[76,82]	18–32%[22,34,52]	18–33%[4,22]	–
	N = 9154[a]	N =?[a]	N = 343[a]	N = 309	
Fatigue	32–90%[8,24,35,41–43,45,47,63,83]	54–85%[50,84]	69–82%[8,22,52]	68–80%[22,53]	73–87%[71,85]
	N = 2888[a]	N = 1435	N = 409	N = 285	N = 116
Breathlessness	10–70%[7,8,11,19,33–36,39–47,61,86–88]	11–62%[50,88]	60–88%[8,22,34,51,52,61]	90–95%[4,22,53,61]	11–62%[55,89]
	N = 10 029[a]	N = 504	N = 948[a]	N = 372[a]	N = 334
Insomnia	9–69%[7,8,11,19,33,39,41–43,45,47]	74%[50]	36–48%[8,52]	55–65%[4,53]	31–71%[55,85,90]
	N = 5606	N = 504	N = 146	N = 150	N = 351
Nausea	6–68%[8,11,19,33–36,39–47,61,91–93]	43–49%[50,94]	17–48%[8,34,52]	–	30–43%[85,95,96]
	N = 9140[a]	N = 689	N = 146[a]		N = 362
Constipation	23–65%[7,11,19,33–35,39–45,47,50,93]	34–35%[50,94]	38–42%[34,52]	27–44%[4,53]	29–70%[97]
	N = 7602[a]	N = 689	N = 80[a]	N = 150	N = 483
Diarrhoea	3–29%[11,33,39–41,43,44,47,61,92,93,98]	30–90%[50,61,98,99]	12%[52]	–	21%[71]
	N = 3392[a]	N = 504[a]	N = 80		N = 19
Anorexia	30–92%[7,8,11,19,33,35,39–46,92,93,100]	51%[50]	21–41%[8,52]	35–67%[4,53]	25–64%[89,96]
	N = 9113	N = 504	N = 146	N = 150	N = 395

1. Minimum–maximum range of prevalence (%) is shown.

2. HD = heart disease; COPD = chronic obstructive pulmonary disease; RD = renal disease.

3. N refer to the total number of patients involved in the studies found for each symptom in a given disease (e.g. there are 372 patients involved in the three studies on pain prevalence in COPD).

4. Superscripted numbers relate to the reference source[b] and indicate the number of studies for each symptom in a given disease (e.g. there are three studies on pain prevalence in COPD patients). In two occasions, a single study reported a prevalence range rather than a single point prevalence—anxiety for COPD and constipation for renal failure. '–' was displayed when no data were found for a specific symptom and condition (e.g. confusion for renal failure).

[a] The number of patients is underestimated or unknown because prevalence figures given by textbooks were considered (for which the number of patients was not provided).

[b] For full reference details, please see original journal article.

Reprinted from Journal of Pain and Symptom Management, Volume 31, Number 1 Solano, J., et al., A comparison of symptom prevalence in far advanced cancer, AIDS, Heart Disease, Chronic Obstructive Pulmonary Disease and Renal Disease, pp. 58-69, Copyright © 2006 U.S. Cancer Pain Relief Committee, with permission from Elsevier, http://www.sciencedirect.com/science/journal/08853924

conducted 'in the last 1–2 weeks of life' (identified as 'group 2' in the original article) (see Table 2.2.3 and Table 2.2.4). Despite the limitations discussed above, studies such as these help to define symptom experience over time and can be useful in service planning. As already discussed, point prevalence data and severity data for symptoms are influenced by, but do not provide detail of, access to quality care.

Data on the prevalence of specific symptoms, even in the setting of malignant disease, is more scarce than expected. With regard to the prevalence of pain, Bonica's landmark review (Bonica, 1985) reported a prevalence of 71% in patients with advanced/metastatic/terminal cancer (Van den Beuken-van Everdingen et al, 2007). In addition to providing prevalence data, Bonica's study highlighted methodological considerations in studies of symptom occurrence, including the presence of serious pain at all stages of cancer, its amenability to effective management, and the variation in pain experience over a day and over longer periods (Greenwald et al., 1987).

Other important studies have presented data relating to the experience of pain in cancer (Hearn et al., 2003; Holtan et al., 2007) and non-cancer (Solano et al., 2006; Murray et al., 2012) settings, or both. Most studies have also noted that effective management of pain can be achieved with adherence to the WHO ladder recommendations for management. An unexpected consequence of understanding available pain prevalence data is that it may also provide reassurance to some individuals as these statistics suggest

Table 2.2.3 Summary of symptom prevalence in cancer *prior* to the last 1–2 weeks of life[a]

	Symptom prevalence in group 1			
	Number of studies	**Number of patients**	**Pooled prevalence (%)**	**95% CI (%)**
N	40	25074		
Fatigue	17	6727	74	(63; 83)
Pain	37	21917	71	(67; 74)
Lack of energy	6	1827	69	(57; 79)
Weakness	18	14910	60	(51; 68)
Appetite loss	37	23112	53	(48; 59)
Nervousness	5	727	48	(39; 57)
Weight loss	17	13167	46	(34; 59)
Dry mouth	20	6359	40	(29; 52)
Depressed mood	19	8678	39	(33; 45)
Constipation	34	22439	37	(33; 40)
Worrying	6	1378	36	(21; 55)
Insomnia	28	18597	36	(30; 43)
Dyspnoea	40	24490	35	(30; 39)
Nausea	39	24263	31	(27; 35)
Anxiety	12	7270	30	(17; 46)
Irritability	6	1009	30	(22; 40)
Bloating	5	626	29	(20; 40)
Cough	24	11939	28	(23; 35)
Cognitive symptoms	9	1696	28	(20; 38)
Early satiety	5	1639	23	(8; 52)
Taste changes	11	3045	22	(15; 31)
Sore mouth/stomatitis	8	2172	20	(8; 39)
Vomiting	24	9598	20	(17; 22)
Drowsiness	16	11634	20	(12; 32)
Oedema	13	3486	19	(15; 24)
Urinary symptoms	15	120111	18	(15; 21)
Dizziness	12	3322	17	(11; 25)
Dysphagia	25	16161	17	(14; 20)
Confusion	17	11728	16	(12; 21)
Bleeding	5	8883	15	(11; 20)
Neurological symptoms	11	10004	15	(10; 23)
Hoarseness	5	1410	14	(7; 26)
Dyspepsia	7	3028	12	(9; 15)
Skin symptoms	7	9177	11	(6; 20)
Diarrhoea	22	16592	11	(7; 16)
Pruritus	14	6676	10	(7; 15)
Hiccup	7	3991	7	(3; 15)

[a] Referred to as 'Group 1' in original study.

CI, confidence interval.

Reprinted from *Journal of Pain and Symptom Management*, Volume 34, Number 1, Teunissen, S.C. et al., Symptom prevalence in patients with incurable cancer: a systematic review, pp. 94–104, Copyright © 2007 U.S. Cancer Pain Relief Committee, with permission from Elsevier, http://www.sciencedirect.com/science/journal/08853924

that there is a proportion of patients with advanced cancer who do not report pain and that although pain is a significant problem for many, it is not an inevitable consequence of a cancer diagnosis. Communication of information about pain to patients and carers benefits from attention to these factors.

Van den Beuken-van Everdingen and co-authors (2007) provided pooled estimates of prevalence for four subgroups of patients based on different stages of the cancer care pathway. They report pooled prevalences of pain of (a) 33% (95% confidence interval (CI) 21–46% (from studies including patients after curative treatment), (b) 59% (95% CI 44–73%) from studies including patients under anti-cancer treatment, (c) 64% (95% CI 58–69%) from studies including patients with disease characterised as advanced/metastatic/terminal, and (d) 53% (95% CI 43–63%) from studies including patients at all disease stages. They also report that for one-third of patients pain was graded as moderate or severe. The pooled estimates of prevalence of pain were greater than 50% for the six cancer groups they examined. Age, continent of origin, and date of study did not contribute to statistically significant variation.

Pain is not only among the most common symptoms in terms of incidence, but it ranks highly with regard to intensity (Tishelman et al., 2007) and distress (Bruera et al., 1991; Portenoy et al., 1994; Hwang et al., 2003). Other common and distressing symptoms for which specific point prevalence data are available include fatigue (Solano et al., 2006; Tishelman et al., 2007), depression (Hotopf et al., 2002; Mitchell et al., 2011), delirium (Leonard et al., 2008), breathlessness (Elkington et al., 2005; Solano et al., 2006; Teunissen et al., 2007; Walke et al., 2007; Currow et al., 2010), disturbed bowel function (Clark et al., 2012), and psychosocial distress (Addington-Hall et al., 1998a; Hynninen et al., 2005; Jacobsen et al., 2005; Averill et al., 2007; Holland et al., 2007; Blinderman et al., 2008; Hill et al., 2008).

The evidence suggests that neuropsychiatric symptoms and syndromes are also particularly common toward the end of life (occurring in up to one in two patients) (Derogatis et al., 1983) and that under-recognition, misdiagnosis (Fallowfield et al., 2001), and under-treatment persist (Lloyd Williams et al., 2003). In the setting of far-advanced cancer anxiety (Roth et al., 2007), sleep disorders (Mercadante et al., 2004), post-traumatic stress disorder (Breitbart, 1995; Leonard et al., 2009), demoralization (Kissane et al., 2001), and suicidal ideation have all been identified as prevalent and distressing neuropsychiatric syndromes.

Symptom occurrence in the last days of life: what symptoms can be expected in the very last days of life?

Much has been written in recent decades about the mandate for optimum care for all dying patients at the very end of life (Field and Cassel, 1997; National Institute for Clinical Excellence, 2004; WHO, 2007; Martin-Moreno et al., 2008) (see also Chapter 1.1). Recently, health-funding bodies, locally and nationally, have invested in comprehensive programmes to assist generalist and specialist clinicians to improve care for patients in the last days of life, regardless of setting or diagnosis. Epidemiological data about symptoms and health-care needs during this period of life can inform care provision and assist in defining priorities for the education of clinicians.

There are several problems inherent in reviewing data regarding symptoms at the very end of life. Fatigue, weakness, and lack of energy along with dyspnoea and pain are reported as highly prevalent in most studies examining symptoms at this time of life (Teunissen et al., 2007) Many of these symptoms and/or the distress associated with them are amenable to treatment and as a result, symptom prevalence data must be interpreted in the context of an understanding that some or many symptoms are amenable to treatment. It is important to note that point prevalence data alone do not give insight into the level of treatment provided. It must be noted that in some studies, data on symptoms such as fatigue and those symptoms related to delirium are conspicuous by their absence. This may result from bias of a particular tool (some tools have excluded fatigue) or, for example, the absence of delirium in an inventory of symptoms at the end of life. The omission of a symptom from a specific tool will unavoidably bias outcomes, so it is important to understand how a symptom assessment tool has been developed.

Reports from hospice programmes and pain studies suggest that despite the prevalence of symptoms, most deaths can be peaceful (Saunders, 1948; Lichter et al., 1990; Seeman, 1992; Hinkka et al., 2001). Although an early but informative study of this time of life was published in 1904 by Osler (Osler, 1904; Hinohara, 1993), studies on symptoms towards the end of life, especially in the very final days of life, have been rare until recently and often limited to small case series that relied on proxy reports. Table 2.2.4 provides pooled prevalence estimates from a comprehensive meta-analysis of cancer-related symptoms in the last 1–2 weeks of life (Teunissen et al., 2007). Symptoms during the last days or weeks of life have also been captured by other studies (Foley et al., 1995; Pritchard et al., 1998).

Longitudinal, population-based data relating to the experience of specific symptoms occurring at the very end of life are essential for planning service provision and setting training and research agendas but have only rarely been published. A study from Western Australia documented patient dyspnoea in 5862 patients who had rated their dyspnoea over time in a routine collection of symptom data in a clinical palliative care setting. Data were reported from patients over time, with a median of 48 days of data collection, up until the day of death. In the last days of life the proportion of patients with 'no dyspnoea' fell to 35% but those who rated dyspnoea as greater than 7 out of 10 rose to 26%. Moderate to severe dyspnoea in patients with respiratory failure was sustained over many months before death, and mild to moderate dyspnoea was also reported in other patients in the months preceding death (Currow et al., 2010). This study is a good example of how data collected in a standardized manner in a clinical setting can be analysed to provide important information about some groups and inform the development of treatment and support interventions, as well as patient, caregiver, and provider educational strategies.

Despite significant advances in palliative care treatments and interventions, there are data that suggest that, at the very end of life, unmet symptom-related health-care needs amenable to palliative care interventions persist (Okuyama et al., 2004; Goodridge et al., 2008; Rustoen et al., 2008; Laugsand et al., 2011). For example, the findings of the Study to Understand Prognosis and Preferences for the Outcomes and Risks of Treatment (SUPPORT) were published in a number of papers in the mid 1990s. This study followed 9105 adults hospitalized in the United States with at least one of nine life-threatening diagnoses. One finding was that proxies reported that 50% of conscious patients were in moderate to severe pain for more

Table 2.2.4 Summary of symptom prevalence in the *last* 1–2 weeks of life[a]

	Symptom prevalence in group 2: patients in the last 1–2 weeks of life				
	Number of studies	Number of patients	Pooled prevalence (%)	95% CI (%)	p[b]
N	6	2219			
Fatigue	2	120	88	(12; 100)	0.506
Weight loss	2	1149	86	(77; 92)	0.023
Weakness	3	477	74	(50; 89)	0.262
Appetite loss	3	2008	56	(15; 92)	0.460
Pain	3	1626	43	(32; 39)	0.004
Dyspnoea	6	2219	39	(20; 62)	0.695
Drowsiness	3	894	38	(14; 70)	0.303
Dry mouth	4	1010	34	(10; 70)	0.794
Neurological symptoms	1	176	32	(26; 40)	0.500
Anxiety	2	256	30	(11; 62)	0.923
Constipation	6	2219	29	(16; 48)	0.747
Confusion	4	1070	24	(6; 62)	0.410
Depressed mood	3	850	19	(9; 36)	0.104
Nausea	6	2219	17	(8; 31)	0.047
Skin symptoms	1	593	16	(14; 20)	0.750
Dysphagia	4	1070	16	(6; 37)	0.825
Insomnia	4	889	14	(3; 44)	0.094
Cough	4	829	14	(3; 43)	0.291
Vomiting	3	799	13	(9; 18)	0.313
Bleeding	1	176	12	(8; 18)	0.667
Oedema	1	90	8	(4; 16)	0.286
Dizziness	2	653	7	(5; 9)	0.264
Irritability	1	90	7	(3; 14)	0.671
Diarrhoea	5	2129	6	(2; 19)	0.258
Urinary symptoms	3	850	6	(5; 8)	0.017
Dyspepsia	2	804	2	(1; 4)	0.111

[a] Referred to as 'Group 2' in original study.
[b] Comparison of median percentages, Group 2 versus Group 1, Mann–Whitney test.

CI, confidence interval.

Reprinted from Journal of Pain and Symptom Management, Volume 34, Number 1, Teunissen, S.C., et al., Symptom prevalence in patients with incurable cancer: a systematic review, pp. 94–104, Copyright © 2007, U.S. Cancer Pain Relief Committee, with permission from Elsevier, http://www.sciencedirect.com/science/journal/08853924

than half the time during the last 3 days of life (SUPPORT Principal Investigators, 1995). Epidemiological studies of cancer patients from other countries reveal similar rates of inadequate pain control (Laugsand et al., 2011) and unmet symptom management needs are also evident for patients with non-cancer, life-threatening conditions (Covinsky et al., 1996; Goodridge et al., 2008; Rustoen et al., 2008). As discussed above, unmet symptom management needs are important research findings; however, as previously emphasized, data must be interpreted in the context of access to skilled care as well as the amenability of symptoms to treatment and the ability of multidisciplinary services to meet complex needs (Meuser et al., 2001).

Another aspect of the physical experience that has been rated as highly important by cancer patients is the area of communication, consciousness, and mental acuity towards the end of life (Steinhauser et al., 2000). Few epidemiological studies have reported on the longitudinal trends in the level of consciousness towards the end of life. The large National Mortality Followback Study in the United States addressed many aspects of health care including the end-of-life experience (Seeman, 1992). This study sought the perceptions of family carers in regard to decedents and, with respect to cognitive function at the end of life, reported that 68.9% of patients 'never or hardly ever' had trouble in recognizing family members or friends during the last year of life (Seeman, 1992). Delirium is reported to frequently accompany the last hours of life for patients with cancer and non-cancer-related illnesses (Conill et al., 1997; Teunissen et al., 2007), but, as with other symptoms, such data must be considered in the context of the availability of effective management (Seeman, 1992; Lawlor et al., 2000).

Trajectories of functional decline towards the end of life: what can be expected over time?

Functional decline in the months before death has been described in several studies, including one by Glaser and Strauss (1968) that described the trajectories of dying. More recently, Lunney et al. (2003) described four general patterns of functional decline (see Fig. 2.2.5). Of note, these 'general patterns' of care needs are supported by detailed epidemiological data, in this case from US Medicare data sets (Lunney et al., 2003). It is important to acknowledge that while general trends exist, these trajectories are not necessarily applicable to individual patients. Functional decline can be viewed to some degree as a 'proxy' for health-care needs in that it has implications for personal care, physical support in the home, and caregiver supports. Clearly, on a national, regional, or institutional level it is important for health-care planning to accommodate the care needs of populations implied by trajectories of functional decline.

On an individual level, this type of epidemiological data about performance status and function can assist in facilitating discussion about an individual's projected symptom experience and can help in answering such questions as: 'Is it likely I will have months lying in bed unable to speak or get up?', 'Is it likely I will need someone to look after me?', or 'Is it likely I will be able to stay at home?'. As an example, it may appear almost redundant to many clinicians to state the general differences between the functional decline and care needs of a patient with Alzheimer's disease and the needs of a patient with acute myeloid leukaemia.

For patients and carers this is most often far from obvious, and rather than being left to draw their own conclusions based on what they have observed in others, in the literature, and/or the media, patients and carers may benefit from timely and skilled communication with a health professional who has a good understanding of common functional trajectories.

Health administrative data sets: how can these be used to assess needs and quality of care?

Some information about population health-care needs at the end of life has been provided by a number of large, well-designed epidemiological studies (Seeman, 1992; Addington-Hall et al., 1995; McNamara et al., 2007; Coupland et al., 2010; Seow et al., 2012). Further information about the longitudinal trajectory of functional and other needs would be helpful for service planning.

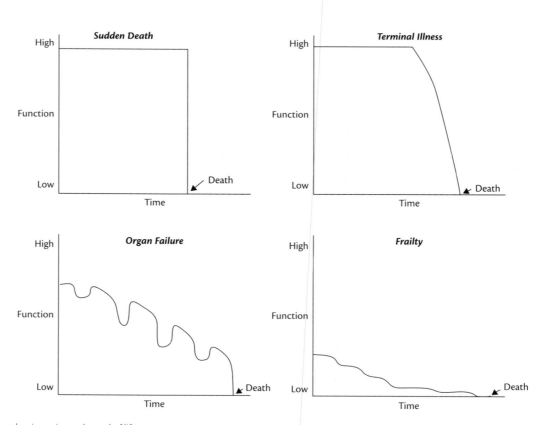

Fig. 2.2.5 Functional trajectories at the end of life.

Reproduced from Lunney, J.R. et al., Profiles of older Medicare decedents, *Journal of the American Geriatric Society*, Volume 50, Issue 6, pp.1108–1112, Copyright © 2002, with permission from John Wiley & Sons, Inc. All Rights Reserved.

With an increase in the potential to analyse large health-care administrative data sets through record linkage, there is increased discussion about the role that information extracted from these datasets can play in assessing the quality of care. Many studies of this nature have been carried out in recent years looking at the period towards the end of life including large epidemiological studies that have provided information about health-care utilization over the period near to the end of life. Although a full review of these studies is beyond the scope of this section, these include studies looking at costs of care (Fassbender et al., 2005; Yabroff et al., 2007), palliative care service use (Fassbender et al., 2005; Rosenwax et al., 2006), place of death (McNamara et al., 2007), and hospital and community health experiences including physician visits, procedures, intensive care admissions, emergency department presentations, and length of stay in hospital (Kaul et al., 2011; Unroe et al., 2011).

A recent Canadian study illustrates the types of findings possible in these studies. This study examined the public provider costs associated with the last 6 months of life for all cancer deaths in Ontario. Investigators found that 75% of costs associated with end of life and palliative care were incurred in the acute hospital setting (Walker et al., 2011). Other investigators found that 26.6% of costs were borne by family/carers (Dumont et al., 2010).

Increasingly, investigators have sought to explore the question of how to use data points within health administrative data sets to develop indicators of quality of care at the end of life and, to achieve this, have used methods including seeking expert opinion and patient and carer feedback about such indicators through focus groups (Earle et al., 2005; Grunfeld et al., 2008). It is becoming clearer with time that indicators could, with widespread use and further work on appropriate benchmarks for various regions, be used within and among health services to inform planning and predict service needs (e.g. home care, emergency room services, etc.) (The Dartmouth Atlas of Health Care, 2007). The ability of indicators in these data sets to truly capture the appropriate endpoints relating to quality of care remains complicated. Limitations include the challenge inherent in non-subjective indicators to provide a clear representation of many aspects of the patient's experience. These data sets cannot generally answer questions such as whether patients' preferences were honoured, and whether patients and carers were satisfied with care (Grunfeld et al., 2008). In summary, while there is a wealth of data related to health-care utilization there is a need to both refine validated quality indicators, and to develop systems to measure and record patient-reported outcomes to ensure information is meaningfully recorded to inform patient-centred care (Grunfeld et al., 2008; Higginson, 2013).

Caregiver concerns

A single death affects many others in terms of informal caregiving and grief (see Chapter 17.6). Documentation of the caregiver's experience towards the end of life is therefore an important aspect of the epidemiology of the end-of-life experience.

Many caregivers willingly provide care, and indeed report that they find the role of carer a rewarding and an important part of family experience (Andrén et al., 2008). Notwithstanding this, research conducted across diagnoses and in various countries has tended to focus on the significant demands and burdens that arise from caring for patients with life-threatening illnesses and despite the positive aspects of the role, one in 13 carers in one study (7.4%) indicated that they would not take on the caring role again (Currow et al., 2011). Caregiving has been shown to affect both the physical (Christakis et al., 2006) and psychological (Zivin et al., 2007) health and the social and financial (Carmichael et al., 1998; Emanuel et al., 2000; Berecki-Gisolf et al., 2008) situation of caregivers (Aoun et al., 2005; Burton et al., 2012). Population-based sampling such as that undertaken by Addington Hall et al. (1998b) can provide important information about carers of patients with a particular diagnosis. For instance, the study by Addington-Hall et al. presents data from a representative sample of carers for a person who died from stroke and state that 43% of carers reported to have needed more assistance with personal care and 31% reported unmet needs regarding financial issues. For further information about caregivers, readers are referred to Chapters 6.1, 6.2, and 16.1 and to studies such as the 1999 National Long Term Care Study (NLTCS) (Wolff et al., 2007) and the SUPPORT study (Covinsky et al., 1996).

In addition to the impact of caregiving on physical and psychological health, from a societal and epidemiological perspective, the financial and social impact of caregiving is also significant. As an example, in the SUPPORT study, in which care in the United States was investigated, it was reported that 31% of families caring for patients near the end of life lost most or all of the family's savings and, in 20% of cases, the caregiver had to resign from work or make another major life change to continue to provide care (Covinsky et al., 1996). Informal carers and their households are certainly at risk of suffering loss of income, and indeed epidemiological studies have demonstrated the significant impact that caregiving has on workforce participation (Carmichael et al., 1998; Berecki-Gisolf et al., 2008). Such data raise questions about availability of resources and policy to address the needs of carers. The importance of assessing the impact of caregiver interventions on carer burden beyond financial and health concerns is supported by existing literature. There is evidence suggesting that carers regard information, emotional support, practical care, and patient comfort as most important (Addington-Hall et al., 1998b; Burton et al., 2012).

The array of studies reporting on the needs and experiences of caregivers from high-income countries contrasts with the paucity of data relating to this from low-income countries. While less research has been done in low-income areas, an interesting small study by Grant et al. reported that for advanced cancer 'the emotional pain of facing death was the prime concern of Scottish patients and their carers, while physical pain and financial worries dominated the lives of Kenyan patients and their carers' (Grant et al., 2003). While more data are needed worldwide on the caregiver's experience, the overlapping needs of caregivers and the contrasting needs reported in this study provide some insight into the spectrum of needs and the disparities that exist among caregivers.

Cultural experiences and the existential context

Death is laden with emotional, social, and cultural significance (see Chapter 2.5). A diverse spectrum of beliefs exists about the spiritual/existential and cultural aspects of death and the period prior to, and after, death. Despite much being discussed in the popular media and the fact that many hold strong beliefs relating to this time of life, and the time before and after death, there is a paucity of epidemiological data concerning perceptions about the 'metaphysical' domains of experience near to the end of life with few publications in the peer-reviewed literature. Cultural factors are important in relation to symptom experience, distress, and communication at the end of life and addressed elsewhere in this textbook. Well-designed epidemiological studies investigating cultural aspects of the end-of-life experience within and across different social, geographical, and cultural groups would serve to illuminate this aspect of the end-of-life experience.

Conclusion

The study of the epidemiology of the end-of-life experience is an evolving and important field with an increasing number of studies being published that shed light on the experiences of those within populations who are nearing the end of life, and the experiences of caregivers. The use of validated tools, carefully designed studies, and record linkage will, it is hoped, shed more light on this important area over time. It is important for epidemiological enquiry that the symptoms and health-care needs at the end of life be a subject of focused study throughout the world if health policy is to truly reflect the spectrum of needs of individuals who are near to the end of life.

Acknowledgements

Professor Ingham's research for this publication was undertaken, in part, with funding support from the Cancer Institute New South Wales Academic Chairs Program. The views expressed herein are those of the authors and are not necessarily those of the Cancer Institute of New South Wales. The authors wish to acknowledge the work of Dr Paula Mohacsi, PhD, MBA, MSc (Ed Studies) RN in the preparation of the manuscript.

Online materials

Complete references for this chapter are available online at <http://www.oxfordmedicine.com>.

References

Gomes, B., Calanzani, N., Curiale, V., Mccrone, P. & Higginson, I. J. 2013. Effectiveness and cost-effectiveness of home palliative care services for adults with advanced illness and their caregivers. Cochrane Database Syst Rev, 6, CD007760.

Higginson, I.J. and Costantini, M. (2008). Dying with cancer, living well with advanced cancer. *European Journal of Cancer*, 44, 1414–1424.

Institute for Health Metrics and Evaluation Interactive Data Visualisations: Global burden of disease interactive cause and risk heat map (2010) [Online] Available at <https://www.healthdata.org/data-visualization/gbd-heatmap>

Institut national d'études démographiques (2013). *Population Maps: Life Expectancy at Birth, All Countries, 2013*. [Online] Available at: <http://www.ined.fr/en/everything_about_population/graphs-maps/interactive-world-maps/>

Lunney, J.R., Lynn, J., and Hogan, C. (2002). Profiles of older medicare decedents. *Journal of the American Geriatric Society*, 50, 1108–1112.

Lynch, T., Clark, D., and Connor, S.R. (2011). *Mapping Levels of Palliative Care Development: A Global Update 2011*. London: Worldwide Palliative Care Alliance.

Solano, J.P., Gomes, B., and Higginson, I.J. (2006). A comparison of symptom prevalence in far advanced cancer, AIDS, heart disease, chronic obstructive pulmonary disease and renal disease. *Journal of Pain and Symptom Management*, 31, 58–69.

Teunissen, S.C., Wesker, W., Kruitwagen, C., de Haes, H.C., Voest, E.E. and de Graeff, A. (2007). Symptom prevalence in patients with incurable cancer: a systematic review. *Journal of Pain and Symptom Management*, 34, 94–104.

World Health Organization (2013d). *The Top 10 Causes of Death. Fact Sheet Number 310* [updated July 2013]. [Online] Available at: <http://www.who.int/mediacentre/factsheets/fs310/en/index.html>

World Health Organization (n.d. b). *Projections of Mortality and Causes of Death, 2015 and 2030. World Bank Income Groups*. [Online] Available at: <http://www.who.int/healthinfo/global_burden_disease/projections/en/index.html>

2.3

Predicting survival in patients with advanced disease

Paul Glare, Christian T. Sinclair, Patrick Stone, and Josephine M. Clayton

Introduction to predicting survival in patients with advanced disease

Diagnosis, treatment, and prognosis have long been recognized as the three cardinal skills of clinical medicine (Hutchinson, 1934). Prior to the twentieth century, when few effective treatments were available for any disease, offering a prognosis was about all the physician could do. Due to progress in diagnosis and treatment in the twentieth century, the need for this kind of prognostication has—thankfully—largely disappeared (Christakis, 1997). In the twenty-first century, the growth of palliative medicine has led to a renaissance of interest in predicting survival in patients with fatal diseases. But nowadays they are chronic, incurable conditions such as advanced cancer, end-organ failures, and dementia, and not acute, medical diseases such as pneumonia.

There are many reasons why palliative care clinicians need to be proficient at prognosis:

◆ It provides patients and their families with information on what to expect so they can set meaningful goals, priorities, and expectations for care.

◆ It is a key technical prerequisite for many clinical decisions.

◆ It determines eligibility for the hospice benefit in the United States and admission to inpatient units in other countries.

◆ It is important for the design and analysis of clinical trials.

Despite the importance of prognosis as a clinical skill in palliative care, most clinicians are not trained how to do it well. Prognostic issues may be covered in a class on 'breaking bad news' which typically uses disclosure of a poor prognosis as an example of difficult physician–patient communication. But most students are not taught how to formulate a prognosis or how to use it appropriately. Being poorly trained in the prognosis skills, it is not surprising that physicians find it difficult to prognosticate and do not like doing it (Christakis and Iwashyna, 1998). They also find it stressful because they believe patients desire too much certainty and accuracy from their predictions. They also feel intimidated by being judged by patients and other clinicians if their prognosis is wrong—although not as badly as for getting the diagnosis wrong. As a result, various norms of prognostication have evolved within mainstream clinical medicine:

◆ Avoid prognosticating.

◆ Wait to be asked rather than volunteering a prediction, especially if the clinical situation is atypical.

◆ Be optimistic, especially if the patient is also optimistic.

◆ Avoid being specific.

◆ Do not use prognostication for survival in treatment decision-making.

These behaviours emphasize the need to improve both education and clinical research in prognosis. There have been advances in the science of prognostication in the past 10 years that are teachable to physicians to improve their confidence to make predictions. Palliative care specialists should have special expertise in this area because it will guide care planning, diagnostic and treatment decisions, as well as communication with patients and families.

In *The Book of Prognostics*, Hippocrates wrote that the physician who was a good prognosticator was highly esteemed among his colleagues and trusted by his patients. This secular perspective contrasts with many religious traditions which insist that only God knows the hour of an individual's death. As a result, in many non-English-speaking cultures, such discussions have traditionally been avoided, although this situation may be gradually changing (Bruera et al., 2000). Patients, family, and staff who wish to defer discussing prognosis to the idea 'God only knows' may use it as a way to culturally identify the acknowledged uncertainty of prognostication.

Even in cultures that accept that predicting survival is allowable, questions are asked about the importance of prognostication. Unlike modern diagnosis and treatment, prognostication remains inherently inaccurate. Nevertheless, we believe prognostication is necessary and inevitable, and in the best interests of all involved. There may even be a moral duty for clinicians to prognosticate (Broeckaert and Glare, 2008), striving to formulate as accurate a prediction as possible, and to communicate it and use it appropriately. This means deeply embedding the clinical acts of prognostication in an open, flexible, dialogical, patient-centred approach (Glare, 2011).

Scientific principles of prognostication

Domains of prognosis

Although the focus of this chapter is on predicting survival, it is important to remember that the word prognosis is defined more broadly by clinical epidemiologists as the 'relative probabilities of the various outcomes of the natural history of a disease' (Sackett et al., 1991). To categorize the many different outcomes of a disease which can be predicted, the '5Ds of prognostication' has been proposed (Fries and Ehrlich, 1981):

- disease progression/recurrence
- death
- disability/discomfort
- drug toxicity
- dollars (costs of health care).

All five of the 'Ds' are relevant to palliative care, and patients may be more interested in predictions other than survival, such as response rates and side effects of palliative therapies (Steinhauser et al., 2000). However, because remaining survival time is so central to establishing patient-centred goals, making decisions about treatment and end-of-life decision-making, the focus of this chapter is on predicting death.

Three components of prognostication

The clinical act of prognostication is in fact a composite of three skills that palliative care clinicians should be competent in. These are formulating the prognosis, communicating the prognosis, and using the prognosis when making clinical decisions. To date, prognosis research has focused on good formulation and communication. With the exception of the Study to Understand Prognosis and Preferences for the Outcomes and Risks of Treatment (SUPPORT) study (The SUPPORT Principal Investigators 1995), there have been few studies of how clinicians use prognostic information when making decisions.

Formulating the prognosis: two approaches

A prognosis can be formulated in one of two ways. The first, called clinical prediction of survival (CPS), involves the use of subjective judgement and formulation of the prognosis in the clinician's head. The other way, referred to as actuarial judgement, relies on statistical data such as median survivals and hazard ratios and eliminates the need for the human judge (Dawes et al., 1989). Research from clinical psychology indicates actuarial judgement is generally superior to clinical judgement in predicting human behaviour (Steyerberg and Harrell, 2002), but this is not yet the case for predicting survival.

Irrespective of how the prognosis is formulated, it may be expressed as a temporal prediction or a probabilistic one. A temporal prediction estimates the time to the event (that is, death) and is normally expressed as a continuous variable (i.e. actual number of days, weeks, or months) but may also be a categorical variable (e.g. < 3 weeks, < 6 months, > 1 year). A probabilistic prediction estimates the chance of surviving to a certain time point, for example, percentage chance of being alive in 6 months.

The question of which is the best way to formulate and express the prognosis raises the topic of research in prognosis and the methodological challenges that are encountered when designing or appraising a prognostic study, and they are very different to the methodological issues arising in a clinical trial of a therapy (Laupacis et al., 1994; Altman, 2009). There are many different research questions in prognosis, including evaluation of predictive factors, development and validation of prognostic models, and systematic reviews of the two. Some of the characteristics of a well-designed study to evaluate the association of a prognostic factor with survival are shown in Box 2.3.1.

Box 2.3.1 Characteristics of well-designed studies to evaluate the association of prognostic factors with survival

- A well-defined study population
- Inception cohort design
- Prognostic factors selected are appropriate and clearly defined
- Sample size is adequate for sufficient statistical power
- Clearly defined end point
- Complete follow-up of all patients
- Data analysis is appropriate to test associations between the study factors and survival
- A measure of agreement between the predicted and actual survival
- The definition of accuracy is explicit and appropriate
- The prediction tested mirrors clinical language or practice (i.e. not hazard ratios).

Reproduce from Altman, D., Systematic reviews of studies of prognostic variables. Systematic reviews in health care: meta-analysis in context, *British Medical Journal*, Volume 323, Issue 7306, pp. 224–8, Copyright © 2001, with permission from BMJ Publishing Group Ltd.

Subjective judgement: clinical prediction of survival

Little is currently known about what goes through a clinician's head when they are using subjective judgement. Are they being truly subjective, are they recalling previous patients similar to the one before them, or are they using a kind of actuarial judgement and weighing clinical and other factors? A survey of Italian oncologists found they mainly utilized tumour-related factors when formulating the prognosis in advanced disease (Tannenberger et al., 2002), even though factors such as performance status, symptom burden, and laboratory tests are more relevant in this setting (Hauser et al., 2006). For the clinician who wishes to be more systematic with their CPS, a semi-structured approach has been posited (Mackillop, 2006), beginning with the general prognosis which is based on the clinical and pathological findings (e.g. median survival of 6 months for stage 4 lung cancer). This is then customized to the patient's clinical situation, taking into account their co-morbidities, symptoms, and laboratory abnormalities, as well as their psychosocial issues.

Studies of the accuracy of CPS in advanced cancer indicate that temporal CPS are typically inaccurate, with less than one-quarter of predictions falling within 33% either side of the actual survival, and most being in the over-optimistic direction (Christakis and Lamont, 2000; Glare et al., 2003). Probabilistic CPS are often more accurate (typically in the 60–75% range) and have less of an optimistic bias. Factors influencing the accuracy of CPS have been evaluated. Improvements may be achieved with repeated estimates or asking multiple clinicians to predict. Few differences have been found between disciplines, although physicians may make better initial predictions and nurses may be better in the last few days of life—perhaps because of the amount of time they spend with the patient (Oxenham and Cornbleet, 1998). Experience matters, but a strong physician–patient relationship has been shown to lower prognostic accuracy (Christakis and

Lamont, 2000). The accuracy of CPS in non-malignant diseases is less well studied, but clinicians may be less likely to overestimate prognosis in these populations. Other terminology from the science of measurement, such as calibration and discrimination are also relevant to survival predictions. Predictions discriminate well if the patients in one prognostic group have a different survival to those in another prognostic group. Predictions are well calibrated if patients with better prognoses live longer than patients with worse prognoses.

In an attempt to improve CPS, national organizations in the United Kingdom and the United States have offered clinicians guidance on this subject. In the United Kingdom, the National Health Service's Gold Standards Framework prognostic indicator guidance consists of general 'triggers' for identifying patients and then some more specific guidance for individual diseases (Gold Standards Framework, 2011). In the United States, where incorrectly recommending hospice can result in charges of fraud, the National Hospice and Palliative Care Organization (NHPCO) has developed guidelines to help physicians determine if American patients meet the 6-month prognosis rule 'if the disease follows its usual course' to be eligible for the hospice benefit. These guidelines have been shown to be not very accurate, especially for patients with non-cancer diagnoses (Fox et al., 1999).

For physicians facing difficulties with formulating a CPS, an alternative approach is to ask oneself the 'surprise question', namely 'Would I be surprised if the patient died in the next . . . ?'. Rather than needing to definitely conclude that the patient is dying, asking if they would be surprised if the patient died before some future time point may be more intuitive and feasible. In a study of 826 patients with breast, lung, or colon cancer being followed at a US university cancer centre, 41% of the 'No, I would not be surprised' patients had died at 12 months, while only 3% of the 'Yes, I would be surprised' group had died (Moss et al., 2010). Patients in the 'No' group in this study were older, more likely to have stage IV disease, more likely to have lung cancer, and more likely to have completed an advance directive.

Actuarial judgement: predictive factors in advanced disease

Performance status

Performance status has long been recognized as a predictor of various oncological outcomes, including survival. Multiple studies in the 1980s and 1990s confirmed that cancer patients with a low score on the Karnofsky Performance Status (KPS) scale—developed in the 1940s to assess the effects of chemotherapy on functional level in cancer patients—had a short survival.

One limitation of the KPS scale is that the definitions for scores below 50 depend on the patient's need for hospitalization. The rapid development of community-based palliative care and home hospice programmes over the past 30 years that strive to keep the patient at home has made the KPS scale difficult to apply in these settings. To overcome this problem, the Palliative Performance Scale (PPS) was developed. Multiple studies have shown that the PPS score is a strong predictor of survival in cancer patients already identified as palliative. A meta-analysis of four studies demonstrated that each PPS level is distinct and without grouping (Downing et al., 2007). A large study of PPS scores in ambulatory cancer patients found that the average PPS score declined slowly over the 6 months before death, starting at approximately 70 and

ending at 40, declining more rapidly in the last month (Seow et al., 2011). Prognostat is a web-based tool for survival prediction in palliative care patients which is based on the PPS (Health Terminology Group, n.d.). It includes a calculator, survival tables, and a nomogram for cancer and non-cancer patients.

Symptoms

Most of the research on the impact of symptoms and survival has involved cancer patients. Various individual symptoms have been consistently associated with poor survival in multiple studies (Vigano et al., 2000). The strongest association is with the anorexia-cachexia complex, which has been called the 'final common pathway of terminal cancer'. Dyspnoea and confusion are also associated with a short survival in most studies. In hospice patients with a better performance status (above 40 on the KPS scale), a high symptom burden helps identify the subset with a worse survival outlook (Reuben et al., 1988).

Somewhat surprisingly, pain is not usually identified as one of the predictors of a poor survival in studies of prognostic factors, even though it is known to be a progressive problem in cancer patients. This discrepancy is likely to be explained by lead time bias. Most of the studies of prognostic factors in advanced cancer do not utilize a true, disease-based inception cohort. Instead they study patients who have been referred to palliative care services or hospice, in whom pain is usually the trigger for referral. In a recent study, the use of strong opioids, rather than pain per se, was shown to be prognostic (Gripp et al., 2007).

Various symptom scores have also been shown to be associated with survival, including the Symptom Distress Score (Degner and Sloan, 1995), Rotterdam Symptom Checklist (Earlam et al., 1996), the Memorial Symptom Assessment Scale (Chang et al., 1998), and the Edmonton Symptom Assessment Scale (Seow et al., 2011). In ambulatory cancer patients with end-stage disease, more than one-third of the cohort reported moderate to severe Edmonton Symptom Assessment Scale scores (i.e. 4–10) for most symptoms in the last month of life. Average scores for pain, nausea, anxiety, and depression scores remained relatively stable over the final 6 months. Conversely, shortness of breath, drowsiness, well-being, lack of appetite, and tiredness increased in severity over time, particularly in the month before death.

The association between symptoms and survival is less well studied in non-cancer patients. A systematic review of the prevalence of 11 common symptoms among end-stage patients with cancer, acquired immunodeficiency syndrome, heart disease, chronic obstructive pulmonary disease (COPD), or renal disease found that symptoms were widely and homogeneously spread across the five diseases (Solano et al., 2006). Pain, breathlessness, and fatigue were found among more than 50% of patients, for all five diseases. The authors concluded that the concept of a 'final common pathway' towards death featuring fatigue, anorexia, weight loss, and dyspnoea applies as much to non-malignant diseases as it does to cancer.

Mood, quality of life, and self-rated health

While several physical symptoms are associated with a poor survival, the impact of psychological symptoms is less clear. A systematic review of depression, cancer, and survival identified 25 relevant studies and concluded that mortality rates were significantly higher in depressed patients, but the effect size was small. Mortality rates were up to 25% higher in patients experiencing depressive symptoms and up to 40% higher in patients diagnosed with major or minor depression. The effect of depression remains after adjustment for other prognostic factors, suggesting that depression may play a causal role (Satin et al., 2009). Intriguingly, accelerated cellular aging as indexed by short telomere length has emerged as a potential common biological mechanism linking various forms of psychological stress and diseases of aging, including cancer (O'Donovan et al., 2012).

Quality of life (QOL) scores generally are not associated with survival, especially when measured with instruments developed for palliative care that focus largely on non-physical domains. The Therapeutic Impact Questionnaire developed in Italy for use in hospice/palliative care, rates four major components of QOL—physical symptoms, function, psychological state, and family and social relationships (Tamburini et al., 1996). Global well-being is also evaluated. Only the patient-rated perception of cognitive function and global well-being showed independent prognostic value. Patients had median survivals of 137, 50, and 17 days for impairment of neither, one, or both scales, respectively.

Self-rated health (SRH) is increasingly being recognized as a valid measure for predicting future health outcomes, including survival. Global SRH, the most commonly used measure to rate overall health, is an important predictor of mortality. An unfavourable assessment of overall health has been associated with increased risk of death, even after controlling for socioeconomic status, physical health, functioning, chronic conditions, and health risk behaviours. In a study of ambulatory advanced cancer patients with a median survival time of 10 months, SRH was the strongest predictor of survival from baseline (Shadbolt et al., 2002). The risk of dying was greatest for patients rating their health as 'poor', intermediate if they rated it 'fair', and lowest if they rated it 'good' or better.

Co-morbidities

Cancer patients often have other diseases or medical conditions in addition to their cancer, especially when they are older. Multiple studies have shown that early-stage cancer patients with co-morbid conditions have worse outcomes than patients without co-morbid ailments. The prognostic impact of co-morbidities is greatest for patients with cancers associated with a long natural history, such as prostate cancer, and least in patients with aggressive cancers, such as lung cancer (Read et al., 2004). Co-morbidities have been shown to influence the survival of critically ill cancer patients (Soares et al., 2005), but have rarely been evaluated in studies of prognostic factors in less severely ill palliative care patients. A notable exception is the SUPPORT prognostic model (Knaus et al., 1995), which included cancer as a co-morbidity in patients with other diagnoses (see later section).

Biomarkers

The possibility of taking a single blood sample to provide a precise, accurate, objective estimate of prognosis is tantalizing to clinicians. Pro-inflammatory cytokines such as interleukin-6 (IL-6) are implicated in the genesis of the anorexia-cachexia syndrome (Lee et al., 2004), and C-reactive protein (CRP) is a readily available, inexpensive blood test that is highly correlated with IL-6 levels for inflammation. Other parameters that have been evaluated include elevations of serum alpha-1-acid glycoprotein, alkaline phosphatase, lactate dehydrogenase, and pseudocholinesterase.

Several simple, objective prognostic scores incorporating CRP levels have been developed in advanced cancer. The Glasgow Prognostic Score uses CRP and albumin levels, with elevated CRP levels and hypoalbuminaemia being awarded prognostic points. It has been shown to predict survival in patients with advanced lung cancer (Forrest et al., 2005) and gastric cancer. The vitamin B_{12}/CRP Index (BCI) takes the product of the serum vitamin B_{12} (in pmol/L) and CRP (mg/mL). A retrospective analysis of BCI scores in Swiss geriatric cancer patients who were terminally ill showed that a high score (> 40,000) was associated with a poor survival, that is, less than a 10% chance of surviving 3 months (Geissbuhler et al., 2000). This finding has been validated by others (Kelly et al., 2007; Tavares, 2010), and shown to be as accurate as CPS (Tavares, 2010).

Biomarkers may be prognostic in other diseases. In heart failure, brain natriuretic peptide (BNP) levels may indicate an increased risk of sudden death (Tannenberger et al., 2002), either alone or combined with troponin levels and CRP. In 44 patients dying suddenly versus 89 other patients who died more slowly within 3 years of first diagnosis of heart failure and ejection fraction less than 35%, multivariate analysis showed that log BNP level was the only independent predictor of sudden death (P = 0.0006), with a cut-off point of log BNP less than 2.11 (130 pg/mL) (Berger et al., 2002).

Prognostic tools and models

Models for cancer patients

There is the potential to combine the simple clinical and laboratory factors described above to provide physicians with accurate information about prognosis. Yet caution is needed in interpreting any studies or systematic reviews on survival prediction and prognostic models. Firstly, it is important to distinguish those based on the general population at large from ones within a defined palliative or hospice population. A strong consideration must be given to the inception cohort issue, which requires patients to be at a uniform, disease-based point in time when the measurements of survival begin. Secondly, even in a defined palliative population, attempting to compare published data to one's own palliative programme requires attention to the demographics and inclusion/exclusion criteria. There is often a difference between patients admitted directly to an acute tertiary palliative care unit and those cared for at home or admitted to a hospice facility. The former admissions are usually for urgent symptom assessment and management and as such, may have shorter survival data due to patient complications and difficult symptoms. Hospices will have a somewhat more stable population at least on admission. Thirdly, prognostic scores with statistical significance will follow a Kaplan–Meier curve for the subset analysed but the location on that curve for each individual's death is less obvious, and is in fact indeterminate without other factors being taken into consideration.

Models for terminally ill cancer patients

Many studies over the past decade have developed multiple regression models to determine the association between prognostic factors and survival in patients with far advanced cancer, but few have tested the predicative accuracy of their final models, a key step in prognostic model building. Some of the better developed models are discussed in more detail here.

The SUPPORT study

The SUPPORT study (Knaus et al., 1995) was designed to identify deficiencies in the care of hospitalized patients with various eventually fatal illnesses. The SUPPORT model was developed for this study, with the aim of providing prognostic information as the cornerstone of improved decision-making about end-of-life care in hospitals. Based on the APACHE system for prognostication in critically ill patients in intensive care units (ICUs), individuals' clinical and physiological parameters were utilized in a complex algorithm that was computer generated and gave a probability for the hospitalized patient being alive in 2 and 6 months' time. Only some of them had cancer, making it difficult to compare this model with others developed in patients with terminal cancer. The mathematical model is complex and not suitable for routine use by the clinician at the bedside. The information provided (chance of being alive in 6 months) is relevant to only a small minority of cancer patients referred to hospice/palliative care. Nevertheless, the SUPPORT study is important because it was the first large study to demonstrate the potential of using actuarial judgement to provide the clinician with accurate prognostic data.

The Palliative Prognostic Index (PPI)

This model was originally developed in Japanese cancer patients enrolled in palliative care programmes (Morita et al., 1999). The PPI is calculated by attributing partial scores to five clinical variables (performance status, oral intake, dyspnoea, delirium, and oedema). In the initial study, the total PPI score was used to define three groups with differing prognoses and these results were subsequently replicated in an independent validation sample. A PPI greater than 4 predicted death within 6 weeks with a positive predictive value (PPV) of 83% and a negative predictive value (NPV) of 71%. A later study by the same group confirmed the effectiveness of the PPI at predicting 6-week survival and also demonstrated that the accuracy of clinicians' estimates was improved if they were provided with PPI scores prior to making a prediction (Morita et al., 2001). Further evidence for the validity of this instrument has been provided by Stone and colleagues (Stone et al., 2008) who reported that among patients referred to their palliative care service in Ireland, the PPI had a PPV for predicting death within 6 weeks of 91% and a NPV of 64%.

The Palliative Prognostic (PaP) score

The predictive model from which the PaP score is derived was developed in Italian home hospice patients with advanced cancer (Pirovano et al., 1999). The model consists of six variables that are easily measured at the bedside, namely Karnofsky performance status, anorexia, dyspnoea, total white blood count, and lymphocyte percentage plus the CPS measured in 2-week intervals out to 12 weeks. These factors were independently predictive of survival, and the model is able to split a heterogeneous sample of patients with far advanced cancer into three groups with differing probabilities of being alive at 30 days (group A > 70%, group B 30–70%, and group C < 30%). To calculate the PaP score, points are allocated for each of the six factors, the points for each being based on their parameters in the model. The individual points are then summed to give a final score, which can range from 0 to 17.5, with higher scores representing worse survival. In the original clinical validation study, group A had a score of 0–5, group B 5.5–11, and group C, 11.5–17.5 (Maltoni et al., 1999).

The PaP score is the most robust prognostic model in hospice and palliative care, having been validated in a variety of populations and settings (Glare and Virik, 2001; Glare et al., 2003, 2004; Naylor et al., 2010; Tarumi et al., 2011). The largest validation study, in a mixed cancer and non-cancer palliative care population at a Canadian acute care hospital, involved 958 patients, 18% of whom had non-cancer diagnoses (Tarumi et al., 2011). In this population, PaP group A had a 78% probability of 30-day survival, group B had a 55% probability, and group C had an 11% probability. These results are in keeping with the original development studies for the PaP and generally support its validity as a prognostic tool in palliative care patients. Although the PaP is the most widely validated of the palliative prognostic scales some investigators have expressed dissatisfaction with its over-reliance on subjective clinician estimates (the clinician's intuitive guess accounts for approximately 50% of the total PaP score) and with the omission of cognitive function (which is known to be a poor prognostic factor) from the scoring algorithm

Prognosis in Palliative care Study (PiPS) models

The PiPS models attempt to address the limitations of the PaP score. A large, prospective, multi-centre study involving over 1000 advanced cancer patients newly referred to palliative care services in England identified 11 core variables (pulse rate, general health status, mental test score, performance status, presence of anorexia, presence of any site of metastatic disease, presence of liver metastases, CRP, white blood count, platelet count, and urea) which independently predicted both 2-week and 2-month survival (Gwilliam et al., 2011). Four other variables had prognostic significance only for 2-week survival (dyspnoea, dysphagia, bone metastases, and alanine transaminase), and eight further variables had prognostic significance only for 2-month survival (primary breast cancer, male genital cancer, tiredness, loss of weight, lymphocyte count, neutrophil count, alkaline phosphatase, and albumin). Separate prognostic models were created for patients without (PiPS-A) or with (PiPS-B) blood results.

These models were able to reliably identify those patients with expected prognoses of 'days', 'weeks', or 'months/years' (St George's, University of London, 2011). The median survival across the PiPS-A categories was 5, 33, and 92 days and survival across PiPS-B categories was 7, 32, and 100.5 days. All four PIPs models performed as well as, or better than, CPS. The area under the curve for all models varied between 0.79 and 0.86. Absolute agreement between actual survival and PiPS predictions was 57.3% (after correction for over-optimism). The models can be used in either competent or incompetent patients and in circumstances when blood results are available and when additional investigations would be inappropriate. The prognostic models were shown to be at least as good as a multi-professional clinical estimate of survival; when blood results were available, the models were significantly better than either a doctor's or a nurse's prediction (but not a multi-professional estimate). The instruments have not yet been independently validated, nor has the performance of the PiPS been compared to the performance of the PaP score or the PPI.

Feliu prognostic nomogram

Feliu and colleagues (Feliu et al., 2011) have developed a nomogram to predict survival of terminally ill cancer patients at 15, 30, and 60 days. The prognostic index is generated from a weighted combination of Eastern Cooperative Oncology Group (ECOG) performance status, albumin, lactate dehydrogenase, lymphocyte counts, and time elapsed between initial diagnosis and development of a terminal disease. The nomogram correctly classified survival in 70% of patients in the development study and in 68% of the validation cohort. The authors tested their nomogram against the PaP score and found the nomogram to be significantly more accurate. A potential limitation of the Feliu nomogram is its reliance on the concept of the 'time to terminal diagnosis'. This is a very subjective concept, potentially open to the same limitations as using CPS in the PaP. To assist validation studies of the nomogram, standardized definitions of the onset of a terminal diagnosis, for example, progression through third-line chemotherapy, are needed.

Prognostic tools for less seriously ill cancer patients receiving palliative care

There is currently no prognostic model for predicting survival from cancer that has been validated in the setting of an outpatient palliative care clinic, where patients often don't have many of the symptoms and other problems incorporated in the above models and often survive for several years. A vast amount of prognostic information is available for individual cancers within the oncology literature but is not easily accessible; PubMed has no single MeSH term for 'prognostic index' (Yourman et al., 2012). A tool that is applicable to the heterogeneous patient population seen in the palliative care outpatient clinic is urgently needed. As more palliative care programmes offer ambulatory clinics for patients with months–years to live, a tool for predicting their survival is an important innovation.

A prognostic tool has been developed for ambulatory patients receiving palliative radiotherapy (Chow et al., 2002). It has subsequently been simplified (Chow et al., 2008), the simplified model utilizing just three variables—primary cancer type, site of metastases, and performance status—to divide patients into three independent prognostic groups with median survivals of 12, 6, and 3 months, respectively. This simple prognostic model may be applicable to the broader palliative care population (Vij et al., 2012).

Prognostic tools and models for other life-limiting diseases

End-organ failures

Congestive heart failure (CHF)

The prognosis of CHF may be as bad, if not worse, than many cancers (see Chapter 15.3). Overall, 1-year and 5-year survival rates in the Framingham Heart Study were 57% and 25% in men and 64% and 38% in women, respectively (Ho et al., 1993). The New York Heart Association (NYHA) classification category is the major gauge of disease severity in CHF, and is the cornerstone of the criteria for hospice admission for CHF in the United States. Based on data from the Framingham Heart Study and other studies, NYHA Class IV (severe symptoms) CHF has a 1-year mortality of 30–40%. However, providing more accurate predictions of 6–12-month mortality has been nearly impossible, due to the unpredictable disease trajectory of CHF. On the one hand it is highly mutable by application of evidence-based therapies, yet it is also marked by a high incidence of sudden death, in the vicinity of 15–20%.

A limitation of the current US hospice admission criteria for CHF is that they are outdated. Written by the NHPCO in 1996, 'optimal treatment' is specified as angiotensin-converting enzyme inhibitors, diuretics, and vasodilators when contemporary optimal treatment includes beta blockers, aldosterone antagonists, and device therapies. The increased use of left ventricular assist devices as 'destination therapy', that is, until death in patients who are non-eligible for transplants, also makes prognostication in CHF increasingly challenging, as do the placement of pacemakers and intra-cardiac defibrillators.

Although it does not predict 6-month mortality, the Seattle Heart Failure Model is a well-validated model that provides an accurate estimate of 1-, 2-, and 3-year survival with the use of easily obtained clinical, pharmacological, device, and laboratory characteristics (Levy et al., 2006; Mozaffarian et al., 2007). Caution should be noted in application in the very elderly, as it is given to greatly overestimating prognosis in this group. A dynamic web version is available which shows changes in Kaplan–Meier survival curves as various parameters are inserted (University of Washington, n.d.). Enhanced Feedback for Effective Cardiac Treatment (EFFECT), a Canadian consortium, has validated another online prognostic model (Canadian Cardiovascular Outcomes Research Team, n.d.).

The prognosis for survival to discharge after cardiopulmonary resuscitation (CPR) is also important, as it is the typical starting point in a discussion of code status. The outcome of in-hospital arrest has not changed since the early 1990s, even though there have been major improvements in the outcome of out-of-hospital cardiac arrest during this period. For the general hospitalized patient experiencing an in-hospital cardiac arrest, a return of spontaneous circulation can be achieved with CPR approximately 50% of the time, but less than 20% of patients survive to discharge (Ehlenbach et al., 2009). The neurological outcomes of those who survived to discharge were generally good, and most patients admitted from home pre-arrest were able to return there. Having multiple co-morbidities pre-arrest is associated with a worse outcome, as are extreme age, poor functional status, and admission from a nursing home.

Chronic obstructive pulmonary disease

COPD also has a poor prognosis with men aged 65 with stage 3 or 4 COPD who continue to smoke dying 10 years before non-smokers without COPD (Shavelle et al., 2009) (see Chapter 15.2). Traditionally, the two most important prognostic factors in COPD have been forced expiratory volume in 1 second (FEV_1) and age. More recently, the level of dyspnoea, graded by the Medical Research Council (MRC) dyspnoea scale, has been found to be a better predictor of survival than the FEV_1 (O'Donnell et al., 2007). For example, a Japanese study of mortality predictors in 227 outpatients with COPD of whom 73% were alive at 5 years found that dyspnoea was significantly correlated to the 5-year survival rate and the level of dyspnoea had a more significant effect on survival than disease severity based on FEV_1 (Oga et al., 2003).

Factors other than age, dyspnoea, and FEV_1 have been evaluated in prognostic models of dyspnoea. The BODE Index incorporates *b*ody mass index (BMI), *o*bstruction (FEV_1 %), *d*yspnoea (MRC dyspnoea scale), and *e*xercise capacity (6-minute walk distance) (Celli et al., 2004). Similarly, the HADO score includes *h*ealth (5-point self-assessment), *a*ctivity (self-reported), *d*yspnoea, and *o*bstruction (FEV$_1$ %) (Esteban et al., 2006). The BODE Index and the HADO Score have both been identified as good predictors of all-cause and respiratory mortality in COPD. In patients with severe COPD (FEV$_1$ < 50%) the BODE Index may be more accurate (Esteban et al., 2010).

Two major clinical issues related to prognosis in COPD are the identification of patients who are eligible for hospice and the outcomes of mechanical ventilation. COPD patients most likely to die within 6–12 months include those with severe, irreversible airflow obstruction, severely impaired and declining exercise capacity and performance status, older age, concomitant cardiovascular or other co-morbid disease, and a history of recent hospitalizations for acute care (Hansen-Flaschen, 2004). Clinicians' predictions in COPD found underestimation of survival after admission to the ICU. For example, the quintile of patients with the lowest expected prognosis (10% probability to survive 6 months) had a group survival of 40% at 6 months (Wildman et al., 2007). The reason for the underestimate is not elucidated in this study but the issue is important for further study as it may impact decisions to admit to the ICU that may be overweighted towards futility arguments. This is an excellent illustration for how prognostication can have profound impacts on policy and utilization of resources, and should be a critical area for more research to serve patients best.

Prognostic models for the frail elderly

Prognosis in the general geriatric population

Failure to consider prognosis in the context of clinical decision-making in the elderly can lead to poor care (see Chapter 16.3). Healthy older patients with good prognosis have low rates of cancer screening, while hospice is underutilized for patients with non-malignant yet life-threatening diseases. Guidelines increasingly incorporate life expectancy as a central factor in weighing the benefits and the burdens of tests and treatments, but prognostic indices offer a potential role for moving beyond arbitrary, age-based cut-offs in clinical decision-making for older adults.

Many geriatric prognostic indices have been published. An excellent recent systematic review of this literature has identified 16 indices that predict risk of mortality from 6 months to 5 years for older adults who do not have a dominant terminal illness such as CHF or dementia, and who are in a variety of clinical settings (Yourman et al., 2012). The review focuses on the accuracy, generalizability, potential for bias, and usability of these indices. To enable clinicians to find the right tool from the 16 available that best fits their patient's situation, the review's authors have created a website which provides an online repository of each of the indices in the review and advice about when to use them (Yourman et al., n.d.).

Dementia patients

The illness trajectory for Alzheimer's dementia follows a generally predictable decline in functional and cognitive status (see Chapter 15.4). The onset of inability to walk unaided indicates the patient is entering the final phase of the illness. However, the final phase of the illness can be protracted and the event that precipitates the death is often unclear. The current NHPCO hospice admission criteria for dementia requires the patient to be stage 7C on the FAST (Functional Assessment Staging Tool; Reisberg 1988) classification system—defined as dementia with impaired activities of daily living (ADLs), incontinence and loss of ambulation—plus the onset of a major medical complication such as aspiration pneumonia, urinary tract infection, or decubitus ulcers in the previous 12 months. Two small studies (Luchins et al., 1997; Hanrahan et al., 1999) have reported that the NHPCO guidelines did appear to identify patients at higher risk of dying within 6 months, but in one study, 30% patients with dementia aged more than 90 years who had been referred to a US hospice programme were still alive 3 years later (Aguero-Torres et al., 1998). Several other studies have found the guidelines had a predictive ability 'no better than chance' (Schonwetter et al., 1998, 2003; Mitchell et al., 2004). Furthermore, many bed-ridden dementia patients do not progress through the earlier stages of the FAST system in an orderly fashion. They are not technically at stage 7C and therefore not hospice eligible. Hospice has been shown to benefit people dying with dementia (Teno et al., 2011), but these studies indicate that prognostication is difficult and may be a barrier to hospice enrolment (Jayes et al., 2012).

In view of the inaccuracy of the NHPCO criteria, several other tools have been developed to improve on them. Of them, the Advanced Dementia Prognostic Tool (ADEPT) has been specifically developed to be more accurate than the FAST 7C criteria used for hospice eligibility, and validated against them (Mitchell et al., 2010). Unlike FAST, ADEPT includes scores for age, male gender, weight loss/BMI, performance status, ADLs, symptoms, and continence. When benchmarked against FAST, it performed slightly better (58% vs 51% accuracy).

Communicating a prognosis

Multiple surveys show most patients with cancer want information about their prognosis (Kutner et al., 1999; Butow et al., 2002; Hagerty et al., 2004, 2005; Parker et al., 2007; Innes and Payne, 2009), whether it be good news or bad (Fallowfield et al., 2002) (see Chapter 6.1). But talking to patients about prognosis is difficult and clinicians are poor at this type of communication. There are large discrepancies between patients' and healthcare professionals' perceptions about how much information is needed, how much information has been given, and what such information means (Hancock et al., 2007). Clinicians tend to underestimate patients' prognostic information needs and overestimate how much they had understood about their illness and its likely outcome (Beadle et al., 2004).

Giving patients prognostic information is also important in terms of the effects it can have on patient outcomes. Advance care planning for patients at the end of life requires frank disclosure about prognosis. In one large cohort study (Wright et al., 2008), explicit discussion of end-of-life issues was associated with less aggressive medical care near death, earlier hospice referrals, and improved outcomes for bereaved family members. Without such explicit prognostic information patients may find themselves being managed in the acute care setting at the end of life rather than a more appropriate environment (Innes and Payne, 2009; Mack and Smith, 2012).

Physicians and patients may, to some extent, enter into a level of collusion about avoiding any discussion of prognosis (The et al., 2000). Consultations tend to focus on treatment options and the results of investigations rather than on questions of prognosis, often involving 'false optimism' about the prospects of recovery. This optimism may be fostered both by doctors' reluctance to give clear information about prognosis and patients' avoidance of asking direct questions.

What prognostic information do patients want?

Patients both crave and dread prognostic information. They are caught between wanting to know what is going on and fearing the answers they might receive. Therefore, they want the prognosis to be given by someone whom they perceive to be an expert, and they find inconsistent information or evasiveness on the part of the professional to be distressing and unhelpful. Patients also want hopeful messages, even when they accept the terminal phase of the illness (Kutner et al., 1999; Kirk et al., 2004). Strategies clinicians may use to facilitate hope when discussing prognosis include retaining professional honesty, avoiding being blunt or giving more detailed information than desired by the patient, pacing of information, respecting patients' need to follow alternative paths/ treatments, and exploring and facilitating realistic goals and wishes where appropriate.

Many studies have stressed the importance of individualizing the content of prognostic discussions, but few patient characteristics have been identified to predict how much information patients want or how such information should be delivered (Kutner et al., 1999). Patients have different needs from one another and individual patients' information needs and preferences can change during the course of their illness. While many want to discuss prognosis when they were first diagnosed with metastatic disease, others want to negotiate with the clinician about when such issues were discussed. In one study, more than half the patients wanted the physicians to initiate discussions about prognosis, less than a quarter only wanted the physician to tell them about survival 'if asked', and approximately 10% of patients never wanted to discuss likely duration of survival (Hagerty et al., 2004). In general, women want more information than men (Fallowfield et al., 2002) and older patients request less information than younger patients. Cultural differences may also be important (Parker et al., 2007). Likewise patients tend to want less information as their underlying disease progresses and they approach the terminal phase of their illness.

How to communicate the formulated prognosis to the patient?

Although patients generally indicate they want information about prognosis, it is not always clear what is the best way to communicate such information. Guidelines and other recommendations for the best way to deliver the information are available (Clayton et al., 2007; Back et al., 2009; Kiely et al., 2010). They stress the importance of communication occurring within the context of a caring, trusting relationship, consistency of information within the multiprofessional team, and the need to communicate prognostic information to other members of the family. As highlighted above, not all patients want to be provided with an estimation of their life expectancy. Hence it is very important to first clarify the person's understanding of their medical situation and the information they desire. Any information provided about prognosis should then be tailored to the individual needs of patients and their families.

Most patients want to be informed of their likely survival duration in a straightforward and clear manner. For patients who would like to be provided with a numerical estimation of their life expectancy the following approach has been advocated for patients with advanced cancer (Kiely et al., 2010). The first step is to use a prognostic tool to estimate the median survival of a group

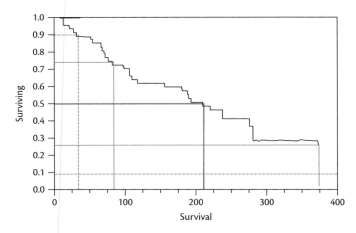

Fig. 2.3.1 Using the median survival to make other probabilistic survival predictions.

with similar characteristics. The survival curve of patients with a variety of advanced cancers typically approximates an exponential function—as would be predicted for a heterogeneous population (see Fig. 2.3.1) (Stockler et al., 2006). In the case that follows, assume that the median survival is 6 months.

◆ Explain that a median survival of 6 months means that 50% will live longer than 6 months.

◆ Use simple multiple of the median to estimate and explain the typical, best case, and worst case scenarios:

• Typical—about half of similar patients would live for somewhere between 3 and 12 months (half to double the predicted median).

• Best case—about 10% of patients could expect to live beyond 2 years (three to four times the predicted median).

• Worst case—about 10% of patients will experience more rapid decline and will die within 1 month (1/6 of the predicted mean).

Using multiples of the median to estimate and provide typical, best, and worst case scenarios as outlined above may offer a way of conveying more realism and hope than a single point estimate of the median survival. Finally after providing patients with information about life expectancy it is important to explore and acknowledge the patient's and family's emotional reaction to the news and to check their understanding about what has been discussed.

Conclusion

Prognostication remains a challenging topic in palliative care. In the past 20 years, much research has been undertaken to identify ways of improving the accuracy and precision of clinicians' estimates and as presented here many tools are now available to improve prognostication.

While we are now in a better position to give the patient 'x % chance of surviving for y weeks/months', we are not yet able to posit any of the existing tools as the ideal one to be recommended for widespread use. Most of the existing tools focus on performance status, symptoms, and simple laboratory markers; while these are helpful, they are no more accurate than the subjective judgements of experienced clinicians. Novel objective prognostic factors need to be identified, and biomarkers such as CRP and the proinflammatory cytokines are the main focus of current research.

Clinical judgement remains important, in our opinion. The clinical data needed to use a tool to calculate the prognosis (e.g. recent laboratory parameters) may not be available, tools may not provide the prognostic information required, and they may not have been validated in the population to which the individual patient belongs. Clinical judgement alone may be sufficient if the issue is acknowledging a probability of dying from an illness in the foreseeable future. The SUPPORT study showed patients will change their planning behaviour once they understand the chance of surviving beyond 6 months is small. Furthermore, models predicting survival should be thought of like any diagnostic test, that is, they should not be interpreted in isolation but as a way of improving the pre-test probability of survival, which is based on clinical judgement.

Even if precise and accurate predictions of survival duration become available, this alone should never drive treatment plans. What ultimately is needed is not so much an accurate prediction of time but an acknowledgement of the possibility of dying, communicated carefully by the compassionate and skilful physician.

Online materials

Additional online materials for this chapter are available online at <http://www.oxfordmedicine.com>.

References

Aguero-Torres, H., Fratiglioni, L., Guo, Z., Viitanen, M., and Winblad, B. (1998). Prognostic factors in very old demented adults: a seven-year follow-up from a population-based survey in Stockholm. *Journal of the American Geriatrics Society*, 46(4), 444–452.

Altman, D. (2001). Systematic reviews of studies of prognostic variables. *BMJ*, 323(7306), 224–228.

Altman, D.G. (2009). Prognostic models: a methodological framework and review of models for breast cancer. *Cancer Investigation*, 27(3), 235–243.

Bachmann, P., Marti-Massoud, C., Blanc-Vincent, M.P., *et al.* (2003). Summary version of the Standards, Options and Recommendations for palliative or terminal nutrition in adults with progressive cancer (2001). *British Journal of Cancer*, 89(Suppl. 1), S107–110.

Back, A., Arnold, R.M. and Tulsky, T.J. (2009). *Mastering Communication with Seriously Ill Patients—Balancing Honesty with Empathy and Hope*. New York: Cambridge University Press.

Bao, Y., Dalrymple, L., Chertow, G.M., Kaysen, G.A., and Johansen, K.L. (2012). Frailty, dialysis initiation, and mortality in end-stage renal disease. *Archives of Internal Medicine*, 172(14), 1071–1077.

Beadle, G.F., Yates, P.M., Najman, J.M., *et al.* (2004). Beliefs and practices of patients with advanced cancer: implications for communication. *British Journal of Cancer*, 91(2), 254–257.

Berger, R., Huelsman, M., Strecker, K., *et al.* (2002). B-type natriuretic peptide predicts sudden death in patients with chronic heart failure. *Circulation*, 105(20), 2392–2397.

Brechtl, J.R., Patrick, P.A., Visintainer, P., and Brand, D.A. (2005). Predictors of death within six months in patients with advanced AIDS. *Palliative & Supportive Care*, 3(4), 265–272.

Brody, K.K., Perrin, N.A., and Dellapenna, R. (2006). Advanced illness index: predictive modeling to stratify elders using self-report data. *Journal of Palliative Medicine*, 9(6), 1310–1319.

Broeckaert, B. and Glare, P. (2008). Ethical perspectives. In P. Glare and N. Christakis (eds.) *Prognosis in Advanced Cancer*, pp. 88–94. Oxford: Oxford University Press.

Bruera, E., Miller, M.J., Kuehn, N., MacEachern, T., and Hanson, J. (1992). Estimate of survival of patients admitted to a palliative care unit: a prospective study. *Journal of Pain & Symptom Management*, 7(2), 82–86.

Bruera, E., Neumann, C.M., Mazzocato, C., Stiefel, F., and Sala, R. (2000). Attitudes and beliefs of palliative care physicians regarding communication with terminally ill cancer patients. *Palliative Medicine*, 14(4), 287–298.

Butow, P.N., Dowsett, S., Hagerty, R., and Tattersall, M.H.N. (2002). Communicating prognosis to patients with metastatic disease: what do they really want to know? *Supportive Care in Cancer*, 10(2), 161–168.

Canadian Cardiovascular Outcomes Research Team (n.d.). *Enhanced Feedback for Effective Cardiac Treatment (EFFECT) Study*. [Online] Available at: <http://www.ccort.ca>.

Capitani, E., Cazzaniga, R., Francescani, A., and Spinnler, H. (2004). Cognitive deterioration in Alzheimer's disease: is the early course predictive of the later stages? *Neurological Sciences*, 25(4), 198–204.

Celli, B.R., Cote, C.G., Marin, J.M., *et al.* (2004). The body-mass index, airflow obstruction, dyspnoea, and exercise capacity index in chronic obstructive pulmonary disease. *The New England Journal of Medicine*, 350(10), 1005–1012.

Chang, V.T., Thaler, H.T., Polyak, T.A. Kornblith, A.B., Lepore, J.M., and Portenoy, R.K. (1998). Quality of life and survival: the role of multidimensional symptom assessment. *Cancer*, 83(1), 173–179.

Chiang, J.-K., Cheng, Y.-H., Koo, M., Kao, Y.-H., and Chen, C.-Y. (2010). A computer-assisted model for predicting probability of dying within 7 days of hospice admission in patients with terminal cancer. *Japanese Journal of Clinical Oncology*, 40(5), 449–455.

Chow, E., Abdolell, M., Panzarella, T., *et al.* (2008). Predictive model for survival in patients with advanced cancer. *Journal of Clinical Oncology*, 26(36), 5863–5869.

Chow, E., Fung, K., Panzarella, T., Bezjak, A., Danjoux, C., and Tannock, I. (2002). A predictive model for survival in metastatic cancer patients attending an outpatient palliative radiotherapy clinic. *International Journal of Radiation Oncology, Biology, Physics*, 53(5), 1291–1302.

Christakis, N.A. (1997). The ellipsis of prognosis in modern medical thought. *Social Science & Medicine*, 44(3), 301–315.

Christakis, N.A. and Iwashyna, T.J. (1998). Attitude and self-reported practice regarding prognostication in a national sample of internists. *Archives of Internal Medicine*, 158(21), 2389–2395.

Christakis, N.A. and Lamont, E.B. (2000). Extent and determinants of error in doctors' prognoses in terminally ill patients: prospective cohort study. *BMJ*, 320(7233), 469–472.

Chuang, R.-B., Hu, W.-Y., Chiu, T.-Y., and Chen, C.-Y. (2004). Prediction of survival in terminal cancer patients in Taiwan: constructing a prognostic scale. *Journal of Pain & Symptom Managemen*, 28(2), 115–122.

Clayton, J.M., Hancock, K.M., Butow, P.N., *et al.* (2007). Clinical practice guidelines for communicating prognosis and end-of-life issues with adults in the advanced stages of a life-limiting illness, and their caregivers. *Medical Journal of Australia*, 186(Suppl. 12), S77, S79, S83–108.

Dawes, R.M., Faust, D., and Meehl, P.E. (1989). Clinical versus actuarial judgment. *Science*, 243(4899), 1668–1674.

Degner, L. and Sloan, J. (1995). Symptom distress in newly diagnosed ambulatory cancer patients and as a predictor of survival in lung cancer. *Journal of Pain & Symptom Management*, 10(6), 423–431.

Downing, G.M., Lau, F., Lesperance, M., *et al.* (2007). Meta-analysis of survival prediction with the Palliative Performance Scale. *Journal of Palliative Medicine*, 23(4), 245–252.

Earlam, S., Glover, C., Fordy, C., Burke, D., and Allen-Mersh, T.G. (1996). Relation between tumor size, quality of life, and survival in patients with colorectal liver metastases. *Journal of Clinical Oncology*, 14(1), 171–175.

Ehlenbach, W.J., Barnato, A.E., and Curtis, J.R. (2005). Epidemiologic study of in-hospital cardiopulmonary resuscitation in the elderly. *The New England Journal of Medicine*, 361(1), 22–31.

Esteban, C., Quintana, J.M., Aburto, M., Moraza, J., and Capelastegui, A. (2006). A simple score for assessing stable chronic obstructive pulmonary disease. *Quarterly Journal of Medicine*, 99(11), 751–759.

Esteban, C., Quintana, J.M., Moraza, J., et al. (2010). BODE-Index vs HADO-score in chronic obstructive pulmonary disease: which one to use in general practice? *BMC Medicine*, 8, 28.

Fallowfield, L.J., Jenkins, V.A., and Beveridge, H.A. (2002). Truth may hurt but deceit hurts more: communication in palliative care. *Palliative Medicine*, 16(4), 297–303.

Feliu, J., Jimenez-Gordo, A.M., Madero, R., et al. (2011). Development and validation of a prognostic nomogram for terminally ill cancer patients. *Journal of the National Cancer Institute*, 103(21), 1613–1620.

Forrest, L.M., McMillan, D.C., McArdle, C.S., Angerson, W.J., Dagg K., and Scott, H.R. (2005). A prospective longitudinal study of performance status, an inflammation-based score (GPS) and survival in patients with inoperable non-small-cell lung cancer. *British Journal of Cancer*, 92(10), 1834–1836.

Fox, E., Landrum-McNiff, K., Zhong, Z., Dawson, N.V., Wu, A.W., and Lynn, J. (1999). Evaluation of prognostic criteria for determining hospice eligibility in patients with advanced lung, heart, or liver disease. SUPPORT Investigators. Study to Understand Prognoses and Preferences for Outcomes and Risks of Treatments. *Journal of the American Medical Association*, 282(17), 1638–1645.

Fries, J.F. and Ehrlich, G.E. (1981). *Prognosis. Contemporary Outcomes of Disease*. Bowie, MD: The Charles Press Publishers.

Geissbuhler, P., Mermillod, B., and Rapin, C.H. (2000). Elevated serum vitamin B12 levels associated with CRP as a predictive factor of mortality in palliative care cancer patients: a prospective study over five years. *Journal of Pain & Symptom Management*, 20(2), 93–103.

Glare, P. (2011). Predicting and communicating prognosis in palliative care. *BMJ*, 343, d5171.

Glare, P., Eychmueller, S., and Virik, K. (2003). The use of the palliative prognostic score in patients with diagnoses other than cancer. *Journal of Pain & Symptom Management*, 26(4), 883–885.

Glare, P. and Virik, K. (2001). Independent prospective validation of the PaP score in terminally ill patients referred to a hospital-based palliative medicine consultation service. *Journal of Pain & Symptom Management*, 22(5), 891–898.

Glare, P., Virik, K., Jones, M., et al. (2003). A systematic review of physicians' survival predictions in terminally ill cancer patients. *BMJ*, 327(7408), 195–198.

Glare, P.A., Eychmueller, S., and McMahon, P. (2004). Diagnostic accuracy of the palliative prognostic score in hospitalized patients with advanced cancer. [Erratum appears in *Journal of Clinical Oncology*, 2005, 23(1), 248]. *Journal of Clinical Oncology*, 22(23), 4823–4828.

Gold Standards Framework (2011). *The GSF Prognostic Indicator Guidance*. [Online] Available at: <http://www.goldstandards-framework.org.uk/cd-content/uploads/files/General%20Files/Prognostic%20Indicator%20Guidance%20October%202011.pdf>.

Gripp, S., Moeller, S. Bolke, E., et al. (2007). Survival prediction in terminally ill cancer patients by clinical estimates, laboratory tests, and self-rated anxiety and depression. *Journal of Clinical Oncology*, 25(22), 3313–3320.

Gwilliam, B., Keeley, V., Todd, C., et al. (2011). Development of prognosis in palliative care study (PiPS) predictor models to improve prognostication in advanced cancer: prospective cohort study. *BMJ*, 343, d4920.

Hagerty, R.G., Butow, P.N., Ellis, P.A., et al. (2004). Cancer patient preferences for communication of prognosis in the metastatic setting. *Journal of Clinical Oncology*, 22(9), 1721–1730.

Hagerty, R.G., Butow, P.N., Ellis, P.M., Dimitry, S., and Tattersall, M.H.N. (2005). Communicating prognosis in cancer care: a systematic review of the literature. *Annals of Oncology*, 16(7), 1005–1053.

Hancock, K., Clayton, J.M., Parker, S.M., et al. (2007). Discrepant perceptions about end-of-life communication: a systematic review. *Journal of Pain & Symptom Management*, 34(2), 190–200.

Hanrahan, P., Raymond, M., McGowan, E., and Luchins, D.J. (1999). Criteria for enrolling dementia patients in hospice: a replication. *American Journal of Hospice & Palliative Care*, 16(1), 395–400.

Hansen-Flaschen, J. (2004). Chronic obstructive pulmonary disease: the last year of life. *Respiratory Care*, 49(1), 90–97.

Hauser, C.A., Stockler, M.R., and Tattersall, M.H. (2006). Prognostic factors in patients with recently diagnosed incurable cancer: a systematic review. *Support Care Cancer*, 14(10), 999–1011.

Health Terminology Group (n.d.). *Prognostat*. School of Health Information Science at the University of Victoria. [Online] Available at: <https://htg.his.uvic.ca/tools/PrognosticTools/PalliativePerformanceScale/Prognostat/index.php>.

Ho, K.K., Anderson, K.M., Kannel, W.B., Grossman, W., and Levy, D. (1993). Survival after the onset of congestive heart failure in Framingham Heart Study subjects. *Circulation*, 88(1), 107–115.

Hudson, A. (1990). Amyotrophic lateral sclerosis: clinical evidence of differences in pathogenesis and etiology. In A. Hudson (ed.) *Amyotrophic Lateral Sclerosis: Concepts in Pathogenesis and Etiology*, pp. 108–143. Toronto: University of Toronto Press.

Hutchinson, R. (1934). Prognosis. *The Lancet*, i, 697.

Hyodo, I., Morita, T., Adachi, I., Shima, Y., Yoshizawa, A., and Hiraga, K. (2010). Development of a predicting tool for survival of terminally ill cancer patients. *Japanese Journal of Clinical Oncology*, 40(5), 442–448.

Innes, S. and Payne, S. (2009). Advanced cancer patients' prognostic information preferences: a review. *Palliative Medicine*, 23(1), 29–39.

Jayes, R.L., Arnold, R.M., and Fromme, E.K. (2012). Does this dementia patient meet the prognosis eligibility requirements for hospice enrollment? *Journal of Pain & Symptom Management*, 44(5), 750–756.

Kaufmann, P., Levy, G., Thompson, J.L., et al. (2005). The ALSFRSr predicts survival time in an ALS clinic population. *Neurology*, 64(1), 38–43.

Kelly, L., White, S., and Stone, P.C. (2007). The B12/CRP index as a simple prognostic indicator in patients with advanced cancer: a confirmatory study. *Annals of Oncology*, 18(8), 1395–1399.

Kiely, B.E., Tattersall, M.H., and Stockler, M.R. (2010). Certain death in uncertain time: informing hope by quantifying a best case scenario. *Journal of Clinical Oncology*, 28(16), 2802–2804.

Kirk, P., Kirk, I., and Kristjanson, L.J. (2004). What do patients receiving palliative care for cancer and their families want to be told? A Canadian and Australian qualitative study. *BMJ*, 328(7452), 1343.

Knaus, W.A., Harrell, F.E., Jr, Lynn, J., et al. (1995). The SUPPORT prognostic model. Objective estimates of survival for seriously ill hospitalized adults. Study to understand prognoses and preferences for outcomes and risks of treatments. *Annals of Internal Medicine*, 122(3), 191–203.

Kutner, J.S., Steiner, J.F., Corbett, K.K., Jahnigen, D.W., and Barton, P.L. (1999). Information needs in terminal illness. *Social Science & Medicine*, 48(10), 1341–1352.

Laupacis, A., Wells, G., Richardson, W.S., and Tugwell, P. (1994). Users' guides to the medical literature. V. How to use an article about prognosis. Evidence-Based Medicine Working Group. *Journal of the American Medical Association*, 272(3), 234–237.

Lee, B.N., Dantzer, R., Langley, K.E., et al. (2004). A cytokine-based neuroimmunologic mechanism of cancer-related symptoms. *Neuroimmunomodulation*, 11(5), 279–292.

Levy, W., Mozaffarian, D., Linker, D., et al. (2006). The Seattle Heart Failure Model: prediction of survival in heart failure. *Circulation*, 113(11), 1424–1433.

Low, J.A., Liu, R.K.Y., Strutt, R., and Chye, R. (2001). Specialist community palliative care services—a survey of general practitioners' experience in Eastern Sydney. *Supportive Care in Cancer*, 9, 474–476.

Luchins, D.J., Hanrahan, P., and Murphy, K. (1997). Criteria for enrolling dementia patients in hospice. *Journal of the American Geriatrics Society*, 45(9), 1054–1059.

Mack, J.W. and Smith, T.J. (2012). Reasons why physicians do not have discussions about poor prognosis, why it matters, and what can be improved. *Journal of Clinical Oncology*, 30(22), 2715–2717.

Mackillop, W.J. (2006). The importance of prognosis in cancer medicine. In M.K. Gospodarowicz, B. O'Sullivan, and L.H. Sobin (eds.) *Prognostic Factors in Cancer*, pp. 3–22. Hoboken, NJ: Wiley-Liss.

Maltoni, M., Nanni, O., Pirovano, M., et al. (1999). Successful validation of the palliative prognostic score in terminally ill cancer patients.

Italian Multicenter Study Group on Palliative Care. *Journal of Pain & Symptom Management*, 17(4), 240–247.

Mandrioli, J., Faglioni, P., Nichelli, P., and Sola, P. (2006). Amyotrophic lateral sclerosis: prognostic indicators of survival. *Amyotrophic Lateral Sclerosis*, 7(4), 211–220.

Martin, L., Watanabe, S., Fainsinger, R., *et al.* (2010). Prognostic factors in patients with advanced cancer: use of the patient-generated subjective global assessment in survival prediction. *Journal of Clinical Oncology*, 28(28), 4376–4383.

Mitchell, S.L., Kiely, D.K, Hamel, M.B., Park, P.S., Morris, J.N., and Fries, B.E. (2004). Estimating prognosis for nursing home residents with advanced dementia. *Journal of the American Medical Association*, 291(22), 2734–2740.

Morita, T., Tsunoda, J., Inoue, S., and Chihara, S. (1999). The Palliative Prognostic Index: a scoring system for survival prediction of terminally ill cancer patients. *Supportive Care in Cancer*, 7(3), 128–133.

Morita, T., Tsunoda, J., Inoue, S., and Chihara, S. (2001). Improved accuracy of physicians' survival prediction for terminally ill cancer patients using the Palliative Prognostic Index. *Palliative Medicine*, 15(5), 419–424.

Moss, A.H., Lunney, J.R., Culp, S., *et al.* (2010). Prognostic significance of the "surprise" question in cancer patients. *Journal of Palliative Medicine*, 13(7), 837–840.

Mozaffarian, D., Anker, S., Anand, I., *et al.* (2007). Prediction of mode of death in heart failure: the Seattle Heart Failure Model. *Circulation*, 116(4), 360–362.

Naylor, C., Cerqueira, L., Costa-Paiva, L.H.S., Costa, J.V., Conde, D.M., and Pinto-Neto, A.M. (2010). Survival of women with cancer in palliative care: use of the palliative prognostic score in a population of Brazilian women. *Journal of Pain & Symptom Management*, 39(1), 69–75.

O'Donnell, D. E., Aaron, S., Bourbeau, J., *et al.* (2007). Canadian Thoracic Society recommendations for management of chronic obstructive pulmonary disease—2007 update. *Canadian Respiratory Journal*, 14(Suppl. B), 5B–32B.

O'Donovan, A., Tomiyama, A.J., Lin, J., *et al.* (2012). Stress appraisals and cellular aging: a key role for anticipatory threat in the relationship between psychological stress and telomere length. *Brain, Behavior, and Immunity*, 26(4), 573–579.

Oga, T., Nishimura, K., Tsukino, M., Sato, S., and Hajiro, T. (2003). Analysis of the factors related to mortality in chronic obstructive pulmonary disease: role of exercise capacity and health status. *American Journal of Respiratory and Critical Care Medicine*, 167(4), 544–549.

Ohde, S., Hayashi, A., Takahasi, O., *et al.* (2011). A 2-week prognostic prediction model for terminal cancer patients in a palliative care unit at a Japanese general hospital. *Palliative Medicine*, 25(2), 170–176.

Oxenham, P. and Cornbleet, M.A. (1998). Accuracy of prediction of survival by different professional groups in a hospice. *Palliative Medicine*, 12, 117–118.

Parker, S. M., Clayton, J.M., Hancock, K., *et al.* (2007). A systematic review of prognostic/end-of-life communication with adults in the advanced stages of a life-limiting illness: patient/caregiver preferences for the content, style, and timing of information. *Journal of Pain & Symptom Management*, 34(1), 81–93.

Piepers, S., van den Berg, J.P., Kalmijn, S., *et al.* (2006). Effect of non-invasive ventilation on survival, quality of life, respiratory function and cognition: a review of the literature. *Amyotrophic Lateral Sclerosise*, 7(4), 195–200.

Pirovano, M., Maltoni, M., Nanni, O., *et al.* (1999). A new palliative prognostic score: a first step for the staging of terminally ill cancer patients. Italian Multicenter and Study Group on Palliative Care. *Journal of Pain & Symptom Management*, 17(4), 231–239.

Rakowski, D.A., Caillard, S., Agodoa, L.Y., and Abbott, K.C. (2006). Dementia as a predictor of mortality in dialysis patients. *Clinical Journal of the American Society of Nephrology*, 1(5), 1000–1005.

Read, W.L., Tierney, R.M., Page, N.C., *et al.* (2004). Differential prognostic impact of comorbidity. *Journal of Clinical Oncology*, 22(15), 3099–3103.

Reisberg, B. (1988). Functional assessment staging (FAST). *Psychopharmacology Bulletin*, 24(4), 653–659.

Reuben, D.B., Mor, V., and Hiris, J. (1988). Clinical symptoms and length of survival in patients with terminal cancer. *Archives of Internal Medicine*, 148(7), 1586–1591.

Sackett, D.L., Haynes, R.B., Guyatt, G.H., and Tugwell, P. (1991). *Clinical Epidemiology. A Basic Science for Clinical Medicine*. Boston, MA: Little, Brown and Company.

Satin, J.R., Linden, W., and Phillips, M.J. (2009). Depression as a predictor of disease progression and mortality in cancer patients: a meta-analysis. *Cancer*, 115(22), 5349–5361.

Schonwetter, R.S., Han, B., Small, B.J., Martin, B., Tope, K., and Haley, W.E. (2003). Predictors of six-month survival among patients with dementia: an evaluation of hospice Medicare guidelines. *American Journal of Hospice & Palliative Care*, 20(2), 105–113.

Schonwetter, R.S., Soendker, S., Perron, V., *et al.* (1998). Review of Medicare's proposed hospice eligibility criteria for select noncancer patients. *American Journal of Hospice and Palliative Care*, 15(3), 155–8.

Selwyn, P.A. and Forstein, M. (2003). Overcoming the false dichotomy of curative vs palliative care for late-stage HIV/AIDS: "let me live the way I want to live, until I can't". *Journal of the American Medical Association*, 290(6), 806–814.

Seow, H., Barbera, L., Sutradhar, R., *et al.* (2011). Trajectory of performance status and symptom scores for patients with cancer during the last six months of life. *Journal of Clinical Oncology*, 29(9), 1151–1158.

Shadbolt, B., Barresi, J., and Craft, P. (2002). Self-rated health as a predictor of survival among patients with advanced cancer. *Journal of Clinical Oncology*, 20(10), 2514–2519.

Shavelle, R.M., Paculdo, D.R., Kush, S.J., Mannino, D.M., and Strauss, D.J. (2009). Life expectancy and years of life lost in chronic obstructive pulmonary disease: findings from the NHANES III Follow-up Study. *International Journal of Chronic Obstructive Pulmonary Disease*, 4, 137–148.

Shaw, A.S., Ampong, M.A., Rio, A., *et al.* (2006). Survival of patients with ALS following institution of enteral feeding is related to pre-procedure oximetry: a retrospective review of 98 patients in a single centre. *Amyotrophic Lateral Sclerosis*, 7(1), 16–21.

Shoesmith, C.L., Findlater, K., Rowe, A., and Strong, M.J. (2007). Prognosis of amyotrophic lateral sclerosis with respiratory onset. *Journal of Neurology, Neurosurgery & Psychiatry*, 78(6), 629–631.

Soares, M., Salluh, J.I., Ferreira, C.G., Luiz, R.R., Spector, N., and Rocco, J.R. (2005). Impact of two different comorbidity measures on the 6-month mortality of critically ill cancer patients. *Intensive Care Medicine*, 31(3), 408–415.

Solano, J.P., Gomes, B., and Higginson, I.J. (2006). A comparison of symptom prevalence in far advanced cancer, AIDS, heart disease, chronic obstructive pulmonary disease and renal disease. *Journal of Pain & Symptom Management*, 31(1), 58–69.

Steinhauser, K., Christakis, N.A., Clipp, E., McNeilly, M., McIntyre, L., and Tulsky, J. (2000). Factors considered important at the end of life by patients, family, physicians, and other care providers. *Journal of the American Medical Association*, 284(19), 2476–2482.

Steyerberg, E. and Harrell, F. (2002). Statistical models for prognostication. In M. Max and J. Lynn (eds.) *Symptom Research: Methods and Opportunities*. [Online] Available at: <http://painconsortium.nih.gov/symptomresearch/>.

St George's, University of London (2011). *The PiPS Prognosticator*. [Online] Available at: <http://www.pips.sgul.ac.uk>.

Stockler, M.R., Tattersall, M.H., Boyer, M.J., Clarke, S.J. Beale, P.J., and Simes, R.J. (2006). Disarming the guarded prognosis: predicting survival in newly referred patients with incurable cancer. *British Journal of Cancer*, 94(2), 208–212.

Stone, C.A., Tiernan, E., and Dooley, B.A. (2008). Prospective validation of the palliative prognostic index in patients with cancer. *Journal of Pain & Symptom Management*, 35(6), 617–622.

Suh, S.-Y., Choi, Y.S., Shim, J.Y., *et al.* (2010). Construction of a new, objective prognostic score for terminally ill cancer patients: a multicenter study. *Supportive Care in Cancer*, 18(2), 151–157.

Tamburini, M., Brunelli, C., Rosso, S., and Ventafridda, V. (1996). Prognostic value of quality of life scores in terminal cancer patients. *Journal of Pain & Symptom Management*, 11, 32–41.

Tannenberger, S., Malavasi, I., Mariano, P., Pannuti, F., and Strocchi, E. (2002). Planning palliative or terminal care: the dilemma of doctors' prognoses in terminally ill cancer patients. *Annals of Oncology*, 13, 1319–1323.

Tarumi, Y., Watanabe, S.M., Lau, F., *et al.* (2011). Evaluation of the Palliative Prognostic Score (PaP) and routinely collected clinical data in prognostication of survival for patients referred to a palliative care consultation service in an acute care hospital. *Journal of Pain & Symptom Management*, 42(3), 419–431.

Tavares, F. (2010). Is the B12/CRP index more accurate than you at predicting life expectancy in advanced cancer patients? *Journal of Pain & Symptom Management*, 40(1), e12–13.

Teno, J.M., Gozalo, P.L., Lee, I.C., *et al.* (2011). Does hospice improve quality of care for persons dying from dementia? *Journal of the American Geriatrics Society*, 59(8), 1531–1536.

Teno, J.M., Harrell, F.E.,Jr., Knaus, W., *et al.* (2000). Prediction of survival for older hospitalized patients: the HELP survival model. Hospitalized Elderly Longitudinal Project. *Journal of the American Geriatrics Society*, 48(5 Suppl.), S16–24.

The, A.M., Hak, T., Koeter, G., and van Der Wal, G. (2000). Collusion in doctor-patient communication about imminent death: an ethnographic study. *BMJ*, 321(7273), 1376–1381.

The SUPPORT Principal Investigators (1995). A controlled trial to improve care for seriously ill hospitalized patients. The study to understand prognoses and preferences for outcomes and risks of treatments (SUPPORT). *Journal of the American Medical Association*, 274(20), 1591–1598.

University of Washington (n.d.). *Seattle Heart Failure Model*. [Online] Available at: <http://www.seattleheartfailuremodel.org>.

Vigano, A., Bruera, E., Jhangri, G.S., Newman, S.C., Fields, A.L., and Suarez-Almazor, M.E. (2000). Clinical survival predictors in patients with advanced cancer. *Archives of Internal Medicine*, 160(6), 861–868.

Vij, B., Stabler, S.M., Thaler, H.T., and Glare, P.A. (2012). External validation of the simple prognostic score in a palliative care clinic at a comprehensive cancer center. *Journal of Clinical Oncology, 2012 ASCO Annual Meeting Proceedings (Post-Meeting Edition)* 30(15 Suppl.), e19566.

Walter, L.C., Brand, R.J., Counsell, S.R., *et al.* (2001). Development and validation of a prognostic index for 1-year mortality in older adults after hospitalization. *Journal of the American Medical Association*, 285(23), 2987–2994.

Wildman, M.J., Sanderson, C., Groves, J., *et al.* (2007). Implications of prognostic pessimism in patients with chronic obstructive pulmonary disease (COPD) or asthma admitted to intensive care in the UK within the COPD and asthma outcome study (CAOS multicentre observational cohort study. *BMJ*, 335(7630), 1132.

Wong, C.F., McCarthy, M., Howse, M.L., and Williams, P.S. (2007). Factors affecting survival in advanced chronic kidney disease patients who choose not to receive dialysis. *Renal Failure*, 29(6), 653–659.

Wright, A.A., Zhang, B., Ray, A., *et al.* (2008). Associations between end-of-life discussions, patient mental health, medical care near death, and caregiver bereavement adjustment. *Journal of the American Medical Association*, 300(14), 1665–1673.

Yourman, L.C., Lee, S.J., Schonberg, M.A., Widera, E.W., and Smith, A.K. (2012). Prognostic indices for older adults: a systematic review. *Journal of the American Medical Association*, 307(2), 182–192.

Yourman, L.C., Lee, S.J., Schonberg, M.A., Widera, E.W., and Smith, A.K. (n.d.). *ePrognosis. Estimating Prognosis for Elders*. [Online] Available at: <http://www.eprognosis.com>.

Yun, Y.H., Heo, D.S., Heo, B.Y., TYoo, T.W., Bae, J.M., and Ahn, S.H. (2001). Development of terminal cancer prognostic score as an index in terminally ill cancer patients. *Oncology Reports*, 8(4), 795–800.

2.4

Defining a 'good' death

Karen E. Steinhauser and James A. Tulsky

Introduction to defining a 'good' death

Woody Allen often commented that he was not afraid to die, but did not want to be there when it happened (Allen, 1983). This is emblematic of our society's ambivalence towards the notion of a 'good death' (Rousseau, 1997; Steinhauser et al., 2001). Its inherent irony is instructive for palliative care clinicians. While death may be inevitable, for patients, it is rarely the goal. Therefore, naming deaths 'good' or 'bad' should be met with caution.

There is a long historical and literary tradition discussing the 'good death'. In some of the best known work on evolution in Western attitudes towards death, social historian Philippe Aries uses cemetery iconography, notary records, wills, art, and literature to explore changing patterns in cultural norms of dying and death over the last 1500 years (Aries, 1980). For example, we learn that contemporary preferences for sudden death or death during sleep stand in contrast to previous eras in which populations literally prayed, in the Anglican Great Litany, not to die, 'suddenly and unprepared' (Aries, 1980; Vig and Pearlman, 2004). Aries' work demonstrates the plasticity of how we view circumstances of death and the relativism of the terminology 'good' and 'bad'.

Extraordinary variation exists in the social construction of the meaning of dying and death and the social organization and cultural norms surrounding end of life (Aries, 1980; Hart et al., 1998; Seale, 1998; Kim and Lee, 2003; DelVecchio Good et al., 2004; Long, 2004; Radley, 2004; Hirai et al., 2006). Recent work describing end-of-life activities in diverse regions such as Japan, North America, the Netherlands and Papau New Guinea, and spanning contemporary, classical, and biblical eras (Seale and van der Geest, 2004) finds that humans create and enact cultural scripts in ways that describe death as either 'good' or 'bad' (Seale and van der Geest, 2004).

While these cited works provide in-depth sociocultural and historical exploration of how we define the meaning of death, the focus of this chapter is on the reappearance in the last 40 years of attempts to define a good death in the medical context, the empirical investigation of the construct, the clinical implications of using the terminology 'good death', and an alternative framework for language defining preferences at end of life.

Context of contemporary exploration of 'good death'

In 1908, William Osler conducted a study of 486 deaths at Johns Hopkins Hospital reporting that 90 patients experienced pain, 11 anxiety, and for the majority, death was 'nothing more than falling asleep' (Kring, 2006). Deaths in this era occurred all across the life course spectrum and were the result of either old age or catastrophic illness with limited medical intervention capable of extending life. Despite the site of Osler's investigation, the majority of deaths at that time did not happen in the hospital.

Rather, deaths in the nineteenth and early twentieth centuries occurred primarily at home with support of family, church, and community (Sudnow, 1967; Aries, 1980; Hart et al., 1998). However, by the second half of the twentieth century the primary site of death had shifted to the hospital. Moreover, by the 1960s, the landscape of death in Western culture had changed dramatically as medicine had experienced a variety of therapeutic and technological revolutions resulting in the capacity to extend life, including antibiotic therapies, artificial nutrition and cardiopulmonary resuscitation. In this latter twentieth-century hospital setting, death's meaning was narrowed primarily to a physiological event. As such, death was defined less as an expected and natural part of the life course and more as a failure of medical technology and intervention (Byock, 1996).

By the late 1950s, social reformers, such as Cicely Saunders, began to critique conventional medical care for dying patients, arguing that hospitals lacked both the specific expertise in palliation of symptoms as well as the multidisciplinary perspective that attended to social, psychological, and spiritual aspects of care (Saunders, 1978). In 1967, after returning to medical school to supplement her nursing, social work, and divinity training, she opened St. Christopher's hospice as a multidisciplinary care centre that emphasized palliative versus curative therapies and promoted quality of life over quantity of life.

Amidst this social reform movement, in-depth inquiry of death and dying began to appear in the medical, nursing, and social science literatures. Seminal qualitative accounts were published in the few years following the opening of St. Christopher's. Prominent sociologists Glaser, Strauss, and Sudnow were among the first to refocus study on end of life and to conceptualize trajectories of dying (Glaser and Strauss, 1965; Sudnow, 1967). Emerging from a tradition of grounded theory, Glaser and Strauss became participant observers in hospital settings and described four 'contexts of awareness surrounding the dying experience: closed awareness, suspicious awareness, mutual pretense, and open awareness' (Glaser and Strauss, 1965). Their conceptualization reflected an era during which patients often were not informed of terminal diagnoses or poor prognoses. Their sociological critiques were heavily counter-cultural in their scrutiny of the power dynamics of the paternalistic hospital culture.

A few years later, Elizabeth Kubler-Ross called further attention to the unmet needs of patients and the personal evolution of people coming to terms with a terminal diagnosis (Kubler-Ross,

1969). Though the stages of grief—denial, anger, bargaining, depression, and acceptance—were never tested empirically, her theory of dying and death is perhaps the best known and most frequently cited to this day. In fact, after her work, investigation of death and dying would receive scant attention until the 1990s.

The subtext of many of these investigations was that conventional medical care settings often played host to 'bad' deaths, typified by excessive use of technology, with patient and family wishes ignored, lack of patient knowledge and autonomy in decision-making, the patient reduced to a physiological system versus whole person, and quality of life devalued.

The hospice movement, both in its British foundations and its importation to the United States, arose within this context and was part of a larger 'death with dignity' movement of the 1960s and 1970s. Those involved in hospice and early palliative care worked to reclaim the experience of dying and death beyond a biomedical event. In this context, a 'good' death was the obverse of the previously described situations. The goals were to increase awareness of end of life as a part of a natural life course and to acknowledge dying patients as whole persons in the context of fuller lives lived, as well as family and community nexus. 'Good death' connoted a model of care more closely matching patient and family preferences, with the terminology designed to serve as a vision of improved experience for dying persons.

Empirical investigations of a 'good death'

Despite the popularity and growth of the hospice movement, widespread, systematic attempts to define a 'good death' empirically did not appear in the medical literature until after the publication of the Study to Understand Prognosis and Preferences for the Outcomes and Risks of Treatment (SUPPORT) findings. This large multi-site study documented poor care of dying patients and their families in five top US medical centres and redefined the landscape of end-of-life and palliative care (The SUPPORT Principal Investigators, 1995). SUPPORT described hospitalized patients dying in pain, without their wishes known, and in isolation. The results provided empirical evidence of what was wrong with hospital deaths.

Care of dying patients became a priority in the United States and organizations such as the American Medical Association, the Veterans Health Administration, and The Robert Wood Johnson Foundation committed funding to improving education and quality of care (Field and Cassel, 1997). Efforts to develop and evaluate hospice and palliative care became expanded in US and international journals. If clinicians and administrators were to provide quality of care and quality of life at the end of life, they must first define quality. If SUPPORT had given empirical evidence of 'bad' deaths, what was the empirical evidence regarding the definition of a 'good' death?

In the 17 ensuing years, over 400 Medline articles include the construct 'good death'. A smaller subset of independent studies have attempted to define the construct through analyses of qualitative and quantitative data gathered from patients, family members, and health-care providers. These have been reviewed systematically in both the medical and nursing literatures (Morris et al., 1986; King and Bushwick, 1994; McNamara et al., 1994; Asch et al., 1995; Layde et al., 1995; Low and Payne, 1996; Payne et al., 1996; Lynn et al., 1997; Ellington and Fuller, 1998; Emanuel and Emanuel, 1998; Singer, Martin, and Kelner, 1999; Steinhauser

et al., 2000a, 2000b; Kristjanson et al., 2001; Mak, 2001; Cohen and Leis, 2002; Curtis et al., 2002; Hanson et al., 2002; Hopkinson and Hallett, 2002; Masson, 2002; Pierson et al., 2002; Ganzini et al., 2003; Kim and Lee, 2003; Tong et al., 2003; DelVecchio Good et al., 2004; Leichtentritt, 2004; Long, 2004; McNamara, 2004; Vig and Pearlman, 2004; Borbasi et al., 2005, 2006; Ferrell, 2005; Goldsteen et al., 2006; Hirai et al., 2006; Kring, 2006; Rietjens et al., 2006; Miyashita et al., 2007a; Hales et al., 2008). While each study lends a unique population or conceptual nuance, some common features exist among attempts to define a 'good death'.

Mutlidimensionality

The social reformers propelling the 'good death' movement of the 1960s and 1970s were responding to the narrowing of the patient experience to the biomedical realm. Recent empirical investigation suggests that perhaps the most important feature to recognize about a 'good death' is its multidimensional nature.

In 2008, Hales et al. reviewed 17 studies defining quality at end of life (Hales et al., 2008). Five of the studies were conducted with health-care providers only; five were conducted among only patient populations, three were studies of non-patient, non-health-care provider populations; and the remaining included both patients and or families, and providers. Seven common broad domains were found: *physical experience, psychological experience, social experience, spiritual or existential experience, the nature of health care, life closure and death preparation,* and *circumstances of death*.

Expectedly, *pain and symptom management* was the most commonly identified theme. Yet, variation exists in how individuals prefer this domain to be addressed. For example, some patients may wish to balance analgesia with lucidity to allow meaningful personal interactions, and thus may tolerate some pain to achieve a higher state of alertness, if necessary. More recent studies suggest that physical dimensions include not only pain and symptoms but attention to *functional status*, which is highly correlated with continued independence and quality of life (Walke et al., 2007).

This body of work confirms that the physiological aspects of end-of-life experience are only a point of departure in overall definitions of a 'good death' or quality at end of life (Steinhauser et al., 2000a). Attention to emotional or *psychological* and *social* well-being are crucial. Patients experience their illness living a variety of roles and inter-relationships that need to be sustained as part of whole-person care. Interestingly, earlier sociological theory proposed that dying patients, and older adults, in general, experienced a natural 'disengagement' as end of life loomed. However, this theory has been debunked by empirical evidence showing the desire for and power of continued role engagement. Although dying patients usually experience physical decline or limitation, they may experience growth in social and emotional areas.

Similarly, attention to *spiritual* or transcendent aspects of experience are reported as central to quality experience and hold opportunity for growth (Daaleman and Nease, 1994; Byock, 1996; Cohen and Leis, 2002). This domain may be expressed in traditional religious terms, via connection with nature or as overall sense of meaning and purpose in life. There is some evidence of it increasing in importance as death nears (Byock, 1996). Of note, the absence of this domain in traditional quality of life measures was a main factor limiting their reliability and validity when applied to the context of dying.

While physical, social, psychological, and spiritual domains had been predicted by some of the pre-empirical literature, several new domains emerged from empirical investigation. These include *preparation for death or end of life, nature of health care, and life completion*. In contrast to settings of 'closed awareness' reported as common in the 1960s, 'good death' investigations of the 1990s and early 2000s suggested many patients with advanced serious illness wanted an opportunity to know what to expect about the course of their illness, to put personal affairs in order, to make financial arrangements and personal business, to not be a burden to family, to prepare their families for the future, and, for some, to plan one's own funeral. It is important to note the contradiction found in the literature whereby populations within the same study report valuing 'dying in their sleep', 'dying suddenly', and 'being prepared' (Vig and Pearlman, 2004).

These studies show that *preparation* is not limited to patients. Families also need to be prepared for what to expect about the course of illness and decision-making.

> I can't tell you how many times, working in the emergency room, [that I saw] families [take a patient home]; this patient was going to die at home. And, when the last breath came, the families panicked. They brought the patient into the emergency room and went through the whole process [resuscitation]. Preparing the family, assessing what they actually know, and figuring out what you have to teach them is essential. [Nurse] (Steinhauser et al., 2000b)

Finally, some have also described the importance of provider preparation, coming to terms with their own fears about mortality and the emotions generated in caring for those who die (Steinhauser et al., 2000a).

Another less expected domain revealed in the 'good death' studies was the *nature of health care*. This domain focused on issues such as the appropriateness of level of technological intervention—levels in keeping with patient and family wishes, as well as communication with health-care providers, knowing how and where to get answers to questions, and overall relationship with the provider (Steinhauser et al., 2000a, 2000b; Perkins et al., 2008). The latter issue of relationship included maintaining patient dignity and treating patients as whole persons rather than as diseases.

Finally, the domain of *life completion* has been central to many investigations conceptualizing a 'good' death (Steinhauser et al., 2000b; Vig and Pearlman, 2004; Hirai et al., 2006; Rietjens et al., 2006). Attributes of completion include life review, closure, coming to peace, resolving conflicts, contributing to others, spending time with family and friends, and saying good-bye. Completion may involve personal reflection or individual spiritual practice, or may be more explicitly communal including family or a wider social circle. Of course many organized religions denote particular rites of spiritual completion for both the dying and the mourner. As with all domains, cues regarding specific expression should come from the patient or family. Within this domain, the attribute of contributing to others reminds family members and providers the importance not only of what patients may need to receive but also what they need to give to experience wholeness as they face the end of their lives.

Importance of role

Studies attempting to define a positive end-of-life experience reveal the importance of role in perception of what constitutes 'good'. For example, studies show that physician perspectives tend to be more narrowly biomedical. And the data suggest a discrepancy in physician versus family and patient ratings of the importance of spirituality and completion attributes such as prayer (Byock, 1996; Cohen and Leis, 2002). In one survey asking participants to rank order nine attributes of end of life, families' and patients' rankings of being at peace and freedom from pain were statistically equal in importance (Steinhauser et al., 2000a). In contrast, physicians rated coming to peace as a distant third. Patients also were more likely to rate higher the importance of mental alertness and a desire not to be a burden to family or society.

In this same study, non-physician providers were more likely than patients to rate as important, 'talking about the meaning of dying'. Family members were more likely than patients to rate the importance of discussing personal fears or meeting with clergy. Again, it is instructive to take cues from patients about how they want to discuss this issue. Qualitative findings suggest patients may wish to discuss purpose and life more than meaning of death.

In a survey of hospice nurses definitions of a 'good death' McNamara and colleagues found that definitions of 'bad' deaths included those in which the patient did not internalize hospice philosophy, leaving staff frustrated (McNamara et al., 1994). Non-internalization included not accepting the imminence of death, allowing non-palliative therapies to continue, and the family wanting 'everything done' despite terminal diagnoses. Such circumstances were thought to compromise a peaceful 'natural' death.

Importance of culture

In addition to individual and family variation in preferences for end of life, cultural scripts also predominate (see Chapter 2.5). While this is expanded upon more fully elsewhere in this textbook, studies relating to minority and majority population variation suggest a desire for clinician awareness of cultural issues, particularly heightened attention to the role spiritual beliefs play in decision-making, and attention to individual interpretation of minority culture scripts (Tong et al., 2003). Within the US population, a growing literature has demonstrated increased preference for life-sustaining therapies among Latino and African American populations (Tulsky et al., 1997). However, in one study African Americans were more likely to 'want all available treatments' but less likely than Caucasian participants to want to be 'connected to machines' (Steinhauser et al., 2000a). These varying responses among groups sensitized providers to patient and family differential interpretation of medical jargon, and true variation in preferences for treatment. As many sources have noted, when working with populations of patients traditionally denied access to care, withdrawing and withholding treatments are met with understandable apprehension.

Much of the empirical work defining a 'good death' has involved English-speaking Western populations in which individual decision-making and autonomy is culturally rewarded. However, more recently, a number of studies have explored the meaning of a 'good death' in a variety of cultural contexts (Munn and Zimmerman, 2006; Rietjens et al., 2006; Miyashita et al., 2007, 2008; Sanjo et al., 2007; Yao et al., 2007; Spathis and Booth, 2008; Murakawa and Nihei, 2009; Nelson et al., 2009; Iranmanesh et al., 2011; Wilches-Gutierrez et al., 2012; Wilson et al., 2009a, 2009b).

For example, Asian cultures with normative scripts including notions of filial piety will display markedly different preferences for treatment and communication on the part of patients and families. A noteworthy study of Korean attitudes towards patient autonomy showed that while 42% of respondents knew of their terminal condition, approximately 22% made treatment decisions primarily on their own with approximately 36% leaving their treatment decisions to others. Higher individual decision-making was associated with lower quality of life and quality of death scores, including assessments of physical and psychological comfort (Mo et al., 2012). More familial or communal decision-making models, though prevalent, are less well represented in the research literature, and therefore deserving of future study.

A study of Mexican culture found increased mortality rates around holidays, such as Christmas and All Saints Day, and accompanying higher ratings of quality of dying at these times (Wilches-Gutierrez et al., 2012). Respondents discussed the belief in a greater presence of religious deities on such holidays, ensuring a more 'beautiful death'. Such interpretations stand in contrast to other cultural scripts which consider holiday deaths to be imbued with a greater sense of loss. Social construction of the meaning of death is varied and often in direct opposition to the palliative care's normative views of grief and loss.

Importance of timing

In addition to cultural variation, clinicians must take note of the importance of timeframe in patient and family preferences. The literature reveals little consensus on what time frame constitutes the end of life. Furthermore, preferences will likely differ by stage of illness and evolve over time with definitions of 'good experience' living with advanced serious illness being distinct from 'good dying', as distinct from a 'good death'. For example, immediately after a diagnosis of metastatic disease *preparation* may include discussions of possible courses of treatment, the combination of curative and palliative therapies, and helping patients remain integrated with normal work and social roles. As illness progresses, preparation may include discussions of decreasing the use of curative therapies and increasing palliative approaches, discussion of hospice, and increased attention to issues of completion. As dying becomes imminent, preparation may involve working with the family about expectations of care, location of care, and education regarding the very end of life.

Developmental stage

Most 'good death' studies have been done within adult populations. The Initiative for Pediatric Palliative Care and the National Hospice and Palliative Care Organization, among others, have spearheaded efforts to improve care of children at the end of life (Feudtner, 2004; Welch, 2008). Towards that end, investigators have gathered perspectives of families and providers to identify whether childhood death can ever be considered 'good', what elements might be associated with better and worse scenarios, and whether these are applicable to the nearly 55 000 childhood deaths in the United States (Feudtner, 2004; Welch, 2008). Full reviews of efforts to improve paediatric palliative care are covered elsewhere in the textbook. We limit our brief discussion to definitions of the construct of good death.

Some of the domains considered essential to 'good' end-of-life experiences in children are similar to those found in adult populations, such as pain and symptom management, emotional and spiritual support, maximizing quality of life, need for family respite, continuity of care across settings, and making care match individual values and preferences (Feudtner, 2004; Welch, 2008). Other domains are similar to adult populations but entail special considerations due to developmental and population complexities of paediatrics. For example, Feudtner outlined the importance of addressing the total population in need; in paediatrics that may include those children born with the expectation of impending death, those who acquire illnesses after birth, and those with a sudden death due to trauma (Feudtner, 2004). The leading causes of death after the age of 1 year include unintentional injuries followed by congenital abnormalities, malignant neoplasms, and intentional injuries. Research also shows the importance of collaborative decision-making and supportive decision-making which in paediatrics includes the family as well as informing and involving children to the extent to which they are developmentally capable and desiring involvement. An additional domain of 'managing trade-offs adroitly' refers to the potential caregiver tension between a desire to limit suffering and take therapeutic risks given a child's age, life yet to be lived, and biological resilience (Feudtner, 2004). Additionally, investigators note the importance of maximizing safety and effectiveness, largely around polypharmacy, and finally, attending to timely introduction of bereavement services. The latter domain acknowledges that nearly all paediatric deaths are viewed by familial caregivers as untimely, adding to the complexity of grief. The sense of a death being on or off time in an expected life course applies to most deaths not experienced during old age. While investigation of the unique developmental needs are obvious in paediatric populations, the field would benefit from additional research examining social construction of the meaning of death across the lifespan and various adult developmental stages (Erikson, 1982).

Importance of diagnosis

Early hospice and palliative care populations were comprised, primarily, of patients with cancer. As such, literary, cultural, and empirical definitions of a 'good death' grew from the experience of living and dying from advanced cancer. Realizing the limitations to generalizability for broader end-of-life populations, investigators began seeking the perspectives of those living with a variety of life limiting illnesses (Steinhauser et al., 2000a, 2000b; Pierson et al., 2002; Walke et al., 2007; Chattoo and Ahmad, 2008; Chattoo and Atkin, 2009; Kaufman, 2011). Though sample size often precluded in-depth investigation of experiences unique to various illness types and disease trajectories, more recent work has been designed specifically to learn about the particular constructions of a 'good death' for those with congestive heart failure, chronic obstructive pulmonary disease, dementia, end-stage renal disease among others (Russ et al., 2007; Gott et al., 2008; Spathis and Booth, 2008). Two studies in heart disease (Gott et al., 2008; Chattoo and Ahmad, 2008; Chattoo and Atkin, 2009) demonstrated that both the heightened levels of uncertainty and increased possibility of sudden death among those with congestive heart failure, posed a challenge to conventional palliative care beliefs regarding values of patient 'open awareness' and even autonomy and individuality. They revealed conflict between cardiologists' culture of 'living with heart failure' and palliative care's attention to 'dying with heart failure' calling for different and more nuanced engagement with patient and illness uncertainty. Similarly, research in patients with chronic obstructive pulmonary disease highlighted notions of uncertainty and reported definitions of 'good' end-of-life care not precluding life-sustaining interventions.

Location of death

The seven domains listed earlier often are referred to under the general rubric of the biopsychosocial and spiritual model of care. The model, as just described, enjoys significant empirical support. In addition, two recent studies expand the notion of elements that contribute to the quality of end of life for patients and families. Casarett and colleagues highlighted advanced cancer patients' preferences for 'supportive services' even over traditional hospice services (Casarett et al., 2008a). Supportive services included vouchers for practical assistance at home, transportation, peer support, meal delivery, case management, and family care. Perkins and colleagues emphasize additional supportive services such as emergency contacts and case management (Perkins et al., 2008). While much of the 'good death' literature was built on investigation into improving care of hospitalized patients, we must recognize that a majority of care in the dying trajectory occurs in the outpatient, home, and community settings. Therefore, newer models of good end-of-life experience must expand beyond the individual inpatient model of care.

The most recent research extending investigation beyond hospital end-of-life experiences has focused on defining a 'good death' in long-term care settings. Studies identify domains such as adequacy of staffing, facility environment and size, and the capacity of staff to 'be there' for residents and family (Munn and Zimmerman, 2006). Other studies identify the importance of creating 'family-like' bonds between staff and residents and family and improved communication. In this setting, definitions of a good death confirm previously identified interpersonal and more quality of life domains and extend those domains to include facets of resident and family experience directly related to quality of care.

In addition, a literature trend is the transition from identifying what constitutes a 'good death' to implementation of such definitions. One of the broadest examples is the efforts by the Department of Veterans Affairs to introduce and fund policy and clinical care initiatives to ensure quality end-of-life care for veterans across their nationwide health-care system (Edes et al., 2007; Casarett et al., 2008b). In these efforts, researchers wrestle with measuring the interconnected yet distinct concepts of 'good death', quality of life at end of life, and quality of care at end of life (Hales et al., 2010).

Opportunity for growth

Ira Byock has described the benefit of adopting a life cycle model when providing care at the end of life (Byock, 1996). The medical model begins assessment and treatment by generating a problem list. From the time a patient presents with symptoms, the clinical interviews and choice of diagnostic testing is determined by these problems. While this approach brings focus and efficiency to diagnostic testing and treatment, it is best suited to acute medicine and has limitations when applied to the context of care of incurably ill patients. Incurably ill patients surely are met with the daunting challenges of physical symptom exacerbation and functional decline; however, a purely problem-based approach offers less guidance in helping patients navigate areas of experience in which

they may experience improvement or growth. A life cycle model assumes death is the natural end of a life course. And, building on the work of human development by Erikson, Bulter, and Cassell, Byock notes the expected developmental tasks associated with this phase of life (Cassell, 1973; Butler, 1974, 1980; Byock, 1996). These tasks include attention to life review, resolution of conflict, forgiveness, acceptance and generativity. Most importantly, this framework allows one to conceptualize end of life, like other phases of the life course, as holding opportunity for growth rather than only the decline predicted by the medical model. Growth will most likely occur in emotional and spiritual domains (and areas like preparation and completion) and is hypothesized to account for discrepancies in patient versus observer ratings of quality of life.

Measuring a 'good death' and quality of death and dying

Attempts to measure a 'good death' can be found among assessment tools specifically reflecting this name, (e.g. The Good Death Questionnaire, The Good Death Inventory) and also in a larger body of work assessing the quality of dying and death (Hales et al., 2008). A recent review showed extensive variation in measures rigor with regard to design and reliability and validity. Of the 18 measures reviewed, half reported no reliability of validity information, five were single-item measures, and fewer than half reported definitions of quality of death and dying. All measures were designed for retrospective accounts of family or professional caregivers. This is the soundest way of assessing last days of life and moment of death in populations with significant percentages unable to respond, yet requires additional efforts to understand direction and strength of proxy bias among domains as well as surrogate characteristics (Steinhauser et al., 2002; Hales et al., 2008). Additionally, most research demonstrates few measures allow for weighting response preferences to match individual circumstances of changing values over time. Measures of sensitivity to change over time also is an area in need of refinement.

Because this chapter focuses on definition and measurement of a 'good death', we have not discussed the vast literature on quality of life or quality of care at the end of life. The former is best suited to periods in the palliative care trajectory preceding periods of imminent dying and allows for real-time, prospective patient-rated assessments (Steinhauser, 2005). Quality of care may rely on patient, family, or provider perspective as well as administrative and organizational data of clinical benchmarks (Ferrell, 2005).

Clinical implications of the term 'good death'

In this article we have reported on research which sought to define a 'good' death. Yet, it is important to discuss the clinical implications of using such language. In one of our studies, 'In search of a good death: observations of patients, families and providers' we concluded that there is no one 'good death' (Steinhauser et al., 2000b). Rather, each end-of-life experience is a process to be negotiated and renegotiated in the context of that patient's and family's values, preferences, and life course. We were strongly cautioned by nurses, for example, that it was important to know there was 'no one right way to die' and warned against implying to patients that 'you're not dying the right way, because you're not dying the way we think you should'.

While early hospice founders used language of a 'good' death to rally reformers to a new vision of care, in recent years the language of a 'good' death often has taken on a denotation of specific expectations of what should occur at the end of life. The zeal driving the early movement has risked imposing a sense of a 'right way' to die. Its components include being free of pain, surrounded by family, free of conflict, acceptance death, stopping curative treatment, being at peace, and preferably dying at home. While those may be components many or most would define as positive, the implication is that one can define a good death, and should achieve it. Unfortunately, though propelled by positive intentions, such definition risks imposing an unintended paternalism. Furthermore, data of patient and family preferences at end of life exhibit far more nuance and variation.

For example, a national survey revealed that only about 50% of respondents ranked dying at home as important (Steinhauser et al., 2000a). In related qualitative research linked to the survey, while many valued dying at home, other patients and families described circumstances of caregiver frailty, superstition, or fear of bad memories as dissuading them from wanting the death to occur at home. Family members and non-physician health-care providers were significantly more likely than patients to identify 'talking about the meaning of dying' as important. And though coming to peace often is highly valued by patients, working to resolve conflicts can be complex and contain periods of great uncertainty, for patients, families, and providers hoping to guide them. And, by the time of death, everything is not always resolved. Again, there is caution to those working with dying patients that these uncertainties and lack of resolution do not represent failures on the parts of patients and families, but merely illustrate rich variation in the way people live their entire lives.

Health-care providers are most likely to be challenged by patients whose conception of a good death includes the use of medically non-beneficial treatments in the setting of clearly imminent death (e.g. parenteral nutrition or attempted cardiopulmonary resuscitation). In some cases, such preferences are reflective of unresolved loss or other emotional distress, and the best response may be empathy and support, which often leads to a change of treatment course. For other patients, these views are rooted in deeply vitalist traditions and are consonant with a broader set of values and goals. When that is true, an honest respect for individual choice compels us to honour such preferences. In the rare cases where health-care providers cannot find a way to reconcile these actions with their own sense of the goals of medicine, mediation via ethics consultation or other processes may be required.

Alternative language—defining goals at end of life

Therefore, rather than promoting a construct of a 'good' death, we favour the language of helping patients and families define and meet goals at the end of life. This paradigm has several advantages. First, in the medical context, we expect that goals vary between individuals. Second, we expect that they may change over time. Therefore, they require ongoing communication and negotiation. Third, the language of goals engages patients as active participants. Drawing from the self-management literature, the clinician may be the expert on the disease process, but the patient is the expert on their life. Fourth, it acknowledges a future orientation and ongoing contributions. Fifth, for the clinician, it is action oriented and moves beyond the idea (not common in palliative care) of having nothing more to offer. There are always additional goals.

Although we favour the paradigm in general, it does have some disadvantages, and points of caution. First, the language of goals may imply achievement and productivity, and risk imposing such expectations on patients. This would be counterproductive. Second, culturally we may think of goals as 'doing'. Yet, we do not want to understate the importance of offering a sense of presence to patients and simply 'being' with them in their illness.

Being with patients and families may involve offering assurance, through words and actions, that the provider will be present through the course of treatment and illness. It may involve deep listening and necessary silences, in the presence of powerful emotions. And, it may involve assurance of commitment to negotiating and renegotiating preferences for care that attend to domains of physical, social, emotional, spiritual well-being as well as issues of preparation and life completion. Together, acknowledging that the quality of end-of-life experience is dependent upon attending to the multiple dimensions of whole persons facing illness in the context of an entire lifetime of values and choices and the web of family and community.

Online materials

Complete references for this chapter are available online at <http://www.oxfordmedicine.com>.

References

Allen, W. (1983). *Without Feathers*. New York: Ballantine Books
Aries, P. (1980). *The Hour of Our Death*. New York: Knopf Publishers.
Butler, R.N. (1974). Successful aging and the role of the life review. *Journal of the American Geriatrics Society*, 22(12), 529–535.
Byock, I. R. (1996). The nature of suffering and the nature of opportunity at the end of life. *Clinics in Geriatric Medicine*, 12(2), 237–252.
Casarett, D., Fishman, J., O'Dwyer, P.J., Barg, F.K., Naylor, M., and Asch, D.A. (2008a). How should we design supportive cancer care? The patient's perspective. *Journal of Clinical Oncology*, 26(8), 1296–1301.
Casarett, D., Pickard, A., Amos Bailey, F., *et al.* (2008b). Important aspects of end-of-life care among veterans: implications for measurement and quality improvement. *Journal of Pain and Symptom Management*, 35(2), 115–125.
Cassell, E.J. (1973). Learning to die. *Bulletin of the New York Academy of Medicine*, 49(12), 1110–1118.
Chattoo, S. and Atkin, K.M. (2009). Extending specialist palliative care to people with heart failure: semantic, historical and practical limitations to policy guidelines. *Social Science & Medicine*, 69(2), 147–153.
Curtis, J.R., Patrick, D.L., Engelberg, R.A., Norris, K., Asp, C., and Byock, I. (2002). A measure of the quality of dying and death: initial validation. *Journal of Pain and Symptom Management*, 24(1), 17–31.
Daaleman, T.P., and Nease, D.E., Jr. (1994). Patient attitudes regarding physician inquiry into spiritual and religious issues. *The Journal of Family Practice*, 39(6), 564–568.
DelVecchio Good, M.J., Gadmer, N.M., Ruopp, P., *et al.* (2004). Narrative nuances on good and bad deaths: internists' tales from high-technology work places. *Social Science & Medicine*, 58(5), 939–953.
Emanuel, E.J. and Emanuel, L.L. (1998). The promise of a good death. *The Lancet*, 351(Suppl. 2), SII21–29.
Erikson, E. (1982). *The Life Cycle Completed: A Review*. New York: Norton.
Ferrell, B.R. (2005). Overview of the domains of variables relevant to end-of-life care. *Journal of Palliative Medicine*, 8(Suppl. 1), S22–29.

Field, M. and Cassel, C. (1997). *Approaching Death: Improving Care at the End of Life*. Washington, DC: Institute of Medicine.

Ganzini, L., Goy, E.R., Miller, L.L., Harvath, T.A., Jackson, A., and Delorit, M.A. (2003). Nurses' experiences with hospice patients who refuse food and fluids to hasten death. *The New England Journal of Medicine*, 349(4), 359–365.

Glaser, B. and Strauss, A. (1965). *Awareness of Dying*. Chicago, IL: Aldine.

Gott, M., Small, N., Barnes, S., Payne, S., and Seamark, D. (2008). Older people's views of a good death in heart failure: implications for palliative care provision. *Social Science & Medicine*, 67(7), 1113–1121.

Hales, S., Zimmermann, C., and Rodin, G. (2010). Review: the quality of dying and death: a systematic review of measures. *Palliative Medicine*, 24(2), 127–144.

Hales, S., Zimmermann, C., and Rodin, G. (2008). The quality of dying and death. *Archives of Internal Medicine*, 168(9), 912–918.

Hirai, K., Miyashita, M., Morita, T., Sanjo, M., and Uchitomi, Y. (2006). Good death in Japanese cancer care: a qualitative study. *Journal of Pain and Symptom Management*, 31(2), 140–147.

Kaufman, S. (2011). Improving quality and outcomes with alternative dialysis modalities. *Nephrology News & Issues*, 25(12), 8, 10.

Kubler-Ross, E. (1969). *On Death and Dying*. New York: Macmillan Publishing.

Leichtentritt, R.D. (2004). The meaning that young Israeli adults ascribe to the least undesirable death. *Death Studies*, 28(8), 733–759.

Long, S.O. (2004). Cultural scripts for a good death in Japan and the United States: similarities and differences. *Social Science & Medicine*, 58(5), 913–928.

Lynn, J., Teno, J.M., Phillips, R.S., *et al.* (1997). Perceptions by family members of the dying experience of older and seriously ill patients. SUPPORT Investigators. Study to Understand Prognoses and Preferences for Outcomes and Risks of Treatments. *Annals of Internal Medicine*, 126(2), 97–106.

McNamara, B., Waddell, C., and Colvin, M. (1994). The institutionalization of the good death. *Social Science & Medicine*, 39(11), 1501–1508.

Miyashita, M., Sanjo, M., Morita, T., Hirai, K., and Uchitomi, Y. (2007). Good death in cancer care: a nationwide quantitative study. *Annals of Oncology*, 18(6), 1090–1097.

Mo, H.N., Shin, D.W., Woo, J.H., *et al.* (2012). Is patient autonomy a critical determinant of quality of life in Korea? End-of-life decision making from the perspective of the patient. *Palliative Medicine*, 26(3), 222–231.

Munn, J.C. and Zimmerman, S. (2006). A good death for residents of long-term care: family members speak. *Journal of Social Work in End-Of-Life & Palliative Care*, 2(3), 45–59.

Murakawa, Y. and Nihei, Y. (2009). Understanding the concept of a 'good death' in Japan: differences in the views of doctors, palliative and non-palliative ward nurses. *International Journal of Palliative Nursing*, 15(6), 282–289.

Pierson, C.M., Curtis, J.R., and Patrick, D.L. (2002). A good death: a qualitative study of patients with advanced AIDS. *AIDS Care*, 14(5), 587–598.

Rousseau, P. (1997). Hope and the terminally ill. *Clinics in Geriatric Medicine*, 5(13), 15.

Saunders, C. (1978). Hospice care. *American Journal of Medicine*, 65(5), 726–728.

Seale, C. and van der Geest, S. (2004). Good and bad death: introduction. *Social Science & Medicine*, 58(5), 883–885.

Singer, P.A., Martin, D.K., and Kelner, M. (1999). Quality end-of-life care: patients' perspectives. *Journal of the American Medical Association*, 281(2), 163–168.

Spathis, A. and Booth, S. (2008). End of life care in chronic obstructive pulmonary disease: in search of a good death. *International Journal of Chronic Obstructive Pulmonary Disease*, 3(1), 11–29.

Steinhauser, K.E., Christakis, N.A., Clipp, E.C., McNeilly, M., McIntyre, L., and Tulsky, J.A. (2000a). Factors considered important at the end of life by patients, family, physicians, and other care providers. *Journal of the American Medical Association*, 284(19), 2476–2482.

Steinhauser, K.E., Clipp, E.C., McNeilly, M., Christakis, N.A., McIntyre, L.M., and Tulsky, J.A. (2000b). In search of a good death: observations of patients, families, and providers. *Annals of Internal Medicine*, 132(10), 825–832.

The SUPPORT Principal Investigators (1995). A controlled trial to improve care for seriously ill hospitalized patients: the study to understand prognosis and preferences for outcomes and risks of treatments (SUPPORT). *Journal of the American Medical Association*, 274, 1591–1598.

Tong, E., McGraw, S.A., Dobihal, E., Baggish, R., Cherlin, E., and Bradley, E.H. (2003). What is a good death? Minority and non-minority perspectives. *Journal of Palliative Care*, 19(3), 168–175.

Tulsky, J.A., Cassileth, B.R., and Bennett, C.L. (1997). The effect of ethnicity on ICU use and DNR orders in hospitalized AIDS patients. *Journal of Clinical Ethics*, 8(2), 150–157.

Vig, E.K., and Pearlman, R.A. (2004). Good and bad dying from the perspective of terminally ill men. *Archives of Internal Medicine*, 164(9), 977–981.

Welch, S.B. (2008). Can the death of a child be good? *Journal of Pediatric Nursing*, 23(2), 120–125.

Wilches-Gutierrez, J.L., Arenas-Monreal, L., Paulo-Maya, A., Pelaez-Ballestas, I., and Idrovo, A.J. (2012). A 'beautiful death': mortality, death, and holidays in a Mexican municipality. *Social Science & Medicine*, 74(5), 775–782.

Wilson, D.M., Fillion, L., Thomas, R., Justice, C., Bhardwaj, P.P., and Veillette, A.M. (2009a). The 'good' rural death: a report of an ethnographic study in Alberta, Canada. *Journal of Palliative Care*, 25(1), 21–29.

Yao, C.A., Hu, W.Y., Lai, Y.F., Cheng, S.Y., Chen, C.Y., and Chiu, T.Y. (2007). Does dying at home influence the good death of terminal cancer patients? *Journal of Pain and Symptom Management*, 34(5), 497–504.

2.5

Ethnic and cultural aspects of palliative care

LaVera Crawley and Jonathan Koffman

Introduction to ethnic and cultural aspects of palliative care

The goal of this chapter is to identify 'differences that make a difference' (Parens, 1998) among individuals and groups when they negotiate institutions and practices for palliative and end-of-life care. Culture is but one of several typologies of difference that has been used to signify diversity among individuals and groups. If narrowly defined from an anthropological perspective, culture can be thought of as that which refers to the 'patterns, explicit and implicit, of and for behaviour acquired and transmitted by symbols, language, and rituals (Kroeber and Kluckholn, 1952). Seen as a 'recipe' for living in the world, this conceptual framework for culture explains the means of transmitting these 'recipes' to the next generation (Donovan, 1986). However, this is a limited understanding of culture that, if used here, risks minimizing discussions of cultural aspects of palliative care to an interpretive list of end-of-life beliefs and practices from a range of so-called cultural groups. This has also been referred to as the 'fact-file' or 'checklist' (Gunaratnam, 2003a) approach that, while informative in regards to interpreting behaviours, symbols, rituals, and other cultural practices of certain ethnic or religious groups that may be important and meaningful at the end of life, runs the risk of encouraging generalizations about individuals and groups based on cultural identity. This in turn may then lead to the development of stereotypes, prejudices, and misunderstandings.

Culture is not static because identity, be it cultural, ethnic, religious, or using other categories, is in a constant process of adaptation and change, often in response to interactions with yet 'others' who are different in multitudes of ways. Culture is not the sole possession of those who are considered 'ethnic' minority groups. All people, the health-care practitioner included, brings his or her own cultural self into the medical or nursing encounter—a self that holds assumptions about the world and engages in practices and behaviours learned from their family and society of origin and, in the case of the health practitioner, from Western scientific and professional ideologies. Cross-cultural or intercultural interactions are not merely interpretative where each party needs only to translate the language, signs, behaviours, or practices of the other. Ideally, these exchanges are also dialogical and relational. All parties enter into some transformational 'third space' (Bhabha, 1988) where meaning is negotiated and new understandings emerge. Therefore programmes in 'cultural competency' that merely utilize an interpretive approach, emphasizing technical competencies utilized during the clinical encounter (such as communication skills), may miss the opportunity to teach skills needed for attitudinal transformations (such as sensitivity and humility) that are critical for 'developing mutually beneficial and non-paternalistic . . . partnerships' with patients and families (Tervalon and Murray-Garcia, 1998).

Understanding identity

In addition to culture, self- or group identification may be based on race, ethnicity, tribal or clan affiliation, nativity, generational status, citizenship, gender, religion, politics, sexual orientation, social and economic class, and other categories (Koffman, 2006). Race, a rather contentious category of identity, has its roots in social Darwinism, and relies heavily on an expectation of perceived (versus real) biological differences between people and populations (*Collins Concise Dictionary*, 2001). Historically, race has been used to describe geographically separated populations (such as the African race), cultural groups (Jews), nationality (the English race), and mankind in general (the human race). Racialized research in science has a long and inglorious history (Gould, 1981; Stepan, 1982). In the mid-nineteenth century, the cephalic index, a method for describing the shape of the skull, became a popular way of describing and dividing races. Under the influence of phrenology, a hierarchy of races was devised with white Europeans at the top and black Africans at the bottom. Intelligence, physique, culture, and morality were all placed in an order, the so-called Great Chain of Being philosophy used to justify slavery, imperialism, anti-immigration policy, and the social status quo (Singh, 1997). Biological determinism also became prominent in medicine and medical practitioners frequently contributed to racialized science (Ahmad, 1993) with the theory of racial hygiene in Nazi Germany being a horrific and notorious example. However, differences that do exist between peoples and populations are very minor and largely reflect superficial physical characteristics such as facial features, hair, or skin colour. Many researchers have therefore now discredited race as being inaccurate and misleading (Karlsen and Nazroo, 2002b).

Less controversial but equally misunderstood is the concept of ethnicity (Chaturvedi, 2001; Afshari and Bhopal, 2002). As a category of identity, it reflects the social grouping of people on the basis of historical or territorial identity or by shared cultural patterns and traditions maintained between generations (Senior and Bhopal, 1994; Crawley, 2005). One's ethnicity can be defined by language, such as the Spanish language that unites Hispanic peoples in Central and South America and the Caribbean who are otherwise separated by geography, history, and politics. It can also be defined by shared ancestry, such as subgroups of diasporic black people who are descendants of slaves from West and Central Africa. There are also subcategories used in identifying certain ethnic groups. For example, among ethnic black people, further delineations can be made by nativity and citizenship: African Americans who are descendants of slaves and of multiple generations born in and holding citizenship in the United States may be ethnically distinct (e.g. in language or culture) from black Haitians, Cubans, Jamaicans, or other descendants of African slaves who reside in the Caribbean, South America, the United Kingdom, or other diasporic locations. Other ways in which people express their identity include kinship by tribal or clan affiliation which can be extremely influential (and potentially volatile) in intergroup dynamics.

Identity is both internally (self-) defined and externally (structurally) imposed (Karlsen and Nazroo, 2002a) which has bearing not only in how an individual or group sees oneself but also in how they are treated by society. Needless to say, the politics and social science of identity is complex. Furthermore, semantic confusion is very common when the concepts of identity are used in clinical and research settings. Race, ethnicity, and culture are often used interchangeably, subject to misuse, or confused with other social metrics, such as social class or education (Hillier and Kelleher, 1996). The manner in which these concepts are used may change due to prevailing fashions and politics (Gunaratnam, 2003b).

Structural factors, defined as rules, roles, and institutions derived from dynamic social, economic, political, and historical processes, may play an important role in creating and maintaining cultural, racial, and/or ethnic identities themselves, or various aspects associated with those identities. An example can be seen with the conflation of ethnic identity with class: in places or situations where institutional racism or other forms of discrimination constrain freedom and development for certain segments of a population, such as on the basis of racial or ethnic visibility, these structural factors may produce patterns (e.g. poverty, poor education, crime) that become erroneously attached to the identity of that group (Karlsen and Nazroo, 2002a). The same can be said for structural factors that privilege other segments of the populations.

To compound the confusion, there is no uniformity in how people are classified across national boundaries. For example, the National Health Service and census in the United Kingdom identify five different categories of 'ethnicity' (white, mixed, Asian, black, or Chinese) that are further broken down into different subgroups based on countries of origin (e.g. Indian, Pakistani, Bangladeshi, or other for Asian; Caribbean, African, or other for black people, etc.) (Office of National Statistics, 2003); while the US census collapses many distinct populations into one dichotomous category of 'ethnicity' (Hispanic or non-Hispanic) and five single broad categories of 'race,' (white, black or African American, American Indian or Alaskan Native, Asian, and Native Hawaiian or Other Pacific Islander) (Office of Management and Budget. Revisions to the standards for the classification of federal data on race and ethnicity. Federal Register, 1997; 62(210): 58782–58790). The South African census uses five population categories based on self-classification (Black African, Colored, Indian or Asian, White, or Other) (Lehohla, 2003). Canada collects census data based on ethnic origins (defined by ancestry) and on a category called 'visible minority' status, defined as 'persons other than Aboriginal persons who are not white in race or colour' (Statistics Canada, 2001). Lastly, there is evidence that many people change their assigned identity over time, as is their prerogative (Bhopal, 1995). US-based research has shown that at least 35% of respondents altered their self-assignment over a year and in the validation study following the 1991 British census, 12% of 'black' people altered their ethnic group, as did 22% of 'other' category (Pringle and Rothera, 1995).

This mutability attests to the fact that people inhabit multiple identities which are expressed or perceived differently as needs and circumstances change (Karlsen and Nazroo, 2002a; Crawley, 2005). The relevance of this discussion for palliative care is to caution the clinician and researcher to be mindful of the difficulties in interpreting events at the bedside or reports in the literature related to culture, race, ethnicity, or other identifiers. Employing clearly and rationally defined demographic categorizations of identity in studying epidemiological patterns of morbidity and mortality has usefulness for policy implications, such as determining what systems of care are needed or measuring inequities in quality of care delivered across population groups. However, employing essentialized notions of preferences or behaviours at the bedside runs the risk of compromising an individual's 'needs and concerns [that] may not conform to preconceived or stereotyped patterns' (Crawley, 2005). What best serves the needs of all patients is knowledge of the particular individual's beliefs, values, preferences, and practices—knowledge gained by asking the patient or family directly or by utilizing resources that promote patient-centred and relationship-centred care.

The special case of immigration

Throughout human history, individuals, families and groups have emigrated from their native homes to other places for many reasons: the prospect of educational, economic or social advantage; the need to escape war, political torture or other conflicts; or the desire to reunite with other family members. Globalization has brought with it an unprecedented increase in the numbers of people who have migrated to developed countries. As of 2010, there were an estimated 214 million immigrants worldwide: nearly 70 million of these immigrants arrived in Europe and over 50 million in North America—an increase of nearly 40% in these regions compared to 20 years earlier (United Nations, Department of Economic and Social Affairs, Population Division, 2009). This trend is expected to continue and to increase. In the United States, for example, it is estimated that by the year 2050, nearly two-thirds of the population will be immigrants.

The International Observatory on End-of-Life Care that monitors the global development of hospice and palliative care services around the world reports that such services are unavailable or are uneven at best in resource-poor and medium-resource countries when compared to European and English-speaking countries (International Observatory on End of Life Care, 2006). Subsequently the immigrant may not have had much exposure to or knowledge of palliative care services provided by hospices or other health-care institutions in their home country. For example, the Observatory documented misperceptions about and stigmas regarding palliative care in Mexico (Clark, 2006). As such, expectations for palliative care may thus be lowered among Mexican immigrants who bring from their country of origin misperceptions or lowered priorities for this type of care (Crawley and Chaudhary, 2006). In addition, some immigrants may find accessing quality care and finding funds for hospice, palliative care, and other end-of-life health services to be a complex and potentially confusing process that may be compounded by unfamiliarity with laws and regulations of the host country. The immigrant's knowledge of and preference for palliative or other health care may be influenced by factors related to immigration itself. For example, refugees and asylum seekers who have experienced violence, or who may have been exposed to torture or other state-sanctioned or war-related trauma, may be mistrustful of government-run health-care or social service institutions and authorities (Gavagan and Martinez, 1997; Gavagan and Brodyaga, 1998). They may also face fears and uncertainties that accompany their experiences as an immigrant.

Immigration also impacts the workforce that provides caregiving for those who are dying. Foreign health-care workers are motivated to leave their native countries for reasons general to all immigrants—educational, economic or social advantage; family reunification—or they may leave due to inadequate health-care infrastructures and technologies (Crawley et al., 2007). The result in some receiving countries is a growing immigrant workforce who bring their own unique cross-cultural issues to health-care delivery systems. On the one hand, an increasingly diverse health-care workforce may help improve outreach to diverse communities, particularly with access issues such as language barriers. On the other hand, these workers will represent a spectrum of acculturation or assimilation of the language, customs, values, and perspectives of the host country. Just as there can be 'native' providers who lack cultural competency and sensitivity towards immigrant patients, there can be those immigrant providers who lack these skills with 'native' patients. Central to this issue is communication capability.

Cultural versus moral relativism

Cultural relativism or multiculturalism is defined as 'a social-intellectual movement that promotes the value of diversity as a core principle and insists that all cultural groups be treated with respect as equals' (Macklin, 1998). In social, economic and political arenas, this is a laudable goal, although it may seem as narrow in the sense of applying limited or narrow definitions of culture or identity as what is discussed above. Efforts for ensuring equitable access to societal goods across all populations, including quality care for the seriously ill and dying, requires attention to salient differences within and among groups. However, blindly embracing this principle does carry an inherent risk of mistaking cultural relativism with moral relativism. Respect for diversity does not mean one should tolerate actions that violate another's human rights. A case example is warranted: a young adult immigrant from Yemen with advanced metastatic cancer required large doses of opioids to control his pain. The patient described his pain as unbearable and requested relief from his physician. The patient's family, traditional Muslims, strongly objected to the prescribing and administering of opioids required to relieve the patient's pain and suffering, quoting scriptures that held that pain was to be endured as test of faith (Al-Jeilani, 1987).

Cultural relativism indeed requires us to respect the role that religious and other cultural beliefs and practices hold; however, it may be difficult to be tolerant of practices if doing so forces us to violate moral principles such as non-maleficence (to avoid doing harm) or beneficence (serving what is in the patient's benefit). If the patient, rather than his family, acknowledged this preference to forego treatment of his pain, then the moral dilemma between the doctor and patient may need to be addressed. In this case, however, the patient did request relief and thus the provider might feel the prima facie obligation to address the patient's request for pain relief with respect for his autonomous right for health-care decision-making. The moral dilemma then, is truly between the patient and his family.

However, one may counter argue that such moral principles are not culturally neutral to begin with and, rather, reflect a Western bias of what counts as right or wrong. Respect for individual autonomy is a Western ideal. Among other populations, the family or community is thought to be the unit of autonomy. For example, among some Asian or Hispanic populations, it is believed that the family should be the decision-maker and in some cases patients should be shielded from information deemed potentially disturbing. This is a classic dilemma brought to ethics committees or consultations for deliberation and an example of why cross-cultural or intercultural interactions should be seen as dialogical and relational. The goal for all parties in such interactions is not to condone or to condemn the 'other' but rather to seek understanding and to co-create resolutions that are mutually acceptable. Understanding goes beyond interpretation of beliefs and values; it also means looking at the structural aspects of a practice: what purpose it serves in the cultural group or society. If a group values family autonomy over individual autonomy while the physician or medical system values the reverse, then a mutually acceptable solution might entail asking the patient if he or she would autonomously prefer the family to make decisions, thereby autonomously relinquishing autonomy. In summary, as ethicist Ruth Macklin has written, blind tolerance, which she calls 'extreme ethical relativism', is not useful. However, Macklin reminds us that neither is Western cultural imperialism. The middle ground is the following: cultural, religious, and ethnic groups should be treated as equals—conforming to the principle of justice as equality—while at the same time this should be balanced with intolerance of practices that are unjust and oppressive (Macklin, 1998).

Differences that make a difference

How we understand the influence of diversity in patterns of advanced disease, illness experiences, responses to treatment, and the use of specialist palliative care services is important given increasing evidence that we are not all equal in death and dying (Oliviere, 1999; Crawley et al., 2000; Karim et al., 2000; Firth, 2001; Koffman and Higginson, 2001; Gunaratnam, 2003a). Race- or ethnic-based disparities in mortality and in diagnosis, quality of care, referral patterns to specialist palliative care, and treatments for pain and other physical symptoms have been documented in many developed countries (Berthoud and Modood, 1997; Harding and Maxwell, 1997; Department of Health, 1998; Farrell, 2000; Karim et al., 2000; Gibson, 2001; Karlsen and Nazroo, 2002a; Koffman et al., 2003, 2005; Mooney, 2003; Smedley et al., 2003; Casas-Zamora and Ibrahim, 2004; Crawley, 2005; Paradies, 2006).

In the United States, a comprehensive review of evidence of unequal treatment, commissioned by the US congress and produced by its Institute of Medicine (IOM), documented race- or ethnic-based inequities in pain and chronic disease management, cancer care, and other clinical care settings and suggested that inequities may be due to patient-level, provider-level, and/or health system-level variables, alone or in combinations (Smedley et al., 2003). Patient-level factors would include ethno-cultural, social, or other beliefs, preferences, or knowledge about health options. According to the IOM study, patient-level factors were thought to be the least likely contributor to disparities. On the other hand, both provider stereotyping and bias, and how health-care systems are organized as well as the degree to which people have access to care were shown to more likely influence health outcomes for minority patients.

The existence of prejudice and stereotyping by health-care providers may be difficult for many non-minority providers to accept, as we all presume to consciously abhor such discriminatory attitudes and behaviours. The important contribution of the IOM report in thinking about this issue was its suggestion that it is not conscious attitudes that drive discrimination but rather those unconscious or implicit attitudes that may compel us when we are under duress. As Fyodor Dostoyevsky stated:

> In every man's memories there are such things as he will reveal not to everyone, but perhaps only to friends. There are also such as he will reveal not to friends, but only to himself, and that in secret. Then finally, there are such as a man is afraid to reveal even to himself, and every decent man will have accumulated quite a few things of this sort. That is, one might even say: the more decent a man is, the more of them he will have. (Dostoyevsky, 2003)

Health system-level factors such as poor access to health-care services have been reported by black and minority ethnic groups in the United States and the United Kingdom (Harding and Maxwell, 1997; O'Neill and Marconi, 2001). This is also an issue for end-of-life care where the impact of ageing on the black and minority ethnic groups now means larger numbers of older members within these communities will require health services for advanced disease. A limited number of reports have levelled criticism of care at the end of life for these communities and poor access to appropriate care. Low rates of cancer were seen as one explanation to account for low uptake of service provision, but the figures were likely to have been inaccurate because of inadequate ethnic monitoring (Aspinall, 1999). The authors concluded 'some black and Asian patients and their carers are very disadvantaged, as they do not know what they are entitled to, and hence what to ask for by way of benefits and services' (Hill and Penso, 1995). More recently, a study in an inner London health authority demonstrated that African Caribbean patients with advanced disease experienced restricted access to some specialist palliative care services compared to white British deceased patients (Koffman and Higginson, 2001), yet an analysis of local provision revealed no lack of palliative care services (Eve et al., 1997). This may be due to poor knowledge and awareness of palliative care and related services (Koffman et al., 2007). This example of under-utilization of palliative care services by the black Caribbean community at the end of life supports other recent research among minority ethnic communities (Farrell, 2000; Skilbeck et al., 2002). The explanations to account for this build on work conducted by Currow and colleagues (Currow et al., 2008) among others (Ahmed et al., 2004; Koffman and Higginson, 2004), all of which may operate in combination, and are highlighted in Fig. 2.5.1. Identifying and eliminating health inequities in the delivery of quality palliative care is a critical mandate. Institutional standards for monitoring and ensuring the cultural sensitivity and competency of the palliative medicine workforce should be employed, as should strategies to increase community-based partnerships. Ultimately, it is incumbent on service providers to redress these disparities by active processes rather than imagining that people who are often already marginalized can improve their own access to services.

Providing equitable, culturally appropriate palliative care

The World Health Organization definition of palliative care specifies two goals: improving quality of life (QOL) of patients and families and preventing and relieving suffering. It identifies three strategies for meeting those goals: early identification, impeccable assessment, and [appropriate] treatment. Lastly, the definition addresses four domains of care: (1) problems related to pain, (2) other physical conditions, (3) the psychosocial, and (4) the spiritual. The remaining sections of this chapter addresses these goals, strategies, and domains in relation to delivering quality palliative care in cross- or multi-cultural settings.

Goals of palliative care in cross-cultural contexts

Quality of life

The World Health Organization defines QOL as 'an individual's perception of their position in life in the context of the culture and value systems in which they live and in relation to their goals, expectations, standards and concerns' (World Health Organization, 2006). When applied to palliative care, the focus is on maximizing the quality within the time remaining in a patient's life. Because quality should be subjectively defined by patients and their families, cultural factors relevant to the individual and their family need to be addressed when assessing their QOL preferences and requirements.

Many QOL assessment instruments include broad areas representing key domains such as physical symptoms, functional status, interpersonal relations, emotional well-being, and the experience of spiritual or existential transcendence. However, the subjective nature of the concept of QOL and instruments used to measure it must also consider variations in meanings of these domains across cultural groups. Recognizing the need to address cultural components in assessing quality, the World Health Organization initiated the WHOQOL project to 'develop an international cross-culturally comparable quality of life assessment instrument' (Murphy et al., 2000).

The psychometric properties of the WHOQOL instrument were tested in several stages and across multi-cultural field sites to ensure cross-cultural validity including:

◆ agreement on the definition of QOL

◆ standardization of questions or items and of scale construction

◆ field testing final instruments.

Both the 100-item instrument (WHOQOL-100) and the shorter 26-item version (WHOQOL-BREF) are available in many

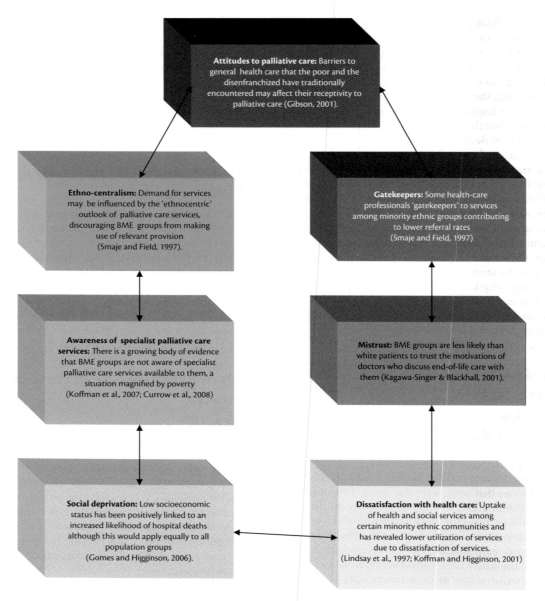

Fig. 2.5.1 Possible explanations to account for under-utilization of specialist palliative care among black and minority ethnic (BME) groups.

languages and can be used clinically for individual patients as well as in cross-cultural research for inter- and intra-group comparisons (World Health Organization, 2006). The initial field sites, located in Australia, Croatia, France, India, Israel, Japan, the Netherlands, Panama, Russia, Spain, Thailand, the United Kingdom, the United States, and Zimbabwe, each adapted the standardized instrument to their population-based needs. To date there are now over 30 sites worldwide and more continue to field test and adapt the instrument to the unique cultural needs of their countries.

Preventing and relieving suffering

Cultural factors mediate the ways in which symptoms associated with advanced disease are identified and interpreted. Examples include the appropriate modes of expression of pain and other symptoms, and the associated suffering, whether an illness and

symptoms are stigmatized, and whether the dependencies that accompany advanced disease are considered an acceptable part of the normal life cycle. The evidence of the influence of cultural and ethnic factors on symptom interpretation is fascinating and frequently raises more questions than it answers. In the 1950s, Zborowski demonstrated differences among old American, Irish, and other migrant communities' perceptions of their pain (Zborowski, 1952). Most recently, Koffman et al. observed significantly higher levels of symptom-related distress among black Caribbean peoples compared with native-born white United Kingdom patients with advanced cancer living in south London. This finding was only partly explained by simple variations in treatment levels between the two groups (Koffman, et al., 2003). Along with other researchers (Lasch, 2002; Cintron and Morrison, 2006), the authors suggest that the language of expressing symptom-related distress may be reinforced by cultural expectations (Koffman et al., 2003). Expressions of suffering have been shown to serve a purpose. It has been observed in some African American communities that suffering is perceived to be redemptive, bringing those who experience it closer to God (Crawley et al., 2000).

In other communities the actual language used to describe distress and suffering has implications for the delivery of palliative care. Krause revealed that the expression in Punjabi, 'Dil *me* girda hai,' used by Panjabis in Bedford, often translates as the 'sinking heart' to reflect a range of psychological and somatic conditions (Krause, 2005). In addition, she suggests that the 'generalized hopelessness' which characterizes depressive disorders in women living in London would not be regarded as abnormal among Hindu, Muslim, and Buddhist women who would regard 'hopelessness' as an aspect of life which can only be overcome on the path to salvation. Ahmed takes the view that while South Asian patients may be well aware of their own psychosomatic symptoms, general practitioners (GPs) (including Asian GPs) tend only to acknowledge physical symptoms and do not recognize psychological distress (Ahmed, 1998). The ongoing challenge is for health-care professionals to explore and acknowledge culturally determined understandings and expressions associated with advanced disease that do not mirror their own.

Strategies of palliative care in cross-cultural settings

Early identification

Problems with late referrals to hospice or for palliative care in general are a concern for all populations. To avoid the appearance of medical abandonment, it is important to integrate the goals of hospice and of palliative care early in the disease process, particularly for those illnesses that are predictably fatal. This is particularly important for immigrants or members of ethnic or cultural communities who may already feel marginalized or vulnerable due to their minority status. Myths or misunderstandings about the goals of palliative care should be addressed where possible early on through culturally effective communication—which can also enable the palliative care team to learn about and incorporate the unique perspectives of the patient into the multidisciplinary management of their care.

Identifying preferences for medical care in advance of untoward or terminal circumstances can be a difficult and emotional process. The decision-making model of advance care planning derived from bioethics practices assumes that choices made by the individual can be arrived at through rational processes that are unchanged by time, shifting social consequences, or disease and illness progression; good advance care planning permits for changes and shifts overtime for an individual or a community. Such a model may only appeal to certain subsets of people, thus limiting the utility of instruments used for advance planning (living wills or durable powers of attorney for health care).

For some groups, speaking about the dying process or planning for death may represent a transgression of a strong cultural taboo and could create additional distress. Other patients, unfamiliar with or mistrustful of the legal system, may misconstrue the purpose or nature of formal advance care planning documents. In all cases, rather than abandon the goals of advance care planning, strategies should be sought that facilitate understanding. For example, a generic discussion to identify a health-care proxy need not be cast as a discussion of death, but rather an opportunity to determine desired roles of various family members and support persons. Discussions about patient preferences for end-of-life care should be culturally and linguistically appropriate and reflect sensitivity to patients' values and beliefs.

Impeccable assessment

Critical to assessing and monitoring palliative care needs is the ability to communicate clearly and effectively. The inability to do so not only affects access to palliative care services but has been shown to be a source of serious problems in clinical consultations and the cause of misunderstandings among patients, family members and health-care providers (Nazroo, 1997; Koffman and Higginson, 2001). Important communication difficulties arise where there is an over-reliance on a patient's relatives acting on their loved ones' or dependants' behalf. While this may well be simpler than accessing an interpreter, it can potentially disadvantage both the doctor and the patient (Crawley et al., 2000).

The family interpreter may filter, abbreviate, or omit very important information, or inform the doctor or the patient what he or she thinks the doctor and patient needs to know. Important medical information may not be understood adequately or conveyed in full (Butow et al., 2011). Further, the use of children as interpreters is considered inappropriate. Details about an illness may be very intimate and it places an unfair burden on them (Yee, 1997). Using friends or untrained lay interpreters from the local community can be even more problematic since there can be issues of confidentiality and fear of gossip in the wider community (Firth, 1997). Moreover, communication is not only an issue of spoken language. It also involves body language, cultural rules as to what is courteous (such as not looking the professionals—especially of the opposite gender—in the eye), and appropriate behaviours in an unequal gender and power relationship (Firth, 2001). People who speak English with a different accent or dialect can also be judged to be less intelligent or fail to be understood or understand what is being said to them (Firth, 1997).

Appropriate treatment

It is widely acknowledged that management of physical and psychological symptoms associated with advanced disease can be difficult in mono-cultural interactions between clinicians and patients because of differences in perspective between Western biomedicine and lay health beliefs and practices. However, the design and assessment of effective health care for culturally diverse patients, both long-term residents and new immigrants and refugees, is even more complicated. New immigrants increasingly come to the United States and the United Kingdom, among other countries, from regions such as Southeast Asia, Latin America, and Africa, and are even more heterogeneous than their European predecessors (Lasch, 2002). Within the same ethnic group, individuals come from all walks of life with differing educational, occupational, and economic status, ties to their country of origin, and geographical background. All these factors affect their ethnic identity and their cultural responses to health and illness. Understanding and controlling patients' symptoms in a health-care system where the dominant imperative is for economic efficiency represents a challenge. When clinicians look to published research to acquaint themselves with the ways in which ethnicity or culture may impinge upon the experience, expression, or behaviours related to responses, they find a vast array of disciplinary lenses and diverse theoretical approaches that are often not made explicit, thus generating inconsistent findings.

Domains of palliative care for culturally diverse populations

Albert Schweitzer is noted to have said 'Pain is an even worse master than death' (Marcus and Arbeiter, 1994, p. 4). Pain is a common and often distressing symptom associated with cancer, with a prevalence of over 90% in the more advanced stages of the disease (Solano et al., 2006). Although treatments to manage this symptom have improved dramatically in recent years, some patients still experience severe pain due to its refractory nature, poor management, or a reluctance to take medication. In recent years, the number of research articles that have examined the interface between pain and ethnicity have increased (Bonham, 2001; Morris, 2001). This has particular relevance given that ethnic and cultural diversity is more common in countries around the world; health-care professionals are now more likely to care for patients from backgrounds that differ from their own.

Whilst pain is an individual experience that may affect people differently, it is also plausible that biological markers which may be shared within a group may contribute to reported pain severity. If this is so, ethnic differences in experiential pain sensitivity could help explain group differences in clinical pain. However, the evidence base that has attempted to explore this complex aspect of pain presents a mixed picture. An early study conducted by Chapman and Jones reported lower heat pain thresholds and tolerance among African American study participants compared to non-white Hispanics (Chapman and Jones, 1944). Whilst other studies present similar findings (Woodrow et al., 1972), more recent (and more sophisticated) studies that have utilized several different methods of assessment to compare pain among African Americans and non-white Hispanics, have not identified marked differences in pain ratings across groups (Edwards and Fillingim, 1999; Campbell et al., 2003).

It is important to recognize that pain has the potential to affect all, regardless of biological, ethnic, or cultural differences. Comparative studies on pain thresholds across population groups—identifying which group experiences more or less pain under given conditions—are potentially racist and without clear clinical value. However, what would be clinically relevant is individual patient assessment of pain levels. While there has been enormous progress in the field of pain in recent years, the actual delivery of care of individuals in pain is still far from adequate. In 1990–1991, a study of 1308 outpatients with cancer noted that 67% reported pain with 62% of those in pain reporting pain severe enough that ability to function was impaired (Cleeland et al., 1994). However, as we focus on pain and why it is too often ineffectively treated, it is evident that certain minority populations are at higher risk for ineffective or sub-therapeutic treatment of pain. Evidence from recent studies, principally conducted in the United States and the United Kingdom, paints the clear picture that one's ethnic background matters in the treatment of cancer pain; the studies' most poignant findings are related to the disparity in treatment of minority ethnic patients compared to their white peers. Moreover, the studies, when reviewed as a group, identify

that these disparities exist across a number of types of health-care facilities and treatment settings, from the community hospital to the nursing home.

The cultural meaning and shaping of pain

Pain is never the sole creation of our anatomy and physiology. Rather, as Morris (2001) suggests, it emerges only at 'the intersection of bodies, minds and cultures'. Pain attributions and meanings may be learnt by the members of a particular culture and then transmitted to others. Cancer-pain 'meanings' have frequently been identified as invoking religious beliefs. For example, recent research among black Caribbean and white British patients observed that beliefs about pain were mediated by religious beliefs that influenced attitudes towards medication and the accommodation of distress; a number of black Caribbean cancer patients regarded their pain as representing a test of religious faith or a justified punishment. In this religious context, these patients believed that cancer suffering was part of life, to be endured in order to enter heaven (Koffman et al., 2008). Although these findings may appear to be inappropriate and even anti-therapeutic (Bendelow and Williams, 1995; Juarez et al., 1999), health-care professionals should remind themselves of Helman's three propositions about pain, all of which have resonance in such a clinical encounter:

1. Not all social or cultural groups respond to pain in the same way.

2. How individuals perceive and respond to pain, both in themselves and others, can be largely influenced by their cultural background.

3. How, and whether, people communicate their pain to health professionals and to others can be influenced by cultural factors (Helman, 2007, p. 185).

Assessment and communication of pain in the clinical encounter

At its core, pain represents a subjective experience. It therefore relies heavily on impeccable assessment and communication between health-care professionals and patients. Although patients from minority ethnic groups share many of the same concerns that limit pain control with majority populations, data from a number of studies suggest that the manner in which pain is communicated varies from one group to the next (Cleeland, 1989; Anderson et al., 2002). Several important issues therefore warrant consideration. First, patients with serious medical conditions such as advanced cancer may under-report their pain and its severity and this may be culturally determined. For example, African American and Hispanic cancer patients have reported stoicism and the belief that their pain is an inevitable part of their illness experience and must be accepted (Juarez et al., 1999). Second, the most frequently studied factor that has been shown to influence pain assessment involves its actual severity. When pain severity is low, patients and health-care professionals report good agreement in rating of this symptom (Grossman et al., 1991; Tait and Chibnall, 1997). However, when patients rate higher levels of pain there is evidence that health-care professionals do not concur with their assessments (Chibnall et al., 1997). In addition, there is also evidence that patients reporting high pain severity also experience prejudiced stereotyping which may be amplified by racism (Tait and Chibnall, 1997).

Like QOL measures, a range of cross-culturally validated instruments for assessing pain can be employed at the bedside.

Pain intensity scales and multidimensional tools have been translated into several languages; however, mere translation of standardized instruments into the language of a given patient may not ensure its efficacy for that patient's cultural group. The selection of a scale or tool should be based on the patient's literacy and ability to understand numerical ratings, images, or sensory, affective and evaluative descriptors used in numerical rating, visual analogue, or multidimensional scales.

Health-care system factors

Racial and ethnic differences in the utilization of health-care services in general and palliative care in particular are well documented (Spruyt, 1999; Koffman and Higginson, 2001; Koffman et al., 2007). Specific examples can also be cited in relation to the management of cancer-related pain. For example, in examining a randomized selection of pharmacies located in New York City, Morrison and colleagues observed that 50% of pharmacies located in neighbourhoods with proportionately larger minority residents did not stock adequate supplies of opioids to treat severe cancer pain (Morrison et al., 2000). In the United Kingdom, several studies have identified disparities in the uptake of specialist in-patient and community-based specialist palliative care among black and minority ethnic groups (Koffman and Higginson, 2001; Ahmed et al., 2004).

Other symptoms

Like pain, symptoms of anxiety, depression and delirium, common in the advanced and terminal stages of dying, may be expressed and understood differently across various ethnic and cultural groups. Symptom formation can be influenced by sociopolitical factors in conjunction with biological and environmental variables. Behaviours considered normative within the psychospiritual belief systems of a given culture (e.g. spirit possession, visions of spirits or ghosts, etc.) may be considered delusional or otherwise pathological within a Western biomedical model. Conversely, certain culture-specific patterns of anxiety or distress that do not fit medical classifications (so-called culture-bound syndromes) may be missed in evaluating the mental health of patients and their families.

Psychosocial domains

Social support networks are crucial factors in the psychological well-being of the seriously ill and the dying patient (Koffman et al., 2012). Within those networks, informal caregivers perform an essential role for both the patient and for the health delivery system. The emphasis on care in the community rather than institutions, and the growing awareness that in some communities, people would prefer to die at home given the choice (Gomes and Higginson, 2006), means that informal caregivers are indispensable partners of health and social care professionals. Many assume responsibilities of care that were previously confined to specialist in-patient settings and community hospitals (Rhodes and Shaw, 1999). Caring for family members is regarded as an important obligation in many ethnic communities (Koffman and Higginson, 2003; Koffman et al., 2012). Further, for many ethnic minority families, caring for dying relatives at home when possible is considered a matter of honour and integrity as well as a means of ensuring the death occurs in a holy place (Spruyt, 1999). Karim et al. refer, in addition to Currow and colleagues, to the stigma and loss of face from not caring for close family relatives (Karim et al., 2000; Currow et al., 2008). In the Hindu tradition, the concepts of karma and sacred duty may place the family of a loved one or dependant under additional stress in order to do the right thing (Firth, 1997). Spruyt found that east London Bangladeshi children became actively involved in the care of dying patient and in interactions with professionals, and had to act as interpreters. This had a negative impact on them subsequently. A number of children were required to give up formal schooling and older sons gave up work to help with care of relatives. When there is home care the burden often falls upon one person, but without ready access to outside support (Spruyt, 1999). For example, in the United Kingdom, multigenerational Pakistani and Bangladeshi families who wish to provide traditional support may also be in situations with high unemployment and poverty, and large families of young children (Blakemore, 2000). Home care is also not without problems when outside help is needed, because many ethnic minorities would regard this as a sense of failure in the eyes of the community, and it may also be regarded as an invasion of privacy (Firth, 2001). Smaje and Field also point out the tensions which can arise when an elderly person needs and demands care from a female relative who may have quite different expectations, especially if the carer also has children born in the host country (Smaje and Field, 1997). However, it is important to bear in mind that expectations of care from family relatives may change in coming years as patterns of family life and social networks evolve through a process of acculturation.

Spiritual domains

The experience of advanced disease can have a profound effect on patients and their family and friends. Indeed, during their illness, many patients may raise questions that relate to their identity and self-worth as they seek to find the ultimate meaning in their life. Some patients attempt to answer these questions by examining their religious or spiritual beliefs. Formal religion is a means of expressing an underlying spirituality, but spiritual belief, concerned with the search for existential or the ultimate meaning in life, is a broader concept and may not always be expressed in a religious way.

Hope is an important spiritual resource that has been correlated with one's ability to adapt and cope with serious illness. Thus it is an essential assessment and intervention tool in palliative care. A comprehensive review of the multidisciplinary theoretical and empirical work on hope has produced the following definition: hope is a future-directed positive emotion or expectation constructed from biological, psychological, and social resources. This understanding of hope, however, is 'culture-bound,' reflecting a specific Western cognitive-temporal and affective-behavioural concept based largely on an expectancy-value psychological model. To date, there is a paucity of studies on hope across cultures and those that exist may be hampered by the use of measurement tools that reflect a specific Western bias. The most commonly reported tool, the Herth Hope Index, was developed in the United States and validated among American patients of European descent who were predominately Christian. This tool is based on a three-factor model that presumes hope is future/time oriented, influenced by expectations, and involves a sense of interconnectedness with self and other. As such, this definition may not capture the unique cultural aspects needed to accurately assess the spiritual needs of patients who hold a different understanding of relationships and responsibilities (i.e. holding a collectivist vs individualist expectation of decision-making or other outcomes). The 'future-directedness' of hope may not translate across cultural groups that hold a different orientation toward time (time as cyclical or circular compared to linear). For example, Chinese folk wisdom or beliefs grounded in Confucianism may promote a stance of hope in the present as opposed to the future; or hope in the ancestral afterlife as opposed to this life. It has been suggested that concepts such as optimism or keeping faith, rather than hope, may be more culturally appropriate for people holding traditional Chinese values. Understanding the diverse multicultural norms around hope is especially salient among individuals and groups that favour non-disclosure of terminal or other bad prognostic information in order to preserve 'hope'. Identifying what hope means to these patients and families will allow providers to incorporate a culturally responsive model of hope and to identify appropriate strategies for its promotion among multicultural patient populations.

Conclusion

The palliative care movement has assumed a role in addressing the health and social care needs of patients and families facing the inevitability of death. It has only been recently that attention has focused on the importance of providing care for increasingly diverse societies, including in the United States, United Kingdom, Canada, Australia, and New Zealand among others. This has now become a demographic imperative. This chapter has shown that the language of understanding difference is complex yet fascinating. When considering its influence in the provision of care at the end of life and during bereavement, perhaps we should hold a double lens: one that applies a framework of equity to understand and serve population needs of specific communities; and another that never loses sight of the individuals and families before us—those with clinical, psychosocial, and spiritual needs and concerns that may not conform to preconceived or stereotyped patterns. Always, we should be mindful that an individualized approach to palliative care with a focus on quality is paramount for any patient, regardless of their ethnic or cultural background.

Online materials

Complete references for this chapter are available online at <http://www.oxfordmedicine.com>.

References

Ahmed, N., Bestall, J.C., Ahmedzai, S.H., Payne, S.A., Clark, D., and Noble, B. (2004). Systematic review of the problems and issues of accessing specialist palliative care by patients, carers and health and social care professionals. *Palliative Medicine*, 18(6), 525–542.

Butow, P.N., Goldstein, D., and Bell, M.L. (2011). Interpretation in consultations with immigrant patients with cancer: how accurate is it? *Journal of Clinical Oncology*, 29(20), 2801–2807.

Currow, D.C., Agar, M., Sanderson, C., and Abernethy, A.P. (2008). Populations who die without specialist palliative care: does lower uptake equate with unmet need? *Palliative Medicine*, 22(1), 43–50.

Gibson, R. (2001). Palliative care for the poor and disenfranchised: a view from the Robert Wood Johnson Foundation. *Journal of the Royal Society of Medicine*, 94, 486–489.

Gomes, B. and Higginson, I.J. (2006). Factors influencing death at home in terminally ill patients with cancer: systematic review. [Erratum appears in *BMJ*, 2006, 332(7548), 1012]. *BMJ*, 332(7540), 515–521.

Kagawa-Singer, M. and Blackhall, L.J. (2001). Negotiating cross-cultural issues at the end of life: 'You got to go where he lives'. *Journal of the American Medical Association*, 286(23), 2993–3001.

Koffman, J., Burke, G., Dias, A., Ravel, B., Byrne, J., Gonzales, J., and Daniels, C. (2007). Demographic factors and awareness of palliative care and related services. *Palliative Medicine*, 21(2), 145–153.

Koffman, J. and Higginson, I.J. (2001). Accounts of carers' satisfaction with health care at the end of life: a comparison of first generation black Caribbeans and white patients with advanced disease. *Palliative Medicine*, 15(4), 337–345.

Koffman, J. and Higginson, I.J. (2004). Dying to be home? A comparison of preferred place of death of first generation black Caribbean and native-born white patients in the United Kingdom. *Journal of Palliative Medicine*, 7, 628–636.

Lindsay, J., Jagger, C., Hibbert, M., Peet, S., and Moledina, F. (1997). Knowledge, uptake and the availability of health and social services among Asian Gujarati and white persons. *Ethnicity and Health*, 2, 59–69.

Smaje, C. and Field, D. (1997). Absent minorities? Ethnicity and the use of palliative care services. In J. Hockey and N. Small (eds.), *Death, Gender and Ethnicity*, pp.142–165. London: Routledge.

2.6

The economic challenges of palliative medicine

Thomas J. Smith and J. Brian Cassel

Introduction: the reasons to do palliative care

The compelling reasons for palliative care continue to be better symptom management, better advanced care planning and medically appropriate goal setting, and transitions to hospice care (Morrison and Meier 2004). Since the first edition of this book, over 80% of hospitals in the United States now have palliative care programmes (Center to Advance Palliative Care, 2014), the United Kingdom has strongly endorsed palliative care in the End of Life Care Strategy as a way to allow more patients to die at home with better quality of care (Department of Health, 2008), and the American Society of Clinical Oncology has endorsed concurrent palliative care for all seriously ill cancer outpatients (Smith et al., 2012a). Other new-found compelling reasons include better survival with hospice care, better survival with concurrent palliative care, and lower cost to hospitals and government and insurance funders. In every study to date, hospice and palliative care have been associated with equal or better survival and lower cost. A compilation of the available studies, in Fig. 2.6.1, shows that the group that receives palliative care has lower in-hospital or total costs.

In this chapter, we will define the various types of cost and clinical studies and discuss the available data about the economic challenges of palliative care, how to apply the available data, how to collect and present some useful and useable data, and new directions for research. We have summarized the key learning points in Box 2.6.1.

Why is cost important?

The United States is an example of uncontrolled health spending. Currently the United States spends 18% of the gross domestic product (GDP) on health care, which translates into $8000 per person per year; Canada and most other countries spend $4000–5000 per person per year and have equivalent health outcomes (Organisation for Economic Co-operation and Development, 2012). Insurance premiums for a family of four have risen from $6000 in 2000 to over $15,000 in 2011, with co-payments rising from $1000 to over $4000 (Claxton et al., 2010). There are over a million medical bankruptcies each year, with over half amongst insured people (Himmelstein et al., 2009). Almost one-quarter of Medicare spending (the single payer system for those over age 65) is in the last year of life and over 9% in the last month of life

(Riley and Lubitz, 2010). There is great variation in end-of-life care in the United States, such that over half of patients die in the ICU at some hospitals, and the use of hospice care varies from 20% to 40%, when it should be over 60% (The Dartmouth Institute for Health Policy and Clinical Practice, 2014).

Other countries have different issues. In the United Kingdom, and much of the world, the dramatic rise of deaths in the hospital has driven up health-care costs. Before the Second World War this rarely happened but at present 58% of people die in hospital, which has increased the need for beds, with attendant costs (Gardiner et al., 2013). The barriers to better palliative care are familiar: lack of discussions about palliative care, avoidance of discussions to maintain false hope, and lack of mechanisms for a smooth transition (Gott et al., 2011). Over half of all complaints about medical care in the United Kingdom relate to poor end-of-life care, which the National Health Service (NHS) is addressing with the End of Life Care Programme. In the Middle East and countries like Portugal there has been an even more rapid shift, with over half of all patients now dying in hospital within the past generation, which is simply unsustainable financially. In most cultures, when people are given a choice, they prefer to die at home. Despite the large percentage of deaths in UK hospitals, current UK data show an increase in deaths at home and decline in deaths in hospital, which suggests that such programmes can be successful (Gomes et al., 2012).

Types of cost studies and how they are used in decision-making

The traditional ways of balancing cost and health outcomes are reviewed briefly in Table 2.6.1. In decades past, clinical outcomes alone were sufficient. But with palliative drugs now costing over $100,000 a year it is critical that we ascertain if the benefit is affordable. Some examples include palliative sipuleucel-T for metastatic castrate-resistant prostate cancer (survival benefit 4 months, cost US$90,000), and palliative treprostinil (Remodulin®, US$120,000/year) and epoprostenol (Flolan® US$100,000/year) for pulmonary hypertension, with better exercise tolerance, but no clear cut improvement in overall survival (Macchia et al., 2011). It is clear that the problems of balancing cost and effectiveness will persist.

Clinical outcomes alone

When a drug is much better than any other treatment, for instance, imatinib mesylate (Gleevec®) in the treatment of chronic

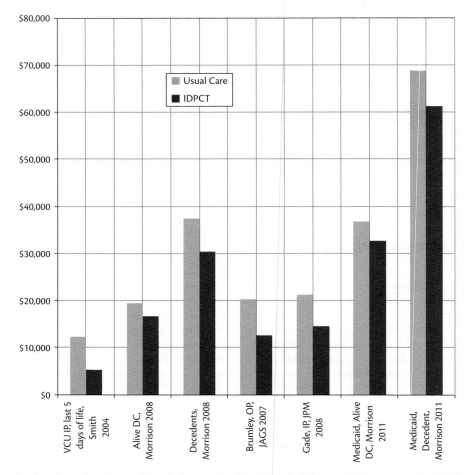

Fig. 2.6.1 Representative studies that show reduced costs with palliative care. Key: IDPCT, interdisciplinary palliative care team; VCU IP, Virginia Commonwealth University Inpatient Unit; DC, discharges; Decedents, patients who died during that admission; OP, outpatients randomized to usual care versus usual care and interdisciplinary palliative care team; IP, inpatients randomized to usual care versus usual care plus and interdisciplinary palliative care team; Medicaid, Alive Medicaid-eligible patients discharged alive. The Gade and Brumley trials are randomized controlled trials.

Box 2.6.1 Key learning points about palliative care finances

The imperatives for palliative care include financial issues, but the main goal is better patient care.

The evidence for cost savings or cost avoidance in hospice is strong.

The evidence for cost savings and cost avoidance in acute palliative care is strong, particularly in integrated health systems such as a national health insurance or health maintenance organization.

The economic outcomes of palliative care programmes are not limited to cost-avoidance and include cost savings, best use of scarce resources such as the intensive care unit (ICU), good will, and profit.

Data that illustrate good care and positive financial impact on the institution are relatively simple to collect.

---

myelogenous leukaemia or gastrointestinal stromal tumour, medical care decisions are clear-cut. It is a lifesaving drug but the cost ranges from $32,000 to $98,000 per year depending on dose. With such blockbuster drugs, the only real issue is how to make room in the budget; another issue is that patients who bear some or all of the financial cost will stop taking expensive drugs in an economic downturn (Kelley and Venook, 2010). The second and third drugs on the market for the same indication were priced even higher and to date there has been no price competition (Tuma, 2007), so alternative strategies on cost control will continue to be needed. The NHS in England is trying several, including 2 free months of the drug (paid for by the manufacturer), and the NHS only pays if the drug is successful (Rawlins et al., 2010; Yong et al., 2010).

Cost alone

Very few, if any, new drugs cost less than the treatment they replace. Knowing that a drug or treatment is inexpensive does not help decision-makers without some indication that a treatment actually works. For example, a widely used anti-nausea remedy lorazepam (Ativan®), diphenhydramine (Benadryl®) and haloperidol gel ('ABH gel') costs pennies for each dose, but is not absorbed, so cannot be effective (Smith et al., 2012b).

Cost minimization

Cost minimization combines clinical results with cost. Two equally effective strategies are compared, and the one that has

Table 2.6.1 Types of studies and application to palliative care

Type of study	Advantages and disadvantages	Application to palliative care
Clinical outcomes alone	Easy to perform Ignores costs	Traditional way to make decisions, e.g. imatinib mesylate (Gleevec®) works for chronic myelogenous leukaemia. Find a way to pay for it
Cost alone	Ignores clinical outcomes	Rarely used to make decisions, unless the medical outcomes are similar (cost minimization, below)
Costs and clinical outcomes together		
Cost minimization: assumes two strategies are equal; lowest cost strategy is preferred	Easy to do if there are direct comparisons	For instance, if methadone gives equivalent pain relief to sustained-release morphine, then use the less expensive option
Cost-effectiveness: compares two strategies; assigns $ per additional year of life (LY) saved by strategy	Requires a trial that directly compares strategies, and economic analysis alongside that trial. 'Only accept treatments that gain a year of life for under $100,000/LY	Palliative care usually adds no additional LYs, so rarely applicable. May be most appropriate in chemotherapy or other interventions that prolong life
Cost utility: assigns $ per additional LY saved by strategy, then estimates the quality of that benefit in $/quality-adjusted life year (QALY).	Compares two strategies, with their quality of life comparisons converted to utility, or the value placed on time in a health state, e.g. time spent on chemotherapy = 0.7 compared to a healthy individual whose utility = 1.0	There are few interventions that make a large difference in utility Also, there is rarely one simple yardstick of utility that covers all health states.
Cost–benefit: compares two strategies but converts the clinical benefit to money, e.g. a year of life is worth $100 000	Possible but rarely done due to difficulty in assigning $ value to human life	Would almost certainly be unfavourable to most palliative interventions, as patients rarely work or generate income
Special considerations		
Cost avoidance: measure the costs saved by not doing procedures, or by moving from an expensive place of care to a less expensive place	Can be easy to calculate (moving from ICU bed to regular or hospice bed) or difficult (avoided CAT scans, for which there is no financial record)	Hospital-based programmes routinely show cost savings to the health system. Important to know who is avoiding the cost and who may be absorbing the cost. For instance, if palliative care transfers sick patients to hospice, it will save the hospital money but cost the hospice money if the daily costs are above the per diem given to the hospice organization, typically US$150 per day (Passik et al., 2004)
Opportunity cost: the cost of performing one action rather than another. For instance, the opportunity cost of a patient staying in the ICU when appropriate for palliative care end of life is the high cost of that day plus the lost revenue of the ICU day plus the lost opportunity if a potential patient did not get appropriate trauma or ICU care	Harder to calculate	Familiar concept to most CEOs. They may quickly realize that gaining 200 ICU bed days a year by transferring appropriate patients 1 day sooner would generate $1100/day × 200 days, and prevent the hospital from being on Emergency Room diversion.

the least total cost is preferred. An example is drugs which are designed simply to replace expensive drugs with equivalent ones. In palliative care, Bruera and colleagues showed that methadone was equal to sustained-release morphine in the relief of pain (Bruera et al., 2004); the choice should depend on which is less expensive. This approach is not without flaws. First, it requires that there be a direct comparison of the drugs or technologies. Second, it may put too much emphasis on immediate treatments costs alone, and not enough on long-term costs; for instance, if ABH gel is less expensive than other more effective anti-nausea drugs, one hospitalization for refractory nausea would outweigh hundreds of pounds of savings on the cheaper but less effective remedy (Smith et al., 2012b).

Palliative and supportive care, including home and inpatient hospice care, is a good example of cost minimization. If we assume that survival is equal and the care is at least as good and costs are lower, then we should choose hospice and palliative care. Palliative care consultation improves appropriate hospice enrolment. Morrison et al. compared 1427 patients who did not have a palliative care consult with 296 patients who did, matched in every other respect, and found that if the palliative care team were involved, 30% of hospice eligible patients were discharged to hospice compared with just 1% of patients not seen by palliative care (Morrison et al., 2011). Patients enrolled in palliative care programmes at Sutter Health enrolled in hospice 47% of the time, compared to 20% of similar patients (Meyers et al., 2004,

2011). Appropriate transition to hospice not only improves care (Peppercorn et al., 2011), but is also associated with longer survival (Connor et al., 2007) and lower costs (Pyenson et al., 2004). The most recent data show that hospice saves US Medicare about US$2309 in the last year of life compared to conventional care, and that the savings increase the longer hospice is used (Taylor et al., 2007).

Cost-effectiveness

This method compares two known strategies in both effectiveness (years of additional life gained) and cost, then assigns a cost per additional year of life (LY) saved by the best ('dominant') strategy. For instance, adjuvant chemotherapy for a 45-year-old woman with early-stage breast cancer would be expensive, but would add 5.1 months of additional life at a cost of about $15,000 per year (Hillner and Smith, 2007). Expensive therapies can be 'cost-effective' too if they provide substantial benefit. For instance, trastuzumab (Herceptin®) for adjuvant treatment of breast cancer patients is expensive (over $50,000 in all countries) but the 50% relative reduction in recurrence risk and 1.5 additional years for the average patient makes the cost-effectiveness ratio of $14,000 to $40,000/LY acceptable (Kievit et al., 2005).

There are several assumptions about this method that make it difficult to apply in the real world. First, it implies a limit to resources such that there must be some 'cap' on the cost-effectiveness ratio. The World Health Organization has defined 'reasonable' cost-effectiveness as interventions with a cost-effectiveness ratio that is less than the per capita GDP (Lillemoe et al., 1993; World Health Organization, 2001). Second, it assumes that a single week of added life for 52 persons equals 1 full year of life for another person. Third, it assumes that all people are somehow in the same health system and share a single set of values. Fourth, it requires someone to fund these difficult studies to generate cost-effectiveness data, when many patients are only interested in cure, doctors have a strong interest in benefit, and drug companies are interested in profit, and not usually social justice. Currently, the United Kingdom, Australia, Canada, and most countries use explicit cost-effectiveness to determine insurance coverage, but the United States does not.

Another issue is the question of 'whose costs' are being saved. In the United States and other countries with large hospital infrastructures and large third-party funder markets (e.g. Germany), one must keep in mind that money is changing hands several times. One can reduce hospital costs in ways that do not affect the amount paid to the hospital by the funders. In instances where funders do cut costs, typically this means lower revenue to providers (hospitals and doctors).

Palliative care brings an additional challenge in that very few palliative treatments make people live longer so that additional LYs are not saved. Nearly all the available studies show equal survival, with only one showing improved survival of 2.7 months with concurrent oncology and palliative care (Temel et al., 2010), with about $2000 less overall cost (Greer et al., 2012).

Cost utility adds adjustments for quality of life

In cost-utility analysis the quality of life in a given state of disease or treatment ('health state'), is converted to a utility ratio where 1 equals perfect health and 0 equals death. For example, a patient whose pain has been relieved may have a utility range of 0.90 of 1.00, whereas a patient with continued pain may have a utility range of 0.50. The utility ratio converts 'cost-effectiveness' into cost per quality-adjusted life year (QALY). For example, an intervention that costs $100,000 per year of life gained would be converted to $50,000 per QALY if the treatment doubled the patient's utility score from 0.5 to 1.0. This intervention, however welcomed, would not save money but would cost an additional $50,000 to save an additional QALY with the intervention.

There are several difficulties with the cost-utility method. One is assigning proper utility ratios to the various health states. Controversy exists as to the most appropriate source of values: patients, healthcare workers, or the general population (society) due to differences in perspective. Patients and clinicians place greater emphasis on the issues that matter most to them, such as life, morbidity, or expense. For example, patients are more likely than clinicians to accept toxic treatments in exchange for minor clinical benefits, and a 1% chance of cure or 10% chance of symptom relief may be sufficient for them to choose treatment over supportive care (reviewed by Russell et al., 1996). The most objective source is probably lay people (jurors) whose money is being used (Russell et al., 1996; Smith et al., 2005); the difficulty lies in educating them properly in all aspects of a patient's experience, for example, emotional turmoil, treatment toxicity, inconvenience, and other physical and psychosocial stressors.

A second problem is the magnitude of palliative care interventions, which is usually not enough to change overall ('global') quality of life or utility values. A recent exception was the randomized trial of palliative care alongside usual oncology care versus usual oncology care alone which showed a substantial difference in global quality of life (Zimmerman et al., 2012). Whether the magnitude is enough to change utility scores has not been studied.

Several recent cost-effectiveness or cost-utility studies have produced results that will be of use to decision-makers. Single-fraction radiation for painful bone metastases instead of the usual six treatments was as effective and cost substantially less (van den Hout et al., 2006). Shorter-fraction regimens for palliative treatment of lung cancer, 2×8 Gy versus 3×10 Gy, showed the opposite effect; the cost-utility ratio for the 10×3 Gy schedule versus the 2×8 Gy schedule was acceptable at $40,900/QALY. The longer regimen had an acceptable cost-effectiveness ratio because people lived longer with the 10×3 Gy treatment, offsetting the higher treatment cost (Mason et al., 2011). In countries with nationalized healthcare systems, the QALY is more important and more frequently used (e.g. in the United Kingdom with its NHS) than in other countries such as the United States where there is neither a single, nationalized healthcare system providing care, nor a single, nationalized payer.

Cost–benefit

This method compares two interventions then assigns a monetary value to the added clinical benefit of the best strategy, based on the overall economic productivity of an individual. Therefore, a treatment that costs $50,000 to prolong life 1 year would be acceptable if the person could produce $50,000 of economic worth in that year, but not if the person only produced $10,000 that year. This kind of analysis, while useful in business decisions, is rarely used in clinical studies because of the difficulties in assigning a monetary value to a human life, especially if that value is tied to an individual's socioeconomic status. Since palliative care patients rarely produce income, even if their symptoms are well controlled, palliative care interventions would be at a distinct disadvantage.

Cost avoidance

This concept has been widely used as an economic argument for palliative care. If a patient can be moved from a US$5000/day ICU bed to a US$1500/day palliative care bed, with equal or better care that meets the patient's goals, *a US$3500 cost will have been avoided each day for each patient*. Taken in aggregate, these costs can be substantial and more than offset palliative care programme costs. For instance, palliative care programmes have reported only a small profit, but annual savings of over US$1 million due to 'cost avoidance' defined as costs saved by transferring a patient from a high-cost venue to a low-cost one, such as from ICU to a regular hospital bed (Brumley et al., 2007; Gade et al., 2008; Smith and Cassel, 2009; Morrison et al., 2011). Similarly, not doing 50 computed tomography (CT) scans each year by careful matching of the goals of care with the diagnostic tests could save up to US$2500 × 50 = US$125,000. In a cost-based system such as national health insurance or diagnosis-related group (DRG) payment system, this would be a desired outcome; however, in a profit-based system this could represent substantial lost profit.

Cost avoidance is relatively easy to measure from usual data bases in US hospitals if there are comparable patients to match before the intervention, because billing systems record what was actually done. A simple historical analysis would show that more patients receive comfort care once a palliative care (PC) programme is established than under standard care. However it is much more difficult to quantify patient-level (or day-level) hospital cost savings in other countries, such as England, where fewer hospitals have invested in systems to do patient-level (or episode-level) cost accounting and cost allocation. In such countries or scenarios, the simplest way to collect data about cost savings is a notebook of 'avoided tests' after palliative care consult, for example, for the first 50 PC consult patients, 50 planned CTs or similar procedures were cancelled. Or to use hospital data on the frequency, duration, and intensity of hospitalizations per patient, comparing PC and non-PC patients.

Large insurers have noted the benefits of enhanced palliative care. In a series of landmark observational trials, researchers at Aetna introduced an expanded access 'Compassionate Care Programme'. They identified cancer patients being treated for terminal conditions through their billing patterns, offered expanded access hospice without having to give up conventional treatment, and offered 24-hour daily help with symptoms by a nurse call-in line. Patients were also assigned a care manager. Hospice use doubled, hospice days doubled, hospital and ICU admissions were dramatically reduced (Spettell et al., 2009), and costs were reduced 22% in the last 40 days of life (Krakauer et al., 2011). Whether the change in resources and costs is due to the PC consult by itself, or the underlying reasons for the PC consult (change in medical goals, change in family or patient perspective, change in physician perspective) cannot be answered from the available data. Since these studies have now been replicated in numerous settings, it seems unlikely that the reduction in resources and costs is unrelated to PC consultation; but, one cannot ascribe all the change to the consultation itself. In the case of PC, the retrospective correlational studies correlate well with the available randomized clinical trials that show equal survival with substantial cost savings (Smith and Cassel, 2009).

Additional considerations

There are a few important other considerations in the economics of PC. The first is *perspective*: whose money is being spent, on whom? In general, health economists take the societal viewpoint; that is, society has limited resources and wants to spend it to gain the most health for the most people. This runs directly counter to the individual viewpoint that only one person's health—'mine'—matters. The societal impact would also take into account work and time lost, and all the additional costs of care that are absorbed by families. Since studies often cannot take all these into account, a common compromise is to take the view of a health system or funder, for example, the NHS in the United Kingdom or Canada or a large insurer in the United States. As an example, a palliative care programme that accepts patients from the hospital will lower the hospital costs; if however, that palliative care programme transfers these patients to hospice, and the patients continue to use more care (IVs, pain medicines, diagnostic tests) then hospice costs increase even though the total costs decrease (Passik et al., 2004). Palliative care programmes for inpatients have consistently shown cost savings of 25–60% (Smith et al., 2003; Naik, 2004; Morrison et al., 2008, 2011).

A second concern is *opportunity cost*, simply defined as the additional revenue that could be gained if money had been used in a different way (this will only be relevant in health systems where third-party revenue is at stake). For instance, an ICU bed that is filled by someone who is not getting better may force the hospital into diversion. In a natural experiment, Oregon Health Center found that every hour of Emergency Room diversion cost the hospital system over $1100 *per hour* in profit, the opportunity cost of diversion. Transferring patients from the ICU to a more appropriate venue may give cost avoidance of $2500/day, *and* open that bed for an additional patient (McConnell et al., 2006). The opportunity cost of filled ICU beds is a sound financial concept that is understandable to most chief executives; if a palliative care programme assists in the transfer of 200 patients 2 days earlier, then the medical staff will have 400 more ICU bed days available.

A third concern is *mortality* in the hospital. If a hospital has a robust palliative care programme, will patients come there, die, and worsen the hospital mortality statistics? The two reports available strongly suggest that mortality is not increased in programmes that have the best palliative care systems (Elsayem et al., 2004; Cassel et al., 2010a).

A fourth issue is who funds palliative care specialists. In the United States, the Veterans Administration healthcare system and the Kaiser Permanente system, both of which have annual healthcare expenditure budgets and do not rely primarily on revenue from third parties, have invested millions of dollars in funding specialists, teams and palliative care units. In other US hospitals, a mixture of direct clinical revenue for specialists and a subsidy from the hospital together fund the teams (see Morrison et al., 2008). In terms of hospice provision, the US Medicare Hospice Benefit provides a reliable funding stream for patients in hospice and hospice touches over 40% of deaths in the United States (National Hospice and Palliative Care Organization, 2013). Other countries have struggled to provide an adequate funding stream for hospice—for example, in the United Kingdom, a large portion of hospice expenses are paid for through charity, and hospice touches far fewer of the deaths.

The available clinical and economic data

We have organized the available randomized clinical trial data into one table of important clinical effectiveness and cost data (Table 2.6.2). No trial has shown worse care or an increase in costs, or any sort of harm to patients.

Clinical effectiveness

The effectiveness data for palliative care is now sufficient for the American Society of Clinical Oncology to recommend concurrent palliative care alongside usual oncology care for all seriously cancer patients (Smith et al., 2012a). The most recent randomized clinical trial from Canada confirms and extends these findings (Zimmerman et al., 2012). The only negative randomized clinical trials used a model of consultant care outside the usual care team, such that only about 20% of recommendations were followed

Table 2.6.2 Randomized trials of palliative care

Author, year, intervention type	Outcomes					
	Symptoms	**Quality of life**	**Mood**	**Satisfaction**	**Resource use**	**Survival**
Pantilat et al., 2010 Study performed 2002–2003 Consultant MD model[a]	No difference	Not measured	Depression not reported, anxiety no difference	Not measured	Not measured	Not measured
Rabow et al., 2004 Consultant MD model	Less dyspnoea, $P = 0.01$, no change in pain	No difference	Less anxiety ($P = 0.05$), no change in depression ($P = 0.28$)	No difference	No difference	Not measured
Brumley et al., 2007 Interdisciplinary palliative care team (IPCT)	Not measured	Not measured	Not measured	Improved, $P < 0.05$	Cost $12,670 vs $20,222, $P = 0.03$ Hospital days reduced by 4.36 ($P < 0.001$)	No difference
Gade et al., 2008 IPCT	No difference	No difference	No difference	IPCS patients reported greater satisfaction with their care experience ($P = 0.04$) and providers' communication ($P = 0.0004$)	Total mean health costs $6766 lower (IPCS: $14,486; UC: $21,252, $P < 0.001$). Net cost savings of $4855 (staffing costs) per patient ($P < 0.001$).	No difference
Bakitas et al., 2009 Nursing education intervention	Improved $P = 0.06$	Improved $P = 0.02$	Improved $P = 0.02$	Not measured	No difference	No difference
Temel et al., 2010 IPCT	Improved $P = 0.04$	Improved $P = 0.03$	Less depression $P = 0.01$	Not measured	Less aggressive care $P = 0.05$ Costs about $2200 less per patient with PC	11.6 vs 8.9 months $P = 0.02$
Meyers et al., 2011 Three education sessions in the first month to learn problem-solving skills	Not measured	Patients: no difference. Caregivers: declined at less than half the rate of control, $P = 0.02$	No difference	Not measured	Not measured	Not measured
Zimmerman et al., 2012 Cluster randomized trial of palliative care alongside usual oncology care	Improved	Improved	Improved	Not reported	Not yet reported	Equal

[a] The model was a consultant physician who was not a member of the team and made recommendations which were not followed the majority of the time. The primary care provider followed recommendations for opioid prescription in 8% of cases, and antidepressant prescription only 17% of cases. This may partly explain the lack of effect

AD, advance directive; ED, emergency department; IPCS, interdisciplinary palliative care service; IPCT, Interdisciplinary palliative care team; OR, odds ratio; PC, palliative care; UC, usual care.

Source: data from personal communication, Steve Pantilat MD, May 2, 2011.

(Pantilat et al., 2010); we would not reject a trial of a new drug if compliance were only 20%.

The impact of hospice and palliative care on cost of care

Hospice was designed to improve care, not save money, but a good side effect has been cost control. The original Medicare hospice benefit was developed with the intent to improve care, not save money, but was required to be 'revenue neutral' (or, not cost Medicare any additional money). As noted above, hospice care saves money compared to usual care at the end of life, and the longer hospice is used, the more money is saved (Taylor et al., 007).

The available studies of palliative care strongly suggested substantial cost savings as shown in Fig. 2.6.1. Originally, Smith et al. reported over 60% hospital cost savings when patients died under the care of the palliative care team, matched to other patients who died in the hospital (Smith et al., 2003; Naik, 2004). The same group subsequently reported substantial reductions in all symptoms measured, if present, within 48 hours suggesting that the care was equal or better than usual care (Khatcheressian et al., 2005). Elsayem and colleagues at M.D. Anderson Cancer Center reported good symptom control accompanied by a dramatic decrease in costs (Elsayem et al., 2004). More recently, Morrison and colleagues showed that in New York State, hospitals with palliative care programmes increased appropriate referrals to hospice by tenfold, and saved over $5000 per admission (Naik, 2004; Morrison et al., 2008).

There are now several randomized trials that show substantial improvements in care associated with equal or reduced costs, as shown in Table 2.6.3. The data from the two randomized trials

Table 2.6.3 Practical palliative care measures and how to collect them

Measure	Data source	Units	Comment
Clinical			
Pain scores	Symptom assessment scale	Visual or linear scale in common use	Use what is in common use at the institution, so that PC scores can be compared to other unit scores.
Other symptom scores, e.g. fatigue, dyspnoea	Symptom assessment scale	Edmonton, Memorial or similar symptom assessment scale	Most other units will not collect data, so PC can accelerate change by showing benefit
Patient and family satisfaction	Survey instruments		Most commercial patient satisfaction firms do not survey decedent families
Stories of patient and family satisfaction	Collected thank you notes and letters		Stories are really important to catch someone's attention. Insert in text boxes in all newsletters. Copy and send to CEO monthly
Economic and other			
Profit margin	Health system financials	Amount contributed to the health system	Most PC programmes will not generate profit, but it is important to be 'cost neutral' to the health system. If the loss is small, it can be made up by contributions
Cost avoidance	$/day saved by transfer to PC team or unit, with resources matched to goals of care	Amount saved for the health system	Each day of transfer from a high-cost to low-cost venue may save $1500 or more. In addition, it will free up the high-cost ICU beds or ED space.
Referrals	By month and year	New patients to the service New patients referred specifically to PC Recurring patients	Documents the amount of work done in understandable terms May document new patients brought to system by PC (new business)
Length of stay	Inpatient LOS for those patients seen by PC team	Days	There may not be much difference. It is important to show that LOS is not increased by PC compared to usual care, in most health-care systems
ICU transfers	All transfers, and LOS before/after	Measure all transfers from ICU after PC consultation	This frees valuable ICU time
Direct ED admissions	All consultations and direct admissions	Measure the LOS, costs of ED consults and admissions	May show a shorter LOS and lower cost than similar patients who are admitted to general service then later to PC
Research grants and funds	Report all submissions and successful requests	All, including $ requested and received	This is a common measure of success for many programmes housed in academic programmes
Scholarly works		Papers, abstracts, presentations	This is the most understandable measure of academic success
Charitable contributions			This may offset losses. Most PC programmes work well with their institutional development officers for fund raising

ED, emergency department; ICU, intensive care unit; LOS, length of stay; PC, palliative care.

Table 2.6.4 Model presentation for palliative care

Clinical	Economic
All symptoms improved from day 1 to day 3 1st day comparison day	1. 1800 consultations done hospital-wide fiscal year 2012
	2. 350 outpatient new consultations and 1000 repeat visits
	3. 5.2 of 6 palliative care beds filled daily
	4. Profit overall $20,000
	5. Profit on direct admissions from ER, clinic, hospice $250,000; losses on transfer cases $230,000
	6. Cost avoidance $900,000
	7. Professional income of $150,000, covering 60% of salaries
	8. Additional ICU capacity of 250 bed days
	9. Charitable contributions $250,000
	10. Grant funding $400,000
	11. 5 papers; 3 abstracts; 6 regional/national presentations
	12. Two awards for exemplary service

done within the Kaiser Permanente health maintenance organization were so compelling, with better care and $4500–7000 savings per person, that this is now standard care at all their hospitals (Brumley et al., 2007; Gade et al., 2008). The study of non-small cell lung cancer patients randomized at presentation to usual oncology care versus usual oncology care plus concurrent care demonstrated substantially improved quality of life, quality of care, better survival (Temel et al.,2010), and a cost saving of over $2000 per person (Greer et al., 2012). Patients with multiple sclerosis who received palliative care, cost the UK NHS £1200 less than their peers who did not receive it, even incorporating the cost of the care (Higginson et al., 2009) and had better clinical outcomes during and after the trial for up to 6 weeks (Currow et al., 2011).

How to collect and present useable data

A key question before collecting data is to decide beforehand on its use. Is the interested party interested in passing accreditation, improving market share, improving patient satisfaction, reducing health system costs, or increasing profits? The goal will dictate what data to collect and how to present it. In collecting and presenting the data, we have found that the simplest approach is the most effective. Most administrators want to know that the programme is successful, defined as providing good care, keeping busy, and not losing too much money.

We advise programmes to collect useful data that are being requested, and no more. Some common metrics are listed in Table 2.6.3. To collect more data than is actually used, takes time, effort, and money that would be better spent doing clinical care or research.

Presentation of the data should be as simple as possible. We have found that a simple 'improved care at no extra cost' approach is well received, as shown in Table 2.6.4. Again, most administrators will not be expecting palliative care to make a large profit. The goal of this report is fairly and accurately to reflect the activity and impact of the programme.

New directions

Palliative care is now well established as a necessary part of modern clinical care that can improve quality of life and quality of care and can save money. Additional research is needed to confirm results in different diseases, especially non-cancer (Farquhar et al., 2011; Higginson et al., 2011). As a field, we must determine a simple, easy to understand metric of the net benefits and burdens of palliative care in order for funders to justify new and continuing investments (Currow et al., 2011).

Resources

Palliative Care Leadership Center Curriculum (PCLC)—Center to Advance Palliative Care. The PCLC curriculum addresses issues relevant to each stage of palliative care programme development: structural, organizational, and financial. See 'Module 3: Making the Financial Case', available at <http://www.capc.org/palliative-care-leadership-initiative/curriculum>. This curriculum shows a programme how to build a financial case for palliative care, alongside the clinical case. There are core, custom, and advanced modules available.

Inter-Institutional Collaborating Network On End Of Life Care (IICN) website: 'free access to over 4,000 pages of high-quality education materials about end-of-life care, palliative medicine, and hospice care, including the full text of several books'. This includes a very helpful guide to starting PC programmes: TriCentral Palliative Care Programme Toolkit, available at <http://www.growthhouse.org/palliative/>.

Online materials

Complete references for this chapter are available online at <http://www.oxfordmedicine.com>.

References

Bakitas, M., Lyons, K.D., Hegel, M.T., et al. (2009). Effects of a palliative care intervention on clinical outcomes in patients with advanced cancer: the Project ENABLE II randomized controlled trial. *Journal of the American Medical Association*, 302(7), 741–749.

Brumley, R., Enguidanos, S., Jamison, P., *et al.* (2007). Increased satisfaction with care and lower costs: results of a randomized trial of in-home palliative care. *Journal of the American Geriatrics Society*, 55(7), 993–1000.

Cassel, J.B., Hager, M.A., Clark, R.R., *et al.* (2010a). Concentrating hospital-wide deaths in a palliative care unit: the effect on place of death and system-wide mortality. *Journal of Palliative Medicine*, 13(4), 371–374.

Center to Advance Palliative Care (2005). *Impact Calculator.* [Online] Available at: <http://www.capc.org/impact_calculator_basic/>.

Center to Advance Palliative Care (2014). *Palliative Care Tools, Training & Technical Assistance.* [Online] Available at: <http://www.capc.org>.

Connor, S.R., Pyenson, B., Fitch, K., Spence, C., and Iwasaki, K. (2007). Comparing hospice and nonhospice patient survival among patients who die within a three-year window. *Journal of Pain and Symptom Management*, 33(3), 238–246.

Currow, D.C., Abernethy, A.P., Bausewein, C., Johnson, M., Harding, R., and Higginson, I. (2011). Measuring the net benefits of hospice and palliative care: a composite measure for multiple audiences-palliative net benefit. *Journal of Palliative Medicine*, 14(3), 264–265.

Gade, G., Venohr, I., Conner, D., *et al.* (2008). Impact of an inpatient palliative care team: a randomized control trial. *Journal of Palliative Medicine*, 11(2), 180–190.

Higginson, I.J., Costantini, M., Silber, E., Burman, R., and Edmonds, P. (2011). Evaluation of a new model of short-term palliative care for people severely affected with multiple sclerosis: a randomised fast-track trial to test timing of referral and how long the effect is maintained. *Postgraduate Medical Journal*, 87(1033), 769–775.

Morrison, R.S., Dietrich, J., Ladwig, S., Quill, T., Sacco, J., Tangeman, J., and Meier, D.E. (2011). Palliative care consultation teams cut hospital costs for Medicaid beneficiaries. *Health Affairs*, 30(3), 454–463.

Morrison, R.S., Penrod, J.D., Cassel, J.B., et al. (2008). Cost savings associated With US hospital palliative care consultation programmes. *Archives of Internal Medicine*, 168(16), 1783–1790.

National Hospice and Palliative Care Organization (2013). *NHPCO's Facts and Figures: Hospice Care in America, 2013 Edition.* [Online] Available at: <http://www.nhpco.org/sites/default/files/public/Statistics_Research/2013_Facts_Figures.pdf >.

Pyenson, B., Connor, S., Fitch, K., and Kinzbrunner, B. (2004). Medicare cost in matched hospice and non-hospice cohorts. *Journal of Pain and Symptom Management*, 28(3), 200–210.

Rabow, M.W., Dibble, S.L., Pantilat, S.Z., and McPhee, S.J. (2004). The comprehensive care team: a controlled trial of outpatient palliative medicine consultation. *Archives of Internal Medicine*, 164(1), 83–91.

Smith, T.J. and Cassel, J.B. (2009). Cost and non-clinical outcomes of palliative care. *Journal of Pain and Symptom Management*, 38(1), 32–44.

Smith, T.J., Coyne, P., Cassel, J.B., *et al.* (2003). A high volume specialist palliative care unit and team may reduce in-hospital end of life care cost. *Journal of Palliative Medicine*, 6, 699–705.

Smith, T.J., Temin, S., Alesi, E., *et al.* (2012a). American Society of Clinical Oncology provisional clinical opinion: the integration of palliative care into standard oncology care. *Journal of Clinical Oncology*, 30(8), 880–887.

Spettell, C.M., Rawlins, W.S., Krakauer, R., *et al.* (2009). A comprehensive case management programme to improve palliative care. *Journal of Palliative Medicine*, 12(9), 827–832.

Temel, J.S., Greer, J.A., Muzikansky, A., *et al.* (2010). Early palliative care for patients with metastatic non small-cell lung cancer. *The New England Journal of Medicine*, 363(8), 733–742.

Zimmerman, C., Swami, N., Rodin, G., *et al.* (2012). Cluster-randomized trial of early palliative care for patients with metastatic cancer. *Journal of Clinical Oncology*, 30(Suppl.), Abstract 9003.

SECTION 3

Service delivery issues in palliative care

Barriers to the delivery of palliative care

Barry J.A. Laird

Introduction to barriers to the delivery of palliative care

There are several key barriers to the delivery of palliative care (Lynch et al., 2010). Probably one of the first aspects to be considered a barrier is the definition of 'palliative care'. The World Health Organization (WHO) defines palliative care as:

an approach that improves the quality of life of patients and their families facing the problem associated with life-threatening illness, through the prevention and relief of suffering by means of early identification and impeccable assessment and treatment of pain and other problems, physical, psychosocial and spiritual. Palliative care:

- provides relief from pain and other distressing symptoms
- affirms life and regards dying as a normal process
- intends neither to hasten or postpone death
- integrates the psychological and spiritual aspects of patient care
- offers a support system to help patients live as actively as possible until death
- offers a support system to help the family cope during the patient's illness and in their own bereavement
- uses a team approach to address the needs of patients and their families, including bereavement counselling, if indicated
- will enhance quality of life, and may also positively influence the course of illness
- is applicable early in the course of illness, in conjunction with other therapies that are intended to prolong life, such as chemotherapy or radiation therapy, and includes those investigations needed to better understand and manage distressing clinical complications. (WHO, 2014)

However, what health professionals and patients consider palliative care may differ both between these groups and/or within them. Some may still regard palliative care as end-of-life care only or associated with cancer. The ideology of palliative care being a concept with which to approach management of patients may still not be fully understood. Furthermore, the differences between generalist and specialist palliative care may also contribute to confusion.

Irrespective of semantics, currently palliative care reaches only a small fraction of those who could benefit from it. Of particular concern is that this situation is likely to become worse.

According to the WHO, in 2008, 7.6 million people died of cancer (approximately 13% of all deaths). Of these, approximately 70% occurred in low- or middle-income countries where palliative care services may be less available. Although survival rates for cancer continue to improve in several key tumour groups, cancer-specific mortality as a proportion of deaths is expected to increase, largely due to a shift from communicable diseases to non-communicable diseases over the next 25 years (Mathers and Loncar, 2006). As a result, death from cancer is going to affect more people and palliative care has to be able to meet the increased demand.

Although palliative care as a concept has largely been embraced throughout the world, its implementation into routine clinical care is lacking. There are many reasons for this but fundamental to improving palliative care access for everyone, is the argument that palliative care should be considered as a human right.

One of the main justifications for this approach is that if palliative care were designated a human right, this would provide the necessary, non-negotiable, impetus for global health policymakers to implement palliative care (Gwyther et al., 2009). Furthermore, it would mean that the obligations for meeting human rights in general, would be adopted for palliative care. This would have several key implications: existing palliative care services which lack the foundation of a secure funding source would have greater bargaining power to obtain robust funding while countries with limited or no services would be encouraged to address this.

The WHO is the key group necessary to develop palliative care worldwide. Strategies developed by the WHO and mirrored by the European Association of Palliative Care (EAPC), the International Association of Hospice and Palliative Care (IAHPC), and the Worldwide Palliative Care Alliance (WPCA) aim to help countries advance palliative care services (Gwyther et al., 2009). Areas of focus include:

- improving drug availability
- education
- policy development
- quality of care
- research.

Essential to the change from palliative care being a principle available to the few, to being available to all, and a human right, is the need to address the many barriers to the efficient and effective delivery of high-quality palliative care. These vary with factors such as geographical setting, economic resources, and the availability of education and training. In this chapter, an overview of these issues is provided, beginning with a global perspective, progressing through social, and organizational, issues, to professional and individual barriers.

Global and economic barriers

Global barriers

The International Observatory on End of Life Care has been monitoring global palliative care development since 2003. Although not wholly exhaustive, a picture of palliative care development on a worldwide scale is slowly emerging. In 2008, Wright and colleagues presented a map of global palliative care development with the aim of categorizing the extent of palliative care services (Wright et al., 2008). From this, it was identified that approximately 50% of the world's countries had a palliative care service; however, only 15% of countries had an integrated palliative care service. This begs the question, what barriers exist globally to prevent palliative care being more widely available?

Advancing palliative care as basic human right may help to improve palliative care access. The role of international palliative care organizations is key to breaking barriers. These include the Asia Pacific Hospice Palliative Care Network, the African Palliative Care Association, the EAPC, the IAHPC, the National Hospice and Palliative Care Organization (United States), and Help the Hospices (United Kingdom). Efforts have also been cemented by the advent of the World Hospice and Palliative Care Day, in 2005.

Building on these strong foundations is the WPCA. Established in 2004, the WPCA is a coalition of key national groups whose aim is the advancement of palliative care towards the ultimate goal of universal access to affordable, high-quality palliative care (Praill and Pahl, 2007). It has been recognized that there is disparity between services nationally and internationally. Furthermore, services are often poorly resourced and of insufficient numbers to meet the increasing needs placed upon them. The WPCA's role is advisory with the remit of developing a better understanding of palliative care policy and disseminating good practice.

Only with greater information about palliative care services, dissemination of good practice, and assistance with policy development can key global barriers to palliative care be broken down.

Economic barriers

Basic health care is becoming less accessible to many (Hsiao and Liu, 1996). This is due to rising drug and health-care costs, in addition to an increased global demand on health-care services; particularly due to the aging population and longer life expectancy.

Palliative care is not immune to these economic constraints; however, one advantage palliative care has compared to other areas of medicine is that the basic drugs needed for symptom control are relatively inexpensive. It has also been shown that pain-relieving medication costs a greater proportion of monthly household income in the developing countries than is the case in the developed world (De Lima et al., 2004). The main economic barrier is resourcing palliative care providers. The intensive medical and nursing support that typifies palliative care is resource heavy.

As non-communicable diseases take precedence, associated with chronicity, there is a marked burden on the health-care system. Developing palliative care services on top of an already burdened health-care system is challenging. Of interest is that in some countries government expenditure on health care has an inverse relationship with wealth. This means that developing countries which have a high demand for palliative care services also have a high demand for basic health care.

Although better, palliative care services in developed countries are not perfect. For example, in the United States, in the Medicare programme, to qualify for referral to palliative care a patient requires certification of terminal illness, usually only permissible near the end of life; in the United Kingdom, which is a world leader in palliative care, the speciality relies heavily on charitable funding, with full National Health Service integration and financial support not established.

In some countries, an inherent lack of health funding means that key priorities (clean drinking water, vaccination against communicable disease, and so on) are addressed while 'less important' areas such as palliative care are neglected. This is also compounded by unstable governments within countries—frequent changes in ruling parties means that varying health policies are adopted (Lynch et al., 2009).

There is also a variation in the types of palliative care funding that are supported. More cost-efficient areas such as hospice, hospital, or general palliative care can be favoured over more expensive options, such as home care. Health-care provision has also to compete against other areas of social demand. For example, in some countries unemployment, poverty, and war mean that palliative care per se is of low priority. The main focus is on caring for patients in the dying phase, with other areas of palliative care being neglected.

Clearly, areas such as palliative care and health-care provision for chronic and incurable disease are low priorities for some developing countries. Nevertheless there are beacons of palliative care excellence in some developing countries. In Uganda and in Kerala (South India) there is excellent palliative care service provision despite low socioeconomic status (Jagwe and Barnard, 2002). It is grounds for optimism that such networks are possible in the developing world and that they are able to provide models for other countries.

Drug availability

Although palliative care patients can require the use of many drugs, fundamental to the armamentarium are opioids. There can be limitations through government policy restrictions on opioid use and rigid prescribing regulations. There is also a disparity in the cost of opioids between countries which can also result in widespread variation in opioid use. This is all compounded by stigmatization; that use of opioids is still associated in some countries with addiction, side effects, and the end of life.

Inadequate access to opioids and other essential symptom control medication is still one of the primary barriers to global palliative care development. Pain is the most common symptom in cancer patients and the publication of the WHO analgesic ladder for cancer pain relief in 1986 aimed to provide an easily followed and globally applicable algorithm for pain (Azevedo Sao Leao Ferreira et al., 2006). While the majority of cancer pains can be controlled using this ladder, a key barrier is the limited availability of opioids. In terms of medication, morphine is relatively inexpensive but it is still not available to millions who need it.

Reluctance to prescribe opioids by health-care professionals is another factor which has limited their use in palliative care.

To combat all areas aspects affecting drug availability, the WHO has highlighted key points for development: education, government policy, drug availability, and the implementation of palliative care services throughout society (Stjernsward et al., 2007). Clearly further work is need to improve popular, professional, and government understanding about opioids, while education is needed to impart the principles of palliative care prescribing and opioid use to health-care professionals.

Social barriers

Ethnicity

One of the key challenges in a multicultural society, particularly in the Western world, is the integration of palliative care appropriately into groups with different cultural backgrounds. It is known that uptake of palliative care services by patients in minority ethnic groups is less than those patients who make up the majority of the population (Ward et al., 2004). Nevertheless, it is important that palliative care reaches out to these groups as they have the same (and sometimes greater need) for palliative care than majority groups. For example, in people with different religious backgrounds, most palliative care services will struggle to deliver appropriate care (Francoeur et al., 2007). There may be several reasons for this which need to be addressed including limitations on resources, institutional, and sometimes personal, racial, or religious discrimination. There may also be limited awareness among health professionals of cultural or religious issues which could impact on the patient's attitude to palliative care. There may also be limited awareness among patients as to the role of hospices and challenges in discussing death with these groups. Recent migrants, those with language or other communication difficulties, and no family advocate present particular challenges (Worth et al., 2009).

Elderly

The number of people dying in care homes in the developed world is steadily increasing so it is important that this group receive appropriate palliative care. However, residential care, particularly in the elderly, has been described as the last frontier for palliative care (Phillips et al., 2006). Palliative care is strongly advocated, however patients who are in long-term care homes do not always receive good end-of-life care, and indeed it is challenging to provide this. A systematic review suggested there were three main causes: delivery system barriers intrinsic to long-term care settings, barriers related to financial issues, and barriers due to regulatory factors (Huskamp et al., 2012).

One of the ways that palliative care can be improved is to develop the role of a link nurse, a trained nurse with specific palliative care skills, including a role in education. Nevertheless, barriers do exist to the efficient use of link nurses such as lack of management support, frequent changes in the workforce, and lack of adequate preparation (Hasson et al., 2008).

The elderly are also more likely to die in hospital settings in general, so ensuring there is appropriate palliative care access is key. The main challenges to providing this include attitudinal differences in the elderly, a lack of resources, and lack of clarity as to which health-care professionals may be most appropriate to provide care for them (specialist versus general palliative care providers, i.e. care of the elderly physicians) (Gardiner et al., 2011).

Homeless

This group of patients can be a particular challenge in palliative medicine and as the number of homeless people is increasing, this is an area where palliative care needs to be accessible. There are, however, barriers which can prevent the appropriate delivery of palliative care to this group of patients. Homeless people have more physical problems (chronic health problems and increased physical and sexual abuse) which are often compounded by lack of access to health services (Rousseau, 1998). The problem of illicit drug use, which tends to be more common among this group of patients, presents some specific challenges in accessing palliative care. These have been identified as concerns from patients such as how withdrawal from drugs will be managed, and a lack of trust in health-care providers (and vice versa), as well as concerns about prejudice (McNeil and Guirguis-Younger, 2012).

Community

Community health professionals have a major role in delivering palliative care, particularly as a large proportion of patients with life-limiting illness wish to die at home. A Japanese survey of community physicians showed that the majority (92.4%) expressed a willingness to provide palliative care, but this would be limited to consultation (83.4%) and referral to a palliative care service (86.8%) (Peng et al., 2013). Only 42.2% were willing to provide home visits. Home visits were more likely to be provided if physicians were family medicine specialists and older than 50 years. It is of interest that the presence of palliative care knowledge did not influence the likelihood of a home visit. The main barriers to effective palliative care delivery by general practitioners were examined in a study from the Netherlands. These included organizational barriers, coordination of care, knowledge, time constraints, and communication difficulties (Groot et al., 2007).

It is also important that advanced care planning is implemented in primary care settings, particularly as patients often prefer to die at home. However, barriers that exist include prognostic uncertainty, limited collaboration with secondary care, a desire to maintain hope, and resistance to a 'tick-box approach' to health care (Boyd et al., 2010). Challenges also occur in providing palliative care in rural versus urban settings. Nurses working in rural settings providing palliative care were more confident in their abilities, but spent more time travelling, than their urban counterparts (Kaasalainen et al., 2011).

Prisoners

Just as the population is becoming older, so is the prison population. In keeping with this, an increasing number of inmates will die in prison from chronic malignant and non-malignant disease. Challenges in caring for these patients at the end of life are, in general, similar to those in the community; however, health-care systems can vary.

For some, prison may afford more regular contact with health care than in the community. In some cases excellent hospice programmes exist within prisons. Clearly, this varies widely within and between countries; however, in the developed world, there is generally some form of established system.

People in prisons are in general poor, and have often suffered from a lack of adequate health care before incarceration. In countries where there has been a trend towards increased sentences, determinate sentences, and mandatory minimum sentences, the average age of the prisoners has also increased. Together these often result in the prisoners suffering from several medical problems and disorders—such as chronic obstructive pulmonary disease (COPD), coronary disease, end-stage renal and liver disease, hypertension, and diabetes—and often in need of palliative care (Linder and Meyers, 2007). Increasing numbers of convictions for drug possession and use have also led to an increase the number of prisoners suffering from HIV and AIDS due to drug injection. AIDS has become the leading cause of death in prisons in the developed world. Patients suffering from HIV and AIDS need complex treatment and access to palliative care, and the high numbers of these patients in prisons represents a major challenge.

The poor socioeconomic background of many prisoners also often means increased issues with learning difficulties and limited reading skills. While giving more patient information and an open discussion with the patient has been the focus of palliative care in general, difficulties in reading, understanding, and acting on health information can be limiting for prisoners. The result may be misunderstandings, frustration, and poorer health outcomes. Dying prisoners may need increased medical attention, extended visiting hours with family, access to special foods, and relaxation from routine duties. Some prisoners can be transferred to hospice units at the end of life, where better end-of-life care can be provided. However, this often results in the dying prisoners being further away from their families (Dubler, 1998).

Staff caring for terminally ill inmates may face barriers such as limited facilities, restricted access to medication, and limited autonomy (Linder and Meyers, 2007). In addition, there may be limited specialist palliative care skills among health professionals working in the prison, and more often it will be general staff who provide this service. Nevertheless, in some developed countries there is often good collaboration between palliative care services in the community who support colleagues working in prison health-care systems. Such systems support palliative care in the prison setting to improve slowly.

End-of-life care requires a trusting alliance between the care providers and the patient. To achieve such a relationship in prison is challenging. In contrast to the general population, prisoners do not assume that the system is acting in their best interests. Dying prisoners may not be convinced that decisions to limit care and permit death have been preceded by the full range of efforts to extend and support life.

Professional barriers

There are many factors related to the practices of health- and social-care professionals that impact on the quality of end-of-life care and referral to appropriate palliative care services.

Attitudes

Although palliative care has long been associated with cancer, barriers exist to integrating palliative care into oncology (Abrahm, 2012). Abraham has argued that there are several key reasons for this. Firstly, there is a degree of learned helplessness from oncologists who have been used to a culture where there is a lack of effective medication with which to manage symptoms. Secondly, there may be lack of adequate communication skills to deal with difficult situations. Another aspect which can impair the integration of palliative care into oncology is compassion fatigue. Grief oncologists feel develops from years of caring for patients who despite best efforts succumb to their illness. This may contribute to 'burn out'.

Oncologists may be of the opinion that they already provide 'palliative care' but their skills can be optimized through time spent working with a specialist palliative care team (Wiebe and Von Roenn, 2010). Limitations can be addressed by ensuring that palliative care training is available to oncologists and this may in part reduce compassion fatigue, while improving palliative care delivery to cancer patients. These steps may afford an increased integration of palliative care and oncology.

Palliative care may be underused in patients with haematological malignancy. A systematic review demonstrated that patients with these malignancies were less likely to receive palliative care than those with other cancers (Howell et al., 2011). Possible explanations include ongoing management by the haematology team, and consequently strong bonds between staff and patients, and challenges with transitions (e.g. withdrawal of blood product support).

A structured transition to a palliative care approach for patients although advocated, is not always evident. One study suggested that prognosis was not always discussed with patients while consensus among the clinical team that a palliative approach should now be the main focus of care was not always achieved in practice (Gott et al., 2011). Furthermore, discussions regarding the adoption of a palliative care approach were not often held with patents, resulting in patients being discharged with unrealistic expectations regarding prognosis. Physicians are often supportive of a palliative care approach, the main barrier for patients being prognostic uncertainty (Snow et al., 2009).

Barriers that were identified included difficulty in 'standing back' in acute hospital settings and professional hierarchies impeding junior medical and also nursing staff from being involved in patient management decisions.

Another barrier to the implementation of palliative care is, when there has been a delay in diagnosis (due to a problematic doctor–patient relationships, a feeling of helplessness, strong emotions from patients and families, and time restraints) (Slort et al., 2011).

Although palliative care is not solely associated with end-of-life care, this is an area where specific barriers particularly exist. Three specific areas were identified in a study conducted to assess the views of palliative care professionals (Feeg and Elebiary, 2005). These included a reluctance of other health professionals to refer to palliative care, a lack of familiarity with the availability and suitability of hospice teams, and the association of hospice care with death.

To improve access to palliative care services in the acute hospital setting several key aspects have been identified, including visibility on the wards, informal routes of access, and consensus on the remit of specialist palliative care services (Ewing et al., 2009). In end-of-life care, several further key barriers exist, for example, inadequate medical education, professional uncertainty regarding the difference between stopping life-sustaining treatment and active euthanasia, difficulty in diagnosing dying, and a perception that death is a professional failure. Another issue is that when patients are transferred to a hospice setting for end-of-life care this segregation from familiar health-care providers may provoke anxiety and in itself be a barrier to the delivery of optimal palliative care (Meier et al., 1997).

Treating fellow health professionals can also be a barrier to the delivery of palliative care. One study examined how the challenges of treating doctors who are palliative care patients identified barriers to implementing palliative care (Noble et al., 2008). These include difficulty in health professionals assuming the patient role, raising barriers to psychosocial aspects of care, and late referral to services.

In general, patients with a non-cancer diagnosis have less access to palliative care than patients with a cancer diagnosis. The End of Life Care Strategy in the United Kingdom raised the profile of end-of-life care, suggesting increased planning and delivery is needed to ensure individuals can choose where and how they die. Several reasons exist as to why end-of-life care access is more difficult in non-cancer patients including differing disease trajectories and care planning, all on a background of appropriate funding. These areas are explored further in relation to specific conditions in 'Barriers in key disease groups' (Addicott, 2012).

General barriers to providing palliative care in non-cancer disease include lack of clarity regarding prognosis, hegemony of the curative approach, avoiding words, and the desire to cheat death (Mahtani-Chugani et al., 2010). Indeed provision of palliative care should be tailored to the trajectory of the individual patient.

Knowledge

Lack of knowledge is a key barrier to palliative care among health professionals. This has been compounded by confusion regarding terminology (specialist versus general palliative care), whether or not patients need to be near the end of life, and even whether palliative care is appropriate for non-malignant, life-limiting disease.

Whist all of these may apply there can be great variation between services which adds to confusion.

Clearly, in an ideal world, differences would not exist; however, it is important that health professionals are aware of the nuances of their local palliative care service. There is an impetus on palliative care services to provide clear guidance on who is appropriate to refer, different services that are available, and also the appropriate time to refer patients. The latter is particularly relevant in the United States since to be eligible for specialist palliative care under Medicare, patients generally need to have a life expectancy of less than 6 months (Brickner et al., 2004).

Which patients are deemed appropriate for palliative care referral can vary between health professionals. One study suggested nursing staff were more likely than medical staff to identify palliative care needs in non-malignant disease; however, this disparity lessened as the patient neared death (Gott et al., 2001). Differences also exist between specialties—for example, oncologists are more likely to refer to palliative care services than other specialists, such as cardiologists.

Barriers in key disease groups

Cardiac disease

Cardiac failure is one of the main areas where palliative care is important (see Chapter 15.3). It is associated with quite marked symptoms including fatigue, breathlessness, and decreased quality of life. In addition to providing good symptomatic relief, palliative care can also provide patient and family support, while assisting in the complex decision-making process that occurs near the end of life. Despite supporting evidence that palliative care is

of benefit in patients with cardiac failure, it remains underused (Lemond and Allen, 2011). As with other conditions, prognostic uncertainty is a barrier to access to palliative care in cardiac failure. Furthermore, inexperience among health professionals can contribute to a lack of palliative care access in patients with cardiac failure (Lemond and Allen, 2011).

Respiratory disease

There is a need for the multidisciplinary approach that is used in palliative care to be implemented in chronic respiratory disease. Reluctance to negotiate end-of-life decisions and a perceived lack of understanding among patients and carers regarding the illness trajectory are regarded as key barriers in end-stage respiratory disease (Spence et al., 2009). There is a lack of evidence and guidelines to support palliative care in chronic respiratory disease in comparison to cancer patients (Hardin et al., 2008).

HIV/AIDS

Patients with HIV/AIDS face some similar difficulties to those coping with chronic cardiac failure and COPD, in that prognostication is difficult and communication with professionals involved in care may not be well enough developed to encompass end-of-life issues in a meaningful way (see Chapter 15.1).

In addition, the stigma of the disease can act as a barrier to effective palliative care, as can negative attitudes to homosexuality or substance abuse (Rondahl et al., 2003). Patients with HIV/AIDS often have a heavy, heterogeneous symptom burden which even experienced palliative care practitioners may feel ill-equipped to manage and patients may prefer specialist HIV/AIDS services for this reason.

There are also major issues involved in the care of those who are bereaved and orphaned (Clark et al., 2007). The case of HIV/AIDS care emphasizes the need for palliative care to sit alongside active treatment with highly active retroviral therapy which can itself cause pain and other symptoms.

If palliative care in HIV/AIDS is to be equitable and effective, services need to minimize discrimination, facilitate ongoing improvement in palliative care knowledge and skills for health-care professionals, produce clear referral criteria for specialist palliative care services, and ensure that high-quality palliative care is available whatever the setting (Harding et al., 2005).

Renal failure

Patients who are receiving dialysis have multiple symptomatic needs including pain, fatigue, mood disorders, and cognitive impairment (see Chapter 15.6). It is also difficult to provide accurate prognoses in this group of patients, due to varying disease trajectories, despite this being a clear need of patients. Palliative care input to this group of patients generally occurs infrequently (Kurella Tamura and Cohen, 2010).

Conclusion

Despite the multiple barriers that exist to the delivery of palliative care, there are grounds for optimism. Palliative care as a concept appears to be well understood and received, suggesting this barrier in part been has overcome (Hanratty et al., 2006). The WHO has promoted policies and advice for the rational implementation of pain relief and palliative care (Stjernsward et al., 1996). Palliative care is now seen as an accepted part of management in many non-malignant, life-limiting conditions and at least basic palliative care education is given to health professionals. As increasing areas develop where palliative care is required, it is important that barriers are overcome to ensure that palliative care as a foundation of good health care is realized.

Acknowledgements

Text extracts from World Health Organization, *WHO Definition of Palliative Care*, available from http://www.who.int/cancer/palliative/definition/en/, Copyright © 2014, reproduced with permission of the World Health Organization.

References

Abrahm, J.L. (2012). Integrating palliative care into comprehensive cancer care. *Journal of the National Comprehensive Cancer Network*, 10, 1192–1198.

Addicott, R. (2012). Delivering better end-of-life care in England: barriers to access for patients with a non-cancer diagnosis. *Health Economics, Policy and Law*, 7, 441–454.

Azevedo Sao Leao Ferreira, K., Kimura, M., and Jacobsen Teixeira, M. (2006). The WHO analgesic ladder for cancer pain control, twenty years of use. How much pain relief does one get from using it? *Supportive Care in Cancer*, 14, 1086–1093.

Boyd, K., Mason, B., Kendall, M., *et al.* (2010). Advance care planning for cancer patients in primary care: a feasibility study. *British Journal of General Practice*, 60, e449–458.

Brickner, L., Scannell, K., Marquet, S., and Ackerson, L. (2004). Barriers to hospice care and referrals: survey of physicians' knowledge, attitudes, and perceptions in a health maintenance organization. *Journal of Palliative Medicine*, 7, 411–418.

Clark, D., Wright, M., Hunt, J., and Lynch, T. (2007). Hospice and palliative care development in Africa: a multi-method review of services and experiences. *Journal of Pain and Symptom Management*, 33, 698–710.

De Lima, L., Sweeney, C., Palmer, J.L., and Bruera, E. (2004). Potent analgesics are more expensive for patients in developing countries: a comparative study. *Journal of Pain and Palliative Care Pharmacotherapy*, 18, 59–70.

Dubler, N.N. (1998). The collision of confinement and care: end-of-life care in prisons and jails. *Journal of Law, Medicine & Ethics*, 26, 149–156.

Ewing, G., Farquhar, M., and Booth, S. (2009). Delivering palliative care in an acute hospital setting: views of referrers and specialist providers. *Journal of Pain and Symptom Management*, 38, 327–340.

Feeg, V. D. and Elebiary, H. (2005). Exploratory study on end-of-life issues: barriers to palliative care and advance directives. *American Journal of Hospice and Palliative Care*, 22, 119–124.

Francoeur, R.B., Payne, R., Raveis, V.H., and Shim, H. (2007). Palliative care in the inner city. Patient religious affiliation, underinsurance, and symptom attitude. *Cancer*, 109, 425–434.

Gardiner, C., Cobb, M., Gott, M., and Ingleton, C. (2011). Barriers to providing palliative care for older people in acute hospitals. *Age and Ageing*, 40, 233–238.

Gott, M., Ingleton, C., Bennett, M.I., and Gardiner, C. (2011). Transitions to palliative care in acute hospitals in England: qualitative study. *BMJ*, 342, d1773.

Gott, M.C., Ahmedzai, S.H., and Wood, C. (2001). How many inpatients at an acute hospital have palliative care needs? Comparing the perspectives of medical and nursing staff. *Palliative Medicine*, 15, 451–460.

Groot, M.M., Vernooij-Dassen, M.J., Verhagen, S.C., Crul, B.J., and Grol, R.P. (2007). Obstacles to the delivery of primary palliative care as perceived by GPs. *Palliative Medicine*, 21, 697–703.

Gwyther, L., Brennan, F., and Harding, R. (2009). Advancing palliative care as a human right. *Journal of Pain and Symptom Management*, 38, 767–774.

Hanratty, B., Hibbert, D., Mair, F., *et al.* (2006). Doctors' understanding of palliative care. *Palliative Medicine*, 20, 493–497.

Hardin, K.A., Meyers, F., and Louie, S. (2008). Integrating palliative care in severe chronic obstructive lung disease. *COPD*, 5, 207–220.

Harding, R., Easterbrook, P., Higginson, I.J., *et al.* (2005). Access and equity in HIV/AIDS palliative care: a review of the evidence and responses. *Palliative Medicine*, 19, 251–8.

Hasson, F., Kernohan, W.G., Waldron, M., Whittaker, E., and McLaughlin, D. (2008). The palliative care link nurse role in nursing homes: barriers and facilitators. *Journal of Advanced Nursing*, 64, 233–242.

Howell, D.A., Shellens, R., Roman, E., Garry, A.C., Patmore, R., and Howard, M.R. (2011). Haematological malignancy: are patients appropriately referred for specialist palliative and hospice care? A systematic review and meta-analysis of published data. *Palliative Medicine*, 25, 630–641.

Hsiao, W.C. and Liu, Y. (1996). Economic reform and health—lessons from China. *The New England Journal of Medicine*, 335, 430–432.

Huskamp, H.A., Kaufmann, C., and Stevenson, D.G. (2012). The intersection of long-term care and end-of-life care. *Medical Care Research and Review*, 69, 3–44.

Jagwe, J.G. and Barnard, D. (2002). The introduction of palliative care in Uganda. *Journal of Palliative Medicine*, 5, 160–163.

Kaasalainen, S., Brazil, K., Wilson, D.M., *et al.* (2011). Palliative care nursing in rural and urban community settings: a comparative analysis. *International Journal of Palliative Nursing*, 17, 344–352.

Kurella Tamura, M. and Cohen, L.M. (2010). Should there be an expanded role for palliative care in end-stage renal disease? *Current Opinion in Nephrology and Hypertension*, 19, 556–560.

Lemond, L. and Allen, L.A. (2011). Palliative care and hospice in advanced heart failure. *Progress in Cardiovascular Diseases*, 54, 168–178.

Linder, J.F. and Meyers, F.J. 2007. Palliative care for prison inmates: 'don't let me die in prison'. *Journal of the American Medical Association*, 298, 894–901.

Lynch, T., Clark, D., Centeno, C., *et al.* (2010). Barriers to the development of palliative care in Western Europe. *Palliative Medicine*, 24, 812–819.

Lynch, T., Clark, D., Centeno, C., *et al.* (2009). Barriers to the development of palliative care in the countries of Central and Eastern Europe and the Commonwealth of Independent States. *Journal of Pain and Symptom Management*, 37, 305–315.

Mahtani-Chugani, V., Gonzalez-Castro, I., De Ormijana-Hernandez, A.S., Martin-Fernandez, R., and De La Vega, E.F. (2010). How to provide care for patients suffering from terminal non-oncological diseases: barriers to a palliative care approach. *Palliative Medicine*, 24, 787–795.

Mathers, C.D. and Loncar, D. (2006). Projections of global mortality and burden of disease from 2002 to 2030. *PLoS Medicine*, 3, e442.

McNeil, R. and Guirguis-Younger, M. (2012). Illicit drug use as a challenge to the delivery of end-of-life care services to homeless persons: perceptions of health and social services professionals. *Palliative Medicine*, 26, 350–359.

Meier, D.E., Morrison, R.S., and Cassel, C.K. (1997). Improving palliative care. *Annals of Internal Medicine*, 127, 225–230.

Noble, S.I., Nelson, A., and Finlay, I.G. (2008). Challenges faced by palliative care physicians when caring for doctors with advanced cancer. *Palliative Medicine*, 22, 71–76.

Peng, J.K., Chiu, T.Y., Hu, W.Y., Lin, C.C., Chen, C.Y., and Hung, S.H. (2013). What influences the willingness of community physicians to provide palliative care for patients with terminal cancer? Evidence from a nationwide survey. *Japanese Journal of Clinical Oncology*, 43, 278–285.

Phillips, J., Davidson, P.M., Jackson, D., Kristjanson, L., Daly, J., and Curran, J. (2006). Residential aged care: the last frontier for palliative care. *Journal of Advanced Nursing*, 55, 416–424.

Praill, D. and Pahl, N. (2007). The worldwide palliative care alliance: networking national associations. *Journal of Pain and Symptom Management*, 33, 506–508.

Rondahl, G., Innala, S., and Carlsson, M. (2003). Nursing staff and nursing students' attitudes towards HIV-infected and homosexual HIV-infected patients in Sweden and the wish to refrain from nursing. *Journal of Advanced Nursing*, 41, 454–461.

Rousseau, P. (1998). The homeless terminally ill and hospice & palliative care. *American Journal of Hospice and Palliative Care*, 15, 196–197.

Slort, W., Blankenstein, A.H., Deliens, L., and Van Der Horst, H.E. (2011). Facilitators and barriers for GP-patient communication in palliative care: a qualitative study among GPs, patients, and end-of-life consultants. *British Journal of General Practice*, 61, 167–172.

Snow, C.E., Varela, B.R., Pardi, D.A., Adelman, R.D., Said, S., and Reid, M.C. (2009). Identifying factors affecting utilization of an inpatient palliative care service: a physician survey. *Journal of Palliative Medicine*, 12, 231–237.

Spence, A., Hasson, F., Waldron, M., *et al.* (2009). Professionals delivering palliative care to people with COPD: qualitative study. *Palliative Medicine*, 23, 126–131.

Stjernsward, J., Colleau, S.M., and Ventafridda, V. (1996). The World Health Organization Cancer Pain and Palliative Care Program. Past, present, and future. *Journal of Pain and Symptom Management*, 12, 65–72.

Stjernsward, J., Foley, K.M., and Ferris, F.D. (2007). The public health strategy for palliative care. *Journal of Pain and Symptom Management*, 33, 486–493.

Ward, E., Jemal, A., Cokkinides, V., *et al.* (2004). Cancer disparities by race/ethnicity and socioeconomic status. *CA: A Cancer Journal for Clinicians*, 54, 78–93.

Wiebe, L.A. and Von Roenn, J.H. (2010). Working with a palliative care team. *Cancer Journal*, 16, 488–492.

Worth, A., Irshad, T., Bhopal, R., *et al.* (2009). Vulnerability and access to care for South Asian Sikh and Muslim patients with life limiting illness in Scotland: prospective longitudinal qualitative study. *BMJ*, 338, b183.

Wright, M., Wood, J., Lynch, T., and Clark, D. (2008). Mapping levels of palliative care development: a global view. *Journal of Pain and Symptom Management*, 35, 469–485.

World Health Organization (2014). *WHO Definition of Palliative Care*. [Online] Available at: <http://www.who.int/cancer/palliative/definition/en/>.

3.2

Palliative care delivery models

Irene J. Higginson

Introduction to palliative care delivery models

Since the initiation of modern hospice and palliative care, led by Cicely Saunders in the United Kingdom, then Vittorio Ventafridda in Europe and Balfour Mount in Canada, palliative care has evolved and is now integrated into mainstream medicine in many countries, with a network of services, the development of a medical specialty or sub-speciality, and creation of academic departments to build knowledge and practice.

In high-income countries, those aged 60 and older bear 35% of the disease burden, a disproportionately high percentage relative to the population distribution, with the leading causes all being chronic diseases (World Health Organization, 2008). As the population in developed countries ages, the disease burden will only increase further and will challenge their health-care systems. Advances in cancer and other treatments leads to patients living longer and experiencing more co-morbidities (Sullivan et al., 2011). Developed countries have to cope with the increasing demand for palliative care services amidst soaring health-care expenditures, tight budgets, and rising patient expectations (Harding et al., 2003; Harding and Higginson, 2005). Each system would have to develop and improve their current palliative care system to meet their future population's needs. As developed countries have varied health financing and delivery structures, contrasting the different models would allow lessons to be distilled that could be applicable to other systems. Thus, palliative care has received growing attention from patients, health-care professionals, and health-care providers in recent years.

Adapted to diverse health-care systems, palliative care services have been developed in more than 100 countries throughout the world. Although originally conceived as something concerned only with the end of life, palliative care has now become more integrated, with services offered throughout the disease trajectory (see Fig. 3.2.1). This chapter considers the different service delivery models and some of the evidence of their effectiveness.

Generalist versus specialist palliative care

One of the challenges for palliative care is the high prevalence of conditions that need palliative care. Every year there are around 53 million deaths worldwide. Of these approximately 80% have a period of progressive illness and/or disability, when the disease becomes unresponsive to curative treatment. Murtagh et al., comparing methods of needs assessment of palliative care, identified that between 69% and 82% of those who die need palliative care (Murtagh et al., 2014). Almost every clinician in health care will encounter patients at or approaching the end of life, those with progressive and symptomatic illness, and bereaved families. Thus, because palliative care needs to be part of every clinician's duties, and because specialist palliative care could not and may not need to expand to care for everyone who has progressive illness or is reaching the end of their life, there is often a distinction between what is called 'generalist' palliative care and specialist palliative care. The former concerns clinical care for all people who have progressive, life-limiting, or end-of-life conditions while specialist palliative care is offered by specialists, and is concerned with patients with the more complex needs.

Generalist palliative care is usually defined as palliative care provided for those affected by life-limiting or progressive illness as an integral part of standard clinical practice by any health-care professional that is not part of a specialist palliative care team (Shipman et al., 2008). In the community, generalist palliative care is provided by primary care teams, district nurses, nursing and residential home care staff, and other community support services. In hospitals, it is provided by general medical and surgical teams, and specialists for specific diseases or circumstances, such as oncology, respiratory, renal, intensive care, and cardiac teams (Shipman et al., 2008). Condition-specific specialist nurses often work across the interface between hospital and community (Aspinal et al., 2012).

In some countries, such as the United Kingdom, improving generalist palliative and end-of-life care has been a major focus of health policy. The UK Department of Health End of Life Care Strategy sought to 'bring about a step change in access to high quality care for all people approaching the end of life' in all care settings (Department of Health, 2008). This is to be achieved with a whole system and care pathway approach for commissioning and providing integrated services, improving coordination. It specifically stated that it involved workforce development including education and training for generalists as well as specialists.

Specialist palliative care is palliative care provided by those who have undergone specific training and/or accreditation in palliative care/medicine working in the context of an expert interdisciplinary team of palliative care health professionals.

Specialist palliative care may be provided by inpatient palliative care units (PCUs) or hospices, hospital palliative care teams, community palliative care or hospice teams, and paediatric specialist palliative care teams. Increasingly, specialist palliative care services need to meet standards developed nationally, work exclusively in palliative care, and have staff who have completed specialist training.

However, a distinction made on the nature of the service is not enough, there needs to be a distinction on the basis of patient and/

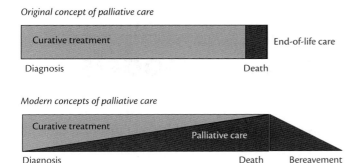

Original concept of palliative care

Modern concepts of palliative care

Fig. 3.2.1 How services for palliative care have moved from rectangles to triangles.

or family circumstances and need. A common distinction is the complexity of patients and families. Generalists will provide care for everyone with less complex needs. Specialists in palliative care have a higher level of expertise in complex symptom management, spiritual support, psychosocial support, cultural support, and grief and loss support, and thus care for patients and families with the higher levels of these needs.

Specialist palliative care services usually have three components: (1) directly provide care for the more complex patients and families, (2) provide education and support to generalists, and (3) undertake or collaborate in research to improve the care for patients and families in the future. The provision of education is widely accepted as a role for specialist palliative care, although the nature and level of support is not well defined. The requirement to undertake research is more recent, and at present is not universally provided by all hospices and palliative care teams. The proportion and detailed circumstances of those patients and families with the more complex needs that require 'specialist' rather than 'generalist' palliative care is also not well defined and varies both within and between countries, and within and between diseases (Oliver and Webb, 2000; Johnson et al., 2008, 2011; To et al., 2011).

Currow and colleagues attempted to estimate population wishes for specialist palliative care, and also levels of need among people with diseases other than cancer (Currow et al., 2004, 2008). They found limited levels of unmet need for specialist palliative care according to bereaved relatives. However, the levels of unmet need depend on knowledge of what palliative care can offer, which is varied, especially in some populations and cultures (Calanzani et al., 2013). Research in specific non-cancer populations not referred to palliative care has identified levels of symptoms and problems similar to those among cancer patients who were referred to specialist care, suggesting inequity of provision exists at least in some settings and diseases (Solano et al., 2006; Murray et al., 2007; Selman et al., 2007; Harding et al., 2009; Gysels and Higginson, 2011; Bajwah et al., 2012). Daveson et al., in a population-based survey in seven European countries involving 9344 respondents, found two prominent themes in the responses to open comments: (1) a need for improved quality of end-of-life and palliative care, and access to this care for patients and families; and (2) the recognition of the importance of death and dying, the cessation of treatments to extend life unnecessarily, and the need for holistic care to include comfort and support. The public appeared to recognize the importance of death and dying and were concerned to prioritize quantity of life over quality of life,

also calling for improvement in palliative and end-of-life care services (Daveson et al., 2014).

Joint working and interface between specialist and generalist palliative care is also important. The wide range of health needs of people with progressive or far advanced diseases often requires collaboration and co-working between many sectors, such as specialists in care for older people, oncology, disease specialists, and palliative, primary, and social care. Such joint models are newly emerging in many fields, such as earlier integration with oncology and palliative care—with joint clinics and other initiatives. Such models include outpatient palliative care services, integrated with oncology (Temel et al., 2010); a breathlessness support service run jointly between palliative care and respiratory medicine (Bausewein et al., 2012); and a new short-term service for patients severely affected by multiple sclerosis (MS), offered jointly between neurology and palliative care (Edmonds et al., 2010; Higginson et al., 2011).

Models of specialist palliative care delivery

Delivery of specialist palliative care differs slightly throughout the world but similar structures have evolved: inpatient palliative care is provided in dedicated PCUs or hospices, specialist palliative care teams offer palliative care consultations either in the hospital or in the community within home care programmes, and increasingly outpatient, day care, and respite services. The following subsections consider the most common established and emerging models, and to a limited extent their evidence base. Note that several PCUs offer a combination of services—for example, most inpatient PCUs and hospices also offer other services, such as, if they are based in the community, home care and day care, or if based in a hospital, hospital consultation. It is not that one specific service is better than or preferable to another: community support is essential as evidence consistently shows that most patients want to be cared for at home for as long as possible and often to die there (Gomes et al., 2012b, 2013b) and yet more than half of deaths in most countries occur in hospitals (Cohen et al., 2008; Gomes et al., 2012a).

Inpatient palliative care units and inpatient hospices

The European Association for Palliative Care (EAPC), in its white paper on standards and norms, defines a PCU as a department specialized in the treatment and care of palliative care patients (Radbruch et al., 2010). It can be a stand-alone service (as with many of the inpatient hospices in the United Kingdom) or a ward or unit within or adjacent to a hospital (as is common, for example, in Germany, some parts of Canada, among others). The aim of PCUs and hospices is to alleviate disease and therapy-related discomfort and, if possible, to stabilize the status of the patient and offer patient and carers psychological and social support in a way that allows for discharge or transfer to another care setting.

In her early writing on hospices, Dame Cicely Saunders emphasized the importance of environment—that a hospice should be welcoming, calm, and cheerful, in contrast to most acute hospital wards (Saunders, 2001). St Christopher's Hospice, founded by Dame Cicely Saunders in 1967, followed this guidance, with gardens, a welcoming atmosphere, and sense of peace and cheerfulness.

PCUs and inpatient hospices admit patients whose condition (physical, emotional, social, and spiritual) would benefit from specialist multiprofessional palliative care. Patients can be admitted for a few days to several weeks; their medical, nursing, psychosocial, or spiritual problems determine this. As mentioned earlier, these units may also provide other services.

Evidence about the effectiveness of specialist PCUs and inpatient hospices suggests that they provide benefits in terms of symptom management, and in particular higher satisfaction with the quality of care from patients and families (Higginson and Evans, 2010). Much of the early evaluation concerned St Christopher's hospice, with quasi-experimental designs showing improved symptom management and satisfaction. Later a randomized trial of a PCU ward found few differences in symptoms but a difference in family satisfaction, although there was contamination between arms, but other studies suggested a benefit of inpatient hospices (Higginson et al., 2003; Gysels and Higginson, 2004). The satisfaction of patients and families with inpatient hospices is much higher than for conventional care, especially hospitals. A national survey of 18 000 bereaved relatives in the United Kingdom in 2011 found that inpatient hospices were reported as outstanding or excellent by 59%, contrasted with 32% for hospitals (NHS Medical Directorate End of Life Care, 2012).

Hospice: a word with different international meanings

The term hospice has different meanings internationally. This has partly arisen because in Latin-root languages hospice sometimes has a very similar meaning to hospital. So Balfour Mount, seeing an alternative word in French-speaking Canada, coined the word palliative, which is more often used nowadays. In many countries, for example, the United Kingdom, the function of an inpatient hospice and a PCU are similar. But, in other countries, a distinction exists—in Germany, for example, patients will be admitted to a PCU for crisis intervention and to an inpatient hospice for end-of-life care (Radbruch et al., 2010). In some countries (e.g. the United States), a hospice, in contrast to a PCU, is a free-standing service which is predominantly home care.

Palliative care consultation teams

Consultation teams provide an additional layer of support and advice for patients and families, working with existing professionals. They can be focused predominantly on hospital patients, or patients at home or both.

Hospital teams

Hospital palliative care support teams provide specialist palliative care advice and support to other clinical staff, patients, and their families and carers in the hospital environment (Radbruch et al., 2010). They offer formal and informal education, and liaise with other services in and out of the hospital. Hospital palliative care support teams are also known as hospital supportive care teams. A core aim is the alleviation of multiple symptoms experienced by patients, and for this the team members will advise on management and sometimes prescribe directly. Teams usually also offer support and education for existing staff, including on pain and symptom assessment and control, holistic care, and psychosocial support. They are usually involved in seeing the patients in all areas of the hospital (Radbruch et al., 2010).

Evidence regarding the effectiveness of hospital palliative care teams comes mainly from quasi-experimental studies. Outcomes considered included symptoms, quality of life, time in hospital, total length of time in palliative care, or professional changes, such as prescribing practices. Most studies indicate a small positive effect of the hospital team, compared to usual care (Higginson et al., 2002; Higginson and Evans, 2010). Multiprofessional teams with more skilled staff may offer greater benefits (Finlay et al., 2002).

Home care teams

Home palliative care teams provide specialized palliative care to patients who need it at home and support to their families and carers at the patient's home. They also provide specialist advice to general practitioners (GPs), family doctors, nurses, and others caring for the patient and family at home (Radbruch et al., 2010). Commonly they reach out to patients in the community wherever they are, including in nursing and residential homes.

The home palliative care team will visit patients and their families in the community at the request of other community professionals, and provides an additional layer of support and help. It has an advisory and mentoring function, and offers its expertise in pain therapy, symptom control, palliative care, and psychosocial support (Radbruch et al., 2010). Advice and support by the home palliative care team is also provided directly to the patient and family, in particular helping with coordination of care, emotional, social, and spiritual support. The extent to which the palliative care team directly decides what treatments should be provided, or advises the GP regarding this, varies. The most usual model is to advise, but in some instances, because the case is complex or because the GP prefers this, the team takes over prescribing for the patient.

Less frequently in many settings, except home hospice care, the home palliative care team provides 'hands-on' direct care, sometimes taking over care (as in the hospice model in the United States) or in collaboration with the GP and other primary care workers. This model approaches that of 'hospice' at home—where all care is provided to patients at home (Grande et al., 2004).

There is very good evidence, from systematic reviews and original studies, regarding the benefits of home specialist palliative care teams. The most recent Cochrane review identified 23 studies, of which 16 were randomized controlled trials, including 37 561 participants and 4042 family caregivers. The patients cared for mostly had advanced cancer but some had congestive heart failure, chronic obstructive pulmonary disease, HIV/AIDS, MS, and other conditions. Meta-analysis showed that a home specialist palliative care team more than doubled the odds of dying at home compared to the conventional care (odds ratio 2.21, 95% confidence interval 1.31–3.71; P = 0.003). In addition, narrative synthesis showed evidence of small but statistically significant beneficial effects of home palliative care services compared to usual care on reducing symptom burden for patients (Gomes et al., 2013a).

Palliative care outpatient services

Palliative outpatient clinics offer consultation for patients living at home who are able to visit the clinic. Palliative outpatient clinics can be offered from hospital or inpatient PCUs or hospitals. There is an increasing variety of such services, with outpatient services being offered jointly with oncology, respiratory medicine, or neurology services. They often meet the need to integrate services and can help to introduce patients earlier to palliative care in a non-threatening way, providing help with, for example, specific symptoms or advance care planning. To date, however, evaluations are few and these are much needed for the future.

Day care

Day hospices or day care centres are spaces in hospitals, hospices, PCUs, or the community especially designed to provide additional support to patients in the community and their families. For units that have inpatient beds, sometimes the inpatients will also attend day care, especially those who are well enough and are planning to go home. Patients are usually eligible for day care only if they are already in the care of a home palliative care team, affiliated with that particular centre. The nature of services offered varies along a continuum from the more medical/health orientated to the more social and recreational. Quite often day centres offer a variety of complementary therapies.

Evaluations regarding the comparative effectiveness of day care are limited, and those to date have not shown great benefits for the more 'social models' of day care, although it is possible that the outcomes may have been inadequate (Douglas et al., 2000, 2003; Higginson et al., 2010). Although patients in non-comparative studies report high satisfaction with day care, these benefits are not seen when studies use a control group or quasi-experimental design. A recent comparative evaluation of day care appeared to suggest that hope was improved, and more research on this aspect is needed (Guy et al., 2011).

Short-term integrated palliative care

A new model of specialist palliative care is developing in response to the changing needs of patients. In general, palliative care services have accepted patients and kept them 'on their books', even if not as inpatients, until the person died. But better integration with existing services, earlier involvement of palliative care specialists, and providing care for patients with longer trajectories of illness (in both cancer and non-cancer conditions) requires new models of palliative care. In response, the model of short-term integrated palliative care has been developed and trialled at the Cicely Saunders Institute in London and elsewhere.

First developed in the care of people with MS, the integrated service has a definite goal to see patients for a limited time, to set things in order, and then discharge them to the care of existing services. For people severely affected by MS this was usually no more than three visits/contacts. After this, 90% of those referred were discharged to local community and existing services, and 10% were referred to continuing palliative care. The outcomes at 6 weeks and 12 weeks in a phase II randomized trial, showed improved symptom control and reduced caregiver burden (Higginson et al., 2006, 2008, 2009, 2011). Fig. 3.2.2 shows how the service links to others. It is an emerging model of care that now needs further evaluation in demonstration projects and trials.

Principles and structures common to specialist palliative care services

Several principles are common to all the palliative care services. These include attention to the individual and total (physical, emotional, social, and spiritual) needs of the person, and considering the patient and the family as the unit of care (Saunders,

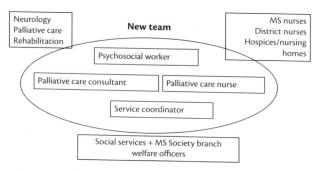

Fig. 3.2.2 Model of short-term early palliative care in multiple sclerosis (MS).

2001; Davies and Higginson, 2004a, 2004b; Radbruch et al., 2010). There is a focus on excellent communication and coordination. Gaertner and colleagues developed with local experts a template for palliative care consultations in a comprehensive cancer centre delineating detailed information of infrastructure, general underlying principles, goals of the palliative care intervention (including symptom assessment and management), and empowerment through patient participation and autonomy (Gaertner et al., 2011). These aspects are captured in some of the common outcome measures specifically developed to assess palliative care, such as the Palliative Care Outcome Scale (Bausewein et al., 2011; Higginson et al., 2012), the Edmonton Symptom Assessment Scale (Watanabe et al., 2012), and the Support Team Assessment Schedule (Bausewein et al., 2011).

Professionals involved

Multiprofessional staffing is central to all palliative care services, as these are needed for the wide ranging problems of patients and families (Fig. 3.2.3) (Davies and Higginson, 2004a, 2004b). Specialist palliative care physicians and palliative care nurses are usually part of all services but other professionals such as social workers, pharmacists, psychologists, physiotherapists, occupational therapies, and chaplains or faith leaders are often involved, especially in inpatient units. The variety of team compositions is certainly related to organizational and resource issues. However, in view of the physical, psychosocial, and spiritual needs of palliative care and its holistic approach, inclusion of professionals other than doctors and nurses should be stressed as palliative care develops for the future.

Target population

The dominant group of patients receiving palliative care services are those with advanced cancer (Gomez-Batiste et al., 2010; Duursma et al., 2011; Farquhar et al., 2011; Gaertner et al., 2012; Jongen et al., 2012; Paiva et al., 2012). More recently, newly diagnosed lung cancer (Temel et al., 2010), glioblastoma (Pace et al., 2012), and prostate cancer (Yennurajalingam et al., 2012) were the focus. Palliative care has begun to extend to include patients with non-malignant disease such as severely affected by MS (Higginson et al., 2009; Edmonds et al., 2010; Higginson et al., 2011), advanced heart failure (Schwarz et al., 2012), advanced respiratory disease or symptoms of breathlessness (Farquhar et al., 2011; Bajwah et al., 2012; Bausewein et al., 2012), or advanced chronic disease (predominantly neurological disease and cancer) (Fernandes et al., 2010).

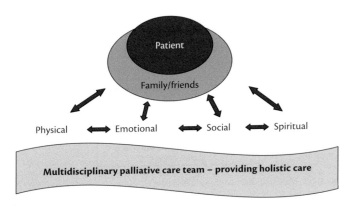

Fig. 3.2.3 Multidisciplinary palliative care team to respond to holistic patient and family needs.

Conclusion

Palliative care service delivery models operate across all the settings where patients need support. There is a distinction between general palliative care (provided by all clinicians) and specialist palliative care (provided by those with specific training and unique interest in palliative care for the more complex patients). Some models of service—home and hospital consultation teams, inpatient PCUs, and inpatient hospices—are well established and have a strong evidence base. Newly emerging models, with greater integration and short-term and outpatient palliative care, are promising and are beginning to be offered but require evaluation. Some principles and values are common, including a holistic, multi-professional approach based on need, which responds to the individual needs of the patient and their family and considers the patient and family the unit of care.

Online materials

Complete references for this chapter are available online at <http://www.oxfordmedicine.com>.

References

Bausewein, C., Le Grice, C., Simon, S., and Higginson, I. (2011). The use of two common palliative outcome measures in clinical care and research: a systematic review of POS and STAS. *Palliative Medicine*, 25, 304–313.

Cohen, J., Bilsen, J., Addington-Hall, J., *et al.* (2008). Population-based study of dying in hospital in six European countries. *Palliative Medicine*, 22, 702–710.

Daveson, B.A., Alonso, J.P., Calanzani, n., *et al.* (2014). Learning from the public: citizens describe the need to improve end-of-life care access, provision and recognition across Europe. *European Journal of Public Health*, 24(3), 521–7.

Davies, E. and Higginson, I.J. (2004b). *Palliative Care: The Solid Facts.* Copenhagen: World Health Organization.

Gomes, B., Calanzani, N., Curiale, V., McCrone, P., and Higginson, I.J. (2013a). Effectiveness and cost-effectiveness of home palliative care services for adults with advanced illness and their caregivers. *The Cochrane Database of Systematic Reviews*, 6, CD007760.

Gomes, B., Calanzani, N., Gysels, M., Hall, S., and Higginson, I. J. (2013b). Heterogeneity and changes in preferences for dying at home: a systematic review. *BMC Palliative Care*, 12, 7.

Gomes, B., Higginson, I. J., Calanzani, N., *et al.* (2012b). Preferences for place of death if faced with advanced cancer: a population survey in England, Flanders, Germany, Italy, the Netherlands, Portugal and Spain. *Annals of Oncology*, 23, 2006–2015.

Gomez-Batiste, X., Porta-Sales, J., Espinosa-Rojas, J., Pascual-Lopez, A., Tuca, A., and Rodriguez, J. (2010). Effectiveness of palliative care services in symptom control of patients with advanced terminal cancer: A Spanish, multicenter, prospective, quasi-experimental, pre-post study. *Journal of Pain and Symptom Management*, 40, 652–660.

Harding, R. and Higginson, I.J. (2005). Palliative care in sub-Saharan Africa. *The Lancet*, 365, 1971–1977.

Higginson, I.J., Finlay, I.G., Goodwin, D.M., *et al.* (2003). Is there evidence that palliative care teams alter end-of-life experiences of patients and their caregivers? *Journal of Pain and Symptom Management*, 25, 150–168.

Higginson, I.J., McCrone, P., Hart, S.R., Burman, R., Silber, E., and Edmonds, P.M. (2009). Is short-term palliative care cost-effective in multiple sclerosis? A randomized phase II trial. *Journal of Pain and Symptom Management*, 38, 816–826.

Murtagh, F.E., Bausewein, C., Verne, J., Groeneveld, E.I., Kaloki, Y.E., and Higginson, I.J. (2014). How many people need palliative care? A study developing and comparing methods for population-based estimates. *Palliative Medicine*, 28(1), 49–58.

Shipman, C., Gysels, M., White, P., *et al.* (2008). Improving generalist end of life care: national consultation with practitioners, commissioners, academics, and service user groups. *BMJ*, 337, a1720.

Temel, J.S., Greer, J.A., Muzikansky, A., *et al.* (2010). Early palliative care for patients with metastatic non-small-cell lung cancer. *The New England Journal of Medicine*, 363, 733–742.

To, T.H., Greene, A.G., Agar, M.R., and Currow, D.C. (2011). A point prevalence survey of hospital inpatients to define the proportion with palliation as the primary goal of care and the need for specialist palliative care. *Internal Medicine Journal*, 41, 430–433.

3.3

Palliative care in the emergency department

Paul L. DeSandre and Karen May

Introduction to palliative care in the emergency department

Training and practice in emergency medicine prioritizes acute illness and life-prolonging interventions. As the elderly population continues to grow, more patients with crises related to illness and debility are expected to rely on emergency departments for help. Severely ill and functionally impaired elderly patients seek emergency care not only for physical concerns, but also for concerns related to psychological or financial distress, and access to care (Grudzen et al., 2010). Clinicians may feel ill-equipped to provide the necessary care for these patients, but they recognize the importance in providing this care (Smith et al., 2009; Stone et al., 2011). There is increasing evidence of the benefit of early palliative care intervention in acute care settings (Campbell and Guzman, 2003; Lustbader et al., 2011).

As the entry point to the hospital and often the health-care system, the emergency department is uniquely positioned for early identification of patients with unmet palliative care needs (Mahony et al., 2008). In addition, the emergency department is often a staging area for negotiating the difficult decisions surrounding life-sustaining interventions and an environment where sudden life-altering events are managed. In recognition of the need to evolve expertise in managing these critical concerns in patient care, there is wide support for improving palliative care practices in the emergency department (American College of Emergency Physicians, 2014; National Consensus Project for Quality Palliative Care, 2013; Emergency Nurses Association, 2013).

Models have been proposed for encouraging the integration of palliative care practices into routine care in the emergency department (Grudzen et al., 2011). Also, resources are available and continue to develop for improving education, clinical care, and research (Education in Palliative and End of Life Care—Emergency Medicine, 2010) Center to Advance Palliative Care, 2011). This chapter will introduce these principles and provide structured approaches to the care of patients with palliative care needs in the emergency department.

Rapid palliative care assessment in the emergency department

The initial assessment of all patients presenting to the emergency department is a triage process based on the level of acuity to direct care to the most critical patients first. Patients with significant unmet palliative care needs may present to the emergency department at any stage of illness and at any level of acuity. The emergency clinician must recognize these patients as early as possible, and assure that their care is not only efficient and effective, but also concordant with the goals of the patient and the family. Two tools have been developed to rapidly guide care in the emergency department. The first developed as an initial screen for palliative care needs in stable patients, the Screen for Palliative and End of Life Care Needs in the Emergency Department (SPEED) assessment tool. The second is the mnemonic 'ABCD', which was developed to assist in the approach to patients in critical condition.

The SPEED tool is designed for use as a brief multidimensional symptom assessment for quick administration in the emergency department. It is a 13-question assessment tool adapted from the previously developed NEST assessment tool (Emanuel et al., 2001). It can be performed rapidly by anyone on the care team (physician, nurse, chaplain, social worker, or other health-care worker), but may have particular utility at the point of triage. This is the first tool designed for use in the emergency department and tested favourably for both reliability and validity in screening for palliative care needs of cancer patients (Richards et al., 2011). SPEED addresses five major domains of palliative care needs: physical, therapeutic, psychological, social, and spiritual. A preliminary study applied the SPEED instrument to 1842 patients in routine emergency department triage and found nearly half of the patients had at least moderate to severe pain, and approximately one-quarter of the patients had at least moderate difficulty with care needs at home, difficulty with medications, were feeling overwhelmed, and had difficulty getting medical care that fitted their goals (Quest et al., 2011). These findings support other emergency department-based efforts to identify patients with unmet palliative care needs (Mahony et al., 2008; Waugh, 2010; Glajchen et al., 2011; Grudzen et al., 2011) with the advantage of brevity and simplicity of application.

Patients arriving at the emergency department in critical condition at the final stages of chronic progressive illnesses are a complex challenge. Despite the inherent chaos of the environment, the emergency clinician must immediately intervene within the context of the patient's illness and goals of care. Therefore, a simultaneous rapid palliative care assessment must occur concurrently with temporizing medical interventions until either goals are clear or life-sustaining interventions are necessary, despite a lack of clarity.

Table 3.3.1 ABCD critical care intervention mnemonic

A	Advance directive:
	Check available records or reports from paramedics or family
B	Better symptom control:
	Attend to symptoms while avoiding invasive interventions to allow time to evaluate whether more invasive interventions would achieve intended goals
C	Caregivers:
	Provide reassurance to patient
	Contextualize patient goals and recent functional and medical changes to foster reasonable discussion of medical decision-making.
D	Decision-making capacity:
	Assess patient's ability to reliably engage in dialogue about medical goals and interventions.

Adapted with permission from Emanuel, L.L., von Gunten, C.F., Ferris, F.F., eds. *The Education in Palliative and End-of-life Care (EPEC) Curriculum: Emergency Medicine*: © The EPEC Project, 1999, 2003.

The mnemonic, ABCD, was developed by the Education in Palliative and End of Life Care for Emergency Medicine (EPEC-EM) project (EPEC, 2010) to assist in these situations and is summarized in Table 3.3.1. This approach provides a framework to assess and address the immediate symptom needs of the patient while simultaneously acquiring information to guide medical interventions that can reasonably achieve the goals of the patient and family (B in the mnemonic). There are three remaining elements of the mnemonic: existence of an advance directive (A); the presence of a knowledgeable caregiver (C); and the capacity of the patient to participate in medical decision-making (D). These factors allow the medical provider to place the patient's current condition in the context of the underlying illness, recent functional decline, and goals for medical care. This information can be used to provide recommendations for reasonable medical interventions within the value system of the patient and family.

Rapid titration of opioids in cancer pain

Patients with malignancy often present to the emergency department with uncontrolled pain (Vandyk et al., 2012). Overall, pain is also the most common reason patients seek emergency care, yet analgesics are underutilized, and delays to treatment are common (Todd et al., 2007). Historically, there have been barriers to optimal pain management in the emergency department, including lack of training (Lamba et al., 2012), inadequate assessment (Stalnikowicz et al., 2005), misinterpretation of reasons for seeking care (Wilsey et al., 2008), and disparities in treatment practices among clinicians (Cone et al., 2003; Pletcher et al., 2008). Therefore, patients coming to the emergency department with severe breakthrough cancer pain may be justifiably fearful that their pain may not be addressed in a timely or adequate manner.

Assessing severity of malignant pain in the emergency department using a standardized pain scale such as the numerical rating scale, is an important first step (Todd, 2005). Severe pain in malignancy has been referred to as a 'cancer pain emergency' and rapid titration of parenteral opioids has been demonstrated to provide effective *and safe* control of pain while concurrently addressing

other diagnostic concerns (Hagen et al., 1997; Mercadante et al., 2002; Soares et al., 2003). In addition to severity, initial assessment of cancer pain must also quickly identify underlying patient characteristics, such as prior exposure to opioids or underlying organ dysfunction, which would alter initial dose calculations. Also, new or progressive pain with the potential for emergent interventions, such as spinal cord compression with motor dysfunction, must be pursued concurrently.

In an effort to encourage emergency clinicians to provide timely and effective intervention, a five-step approach was originally introduced through the EPEC-EM curriculum and is based, in part, on recommendations from the American Pain Society (Miaskowski et al., 2005, pp. 39–48; EPEC, 2010; DeSandre and Quest, 2009) (see Table 3.3.2).

Communications in the emergency department

Navigating patients and families through the chaotic experience of the emergency department and negotiating reasonable plans for medical care is a skill required of all emergency clinicians. When patients and families are faced with situations related to mortality in the emergency department, communication requires particular sensitivity and focus. Structured approaches can improve communication by reducing clinician distress in these difficult situations (Baile et al., 2000). A structured approach can be used to address three important scenarios in the emergency department: (1) rapidly establishing goals of care, (2) death disclosure, and (3) family presence during cardiopulmonary resuscitation (CPR) (if it is assessed as appropriate to initiate CPR).

Goals of care

Goal setting is a routine practice of emergency care. Patients present to the emergency department at all phases of illness, and the emergency department is often the staging area for complex medical decisions that set a trajectory for future interventions. Patients are placed on ventilators, sent to surgery, admitted to intensive care units, and sometimes supported symptomatically as they die. Patient and clinician goals must ultimately align in order to ensure medical interventions are likely to be beneficial. Prior to any diagnostic test or medical intervention in the emergency department, the clinician anticipates an outcome. If a test or intervention would not change the outcome, then it would not be medically reasonable to proceed. Other interventions may be more reasonable, in order to limit suffering, or ensure a person can die in a peaceful environment.

'Goals of care' have been defined as 'physical, social, spiritual, or other patient-centered goals that arise following an informed discussion of the current disease(s), prognosis, and treatment options' (Weissman and Meier, 2011). There are several perceived barriers facing emergency clinicians needing to address goals of care prior to intervening with diagnostic evaluations or therapies. Unlike more time-intensive approaches, the purpose of discussing a patient's goals of care in the emergency department often seeks to answer questions about interventions, such as whether or not a ventilator or the intensive care unit will achieve the most appropriate clinical outcome. While it is clear that family meetings are an effective communication strategy for many complex medical decisions (Hudson et al., 2009), emergency clinicians may

Table 3.3.2 A strategy for rapid titration of opioids in cancer pain emergencies

Step 1: assess	◆ Familiar pain or uncharacteristic pain?
	◆ Cancer related or unrelated?
	◆ Progressive baseline pain (> 12/24 hours) or breakthrough pain?
	◆ Medications, dosages, and responses over past 24–48 hours?
	◆ Severity:
	  • if ≥ 7/10 or equivalent and fully alert, initiate step 2
	  • if < 7/10 or not fully alert, further assessment is warranted

Step 2: treat severe pain[a]	Opioid naïve: ◆ Dose: 0.1 mg/kg intravenous morphine or equivalent[b] Opioid tolerant (> 60 mg morphine or equivalent per day for at least 1 week): ◆ Dose: 5–15% of daily morphine equivalents IV[b]
Step 3: reassess (15 minutes if intravenous; 30 minutes if subcutaneous)	◆ Apply same pain scale assessment ◆ Assess for unwanted side effects such as somnolence, nausea, or confusion
Step 4: achieve adequate pain control	◆ If still > 7/10 or equivalent, administer double initial dose[c] ◆ If < 50% improvement, administer same dose[c] ◆ Repeat steps 3 and 4 until pain is adequately controlled or unwanted side effects limit further escalation.

Step 5: disposition and follow-up plan	◆ Consider hospital admission:
	  • inadequate control of pain
	  • persistent side effects
	◆ Collaborate for outpatient continuity (consultants and/or primary providers)

[a] Patients with renal, hepatic, or pulmonary dysfunction should have initial dose reduction of 25–50% or more depending on clinical judgement.
[b] May use subcutaneous route if intravenous unavailable.
[c] Patient is fully alert and without unwanted side effects.

Source: data from Education in Palliative and End-of-life Care (EPEC), *Education in Palliative and End of Life Care: EPEC for Emergency Medicine*, Copyright © 2008; DeSandre, P. and Quest, T., Management of Cancer-Related Pain, *Emergency Medicine Clinics of North America*, Volume 27, Issue 2, pp.179–194, Copyright © 2009; and Miaskowski, C. et al., Guideline for the Management of Cancer Pain in Adults and Children, pp.39–48, in *APS Clinical Practice Guidelines Series*, No. 3., American Pain Society, Glenview, Illinois, USA, Copyright © 2005.

feel ill-prepared for such meetings in the emergency department or the clinical situation is changing too rapidly for a family meeting to occur.

Similar to the guidelines for conducting a family meeting (Hudson et al., 2008), one strategy for effective goals of care discussions in the emergency department uses a seven-step approach:

1. getting started
2. assess what is known
3. explore expectations and hopes
4. suggest goals
5. recommend
6. confirm
7. plan (EPEC, 2010).

Step 1: getting started

Like other communication strategies, start by acquiring sufficient information and limiting environmental distractions in order to conduct the meeting effectively. Have the questions clear in your mind, have the necessary family and support staff present or on the phone, and introduce everyone involved in the meeting along with their relationship to the patient or role in clinical care. Start with reassurance, such as, 'In an effort to provide the best possible care for. . ., we need to determine which investigators and interventions would be most beneficial'.

Step 2: what is known?

In order to proceed from a common perspective, it is important that the patient or family have a similar understanding of the disease and the prognosis. If there are questions or a lack of clarity, it may be necessary to provide or obtain additional information before proceeding further.

Step 3: what is expected or hoped for?

Whenever possible, the patient's goals should be communicated directly from the patient either verbally or in the form of an advance directive. Eliciting the patient's perspectives may be challenging if the patient has lost the capacity to interact, has never communicated these concerns to their family previously, or both. Often, the patient has spoken to family about conditions they would find acceptable or unacceptable, such as 'I want to be at home with my family when I die', or 'I never want to be left on a machine if I won't recover'. In order to preserve autonomy and objectivity, in such situations, it is helpful to ask the family questions from the perspective of the patient, and to imagine what the patient would want or not want in particular scenarios. If the family is unable to imagine or report the patient's direct perspectives, it may be more useful to ask the family if the patient has ever spoken about others who have died or been critically ill in ways the patient found acceptable or unacceptable. Was hospice involved? Were they held on life-sustaining interventions beyond what appeared reasonable? Was there evidence of suffering? Were there things the patient wished were different? Importantly the question 'What do you want for. . . ?' should never be asked. Instead, 'What would be acceptable for. . . under these circumstances?' assuming that there are viable clinical options.

A common fear among emergency clinicians is that questions about hopes and expectations may lead to responses such as 'do everything'. A productive approach to understanding this general hope is to redirect the focus onto specific burdens and benefits of particular interventions. For example, some patients may want to sustain biological existence regardless of the likelihood of ever achieving awareness. This is very uncommon. For most patients and families, 'everything' often refers to any interventions whose benefits would outweigh adverse outcomes and is most often focused in the minds of families on physical comfort. For persistent requests for high-burden interventions that are unlikely to achieve patient goals, a 'harm reduction strategy' is recommended. This approach attempts to support reasonable medical interventions within the context of patient-centred goals (Quill et al., 2009).

Step 4: suggest goals

In order to offer reasonable suggestions for goals, the emergency clinician should frame the suggestions in the context of prognosis of hours to days, days to weeks, weeks to months, or months to years. An example might be, 'People close to death often are most concerned with assuring comfort, peace, and dignity in their dying process' or 'People with only weeks to months to live often focus on avoiding the risk of dying in an intensive care unit, and may consider treatments that are not too high of a burden, such as a trial of intravenous antibiotics'.

If the expectations or hopes communicated are medically unachievable, reframing hope towards medically achievable goals can be an effective strategy. Examples include controlling physical symptoms, providing access to emotional or practical support, and assuring dignity (Clayton et al., 2005).

Step 5: make a recommendation

Clear recommendations from the emergency clinician can be a powerful source of comfort for patients and families. The recommendations should be based on medically achievable goals from the patient's perspective whenever possible. For example, a patient may present to the emergency department with advanced cancer and severe functional impairment who is demonstrating ventilatory insufficiency, but had previously communicated they never wanted to 'die on machines'. If the patient is unlikely to ever achieve ventilator independence or survival off a ventilator, then a recommendation to focus on controlling dyspnoea and avoiding intubation will be more concordant than a recommendation to proceed with intubation. Likewise, if the same patient were at risk for imminent cardiac arrest and death, an understanding of likely outcomes of CPR would inform your recommendations. Patients and families often have unrealistic understanding of CPR (Heyland et al., 2006). Cardiac arrest itself portends an extremely poor prognosis, and patients with advanced illness with poor function at baseline are unlikely to survive CPR and almost certainly will not regain pre-arrest levels of function (Ebell et al., 1998; Ewer et al., 2001; Peberdy et al., 2003; Reisfield et al., 2006; Young 2009; Sasson et al., 2010). For patients who survive attempts at CPR with such severe underlying disease, dependence on life-sustaining interventions through end of life is the expectation. Therefore, a recommendation in this setting is to avoid CPR.

Step 6: confirm understanding

Once goals and recommendations are established, consensus dictates any immediate interventions. Summarize the available medical options to support the patient's goals, and assure understanding and agreement. If no consensus can be achieved reasonably, the emergency clinician may need to initiate specific life-sustaining interventions to allow the family time to process what is happening to the patient. In such complex situations, further communication with the family will be necessary after the initial attempts to medically stabilize the patient.

Step 7: plan

A clear plan of care sets the course for appropriate disposition and follow-up. The emergency clinician may focus initially on symptom management while other needs, such as psychosocial distress, are being addressed by other interdisciplinary professionals. If life-sustaining interventions are initiated in the emergency department, then a timeframe and conditions for future discussions should be established.

Death disclosure

Informing a family of the devastating news that a loved one has died is particularly challenging in the emergency department, where the death is often relatively unexpected or sudden. Emergency clinicians may feel uncertain of the best approach, yet they are required to have these extraordinarily sensitive conversations routinely (Stone et al., 2011). Death disclosure is a form of breaking bad news, and educational models exist to teach these skills in the emergency department (Quest et al., 2002; Benenson and Pollack, 2003; Hobgood et al., 2005). Each of these models share four common elements:

♦ attending to survivors on arrival to the emergency department

♦ unequivocal communication of the death

♦ allowing for and reflecting on the emotional response

♦ offering survivors to view the body of the deceased (Quest, 2008).

A nine-step approach incorporates these elements from the educational models and is recommended for managing death disclosure in the emergency department (EPEC, 2010).

Step 1: preparation

When a family arrives in the emergency department, they may not be aware that the patient has died. In order to limit additional emotional trauma to the family, staff should be prepared to receive them on arrival while the clinician is informed of their presence. The room should be quiet and private with adequate seating, away from other emergency department traffic, and equipped with facial tissues. The emergency clinician should be prepared to immediately respond having all available information (including the patient's full name), and assure that the body is being cleaned and prepared for viewing by the family. Relevant staff such as the physician, nurse, social worker, and chaplain should enter the room together. Mobile phones or pagers should be handed over to colleagues until after the death disclosure.

Step 2: engagement

While universal introductions are essential, when entering the room, the appropriate sense of gravitas must be evident. The initial introductions must state the full name of the patient and all involved staff, while unequivocally identifying the primary survivor and the relationship to the patient. If there are children present, depending on their age and maturity, it might be best to communicate first to the parent separately from the children, then collaborate to determine how best to communicate with them.

Sit down, preferable closest to the primary survivor (whether or not they choose to sit down). Maintain awareness of body language to communicate respect, cultural sensitivity, and engagement.

Step 3: transition

The preferred opening communication to a sudden death in the emergency department is to provide information about the immediate circumstances prior to the patient's death. One approach may be, 'I'm not sure what you know about what has happened, but I'm afraid I have some bad news about [identify deceased patient by name and relationship to the survivor]. . . ' or 'I'm not sure if you are aware that [deceased patient's name] was involved in a serious accident . . . '.

Step 4: 'dead' or 'died'

It is imperative that any euphemisms be avoided at this stage. Survivors are predictably in a state of emotional shock from the transition statements, so unequivocal language must follow to avoid misperception. An example of clear communication would be, 'I'm sorry to tell you that [patient's full name] has died'.

Step 5: reaction tolerance

Emotional response to devastating news is an unpredictable and individual experience. It may be highly expressive as agony or anger, or it may be profoundly withdrawn or stunned. Allowing time, presence, and empathic but clear communication should quickly stabilize the situation and direct further explorations.

Understanding and engaging empathic responses is a skill that can be both taught and practised. Many clinicians may be uncomfortable with the risk of creating an emotionally uncomfortable situation while in the emergency department. With preparation and practice, emergency clinicians can engage in these necessary interactions with both efficiency and compassion. One useful technique for communicating empathy can be performed in under 40 seconds while improving satisfaction and decreasing the anxiety of the emotional experience for the patient (Fogarty et al., 1999):

◆ Acknowledge:
  • 'This is not what you were expecting.'
  • 'You seem angry.'
◆ Legitimize:
  • 'Many people in this situation would feel angry.'
◆ Explore:
  • 'Can you tell me what you are most concerned about right now?'
◆ Empathize:
  • 'I wish the news were better.'
◆ Commit:
  • 'I will make sure we have a good plan in place before you leave today.'

Step 6: information

The surviving family hopes for a lack of suffering. Although it may not be possible to empirically report on the patient's experiences, it is reasonable to assume that the patient was not experiencing physical suffering once unconscious. If the death was violent or otherwise a difficult death, the clinician can speak to the importance of the interventions used to control pain and suffering prior to death.

Information about the patient's underlying medical conditions is often needed to understand and report on the likely cause of death, and may help provide additional closure if related to a known illness. An approach might be, 'To better understand what happened to [deceased patient's name], may I ask you some questions about his/her medical history? I can also tell you what we know and answer any questions you may have'.

Step 7: viewing

Family typically will choose to view the deceased person, and it should be offered. It may work best to have support staff guide the family into the room, and assure ongoing availability nearby.

Step 8: conclusion

Prior to leaving the family, the clinician should offer condolences and provide contact information for any additional questions.

If the deceased is a child, support staff can offer to provide the bereaved something tangible from the child, such as a lock of the child's hair to take with them.

Step 9: self and staff care

Death experiences in the emergency department can be exhausting for everyone involved, particularly if a child has died, or if the death was violent, or if the death triggers transference of personal memories for clinicians or other staff. It can be helpful to ask involved staff how they are managing and to verbalize feelings or distress. Staff should consider a routine debriefing just after the death disclosure and possibly after work, or with other friends and family or with a trusted third party.

Family presence during resuscitation

There is increasing acceptance for allowing family presence during resuscitation in the emergency department in both adults and paediatrics (Kleinman et al., 2010; Morrison et al., 2010). Parents in particular want to be given the choice to be present at the bedside of their child during CPR and those who have lived through the experience were grateful and would repeat the experience if faced with it again. Although family members generally do not create interference, there remains significant apprehension among clinicians and variability in practice. Clinicians vary in their level of comfort or even their perceptions of the appropriateness of including family members in a resuscitation event. Policies encouraging the use of family presence during resuscitation are recommended to promote more uniformity in practice (Dingerman et al., 2007; Tinsley et al., 2008; Dudley et al., 2009).

Although no consensus guidelines are available to provide universal recommendations, certain common themes have emerged from the literature to guide practice (Boudreaux et al., 2002; Agard, 2008; Doolin et al. 2011). First, although family presence should certainly be encouraged, the situation may dictate whether or not to proceed. Certain conditions should be met to assure comfort of the family members and the medical team. The number of family members may need to be limited during the initial phases of resuscitation, while 'final goodbyes' may be encouraged by a controlled process of bringing in other family members as the patient ceases to respond to reasonable resuscitative efforts. A 'family support person' should be identified from the staff, freed of other clinical responsibilities to remain with the family members throughout the resuscitation. The family support person can be a social worker, chaplain, or nurse. They should be trained sufficiently to guide the family members through the medical process by interpreting events and provide psychosocial support, while monitoring behaviours and assuring a controlled situation (Farah et al., 2007).

Given the common discomfort expressed by clinicians regarding family presence, a stepwise structure may help to guide clinicians while also meeting the needs of the staff and the family.

Step 1: introduction

As the essential family members are brought into the room by the family support person, the family support person should introduce the family members. The resuscitation team leader should then introduce themselves as the 'doctor responsible for the care of your [state relationship to the patient, such as "husband"]'.

Step 2: status

Either the resuscitation team leader or a delegate reviews the situation and current status in clear and concise terms. For example, 'Your husband's heart has stopped beating and we are trying to restart the heart'.

Step 3: prognosis

Given the high likelihood of death in cardiac arrest, it is prudent to warn the family members of the seriousness of the situation. A statement such as, 'As you can see, this is an extremely serious situation, and we are worried that your husband may not survive'.

Step 4: plan

State the plan of further care, such as, 'We are giving him powerful medications and electricity to try to restart his heart'.

Step 5: provide

Provide standard resuscitation as indicated by the situation.

Step 6: review

A. Return of spontaneous circulation:

   a. Review: provide a quick summary of the events leading to return of spontaneous circulation.

   b. Plan: state what will be done to maintain the patient's condition while attempting to move the patient to the intensive care unit for further interventions.

B. No return of spontaneous circulation:

   a. Overview: provide a brief summary to serve as a warning communication. For example, 'Mr Jones' heart has stopped and he is not responding to therapy'.

   b. Review: in anticipation of stopping the resuscitation due to lack of response, summarize all the relevant interventions that have been performed to create a clear picture of the course of events for the staff and the family members. An example might be, 'Please allow me to review the course of events. We have a secure airway with good lung ventilation. We have performed effective chest compressions for 30 minutes. With refractory ventricular fibrillation, we have attempted defibrillation multiple times, given a total of 3 mg adrenaline and 300 mg amiodarone, yet we have not achieved spontaneous circulation and (Mr Jones) is now demonstrating asystole on the monitor'.

   c. Recommendations: while continuing resuscitative efforts, the team leader may consider asking for any other recommendations from other team members. This establishes team concordance and assures that all reasonable medical efforts have been performed to the level of comfort of the entire team, as witnessed by the family.

   d. Transition: in a firm but compassionate manner, prepare the family members for the discontinuation of resuscitation. It may be appropriate at this time to tell the family that the heart is not responding. It may also be an important opportunity for any essential family to come into the room to see or touch the patient before death is pronounced.

   e. Pronouncement: the formality of a death pronouncement not only defines a clear time of death to the staff, but it also communicates the unequivocal truth for the family that the patient has died. For example, 'With consensus, the patient is pronounced dead at 22:17 hours'.

   f. Condolence: create silence and the space to grieve by turning off all alarms and monitors, offering condolences to the family, and offering to speak to any remaining family outside of the resuscitation room.

Step 7: acknowledge

It is essential to acknowledge with gratitude the difficulty of the event, the skill of the staff, and effort put forth to attempt to save the life of the patient. For example, 'Thank you team. This is never easy. I appreciate your skill and hard work'.

Step 8: inform

Either offer to inform the remaining family independently, or offer to bring the family members in the room to the others to inform them of the patient's death. As with other death disclosures, this would be an appropriate time to gather additional medical information to better understand the cause of death.

Step 9: self and staff care

The same principle applies as with death disclosure (see earlier subsection). Debriefing after attempts at resuscitation is an excellent method of assuring that all concerns about the resuscitation are addressed. It is also an important time for self-reflection and staff assessment prior to returning to patient care.

Online materials

Additional online materials for this chapter are available online at <http://www.oxfordmedicine.com>.

References

Agard, M. (2008). Creating advocates for family presence during resuscitation. *Medsurg Nursing*, 17(3), 155–160.

American College of Emergency Physicians (2014). *Ethical Issues at the End of Life*. [Online] Available at: <http://www.acep.org/Clinical---Practice-Management/Ethical-Issues-at-the-End-of-Life/>.

Baile, W., Buckman, R., and Lenzi, R., *et al.* (2000). SPIKES—a six-step protocol for delivering bad news: application to the patient with cancer. *Oncologist*, 5(4), 302–311.

Benenson, R. and Pollack, M. (2003). Evaluation of emergency medicine resident death notification skills by direct observation. *Academic Emergency Medicine*, 10, 219–223.

Boudreaux, E., Francis, J., and Loyacano, T. (2002). Family presence during invasive procedures and resuscitations in the emergency department: a critical review and suggestions for future research. *Annals of Emergency Medicine*, 40, 193–205.

Campbell, M. (2007). How to withdraw mechanical ventilation: a systematic review of the literature. *AACN Advanced Critical Care*, 18(4), 397–403.

Campbell, M., Bizek, K., and Thill, M. (1999). Patient responses during rapid terminal weaning from mechanical ventilation: a prospective study. *Critical Care Medicine*, 27, 73–77.

Campbell, M. and Guzman, J. (2003). Impact of a proactive approach to improve end-of-life care in a medical ICU. *Chest*, 123(1), 266–271.

Center to Advance Palliative Care (2011). *Improving Palliative Care in Emergency Medicine*. [Online] Available at: <http://www.capc.org/ipal/ipal-em>.

Chan, J., Treece, P., Engleberg, R., et al. (2004). Association between narcotic and benzodiazepine use after withdrawal of life support and time to death. *Chest*, 126, 286–293.

Clayton, J., Butow, P., Arnold, R., and Tattersall, M. (2005). Fostering coping and nurturing hope when discussing the future with terminally ill cancer patients and their caregivers. *Cancer*, 103(9), 1965–1975.

Cone, D., Richardson, L., Todd, K., et al. (2003). Health care disparities in emergency medicine. *Academic Emergency Medicine*, 10(11), 1176–1183.

Curtis, J. (2005). Interventions to improve care during withdrawal of life-sustaining treatments. *Journal of Palliative Medicine*, 8(Suppl. 1), S116–31.

DeSandre, P. and Quest, T. (2009). Management of cancer-related pain. *Emergency Medicine Clinics of North America*, 27(2), 179–194.

Dingerman, R., Mitchell, E., Meyer, E., et al. (2007). Parent presence during complex invasive procedures and cardiopulmonary resuscitation: a systematic review of the literature. *Pediatrics*, 120(4), 842–854.

Doolin, C.T., Quinn, L.D., Bryant, L.G., et al. (2011). Family presence during cardiopulmonary resuscitation: using evidence-based knowledge to guide the advanced practice nurse in developing formal policy and practice guidelines. *Journal of the American Academy of Nurse Practitioners*, 23(1), 8–14.

Dudley, N., Hansen, K., Furnival, R.A., et al. (2009). The effect of family presence on the efficiency of pediatric trauma resuscitations. *Annals of Emergency Medicine*, 53(6), 777–784.

Ebell, M., Becker, L., Barry, H., and Hagen, M. (1998). Survival after in-hospital cardiopulmonary resuscitation: a meta-analysis. *Journal of General Internal Medicine*, 13(12), 805–806.

Education in Palliative and End of Life Care (2010). *EPEC for Emergency Medicine*. [Online] Available at: <http://epec.net/epec_em.php>.

Emanuel, L., Alpert, H., and Emanuel, E. (2001). Concise screening questions for clinical assessments of terminal care: the needs near the end-of-life care screening tool. *Journal of Palliative Medicine*, 4(4), 465–474.

Emergency Nurses Association (2013). *Palliative and End-Of-Life Care in the Emergency Department*. Position statement. [Online] Available at: <http://www.ena.org/SiteCollectionDocuments/Position%20Statements/PalliativeEndOfLifeCare.pdf>.

Ewer, M., Kish, S.K., Martin, C.G., Price, K.J., and Feeley, T.W. (2001). Characteristics of cardiac arrest in cancer patients as a predictor of survival after cardiopulmonary resuscitation. *Cancer*, 92(7), 1905–1912.

Farah, M., Thomas, C., and Shaw, K. (2007). Evidence-based guidelines for family presence in the resuscitation room. *Pediatric Emergency Care*, 23(8), 587–591.

Fogarty, L., Curbow, B.A., Wingard, J.R., McDonnell, K., and Somerfield, M.R. (1999). Can 40 seconds of compassion reduce patient anxiety? *Journal of Clinical Oncology*, 17(1), 371–379.

Glajchen, M., Lawson, R., Homel, P., et al. (2011). A rapid two-stage screening protocol for palliative care in the emergency department: a quality improvement initiative. *Journal of Pain and Symptom Management*, 42(5), 657–662.

Grudzen, C., Richardson, L.D., Morrison, M., Cho, E., and Morrison, R.S. (2010). Palliative care needs of seriously ill, older adults presenting to the emergency department. *Academic Emergency Medicine*, 17(11), 1253–1257.

Grudzen, C., Stone, S., and Morrison, R. (2011). The palliative care model for emergency department patients with advanced illness. *Journal of Palliative Medicine*, 14(8), 945–950.

Hagen, N., Elwood, T., and Ernst, S. (1997). Cancer pain emergencies: a protocol for management. *Journal of Pain and Symptom Management*, 14(1), 45–50.

Heyland, D., Frank, C., Groll, D., et al. (2006). Understanding cardiopulmonary resuscitation decision making: perspectives of seriously ill hospitalized patients and family members. *Chest*, 130(2), 419–428.

Hobgood, C., Harward, D., Newton, K., and Davis, W. (2005). The educational intervention 'GRIEV_ING' improves the death notification skills of residents. *Academic Emergency Medicine*, 12, 296–301.

Hudson, P., Quinn, K., O'Hanlon, B., and Aranda, S. (2008). Family meetings in palliative care: Multidisciplinary clinical practice guidelines. *BMC Palliative Care*, 7, 12.

Hudson, P., Thomas, T., Quinn, K., and Aranda, S. (2009). Family meetings in palliative care: are they effective? *Palliative Medicine*, 23(2), 150–157.

Kleinman, M., de Caen, A., and Chameides, L., et al. (2010). Part 10: Pediatric basic and advanced life support: 2010 International Consensus on Cardiopulmonary Resuscitation and Emergency Cardiovascular Care Science With Treatment Recommendations. *Circulation*, 122, S466–S515.

Lamba, S., Pound, A., Rella, J., and Compton, S. (2012). Emergency medicine resident education in palliative care: a needs assessment. *Journal of Palliative Medicine*, 15(5), 516–520.

Lustbader, D., Pekmezaris, R., and Frankenthaler, M., et al. (2011). Palliative medicine consultation impacts DNR designation and length of stay for terminal medical MICU patients. *Palliative & Supportive Care*, 9, 401–406.

Mahony, S., Blank, A., Simpson, J., et al. (2008). Preliminary report of a palliative care and case management project in an emergency department for chronically ill elderly patients. *Journal of Urban Health*, 85, 443–451.

Mercadante, S., Villari, P., Ferrera, P., Casuccio, A., and Fulfaro, F. (2002). Rapid titration with intravenous morphine for severe cancer pain and immediate oral conversion. *Cancer*, 95(1), 203–208.

Miaskowski, C., Cleary, J., Burney, R., and Coyne, P., et al. (2005). *Guideline for the Management of Cancer Pain in Adults and Children*. APS Clinical Practice Guidelines Series, No. 3. Glenview, IL: American Pain Society.

Morrison, L., Kierzek, G., and Diekema, D.S., et al. (2010). Part 3: Ethics: 2010 American Heart Association Guidelines for Cardiopulmonary Resuscitation and Emergency Cardiovascular Care. *Circulation*, 122, S665–S675.

National Consensus Project for Quality Palliative Care (2013). *Clinical Practice Guidelines for Quality Palliative Care* (3rd ed.). Pittsburgh, PA: National Consensus Project for Quality Palliative Care.

Peberdy, M., Kaye, W., Ornato, J.P., et al. (2003). Cardiopulmonary resuscitation of adults in the hospital: a report of 14720 cardiac arrests from the National Registry of Cardiopulmonary Resuscitation. *Resuscitation*, 58(3), 297–308.

Pletcher, M., Kertesz, S., Kohn, M., and Gonzales, R. (2008). Trends in opioid prescribing by race/ethnicity for patients seeking care in US emergency departments. *Journal of the American Medical Association*, 299(1), 70–78.

Quest, T., Gisondi, M., Engle, K., et al. (2011). *Implementation of the Screening for Palliative Care Needs in the Emergency Department (SPEED) Instrument in Two Emergency Departments*. Presented at the Society for Academic Emergency Medicine Annual Meeting, Boston, MA.

Quest, T., Marco, C., and Derse, A. (2009). Hospice and palliative medicine: new subspecialty, new opportunities. *Annals of Emergency Medicine*, 54(1), 94–102.

Quest, T., Otsuki, J.A., Banja, J., Ratcliff, J.J., Heron, S.L., and Kaslow, N.J. (2002). The use of standardized patients within a procedural competency model to teach death disclosure. *Academic Emergency Medicine*, 9, 1326–1333.

Quest, T.E. (2008). The hardest news: death disclosure in the emergency department. *Medscape Journal of Medicine*, 10(8), 194.

Quill, T., Arnold, R., and Back, A. (2009). Discussing treatment preferences with patients who want 'everything'. *Annals of Internal Medicine*, 151(5), 345–349.

Reisfield, G., Wallace, S.K., Munsell, M.F., Webb, F.J., Alvarez, E.R., and Wilson, G.R. (2006). Survival in cancer patients undergoing in-hospital cardiopulmonary resuscitation: a meta-analysis. *Resuscitation*, 71(2), 152–160.

Richards, C., Gisondi, M., Chang, C., *et al.* (2011). Palliative care symptoms assessment for patients with cancer in the emergency department: validation of the Screen for Palliative and End-of-Life care needs in the Emergency Department instrument. *Journal of Palliative Medicine*, 14(6), 757–764.

Sasson, C., Rogers, M., Dahl, J., and Kellermann, A. (2010). Predictors of survival from out-of-hospital cardiac arrest: a systematic review and meta-analysis. *Circulation: Cardiovascular Quality and Outcomes*, 3(1), 63–81.

Schmid, M., Kindlimann, A., and Langewitz, W. (2005). Recipients' perspective on breaking bad news: how you put it really makes a difference. *Patient Education and Counseling*, 58(3), 244–251.

Smith, A., Fisher, J., and Schonberg, M., *et al.* (2009). Am I doing the right thing? Provider perspectives on improving palliative care in the emergency department. *Annals of Emergency Medicine*, 54(1), 86–93.e1.

Soares, L., Martins, M., and Uchoa, R. (2003). Intravenous fentanyl for cancer pain: a 'Fast Titration' protocol for the emergency room. *Journal of Pain and Symptom Management*, 26(3), 876–881.

Stalnikowicz, R., Mahamid, R., Kaspi, S., and Brezis, M. (2005). Undertreatment of acute pain in the emergency department: a challenge. *International Journal for Quality in Health Care*, 17(2), 173–176.

Stone, S., Mohanty, S., Grudzen, C.R., *et al.* (2011). Emergency medicine physicians' perspectives of providing palliative care in an emergency department. *Journal of Palliative Medicine*, 14(12), 1333–1338.

Tinsley, C., Hill, J., Shah, J., *et al.* (2008). Experience of families during cardiopulmonary resuscitation in a pediatric intensive care unit. *Pediatrics*, 122(4), e799–804.

Todd, K., Ducharme, J., and Choiniere, M., *et al.* (2007). PEMI Study Group. Pain in the emergency department: results of the pain and emergency medicine initiative (PEMI) multicenter study. *Journal of Pain*, 8, 460–466.

Todd, K.H. (2005). Pain assessment instruments for use in the emergency department. *Emergency Medicine Clinics of North America*, 23(2), 285–295.

Vandyk, A., Harrison, M.B., Macartney, G., Ross-White, A., and Stacey, D. (2012). Emergency department visits for symptoms experienced by oncology patients: a systematic review. *Support Care Cancer*, 20(8), 1589–1599.

Waugh, D. (2010). Palliative care project in the emergency department. *Journal of Palliative Medicine*, 13(8), p. 936.

Welch, S. (2010). Twenty years of patient satisfaction research applied to the emergency department: a qualitative review. *American Journal of Medical Quality*, 25(1), 64–72.

Weissman, D. and Meier, D. (2011). Identifying patients in need of a palliative care assessment in the hospital setting; a consensus report from the Center to Advance Palliative Care. *Journal of Palliative Medicine*, 14(1), 17–23.

Wilsey, B., Fishman, S.M., Ogden, C., Tsodikov, A., and Bertakis, K.D. (2008). Chronic pain management in the emergency department: a survey of attitudes and beliefs. *Pain Medicine*, 9(8), 1073–1080.

Young, G. (2009). Neurologic prognosis after cardiac arrest. *The New England Journal of Medicine*, 361, 605–611.

3.4

Palliative care in the nursing home

Jane L. Phillips, Annmarie Hosie, and Patricia M. Davidson

Introduction to palliative care in the nursing home

Internationally, ageing, technological advances, evolving patterns of disease and disability, and changes in family structures have resulted in nursing homes becoming the final residence for many frailer older people. Many terms are used to describe the nursing home setting, including 'care homes', 'residential homes', 'residential aged care facilities', and 'aged care', 'skilled-care', or 'long-term care facilities'. In this chapter 'nursing homes' are defined as collective institutional settings where continuous care is provided for older people throughout the 24-hour period, 7 days a week on an ongoing basis (Hall et al., 2011). Much of the on-site assistance with activities of daily living in nursing homes is predominately provided by an unregulated or minimally trained carer workforce with registered nurse supervision. Professional nursing and medical care is provided either by on-site or visiting doctors, nurses, and allied health professionals from external services.

In the United States, there are currently 1.6 million older people living in nursing homes ('residents') (Ouslander and Berenson, 2011). The unprecedented demand for institutional care by people aged over 85 years is likely to continue to increase and has significant cost implications and considerations for the health workforce. In Australia alone, during 2009 to 2010, a one billion dollar increase in the aged care budget was needed to fund an additional 4550 nursing home beds just to meet existing demand (Australian Institute of Health and Welfare, 2011). In the United Kingdom, 15 700 nursing homes currently provide care to over 400 000 residents (Mathie et al., 2012). In Canada, nursing home beds now exceed the number of acute care beds (Canadian Institute for Health Information, 2007). Given these trends nursing homes will continue to be major providers of palliative care for the frail aged and for people whose complex care needs exceed available community resources and capacity of family caregivers.

Admission to a nursing home is frequently the consequence of caregiver burden or living alone, care needs exceeding available community resources, or needing end-of-life care (Seymour, 2011). Currently, the majority of all residents are aged over 85 years, with three-quarters having high care needs related to behaviours, activities of daily living, or complex health-care needs (Australian Institute of Health and Welfare, 2011). Whereas residents once lived in nursing homes for longer periods, over a third (38%) now die within a year of admission, with a quarter of these

deaths occurring within the first 6 months (Australian Institute of Health and Welfare, 2011). Between 16% and 30% of all deaths in the developed world now occur in nursing homes: United States, 24% (Goldberg and Botero, 2008); United Kingdom, 17% (Tebbit, 2008); Canada, 30% (Motiwala et al., 2006); and Australia, 16% (Australian Government Department of Health and Ageing, 2010). Despite this unprecedented demand, disparities in resources and infrastructure (Brennan, 2007) continue to impact on residents' access to palliative care.

This chapter details the palliative care needs of older people living in nursing homes and the challenges and opportunities to deliver better end-of-life care to this population; and proposes utilizing the Chronic Care Model as a framework for delivering the elements of a *palliative approach* to improve care outcomes for residents and their families.

Demography and epidemiology of dying in a nursing home

With advancing age comes an increased incidence of chronic co-morbidities, such as stroke, heart failure, chronic obstructive pulmonary disease, degenerative neurological disease, arthritis, dementia, frailty, visual impairment, and hearing loss (World Health Organization, 2011). The six leading causes of death of people aged over 65 years in the United States are heart disease (44%), cancer (29%), stroke (11%), chronic obstructive pulmonary disease (8%), influenza and pneumonia (4%), and diabetes (4%) (Federal Interagency Forum on Aging-Related Statistics, 2008). Approximately two-thirds of all US nursing home residents have two or more co-morbidities (Wolff et al., 2002), with approximately half having a diagnosis of dementia, while in the United Kingdom it is estimated that 40% of all older people admitted to nursing homes have dementia (British Geriatrics Society, 2012). Alzheimer's disease is now the seventh leading cause of death in the United States (Alzheimer's Association, 2011), and people with dementia are more likely to die in a US nursing home, compared to people dying with cancer and/or from other conditions (66% vs 20% vs 28%, respectively) (Alzheimer's Association, 2011).

Alongside the prevalence of multiple chronic conditions, many residents have unrelieved symptoms, have lower use of hospice care and more hospitalization, are the recipients of poor communication, have less capacity and opportunity to participate in advance care planning, and experience more family dissatisfaction (Oliver et al., 2004; Munn et al., 2006). Residents with advanced dementia are often unable to communicate their needs or participate in decision-making and rely on substitute decision-makers (van der Steen, 2010). They are also more likely than residents with cognition to experience pneumonia and/or eating difficulties (van der Steen, 2010). Residents with cognition have expressed concerns that they often have too little involvement in decision-making, limited access to someone to discuss their concerns, limited access to appropriate information, and that tests and results are often not clearly explained (Wetle et al., 2005).

Older people with dementia nearing the end of life experience significant symptom burden including, but not limited to, pain, breathlessness, discomfort, restlessness, agitation, difficulty swallowing, aspiration, and pressure ulcers (Mitchell et al., 2009; van der Steen, 2010). Up to 83% of people living with dementia in nursing homes experience pain, while between 12% and 32% experience breathlessness at some point in their disease process (Mitchell et al., 2009). Similar to other illness trajectories, these symptoms frequently increase as death approaches (Mitchell et al., 2009). Consequently, many deaths in nursing homes are not considered to be a good death, that is, a death 'free from avoidable distress and suffering for patients, families and caregivers; in general accord with patients' and families' wishes; and reasonably consistent with clinical, cultural and ethical standards' (Field and Cassel, 1997, p. 24). Over the past decade there has been increasing recognition and acceptance of the need to extend palliative care to underserved populations such as nursing home residents.

Challenges

Despite the burden of co-morbidities and prevalence of distressing symptoms in this population, there is still minimal integration of geriatric care, chronic disease management, and palliative care in either the clinical or research context. Advanced dementia has a long and unpredictable illness trajectory, setting it apart from other terminal illnesses. A focus on 'healthy ageing' has made it difficult to draw attention to the policy and practice changes required in nursing homes to provide palliative care (Abbey et al., 2006), while organizational and clinical factors impact on the capacity of nursing homes to manage residents' chronic diseases and their subsequent end-of-life care (Seymour, 2011). There are also few evidence-based guidelines (Australian Department of Health and Ageing and National Health and Medical Research Council, 2006) to assist aged care clinicians effectively manage the multiple co-morbidities experienced by an older, frailer nursing home population (Weiss et al., 2007). The evidence-based guidelines that do exist rarely acknowledge how to effectively manage more than one chronic and complex illness or consider drug–drug and drug–disease interactions in older people (Weiss et al., 2007).

Complex operating environment ripe for reform

Nursing homes have developed separately to palliative care in spite of the importance of these needs (Hockley et al., 2010). Nursing homes are complex care environments, largely constructed as an 'industry' as opposed to a 'service', as a result of many of them functioning in private business models. In many countries, increasing longevity has prompted the transition of nursing homes from a welfare model towards a user pays system, with an economic emphasis to minimize labour costs and maximize

profits. A meta-analysis using data from both observational and randomized control trials found that an organization's financial operating status impacted on some aspects of nursing home quality, with not-for-profit homes having more or higher quality staffing compared to for-profit nursing homes; and that not-for-profit nursing homes delivered higher quality care on average compared to for-profit homes (Comondore et al., 2009). Business models and predominance in the private sector have meant reform within this care sector has been difficult to achieve and monitor, with significant change only occurring in response to legislation (Chenoweth and Kilstoff, 2002). However, not all legislative change has impacted positively on residents' outcomes. In countries such as Australia where the legislative need for 24-hour care provided by a registered nurse has been repealed, the resident to registered nurse ratio has been significantly altered (Angus and Nay, 2003). As a result, older people admitted to Australian nursing homes are now largely cared for by unregulated workers (Richardson and Martin, 2004) supported by a smaller ratio of registered nurses, who are relegated increasingly to management duties (Angus and Nay, 2003). This workforce profile presents challenges when palliative care demands a skilled nursing response and resident and family care needs are increasingly complex. These changes in skill mix have also increased the demands on the acute care sector.

Medical care in nursing homes varies considerably across countries and is largely shaped by funding mechanisms and local policy. In the majority of countries, medical care is provided by doctors employed directly by the nursing home (Donald et al., 2008), whereas in the United Kingdom and Australia, general practitioners (GPs) are the main providers of medical care to nursing home residents on a fee-for-service basis (Gadzhanova and Reed, 2007). However, the visiting GP model presents challenges, as the time-consuming nature of nursing home visits, especially when residents are scattered across multiple facilities, onerous documentation, and poor remuneration all impact on GPs' willingness to provide medical care in this setting (Glendinning et al., 2002; Gadzhanova and Reed, 2007). There is growing concern that medical services to nursing homes are inadequate to meet current needs, let alone future demands, with many nursing homes finding it increasingly difficult to secure medical care (Glendinning et al., 2002; Gadzhanova and Reed, 2007).

From the consumer perspective, many residents and/or their families are often forced to establish a relationship with a new GP when admitted to a nursing home, largely because they have been admitted to a nursing home in a geographical area not serviced by their usual GP, their usual GP doesn't have formal links with the nursing home, and/or doesn't provide a nursing home service (Gadzhanova and Reed, 2007). In the United Kingdom, this challenge has been partially addressed through nursing home management entering into ad hoc remuneration arrangements with GPs to secure ongoing medical care for their residents (Glendinning et al., 2002). Limited access to timely medical care often precludes development of appropriate processes to identify and manage each resident's decline (Wetle et al., 2005) and contributes to unnecessary and often distressing hospital admissions (Ahronheim et al., 1996).

Reducing avoidable hospitalizations

In 2005, there were potentially $3.1 billion of avoidable US hospitalizations, with 85% of these total costs related to nursing home residents being transfers to acute care (Ouslander and Berenson, 2011). In the United States, higher health-care expenditure in the last 6 months of life is associated with decline in functional status, ethnicity, certain chronic conditions, and lack of nearby family support, regardless of regional characteristics (Kelley et al., 2011). Poor transitional care processes also contribute to substantially high readmission rates for residents (Quinn, 2011). It is estimated that one in four older people admitted to a US nursing home directly from hospital has an acute care readmission within 30 days (Ouslander and Berenson, 2011). Hospitalization for older people is dangerous and associated with reduced function, and increased morbidity and mortality (Ouslander and Berenson, 2011). Over the past decade reducing nursing home hospitalization rates has been a policy priority across the developed world (Grabowski et al., 2008), largely driven by the need to reduce both the adverse effects of hospitalization and excessive health-care costs (Kelley et al., 2011). Averting this trend requires multifaceted interventions that strategically build the capacity of nursing homes to better align the resident's goals of care with hospitalization decisions and in the process, change institutional patterns of care, physician practice patterns, and resident and family preferences (Kelley et al., 2011).

Access to hospice and specialist palliative care input

In the United States, the Medicare Hospice Benefit supports the delivery of hospice care across all care settings, including nursing homes where just over a third (36%) of all beneficiaries reside. Three-quarters (76%) of US nursing homes now have an established contract with a hospice provider (Gozalo and Miller, 2007). Hospice care increases the resident's access to palliative care expertise and care protocols, improved pain management (Miller et al., 2002), reduces hospitalization rates during the last month of life (Gozalo and Miller, 2007), and reduces the number of residents who die in hospital (Munn et al., 2006; Gozalo et al., 2008). In contrast, hospitalized patients with dementia are more likely than non-demented patients to have a longer terminal stay (Guijarro et al., 2010) and less likely to receive palliative treatment or have their families involved in decision-making (Afzal et al., 2010). Despite the positive benefits of access to hospice care, the US hospice care eligibility restrictions frequently result in late referrals, especially if families don't fully understand the role and advantages of engaging hospice services (Wetle et al., 2005).

Hospice enrolment substantially reduces care costs (22%) for residents, with shorter nursing home admissions (≤ 90 days) and a small cost reduction (8%) for residents with cancer who have longer stays (> 90 days). Whilst hospice care is cost-neutral for people with dementia, it increases care costs (10%) for people with a diagnosis other than cancer or dementia due to diagnostics (Gozalo et al., 2008). However, access to hospice care is influenced by disease type and proximity to services, with residents with a cancer diagnosis and who live in relatively close proximity to a hospice more likely to be enrolled in hospice (Gozalo and Miller, 2007), than residents with dementia (Munn et al., 2006). In countries with universal health care, access to specialist palliative care services for nursing home residents is underpinned by a population-based approach, where specialist teams provide a consultative service for residents with more complex palliative care needs (Palliative Care Australia, 2005a). However, access to these specialist palliative care teams similarly varies due to geographical or resource allocation barriers.

Opportunities

Promoting a palliative approach in nursing homes

Nursing homes now lie at the interface between continuing care and palliative care (Froggatt, 2001) and increasingly function as slow-stream hospices (Phillips et al., 2006). Given this changing role there is a need to develop new models of care that promote a palliative approach in the nursing home setting. A palliative approach is care that has the potential to improve the quality of life for older people with any life-limiting condition, and their families, by reducing their suffering through early identification, impeccable assessment, and treatment of pain, physical, psychological, social, cultural, and spiritual needs (Australian Department of Health and Ageing and National Health and Medical Research Council, 2006). A palliative approach ensures care is tailored to address residents' and their families' needs, well before the last days or weeks of life. Focusing attention on a palliative approach helps achieve the best possible quality of life for older people and their families by facilitating: (1) evidence-based symptom management; (2) appropriate decision-making support and goal setting, including advance care planning; (3) access to practical aid, community resource, and specialist palliative care advice or support as required; and (4) collaborative and seamless end-of-life care within the nursing home (Davidson and Phillips, 2012).

A palliative approach enables a larger proportion of older people to live and die comfortably in this care setting, as opposed to being transferred to acute care (Reymond et al., 2011). Implementing a palliative approach requires nursing homes to focus on strategies to better manage residents' symptoms, develop an ethos of care that openly acknowledges that death frequently occurs in this setting, attend to residents' spiritual needs, offer caring and appropriate information to residents and their families, attend to the needs of residents' families and friends, and be mindful of the needs of staff (Sander and Russell, 2001). Adopting a palliative approach to care is of equal, if not of more value, to the family than to the person dying (Kristjanson et al., 1996). Given the prevalence of dementia in this population, attending to a resident's substitute decision maker's needs is a high priority, especially as the quality of care at the end of life may be an important predictor of bereavement outcomes (Gauthier and Gagliese, 2012).

A recent Cochrane review (Hall et al., 2011) examining multi-component interventions to enhance the provision of a palliative approach in nursing homes identified weak evidence for the following three elements of care: (1) communication, with a focus on identifying residents who would benefit from a specialist palliative care referral and negotiating this with their treating doctor and family (Casarett et al., 2005); (2) the development of palliative care leadership teams, technical assistance meetings for team members, education in palliative care for all staff, and feedback on performance (Hanson et al., 2005); and (3) targeted symptom control strategies to improve discomfort (Kovach et al., 1996). In addition to these three elements a palliative approach in nursing homes also requires a commitment to: (1) person-centred care; (2) creating a palliative care team for each resident based on need; (3) optimizing symptom control; (4) advance care planning; and (5) timely recognition of dying.

Person-centred care

Person-centred care places the resident at the centre and recognizes individual differences, preferences, and cultural diversity, with cultural and religious beliefs and practices surrounding death and dying integral to providing a person-centred palliative approach to older people in nursing homes (Clark and Phillips, 2010). Mead and Bower (2000) have identified five distinct patient–provider relationship dimensions that shape patient-centred care, which can be equally applied to resident care, including the: (1) bio-psychosocial perspective; (2) 'resident as person'; (3) sharing power and responsibility; (4) therapeutic alliance; and (5) 'physician as person'. Influential factors relating to the resident, health professional, consultation, professional context, and societal 'shapers' all need to be acknowledged and taken into consideration to achieve person-centred care (Mead and Bower, 2000).

When considering a person-centred palliative approach, key priorities of residents nearing the end of life with decision-making capacity are: (1) being active to the very last; (2) having one's will respected and being allowed to die; (3) not being in pain; and (4) being amongst persons close to one (valediction and showing respect) (Pleschberger, 2007). When asked about their end-of-life care expectations, residents with decision-making capacity indicated that they hadn't spoken to aged care personnel about this issue but assumed that their family or primary care physician would take responsibility for making these decisions (Mathie et al., 2012). Other than with decision-making capacity, other factors that influenced residents' ability to discuss end-of-life care was their level of acceptance of living in a nursing home, family involvement in making decisions, and self-efficacy about their capacity to influence everyday decision-making (Mathie et al., 2012). Families have expressed concerns that they were unaware the resident was nearing the end of their life and that dying residents' needs weren't sufficiently addressed, because of difficulties accessing medical care and the limited palliative care capabilities of aged care personnel (Miller et al., 2004; Wetle et al., 2005). While little is known about the end-of-life wishes of residents with cognitive impairment, evidence from the literature suggests that a 'good death' from their families' perspective is a combination of good symptom management, clear decision-making, good preparation for death, completion and affirmation of the whole person, and a smooth transition from usual care to terminal care (Bosek et al., 2003; Gibson and Gorman, 2010).

Creating a palliative care team for each resident based on need

Providing a palliative approach requires the creation of a care team for each resident based on their individual needs. For the majority of residents, the primary aged care team (nurses, care assistants, GPs/physician, family, divisional therapists, and volunteers) can readily provide this care. Residents with complex care needs can benefit from input from external specialists, such as the specialist palliative care, aged care, or psycho-geriatric services (Casarett et al., 2005). In some situations, establishing a shared care model of palliative care, that includes primary health, community-based services, as well as external specialist services, is required to address the resident's and their family's palliative care needs (NSW Health, 2011). Strengthening the linkages between care providers may help to reduce avoidable hospitalizations, especially if community-based health professionals can effectively meet the resident's care needs (Ouslander and Berenson, 2011). There is emerging evidence that a single palliative care assessment shortly after nursing home admission may be the most effective format for optimizing the resident's palliative care outcomes. A recent non-blinded prospective comparison trial involving older people (n = 81) living in three US assisted living facilities found that palliative care assessments conducted at 3-monthly intervals were no better than a single early palliative care assessment in improving palliative care outcomes (Jerant et al., 2006).

Effective team communication is integral to a palliative approach, with case conferencing being an ideal forum to facilitate the delivery of multidisciplinary care. This approach brings together relevant health professionals and the resident's primary decision-makers, usually family members, to discuss the current stage of illness and agree on a person-centred management plan based on best available evidence (Abernethy et al., 2006; Phillips et al., 2013). Case conferencing can improve care outcomes for older people with advanced dementia living in nursing homes through better communication, coordination and engagement of relevant health professionals, residents and their families in a collaborative care planning process, promotion and adoption of more appropriate symptom management strategies, reducing unnecessary hospitalizations, and promoting seamless transitions, if hospitalization is required (Phillips et al., 2013).

Optimizing symptom control

Adopting a palliative approach requires that the symptoms of residents be assessed and managed in a timely and appropriate manner. This is crucial given the symptom burden in this population with approximately (60%) of residents estimated to have dementia, half (40–50%) experiencing pain, and 40% being classified as depressed (The Royal Australian College of General Practitioners, 2006). Older residents with non-malignant diseases and those with cognitive impairment are most at risk of inadequate assessment and management of pain in all care settings, including nursing homes (Abbey et al., 2004). As a commitment to impeccable assessment is an integral component of a palliative approach (World Health Organization, 2003), ensuring aged care providers have access to validated symptom assessment tools that are both sensitive to the needs of older people with multiple co-morbidities and high levels of cognitive impairment is crucial. Selecting assessment tools that are reliably and easily administered by a diverse and largely unskilled carer workforce is also an important consideration (see Chapter 7.1).

Polypharmacy and cognitive, behavioural, and swallowing problems make medication administration in this setting a complex, time-consuming, and potentially hazardous activity, especially if the nurse is unfamiliar with the resident (Thomson et al., 2009). Polypharmacy and adverse drug reactions are common in the nursing home setting, with residents being prescribed an average of ten medications (Patterson et al., 2010). While various strategies have been initiated at an international, national, state, and local level to improve the quality of prescribing and reduce medication errors in nursing homes (Hughes et al., 2011), few clinical trials have evaluated systematic withdrawal of medications among older people (Beer et al., 2011).

The time-consuming nature of medication administration as residents lose their ability to swallow may also influence decisions to insert a feeding tube for a nutrition and medication administration route, with a complex mix of financial, organizational, demographic, and ethnic factors, as opposed to best evidence (Mitchell et al., 2003), also impacting on feeding tube insertion decisions. Yet, there is little evidence that enteral tube feeding confers any survival benefit for people with advanced dementia and there is little data about its adverse effects (Sampson et al., 2009). In some countries, system-wide incentives are promoting inappropriate use of tube feeding, undermining residents' safety and quality of life (Finucane et al., 2007).

Advance care planning

Whilst death is frequent in nursing homes, advance care planning has traditionally not been raised or discussed in an open and honest manner with residents and their families. In the absence of an up-to-date advanced care plan or previous conversations with the resident and/or their family, aged care personnel often feel compelled to transfer the resident to hospital, as they may be unsure of the resident's wishes, as well as being ill-prepared or unable to manage specific clinical situations. It is estimated that approximately 40% of residents with advanced dementia receive at least one burdensome treatment in the last 3 months of life because they don't have a documented advance care plan (Mitchell et al., 2009). Many of these inappropriately used invasive treatments compromise comfort for little or no survival benefit, whilst impacting adversely on family satisfaction with care (Meier et al., 2001; Givens et al., 2010).

Proactive advance care planning conversations in the nursing home setting offer the multidisciplinary care team, residents, and their family an opportunity to: (1) identify an appropriate substitute decision-maker; (2) clarify resident's values and preferences over time; and (3) to consider what action they would take when the resident's health deteriorates (Sudore and Fried, 2010). These structured conversations are also critical to reducing unnecessary hospital re-admissions (Quinn, 2011). A US study has demonstrated that conducting a structured interview to identify residents with palliative care needs resulted in residents being more likely to be enrolled in hospice within 30 days and fewer acute care admissions. Residents' families also rated the care provided more highly than those receiving usual care (Casarett et al., 2005). In another study, conducting a brief 15-minute advance care planning conversation with families of the resident with advanced dementia's transition to nursing home also increased families' satisfaction with care (Engel et al., 2006).

Timely recognition of dying

In the nursing home setting, death typically follows one of four final pathways: (1) a sudden death; (2) a death following a terminal illness; (3) a death following an acute episode; or (4) a death following a process of general deterioration (Sidell et al., 1997). While older people in the community in the year preceding death experience varying levels of disability, ranging from severe to no disability, the predictable pattern of deterioration identified for residents with advanced dementia is a trajectory of persistently severe disability (Gill et al., 2010). A pattern of deterioration occurring over months and sometimes years adds to the uncertainty of determining exactly when a transition to a palliative approach is indicated for a resident. Reserving palliative care for residents who are dying is of limited value, for the majority of residents will

have experienced symptoms and distress as part of their slow and gradual decline (Lynn and Adamson, 2003).

The ambiguity created by this discordance impacts on aged care providers' ability and confidence to accurately determine when palliative care is indicated. In the United Kingdom, the National Health Service has recommended that primary care providers consider the 'surprise question', that is: 'Would I be surprised if this person were to die in the next 6–12 months?' (Lynn and Adamson, 2003). Despite concerns about the suitability of this approach for people with heart failure and chronic obstructive pulmonary disease (COPD) being raised (Small et al., 2010), if used as a screening question, the 'surprise question' can prompt the multidisciplinary team to review the resident's care needs and plan accordingly (Murray and Boyd, 2011).

In planning for the resident's end-of-life care, consideration needs to be increasingly given to deactivate implantable cardioverter-defibrillators, which produce painful shocks at the end of life and are distressing for the family to witness (Goldstein et al., 2010). Similar to hospices, nursing homes need policies and procedures to proactively identify residents with these devices and to ensure that there is an appropriate deactivation plan for when it is deemed appropriate to do so. Conversations about managing these devices needs to be documented in the resident's medical records and goals of care, including such details as how this device will be managed at the end of life, who will be responsible for deactivating the device, and ensuring the device's deactivation instructions are accessible within the nursing home (Goldstein et al., 2010).

A proposed framework for implementing a palliative approach

While there is a growing body of evidence to guide the delivery of palliative care in nursing homes, many aged care providers find it difficult to implement and apply a palliative approach in a systematic and strategic manner. The Chronic Care Model (Wagner et al., 2001) is a useful conceptual model to identify the action required at the consumer (resident and family), health professional, and system levels to strengthen the provision of a palliative approach in nursing homes. The Chronic Care Model has previously been used by a diverse range of health-care organizations to improve health-care delivery to people with chronic and complex illnesses (World Health Organization, 2002). Applying the Chronic Care Model in nursing homes would ensure that the needs of residents and their families remain the focus of care (Fig. 3.4.1 and Table 3.4.1), whilst acknowledging the fundamental importance of the following:

1. Enabling positive policies that promote the delivery of a palliative approach at the systems level, along with executive support and sponsorship at the organizational level.

2. An adequately prepared workforce with the prerequisite geriatric and palliative care capabilities, plus a commitment to maintaining an adequate workforce skill mix in nursing homes to respond to the population's changing clinical profiles.

3. Supporting collaborative partnerships across care settings to better meet the needs of residents, especially those with complex care or symptom control needs.

4. Access to decision support tools for aged care nurses, care assistants and GPs so they are able to provide evidence-based care and identify when expert assistance ought to be sought.

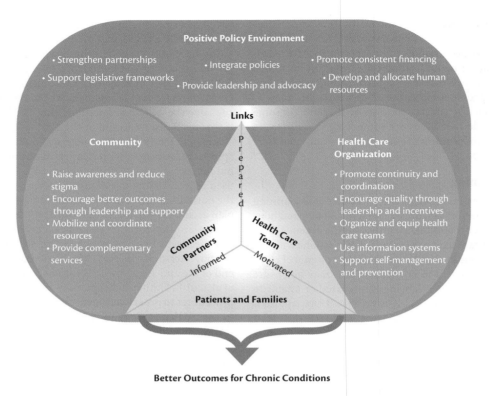

Fig. 3.4.1 The WHO Chronic Care Model—'Better Outcomes for Chronic Conditions'. The WHO Chronic Care Model helps identify the action required to integrate a palliative approach into the nursing home sector by addressing the key elements required for change at the systems level (see also Table 3.4.1).
Reprinted with permission from World Health Organization, 'Innovative Care for Chronic Conditions: Building Blocks for Action', p. 72, in World Health Organization, WHO Definition of Palliative Care, Copyright © World Health Organization 2002, available from http://www.who.int/cancer/palliative/definition/en/

5. Access to clinical information systems, including point-of-care evidence, electronic health records, and electronic prescribing systems to support care delivery.

6. Empowering consumers to take greater responsibility for their health by focussing on engaging residents with capacity and their families in the care planning and decision-making process.

Positive public policy

There are numerous opportunities to reorientate health-care systems through positive public policy to better support the delivery of a palliative approach in nursing homes. For example, while historically US policies such as nursing home regulations which emphasize rehabilitation, a 6-month life expectancy being a hospice eligibility criterion, and external monitoring of hospice referral patterns and contractual relationships between nursing homes and hospice providers were all considered appropriate, these policies are now effectively limiting the enrolment of residents in hospice programmes (Hoffmann and Tarzian, 2005). Similarly, given the uncertain illness trajectory of many residents, the incentive for US hospice providers not to exceed the aggregated payment cap for its beneficiaries is another potential hospice enrolment barrier (Stevenson and Bramson, 2009).

Current nursing home funding regulations also reinforce a task-orientated approach to care delivery, making it difficult to tailor care to meet each resident's individual needs. The frailty and complexity of a resident's care needs demand that care subsidies reflect the actual level of care required. Only with adequate reimbursement will nursing homes be able to employ enough

appropriately trained professionals, including nurses and care assistants, to meet the complex health needs of residents.

An environment of increasing technological complexity, where older people with higher acuity are increasingly being managed within nursing homes for shorter periods of time before dying now demands that a palliative approach be implemented from the moment a person enters a nursing home (Phillips et al., 2007) and be acknowledged as an integral responsibility of the sector. Yet, the fragmented nature of most health systems ensure that traditionally there has frequently been little connection and integration of aged care services and health (Australian Government Department of Health and Ageing, 2010). In Australia, for example, while quality standards for aged (Aged Care Standards Agency, 2001) and palliative care (Palliative Care Australia, 2005b) both exist, neither currently acknowledges the unique and often complex palliative care needs of older people in nursing homes. In the United Kingdom, there has been better alignment of aged and palliative care standards, with a set of national minimum standards that regulate palliative care in nursing homes, while in France there is a legal requirement that palliative care be implemented in all nursing homes (Froggatt and Reitinger, 2013).

A recent mapping exercise across Europe identified over 60 initiatives to support the development of palliative care in nursing homes (Froggatt and Reitinger, 2013). Whilst the diversity of these initiatives reflects differing priorities and opportunities, it affirms the importance of a palliative approach for residents and their families. A summary of these 60 initiatives is available at <http://www.lancaster.ac.uk/shm/research/ioelc/projects/eapc-taskforce-ltc/ltc_initiatives.pdf>. Unfortunately, many of

Table 3.4.1 The Chronic Care Model as applied to improving palliative care outcomes for nursing home residents

Chronic care domains	Elements	Action required
Positive policy environment	Strengthen partnerships	Encourage engagement and input from specialist services
		Promote inter-sectorial collaboration through clinical networks
	Support legislative frameworks	Link standards to funding and accreditation
		Establish minimum registered nursing to resident ratios
	Integrate policies	Align nursing home and palliative care standards
		Promote advance care planning
	Provide leadership and advocacy	Promote and support priority-driven research
		Build health workforce palliative approach capabilities
	Promote consistent financing	Remove perverse incentives
	Develop and allocate human resources	Appropriate ratio of registered nurses
Community	Raise awareness and reduce stigma	Greater community engagement into nursing homes
		Reduce ageism
		Value the care provided in nursing home
	Encourage better outcomes through leadership and support	Promote a palliative approach in the community
		Workforce continuing professional development
	Mobilize and coordinate resources	Pre-admission nursing home clinics
		Establish advance care planning clinics
	Provide complementary services	Embed palliative care volunteers in nursing homes
Health-care organization	Promote continuity and coordination	Promote person-centred care
		Facilitate 'pop-up' shared palliative care teams
		Ensure specialist input for residents with complex needs
		Establish multidisciplinary case conferencing
	Encourage quality through leadership and incentives	Build workforce palliative care capacity
		Role redesign—nurse practitioners and medical input
	Use information systems	Evidence-based guidelines
		Electronic health records
		Appropriate symptom assessment tools
	Support self-management and prevention	Engage residents and families in advance care planning

these initiatives were undertaken as time-limited 'projects' and have not been sustained due to lack of ongoing funding or organizational support (Froggatt and Reitinger, 2013). Demonstrating that like any reform, embedding a palliative approach in the nursing home setting requires improved alignment of relevant legislation, policies, and standards, supported by appropriate funding.

Community

The general reluctance at a societal level to discuss death and dying also shapes the level of community awareness of palliative care and more specifically, the applicability of a palliative approach for residents. Promoting awareness of a palliative approach across the community will make it easier in the future for aged care providers to discuss this issue with residents and their families. Proactively disseminating information about a palliative approach and advance care planning to prospective residents and families contemplating the transition to nursing home care supports appropriate care (Lowe et al., 2003). This empowering aspect of a palliative approach helps foster greater awareness amongst the resident and their family of the model of care that is offered within the nursing home and the level of support available to address their end-of-life care needs. It also promotes the creation of more supportive care environments and gently encourages better understanding and capacity of aged care providers and families to deal with death and dying (Kellehear, 1999). In Australia, the recent announcement of a national advance care planning advisory service to actively engage and support aged care providers and GPs to initiate advance care planning discussion with residents and families, will raise awareness of the palliative care needs of residents and the importance of regularly reviewing the goals of care as their health deteriorates.

Volunteers

Nursing homes have traditionally often been isolated from the wider community, but there is an increasing need for them to seek greater community engagement. A structured and well-managed active volunteer programme is one way of engaging interested and suitable community members in the operation of the nursing home. Volunteers are an important adjunct to the interdisciplinary palliative care team (McKinnon, 2002). In specialist palliative care services, these unpaid workers undertake a range of practical, administrative, and supportive care activities in accordance with local service needs, their personal capabilities, and preferences (Palliative Care Victoria, 2010). Extending or establishing a volunteer programme in nursing homes could enhance the delivery of a palliative approach to older people nearing their end of life.

Building workforce capacity

In addition to adequate staffing, appropriate equipment, good medical support, and greater involvement with specialist palliative care teams, building the palliative approach capacity of aged care professionals is an essential element towards improved care for nursing home residents (Phillips, 2008). Over the past decade, many initiatives at both the local organizational and national level have been implemented to expand the aged care workforce's palliative approach competencies (Froggatt, 2001) through: (1) specialist support and ad hoc education; (2) tailored palliative care education programmes, delivered either face to face or online; (3) building clinical champion capabilities; or (4) a combination of specialist support and tailored education (Avis et al., 1999: Phillips, 2008).

Building the aged care workforces' palliative approach capabilities require a strategic commitment to increasing the palliative content in the vocational, undergraduate, and post-graduate health workforce curricula. A range of continuing professional education opportunities are also needed for registered health professionals to increase their symptom assessment and medication management competencies, particularly related to administering opiates; comfort and confidence to initiate and engage in end-of-life conversations and to discuss death, knowing when to initiate a palliative approach and recognizing dying; and communicating effectively with residents and their families about a palliative approach. Any continuing professional education programme implemented for aged care needs to be configured to be responsive to workforce turnover.

Health-care organization

Organizational elements identified as being critical to success for introducing a palliative approach into nursing homes include: (1) strong and committed leadership; (2) active involvement of the medical director; (3) availability of a nurse with palliative care expertise to guide and support the implementation; (4) presence of an onsite clinical champion; (5) combining a 'bottom-up' and 'top-down' approach to organizational change; (6) implementing change in small manageable increments; (7) inclusion of all staff in the effort; (8) regular meetings where discussions of palliative care occur; (9) maintenance of dying residents within the existing unit structures; and (10) capacity to use the programme as a benchmark of quality care and regulatory compliance (Strumpf et al., 2004). The ability of nursing homes to provide a palliative approach will be influenced by all of these factors.

Reorganizing the health-care workforce

A recent literature review identified several models of primary medical care configured to optimize outcomes in the nursing home setting, including the following:

1. Enhanced medical care provided by lead practices.

2. Provision of modest incentive payments to support lead practices to provide anticipatory care to specific nursing homes through a service level agreement.

3. Attached primary care services: general practices within a defined geographical area agreeing to be linked to specific nursing homes and to provide weekly visits, anticipatory care, and regular reviews.

4. Dedicated primary care service: the local primary care organization establishes a dedicated primary care multidisciplinary specialist service to provide primary care services to local nursing homes which focus on medical care and capacity building, including a focus on end-of-life care planning for people requiring palliative care.

5. Integrated primary and secondary care service: the establishment of a multidisciplinary team, composed of an advanced practitioner nurse, GP, and consultants to deliver comprehensive medical care to older people in nursing homes (Donald et al., 2008).

Nurse practitioners are increasingly being utilized in underserved populations, including older people in nursing homes (Aigner et al., 2004). Assessing the impact of nurse practitioners in nursing homes had largely been undertaken using non-randomized trials including before and after studies (Christian and Baker, 2009), with an absence of raw data being reported preventing meta-analysis. While few studies have focused specifically on palliative care nurse practitioners, a reduction in hospitalization rates and transfers to hospital emergency departments for assessment, reduced lengths of stay for hospitalized nursing home residents, and cost savings (Christian and Baker, 2009), suggests that developing the nurse practitioner role offers exciting opportunities to improve residents' palliative care outcomes. Any intervention designed to evaluate the effectiveness of this role ought to be robustly tested and able to generate level 1 evidence to inform future practice. Robust evaluation of all health workforce redesign initiatives is required to determine their cost-effectiveness and capacity to improve care outcomes for older people in nursing homes.

Decision supports

Various symptom-based guidelines have been developed to support the delivery of evidenced-based care and to assist nursing homes to develop and apply suitable policies and procedures (Abbey et al., 2006). The 'Gold Standards Framework for Care Homes' has been promoted in the United Kingdom (Hockley et al., 2010), while evidence-based palliative approach guidelines have been developed for Australia (Australian Department of Health and Ageing and National Health and Medical Research Council, 2006). These decision support tools have contributed to culture change within the aged care sector and resulted in increases in advanced care planning documentation and a reduction in avoidable hospitalization and hospital deaths (Hockley et al., 2010;

Reymond et al., 2011; Horey et al., 2012). These positive trends need to be confirmed using more robust research designs, such as prospective controlled trials (Phillips et al., 2011).

The introduction of information and communications technology solutions into nursing homes globally aims to improve their effectiveness and efficiency within the sector. These technological advances provide opportunities for better decision support, access to counselling and mentorship, communication across care settings, between health-care professionals and between residents, their caregivers, and the multidisciplinary team (Tung et al., 2011; Green and Levi, 2012). The introduction of electronic health records in Australian nursing homes has improved the convenience and efficiency of essential health data processing and empowered aged care providers (Zhang et al., 2012).

Research strategy

Despite the challenges of conducting research in nursing homes (Thompson and Chochinov, 2006), over the past decade there has been an increase in the number of palliative care studies undertaken in this care setting. Yet, as evidenced in this chapter, few of these studies have been designed to generate the high levels of evidence required to change practice (Hall et al., 2011). As a rapidly evolving sub-speciality there is a need to strengthen the palliative care evidence base (Currow et al., 2009). This requires an investment in priority-driven research that will systematically build this evidence base, and to progress from descriptive to interventional research (Sigurdardottir et al., 2010). Research ought to focus on the needs of consumers (older people and their families), providers (aged care and palliative care professionals), and system (nursing homes, policy and reform), in priority areas including:

1. *Consumers*: symptom prevention, recognition, assessment, and management, particularly for people with limited communication, dementia, and frailty (van der Steen, 2010); de-prescribing for older people (Beer et al., 2011); effectiveness of decision support tools and case conferencing for nursing home populations (Phillips et al., 2011); and predictors of older people at high risk of suffering at the end-of-life (Sigurdardottir et al., 2010).

2. *Providers*: effectiveness of interventions to improve the palliative care expertise of aged care providers, and the aged care expertise of palliative care providers (Hall et al., 2011).

3. *Systems*: setting quality standards in palliative care (Sigurdardottir et al., 2010); better aligning policies, standards, and accreditation; eligibility and reimbursement items to promote a palliative approach in nursing homes (Hoffmann and Tarzian, 2005); service intensity, and quality of care across settings (Stevenson and Bramson, 2009); and comparisons of service delivery models (Sigurdardottir et al., 2010).

Undertaking international comparisons of treatment, care, and outcome benefits in different health-care systems, and transnational studies using the same instruments, are required to increase our understanding of the generalizability of the approaches adopted (van der Steen, 2010). Health-care research is required to guide development of models of care (Sigurdardottir et al., 2010) that promote the delivery of a palliative approach. As the palliative care evidence base expands, translating evidence into practice is increasingly important, as evidence-based practice has the potential to redress inconsistencies in care and to improve care delivery, regardless of care setting, and is a key driver for health-care reform (Grimshaw and Eccles, 2004).

Conclusion

Increasing longevity and rising prevalence of chronic and co-morbid illnesses ensure that although more people now live longer with progressive life-limiting illnesses they experience significant disability before dying. Enabling nursing homes to better meet the needs of older people and their families requires multifaceted interventions targeting change at the policy, organizational, health professional, and consumer levels. The Chronic Care Model provides a framework for systematically addressing the policy, community, and health services organizational actions required to ensure the delivery of best evidence-based palliative care in nursing homes.

A palliative approach as a philosophy of care promotes older people's function, whilst maintaining dignity and minimizing discomfort and suffering of older people in nursing homes and their families, making it a policy priority. Integrating a palliative approach from an older person's transition into a nursing home would help to ensure that the many symptoms experienced as a result of multiple co-morbidities don't go undetected or undertreated; and that the unique needs of older people who experience communication problems due to disability or dementia are better acknowledged and catered for. Aligning a palliative approach with the Chronic Care Model offers the opportunity to systematically address the challenges of providing best evidence-based palliative care in this setting, and improve end-of-life care outcomes for older people residing in nursing homes and their families and caregivers.

References

Abbey, J., Froggatt, K., Parker, D., and Abbey, B. (2006). Palliative care in long-term care: a system in change. *International Journal of Older People Nursing*, 1, 56–63.

Abbey, J., Piller, N.B., De Bellis, A., *et al.* (2004). The Abbey pain scale: a 1-minute numerical indicator for people with end-stage dementia. *International Journal of Palliative Nursing*, 10, 6–13.

Abernethy, A.P., Currow, D.C., Hunt, R., *et al.* (2006). A pragmatic 2 x 2 x 2 factorial cluster randomized controlled trial of educational outreach visiting and case conferencing in palliative care-methodology of the Palliative Care Trial [ISRCTN 81117481]. *Contemporary Clinical Trials*, 27, 83–100.

Afzal, N., Buhagiar, K., Flood, J., and Cosgrave, M. (2010). Quality of end-of-life care for dementia patients during acute hospital admission: a retrospective study in Ireland. *General Hospital Psychiatry*, 32, 141–146.

Aged Care Standards Agency (2001). *Accreditation Guide for Residential Aged Care Services*. Canberra: ACSA Ltd.

Ahronheim, J.C., Morrison, R.S., Baskin, S.A., Morris, J., and Meier, D.E. (1996). Treatment of the dying in the acute care hospital: advanced dementia and metastatic disease. *Archives of Internal Medicine*, 156, 2094–2100.

Aigner, M.J., Drew, S., and Phipps, J. (2004). A comparative study of nursing home resident outcomes between care provided by nurse practitioners/physicians versus physicians only. *Journal of the American Medical Directors Association*, 5, 16–23.

Alzheimer's Association (2011). Alzheimer's disease facts and figures. *Alzheimer's & Dementia* 7, 1–68.

Angus, J., and Nay, R. (2003). The paradox of the Aged Care Act 1997: the marginalisation of nursing discourse. *Nursing Inquiry*, 10, 130–138.

Australian Department of Health and Ageing and National Health and Medical Research Council (2006). *Guidelines for a Palliative Approach in Residential Aged Care: Enhanced Version—May 2006*. Canberra: Australian Government.

Australian Government Department of Health and Ageing (2010). *Supporting Australians to Live Well at the End of Life: National Palliative Care Strategy*. Canberra: Department of Health and Ageing.

Australian Institute of Health and Welfare (2011). *Residential Aged Care in Australia 2009-10: A Statistical Overview*. Aged Care Statistics Series No. 35. Canberra: Australian Institute of Health and Welfare.

Avis, M., Greening Jackson, J., Cox, K., and Miskella, C. (1999). Evaluation of a project providing community palliative care support to nursing homes. *Health and Social Care in the Community*, 7, 32–38.

Beer, C., Loh, P., Peng, Y.G., Potter, K., and Millar, A. (2011). A pilot randomized controlled trial of deprescribing. *Therapeutic Advances in Drug Safety*, 2, 37–43.

Bosek, M.S.D.W., Lowry, E., Lindeman, D.A., Burck, J.R., and Gwyther, L.P. (2003). Promoting a good death for persons with dementia in nursing facilities: family caregivers' perspectives. *JONA'S Healthcare Law, Ethics and Regulation*, 5, 34.

Brennan, F. (2007). Palliative care as an international human right. *Journal of Pain and Symptom Management*, 33, 494–499.

British Geriatrics Society (2012). *Failing the Frail: A Chaotic Approach to Commissioning Healthcare Services for Care Homes*. London: British Geriatrics Society.

Canadian Institute for Health Information (2007). *Health Care Use at the End of Life in Western Canada*. Ottawa: Canadian Institute for Health Information.

Casarett, D., Karlawish, J., Morales, K., Crowley, R., Mirsch, T., and Asch, D.A. (2005). Improving the use of hospice services in nursing homes. *Journal of the American Medical Association*, 294, 211–217.

Chenoweth, L. and Kilstoff, K. (2002). Organizational and structural reform in aged care organisations: empowerment towards a change process. *Journal of Nursing Management*, 10, 235–244.

Christian, R. and Baker, K. (2009). Effectiveness of nurse practitioners in nursing homes: a systematic review. *JBI Library of Systematic Reviews*, 30, 1359–1378.

Clark, K. and Phillips, J.L. (2010). Culture and ethnicity in end of life care. *Australian Family Physician* 39, 210–213.

Comondore, V.R., Devereaux, P., Zhou, Q., *et al.* (2009). Quality of care in for-profit and not-for-profit nursing homes: systematic review and meta-analysis. *BMJ*, 339, b2732.

Currow, D.C., Wheeler, J.L., Glare, P.A., Kaasa, S., and Abernethy, A.P. (2009). A framework for generalizability in palliative care. *Journal of Pain and Symptom Management*, 37, 373–386.

Davidson, P.M., and Phillips, J.L. (2012). Palliative care in chronic illness. In M. O'Connor, S. Lee, and S. Aranda (eds.) *Palliative Care Nursing: A Guide to Practice* (3rd ed.), pp. 291–307. Melbourne: Ausmed.

Donald, I.P., Gladman, J., Conroy, S., Vernon, M., Kendrick, E., and Burns, E. (2008). Care home medicine in the UK—in from the cold. *Age and Ageing*, 37, 618–620.

Engel, S.E., Kiely, D.K., and Mitchell, S.L. (2006). Satisfaction with end-of-life care for nursing home residents with advanced dementia. *Journal of the American Geriatrics Society*, 54, 1567–1572.

Federal Interagency Forum on Aging-Related Statistics (2008). *Older Americans 2008: Key Indicators of Well-Being*. Washington, DC: US Independent Agencies and Commissions.

Field, M.J. and Cassel, C.K. (eds.) (1997). *Approaching Death: Improving Care at the End of Life*. Washington: DC: Institute of Medicine.

Finucane, T.E., Christmas, C., and Leff, B.A. (2007). Tube feeding in dementia: how incentives undermine health care quality and patient safety. *Journal of the American Medical Directors Association*, 8, 205–208.

Froggatt, K. (2001). Palliative care and nursing homes: where next? *Palliative Medicine*, 15, 42–8.

Froggatt, K., and Reitinger, E. (2013). *Palliative Care in Long-Term Care Settings for Older People*. EAPC Taskforce 2010–2012 Report. [Online] Available at: <http://www.eapcnet.eu/ Portals/0/Organization/Long%20term%20care%20settings/ FinalReportLongTermCareSettings_2013.pdf>.

Gadzhanova, S., and Reed, R. (2007). Medical services provided by general practitioners in residential aged-care facilities in Australia. *Medical Journal of Australia*, 187, 92–4.

Gauthier, L. R., and Gagliese, L. (2012). Bereavement interventions, end-of-life cancer care, and spousal well being: a systematic review. *Clinical Psychology: Science and Practice*, 19, 72–92.

Gibson, M., and Gorman, E. (2010). Contextualizing end-of-life care for ageing veterans: family members' thoughts. *International Journal of Palliative Nursing*, 16, 339.

Gill, T.M., Gahbauer, E.A., Han, L., and Allore, H.G. (2010). Trajectories of disability in the last year of life. *The New England Journal of Medicine*, 362, 1173–1180.

Givens, J.L., Jones, R.N., Shaffer, M.L., Kiely, D.K., and Mitchell, S.L. (2010). Survival and comfort after treatment of pneumonia in advanced dementia. *Archives of Internal Medicine*, 170, 1102–1107.

Glendinning, C., Jacobs, S., Alborz, A., and Hann, M. (2002). A survey of access to medical services in nursing and residential homes in England. *The British Journal of General Practice*, 52, 545.

Goldberg, T.H. and Botero, A. (2008). Causes of death in elderly nursing home residents. *Journal of the American Medical Directors Association*, 9, 565–567.

Goldstein, N., Carlson, M., Livote, E., and Kutner, J. S. (2010). Brief communication: management of implantable cardioverter-defibrillators in hospice: a nationwide survey. *Annals of Internal Medicine*, 152, 296.

Gozalo, P.L. and Miller, S.C. (2007). Hospice enrollment and evaluation of its causal effect on hospitalization of dying nursing home patients. *Health Services Research*, 42, 587–610.

Gozalo, P.L., Miller, S.C., Intrator, O., Barber, J.P., and Mor, V. (2008). Hospice effect on government expenditures among nursing home residents. *Health Services Research*, 43, 134–153.

Grabowski, D.C., Stewart, K.A., Broderick, S.M., and Coots, L.A. (2008). Predictors of nursing home hospitalization: a review of the literature. *Medical Care Research & Review*, 65, 3–39.

Green, M.J. and Levi, B.H. (2012). The era of 'e': the use of new technologies in advance care planning. *Nursing Outlook*, 60, 376–383 e2.

Grimshaw, J. and Eccles, M. (2004). Is evidence-based implementation of evidence-based care possible? *Medical Journal of Australia*, 180, S50–S51.

Guijarro, R., San Román, C.M., Gómez-Huelgas, R., *et al.* (2010). Impact of dementia on hospitalization. *Neuroepidemiology*, 35, 101–108.

Hall, S., Kolliakou, A., Petkova, H., Froggatt, K., and Higginson, I. J. (2011). Interventions for improving palliative care for older people living in nursing care homes. *Cochrane Database of Systematic Reviews*, 3, CD007132.

Hall, S., Petkova, H., Tsouros, A.D., Costantini, M., and Higginson, I. (eds.) (2011). *Palliative Care for Older People: Better Practices*. Copenhagen: WHO, Regional Office for Europe.

Hanson, L.C., Reynolds, K.S., Henderson, M., and Pickard, M.D. (2005). A quality improvement intervention to increase palliative care in nursing homes. *Journal of Palliative Medicine*, 8, 576–584.

Hockley, J., Watson, J., Oxenham, D., and Murray, S.A. (2010). The integrated implementation of two end-of-life care tools in nursing care homes in the UK: an in-depth evaluation. *Palliative Medicine*, 24, 828–838.

Hoffmann, D.E. and Tarzian, A.J. (2005). Dying in America—an examination of policies that deter adequate end-of-life care in nursing homes. *Journal of Law, Medicine & Ethics*, 33, 294–309.

Horey, D.E., Street, A.F., and Sands, A.F. (2012). Acceptability and feasibility of end-of-life care pathways in Australian residential aged care facilities. *The Medical Journal of Australia*, 197, 106–109.

Hughes, C., Lapane, K., and Kerse, N. (2011). Prescribing for older people in nursing homes: challenges for the future. *International Journal of Older People Nursing*, 6, 63–70.

Jerant, A.F., Azari, R.S., Nesbitt, T.S., Edwards-Goodbee, A., and Meyers, F.J. (2006). The palliative care in assisted living (PCAL) pilot study: successes, shortfalls, and methodological implications. *Social Science & Medicine*, 62, 199–207.

Kellehear, A. (1999). *Health Promoting Palliative Care*. Melbourne: Oxford University Press.

Kelley, A.S., Ettner, S.L., Morrison, R.S., Qingling, D., Wenger, N.S., and Sarkisian, C.A. (2011). Determinants of medical expenditures in the last 6 months of life. *Annals of Internal Medicine*, 154, 235–42.

Kovach, C.R., Wilson, S.A., and Noonan, P.E. (1996). The effects of hospice interventions on behaviors, discomfort, and physical complications of end stage dementia nursing home residents. *American Journal of Alzheimer's Disease and Other Dementias*, 11, 7–15.

Kristjanson, L.J., Sloan, J.A., Dudgeon, D., and Adaskin, E. (1996). Family members perceptions of palliative cancer care: predictors of family functioning and family members' health. *Journal Palliative Care*, 12, 10–20.

Lowe, T.J., Lucas, J.A., Castle, N.G., Robinson, J.P., and Crystal, S. (2003). Consumer satisfaction in long-term care: state initiatives in nursing homes and assisted living facilities. *The Gerontologist*, 43, 883–896.

Lynn, J. and Adamson, D. M. (2003). *Living Well at the End of Life: Adapting Health Care to Serious Chronic Illness in Old Age*. White Paper. Santa Monica, CA: RAND Health.

Mathie, E., Goodman, C., Crang, C., *et al*. (2012). An uncertain future: the unchanging views of care home residents about living and dying. *Palliative Medicine*, 26, 734–743.

McKinnon, M.M. (2002). The participation of volunteers in contemporary palliative care. *The Australian Journal of Advanced Nursing*, 19, 38–44.

Mead, N., and Bower, P. (2000). Patient-centredness: a conceptual framework and review of the empirical literature. *Social Science & Medicine*, 51, 1087–1110.

Meier, D.E., Ahronheim, J.C., Morris, J., Baskin-Lyons, S., and Morrison, R.S. (2001). High short-term mortality in hospitalized patients with advanced dementia: lack of benefit of tube feeding. *Archives of Internal Medicine*, 161, 594.

Miller, S., Mor, V., Wu, N., Gozalo, P., and Lapane, K. (2002). Does receipt of hospice care in nursing homes improve the management of pain at the end-of-life? *Journal of the American Geriatrics Society*, 50, 507–515.

Miller, S.C., Teno, J.M., and Mor, V. (2004). Hospice and palliative care in nursing homes. *Clinics in Geriatric Medicine*, 20, 717–734.

Mitchell, S.L., Teno, J.M., Kiely, D.K., *et al*. (2009). The clinical course of advanced dementia. *The New England Journal of Medicine*, 361, 1529–1538.

Mitchell, S.L., Teno, J.M., Roy, J., Kabumoto, G., and Mor, V. (2003). Clinical and organizational factors associated with feeding tube use among nursing home residents with advanced cognitive impairment. *Journal of the American Medical Association*, 290, 73–80.

Motiwala, S.S., Croxford, R., Guerriere, D.N., and Coyte, P.C. (2006). Predictors of place of death for seniors in Ontario: a population-based cohort analysis. *Canadian Journal on Aging/La Revue canadienne du vieillissement*, 25, 363–371.

Munn, J.C., Hanson, L.C., Zimmerman, S., Sloane, P.D., and Mitchell, C.M. (2006). Is hospice associated with improved end-of-life care in nursing homes and assisted living facilities? *Journal of the American Geriatrics Society*, 54, 490–495.

Murray, S. and Boyd, K. (2011). Using the 'surprise question' can identify people with advanced heart failure and COPD who would benefit from a palliative care approach. *Palliative Medicine*, 25, 382–382.

NSW Health (2011). *Paediatric Palliative Care Planning Framework 2011–2014*. Sydney: NSW Government.

Oliver, D.P., Porock, D., and Zweig, S. (2004). End-of-life care in U.S. nursing homes: a review of the evidence. *Journal of the American Medical Directors Association*, 5, 147–155.

Ouslander, J.G. and Berenson, R.A. (2011). Reducing unnecessary hospitalizations of nursing home residents. *The New England Journal of Medicine*, 365, 1165–1167.

Palliative Care Australia (2005a). *A Guide to Palliative Care Service Development: A Population Based Approach*. Canberra: Palliative Care Australia.

Palliative Care Australia (2005b). *Standards for Providing Quality Palliative Care for All Australians*. Canberra: Palliative Care Australia.

Palliative Care Victoria (2010). *Victorian Volunteer Survey*. Melbourne: Palliative Care Victoria.

Patterson, S.M., Hughes, C.M., Crealey, G., Cardwell, C., and Lapane, K.L. (2010). An evaluation of an adapted U.S. model of pharmaceutical care to improve psychoactive prescribing for nursing home residents in Northern Ireland (Fleetwood Northern Ireland Study). *Journal of the American Geriatrics Society*, 58, 44–53.

Phillips, J., Davidson, P. M., Kristjanson, L. J., Jackson, D., and Daly, J. (2006). Residential aged care: the last frontier for palliative care. *Journal of Advanced Nursing*, 55, 416–424.

Phillips, J.L. (2008). *Navigating a Palliative Approach in Residential Aged Care Using a Population Based Focus*. PhD dissertation. University of Western Sydney.

Phillips, J.L., Davidson, P.M., Ollerton, R., Jackson, D., and Kristjanson, L. (2007). Commitment and compassion: Survey results from nurses and care assistants working in residential aged care. *International Journal of Palliative Nursing*, 13, 282–290.

Phillips, J.L., Halcomb, E.J., and Davidson, P.M. (2011). End-of-life care pathways in acute and hospice care: an integrative review. *Journal of Pain and Symptom Management*, 41, 940–955.

Phillips, J.L., West, P.A., Davidson, P.M., and Agar, M. (2013). Does case conferencing for people with advanced dementia living in nursing homes improve care outcomes: evidence from an integrative review? *International Journal of Nursing Studies*, 50, 1122–1135.

Pleschberger, S. (2007). Dignity and the challenge of dying in nursing homes: the residents' view. *Age and Ageing*, 36, 197–202.

Quinn, T. (2011). Emergency hospital admissions from care-homes: who, why and what happens? A cross-sectional study. *Gerontology*, 57, 115–120.

Reymond, L., Israel, F.J., and Charles, M.A. (2011). A residential aged care end-of-life care pathway (RAC EoLCP) for Australian aged care facilities. *Australian Health Review*, 35, 350–356.

Richardson, S. and Martin, B. (2004). *The Care of Older Australians: A Picture of the Residential Aged Care Workforce*. Adelaide: The National Institute of Labour Studies Flinders University.

Sampson, E.L., Candy, B., and Jones, L. (2009). Enteral tube feeding for older people with advanced dementia. *Cochrane Database of Systematic Reviews*, 2, CD007209.

Sander, R. and Russell, P. (2001). Caring for dying people in nursing homes. *Nursing Older People*, 13, 21–26.

Seymour, J.E.A.K. (2011). Do nursing homes for older people have the support they need to provide end-of-life care? A mixed methods enquiry in England. *Palliative Medicine*, 25, 125–138.

Sidell, M., Katz, J., and Komaromy, C. (1997). *Death and Dying in Residential and Nursing Homes for Older People: Examining the Case for Palliative Care*. Report for the Department of Health. Milton Keynes: The Open University.

Sigurdardottir, K.R., Haugen, D.F., van der Rijt, C.C.D., *et al*. (2010). Clinical priorities, barriers and solutions in end-of-life cancer care research across Europe. Report from a workshop. *European Journal of Cancer*, 46, 1815–1822.

Small, N., Gardiner, C., Barnes, S., *et al*. (2010). Using a prediction of death in the next 12 months as a prompt for referral to palliative care acts to the detriment of patients with heart failure and chronic obstructive pulmonary disease. *Palliative Medicine*, 24, 740.

Stevenson, D.G. and Bramson, J.S. (2009). Hospice care in the nursing home setting: a review of the literature. *Journal of Pain and Symptom Management*, 38, 440–451.

Strumpf, N.E., Tuch, H., Stillman, D., Parish, P., and Morrison, N. (2004). Implementing palliative care in the nursing home. *Annals of Long-Term Care*, 12, 35–41.

Sudore, R.L. and Fried, T.R. (2010). Redefining the 'planning' in advance care planning: preparing for end-of-life decision making. *Annals of Internal Medicine*, 153, 256–261.

Tebbit, P. (2008). *Capacity to Care: A Data Analysis and Discussion of the Capacity and Function of Care Homes as Providers of End-of-Life Care*. London: National Council for Palliative Care.

The Royal Australian College of General Practitioners (2006). *Medical Care of Older Persons in Residential Aged Care Facilities*. Melbourne: The Royal Australian College of General Practitioners.

Thompson, G.N., and Chochinov, H.M. (2006). Methodological challenges in measuring quality care at the end of life in the long-term care environment. *Journal of Pain & Symptom Management*, 32, 378–391.

Thomson, M.S., Gruneir, A., Lee, M., *et al.* (2009). Nursing time devoted to medication administration in long-term care: clinical, safety, and resource implications. *Journal of the American Geriatrics Society*, 57, 266–272.

Tung, E.E., Vickers, K.S., Lackore, K., Cabanela, R., Hathaway, J., and Chaudhry, R. (2011). Clinical decision support technology to increase advance care planning in the primary care setting. *American Journal of Hospice Palliative Care*, 28, 230–235.

Van der Steen, J.T. (2010). Dying with dementia: what we know after more than a decade of research. *Journal of Alzheimer's Disease*, 22, 37–55.

Wagner, E.H., Austin, B.T., Davis, C., Hindmarsh, M., Schaefer, J., and Bonomi, A. (2001). Improving chronic illness care: translating evidence into action. *Health Affairs*, 20, 64–78.

Weiss, C.O., Boyd, C.M., Yu, Q., Wolff, J.L., and Leff, B. (2007). Patterns of prevalent major chronic disease among older adults in the United States. *Journal of the American Medical Association*, 298, 1160–1162.

Wetle, T., Shield, R., Teno, J., Miller, S.C., and Welch, L. (2005). Family perspectives on end-of-life care experiences in nursing homes. *The Gerontologist*, 45, 642–650.

Wolff, J.L., Starfield, B., and Anderson, G. (2002). Prevalence, expenditures, and complications of multiple chronic conditions in the elderly. *Archives of Internal Medicine*, 162, 2269.

World Health Organization (2002). *Innovative Care for Chronic Conditions: Building Blocks for Action*. Geneva: WHO.

World Health Organization (2003). *WHO Definition of Palliative Care*. [Online] Available at <http://www.who.int/cancer/palliative/definition/en/>.

Zhang, Y., Yu, P., and Shen, J. (2012). The benefits of introducing electronic health records in residential aged care facilities: a multiple case study. *International Journal of Medical Informatics*, 81, 690–704.

SECTION 4

The interdisciplinary team

4.1

The core team and the extended team

Dagny Faksvåg Haugen, Friedemann Nauck, and Augusto Caraceni

Introduction to the core team and the extended team

Teamwork is an essential component of palliative care. This chapter gives a short overview of the pleasures and challenges of teamwork, and presents and discusses the interdisciplinary palliative care team.

What is a team?

A team may simply be defined as two or more people working together. However, working together is not sufficient to make a pair or a group of people into a team. A widely used definition describes a team as 'a small number of people with complementary skills who are committed to a common purpose, performance goals, and approach for which they hold themselves mutually accountable' (Katzenbach and Smith, 1992). Team members work in an interdependent manner.

Health-care teams

Teams make it possible for health-care professionals to work closely together. *Multiprofessional* teams are employed in areas where patients have extensive and complex needs. Multiprofessional simply means that team members have different professional backgrounds. A multiprofessional team may be multidisciplinary or interdisciplinary.

In a *multidisciplinary* team all team members have their own clearly defined place in the care regimen (Cummings, 1998; Crawford and Price, 2003). Although each professional may provide vital information towards decision-making, generally only one person, usually a physician or nurse, makes the treatment decisions. A common decision-making process demands an *interdisciplinary* approach.

The interdisciplinary team

An interdisciplinary health-care team is described as 'an identified collective in which members share common team goals and work interdependently in planning, problem solving, decision-making, and implementing and evaluating team-related tasks' (Drinka, 1994).

This description will be valid for most interdisciplinary teams, but they still differ with respect to the following:

+ Size
+ Mix of professions
+ The degree of integration or closeness of working between team members
+ The extent of collective responsibility, that is, the extent to which the team as a collective is responsible and held accountable for providing the service
+ Membership of the team—who is and who is not a member, and what membership means
+ The patient pathway through the team—time and process
+ Decision-making
+ Management and leadership (Øvretveit 1996).

Advantages of teamwork

Health-care teams are more effective than single practitioners and may improve both the quality and quantity of services (Øvretveit, 1996; Mickan, 2005; Lemieux-Charles and McGuire, 2006). Teamwork improves communication and coordination and allows for maximal diversity of professional expertise. These factors lead to organizational benefits like reduced hospitalization time and costs, reduced unanticipated admissions, and better accessibility for patients.

In fact, successful teams may possess combinations of skills that no single individual may demonstrate on his or her own (Crawford and Price, 2003). The type and diversity of clinical expertise involved in team decision-making has been shown to be a major factor accounting for teams' improvements in patient care and organizational effectiveness (Blomqvist, 2004; Lemieux-Charles and McGuire, 2006).

Objectives

The interdisciplinary team should try to achieve the following objectives:

+ Accurate and speedy assessment
+ Effective, integrated treatment and care
+ Efficient communication with the patient and the family, with other professionals and institutions, and within the team itself
+ Audit of the team's activities and outcomes.

Team members may give each other valuable feedback and support. On the other hand, working closely together may also precipitate conflicts more easily.

Team performance

Team performance is influenced by factors relating to the *structure* of the team and to *processes* involved in team functioning (Table 4.1.1) (Mickan and Rodger, 2000; Blomqvist, 2004; Mickan and Rodger, 2005; Lemieux-Charles and McGuire, 2006). The structural factors include organizational aspects as well as characteristics of the group and the individual team members.

Team size and membership: core and extended teams

By definition, a team is a small number of people (Katzenbach and Smith, 1992), usually no more than 15, and often between five and ten. A team of five or six full-time members has been suggested as ideal (Kane, 1975). Unresolved differences are better tolerated in larger teams, but it takes more time to reach decisions. Around 20 seem to be the maximum number of team members consistent with efficient teamwork (Kane, 1975; Lemieux-Charles and McGuire, 2006; Maddocks, 2006).

Membership defines the team's boundaries. The most common membership distinction is between *core* and *associated*, the latter belonging to the extended team (Øvretveit, 1990, 1996). Core members are usually full-time members governed by the team policy and managed by the team leader. Associate can mean part-time in the team, not governed by team policy, and having managers outside the team. Each team member must have a distinct and necessary role within the team (Mickan, 2005).

Knowledge and skills

All team members have to be specialists and confident in their own fields to be valid 'instruments' in the interdisciplinary 'orchestra'. However, it is also necessary to have a clear understanding of the other team members' expertise and contributions. Each health-care discipline has its own 'cognitive map' consisting of its conceptual basis, terminology, observational approaches, and theoretical framework. Working together in a team requires some degree of understanding of the 'maps' of the other team members (Reese and Sontag, 2001; Blomqvist, 2004).

Attitudes

Even more important are the attitudes of the team members (Reese and Sontag, 2001; Crawford and Price, 2003). The tendency to believe that one's own way of framing problems or solutions is the best is a common obstacle to good teamwork (Blomqvist, 2004).

Philosophies of teamwork

The team members' attitude to teamwork is rooted in their understanding of what teamwork really means. Team members' interpretations of teamwork have been shown to be just as important as organizational and group dynamic constraints (Freeman et al., 2000). Freeman and co-workers identified three philosophies of teamwork:

◆ The *directive* philosophy is based on the assumption of hierarchy in the team. One person takes the lead by virtue of status and power and directs the actions of the other team members.

◆ The *integrative* philosophy assumes that each professional's contribution has equal value. All team members are seen as team players, and communication and discussions within the team are given vital importance.

◆ The *elective* philosophy of teamwork is held by professionals who prefer clear and distinct team roles to operate autonomously and only relate briefly to other team members when they see a need for it themselves.

Team processes

Team processes describe how the team handles tasks and interpersonal dynamics to produce the desired outcome (Table 4.1.1) (Mickan and Rodger, 2000).

The development of a team

Research on group processes has shown that teams often go through typical phases in their development (Tuckman, 1965; Katzenbach and Smith, 1992; Payne, 2006).

Forming is the first phase when the group constitutes itself and faces its task for the first time. The team members feel insecure and test out behaviour in the group. The group is dependent on a formal leader. In this phase it is important to develop rules and methods for the work on the team and define the tasks for each team member.

Storming is the characteristic phase of turbulence, critical opposition, and power struggle which often follows once the team is established. Conflicts arise between subgroups, and differences in opinion and competition between team members appear.

Norming characterizes the next phase when the team players finally agree on rules and adapt to common norms. The members resist conflicts and get a feeling of belonging together. There is an open exchange of opinions and feelings, and cooperation develops.

Performing or *adjourning* should be the final, lasting stage of team development. By now the team has developed functional processes for problem solving. The team members know their roles, support each other, and devote their energy to fulfilling the team's objectives (Tuckman, 1965).

This simplified, schematic description is not valid for every team (Drinka, 1994). Still, these common steps might be a help to understand team dynamics and guide your team in the right direction.

Roles of team members

A role is understood as the expectations the individual has of what they are supposed to do in their work, but also what others expect

Table 4.1.1 Characteristics of effective teamwork

Organizational structure	Individual contribution	Team process
Clear purpose	Self-knowledge	Coordination
Appropriate culture	Trust	Communication
Specified task	Commitment	Cohesion
Distinct roles	Flexibility	Decision-making
Suitable leadership		Conflict management
Relevant members		Social relationships
Adequate resources		Performance feedback

Reproduced from Mickan S and Rodger S, Characteristics of effective teams: a literature review, Australian Health Review 2000, Volume 23, pp. 201–8, Copyright © 2000 with permission from CSIRO PUBLISHING, <http://www.publish.csiro.au/nid/270/paper/AH000201.htm>.

from the person (Blomqvist, 2004). The role is linked tightly to the professional identity and gives the owner certain duties and privileges. Role ambiguity and role conflicts threaten teamwork and must be sorted out (Kane, 1975). Clarification of roles first of all concerns the *professional roles* in the team. Who should take on which tasks? Role overlap might lead to competition, or that several team members work on the same task. Some role overlap, however, may be beneficial and actually increase the team's resources, as long as this is agreed upon by all team members (Reese and Sontag, 2001; Crawford and Price, 2003).

In addition to the professional role, other roles will develop in a team. Every team member has a *personal role* rooted in their sex, age, ethnical background, and socioeconomic state (Kane, 1975). In addition, other *formal roles* may be given, like team leader or supervisor.

Informal roles reflect the individual team member's personality and style which have given them a certain position in the group. These informal roles may be more or less conscious and articulated, but roles like 'mother', 'clown', 'messy head', and 'saviour' may be familiar.

Leadership

Team leadership concerns three aspects: management, handling of professional challenges, and motivation and policy. *Management* (administration) is important, but not necessarily a job for the team leader. Although the physician will be responsible for the medical treatment, *professional, task-centred leadership* in the interdisciplinary team should vary from case to case, depending on the nature of the needs of the individual patient and family (Cummings, 1998). The *team leader* should guide the team in the right direction, by:

◆ keeping purpose, goals, and approach relevant and meaningful

◆ building commitment and confidence

◆ strengthening the mix and level of skills

◆ managing external relations, removing obstacles

◆ creating opportunities for others

◆ doing real work (Katzenbach and Smith, 1992).

Leadership is a combination of goal-oriented and interpersonal skills (Kane, 1975; Øvretveit, 1990; Barczak, 1996).

Øvretveit states that the quickest way to establish a close and effective team is to start with a clearly defined team leader role: 'I do not know of any teams which have close teamwork and have survived changes of membership without a clear team leader position. One of the biggest mistakes is to believe that interprofessional and interagency conflicts, rivalries and protectionism can be avoided by not defining a team leader role' (Øvretveit 1990).

Communication and cohesion

Communication is the means through which the team members interact and the work gets done (Jünger et al., 2007). Communication is equally important within the team and between the team and the organization: patients, family members, other health-care professionals, and managers (Kane, 1975; Mickan and Rodger, 2000; Müller and Kern, 2006). Although challenging at times, the patient's and family's right to confidentiality should always be respected and appropriate consent obtained.

Ongoing communication requires commitment of time and energy and is enhanced through physical proximity of offices, common records, and frequent, structured meetings (Katzenbach and Smith, 1992). Meetings provide the main forum and structure within which a team works. Team conferences for assessment, planning, and evaluation of patient care should be held at least weekly, and should be planned carefully, including time for reflection and review (Macmillan et al., 2006).

Cohesion is a feeling of belonging which gives the team members shared enjoyment and pride in their achievements and a wish to remain within the team (Mickan and Rodger, 2000, 2005). This commitment and involvement is generated by working together over time, and is supported by good performance feedback, success in adversity, good communication, and conformity to norms (Vinokur-Kaplan, 1995; Mickan and Rodger, 2000). In their study of Australian health-care teams, Mickan and Rodger found communication and cohesion as two of the categories most able to distinguish effective teams. The other four categories were mutual respect, goals, purpose, and leadership (Mickan and Rodger, 2005).

Decision-making

Decision-making skills are a basis for effective teamwork and a main responsibility for the leader (Kane, 1975). All team members need to contribute to the team's decisions.

Decision-making includes describing the problem, presenting and discussing alternative solutions, prioritizing and choosing among the alternatives, and finally assigning and accepting responsibility and deciding a time frame. In the palliative care team, agenda setting as well as decision-making ultimately must be guided by the patient's and family's needs, wishes, and preferences (Council of Europe, 2003; Maddocks, 2006).

Conflict-solving

Any work group may be subject to stresses and conflicts. Diversity of professional backgrounds presents an additional challenge (Cummings, 1998; Reese and Sontag, 2001; Crawford and Price, 2003). All aspects of teamwork discussed so far may give rise to conflicts. In addition, external factors—scarcity of resources, organizational changes, and work-related strain like working with the terminally ill—may add to the stress. Ability at conflict-solving is an important feature of any successful team (Kane, 1975; Lemieux-Charles and McGuire, 2006).

Any conflict arising in the team should be taken seriously and identified as soon as possible. Investigating the root of the problem is usually more rewarding than focusing just on the symptoms. Possible solutions must be discussed and the necessary steps taken to reach the desired outcome, including clarifying who must be involved (Speck, 2006).

Clinical supervision is recognized as a valuable tool for professional growth and support and should be available to the interdisciplinary team. Supervision has an important role in preventing and solving team conflicts (van Staa et al., 2000; Speck, 2006).

Team building

Teams are dynamic. Appropriate team structures facilitate the development of team processes, but as teams evolve, team processes often shape the structures within which they function best (Mickan and Rodger, 2000). Accordingly, both team structure and processes should be considered when building effective teams (Table 4.1.1).

Shared learning and getting to know each other by spending time together are the core aspects of 'team building' activities (Payne, 2006). A work climate characterized by good social relationships, personal recognition, feedback, and humour influences positively team members' psychological well-being, organizational commitment, and belief in the team's effectiveness (Mickan and Rodger, 2000).

The palliative care team

Teamwork is an inherent feature of palliative care. The palliative care team is an interdisciplinary health-care team with its own characteristics and challenges.

A palliative care team is usually understood as a clinical team, although many teams also are engaged in teaching, service development, and research. The palliative care team should be found in any setting providing specialist palliative care.

The palliative care team: defined and flexible

To be a team, the team members need to be defined (Drinka, 1994; Lemieux-Charles and McGuire, 2006). This is vital for the communication and collaboration within the team, but also for the organization served by the team. A palliative care team should be identified clearly by the name of the team or the programme, and its members should be outlined clearly.

While efficient teamwork demands a defined core team, palliative care also needs to be flexible (Maddocks, 2006). The extended 'team' may consist of some members from the palliative care staff team or consult team in addition to family members, hospital physician, general practitioner, home care nurse, volunteer, etc. In this way a palliative care team is not static. However, although flexibility is needed, loose team boundaries may lead to drifting team members becoming multidisciplinary instead of interdisciplinary.

The core team

Most recommendations for the organization of palliative care services define a core palliative care team consisting of a physician, preferably a consultant in palliative medicine, and a specialist nurse (National Institute for Clinical Excellence, 2004; Doyle, 2009). The UK recommendations specify the physician being supported by other medical staff including junior staff who may be on rotations, and also include secretarial/administrative support in the core team (National Institute for Clinical Excellence, 2004; Booth et al., 2009). Guidelines from the United States include a social worker and chaplain in the core team (National Consensus Project for Quality Palliative Care, 2013).

Having placed the nurse and physician at the core of the palliative care team simply reflects that these are the two professions most often needed by people with advanced, life-threatening disease. Accordingly, the nurse and the physician usually work full time on the team, while other team members often will be part-time or attached staff.

The extended team

The extended palliative care team ideally should be designed to be able to address all the needs of the patients and families served by the team. The team should include psychology, social work, and chaplaincy expertise, and access to specialist pain management, physiotherapy, occupational therapy, and dietetics (Palliative Care

Australia, 2003; National Institute for Clinical Excellence, 2004; Norwegian Association for Palliative Medicine, 2004; National Consensus Project for Quality Palliative Care, 2013). Pharmacy expertise is likely to be increasingly important. A number of other health-care providers and therapists may be included as needed (MacMillan et al., 2006; Doyle, 2009). The team must be skilled in care of the patient population to be served (Palliative Care Australia, 2003).

Are the patient and the family team members?

Palliative care interventions must be given with the patient's consent and in accordance with their wishes. The patient may thus be considered a member of the extended team, even if they do not take part in all team conferences (Doyle, 2009).

Likewise, the members of the patient's family can be considered members. They have an important role in the overall care of the patient, and their opinions should be included when formulating plans for treatment and care (Doyle, 2009).

The palliative care staff team

Historical perspective

The establishment of St Christopher's Hospice in London by Dame Cicely Saunders in 1967 is regarded as the foundation of the modern hospice movement (Saunders, 2000). Multiprofessional teamwork was regarded an essential cornerstone of holistic hospice care. Experience has shown that hospice care can be established and implemented in many settings and cultures and in countries with widely different resources (Saunders, 2000).

The dramatic change of focus made it necessary to establish the first hospices outside the acute hospital setting (Dunlop and Hockley, 1998; Hockley, 1999). Gradually the pendulum has swung back. Deficiencies in terminal care for hospital patients prompted the surgeon Balfour Mount to establish the first palliative care unit at the Royal Victoria Hospital in Montreal in 1975 (Mount, 1976).

In some countries, inpatient hospices are very different from palliative care units in terms of funding, length of patient stay, and main task of care (end-of-life care versus crisis intervention and symptom control), while in others they are much more alike. Some countries have chosen not to have 'hospice' as an organizational element—either because of the term's historical associations, or because it is not specific for the contents or quality of the service provided (Norwegian Association for Palliative Medicine, 2004).

Staff teams in hospices and palliative care units

Most members of the palliative care staff team will be defined as core members (National Institute for Clinical Excellence, 2004). This is necessary to provide comprehensive care addressing all the patients' and families' needs.

Recommendations for staffing

The high complexity of problems and the extensive nursing needs demand a higher ratio of staff per patient in hospices and palliative care units, as compared to most other institutional wards. Staffing levels are also influenced by disease panorama and needs for special skills (patients with advanced neurological disease like motor neurone disease are generally very resource intensive), demographics (younger people and families with children often require more support), number of admissions and rate of turnover, and cultural factors (e.g. need for interpreters and more time-consuming conferences) (Palliative Care Australia, 2003). Care for the dying includes care for their relatives, which often is time-consuming and may require the attention of the whole team.

Recommendations for staffing vary between countries (Council of Europe, 2003; Palliative Care Australia, 2003; National Institute for Clinical Excellence, 2004; Norwegian Association for Palliative Medicine, 2004; Doyle, 2009; Radbruch et al., 2010; National Consensus Project for Quality Palliative Care, 2013).

The extended interdisciplinary medical team

Specialist palliative care may be advanced medical treatment, highlighted in academic palliative medicine units in tertiary hospitals, admitting the most complex cases (El Osta and Bruera, 2006). These units need an extended interdisciplinary medical team to handle any emergencies or complications that may arise. The core staff team should include all relevant professions, including nurses with different specialties. A number of medical specialties must be linked to the team and accessible for consult at short notice. Relevant specialties include orthopaedics, infectious diseases, advanced pain medicine, oncology, urology, gastrointestinal surgery, and psychiatry.

Palliative care units in nursing homes and residential homes

Even though it is undisputed that palliative care should be provided in the settings of care for older people (Davies and Higginson, 2004), this field is poorly developed. However, some European countries have an active policy to establish palliative care units in nursing homes (Francke and Kerkstra, 2000; Norwegian Association for Palliative Medicine, 2004). Many of the patients admitted to these units have palliative care needs due to chronic diseases typical of old age. This creates additional requirements for the staff, for example, pain assessment and symptom control in demented patients and knowledge in a wide variety of chronic and/or neurological diseases. When setting up the team, expertise in geriatrics/nursing home medicine and geriatric nursing should be included.

The palliative care consult team

As hospice practice developed in the UK, many patients admitted to hospices for symptom control were able to be discharged back to their own homes. This precipitated the need for hospices to develop their own home-care teams. From the end of the 1970s, palliative care started to come full circle back into acute care with the formation of hospital palliative care teams.

The typical consult team is found in acute care hospitals (Booth et al., 2009), but teams may operate in different settings, and are especially important as links between the different levels of the health-care system.

Hospital-based palliative care teams

The move of hospice care to acute care hospitals started with the consult teams at St. Luke's Hospital in New York (1974) and St Thomas's Hospital in London (1977) (O'Neill et al., 1992). At that time, 50–60% of all deaths occurred in hospitals, as is still the case in many developed countries today. In later years, services providing palliative care for patients admitted to acute care facilities have developed as an important part of specialist palliative care in many countries.

Team composition and tasks

Team composition depends on the purpose and goals of the service. These are influenced by the hospital characteristics, the patient populations to be served, additional palliative care services inside or outside the hospital, finances, and existing national standards.

Palliative care teams may be linked to a palliative care unit or may operate in hospitals not having palliative care inpatient facilities (Mount, 1976; O'Neill et al., 1992; Norwegian Association for Palliative Medicine, 2004; El Costa and Bruera, 2006).

The following aims are common for most consult teams (Dunlop and Hockley, 1998; Hockley, 1999):

- To work alongside the hospital ward team by advising on symptom control and psychosocial/spiritual issues
- To support relatives in difficult situations
- To support staff in difficult decisions and grief
- To educate staff in palliative care
- To liaise with hospice /other palliative care services and home care services.

Hospital teams usually have several levels of intervention, from a consulting role to shared care and eventually transfer of care:

- Advice and guidance to professionals on the ward team without direct contact with patient.
- Single visit for assessment and advice on further plans for care, preferably with referrer. Further contacts specifically at referrer's request.
- Short-term interventions with patients or families for specific problems.
- Ongoing contact due to multiple, complex problems requiring regular specialist assessment and interventions. In this case the team might temporarily take over patient responsibility.

Consultations are also provided for cancer patients still receiving disease-modifying treatment and patients with non-malignant conditions. This gives the palliative care team a unique role as the interface between palliative medicine and other medical specialties (Glare et al., 2003). Speaking in terms of teams, the consultant, advanced nurse practitioner or other members of the consult team will be part of the extended medical team in the intensive care unit, the department of oncology, and other hospital wards. This is especially important to promote integration of palliative care early in the disease trajectory (Temel et al., 2010).

Community teams

Community teams may be hospital based or community based. Home-care teams must have clear objectives and guidelines for the level of intervention, to ease the cooperation with primary care services.

Services providing extended specialist palliative nursing, medical, social and emotional support, and care in the patient's home, are often known as 'hospice-at-home' (National Institute for Clinical Excellence, 2004). Care may be provided as crisis management or for longer periods of time. By establishing a full range hospice at home, the team assumes full control of the patient and works like a staff team. In such cases, responsibility must be clearly defined and assigned.

Community teams may also serve nursing homes (El Osta and Bruera, 2006), or larger communities may have special teams serving these institutions.

Outcomes of hospital palliative care teams

Although there is a need for more and better quality research in palliative care, palliative care teams have been shown to improve symptom control (Ellershaw et al., 1995; Higginson et al., 2002; Cintron and Meier, 2006; Higginson and Evans, 2010), increase patient and carer satisfaction (Hearn and Higginson, 1998), and have an impact on communication and psychosocial aspects of care (Ellershaw et al., 1995; Hearn and Higginson, 1998; Glare et al., 2003; Jack et al. 2004; Vernooij-Dassen et al., 2007).

Planning the team

The majority of palliative care teams have started from an enthusiastic individual convinced of the needs for and usefulness of specialist palliative care. Although probably no team may come into being without at least one such committed person, a structured planning process will save time and frustration (Dunlop and Hockley, 1998).

The size and composition of the team should be based on a thorough needs assessment which in turn leads to clear task objectives and careful job descriptions. In many cases, the team will be formed from practitioners already employed by the institution, brought together from different departments and grouped into a team. This situation is not ideal and calls for a dedicated team leader, well-defined roles for the team members, and strong support from the institution's management and organization.

Evaluating the team

Audit of the team's activities and outcomes is one of the objectives of interdisciplinary teamwork (Hunt et al., 2004). This demands clearly defined, attainable and measurable goals (Lemieux-Charles and McGuire, 2006). Keeping good records and compiling statistics are first steps to evaluate the service.

Clinical and organizational audit is described in Chapter 19.9. Audit and quality measurement may be applied to three levels of teamwork, and palliative care teams should formulate goals regularly within these three domains:

◆ Structure

◆ Processes

◆ Outcomes.

Structural factors include having job descriptions, systems for referral and feedback, telephone access, symptom assessment tools, and other organizational elements in place.

Processes refer to how the structural elements are used and the teamwork is performed:

◆ The patient pathway through the team—number of referrals, referral time, time expenditure, use of symptom assessment tools, family meetings, etc.

◆ Communication and documentation—record keeping, discharge summaries, network meetings.

◆ Internal processes of teamwork—team functioning, performance and effectiveness—which may be measured by a number of validated tools (Fulmer and Hyer, 1998).

Outcomes relate to results obtained through the team's efforts, auditing the effects of actual interventions in changing ward practice, improving symptom control, patient and family satisfaction, patient and family understanding of disease progression, etc. A large number of questionnaires and outcome scales have been developed to this end (Hunt et al., 2004) (see Section 7).

The interdisciplinary teaching team

Every health-care practitioner is a lifelong learner, and every palliative care team should provide an environment for learning and development for its members. Equally important, is that everyone acting as a specialist practitioner automatically becomes a teacher and a role model.

The advisory role of the palliative care consult team makes it easy to turn almost all clinical contacts into teaching opportunities. The first visit for comprehensive assessment provides an ideal situation to demonstrate communication techniques and involve the junior doctor and ward nurse or general practitioner and home care nurse in discussions on assessment and treatment (Dunlop and Hockley, 1998; Cintron and Meier, 2006). Case discussions, ward rounds, and staff meetings provide similar opportunities. Changes in medication or other treatments should always be discussed with the staff. These are extremely important steps to ensure provision of basic palliative care in all the services the team comes into contact with, inside or outside the hospital.

Every palliative care team must also engage in formal educational sessions. This means that 'teaching the teachers' must be included in the team training. Common, interdisciplinary educational sessions facilitate shared learning for professional groups working together. Separate teaching for each group is also needed, but even so the interdisciplinary approach should be emphasized, for example, in case presentations (Council of Europe, 2003; Jeffrey, 2003; Lawrie and Lloyd-Williams, 2006).

The interdisciplinary research team

Every palliative care team should strive to improve its work through research and development. Unfortunately research often has to give way to pressing clinical activities, and there is a lack of funding and academic chairs and departments in the field. Nevertheless palliative care research is increasing, including some exciting international collaborations.

Translational research, trying to answer questions originating in the clinical as well as in the molecular setting by combined approaches, is one example of true interdisciplinary work (Kaasa and Dale, 2005).

Online materials

Complete references for this chapter are available online at <http://www.oxfordmedicine.com>.

References

Booth, S., Edmonds, P., and Kendall, M. (2009). *Palliative Care in the Acute Hospital Setting: A Practical Guide.* Oxford: Oxford University Press.

Cintron, A. and Meier, D.E. (2006). The palliative care consult team. In E. Bruera, I. Higginson, D. von Gunten, and C. Ripamonti (eds.) *Textbook of Palliative Medicine*, pp. 259–265. Boca Raton, FL: CRC Press.

Crawford, G.B. and Price, S.D. (2003). Team working: palliative care as a model of interdisciplinary practice. *Medical Journal of Australia*, 179, 32–34.

Cummings, I. (1998). The interdisciplinary team. In D. Doyle, G.W.C. Hanks, and N. MacDonald (eds.) *Oxford Textbook of Palliative Medicine* (2nd ed.), pp. 19–30. Oxford: Oxford University Press.

Doyle, D. (2009). *Getting Started: Guidelines and Suggestions for Those Starting a Hospice / Palliative Care Service* (2nd ed.). Houston, TX: IAHPC Press. Available at: <http://hospicecare.com/about-iahpc/publications/manuals-guidelines-books/getting-started/>.

Drinka, T.J.K. (1994). Interdisciplinary geriatric teams: approaches to conflict as indicators of potential to model teamwork. *Educational Gerontology*, 20, 87–103.

Dunlop, R.J. and Hockley, J.M. (1998). *Hospital-Based Palliative Care Teams: The Hospital-Hospice Interface* (2nd ed.). Oxford: Oxford University Press.

El Osta, B. and Bruera, E. (2006). Models of palliative care delivery. In E. Bruera, I. Higginson, D. von Gunten, and C. Ripamonti (eds.) *Textbook of Palliative Medicine*, pp. 266–276. Boca Raton, FL: CRC Press.

Higginson, I.J. and Evans, C.J. (2010). What is the evidence that palliative care teams improve outcomes for cancer patients and their families? *The Cancer Journal*, 16, 423–435.

Jack, B., Hillier, V., Williams, A., and Oldham, J. (2004). Hospital based palliative care teams improve the insight of cancer patients into their disease. *Palliative Medicine*, 18, 46–52.

Jeffrey, D. (ed.) (2003). *Teaching Palliative Care: A Practical Guide.* Oxford: Radcliffe Medical Press Ltd.

Jünger, S., Pestinger, M., Elsner, F., Krumm, N., and Radbruch, L. (2007). Criteria for successful multiprofessional cooperation in palliative care teams. *Palliative Medicine*, 21, 347–354.

Katzenbach, J.R. and Smith, D.K. (1992). *The Wisdom of Teams.* Boston, MA: Harvard Business School Press.

Lawrie, I. and Lloyd-Williams, M. (2006). Training in the interdisciplinary environment. In P. Speck (ed.) *Teamwork in Palliative Care: Fulfilling or Frustrating?*, pp. 153–165. Oxford: Oxford University Press.

Lemieux-Charles, L. and McGuire, W.L. (2006). What do we know about health care team effectiveness? A review of the literature. *Medical Care Research and Review*, 63, 263–300.

MacMillan, K., Emery, B., and Kashuba, L. (2006). Organization and support of the interdisciplinary team. In E. Bruera, I. Higginson, D. von Gunten, and C. Ripamonti, (eds.) *Textbook of Palliative Medicine*, pp. 245–250. Boca Raton, FL: CRC Press.

Mickan, S.M. (2005). Evaluating the effectiveness of health care teams. *Australian Health Review*, 29, 211–217.

Mickan, S. and Rodger, S. (2000). Characteristics of effective teams: a literature review. *Australian Health Review*, 23, 201–208.

Mickan, S.M. and Rodger, S.A. (2005). Effective health care teams: a model of six characteristics developed from shared perceptions. *Journal of Interprofessional Care*, 19, 358–370.

National Consensus Project for Quality Palliative Care (2013). *Clinical Practice Guidelines for Quality Palliative Care* (3rd ed.). Pittsburgh, PA: National Consensus Project for Quality Palliative Care. Available at: <http://www.nationalconsensusproject.org/Guidelines_Download2.aspx>.

National Institute for Clinical Excellence (2004). *Improving Supportive and Palliative Care for Adults with Cancer: The Manual.* London: National Institute for Clinical Excellence.

Øvretveit, J. (1996). Five ways to describe a multidisciplinary team. *Journal of Interprofessional Care*, 10, 163–171.

Palliative Care Australia (2003). *Palliative Care Service Provision in Australia: A Planning Guide* (2nd ed.). Canberra: Palliative Care Australia.

Radbruch, L., Payne, S., and the Board of Directors of the EAPC (2010). White Paper on standards and norms for hospice and palliative care in Europe: part 2. Recommendations from the European Association for Palliative Care. *European Journal of Palliative Care*, 17(1), 22–33.

Speck, P. (2006). Maintaining a healthy team. In P. Speck (ed.) *Teamwork in Palliative Care: Fulfilling or Frustrating?*, pp. 95–115. Oxford: Oxford University Press.

4.2

Teaching and training in palliative medicine

Karen Forbes and Jane Gibbins

Introduction to teaching and training in palliative care

Patients die in almost all areas of medicine; it is therefore essential for doctors to be equipped with the knowledge, skills, attitudes, and behaviours necessary to look after patients who need care at the end of life. Both generalists caring for patients with advanced disease, and health-care professionals specializing in palliative medicine require training to enable them to provide the best care for all patients. Whilst there has been progress in providing and improving educational opportunities in palliative care for physicians at all stages of their training, it is suggested that training deficits still lead to many patients receiving poor care at the end of life (Department of Health, 2008; Bui, 2012).

Training needs

The National Council for Palliative Care in the United Kingdom suggests that palliative care is provided by 'two distinct categories of health and social care professionals', those who provide day-to-day care for patients, and those who specialize in palliative care (National Council for Palliative Care, 2012). It is suggested that a 'significant minority' of patients will need specialist palliative care; the remainder need their usual carers to have the necessary skills to provide good 'generalist' palliative care. Training needs for specialists in palliative medicine and those caring for patients within other specialties or in the community will differ, but it has long been recognized that the foundations of the necessary competencies need to be laid down during undergraduate medical training for all future doctors:

> Unlike other specialties, palliative medicine is not concerned with facts and skills needed by a few practitioners but those needed by every doctor, whether generalist or specialist, reminding us that palliative care is the right of every patient and its provision the responsibility of every doctor. (Doyle, 1996)

The literature on palliative care teaching has evolved. Papers on teaching to medical undergraduates were followed only more recently by studies on postgraduates, and education for specialists still features less frequently.

Education for medical undergraduates

Early reports focus on the inadequacy of teaching and the need for the inclusion of teaching about death and dying in curricula (Barton, 1972; Hull, 1991). Subsequent publications are commonly surveys of the teaching available (Field, 1984; Dickinson and Mermann, 1996; Field and Wee, 2002) or present the case for including such teaching and then describe the course developed in the authors' institutions. Initially such papers were descriptive, however once the need for such teaching was acknowledged fully, papers emerged discussing how such teaching should be delivered and by whom and then arguing for the teaching to be evaluated.

A number of authors have carried out sequential surveys of palliative care education within medical schools. Dickinson, and Dickinson and Mermann mailed questionnaires to the deans of all medical schools in the United States at 5-yearly intervals from 1975 to 2010. Increasing incorporation of teaching was demonstrated over the time period, with 100% and 99% offering teaching about death and dying and palliative care respectively in 2010. Whilst the number of separate courses has increased over time, only 21% of schools ran such a course in 2010, the majority offering more integrated teaching, taught in 76% of schools by a multidisciplinary team. In 2010, 28% of schools had a 'terminally ill patient' address the class, and 67% of students spent time with hospice patients. The average number of hours of palliative care teaching was 12 (Dickinson and Mermann, 1996; Dickinson, 2011).

In 2000, Oneschuk and colleagues reported a comparative questionnaire survey of all 16 medical schools in Canada, all 30 in the United Kingdom, and 129 schools selected randomly from the United States and Western Europe; 67% responded. Whilst 64% of schools in the United Kingdom reported palliative medicine experience was part of the core curriculum, this was the case for only 11% of schools in the United States, 14% in Canada, and 19% of schools in Western Europe. Optional experience in palliative medicine was offered in 82% of UK, 71% of Canadian, 62% of American and 30% of Western European schools. Teaching using small discussion groups and case-based learning in small groups was reported for the majority of schools in the United Kingdom and Canada. Other schools continued to use predominantly lecture-based teaching. Oneschuk and colleagues noted that courses were often run by a single academic faculty member and suggested the number of both educational programmes and faculty members needed to increase for palliative care education to improve (Oneschuk et al., 2000). In a more in-depth survey of Canadian medical schools in 2001, Oneschuk and colleagues concluded that there were still barriers to implementing palliative care education and there was a need for increased student exposure, curriculum and faculty development, and student assessment and evaluation (Oneschuk et al., 2004). Gibbins et al. came to similar conclusions in the United Kingdom (Gibbins et al., 2009).

Field, and then Field and Wee, surveyed all UK medical schools in 1983, 1992, and 2000–2001. The 1983 questionnaire survey indicated that all but four medical schools delivered some teaching on death and dying, but for some this might be a single lecture (Field, 1984). In 1992, all schools taught most of the subjects relevant to palliative medicine. Some students experienced visits to palliative care units or hospices, although only a few schools required this as part of the core curriculum. In 2000–2001, Field and Wee concluded 'the amount of such teaching varied widely and appeared in the curriculum in a variety of manners, times and places'; however, they suggested the integration of palliative care into curricula was positive and should encourage students to apply their palliative care knowledge in other areas of medicine (Field and Wee, 2002).

Undergraduate curriculum development

By 1980, the objectives of teaching on death and dying were relatively consistent in all US medical schools providing teaching; however, the 'course content, faculty and patient roles, learning resources, and involvement in curriculum research did not evidence a systematic development' (Smith et al., 1980). Teaching in palliative care was driven mainly by interested faculty, and indeed Gibbins et al. have found that a 'champion' is crucial to the successful integration of palliative care into, often crowded, undergraduate curricula (Gibbins et al., 2009). National and international palliative care associations often responded to the resulting heterogeneity of teaching by developing national curricula, and finally national or governmental regulatory bodies issued standards related to accreditation of medical schools or the standard a new graduate must achieve which, in turn, drove further development of curriculum, teaching, and assessment.

Undergraduate palliative care curricula

The deans of the Canadian medical schools published a curriculum for the teaching of palliative care to Canadian undergraduates in 1993 (MacDonald et al., 1993). The American Academy of Hospice and Palliative Medicine (AAHPM) first published *Hospice and Palliative Medicine: Core Curriculum and Review Syllabus* in 1998 (Schonwetter et al., 1999). Since 2000, the Liaison Committee for Medical Education, which accredits US and Canadian medical schools, has included end-of-life care as an educational objective in its standards (Liaison Committee on Medical Education, 2013) but made no recommendations as to how these standards should be met. In the United States, the Education for Physicians on End-of-life Care (EPEC) Project began in 1997, aligned with the American Medical Association (Robinson et al., 2004). It proposes a curriculum, trains the trainers, and provides educational resources. Educating Future Physicians in Palliative and End-of-Life Care (EFPPEC) was a similar project in Canada. The EFPPEC website announces it completed its remit in 2008, although resources such as an undergraduate curriculum remain available (EFPPEC, 2008). Both projects have influenced both undergraduate and postgraduate palliative medicine education. In Australia, the Department of Health and Ageing has funded a multidisciplinary Palliative Care Curriculum for Undergraduates (PCC4U) project, in 2011–2014, which is reported to be in use in ten out of 20 medical courses (PCC4U, 2013).

The Association for Palliative Medicine for the United Kingdom and Ireland (APM) published its first curriculum in 1993 (APM, 1993). This curriculum was divided into three sections outlining the curriculum requirements for medical students, for non-specialists, and for those undergoing specialist training. The publication of *Tomorrow's Doctors* in 1993 (General Medical Council (GMC), 1993) required, for the first time, that learning about caring for the dying was included in UK medical undergraduate teaching. In *Tomorrow's Doctors* (2003) the GMC set out the knowledge, skills, attitudes and behaviours expected of new graduates in medicine, and included the recommendation that graduates must know about and understand the principles of 'palliative care, including care of the terminally ill' (GMC, 2003). A consensus syllabus subsequently updated the 1993 APM curriculum through a Delphi study of palliative care experts (Paes and Wee, 2008).

The United Kingdom, United States, and Australasia are recognized as having led the development of teaching in palliative care. In 2007, a European task force on medical education presented the *Curriculum in Palliative Care for Undergraduate Medical Education—Recommendations of the European Association for Palliative Care* (European Association for Palliative Care (EAPC), 2007), although palliative medicine was integrated into undergraduate curricula in German medical schools, for example, only in 2013 (Schiessl et al., 2013). However, curricula are being developed elsewhere, even in countries and regions where palliative care services have been established more recently, for example, a consensus syllabus for undergraduate medical education was published in Japan in 2012 (Kizawa et al., 2012).

Planning undergraduate teaching

The Palliative Education Assessment Tool was developed to 'facilitate curricular mapping of palliative care education' (Meekin et al., 2000). It is suggested seven domains (palliative care, pain, neuropsychological symptoms, other symptoms, ethics and the law, patient/family/non-clinical caregiver perspectives on end-of-life care, and clinical communication skills) should be represented in any undergraduate curriculum. In setting up or reviewing an undergraduate course, this tool could allow faculty to map existing provision, including, in an increasingly multidisciplinary health-care environment, teaching delivered by other health-care professionals, which might otherwise not be obvious. Alternative methods of needs assessment might be using a Delphi technique, focus groups of staff and students, previous student evaluations, or faculty expert opinion. Having identified gaps, teaching and learning experiences to address them can be designed and implemented.

Many undergraduate curricula specify the knowledge, skills, and attitudes that students must acquire prior to qualification. Latterly, most curricula have moved from a knowledge, skills, and attitudes focus towards competency-based objectives. Competencies are a set of observable and measurable behaviours encompassing the combined knowledge, skills, abilities, and personal attributes that make someone able to carry out a given task or do a given job. In designing teaching, the desired learning objectives/outcomes, or competency statements for the student should be made clear. Objectives drive assessment and assessment drives learning, so objectives should be specific, measurable, achievable, relevant, and timely (SMART) and, particularly for competency-based assessment, should make explicit what the student needs to be able to do, under what circumstances, how well, and when.

Methods of teaching

A variety of approaches to teaching have been taken at different times within different medical school curricula. For many schools, teaching was not part of the core curriculum, and students gained only optional palliative care experience. Many schools continued to deliver a small number of lectures or tutorials. Others were more innovative and introduced learning about death and dying at other opportunities, for example, at the time of anatomy dissection (Marks and Bertman, 1980) or communication skills teaching (Charlton, 1993). As palliative medicine and end-of-life care have gained increasing credibility, more diverse and imaginative teaching methods have been employed. Knowledge-based learning objectives can be acquired through lectures, tutorials, and group discussions. Skills can be encouraged through problem-based learning, role-play (Torke et al., 2004), goldfish bowl discussions (Jeffrey, 2002), consultations with simulated patients (actors) (Kahn et al., 2001), and supported observed hospice visits and clinical attachments.

Knowledge-based learning outcomes and some practical and problem-solving skills are relatively straightforward to teach. Competency-based palliative care objectives are more complex and may need to be met in a number of more inventive or novel ways. Pain and symptom management have been taught with psychological and ethical issues, and teamwork within facilitated multiprofessional workshops involving family caregivers (Wee et al., 2001). In some schools, students are paired with a patient with cancer over a prolonged period (Maughan et al., 2001). Students spend time with patients and their families, attending appointments, investigations, and visiting them at home. Students' learning is supported through tutorials and written reflective portfolios. Whilst such learning is usually evaluated highly, supporting students is important and may be particularly difficult for those students who have personal experience of illness or bereavement. More recent approaches include involving bereaved family members in teaching communication skills (Schillerstrom et al., 2012); the use of literature, drama, and film to teach palliative care competencies (Ring and Reilly, 2003; Dietz et al., 2012; Jeffrey et al., 2012); and the use of combinations of e-learning and simulation to teach spiritual and cultural aspects of care (Ellman et al., 2012).

Teaching attitudes is complex. The *Oxford Dictionary of English* defines 'attitude' as 'a settled way of thinking or feeling' ('Attitude', 2013). Professional attitudes are important in many areas of medicine, but perhaps particularly so in palliative and end-of-life care, where attitudes such as seeing death as failure, therapeutic nihilism in patients with cancer or other end-stage disease, wishing to avoid dying patients, and fears about opioids can all influence patient care adversely. The literature suggests that end-of-life issues are not discussed within the culture of the working environment, and so these attitudes may remain unaddressed (SUPPORT Investigators, 1995; Fitzsimons et al., 2007; Gibbins et al., 2010, 2011).

Lloyd-Williams and Dogra explored the attitudes of second year medical students using a non-validated questionnaire before and after a six-hour course about palliative care comprising

lectures, small group teaching, videos and case based discussions (Lloyd-Williams and Dogra, 2004). One hundred and forty-nine students completed the questionnaire which revealed positive attitudes towards caring for chronically ill and dying patients before and after the teaching, and a significant improvement in views of the hospice. These students were surveyed prior to significant exposure to patients and thus their attitudes were theoretical rather than based on experience. Attitudinal change may occur with increased knowledge alone, but it may require also role modelling and facilitated discussion and reflection following clinical or educational encounters. We have described changing students' attitudes towards opioids using e-learning tutorials which prompted reflection, for example (Forbes and Gibbins, 2010).

Postgraduate training in palliative medicine

The UK Department of Health set out a useful classification of healthcare staff who required training to improve palliative care for patients within its End-of-life Care Strategy. These were:

- Group A—staff who work in specialist palliative care and hospices.

- Group B—staff who frequently deal with end-of-life care as part of their role, for example, secondary care staff who work in the emergency department, acute medicine, respiratory medicine, care of the elderly, cardiology, oncology, renal medicine, intensive care, and those who work with patients with long-term neurological conditions.

- Group C—staff who work within other services and who have to deal with end-of-life care infrequently (Department of Health, 2008).

All staff need training in communication skills, assessing a patient's needs and preferences, advance care planning and symptom control. Clearly staff in group A will have their own specialist curricula, and those in group C need mainly to be aware of palliative care issues and empowered to recognize that a patient might be approaching the end of life and where to gain support.

A Royal College of Physicians' (RCP) working party in the United Kingdom suggested that it is the group B professionals whose palliative care continuing professional development is most important; in particular, they need advanced communication skills because they initiate discussions about issues at the end of life (RCP Working Party et al., 2012). Within this group we suggest that recently qualified doctors are generally the clinicians who spend most time with patients with palliative care needs; their early post-qualification period is, therefore, an important time for them to put their undergraduate training into practice and to consolidate their palliative care skills.

Many newly qualified doctors report being unprepared to care for patients with end-of-life and palliative care needs; they lack confidence in breaking bad news, empathizing, discussing prognosis and symptom control (Charlton and Smith, 2000), and managing distress and social issues (Bowden et al., 2013). They often report having received little or no training at medical school, or that it was inadequate for their role, and they want to learn more. For example, in a survey of all first year graduates in the UK (43% response rate, $N = 2062$), 71% felt they needed more teaching about symptom control and 41% in communication skills in caring for patients with cancer (Cave et al., 2007). In the United States, the authors of a survey of 972 internists and family practitioners concluded that although these physicians provide palliative care, they feel their skills are lacking (Farber et al., 2004). A telephone survey of 1455 students, 296 junior doctors, and 287 senior clinicians from accredited medical schools with response rates of 62%, 56%, and 41% respectively revealed that juniors 'are systematically protected from, or deprived of, opportunities to learn from caring for dying patients. When they do participate in this care, they lack role models with expertise to learn from, as well as feedback and support that facilitate clinical growth'. Many of the respondents did not perceive that dying patients were considered 'good teaching cases'. Students and juniors felt unprepared to provide, and senior and junior doctors unprepared to teach, many key components of good care for the dying; only 17% of senior clinicians reported having taught some aspect of end-of-life care in the past year (Sullivan et al., 2002).

The literature suggests that junior doctors in different countries learn palliative care experientially. A study in Switzerland found 'learning by doing counts strongly for palliative care'; doctors who had more experience with situations involving palliative care had significantly higher competency scores than those with less experience (Mulder et al., 2008). A US study of 20 house-staff reported that formal education in palliative care was not a major source of learning; staff learned mostly on the job, by observing attending physicians, and by making mistakes (Schulman-Green, 2003). Gibbins et al. have reported that students gain little exposure to patients at the end of life during their training, despite increasing curriculum time for palliative care, and report learning by 'trial and error . . . on the job' once they qualify, with nursing staff and hospital palliative care teams being important informal teaching resources (Gibbins et al., 2011).

Few studies consider the skills of senior hospital doctors in caring for patients at the end of life. Many senior consultants have received little or no training in palliative care as undergraduates; they will have learnt by observing others in practice, perhaps from professionals with even less training (Schulman-Green, 2003). Qualitative interviews and focus groups reveal that even caring specialist clinicians find it difficult to face their patients' palliative care needs and to discuss end-of-life issues with them (Fitzsimons et al., 2007). This is significant, since these clinicians will serve as role models to students and junior doctors, potentially informing them, through the 'hidden' curriculum, that palliative care issues can, or should, be avoided. Whilst students, for example, acknowledged learning from end-of-life courses, they found 'patient care experiences guided by teams that acknowledged deaths, role-modelled end-of-life care, and respected students' participation in patient care' far more useful (Ratanawongsa et al., 2005). It is interesting to note that in the RCP Working Party's document on continuing professional development, two-thirds of physicians had not attended any end-of-life care educational event in the last 2 years. Respondents were very confident in their ability to recognize when a patient was approaching the end of life, discuss this with the patient and family, break bad news, control pain, and withhold and withdraw treatment (RCP Working Party, 2012). These results are surprising given ongoing reports of poor care, but are reports of self-rated confidence only, without any proxies for actual skills. It is likely that at least some of these physicians were unaware of their own incompetence. The working party recommended that all physicians caring for patients with palliative care needs attend at least one relevant training event every 5 years.

The literature considering the training of primary health-care or family practice doctors is not extensive, and is often about UK general practitioners (GPs). The skills and training of this group of doctors are important as most patients who know they have life-limiting illness wish to die at home (Gomes et al., 2013). A significant part of early GP training takes place in hospital in the United Kingdom. In a UK-wide postal survey, Low and colleagues reported that while 60–70% of GP trainees had received training in control of pain and other symptoms, only 40–50% had received communication skills training, teaching about bereavement care, or the use of syringe drivers. The median number of patients with palliative care needs they had cared for during their training was five (Low et al., 2006). For most, their deficiencies in training were only remedied once they entered their year in primary care towards the end of their GP training. Their hospital training had thus not provided relevant palliative care training.

Becoming a specialist in palliative medicine

Palliative medicine is recognized in different ways in different countries, for example, in Australia, New Zealand, Hong Kong, and Taiwan it is fully certified. The American Board of Medical Specialties recognized the subspecialty of Hospice and Palliative Medicine in the United States as recently as 2006. In Europe, palliative medicine has specialist status in only two countries, the United Kingdom (since 1987) and Ireland (1995). In five other countries, it is regarded as a subspecialty, that is, doctors seek a second specialization following full certification in another specialty; these countries are Poland (since 1999), Romania (2000), Slovakia (2005), Germany (2006), and France (2007). As of 2006, ten other European countries were discussing certification (Centeno et al., 2007).

Where specialist training is well developed, national bodies have usually agreed on competency-based curricula for specialist palliative care. In the United States, the Accreditation Council for Graduate Medical Education (ACGME) is responsible for accrediting post-MD training programmes. It accredits fellowship training programmes in palliative medicine, but the AAHPM advises on the necessary competencies. In the United Kingdom, such curricula are approved by the GMC, and training programmes are overseen by a specialty training committee of the RCP. Similarly, the Royal Australasian College of Physicians lays out the competency requirements for training in Australia and New Zealand. In many other countries, there are no competency frameworks for training in palliative medicine.

Assessment of palliative care competencies

It is useful to consider models of how learners achieve and demonstrate competencies in reviewing the literature pertaining to education in palliative care. In 1990, Miller proposed a model for the assessment of clinical skills, competence, and performance, depicted as Miller's pyramid (Miller, 1990). As a learner's competence increases, they are able to demonstrate that they 'know' what they should do, then 'know how' they should do something; next they can 'show how' to do a skill or task and finally they can perform or 'do' it in practice. Fig. 4.2.1 shows examples of the assessment methods used at each level of the pyramid.

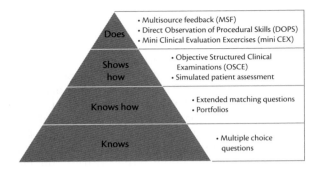

Fig. 4.2.1 Miller's pyramid.

Adapted from Miller GE, Assessment of clinical skills/competence/performance, *Academic Medicine*, Volume 65, Issue 9, pp. s63–67, Copyright © The Association of American Medical Colleges, with permission from Lippincott, Williams and Wilkins.

Assessment of undergraduates

Lempp and colleagues suggest that students remain 'orientated strongly towards examinations which are useful in ensuring proficiency in clinical skills but may detract from other learning' (Lempp et al., 2005). Gibbins et al.'s study confirmed this in palliative care (Gibbins et al., 2011). In 2002, only six of 24 UK medical schools assessed teaching about death, dying, and bereavement with some form of examination (Field and Wee, 2002), and a 2008 survey suggested only 30% of US medical schools assessed palliative care outcomes during student clerkships (Van Aalst-Cohen et al., 2008). Where students are assessed, predominantly knowledge-based outcomes are examined, however many schools have introduced objective structured clinical examinations which allow students to demonstrate how they put knowledge into practice and allow assessment of, for example, communication skills and students' attitudes towards patients with end-stage or life-limiting disease. Since students tend to see areas of curriculum content that are not examined as less important than areas that are, assessment of palliative care skills is critical in improving students' and doctors' attitudes towards, and skills in, palliative care.

Assessment of postgraduates: non-specialists

Much continuing professional development in palliative care is evaluated rather than assessed. Where trainees have learning objectives relevant to palliative care within their specialist curricula, these will usually be assessed in similar ways to their other learning objectives, predominantly through knowledge tests and workplace-based assessments. In the United Kingdom there are a number of postgraduate medical degree qualifications in palliative care or medicine available at Diploma and Master's level, however these are optional academic rather than clinical qualifications, and are therefore assessed through essays, presentations, publications, and dissertations, rather than clinically.

Assessment of specialist training in palliative medicine

Accrediting bodies have a responsibility to ensure that doctors awarded specialist qualifications are competent to care for patients, and therefore their training and assessment of competencies must be robust. Whilst competency-based training might be seen as complete once a trainee has gained the necessary competencies, many programmes specify a minimum length

of training also. The United Kingdom probably has the most extensive programme, requiring 4 years of training. The Royal Australasian College of Physicians Chapter of Palliative Medicine Education Committee requires trainees to complete 3 years of training. Fellowship training in the United States is for 1 year. The structures of these programmes differ, however the way that trainees demonstrate their competencies is similar. Most trainees must have satisfactory educational supervisor reports and complete a variety of workplace-based assessments, which allow them to demonstrate their competence in clinical practice, that is, at the 'does' level of competence within Miller's pyramid. In the United States, the Hospice and Palliative Medicine Competencies Project work group has laid out a set of measurable outcomes for hospice and palliative medicine competencies. These, as for other curricula, should 'represent those for the minimally competent specialist palliative care physician, not the expert'. The group refers to the Dreyfus model of skill acquisition where the novice develops into the advanced beginner, before becoming competent, then proficient, then an expert (AAHPM, 2009). These outcomes link to a clearly blue-printed and extensive toolkit of assessment methods, which include fellow self-assessments, attending physician and faculty assessments, chart reviews, assessments of communication skills and professionalism, academic, and palliative medicine structured portfolios and multisource (360°) feedback (AAHPM, 2009).

In the United Kingdom and Australasia, trainees must complete successful case-based discussions (CBDs) and mini-clinical evaluation exercises (mini-CEXs). Mini-CEXs are supervised learning events where an educational supervisor observes the trainee interacting with a patient and/or family, scores the encounter, and provides feedback to the trainee. In the United Kingdom, trainees also have to complete a number of relevant DOPS (direct observation of procedural skills), structured audit and teaching assessments, and seek and reflect upon multisource feedback from the multidisciplinary team. Knowledge is assessed also by trainees being required to pass a best-of-five multiple choice question specialty certificate examination.

Evaluation of palliative care teaching

In a similar way to Miller's pyramid of competence, Kirkpatrick's four-levels model describes how increasingly complex behavioural changes can be evaluated (Kirkpatrick, 1979). The considerations are: at level 1, the learner's reaction to teaching; at level 2, the changes in knowledge, attitudes, and skills the learner has acquired; at level 3, the degree to which participants apply what they learned during training in practice; and at level 4, whether desired outcomes occur because of the learning acquired, at learner or organizational level.

In 1997, MacLeod and James cautioned against a view of palliative care education as too complex, precious, and problematic to evaluate (MacLeod and James, 1997). For some time these issues seemed to hamper good evaluation of palliative care and relegate it to level 1 of Kirkpatrick's evaluation model, that is, the learners' reaction, usually satisfaction with teaching. Palliative care teaching is generally rated highly in studies, but robust evaluation requires more than students enjoying the teaching. Various studies have sought to demonstrate that teaching has led to students gaining knowledge and skills. Knowledge is relatively easy to test;

this is often done using a pre-and post-course assessment model. Whilst it is not surprising that knowledge scores improve immediately after teaching, some authors have repeated assessments to see if these improvements are sustained over time. Assessment and evaluation are not being used synonymously here; an individual may be assessed to see if their knowledge scores have increased following teaching, a group of students' assessments scores may be used to evaluate the effectiveness of that teaching.

Von Gunten and colleagues assessed the knowledge scores of 593 third year students following a taught and experiential palliative care course (von Gunten et al., 2012). Data were available for 487 students before and after the course and at year 4. Students demonstrated a statistically significant increase in knowledge scores (by 23%); these scores had fallen by 6% in the year following teaching. Goldberg and colleagues compared graduating students' knowledge after a 1-week clinical rotation in palliative medicine in addition to the 'interactive didactic' sessions the previous year's graduates had received. Disappointingly, the students' mean knowledge scores were similar (Goldberg et al., 2011).

The large number of medical students makes assessing palliative care skills in clinical practice difficult logistically. Burden to patients and lack of validated tools undoubtedly deter educators from evaluating teaching outcomes in clinical practice in postgraduates, also. Teaching is often evaluated, therefore, by asking participants to rate their confidence and self-assessed competence in carrying out relevant skills, for example, prescribing or communicating with patients and their families. In general, students' confidence and perceived competence improve with palliative care teaching. In medical students who often have little contact with patients approaching the end of life, such judgements may mean little, and what graduates say they will do in theory may not be translated into practice.

Doctors may be poor judges of their own competence; as part of a randomized controlled trial, Dickson and colleagues compared 143 internal medicine trainees' self-assessed ratings of competence with their patients', patients' families', and clinician-evaluators' scores on a questionnaire on the quality of end-of-life communication (Dickson et al., 2012). There was no correlation between these quality scores and the doctors' perceived competence. More worryingly, there was correlation for 'treatment discussions' only, and here the more confident the trainee, the lower the families' ratings were. The authors conclude that 'efforts to improve communication about end-of-life care should consider outcomes other than physician self-assessment to determine intervention success'. There is some evidence that doctors overestimate their own competence. In a carefully carried out evaluation of a faculty development programme in palliative care, delegates were asked to rate their attitudes and knowledge about end-of-life care practices, and their ability to teach aspects of palliative and end-of-life care (Sullivan et al., 2005). The authors used an unusual and potentially very useful approach. They administered questionnaires both before and after teaching, but they asked delegates to rate their pre-programme attitudes and knowledge again after the teaching. As they had expected, delegates rated their pre-course abilities more highly before teaching and reappraised their responses following teaching, that is, before the teaching they did not know fully what they did not know. Delegates rated the teaching highly and qualitative comments suggested changes in approaches to patient care; however,

questionnaires to assess changes in pain and symptom management, whilst showing positive trends, did not meet the authors' criteria for statistical significance.

Questionnaires have been developed to evaluate some of the attitudes relevant to palliative care, such as the thanatophobia (fear of death and dying) scale (Merrill et al., 1998), or knowledge about opioids and the management of pain in patients at the end of life (Elliott et al., 1995). However, there are challenges with such questionnaires. The thanatophobia scale includes statements such as 'dying patients make me feel uneasy', 'when patients begin to discuss death, I feel uncomfortable', 'I feel helpless when I have terminal patients on my ward'. Clinicians caring for dying patients may feel uneasy, uncomfortable, or helpless when talking to or treating patients who are dying or 'terminal'; however, we do not know from the literature whether such 'fears' have a negative impact on doctors' care for patients. More recently, Mason and Ellershaw have developed and studied the psychometric properties of the Self-Efficacy in Palliative Care (SEPC) scale to assess students' perceived confidence in communication, symptom management, and multiprofessional team working, important skills in palliative care. It is based on 'Bandura's theory' which hypothesizes the greater the individual's perception of efficacy (confidence) in a skill and the more rewarding the outcome expectancy, the more likely the individual is to perform the skill or behaviour. This scale has been studied with 140 medical students in one institution before and after teaching about palliative care, and showed an increase in their perceived skills of communication, symptom management and multi-professional team working (Mason and Ellershaw, 2004). Utilizing the SEPC scale and the thantophobia scale the same authors report that, following a 2-week education and clinical placement programme in palliative care, students' beliefs in their ability to practise and their attitude towards palliative care improved significantly (Mason and Ellershaw, 2008). They conclude, 'in accordance with the study's theoretical driver, it is reasonable to propose that the engaged active learning will have a positive effect on the future care of dying patients'. Further work is needed to determine whether the SEPC scale is a robust measure of the outcome of palliative care education in medical students, taking into account doctors' abilities in assessing their own efficacy and competence as described above.

Evaluation: does teaching and learning in palliative care improve patient care?

The best evaluation of palliative care teaching would be that it was shown to improve patient care. This is, of course, the crux of the problem. Ury and colleagues examined pharmacy records and demonstrated improved prescribing practices for pain following an educational intervention, suggesting that attitudes towards opioids and fears about addiction and so on had been changed by education (Ury et al., 2002). However, whether patients' pain outcomes were improved was not examined. Miller and Wee suggest we may need to consider indirect indicators of effective palliative care teaching rather than patient care outcomes; they suggest improvements in appropriate referrals from junior doctors to specialist palliative care teams or the inclusion of palliative care topics within their teaching by the wider medical school teaching community (Miller and Wee, 2006). Whilst these may be useful outcomes, they remain measurable proxy outcomes.

Conclusion

Curriculum development and delivery in palliative care education has come a long way. Despite this, patients at the end of their lives are still let down by doctors without the necessary skills to care for them. A number of challenges remain. Whilst students are receiving more curriculum time in palliative care, they need exposure to and real clinical experience with patients approaching the end of their lives. Junior doctors need support from seniors who acknowledge patients' needs, role model good communication and care, and facilitate their juniors' reflection and learning from these encounters. Perhaps in turn they can become the seniors who acknowledge and celebrate the rewards of caring for patients who cannot be cured, rather than continuing to teach, through hidden and informal curricula, the culture of focus on cure.

We know the research to validate *clinical* outcome measures in palliative care is difficult because of the well-documented problems with research in this patient population. The paucity of robust clinical outcome measures and the multiple potential confounding factors make evaluating the clinical impact of palliative care teaching perhaps even more testing. This does not mean we should not try. In an evidence-based world, our main challenge is to encourage and develop innovative clinical and research partnerships to design, deliver, and evaluate educational packages to demonstrate how education in palliative care best benefits patients and their families.

Online materials

Complete references for this chapter are available online at <http://www.oxfordmedicine.com>.

References

American Association of Hospice and Palliative Medicine Project Phase 2 Work Group (2009). *Measurable Outcomes for Hospice and Palliative Medicine Competencies, Version 2.3*. [Online] Available at: <http://www.aahpm.org/fellowship/default/competencies.html>.

Association for Palliative Medicine of Great Britain and Ireland (1993). *Palliative Medicine Curriculum*. Southampton: APM.

Bowden, J., Dempsey, K., Boyd, K., Fallon, M., and Murray, S.A. (2013). Are newly qualified doctors prepared to provide supportive and end-of-life care? A survey of Foundation Year 1 doctors and consultants. *Journal of the Royal College of Physicians of Edinburgh*, 43, 24–28.

Bui, T. (2012). Effectively training the hospice and palliative medicine physician workforce for improved end-of-life healthcare in the United States. *American Journal of Hospice and Palliative Care*, 29, 417–420.

Cave, J., Woolf, K., Dacre, J., Potts H.W., and Jones, A. (2007). Medical student teaching in the UK: how well are newly qualified doctors prepared for their role caring for patients with cancer in hospital? *British Journal of Cancer*, 97, 472–278.

Centeno, C., Noquera, A., Lynch, T., and Clark, D. (2007). Official certification of doctors working in palliative medicine in Europe: data from an EAPC study in 52 European countries. *Palliative Medicine*, 21, 683–687.

Department of Health (2008). *The End of Life Care Strategy: Promoting High Quality Care for all Adults at the End of Life*. [Online] Available at: <https://www.gov.uk/government/uploads/system/uploads/attachment_data/file/136431/End_of_life_strategy.pdf>.

Dickinson, G.E. (2011). Thirty-five years of end-of-life issues in US medical schools. *American Journal of Hospice and Palliative Medicine*, 28, 412–417.

Dickson, R.P., Engelberg, R.A., Back, A.L., Ford, D.W. and Curtis, J.R. (2012). Internal medicine trainee self-assessments of end-of-life communication skills do not predict assessments of patients, families, or clinician-evaluators. *Journal of Palliative Medicine*, 15, 418–426.

Doyle, D. (1996). Education in palliative medicine. *Palliative Medicine*, 10, 91–92.

Educating Future Physicians in Palliative and End-of-Life Care (2004). *Undergraduate Curriculum for Medical Education in Palliative and End-of-Life Care*. [Online] Available at: <http://www.afmc.ca/efppec/docs/pdf_2006_ug_curriculum_fact_sheet.pdf>.

European Association for Palliative Care Task Force on Medical Education (2007). *Curriculum for Palliative care in Undergraduate Medical Education: Recommendations of the European Association for Palliative Care*. [Online] Available at: <http://www.eapcnet.eu/LinkClick.aspx?fileticket=VmnUSgQm5PQ%3D>.

Field, D. and Wee, B. (2002). Preparation for palliative care: teaching about death, dying and bereavement in UK medical schools 2000–2001. *Medical Education*, 36, 561–567.

Fitzsimons, D., Mullan, D., Wilson, J., *et al.* (2007). The challenge of patients' unmet palliative care needs in the final stages of chronic disease. *Palliative Medicine*, 21, 313–322.

General Medical Council (2003). *Tomorrow's Doctors*. London: General Medical Council.

Gibbins, J., McCoubrie, R., and Forbes, K. (2011) Why are newly qualified doctors unprepared to care for patients at the end of life? *Medical Education*, 45, 389–399.

Gibbins, J., McCoubrie, R., Maher, J., and Forbes, K. (2009). Incorporating palliative care into undergraduate curricula: lessons for curriculum development. *Medical Education*, 43, 776–783.

Gibbins, J., McCoubrie, R., Wee, B., Maher, J., and Forbes, K. (2010) 'Recognising it's part and parcel of what they do'; teaching palliative care to medical undergraduates in the UK. *Palliative Medicine*, 24, 299–305.

Gomes, B., Calanzani, N., Gysels, M., Hall, S. and Higginson, I.J. (2013). Heterogeneity and changes in preferences for dying at home: a systematic review. *BMC Palliative Care*, 12, 7.

Liaison Committee on Medical Education (2013). *Functions and Structure of a Medical School: Standards for Accreditation of Medical Education Programs Leading to the M.D. degree*. [Online] Available at: <http://www.lcme.org/functions.pdf>.

MacDonald, N., Mount, B., Boston, W., and Scott, J.F. (1993). The Canadian palliative care undergraduate curriculum. *Journal of Cancer Education*, 8, 197–201.

MacLeod, R.D. and James, C.R. (1997). Improving the effectiveness of palliative care education. *Palliative Medicine*, 11, 375–380.

Mason, S. and Ellershaw, J. (2004). Assessing undergraduate palliative care education: validity and reliability of two scales examining perceived efficacy and outcome expectancies in palliative care. *Medical Education*, 38, 1103–1110.

Mason, S. and Ellershaw, J. (2008). Preparing for palliative medicine: evaluation of an education programme for fourth year medical undergraduates. *Palliative Medicine*, 22, 687–692.

Meekin, S.A., Klein, J.E., Fleischman, A.R., and Fins, J.J. (2000). Development of a palliative education assessment tool for medical student education. *Academic Medicine*, 75, 986–992.

Miller, G.E. (1990). Assessment of clinical skills/competence/performance. *Academic Medicine*, 65, s63–s67.

National Council for Palliative Care (2012). *What is Palliative Care?* [Online] Available at: <http://www.ncpc.org.uk/palliative-care-explained>.

Palliative Care Curriculum for Undergraduates (2013). *Progress Report 4*. [Online] Available at: <http://www.pcc4u.org/images/pdf/project-report/pcc4u_project_report_20130531.pdf>.

Robinson, K., Sutton, S., von Gunten, C.F., *et al.* (2004). Assessment of the Education for Physicians on End-of-life Care (EPEC) Project. *Journal of Palliative Medicine*, 7, 637–645.

Royal College of Physicians, National End of Life Care Programme, Association for Palliative Medicine of Great Britain and Ireland (2012). *Improving End-of-Life Care: Professional Development for Physicians. Report of a Working Party.* London: Royal College of Physicians.

Schonwetter, R.S., Hawke, W., and Knight, C.F. (eds.) (1999). *Hospice and Palliative Medicine Core Curriculum and Review Syllabus.* Chicago, IL: American Academy of Hospice and Palliative Medicine.

SUPPORT Investigators (1995). A controlled trial to improve care for seriously ill hospitalised patients: the study to understand prognoses and preferences for outcomes and risks of treatment. *Journal of the American Medical Association*, 274, 1591–1598.

Van Aalst-Cohen, E.S., Riggs, R., and Byock, I.R. (2008). Palliative care in medical school curricula: a survey of United States medical schools. *Journal of Palliative Medicine*, 11, 1200–1202.

4.3

Nursing and palliative care

Deborah Witt Sherman and David C. Free

Introduction to nursing and palliative care

Although nursing is one of the oldest of the arts, it is one of the youngest of the professions. The origin of the word 'nursing' is derived from the Latin word *nutrire*, which means 'to nourish'. The word 'nurse' has its roots in the word *nutrix*, which means 'nursing mother'. Over the centuries, the meanings of these terms have broadened to encompass the training and education of a person who not only cares for the sick and dying, but also who cares for families, communities, and for humanity (Donahue, 1985).

Nursing has long been defined as both an art and a science. Nursing has moved beyond knowledge gained by reliance on tradition, trial and error, or authoritative statements of experts, to the generation of knowledge based on logical analysis and scientific inquiry. As a humanistic science, the purpose of nursing is to describe, explain, predict, and control phenomenon central to its concern, that of people and our world. The art of nursing is the creative use of the science of nursing for human betterment (Rogers, 1992).

Nursing has been an integral part of societal movements involved in the existing culture, while shaping and being shaped by culture (Donahue, 1985). Although dying and death are universal and part of the human condition, illness and death often can be delayed by science and medical technology. Life-prolonging therapies have assisted individuals to live longer with life-threatening illness, although death ultimately occurs. It has been understood that the care of those with life-limiting illness requires the best of modern science, along with an appreciation of emotional, social, and spiritual needs, and ways to alleviate any associated suffering.

As individuals are living longer with life-threatening or chronic illness, practitioners have realized that patients and families have needs and concerns that begin at the time of diagnosis, and that comprehensive care is needed from the time of diagnosis forward. Furthermore, care must be extended to families during the illness experience, through the death of the patient, and throughout the bereavement period for families. It also has become apparent that patients and their families, who are experiencing all types of life-limiting illnesses, and not only those affected by cancer, need this type of care.

Palliative care may be best understood as evolving from the original model of hospice care, but more explicitly endorses a combination of disease-modifying and supportive therapies intended to promote the well-being of patients and families experiencing serious, chronic, progressive and life-limiting or life-threatening illness. Palliative care not only focuses on pain control and symptom management, but also addresses the emotional, social, cultural, and spiritual needs of patients and families at any time during the illness trajectory, and unlike hospice care, is provided in the context of curative therapies. The ultimate goal of palliative care is to support the best possible quality of life for patients and their families (National Consensus Project for Quality Palliative Care, 2009). The concept of palliation is not new however. The term *palliate* has been seen in early records dating from the fourteenth century. It was in the eleventh century when the first hospices are believed to have originated, initially as refuges for weary travellers and religious pilgrims to Jerusalem in the Crusades, and later, to provide care for the sick and the dying (Connor, 1998).

Nurses, who are educated in palliative care nursing, 'facilitate the caring process through a combination of science, presence, openness, compassion, mindful attention to detail, and teamwork' (Coyle, 2006, p. 5). As members of the interdisciplinary palliative care team, nurses, physicians, social workers, and other health professionals each bring their own specialized competence and expertise gained through education, credentialing, and experience. Through interprofessional collaboration, an effective and compassionate plan of care is developed based on the best scientific evidence available, clinical judgement, and a recognition of the wishes and preferences of the patient and family, known as evidence-based practice.

With close to 19.4 million nurses globally, nursing is the world's largest profession (World Health Organization, 2011). Consistently ranked the most trusted profession both in America (Gallup Incorporated, 2010) and internationally, nurses have a tremendous potential to reform health care and ensure quality care for seriously ill patients and their families. Nurses understand the individual's need for control and can emphasize the patients' and families' active participation in decision-making. Nurses' discussions with patients and families can 'replace uncertainty with certainty, hopelessness with faith and despair with empowerment. Palliative care nursing is an exquisite blend of aggressive management of pain and symptoms associated with disease and its treatment, coupled with holistic and humanistic caring' (Sherman and Matzo, 2006, p. xx). Palliative care nursing requires the integration of empirical, aesthetic, personal, and ethical knowledge in providing patient- and family-centred holistic care. This integration of nursing knowledge assists nurses in reshaping societal perspectives regarding illness, dying, and death. Nurses understand that, when individuals move beyond fear, there is an opportunity for healing and continued growth for patients and families, even as death approaches.

Integration of knowledge in palliative care nursing

According to Coyle, the statement 'I failed to care for him properly because I was ignorant' (Coyle, 2006, p. 5) speaks to the need for health professionals, including nurses, to be educated in palliative care. The knowledge base of a discipline includes information, facts, principles, and theories that are organized according to the beliefs of the discipline. Throughout nursing history, knowledge has been obtained through tradition, expert opinion, borrowed knowledge from other disciplines, and role modelling. Based on an analysis of the conceptual and syntactical structure of nursing knowledge, Carper identified four fundamental patterns of knowing: empirical, aesthetic, personal, and ethical knowing (Carper, 1978).

Empirical knowledge

As nursing has developed as a profession, it has been both recognized and accepted that nursing practice must be based on empirical knowledge, or the science of nursing, which involves problem solving, logical reasoning, and scientific inquiry. Empirical knowledge draws upon a reality that can be observed and measured, and therefore verified by others (Carper, 1978). Qualitative and quantitative research builds and tests theories and provides important insights regarding the health of individuals, families, and communities and the dynamic relationships with the environment. More specifically, nursing is interested in the lives of people in particular environments and their diverse perspectives on promoting health, preventing illness, and managing disease. The goal is to move to greater levels of health and wellness and to improve quality of life. The development, testing, validation, and application of theories through research provide the evidence that informs evidence-based practice. The concept of praxis is often used in nursing to describe the interactive relationship between research and practice—each informing the other (Rolfe, 2006).

With the adoption of evidence-based practice as the standard in medicine and nursing, all levels of evidence from lower levels of evidence such as expert opinion through to the meta-analyses of randomized controlled trials provide the empirical knowledge needed to guide nursing practice in general, as well as in palliative care. The combination of evidence-based practice with humanistic and compassionate care represents the imperative to integrate the science and the art of nursing.

Aesthetic knowledge

Aesthetic knowledge or the art of nursing involves a deep appreciation of the meaning of a situation. Aesthetic knowing is made visible through the actions, conduct, attitudes, narrative, and interactions of the nurse in relation to others. It involves participating in or experiencing another's feelings and the ability to envision valid ways of helping in relation to desired outcomes and the goals of care. Aesthetic knowledge enables a nurse to envision the possibilities and to know what to do and how to be in the moment. Aesthetic knowledge supports the dynamic integration of parts into a whole (Carper, 1978). In the care of those with life-limiting or chronic illness, aesthetic knowledge enables the nurse to see the entire situation related to the interplay of physical, emotional, social, cultural, and spiritual needs and to develop a plan of care that focuses on the whole person within the context of their

family and community. Evidence-based practice involves not only empirical knowledge but also an understanding of the meaning of the situation, which further informs clinical judgement.

Personal knowledge

In addition to the integration of empirical and aesthetic knowledge, the clinician also integrates their personal and professional experiences in the form of personal knowledge. Personal knowledge refers to the inner experience of becoming a whole and genuine person. Personal knowing encompasses knowing one's own self and others (Carper, 1978). Empiric theories can be learned, but their meaning for the individual comes from personal reflection and experience. Personal knowing occurs through entering the world of the person being cared for, understanding their world, and responding to them. Personal knowledge is therefore concerned with the quality of interpersonal contacts, promoting therapeutic relationships, and providing individualized care. Personal knowledge also involves personal integrity and honesty, as well as enthusiasm, courage, and imagination (Carper, 1978). As palliative care clinicians, nurses reflect on their personal and family experiences with illness, loss, and grief, as well as on the experiences of patients and families for whom they have cared. With personal knowledge, nurses respond in loving, and supportive ways to the suffering of patients and families.

Ethical knowledge

Ethical knowledge must be integrated in palliative care. Ethical knowledge or the moral component of nursing is concerned with the right action within a situation. It includes voluntary actions that are deliberate and subject to judgement as right or wrong. Ethical knowing in nursing requires both experiential knowledge and knowledge of the formal principles, ethical codes, theories, and local, state, and federal laws that relate to or govern the discipline and society. It involves advocating for the patient. Ethical knowledge provides insight about which choices are possible and why. It provides direction towards choices that are good, sound, responsible, or just (Carper, 1978). In palliative care nursing, ethical knowledge is very important in assisting patients and families in making end-of-life decisions. Palliative care nurses are often members of ethics committees and grapple with ethical dilemmas in clinical situations.

Emancipatory knowledge

The concept of emancipatory knowledge, a fifth way of knowing, was introduced in 2010 (Kagan et al., 2010). It denotes an awareness of social injustices and disparities, and the ability to investigate their sources, and bring about the changes needed to correct the systemic and underlying causes of injustice and oppression that impact health and society. Each individual pattern of knowing—empirical, aesthetic, personal, ethical, and emancipatory—is necessary, but insufficient alone for achieving the goals of nursing. All of the ways of knowing are important in defining the whole. This is illustrated by considering the response to a common question: 'Which nursing intervention is best to relieve pain?' An *empirical* study can test hypothetical relationships among methods of pain management, each of which is influenced by *aesthetic* meanings of relieving pain, *personal* meanings concerning the experience of pain, *ethical* values that influence how and when pain relief is given and received, and *emancipatory* factors that address social injustices and inequities that might affect equitable access to the treatment of pain (Carper, 1978). Failure to integrate knowledge within all of the patterns of knowing leads to uncritical acceptance, narrow interpretation, and partial utilization of knowledge. When this occurs, the ways of knowing are used in isolation from one another and the potential for synthesis of the whole is lost. When removed from the context of the whole of knowing, empirics produces control and manipulation; aesthetics produces indulgence in self-serving expressions and lack of appreciation for the meaning in a context; personal knowing produces isolation and self-distortion; ethics produces rigid doctrine and insensitivity to others (Carper, 1978); while emancipatory knowing alone could lead to aimless and ineffective activism. Palliative care nursing, therefore, involves the integration of all patterns of knowing to alleviate suffering and create an opportunity in which illness, dying, and death may become a time of healing or being made whole. In the formal education or continuing education of nurses in palliative care, it is important to recognize the integration of empirical, aesthetic, personal, ethical, and emancipatory knowledge so that nurses can 'practice what they know' and provide a holistic patient- and family-centred plan of care that is effective, evidence-based, compassionate, and equitable.

Palliative care nurses: responding to changing health-care needs

Across the world, there are aging populations, an increase in the incidence and prevalence of HIV/AIDS and cancer, and people living longer with prolonged advanced and chronic illness. The evolution of the field of palliative care has been a response to the changing profile of illness, dying, and death in the twentieth century (Stjernswärd and Pampallona, 2004). In the United States, for example, the number of Americans with serious or life-limiting illness is expected to double in the next 25 years with the aging of the baby-boomers (Morrison et al., 2011). Globally, the percentage of the total population over age 60 is expected to double from 11% to 22%, and the number of elderly over age 80 is expected to increase by a factor of 26 by 2050 (Bloom et al., 2011). In the decades to come, there will be an international imperative to care for aging populations, particularly as palliative care continues to expand its focus upstream from end-of-life care to the care of the patients and families experiencing serious, chronic, progressive, and life-limiting or life-threatening illness.

The increasing demand for palliative care services in the United States has been evidenced by the growth in hospital palliative care teams in the past 10 years. A decade ago, there were virtually no palliative care programmes in US hospitals. Today, palliative care teams can be found in 63% of the nation's hospitals that have 50 beds or more. As such, access to palliative care in US hospitals has more than doubled in the past 5 years (Morrison et al., 2011). Hospice care, as part of the continuum of palliative care, has also experienced a rapid growth in the United States in response to demand. From 1984 to 2010, there was a 110-fold increase in the number of hospices participating in Medicare in the United States, rising from 31 to 3407 (National Hospice and Palliative Care Organization). Worldwide estimates suggest that over 300 million people or 3% of the global population have either palliative or end-of-life care needs each year (Skilbeck and Payne, 2005). The steady rise in the number of patients and families

accessing hospice and palliative care services not only supports this projection of an increased future need (National Hospice and Palliative Care Organization), but also portends an increased need for adequately prepared generalist and specialist nurses in order to provide the care. There has been concern about the ability to meet this projected significant growth in the need for hospice and palliative care services with adequately educated and trained nurses.

In the past, the education of nurses in end-of-life care has been inconsistent at best, and was neglected for the most part, in both undergraduate and graduate nursing curricula (American Association of Colleges of Nursing (AACN), 1998). In 1997, the International Council of Nurses issued a mandate that nurses have a unique and primary responsibility to ensure the peaceful death of patients. In response, the AACN convened a round table of expert nurses to identify the precepts underlying hospice and palliative care. Round-table experts concurred that these precepts should be foundational to the educational preparation of nurses. Based on these precepts, the document, entitled *Peaceful Death*, was developed, which outlined baccalaureate competencies for palliative/hospice care and content areas where competencies can be taught (AACN, 1998). At the same time, the American Nurses Association formulated a position statement regarding the promotion of comfort and relief of pain of dying patients, reinforcing nurses' obligation to promote comfort and ensure aggressive efforts to relieve pain and suffering. National, state, and local indicators also pointed to the need for all nurses to have generalist-level knowledge of palliative care.

Generalist and specialist level of palliative care nursing

Nursing practice is differentiated according to the nurse's educational preparation, and licensure, which ranges from basic/generalist level through an advanced level of competency. Certified at the basic level of competency, the nurse may be licensed as a licensed practical nurse or registered professional nurse who has gained competencies in palliative and hospice care through their general educational programmes, professional work experiences, and ongoing continuing education. By virtue of graduate education and related clinical expertise, the advanced practice palliative care nurse is a specialist who demonstrates greater depth and breadth of knowledge and skill in theory, research, and practice reflected in the standards of care of palliative care and hospice nursing (Hospice and Palliative Care Nurses Association, 2002).

General registered nurses

In the United States, the current expectation is that all registered nurses have a basic or generalist level of knowledge and competency in palliative care. This includes a holistic approach to care including pain and symptom assessment and management, cultural competence, effective communication skills, recognition of ethical and legal aspects of care, and knowledge regarding care of the imminently dying patient. To ensure that all nurses have generalist level knowledge of palliative care, several educational initiatives have occurred. Since 2000, initiatives have included the integration of palliative care content in nursing textbooks, including the seminal textbook *Palliative Care Nursing: Quality Care to the End of Life* (Matzo and Sherman, 2010) and the *Oxford Textbook of Palliative Nursing* (Ferrell and

Coyle, 2010). Furthermore, there has been the integration of palliative care content in associate degree, baccalaureate, and graduate programmes through a project known as ELNEC (End-of-Life Nursing Education Consortium). ELNEC was established in 2000 with initial funding from the Robert Wood Johnson Foundation to develop a national curriculum to address the fact that most nursing students were not receiving adequate training and preparation for end-of-life care during their basic nursing education. Nearly 14,000 nurses and other health-care professionals from the United States and other countries have received ELNEC training to date to provide quality care to seriously ill and dying patients and their families. Those who have received training since the establishment of the ELNEC Train-the-Trainer programme have gone on to train 390,000 additional nurses and other providers in their respective institutions and organizations. Some developed countries are leading the way in terms of integrating palliative care education into their basic nursing education curricula. One notable example is Israel, where all general nursing programmes include a full unit of palliative care nursing.

Specialist palliative care nurses

Specialist palliative care nurses are also being educated and trained. These advanced practice nurses (APNs) must have the appropriate educational preparation to assume responsibility for health-care decisions and are acknowledged as core members, and often leaders of the palliative care team. In 1998, the first Advanced Practice Palliative Care Nurse Practitioner programme in America was begun at New York University in New York, under the leadership of Dr Deborah Witt Sherman. Subsequently, Dr Sherman took this Master's curriculum to Tenshi College in Japan. The first Palliative Care Clinical Nurse Specialist (CNS) programme was begun at Ursuline College in Ohio under the leadership of Dr Denise Sheehan. According to the 2008 AACN Consensus Model for APNs (APRN Consensus Work Group & National Council of State Boards of Nursing APRN Advisory Committee, 2008), advanced practice level preparation for any specialty must be accomplished initially through education in one of four APN roles: CNS, Certified Registered Nurse Anesthetists (CRNA), Certified Nurse Midwives (CNMs), or Certified Nurse Practitioner (CNP) programmes. APNs must also be educated in at least one of six possible population foci: family, adult-gerontology, paediatrics, neonatal, women's health, or psych/mental health.

Today, over 15 nursing schools in America offer specialist/graduate-level palliative care education by combining palliative care with other advanced practice master's programmes such as an adult health, geriatric nursing or paediatric nursing (Hospice and Palliative Nurses Association (HPNA), 2013). While advanced preparation in palliative and hospice nursing can be accomplished in the context of a Master's degree programme as a sub-specialty, it can also be accomplished by completing one of the available post-Master's certificate programmes in palliative care offered at several American schools (HPNA, 2013). Through clinical experience and continuing education in palliative care, APNs in other specialties may also become eligible to take the advanced practice palliative care certification examination, provided they have the required minimum of 500 hours of supervised clinical practice specifically in the area of palliative care. Additionally, a Doctor of Nursing Practice (DNP) programme with a palliative care focus option recently became available at the University of South Alabama. In addition to the US and Japan, Advanced Practice Palliative Master's programmes are offered in other countries, such as the United Kingdom and Australia.

In the United States and other countries, hospice and palliative care nurses associations have supported the evolution of palliative and hospice nursing. Certification at the generalist and advanced practice levels of palliative and hospice nursing continues to be a critical focus of these organizations. For example, since early 2001, in the United States, the number of registered nurses credentialed at the basic level has risen from 7000 to 11,600 (National Board for Certification of Hospice and Palliative Nurses (NBCHPN)). As of March 2012, 18,000 individuals have been certified in the United States by the NBCHPN as nursing assistants, licensed practical nurses, registered nurses, and APNs.

It is recognized internationally that certification in hospice and palliative care nursing is valued because the individual nurse:

◆ has a tested and proven competency across the spectrum of palliative care and hospice nursing care

◆ has access to a national network of experienced and knowledgeable palliative care and hospice nurses

◆ has demonstrated a commitment to his or her specialty practice by pursuing certification

◆ has demonstrated dedication of professional development in his or her nursing career

◆ is an asset to his or her employer in an atmosphere of increasing awareness regarding quality in health care (Lentz and Sherman, 2006).

The scope and standards of palliative care and hospice nursing

The scope of palliative and hospice nursing continues to evolve as the art and science of palliative care develop. The philosophical precepts of palliative and hospice care emphasize the importance of holistic care offered to patients and families across the life span and in diverse health-care settings. As such, palliative and hospice nurses provide evidence-based care that addresses the physical, emotional, social, and spiritual/existential needs of patients and their families, with the primary goal of promoting quality of life through the relief of suffering along the illness trajectory. Palliative care nursing is provided to patients and families in acute care hospital units; inpatient palliative care units; inpatient, home, or residential hospices; ambulatory palliative care clinics; long-term care facilities and assisted living facilities; prisons; and private practices (Hospice and Palliative Care Nurses Association, 2002).

Relief of suffering and the possibility of improved quality of life for individuals and families are enhanced by:

◆ providing effective pain and symptom management

◆ addressing psychosocial and spiritual needs of patient and family

◆ incorporating cultural values and attitudes in developing a plan of care

◆ creating a healing environment to promote a peaceful death

◆ supporting those who are experiencing loss, grief, and bereavement

- promoting ethical and legal decision-making
- advocating for personal wishes and preferences
- utilizing therapeutic communication skills in all interactions
- facilitating collaborative practice
- ensuring access to care and community resources through influencing/developing health and social policy
- contributing to improved quality and cost effective services
- creating opportunities and implementing initiatives for palliative care education for patients, families, colleagues, and community
- participating in the generation, testing, and/or evaluation of palliative care knowledge and practice (Hospice and Palliative Care Nurses Association 2002).

Advanced Practice Palliative Care Nurses, who have advanced knowledge and skill in palliative care, play a vital role by assessing, implementing, coordinating, and evaluating care throughout the disease trajectory, as well as counselling and educating patients and families, and facilitating continuity of care between hospital and home. APNs also obtain knowledge about ethical issues facing individuals and families, and develop strategies to assist them in defining expected goals of care, as well as accessing and coordinating appropriate care. In addition to clinical expertise, APNs may assume leadership roles in practice, education, research, and administration, which further advance palliative and hospice care as a nursing specialty.

By articulating the scope and standards of professional nursing practice, the specialty defines its boundaries, informs society about the parameters of nursing practices, and develops the regulations for the specialty. As in all nursing specialties, nurses must practice within the scope of their specialty, as outlined by regulation, a professional code of ethics, and professional practice standards (Hospice and Palliative Care Nurses Association, 2002).

The standards of care reflect the values and priorities of palliative care nursing and provide a framework to evaluate practice (Box 4.3.1). These standards are authoritative statements, written in measurable terms, which define the palliative care nurses' responsibilities and their accountability to the public regarding patient/family outcomes. The standards of professional performance describe the competent professional role behaviours of palliative and hospice nurses, including activities related to quality of care, performance appraisal, education, collegiality, ethics, collaboration, research, and resource utilization (Hospice and Palliative Care Nurses Association, 2002). The nursing process includes clinical decision-making and encompasses all actions of the nurse in the care of patients and families. Although the standards, which express the philosophical beliefs of palliative care nursing, remain stable over time, the criteria intrinsic to each standard changes as scientific knowledge and technology are advanced. The standards of care are written both at the basic and advanced practice levels and reflect the nursing process, which involves assessment, diagnosis, outcomes identification, planning, implementation, and evaluation.

Foundational to the standards of care are the following tenets:

- Care should be age appropriate and culturally sensitive.
- A safe environment is to be maintained.

- Education of patients and families is essential.
- Coordination and continuity of care across settings and caregivers must occur.
- Communication and the management of information must be effective (Hospice and Palliative Care Nurses Association 2002).

Competency frameworks have evolved largely from Bloom's learning taxonomy (Bloom, 1956) and take into account how knowledge attainment and skill development occur incrementally based on education and experience. A number of jurisdictions including the United States, Canada, Ireland, United Kingdom, New Zealand, and Australia have developed and, in many cases, validated palliative care nursing competency frameworks. These competency frameworks have been linked to nursing curriculum development in each respective country in order to establish and advance the skills, competencies, values, and standards of care for palliative care nursing (Connolly and Charnley, 2012).

Nurse-generated palliative care research

The science of palliative care and hospice nursing focuses on the generation of basic and applied knowledge in describing, explaining, predicting, and controlling phenomena related to the care of individuals with serious, chronic, progressive, and life-limiting or -threatening illness and their families. The ultimate goal of nursing research is to improve the care of patients and families in areas of symptom management, psychological responses to illness, and the family caregiver experience (Ferrell, 2010). Qualitative studies in palliative and hospice care are important to understanding the subjective experiences of patients and their families and in developing theories for further testing. Quantitative studies are essential for testing theories, determining the incidence, prevalence, and severity of symptoms, and evaluating models of care and palliative care and hospice interventions.

Nurses have historically contributed to the advancement of research and science. Florence Nightingale, known as the 'mother of nursing', was identified as the first nursing researcher as she kept detailed and systemic records of her observations and understood the value of data in informing nursing practice. Early palliative care nurse researchers included Jeanne Quint Benoliel, who in the 1960s, established a programme of research focused on the subjective experience of patients following a diagnosis of life-threatening illness. In the 1970s, Ida Martinson studied the care of dying children, while in the late 1980s, Marilyn Dodd conducted research on patients' self-care management of adverse effects of. In 1992, Elizabeth Clipp examined health transitions and the complexity of human functioning (Lunney, 2011).

Over last 25 years, nursing research has made significant contributions to science. With the establishment of the National Institutes of Nursing Research in 1997 as an Institute within the US National Institutes of Health, interprofessional colleagues, including nurse researchers, have examined phenomenon relevant to the specialty of palliative and hospice care. Similar research institutes in the United Kingdom, Canada, and Australia provide the international community with findings that inform evidence-based practice. Nursing researchers and scholars in academic institutions, particularly research universities and academic medical centres, are submitting research proposals for federal and foundation funding to advance the science of palliative care.

Box 4.3.1 The standards of care for palliative care and hospice nursing at the basic and advanced practice levels.

Standard I: assessment

At the basic level of competence, the palliative care nurse collects individual and family data. At the advanced practice level, the palliative care nurse conducts in-depth and comprehensive assessment based on a synthesis of individual and family health data. Data collection involves information from multiple sources. Assessment is systematic and ongoing. Assessment includes a comprehensive health history, review of systems, physical examination, determination of functional status, information from laboratory data or diagnostic tests, identification of goals of care, and determination of patients' and families' emotional status, spiritual well-being, coping techniques, and resources. The assessment data are prioritized and documented (HPNA, 2002).

Standard II: diagnosis

At the basic level of competence, the palliative care nurse analyses the assessment data in determining nursing diagnoses. At the advanced practice level, the palliative care nurse utilizes an accepted framework that supports palliative care nursing knowledge. Clinical judgement is used in critically analysing data in the formulation of differential medical diagnoses and nursing diagnoses. Diagnoses are derived from multidimensional sources of data; are validated with the patient, family, and interdisciplinary team; actual or potential responses to alterations in health are identified; problems that may be prevented, resolved, or diminished by nursing interventions are identified; and are communicated and documented in the medical record (HPNA, 2002)

Standard III: outcome identification

The palliative care nurse educated at the basic level identifies expected outcomes relevant to the patient and family in collaboration with the interdisciplinary team. The palliative care nurse educated at the advanced level identifies outcomes based on the critical analyses of both complex assessment data and diagnoses. Expected outcomes are mutually formulated with the patient, family, interdisciplinary team, and other health-care providers, when appropriate. Outcomes are culturally sensitive and reflect the patient's and family's values, beliefs, and preferences. Expected outcomes are realistic in accordance with the goals of care and evidence-based practice. Expected outcomes reflect continuity of care across all settings from admission through family bereavement. At the advanced practice level, the palliative care nurse also determines risks, benefits, and costs, as well as modifying the outcomes based on changes in the patients' and families' health status (HPNA, 2002).

Standard IV: planning

At the basic level of competency, the palliative care nurse develops a plan of care that includes interventions to attain the expected health-related outcomes. At the advanced practice level, the palliative care nurse develops a comprehensive plan of care that prescribes evidence-based interventions and reviews the risks and burdens with patients, families, and in consultation with other providers. The plan of care is individualized to the needs, desires, and resources of the patient and family, and is developed in collaboration with members of the interdisciplinary team. The plan is dynamic and is updated regularly, yet provides continuity of care. At the advanced practice level, the palliative care nurse develops strategies that promote quality of life through independent clinical decision-making and provides direction and guidance to other members of the interdisciplinary team (HPNA, 2002).

Standard V: implementation

At the basic level, the palliative care nurse implements the interventions ordered by the physician or APN. These interventions involve the provision of direct care, which facilitate self-care; maximize, restore, or maintain function; enhance well-being; support healthy patterns of living; and provide emotional support and the relief of symptoms. At the advanced level, the palliative care nurse prescribes, orders, or implements medical and nursing interventions. Interventions are evidence-based, implemented in a safe, timely, and ethical manner, and modified based on continual assessment of the patient's or family's response. At the advanced practice level, palliative care nurses supplement interventions at the basic level with sophisticated skills in data synthesis; they may negotiate health-related services and additional specialized care, provide consultation, employ complex strategies, oversee interventions and teaching modalities to promote and maintain health, and makes appropriate referrals (HPNA, 2002).

Standard VI: evaluation

The palliative care nurse educated at the basic level evaluates patients' and families' progress in attaining expected outcomes. At the advanced level, the palliative care nurse critically appraises and comprehensively evaluates all relevant data related to attainment of expected outcomes and goals of care. At the advanced level, palliative care nurses incorporate advanced knowledge, practice, and research into the evaluation process and assume responsibility for the process. Evaluation is systematic, criterion-based, ongoing, and reviewed with other members of the interdisciplinary team. Revisions in the diagnosis, expected outcomes, and plan of care are documented and communicated to the patient, family, and other team members to ensure continuity of care (HPNA, 2002).

Source: data from Hospice and Palliative Care Nurses Association, *Competencies for advanced practice hospice and palliative care nurses*, Kendall/Hunt Publishing Company, Dubuque, Iowa, USA, Copyright © 2002 by the Hospice and Palliative Nurses Association.

In 1998, the Hospice Nurses Foundation in the United States also became a funding agency for palliative care nursing research and published its first research agenda for 2009 to 2012 to investigate the symptoms of dyspnoea, constipation, and fatigue (HPNA, 2012). The HPNA research agenda for 2012 to 2015 (HPNA, 2012) is based on the *Clinical Practice Guidelines for Quality Palliative Care*, developed through the National Consensus Project (National Consensus Project for Quality Palliative Care, 2009). Although there are eight domains of palliative care propounded in the *Clinical Practice Guidelines*, the HPNA research agenda focuses scientific inquiry on the first three domains, specifically on structure and processes of care, physical aspects of care, and psychological and psychiatric aspects of care. The domain of structure and processes of care considers the optimal membership of interdisciplinary teams, the focus on the patient and family as the unit of care, and the locations and models of care delivery. The research agenda related to physical aspects of care focuses on issues related to symptom management and the decline of individuals with multiple co-morbid conditions, as well as a focus on the physical care of patients in special populations. Within the psychological and psychiatric domain, the focus of inquiry is on the needs of individuals with serious mental illness (HPNA, 2012). Other funding agencies are interested in ways of promoting interprofessional education, the value of professional specialty certification, the integration of palliative care concepts into standard care across health communities, the value of concurrent curative with palliative care, and the use of research findings to shape health policy (HPNA, 2012).

As generalists or specialists in palliative and hospice care, all nurses have the opportunity to participate in research dependent on their level of education. Nurses at all levels can identify clinical problems specific to the specialty, serve as members of the research team, participate in data collection for pilot projects, surveys, or formal studies, critique research findings to determine the application of findings in practice and in the development of standards of care and the development of policies (Lunney, 2011).

In collaboration, nursing scientists and clinicians are responsible for evidence-based practice as the empirical findings of research inform clinical practice. The quantity and quality of research are evident in the number of scholarly publications and presentations at national and international palliative care conferences. For example, 14% of the 1073 palliative care English-language, peer-reviewed research articles published in 2010 and found through the CINAHL database identify nurses as either first or co-authors (Lunney, 2011). Nurse researchers, as principal investigators, often lead the interprofessional research team where each provide their specialized perspective to identifying relevant research problems, and offer expertise in quantitative or qualitative research methodologies. As a research team, nurses, physicians, and other health professionals consider ways of overcoming the barriers to recruitment and challenges to retention of such vulnerable populations as individuals who are seriously ill and dying and their family members. All health professionals must be committed to research collaboration to move forward the science of palliative and hospice care as a specialty.

The value of palliative care nursing

APNs play a pivotal role in palliative care (Sherman and Cheon, 2012). Several articles and research studies have examined the role of the palliative care APN. Many of the early studies were conducted outside the United States. Based on a study conducted in Switzerland, Hurlimann et al. (2001) reported that CNSs in palliative care influence patient care by direct care, bedside teaching, and case reviews. Jack et al. (2003) conducted a qualitative study to investigate the role of the CNS within a palliative care team in an acute care hospital setting in the United Kingdom. The results, based on interviews of 23 nurses and physicians, indicated that palliative care Nurse practitioners (NPs) offer support and advice to colleagues, as well as education, which improves the quality of care. Corner et al. (Kuebler, 2004) conducted a longitudinal study in England, which enrolled 76 patients and assigned them to 12 Macmillan palliative care nurses over a 28-day period. Based on the EORTC Quality of Life Questionnaire, significant improvements in emotional and cognitive functioning and in patient anxiety scores, measured by the Palliative Care Outcomes Scale, were reported from baseline to day 7. Patient records further indicated overall positive outcomes of care from Macmillan specialist palliative care interventions in 55% of the cases.

Quaglietti et al. (2004) propose that APNs are uniquely positioned to 'bridge' the gaps in health care based on their independent practice, varied practice sites, and improving reimbursement patterns. Studies have also been conducted regarding the effectiveness of specific roles of nurses in improving the quality of life of patients with life-threatening diseases. Aiken et al. (2006) conducted a randomized trial comparing the PhoenixCare demonstration programme of palliative care and coordinated care/case management for serious chronically ill patients with chronic heart failure ($N = 130$) and chronic obstructive pulmonary disease ($N = 62$), with an equal number of controls who received active treatment from the managed care organizations. Registered nurse case managers provided intensive home-based case management to address disease and symptom management, prepare for end of life, assess physical and mental functioning, and utilization of medical services by patients and families. The results indicated that patients in the intervention group had lower symptom distress, greater physical function, higher self-rated health, and better outcomes on self-management of illness. This novel model of patient care, which combined greatly enhanced palliative care with ongoing managed care organization treatment, was associated with improved quality of life for patients with serious chronic illness.

Additional US studies have clearly demonstrated some of the benefits of APNs in palliative care. Bookbinder and colleagues (Bookbinder et al., 2011) have suggested that NP-based delivery models can increase access to and the availability of specialist-level palliative care in the community. A recent palliative care clinic pilot study (Owens, et al., 2011) demonstrated that NPs by experience and education are ideally suited to manage both primary and palliative care needs of individuals. Other studies (Bakitas, et al., 2009; Dyar et al., 2012) have found that APN interventions in palliative care were not only well received by patients and families, but also demonstrated measurable improvement in patients' quality of life and mood.

The health-care cost-effectiveness and quality of care for NPs in general has been well demonstrated (American Academy of Nurse Practitioners, 2010; Newhouse et al., 2011). The cost-effectiveness of in-hospital and home-based palliative care has been clearly shown by a reduction in health-care spending for America's sickest and most costly patient populations (Brumley et al., 2007; Penrod et al., 2010). However, there are a limited number of studies that specifically focus on the cost-effectiveness of APNs in palliative care. Nonetheless, nurse coordination of palliative care has been shown to maintain the level of clinical care and outcomes, while saving costs. One study reported a 40% cost savings with nurse-led palliative care (Payne et al., 2002). Further studies are warranted to provide information on cost-effectiveness in the context of quality care, and to obtain further evidence regarding the patient and family outcomes related to care provided by hospice and palliative care nurses, and particularly by those at the advanced practice level. While palliative care has become an economic imperative in reducing the health-care costs, palliative care is, more importantly, 'a humanistic imperative to insure that quality of life is promoted during all phases of the illness experience for both patients and their family caregivers' (Sherman and Cheon, 2012).

Palliative care nurses as health educators and public health advocates

According to Payne, 'Nurses have been and continue to be important in spearheading, introducing and developing hospice and palliative care services internationally' (Payne et al., 2002, p. 21) One of the key roles in the development, advancement and performance of the palliative care nursing is that of educator. The role of the palliative care nurse as educator ideally involves a variety of communications and interactions that may encompass any and all of the following: patient care and families, other health and social care providers, nursing students, institutional decision and policy makers, ethics consultants, community stakeholders and organizations, and political officials.

In the academic setting, palliative care nurses advance the specialty through curriculum development and the inclusion of palliative care teaching units and concepts, as well as through palliative care-focused research, dissemination, knowledge transfer, and research utilization. Palliative care nursing education is being enhanced and made more accessible through programmes such as the ELNEC Train-the-Trainer, which facilitates the dissemination of nursing knowledge to nurses and other colleagues both domestically and abroad (Paice et al., 2007).

In clinical practice settings, palliative care nurses have a role as health educators in promoting optimal patient and family well-being through teaching activities such as pain and symptom management; patient rights and decision-making; informing families of community and social support services; and teaching about other therapies, interventions, and self-care. Palliative care nurses as health-care team members mentor and teach other members of the interdisciplinary team regarding evidence-based approaches in palliative care.

Palliative care nurses are also public health advocates given that palliative care is a public health concern. 'Since death has a universal incidence, the incidence, de facto, makes it a public health concern' (Foley, 2003, p. 25). The aforementioned shifts in population and disease demographics, as well as the aging, dying, and palliative care needs of the 'baby boom' generation will place a strain on health-care systems and resources and will represent one of the key public health challenges of the century (Gott and Ingleton, 2011). The characteristics often seen in public health priorities are now seen with palliative and end-of-life care, such as

major impact, high social and financial burden, and the potential to mitigate illness-related suffering for patients and families (Rao et al., 2002; Foley, 2003).

Globally, here is a tremendous need for increased access to quality palliative care. Only 1 billion people worldwide have access to opioids and some form of palliative care services, particularly in North America, Europe, Australia, and New Zealand. However, more than 5 billion people do not have access to basic pain and symptom management medications and services. The lack of access to pain relief and palliative care an urgent global public health crisis, particularly the lack of equitably access in underdeveloped countries (San Diego Hospice, 2012). By virtue of their numbers, experience, education, time spent at the bedside, and insight into the lived experiences of patients and families, nurses have the potential to play a prominent role in as public health advocates for palliative care at the local, national, and global level (Payne et al., 2009). As both citizens and patient advocates, palliative care nurses work with key decision- and policymakers to inform them about the importance and effectiveness of quality, accessible, and equitable palliative care to improve outcomes, cost-effectiveness (Morrison et al., 2008; Penrod et al., 2010), and to ensure the preservation of basic human rights and dignity. In doing so, palliative care nurses continually serve as advocates for patients, families, and communities, in promoting global health and well-being (Payne et al., 2002) through micro and macro level activities and engagement.

As public health advocates, the role of the palliative care nurse involves the following:

♦ Coordination and continuity of care across settings and caregivers

♦ Education of patients, families, and providers

♦ Promoting and upholding palliative care as a basic human right

♦ Establishing networks of providers

♦ Increasing equity and access to palliative and end-of-life care in developed, and particularly in underdeveloped or resource-poor countries

♦ Developing and enhancing palliative care delivery models

♦ Increasing access to opioids and other symptom management modalities

♦ Increased public and political awareness

♦ Developing integrated care pathways

♦ Actively participating in public policy development, engagement, and social/political activism (Payne et al., 2009).

In addition, palliative care nurses advocate for a new perspective, which includes a focus on health and its promotion, even in the face of serious illness. Palliative care nurses assist patients and families in living life each day to the fullest, with the enhancement and maximization of their potential and the achievement of health even within the context of illness (Skilbeck and Payne, 2005).

Visions for palliative and hospice nursing

Nursing is a way of being in the world which involves a desire to support and care for others and the intention to heal. Nurses witness the suffering of people and are drawn towards them very often in informal caregiving roles as family members, friends, or members of a community, as well as in professional roles. In witnessing suffering and death, there is often an awakening of nurses' own sense of mortality. Nurses learn of the preciousness of each day, the struggles to find meaning in life and death, as well as the opportunities to transcend the mundane and realize a connection to something larger than self. Though nurses may view living and dying through different lenses because of different cultural or spiritual perspectives, nurses' intentions remain focused on doing good, preventing harm, and being fair and just as they care competently and compassionately for others. As nurses mature as people and in their role as nurses, the egocentric 'I' shifts to a 'We'. The pain or joys of others are felt in a nurse's heart and their intellect strives to gain the knowledge and skills necessary to offer care to the whole person—mind, body, and spirit. Nurses seek to understand the world not only through formal education, but also through their life experiences as they learn about themselves and observe others. Indeed, patients and families often demonstrate a sense of resiliency in the face of adversity and teach others how to die with grace and dignity.

Nurses strive to understand the societal changes occurring at international, national, regional, and local levels that influence health and well-being. Nurses seek to make a difference in the lives of their patients, families, and communities as they work towards human betterment and goals that promote the greater good. The future vision for palliative care and hospice nursing rests on the belief that nurses are a valuable resource in national efforts to improve care and quality of life for patients and their families living with advanced, life-limiting illness. It is through collaborative efforts that the roles of hospice and palliative care and hospice nurses will be fully actualized. Professional organizations in nursing, medicine, hospice, and palliative are called upon to engage in dialogue about the role of APNs, and opportunities and strategies to advance the role. Nursing educators must become knowledgeable about palliative care and develop continuing education programmes, which support palliative care and hospice nursing competencies. Researchers are called upon to continue examining the effects of palliative care education, interdisciplinary palliative care teams, the impact of palliative care generalist and specialist nurses, and the safety, quality, and cost-effectiveness care provided APNs in palliative care. Models of palliative and hospice care delivery in rural areas, in the community, at home, in skilled nursing facilities, and hospital settings, and their impact of patients, families, goals of care, advance care planning, and quality of life are needed. APNs who practise in palliative care and hospice are called upon to document and disseminate the health-care outcomes and engage in interdisciplinary research and translate research findings into practice (Promoting Excellence in End of Life Care, 2002).

Payers of health-care services are called upon to recognize the specialty of palliative care, and provide APNs with adequate and consistent compensation that is commensurate with APNs scope of practice, authority, and responsibility, regardless of practice setting. Regulatory agencies, such as state, national, regional and global nursing organizations, are called upon to work collaboratively and consistently to recognize the scope and standards of advanced practice palliative care nursing. Insurers and legislators are called upon to remove barriers that prevent APNs from practising to the full extent of their education and training, to address challenges related to APN billing processes, and to eliminate inequalities in reimbursement rates for APN services. Health-care systems and providers are also asked to develop or expand practice opportunities for APNs in all settings that care for patients who may experience life-threatening illness. Health-care systems are called upon to develop and maintain interdisciplinary palliative care teams, establish effective policies related to the ethical and evidence-based provision of palliative and end-of-life care, and to work towards the goal of achieving certification where possible, such as through the Joint Commission's new Advanced Certification Program for Palliative Care in the United States.

The vision for palliative care and hospice nursing will be actualized through the collective efforts and commitment of nurses at all levels of practice. Nurses' full potential in health care will be fulfilled by a combination of exceptional knowledge in nursing, clinical skill, sensitivity, originality, ambition, desire, and self-respect. Nurses must continue to nurture their intellect, creativity, and spirit; rely on their own authority and ability to self-govern the profession; value the integrity of human wholeness by offering care which integrates empirical, aesthetic, personal, ethical, and emancipatory knowledge; and have faith and confidence in their personal and professional abilities. Indeed, a universe of infinite potentials arises for palliative care and hospice nurses as they 'Dream Big' and create a reality that improves the quality of care and quality of life of patients with life-threatening illness and their families.

Online materials

Complete references for this chapter are available online at <http://www.oxfordmedicine.com>.

References

Aiken, L., Butner, J., Lockhart, C., *et al.* (2006). Outcome evaluation of a randomized trial of the PhoenixCare Intervention: program of case management and coordinated care for the seriously chronically ill. *Journal of Palliative Medicine*, 9, 111–126.

American Association of Colleges of Nursing (1998). *Peaceful Death: Recommended Competencies and Curricular Guidelines for End-of-Life Nursing Care*. [Online] Available at: <http://www.aacn.nche.edu/elnec/publications/peaceful-death>.

APRN Consensus Work Group & National Council of State Boards of Nursing APRN Advisory Committee (2008). *The Consensus Model for APRN Regulation: Licensure, Accreditation, Certification, & Education*. [Online] Available at: <https://www.ncsbn.org/Consensus_Model_for_APRN_Regulation_July_2008.pdf>.

Carper, B.A. (1978). Fundamental patterns of knowing in nursing. *Advances in Nursing Science*, 1, 13–23.

Coyle, N. (2006). Introduction to palliative care nursing. In B.R. Ferrell and N. Coyle (eds.) *The Textbook of Palliative Nursing* (eds.), pp. 5–12. New York: Oxford University Press.

Donahue, M. (1985). *Nursing: The Finest Art*. St Louis, MO: The C.V. Mosby Company.

Hospice and Palliative Nurses Association (2002). *Competencies for Advanced Practice Hospice and Palliative Care Nurses*. Dubuque, IA: Kendall/Hunt Publishing.

Hospice and Palliative Nurses Association (2012). 2012–2015 *Research Agenda*. Pittsburgh, PA: HPNA.

Hospice and Palliative Nurses Association (2013). *Graduate Program Listing*. [Online] Available at: <http://www.hpna.org/DisplayPage.aspx?Title=Graduate%20Program%20Listing>.

Jack, B., Oldham, J., and Williams, A. (2003). A stakeholder evaluation of the impact of the palliative care clinical nurse specialist upon doctors and nurses within an acute hospital setting. *Palliative Medicine*, 17, 283–288.

Lentz, J. and Sherman, D.W. (2006). Professional organizations and certifications in hospice and palliative care. In M. Matzo and D.W. Sherman (eds.) *Palliative Care Nursing: Quality Care to the End of Life* (2nd ed.), pp. 117–132. New York: Springer Publishers.

Lunney, J. (2011). Hospice and palliative nursing research: 25 years of progress. *Journal of Hospice & Palliative Nursing*, 13, S3–S7.

Matzo, M., and Sherman, D.W. (eds.) (2010). *Palliative Care Nursing: Quality Care to the End of Life* (3rd ed.). New York: Springer Publishers.

Morrison, R.S., Augustin, R., Souvanna, P., and Meier, D.E. (2011). America's care of serious illness: a state-by-state report card on access to palliative care in our nation's hospitals. *Journal of Palliative Medicine*, 14, 1094–1096.

Morrison, R.S., Penrod, J.D., Cassel, J.B., *et al.* (2008). Cost savings associated with US hospital palliative care consultation programs. *Archives of Internal Medicine*, 168, 1783–1790.

National Consensus Project for Quality Palliative Care. (2009). *Clinical Practice Guidelines for Quality Palliative Care* (2nd ed.) Brooklyn, NY: National Consensus Project for Quality Palliative Care. Available at: <http://www.nationalconsensusproject.org/guideline.pdf>.

Paice, J.A., Ferrell, B.R., Coyle, N., Coyne, P., and Callaway, M. (2007). Global efforts to improve palliative care: the international end-of-life nursing education consortium training programme. *Journal of Advanced Nursing*, 61, 173–180.

Penrod, J.D., Deb, P., Dellenbaugh, C., *et al.* (2010). Hospital-based palliative care consultation: effects on hospital cost. *Journal of Palliative Medicine*, 13, 973–979.

Quaglietti, S., Blum, L., and Ellis, V. (2004). The role of the adult nurse practitioner in palliative care. *Journal of Hospice and Palliative Nursing*, 6, 209–214.

Sherman, D.W. and Matzo, M. (2006). Preface. In M. Matzo and D.W. Sherman (eds.) *Palliative Care Nursing: Quality Care to the End of Life*, pp. xix–xx. New York: Springer Publishers.

Stjernswärd, J. and Pampallona, S. (2004). Palliative medicine: a global perspective. In D. Doyle, G. Hanks, N. Cherny, and K. Calman (eds.) *Oxford Textbook of Palliative Medicine*, pp. 1227–1245. Oxford: Oxford University Press.

Social work in palliative care

Terry Altilio and Nina Laing

Introduction to social work in palliative care

In 2001, Dame Cicely Saunders authored a commentary entitled *Social Work and Palliative Care—The Early History*. She documents the integration of social work in hospitals in the United Kingdom as early as 1905 and describes her own experience in the 1940s when she trained as an almoner (medical social worker), complementing her nursing education and predating her decision to become a physician. During 1905, in the United States, Massachusetts General Hospital would be the first hospital to employ social workers. This was consequent to the vision and commitment of Richard Cabot, a physician who observed that social and psychological issues were intimately entwined with medical care and health (Gehlert, 2012). Saunders links the reciprocal and enriching work of social work authors by honouring the work of Ruth Abrams, who, as early as 1945, published in *The New England Journal of Medicine* a study of 200 people with cancer receiving end-of-life care. She writes of her discovery of Alison Player's (1954) article 'Casework in Terminal Illness' and credits Margaret Torrie, a social worker in the United Kingdom, with founding Cruse Bereavement Care, a national organization that continues to provide bereavement care at no cost. Additional articles reflecting early social work contributions include Aitken Swan's (1959) report of interviews with families of 200 people with cancer cared for at home and Bailey's (1959) survey of the social needs of 155 people with lung cancer. Lastly, Dame Cicely tributes Zelda Foster, whose writings influenced the care of terminally ill veterans and their families, an impact that extended much beyond the Veteran Hospitals.

This early link of palliative social work clinicians in the United Kingdom and the United States provided a foundation for the evolving specialty which continues to be enriched by social work practitioners across the world. The international nature of the specialty was reflected in the Social Work Summit held in 2005 at the National Association of Social Workers (NASW) in Washington, DC. The Summit included clinicians, researchers, and educators. The *Oxford Textbook of Palliative Social Work* published in 2011 includes an international section honouring the skills, resilience, and diversity of the social work contribution to palliative care around the world. In addition, in the United States, NASW competencies have been established by NASW and in 2007, a monograph titled *What Social Workers Do* was published by the National Hospice and Palliative Care Organization. In Canada, research was undertaken to validate competencies (Bosma et al., 2009) and in the United Kingdom the work of Beresford and colleagues (2007) enhanced our understanding of service users' perceptions of specialist palliative social work.

Palliative care: the convergence

The definition of palliative care selected for this chapter is the most recent World Health Organization definition (World Health Organization, n.d.). In the United States, the National Consensus Project for Quality Palliative Care (2009) defines a similar scope which is informed by guidelines describing core precepts and structures.

Both documents reflect a commitment to psychosocial and spiritual aspects of care. As with other disciplines, the immediate focus of social work intervention and advocacy is often determined by the urgency of needs, resources available, and the challenges presented by social, political, and economic factors. Thus around the globe the contributions of social work will vary. In some settings, palliative social workers may integrate the psychosocial and spiritual aspects of pain and symptom management as a focus of assessment and intervention. However, in many parts of the world where access to opioids is limited, the primary mandate may be advocacy focused on improving access to medications for patients who suffer with unremitting pain during illness and at the end of life. In some settings the commitment to autonomy is actualized by social work participation in the comprehensive work of advance care planning while in other settings this focus on the future may be incongruous with social, spiritual, or cultural values.

Social work and its synergy with palliative care

No matter where in the world social workers practise, there is a unifying code of ethics that speaks of values inherent in the profession many of which are reflected in core principles of palliative and end-of-life care. In 2004, the International Federation of Social Workers (IFSW) and the International Association of Schools of Social Work (IASSW) approved a joint document *Ethics in Social Work, Statement of Principles*. As in palliative and end-of-life care, overarching principles and values frame social work practice and are reflected in the following definition:

> The social work profession promotes social change, problem solving in human relationships and the empowerment and liberation of people to enhance well-being. Utilising theories of human behaviour and social systems, social work intervenes at the points where people interact with their environments. Principles of human rights and social justice are fundamental to social work. (IFSW and IASSW, 2004, p. 1)

As the concepts of relationship, human rights, empowerment, and social justice are operationalized, we begin to identify the perspective and expertise that social workers bring to palliative practice. Respect for the inherent worth and dignity of all people is related to supporting their physical, psychological, emotional and spiritual integrity, and well-being. Autonomy and participation are linked to a respect for strength and resilience, and treating the whole person within their environments. The social justice focus extends both to the individual and to society as a whole and in elucidating this value; the inherent commitment to diversity and to advocacy is reflected. While the nature of advocacy may be influenced by the population served and the part of the world in which social workers practice, the social justice mandate and commitment to the under-served does not dissipate but rather changes in focus and form. This joint document guides professional conduct and speaks to many common values such as competence, integrity, confidentiality, compassion, accountability, empathy, and critical thinking.

Social work: assessment and intervention

As with other disciplines, social workers listen, think critically, and respond from the perspective of their training. While all palliative care clinicians are expected to provide emotional support and attend to the psychological, social, and spiritual needs of patients and families, there are unique skills brought by each discipline and from these skills flow consequent responsibilities. The ability to identify psychosocial or spiritual distress, while a generic competency of palliative clinicians, does not necessarily assume the skills to intervene, especially in more complex situations. Therefore it is essential to know when to enlist the expertise of interdisciplinary colleagues.

Social work assessment emanates from a systems approach and a view of the person in the multiple environments, internal and external, which influence and inform their experiences. Social workers are therefore, by training, inclined to observe the influence of factors such as illness, medical systems, practical challenges, thoughts and feelings, symptoms, and disability, not only on the person, but on their family constellation and equilibrium. In addition to the environmental perspective the precept 'starting where the client is' (Goldstein, 1983) invites a process of exploration and inquiry whether through tools or conversation. This implicitly demands that we 'listen' to the multilayered communication that frames the patient's story and subsequently focuses intervention. Concurrently this inquiry, which extends beyond the medical to the emotional, social and spiritual life of the patient and their family, leads to a thoughtfulness about the boundaries of confidentiality.

Confidentiality

Inviting a patient to relate aspects of their personal narrative requires sensitivity to confidentiality given the team nature of palliative care. Information that is shared is often private, personal, and family-related, and patients and families are often unaware that information is shared. Hence implicit consent cannot be assumed. Respect for confidentiality and autonomy mandates that team members request consent to share intimate personal aspects of their lives beyond the medical when necessary. For some clinicians, information wields power, for others it represents an exclusive relationship with the patient, and still for others the need to know comes from simple curiosity.

In a specialty based in respect across disciplines, 'a test of trust' rests in an acceptance that honouring patient confidentiality and autonomy means that clinicians receive information that is necessary to do their work and that some information may be held confidential both in team meetings and in documentation (Randall and Downie, 1999; Monroe, 2005). Best practice methods suggest that we inform people that to get optimal care information does need to be discussed at a team level with the patient's permission. Additionally, encounters between a health care professional and patient or family requires a dated entry in the clinical record.

Assessment

Consequent to the environmental perspective, social work attunes to culture, and patient and family's biopsychosocial-spiritual history to identify areas of strength, resilience, and challenge. This helps to grasp the larger context within which illness developed (Cadell et al., 2011). The assessment process may include screening and/or assessment tools. Alternatively, it may be based in questions and conversation designed to validate the person and family beyond the illness, discover or elaborate areas of concern, sources of distress, and practical needs. At the heart of assessment is relationship, communication, verbal and non-verbal, and critical thinking which guides the process. As such, assessment is also an intervention informed by expertise and based in the listening and respect for the experience and perceptions of the patient, family caregivers, and family. The critical thinking that informs questions and comments often serves to uncover the meanings or interpretations attributed by patient and family to the various aspects of the illness experience. Inquiry about mood, sleep, or pleasure may assist in identifying patients who are anxious or depressed, fatigued, or in pain, leading to an interdisciplinary treatment plan which integrates knowledge of evidence, patient and family receptiveness, and available resources. Social workers with knowledge of symptoms bring valuable observations to medical and nursing colleagues for the purpose of exploring aetiology and crafting a treatment plan responsive to the multiple factors that often inform the symptom experience of seriously ill patients (Block, 2006; Cagle and Altilio, 2011; Walsh and Hedlund, 2011). An assessment process embedded in environment and relationship is adapted to the cultural variables that infuse the lives of patient, family, and clinician as well as the institutions in which care is provided.

Culture

Congruent with a focus on environment and strengths, social work assessment includes attention to the role and influence of culture. Culture can be understood as the integrated collection of socially determined and socially transmitted customs and beliefs, which shape the values of a given group of people and influence how they behave and interpret the world around them (Kemp, 2005; Young-Laing, 2009). Therefore, how an individual understands pain and suffering, caregiving, life-threatening illness, and spiritual and social functioning, for example, can be inextricably linked to their cultural background.

While the expectation of social workers and other practitioners is to develop a practice that is responsive to cultural variation, in practice, respect for cultural differences is a continuing and evolving process. Clinicians develop an awareness that they are not culturally 'neutral', accepting that we bring to bear not only our individual culture, but also, the culture of our profession or institution and all its corresponding biases, preferences, customs, and beliefs. This attentiveness to self-awareness is an integral aspect of social work training and leads to an understanding of how our cultures influence how we receive patients, or conversely, how they may receive us and how this cultural exchange could impact the evolving relationship. Achieving good clinical outcomes in the setting of such a cross cultural exchange requires sensitivity, respect, knowledge, and the humility to ask for guidance from patients and families (Kemp, 2005).

Many practitioners possess generalist understanding of the role of culture in health care. It is also essential to become familiar with the cultural practices and beliefs of specific populations served, both from personal encounters and enquiry as well as from the literature in order to utilize these insights to intervene clinically (Kemp, 2005; Young-Laing, 2009). At the same time clinicians work to avoid a reductionist approach which stereotypes or falsely imposes the role of culture in lieu of more careful individualized assessment of the client–family–practitioner dynamic. Despite common attitudes and behaviours, there is often heterogeneity among cultures and within families and social work observation and enquiry about the family system works to identify such variation. There can be for example, great variation between generations in the perceived authority of a physician which might impact communication style and lead to familial conflict regarding treatment planning or decision-making.

Language differences abound and are an aspect of culture which can often present as a barrier to accessing quality care. Social work attunes to the many variables at play when the clinical team decides how to access translation services. When available, skilled professional interpreters may provide as close to verbatim translation as possible (Butow et al., 2011). Yet, even then, the subtleties of communication can literally be lost in translation and meanings misconstrued. Interpreters who are prepared by the clinical team can be most effective in carrying out their roles. For example, a patient may use the word 'tumour', but never the word 'cancer', something an interpreter should know in advance so as not to risk causing unintended harm. In the absence of professionals who speak the language, trained interpreters, or technological interpreter assistance, family members are often looked upon for assistance. While sometimes necessary, this option creates the possibility that family dynamics, personal beliefs, or individual discomfort with sensitive or difficult discussions could lead to distorted messages, things left unsaid or improperly interpreted with the unintended consequence of increased distress for both the family 'interpreter' and the family system. Equally important is the reality that the treatment team cannot know what is actually being communicated within the family.

Ultimately, culturally informed practice can illuminate and enrich the clinician–patient–family dynamic, identify areas of confusion, and/or clarify perceptions of illness and treatment. Clinicians often discover a path to culturally syntonic ways to intervene and perhaps identify resources within the cultural community, which contribute to positive clinical outcomes and sustain the patient and family as they transition back into their community. This potential reflects the systems approach which is integral to social work and attends to the interaction of people and the many systems of which they are a part. Respect for the power and potential of systems leads to a special affinity for the value and opportunity in team work and family conferencing, two core processes of palliative care.

Family meetings

Palliative care, at its most comprehensive seeks to address the needs of the whole patient, which in many instances includes family who provide continuity and assist in contextualizing the life of the patient. In the most generic sense, family encompasses biological families, families of creation, friends, and other persons of importance the patient identifies as belonging to their extended network. The family also becomes a unit of care as their needs and experiences are often intertwined with that of the patient. As a result, a family meeting can prove to be a powerful intervention to address the multifaceted needs of both the patient and family.

Family meetings are an important tool to enhance dialogue, provide information, respond to emotional distress, and marshal resources to help problem-solve, make decisions, and establish goals of care. Meetings can also help to substantiate a therapeutic relationship, explore patient and family experiences, and create an opportunity for the team to learn about the patient, and the shared values and beliefs which can prove invaluable in providing quality care (Altilio et al., 2008). Consequent to the complexity and the potential for positive outcomes, a well-planned family meeting often takes preparation ahead of time (Cohen Feinberg et al., 2011). By starting where the patient is, social workers utilize their assessment skills to help the team prepare for a meeting.

Understanding who has requested the meeting and the reason it is being held often guides decisions about who will facilitate and who needs to attend; which family members and which practitioners are essential to the process and expected outcomes. These decisions are rooted in sound clinical judgements including respect for cultural values. For example, outcomes are enhanced when the perceived authority of physicians is acknowledged, marshalled, or mitigated, depending on the needs and particular circumstances of the patient. The patient who experiences their care as fragmented or perceives conflicting messages from team members may benefit from a large cohort of involved practitioners in attendance. Alternatively, the patient who struggles to trust or is intimidated by the power of perceived experts may be best served by careful selection of a limited number of clinicians.

While many medical specialists such as intensivists and oncologists are trained to facilitate family meetings, social workers are often the most comfortable and skilled in group and family dynamics. Although social workers are adept at facilitating discourse, negotiation and skilled communication is only made relevant by careful 'listening' on multiple levels. The clinician serving as a 'silent participant' and 'participant observer' of family and group dynamics and communication processes has a responsibility to complement and enhance the process. Interventions designed to facilitate dialogue, interpret non-verbal communications or clarify confusion are chosen based on active ongoing clinical assessment of the patient and family process both within itself and in relation to the clinical team.

During family meetings, social workers use multiple interventions. They may utilize supportive counselling techniques, cognitive reframing, and anticipatory guidance to assist patients and families as they integrate complex information spoken in the language of medicine and struggle to make decisions which impact the present and the future. They may invite expression of emotion, explore thought and meaning, and enhance informed decision-making and problem-solving as patients and families anticipate and prepare for outcomes or experiences which are unfamiliar and uninvited.

The listening skills implicit in social work training are essential to positive outcomes in family meetings. Indeed, listening is one of the more vital behaviours during a family meeting. The intensive care unit (ICU) is a setting in which family meetings are an assumed part of daily care and therefore much research has focused on palliative and end-of-life care in the ICU and communication with families. While the ICU represents only a portion of the settings in which palliative care is provided, some of the outcomes may have broader implications. Studies suggest that family members feel more positive about communications with physicians when more time is spent listening to the family than speaking to them (McDonagh et al. 2004). Additionally, there have been several studies evaluating the impact of communication in the ICU on the mental health outcomes of family members of patients receiving end-of-life care. While study in this area is ongoing, existing research suggests that there may be a connection between satisfaction with communication and improved mental health outcomes for family members after death (Azoulay et al., 2005; McCormick et al., 2007; Wright et al., 2008; McCormick, 2011). While exclusive to the ICU, this research supports a hypothesis that attention paid by all disciplines to the process of family meetings serves patients and families in the immediate and beyond and thus may be thought of as a pre-bereavement intervention.

Social work: role and responsibility in team

Palliative care as a team-based specialty engages multiple disciplines and different schools of thought in an effort to approach the varied needs of patients. Depending on the setting and resources available, a team can vary in size and constellation. In many practices, the 'person in environment' concept expands team to include family, community resources, and spiritual communities. Single practitioners may develop 'teams of creation' with floating memberships serving the needs of individual patients and families. Even in settings where there are more robust palliative care teams, the needs of the patient and family may be best met by an inclusiveness which invites participation by others who are integral to the patient's life, such as a long-term community physician, a treating oncologist, or a member of the clergy who has known the patient over time.

While a team-based approach is a key component to quality palliative care, how teamwork is translated into practice can vary according to the model chosen and the skills and training of the team members. The interdisciplinary model rests on synergistic and interdependence of clinicians who come with the unique expertise of their chosen profession as well as shared skills. Most palliative care clinicians recognize that individuals do not parcel out their spiritual, psychological, social, and medical needs but often present an integrated experience that requires clinician flexibility, role sharing, and knowledge both of one's own skills and those of others. Consequently, clinicians know when to consult for guidance and when to refer to other team experts. An interdisciplinary team is one in which a cohort of professionals with distinct roles and responsibilities act in concert with one another to produce successful outcomes (Crawford and Price, 2003). By creating an adaptive and interactive team environment, the expectation is that the team as a unit will achieve outcomes that exceed those possible if each practitioner were acting as an individual (Crawford and Price, 2003). However, for an interdisciplinary team to function at its best, it requires mutual respect for the different professionals involved, an environment of trust and safety, a willingness to challenge one another, and a recognition that our varied expertise means that we see patients and problems from differing perspectives.

Within the construct of team, social workers are often uniquely positioned consequent to their training in group dynamics, advocacy, and communication. These skills are essential when working with patients and families, and also when functioning as both a participant and an observer within the group dynamic of team. A social worker will listen and assess from a skill set which often identifies barriers, environmental issues, and patient, family, team, and system dynamics which may either potentiate or impede the goals of patients and families. Plans of care and treatment approaches can then be fashioned from a strengths-based perspective and with an awareness of the unique circumstance of the individual patient and family.

Patient family narrative: an illustration

Whether intervening within a family meeting, exploring decisions related to advance directives or resuscitation, discussing practical needs, or exploring the suffering component of pain, social work interventions have the potential to impact present treatment plans and to influence legacy if death is the ultimate outcome.

Lilie is the 46-year-old mother of Kevin, age 10 and Jamal, age 15. She came from the Virgin Islands to the United States seek medical care after having been diagnosed with breast cancer at the age of 39. She has two sisters in New York. For the past 5 years disease-modifying therapies have contributed to a quality of life that has enabled her to parent her sons, negotiate a fifth-floor, walk-up apartment, and maintain her independence and privacy. When diagnosed with metastatic disease to the bone, unremitting pain necessitated hospital admission and consultation with the palliative care team. Complementing the active pharmacological management of pain, social work assessment included the following:

◆ Understanding the impact of increasing pain and impaired physical functions on Kevin and Jamal, the family structure, and equilibrium.

◆ Exploring the emotional, cognitive, and spiritual aspects of Lilie's pain experience to offer interventions which complement radiation treatments and pharmacotherapy.

◆ Considering the existential, emotional, and cognitive impact as the medical treatments she came to the United States to seek become unable to extend her life.

◆ Exploring practical needs and resources to support her goals related to parenting and sustained function.

◆ Exploring Lilie's values, beliefs, and parental choices related to disclosure of prognosis to her extended family and children; her thoughts about future guardianship and care.

During lengthy hospitalizations Lilie forged a valued and reciprocal relationship with the oncology team. She maintained the structure of her family by parenting from the bed, directing Jamal in his care of Kevin. While she initially chose not to engage family to assist with her children, she consented to social work contact with Kevin's school yet would not allow disease- or prognostic-related information to be shared with her children or extended family. In the course of medical treatment, a lumbar puncture provided an opportunity for the social worker to assist with related distress and pain through a focused breathing imagery exercise which provided relief from procedure-related pain and validated her internal locus of control. It also led Lilie to re-awaken an artistic side of herself she had temporarily lost to disease and pain. She returned to writing poetry and expressing herself through music. She allowed her children to participate in joint videotaped music therapy sessions during which she wore island dress, sang, and played the drums. Concurrent with her choice to withhold information about the extent of illness, she engaged in shared therapeutic work which created a legacy. Her lyrics included the theme of 'going to the top of the mountain' which was understood to be a metaphor for transition and death.

Lilie's disease spread within her bones. As her body became increasingly fragile so did the structure of her family system as she became less able to orchestrate. As she experienced the fragility of her body and was informed of the risk of fractures she realized emotionally and cognitively that she could not return home and allowed the social worker to contact her sisters, extending the system of support. Jamal continued in his parenting role and asked direct questions driven by his observations of his mother's increased debility. Jamal's direct questioning, ongoing psycho-education, and an evolving trust in the social worker and clinical teams created the therapeutic environment wherein Lilie allowed some of Jamal's questions to be answered.

Lilie suffered a pathological fracture of the humerus while being moved by the staff she had come to trust and depend on as she became more disabled. This crisis event occurred amidst subtle signs of an emerging delirium that had not been recognized and created a crisis of relationship and trust with Lilie reporting to family that staff had hurt her and were withholding pain medications. This accusation caused suffering and anger both in the family system and the professional caregivers who cared deeply for Lilie. As the delirium was recognized, pharmacotherapy was initiated. A family meeting was organized to assist family and staff to consider the influence of the delirium on Lilie's perceptions and interpretations of the intent and meaning of staff's behaviours. Lilie's attribution of intentional harm on the part of staff became better understood when days before she died she spontaneously shared with the social worker 'woman to woman' that she had been physically abused by her former husband, an aspect of personal history that had been held private and protected.

Conclusion

Social workers practise in diverse settings and have the opportunity to move palliative care values and processes beyond hospitals and hospices to nursing homes, prisons, and senior centres. While most patients and families grasp the role of physicians, nurses, and chaplains, the functions of social work in health care is often less clear. Palliative care social work skills are a rich opportunity to serve patients, families, teams, and institutions. While social work clinicians may practise from different theoretical models, the work of discovering the individual's perception of their experience is universal. Rather than *informing*, 'starting where the client is' means that we invite patients and families to share what *they* see, their perceptions as well as the meaning they attribute to what has happened in their lives. Listening to the views of others is a primary focus for the social work discipline whose impact is anchored in the critical thinking that informs communication and the interventions they choose.

Social work clinicians whether engaged in direct practice, programme planning, teaching, or research now have access to a burgeoning literature, learning resources, competencies, leaders, and advocates to continue the reciprocal process on learning and enriching the shared work of palliative care. Patients and families living with life-threatening illness are amongst the most vulnerable both to our power and to the skills and compassion we bring to their care. This is a compelling ethical and moral mandate to be the best that we can be.

Online materials

Additional online materials and complete references for this chapter are available online at <http://www.oxfordmedicine.com>.

References

Aitken-Swan, J.(1959). Nursing the late cancer patient at home; The family's impressions. *The Practitioner*, 183, 64-65.

Altilio, T. and Otis-Green, S. (eds.) (2011). *Oxford Textbook of Palliative Social Work*. New York: Oxford University Press.

Azoulay, E., Pochard, F., Kentish-Barnes, N., et al. (2005). Risk of post-traumatic stress symptoms in family members of intensive care unit patients. *American Journal of Respiratory Critical Care*, 171(9), 987–994.

Beresford, P., Adshead, L., and Croft, S. (2007). *Palliative Care, Social Work and Service Users: Making Life Possible*. Philadelphia, PA: Jessica Kingsley Publishers.

Bosma, H., Johnston, M. and Cadell, S., et al. (2009) Creating social work competencies for practice in hospice palliative care. *Palliative Medicine*, 23, 1–9.

Cagle, J.G., and Altilio, T. (2011). The social work role in pain and symptom management. In T. Altilio and S. Otis-Green (eds.) *Oxford Textbook of Palliative, Social Work*, pp. 271–286. New York: Oxford University Press.

Cohen Feinberg, I., Kawashima, M., and Asch, S.M. (2011). Communication with families facing life-threatening illness: a research-based model for family conferences. *Journal of Palliative Medicine*, 14(4), 421–427.

Crawford, G.B. and Price, S.D. (2003). Team working: palliative care as a model of interdisciplinary practice. *Medical Journal of Australia*, 179(6 Suppl.), S32–34.

Gehlert, S. (2012). The conceptual underpinnings of social work in health care. In S. Gehlert and T.A. Browne (eds.) *Handbook of Health Social Work*, pp. 3–20. Hoboken, NJ: John Wiley and Sons, Inc.

International Federation of Social Workers and International Association of Schools of Social Work (2004). *Ethics in Social Work, Statement of Principles*. Available at: <http://www.iassw-aiets.org/uploads/file/20130506_Ethics%20in%20Social%20Work,%20Statement,%20IFSW,%20IASSW,%202004.pdf>.

Kemp, C. (2005). Cultural issues in Palliative Care. *Seminars in Oncology Nursing*, 21(1), 44–52.

McCormick, A.J. (2011). Palliative care social work in the intensive care unit. In T. Altilio and S. Otis-Green. (eds.) *Oxford Textbook of Palliative Social Work*, pp. 53–62. New York: Oxford University Press.

McCormick, A.J., Engelberg, R., and Curtis, J.R. (2007). Social workers in palliative care: Assessing activities and barriers in the intensive care unit. *Journal of Palliative Medicine*, 10(4), 929–937

National Association of Social Workers (NASW) (2004). Standards for palliative and end-of-life care. [Online] Available at: <http://www.socialworkers.org/practice/bereavement/standards/standards0504New.pdf>.

Raymer, M., and Gardia, G. (2007). *What Social Workers Do: A Guide to Social Work in Hospice and Palliative Care*. Alexandria, VA: NHPCO.

Saunders, C. (2001). Social work and palliative care—the early history. *British Journal of Social Work*, 31, 791–799.

Walsh, K. and Hedlund, S. (2011). Mental health risk in palliative care: the social work role. In T. Altilio and S. Otis-Green (eds.) *Oxford Textbook of Palliative Social Work*, pp. 181–191. New York: Oxford University Press.

World Health Organization (n.d.). *WHO Definition of Palliative Care.* [Online] Available at: <http://www.who.int/cancer/palliative/definition/en/>.

Wright, A., Zhang, B., Ray, A., *et al.* (2008). Associations between end of life discussions, patient mental health, medical care near death and caregiver bereavement adjustment. *Journal of the American Medical Association*, 300(14), 1665–1673.

Young-Laing, B. (2009). A critique of Rothman's and other standard community organizing models: toward developing a culturally proficient community organizing framework. *Community Development*, 40(1), 20–36.

The role of the chaplain in palliative care

George Handzo and Christina M. Puchalski

Introduction to the role of the chaplain in palliative care

Spiritual care is an essential domain of palliative care (National Consensus Project, 2004). Spirituality is the essence of one's humanity and therefore a key factor in how people cope with illness and find healing and a sense of coherence (Norris et al., 2013). As Teilhard de Chardin wrote, 'We are not human beings having a spiritual experience; we are spiritual beings have a human experience' (de Chardin, 1976). This is why spiritual care and chaplaincy exist in health care and particularly in palliative care. Health care was founded on compassionate principles with attention to the whole person and emphasis on healing. In the twentieth century, with the rise in science and technology, the care of the patient became more focused on disease and cure. Today, health care is reclaiming its holistic roots, recognizing that the care of the patient requires attention to all dimensions of the patient's life—body, mind, and spirit. Nowhere is this truer than in the practice of palliative and end-of-life care.

Palliative care, as defined by the World Health Organization, 'is an approach that improves the quality of life of patients and their families facing the problems associated with life-threatening illness, through the prevention and relief of suffering by means of early identification and impeccable assessment and treatment of pain and other problems, physical, psychosocial, and spiritual' (World Health Organization, n.d.). This definition is notable for including spirituality as a potential area for diagnosis and treatment. Furthermore, the concept of suffering is included and embraces not just physical pain but also spiritual and existential domains. Thus, palliative care done well must include and take into account the spiritual dimension of the patient, the family, and, we would argue, the clinicians and other caregivers.

In 2004, the National Consensus Project for Quality Palliative Care was created as a task force of the American Academy of Hospice and Palliative Medicine to define and promote clinical practice guidelines for quality palliative care (National Consensus Project, 2004). It determined that spiritual, existential, and religious care is a required domain of care. However, in practice, clinicians did not know how to implement such care. Was this care only to be done by clergy or chaplains? What was the role of other clinicians? To address this issue, a National Consensus Conference (NCC), Improving the Dimension of Spiritual Care within Palliative Care, convened in 2009 (Puchalski et al., 2009). The consensus group developed models and guidelines for interprofessional spiritual care. It determined that all members of the health care team are responsible for addressing patients' spiritual issues within the biopsychosocial-spiritual framework (Sulmasy, 2002). The conference highlighted the importance of board-certified or board-eligible chaplains as the spiritual care experts and essential members of palliative care and other care teams.

The NCC also highlighted the role of spirituality as part of the professional development of all clinicians. Teilhard de Chardin (1976) reminds us that we are all spiritual beings no matter what our role is in health care. The spirituality of the care professional can impact how that person understands health and illness and how they interact with their patients. In fact, as was proposed in the NCC, healing occurs within the context of the relationship between clinician and patient and between chaplain and patient. Spiritual care recognizes this key element of care—the compassionate and caring relationship between any clinician/chaplain and patient is central to whole person care.

Background

The strong contribution of spirituality and religion to health is well documented (Jenkins and Paragament, 1995; Cohen et al., 1996; Tsevat et al., 1999; George et al., 2000; Gail and Comblatt, 2002; Puchalski, 2008; Koenig et al., 2012). Spirituality and religion have also been documented as strong contributors to how people cope with illness and suffering (Pargament, 1997; Balboni et al., 2007; Delgado-Guay et al., 2011). Traditionally, questions have surrounded the application of this knowledge and have focused on the issue of whether spiritual care or spiritual interventions in the process of delivering health care make a difference in coping or whether spirituality is so entwined in the humanity of all people that it is impervious to any intervention, especially during times of stress. There has now been significant research that provides evidence that providing for spiritual and religious needs yields benefits both to the patient and to the health care system. For example, Balboni and colleagues (2011) found that the majority of patients with advanced cancer report a significant spiritual issue. When patients' spiritual needs were met during hospital care, they were less likely to die in an intensive care unit and likely to spend more time in hospice (Balboni et al., 2011).

Another study found that 41% of inpatients desired a discussion of religious/spiritual (R/S) concerns while hospitalized, but only half reported having such a discussion. Overall, 32% of inpatients reported having a discussion of their religious/spiritual concerns.

Religious patients and those experiencing more severe pain were more likely both to desire and to have discussions of spiritual concerns. Patients who had discussions of religious/spiritual concerns were more likely to rate their care at the highest level on four different measures of patient satisfaction, regardless of whether or not they said they had desired such a discussion (Williams et al., 2011). Ai and colleagues found strong evidence for a link between spiritual struggle and poor health outcomes (Ai et al., 2010). Their work suggests that addressing spiritual struggle with patients might improve health-care outcomes.

While the relationship of spirituality and health has long been generally accepted and is now increasingly documented quantitatively, the issue of if and how to best address religious and spiritual concerns has not been clear. Historically, and often still today, the care of religious and spiritual needs has been delegated to faith communities. This model of care, which is still widely used, while providing for the needs of those who belong to organized religious communities, has several deficiencies. Generally, no care is provided for those who do not identify with an organized religious community (Fitchett et al., 2000). One study documented that only 42% of hospitalized patients could identify a spiritual counsellor to whom they could turn (Sivan et al., 1996). Furthermore, the diversity of religious and cultural backgrounds in many health-care settings has increased to the point where people of many groups are not having even their religious needs met.

To address some of these deficiencies there has been a rise in professional chaplaincy care. Recent work comparing chaplaincy care in the United States, the United Kingdom, and Australia concluded that chaplaincy practice in all three countries is moving towards a more multifaith, patient-centred model which, coincidentally, is much more aligned with the preferred role of chaplaincy in palliative care (Orton, 2008). In general, clergy provide religious-specific care while chaplains provide spiritual care within a medical setting, allowing chaplains to meet the needs of religious and non-religious patients and also to extend spiritual care to issues specifically related to medical care, for example, advance directives, family meetings, and addressing spiritual distress in the context of illness.

Training for chaplains

To support this new model, professional chaplains have been clinically and academically trained. In North America, especially the United States, the training for chaplains is foundationally a clinical training programme, clinical pastoral education (CPE), whereas the foundational training for chaplains in Europe is received in an academic setting. Chaplains in North America have the opportunity to become 'board certified' based on a set of clinical competencies. CPE is conducted in clinical settings and focuses on training chaplains in listening skills, forming relationships in order to support patients, and functioning as a member of the health-care team. Chaplains are taught to minister to patients of any faith or no faith as opposed to the traditional model of ministering only to patients of the chaplain's own faith tradition. Since 2013, North American chaplains are able to obtain subspecialty certification in palliative care chaplaincy. In North America, certified chaplains subscribe to a Code of Ethics which, among other things, prohibits proselytizing (Association of Professional Chaplains, 2000). The net result of this training is to recognize and distinguish professional health-care chaplaincy as a discipline separate from other forms of ministry.

Current standards for health-care chaplaincy

The context for chaplaincy in Europe, North America, and Australia can seem different from each other, but most regions of the world where health-care chaplaincy is fairly well developed have standards of practice that are largely congruent (European Network of Health Care Chaplains, 2002; Australian Health and Wellness Association, 2004; College of Health Care Chaplains, 2007; Association of Professional Chaplains, 2009), though the United States and Australia are more particular and clinically oriented.

Spiritual care in palliative care

Chaplaincy is a key component of the interprofessional spiritual care model developed at the NCC in 2009 (Puchalski et al., 2009). Spiritual care in palliative care is based on several premises:

- All staff will be trained in and participate in spiritual care at some level appropriate to their discipline.

- All patients will have spiritual care fully integrated into their care through spiritual screening, spiritual history, a spiritual assessment if indicated, and the inclusion of spiritual needs in their care plan.

- A professional chaplain with specific training in delivering multifaith as well as non-faith specific spiritual care in palliative care will be the spiritual care lead on the team.

Definitions

One of the major issues in this area of practice is a lack of clear definitions. One of the tasks of the NCC on Spiritual Care in Palliative Care in 2009 was to develop a consensus definition of spirituality:

> Spirituality is the aspect of humanity that refers to the way individuals seek and express meaning and purpose and the way they experience their connectedness to the moment, to self, to others, to nature, and to the significant or sacred. (Puchalski et al., 2009, p. 887)

This definition was agreed to by a large group from many faith and non-faith traditions and philosophical backgrounds and disciplines. The focus on 'meaning and purpose' and 'connectedness' are themes in most definitions of spirituality.

Religion is one expression of spirituality:

> Religion is an organized system of beliefs, practices, rituals, and symbols designated (a) to facilitate closeness to the sacred or transcendent (God, higher power, or ultimate truth/reality), and (b) to foster understanding of one's relationship and responsibility to others living in a community. (Koenig et al., 2001, p. 18)

But there are other expressions including nature, art, and humanism, among others.

Another ambiguity in the field is the frequent conflation of 'spiritual care', 'chaplaincy care', and 'pastoral care'. The US Association of Professional Chaplains and others have adopted the following distinctive definitions:

Spiritual care

> Interventions, individual or communal, that facilitate the ability to express the integration of the body, mind, and spirit to achieve

wholeness, health, and a sense of connection to self, others, and[/or] a higher power. (Health Ministries Association, 2005)

Chaplaincy care

Care provided by a board certified chaplain or by a student in an accredited clinical pastoral education program, e.g., ACPE. Examples of such care include emotional, spiritual, religious, pastoral, ethical, and/or existential care. (Peery, 2009)

Pastoral care is now understood as a term that comes out of the Christian tradition and generally describes the care given by a faith leader to members of his or her community (LaRocca-Pitts, 2006). As such, it is inconsistent with the current multifaith emphasis.

All members of the health-care team participate in spiritual care to some degree as they all participate in psychosocial and to some degree physical care. Chaplaincy care encompasses those functions which require the spiritual care specialist on the team with the degree of training required. Pastoral care under this definition could be part of what the particular chaplain does when he/she is caring for people from his/her own faith tradition. Otherwise, it is generally part of what Christian clergy do when they care for their own congregants. Pastoral care is still the term used in many parts of the world to encompass what are here called chaplaincy care and maybe even spiritual care. We believe that the definitions proposed here, besides being more commonly accepted, clear some confusion and are useful to the present model and the principles of palliative care.

Model for chaplaincy in palliative care

In the model of interprofessional spiritual care, the role of the chaplain is to be spiritual care lead on the team and, as such, the spiritual care specialist (Handzo and Koenig, 2004). All other members of the team are spiritual care generalists. Thus, social workers would be spiritual care generalists just as chaplains are also emotional care generalists. However, spiritual issues requiring complicated interventions would be referred to the chaplain just as social/emotional issues requiring complicated interventions would be referred to the social worker. This model for spiritual care is aligned with other processes of clinical care.

In a typical case, a patient entering a health-care facility would be screened for spiritual distress along with the rest of his or her screening processes. An algorithm would govern whether or not the patient is referred to a chaplain as a result of that screening. The patient would also receive a spiritual history as part of their total history by the clinicians who develop treatment or care plans. The goal of the spiritual history would be to help the clinician understand their patient in a whole-person context, to identify spiritual resources of strength, and to identify spiritual distress.

Protocols may be helpful to determine whether the patient needs a referral to a chaplain or whether any spiritual needs could be addressed directly by the clinician. Those patients whose screening or history indicates the possibility of spiritual distress would receive a full spiritual assessment by a professional, trained chaplain. The patient's spiritual needs would be included in the patient's treatment or care plan and the patient's discharge plan. This model aligns with current best practice

in health-care chaplaincy (Handzo, 2006; Peery, 2012) as well as best practice in spiritual care in palliative care (Puchalski et al., 2009).

Since the chaplain is the lead on this process, it is the chaplain's responsibility to design the infrastructure that supports this process, oversee its integration, and make sure that other staff are fully trained in its use. The chaplain needs to institute and continually improve systems for spiritual screening, history taking, and assessment including diagnoses, spiritual treatment, and discharge plans.

Spiritual screening

If chaplaincy resources are going to be focused on patients in spiritual need rather than simply those who want to see a chaplain, the goal should be to set up systems which allow chaplains to connect with those in distress as quickly as possible.

The key to this strategy is an effective screen for spiritual distress on admission. According to Fitchett and Canada (2010), screening utilizes one or two questions to find out whether a patient is experiencing serious religious or spiritual distress that then requires an immediate referral to a chaplain.

In the United States, spiritual and religious screening questions are often restricted to asking how the patient wants their religion listed and whether they want to see a chaplain. These questions are focused on identifying those who want to see a chaplain as opposed to those who need to see a chaplain. There is some indication that those with spiritual distress are less likely to ask for a chaplain than others (Fitchett, 1999). For these reasons, the question, 'Do you want to see a chaplain?' should not be used.

The screening questions devised and tested by Fitchett and Risk (2009) are recommended. At this time, they are the only questions with a published validation study (see Table 4.5.1).

Another possible screen is the one question, 'Are you at peace?' tested by Steinhauser and her colleagues (2006). However, while this screen shows some promise in identifying spiritual distress, it has only been tested with patients at the end of life and only as a research tool.

Table 4.5.1 Screening questions

The screening questions are:	
1.	Is religion/spirituality important to you as you cope with your illness? (Yes/No)
2. (If 'yes' to #1)	How much strength/comfort do you get from your religion/spirituality right now?
	a. all that I need
	b. somewhat less than I need
	c. much less than I need
	d. none at all
	Answers 'c' or 'd' should trigger an automatic referral to chaplaincy
3. (If 'no' to #1)	Has there ever been a time when religion and spirituality was important to you? (Yes/No)
	'Yes' should trigger an automatic referral to chaplaincy

Source: data from Fitchett, G and Risk, J. L., Screening for spiritual struggle, *Journal of Pastoral Care and Counseling*, Volume 62, Issue 1–2, pp. 1–11, Copyright © 2009.

The role of the chaplain in setting up the screening process is to educate staff about why these questions are important and how to make referrals. Given the nature of the screen, there is no need for staff to be trained in clinically interpreting screening results.

Spiritual history

Like screening, history taking is a routine part of admitting a patient to a hospital. Standards for physicians, nurses, and others on the team support the inclusion of spirituality as part of the clinical history. For instance, the American College of Physicians notes that it is the physician's responsibility to attend to all dimensions of the patient's suffering—the psychosocial and spiritual suffering as well as the physical (Karlawish et al., 1999; Lo et al., 1999). As discussed in the NCC, attending to spiritual suffering requires inquiry into spirituality of patients and thus within the clinical history a spiritual history should be included. The history should include an assessment of spiritual symptoms as well. Up until recently, one barrier to this inclusion has been the lack of an evidence-informed spiritual history tool. One history tool, FICA (Puchalski, 2006; Puchalski and Romer, 2000), which is widely used in different clinical settings, has been reviewed (Borneman et al., 2010). The basic format of the FICA tool is shown in Table 4.5.2.

In practice, some primary caregivers feel uncomfortable talking to patients about this domain of the patient's life. Currently this tool is used widely in clinical settings by clinicians who do clinical histories and develop treatment plans. Some chaplains utilize the tool but it is intended for physicians, nurses, social workers, physical therapists, and so on.

The majority of medical schools in the United States have spiritual history taking as part of their curriculum and there is growing interest internationally in this area (Puchalski et al., 2012). On health-care teams the professional chaplain should be involved in ongoing education on spiritual issues with physicians, nurse practitioners, and others who take histories in how to talk to patients about these issues. Most patients want their caregivers

Table 4.5.2 Spiritual history tool

F	'Do you consider yourself spiritual or religious?' or 'Do you have spiritual beliefs that help you cope with stress?' If the patient responds 'No,' the health care provider might ask, 'What gives your life meaning?' Sometimes patients respond with answers such as family, career, or nature
I	'What importance does your faith or belief have in our life? Have your beliefs influenced how you take care of yourself in this illness? What role do your beliefs play in regaining your health?'
C	'Are you part of a spiritual or religious community? Is this of support to you and how? Is there a group of people you really love or who are important to you?' Communities such as churches, temples, and mosques, or a group of like-minded friends can serve as strong support systems for some patients
A	'How would you like me, your healthcare provider, to address these issues in your healthcare?'

Reproduced from The George Washington Institute for Spirituality and Health, *FICA Spiritual History Tool*, available from http://smhs.gwu.edu/gwish/clinical/fica/spiritual-history-tool, Copyright © C. Puchalski, with permission of the author.

to take account of their religious and spiritual beliefs and values in planning their care as was shown in the FICA validation study (Borneman et al., 2010). Numerous surveys have also demonstrated that the majority of patients want their physicians to address patients' spirituality and integrate it into patients' treatment plans (Ehman et al., 1999; McCord et al., 2004). Training materials are available for the FICA tool through the George Washington Institute for Spirituality and Health (<http://www.gwish.org>).

Diagnostic categories

The NCC recommended that all clinicians respond to spiritual distress with the same intensity as to physical pain (Puchalski et al., 2009). The NCC further recommended diagnostic categories for spiritual distress and developing a taxonomy for spiritual distress, including specific and tested treatment plans.

As in other areas of clinical care, a clinician can suggest a preliminary diagnosis based on that clinician's spiritual history. This diagnosis would drive a referral, in this case, to the professional chaplain. The chaplain, like any other specialist, would amend or confirm the diagnosis as warranted based on that chaplain's spiritual assessment.

One set of diagnoses has been posited in the National Comprehensive Cancer Center's Distress Management Guidelines (National Comprehensive Cancer Network, 2012). These guidelines have been vetted yearly for over a decade with providers including many chaplains at NCCN member institutions and deemed appropriate. The diagnoses include:

- guilt
- hopelessness
- grief
- concerns about death and afterlife
- conflicted or challenged belief system
- loss of faith/doubts
- concerns about meaning/purpose in life
- concerns about relationship to deity
- conflict between religious beliefs and recommended treatment
- conflict with/loss of religious community.

Spiritual assessment

Fitchett and Canada (2010) define a spiritual assessment as:

A more extensive [in-depth, on-going] process of active listening to a patient's story as it unfolds in a relationship with a professional chaplain and summarizing the needs and resources that emerge in that process. The summary includes a spiritual care plan with expected outcomes which should be communicated to the rest of the treatment team.

There is currently no widely accepted or validated chaplain spiritual assessment tool. Further, while whatever outline is used needs to cover some basic issues, the essential requirement is for all chaplains and chaplaincy students within an institution to use the same format so that it can be integrated into the medical record and so other staff learn what to expect from a chaplain note.

One option for assessment is presented by Brent Peery (2012) and is based on outcome-oriented chaplaincy. This assessment includes the following:

◆ Needs: relationship with God, support system, meaning/determinism, forgiveness, advance care planning, emotional/relational issues, grieving, other spiritual needs

◆ Hopes: relationship with God, forgiveness, God as comforter, support

◆ Resources: relationship with God, religious/spiritual practices, community support, other.

Another similar system is proposed by Donovan (2012). Pruyser (1976) and Fitchett (2002) have proposed more extensive outlines which have been extensively used over the years.

An outline of issues that could be covered in a spiritual assessment by a chaplain would include the following:

◆ Determinism/meaning:
  • Is everything that happens determined by God?
  • If not, how/why do 'bad things' happen?
  • How does this cause translate into meaning?
  • Differentiating illness as gift or punishment

◆ Grief:
  • Spiritual/existential losses
  • Loss of sense of immortality
  • Loss of sense that God will protect you from all harm

◆ Despair:
  • Rooted in sense of abandonment/hopelessness
  • God does not let 'bad things happen to good people'

◆ God the Judge versus God the Comforter:
  • Is God a 'judging' God?
  • Does God punish people while they are still alive?
  • Or is God primarily a 'comforting' God?
  • Is God's primary role to support people through hard times?

◆ Forgiveness:
  • Sin is what the patient perceives it to be
  • Important to not impose caregiver values and beliefs
  • Religions have distinct ways of expiating sin
  • Explore forgiveness ritual
  • Suffering itself may be seen as a way to 'work off' sins.

Referrals to chaplains

As is done with many other disciplines, referrals to a chaplain in some circumstances should be automatic and even automated if that is possible. The minimal standard in any circumstance is for the chaplain to see every patient who evidences spiritual distress on screening or history. If the palliative care service is small enough and/or the chaplaincy coverage is robust enough, any referral to the palliative care service can automatically generate a referral to the chaplain. This situation does not imply that spiritual screening

or history taking do not need to be done. As with other services, screening functions to direct the chaplain to those with significant need and the history still serves to help the primary care provider come to know the patient in all domains. In any case, the patient and family can refuse the chaplain. However, the chaplain's visit should always be presented as a regular service that is part of what palliative care offers rather than an add-on that is not necessarily central to the team's scope of practice. The inclusion of the chaplain should always be considered when planning a patient/family meeting to discuss care plans and in planning interventions with especially disruptive families.

Tasks of the chaplain

While chaplains certainly are the specialist in helping patients, families, and staff discover and use their spiritual and religious resources in the service of their healing, their most basic skill is listening and fostering clear communication. Learning to listen without bias and reflect what the patient or family member is saying accurately is a central focus of CPE. Chaplains are often regarded by patients and family members as neutral parties. Some options for leveraging this training and skill include the following:

◆ Facilitating goals of care discussions/family meetings
◆ Facilitating palliative care meetings
◆ Facilitating communication when bad news is being delivered
◆ Being present with family members after a death.

In the United States, the chaplain is often regarded as the 'culture broker' on the team (Joint Commission, 2006). As the culture broker, the chaplain assists the patient, family, and health-care team bridge any cultural, ethnic, or religious issue which may hinder communication between and among them. As experts in helping people identify and articulate their beliefs and values, chaplains have expertise in identifying and helping teams accommodate the cultural beliefs and practices families have. It is also part of the chaplain's role to be aware of the religious resources in the community which can be called on as needed.

As already mentioned, the chaplain should be involved in educating other staff on spiritual and religious issues including training staff on administering spiritual screening and spiritual history protocols. Staff education is also appropriate before major religious holidays which might be observed by patients and families so that staff know what to expect in terms of patient and family customs, diet, and other special activities around the particular holiday. The chaplain also provides spiritual care to the clinical team. Clinicians can be affected by the stress of caring for ill patients, conflicts about providing care to patients that clinicians might feel is 'futile', and burnout from over-caring. Spirituality is a critical aspect of clinicians' professional development (Puchalski et al., 2009; Puchalski and Guenther, 2012) because it underlies the vocation clinicians have to service others but it also provides internal resources for support and reflection for clinicians. Chaplains are important resources to clinicians and other caregivers.

Chaplains are unique in that, like community clergy, they are charged with the professional care of those in their own community. That is, the chaplain is the chaplain to the staff as well as to the patients and families (Association of Professional Chaplains, 2009). In this role, the chaplain can help the team, individually and as a group, process its own spiritual issues and help use its spiritual strengths to provide better care (Puchalski et al., 2009). These activities could include memorial services, meditations as part of staff meetings, spirituality groups for staff, debriefing, and individual counselling.

Chaplain interventions

There is no accepted taxonomy of chaplaincy interventions with patients and families especially as tied to assessments and outcomes. Peery (2012) has proposed an extensive list which covers the universe of what chaplains do. Some research on a selected population also exists (Handzo et al., 2008). As indicated earlier, much of what chaplains do falls under the general rubric of reflective listening and emotional support. Professional chaplains do not generally engage in teaching patients about belief unless the patient specifically asks for it. Any intervention a chaplain would make under the broad category of counselling is, likewise, focused on helping the patients and family members come to their own understandings and conclusions rather than giving them answers.

The chaplain's skill in communication and emphasis on listening and non-judgemental presence comes into play in helping patients and caregivers deal with spiritual distress. The chaplain's primary goal in these situations is to help the patient find their own meaning and discover their own resources through listening to and reflecting their individual life story. The chaplain might use appropriate readings or music to assist in this process. For patients who would like ongoing counselling, the chaplain might refer to community resources such as community clergy, pastoral counsellors, or spiritual directors.

All chaplains are also trained in religious interventions. These fall into two categories. The first is those that the chaplain does as a clergyperson with a person of his or her own faith group. In this case, the chaplain is operating as a clergyperson of that faith group. The second group includes interventions which do not necessarily require the chaplain and the patient to be of the same faith group. For instance, professional chaplains are trained to pray with people of any faith. They also can often read from the patient's sacred texts or help the patient find music or other spiritual resources. Chaplains also occasionally officiate at weddings and funerals—sometimes for patients of their own faith and sometimes not.

Conclusion

Spirituality has been shown to be important in the care of patients, especially those with serious and chronic illness. Data shows an impact of spirituality as well as religious beliefs and practices on health-care outcomes as well as medical decision-making. Spiritual care also describes a whole-person model of care that supports the provision of respectful, compassionate care that honours the inherent dignity of all who receive as well as provide care. Thus spirituality is important for patients as well as family and professional caregivers. Standards for palliative care include spiritual care as a required domain of palliative care. Models and recommendations have been developed to facilitate interprofessional spiritual care where all members of the team attend to the spiritual issues of patients with the professional chaplain being the expert in spiritual care. Health-care providers should be performing a spiritual screening or history with patients to help identify the need for chaplain referral, patient and family spiritual distress or suffering, as well as patient and family spiritual resources of strength. Chaplains function as the spiritual care lead on the team. They do a more intensive assessment and help clinicians with diagnosis of spiritual distress as well as treatment plans regarding spirituality. Chaplains work with patients and families to help them with their spiritual distress or their spiritual issues. Chaplains also provide spiritual care to the team. Chaplains are an essential member of the interdisciplinary care team and should be integrated on all palliative care teams.

Online materials

Complete references for this chapter are available online at <http://www.oxfordmedicine.com>.

References

Ai, A.L., Pargament, K.I., Kronfol, Z., Tice, T.N., and Appel, H. (2010). Pathways to post-operative hostility in cardiac patients: mediation of coping, spiritual struggle and interleukin-6. *Journal of Health Psychology*, 15, 186–195.

Association of Professional Chaplains (2009). *Standards of Practice for Professional Chaplains in Acute Care*. [Online] Available at: <http://www.professionalchaplains.org/files/professional_standards/standards_of_practice/standards_practice_professional_chaplains_acute_care.pdf>.

Balboni, T., Balboni, M., Paulk, M., *et al.* (2011). Support of cancer patients' spiritual needs and associations with medical care costs at the end of life. *Cancer*, 117(23), 5383–5391.

Borneman T., Ferrell B., and Puchalski C. (2010). Evaluation of the FICA tool for spiritual assessment. *Journal of Pain and Symptom Management*, 20(2), 163–173.

Delgado-Guay, M., Hui, D., Parsons, H., *et al.* (2011). Spirituality, religiosity, and spiritual pain in advanced cancer patients. *Journal of Pain and Symptom Management*, 41(6), 986–994.

Donovan, D.W. (2012). Assessments. In S. Roberts (ed.) *Professional Spiritual and Pastoral Care: A Practical Clergy and Chaplain's Handbook*, pp 42–60. Woodstock, VT: Skylight Paths Publishing.

Ehman, J.W., Ott, B.B., Short, T.H., Ciampa, R.C., Hansen-Flaschen, J. (1999). Do patients want physicians to inquire about their spiritual or religious beliefs if they become gravely ill? *Archives of Internal Medicine*, 159(15), 1803–1806.

Fitchett, G. (1999). Screening for spiritual risk. *Chaplaincy Today*, 15(1), 2–12.

Fitchett, G. (2002). *Assessing Spiritual Needs: A Guide for Caregivers*. Lima, OH: Academic Renewal Press.

Fitchett, G. and Canada, A. L. (2010). The role of religion/spirituality in coping with cancer: evidence, assessment, and intervention. In J.C. Holland (ed.) *Psycho-Oncology* (2nd ed.), pp. 440–446. New York: Oxford University Press.

Fitchett, G., Meyer, P.M., and Burton, L.A. (2000). Spiritual care in hospital: who requests it? Who needs it? *Journal of Pastoral Care*, 54(2), 173–186.

Fitchett, G. and Risk, J.L. (2009). Screening for spiritual struggle. *Journal of Pastoral Care and Counseling*, 62(1, 2), 1–11.

George, L.K., Larson, D.B, Koenig, H.G., and McCullough, M.E. (2000). Spirituality and health: what we know, what we need to know. *Journal of Social and Clinical Psychology*, 19(1), 102–116.

Handzo, G. (2006). Best practices in professional pastoral care. *Southern Medical Journal*, 99(6), 663–664.

Handzo, G.F., Flannelly, K.J., Kudler, T., *et al.* (2008). What do chaplains really do? II. Interventions in the New York Chaplaincy Study. *Journal of Health Care Chaplaincy*, 14(1), 39–56.

Handzo, G.F. and Koenig, H.G. (2004). Spiritual care: whose job is it anyway? *Southern Medical Journal*, 97(12), 1242–1244.

Jenkins, P.A. and Pargament, K.I. (1995). Religion and spirituality as resources for coping with cancer. *Journal of Psychosocial Oncology*, 13, 51–75.

Joint Commission Publications (2006). *Providing Cultural and Linguistically Competent Care*. Oak Brook, IL: Joint Commission Publications.

Karlawish, J., Quill, T., and Meier, D. (1999). A consensus-based approach to providing palliative care to patients who lack decision-making capacity. ACP-ASIM end-of-life care consensus panel. *Annals of Internal Medicine*, 130, 835–840.

Koenig, H.G., King, D.E., and Carson, V.B. (2012). *Handbook of Religion and Health* (2nd ed.). Oxford: Oxford University Press.

Lo, B., Quill, T., and Tulsky, J. (1999). Discussing palliative care with patients. ACP-ASIM end-of-life care consensus panel. *Annals of Internal Medicine*, 130, 744–749.

McCord, G., Gilchrist, V.I., Grossman, S.D., *et al.* (2004). Discussing spiritual issues with patients: a rational and ethical approach. *Annals of Internal Medicine*, 2(4), 356–361.

National Comprehensive Cancer Network (2012). *Distress Management Guidelines*. [Online] Available at: <http://www.nccn.org/professionals/physician_gls/f_guidelines.asp>.

National Consensus Project (2004). *Clinical Practice Guidelines for Quality Palliative Care*. [Online] Available at: <http://www.national-consensusproject.org/Guidelines_Download2.aspx>.

Norris, L., Walseman K., and Puchalski, C.M. (2013). Communicating about spiritual issues with cancer patients. In A. Surbone, M. Zwitter, M. Rajer, and R. Stiefel (eds.) *New Challenges in Communication with Cancer Patients*, pp. 91–104. New York: Springer.

Orton, M. (2008). Emerging best practice pastoral care in the UK, USA and Australia. *Australian Journal of Pastoral Care and Health*, 2(2), 1–28.

Pargament, K.I. (1997). *The Psychology of Religion and Coping: Theory, Research, Practice*. New York: The Guildford Press.

Peery, B. (2012). Outcome oriented chaplaincy: intentional caring. In S. Roberts (ed.) *Professional Spiritual and Pastoral Care: A Practical Clergy and Chaplain's Handbook*, pp. 342–361. Woodstock, VT: Skylight Paths Publishing.

Pruyser, P. (1976). *The Minister as Diagnostician*. Philadelphia, PA: Westminster, John Knox Press.

Puchalski, C. (2006). Spiritual assessment in clinical practice. *Psychiatric Annals*, 36(3), 150–155.

Puchalski, C. and Guenther, M. (2012). Restoration and re-creation: spirituality in the lives of healthcare professionals. *US National Library of Medicine National Institutes of Health*, 6(2), 254–258.

Puchalski, C. and Romer, A.L. (2000). Taking a spiritual history allows clinicians to understand patients more fully. *Journal of Palliative Medicine*, 3(1), 129–137.

Puchalski, C.M., Virani, R., Ferrell, B., *et al.* (2009). Improving the quality of spiritual care as a dimension of palliative care. *Journal of Palliative Medicine*, 12(10), 885–904.

Sivan, A., Fitchett, G., and Burton, L. (1996). Hospitalized psychiatric and medical patients and the clergy. *Journal of Religion and Health*, 36(3), 455–467.

Sulmasy, D.P. (2002). A biopsychosocial-spiritual model for the care of patients at the end of life. *Gerontologist*, 42(3), 24–33.

Williams, J., Meltzer, D., Arora, V., Chung, G., and Curlin, F. (2011). Attention to inpatients' religious and spiritual concerns: predictors and association with patient satisfaction. *Journal of General Internal Medicine*, 26(11), 1265–1271.

4.6

Occupational therapy in palliative care

Jill Cooper and Nina Kite

Introduction: what occupational therapists do and where they work

Occupational therapy aims to help patients achieve their optimum independence in activities that are important to them by using specific treatments and interventions.

In day-to-day use the term 'occupation' refers to an individual's job. But in the context of occupational therapy, occupation refers to:

- self/personal care, which applies to all activities we carry out in order to look after ourselves
- productivity, which incorporates work-related roles and domestic activities
- leisure, which refers to hobbies, sports, and general interests (Hammell, 2009).

Within palliative care, occupational therapists work in a variety of settings including the hospital, community, and hospice and form a significant part of the interdisciplinary team (Squire, 2011). As health systems and resources develop and change, occupational therapy palliative care services are often focused more in the community (Kealey et al., 2005).

As well as playing a vital role in planning for safe discharge home and assessing and prescribing equipment to enable safety and independence, occupational therapists carry out treatment sessions to help patients manage their symptoms and be as independent as possible (Booth et al., 2011).

Occupational therapy services should be accessible for all patients with life-limiting diseases in all settings and at every stage of their illness.

Foundations underpinning occupational therapy

Occupational therapy interventions are underpinned by the following core skills:

- Collaboration with the patient: building a collaborative relationship with them that promotes reflection, autonomy, and engagement in the therapeutic process.
- Assessment: assessing and observing functional potential, limitations, ability, and needs, including the effects of physical and psychosocial environments.

- Enablement: enabling people to explore, achieve, and maintain balance in their activities of daily living in the areas of personal care, domestic, leisure, and productivity as described above.
- Problem-solving: identifying and solving problems in day-to-day life (also referred to as occupational performance).
- Using activity as a therapeutic tool: using activities to promote health, well-being, and function by analysing, selecting, synthesizing, adapting, grading, and applying activities for specific therapeutic purposes.
- Group work: planning, organizing, and leading activity groups.
- Environmental adaptation: analysing and adapting environments to increase function and social participation (Creek, 2003).

The foundations of occupational therapy are based within a person-centred approach. This involves the occupational therapist actively listening, encouraging the person to express their wishes and goals, and showing empathy to hear and understand their expectations of the service and points of view (Sumsion and Law, 2006). Overall, it involves working together to achieve what the person wants to achieve (Cooper, 2006).

In palliative care, this requires flexibility to reflect changing needs, for example, as a person becomes more fatigued and dependent, occupational therapy interventions may move away from teaching strategies to manage washing and dressing, and instead focus on liaising with social work or community colleagues to organize a package of care.

It is important to note that occupational therapy is symptom led rather than disease led. Although crisis intervention cannot always be avoided, the occupational therapist will work with the patient and carers to anticipate problems that may arise. The patient does not have to accept the advice or equipment at that early stage, but they will have been made aware of it and can contact the occupational therapist in the future if they deteriorate and require input.

Environment and equipment

The patient and their carers have to live within a physical, social, and emotional environment and great care needs to be taken when adjusting this to enable them to cope at home. For example, a patient's bedroom may be upstairs, but if they have extreme weakness or fatigue, they may not be able to manage the stairs.

Therefore, there might need to be environmental changes such as a patient living downstairs.

Whilst the occupational therapist often provides equipment to help patients manage at home, this must be carefully assessed so they are not cluttered with too much equipment. Apart from overloading them with too much, the risk of altering the environment has huge implications on how the rest of the family manage and how it will affect their memories of the patient's later stages of life at home (see Table 4.6.1).

Planning for safe discharge home

Higginson (2003) reported that of the 56% of palliative care patients who identify home as their preferred place of death, only

Table 4.6.1 Equipment and aids available following occupational therapy assessment, education on their use, and provision (Miller and Cooper, 2010)

Difficulty with	Possible aids and adaptations
Bed transfers	◆ Back rest to support patient in a sitting position ◆ Mattress variator to assist lying to sitting ◆ Leg lifter to enable the patient to lift legs into bed ◆ Blocks to raise bed height ◆ Use of sliding sheets for positioning and moving ◆ Specialist hospital profiling bed, electrically operated and generally required if nursing care is needed ◆ Hoist and slings for safe transfers
Toilet transfers	◆ Toilet seats of varying height and design that are safely fitted and removed ◆ Frames to fit around the toilet and provide patients with something to push up from ◆ Strategically placed grab rails ◆ Other equipment such as commode, male and female urinals
Bath or shower transfers	◆ Range of bathboards that can be easily fitted to assist with transfers ◆ Hydraulically operated bath seats which lift patients in and out of the bath ◆ Strategically placed grab rails ◆ Shower seats, either freestanding or wall-fixed
Chair transfers	◆ Range of blocks to raise chairs and settees ◆ High back, orthopaedic chair with firm armrests and of correct height for safe transfers ◆ Riser recliner armchair enabling patient to sit with legs elevated and sometimes with an option to help them stand from sitting
Transferring in/out of car	◆ Sliding boards may be appropriate here but require full individual assessment and training
Mobility	◆ Joint working with physiotherapist to establish safest mobility techniques ◆ Wheelchairs with detachable sides to enable sliding board transfers. Wheelchair must have correctly fitted and adjusted footrests heights, seat dimensions, and pressure cushion if required
Walking aids whilst carrying out daily activities	◆ If patient uses a frame or stick, they may need a caddy that fits to the frame so that they can carry items, or a trolley on which to carry them
Stairs	◆ Installation of addition handrails or banisters for safety ◆ Stairlifts can be hired or bought privately but this can be expensive and the occupational therapist needs to give advice on this. Social services grants are time-consuming and may not be appropriate ◆ Through-floor lifts are extremely expensive and disruptive when being fitted and it might more practicable to arrange one-floor living or 'micro environment'
Meal preparation	◆ Kitchen aids including jar openers, non-slip mats, specialist cutlery, and adapted crockery and equipment can help in maintaining safety in the kitchen
Personal care	◆ Long-handled equipment such as shoehorns and sponges can help the patient reach their lower extremities. Other adapted equipment helps with poor grip such as button hooks, elastic shoelaces, Velcro fastenings instead of zips and buttons
Manual handling	◆ Hoists, electric and manual, free standing, and ceiling track may be required for safe transfers ◆ Additional equipment includes sliding sheets and transfer boards ◆ All of these require annual training and specialist knowledge and skills
Specific difficulties: spinal cord compression, at risk of falls	◆ Assessment for safety in transfers, identifying need for equipment such as hoist, sling, pressure relief, sliding board, wheelchair and planning for a complex discharge to a suitable place of care if home is not feasible ◆ Falls risk requires assessment for actual and potential hazards and addressing the practical problems

26% achieve this. Enabling patients to die at home requires a well-coordinated, interprofessional team including the discharge coordinator, occupational therapist, ward staff, district nurse, and community support agencies. It is essential that the patient has as seamless a transition as possible between settings of care especially when returning home. This requires establishing what the patient and, separately, their carers want, liaising with community teams, and ordering all the equipment and services. It takes an enormous amount of time and effort by everyone, particularly for complex interventions.

The key responsibilities of the occupational therapist within discharge planning include assessment of the environment, either with or without the patient depending on the circumstances. This will identify access into the property, whether there are difficult steps or doorways, and how professionals and carers will be able to get in if the patient cannot answer the door. The essential facilities such as toilet, washing, and sleeping areas are assessed and whether equipment is required to make returning home feasible.

Meeting carers and families in their own homes often enables them to disclose information which they would not otherwise share with health-care professionals. This helps in establishing the trust and rapport to support and work with them as well as establishing how the services can meet their requirements.

If all the assessments and arrangements have taken place before a hospital admission or discharge is required, it should be seen as a valuable service and treatment option which was offered to the patient and carers. The carers can see that every avenue was explored to try and return the patient home, even if it did not actually take place.

Management of cognitive and perceptual impairments

Cognitive and perceptual deficits, including confusion, manifest themselves in a number of ways. They may be as result of a brain tumour, infection, side effects of medications, central nervous system metastases, or chemical imbalance such as hypercalcaemia. Furthermore, they may be temporary, fluctuating, or permanent.

Although there are numerous standardized assessments which identify neurological deficits such as memory, planning, and problem-solving, their use is almost always inappropriate in palliative care as they are so time-consuming and tiring for the patient. Re-assessment may only confirm to the patient that they are deteriorating.

The occupational therapist observes the patient during functional activities such as washing, dressing, and meal preparation, which then helps them identify any deficits and implications for safety and independence. For example, when a patient is unsafe cooking with gas, handling hot items, and forgetting to take medication, the occupational therapist can address these issues practically. Fluctuating or deteriorating cognitive levels can be extremely distressing for both patients and carers, and the aim of the occupational therapist is to assist the carers in coping with this and maximize the time the patient can be supported at home.

Practical strategies such as the use of memory aids can be explored, and advice can be given about the level of supervision the patient may require, and whether they are safe to be left alone at home.

Rehabilitation in palliative care

The ethos of occupational therapy compliments the World Health Organization's key principles of palliative care:

- ◆ Relief from pain and other distressing symptoms
- ◆ Psychological and spiritual care
- ◆ A support system to help patients live as actively as possible in the face of impending death
- ◆ A support system to sustain patient's friends and family during illness and bereavement (World Health Organization, n.d.).

Dietz (1981) describes rehabilitation in cancer care as comprising four distinct aspects, the last being palliative rehabilitation. Palliative rehabilitation involves assisting with symptom control and providing comfort and support to patients with advanced disease. The focus continues to be on optimizing independence.

This reinforces how, within the palliative care setting, it is essential that the occupational therapist maintains a flexible approach regarding the varying symptoms that the patient may exhibit as a result of advanced disease and adapting goals as a person's clinical condition changes.

Skills required to manage activities of daily living

A person needs to have certain levels of physical, emotional, and social skills to function independently. When there are problems in any of these areas, the occupational therapist needs to analyse the problems so that they can be addressed with treatment programmes, adaptation, and equipment. These may include the following:

- ◆ Motor skills which involve the functional use of muscle strength and tone, range of movement, endurance, stamina, and fine and gross motor skills. Disease-related symptoms might result in prolonged periods of inactivity leading to muscle wastage, weight loss, generalized weakness or even weight gain or oedema as a result on steroids.
- ◆ Sensory skills which involve identification and interpretation of external and internal sensory stimuli, including pain, altered sensation, balance deficits and visual disturbances.
- ◆ Cognitive skills for which deficits may be as a result of tumour growth, either primary or secondary, or side effects of drugs used for symptom control. The individual may present with altered levels of arousal or exhibit impairment of memory, planning, problem-solving, and communication.
- ◆ Intrapersonal skills where advanced disease may affect an individual's self-image and identity, which in turn may affect how they behave and participate in occupation.
- ◆ Interpersonal skills where individuals may experience a loss of control and may feel they are unable to fulfil their existing roles such as mother, breadwinner, or employee. This can have an enormous impact on self-esteem.
- ◆ Self-maintenance occupations, which refer to activities that one regularly carries out to take care of oneself such as toileting, washing and dressing, feeding and sleeping. Usually these would be carried out with a degree of privacy and the individual is likely to have their own routine. Some people may place enormous value

and meaning on performing these activities independently. If they decline help at home, the occupational therapist then focuses on risk assessment, provision of equipment to facilitate independence and safety, and education in compensatory strategies.

◆ Productivity occupations, in which the individual supports themselves, for example, shopping, cooking, as well as paid employment, housework, and studying.

◆ Leisure occupations, which relate to all activities carried out for pleasure and enjoyment. It is essential that meaningful leisure pursuits are identified and adapted to enable greater participation so that the person can continue with these (Miller and Cooper, 2010).

Goal setting and grading activities

Goal setting is a vital component of therapeutic interventions and its value has been demonstrated within the palliative care setting as a means of focusing the interdisciplinary team (Jennings, 2010). Through collaboration with the patient and their carers, the occupational therapist sets specific, realistic, achievable, and measurable goals for what the patients wants to achieve.

By applying grading techniques to an activity, the occupational therapist can adjust it depending on how the patient is managing. This is done by adapting the environment such as moving furniture or providing equipment. Additionally, techniques such as backward and forward chaining may be used. Backward chaining requires the occupational therapist to complete all the necessary steps, for example, in showering the patient and let them complete the last step. Forward chaining means that the patient completes the first step and the occupational therapist completes the remainder of the activity. Increasing the number of steps which the patient can manage helps build up their stamina and skills. Similarly, if a person deteriorates, a staged decline can be planned to help them adjust to changing circumstances.

Safety is a vital issue which must not be taken lightly. Safety can be improved by providing appropriate equipment, but the patient and carers may be put at risk if a thorough assessment is not carried out and all the potential hazards taken into consideration. For example, a motorized wheelchair or stairlift might sound as though it would be the answer to someone's mobility problems, but the person's cognitive skills, physical balance, abilities, general stamina, and financial situation would all need very careful assessment by the occupational therapist.

Occupational therapy in the management of symptom clusters

Symptom clusters relate to three or more related symptoms that may interact with each other and have a significant effect on the patient's quality of life (Esper and Heidrich, 2005). The combination of anxiety, breathlessness, and fatigue results in such a symptom cluster (Gilbertson-White et al., 2011) and the management of anxiety has a positive impact on the other two symptoms.

Anxiety management and relaxation sessions

It is normal for everyone to experience some degree of anxiety, and in fact by its very existence, it aids everyday survival and performance in certain situations. This natural response is referred to as the 'fight or flight' response which, when activated, enables us to confront and fight the danger or run away from it. Although anxiety may be viewed as an entirely appropriate reaction to advanced disease, prolonged anxiety can cause problems in carrying out day-to-day activities. Therefore, occupational therapy needs to treat the symptom. Exacerbating factors may include pre-existing psychiatric conditions, poorly controlled pain, medication toxicities, and psychological and spiritual issues.

Relaxation is one of the main strategies for managing anxiety and aims to:

◆ understand and recognize the individual's level of anxiety

◆ understand the need for relaxation and recognize certain situations that may trigger tension

◆ experience a variety of relaxation techniques thus enabling the individual to choose the most appropriate one

◆ appreciate the importance of planning time for relaxation as part of the individual's daily activities and lifestyle

◆ improve quality of sleep and performance of physical skills

◆ increase self-esteem and confidence

◆ ease relationships with others

◆ channel and control effects of anxiety and avoid unnecessary fatigue.

Relaxation programmes vary depending on resources available; however, a basic outline would include education and practice using techniques, some of which are outlined in Table 4.6.2.

The focus, as with all occupational therapy interventions, is to promote independence and challenge the loss of control which can occur when patients have to deal with life limiting conditions.

Breathlessness management

Although breathlessness is a common symptom in lung cancer patients, severe breathlessness also affects approximately 30% of the palliative care population in the last weeks of life (Currow et al., 2010). It is a subjective sensation and the overall physical and psychological implications are immeasurable. Interdisciplinary input is vital to manage the patient efficiently as breathlessness needs to be assessed and managed according to the individual's needs. Three main aims of management are to:

1. explore the meaning of the symptom to the patient and carers and families

2. enable activity so that they can achieve optimum independence and control despite their debilitating symptom

3. help patients manage any anxiety and panic attacks, including teaching relaxation techniques as part of the management programme.

Enabling activity for breathless patients

Pacing activities may sound simple but it is often complex (Cooper, 2006: Booth et al., 2011). By working with the patient to use energy conservation, they can take part in activities which they value. Energy conservation is the deliberate planned management of one's personal energy resources in order to prevent their depletion (Barsevick et al., 2002). It includes the following techniques for patients to manage daily activities and cope with breathlessness.

Table 4.6.2 Relaxation programme

Programme	Technique
Assessment	Do you have any previous experience of relaxation? How does anxiety affect your daily life? What are your expectations of relaxation?
Body charts and awareness	Mark on body chart the specific areas of physical tension Discuss increasing awareness of how the body feels when it is tense
Establish programme	Agree treatment plan over set number of sessions, to be reviewed and results recorded at each session
Progressive muscular relaxation	Sequential technique in which each muscle group is tensed then relaxed Structured session in which the individual does not use their imagination but follows logical set of exercises
Passive neuromuscular and release-only relaxation	Releasing tension from muscle groups The individual identifies the muscles which are tense without actively tensing muscles
Autogenic relaxation	A systematic programme which teaches the body and mind to respond to verbal commands to relax
Guided visualization	The participant actively uses their imagination and positive images to induce a feeling of well-being and relaxation
Unguided visualization	This allows more freedom for the imagination, empowering the individual to select their scene or sequence of events to visualize
Challenging negative thought patters	Individual is encouraged to use positive phrases such as 'choose' and 'can' rather than focusing on negative ones which increase stress such as 'should, must, ought to'

Source: data from Ewer-Smith, C., Patterson S., The use of an occupational therapy programme within a palliative care setting, *European Journal of Palliative Care*, Volume 9, Issue 1, pp. 30–33, Copyright © 2002 Hayward Medical Communications, a division of Hayward Group Ltd.

The five Ps:

◆ Prioritize—consider which activities are important to you each day, and prioritize those for which you would like to conserve your energy.

Try to cut out unnecessary tasks in order to conserve your energy.

◆ Plan—organize your activities as effectively as possible in order to conserve as much energy as you can.

Consider which times of the day are best for you to be active or at rest.

Try not to do too much in any one day and plan your activities for the week ahead wherever possible.

◆ Pace—it is important to balance periods of activity with periods of rest. You may need to rest during an activity and allow yourself a little extra time to get things done.

◆ Position—work out a position that is comfortable for you when you feel breathless and practise this so that you can help yourself.

Think about your posture and try to maintain this so that you avoid becoming uncomfortable and conserve your energy.

◆ Permission—Give yourself permission *not* to do activities which result in your becoming breathless and tired.

Instead of thinking along the lines of 'I must', 'I ought', try and challenge this negative thinking and way you view this and say to yourself 'I choose to', or 'I wish to do' instead (Ewer-Smith, 2002).

Personal plan for coping with breathlessness

Breathlessness is an anxiety-provoking symptom for both the patient and those who witness it and education is the key to coping with this (Cox, 2002). Once the occupational therapist and other team members have established the most effective way of coping with the individual's problems, a personal plan can be developed to help the patient and carers regain control during such an episode. This includes establishing the following:

◆ How to practice breathing control. This depends entirely on the individual, whether they need oxygen, or a nebulizer, and what technique suits them such as how to position their shoulders.

◆ What to do when they are breathless. Following thorough assessment, the patient will be advised what they need to do, whether to rest, use oxygen, or how to help the upper chest relax.

◆ Positions to use when breathless. The individual may find sitting upright, leaning forward or backwards, or lying on their side most comfortable and the best position for them will be emphasized on the personal plan.

◆ Exercising. What level of gentle exercise will help them.

◆ Breathing control whilst walking. Following thorough assessment, advice will be given on which breathing techniques will help.

◆ Managing daily activities. The occupational therapist will assess whether equipment and different strategies and techniques are required and advise accordingly.

◆ Equipment. A wheelchair may be useful for conserving energy, and other equipment to save energy in the kitchen, bathroom, and around the house may be of help.

These approaches will not totally alleviate breathlessness but can make it easier to manage (Booth et al., 2011).

Fatigue management

Cancer-related fatigue affects more than 70% of patients in palliative care (Ahlberg et al., 2003). It presents as exhaustion and a lack of energy and prevents them taking part in everyday activities which they often previously managed independently. It may also result in insomnia or disturbed sleep patterns, cognitive deficits such as memory difficulties, reduced attention span, and affect their psychological well-being, resulting in impatience and mood swings. It is a multidimensional symptom affecting the patient's physical, social, cognitive, and emotional well-being

The principles of fatigue management are exercise, pharmacological interventions, complementary therapies, and adjustment strategies using psychological and education approaches.

The role of the occupational therapist within fatigue management centres on educative, rehabilitative, and compensatory interventions (Lowrie, 2006) and uses many of the principles already discussed within the anxiety and breathlessness sections:

◆ Fatigue diaries may be used to identify the patient's current level of functioning, highlight which activities and occupations they most value, and establish goals and priorities.

◆ Educating the patient and carers about the nature of fatigue symptoms and means of management can alleviate anxiety and help them to understand this common side effect.

◆ Energy conservation techniques can be explored with the patient and taught, as described within the enabling activity section of breathlessness.

◆ Patients should be encouraged to use goal setting as a means of setting realistic goals by breaking down tasks into smaller, more manageable components, thus enhancing the patient's perception of control.

◆ Equipment can also help alleviate fatigue, as shown in Table 4.6.1.

Memory problems

The patients themselves or their carers may notice short-term memory problems, impaired attention and planning, and problem-solving difficulties. This can impact on the patient's ability to maintain independence with activities which they value and potentially affect their relationships with others. Occupational therapists can advise the patient and carers about minimizing distractions when participating in an activity, assess the implication of such cognitive deficits upon safety, and look into simplifying activities so as to minimize the demands.

Outcome measures

Using outcome measures enables the occupational therapist to measure changes that have occurred as a direct result of intervention although it must be acknowledged that the patient is often seen by a number of members of the interprofessional team so change cannot be solely attributed to one team member.

Outcome data can show areas that need development, as well as areas of particular strength within a service.

Rather than just wanting an outcome measure for the sake of it, Eva (2006) advises that the occupational therapist must be clear about what it is they want to measure. Occupational therapists must be precise about the rationale underpinning the use of an outcome measure and be aware of both the administrative burden and the fact that they are dealing with deteriorating conditions in palliative care.

Goal setting can be used as long as goals are SMART, that is, specific, measurable, attainable, realistic, and time bound. These can be clearly measured and will provide useful meaningful information regarding their progress and success.

The Canadian Occupational Performance Measure (COPM) (Law et al., 2005) is a client-centred, individualized measure of the impact of physical, sociocultural, mental, and spiritual aspects of occupational functioning. The patient identifies areas of difficulty within the areas of self-care, productivity, and leisure and rates them on a scale of 1–10. Five of these functional problems then become the focus for rehabilitation and determine rehabilitation goals which are then evaluated over a period of time. Its success has been limited in palliative care as the patient, by nature of the life-limiting illness, will deteriorate (Norris, 1999).

The AusTOMs (Unsworth and Duncombe, 2004) is an Australian therapy outcome measure which measures 12 scales for occupational therapy which broadly reflect a patient's status across four domains of health and functioning and are rated by the occupational therapist not the patient. The ratings are based on clinical judgement using knowledge of the patient and how they are functioning. Again, its success may be limited by the palliative nature of patients.

These detailed individual assessments are in contrast to the World Health Organization Performance Scale and the Karnofsky Performance Scale (Cancer Research UK, 2013), which are broad indicators used in clinical research trials. The World Health Organization Performance Scale has categories from 0 to 4, '0' being fully active through to '4' being bed or chair dependent, requiring full care. The Karnofsky Performance Scale ranges from 100, at which there is no evidence of disease and the scale descends down to 10, at which the individual is very ill and unlikely to recover. For the purpose of the occupational therapy assessment, these lack the specific detail required for individual programmes and treatment plans.

Measuring outcomes with numerical scores can show a snapshot of effectiveness, that is, quantitative scores, but will not give in-depth information about how the patient is managing. However, qualitative outcomes provide more meaningful data to the occupational therapists but this may not be of interest to those parties who simply want numbers and scores.

Occupational therapists working in palliative care have not found a completely successful outcome measure, mainly because they have to manage the contrast between enhancing the value and meaning of a person's remaining life while simultaneously supporting approaching death (Eva, 2006).

Conclusion

Occupational therapy aims to enhance the patient's and their carers' quality of life through taking part in activities or occupations that are important to and valued by them. This is achieved by education, equipment provision and adaptations, and treatment programmes. This helps the patient to gain as much control and choice as possible at the advanced and palliative stages of disease.

Whilst the occupational therapist has unique skills and role, they are a vital member of the interdisciplinary team and strive to deliver holistic care for the patient and carers during the final stages of their illness.

Online materials

Complete references for this chapter are available online at <http://www.oxfordmedicine.com>.

References

Booth, S., Moffat, C., Farquhar, M., Higginson, I.J., and Burkin, J. (2011). Developing a breathlessness intervention service for patients with palliative and supportive care needs, irrespective of diagnosis. *Journal of Palliative Care*, 27(1), 28–36.

Cooper, J. (2006). Occupational therapy in the management of breathlessness. In J. Cooper (ed.) *Occupational Therapy in Oncology and Palliative Care* (2nd ed.), pp. 51–60. Chichester: Wiley.

Currow, D.C., Smith, J., Davidson, P.M., Newton, P.J., Agar, M.R., and Abernethy, A.P. (2010). Do the trajectories of dyspnoea differ in prevalence and intensity by diagnosis at the end of life? A consecutive cohort study. *Journal of Pain Symptom Management*, 39(4), 680–690.

Gilbertson-White, S., Aouizerat, B.E., Jahan, T., and Miaskowski, C. (2011). A review of the literature on multiple symptoms, their predictors, and associated outcomes in patients with advanced cancer. *Palliative & Supportive Care*, 9(1), 81–102.

Jennings, A. (2010). Palliation in breathlessness: a combined approach is needed. *European Journal of Palliative Care*, 17(4), 162–166.

Kealey, P. and McIntyre, I. (2005). An evaluation of the domiciliary occupational therapy service in palliative cancer care in a community trust: a patient and carers perspective. *European Journal of Cancer Care*, 14(3), 232–243.

Lowrie, D. (2006). Occupational therapy and cancer related fatigue. In J. Cooper (ed.) *Occupational Therapy* in *Oncology and Palliative Care* (2nd ed.), pp. 61–82. Chichester: Wiley

Squire, N. (2011). Contribution of occupational therapy to the palliative care team: results of a pilot project. *European Journal of Palliative Care*, 18(3), 136–139.

Sumsion, T. and Law, M. (2006). A review of evidence on the conceptual elements informing client-centred practice. *Canadian Journal of Occupational Therapy*, 73(3), 153–162.

Unsworth, C.A. and Duncombe, D. (2004). *AUSTOMS for Occupational Therapy* (2nd ed.). Victoria: LaTrobe University.

World Health Organization (n.d.). *WHO Definition of Palliative Care*. [Online] Available at: <http://www.who.int/cancer/palliative/definition/en/>.

4.7

Music therapy in palliative care

Clare O'Callaghan

Music is intricately woven into the fabrics of life and takes on deeper significance during times of transition, loss, and grief.

Reproduced from Magill, L. Art therapy and music therapy, p. 425, in Holland J.C. et al. (eds) *Psycho-oncology*, Second Edition, Copyright © 2010, by permission of Oxford Unversity Press Inc.

Introduction to music therapy in palliative care

Music therapists offer musical experiences to improve comfort and enhance the lives of palliative care patients and their families. Music's helpful role in dealing with transition and loss is long evident in tribal rituals and religious and community practices (Laderman and Roseman, 1996). In the 1970s, pioneering music therapists Lucanne Magill and Susan Munro respectively brought live music to patients at Memorial Sloan Kettering Cancer Center, New York, and The Royal Victoria Hospital Palliative Care Unit, Montreal. Music therapists now contribute to holistic patient care in palliative inpatient and home-based services, and other settings caring for people with degenerative conditions, throughout the world.

In palliative care, music therapy can be defined as the creative and professionally informed use of music in a therapeutic relationship with people identified as needing physical, psychosocial, or spiritual help, or desiring further self-awareness, to enable increased life satisfaction and quality. Music therapists, who are university trained and accredited by national registration committees, can often extend the way that music enhances patients' well-being and their connection with who and what matters in their lives. The musical elements and evolving therapeutic relationship can underlie helpful, sometimes transformative experiences. The focus is on therapeutic process rather than musical products and participants do not have to have musical backgrounds to benefit. Music therapists invite patients and families to explore and choose music therapy methods. The therapeutic relationship informs how the music is shared and created. It can be distinguished from music thanatology which is the provision of 'prescriptive music, using harp and voice at bedside' with the compassionate musician's presence (Cox and Roberts, 2007, p. 80). This chapter will describe ways in which music therapists work in palliative care, clarify research supporting its efficacy, and offer strategies for how caregivers may offer music to support palliative care patients when music therapists are not available.

Music therapy in adult contexts: assessment, methods, and effects

Various descriptions of music therapy in palliative care with adult patients, families (including anyone significant in their lives), and staff carers are available (Munro and Mount, 1978; Munro, 1984; Dileo and Loewy, 2005; Hilliard, 2005). Music therapists typically receive referrals from staff, patients themselves, or their families. As patients' conditions fluctuate, sessions may be flexibly scheduled, range from minutes to over 1 hour, and can be offered occasionally to almost daily. Therapists can visit patients at bedsides in hospitals and homes bringing accompanying instruments, sheet music, or recorded music. The author often brings sheet music with up to 7000 songs and classical pieces that she can spontaneously play on an electric piano. Music therapy groups may also be conducted in day hospices, inpatient palliative care, or nursing home settings. Many music therapy departments incorporate extensive recorded music libraries, audio equipment, and tuned and untuned instruments.

Upon meeting patients, the music therapist's assessment includes determining the patient's music preferences, the relevance of music throughout their lives, and biopsychosocial needs or spiritual and aesthetic interests that may be addressed through music therapy. Music therapy methods offered to patients and their families can include (a) replaying the music of their lives, including live performance (by therapist and/or participant), music listening, music and life review, and lyric substitution in familiar songs; (b) exploring 'new' music, including therapeutic song writing, music improvisation, and unfamiliar music; (c) guided use of music, such as relaxation inductions with live or recorded music; and (d) music-based gift or legacy creation, such as song compositions and music-based audio-visual recordings. Ways in which music therapists can support patients and families are listed in Table 4.7.1.

Table 4.7.1 Some music therapy aims in palliative care

Supportive validation	One's feelings and thoughts
	Of a life that has been and is still being well lived
	One's self-worth; spiritual way of being
	Contemplation; a time to 'be'
Increased self-awareness to aid coping	Self-discovery
	Reawakening or reworking of an earlier awareness
Symptom relief and relaxation	Including pain, tension, dyspnoea, nausea, insomnia, restlessness
Connectedness	Those with cognitive impairment
	Those with language barriers and communication difficulties
	Expanded opportunities for interactions with family members, friends, other patients, staff
Aesthetic and spiritual experience	Pleasure
	Diversion; normalcy
	Creative expression
	Transcendence
Support expression of grief, bereavement	Dealing with loss: acceptance of one's own way; reframing regret; helpful catharsis
	Increasing confidence and strength for moving forward

Replaying the music from one's life

Patients often choose to experience music that elicits emotions, messages, or memories of places, events, and people that they want to feel connected with, and supported or inspired by. One patient, for example, consistently asked the music therapist to sing '(You are the) Wind Beneath My Wings'[a] because, she said, no one had ever told that they loved her. Identifications with lyrics associated with themes such as adversity, loss, and hope, and singers who have lived with life-threatening conditions, can enable one to feel understood and part of a wider human experience. People project into music and take from it what is needed because music is polysemous: it can be interpreted in multiple ways. For example, while 'Sailing'[b] may simply evoke happy youthful memories for one patient, another may repeatedly request the song to connect with the lyrics. Music can nurture or sustain in unexpected ways. The day before he died, a patient requested that the music therapist play 'The Prayer'[c] on the electric piano, and then asked for the lyrics so that he could sing it sometime. Although unable to outwardly sing, the invigorating and life-affirming properties of music still allowed him to connect with his non-patient musician identity: he could imagine singing until he died, and possibly felt hope 'singing' the song's lyrical plea of guidance to a safe place.

Patients often request songs once sung by parents or other important people, which can evoke supportive feelings of nurturance. They may also request songs sung at school, that signified courtships, were enjoyed at dances, parties, musical theatre, or concerts, or have spiritual meaning, affirm faith, and enable prayerful contemplation. Music can powerfully elicit emotions and images associated with earlier times. Patients may listen, sing along, or share memories, laughter, and tears, sometimes with their families, other patients, and staff. Elicited stories about their musical memories can reflect the important 'dignity-conserving perspective', 'continuity of self' (Chochinov, 2012, p. 14). Music-based reminiscence can improve communication between patients and those close to them, validate their lives, enhance insight, ethnic and cultural affirmation, and improve self-esteem, sense of worth, and identity (Forrest, 2000). Regrets may also be reframed and reconsidered. Through computerized music scrapbooking, young cancer patients have also arranged meaningful song fragments into new musical works which validate and express important sentiments (Robyn Booth, personal communication, 1 November 2006). Patients' life stories and favourite musical pieces can also be audio-recorded as legacies, perhaps combined with accompanying photo albums. Patients who cannot verbally communicate, for example, through motor neurone disease, can especially find this a meaningful way of sharing their non-patient identity with visitors and staff.

Physical reactions to music therapy may also reveal vital parts of a patient's personhood, arguably reflecting 'dignity-conserving care' (Chochinov, 2012, p. 36). This was evident, for example, in day hospice music therapy groups when one patient held onto a glass of wine in one hand, her wheelchair with the other, and stood up and danced while others waltzed to recorded band music; a seated 90-year-old whose feet could still manoeuvre Scottish highland gigue steps; and when a patient could sing perfectly despite expressive aphasia due to a brain tumour. Music therapy experiences can affirm one's life roles, community contributions, and extend self-awareness and ability to meaningfully express. This is especially evident when patients engage in song lyric substitution, as the music can give impetus to one's creation of personal lyrics, and the hearing of one's meaningful expressions mirrored back through song can soothe, affirm, and inspire self-pride. A particularly useful song for inviting patients to substitute lyrics to is 'One Day at a Time'.[d] When experiencing music one's non-discursive (non-verbal) level of awareness may also be accessed and experienced as a felt, mindful, or a symbolic sensation, possibly enabling longed-for relaxation or peacefulness. This often seems apparent when patients ask for a favourite piece of music to be played repeatedly, or when patients comment, 'You can stay here all day' when the music therapist softly plays their preferred music at their bedsides. The balance of music, discussion, and counselling is therefore monitored and variable in sessions because initiating verbal reflections may shift a patient's focus from a restful or transformative 'feelingful' mode to a less helpful cognitive state.

Patients and families

Music therapy can enable an intimate and comfortable context for patients and families to convey supportive and validating messages through choosing music to enjoy and relax with together and share elicited memories. Affirming messages may also be non-verbally expressed through 'knowing' looks and smiles, hand-holding, massaging touch, embraces, shared singing, and dancing rhythmically with the music, which can involve kicking legs or holding and moving hands together, even when one is in a bed or bed-chair. Music therapy may also help to sustain family members maintaining long vigils at patients' bedsides at the end of their lives. When barely rousable, patients may still smile or squeeze their loved one's hand to acknowledge a significant song and statement, and when non-rousable, family may continue to communicate with their loved ones through asking for meaningful songs (e.g. 'Love will Go On'[e]) and hymns (e.g. 'Amazing Grace'), and singing or sharing memories. Such good memories of how patients are cared for can ease distress in bereavement (Reid et al., 2006). Music therapy in multi-bed rooms can also inspire shared involvement of patients, families, visitors, and staff in uplifting ways, and through singing together or sharing music-based stories, acknowledge each other's value.

Combining music with allied therapies may also broaden therapeutic benefits of both modalities. For example, patients can use music with physiotherapy exercises, and art therapists have helped patients to create CD covers for songs composed in music therapy and to integrate important aspects of patients' musical backgrounds into their art legacies. Music therapy alongside art therapy in an aesthetically tranquil hospice setting connected with surrounding bush-land contributes to a 'generative community environment' which can enable patients to feel 're-empowered', to creatively regain a sense of identity, and to connect with their faith in a 'sacred place' (Glenister, 2012, p. 91).

Exploring 'new' music

Therapeutic song writing

Through therapeutic individual or group song writing patients and families can express important sentiments in a contained and quick way. People can express what may be difficult to verbalize, and the creative effort may bring pride, spiritual comfort, self-affirmation, or cathartic relief (O'Callaghan, 2005). A music therapist also found that helping cancer patient to create an opera helped them to feel calm, healed, proud, and express fears and grief (O'Brien, 2006). Patients with cognitive impairment can also write songs as therapists provide necessary structure such as multiple choices of lyrics, melodic fragments, harmonies, and tempos. Adding musical accompaniment may extend the therapeutic effect of verbal expressions, because music is a mnemonic and can reinforce emotional meaning. To help palliative care patients write songs: (a) the music therapist invites a patient or family member to consider a topic and then helps them to brainstorm lyrical ideas through encouraging free association or offering prompts and questions; (b) the therapist and patient then group and transform the ideas into a song lyric structure; (c) the therapist invites suggestions for musical elements (melody, harmony, rhythms speed, genre, volume) or offers musical alternatives, line by line, for the patient to choose from, and (d) the therapist, patient, or an extended group record the completed song (O'Callaghan et al., 2009).

Palliative care patients may write songs about their illness journey, for someone important, the general community, or their faith, and experience relationship closure, self-expression, spiritual enhancement, and life review (Dileo and Magill, 2005). Analysis of lyrics of 64 songs written by 39 palliative care patients in music therapy revealed that the patients used song writing to express messages, self-reflections, compliments, memories, imagery, prayers, and reflect about adversity and their significant others, including pets (O'Callaghan, 1996a). Another analysis of 35 songs written by 27 cancer inpatients for their children found that parents' song lyrics included their memories of times spent with their children; messages of love, compliments, and/or hopes for the children; existential beliefs, such as being available for the children now and in the afterlife; and supportive suggestions, such as who the children can turn to for future support (O'Callaghan et al., 2009). Arguably, these findings indicate that therapeutic songwriting may support parent–child connectedness during the parents' illnesses (O'Callaghan and Jordan, 2011) and, if the parent sadly dies, the child's coping through bereavement as positive associations with the deceased help the bereaved (Raphael, 1984). This is important given the scant information about how to support parents and their children through palliative care (Saldinger et al., 2004).

Improvisation

In music therapy improvisation, the music therapist and participant/s may improvise together on tuned (e.g. keyboard, metallophone, xylophone) or untuned (e.g. drums, rain sticks) instruments, with or without vocalizations. A simple, often effective way of introducing tuned instrument improvisation to patients is through the pentatonic scale. This is a group of five notes which always sound harmonious when the notes are played together. Within this musical relationship, the client musically expresses aspects of their creative self, and the therapist's improvised musical reflections (mirroring) can affirm and extend the participant's musical and holistic way of being. These creative musical experiences can be enjoyable, 'freeing', and transform one's way of cognitively and feelingfully experiencing the world. The ongoing musical dialogue can affirm that the client has been heard and is known, inspiring further creativity, which may lead to further adaptive self-awareness. This has been illustrated in work with a gentleman with motor neurone disease (Salmon 1995) and with HIV-positive men (Hartley, 1999).

Concerts, music appreciation

Music therapists may also organize concerts and music appreciation sessions, where the therapist presents information about singers, bands, or musical genres in response to patients' requests, for those seeking to pursue novel, interesting, and educative experiences for as long as they can. Concerts may include patient, family, or staff performers or good musicians from the community.

Guided use of music

Relaxation inductions and music, and instructions for the use of music, may be used to help patients manage symptoms and feel less stress, including when undergoing scans or procedures. Good relaxation induction scripts are widely available and some include suggestions for music usage (Grocke and Wigram, 2007).[1] When patients are tense and very ill the author sometimes finds that a short relaxation induction followed by about 5–15 minutes of live music can be helpful, for example, 'The Swan',[f] 'Watermark',[g] the *Deer Hunter* 'Cavatina',[h] the *Moonlight Sonata* first movement and *Sonata Pathétique* second movement by Beethoven, and Nocturne in E flat by Chopin. Musical elements need to be steady without extreme variations in tempo, rhythms, and dynamics (loud/soft).

Preferred music is most associated with relaxation response (Stratton and Zalanowski, 1984) and pain reduction (Mitchell and MacDonald, 2006). Music alters mood through activating neural areas involving arousal, pleasure, dopamine production, and opioid transmission, more broadly than those elicited by language

(Levitin, 2006). Theoretical rationales for pain reduction in music therapy include direct physiological response to music stimuli that alter neural components of pain sensation, as well as cognitive and emotional changes aligned with increased self-awareness, thereby altering one's sense of the meaning, and thus perception, of pain (O'Callaghan, 1996b). When playing music to distract from symptoms, therapists often use the isoprincipal, musically matching patients' physical and emotional states, and gradually shifting the musical elements as patients move into more desired states, for example, slowing music down as breathing rate slows with relaxation. When participants have control over the music experienced in sessions, adverse effects are rare.

Specific populations

Children and adolescents

Music is often a central part of children's and adolescents' lives. It enables young cancer patients a connection with 'normalcy' and offers a vehicle for releasing emotions and energy, connecting with family and friends, and identity development (O'Callaghan et al., 2011, 2012). Music therapy can also help to alleviate young patients' distress and symptoms (O'Callaghan et al., 2011), improve coping with aversive procedures like radiotherapy (Barry et al., 2010), as well as improve their mood (Barrera et al., 2002), coping, and initiation behaviours (Robb et al., 2008). Music therapists tailor interventions to the young patients' cognitive abilities and emotional states. Those unable or unwilling to discuss feelings may symbolically express and find self-understanding, such as when a 'miserable and depressed' 8-year-old child was able to express grief and give a message to her best friend through song writing shortly before her death (Daveson and Kennelly, 2000), and when two 13-year-old-patients with brain tumours undergoing radiotherapy required less anxiolytics after experiencing improvisation, song writing, or therapeutic music lessons (O'Callaghan et al., 2007). Families may also have normalized and 'fun' experiences, for example when 4-year-old Peter smiled after a blanket was put on and gently pulled from his face during a Swedish playsong the day before he died (Aasgaard, 2001), and when a grandmother said that the happiest she had ever seen her 14-year-old grandson with AIDS was when he received a trumpet from a hospice on which the music therapist gave him lessons (Hilliard, 2003).

Cognitive impairment

Cerebral areas and neural systems activated during some musical activities are 'relatively independent from the areas used for verbal tasks' (Sergent et al., 1992, p. 108). Furthermore, long-term memories of music are relatively preserved in people with cognitive impairment. Therefore, the therapeutic use of both language and music are more likely to activate preserved neural function in palliative care patients who have brain impairment than when caregivers use language alone. Using both music and verbal language with people with brain impairment expands opportunities for them to have an aesthetic experience and meaningful connections with others. This includes patients with brain cancer and dementing conditions who can sometimes still sing, play instruments, write songs, and share music related interests, reminiscences, and humour with patients and families.

Music improvisation and familiar music can also provide a highly interactive medium for working with patients in low-awareness states following profound brain injury who display minimal and inconsistent spontaneous responses. The diagnosis of 'vegetative state' in one patient, following a severe anoxic brain injury in a cardiac arrest, was revised to a 'minimally conscious state' following purposeful, non-verbal responses in music therapy. Her family, who 'knew she was in there', then worked with the music therapist to find ways that they could leisurely share music with her (Magee, 2005). This work is described as 'neuropalliative rehabilitation'.

Ethnic minorities

Music therapists try and offer a wide variety of musical styles from many cultures. Patients unfamiliar with the dominant language in their care setting may experience reduced isolation, validation, and joy as they experience songs from their language of origin. Culturally significant music may also help patients to reconfirm their identity within their wider socio-historical and ethnic heritage, assist their expression of pain, grief, and memories, and support their preparation for death and their family members' grieving (Forrest, 2000).

Bereavement

Caregivers' music therapy memories shared with deceased family members indicates pre-loss music therapy's role for healthy grieving (Lindenfelser et al., 2008; Magill, 2009). For example, a grandmother caring for her four grandchildren said that memories of family song writing sessions before their mother (her daughter) had died allowed them to remember 'some good feelings, not all sad' (O'Callaghan et al., 2013).

Music therapy groups for 18 bereaved adolescents incorporating song writing, improvisation, or song listening and discussion gave the participants permission to grieve which helped them to feel better (McFerran et al., 2010). Therapeutic song writing also helped six bereaved children to accept loss, and express emotions and memories connected with their loved ones (Roberts, 2006).

Music-based care and the relevance of music therapists

Palliative care workers are encouraged to invite patients and families to consider using music for self-care whenever possible and music-based care suggestions are outlined in Box 4.7.1. Employment of music therapists is, however, recommended for extending music's capacity to enhance life quality. This is enabled through the therapeutic relationship and music therapists' knowledge of theoretically informed and evidence-based methods.

Therapeutic relationship in music therapy

The music therapist's supportive presence may be conceptualized as providing a 'sounding board' or a musical 'human mirror'. Winnicott suggested that in psychotherapy the therapist 'reflects back' aspects about the patient, enabling the person to exist 'as an expression of I AM, I am alive, I am myself' (Winnicott, 1971, p. 56). In music therapy, the patient may be 'reflected back' in a multisensorial manner, that is, musically, verbally, and non-verbally, expanding the potential for creative reintegration and new awareness. Improvisations and familiar music in music therapy are always experienced anew, creatively perceived and expressed, potentially transducing into helpful ways of viewing and coping

Box 4.7.1 Suggestions for staff caregivers offering music in palliative care

◆ Patient choice is imperative, including type of music, its volume, when and where it is listened to, and for how long. Ensure patients can control volume and turn their music off whenever possible; regularly offer to help music access (or to turn it off) when patients are unable to operate music systems when they have a disability. Once a person with anarthria and physical disability from motor neurone disease spelled out on the e-tran board (with eye movements) that the music therapist needed to take her CD player away because busy staff put headphones on her ears and did not inquire about the volume before leaving.

◆ One's preferred music is most associated with relaxation. Hence music therapists do not advocate the indiscriminate use of 'piped' music in palliative care settings: what one person finds helpful may be aggravating for another.

◆ Suggest that patients bring their own music, labelled with their name when coming for inpatient stays or procedures (e.g. iPods/CDs) and have CD players and headphones available as necessary.

◆ When patients intend using music for aversive procedures, suggest that they consider how they would feel if the experience contaminated their enjoyment of that same music in the future. Some people find using preferred music to help them through an unpleasant experience does not impact upon their future enjoyment of that music, while others need to avoid it in the future.

◆ Encourage 'normal' family interactions through sharing music as appropriate. For example, parent inpatients may play children's music CDs/playlist during young children's visits; families can bring instruments to play into inpatient settings; hospices may a have guitar, harmonica, or keyboard available for patients and families to play. Suggest that family members and friends bring in patients' favourite CDs into hospital and listen to music together, or offer to buy a favourite CD instead of flowers. In home-based palliative care, suggest that patients and families consider listening to old music collections; help them consider ways of getting to concerts/ bands if they are concert goers (e.g. borrowing a wheelchair; contacting concert venues about wheelchair access and convenient car parking availability).

◆ Encourage the development of music libraries with diverse music choices in hospital settings that patients/families can access. Perhaps include CD 'samplers' or playlists on MP3 players which offer a range of music styles so that patients and families can explore unfamiliar types of music that may be helpful. As people become more unwell music preferences may change.

◆ Invite patients, perhaps with their families, to consider making CDs or playlists of the musical highlights of their lives. Memories or messages related to the music can be also put on the CD. These 'musical life reviews' can elicit affirming conversations and can be given as gifts.

◆ Inquire about and talk to patients about their music interests which indicates interest in the 'person' beyond the patient. Sometimes talking about music can be just as enjoyable as listening to it.

◆ Consider the presentation of live concerts or background music sensitively in public palliative care settings. Live concerts in palliative care settings, including accomplished musicians and music students, and even patients and families themselves, can be normalizing, interesting, and enjoyable. Performers may suggest that patients and families need to feel free to leave the concerts as needed. Live acoustic ambient music to enhance the environment may be offered in areas where people can move to and from (e.g. foyers). Volume should not be too loud: normal conversations need to be still audible. Avoid presenting music with loss and death themes in this context. Instrumental music, for example, acoustic classical guitar or piano, may be good. Inviting anonymous written feedback to be placed in strategically located feedback boxes can help with understanding what music is appropriate for the context.

◆ When patients have cognitive impairment (e.g. adynamic, memory loss) regularly offer music.

◆ Some patients with memory loss find listening to the same music repeatedly enjoyable.

◆ If patients and families appear 'sad' listening to music this is often ok, especially if they have requested the music. It is important that they can feel free to turn the music off (or leave a concert) if they wish. Consider whether to inquire about the emotion and offer support or leave them to contemplatively be. If a patient or family member is concerned about their music reaction perhaps reassure that varied (and different) responses to music can be normal when one is dealing with serious illness. It is possible that the person is experiencing the 'pleasurable sadness' paradox, that is, enjoying listening to music that evokes sadness alongside positive feelings.*

◆ Consider the potential effects of your personal music usage on the wards on overhearing patients and staff.

◆ When patients are unarousable at the end of life, family members may be invited to put soft music on in the room that they believe that patient would like, and softly hum or sing one of their favourite songs, hymns, or melodies. Reassure them that it does not matter if they don't remember the words.

*Source: data from Vuoloski, J.K., Thompson, W.F., McIlwain, D., and Eerola, T. Who enjoys listening to sad music and why? *Music Perception*, Volume 29, pp. 311–317, Copyright © 2012 by The Regents of the University of California. All rights reserved.

with illness experience. The therapeutic impetus encapsulated in live musical involvement with a trained music therapist cannot be underestimated as the therapist validates and often improves people's experiences through reflective listening and supportive musical and verbally insight-oriented dialogue.

As patients move closer to death, however, expecting significant psychotherapeutic changes may be inappropriate. The therapist may still softly play the music that has previously enriched the patient's life, and assist family members and friends to continue their supportive presence or expression of messages. This is especially evident, for example, when the music therapist accompanies a spouse singing a favourite courtship song to their dying partner, when children of dying patients ask for songs that they remember their parents loved watching them dance to in school concerts, and when the therapist accompanies family members sing hymns during bedside vigils, such as when one patient's favourite, 'Here I am Lord',[i] was being sung by her children as she took her final breath.

Research and evidence

Extensive music therapy research has been conducted within this field, exemplified by three Cochrane reviews[2] in music therapy palliative care (Bradt and Dileo, 2010), oncology (Bradt et al., 2011), and dementia (Vink et al. 2011). There is also a review, spanning 1983–2009, of 61 research projects in music therapy, cancer, and palliative care encompassing 32 objectivist (quantitative), 26 constructivist (qualitative), and ten mixed methods publications. This latter review found considerable evidence for music therapy improving the life quality of patients and family and staff caregivers in myriad ways. For example, randomized controlled trials (RCTs) and non-controlled quantitative studies showed findings of improved mood, relaxation, spiritual well-being, comfort, and reduced pain, distress, depression, pain, anxiety, isolation, and boredom. Qualitative research findings revealed that music therapy can be a positive social, emotional, and spiritual experience, which provides opportunity for creativity, healing, aesthetic meaning, expanded identity, and it can affirm one's sense of aliveness. Family and staff caregivers also find witnessing and experiencing music therapy's effects personally helpful. (See O'Callaghan (2009) for summaries of these studies and references.)

A Cochrane review meta-analysis on five end-of-life care studies (175 participants) found statistically significant findings in three studies for improved quality of life scales in three domains: functional, psycho-physiological, and social/spiritual well-being (Bradt and Dileo, 2010, p. 2). For example, in one RCT, which examined music therapy's effect on 25 hospice inpatients, anxiety, pain, tiredness, and drowsiness were significantly reduced in the music therapy intervention group compared to the volunteer visitor control group (Horne-Thompson and Grocke, 2008). Another Cochrane review, which examined the effect of music therapy and pre-recorded music listening interventions on physical and psychological outcomes in cancer patients, included 30 trials (1891 participants) (Bradt et al., 2011). The meta-analysis findings also suggested that music may improve life quality and mood, and reduce anxiety and pain. In one RCT, for example, which included 62 patients receiving autologous stem cell transplants for haematological malignancies, the music therapy group scored significantly lower on the anxiety/depression and total mood disturbance score compared with the controlled standard care group (Cassileth et al., 2003). The authors of both these Cochrane reviews, however,

warned that the findings need to be viewed cautiously as most of the studies included high bias risks (Bradt and Dileo, 2010; Bradt et al., 2011). Within Cochrane reviews, findings of 'high bias risk' can mean that one of four criteria for dealing with internal risk domains were not met, that is, (a) adequate randomization, (b) allocation concealment, (c) detail about incomplete outcomes, and (d) blinding of participants, service providers, and assessors (Higgins and Altman, 2008). As, 'it is not possible in music therapy studies to blind participants and those providing the interventions' (Bradt and Dileo, 2010, p. 5), perhaps if the first three mentioned criteria are met (randomization, allocation concealment, and incomplete outcomes addressed) and the assessor is blinded, music therapy trials should be rated as producing high enough quality findings.

Arguably, RCTs and other quantitative studies included in these Cochrane reviews do not produce superior findings to well-conducted qualitative research when investigating music therapy's effect on subjective experiences in palliative care. In RCTs, alongside the problem of non-blinding potentially biasing outcomes, the control of variables is also difficult because (a) music therapy is not a standardized treatment, (b) patient–carer relationships are associated with therapeutic gain (Kain et al., 2004), and (c) conducting studies on representative samples with even distribution of confounders in treatment groups is difficult, especially with small samples. Hence it is suggested that quantitative research only allows logical or conceptual rather than predictive generalizations, just like qualitative research does. Qualitative research on music therapy research questions in palliative care is preferred by some researchers because (a) it can be unethical to withhold (or delay) potentially supportive care through RCTs when patients are assigned to non-experimental groups (Keeley, 1999); (b) RCTs include standardized measurement scales which may provide information important to the researcher but not patients (McGrath, 2000); (c) RCTs do not necessarily support palliative care principles of patient- and family-centred care (Kvale and Bondevik, 2008): patient-centred practice emerges from listening to patients' reflections; and (d) existing outcome tools are not sensitive enough to detect many of the benefits reported in qualitative studies.

Constructivist (qualitative) research approaches can collect patients' and caregivers' idiosyncratic voices, identifying what they find important. Grounded theory methodology, for example, informed a multisite study which uncovered how 100 oncology staff members, who witnessed music therapy on their wards, were often incidentally supported by music therapy and, as a result, perceived improvements in their care of patients (O'Callaghan and Magill, 2009). Grounded theory methods were also used in a study conducted with six patients with chronically progressive multiple sclerosis. Music therapy provided opportunities for the patients to challenge their disabled identities. Improvisation either validated or reminded them of physical loss, and songs supported coping strategies to deal with the condition's emotional impact (Magee and Davidson, 2004).

Closure

Previously, people lived with shared understandings and ways of how to die and mourn. In contemporary, more individualistic societies people use more privatized ways of dealing with loss (Walter,

1994). Music therapists invite palliative care patients and caregivers to explore how musical attachments from their lifetimes and creative experiences with less familiar music can alleviate physical and emotional distress; nurture and sustain; validate one's unique contribution; restore or continue meaningful connection with who and what is important; and enable new realizations and joy through aesthetic or transcendent experiences. Some of the most profound moments in music therapy are when people apparently experience 'happiness' and 'sadness' in an alternate or simultaneous manner as they relive and reintegrate memories alongside a knowing that their mortal end is near. Almost always, patients want the music to continue. Music can 'carry mourning too heavy for words and preaching' (Roy, 2001, p. 132), provide a familiar 'holding space' (Berger, 2006), and be a vehicle for release. Music therapists are vital members of palliative care teams who are helping to enrich people's lives transitioning from corporeal existence, and the family members, friends, and caring staff accompanying their passage.

Notes

1. Some music therapists with specialized training offer patients with good energy and cognitive capacity the Bonney Method of Guided Imagery and Music. After a relaxation induction clients describe their imagery during musical listening, and then verbally or artistically process their reactions in order to increase self-understanding and personal growth.

2. A Cochrane review is a systematic assessment of a health-care intervention consisting of a systematic review of literature related to the intervention and, if appropriate, a meta-analysis of eligible trials (Higgins and Green, 2008). Cochrane reviews are widely regarded as providing gold standard research findings in health care.

References for songs/music mentioned in chapter (piano versions)

a 'Wind Beneath My Wings' (1982), by Jeff Silbar and Larry Henley.
b 'Sailing' (1972), by Gavin Sutherland.
c 'The Prayer' (1998), by David Foster.
d 'One Day at a Time' (1974), by Marijohn Wilkins and Kris Kristofferson.
e 'Love Will Go On' (1997), by James Horner and Will Jennings.
f 'The Swan', by Saent-Saens (1835–1921).
g 'Watermark' (1988), by Enya.
h *The Deer Hunter* 'Cavatina' (1978), by Stanley Myers.
i 'Here I am Lord' (1981), by Dan Schutt.

Online materials

Complete references for this chapter are available online at <http://www.oxfordmedicine.com>.

References

Aasgaard, T. (2001). An ecology of love: aspects of music therapy in the pediatric oncology environment. *Journal of Palliative Care*, 17(3), 177–181.
Berger, J.A. (2006). *Music of the Soul: Composing Life out of Loss*. New York: Routledge.

Bradt, J. and Dileo, C. (2010). Music therapy for end-of-life care. *Cochrane Database of Systematic Reviews*, 1, CD007169.
Bradt, J., Dileo, C., Grocke, D., and Magill, L. (2011). Music interventions for improving psychological and physical outcomes in cancer patients. *Cochrane Database of Systematic Reviews*, 8, CD006911.
Cassileth, B., Vickers, A., and Magill, L. (2003). Music therapy for mood disturbance during hospitalization for autologous stem cell transplantation. *Cancer*, 98, 2723–2729.
Chochinov, H.M. (2012). *Dignity Therapy: Final Words for Final Days*. New York: Oxford University Press.
Daveson, D. and Kennelly, J. (2000). Music therapy in palliative care for hospitalised children and adolescents. *Journal of Palliative Care*, 16, 35–38.
Dileo, C. and Loewy, J. (eds.) (2005). *Music Therapy at the End of Life*. Cherry Hill, NJ: Jeffrey Books.
Forrest, L.C. (2000). Addressing issues of ethnicity and identity in palliative care through music therapy practice. *Australian Journal of Music Therapy*, 11, 23–37.
Glenister, D. (2012). Creative spaces in palliative care facilities: tradition, culture, and experience. *American Journal of Hospice and Palliative Medicine*, 29(2), 89–92.
Hartley, N. (1999). Music therapists' personal reflections on working with those who are living with HIV/AIDS. In D. Aldridge (ed.) *Music Therapy in Palliative Care: New Voices*, pp. 105–125. London: Jessica Kingsley Pty Ltd.
Hilliard, R. (2005). *Hospice and Palliative Care Music Therapy: A Guide to Program Development and Clinical Care*. Cherry Hill, NJ: Jeffrey Books.
Horne-Thompson, A. and Grocke, D. (2008). The effect of music therapy on anxiety in patients who are terminally ill. *Journal of Palliative Medicine*, 11, 582–590.
Magill, L. (2009). Caregiver empowerment and music therapy: through the eyes of bereaved caregivers of advanced cancer patients. *Journal of Palliative Care*, 25, 68–75.
Magill, L. (2010). Art therapy and music therapy. In J.C. Holland, W.S. Breitbart, P.B. Jacobsen, M.S., Lederberg, M.J. Loscalzo, and R. McCorkle (eds.) *Psycho-Oncology* (2nd ed.), pp. 22–28. Oxford: Oxford University Press.
McFerran, K., O'Grady, L., and Roberts, M. (2010). Music therapy with bereaved teenagers: a mixed methods perspective. *Death Studies*, 34, 541–565.
Munro, S. (1984). *Music Therapy in Palliative/Hospice Care*. St Louis, MO: Magnamusic-Baton.
Munro, S. and Mount, B.M. (1978). Music therapy in palliative care. *Canadian Medical Association Journal*, 119, 1029–1034.
O'Callaghan, C. (2009). Objectivist and constructivist music therapy research in oncology and palliative care. *Music and Medicine*, 1(1), 41–60.
O'Callaghan, C. and Jordan, B. (2011). Music therapy supports parent-infant attachments affected by life threatening cancer. In J. Edwards (ed.) *Music Therapy in Parent-Infant Bonding*, pp. 191–207. Oxford: Oxford University Press.
O'Callaghan, C. and Magill, L. (2009). Effect of music therapy on oncologic staff bystanders: a substantive grounded theory. *Journal of Palliative and Supportive Care*, 7, 219–228.
Salmon, D. (1995). Music and emotion in palliative care: assessing inner resources. In C.A Lee (ed.) *Lonely Waters: Proceedings of the International Conference, Music Therapy in Palliative Care*, pp. 71–84. Oxford: Sobell House.

4.8

The contribution of the dietitian and nutritionist to palliative medicine

Rosemary Richardson and Isobel Davidson

Introduction to the contribution of the dietitian and nutritionist to palliative medicine

Nutritional management of patients receiving palliative care is now accepted as an explicit element of care (Finlay, 2001). This includes attempting to manage the nutritional consequences of anorexia and cachexia which are often considered by health-care professionals as milestones of disease progression. Traditionally, the input from those providing palliative care relating to nutrition is one of ethics and centres on the decision to provide food and fluid as treatment or basic care. However, dietary advice spans the entire palliative care spectrum and serves to enhance quality of life as well as nutritional status (Thoresen et al., 2011). Many patients present with and are distressed by the presence of symptoms that affect their ability to eat 'normally', for example, dysphagia, taste changes, xerostomia, and dementia. The consequent deterioration and alteration in nutritional intake promotes weight loss, fatigue, and is associated with poor functional status (see Fig. 4.8.1).

The role of the dietitian may appear simple in attempting to provide sufficient energy to prevent weight loss, but the complexity of the disease process and the barrage of symptoms which influence feeding behaviour profoundly are numerous. In addition, our improved understanding of the metabolic sequelae of disease highlights further the futility of approaches that merely seek to increase patients' nutritional intake (either enterally or parenterally) in an attempt to replete body mass. More realistic goals in nutritional management are nutritional support to maintain body weight and assist in symptom control to optimize physical well-being and support positivity and hope (Seibaek et al., 2011). The key nutritional strategies that may be used to ameliorate or manage symptoms (see Table 4.8.1) have resulted in the recognition of nutrition as a component of holistic palliative care. While research indicates a clear association with loss of body mass and quality of life (Thoresen et al., 2011), the lack of formal and rigorous evaluation (i.e. randomized controlled trials) of nutritional intervention in practice reflects the inherent difficulties of conducting nutritional research in the palliative care environment. The challenge for practitioners remains striking a balance between the application of research evidence and the practical nutritional needs of the individual.

Approaches to increase nutritional intake

Dietary counselling

Dietary counselling should serve to provide the dietitian with an understanding of the patient's nutritional problems, their needs, and an appreciation of limitations and barriers to complying with nutritional advice/prescriptions. Building relationships is an intrinsic, yet vital, component of dietetic consultation. The landscape for dietetic practice has changed significantly and patients are no longer viewed as passive recipients of dietary intervention. Rather they are viewed as partners in their own dietetic management who work in concordance with their dietitian and participate actively in decision-making and goal setting. Therefore, improving and developing communication skills is an essential component of practice and success depends on integrating structure of the consultation and building effective relationships (Kurtz et al., 2003) (see Fig. 4.8.2). Adopting this approach will enable and empower patients to engage actively in their nutritional care (McCorkle et al., 2011) and be conducive to frank and open discussions.

Patients are surprisingly good at providing the information the dietitian wants to hear. While patients may confirm verbally their compliance to nutritional treatment, in utilizing high-level communication skills the practitioner may find adherence may be limited or non-existent. This may account for the disappointing results of one of the few randomized controlled trials that examined the effect of dietary counselling on food intake, body weight, and quality of life in cancer patients (Ovensen et al., 1993). Patients (N = 57) were randomized to receive nutritional counselling (twice a month for 5 months) and offered nutritional supplemental drinks. The control group (N = 48) ate *ad libitum* and had no counselling. Results showed that, when compared with controls, 5 months of dietary counselling increased total energy intake by 15 kcal/day and 0.6 g protein/day and, not surprisingly, no differences in body weight or quality of life were observed. No details of the structure of the counselling interview were provided, other than that its aim was for patients to achieve recommended intakes.

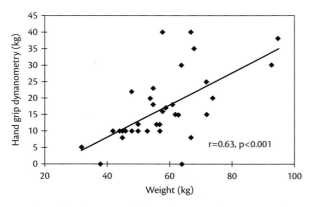

Fig. 4.8.1 Association between weight and grip strength in patients in hospice.

Similarly, a study (Evans et al., 1987) in patients with advanced colorectal and non-small cell lung cancer showed no differences in intake in patients receiving and not receiving dietary counselling.

There remains a paucity of studies that have examined the effect of dietary counselling in palliative care and in the preceding 3 years there appear to be no new additions to the literature. However, a potential proxy of compliance may be to determine a patient's understanding of appropriate nutritional concepts and the outcomes aimed for through intervention. It is worth noting that currently patients seem to have a limited understanding of their condition, approaches being adopted in its management, and a comprehensive understanding of palliative care (Docherty et al., 2008). A patient is more likely to comply if they have a comprehensive understanding of the rationale that underpins a nutritional intervention (Box 4.8.1). Clearly, undertaking further work in this

Table 4.8.1 Nutritional strategies to improve symptom control

Symptom	Causes of decrease in dietary intake	Management
1. Psychological stress/depression	◆ Poor appetite	◆ Antidepressant, psychological support strategies, counselling, complementary therapies (i.e. aromatherapy, reflexology) small frequent meals
2. Altered taste and smell	◆ Food aversions	◆ Dietary counselling and identification of food aversions/preferences
3. Oral thrush/ulceration	◆ Blunting of taste	◆ Pharmacological treatment of symptoms (i.e. nystatin, lignocaine) ◆ Increase use of nutrient-dense cold fluids ◆ Optimize oral hygiene
4. Reduced flow and altered consistency of saliva	◆ Induce gagging and nausea	◆ Use of artificial saliva and hydrating oral gels ◆ To encourage flow of saliva—chew gum or suck on boiled sweets ◆ Optimize oral hygiene
5. Nausea and vomiting	◆ Physical obstruction ◆ Drugs, e.g. opioids ◆ Radio-/chemotherapy	◆ Pharmacological treatment that is effective at mealtimes ◆ Small frequent meals ◆ Avoidance of food aversions ◆ Consume fluids after meals
6. Dysphagia	◆ Physical obstruction/construction	◆ Altered consistency of food semi-solid → puree ◆ Use of nutrient-dense supplements ◆ Consider initiating PEG feeding
7. Respiratory distress	◆ Focus on breathing rather than food intake	◆ Medication before mealtimes ◆ Ensure patient wearing loose clothing ◆ Relaxation exercises ◆ Small meals and present foods that do not require much chewing
8. Early satiety	◆ Cytokine mediated	◆ Maximize availability of food ◆ Small frequent meals ◆ Encourage food consumption when patient feels at their best/less agitated
9. Altered bowel function: (i) Constipation (ii) Diarrhoea	◆ Feeling bloated ◆ Abdominal discomfort ◆ Abdominal discomfort ◆ Fear of symptom leads to food avoidance	◆ Appropriate laxatives ◆ Encourage fluid intake ◆ Encourage consumption of dietary fibre ◆ If possible optimize mobility ◆ Medication: includes anti-diarrhoeas, pancreatic enzyme supplements as appropriate ◆ Temporarily avoid dairy products ◆ Increase intake soluble fibre (e.g. bananas, oranges, oatmeal)
10. Fatigue/lethargy	◆ Neurological ◆ Loss of muscle mass	◆ Maximize intake when patient feels at their best ◆ Avoid foods that require a lot of chewing

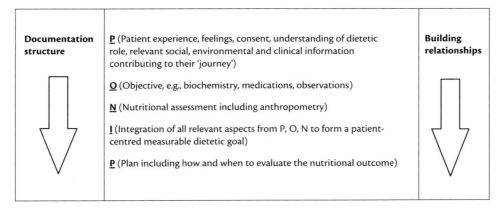

Documentation structure	P (Patient experience, feelings, consent, understanding of dietetic role, relevant social, environmental and clinical information contributing to their 'journey')	Building relationships
	O (Objective, e.g., biochemistry, medications, observations)	
	N (Nutritional assessment including anthropometry)	
	I (Integration of all relevant aspects from P, O, N to form a patient-centred measurable dietetic goal)	
	P (Plan including how and when to evaluate the nutritional outcome)	

Fig. 4.8.2 Consultation structure for effective relationship building.
Source: data from Kurtz S et al., Marrying content and process in clinical method teaching: enhancing the Calgary-Cambridge Guides, *Academic Medicine*, Volume 78, Issue 8, pp. 802–809, Copyright © 2003 Association of American Medical Colleges

area is imperative if oral nutritional interventions are to demonstrate efficacy.

Patients and their informal carers have high expectations of nutritional intervention and have on occasion chosen invasive options such as total parenteral nutrition, with no hope of effect (McCann et al., 1994; Plaisance, 1997). Thoughtful counselling acts to improve patient management and, by putting the patient at the centre of care, allows them to make choices and identify realistic goals. It should be remembered that the Internet is a source of dietary information accessed by many patients and their carers. This may result in alternative therapies being used such as macrobiotic diets, supra dosing of vitamins, and homeopathy. This should be explored in the consultation so that the clinician has a complete picture of what the patient is doing for himself.

Dietary counselling with particularly complex cases involving cachexia-anorexia is a resource-intensive management strategy relying on the knowledge and communication skills of the dietitian. A more effective and efficient strategy may be to promote self-supported management with the patient and carer (Davidson et al., 2012).

Nutritional supplements

Oral nutritional supplements normally provide 1.5 kcal/mL and 0.6 g/mL of protein presented in 200–250 mL cartons and are intended to supplement, not substitute, energy intake from food. Compliance with oral nutritional support regimens was often poor (Akner and Cederholm, 2003) but in recent years this seems to have improved markedly (Hubbard et al 2012). This improvement will result in increased energy intake which in turn may be associated with clinical benefit. Progress in the quality of dietetic consultations may account for this positive shift in compliance to oral nutritional supplements. The role of altered ingestive behaviour should also be taken into account in prescribing the timing of taking oral nutritional supplements.

Timing of consumption

It is well recognized that the control of ingestive behaviour in cachexia influences nutritional intake profoundly. Many patients may have amplification of the satiety cascade (neural and humoral), thereby prolonging the inter-meal interval and

Box 4.8.1 Effective dietary counselling: suggestions for constructing a patient interview

♦ What changes in your diet have there been over the last few months?
  • Quantity
  • Food aversion/taste changes
  • Consistency
  • Diet history.
♦ Do you think nutrition is an important part of your care?
♦ Any symptoms around mealtimes that are troublesome?
  • Pain
  • Respiratory distress
♦ How are you managing with nutritional supplemental drinks?
  • Compliance
  • Change prescription
  • Taste fatigue
♦ Is there any time of the day when you feel at your best?
  • Opportunity to optimize intake.
♦ How is your informal carer (if patient interviewed?)
  • Pressure for patient to eat
  • Anxiety of carer
  • Identify home enteral feeding problems
♦ Are you happy that your nutritional status is monitored?
  • Objectives.

If the patient cannot be interviewed then the carer becomes the source of dietary information.

reducing daily consumption. Indeed, early satiety is frequently reported in patients with a palliative diagnosis (Andrew et al., 2009) to a relatively low gastric volume. One strategy to address this would be to offer energy- and protein-dense supplements before meals (1 hour) when feelings of hunger are strongest. In addition, patients should be discouraged from consuming low nutritive fluids at the beginning of meals such as soups. The rationale for this is to minimize the volumetric effect of fluids on satiety. While this approach is based on the translation of pathophysiology to practice, it remains to be evaluated in the clinical situation (Bell et al., 2003).

There are some concerns that consumption of supplements before meals would result in energy compensation at mealtimes, thus reducing overall daily intake. Interestingly, in a study (Rolls et al., 1991) that examined the effect of nutritive pre-loads (high fat, high carbohydrate) on meal consumption in elderly subjects and younger controls, the elderly subjects did not compensate for the pre-load. These results are encouraging, given that the majority of patients in palliative care are elderly; however, in this study no subject had metabolically active disease which influences both sides of the energy balance equation detrimentally.

Nutritional modulation

A characteristic feature of cachexia, despite its primary cause, is the presence of systemic inflammation. A consequence of this, in addition to loss of functional tissue, is reduced motivation to eat and the ineffective utilization of nutrients. Thus, in conditions where the inflammatory response is more profound, the associated anorexia may be more resistant to interventional strategies and the accretion of lean body mass becomes an impossible goal. In recent years there has been considerable interest in the use of nutrients with putative anti-inflammatory properties that attenuate cachexia and promote anabolism to improve body composition. The primary aim of this treatment modality is to improve survival and quality of life where functional ability is a key component.

Work in patients with advanced pancreatic cancer (Richardson et al., 2001) examining the effect of a fish oil-enriched supplement (eicosapentaenoic acid (EPA), energy and protein dense) on total dietary intake was initially very promising. Nutrient intake (meals and supplement) was significantly greater in those patients receiving the fish oil, than in the group randomized to energy and protein supplements alone. Results from 200 patients with pancreatic carcinoma supplemented with 2 g of EPA revealed net gain of weight and lean tissue. Despite these early successes, more recently a study (Fearon et al., 2006) of over 500 cachectic patients (gastrointestinal and lung cancer) supplemented with either 2 or 4 g/day of EPA indicated no significant treatment benefit in terms of weight or survival. This is supported by other work (Bruera et al., 2003) in a more heterogeneous cachectic group showing EPA had no significant benefits on energy intake and nutritional status. The literature continues to provide unequivocal results with respect to n-3 fatty acid supplementation. A recent double-blind, placebo controlled trial (Finocchiaro et al., 2012) intervening with both EPA and docosahexaenoic acid provided evidence of better preservation of body weight status and anti-inflammatory effects in lung cancer patients receiving chemotherapy.

There remains insufficient evidence to support a clear benefit to n-3 fatty acid supplementation in advanced disease (Ries et al., 2011). However, it may have a role in maintaining nutritional status and limiting the effects of active treatment in palliative therapy in specific homogeneous clinical populations.

Patient acceptance

Taste and smell

Physiological stimulation of gustation and olfaction by food in healthy individuals appears primarily to be a positive influence on intake, so long as the food itself is palatable. Hence chemosensory changes which accompany advanced disease have a significant impact on the quantity and quality of nutrients ingested (Hutton et al., 2007) and predict poorer functional status and quality of life.

Factors that contribute to aberrations in taste and smell are rooted in treatment modalities (drug treatment, radiotherapy), but are less understood in the disease process itself (Lennie et al., 2006; Vance and Burrage, 2006). Perceived changes in taste and smell reported by patients in palliative care, however, are not uniform which makes provision of general advice difficult. To improve compliance in taking supplements, patients should be offered a range of flavours and this also applies to 'normal' diet. This strategy may prevent the development of sensory specific satiety (Rolls and Rolls, 1996) and limits the negative impact of chemosensory changes on nutrient quality.

Promoting dietary intake

Maintaining dietary intake to meet requirements can be particularly difficult in the palliative stage for both practitioner and patient. Health-care professionals must appreciate that eating-related distress is evident in both patients and their family. Frequently food presented needs modification in consistency, attractiveness, and portion size. Symptoms such as pain can reduce dietary intake. In addition, the pressure that the informal carer can put on the patient to eat often goes unrecognized (Strasser et al., 2007).

> My husband is doing his best he cooks my favourite foods and brings it to me on a tray. It's too much, I just can't eat it so I scoop half of it into a bag. [Cancer patient]
>
> At first cooking was difficult; since developing Parkinson's we have radically changed what we eat. [Parkinson's patient]

These issues should be explored during dietary counselling.

Individual attention to detail is important in encouraging dietary intake and many issues are addressed in Table 4.8.1. It is important to make sure the patient is comfortable (e.g. correct positioning, toileting) and the environment is conducive to eating (e.g. catheter bag covered, table/tray attractively presented).

Dysphagia

Patients who may develop dysphagia include those with motor neuron disease, Alzheimer's disease, progressive multiple sclerosis, and Parkinson's disease and is particularly well documented in those with head and neck cancer (Roe et al., 2007). The severity of dysphagia varies considerably. Some patients may have mild swallowing problems requiring minor food modification (texture modification).The recently updated descriptors for texture modified diets (British Dietetic Association, 2009) provide guidelines for all modifications required for patients with swallowing impairment. It should be remembered that the liquid content of modified diets tends to be high and acts to dilute the nutrient content. Macronutrient and micronutrient fortification is often required. Whereas others with severe dysphagia may be unable to tolerate even very little oral intake. For those patients who are unable to swallow enough to maintain hydration or nutrition, placement of a percutaneous endoscopic gastrostomy (PEG) tube may be considered, but long-term treatment goals must be identified.

Home artificial nutrition

The majority of palliative care patients on home feeding are prescribed enteral nutrition (nasogastric and PEG). Implementation of home artificial nutrition support requires significant education and training of the patient and/or their carer. Meticulous discharge planning, communication between the care team, and a structured monitoring process are key elements to making home enteral nutrition an acceptable treatment modality. In a recent survey, the primary reason for instituting home artificial nutrition was found to be to support patient well-being and not, as one might expect, to prolong life (Orreval et al., 2009). The informal carer is most likely to take responsibility for maintaining patency of the feeding tube, feed administration, and routine mentoring.

Prior to starting feeding or sending patients home on feeding, the patient's home should be visited to evaluate practical issues such as:

◆ What storage space is available to stock feed and related consumables (e.g. giving sets)?

◆ Can a drip stand be moved freely round the house? Steps and loose carpets may increase the patient's risk of tripping

◆ Communication support issues.

Nutritional assessment

A precursor to assessment is nutritional screening and the Malnutrition Universal Screening Tool (MUST) is a validated tool used widely in clinical practice (Elia and Stratton, 2012). This screening tool has been designed to identify adults who are underweight or at risk of malnutrition. Screened patients identified at risk of becoming malnourished may be referred to a dietitian who will undertake a full nutritional assessment.

This assessment not only involves determination of nutrient intake (dietary and/or artificial nutritional support), a procedure generally well accepted by the patient, but should also include sequential monitoring of the patient's nutritional status. The latter provides information relating to the progression or attenuation of loss of body mass. Sensitivity to the patient when undertaking the assessment is paramount. If a patient is in the terminal stage of their disease, is immobile, and/or severely demented, undertaking a nutritional assessment may be inappropriate. However, if the patient's stage of cachexia can be appropriately classified (Fearon et al., 2011) this may prove useful in identifying when dietetic interventions are likely to be of greatest benefit.

Body weight

An individual's body weight can be compared with tables (Metropolitan Life Foundation, 1983) which provide 'normal' values for individuals of the same sex, age, and height. However, consideration of recent weight loss (i.e. past 3 months) allows an insight into the magnitude and progression of weight loss. Sarcopenic obesity is now common. It is important to respect the patient's wishes, in that some might not wish their weight to be monitored, and these should be respected. However a recent UK-wide hospice study indicates that there is a clear reluctance of staff to instigate weighing for fear of upsetting patients (Watson et al., 2010). This is despite 96% of patients reporting that this procedure had never upset them and 74% of patients weighing themselves at home.

Weight loss as % of 'used' body weight:

$$\% \text{ weight loss } = \frac{\text{used body weight (kg)} - \text{current weight}}{\text{usual body weight}} \times 100$$

This approach allows the patient to provide their own reference value. An unintentional weight loss of 10% in 3 months is indicative of significant weight loss and 20% of protein energy undernutrition (Kinney, 1988).

Body mass index

Another method of using weight as a nutritional parameter is to express height as a power index of weight:

$$\text{body mass index (BMI) units } (\text{kg/m}^2) = \frac{\text{Weight (kg)}}{\text{Height}^2 (\text{m})}$$

◆ A BMI less than 20 is indicative of mild undernutrition

◆ A BMI less than 18 is indicative of moderate undernutrition

◆ A BMI less than 16 is indicative of severe undernutrition.

The assessor should be aware that the presence of oedema or ascites may mask the degree of undernutrition and care in interpretation of weight data is required. In addition, an overweight patient can be malnourished and may also have significant loss of muscle mass (sarcopenic obesity).

Arm anthropometry

Triceps skinfold thickness provides an indication of fat reserves. This measurement is taken using skinfold calipers at the mid-point between the acnomium process and the olecranon and results are compared with standard values (Jelliffe, 1996).

An indication of skeletal muscle mass may be obtained from subtracting the skinfold thickness from the mid-upper arm circumference. This technique assumes the upper arm is a perfect circle.

$$\begin{aligned} \text{Arm muscle circumference (AMC)} \\ = \text{mid-upper arm circumference (MUAC)} \\ - (\text{triceps skinfold} \times \pi) \end{aligned}$$

The upper arm is easily accessible and less prone to oedema. Information on arm anthropometry should be considered with weight data.

Handgrip dynamometry

Weakness, asthenia, and fatigue are common symptoms of palliative care patients. While weight and arm anthropometry provide quantitative information relating to body mass, handgrip dynamometry is a functional marker of mass and, in end-of-life patients, correlates with body weight (Fig. 4.8.1). If the aim of nutritional intervention is to improve lean body mass, it is important that both the quantity and quality of this tissue increases. This non-invasive technique involves determination of patients maximal grip strength (Windsor and Hill, 1988).

However, it should be remembered that in the presence of a systemic inflammatory response, improvements in body mass are generally not achievable. The overriding component of nutritional management in palliative care is ensuring the wishes of the patient and family are fulfilled. Today, patients and relatives are more informed than ever before and many actively seek information relating to disease and management. This means that the boundaries of practice for health-care professionals have shifted and this is a continuous dynamic process. Now more than ever there is a need for professionals to integrate their understanding of clinical science and current research to inform their practice. The science of cachexia treatment options and research are discussed in detail in Chapter 10.5.

Online materials

Complete references for this chapter are available online at <http://www.oxfordmedicine.com>.

References

Andrew, I., Waterfied, K., Hildreth, A., *et al.* (2009). Quantifying the impact of standardized assessment and symptom management tools on symptoms associated with cancer-induced anorexia cachexia syndrome. *Palliative Medicine*, 23, 680–688.

British Dietetic Association and the Royal College of Speech and Language Therapists (2009). *National Descriptors for Texture-Modification in Adults*. Birmingham: British Dietetic Association.

Davidson, I., Whyte, F., and Richardson, R.A. (2012). Self-management in palliative medicine. *Current Opinion in Supportive and Palliative Care*, 6, 432–437.

Docherty, A., Owens, A., Asadi-Lari, M., *et al* (2008) Knowledge and information needs of informal caregivers in palliative care: a qualitative systematic review. *Palliative Medicine*, 22, 153–157.

Elia, M. and Stratton, R.J. (2012). An analytical appraisal of nutrition screening tools supported by original data with particular reference to age. *Nutrition*, 28, 477–494.

Fearon, K.C.H., Strasser, F., Anker, S.D., *et al.* (2011). Definition and classification of cancer cachexia: an international consensus. *The Lancet Oncology*, 12, 489–495.

Finocchiaro, C., Segre, O., Fadda, M., *et al.* (2012). Effect of n-3 fatty acids in patients with advanced lung cancer: a double blind placebo controlled study. *British Journal of Nutrition*, 108, 327–333.

Hubbard, G.P., Elia, M., Holdaway, A., *et al.* (2012). A systematic review of compliance to oral nutritional supplements. *Clinical Nutrition*, 31, 293–312.

McCorkle, R., Erolano, E., Lazeby, M., *et al.* (2011) Self-management: enabling and empowering patients living with cancer as a chronic illness. *CA: A Cancer Journal for Clinicians*, 61, 50–62.

Orreval, Y., Tishelman, C., Permert, J., and Cederholm, T. (2009). The use of artificial nutrition among cancer patients enrolled in palliative home care services. *Palliative Medicine*, 23, 556–564.

Ovensen, L., Allingstrup, L., Hannibal, J., Mortensen, E.L., and Hansen, O.P. (1993). Effect of dietary counselling on food intake, body weight, response rate, survival and quality of life in cancer patients undergoing chemotherapy: a prospective, randomised study. *Journal of Clinical Oncology*, 13, 2043–2049.

Ries, A., Trottenberg, P., Elsner, F., *et al.* (2011). A systematic review on the role of fish oil for the treatment of cachexia in advanced cancer: an EPCRC cachexia guidelines project. *Palliative Medicine*, 26, 294–304.

Seibaek, L., Petersen, L.K., Blaakaer, J., *et al.* (2011). Hoping for the best, preparing for the worst: the lived experiences of women undergoing ovarian cancer surgery. *European Journal of Cancer Care*, 21, 360–371.

Strasser, F., Binswanger, J., Cerny, T., and Kesselring A. (2007). Fighting a losing battle: eating distress of men with advanced cancer and their female partners. A mixed-methods study. *Palliative Medicine*, 21, 129–137.

Watson, M., Coulter, S., McLoughlin, C., *et al.* (2010). Attitudes towards weight and weight assessment in oncology patients: survey of hospice staff and patients with advanced cancer. *Palliative Medicine*, 24, 623–629.

4.9

Physiotherapy in palliative care

Anne M. English

Introduction to physiotherapy in palliative care

Palliative care and rehabilitation both focus on the concept of helping people to maximize their potential and live as well as they can, given their circumstances.

Physiotherapy is defined as a health-care profession concerned with human function and movement, thereby maximizing people's quality of life. It is a constantly evolving profession that strives towards excellence and consistency within clinical practice (Chartered Society of Physiotherapy (CSP), 2005). It is a science-based profession and takes a person-centred approach to health and well-being which includes the patient's general lifestyle and uses physical approaches to promote, maintain, and restore physical, psychological, and social well-being. It is committed to applying, evaluating, and reviewing the evidence that underpins and informs its practice and delivery (CSP, 2013).

Physiotherapists practise independently, as first-contact practitioners and as part of the multidisciplinary team (MDT). They help to encourage, develop, and facilitate independence, working with people to optimize their functional ability and potential (CSP, 2011). They address problems of impairment and manage recovering, stable, and deteriorating conditions, treating a wide range of physical conditions of people with varying health status (relating both to physical and mental health) (CSP, 2005).

The role of the physiotherapist in palliative care includes assessment, symptom management, function and rehabilitation, education and communication, prevention, and psychological aspects of care. The physiotherapist plays an important role in the MDT in cancer care. Effective MDT working should result in care being considered by professionals with specialist skills and knowledge in the relevant aspects of each cancer type (National Cancer Action Team, 2010). Evidence also supports a multiprofessional approach to patients with neurological conditions, suggesting that neurology, rehabilitation, and palliative care services should be closely linked in order to support patients from diagnosis to death, and physiotherapists are recognized as being involved at different stages of neurological illness trajectory (National End of Life Care Programme, 2010).

Working alongside the patient in a one-to-one relationship provides the opportunity for the physiotherapist to explore further the patient's misconceptions and hesitantly voiced fears. Understanding the physical processes involved can reduce the patient's anxiety and distress. The provision of management strategies empowers the patient to regain control over aspects of their condition, at a time when they are often experiencing helplessness and loss of independence. Carers and family members should also play an active part in caregiving.

Assessment and communication

Patient assessment identifies problems and enables the patient and physiotherapist to agree on realistic goals, formulate a treatment plan, and decide on appropriate outcome measures. Rehabilitation assessment in relation to cancer can be recognized in four stages—preventative, restorative, supportive, and palliative (Dietz, 1980)—and are recognized as essential components of the patient pathway (National Institute for Health and Care Excellence (NICE), 2004). A four-level model has been suggested, recognizing those professionals who should be involved at each level, their function, and their level of expertise (Rankin et al., 2008). Early referral is important to allow anticipation of problems and put coping strategies in place. All goals must be patient centred, measurable, and achievable. They may be simple or complex (e.g. 'to attend my grandson's wedding'). Reassessment and redefining of goals may be necessary on a daily basis as the patient's condition can fluctuate rapidly. Knowledge regarding evidence-based principles of falls management is essential in order to be aware of risks and plan appropriately. A proportion of falls in palliative settings may be preventable and avoidable with regular risk assessment (Help the Hospices, 2010).

The importance of good communication skills in cancer and palliative care is widely recognized and advanced communication skills training is now available (NICE, 2004). Physiotherapists work closely with patients and may be asked difficult questions about prognosis or disease progression. It is important that they have the knowledge and skills to cope in such situations.

Challenging and complex problems

Patients with palliative care needs present multifaceted problems associated with an increasing range of underlying pathologies in a wide range of care settings (Allied Health Professions Palliative Care Project Team, 2004).The physiotherapist is involved in the treatment of patients with active and progressive conditions which may include cancer, HIV/AIDS, neurological, cardiac, chronic respiratory, endocrine diseases, and dementia.

Patients with respiratory problems

Dyspnoea

Breathlessness is a devastating and common symptom in patients with cancer and other advanced progressive illnesses (Fallon and

Hanks, 2006). It is difficult to manage and physiotherapists need a clear understanding of the nature of breathlessness in order to support their patients. A breathlessness assessment must be patient centred, holistic, and an ongoing process. Outcome measures may be subjective, and reliable scales such as the visual analogue scale, numerical rating scale, and modified Borg scale (Borg 1978) may be used to measure the sensation of breathlessness in patients with cancer. Measurements may be taken at first contact with the patient and then at agreed times during and on completion of treatment. A holistic breathlessness assessment may look at timing and frequency of breathlessness, what makes it better or worse, and explores the feelings associated with it (Corner and O'Driscoll, 1999).

Restrictive disorders, for example, primary and secondary lung cancers, mesothelioma, pulmonary fibrosis, and neuromuscular diseases, are characterized by reduced lung volume, poor compliance, and increased work of breathing. Obstructive disorders, for example, chronic obstructive pulmonary disease (COPD), bronchiectasis, and cystic fibrosis, cause increased work of breathing and airflow resistance (Hough, 2001).

Breathlessness is a frightening and unpleasant sensation experienced by many patients with various diagnoses. The effectiveness of a breathlessness service for treatment of lung cancer is recommended by NICE (2011), and suggested by Hately et al. (2003). Management may include airway clearance, breathing control, positioning, cognitive behavioural therapy, fan therapy, pacing (controlling breathing while walking or climbing stairs), prioritizing (choosing the most important activities that need to be done), relaxation, energy conservation, provision of walking aids, and education. Auscultation, pulse oximetry, a thorough history of the patient's medication, including inhalers, nebulizers, and the use of oxygen, are all important (Hough, 2001). Breathless patients automatically adopt positions that ease their breathing. This reduces the work of breathing and sensation of breathlessness. Useful recovery positions are sitting forward while resting forearms on thighs, forward lean standing, and relaxed sitting. Resting positions include forward lean sitting (see Fig. 4.9.1) and high side lying (i.e. lying on the side, knees slightly bent, rolled slightly forward, using three or four pillows to raise the shoulders, one pillow

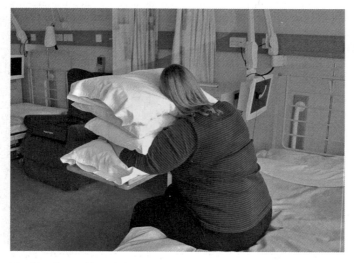

Fig. 4.9.1 Forward lean sitting.

to support the head and neck) (Leyshon, 2012). Breathing control involves the use of the lower chest and upper abdomen therefore encouraging better use of the diaphragm. As the patient becomes more proficient they should be able to control the rate and depth of breathing to suit their needs.

Anxiety and emotions are closely associated with breathlessness and impact negatively on a wide range of other symptoms. Bausewien et al. (2008) conclude there are moderate levels of evidence to support breathing training including ways of managing anxiety in breathless patients. There is also strong evidence to support chest wall vibration and neuroelectrical muscle stimulation to relieve breathlessness in people with COPD (Bausewien et al., 2008).

Relaxation has been shown to reduce heart rate, respiratory rate, oxygen consumption, and blood pressure in breathless patient (Gosslink, 2003). It can also be used to reduce anxiety and to aid control of negative thoughts. Regular practice enables the patient to recall the technique and recreate the feeling of relaxation (Payne, 2000).

A handheld fan directed to the face may also help to reduce the sensation of breathlessness in some breathless patients (Galbraith et al., 2010).

In patients with chronic obstructive airways disease, pulmonary rehabilitation programmes are recommended, with a view to improving exercise capacity, dyspnoea, health status, and psychological well-being (Bolton et al., 2013). There are high levels of evidence to support pulmonary rehabilitation in people with COPD (Bolton et al., 2013). Pulmonary rehabilitation is described as an interdisciplinary programme of care, individually designed to optimize physical and social performance and autonomy. It has been shown to relive dyspnoea and fatigue, improve emotional function, and enhance the patient's control over their condition (Lacasse et al., 2006). Following an exacerbation of their COPD, pulmonary rehabilitation appears to be a very effective and safe intervention (Puhan et al., 2011). Pulmonary rehabilitation programmes include individual exercise programmes and education delivered by the interdisciplinary team (NICE, 2011). Programmes lasting 6–12 weeks are recommended (Bolton et al., 2013).

Management of respiratory secretions

Traditional physiotherapy techniques (e.g. chest wall shakings and vibrations) are used with caution in palliative care and these interventions would be contraindicated for patients with osteoporosis, bone metastases, and haemoptysis (Hough, 2001). Active cycle of breathing, assisted cough, and positioning are used on a regular basis by physiotherapists. Active cycle of breathing is an airways clearance method used to loosen secretions. It includes a combination of breathing control, thoracic expansions, and forced expiratory technique, facilitating expectoration (Bott et al., 2009). Research evidence favours active cycle of breathing over most alternatives for short-term improvement of secretion clearance in patients with COPD, bronchiectasis, and cystic fibrosis (Lewis et al., 2012). Adequate humidification and hydration is essential to encourage secretion clearance and a nebulizer may be helpful.

The use of respiratory suction, especially at the end of life, is a controversial subject and is difficult to research. Noisy breathing is thought to be caused by accumulation of secretions in the upper airways; however, this remains unproven. Oropharyngeal suction, if applied, should always be carried out with extreme caution, as it may be distressing for the patient. Evidence suggests that positional changes and regular mouth care are more appropriate (Wee and Hillier, 2010). Relatives at the bedside may find this stage distressing and good communication skills by the physiotherapist are essential.

Cough

Patients with neuromuscular disorders (e.g. motor neurone disease (MND)) experience a number of respiratory problems. Poor lung compliance and consequently reduced lung volumes hinder the ability to cough effectively. There is a direct link between maximal inspiratory pressure and cough flow, demonstrating the importance of inspiratory muscle strength (Kang et al., 2006). An efficient and inexpensive piece of equipment, the lung volume recruitment (LVR) bag can be used to develop a breath stacking system, resulting in increased cough effectiveness (Armstrong, 2009). The LVR bag can be used up to four times per day or as required (see Fig. 4.9.2). To increase the expiratory force of a cough, a combination of a manually assisted cough and a cough assist machine may be used. The cough assist or mechanical in-exsufflator assists sputum clearance by the use of both positive and negative pressure. Gradual application of positive pressure to the airways is quickly changed to a negative pressure. This pressure change produces a high expiratory flow rate and stimulates a cough (Anderson, 2005). Physiotherapy techniques combined with this, enable secretions to come into the mouth and be wiped or suctioned away.

Cardiac failure

Cardiac failure is becoming more prevalent as people live longer and breathlessness is one of the early symptoms patients experience (Nicholas, 2004). Palliative care plays an important role in improving the quality of life of patients with heart failure, and therefore presents a challenge for physiotherapists to develop future services for these patients; however, heart failure patients have limited access to palliative care services (Harrison et al., 2012). Non-pharmacological interventions to manage breathlessness may include breathing retraining, pacing and prioritizing,

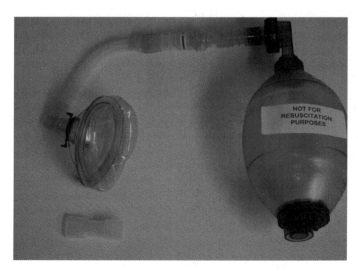

Fig. 4.9.2 Lung volume recruitment bag.

relaxation, a handheld fan, exercise and provision of walking aids and equipment, and psychological interventions (Gadoud et al., 2013). Rehabilitation is focused on exercise programmes to address cardiorespiratory deconditioning and maintenance of muscle bulk (Rees et al., 2009).

Patients with neurological problems

Patients may present with a wide range of different conditions, such as spinal cord compression (SCC), peripheral neuropathies, and cerebral tumours. The disease trajectory of brain tumour patients can vary as symptoms change over a short period of time. The rehabilitation professional must consider the fluctuation in symptoms and patient ability, the ultimate goal is maintaining independence and improving quality of life (Carr et al., 2008). Patients with long-term neurological conditions also come under the palliative umbrella and the importance of controlling symptoms and offering social, psychological, and spiritual support is described (Department of Health, 2005). These patients may have similar symptoms to cancer patients but, due to longer illness trajectories, will experience these symptoms over a greater period of time. Such diseases include multiple sclerosis, Parkinson's disease, MND, and muscular dystrophies.

Physiotherapists have a wide knowledge base and expertise in movement analysis and functional assessment, enabling them to develop individual treatment plans and agree the most appropriate interventions with the patient.

Active assisted exercises and passive movements are helpful in maintaining joint range, preventing muscle shortening and contractures, and reducing spasticity and pain. Patients are encouraged to maintain good posture when sitting and mobilizing. The physiotherapist assists with normal movement patterns, balance, gait analysis, and movement control. Training is given in use of appropriate mobility aids and sometimes the use of a tilt-table is helpful to enable standing to aid ventilation, bladder and bowel function, and most importantly psychological well-being.

Introduction of a wheelchair may be difficult for the patient, as it represents changes in lifestyle and dependency. Advice should be given on transfers into, rising from, and sitting in the wheelchair, maintenance of cushions, and safety for both patient and carer when manoeuvring the chair.

Spinal cord compression

Patients with advanced cancer may develop metastatic cord compression and this often indicates advanced disease. For many patients it may represent the final stage of their illness, and they will need help and support in adapting to a drastic reduction in functional ability and in developing future coping strategies (Lee et al., 2012). The physiotherapist is often ideally placed to note the early signs of SCC and alert the team concerned with future management of this oncological emergency.

In the unstable spine, surgery may be indicated to decompress the tumour and maintain stability, and the physiotherapist will be a core member of the post-surgical team. If unfit for surgery, radiotherapy may be the treatment of choice (Al-Hakim et al., 2006). If SCC occurs, it results in loss of varying degrees of motor, sensory, and autonomic function below the level of compression.

Physiotherapy may consist of balance training, development of upper body strength, instruction in transfers, and use of a wheelchair. Relatives and carers will also require instruction in appropriate techniques. Provision of braces, splints, and walking aids may enable the patient to be as independent and comfortable as possible.

Fatigue

Fatigue is described as a persistent, subjective feeling of tiredness, weakness, or lack of energy, which may be physical or psychological, and is related to cancer or advanced chronic illness (National Comprehensive Cancer Network, 2010).

The effects of cancer-related fatigue are well documented, affecting between 70% and 100% of patients. Fatigue is a common and stressful symptom experienced by patients, and will impact greatly on quality of life (Watson and Mock, 2004). Physical exercise seems to have some benefit in the reduction of fatigue associated with cancer (Cramp and Daniel, 2008). A systematic review (Cramp and Byron-Daniel, 2012) suggests that physical exercise, for example, aerobic walking and cycling, may help to reduce fatigue during and after cancer treatment. This evidence relates specifically to patients with prostate or breast cancer. Hayes et al. (2009) recommend aerobic exercise three to five times weekly for 20–30 minutes in active patients and daily exercise for deconditioned patients.

Exercise

Exercise is known to have many physiological and psychological benefits and is a well-established intervention in palliative care (Oldervoll et al., 2006). Inclusion of physiotherapy-led exercise within cancer pathways can reduce and help to prevent disability (Headley et al., 2004). Exercise may be individual or group, must be safe, have known benefits, and take into account the patient's age, present condition, past medical history, and nutritional status. Positive effects include improvement in muscle strength, balance, endurance, joint range, functional capacity, and reduction in anxiety and depression. Patients presenting with conditions such as anaemia, bone metastases, respiratory insufficiency, and musculoskeletal problems must be carefully assessed, as exercise may be contraindicated. Exercise at end of life should be little and often and goal focused, for example, transferring bed to chair.

Cancer cachexia guidelines and classification are discussed in Chapter 10.5. Fearon et al. (2013) suggest that the management of cachexia is limited and complex. The physiotherapist may become involved in cachexia management. Maddocks et al. (2012) suggest the use of therapeutic exercise as a sound rationale in patients in advanced disease, with a potential to maintain or slow the loss of physical function (see Chapter 10.5).

Pain

The experience of pain is multifactorial and encompasses physical, psychological, emotional, social, and spiritual components (Robb and Ewer-Smith, 2008). Physiotherapists play a major role in pain management and rehabilitation is now considered an essential component of care (NICE, 2004). It is important to involve the patient and carers in treatment planning and goal setting using a patient-centred approach. The aim is to relieve pain and improve function using the best available evidence. A common response to pain is developing pain behaviours, for example, avoiding activities. Pain avoidance is an important part of pain management. Inactivity leads to a cycle of deconditioning, increased muscular tension, joint stiffness, possible contractures, and muscle shortening leading to an increase in pain. Appropriate positioning of patients helps reduce stress on weakened joints and muscles and prevent development of pressure areas. Fracture sites, weakened muscles, and deformities may be immobilized and braced by provision of splints, collars, and various supports.

Physiotherapists may work as part of a MDT ensuring the delivery of high-quality, effective care for people with dementia (NICE, 2006). Physiotherapists may be involved in mobility, falls prevention, exercise, and pain management (Christofoletti et al., 2008). In the advanced stages of the disease, physiotherapists may be working passively, as the patient may not remember or understand the instructions given to them (Pace et al., 2011). In end-of-life care, physiotherapists may advise on positioning, seating, and managing painful contractures (Oddy, 2011).

Physiotherapy techniques to manage pain may include exercise, re-education of posture, relaxation, transcutaneous nerve stimulation (TENS), acupuncture, heat, ice, and massage. Touch is probably the oldest method of relieving pain and discomfort and massage may be used to reduce muscle spasm, relieve pain, and aid relaxation. Soft tissue mobilization is widely practised and includes myofascial techniques and connective tissue massage (British Pain Society, 2010) (see Chapter 9.12).

Nausea, loss of appetite, and constipation

TENS and acupuncture may be used to relieve nausea using the Neiguan antiemetic acupuncture point (Fønnebø, 2011) (see Chapter 9.12).

It has been demonstrated that patients receiving regular physiotherapy of more than 10 minutes daily, experience a significant reduction in appetite disturbance (Laakso, 2003).

Evidence also suggests that there is an increased risk of constipation in people walking less than 0.5 km daily and a squatting position has been shown to facilitate efficient funnelling of the pelvic floor favouring defecation (Kyle, 2007). This can be simulated by provision of a simple step on which to rest the feet, when the patient is seated on the toilet. Raising the knees above the level of the hips, combined with relaxed deep breathing and a gentle rocking motion, may help ease the process of bowel evacuation and relieve constipation.

Chronic oedema

Physiotherapy skills contribute to the team management of lymphoedema and palliative physiotherapists may choose to train to graduate diploma level in lymphoedema management. A swollen limb is a heavy limb, placing stresses on weakened muscles and joints, affecting both posture and mobility. Gravitational oedema may develop in an immobile, dependent limb. Failure of the muscle pump will reduce venous return and increase the load on a struggling, one-way, lymphatic drainage system.

Self-management, using the following four cornerstones of lymphoedema treatment, is taught to patients and/or carers (Mortimer and Todd, 2007):

- ◆ Meticulous skin care
- ◆ Graded exercise and movement

◆ Compression, in the form of hosiery, specialized garments, or bandaging

◆ A modified massage technique which encourages lymph drainage.

This may offer the patient some degree of control but they must be empowered to accept such control. In advanced disease, palliative bandaging is used to control lymphorrhoea and to support the affected tissues.

Lymphoedema management includes breathing exercises. Inspiration has a major effect on thoracic lymphatic drainage and sudden increases in intra-abdominal pressure, for example, coughing, sighing, and laughing, will greatly increase abdominal drainage and empty the cisterna chyli (Twycross et al., 2000).

Conclusion

Physiotherapy in the field of oncology and palliative care is a continuously evolving and developing speciality in cancer and other non-malignant disease (Association of Physiotherapists in Oncology and Palliative Care (ACPOPC), 2009). Rehabilitation is now considered a crucial aspect of the patient pathway in which the physiotherapist plays a pivotal role (NICE, 2004). Many physiotherapists work as sole practitioners and need peer support, clinical supervision, and opportunities for continuing professional development. Membership of ACPOPC is recommended to assist the development process. Physiotherapists working in this speciality may choose to extend their practice to include other skills such as communication training, acupuncture, and lymphoedema management. Physiotherapy students on palliative placements benefit because they experience a diverse range of life-limiting conditions and gain valuable experience. The need for further research remains, however there is already a significant body of evidence to support the importance of physiotherapy in palliative care and the physiotherapist's valuable contribution to the interdisciplinary team.

Online materials

Complete references for this chapter are available online at <http://www.oxfordmedicine.com>.

References

Armstrong, A. (2009). Developing a breath stacking system to achieve lung volume recruitment. *British Journal of Nursing*, 18(19), 1166–1169.

Bausewien, C., Booth, S., Gysels, M., and Higginson, I. (2008). Non-pharmacological interventions for breathlessness in advanced stages of malignant and non-malignant diseases. *Cochrane Database of Systematic Reviews*, 2, CD005623.

Bolton, C.E., Bevan-Smith, E.F., Blakey, J.D., *et al.* (2013). British Thoracic Society guideline on pulmonary rehabilitation in adults. *Thorax*, 68(Suppl. 2), ii1–30.

Bott, J., Blumenthal, S., Buxton, M., *et al.* (2009). Guidelines for the physiotherapy management of the adult, medical, spontaneously breathing patient. *Thorax*, 64(Suppl. 1), i1–51.

Chartered Society of Physiotherapy (2005). *Core Standards of Physiotherapy Practice*. London: Chartered Society of Physiotherapy.

Cramp, F. and Daniel, J. (2008). Exercise for the management of cancer related fatigue in adults. *Cochrane Database of Systematic Reviews*, 2, CD006145.

Fearon, K., Arends, J., and Baracos, V. (2013). Understanding the mechanisms of treatment options in cancer cachexia. *Nature Reviews. Clinical Oncology*, 10(2), 90–99.

Headley, J.A., Ownby, K.K., and John, L.D. (2004). Effect of seated exercise on fatigue and quality of life in women with advanced breast cancer. *Oncology Nursing Society*, 31(5), 977–983.

Hough, A. (2001). *Physiotherapy in Respiratory Care. An Evidence-Based Approach to Respiratory and Cardiac Management* (3rd ed.). Cheltenham: Nelson Thornes.

Maddocks, M., Murton, A.J., and Wilcock, A. (2012). Therapeutic exercise in cancer cachexia. *Critical Reviews in Oncogenesis*, 17(3), 285–292.

National Cancer Action Team (2010). *Characteristics of an Effective Multi-Disciplinary Team*. London: National Health Service.

National Institute for Health and Care Excellence (2004). *Improving Supportive and Palliative Care for Adults with Cancer*. London: NICE.

National Institute for Health and Care Excellence (2011). *The Diagnosis and Treatment of Lung Cancer*. London: NICE.

Rankin, J., Robb, K., Murtaugh, N., Cooper, J., and Lewis, S, (2008). *Rehabilitation in Cancer Care*. Chichester: Wiley Blackwell.

Rees, K., Taylor, R.R.S., Singh, S., Coats, A.J., and Ebrahim, S. (2009). Exercise based rehabilitation for heart failure. *Cochrane Database of Systematic Reviews*, 4, CD003331.

4.10

Speech and language therapy in palliative care

Tim Luckett and Katherine L.P. Reid

Introduction to speech and language therapy in palliative care

Palliative care is an emerging speciality area within the field of speech and language therapy (SLT), with only a small number of specialist positions appointed. Patients with palliative care needs are most often referred to SLTs on the basis of needs associated with their diagnosis (e.g. motor neurone disease (MND)/ amyotrophic lateral sclerosis (ALS)) rather than phase of illness. A search of electronic literature databases returns only a handful of articles on SLT in palliative care, most of which are commentaries rather than research reports (Frost, 2001; Pollens, 2004; Eckman and Roe, 2005; Myers, 2010; Javier and Montagnini, 2011). This belies the fact that many patients in the palliative phase suffer problems with swallowing (dysphagia) and communication, the core domains of SLT practice. The limited presence of SLTs in palliative care means it is likely that swallowing and communication problems go under-recognized and under-treated. Successful management of these problems can have significant impacts on quality of life (QOL) (Kulbersh et al., 2006; Hill, 2010), the ultimate goal of palliative care (World Health Organization, n.d.).

Communication diagnoses common in palliative care include:

- dysphasia/aphasia—a difficulty understanding and/or using spoken or written language
- dysarthria—impaired speech due to muscle weakness
- dyspraxia/apraxia of speech—a difficulty forming speech sounds and words due to impaired motor programming
- dysphonia—voice impairment (e.g. weak, hoarse).

It is important to recognize that these problems are distinct; any given person may present with one or a number of them.

In the swallowing domain, SLTs primarily focus on dysphagia in the oropharyngeal stage, with common symptoms including coughing or choking on solids and/or liquids, increased time to eat or drink, and discomfort/pain when swallowing.

This chapter will describe SLT needs commonly associated with a range of life-limiting conditions, together with the latest evidence for clinical practice and service delivery. We begin by summarizing overarching principles and considerations that are shared regardless of the underlying pathology.

A palliative approach to speech and language therapy assessment and management

Palliative goals

Goals of assessment and management in the palliative phase are generally to optimize and maintain communication and swallowing for as long as possible in the context of declining health. But the story is not always one of inexorable decline; there may sometimes be a need to rehabilitate functioning following a medical emergency (e.g. cerebrovascular accident) or treatment with adverse effects (e.g. radiotherapy). As a general rule, interventions aimed at maintaining or improving functioning in communication and swallowing should be undertaken only when there is a reasonable expectation that these domains will positively influence psychosocial well-being or QOL more generally. For example, while (as for any client group) management of dysphagia may be aimed at ensuring nutrition and preventing aspiration, a palliative approach would require that the burden of assessment and management be weighed against likely net benefits to QOL (see below and Chapter 10.1).

The UK's Royal College of Speech and Language Therapists (RCSLT) recommends that SLT in palliative care be guided by the following principles:

- Assess only as required to provide the answers to plan management
- Minimal intervention for maximum gain
- Maintain function where possible
- Improve function if appropriate and realistic
- Utilize compensatory strategies, diet modifications, and safe swallow strategies
- Work as member of a multidisciplinary team (MDT)
- Provide holistic, individual-centred care
- Facilitate communication between individual and team
- Provide education and information
- Advise on risk–benefit evaluation (RCSLT, 2006).

Ensuring a person-centred, multidisciplinary approach to client care

SLTs should seek to assess and manage functioning in a holistic manner that considers biobehavioural contributors and sequelae within the context of each client's cognitive and sensory functioning, symptom profile, broader health status, and personal preferences and needs. Complex care needs arising from multiple comorbidities are commonplace in the palliative setting and require a comprehensive, multidisciplinary approach. SLTs will typically contribute to case management either as a member of an MDT or via consultation (see Chapter 4.1 for a summary of other disciplines commonly involved in palliative care). Of these two models, membership of an MDT generally affords greater opportunity to contribute to care plan development. Care plans outline a given client's individualized goals of assessment and management together with the necessary interventions and multidisciplinary roles required to attain these. The prominence of communication and swallowing will vary according to the urgency of other needs as well as client and family priorities for care. Delivery of SLT should be integrated with other services as parsimoniously as possible to minimize client travel and other burdens. SLTs will need to work with the whole team to implement interventions and support decision-making. Members of the MDT with whom SLTs work especially closely include dieticians to ensure adequate and safe nutrition, physiotherapists to monitor chest conditions, and occupational therapists to access alternative communication devices and devise appropriate set-up for meals.

Assessment and management of problems in communication

Regardless of diagnosis, people in the palliative phase of illness often suffer communication problems due to general weakness, fatigue, and side effects from medication (MacDonald and Armstrong, 2010). Communication is important for advance care planning, decision-making, and psychosocial well-being of both the patient and family as they progress along the disease trajectory. Enabling clients to participate in decision-making about their care is one of the SLT's major roles in the palliative setting (Pollens, 2004).

Assessment and management of communication problems often takes place within the context of limitations in hearing and cognitive functioning, especially where patients are elderly. Optimizing the preconditions for effective communication (e.g. by means of a hearing aid) is essential before implementing interventions targeted at specific deficits.

Problems in speech and voice

Speech production relies on the coordinated processes of respiration, phonation, resonation, articulation, and neurological integration (Kantner and West, 1941): air from the lungs (respiration) passes through the vibrating vocal chords (phonation) to produce sound that is modified in the pharynx, mouth, and nose (resonation) and shaped by the tongue, teeth, and lips (articulation) to produce speech. Declining health status and deconditioning towards the end of life often impact breath control and speech musculature even when these are not directly impaired by underlying pathology.

Voice disorders are generally classified as dysphonia or dysarthria (Cohen et al., 2009). Dysphonia refers to impairment in phonation caused by a deficit in the larynx ('voice box'). It is common in the elderly regardless of health status, especially in the form of presbyphonia, which refers to weakness of voice, change in pitch, decreased projection, vocal fatigue, increased effort to speak, and altered quality of the voice arising from ageing of the larynx. Dysphonia is often worsened in these cases by compensatory strategies such as straining, the remediation of which forms the focus of SLT. Voice therapy aimed at improving efficiency of voicing has been shown to increase voice-related QOL in elderly clients (Berg et al., 2008), and the benefits are likely to be even greater for people with poor health status in whom compensatory strategies may be fatiguing. Conversely, surgical approaches that are sometimes used to treat dysphonia in other groups are less likely to be appropriate in the palliative population.

Dysarthria and apraxia of speech are more common in certain health conditions and will be considered in the next section.

Problems with language

Language refers to systems of symbols that give meaning to speech or other, non-verbal forms of communication (e.g. writing). Language disorders acquired through illness are collectively described as dysphasia/aphasia (terms often used synonymously). Language problems can rise separately or concurrently in the abilities to use or understand language, referred to as expressive and receptive dysphasia respectively.

Problems with communication

Where speech or language, or both, become inadequate for communication due to lack of intelligibility, loss of voice, or inadequate ability to retrieve and use words, SLT may focus on supplementing or replacing these with augmentative or alternative communication (AAC). AAC can take either a low-tech or a high-tech form. Examples of low-tech AAC include paper-based communication charts containing words or pictures that the person can point to. These can either be customized to the particular communication needs of the patient or rely on generic templates that include standard requests in the hospital or home setting. A number of high-tech computerized versions are now available including iPad applications (apps) that rely on input via picture/word selection or typing and produce auditory output (see Fig. 4.10.1). These are now available for loan and subsequent purchase in some service settings. The social acceptability of the iPad has done much to overcome the stigma of AAC; friends and family are often interested in the technology and keen to participate in communication attempts. While there are now a range of free AAC apps for both children and adults, those that are more expensive generally allow greater customization and chance of communication success.

Assessment and management of dysphagia

Assessment and management of dysphagia is alone among the SLT domains in having serious medical implications and should be undertaken only by SLTs who have undergone specialist training at either an undergraduate or postgraduate level.

Langmore et al. (2009) recommend that the following should be considered signs and symptoms for increased risk of dysphagia and aspiration that prompt assessment or re-assessment:

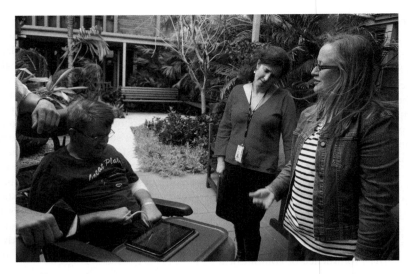

Fig. 4.10.1 A model of care for speech and language therapy.

◆ Persistent throat clearing or coughing during or after eating or drinking

◆ Symptoms such as general weakness and mental status changes

◆ Changes in medical diagnosis such as recent stroke or thyroid disease

◆ Introduction of new medications, particularly if these are likely to impact on level of consciousness or used to treat oropharyngeal symptoms (e.g. oral pain medication for throat cancer)

◆ Recurrent aspiration pneumonias

◆ Significant weight loss of greater than 5–10% or recurrent episodes of dehydration (Langmore et al., 2009).

Other signs to watch for include increased shortness of breath, taking longer than usual to eat or drink, pain/discomfort on swallowing, and difficulty initiating a swallow.

A palliative approach to SLT means that invasive instrumental assessments (endoscopy) and, to a lesser extent, radiological examination (videofluoroscopy/modified barium swallow) tend to be indicated less commonly than for non-palliative client groups. The American Speech-Language-Hearing Association (ASHA) recommends that instrumental assessment not be undertaken where:

1. the client is too medically unstable to tolerate a procedure

2. the client is unable to cooperate or participate (e.g. dementia), or

3. an instrumental examination would not change clinical management (ASHA, 2000).

Alongside other MDT members, SLTs are responsible for supporting clients and families to make shared decisions regarding their care in full knowledge of the burden, risks, and benefits of different approaches to assessment and management, including the option of taking no action at all. ASHA has published guidelines for ethical decision-making relating to dysphagia (ASHA, 2002). Decisions regarding artificial nutrition and hydration in terminal illness are particularly controversial (Goodhall, 1997; Landes, 1999; Huang and Ahronheim, 2000; Wasson et al., 2001; Lipman, 2004; Bozzetti, 2008). Engaging the patient in advance care planning while (s)he still has cognitive capacity will make decision-making less onerous for families if such capacity is lost (Gillick, 2006). Where patients make an informed choice to risk dehydration, malnutrition, and/or aspiration rather than be fed by nasogastric or percutaneous endoscopic gastrostomy tube, management may be aimed primarily at maximizing eating enjoyment while making the best of suboptimal strategies for avoiding these risks to minimize negative impacts on QOL.

Strategies for reducing the risk of aspiration can be classified as compensatory, rehabilitative, or compensatory/rehabilitative (Langmore et al., 2009). Compensatory approaches include changes to the consistency of food and drink (e.g. thickened liquids), postural changes (e.g. sitting upright; 'chin tuck' (Hardy and Morton Robinson, 1999)), alterations in swallowing behaviour (e.g. repeated swallowing, coughing afterwards), or external manipulations (e.g. using a spoon for liquids) aimed at supporting the oropharyngeal stage of swallowing, protecting the airway, and/or ejecting aspirated material. Rehabilitative strategies are aimed at improving the speed, strength, and timeliness of swallowing, and include therapeutic exercises for the tongue, larynx, or pharynx.

Compensatory/rehabilitative strategies are those that are compensatory when introduced but may lead to improved swallowing without continuing intervention in the longer term. These include manoeuvres requiring effort from the client (e.g. super-supraglottic swallow) and increased sensory stimulation (e.g. using ice, sour taste, or electrical stimulation). Aspiration is also less likely where oral and pulmonary hygiene is of a high standard (Langmore et al., 1998).

Box 4.10.1 The Choking Prevention Program

The Choking Prevention Program is an afternoon workshop offered to palliative patients and their carers or nursing staff in Tasmania, Australia. It involves education about the mechanism for choking and risk factors. Then families/carers are trained on what action to take if someone chokes, how to mix thickened fluids and decrease food texture, and how best to position for eating/drinking. A recipe book is provided together with information handouts. Advance care planning is then discussed, with a focus on preferred action to be taken if a choking episode occurs and the benefits and disadvantages of enteral feeding. Often, patients elect to modify their diet and use postures but also continue taking small quantities of food or liquids in their usual consistencies (e.g. sips of tea in the afternoon). In the event of choking, the majority of patients and their families decide that they would like basic measures (i.e. postural adjustment, pressure to the back then chest) but that they do not wish to be resuscitated if they stop breathing. Feedback from families and patients suggest that the Choking Prevention Program alleviates anxiety related to swallowing problems at the end of life.

Over and above avoiding aspiration, aims of SLT intervention for dysphagia in palliative patients often include enhancing enjoyment of eating and drinking, improving nutrition, lessening fatigue, reducing the time spent on meals and taking medications, and reducing anxiety relating to choking. Recent studies also suggest that keeping patients hydrated may be helpful in managing delirium, a common and distressing problem in people at the palliative phase (Galanakis et al., 2011). A palliative patient recommended to take thickened liquids by one of the current authors described the benefits as follows: 'Thank goodness I can drink a glass of water with comfort now. Without that [the thickener], it takes your breath away and it hurts a bit and it (the thickener) doesn't taste of anything.' As well as being flavourless, new-generation thickeners are easy to mix (stir for 30 seconds) and give a smooth, even texture in any temperature or type of liquid that is stable for 24 hours. See Box 4.10.1 for an example of a programme aimed at reducing anxiety related to choking.

Disease-specific considerations in speech and language therapy assessment and management

In addition to the general principles introduced above, assessment and management of communication and swallowing will need to address issues that are specific to particular health conditions encountered in the palliative setting. These are summarized in the following sections, together with case studies from the authors' experience that have been formulated to protect patient identities.

Head and neck cancer

The potential for SLT to contribute to supportive care in cancer has been acknowledged in national guidelines (National Institute for Clinical Excellence, 2004). People with advanced cancer of any type may experience communication and swallowing problems, and dysphagia is predictive of survival (Vigano et al., 2001). Most commonly, however, SLT is indicated for cancers of the head and neck, where both disease and treatment may have profound impacts on the ability to speak and/or swallow (Logemann et al., 1997). A chart audit of hospice patients with head and neck cancer identified that 53% of patients had communication difficulties and 74% dysphagia (Forbes, 1997).

Assessment and management of patients with head and neck cancer often takes place within the context of particular psychosocial predictors and sequelae. It is more common in men, in whom it is associated with socioeconomic disadvantage and continuing heavy alcohol use (Deleyiannis et al., 1996; Conway et al., 2010). Psychosocial problems may become exacerbated in cases where either disease or treatment, or both, is disfiguring (Katz et al., 2003). Lack of management adherence is sometimes raised as a concern but seems to be less of a problem where SLT needs are assessed at a multidisciplinary clinic, at least in early-stage disease (Starmer et al., 2011).

Surgical removal of part or all of the tongue in the treatment of oral cancer is likely to reduce speech intelligibility, especially when the tip of the tongue is affected (Cohen et al., 2009). Where surgery is extensive, SLT may be needed to teach compensatory manoeuvres aimed at modifying intonation, pitch, vocal intensity, and rate of speech (Skelly et al., 1971). Where swallowing is compromised by surgical removal of part of the tongue, head tilting can be used to transit food via gravity (Newman, 2009). Sensory feedback may also be negatively impacted by surgery; in these cases, it may help to exaggerate stimuli by adjusting the size/temperature of the bolus or artificially increasing pressure on the tongue (e.g. using a spoon). SLTs may sometimes work with a prosthodontist to design and support use of a prosthesis.

Rehabilitation of voice and speech in clients who have undergone laryngectomy for laryngeal cancer may make use of oesophageal speech, artificial larynx, or tracheo-oesophageal voice restoration. A study by the United States Department of Veterans Affairs found artificial larynx to be the most frequently used option following laryngectomy, despite being judged the least intelligible (Hillman et al., 1998). The appropriate option for each client will vary according to personal choice, post-treatment tissue changes and complications, behavioural and psychosocial variables, and the availability of SLTs to support rehabilitation (Cohen et al., 2009). SLTs will need to work closely with the medical team and client both pre- and postoperatively to support decision-making and rehabilitation. Because treatment via radiotherapy or chemotherapy is more aggressive when aimed at cure, the most severe acute adverse effects may not be commonly encountered in the palliative setting. However, where curative treatment is unsuccessful or the cancer recurs, SLTs may need to assess and contribute to management of sequelae from long-term impacts of high-dose radiation, including dental decay, subcutaneous fibrosis, oesophageal stenosis, hoarseness, and damage to the middle or inner ear (Manikantan et al., 2009). Where radiotherapy is palliative, a balance is sought between benefits to functioning and QOL resulting from reduction in tumour versus adverse effects such as mucositis and xerostomia (Agarwal et al., 2008). Pre-assessment of swallowing prior to treatment is useful in identifying clients at risk of long-term dysfunction so that information and management can be tailored accordingly (Patterson and Wilson, 2011). Prophylactic swallowing exercises prior to radiotherapy may also be helpful but require further evaluation, especially where radiotherapy is palliative (Roe and Ashforth, 2011).

Brain tumours

In brain tumours, assessment and management of communication and swallowing difficulties often occur within the context of changes in cognitive functioning and, sometimes, personality and social behaviour. Despite the poor prognosis associated with most brain tumours, evidence from a small-scale study suggests that swallowing difficulties may be as responsive to rehabilitation as in stroke (Wesling et al., 2003). Where dysphagia occurs in the weeks prior to death, decision-making about appropriate management will be more complicated (Pace et al., 2009; Sizoo et al., 2010). Communication impairment in brain tumours may include dysphasia, dysarthria, dyspraxia of speech, disfluency, and dysphonia. Intervention may take the form of rehabilitation, the teaching of compensatory strategies to the patient and carers, and education regarding the impairment. Acquired dyspraxia of speech is linked to either cortical or subcortical damage, or both, in the language-dominant hemisphere of the brain (McNeil et al., 2009). Approaches to rehabilitation of dyspraxia can be grouped into (a) articulatory-kinematic, (b) rate/rhythm control treatments, and (c) inter-systemic facilitation/reorganization treatments (Wambaugh et al., 2006a, 2006b). Most evidence for these approaches comes from studies with stroke patients and is most substantial for articulatory-kinematic treatment, which uses a combination of repeated motoric practice, modelling-repetition, integral stimulation, and articulatory cueing.

Brain tumours are among the few cancer types that occur in children and adolescents, with one study reporting an 81% prevalence of problems in SLT domains (Goncalves et al., 2008). Palliative care for children is distinguished by the unique psychosocial implications of life-limiting illness for clients and families in this group (Moody et al., 2011). See Box 4.10.2 for a case study of a client with a brain tumour.

Lung cancer and respiratory disease

Problems with dysphagia and communication are common where there is deterioration in lung function. A developing body of literature suggests a tight neural coupling between the central control of respiration and swallowing which may be disrupted by ageing, neurological disease, respiratory disease, or cancer (Martin-Harris, 2008).The normal breathing pattern during swallowing is inspiration, which aids propulsion of food/drink into the pharynx, a pause in breathing (apnoea) during the swallow, followed by expiration, which helps clear any residue in the airway. Poorly controlled pre-swallow inspiration can lead to material being breathed into the airway. Particularly if a patient is short of breath, it is not uncommon for the swallow to be followed by inspiration due to respiratory drive, increasing the risk of material being drawn into the airway.

Whilst not among the most common symptoms in lung cancer, dysphagia tends to worsen over time (Lovgren et al., 2008). In addition to the mechanism just outlined, dysphagia may also occur as a result of chemoradiation, where there is phase II evidence for efficacy of the human recombinant keratinocyte growth factor, palifermin (Schuette et al., 2012).

> **Box 4.10.2** Brain tumour case study
>
> AB was a 62-year-old woman with a history of glioblastoma. She was living at home and referred to SLT due to word-finding difficulties and intermittent coughing on liquids. Assessment found mild oropharyngeal dysphagia and mild dysphasia with delayed processing, which progressed to moderate dysphasia over the next few weeks. The patient and family were given information regarding dysphagia signs, symptoms, and possible interventions both immediate and into the future. AB responded to the use of head flexion, which eliminated coughing on fluids, and began taking her medication with semi-solids (yoghurt) to increase ease of swallowing. For communication, AB and her family were trained in using an iPad with an AAC app, which she used in both the community and at hospital. The menu was customized to include pictures and phrases relating to her children/grandchildren and trips to the hairdresser.

Up to one-third of patients with advanced chronic obstructive pulmonary disease (COPD) experience dysphagia, often with silent aspiration; this is often a precursor to an exacerbation and hospital admission (Reid, 1998). SLT in COPD patients has demonstrated significant improvement in self-management and swallowing-related QOL, including decreased burden of dysphagia, physical problems of dysphagia, and managing diet options and food selections (McKinstry et al., 2010).

Hoarseness is a common symptom in patients with COPD secondary to gastro-oesophageal reflux disease (Rouev et al., 2005), xerostoma (Roh et al., 2006), or inhaled corticosteroids (Williamson et al., 1995). Disturbances in airflow volume and rate found in COPD also contribute to decreased vocal volume and shorter message length (Martin-Harris, 2000). These problems may also occur in patients with lung cancer, together with vocal cord paralysis (Benninger et al., 1998). Non-invasive interventions by the SLT for vocal paralysis include pushing exercises to improve vocal cord approximation, AAC, and education on how to most effectively manage the impairment. See Box 4.10.3 for a case study concerned with lung cancer.

Dementia

People with dementia present a particularly challenging client group for both practical and ethical reasons. By definition, assessment, management, and decision-making must take place within the context of decreased cognitive function. Problems with swallowing typically begin in the later stages of dementia, by which time patients have often become resistant to care (Feldman and Grundman, 1999). By the time end-stage dementia is reached, almost all intentional communication will have been lost, and assessment must rely on observation alone. Weight loss often persists despite receiving food and fluids. In frontotemporal lobe dementia, the risk of aspiration from neurological deficits may be exacerbated by compulsive eating and food gorging (Langmore et al., 2007).

Intervention for dysphagia in dementia may include diet and posture modification as well as changes in feeding technique and environmental factors. Quite apart from any physiological problems with swallowing, patients may have difficulty maintaining hydration and nutrition due to cognitive and behavioural factors (e.g. an inability to recognize food or liquid in the mouth; refusal to open

Box 4.10.3 Lung cancer case study

CD was a 47-year-old man with advanced lung cancer who presented with difficulty swallowing, weak breathy voice, and fatigue. He was referred to palliative care primarily for reconditioning and pain control. On initial assessment, CD was drowsy secondary to pain medication, and his voice was so weak the listener had to place his/her ear beside his mouth to hear. CD's swallow was moderately to severely impaired, with difficulty chewing textured solids, a moderate delay in initiating a swallow, and a weak cough. He was recommended to take moderately thickened fluids and a purée diet. CD received oxygen during meals to decrease his shortness of breath due to the swallowing apnoea and fatigue. The medical and nursing members of the team worked to find pain control that minimized drowsiness. On review, CD was alert and his swallowing had improved. He progressed to nectar-thickened fluids and a soft diet. CD was keen to improve his voice, so a number of pushing techniques were trialled to improve the approximation of the vocal cords. Pushing down on a chair was found to be particularly effective, which CD began practising during automatic speech (e.g. counting), words, and phrases. Over a 3-week period, CD progressed to being able to have a conversation with someone sitting across the room. After 20 minutes, he became fatigued and made use of a pen and paper to communicate. With a regime of rest periods, CD was able to use his voice throughout the day. His swallowing also improved to the extent he was able to manage a small volume of thin fluids when accompanied by head flexing. Prior to his discharge home, CD and his family were trained in the use of thickened fluids and texture modification as well as what action to take in the event of a choking episode.

Box 4.10.4 Dementia case study

EF was an 87-year-old man with advanced dementia (Alzheimer's disease) who presented with difficulty eating, drinking, and communicating with his family. A swallowing assessment revealed moderate oropharyngeal dysphagia, characterized by difficulty forming a bolus and moderate to severe delay initiating the swallow for food, and clinical signs of aspiration on thin fluids. Intervention included removing distractions when eating, pressing the tongue down with a spoon to cue to the presence of food in the mouth, a puree diet, and the use of 3 teaspoons of lemon juice (thick) before the meal to stimulate the swallow (Pelletier and Lawless, 2003). While the patient responded to requests to use neck flexion and small sips of fluid, he was unable to retain this information without supervision and was placed on mildly thickened fluids. EF was particularly fond of lemonade so, using new-generation thickeners, his family mixed a jug for him so he could have this through the day. This improved his fluid intake. An advance care directive was discussed with the family. When informed about the evidence that enteral feeding does not increase life expectancy or QOL in advanced dementia, the family elected to continue with hand oral feeding into the future.

EF's family were instructed on how to more effectively communicate with him using pictures from home, short sentences, gesture, and tone of voice for meaning and emphasis. To ease the frustrations of communicating, suggestions were made for alternative activities that the family could do with EF that did not require verbal communication in consultation with the occupational therapist (e.g. organizing a box of nuts and bolts).

mouth) (Wasson et al., 2001). Whilst there is evidence that artificial nutrition and hydration neither prevents aspiration nor improves survival or other clinical outcomes (Ganzini, 2006; Sorrell, 2010), tube feeding in advanced dementia remains widespread. Many health professionals, including SLTs, may lack awareness that a palliative approach is indicated in advanced dementia (Vitale et al., 2011). In residential aged care, economic and practical factors may also be influential, as the cost of hand-feeding often outweighs that of artificial nutrition (Lipman, 2004). Educating health professionals and families about the appropriateness of a palliative approach and supporting them in making the transition to comfort care may be the priority at this stage of the disease trajectory.

Speech and language deficits vary according to dementia type (Ross et al., 1990). Cortical dementias such as Alzheimer's disease and Pick's disease are associated with disturbances of language function whereas subcortical dementias such as progressive supranuclear palsy affect the motor aspects of speech. Patients with vascular dementias often have dysarthria with or without language difficulties, depending on the site of the infarcts. Language problems in early dementia are characterized by a difficulty in recalling names or words (anomia), which results in reduced speech fluency and use of circumlocution; these problems worsen as dementia progresses until even the names of immediate family are difficult to recall (Ashley et al., 2006). Therapy is aimed at supporting communication through the use of AAC, situational cues and routines, as well as encouraging family and other caregivers

to enhance verbal communication with gestures, visual cues, and slower speech. Memory books, consisting of autobiographical and daily schedule information, together with prompts to overcome barriers have been found to improve quality of communication between aged care residents with dementia and staff in a cluster randomized trial (Bourgeois et al., 2001). See Box 4.10.4 for a case study concerned with dementia.

Degenerative neurological conditions

A range of degenerative neurological conditions such as MND/ALS, multiple sclerosis, Huntington's disease, and Parkinson's disease can impact communication and swallowing. Dysarthria is the most common speech impairment but differs between conditions with regard to onset, type, and progression (Cohen et al., 2009). Acquired dyspraxia of speech may sometimes be the first sign of neurodegenerative disease (Duffy, 2006). Patients with Parkinson's disease and especially MND/ALS will be likely to require AAC as the disease progresses. For patients in the latter group, AAC may need to become progressively more high tech as physical capacity declines, starting with typing and touchscreens before moving to head-tracking and eye-tracking technologies. A limited, low-tech alternative in the final stages of illness is to use eye-gaze to signal 'yes' or 'no'. In the future, there is hope that people with no physical capacity at all will have recourse to computer-based solutions that make use of brain rather than muscle activity (Allison et al., 2007).

In addition to swallowing problems shared with other diagnoses discussed in this chapter, people with degenerative neurological conditions may present with problems with the oral phase of swallowing due to muscle weakness and excessive saliva, resulting in problems with chewing and social stigma associated with dribbling (Squires, 2006). The disproportionate energy required to eat and drink means that 'little and often' may be the best approach to intake of food and fluids.

Cerebrovascular accident (stroke)

The SLT domain most specifically implicated in stroke is language, with dysphasia occurring in between 22% and 38% of cases (Pedersen et al., 1995; Kyrozis et al., 2009; Dickey et al., 2010). With regard to speech, dysarthria is more common than dysphonia and is worse where the stroke is bilateral, resulting in slow speech, imprecise articulation, and strained voice quality similar to MND; loudness, pitch, and vocal intensity and stress patterns may also be affected (Cohen et al., 2009). Stroke is also the most common cause of acquired dyspraxia of speech, which (as in other conditions) occurs especially frequently in patients who also have dysphasia (Duffy, 2005).

Problems with dysphagia following stroke are predicted by aspiration within the first 72 hours (Ickenstein et al., 2012). Where stroke leads to hemiparesis, the client should be encouraged to turn his/her head to the weak side to divert food down the stronger side of the larynx (Newman, 2009).

Stroke is less commonly the reason for referral to palliative care than a comorbidity endured by people referred for other reasons. Patients referred as a result of stroke often have limited consciousness, and intervention may consist simply of mouth care or comfort feeding (West et al., 2005; Foley et al., 2008; Brady et al., 2012).

Advancing the field of speech and language therapy in palliative care

Addressing the paucity of rigorous research literature is a priority if SLT in palliative care is to become evidence based in order to justify funding and resources. Research in palliative care is undergoing a period of rapid growth (Kaasa and Radbruch, 2008), and SLTs would be well advised to participate in collaborative research groups and other capacity-building initiatives available within the sector more generally. The multidisciplinary nature of palliative care makes it essential that research aimed at answering clinical questions of interest to SLT involves researchers from other disciplines to optimize usefulness and enhance dissemination and translation into practice. As for other symptoms, there is a need to harmonize measurements of communication and swallowing to enhance comparability between studies. For example, a review of speech and voice outcomes following chemoradiation for head and neck cancer found 18 assessment tools had been used in 20 studies (Jacobi et al., 2010).

In practice, there is a need to increase accessibility and referral to SLT for people with life-limiting illness. In the United States, patients enrolled in the Medicare hospice benefit are eligible to receive SLT and other allied health services without additional cost (Centers for Medicare and Medicaid Services, 2010). But even in universal health-care systems, the availability of SLT in palliative care services is variable. Health-care insurers often cover SLT only when the patient has a specific diagnosis. This neglects the fact that patients with life-limiting illness of any kind may require support for communication and swallowing due to weakness, fatigue, and side effects from medication.

Finally, there is a need to develop understanding and capacity in the SLT workforce relating to the palliative approach. Specialist training programmes and SLT support networks are at present limited. In the United Kingdom, an SLT special interest group in palliative and supportive care works in partnership with the RCSLT to develop clinical guidelines and policies and provide opportunities for education (Eckman and Roe, 2005). In Australia, efforts have been made to introduce palliative care to the SLT curriculum at an undergraduate level (Mathisen et al., 2011). A personal communication from ASHA (3 October, 2012) identified no similar initiatives underway in the United States.

Conclusion

This chapter has summarized communication and swallowing problems commonly encountered in people with life-limiting illness, together with approaches to assessment and management. More research is needed to inform appropriately integrated, person-centred models of SLT provision that enable problems with communication and swallowing to be addressed alongside other symptoms and psychosocial and practical needs.

Online materials

Complete references for this chapter are available online at <http://www.oxfordmedicine.com>.

References

American Speech-Language-Hearing Association (2000). *Clinical Indicators for Instrumental Assessment of Dysphagia.* Rockville, MD: ASHA.

American Speech-Language-Hearing Association (2002). *Dysphagia Policies and Ethical Decision Making: Policy.* Rockville, MD: ASHA.

Ashley, J., Duggan, M., and Sutcliffe, N. (2006). Speech, language, and swallowing disorders in the older adult. *Clinics in Geriatric Medicine*, 22, 291–310; viii.

Brady, M.C., Kelly, H., Godwin, J., and Enderby, P. (2012). Speech and language therapy for aphasia following stroke. *Cochrane Database of Systematic Reviews*, 5, CD000425.

Cohen, S., Elackattu, A., Noordzij, P., Walsh, M.J., and Langmore, S.E. (2009). Palliative treatment of dysphonia and dysarthria. *Otolaryngologic Clinics of North America*, 42, 107–121.

Duffy, J.R. (2005). *Motor Speech Disorders: Substrates, Differential Diagnosis, and Management.* St. Louis, MO, Elsevier Mosby.

Duffy, J.R. (2006). Apraxia of speech in degenerative neurological disease. *Aphasiology*, 20, 511–527.

Foley, N., Teasell, R., Salter, K., Kruger, E., and Martino, R. (2008). Dysphagia treatment post stroke: a systematic review of randomised controlled trials. *Age & Ageing*, 37, 258–64.

Frost, M. (2001). The role of physical, occupational, and speech therapy in hospice: patient empowerment. *American Journal of Hospice & Palliative Medicine*, 18, 397–402.

Ganzini, L. (2006). Artificial nutrition and hydration at end of life: ethics and evidence. *Palliative & Supportive Care*, 4, 135–143.

Hardy, E. and Morton Robinson, N. (1999). *Swallowing Disorders Treatment Manual.* Austin, TX: Pro-Ed.

Hill, K. (2010). Advances in augmentative and alternative communication as quality-of-life technology. *Physical Medicine & Rehabilitation Clinics of North America*, 21, 43–58.

Langmore, S.E., Grillone, G., Elackattu, A., and Walsh, M. (2009). Disorders of swallowing: palliative care. *Otolaryngologic Clinics of North America*, 42, 87–105.

MacDonald, A. and Armstrong, L. (2010). The contribution of speech and language therapy to palliative medicine. In G. Hanks, N.I. Cherny, N.A. Christakis, M. Fallon, S. Kaasa, R.K. and Portenoy (eds.) *Oxford Textbook of Palliative Medicine* (4th ed.), pp. 234–242. Oxford: Oxford University Press.

Manikantan, K., Khode, S., Sayed, S.I., *et al.* (2009). Dysphagia in head and neck cancer. *Cancer Treatment Reviews*, 35, 724–732.

McNeil, M.R., Robin, D.A., and Schmidt, R.A. (2009). Apraxia of speech: definition, differentiation, and treatment. In M.R. McNeil (ed.) *Clinical Management of Sensorimotor Speech Disorders* (2nd ed.), pp. 311–344. New York: Thieme.

Newman, K. (2009). Speech and language therapy techniques in end of life care. *End of Life Care*, 3, 8–13.

Pollens, R. (2004). Role of the speech-language pathologist in palliative hospice care. *Journal of Palliative Medicine*, 7, 694–702.

Royal College of Speech and Language Therapists (2006). *Communicating Quality 3*. London: Royal College of Speech and Language Therapists.

Sorrell, J.M. (2010). Use of feeding tubes in patients with advanced dementia: are we doing harm? *Journal of Psychosocial Nursing and Mental Health Services*, 48(5), 15–18.

Squires, N. (2006). Dysphagia management for progressive neurological conditions. *Nursing Standard*, 20, 53–57.

Wambaugh, J.L., Duffy, J.R., McNeil, M.R., Robin, D.A., and Rogers, M. (2006a). Treatment guidelines for acquired apraxia of speech: a synthesis and evaluation of the evidence. *Journal of Medical Speech-Language Pathology*, 14, xv–xxxiii.

Wambaugh, J.L., Duffy, J.R., McNeil, M.R., Robin, D.A., and Rogers, M. (2006b). Treatment guidelines for acquired apraxia of speech: treatment descriptions and recommendations. *Journal of Medical Speech-Language Pathology*, 14, xxxv–lxvii.

Wasson, K., Tate, H., and Hayes, C. (2001). Food refusal and dysphagia in older people with dementia: ethical and practical issues. *International Journal of Palliative Nursing*, 7, 465–471.

West, C., Hesketh, A., Vail, A., and Bowen, A. (2005). Interventions for apraxia of speech following stroke. *Cochrane Database of Systematic Reviews*, 4, CD004298.

The contribution of art therapy to palliative medicine

Michèle J.M. Wood

Introduction: what is art therapy?

Art therapy is an umbrella term for a range of approaches that use visual art media within a psychotherapeutic relationship. Art therapy enables someone to explore personal issues by expressing thoughts, feelings, and other significant issues non-verbally, and thereby provides an alternative to spoken language, aiding better communication and symbolic representation. The art therapist's task is to facilitate the patient's expressive capacities, and help him or her reflect upon what they have produced, including their chosen media and style of working. Art therapy does not aim to distract or divert a person from their difficulties but through encouraging an experience of creativity these difficulties can be perceived and worked with in a new way. The purpose of art therapy is to empower the patient to develop and flourish on a personal level, even at the end of life.

The loss of control in many areas of patients' lives is an inevitable consequence of illness, and one that art therapy aims to address. The physicality of art therapy, where an individual must actively engage with the materials to produce a picture or object, provides an experience that reinforces the person's ability to make choices and their sense of their own vitality. The artwork represents not only something of the patient's mental state but also, by capturing in its marks and traces the movement and pressure of the patient's pencil, brush, or finger, it represents something of their physical condition too. This articulation through the artwork of the mind–body relationship is intrinsic to art therapy. It has been suggested that art therapy's potency resides in this link (Borgmann, 2002; Collie et al., 2006; Siegel, 2009; Stern, 2010), so that art therapy is ideally placed to respond to the psychological effects of physical trauma (Gantt and Tinnin, 2009).

An important aspect of art therapy is that it provides an opportunity to express emotions that may feel unacceptable to the patient. The patient may have stifled feelings of anger, envy, and sadness for fear of upsetting their family or staff. In art therapy, pounding clay, pouring paint, and scribbling violently on paper gives the patient permission to express strong feelings, and the presence of the therapist ensures the patient is not left alone with their distress. Art therapy also allows for the development and expression of more positive feelings such as tenderness, hope, or beauty. The breadth of emotional expression possible through art therapy demands a working environment that provides confidentiality and in which the patient can feel free to be vulnerable. A separate therapy or quiet room designated for art therapy sessions is ideal. There is growing discussion regarding the therapeutic importance of creative spaces within palliative care settings. For example, Glenister suggests a link between the creativity that can be facilitated within such environments and optimal spiritual care (Glenister, 2012).

Art therapy and creative art: similarities and differences

It is important to distinguish art therapy from creative arts activities (Pratt and Thomas, 2007; Hartley and Payne, 2008). Although there are some areas of overlap, art therapy and creative arts projects have different yet complementary functions within palliative care. Both engage the patient in actively using art media and provide a focus and sense of purpose. Both result in an increased sense of control, self-confidence, and make a positive contribution to patients' quality of life. Creative arts projects may aim to help the patient produce artwork for sale, or to bequeath to relatives. Although the artwork produced in art therapy may on occasion have a similar outcome, its focus is different. As patients strive to express and explore their inner emotional landscape through their art there is no expectation that work should be aesthetically 'good' in a conventional sense, or viewed outside the therapy space. Consequently, the artwork may have a rough undeveloped quality to it.

The manner in which the artwork is made offers additional expression for the patient, and deepens communication with the therapist. The need to witness the patient's art-making process is one reason for the therapist's presence in the sessions. Although an aim of art therapy is to facilitate psychological adjustment by the patient to their changed health through this multifaceted communication, the permanent nature of the artwork means that its significance can continue to be unpacked from session to session and outside of the therapeutic relationship. Patients have been known to use their pictures to communicate with friends, family (Luzzatto et al., 2003) other patients in similar situations (Connell, 1998; Wood, 2005), and their doctors and other members of the interdisciplinary team.

Art therapists, artists in residence, and art tutors can and do work alongside each other in many establishments; their combination of skills is particularly effective where their differences are understood. While both encourage the patients' creativity and improve the overall milieu of the health-care environment, art therapy works with the psychological and emotional needs of the patient, which includes their barriers to creativity and their difficulties with self-expression. It can be hard for a patient or a professional to know whether art therapy or recreational art is more appropriate. Most art therapists provide assessment sessions in which the patients' needs may be discerned. Case 1 describes the dual functioning of art making in a palliative care setting showing the different roles played by art therapy and art activity for a woman with motor neurone disease.

Case 1: 'Rosemary' by Jackie Coote, art therapist

Whilst working in a large London hospice I was introduced to Rosemary, who had recently been diagnosed with motor neurone disease. Having become paralysed down one side of her body and rapidly losing the power of speech she had expressed a wish to 'paint her feelings'. She was, by the time I met her, using an electronic writer to communicate and only had the use of her right arm. Anything she 'said' was through the writer. Although unfamiliar with the use of art materials, she engaged in the process very quickly, allowing herself to paint freely. She began to look forward to 'the unexpected', which presented itself to her in each session, like the painting she referred to as her 'Devastated Woodland—half dead, struggling for survival' (Fig. 4.11.1). She was able to relate the image to her feelings about her own situation. Her 'fun' painting became a way to address serious issues around her encroaching illness. Through it she began to express her thoughts and feelings about the adjustments she had to make, not just physically, but psychologically. Through her images she was able to express her painful recognition of change and loss. With the loss of spontaneity and inflexion in speech, Rosemary's painting became her 'voice'. Her choice of materials would often indicate her tone and mood. On one occasion she chose bright, cheerful colours, but the black paper she used reflected her underlying melancholy, and the resulting picture helped her to recognize the tendency to 'put on a cheerful front' when all behind it was not well.

In the course of using art therapy to express difficult and painful feelings, Rosemary discovered another side to her image making. She began to paint alone in her room. This work took on a 'painterly' quality. She painted gardens resembling images from

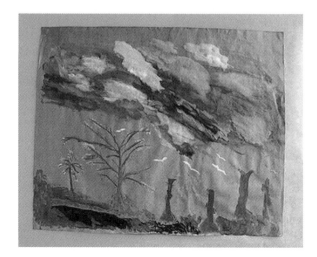

Fig. 4.11.1 Rosemary's 'Devastated Woodland'.

the *Arabian Nights* that contained a sense of richness and fertility. Staff and other patients would come and see what she had been doing each day, and her self-esteem increased considerably. Her images enabled her to become empowered at a time of increasing powerlessness and dependency. With the increase in Rosemary's use of her newly found creative skills, it became important to differentiate between her 'public art' and her 'private art'. She needed reassurance that she still had a private and safe space in the art therapy sessions where she could pour out what she called her 'madness'. She seemed at this point to have moved into a third and what was to be the final phase of the art therapy sessions where, as her body deteriorated, the emotional floodgates opened. Fear, grief, anger, hatred, and despair appeared in the images before us. Her art therapy sessions provided the container necessary to hold the overwhelming grief she poured out in torrents. It was the coping strategy she needed in order to carry on throughout the rest of the day.

Who would benefit from art therapy?

Art therapists work in a range of settings: patients' own homes, prisons, day care units, specialist inpatient units, hospices, and private practice (Bell, 1998; Beaver, 1998; Wald, 2004; Waller and Sibbett, 2005; Oster et al., 2006; Agnese et al., 2012). People with a wide range of conditions including HIV/AIDS, rheumatoid illness, multiple sclerosis, cancer, dementia, and Niemann–Pick's disease have been reported as benefiting from art therapy (Wood, 2004). The range of conditions and variety of settings in which art therapy is offered indicate something of the multiple contributions art therapy can make to patients' care. Whilst recognizing this breadth of application, is it possible to discern which conditions or types of patients would benefit most? Since art therapy is a means of facilitating communication, it is particularly useful for patients, their family, or carers, who are having difficulty with usual modes of communication. Such difficulties can be physical, cognitive, emotional, or even spiritual in origin, and thus provide different starting points and ways of working for the therapist. Case 1 clearly illustrates how art therapy can extend a patient's capacity to manage their emotions, and communicate with others despite physical decline. Similarly, the person with AIDS dementia may no longer be able to coherently discuss their fears and anxieties but may be able to use the qualities available in art to express themselves and relieve their frustrations. In this case, the art therapist may not focus on discussion or interpretation (Wood, 2002). By contrast, where there are emotional difficulties the therapist may well explore in depth the patient's associations to their image and their behaviour. Coote illustrates this in her work with an attention-seeking patient where art therapy allowed the expression of bitterness and resentment, unrecognized aspects of the patient's inner self (Coote, 1998). Connell gives an example of how art therapy was used to address and work through a patient's spiritual struggles (Connell, 1998). The importance of spiritual aspects of art therapy is also discussed by Bell (2011). Trauger-Querry and Haghighi describe an approach using art therapy and music therapy in the reduction of pain (Trauger-Querry and Haghighi, 1999).

Young children, whose developing capacities for verbal expression limit their use of talking therapies, are an obvious group for art therapy, as art and drawing are more familiar means of self-expression (Teufel, 1995). Farrell Fenton, an art therapist with children and young people who have cystic fibrosis, suggests that art therapy works on two levels simultaneously: by providing a means of emotional catharsis while at the same time harnessing the young person's coping strategies (Farrell Fenton, 2000).

Many factors including social status, educational levels, and ethnic backgrounds influence the patient's comfort in expressing and addressing their emotional responses to illness with health professionals. In my experience of serving an ethnically diverse population, art therapy can be a welcome tool for patients negotiating their experiences of illness and treatment in a language and cultural setting that is not their own. Art therapy can strengthen their 'voice' and validate their experiences. While it is important to offer people from all cultural backgrounds access to art therapy, staff should be mindful of the complexity of their patients' cultural values and the ways in which these may vary within groups. One example found in some orthodox branches of Judaism, Islam, and Christianity is the issue of aniconism, where making any representation of the human form is prohibited (Khan, 2012). While such beliefs do not preclude a person from participating in art therapy, understanding the religious and cultural underpinnings of their relationship with visual imagery is vital.

Art therapists as part of the palliative care team

Art therapists usually work under the auspices of the counselling or psychosocial teams and as part of the wider multiprofessional palliative care team (Jones and Browning, 2009; Jones et al., 2013). Referrals to art therapy arise from a close consideration of patients' needs by the team, and in cases where a patient requires emotional support but is unable or unwilling to access counselling, art therapy may be suggested. For example, I work as part of the patient and family support team in a specialist palliative care unit alongside counsellors, social workers, chaplains, and family therapists. Referrals can be made to anyone of us individually, or to our team itself for further assessment of the patients' psychosocial needs. How the different disciplines of the palliative team work together is a matter for consideration, and in particular art therapy's part in this. For example, should a patient have art therapy at the same time as counselling or other emotional/psychological therapies? Art therapy works at verbal and non-verbal levels and while it may be possible for an art therapist to work in conjunction with a counsellor or psychologist this must be based on careful assessment of the patient's needs. It may be that someone begins with art therapy and then moves on to work with another discipline such as music therapy or chaplaincy. Coordination and communication amongst the professionals is key to successful outcomes for the patient.

Art therapists are often employed on fractional or sessional contracts, with the result that they may not always be able to attend team meetings. However, their contributions to patients' care should be conveyed to colleagues in written form as patients' records, in case reports and summaries. Where staff time is limited, art therapists, counsellors, and social workers do represent each other in team discussions to convey the emotional aspects of their patients' care. In the United Kingdom, specific guidelines have been written to enhance an understanding of the role of sessional arts therapies staff (Pratt and Thomas, 2007).

Funding of art therapy is often a major problem. When there are constraints on funding for palliative care services these will often be felt by art therapists, whose contribution may be more readily considered disposable and 'value-added' rather than core to patient care. This issue of funding is probably the main challenge for art therapy in palliative care, since it can confine art therapists to fractional contracts which limit their work, and prevent access to the sorts of research and continuing professional development opportunities enjoyed by their medical, nursing, and allied health professional colleagues.

Are there any hazards of art therapy?

The hazards due to art therapy are minimal but the following pitfalls are worth mentioning. There can be a concern from some staff that the expression of feelings through image-making may unleash a flow of emotion that will overwhelm the patient and those around them. Usually, these concerns dissipate when it is realized that the processes and boundaries of art therapy prevent this from happening. The patient never fully relinquishes control, but through the manipulation of the art materials their usual defences can give way to more symbolic expressions of feeling states (see Case 2). The therapist's skill in working safely and effectively ensures that difficult feelings are contained, addressed, and resolved.

The therapeutic value of art therapy may be undermined if the position of the art therapist in relation to the interdisciplinary team is not respected or clearly understood. One example of this can be seen when art therapy sessions are interrupted for procedures or questions that could be done at another time. Another example is where communication between the art therapist and their colleagues is not valued and there is an unnecessary replication of work with the patient or family.

Another hazard of therapeutic work, and indeed of all work in palliative care, relates to the emotional well-being of staff (Hardy, 2001). Therapists need to ensure that they themselves are adequately supported through the use of supervision, supportive teamwork, and possibly their own personal therapy. All these strategies have proved to be beneficial in guarding against staff burnout and inappropriate behaviour. Art therapy itself is often used for staff support and can facilitate a valuable level of creativity, communication, and expression in tired staff teams (Belfiore, 1994; Nainis, 2005).

On a practical level, the hazard posed to patients by the art materials does need to be considered. Most materials used in art therapy are non-toxic, but where materials could pose a risk (e.g. fixative) therapists ensure that usual health and safety precautions are taken. In cases where cross-infection between patients may be an issue it is standard practice that separate sets of equipment are used.

Evaluating art therapy

The anecdotal literature consisting of accounts by practitioners and patients themselves on the value of art therapy for people with life-threatening, -limiting, or terminal conditions suggests potential benefits of art therapy, which are outlined in Box 4.11.1 (Hill, 1948; Teufel, 1995; Pratt and Wood, 1998; Jones, 2000; Waller and Sibbett, 2005; Stein, 2006; Solomons, 2007; Malchiodi, 2012). Systematic research into art therapy is only just emerging as

Box 4.11.1 Outcomes of art therapy

- Development of a creative attitude by the patient towards their circumstances
- An increased sense of control
- Better communication
- Wider range of expressive capabilities
- Increased insight into patient's own behaviour
- Body image issues addressed
- A cathartic release of emotive issues
- Increased self-esteem and self-efficacy
- Increased ability to confront existential questions and relieve spiritual distress
- Development of positive coping strategies and an increase in coping resources
- Reduction in experiences and reports of physical pain
- Increased quality of life

practitioners and academics begin to investigate its various interventions, outcomes, and therapeutic efficacy. A recent systematic review of studies on art therapy and the management of symptoms in adults with cancer took a close look at the research studies for this population (Wood et al., 2011). It found that most studies were small scale, had methodological limitations, and the disparities between definitions of art therapy and diversity of patient groups prevented evaluation. However, there was some evidence that art therapy might have a beneficial effect on reducing fatigue, tiredness, and psychological and spiritual distress, and in promoting coping. The authors concluded more work was warranted in exploring these benefits further. Since that review, newer studies have favourably evaluated the perceived helpfulness of art therapy to support those undergoing cancer treatment (Forzoni et al., 2010; Agnese et al., 2012) and the benefits of an art therapy intervention for terminally ill patients in hospital in Taiwan (Lin et al., 2012).

Adjusting to multiple losses (purpose, health, and social position), and facing one's own mortality, is equally central to care of the elderly. There has been much work done by art therapists with this population who are often cared for outside of palliative settings. One UK-based study (Rusted et al., 2006) evaluated art therapy with people suffering from dementia using a control group design where the control situation was a standard day centre, mixed activity social group. The researchers found that there was a significant difference between the patients participating in art therapy and those in the control group.

How quickly can the benefits of art therapy be seen?

Patients are referred to art therapy for a variety of reasons and at differing stages of their journey from diagnosis to terminal care. What is clear from many practitioners' reports is that patients with life-threatening and terminal illnesses are motivated to make the most of the time they have left. There is evidence (Balloqui, 2005; Nainis et al., 2006) that even a single session can be of value, as Case 2 shows.

Case 2: 'Robert'

Robert, a man in his early 30s, was diagnosed with AIDS and was in hospital for respite care and symptom control. He had a detached and objective approach to his diagnosis and liked to be informed of all medical facts. When we met, he had announced to staff he no longer wished to discuss his condition.

Robert began the art therapy session by being somewhat surprised by the range of art materials available, and that we had a whole hour together. He said he was unsure about what to do, and I invited him to experiment with the materials to see what marks they made, and what he liked using. Robert said he was anxious about making a fool of himself and of making a mess; he wanted to do things properly. We talked about this initially in relation to his life outside the hospital, and then how he felt about making an image with me watching. Once we had acknowledged these concerns Robert began to draw.

Robert worked with some skill and concentration. As he worked he began to cry. Initially he was embarrassed, but did not stop himself. In fact he was glad to cry. He said that he had not realized he could still feel the things the drawing had brought to mind. He allowed himself to cry freely as he continued with his picture (Fig. 4.11.2). His starting point had been to draw an image of the leaves on the tree outside his bedroom window. However, despite attempts to draw autumn leaves he found himself only able to make them green. He noticed that he concentrated on the veins of the leaves, and made a link with his constant examination of his own veins, which he did to monitor his health. We talked about his green leaves being separate from the tree in the background,

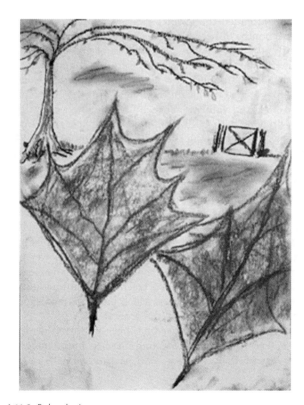

Fig. 4.11.2 Robert's picture.
Reproduced with permission from Wood MJM, 'Art therapy in one session: working with people with AIDS', *Inscape* Winter 27–33, Copyright © 1990 YU INSCAPE.

and his feelings of being plucked from the tree of life before his autumn years.

The tree he had drawn was beginning to blossom, and Robert felt very positive about it. The scene in the background was one that he had drawn several times before when he was a schoolboy. He remembered growing up in the countryside and talked of the dreams he had then for his adult life. Aspirations he regretted that would never now be fulfilled. Robert noticed that he had omitted a fence, which meant that the gate was useless. There seemed to be nothing separating him from the unknown place that lay beyond this field.

At the end of the session Robert reported feeling exhausted but light inside as though a burden had been lifted. This session had enabled Robert to connect with the grief he felt about having AIDS. Although we talked about some of the issues raised in the picture, the main focus was allowing him to feel and to cry. His announcement to staff indicated that he had gone as far as he could with words. This one-off session prompted a positive change in Robert that was noticed by hospital staff and his partner.

Art therapy and support for the carers and those bereaved

Palliative care aims to support not only the patient but also those who are close to them. Support is often provided at hospices for partners, spouses, children, and other family members and friends while the patient is ill and after the patient has died. Case 3 illustrates this.

Case 3: 'Caroline'

'Caroline' attended the hospice's carers' support group during the final months of her older sister's life. She found it helpful to talk with other carers about the stresses of giving up her home and time to support her sister, and Caroline acknowledged how easily she lost sight of her own needs. The art therapy element of the group provided the means by which Caroline could represent, reflect upon, and validate her feelings. She often used different media, drawing with traditional materials, photographing these drawings, and developing them digitally using her iPad. When Caroline's sister died she continued to attend the group, on one occasion bringing with her a seedpod she had found when clearing out her sister's belongings. Caroline used this as the basis for a picture, working both digitally and traditionally, and created a short animation. The animation represented the transformation of the seedpod, which scattered its seeds while Caroline glued it to the paper. What had begun for Caroline as a simple idea to characterize her sister's love of natural objects became a powerful symbol, and part of her process of grieving. Caroline sang Gershwin's aria 'Summertime' as the musical track for her animation; a song the sisters had enjoyed together, which had remained significant for her sister, and one played at the funeral.

Art therapy with the bereaved has been well documented over the past 20 years and in some settings has become an integral part of bereavement services (Simon, 1981; McIntyre, 1990; Pratt, 1998).

Conclusion

Art therapy is being practised in many parts of the world with adults and children living with life-threatening and terminal illnesses. There is a continuing recognition that art therapy does positively benefit patients, their carers, and the professional team. The flexibility of art therapy to address a wide scope of issues ranging from pain to a patient's search for meaning makes it a valuable aspect of palliative care. To ensure that the benefits of art therapy are more clearly understood and that its efficacy is maximized there needs to be an increasing investment in research into this discipline.

Acknowledgment

Case 2: 'Robert' adapted with permission from Wood MJM, 'Art therapy in one session: working with people with AIDS', *Inscape* Winter 27–33, Copyright © 1990 INSCAPE.

Online materials

Additional online materials and complete references for this chapter are available online at <http://www.oxfordmedicine.com>.

References

Agnese, A., Lamparelli, T., Bacigalupo, A. and Luzzatto, P. (2012). Supportive care with art therapy, for patients in isolation during stem cell transplant. *Palliative & Supportive Care*, 10, 91–98.

Beaver, V. (1998). The butterfly garden: art therapy with HIV/AIDS prisoners. In M. Pratt and M.J.M. Wood (eds.) *Art Therapy in Palliative Care: The Creative Response*, pp. 127–139. London: Routledge.

Belfiore, M. (1994). The group takes care of itself: art therapy to prevent burnout. *The Arts in Psychotherapy*, 21(2), 119–126.

Collie, K., Bottorff, J.L., and Long, B.C. (2006). A narrative view of art therapy and art making by women with breast cancer. *Journal of Health Psychology*, 11(5), 761–775.

Connell, C. (1998). *Something Understood: Art Therapy in Cancer Care*. London: Wrexham Publications.

Farrell Fenton, J. (2000). Cystic fibrosis and art therapy. *The Arts in Psychotherapy*, 27(1), 15–25.

Gantt, L. and Tinnin, L.W. (2009). Support for a neurobiological view of trauma with implications for art therapy. *The Arts in Psychotherapy*, 36(3), 148–153.

Glenister, D. (2012). Creative spaces in palliative care facilities tradition, culture, and experience. *American Journal of Hospice and Palliative Medicine*, 29(2), 89–92.

Hartley, N. and Payne, M. (eds.) (2008). *Creative Arts in Palliative Care*. London: Jessica Kingsley Publishers.

Jones, G. (2000). An art therapy group in palliative cancer care. *Nursing Times*, 96(10), 42–43.

Jones, G. and Browning, M. (2009). Supporting cancer patients and their carers: the contribution of art therapy and clinical psychology. *International Journal of Palliative Nursing*, 15(12), 609–614.

Jones, L., Fitzgerald, G., Leurent, B., *et al.* (2013). Rehabilitation in advanced, progressive, recurrent cancer: a randomized controlled trial. *Journal of Pain and Symptom Management*, 46(3), 315–325.e3.

Lin, M.H., Moh, S.L., Kuo, Y.C., *et al.* (2012). Art therapy for terminal cancer patients in a hospice palliative care unit in Taiwan. *Palliative & Supportive Care*, 10(1), 51–57.

Malchiodi, C.A. (ed.) (2012). *Art Therapy and Health Care*. New York: Guilford Press.

Nainis, N., Paice, J.A., Ratner, J., Wirth, J.H., Lai, J., and Shott, S. (2006). Relieving symptoms in cancer: innovative use of art therapy. *Journal of Pain and Symptom Management*, 31(2), 162–169.

Oster, I., Svensk, A.C., Magnusson, E., *et al.* (2006). Art therapy improves coping resources: a randomized, controlled study among women with breast cancer. *Palliative & Supportive Care*, 4(1), 57–64.

Pratt, M. and Wood, M.J.M. (eds.) (1998). *Art Therapy in Palliative Care: The Creative Response*. London: Routledge.

Rusted, J., Sheppard, L., and Waller, D. (2006). A multi-centre randomized control group trial on the use of art therapy for older people with dementia. *Group Analysis*, 39(4), 517–536.

Solomons, D. (2007). *An Art Therapy Journey: Begun in 2005*. Scotland: Marie Curie Cancer Care.

Wald, J. (2004). Hospice in the home: a case study in art therapy. In R. Perry Magniant (ed.) *Art Therapy with Older Adults*, pp. 224–231. Springfield, IL: Charles C Thomas.

Waller, D. and Sibbett, C. (eds.) (2005). *Art Therapy and Cancer Care*. Maidenhead: Open University Press.

Wood, M.J.M. (2002). Researching art therapy with people suffering from AIDS related dementia. *Arts in Psychotherapy*, 29(4), 207–219.

Stoma therapy in palliative care

Jane Ellen Barr

Introduction to stoma therapy in palliative care

Patients with ostomies, wounds, or incontinence in the setting of a serious or life-threatening illness experience numerous challenges, including distress related to pain and other symptoms, psychological disturbances, and family concerns. Expert management of these conditions and their many complications is an essential part of a comprehensive palliative plan of care. In many countries, nurse specialists with advanced training in the management of ostomies, wounds, or incontinence are available as consultants or as members of a specialist palliative care team. These professionals—known variably as stoma nurse specialists; enterostomal therapists; ostomy specialists; wound, ostomy, and continence nurses; or other terms—can improve health care and quality of life for selected patients across venues of care that include hospital, home, long-term care, hospice, and specialized settings. If a stoma nurse specialist is available, he or she may have a key role in directing decision-making and care management related to these problems, evaluating and controlling symptoms that cause patients and families suffering, and providing psychosocial and spiritual support.

Caring for the patient with faecal or urinary diversion

The prevalence of faecal or urinary diversion in populations with advanced illness is unknown, and there is little information about how an ostomy affects care needed at the end of life. Disease progression may affect a patient's ability to continue to manage ostomy self-care. Most patients are encouraged to become independent in ostomy care from the time of their surgery. As health deteriorates, continued self-care may require simplifying pouching systems and accessories. Often, however, self-care activities become compromised and it is necessary to have caregivers assist with care. The stoma specialist may need to identify caregivers who are able and willing to assist and then provide critical training, such as that required to manage pouching systems or drain a continent diversion.

Advanced disease also may create new complications even in those whose course has been stable for a long time. Changes in the peristomal plane (the area under the solid skin barrier and tape of the pouching system, extending out approximately 4 inches (10 cm) from the base of the stoma (Rolstad and Boarini, 1996)) may evolve, requiring stoma care adjustment to prevent bleeding, leakage, and peristomal irritation. The development of constipation, diarrhoea, or bowel obstruction may require special attention. In a worst-case scenario, progression of disease may result in the need for emergent ostomy surgery near life's end.

Palliative ostomy surgery

Surgery to place an ostomy typically is necessitated by a serious complication affecting the intestine or colon. It is intended to decompress bowel obstruction or divert intraluminal contents proximal to an intestinal perforation or a rectovaginal, rectovesical, or enterocutaneous fistula. These complications may be related to the primary disease, usually cancer, to disease-modifying therapy such as pelvic radiation, or to an intestinal disorder unrelated to the terminal illness or its treatment.

The stoma specialist has a key role in palliative ostomy surgery, as with all ostomy surgery. He or she may be involved in stoma site selection, and both pre- and postoperative teaching and management, including pouch selection.

Autonomy, assistance, and dependence in ostomy care

With advanced disease, the person who has had an ostomy often experiences a conflict between the desire to maintain independence in self-care and the inability to face the physiological challenges of debilitating illness. The latter challenges may include motor, sensory, vision, and cognitive defects (Tilley, 2012). In some situations, independence can be maintained by simplifying ostomy care with use of drainable pouches with Velcro® closure or clips, pouches with pre-cut or mouldable skin barriers, closed-end disposable pouches, one-piece pouching systems, or newer two-piece pouching systems with adhesive systems rather than flanges which requires less manual dexterity and strength to apply. A professional specializing in ostomy management is best suited to evaluate the specific needs of the patient, make recommendations, and provide the training necessary to transition to a new system.

At times, it is necessary for a caregiver to assume total responsibility for ostomy care. Planning for this change should be discussed with the patient, if possible. Ideally, the caregiver who becomes responsible would be both the person preferred by the patient and the one most capable to learn and implement the care. Ostomy teaching of the caregiver should begin early, giving the caregiver enough time to adjust. The specific education and training provided to the caregiver generally includes stoma care or diversion intubation. The caregiver's ability to cope with this added burden of care should be assessed and support should be provided. If a caregiver needs to assume full responsibility, specific approaches may simplify care and be preferable, such as the use of closed-end disposable drainable pouches (for faecal diversion) or the use of urostomy pouches or continent urinary diversions that attach to the bedside.

Principles of pouching

Obtaining a good ostomy seal against the peristomal plane, and thereby preventing leakage that could damage peristomal skin integrity, may become increasingly challenging as health deteriorates. The peristomal plane may be changed by weight loss or weight gain, which may result in new abdominal folds and creases, or by a change in the contour of the abdominal wall caused by ascites, tumour growth, varicosities related to portal hypertension, or other conditions. Selecting the right pouching system to obtain a good seal and prevent leakage requires expert assessment of the peristomal plane while the patient is in a lying, sitting, and standing position. In all positions, the stoma specialist assesses the skin for firmness, softness, or unevenness caused by scars, folds, or tumours. Further assessment of the abdominal contour is made, and the peristomal area is inspected to determine whether it is flat, recessed, or protruded. The stoma profile also is assessed.

There are several key principles to follow in pouching an ostomy:

- The pouching system should contain a skin barrier, to prevent the peristomal skin from effluent, and a pouch to contain the effluent.

- The stoma opening in the skin barrier should be the same size and shape as the stoma or equal to or no greater than 1/8 inch (0.3 cm) larger than stoma size.

- The skin barrier type should be chosen based on type of effluent. In faecal diversion, when effluent is liquid and with high amount of digestive enzymes, extended-wear barriers should be chosen. If stool output is formed, standard-wear barriers will provide adequate wear time. Urinary diversions will also get a better wear time with extended-wear skin barriers.

- Flat pouching systems are considered firm or flexible. Firm systems, which have flanges that cannot bend or mould to the contour of the peristomal area, will provide needed support if the peristomal skin is soft or flabby. Flexible systems, which have adhesive and no flange, can be one piece or two piece, and are useful if the peristomal plane is round, firm, or protrudes (e.g. from ascites or peristomal hernia) because it will contour to the shape.

- Convex skin barriers improve the seals when stomas have retracted below skin level and are another option when the peristomal plane is soft or flabby or when the convexity is needed to fill scarring, folds, or creases.

- The stoma profile also gives guidance in selecting a skin barrier and pouching system: a flat skin barrier can facilitate a seal in flush stomas. A convex barrier can be used with stomas that are flush, retracted, or retracted with peristalsis. A flexible skin barrier without flanges is safest for prolapsed stomas to prevent injury.

- The skin barrier should mirror the distinctiveness of the peristomal area. If the peristomal area has creases or scars, skin barrier pastes or washers can be used to fill in the defects and uneven areas.

- When changing the pouching system, the back of the skin barrier should be assessed for any 'hidden leaks' where effluent is on the wafer but has not extended from the skin barrier's adhesive (tape). This is to help establish the wear time of the pouching system and to help assess if any changes are needed to obtain a good seal.

Stoma and peristomal complications

As health status deteriorates, stoma and peristomal skin complications are more likely to occur. Patients with advanced disease who receive newly created stomas are at relatively higher risk for mucocutaneous separation or retraction. Those who have lived with an ostomy may develop long-term complications, such as caput medusa, hernia, or prolapse. These stoma complications can result in poorly fitting and leaking pouching systems, with resultant impaired peristomal skin integrity leading to disorders such as irritant dermatitis or candidiasis.

Stomal and peristomal impairments are important stressors, and may occur in parallel with numerous other problems related to progressive illness. They can augment mood disturbance and social isolation, and profoundly undermine quality of life.

In populations with cancer, palliative ostomy surgery may be required in an area that was previously irradiated. Both radiation injury and recurrent malignancy makes stoma construction difficult. As a result, a postoperative complication, stoma retraction, may occur. With retraction, the stoma is pulled below skin level. Pouching options and adjustments to obtain a good seal may include use of convexity, support belts, and binders.

Mucocutaneous separation is detachment of the stoma from the peristomal skin and can be partial or circumferential, superficial or deep. It often precedes stomal retraction. The risk of mucocutaneous separation after surgery is relatively higher in patients who are in less than optimal condition, such as may occur with immunocompromise or poor nutrition. In most cases, the management of mucocutaneous separation is conservative, focusing on measures to support wound healing when possible. The separation is filled with an appropriate dressing, either to maintain a moist environment or to absorb drainage. The goal is to facilitate granulation tissue formation and re-epithelization of the defect. The skin barrier of the pouching system fits over the filled area to provide protection from the effluent. When the separation heals, other potential complications, such as stenosis and retraction, may occur. Convex skin barriers are not recommended in the presence of mucocutaneous separation as they may increase separation at the stoma and skin junction. When separation is below fascia, surgery is indicated.

Peristomal hernia, a bulge around the stoma as a result of loops of bowel protruding through the fascial defect around the stoma and into the subcutaneous tissue, can result from any cause of increased intra-abdominal pressure. Pouching systems should be changed to flexible systems that mould to the shape of the peristomal plane. Hernia support belts may increase comfort and offer cosmetic benefits by decreasing bulge. Patients who have been irrigating a colostomy are instructed to stop this activity. Use of bulk laxatives and stool softeners often assist with bowel regulation as needed.

Stoma prolapse is a telescoping of the bowel through the abdominal stoma site. It can occur as a result of increase intra-abdominal pressure due to ascites, tumour, or other condition, and often is associated with stomal mucosa oedema. The enlarged stoma is at risk for trauma if a rigid pouching system with a flange is used. Therefore, especially at the end of life, management is often conservative, and involves the selection of a flexible, flangeless pouching system that can accommodate the width and length of the stoma without causing trauma to the stoma. The patient or caregiver can be taught how to reduce the prolapse by lying in a supine position to decrease intra-abdominal pressure, applying a cold pack to the pouch over the stoma to reduce the oedema, and then applying light pressure to the distal portion of the stoma, thereby returning the stoma to its intraperitoneal place. The patient can wear a binder specifically made to include a prolapse flap to keep the stoma reduced during normal activities of living. Should the prolapsed bowel become incarcerated, ischaemia can occur. If pain is severe or infarction occurs, surgical intervention may be necessary.

Patients with advanced liver disease (e.g. from malignancy, cirrhosis, or portal hypertension) may develop a stoma complication known as caput medusa. This condition presents as bluish-purple discoloration of the skin caused by dilatation of the cutaneous veins around the stoma (peristomal varices) (Lo et al., 1984). The varices are large portosystemic collateral veins that appear around the stoma and are related to portal hypertension from where the portal venous system communicates with the systemic circulatory system. Any trauma to the stoma may result in profuse bleeding, which may appear in the pouch itself or occur at the time of the pouch change. Management focuses on controlling the bleeding: direct pressure, cold cloth, topical haemostatic agents (silver nitrate, thrombin), or suture ligation. Patient should be taught measures to prevent bleeding episodes, such as gentle appliance care with removal and washing. Firm, rigid, or convex pouching systems should be avoided. In severe cases, sclerotherapy or surgical intervention to ligate the portosystemic channels or create a portosystemic shunt to lower pressure may be indicated.

Two of the most common peristomal skin complications, irritant dermatitis and candidiasis, are related to pouching problems. Peristomal irritant dermatitis is caused by exposure to stool or urine of peristomal skin under the skin barrier. This condition presents as erythema or a macular rash that progresses to moist, shallow, peristomal denudement and erosions if exposure to irritant continues. The patient may complain of pain, itching, or burning in the peristomal area beneath the skin barrier. Management focuses on correcting the cause by properly measuring and selecting a pouching system that takes into consideration the stoma profile, abdominal contours, and skin surface, by adjusting the frequency of change, and by teaching proper pouching procedures to patients and caregivers. The skin impairment is treated using the 'crusting technique': applying skin barrier powder which is then covered with liquid barrier film with each pouching system change until skin heals.

Peristomal candidiasis is caused by the proliferation of *Candida albicans* in the warm, moist, dry environment beneath the skin barrier. Risk factors for candidiasis are increased with treatments or side effects of treatment such as long-term antibiotic administration, cancer, chemotherapy, and immunosuppressive drug therapy. The primary lesion is a pustule on an erythematous base that evolves into sharply demarcated, eroded patches with small peripheral satellite papules and marginal scaling. The patient may complain of burning and itching, and often leaking pouching systems. Management includes applying topical antifungal therapy, such as miconazole (which treats *Candida* and tinea) or nystatin (which treats *Candida*). Liquid barrier film needs to be applied over antifungal powder to obtain a good skin barrier seal. The infection should be eliminated in about 1 week, but treatment should be continued for another 2 weeks to avert the potential for recurrence. If other sites are noted to be infected, such as the inguinal region or the anxilla, the patient should also be treated with systemic antifungal therapy (e.g. fluconazole).

Continent diversions

Selected patients with colon cancer, inflammatory bowel disease, familial polyposis, or bladder cancer may be able to benefit from more advance surgical techniques that eliminate the need for incontinent faecal or urinary diversions and the wearing of external pouching systems. Continent faecal and urinary diversions are managed by intubation of the pouch or reservoir created during the surgery. In a person with advanced disease who can no longer intubate their own continent diversion, the caregiver may need to learn the technique. Urinary reservoirs are often intubated every 4 hours during day and once at night; faecal reservoirs are intubated four times daily and before bedtime. If the caregiver cannot manage the technique or frequency of intubation, a catheter may be inserted into the reservoir and attached to bedside drainage. If leakage occurs from the continent diversion, it can be pouched in a manner similar to a conventional urinary or faecal diversion. Urinary reservoirs that have increased mucous production may need to be irrigated once or twice daily with water or normal saline, with or without acetylcysteine. In faecal reservoirs, lukewarm water can be instilled into the internal pouch to thin out the stool if necessary to empty the reservoir.

Management of gastrointestinal symptoms in a patient with a stoma

Whenever prescribing or administering medications to a patient with an ostomy, it is important to know the type of ostomy (colostomy, ileostomy) and what amount of bowel was removed or bypassed during the surgery. Patients with right-sided colostomy or an ileostomy with rapid transit time and high liquid output should avoid enteric-coated or sustained -release products.

Patients with a faecal stoma can experience bowel irregularities or complications such as constipation or diarrhoea. Ostomy patients who require opioid analgesics should be assessed for regular bowel functioning. When severe constipation is suspected, a digital assessment with a lubricated gloved finger into the stoma may be indicated to check for impaction. Preventing constipation is important, just as in patients without stomas. Patients and caregivers should be instructed on behavioural interventions, such as exercise as tolerated, and dietary interventions, such as maintaining hydration by drinking fluids or increasing bulk in the diet if appropriate. Laxatives should be prescribed as indicated. If a colostomy becomes impacted, an oil retention fleet enema (administered through a stoma cone), followed by a colostomy irrigation, may be tried. Ileostomy patients do not usually have constipation problems, but bowel functioning should also be assessed. In advanced cancers, whether the patient has an ileostomy or colostomy, partial or complete intestinal obstruction must be considered with irregular bowel functioning.

Just as patients can experience constipation, the person living with a stoma may also have management difficulties related to diarrhoea. Diarrhoea can be a result of too many laxatives, faecal impaction, *Clostridium difficile* infection, or medications such as chemotherapeutic agents. Assessment to determine the cause is crucial since treatment is based on the aetiology. When diet management can have an impact on decreasing frequency of bowel movements, patients and caregivers can be taught about foods that thicken stool such as dried fruit, bananas, boiled rice and pastas, creamy peanut butter, and marshmallows.

Palliative wound care

Prevention of pressure ulcers

The risk of pressure ulcers increases in populations with advanced illness. Risk factors include malnourishment, cachexia, dehydration, chair-bound or bed-bound status, and multisystem failure with resultant poor tissue perfusion to skin. Pressure ulcers can decrease comfort, rest, and quality of life for the person and family. The patient and caregivers should be educated on basic measures to prevent pressure ulcers, such as use of appropriate support surfaces, need for turning and positioning, maintaining clean and dry skin, and use of skin and positioning products to protect high-risk areas. The patient and their family should be assured that pain medication will be provided as needed to keep the patient comfortable during care, such as position changes. Research is needed to clarify the extent to which pressure ulcers are preventable. The term skin failure has emerged in the literature related to impaired skin and tissue integrity near death. Skin failure is defined as death of the skin and underlying tissue resulting from hypoperfusion secondary to multisystem organ failure which occurs as part of the dying process (Langemo and Brown, 2006). Patient, caregivers, and health-care providers need to discuss and agree on the preventive and management plans for each individual person to prevent or treat skin failure. 'Palliative wound care', which follows the basic principles of wound management, such as cleansing, debridement, and creating an optimal moist environment, may lead to very positive results, decreasing the risk of pain and improving quality at life's end. Some patients are cured, a goal of curative wound care protocols (Ennis and Meneses, 2005), which can be viewed as a benefit in improving a patient's overall quality of life (Tippett, 2005). For others, wound healing is an unrealistic goal, either because of poor clinical conditions or local wound factors. Realistic goals may include creating a stable wound with relief of pain, eliminating odour, managing drainage, preventing infection, and maintaining the person's optimal level of function.

Malignant wounds

Malignant fungating wounds occur when an underlying tumour extends through the epithelium. The lesions might be the result of a primary cancer or a metastasis to the skin (O'Brien, 2012). As the tumour increases in size, vessels may rupture or become occluded, with resultant tissue necrosis, infection, and a high output of odorous drainage. Malodour results from bacteria, both aerobic and anaerobic, that reside in necrotic wound tissue.

Fungating lesions are physically and emotionally difficult for the patient and caregivers to manage. They can have a tremendous negative impact on the patient, deepening the sense of helplessness, poor self-image, and isolation from family and friends because of the malodour. Care is focused on symptom management. By decreasing bioburden and necrotic tissue on the fungating lesion, the amount of exudate and odour is often controlled. Topical management includes cleaning the lesion with antibacterial soap and water (often in a shower, if patient can tolerate this), applying topical antimicrobials such as metronidazole crushed tablets or metronidazole gel, and using dressings to facilitate autolytic debridement, exudate absorption, and pain management. When bleeding is a problem, calcium alginate dressing is applied for its haemostatic properties. Hydrofibres and foam dressing also are used to control exudate. Silicone-backed foam dressing may decrease pain and prevents added trauma on removal, in addition to its absorptive effects. Silver and medihoney dressings can also be used for their antimicrobial benefits. The therapeutic effects of honey-based dressings include anti-inflammatory properties that reduce pain and scarring, antibacterial properties that aid in reducing odour, and debridement properties that reduce necrotic tissue (which also helps to decrease odour) (Pieper, 2009).

Herpes zoster

Commonly known as shingles, herpes zoster results from the reactivation of the varicella-zoster virus in a patient who is often immunocompromised. The clinical presentation includes fluid-filled vesicular lesions in a unilateral dermatomal distribution (Wilson, 2007). Management includes use of antiviral medications (aciclovir, valaciclovir, or famciclovir) to decrease the duration of the herpes zoster rash and the severity of pain. The antiviral medications works best when administered to the patient while new lesions are being formed, and no later than 72 hours after the eruption of the rash. Initially, when lesions are moist and draining, topical dressings such as foams with silicone backings provide for absorption, and may decrease pain (Serena and Fry, 2006).

Conclusion

Palliative ostomy and wound care strives to meet the majority of patient's physical and mental health needs in an interdisciplinary team approach. Attention to the patient's and their family's unique needs, culture, values, and preferences are paramount. Focus is on improved quality of life and the provision of effective and efficient patient- and family-centred care. Emphasis is on pain and symptom management, communication, emotional and spiritual support, improved quality of life, and better patient and family satisfaction.

References

Ennis, W.J. and Meneses, P. (2005). Palliative care and wound care: 2 emerging fields with similar needs for outcome data. *Wounds*, 17(4), 99–104.

Langemo, D.K. and Brown, G. (2006). Skin fails too: acute, chronic, and end-stage skin failure. *Advances in Skin and Wound Care*, 19(4), 206–212.

Lo, R.K., Johnson, D.T., and Smith, D.B. (1984). Massive bleeding from an ileal conduit caput medusa. *Journal of Urology*, 131, 114.

O'Brien, C. (2012). Malignant wounds. *Canadian Family Physician*, 58, 272–274.

Pieper, B. (2009). Honey based dressings and wound care: an option for care in the United States. *Journal Wound Ostomy Continence Nursing*, 36(1), 60–66.

Rolstad, B. and Boarini, J. (1996). Principles and techniques in the use of convexity. *Ostomy Wound Management*, 42, 24–32.

Serena, T.E. and Fry, R. (2006). Use of an atraumatic dressing in the treatment of a painful wound resulting from herpes zoster. *Ostomy/Wound Management*, 52(12), 14–16.

Tilley, C. (2012). Caring for the patient with a fecal or urinary diversion in palliative and hospice settings: a literature review. *Ostomy/Wound Management*, 58(1), 24–34.

Tippett, A.W. (2005). Wound at the end of life. *Wounds*, 17(4), 91–98.

Wilson, D.D. (2007). Herpes zoster prevention, diagnosis, and treatment. *The Nurse Practitioner*, 32(9), 19–24.

4.13

Clinical psychology in palliative care

Anja Mehnert

Introduction to clinical psychology in palliative care

Psychological interventions can address a wide spectrum of objectives in palliative care and together aim to reduce psychosocial distress and maintain quality of life in patients and their caregivers. Some of these interventions help the patient and family cope with the fear of death and dying, manage anxiety, and reduce feelings of isolation, sadness, despair, and depression. These affective states closely interact with the physical symptom burden and often track with the deterioration of the illness. Other psychological approaches address problems associated with changes in relations and social roles, increasing dependency, the need to adjust to often impaired functional status, and existential concerns such as the search for meaning in life, hope, sense of dignity, grief, and spirituality. For the practitioner, the provision of psychological care as part of the palliative care team approach is characterized by high time demands, the need for flexibility and cultural competence, the ability to assist with decision-making, and facility with a variety of psychotherapeutic skills including the ability to support non-verbal communication (Irwin and von Gunten, 2010).

Psychological distress and mental disorders in patients with advanced disease

Response to stressors

Recent clinical and research models of comprehensive patient care endorse the integration of palliative care early in the disease trajectory, during the period that disease-modifying and other life-prolonging therapies are actively pursued (Irwin and von Gunten, 2010). The palliative care continuum therefore includes acute illness, chronic illness, and end-of-life/hospice care, as well as bereavement care. This model subsumes the course of psychosocial distress in patients and caregivers, and underscores the significance of their supportive care needs.

The ability to cope with illness and adapt to the challenges it presents is influenced by the changing severity of stressors over time, psychological and psychosocial processes that mediate and modulate response, and the potential occurrence of comorbid disorders. During the trajectory of a life-threatening disease such as cancer, patients are confronted with a variety of biological and psychosocial stressors. Figure 4.13.1 illustrates a model of pathways of distress for cancer adapted from the work of Li et al.,

(2010). This model includes cancer and treatment-related stressors and psychosocial stressors, moderating individual and interpersonal factors, and a range of psychological and behavioural stress responses that have guided clinical psychological research in palliative care through recent years. According to the model, biological stressors arising from the disease and its multimodal treatments include pain and severe physical symptom distress, as well as neurobiological changes that are likely to influence psychological and behavioural stress responses and mental disorders (Li et al., 2010). Medical factors associated with psychological distress, particularly with increased anxiety, include metabolic conditions (e.g. hypo- and hypercalcaemia), neurological conditions (e.g. pain, central nervous system neoplasms), endocrine factors (e.g. hyper- and hypothyroidism), cardiovascular conditions (e.g. arrhythmia, cardiomyopathy), pulmonary conditions (e.g. hypoxia, pulmonary embolism, asthma), and medications (e.g. corticosteroids, bronchodilators, antibiotics, interferon, withdrawal states) (Breitbart et al., 1995; Pessin et al., 2008; Levin and Alici, 2010).

The psychosocial consequences of disease progression result in a range of challenges for both the patient and the caregiver. Advanced disease often is accompanied by functional impairments, dependency, and changes in appearance that can represent a threat to the sense of control, as well as the identity and the sense of dignity of a patient (Chochinov et al., 2009). Patients and caregivers also often face uncertainty and changes in relationships, attachment security, and social roles (Tan et al., 2005; Rodin et al., 2007). They simultaneously have to deal with the organization of care, difficult treatment decisions, changes in their life trajectory and life goals, and (anticipatory) loss and grief. Individual and interpersonal characteristics, such as age or education, life stage, personality patterns, coping strategies, family functioning, available and perceived social support, prior experience with illness and life crisis, and spiritual resources, can both influence and moderate the perception of stressors and the occurrence of psychosocial distress and mental disorders (Li et al., 2010).

In the context of advanced disease, physical symptom distress and psychological distress are closely interrelated. The continuum of psychological and behavioural stress responses consist of a wide range of emotional states experienced by patients and their caregivers. These include worry, anxiety, fear of death, feelings of helplessness, regret, shame, guilt or anger, sadness, demoralization, loss of meaning and hope, and (anticipatory) grief. A large

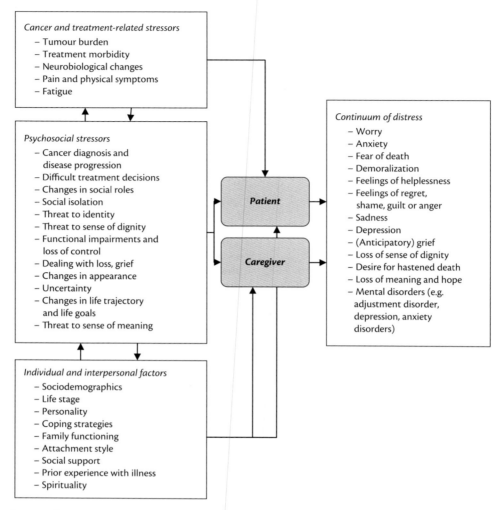

Fig. 4.13.1 Model of pathways to distress.

Adapted from Li, M. and Hales, S.R.G., 'Adjustment Disorders' in Holland, J et al. (Eds.), *Psycho-Oncology*, 2nd edition, pp. 303–310, Oxford University Press, New York, USA, Copyright © 2010, by permission of Oxford University Press USA.

body of evidence suggests that psychological distress can range from normal adaptive emotions through to higher levels of severe and clinically significant symptoms that fulfil standardized diagnostic criteria for an adjustment disorder, anxiety disorder, or depression (Ziegler et al. 2011). Some patients experience a loss of sense of dignity, suicidal thoughts and desire for hastened death, particularly during the end-of-life phase.

Common disorders and phenomena

Adjustment disorder

Adjustment disorder is defined as emotional and/or behavioural symptoms that are in excess of what would normally be expected from exposure to a given stressor (American Psychiatric Association, 2000). Adjustment disorders are characterized by a variety of clinically relevant emotional or behavioural symptoms arising from a specific stressful event such as the diagnosis or recurrence of a life-threatening illness. They are among the most common psychiatric diagnoses in oncology (Miovic and Block, 2007; Passik et al., 2008; Li et al., 2010). Frequent subtypes comprise adjustment disorder with depressed mood, anxiety or

mixed anxiety and depressed mood. Prevalence rates for adjustment disorders range from 11% to 35% (Kugaya et al., 2000; Akechi et al., 2004; Kirsh et al., 2004; Miovic and Block, 2007; Mitchell et al., 2011).

A specific form of non-specific distress, the *demoralization syndrome*, has been described by de Figueiredo and Frank (de Figueiredo and Frank, 1982; de Figueiredo, 1993). The demoralization syndrome is characterized as a person's inability to cope effectively with a stressful event and a loss of sense of mastery. Kissane et al. (2001) and Clarke and Kissane (2002) defined the demoralization syndrome as a clinically relevant syndrome of particular relevance for patients with severe and advanced physical illness, which is characterized by existential distress and despair, and could be diagnosed according to the following criteria: (a) affective symptoms of existential distress, including hopelessness or loss of meaning and purpose in life; (b) cognitive attitudes of pessimism, helplessness, sense of being trapped, personal failure; (c) absence of drive or motivation to cope differently; (d) associated features of social alienation or isolation and lack of support, and (e) allowing for fluctuation in emotional intensity, these phenomena persist across more than 2 weeks. Furthermore, a major depressive or other psychiatric disorder is not present as the primary condition (Kissane et al., 2001). Severe physical illnesses are particularly demoralizing due to their threat to the integrity of the body and the mind, as well as a person's mastery and control (Clarke and Kissane, 2002). Given the frequency of illness-associated experiences of dependence, reduction of social roles and isolation in the face of an uncertain prognosis, populations with advanced illness are particularly vulnerable to stress responses generated from feelings of helplessness and hopelessness, despair and demoralization (Mullane et al., 2009; Mehnert et al., 2011; Vehling et al., 2012b).

Anxiety disorder

Anxiety disorder is characterized by specific cognitive, affective and behavioural/physiological symptoms, such as excessive anxiety and worry, difficulties controlling the worry, difficulty concentrating, irritability, and shortness of breath or chest pain. Subtypes include generalized anxiety disorder, panic disorder, and post-traumatic stress disorder. Using clinical psychiatric interviews, an anxiety disorder was found in 6% to 14% in patients with advanced disease (Miovic and Block, 2007; Mitchell et al., 2011; Vehling et al., 2012a). Using screening measures, much higher prevalence rates of anxiety and significant anxiety symptoms—up to 48%—have been noted (Roth and Massie, 2007; Teunissen et al., 2007; Roy-Byrne et al., 2008; Delgado-Guay et al., 2009; Kolva et al., 2011). With progressive disease, higher symptom burden (e.g. nausea, pain, and dyspnoea), and the physical deterioration, the prevalence of anxiety increases (Delgado-Guay et al., 2009; Kolva et al., 2011). Maladaptive cognitions are also associated with increased anxiety. Patients with advanced disease facing death may be plagued by recurrent unpleasant thoughts, including fears of toxic treatments, pain, further disease progression, social isolation, dependency on others, and death (Roth and Massie, 2007; Passik et al., 2008; Levin and Alici, 2010).

Depressive disorder

Depressive disorder is characterized by specific core symptoms, namely a persistent depressed mood or loss of pleasure. Other symptoms are related to psychomotor changes, and both cognitive and somatic complaints. Depression is a common disorder. Surveys reveal overall rates of depressive symptomatology that range from 14% to 37% in populations with advanced disease (Massie, 2004; Miovic and Block, 2007; Pessin et al., 2008; Delgado-Guay et al., 2009; Wasteson et al., 2009; Lo et al., 2010; O'Connor et al., 2010; Mitchell et al., 2011; Mellor et al., 2013). In severely and terminally ill patients, the prevalence is higher, especially when the illness is associated with limited functionality, insecure attachments, and additional disease burden such as pain (Chochinov et al., 1994; Breitbart et al., 1995; Rodin et al., 2009). For example, depressive symptomatology was found in up to 77% among cancer patients, up to 82% among patients with AIDS, up to 71% among patients with chronic obstructive pulmonary disease, and up to 36% among patients with heart disease (Solano et al., 2006). Other risk factors for depressed mood include younger age, a family and individual history of depression, low perceived social supports, low optimism and low self-esteem, poorer social functioning and a history of stressful or traumatic life events (Miller and Massie, 2010).

Sadness is common and appropriate as part of a human grief response when confronted with terminal illness and the approaching of the end of live (Pessin et al., 2008). In practice, this normal response must be distinguished from clinical depression, which is an adverse condition that causes additional physical and psychosocial burden for these patients (Mellor et al., 2013).

Suicidality and desire for hastened death

Uncontrollable pain, depression, feelings of helplessness and hopelessness, delirium, high unrelieved physical symptom burden, low family support, and being a burden to others are major factors in the desire for hastened death (Hudson et al., 2006; Rodin et al., 2009; Breitbart et al., 2010; Rosenstein, 2011). Occasional thoughts of suicide in patients with advanced disease often represent an attempt to regain a sense of control in a situation experienced primarily as uncontrollable. Studies show that suicidal thoughts occur on average in 15% of patients with advanced cancer, with a wide range between 1.5% and 51% (Henderson and Ord, 1997; Druss and Pincus, 2000; Akechi et al., 2001, 2002, 2010; Rasic et al., 2008). However, few patients experience persistent suicidal thoughts and express the desire for hastened death, particularly in the pre-terminal and terminal stage of the disease.

Khan and colleagues have pointed out that the loss of the will to live in patients with advanced disease may arise from diverse processes, such as the acceptance of death, the lowering of mood, demoralization, or changes in important relationships with caregivers and health-care professionals (Khan et al., 2010). Hudson and colleagues found that the reasons for desire for hastened death were often multiple and complex, and categorized the associated processes as (a) an expression of feelings and current reactions to their circumstances, such as the loss of autonomy and the sense of dignity; (b) a communication of distress and suffering and/or a communication to explore options for relieving their distress; (c) seeking of information about suicide or euthanasia; and (d) specifically seeking health professional assistance with hastened death or acknowledging an intent for suicide (Hudson et al., 2006).

When patients express a desire for death or suicidal intent, the assessment of the suicide risk and the early administration of appropriate treatments, including psychiatric interventions, are critical. Breitbart (1990) and Pessin et al. (2008) have emphasized the importance of a careful and comprehensive evaluation of suicidal thoughts, plans, and current intentions using an empathetic approach. They recommend evaluating the patient's understanding of his/her symptoms, and assessing the mental status, vulnerability, pain control, support system, recent losses, prior psychiatric history including alcohol and substance abuse, and prior suicide attempts and threats. The evaluation should clarify the need for observation and the formulation of a short-term and long-term treatment plan

It is important to pursue an integrated therapeutic approach when managing suicidal ideation in the palliative care setting. Given the associations between suicidal thoughts and emotional suffering from unrelieved pain and physical symptoms, feelings of being a burden to family and dependency on others, and the fear of impending death from advanced disease, one or more of these issues may require targeted interventions. The rapid and effective management of physical and psychological symptoms, for example, may quickly reduce distress and improve suicidal ideation in the majority of patients. Both pharmacological and psychosocial interventions may address depression, feelings of helplessness and hopelessness, demoralization, and loss of meaning in life. Efforts to sustain supportive relationships with caregivers and health professionals also can help patients to regain quality of life.

Psychosocial distress in family caregivers

Psychosocial distress does not only affect patients. Interventions also may be needed to address the distress or disorders experienced by family, friends, and other caregivers. Patients with progressing disease and their caregivers both face the need to accept transition from an emphasis on disease-modifying therapy to an emphasis on palliative care alone. Particularly in the context of advanced illness or impending death, caregivers play an important and challenging role, providing emotional and social support for the patient, helping with medical needs, and meeting increasingly complex instrumental needs such as running the household and work. Furthermore, caregivers may be called upon to assist professionals in making difficult treatment decisions, and these occurrences may be experienced as highly stressful (Huang et al., 2012). When treatments have uncertain benefits and burdens, or the goals of care are ill-defined, conflict may erupt between the patient and caregivers, or between caregivers and health-care providers. Many studies have observed associations between high levels of emotional distress in caregivers, or anticipatory grief, and signs of clinical instability, sudden health changes, or end-stage disease in patients; distress also is magnified when patients experience depression or progressive cognitive impairment. During bereavement, support offers for caregivers include supportive counselling, psychodynamic and interpersonal psychotherapies, cognitive behavioural therapy (CBT), and family therapy (Lichtenthal et al., 2010).

Diagnosis and assessment of psychological distress and mental disorders

The assessment of psychological distress and diagnosis of mental disorders pose a range of clinical challenges in populations with serious or life-threatening illness. Given the complex medical issues and treatment interactions, the aetiology of both physical and psychological symptoms often remains unclear. In some patients, elevated levels of psychological distress or a mental disorder represent premorbid conditions that have continued or worsened with onset and progression of the medical illness. In the much larger proportion of patients, psychological distress represents a response to the life-threatening disease, the deterioration of their health, and the multimodal medical treatments (Kelly et al., 2006).

A relatively small proportion of patients with psychosocial distress or a mental disorder are identified by the health-care team early and referred to receive psychosocial support (Passik et al., 1998; Fallowfield et al., 2001; Kelly et al., 2006). Recommendations are needed to improve the opportunity for early intervention. To some extent these recommendations focus on the interpretation of selected symptoms in the context of advanced illness. It often remains unclear whether a particular symptom, such as difficulty concentrating or weight loss, is a consequence of a treatment such as chemotherapy, or a symptom of a mental disorder such as depression. Many authors recommend that the psychiatric and psychosocial assessment focus on cognitive and psychological symptoms, such as hopelessness or guilt, rather than on somatic symptoms (Passik et al., 2000; Pessin et al., 2005). This is echoed by diagnostic manuals, such as the American Psychiatric Association's *Diagnostic and Statistical Manual of Mental Disorders*. It is often

impossible, however, to differentiate the aetiology of symptoms in patients with advanced disease and multiple symptom burden, and excluding somatic symptoms in the diagnostic assessment risks further an underestimation of mental disorders such as depression (Pessin et al., 2005). In contrast, other diagnostic approaches include all symptoms regardless of their aetiology, and this probably leads to an over-identification of mental disorders (Cassem, 1990). Endicott has suggested a substitutive approach, in which somatic symptoms are replaced in the assessment of depression in patients with somatic diseases (Endicott, 1984). However, even this approach can lead to difficulties in distinguishing psychological symptoms that indicate elevated distress versus a normal adaptive emotional response to the end of life. For example, some catastrophizing thoughts or hopelessness may be present in patients with poor prognosis or in a terminal stage of the disease, yet not be associated with high distress.

During recent years, a range of brief and ultra-brief screening tools have been developed for the assessment of psychological distress in the medically ill. Kelly and colleagues have reviewed these tools and other approaches for measurement of psychological distress in palliative care (Kelly et al., 2006). Single-item screening instruments have been proposed as a useful approach in many conditions. Chochinov and colleagues suggested a single screening item approach ('Are you depressed?') for depression (Chochinov et al., 1997). The National Comprehensive Cancer Network (NCCN) in the United States has established the distress thermometer, a single-item measure to measure distress and associate it with one or more experiential domains (NCCN, 2003), and a single-item approach to identify spiritual distress at the end-of-life was published by Steinhauser et al. (2006).

A longer depression assessment has been developed by Pessin and colleagues (Pessin et al., 2005), based on the responses to the following questions:

- ◆ Anhedonia: *Have you lost interest or pleasure in the things you used to enjoy? Is there anything that you are still able to enjoy?*

- ◆ Depressed mood: *How has your mood been? Have you been feeling sad, depressed, or down? What are you feeling sad about?*

- ◆ Worthlessness and guilt: *Do you worry about being a burden to your family? Do you feel that your life is worthless right now?*

- ◆ Suicidal ideation: *Most patients have some thoughts about death; have you had any? Do you feel that life is not worth living? Do you find yourself thinking about death a lot or think you would be better off dead?*

- ◆ Suicidal plan: *Have you stopped taking care of yourself? Have things gotten so bad that you have thought about hurting yourself or ending your life sooner?*

- ◆ Hopelessness: *How are you feeling about the future right now? Are there things that you are looking forward to?*

- ◆ Insomnia or hypersomnia: *How is your sleep? Do you have trouble falling asleep? Staying asleep? Do you wake up frequently in the night? Do you find when you can't sleep that you are up feeling sad or worrying? Or do you find that the opposite happens, that you are sleeping too much?*

- ◆ Appetite: *How has your appetite been? Does food taste good to you? Would you eat more if you were physically able?*

- ◆ Concentration and indecision: *How has your thinking been? Do you have trouble thinking or remembering things? Do you have difficulty making decisions?*

◆ Fatigue and loss of energy: *How is your energy level? Do you notice that your mood affects your energy level?*

◆ Psychomotor retardation and agitation (clinicians should note behaviour): *Have you noticed you feel slowed down? Have you been moving more slowly than usual? Or do you find the opposite, that you feel fidgety, restless, or keyed-up inside?*

In populations with advanced illness, the time and burden associated with a comprehensive psychological or psychiatric assessment can be challenging for patients, and the assessment may yield information that is difficult to interpret. These negatives should be balanced against the potential positive outcomes that may follow identification and treatment of factors that contribute to distress for the patient and the caregiver. If a brief assessment, even a screening, provides sufficient information to act clinically, it can suffice; if not, additional efforts should be made to acquire information about the source of distress or mental disorder.

Psychological interventions for patients with advanced disease

Clinical psychological/psychotherapeutic care for patients with progressing disease and their caregivers comprises a variety of interventions and techniques, all of which can be integrated into a multidisciplinary care plan (Watson and Kissane, 2011). These include, among others, CBT, cognitive analytic therapy, narrative interventions, relaxation and guided imagery, mindfulness-based interventions, meaning-focused interventions, art therapy, and dignity therapy. Psychotropic medication often is combination with psychotherapeutic interventions for patients with severe distress and should be further clarified with the medical care team.

Psychotherapeutic requirements

The psychotherapeutic work and goals in palliative care settings differ in several respects from psychological interventions for patients with early or curative diseases or physically healthy individuals. First, the time frame for interventions may be limited. Usually, patients can be seen only a few times, depending on the physical condition, the course of the disease, and the inpatient or outpatient setting. The limited time has several implications for the development of a trustful and sustainable therapeutic relationship and psychotherapeutic treatment planning. Treatment planning often depends on the course of the disease and the sometimes quickly changing supportive care needs of patients and/or their caregivers. It requires medical knowledge pertinent to the patient's illness, and information about common medical treatments and their side effects. It also requires close contact and collaboration with the palliative care team, if involved. The often unpredictable course of the disease and changes in the supportive care needs may place high demands on the clinician with regard to flexibility, empathy, and understanding of the patient's situation.

Second, treatment planning for the patient with serious illness must consider that communication with the patient and the caregiver can be hampered not only by severe health conditions, such as delirium, but also by unclear or divergent perceptions about the goals of treatment and the curability of the disease. Temel and colleagues showed that despite having terminal cancer, about one-third of patients newly diagnosed with metastatic non-small cell lung cancer reported that their cancer was curable at baseline, and a majority endorsed getting rid of all of the cancer as a goal of therapy (Temel et al., 2011). In addition, patients experience hope and hopelessness often as closely linked constructs (Sachs et al., 2013). Rodin and Zimmermann used the term 'double awareness' to describe the situation of patients with advanced—yet not terminal—disease and the challenge in dealing with issues of death and dying while remaining engaged in life (e.g. dealing with complex treatment decisions, managing changing relationships) (Rodin and Zimmermann, 2008).

The clinical psychologist is often faced with the difficult task of encouraging patients and caregivers to cope adaptively while promoting acceptance. Support for coping may be focused on helping to maintain hope and quality of life, and reduce psychological stress. Acceptance may require that patients and caregivers face 'realistic' treatment goals and treatment decisions, which themselves have the potential to negatively affect the psychosocial well-being of the patient and the family. The psychologist must be prepared to manage the emotional responses of the patient and the caregiver, which can include frustration and anger, disappointment, despair, (anticipatory) grief, and high levels of distress. These emotions may lead to difficult therapeutic interactions. Finally, clinical psychologists working in palliative care settings must be prepared to deal with personal feelings generated by the closeness to death and dying, their own sense of helplessness, and existential or spiritual questions about the meaning of life and death.

Psychotherapeutic goals and approaches

Supportive psychotherapy

Psychotherapeutic interventions in palliative care usually have a foundation of supportive psychotherapy, on which is built a multimodal approach. Supportive psychotherapy is defined as a therapeutic intervention that aims to help patients and caregivers deal with distressing emotions, and to promote existing resources, strengths, and adaptive coping with the disease (Lederberg and Holland, 2011). In relation to these issues, the objectives of psychotherapeutic interventions include the following (MacLeod, 2008):

◆ Enhancement of adaptive coping efforts

◆ Clarification of misunderstandings and (mis-) expectations

◆ Clarification and/or strengthening of interpersonal relationships

◆ Mobilizing individual and family resources

◆ Reducing psychological symptom burden (e.g. anxiety, depression)

◆ Maintaining hope and life goals

◆ Promoting acceptance

◆ Maintaining a sense of dignity

◆ Finding meaning in life and a sense of peace

◆ Strengthening of self-esteem

◆ Acknowledgement of strengths and achievements in the life of the patient

◆ Reduce feelings of isolation and loneliness of the patients

◆ Acknowledgement of feelings of grief and sadness about loss/saying good bye.

Cognitive behavioural therapy

CBT has been shown to be very effective in treating emotional distress and particularly depression in patients with chronic health conditions (Horne and Watson, 2011). Nonetheless, the approach has been used less often in palliative care settings than in the management of patients with non-life-threatening conditions. However, cognitive techniques, such as cognitive restructuring/reframing, and behavioural techniques, such as activity scheduling and distraction, can help to relief distress from specific symptoms such as anxiety, depression, fatigue, and pain. Contraindications to CBT include organic mental syndromes, schizo-affective disorders, and delirium (Horne and Watson, 2011).

Relaxation and image-based interventions

Relaxation and image-based interventions comprise a wide range of techniques including guided imagery, visualization, and progressive muscle relaxation. These techniques are easy to learn and may help patients regain a sense of control and mastery, develop coping skills for side effects such as fatigue or nausea, and maintain or regain psychological well-being (Lewis and Sharp, 2011). In patients with severe health conditions, however, it should be considered that an intervention such as visualization of the body or body parts can also increase anxiety or even induce panic. Therefore, whether an intervention is appropriate or helpful for a patient should be carefully considered (Lewis and Sharp, 2011).

Mindfulness interventions

Mindfulness interventions, such as mindfulness-based stress reduction (MBSR), have been found useful in patients with life-threatening and advanced diseases (Payne, 2011). These treatments promote (a) self-regulating attention of immediate experience, allowing for greater awareness of mental events in the present moment; and (b) adoption of a curiosity, openness, and acceptance towards one's one experiences in the present moment (Payne, 2011). MBSR has been found to be effective in reducing a variety of unpleasant psychological states such as anxiety and depression, substance abuse, fatigue, insomnia, and fear of recurrence. It may further promote hope and quality of life.

Meaning-centred psychotherapy

Meaning-centred psychotherapy, which comprises specific approaches that promote a sense of meaning and purpose, have been receiving increasing attention in populations with life-threatening diseases. They may be realized as group therapy approaches or individual therapy, and are intended to reduce emotional and spiritual distress and promote hope, courage, and control; mobilize internal resources; and discuss future goals despite limited life expectancy (Breitbart et al., 2012; Nissim et al., 2012). Further aims include strengthening a patient's self-esteem and sense of dignity, to appreciate strengths and past achievements, reduce feelings of isolation, strengthen the relation with the partner and family members, and improve the communication with the professional health-care team (LeMay and Wilson, 2008).

Dignity-centred psychotherapy

Dignity and respect for the patient and his or her care needs represent an essential attitude in palliative care. A sense of dignity for patients encompasses feelings of respect and being worthy despite increasing physical and psychological symptoms; it is often mediated by both intrinsic and extrinsic factors, particularly social interactions (Chochinov and McKeen, 2011). Dignity-centred therapy is particularly designed for patients at the end of life (life expectancy at least 2 weeks). Based on the empirical dignity model by Chochinov et al. (2002), dignity therapy aims to reduce suffering and promote emotional and spiritual well-being, quality of life, and a sense of meaning and purpose by encouraging patients to reflect on their memorable life events (Chochinov and McKeen, 2011). The intervention includes a dignity therapy interview (e.g. 'What are your hopes and dreams for your loved ones?'), and one or two therapy sessions. The interview sessions are transcribed, edited, and read to the patient again and (after corrections) the patient is given the document to share it with family members, friends, or others (Chochinov and McKeen, 2011). Dignity therapy was found to be effective in increasing sense of dignity, improving quality of life and spiritual well-being, and enhancing appreciation through the family based on self-report end-of-life experiences (Chochinov et al., 2011).

'Espero alegre la salida y espero no volver jamás' ['I hope the exit is joyful and I hope never to return'] wrote the Mexican-American painter Frida Kahlo on the last page of her diary next to a drawing, the black angel of death (Le Clézio, 2002)—distressing, touching and honest words which express bitterness, resignation, and perhaps relief and hope for a peaceful death at the end of an extraordinary but painful life. The painter, whose health increasingly deteriorated after life-long physical and mental suffering, needed nursing care and intensive pain management, stands as an example for many terminally ill patients whose lives are changed severely by a progressing disease, which affects all areas of life, including their self-determination. Clinical psychological/psychotherapeutic care for patients with progressing disease and their caregivers is an important part of multidisciplinary palliative care and can promote the acceptance of the life lived, quality of life, hope, well-being, and dignity.

Acknowledgements

Text extracts reproduced from Pessin, H. et al., Clinical assessment of depression in terminally ill cancer patients: a practical guide, *Palliative and Supportive Care*, Volume 3, Number 4, pp. 319–24, Copyright © 2005, with permission from Cambridge University Press.

Online materials

Complete references for this chapter are available online at <http://www.oxfordmedicine.com>.

References

Akechi, T., Okamura, H., Nakano, T., *et al.* (2010). Gender differences in factors associated with suicidal ideation in major depression among cancer patients. *Psycho-Oncology*, 19(4), 384–389.

Akechi, T., Okamura, H., Nishiwaki, Y., and Uchitomi, Y. (2002). Predictive factors for suicidal ideation in patients with unresectable lung carcinoma. *Cancer*, 95(5), 1085–1093.

Akechi, T., Okuyama, T., Sugawara, Y., Nakano, T., Shima, Y., and Uchitomi, Y. (2004). Major depression, adjustment disorders, and post-traumatic stress disorder in terminally ill cancer patients: associated and predictive factors. *Journal of Clinical Oncology*, 22(10), 1957–1965.

American Psychiatric Association (2000). *Diagnostic and Statistical Manual of Mental Disorders* (4th ed., text rev.). Washington, DC: American Psychiatric Association.

Breitbart, W., Poppito, S., Rosenfeld, B., *et al.* (2012). Pilot randomized controlled trial of individual meaning-centered psychotherapy for patients with advanced cancer. *Journal of Clinical Oncology*, 30(12), 1304–1309.

Breitbart, W., Rosenfeld, B., Gibson, C., *et al.* (2010). Impact of treatment for depression on desire for hastened death in patients with advanced AIDS. *Psychosomatics*, 51(2), 98–105.

Chochinov, H.M., Hassard, T., McClement, S., *et al.* (2009). The landscape of distress in the terminally ill. *Journal of Pain and Symptom Management*, 38(5), 641–649.

Chochinov, H.M., Kristjanson, L.J., Breitbart, W., *et al.* (2011). Effect of dignity therapy on distress and end-of-life experience in terminally ill patients: a randomised controlled trial. *The Lancet Oncology*, 12(8), 753–762.

De Figueiredo, J.M. (1993). Depression and demoralization: phenomenologic differences and research perspectives. *Comprehensive Psychiatry*, 34(5), 308–311.

Delgado-Guay, M., Parsons, H.A., Li, Z., Palmer, J.L., and Bruera, E. (2009). Symptom distress in advanced cancer patients with anxiety and depression in the palliative care setting. *Supportive Care in Cancer*, 17(5), 573–579.

Hudson, P.L., Kristjanson, L.J., Ashby, M., *et al.* (2006). Desire for hastened death in patients with advanced disease and the evidence base of clinical guidelines: a systematic review. *Palliative Medicine*, 20(7), 693–701.

Irwin, S. and von Gunten, C. (2010). The role of palliative care in cancer care transitions. In J. Holland, W. Breitbart, P. Jacobsen, M. Lederberg, M. Loscalzo, and R. McCorkle (eds.) *Psycho-Oncology* (2nd ed.), pp. 277–283. New York: Oxford University Press.

Kissane, D.W., Clarke, D.M., and Street, A.F. (2001). Demoralization syndrome—a relevant psychiatric diagnosis for palliative care. *Journal of Palliative Care*, 17(1), 12–21.

LeMay, K. and Wilson, K.G. (2008). Treatment of existential distress in life threatening illness: a review of manualized interventions. *Clinical Psychology Review*, 28(3), 472–493.

Li, M., Hales, S., and Rodin, G. (2010). Adjustment disorders. In Holland, J., Breitbart, W., Jacobsen, P., Lederberg, M., Loscalzo, M., and McCorkle, R. (Eds.), *Psycho-Oncology* (2nd ed.)), 303–310. New York: Oxford University Press.

Lichtenthal, W., Prigerson, H., and Kissane, D.W. (2010). Bereavement: a special issue in oncology. In J. Holland, W. Breitbart, P. Jacobsen, M. Lederberg, M. Loscalzo, and R. McCorkle (eds.) *Psycho-Oncology* (2nd ed.), pp. 537–543. New York: Oxford University Press.

Lo, C., Zimmermann, C., Rydall, A., *et al.* (2010). Longitudinal study of depressive symptoms in patients with metastatic gastrointestinal and lung cancer. *Journal of Clinical Oncology*, 28(18), 3084–3089.

MacLeod, R. (2008). Setting the context: what do we mean by psychosocial care in palliative care? In M. Lloyd-Williams (ed.) *Psychosocial Issues in Palliative Care*, pp. 1–20. New York: Oxford University Press.

Massie, M.J. (2004). Prevalence of depression in patients with cancer. *Journal of the National Cancer Institute. Monographs*, 32, 57–71.

Miller, K. and Massie, M.J. (2010). Depressive disorders. In J. Holland, W. Breitbart, P. Jacobsen, M. Lederberg, M. Loscalzo, and R. McCorkle (eds.), *Psycho-Oncology* (2nd ed.), pp. 311–318. New York: Oxford University Press.

Miovic, M. and Block, S. (2007). Psychiatric disorders in advanced cancer. *Cancer*, 110(8), 1665–1676.

Mitchell, A.J., Chan, M., Bhatti, H., *et al.* (2011). Prevalence of depression, anxiety, and adjustment disorder in oncological, haematological, and palliative-care settings: a meta-analysis of 94 interview-based studies. *The Lancet Oncology*, 12(2), 160–174.

Passik, S.D., Dugan W., McDonald M.V., Rosenfeld B., Theobald, D.E., and Edgerton, S. (1998). Oncologists' recognition of depression in their patients with cancer. *Journal of Clinical Oncology*, 16(4), 1594–1600.

Passik, S.D., Lundberg, J.C., Rosenfeld, B., *et al.* (2000). Factor analysis of the Zung Self-Rating Depression Scale in a large ambulatory oncology sample. *Psychosomatics*, 41(2), 121–127.

Payne, D. (2011). Mindfulness interventions for cancer patients. In M. Watson and D.W. Kissane (eds.) *Handbook of Psychotherapy in Cancer Care*, pp. 39–47. Chichester: John Wiley & Sons.

Pessin, H., Evcimen, Y.A.A., and Breitbart, W. (2008). Diagnosis, assessment, and treatment of depression in palliative care. In M. Lloyd-Williams (ed.) *Psychosocial Issues in Palliative Care*, pp. 129–160. New York: Oxford University Press.

Pessin, H., Olden, M., Jacobson, C., and Kosinski, A. (2005). Clinical assessment of depression in terminally ill cancer patients: a practical guide. *Palliative & Supportive Care*, 3(4), 319–324.

Rasic, D.T., Belik, S.-L., Bolton, J.M., Chochinov, H.M., and Sareen, J. (2008). Cancer, mental disorders, suicidal ideation and attempts in a large community sample. *Psycho-Oncology*, 17(7), 660–667.

Rodin, G., Lo, C., Mikulincer, M., Donner, A., Gagliese, L., and Zimmermann, C. (2009). Pathways to distress: the multiple determinants of depression, hopelessness, and the desire for hastened death in metastatic cancer patients. *Social Science & Medicine*, 68(3), 562–569.

Rodin, G., Walsh, A., Zimmermann, C., *et al.* (2007). The contribution of attachment security and social support to depressive symptoms in patients with metastatic cancer. *Psycho-Oncology*, 16(12), 1080–1091.

Rodin, G. and Zimmermann, C. (2008). Psychoanalytic reflections on mortality: a reconsideration. *Journal of the American Academy of Psychoanalysis and Dynamic Psychiatry*, 36(1), 181–196.

Rosenstein, D.L. (2011). Depression and end-of-life care for patients with cancer. *Dialogues in Clinical Neuroscience*, 13(1), 101–108.

Roth, A.J. and Massie, M.J. (2007). Anxiety and its management in advanced cancer. *Current Opinion in Supportive and Palliative Care*, 1(1), 50–56.

Roy-Byrne, P.P., Davidson, K.W., Kessler, R.C., *et al.* (2008). Anxiety disorders and comorbid medical illness. *General Hospital Psychiatry*, 30(3), 208–225.

Sachs, E., Kolva, E., Pessin, H., Rosenfeld, B., and Breitbart, W. (2012). On sinking and swimming: the dialectic of hope, hopelessness, and acceptance in terminal cancer. *The American Journal of Hospice & Palliative Care*, 30(2), 121–127.

Solano, J.P., Gomes, B., and Higginson, I.J. (2006). A comparison of symptom prevalence in far advanced cancer, AIDS, heart disease, chronic obstructive pulmonary disease and renal disease. *Journal of Pain and Symptom Management*, 31(1), 58–69.

Steinhauser, K.E., Voils, C.I., Clipp, E.C., Bosworth, H.B., Christakis, N.A., and Tulsky, J.A. (2006). "Are you at peace?": one item to probe spiritual concerns at the end of life. *Archives of Internal Medicine*, 166(1), 101–105.

Tan, A., Zimmermann, C., and Rodin, G. (2005). Interpersonal processes in palliative care: an attachment perspective on the patient-clinician relationship. *Palliative Medicine*, 19(2), 143–150.

Temel, J.S., Greer, J.A., Admane, S., *et al.* (2011). Longitudinal perceptions of prognosis and goals of therapy in patients with metastatic non-small-cell lung cancer: results of a randomized study of early palliative care. *Journal of Clinical Oncology*, 29(17), 2319–2326.

Teunissen, S.C.C.M., de Graeff, A., Voest, E.E., and de Haes, J.C.J.M. (2007). Are anxiety and depressed mood related to physical symptom burden? A study in hospitalized advanced cancer patients. *Palliative Medicine*, 21(4), 341–346.

Vehling, S., Koch, U., Ladehoff, N., *et al.* (2012a). Prevalence of affective and anxiety disorders in cancer: systematic literature review and meta-analysis. *Psychotherapie, Psychosomatik, Medizinische Psychologie*, 62(7), 249–258.

Vehling, S., Lehmann, C., Oechsle, K., *et al.* (2012b). Is advanced cancer associated with demoralization and lower global meaning? The role of tumor stage and physical problems in explaining existential distress in cancer patients. *Psycho-Oncology*, 21(1), 54–63.

Wasteson, E., Brenne, E., Higginson, I.J., *et al.* (2009). Depression assessment and classification in palliative cancer patients: a systematic literature review. *Palliative Medicine*, 23(8), 739–753.

Watson, M. and Kissane, D.W. (eds.) (2011). *Handbook of Psychotherapy in Cancer Care*. Chichester: John Wiley & Sons.

Ziegler, L., Hill, K., Neilly, L., *et al.* (2011). Identifying psychological distress at key stages of the cancer illness trajectory: a systematic review of validated self-report measures. *Journal of Pain and Symptom Management*, 41(3), 619–636.

4.14

The contribution of the clinical pharmacist in palliative care

Margaret Gibbs

Introduction to the contribution of the clinical pharmacist in palliative care

Medicines are an essential part of symptom control so it is logical for the palliative care team to include a pharmacist, whose particular expertise is in the safe and effective use of medicines. In the United Kingdom, the National Institute for Health and Care Excellence (NICE) in its guidance *Improving Supportive and Palliative Care for Adults with Cancer* (NICE, 2004) states that the expertise of pharmacists helps to provide the appropriate level of specialist palliative care to patients. Similar documents from the United States, Europe, and Wales have reached the same conclusion (NHS Wales, 2005; National Consensus Project for Quality Palliative Care, 2013) and the UK Palliative Care Funding Review report (Hughes-Hallett et al., 2011) acknowledged the importance of the continued funding for pharmacy services. This chapter reviews the role of clinical pharmacists in palliative care and is based mainly on the situation in the United Kingdom with additional information from other parts of the world.

All hospices with inpatients require a pharmacy supply service but not all include a clinical pharmacist as part of the multidisciplinary team. Clinical pharmacy has been defined as 'that area of pharmacy concerned with the science and practice of rational medication use' (National Consensus Project for Quality Palliative Care, 2013). The traditional training and role of pharmacists started to change in the United Kingdom back in the 1970s following the Noel Hall report (Working Party on the Hospital Pharmaceutical Service, 1970), which encouraged hospital pharmacists to step outside the dispensary and become more involved clinically in the decision-making processes for prescribing. Forty years on, the pharmacy degree, in the United Kingdom, is now a 4-year Master's degree and clinical training occupies the largest part of the curriculum (Wilson et al., 2005). Most hospital pharmacists spend the majority of their time in clinical areas, communicating with other health-care professionals and patients and in 2006, the first cohort of pharmacists qualified as independent prescribers. Many of these now run clinics in hospital and in general practice, seeing their own case load of patients. Pharmacists in the United Kingdom emerge from their training with a different set of skills to those of previous generations and many choose to specialize in a particular therapeutic area within the hospital, primary care, community, or industrial environment. Traditional supply roles associated with the practice of pharmacy have

changed too, becoming more mechanized and delegated more to technical staff. These changes have, in many countries, enabled pharmacists to become more fully engaged members of clinical interdisciplinary teams.

Around 200 pharmacists work as part of palliative care teams in the United Kingdom. A 2002 study (Gilbar and Stefanuik, 2002) indicated that most Canadian teams included a pharmacist (59/69), whilst in Australia the proportion was lower at (42/76). The most recent survey in the United States, in 2012, showed that pharmacists carry out clinical, dispensing, and administrative work in hospice teams (Latuga et al., 2012). The job specification for a palliative care pharmacist can vary greatly with many spending only part of their working week within the speciality. Most UK hospices and hospital teams have a small number of beds, usually not enough to warrant the input of a full-time pharmacist. Community-based services may not have any regular clinical pharmacist input but are supported formally or informally by community or Clinical Commissioning Group (CCG) pharmacists. The 2002 study (Gilbar and Stefanuik, 2002) reported that most pharmacists worked fewer than 20 hours per week in the palliative care service and Canadian pharmacists were more involved clinically, while Australian pharmacists spent more time on administrative and supply functions. The American Society of Health-Systems Pharmacists' Statement outlines the role and responsibilities of a hospice and palliative care pharmacist (Box 4.14.1) and has broad similarities in practice with Canada, Australia, and the United Kingdom (Arter and Berry, 1993; American Society of Health-System Pharmacists, 2002; Gilbar and Stefanuik, 2002).

Several studies have evaluated the effectiveness of the interventions and recommendations of clinical pharmacists working in palliative care and an American study in 2011 (Lee and McPherson, 2006; Wilson et al., 2011) showed that almost 90% of the pharmacists' recommendations were accepted and 80% resulted in the desired clinical outcome.

Clinical pharmacy in the rest of Europe is in an earlier stage of development but a number of European pharmacists are establishing roles in palliative care teams. A palliative care team in Sweden has recently included pharmacists in the team with an improvement seen in stock management, logistics, and resolving pharmaceutical issues (Norrstrom et al., 2010). The value of pharmaceutical input in Japanese and Australian home-care services has been extensively evaluated. In one study from Japan, the value of the input from community pharmacists was marred in some

---

Box 4.14.1 The pharmacist's responsibilities

1. Assessing the appropriateness of medication orders and ensuring the timely provision of effective medications for symptom control.

2. Counselling and educating the hospice team about medication therapy.

3. Ensuring that patients and caregivers understand and follow the directions provided with medications.

4. Providing efficient mechanisms for extemporaneous compounding of non-standard dosage forms.

5. Addressing financial concerns.

6. Ensuring safe and legal disposal of all medications after death.

7. Establishing and maintaining effective communication with regulatory and licensing agencies.

8. Assessing the appropriateness of medication orders and ensuring the timely provision of effective medications for symptom control.

9. Counselling and educating the hospice team about medication therapy.

10. Ensuring that patients and caregivers understand and follow the directions provided with medications.

11. Providing efficient mechanisms for extemporaneous compounding of non-standard dosage forms.

12. Addressing financial concerns.

13. Ensuring safe and legal disposal of all medications after death.

14. Establishing and maintaining effective communication with regulatory and licensing agencies.

Originally published in The American Society of Healthcare Pharmacists (AHSP) Statement on the Pharmacist's Role in Hospice and Palliative, *American Journal of Health-System Pharmacy*, Volume 59, Number 18, pp. 1770–1773, Copyright ©2002, American Society of Health-System Pharmacists, Inc. All rights reserved. Reprinted with permission. (R1408).

---

respect by the financial burden of providing this additional service, although this and another studies, including one carried out over 13 years, showed that pharmacy input was valued by patients (Hussainy et al., 2011; Kato et al., 2011).

The fundamentals of good pharmaceutical care

Pharmaceutical care has been defined as 'the responsible provision of drug therapy for the purpose of achieving defined outcomes that improve the patient's quality of life' (Hepler and Strand, 1990). When pharmacists review or advise on drug regimens, the patient is always at the focus. A traditional mantra for pharmacists is the provision of 'the right drug to the right patient at the right time'. Barber (1995) suggests that individual prescriptions are monitored to maximize effectiveness, minimize risks and costs, and

respect the patient's choices. This patient-centred approach is, of course, fundamental in palliative care so the clinical pharmacist's attention to detail on medication complements all other aspects of care. In order to provide the best care, the clinical pharmacist ensures that the following are provided:

◆ A reliable supply function and regular monitoring of prescribing, including economic reviews

◆ An appropriate medicines management system

◆ Advice and guidance on safe use of drugs of particular relevance to palliative care, for example, syringe driver compatibility

◆ The provision and dissemination of drug-related information both clinical and legislative, for example, involving controlled drugs (CDs).

The following sections will look at these areas in more detail and at how they can be executed most effectively in palliative care.

Supply and monitoring of medication

In the United Kingdom since 1995, hospices with inpatient units have been provided with a budget for their drugs and pharmaceutical services by the commissioners of health services in each locality. Changes are afoot in primary care but the Palliative Care Funding Review (Hughes-Hallett et al., 2011) recommended that current arrangements continue. A contract to provide pharmaceutical services may be set up with a local hospital pharmacy, a community pharmacy, or directly with a wholesaler for the supply function. If a contract is established with a hospital pharmacy, it is normally possible for the hospice to benefit from the advantageous contract prices for the drugs being used in an acute trust. The service should include the functions shown in Box 4.14.2.

An effective supply function is an essential part of the pharmaceutical service and this has, in most environments, become an almost mechanical process with 'original pack' dispensing of blister-packaged tablets or small volumes of liquid preparations. In the United Kingdom, once a pharmacist has screened a prescription for its clinical appropriateness the dispensing can be completed by suitably qualified pharmacy technicians and, in a few larger hospitals, by robotic systems. This means that a clinical pharmacist does not need to be involved directly with the supplies of drugs but needs to set up systems, be confident that they are working, and be made aware of any problems.

Economic issues

The economical use of drugs is important in all health-care settings but it is especially important in hospices, as most are registered charities, in many countries. The majority of drugs used for symptom management are older, relatively inexpensive generic drugs but there are some notable exceptions, such as the bisphosphonates and somatostatin analogues. In a small unit it is very easy for the symptom management for one or two patients who require expensive treatment to make a huge impact on the monthly budget figures. Regular pharmacy meetings to review prescribing patterns can highlight areas of concern, then audit and written guidelines can be constructive tools to ensure the appropriate use of high-cost drugs. The economic benefits of pharmacist involvement have been reported in Japan and Sweden (Lee and McPherson, 2006; Norrstrom et al., 2010).

Box 4.14.2 Functions of a pharmaceutical service to a hospice inpatient unit

Essential

1. A reliable and responsive delivery system with provision for a back-up to provide urgently needed medicines or pharmacist advice out of opening hours.

2. Regular visits from a clinical pharmacist for clinical checking of prescriptions and provision of medicines information.

3. Provision of stock drugs using a regular top-up system, ideally carried out by pharmacy technicians including a regular monitoring system for expiry checks of medicines.

4. Provision of individual patient supplies for the duration of inpatient stay and on discharge.

5. Provision of regular supply of controlled drugs using standard operating procedures.

6. A system for reviewing and updating agreed stock supply.

7. An effective communication system for ordering, managing queries, and supplying information where necessary when the pharmacist is not present.

Desirable

8. Inclusion of pharmacist on clinical governance, risk management, and drug and therapeutics committees within the hospice.

9. Availability of pharmacist to run teaching sessions for hospice staff.

Establishing an agreed stock list for an inpatient unit may evolve into compiling a core formulary. This has been shown to be an effective strategy for reducing cost and improving patient outcomes in one hospice in Kentucky, United States (Snapp et al., 2002). In another study from the United States, it was shown that newer, more expensive pharmacotherapy options were not necessarily more effective than traditional agents, if doses were monitored and titrated by clinical pharmacists (Weschules et al., 2006).

Ideally, any formulary should be evidence based, but the evidence for much of the drug therapy used in palliative care is of a lower level than for other therapeutic areas, at least partly because of the difficulties and perceived difficulties in carrying out randomized controlled trials in terminally ill patients (Steinhauser et al., 2006).

Definition of evidence-based practice

The judicious use of the best available evidence, moderated by patient circumstances and preferences to guide our practice to improve the quality of clinical judgements and facilitate effective health care.

Reproduced from Sackett DL et al., Evidence-based medicine: what it is and what it isn't, *British Medical Journal*, Volume 312, Issue 7023, pp. 71–2, Copyright © 1996 with permission from BMJ Publishing Group Ltd.

Many sets of therapeutic guidelines now exist in the United Kingdom and on the whole, the list of drugs used for symptom control is broadly consistent. Guidance and core formularies have also been developed by palliative and supportive care networks, which were established as a model of integrated service provision alongside cancer networks, in response to *The NHS Cancer Plan* to improve coordination of cancer and palliative care (Department of Health, 2000b). Clinical pharmacists have been involved in many of the network subgroups, coordinating drug treatment and availability. In the United States, the introduction of standardized, evidence-based medication use guidelines is encouraged (Weschules, 2005).

As well as the choice of drugs, the clinical pharmacist can advise on the most appropriate formulation for individual patients. With some exceptions (such as strong opioids and drugs where the avoidance of peak effects in drug blood concentrations may lead to fewer side effects), prescribers are now encouraged to avoid the use of slow-release preparations on economic grounds. In palliative care, our patients' tablet 'burden' can often be a real problem and so use of a more expensive once- or twice-daily preparation, such as slow-release metoclopramide, may be justified.

Managing a drug regimen for a patient who has swallowing difficulties or is being tube fed has pharmaceutical implications. Crushing tablets is to be discouraged, as changing the form of a dose not only takes it outside the terms of its licence, but can also be hazardous as it may change its pharmacokinetics—especially dangerous with a slow-release formulation. Liquid or soluble tablets can be very expensive, so alternative drugs may need to be substituted. The decision to substitute any drug in a situation of stable symptom control has to be considered carefully.

The pharmacist may also alert colleagues to the sensitive issue of discontinuing medication. Effectiveness and tolerability of each medication will be reviewed regularly but decisions on whether a patient nearing the end of life needs to continue with such medication as statins or oral hormonal treatments normally need to be negotiated with the patient and possibly their carers. The goals of care and treatment should be considered in relation to prognosis and the patient's ability to manage their medicines. Initiating drugs with a long onset of action, such as the older antidepressants may not be appropriate if the time to benefit may exceed the patient's life expectancy. These are emotive issues but unfortunately their cost implications can be considerable (Holmes et al., 2006). Moreover, the burden of any side effects at initiation, will have been for no gain.

It is almost inevitable that we have a degree of wastage when drugs are dispensed for patients at the end of their life and although it is a difficult moral issue to destroy what seem to be perfectly sound drugs, we have a statutory responsibility not to re-supply any drugs that have been dispensed to a particular patient to others as we are unable to guarantee their integrity. The only practical way to counter this is to minimize waste by ensuring that appropriate quantities are ordered.

Nurses need also to be aware of the relative costs of dressings and skin and mouth-care preparations. Wound care and mouth care are often challenging areas of palliative care and there is a huge variety of products on the market. With pharmacist input, guidance or decision-making tools can encourage nurses to use the most appropriate and economical choices.

Palliative care in the community

The majority of dying people in the United Kingdom would prefer to die in their own home, although currently only about 20% do so and many are admitted to hospices and more to hospitals in the last days of life (National Council for Palliative Care, 2010). This is a statistic that has rightly occupied a great deal of attention in recent years and strategies are being introduced to improve this. Good end-of-life care at home requires the input of a team of health-care professionals and the role of the pharmacist is expanding. The traditional medicine supply role is of paramount importance but more direct patient care is part of the pharmacist's role in some community teams in the United Kingdom and Australia. Pharmacists are members of the team visiting patients at home, where they can optimize medicines management and reduce medication-related problems (Hussainy et al., 2011). The opportunity to practise as an independent prescriber is a newer role in the United Kingdom and this can speed up access to medicine supply.

Although routine symptom control medicines are prescribed and supplied in the community, the provision of drugs for patients who deteriorate unexpectedly has always been complicated by legislative limits on the ability to hold 'stock' injectable drugs outside pharmacies and hospitals. In addition, many doctors no longer carry their own supply of opioids for security reasons. Medical and nursing cover varies from area to area but the simple lack of availability of the required drugs has led too often to an inappropriate hospital admission, and significant distress, especially during the out-of-hours (OOH) period, which is almost 70% of the week. OOH care in England and Wales underwent a substantial National Health Service (NHS) review in 2000 (Department of Health, 2000a) and other reviews of practice, such as those initiated by Macmillan Cancer Care resulting in the Gold Standards Framework (National Gold Standards Framework (GSF) Centre in End of Life Care, n.d.), have contributed to subsequent re-organization in recent years.

Systems for stocking small quantities of injectable drugs in designated community pharmacies have been set up in various localities. Whilst these schemes are an invaluable back-up, they have not always been a success. This may be because they are not always well publicized to the relevant professionals but, more importantly, there is an inevitable delay in getting the pharmacist and prescription to the pharmacy and back to the patient's house. Underuse of pharmacy schemes leads to expiry of stock. The system should be used in conjunction with immediate access to the necessary drugs by the on-call medical service. Commissioners are responsible for ensuring that there is a safe system in place for providing all the drugs on the national OOH formulary to providers of OOH medical care. A list of essential and desirable drugs is shown in Box 4.14.3. The details of the OOH arrangements need to be agreed locally to suit the geography and population. They should encompass the NICE guidance for improving supportive and palliative care (NICE, 2004), be supported by improved communications, facilitated by introducing the Gold Standards Framework after the publication of *Caring for the Dying at Home* (Thomas, 2003) for community care of the dying, and take into account the Preferred Place of Care (Cohen Fineberg and O'Connor, 2011) initiative.

Clinical pharmacists have been instrumental in establishing so-called just in case schemes where general practitioners (GPs) prescribe a small quantity of injectable drugs for individual patients identified as nearing the end of their life. These drugs can be kept safely in the patient's home in case of a sudden deterioration. In a pilot scheme in Hertfordshire, United Kingdom (Amass

---

Box 4.14.3 Emergency drugs for end-of-life symptom management

Essential (and now on the NHS OOH core formulary)

Strong opioid in injectable form—normally diamorphine or morphine.

Midazolam for sedation.

Cyclizine, haloperidol, levomepromazine for nausea and vomiting.

Glycopyrronium or *hyoscine* for retained secretions.

Desirable

Lorazepam tablets for anxiety and breathlessness.

Oral morphine liquid.

---

and Allen, 2005) over 6 months in 2004, 23 'just in case' boxes were issued, enabling 16 patients to have their symptoms managed and to die at home, which was their expressed preference. Each pack of drugs cost only £10 and the potential saving on an admission to hospital or hospice. Clearly, however, the satisfaction for the patient and their family resulting from good end-of-life care is immeasurable.

Medicines management

The UK Audit Commission introduced the concept of medicines management within its report *A Spoonful of Sugar* in 2001 (Audit Commission, 2001). It aimed to optimize the use of medicines in NHS hospitals, to improve the quality of patient care and rationalize expenditure. Although most hospices are independent of the NHS, the national strategies are normally adopted for the sake of congruity.

Definition of medicines management

Medicines management in hospitals encompasses the entire way that medicines are selected, procured, delivered, prescribed, administered and reviewed to optimize the contribution that medicines make to producing informed and desired outcomes of patient care.

Reproduced with permission from The Audit Commission, *A Spoonful of Sugar: Medicines Management in NHS Hospitals*, Audit Commission Publications, Wetherby, UK, Copyright © 2001, available from http://archive.audit-commission.gov.uk/auditcommission/sitecollectiondocuments/AuditCommissionReports/NationalStudies/nrspoonfulsugar.pdf.

Patient-centred medicines management

When patients have a planned admission to an inpatient unit in the United Kingdom, they are encouraged to bring their current medicines in with them. This has several benefits; it is essential to establish a drug 'history', particularly if symptoms are out of control. It can also clarify whether the patient is actually taking the regimen as prescribed and note what has been used in the past and what the outcomes were. Patients may have a number of symptoms and coexistent pathologies, making it common for them to be taking a large number of medicines, so this is often a time-consuming job involving rummaging through bags full of dispensed medicines. Although the admitting doctor or specialist nurse will normally do this as part of any admissions process, pilot studies have shown that a pharmacy-led medicines review process uncovers issues and is highly acceptable to the patient. Unfortunately, time limitations have not enabled these to become routine.

Bringing in their existing medication also ensures that patients have an ongoing supply, as most units will not have an exhaustive range of stock drugs. It also prevents duplication, reduces waste, and, ultimately, saves money. Not all patients' own drugs can be used so they must be screened for suitability using a checklist, ensuring they are suitably packed, identifiable, not time expired, and labelled correctly for the patient. This also forms part of an audit trail for medicines.

One of the main aims of the NHS medicines management programme is to encourage patients to keep charge of their medicines in a bedside locker and to continue to take them independently. Clearly not all patients admitted to a hospice are suited to self-administration, but those whose admission is for respite or symptom control should be encouraged to do so with multidisciplinary team agreement. Patients need to understand their regimen and manage practical issues such as their ability to open containers, read labels, and appreciate their responsibility for security of their medicines. An agreed assessment process needs to be part of the hospice medicines policy. Almost all patients who are given the chance to self-administer prefer it, because it gives them more control and promotes confidence in managing what may be a complex regimen (Ausburn, 1981). This confidence can be a major contribution to a successful discharge, as many admissions and re-admissions arise because of problems with managing medication. We know that low adherence to instructions with medication affects outcome so patients must be given sufficient information to make an informed choice on the benefits and risks of a therapeutic 'alliance' (Royal Pharmaceutical Society of Great Britain, 1997). Patient counselling by pharmacists promotes understanding of the purpose of each medicine and awareness of potential adverse effects (Al-Rashed et al., 2000). It can also provide an opportunity to discuss practical issues such as the provision of medicines in concordance aids ('dosette boxes'), which may be continued on discharge. Most GP surgeries and pharmacies have a delivery system for prescriptions from surgery to pharmacy and then on to the patient at home.

Community pharmacists establish relationships with their regular patients and their families and have a wider role to play than simply drug supply. In some countries, community pharmacists are responsible for preparing pre-filled syringes for syringe drivers. In the United Kingdom, groups of community pharmacists have undergone additional training in order to support palliative care patients, by setting up prescription monitoring and supply services.

Another important role for palliative care pharmacists is to provide 'seamless' pharmaceutical care for patients as they move from one care setting to another (Scally and Donaldson, 1998). A common NHS electronic patient record system has not been successful, so we rely on a number of different methods of transmitting medication information, some of which are less reliable than others. A medication list will normally be drawn up on discharge and sent to the GP or other doctor looking after a patient, but their community pharmacist can sometimes be left out of the loop and both may be faced with an urgent prescription for an unusual drug unless prior explanation has been provided. Where medicines

---

> **Box 4.14.4** Scenario 1
>
> Susan is 47 years old and has breast cancer with brain and bone involvement. Pain has been the main problem for the past few months but now her increasing weakness is the most distressing part of her daily life. Her analgesic regimen has become very complicated by her being seen by a number of practitioners and more medications being added concurrently without detailed review. On admission to our service she was taking oxycodone modified release and immediate release, regular paracetamol, gabapentin, amitriptyline, diazepam, lidocaine plasters, and using fast-onset fentanyl for incident pain. She was starting to find it too difficult to swallow the oral medications and unsure any more about what was actually helping her pain. We decided to simplify the regimen by stopping the amitriptyline and reducing the diazepam. We changed her gabapentin to pregabalin, which can be taken twice daily instead of three times and advised that she could have the capsules opened and swallow the contents with a little liquid. After a few days, she agreed to a syringe driver so we were able to convert the doses and administer her opioid and a small dose of benzodiazepine via the subcutaneous route. She was able to go home for a few days before she died.

management systems exist, patients' discharge medication will often be dispensed well before the expected discharge. This can present last-minute problems if doses or drugs have been changed in the interim. The importance of timely prescribing and supply to patients, for whom time is limited, needs to be communicated to all health-care professionals providing services. Pharmacists have a major educational role in fulfilling this particular objective (see Box 4.14.4: scenario 1).

Advice and guidance on drugs in palliative care

The relatively new concept of clinical governance was introduced into the NHS with the aim of increasing accountability and quality of care. In common with many other NHS initiatives it has been extended into the voluntary sector and provides a framework for decisions made when considering new treatment options.

Definition of clinical governance

A framework through which [NHS] organizations are accountable for continually improving the quality of their services and safeguarding high standards of care by creating an environment in which excellence in clinical care will flourish.

Reproduced from G. Scally and L.J. Donaldson, Clinical governance and the drive for quality improvement in the new NHS in England, *British Medical Journal*, Volume 317, Issue 7150, Copyright © 1998 with permission from BMJ Publishing Group Ltd.

Pharmacists have a major role in clinical governance issues involving medicines, with many sitting on their hospice Medicines Management or Drug and Therapeutics Groups. The terms of reference of these groups may vary but usually include the review of drugs coming on to the market or drugs being suggested elsewhere for symptom control as well as ensuring the correct application of new drug-related guidance or legislation.

Use of drugs outside their licence

Palliative care practice often involves using drugs outside the terms of their product licence. In order for any new drug to reach the market, the manufacturer must be able to prove that it is a safe and effective treatment. Once this has been proved in a drug development programme, it will be granted a licence for the conditions for which it has been tested. Licensing is both a commercial and medico-legal issue but a doctor may prescribe, a pharmacist may dispense, and a nurse may administer drugs outside the terms of their licence, as long as the drug was being used in accordance with a practice accepted at the time by a responsible body of medical opinion. There is encouragement from UK authorities to discuss the use of medicines outside licence with our patients and although we aim to involve patients in all prescribing decisions, terminology such as 'outside the terms of a drug's licence' may sound more worrying than it need be. Most of the drugs used in this way are long established with well-documented safety and adverse effect profiles, so the main issue is ensuring that there is sufficient evidence for this use, whilst the main issue for patients is to avoid any potential confusion arising from information they may read in the patient information leaflet (PIL), which must be supplied with their dispensed medicines. Hospice pharmacists have written PILs for their own establishment and are usually happy for such information sheets to be used by others. At a small hospice user group this was not an issue of great concern, with patients saying they trusted the health-care professionals to do what they could for them (User Forum, 2012).

Pharmacists regularly advise nurses on the correct methods of administration of drugs. With tube-fed patients or other patients who may find swallowing difficult, it is common practice to consider crushing a tablet or opening a capsule and sprinkling the resultant powder on food or mixing it with a drink. Any of these alterations to the original product renders it outside its licence. Pharmacists have written a number of reference sources to offer advice about the best method of administration of the drug in these circumstances. This may involve changing the drug to an alternative where a licensed liquid or soluble form is available. The use of medicines without any licence is a slightly different issue. It is unlikely that a palliative care unit would wish to use an unlicensed *drug* but we often wish to mix or compound known drugs in unlicensed *formulations* to suit individual patients. Some examples of this are the use of alfentanil injection made into a cutaneous solution that can be sprayed onto the nasal or buccal mucosa and the addition of lignocaine (lidocaine) to a thermoversible gel for the management of painful wounds. Both products are made in regional hospital pharmacies in the United Kingdom. Although US pharmacists are permitted to compound individual preparations for patients, this practice has become very limited in the United Kingdom and is now restricted to a few commercial 'specials' manufacturers and regional, licensed hospital pharmacy manufacturing units. Information on unlicensed medicines is limited, as products have not been subjected to the same regulatory processes as licensed medicines so as much evidence as possible is required that such products are being appropriately and with accountability. Prescribers and pharmacists must both be involved in the decision-making process, using a committee or the clinical governance team to approve and document the rationale for using

unlicensed products. Once sufficient experience has been gained in their use, specialists may start suggesting to generalists that these products be used. The production of referenced information leaflets is important in supporting this. The Brompton Hospitals and some hospices have produced their own leaflets either covering this subject in general or for specific drugs such as the use of haloperidol to treat nausea and vomiting.

Subcutaneous administration of drugs

The use of the subcutaneous route is outside the license for the majority of drugs used in symptom management. The major area of potential problems is where drugs are mixed together in the same syringe. Although the drugs used are familiar and well established, it is not necessarily in a company's financial interests to investigate the compatibility of its injections with those of others. Additionally, many of the drugs we use have lost their patent and are made by generic manufacturers who would be even less inclined to carry out such studies. Pharmacists have been largely responsible for gathering data on the mixing of drugs in syringes for subcutaneous infusions (Dickman and Schneider, 2011). Our knowledge in this area comes from a combination of clinical observation and laboratory tests and ongoing data collection continues to add to this (Palliativedrugs.com, 2014).

Complementary medicines

The use of complementary medicines needs to be considered as a safety issue. Understandably, many patients are concerned about the safety of conventional medicines but there is a perception, fuelled by marketing that if a product is herbal or marketed as 'natural', then it may be safer. There are countless products available

Box 4.14.5 Scenario 2

John is a 68-year-old ex-drug-user who has been on a methadone programme for 8 years. He has developed lung cancer with liver and bone secondaries and is finding it difficult to manage at home alone. He is very vague about his pain relief regimen and called into the hospice overnight to say he was in terrible pain and had just opened the bottle and drunk the whole 100 mL of his oral morphine solution (200 mg) with no effect—analgesic or otherwise. At that time he was prescribed modified-release morphine 100 mg twice daily with 40 mg stats. There is a discrepancy between him, his family doctor, and the drugs team with his reported daily methadone dose and an apparent duplication of prescribing. He has now been admitted to the hospice for symptom control of his pain and nausea. His son asked to speak to the doctor privately as he wants us to know that his dad has been buying street drugs too but feels he would have been unable to do this in the past week or two. We were able to explain to John that unless we were quite clear about what he was taking it would be much more difficult to judge what was helping his pain. He admitted to being very frightened by his pain. I contacted the drugs team to clarify his methadone dose and we decided to leave that as it was and manage his pain separately. After some days with us, he was converted to a fentanyl patch and high strength immediate-release morphine tablets which were easier to monitor when he went home. He managed to return home and although his life continued to be quite chaotic, once home, he reported feeling much better.

supported by testimonials and claims that they work wonders—from improving digestion to curing cancer. When taking a drug history, pharmacists will also make specific enquiries, as patients may not mention complementary therapies because they are not regarded as 'drugs'. The quality of information on complementary medicines is in general not required to be of the same standard as that of conventional medicines, as they are not subject to the same legal controls. This makes it difficult to unpick the evidence. Clinical pharmacists can review the information available critically and offer guidance on potential beneficial and adverse effects of complementary medicines, as well as advising on possible contraindications and drug interactions. Research and data collection on herbal medicines and supplements is enabling us to offer better guidance and the Medicines and Healthcare Regulatory Authority regularly releases bulletins warning of serious safety issues with these medicines. In offering guidance on these products, pharmacists need to carefully word their findings in order to indicate the level of evidence for their statements and to take into account the patient's individual choice to continue with such products.

Practical and pragmatic guidance from the pharmacist is also required for some drug–food interactions that may impact on patients. For example, the ingestion of excessive amounts of vitamin K-containing green vegetables can affect coagulation, but a normal portion of such vegetables on a regular basis presents very low risk. Similarly, the presence of a drinks trolley on hospice wards and day centres prompts pharmacists to alert staff involved in 'administration' to the possible interaction between alcohol and drugs.

Incidents and errors with drugs

Incidents involving drugs account for about 10% of all adverse events reported in NHS hospitals, although over 80% result in no apparent patient harm (National Reporting and Learning Service, 2009). These figures are not necessarily applicable to hospices but the need to review and take appropriate action following adverse drug events is no less important. The ethos of drug error reporting has changed in recent years with a 'no blame' reporting system instigated in many hospitals and the involvement of staff in reporting 'near misses'. The focus is now on *systems* rather than individuals and we are asked to review our practice by the NHS Commissioning Board Special Health Authority in the United Kingdom, which disseminates guidance and safety notices for areas of risk such as the alert on potential for confusion between strengths of opioids (unpublished data). Pharmacists are able to advise on systems for reporting errors and improving safety and are essential members of the group within a hospice that reviews incidents. Writing additional safety steps into policies and sending round awareness bulletins have had positive results in that incidents have not recurred (Anonymous, 2006). Sharing information with other hospice pharmacists has also highlighted common areas for concern and constructive changes, such as persuading a company to improve its packaging, have been achieved.

Provision and dissemination of information

Clinical pharmacy training includes time spent in medicines information centres where pharmacists learn to source and appraise information and research critically to produce unbiased drug reviews. As palliative care expands teams need to keep being updated on drug developments in therapeutic areas other than cancer. Pharmacists can tap into wide resources from regional medicines information services to share updates and reviews

The widespread use of CDs requires particular attention to legislation and regulations. Patients need to be enabled to make choices about their preferred place of care and also to be able to change their minds at short notice. To facilitate this, they need to be able to access their required medicines without delay, yet within the law.

Networking

Like many specialists, most palliative care pharmacists work alone so there is value in communicating with fellow pharmacists for advice and support. Regional and national groups for palliative care pharmacists exist in the United States, Canada, and the United Kingdom, with varying levels of activity. The Scottish Palliative Care Pharmacists Association has created a benchmarking tool for staffing levels of pharmacists, coordinates research, produces guidance, and has a strategic role within the Scottish Health Service. As most work some distance from colleagues, the Internet has become invaluable as a means of sharing information. Multidisciplinary web-based discussion groups have been set up with pharmacists being the third largest professional group participating (after doctors and nurses), and a UK palliative care pharmacists network has now been formed.

Conclusions

The role of a clinical pharmacist in a palliative care team is an especially rewarding and fulfilling one as it presents so many opportunities to utilize specific skills. One needs broad outlook, a flexible and pragmatic approach, and willingness to contribute to judgements based on what is best for any given patient, without always having the highest level of evidence to support some decisions. As palliative care opens up to more patients with non-malignant, life-limiting diseases, there is a need to be aware of a wider range of drug regimens and their implications and to educate as many colleagues as possible to the safe and effective use of drugs in patient-centred palliative care. It is difficult to imagine working in a more privileged environment than one where teams are dedicated to providing the best possible end-of-life care.

Online materials

Additional online materials and complete references for this chapter are available online at <http://www.oxfordmedicine.com>.

References

American Society of Health-System Pharmacists (2002). AHSP statement on the pharmacist's role in hospice and palliative care. *American Journal of Health-System Pharmacy*, 59(18), 1770–1773.

Dickman, A. and Schneider, J. (2011). *The Syringe Driver: Continuous Subcutaneous Infusions in Palliative Care*. Oxford: Oxford University Press.

Hussainy, S., Box, M., and Scholes, S. (2011). Piloting the role of a pharmacist in a community palliative care multidisciplinary team: an Australian experience. *BMC Palliative Care*, 10, 16.

Kato, T. (2011). The role of home palliative care by health insurance pharmacy. *Japanese Journal of Cancer and Chemotherapy* 38(Suppl.)1, 56–58.

Lee, J. and McPherson, M. (2006). Outcomes of recommendations by hospice pharmacists. *American Journal of Health-System Pharmacy*, 63, 2235–2239.

Norrstrom, B., Cannerfelt, I.B., Frid, H., Roos, K., and Ramström, H. (2010). Introduction of pharmaceutical expertise in a palliative care team in Sweden. *Pharmacy World & Science*, 32(6) 829–834.

Palliativedrugs.com (2014). *Which Syringe Driver Do You Use?* [Survey] [Online] Available at: <http://www.palliativedrugs.com/download/140310_syringedriversurvey_v03_sc_final.pdf>.

Wilson, S., Wahler, R., Brown, J., Doloresco, F., and Monte, S.V. (2011). Impact of pharmacist intervention on clinical outcomes in the palliative care setting. *American Journal of Hospice & Palliative Care*, 28(5), 316–20.

Medical rehabilitation and the palliative care patient

Deborah Julie Franklin and Andrea L. Cheville

Introduction to medical rehabilitation and the palliative care patient

Access to palliative care earlier in patients' disease trajectory has made the preservation of functional mobility and independence increasingly pertinent. This chapter focuses on the role that rehabilitation and rehabilitation medicine interventions play in comprehensive palliative treatment plans. Although this chapter concentrates on practices prevalent in the United States and United Kingdom, the issues it addresses are of global relevance.

Both disciplines place importance on the biopsychosocial model of patient care and employ interdisciplinary teams to develop care plans that respond not just to the physiological but also the psychological and social needs of patients and their caregivers. Both rehabilitation medicine and palliative medicine seek multidimensional outcomes that are not related specifically to disease state, such as the Functional Independence Measure (FIM) or quality of life (QOL) parameters.

Rehabilitation strategies contribute to palliative care by (a) maintaining and, if possible, promoting functional independence during a period of expected systemic decline and (b) providing strategies to prevent or slow deleterious complications such as generalized deconditioning, skin breakdown, and contractures.

The judicious selection of durable medical equipment (DME) is best done in collaboration with rehabilitation specialists who can combine extensive knowledge of available componentry with an understanding of the salient medical and prognostic characteristics of a given patient. Physiatrists, physiotherapists (PTs), and occupational therapists (OTs) will also often work closely with DME suppliers to select optimal adaptive equipment for patients developing progressive dependence at home. These can include automatic lifts, bathing, and toileting aides, and wheelchairs as well as smaller items that facilitate autonomy with self-care (e.g. reachers, buttonhole assists, and sock donners).

Delivery of rehabilitation services in palliative care

Many regional and international rehabilitation organizations have special interest groups that focus on palliative care populations. Among physicians, these include oncological rehabilitation groups, geriatric-focused groups, and pain management specialists. Many of these groups are now producing evidence-based care guidelines for treating patients with advanced disease (Sliwa and Marciniak, 1998) or participating in clinical trials assessing the efficacy of their techniques in this population (Dimeo et al., 1998).

Physical medicine and rehabilitation (PM&R), also called physiatry or rehabilitation medicine is the primary medical specialty responsible for the provision of rehabilitation services in the United States. The level of training and competency-based certification required for the delivery of rehabilitation team services varies between countries. In the United States, PTs complete a 2-year master's level degree programme or, more commonly in recent years, a 3-year professional doctorate but can delegate some of their active treatment to physiotherapy assistants or restorative aides.

PTs are asked to attend to issues of strength, endurance, and mobility requiring specialized training. This includes wheelchair skills and other adaptive mobility as well as gait training on increasingly challenging surfaces for ambulatory patients. Programmes should be tailored to reflect the environmental challenges of the home, such as stairs to enter, size of home, location of bed, and bathroom modifications. Transfers to car, van, or adapted vehicle should be reviewed. For patients with inexorably progressive disability, purchase or lease of a vehicle with full wheelchair carrying capacity may be appropriate but should be weighed against cost and limited prognoses. Easy transportation helps patients maintain an involvement in a wider variety of family and community activities.

OTs focus on essential functional activities such as dressing, bathing, toileting, and self-feeding. Many use validated cognitive assessment tools regularly, such as the Montreal Cognitive Assessment (MoCA[R]), a modified Token Test, the Wisconsin Card Sorting Test, or parts of the Wechsler Adult Intelligence Scale, during their initial patient assessment and, if indicated, at subsequent times (Zorowitz and Adamovich, 2000). Earlier in gradually progressing diseases, the input of quantitative neuropsychologists may be used by patients who want to learn strategies for limiting the effect of emerging cognitive deficits. In other situations, neuropsychologists may be asked to help differentiate the memory and attention deficits stemming from untreated depression or anxiety, from symptoms of progressive dementia, or other reversible and irreversible causes of cognitive decline. This information may help to initiate pharmacological management of anxiety, attentional, and arousal deficits as well as mood disorders. Neuropsychometric data may be needed to persuade patients to hand over financial or legal affairs to designated executors, or conversely, to persuade family members that the patient is still able to manage for themselves.

Supportive psychotherapists and counsellors are also core members of all but the sparsest rehabilitation teams. Rehabilitation psychologists have extensive experience in discussing loss of function, acceptance of disability, and illness experience with patients but may need to adjust to the impact of treating terminally ill and actively dying patients.

Social workers and case managers promote access to care by facilitating communication among patients, clinicians, and, where appropriate, funders. They often assist families in applying for financial support from charities to pay for home-care equipment needs or transportation to and from therapy centres.

Although there is an impressive overlap between members and goals of the palliative care and general rehabilitation teams, certain distinctions need to be appreciated when requesting rehabilitation specialists to treat palliative care patients. Most significantly, rehabilitation has traditionally been associated with the restoration of function, which may not be possible in the palliative population. In the palliative care setting, this goal is mostly replaced with the aim of maintaining functional independence for as long as possible. During the 1960s, John Dietz, MD, created one of the first cancer rehabilitation programmes through a collaboration between Memorial Sloan Kettering Hospital and the Rusk Institute of New York University. Dietz is best remembered for introducing a widely used, four-track model for the rehabilitation of patients with cancer:

1. Preventive

2. Restorative

3. Supportive

4. Palliative (Dietz, 1969).

Dietz's fourth track, palliative, produced a mandate to provide rehabilitation services tailored to patients with advanced disease. The efficacy of rehabilitation services at the end of life has been most studied among cancer patients, but rehabilitation care providers have also gained a wealth of experience in the treatment of patients with progressive disabilities such as end-stage organ failure or neurodegenerative diseases. The primary treating team may request a rehabilitation medicine consultation for a comprehensive approach, addressing all associated impairments and resulting disability, or they may choose to prescribe discreet therapeutic interventions administered by PTs, OTs, speech language and respiratory therapists, music therapists, and psychologists. While many of these treatments can be initiated directly by patients and their families in the community, they usually require medical staff to drive requests in a hospital setting.

Several large, well-organized cancer centres in the United States and Europe have established successful in-house rehabilitation programmes to meet the needs of their patients throughout the disease continuum. These centres have served as training programmes for more than two generations of rehabilitation specialists interested in end-of-life care (recognized examples in the United States include the M. D. Anderson Cancer in Texas, the Memorial Sloan Kettering Cancer Center in New York, and the Mayo Clinic in Minnesota). smaller cancer centres have sought to follow suit by funding part-time positions for rehabilitation medicine specialists, or paying for specialized training for therapy staff. The presence of rehabilitation specialists on palliative care teams is often reassuring to patients and their families at a time when they feel restorative services may be withdrawn prematurely. In some cases, palliative care patients may require separate admission to an inpatient rehabilitation programme. Short, targeted rehabilitation stays for palliative care patients may be entirely for family or caregiver training, with little expectation of independent functional gains by the patient. In other cases, a combination of functional gains and caregiver training are used to ensure safety, decrease burden of care, and maximize independence for patients returning home. Rehabilitation units associated with cancer centres have often accumulated decades of expertise in designing realistic and effective treatment plans for patients towards the end of life. Free-standing inpatient rehabilitation facilities that wish to begin treating palliative care patients may need to reinforce programme development with educational opportunities for staff who may not have as much experience in treating patients with advanced disease. The psychological demands of working with patients and their families towards the end of life need to be addressed, particularly for staff who may have chosen rehabilitation because of its focus on recovery.

Inpatient rehabilitation programmes can be offered at various levels of intensity and are designed to offer patients access to concentrated services that would otherwise be difficult to obtain and coordinate. Neuropsychologists, speech language therapists, rehabilitation certified nurses, and, in some cases, orthotists, prosthetists, and equipment vendors work with the treating rehabilitation medicine specialist to return patients to the community. Subacute programmes and skilled nursing facilities offer access to some rehabilitation services but at a lesser intensity. Rehabilitation services are provided routinely as part of home care for patients with many diagnoses. The goals of treatment in the home setting focus on the essentials of self-care, transfers, household ambulation, ascending and descending stairs, and perhaps some early community re-entry for patients, with reduced function, PTs and OTs can provide home assessments and direction for effective management. Lowe et al.'s systematic review provides an effective introduction to the emerging field of therapeutic exercise for cancer patients receiving palliative care (Lowe et al., 2009). Preliminary small studies consistently report functional gains in this population. Results have been replicated for aerobic as well as anaerobic and mixed exercise programmes using gentle bicycle ergometry and/or tailored resistance training. Bicycle ergometry regimens can be based on lower extremity pedalling or upper extremity pedalling. Implementing these interventions requires clearly articulated guidelines for common risks and complications that accompany active interventions in patients with advanced disease. Greater than average knowledge of the pathophysiology of advanced cardiovascular, pulmonary, and renal disease is needed for the selection of individualized interventions. Input from PM&R physicians or others trained in medical rehabilitation is strongly recommended at least at the programmatic planning stages.

Strength, endurance, and functional performance gains can be achieved or maintained through supervised home programmes (Cheville et al., 2012a). Therapists should encourage patients and caregivers to take opportunities for self-management once a programme has been designed. Skilled therapy involvement should be reserved for declines in function warranting reassessment and the introduction of new or altered programmes. For patients able to leave their homes, rehabilitation medicine outpatient visits every

4–8 weeks serve as opportunities for readjusting the overall rehabilitation treatment plan during disease progression. Symptom management including neurolytic procedures for excess spasticity, trigger point injections, advanced wound care, and pharmacological pain management are available through most outpatient rehabilitation medicine practices.

Patients with metastatic bone lesions, hemiparesis, or paraparesis may require customized wheelchairs. Improperly selected seating systems can result in skin breakdown as well as reduced performance. Most rehabilitation centres offer skilled medical equipment selection with medical justification for requested components. The introduction of new equipment often requires a period of supervised training for patients and caregivers. Rehabilitation centres should be able to coordinate delivery of these services through outpatient as well as home visits.

Patients able to seek rehabilitation services at an outpatient facility should be encouraged to do so as the capabilities of an outpatient setting far exceed what can be delivered in the home. Perhaps as importantly, patients may benefit from the social aspects of their visits and the inspiration they may experience from their own gains. However, as their disease progresses, patients may find that travel to the centre becomes too difficult. At such times of transition, outpatient therapists and treating rehabilitation medicine specialists should ensure that patients and their caregivers are equipped with a realistic, home-based maintenance programme.

In the final stages of end-of-life care, the role of rehabilitation services shifts towards preventing injury and the safe delivery of care. Positioning, maintenance of skin integrity, pain control, continence, and safe alimentation become priorities. Therapists may return briefly to teach a previously ambulatory patient and their caregivers wheelchair skills or proper use of mechanical lifts. The impact of rehabilitation services for patients at inpatient hospices has not been widely evaluated, however. However, Yoshioka's 1994 study showed functional gains and improved patient and family satisfaction associated with PT services in an inpatient hospice (Yoshioka, 1994).

Massage refers to the manipulation of superficial muscle groups and tissue. Certain techniques achieve deeper effects through specialized strokes or manoeuvres. Massage contributes to rehabilitation goals by direct mechanical effects as well as reflexive and psychological effects. The mechanical effects include the mobilization of oedema within soft tissue and improvements in vascular perfusion. The term reflexive effect is used to describe the influence of cutaneous stimulation on the autonomic nervous system and the spinal cord. The psychological benefits of massage therapy are reflected in the subjective sense of relaxation and well-being experienced during and after treatment.

More participatory forms of bodywork, such as Feldenkrais, Trager psychophysical integration, and the application of Alexander technique, help to address pain and functional deficits by treating underlying systemic dysfunction. The Feldenkrais method, for example, achieves its goals by increasing conscious awareness of bodily positioning and movement habits. This may be extremely important for patients seeking to limit painful and functional side effects of new hemiparesis or increased tone. Other techniques seek to relieve physical symptoms through a combination of bodily, emotional, and cognitive interventions. Trager psychophysical integration uses gentle mobilization via rhythmic oscillations and rocking with the intention of affecting the subconscious mind as well as the body.

While many types of bodywork require one-to-one patient sessions, several movement therapies can be delivered in a group or class setting. Qigong and t'ai chi can offer low-impact, minimal resistance programmes that improve balance, strength, and endurance (Lee et al., 2007). Modified yoga positions can make the benefits of this several thousand-year-old movement therapy available to even the most medically compromised patients (Farrel et al., 1999; Chen et al., 2007).

Many rehabilitation interventions that are used safely in other patient populations may carry increased risk of injury for patients with advanced disease. Pathological fractures, for instance, can occur without apparent trauma. Armed with this information, patients and givers may choose to proceed with interventions that will improve function and QOL, even if there is accompanying risk. Physicians caring for the patient should be able to provide guidelines and precautions for weight-bearing status, range of motion, cardiovascular parameters, and other limitations if indicated.

Assessment of needs, timing, and integration of interventions and goal setting

Assessment

A strong association between functional status and health-related quality of life (HRQOL) has been established for many disease states. This association is particularly well documented for patients with cancer. As a result, almost all QOL metrics used for cancer patients (e.g. EORTC-QLQ-C30, Functional Assessment of Cancer Treatment (FACT), Functional Living Index Cancer (FLIC), and Cancer Rehabilitation Evaluation System (CARES)) include items that assess functional domains (Heinrich et al., 1984; Schipper et al., 1984; Cella et al., 1993; Osoba et al., 1994). Patients wish to remain functionally autonomous for as long as possible. Eighty-eight per cent of the 301 hospice inpatients that participated in Yoshioka's study expressed a strong desire to recover independent mobility (Yoshioka, 1994). A survey of patients with late-stage disease revealed that the 'loss of ability to do what one wants' was rated highest among end-of-life concerns (Axelsson and Sjoden, 1998). Studies have shown that in some cultural settings, functional decline undermines cancer patients' QOL to the point that they may engage in passive suicidal ideation and ultimately express interest in physician-assisted suicide (Fairclough, 1998; O'Mahony et al., 2005; Mystakidou et al., 2006). In fact, functional status was among the strongest predictors of desire for hastened death and pursuit of euthanasia in several studies (van der Maas et al., 1996; O'Mahony et al., 2005).

As many as 70–80% of cancer patients with advanced disease express interest in receiving rehabilitation services and generally find them useful (Yoshioka, 1994; Cheville et al., 2008). Evidence indicates that substantial improvement can be achieved in multiple domains including mobility, self-care, vocational capacity, and communication (Harvey et al., 1982). Reports describe improved outcomes in both inpatient and outpatient settings among patients with central nervous system (CNS) involvement. In fact, their functional gains are comparable to those of patients with similar impairments of ischaemic and traumatic origin (O'Dell et al., 1998; McKinley et al., 1999, 2000). Hospice inpatients can also improve their mobility indices through standard rehabilitation therapies (Yoshioka, 1994). Mitigation of functional decline through the proactive use of rehabilitation has been demonstrated in patients with inexorably progressive conditions, such as AIDS, progressive multiple sclerosis (MS), and other advanced disease states (Kraft and Alquist, 1996; Hicks, 1999; Yarasheske and Roubenoff, 2001). It is reasonable to generalize these findings and anticipate that functional and QOL maintenance should also be achievable for a proportion of cancer patients as well as those with less well-studied disease processes.

Timing

Joann Lynn and her colleagues have identified trajectories of functional decline in cancer and other illnesses over the last year of life (Lunney et al, 2003). Trajectories are generally characterized by an extended period during which functional capacity remains almost at baseline, with episodes of transient decline in response to disease progression, recurrence, or major disease-modifying therapies. The final phase in advanced disease is often characterized by a dramatic drop in function in the final year or months of life, with marked physical dependency especially in cancer (Cheville et al., 2012b). Many patients arrive at the terminal phase of their disease trajectory having already acquired neuropathies, cognitive deficits, degenerative arthropathies, and other physical impairments that place them at risk of abrupt decline. Determining when to intervene is not always self-evident. The timing of rehabilitation within the complex management of advanced disease is a particularly challenging and under-researched issue. Effective treatments must be delivered expeditiously to patients when they are able to derive the greatest benefits. A number of barriers make it difficult to achieve this goal:

1. Clinicians caring for patients with advanced disease are not necessarily familiar with either the substance or potential benefits of rehabilitation interventions. Consequently, reliable referral patterns are not always established (Beck et al., 2006).

2. Non-rehabilitation clinicians are less likely to screen patients routinely for functional decline. When functional evaluation is not a component of routine care, disability generally receives clinical attention only late in its course, when interventions tend to be less effective.

3. Clinicians may believe that at the stage of illness when disease-modifying therapies are of no further benefit, rehabilitation has similarly little to offer. Ultimately, many non-rehabilitation clinicians have difficulty determining accurately who, when, and why to refer for rehabilitation evaluation and services.

Patient-related barriers also impede the timely involvement of rehabilitation services. Function is not an issue that most patients are accustomed to discussing with their medical caregivers. In fact, they may consider functional decline an inevitable consequence of their condition and not even bring catastrophic declines in their mobility or activity of daily living (ADL) performance to their clinicians' attention (Detmar et al., 2001). Because most rehabilitation interventions require active and ongoing patient participation, patient and support system 'buy in' is essential. Patients must appreciate the need for rehabilitation, recognize future benefit in the process, and perceive meaning in its goals. This level of patient endorsement may occur only after significant functional decline when patients confront dependency.

As delivery of care shifts increasingly from the hospital to the clinic, the need for effective communication both between patients and caregivers as well as patients and their physician will be essential if disability is to be addressed effectively. Failure to address cumulative disability results in patients living at lower levels of function and experiencing more difficulty and distress than is necessary.

Characterizing the magnitude and rate of patients' decline is a challenge. Patients' baseline function, from which they subsequently decline, is also highly variable. Difficulty with an ADL such as dressing or bathing may reflect a drastic and precipitous decline for some patients and virtually no change for others.

It is usually neither fiscally nor logistically possible to have all palliative care patients evaluated by a rehabilitation physician. Elderly patients, or those with multiple co-morbidities and/or a disability at baseline, should be referred for more extensive assessment of their rehabilitation needs. At the very least, such referrals establish a relationship between patients and a rehabilitation team that can be developed in the future. The timing for referral of patients without these risk factors can be based on:

◆ any new or significant basic or instrumental activity of daily living (IADL) difficulty

◆ any new or significant decrease in household or community mobility

◆ frail, ill, or disabled caregiver

◆ recent hospitalization of significant change in medical status (e.g. a period of bed rest, pathological fracture)

◆ symptom (e.g. pain, dyspnoea) interference with function.

Goal setting: foundation, components, and barriers
Foundation

The link between physical impairment and disability has been studied in different populations with advanced disease. In stage IV breast cancer, for example, the most common physical impairments include paraplegia, steroid myopathy, and joint pains (Cheville et al., 2008). These impairments are generally related to disease progression and changes in treatment, and may be associated with abrupt functional decline in the absence of rehabilitation interventions. Pleural or pulmonary compromise can acutely undermine aerobic reserve leading to severe exertional intolerance. Malignant lesions, particularly bone metastases, can undermine the essential supporting structures of the musculoskeletal system. Non-surgical, anti-cancer treatments, including radiotherapy and chemotherapy, can produce disability by injuring muscles and nerves.

Cross-sectional studies in cohorts with advanced lung cancer have demonstrated correlations between fatigue, pain, and functional status (Fox and Lyon, 2006). Pain also correlates strongly with function in other cancer cohorts (Palmore and Cleveland, 1976; Beck et al., 2006). Breakthrough pain, defined as transient increases above baseline that warrant analgesic use, has been identified as an important cause of compromised functional status (Portenoy and Hagen, 1990; Portenoy et al., 1999). A recent longitudinal study established that pain and fatigue ratings, independent of disease progression or the presence of new bone or brain metastases, strongly associate with functional decline

(Cheville et al., 2012b). Therefore, proactive symptom control is an essential component of successful rehabilitation.

The degree to which pain and fatigue engender disability in advanced disease has immediate and practical implications. It has been shown that 75–95% of cancer pain can be controlled through non-invasive means but that these interventions continue to be under-utilized in the home-care setting (Foley, 1985; Levy, 1996; Ferrell et al., 1999; Miaskowski, 2005; McCarberg, 2007). Targeting pain not only addresses an important symptom and source of distress but has the additional documented benefit of limiting functional decline (Hanna et al., 2006).

Studies have determined that patients and their families strive to minimize discussion about caregiving preferences and other disability-related issues, partly because of reluctance to confront the patient's impending decline and partly, in a perhaps misguided effort, to protect one another from psychological stress (Edwards and Forster, 1999; Pecchioni, 2001; Zhang and Siminoff, 2003). Studies that have examined communication patterns between patients and physicians, and between caregiver and physicians, have shown that the needs and desires of patients and caregivers may conflict. Studies of caregivers, after patients' deaths suggest that caregivers would prefer more physician communication regarding the patient's illness (Hanson et al., 1997). These studies indicate that communication preferences cannot be summarized easily. Moreover, they reveal that patients and caregivers may, at times, have diametrically opposed communication needs which in turn can interfere with the selection and implementation of optimal rehabilitation strategies.

Components

Rehabilitation goals should reflect a patient's age, disease, co-morbidities, baseline fitness, and psychological, social, educational, and financial resources. Deitz described four complementary yet distinct function-oriented rehabilitation strategies—preventive, restorative, supportive, and palliative (Dietz, 1969):

1. Preventive rehabilitation seeks to avoid the expected impairments that accompany disease progression. Sitting protocols, for example, limit the physiological impact of prolonged bed rest. The positioning of paralysed limbs and pressure relief techniques are other examples of common preventive interventions. Caregiver education is often highly effective as empowering and informing caregivers can help reduce predictable complications, such as skin breakdown, that result from immobility or poorly managed urinary incontinence.

2. Restorative rehabilitation has as its goal the return of the patient to his or her premorbid level of function. Such approaches are often utilized following intensive oncological or other treatment. Pulmonary rehabilitation can be helpful after thoracotomy or on exacerbation of chronic obstructive pulmonary disease. Other restorative approaches are used to regain upper extremity strength and range of motion after mastectomy or radiation. Structured progressive aerobic conditioning represents a very effective restorative technique for patients undergoing bone marrow transplantation. It can be used judiciously to allow even patients with progressive disease to recover some portion of their premorbid fitness levels.

3. Supportive rehabilitation attempts to optimize functioning in patients with irreversible impairments. Supportive programmes include the multi-modal techniques used to rehabilitate patients after limb salvage procedures such as internal hemi-pelvectomy. Combined interventions focusing on strength, endurance, proprioception, and balance can create functional ambulatory patterns that compensate for impaired limb and pelvic biomechanics.

4. Palliative rehabilitation includes supportive approaches designed to reduce patients' dependence in mobility and self-care activities. Emotional reinforcement and comfort should be provided concurrently. There are many opportunities for effective intervention. Preservation of bowel and bladder continence, for example, is an important goal for patients with advanced disease. Simple rehabilitation interventions can often extend patients' ability to toilet independently until the very terminal stages of cancer. Anasarca and progressive lymphoedema are common among end-stage cancer patients. Palliative rehabilitation approaches such as lymphatic drainage techniques and multi-layer compression bandaging can minimize oedema, thereby enhancing patient comfort and mobility. These measures also function preventatively to reduce the likelihood of local skin breakdown and associated infections.

Barriers

Uncontrolled pain remains one of the best understood components of functional decline in advanced disease. Integration of rehabilitation specialists in palliative care makes it more likely that incident pain precipitated by movement will be identified and managed with pharmacological as well as non-pharmacological interventions. The control of movement-related pain is essential for the maintenance of functional independence. Poor control contributes to a cycle of decreased activity, decreased autonomy, and deconditioning. Lost functional capacity is much harder to restore, particularly in patients with significant disease burden. A proactive approach to baseline and incident pain management thus preserves function as well as contributing to overall HRQOL in patients with advanced disease.

Palliative caregivers and rehabilitation specialists share an interest in achieving pain control in the home setting. Clinical teams often achieve excellent control of baseline pain but have inadequate opportunity to address movement-related, incident pain. Most patients' situations are in the home setting. Their activity profiles generally become more arduous and specific programmes are needed to manage pain induced by typical, at-home activities. Rehabilitation services can play a vital role in establishing an analgesic regimen that supports activity. Pharmacological approaches alone may not suffice. For this reason, an iterative process of refinement is required whereby interventional and pharmacological analgesic approaches coordinate with rehabilitative efforts in responding to the patient's feedback. Patients and their caregivers must be fully engaged in order to learn and practise compensatory strategies and therapeutic exercises. Sources of poor patient participation, such as depression and delirium, must actively be sought and definitely addressed whenever possible.

Rehabilitation's role in reducing incident pain can generally be fulfilled by using the following steps:

1. Ensure that all sources of pain potentially amenable to disease-modifying treatments (e.g. bone metastases, impingement) are addressed.

2. Confirm that baseline or 'at rest' pain is adequately controlled.

3. Establish that patients have recourse to 'as needed' or 'rescue' analgesic dosing for incident or movement-related pain.

4. Collect a realistic profile of the patient's activities following discharge.

5. Educate patients regarding the general approach and the need to attend carefully to incident- or movement-related pain.

6. Trial the full spectrum of activities with current analgesics, soliciting pain ratings for each activity.

7. If incident or movement-related pain intensity exceeds 5 on an 11-point numerical rating scale, retrial with proactive use of 'as needed' or 'rescue' analgesics. Depending on the agent's pharmacokinetics, a full hour may be required after ingestion to achieve maximal serum levels.

8. Retrial painful activities, soliciting pain ratings for each activity.

9. If incident or movement-related pain intensity remains unacceptable, deconstruct painful activities to identify evocative motions and positions.

10. Implement compensatory strategies and determine whether assistive devices and/or orthoses reduce incident pain.

11. Retrial painful activities, particularly when patients are fatigued, and solicit pain ratings for each activity.

12. If pain intensity remains unacceptable, increase 'as needed' medication dosing, change medication and/or add additional medications specifically targeting incident or movement-related pain. If the pain occurs with high frequency, adjustment of patients' baseline regimen may be indicated.

13. If incident or movement-related pain is severe and focal, interventional analgesic approaches may be indicated.

14. If incident or movement-related pain intensity remains unacceptable, continue to iteratively refine the 'as needed' analgesic regimen.

The analgesic principles governing management of incident pain have been detailed by several authors elsewhere and in chapters in Section 9. The main challenge is in achieving an adequate balance between analgesia and unwanted side effects, especially drowsiness when the patient is at rest. Patients and their caregivers should be educated to assess pain needs throughout the day and time breakthrough medication use appropriately. The negative impact of decreased activity that accompanies over-medication should be explained. All patients started on opioid analgesia should be educated about the need for a concomitant bowel programme and should be instructed in several pharmacological and non-pharmacological management strategies. Efficacy of the accompanying bowel programme should be assessed at each outpatient visit and frequently for patients receiving home care. Patients and their caregivers should be encouraged to bring inadequate pain control or troublesome side effects to their care team's attention so that adjustments can be made.

Symptoms other than pain such as dyspnoea, anxiety, nausea, and orthostatic hypotension may also undermine patients' function and autonomy. Using an iterative approach similar to that outlined earlier for pain management, the rehabilitation team can work with patients and their palliative caregivers to ensure that symptoms are controlled during activity. Rehabilitation techniques, compensatory strategies, assistive devices, and orthotics can be used. Activity-associated anxiety similarly can be managed with behavioural techniques and titration of anxiolytics coupled with rehabilitative strategies. Limiting the functional impact of symptoms requires ongoing assessment by therapists during treatment sessions, effective interdisciplinary communication when control is inadequate, and the coordinated efforts of palliative and rehabilitative clinicians.

Medical team leaders for palliative care patients are expected to coordinate with other medical specialties and to share changes in treatment plan or prognoses with rehabilitation clinicians, as these clearly impact on rehabilitation goals, the discharge disposition, and future equipment needs. The rehabilitation team can deploy its resources most effectively when equipped with current and accurate medical information concerning individual patient status.

Rehabilitation strategies for specific palliative care populations

Rehabilitation interventions in palliative care constitute an ongoing integration of rehabilitation services that may have begun with the initial diagnosis or treatment of the patient's underlying disease. Palliative care patients are able to benefit from carefully selected rehabilitation interventions designed to maintain or, in some cases, even restore key elements of independent function. Many of the rehabilitation strategies used to reduce the impairments and disabilities produced by acute and chronic illness offer significant benefit for patients with advanced disease. Rehabilitation units often develop treatment plans based on the six functional domains for FIM scores (Granger et al., 1990, 1993). These are mobility; self-care; sphincter control (bowel and bladder); communication; and social cognition including social interaction, problem-solving, and memory. Goals in these areas can be assigned by any member of the treatment team and discrepancies should be resolved in interdisciplinary team meetings and with input from the patient and their caregivers. Rehabilitation specialists working with patients who are still able to attend outpatient clinics may find themselves operating more independently, but should make every effort to share their treatment plans with all members of the extended treatment team. Although rehabilitation services can be obtained on an ad hoc basis, patients are best served when specific rehabilitation specialists are consistently part of a palliative care team. Medically trained rehabilitation specialists assist in the selection of appropriate goals for patients by combining knowledge of rehabilitation potential with an understanding of the underlying disease processes.

Rehabilitation of palliative care patients with motor deficits

Specific myopathies as well as neurologically mediated motor weakness occur in many patients with advanced disease. Progressive dystrophies, such as Duchenne muscular dystrophy or fascio-scapular-humeral dystrophy, create an increasing reliance on compensatory strategies and adaptive devices for many years prior to a final or more complete phase of dependence.

Patients with these diagnoses and their families have experienced a gradual loss of function over time and may have a wealth of knowledge and equipment that can be built on, as needs increase. Others, in contrast, may experience more abrupt and unexpected onset of motor deficits when vertebral metastases result in paraparesis or a metastatic brain lesion causes hemiplegia. Almost all people also experience a more generalized loss of motor function due to the complex interaction of cardiovascular, nutritional, and musculoskeletal changes associated with prolonged bed rest and frailty. Understanding the aetiology and physiology of impairments that contribute to motor deficits is essential to optimizing rehabilitation interventions.

Certain impairment groups have been the subject of more extensive clinical research. Paraparesis as a result of spinal cord compression (SCC) occurs relatively commonly in patients with metastatic cancer. Traumatic spinal cord injury (SCI) programmes may effectively address the functional needs of comparably impaired palliative care patients with a minimum of retraining. Palliative care populations with SCC require careful modification of SCI protocols as they have different life expectancies and co-morbidities. Common goals include enhancing the paralysed patient's ability to direct care, integrate compensatory strategies, utilize adaptive equipment, and accept realistic goals based on physiological as well as social and environmental constraints. The restoration of motor function in cancer-related SCC is possible in proportion to the duration of deficits prior to treatment usually with radiation or surgery (Guo et al., 2003).

Patients with intracranial processes resulting in motor weakness benefit greatly from the experience rehabilitation specialists have had with stroke and brain injury patients. Studies comparing the outcomes of patients with intracranial lesions who receive rehabilitation services with the outcomes achieved for stroke patients have consistently shown comparable performance in multiple domains (Marciniak et al., 1996). Patients with pure upper motor neuron or mixed upper and lower motor neuron involvement often have increased tone or spasticity that may benefit from neurolytic or pharmacological interventions. Local injections of phenol or botulinum toxin can be used to prevent contractures and joint deformities for patients with advanced disease states as can passive range of motion and splinting programmes.

Lower motor neuron impairments result in focal deficits producing a flaccid paralysis, although leptomeningeal disease can produce more diffuse patterns of lower motor neuron weakness. Lower motor neuron lesions require greater attention to bracing and positioning, to limit pain or further injury to the affected body parts. Understanding the aetiology and pathophysiology of the motor weakness again directs the selection of rehabilitation interventions. The functional benefits of increased tone that can be used to assist with transfers for patients with upper motor lesions is absent in lower motor injury. Earlier introduction of assistive devices rather than pure compensatory strategies may be required. A universal cuff (Fig. 4.15.1) for holding utensils, grooming, and hygiene aids can significantly improve autonomy for patients with hand weakness from a tumour-related compression of the C8 and T1 nerve roots. A balanced forearm orthosis (Fig. 4.15.2) enhances upper extremity function for patients with compromised proximal strength but preserved distal dexterity. Orthotics may be introduced to stabilize vulnerable joints, although their added weight can be counterproductive in the setting of significant weakness.

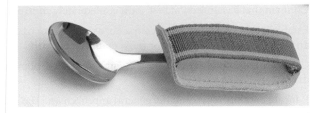

Fig. 4.15.1 Universal cuff 1485.
Image reproduced by courtesy of Patterson Medical Ltd.

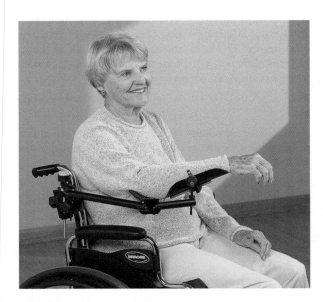

Fig. 4.15.2 Balanced forearm orthosis.
Image reproduced by courtesy of Patterson Medical Ltd.

Isolated 'foot drop' or anterior tibialis weakness can be treated with dynamic or static ankle–foot orthoses (AFO) depending on clinical presentation. In some cases enhanced knee control can be achieved, despite quadriceps, or hamstring weakness, by altering the degree of dorsiflexion or plantarflexion specified in the orthotic prescription. Orthoses can be extended to encompass the knee (KAFO) but the added weight and cumbersome profile limits their utility. Unless a KAFO meaningfully improves a patient's mobility, limiting lower extremity orthoses to distal stabilization with a solid and supportive AFO sufficiently stabilizes and protects the joint to facilitates transfers, even in a patient with flaccid hemiplegia.

Instruction in compensatory strategies enables patients with motor deficits to remain mobile and accomplish self-care activities. Patients are taught to capitalize on the strength of preserved muscle groups and to modify posture and body mechanics to minimize the secondary complications that result from focal weakness. Appropriately selected assistive devices also facilitate mobility and self-care for patients with motor deficits. Reachers, for instance, permit partially paralysed patients to retrieve objects. Devices developed to assist with specific ADLs may reduce the amount of energy expended on specific tasks, such as dressing. Investment in more expensive DME, particularly power wheelchairs, presents a challenging dilemma for patients with advanced disease. Early, proactive identification of emerging deficits allows for equipment to be prescribed for more extended periods. In these cases, prescribing physicians and suppliers should incorporate the expectation of further functional decline into the selection of components. Many amyotrophic lateral sclerosis (ALS)/ motor neuron disease clinics, for instance, begin by providing power wheelchairs with patient-controlled toggle-steering initially, but with the ability to convert to a companion control, as many patients will lose the ability to operate the device safely.

Rehabilitation strategies for sensory deficits

Sensory deficits may be the result of progressive disease such as diabetes, peripheral nerve impingement by tumour, or neurotoxic treatment effects. Damage to proprioceptive and other sensory nerve fibres can have enormous functional impact on standing balance, ambulation, as well as the dexterity needed for many self-care activities. In some cases, sensory deficits can be expected to subside even in advanced disease, if neurotoxic treatments are stopped or there is tumour response to palliative radiotherapy. The devastating sensory and proprioceptive deficits accompanying advanced diabetes, however, are not reversible.

Protection becomes the primary principle in selection of rehabilitation goals and interventions for patients with sensory deficits. Injury to insensate skin must be avoided at all costs, particularly as healing is often impaired due to a number of factors including nutritional status. All patients with insensate skin and their caregivers should be taught a thorough approach to skin inspection and pressure relief through weight shifts and positioning. Exceptional care, including the provision of specialized ortheses, may be necessary as conventional devices may themselves produce non-healing wounds. Moulded AFOs (Fig. 4.15.3) can be trimmed or reshaped if wearing produces skin chafing and sustained irritation. Foam padding can also be added to enhance tolerance. Impaired hand or upper extremity sensation can also lead to non-healing wounds but the relative visibility of these body parts often results in better protection and more prompt treatment. Patients with impaired upper extremity sensation can benefit from consultation with an OT for an introduction to devices that restore some degree of fine motor function in the absence of sensory input. Enlarged utensil handles, buttoners, and even sock donners allow independent performance of ADLs despite impaired sensation, especially if visual function is spared.

Increased reliance on visual cues enables patients with proprioceptive deficits to achieve some degree of compensation. In addition, indirect positional information or proprioceptive feedback can be transmitted through assistive devices such as canes and walkers for patients with primarily lower extremity proprioceptive losses. In addition to proprioceptive feedback, broad-based devices such as walkers and Zimmer frames provide mechanical stabilization for people with impaired balance. The risk of injury from a fall requires careful assessment of when to limit ambulation or at least unsupervised ambulation altogether. Standard, in lieu of wheeled, walkers offer greater stability for frail patients. Many patients achieve greater autonomy and safety by propelling manual wheelchairs rather than walking shorter distances precariously. Nonetheless, the goal of 'walking again' often drives patients to select less safe and efficient forms of mobility. Assistive devices, particularly walkers/rollators/Zimmer frames and wheelchairs can be viewed as publicly embarrassing emblems of disease and declining function. As with the rehabilitation of

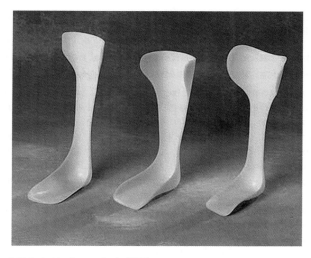

Fig. 4.15.3 Ankle–foot orthosis (AFO).
Images reproduced by courtesy of Patterson Medical Ltd.

acute and chronic conditions, rehabilitation in palliative care requires skilful introduction of solutions that may be unpalatable. Interdisciplinary rehabilitation teams including rehabilitation psychologists have experience helping patients move from wishing for a cure to making the most of remaining abilities. Frequently, underlying depression needs to be addressed pharmacologically as well as psychotherapeutically before rehabilitation strategies can be integrated effectively. The importance of patient and family being integrated with professional management is central and is explored more extensively in our concluding remarks.

Rehabilitation for patients with cerebellar dysfunction or movement disorders

Profound mobility and self-care deficits are associated with the cerebellar injuries and movement disorders that occur as the result of metastatic brain tumours and the paraneoplastic syndromes often associated with ovarian and lung cancer (Clouston et al., 1992; Peterson et al., 1992). Patients with movement disorders such as parkinsonism or other causes of dysmetria, with or without tremor, may benefit from weighted utensils and assistive devices, particularly as motor strength is often preserved in these conditions. Safety awareness and fall prevention must be emphasized repeatedly as denial and other causes of diminished insight often cause patients with ataxia to underestimate the impact of their deficits. Therapists can build on patients' instinctive protective mechanisms, such as adoption of a widened base of support, to establish safe movement patterns. Home and environmental modification can improve safety and prevent falls for all patients with movement disorders, including the more diffuse bradykinesia and loss of protective reflexes seen in advanced dementias. Advanced alcohol-related encephalopathies, hereditary, and non-hereditary spinal cerebellar ataxias, and Huntington's chorea require a sophisticated approach to DME prescription. Wheelchair seating systems, for instance, must be selected to provide maximal postural support without compromising freedom of movement more than necessary. Patient ability to self-propel manually, as well as power mobility may need to be reassessed at intervals. Power mobility settings including speed and responsiveness often can be adjusted to prolong the period of independent mobility in the face of decreasing motor coordination.

Rehabilitation for patients with cranial nerve and mechanical oral motor deficits

Cranial nerve involvement from neoplastic disease, ALS, or MS or other diagnoses can have severe medical and social consequences due to disruption of vision, speech, swallowing, and management of oral secretions. Collaboration with speech therapists, head and neck surgeons, and respiratory therapists may be needed to prevent aspiration pneumonia and ensure adequate oxygenation. Dysphagia and odynophagia can easily compromise nutrition, leading to the various functional and medical problems. Compensatory strategies are available for cognitively intact patients with focal swallowing deficits to help avoid tube feedings or restrictive food consistencies.

Dysarthria can be a devastating symptom for patients who experience a decreasing ability to make their needs known during a period of increasing dependence. In certain cases, intelligibility can be enhanced through compensatory strategies that increase respiratory support for vocalization, by introducing energy conservation techniques and the use of rest breaks. In other cases, augmentative communication devices from simple picture boards and artificial larynxes to computer interfaces that permit word or letter selection are more helpful. Family and caregiver education and training is also essential for diffusing the inevitable frustration of patients who lose the ability to communicate as part of a terminal illness.

Many, but not all, rehabilitation interventions for visual loss, field cuts, or oculomotor compromise remain effective in the palliative care setting. Few patients are going to learn to read Braille during the terminal phases of a disease but many of the other resources developed for the visually impaired in general, such as recorded books, textured organizational tools, and other adaptive equipment, can be used by people with diabetic retinopathy, optic chiasm tumours, or other diagnoses that impair visual function.

Rehabilitation opportunities for patients with cognitive dysfunction

Cognitive deficits increase caregiver burden, create safety concerns, and degrade interpersonal relations. Brain metastases can create deficits such as apraxia, alexia, and aphasia that have wide-reaching impact on numerous areas of independent function. Neurodegenerative processes often impair higher-level cognitive function, short-term memory, and attention, while also creating disturbances in executive function and emotional control. Treating clinicians need to be familiar with algorithms for distinguishing reversible from irreversible causes of cognitive dysfunction among palliative care patients. Urinary tract infections, medication effects, and other reversible causes of delirium are especially prevalent in medically compromised populations. Non-reversible deficits may resemble the more discrete aphasias associated with specific CNS lesions or present as more diffuse cognitive slowing and near-somnolence which can occur as a delayed effect of cranial irradiation.

Speech language therapy and cognitive interventions used for stroke and brain injury patients can result in modest but meaningful functional gains for terminally ill patients. Memory books and computerized prosthetics as well as pharmacological management of agitation or disrupted sleep–wake cycles can improve overall cognitive performance. Training of family, friends, and caregivers is often necessary to ensure continuity and the incorporation of compensatory strategies and other tools. Although time-consuming and only partially effective, these efforts engage patients and their support networks, often creating a sense of helping to make things better at a time that may otherwise be characterized by an overwhelming sense of helplessness and futility.

Rehabilitation strategies for patients with deconditioning

Deconditioning is one of the most widespread physical impairments to occur at the end of life. Many factors including anaemia, dyspnoea, pain, disrupted sleep, nausea, fatigue, orthostatic hypotension, and cachexia result in decreased activity tolerance and accelerate the downward spiral of progressive deconditioning. Rehabilitation interventions for patients with deconditioning in the setting of advanced disease can be divided into approaches that restore or preserve function and those that mitigate the effects of decreased endurance through compensatory strategies and environmental modification.

Therapeutic exercise, particularly for patients with advanced disease, should always be prescribed with careful attention to intensity, modality, and duration as well as the clear articulation of therapeutic goals and necessary precautions. Safe intensities are best understood for patients with advanced cardiac conditions but guidelines are emerging for other diagnoses (Bartels, 2000). Realistic goal selection will determine the choice of modalities although optimal programmes generally mix some proportion of flexibility, aerobic, and resistance or strengthening exercises tailored to the patient's current potential. Active and passive range of motion programmes are important for maintaining the ability to achieve comfortable positioning while also preventing pressure ulcers and limiting joint contractures that may impede hygiene, dressing, and other aspects of self-care. Therapeutic aerobic programmes in patients with advanced cancer have demonstrated the possibility of physiological as well as functional improvement provided that disease progression does not outstrip training effect. A graded conditioning programme can be prescribed for motivated patients. Studies of the efficacy of resistance training and strengthening programmes in androgen-deprived men with prostate cancer have proven the possibility of maintaining or even improving strength in the context of malignancy (Segal et al., 2003). Improved peripheral muscle efficiency often allows patients with pulmonary and cardiac compromise to accomplish more, despite fixed or worsening respiratory and cardiovascular function. Combining strength training with functional activities, such as sit-to-stand transfers is often an efficient way to design exercise programmes for compromised patients with little time or endurance for multi-modal protocols.

Patient safety and, at times, medical liability require careful delineation of exercise precautions. These should include limitations for patients with thrombocytopenia, weight-bearing restrictions for patients with bone metastases, or bracing requirements for patients with spinal instability.

Caregiver support

Palliative care has long recognized that effective interventions require attention to the larger context of patient, family, and social support networks. As disability accrues, these family and social networks may begin providing an increasing proportion of daily care. In their

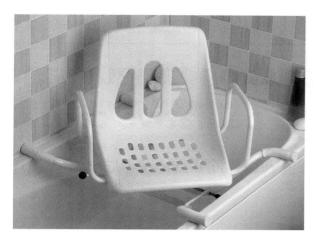

Fig. 4.15.4 Bath chair.
Image reproduced by courtesy of Patterson Medical Ltd.

recent analysis of the needs of family caregivers, Rabow and colleagues identified five burdens that can overwhelm giver resources:

1. Time and logistics

2. Physical tasks

3. Financial costs

4. Emotional and mental health risks

5. Other health risks (Rabow et al., 2004).

Short, focused inpatient rehabilitation stays or intensive teaching prior to discharge from an acute medical service can improve markedly patient safety and decrease caregiver burden. Caregivers should understand the biomechanics of patient transfers that protect both their own and the patient's body. Review of bowel and bladder programmes limits symptomatic and medical complications after discharge and is central to the protection of sacral skin, the prevention of sacral wounds, and minimization of the psychological distress accompanying adult incontinence. Rehabilitation nurses have experience in teaching complex wound care techniques as well as skin protection through pressure relief and positioning. Caregiver training by rehabilitation specialists reduces the risk of injury to patients or their assistants and can conserve time and energy for both by introducing labour-saving devices such as mechanical lifts, stair glides, ramps, wheelchairs, transfer boards, and bathing aides (Fig. 4.15.4). Follow-up training can be provided by home therapists as needs change. Caregiver training also alleviates some of the emotional and psychological stressors that burden patients.

Effective caregiver training includes the patient as much as possible given their current functional capacity. At a minimum, efforts must be made to explain techniques carefully to patients and to maximize their ability to direct their own self-care. Caregivers and, to some extent, patients should be trained to instruct others to allow for intervals of respite care.

Current barriers

All rehabilitation medicine's diagnostic and therapeutic effort is expended on enhancing or preserving patients' capacity for independent mobility, self-care, communication, and cognition. Diseases, their treatments, and their symptoms are only relevant to the rehabilitation paradigm in the manner in which they threaten or potentiate function.

Current clinical practices in palliative care rehabilitation are largely based on the consensus statements for specific disease types (e.g. National Comprehensive Cancer Network), evidence derived from the early or acute stages of disease (e.g. aerobic conditioning during adjuvant chemotherapy), isolated case reports, and common sense. In areas where literature exists, such as acute rehabilitation of cancer patients, study cohorts are generally defined by diagnoses rather than disease stage. Therefore uncertainty remains as to subjects' prospects for disease modification or cure and the proportion of their care delivered with palliative intent. As a result, limited inferences can be made as to the efficacy of rehabilitative interventions in far-advanced disease. At present, honest recognition of rehabilitation's incomplete evidence base in the palliative setting is the best means of preventing inappropriate adherence to therapies of equivocal benefit. The clinician must continuously ground him- or herself by asking, 'Will this improve or better maintain my patient's function?'

Online materials

Complete references for this chapter are available online at <http://www.oxfordmedicine.com>.

References

Beck, L.C., Cheville, A.L., Petersen, T., *et al.* (2006). *Functional Problems in Cancer Patients: Medical Record Documentation and Associated Characteristics*. Paper presented at the American Academy of Physical Medicine and Rehabilitation Annual Assembly, Honolulu, HI.

Cheville, A.L., Kollasch, J., Vandenberg, J., *et al.* (2012a). A home-based exercise program to improve function, fatigue, and sleep quality in patients with stage IV lung and colorectal cancer: a randomized controlled trial. *Journal of Pain and Symptom Management*, 45(5), 811–821.

Cheville, A.L., Troxel, A.B., Basford, J.R., *et al.* (2008). Prevalence and patterns of physical impairments in patients with metastatic breast cancer. *Journal of Clinical Oncology*, 26(16), 2621–2629.

Dimeo, F., Fetsher, S., Lange, W., *et al.* (1998). Effects of aerobic exercise on the physical performance and incidence of treatment-related complications after high-dose chemotherapy. *Blood*, 90, 3390–3394.

Fox, S.W. and Lyon, D.E. (2006). Symptom clusters and quality of life in survivors of lung cancer. *Oncology Nursing Forum*, 33(5), 931–936.

Hanna, A., Sledge, G., Mayer, M.L., *et al.* (2006). A phase II study of methylphenidate for the treatment of fatigue. *Supportive Care in Cancer*, 14(3), 210–215.

Lowe, S.S., Watanabe, S.M., and Courneya, K.S. (2009). Physical activity as a supportive care intervention in palliative cancer patients: a systematic review. *Journal of Supportive Oncology*, 7(1), 27–34.

Lunney, J.R., Lynn, J., Foley, D.J., *et al.* (2003). Patterns of functional decline at the end of life. *Journal of the American Medical Association*, 289(18), 2387–2392.

Mystakidou, K., Parpa, E., Katsouda, E., *et al.* (2006). The role of physical and psychological symptoms in desire for death: a study of terminally ill cancer patients. *Psycho-Oncology*, 15(4), 355–360.

Yoshioka, H. (1994). Rehabilitation for the terminal cancer patient. *American Journal of Physical Medicine & Rehabilitation*, 73, 199–206.

Burnout, compassion fatigue, and moral distress in palliative care

Nathan I. Cherny, Batsheva Werman, and Michael Kearney

Introduction to burnout, compassion fatigue, and moral distress

Work in palliative care and, in particular, end-of-life care is associated with inherent stressors that may impact on the well-being of clinicians working in the field. Work stressors may have diverse impacts on the emotional and professional lives of palliative care and hospice staff; not only to physicians and nurses but to all members of the professional staff and, in some cases, to volunteers as well. Through their impact on professional function, these stressors can adversely affect the effectiveness and quality of care and may compromise the ability to sustain a career in palliative care.

Clinicians involved in the provision of palliative care constantly confront professional, emotional, and organizational challenges. These challenges, especially when workplace support is limited, can make clinicians vulnerable to experiencing one or more of three well-described interrelated syndromes—burnout, compassion fatigue, and moral distress—each of which can lower the threshold for the development of the others (Sundin-Huard and Fahy, 1999; Keidel, 2002; Hamric et al., 2006; Pendry, 2007; Alkema et al., 2008; Newell and MacNeil, 2010; Maiden et al., 2011; Slocum-Gori et al., 2013) (Fig. 4.16.1).

Burnout results from stresses that arise from the clinician's interaction with the work environment (Maslach et al., 2001), compassion fatigue evolves specifically from the relationship between the clinician and the patient (Booth, 1991), and moral distress is related to situation in which clinicians are asked to carry our acts that run contrary to their moral compass. Clinicians who care for dying patients are at risk of all of these (Rohan, 2005) and they can be emotionally, personally, and professionally devastating. It is vital, therefore, that palliative care clinicians are aware of these potential problems and with strategies to mitigate risks and to manage them when they present either in their own individual lives or in the work environment.

Burnout

The burnout syndrome is characterized by losing enthusiasm for work (emotional exhaustion), treating people as if they were objects (depersonalization), and having a sense that work is no longer meaningful (low personal accomplishment). It relates to work (particularly human service work) and it is often present when individuals work under constant pressure. *Emotional exhaustion* refers to feelings of being overextended and depleted of one's emotional and physical resources. Exhaustion prompts efforts to cope by distancing oneself emotionally and cognitively from work (Maslach and Leiter, 2008). *Depersonalization* refers to negative, callous, cynical, or excessively detached responses to various aspects of the job and is another form of distancing (Maslach and Leiter, 2008). *Lack of personal accomplishment* refers to feelings of being ineffectual and underachieving at work.

These feelings may arise from a lack of resources (e.g. critical information, tools, or time) to get the work done, from overload, or from specific other stressors which may be directly related to emotional exhaustion and depersonalization or be independent of them (Maslach et al., 2001; Maslach and Leiter, 2008). Burnout tends to spread gradually and continuously over time unless circumstances alter or active steps are taken to address the factors contributing to work stress.

Better understanding of burnout can be gained by an understanding of its opposite: job engagement. Job engagement is characterized by energy, involvement, and efficacy in the workplace. Many clinicians working in palliative care express a sense of competence, pleasure, and control in their work (Vachon, 1995, 2008). Factors contributing to this desirable professional/emotional situation include feeling professionally competent and able to cope with challenges, having sustainable workload, feelings of choice and control, appropriate recognition and reward, having a supportive work environment, being treated fairly, and having a strong appreciation of the meaning and value of one's work.

Farber (Farber, 2000; Montero-Marin et al., 2009) proposed three different subtypes of burnout: 'frenetic', 'under-challenged',

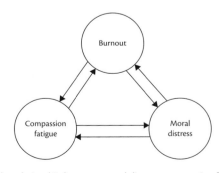

Fig. 4.16.1 The relationship between moral distress, compassion fatigue, and burnout.

and 'worn-out'. The *frenetic type* is overinvested and works extremely hard (to the sacrifice of other personal needs) and is frustrated and distressed by the lack of proportionate satisfaction: success, reward, or appreciation. The *under-challenged type* is indifferent as a result of insufficient challenge, stimulation, or meaning from work. The *worn-out* type is neglectful as a result of having been overwhelmed by too much work stress and lack of proportionate satisfaction, success, reward, or appreciation for the stresses that are endured.

Symptoms and signs of burnout

Burnout ca-n effect individuals or, sometimes, whole teams. Some of the common presenting symptoms are described in Box 4.16.1.

Factors that contribute to burnout

The actors that contribute to burnout are complex and are often interrelated.

Box 4.16.1 Symptoms and signs of burnout

Individual

- Overwhelming physical and emotional exhaustion
- Feelings of cynicism and detachment from the job
- A sense of ineffectiveness and lack of accomplishment
- Avoidance of emotionally difficult clinical situations
- Irritability and hypervigilance
- Interpersonal conflicts: over-identification or over-involvement
- Perfectionism and rigidity
- Poor judgement: professional and personal boundary violations
- Social withdrawal
- Numbness and detachment
- Difficulty in concentrating
- Questioning the meaning of life
- Questioning prior religious beliefs: sleep problems, intrusive thoughts, and nightmares
- Addictive behaviours
- Frequent illness: headaches, gastrointestinal disturbances, immune system impairment.

Team

- Low morale
- High job turnover
- Impaired job performance (decreased empathy, increased absenteeism).

Source: data from Maslach, C., et al., Job burnout. *Annual Review of Psychology*, Volume 52, pp. 397–422, Copyright © 2002 and Vachon, M. L., Staff stress in hospice/palliative care: a review, *Palliative Medicine*, Volume 9, Number 2, pp. 91–122, Copyright © 1995.

Workload

Workload has been identified as a major stressor for palliative care clinicians (Newton and Waters, 2001; Payne, 2001; Rokach, 2005) especially in settings of staff shortages and financial restraint. Dealing with dying patients and their families, excessive caseload of challenging patients and families, inadequate supports, excessive bureaucracy, and lack of time to talk to patients have all been identified as workload stressors. The greater the mismatch between the person and the work environment, the greater is the likelihood of burnout (Maslach and Leiter, 2008). A clear relationship between nursing shortages, understaffing, and burnout among nurses has been demonstrated (Toh et al., 2012).

Control (and training)

A sense of personal control helps people maintain emotional stability and cope with challenges in life. Perceived lack of control and actual lack of control over aspects of one's professional life are both associated with burnout (Glass et al., 1993). Lack of control may be intrinsic, related to lack of competence to cope with the challenges of patient care, self-care, or professional team dynamics. Extrinsic lack of control may relate to organizational structure or style within the work environment.

When clinicians are expected to take responsibility with inadequate training they may experience extreme lack of control. Among palliative care clinicians this may occur if they lack knowledge in interpersonal or communication skills or specific management skills in palliative care. Clinicians with inadequate training in skilled communication (Shimizu et al., 2003; Travado et al., 2005; Bragard et al., 2010), stress management (Bragard et al., 2006), recognition and management of compassion fatigue (Slocum-Gori et al., 2013), conflict resolution (Montoro-Rodriguez and Small, 2006), and symptom control all have a higher risk of burnout (Keidel, 2002; Cherny and Catane, 2003; Bar-Sela et al., 2012; Caruso et al., 2012; Fang et al., 2012).

Extrinsic lack of control may relate to any one or a combination of the following factors: work conditions, scheduling of work hours, patient allocation, patient load, clinical decisions, or organization decisions. Nurses, social workers, and other para-medical staff often feel disempowered, especially in the setting of hierarchical (or vertical) team management styles and in particular by authoritarian decision-making by physician partners who ignore or minimize the significance of their input or judgements.

Interprofessional and team issues

Team conflict, particularly between doctors and nurses or among nurses or between other members of the care team all contribute to burnout (Payne, 2001; Garman et al., 2002; San Martin-Rodriguez et al., 2005; Estryn-Behar et al., 2007; Brinkert, 2010; Bowers et al., 2011; Lasebikan and Oyetunde, 2012). Characteristics commonly seen in poorly functioning interdisciplinary care teams include lack of collaborative practice among professionals, strong hierarchical characteristics, lack of a shared philosophy of care, stifled expression of concerns, and strong professional territoriality. Often conflicts are generated by lack of common understandings of the prevailing goals of care, role diffusion issues, or differences of opinion regarding the appropriate clinical management or issues related to management style (San Martin-Rodriguez et al., 2005; Brinkert, 2010).

Values

Attitudes of clinicians towards palliative care and communication impact how care is implemented (Cherny and Catane, 2003; Lloyd-Williams and Dogra, 2003; Schreiner et al., 2004; Addington-Hall and Karlsen, 2005; Cherny, 2010). There is evidence demonstrating that the degree of congruity between personal values and the values central to the work environment predict for feelings of energy, involvement, and efficacy which are essential for job engagement (Leiter, 2008; Leiter et al., 2009). For instance, oncologists who do not highly value the psychosocial aspects of care and investment in the relief of physical, psychological, and spiritual distress report greater burnout (Cherny and Catane, 2003) and describe a greater degree of burnout, a sense of failure at not being able to alter the course of the disease (Jackson et al., 2008) when working with palliative care patients.

Moral distress (see later section) arising from situations in which one is expected to perform duties that run contrary with one's moral compass may be a major stressor contributing to distress and burnout (Sundin-Huard and Fahy, 1999). Indeed, one of the factors contributing to moral distress derives from having difficulty getting up to one's own standards or to an idealized, and often unattainable, vision of palliative care for the provision of a 'good death'.

Reward

Limited or inadequate financial rewards for the extremely challenging work of palliative care can contribute to burnout. Lack of reward may also relate to the lack of institutional reward to support the development of palliative care services or to provide for the psychosocial and supervision requirements of the clinical staff.

Emotion-work variables

Caregivers dealing with patients who die, particularly those who have had long-term relationships with their clients may experience feelings of grief, loss, or chronic grief (Vachon, 1999; Merluzzi et al., 2011). Coping with grief reactions may be challenged when patients or their children are young, when the distress and symptoms of the patient were not well controlled, and when staff feel that they were unable to deliver the best possible care to the patient when the death was contextually inappropriate such as deaths arising from the side effects of treatment. Repeated intense involvement with the distress of patients and their families in the time leading up to and after the death can traumatize health-care providers and contribute to 'the compassion fatigue syndrome' (Keidel, 2002; Rourke, 2007; Slocum-Gori et al., 2013) (see later) with its consequences which may include avoiding contact with patients, a negative self-assessment of performance, and a host of other responses that may adversely impact on personal and professional well-being and function.

Intrinsic to the challenge of providing palliative care is a delicate balance of maintaining warm supportive contact to those facing death while at the same time finding ways of not being overwhelmed by the patient's suffering, and by the challenges and burden of trying to ease that suffering.

Extrinsic factors

Palliative care staff may also have personal sources of pressure outside the work environment. These include family, financial health, and societal pressures, limited supports, and problems with interpersonal relationships unrelated to their roles as carers (Keidel, 2002). Professional caregivers with more responsibility for their own children or elderly parents, report more stress (Kash et al., 2000). For both women and men, the greater the number of children at home, the more difficulty with work-life balance and emotional exhaustion (Keeton et al., 2007). Being single, however, is also an independent risk factor for burnout (Ramirez et al., 1996).

Personality factors

Overinvested, highly motivated health professionals with intense investment in their profession are at a greater risk for the development of burnout (Leiter and Maslach, 2005; Anewalt, 2009). They become overinvolved and are constantly exposed to experiences of loss, awareness of their own mortality, and the termination of intense relationships (Keidel, 2002). Clinicians with this trait often display diminished awareness of their own physical and emotional needs, thus contributing to a self-destructive pattern of overwork (Anewalt, 2009). This may express itself in a 'psychology of postponement', in which they repeatedly defer attending to their significant relationships and other sources of personal reward until all the work is done or the next professional challenge is achieved (Spickard et al., 2002). A compulsive triad of an exaggerated sense of responsibility, doubt, and guilt can have an enormous impact on clinicians' professional, personal, and family lives (Spickard et al., 2002; Shanafelt et al., 2006).

Demographic variables associated with burnout

Age

Younger caregivers report more stressors and exhibit more manifestations of stress and fewer coping strategies (Vachon, 1995); they are more prone to burnout and stress reactions (Graham et al., 1996; Ramirez et al., 1995, 1996; Kash et al., 2000; Taylor et al., 2005; Kuerer et al., 2007). In contrast, some studies have found that caregivers with more years of experience are less likely to report stress-related symptoms and burnout (Vachon, 1995; Whippen et al., 2004); this, however, has not been a consistent finding (Allegra et al., 2005).

Gender

The data on gender as a risk factor is conflicted and inconclusive. Although most studies show women to be at higher risk for burnout and mental health problems (Graham et al., 1996; Kash et al., 2000; Kuerer et al., 2007), two surveys on the mental health of UK National Health Service physicians (880 consultants in 1994 compared with 1308 in 2002) found male and middle-aged consultants to be particularly at elevated risk (Taylor et al., 2005).

Epidemiology of burnout in oncology and palliative care

There has been considerable research into the epidemiology of burnout in palliative care (Masterson-Allen et al., 1985; Bram and Katz, 1989; Nash, 1989; Mallett et al., 1991; Ramirez et al., 1995; Vachon, 1995, 1999; Keidel, 2002; Swetz et al., 2009; Ostacoli et al., 2010; Pereira et al., 2011; Huynh et al., 2012; Slocum-Gori et al., 2013) and in oncology (Costantini et al., 1997; Kash et al., 2000; Lyckholm, 2001; Whippen et al., 2004; Allegra et al., 2005; Asai et al., 2006; Sherman et al., 2006; Balch and Copeland, 2007;

Kuerer et al., 2007; Arigoni et al., 2008; Liakopoulou et al., 2008; Alacacioglu et al., 2009; Mukherjee et al., 2009; Ostacoli et al., 2010; Shanafelt and Dyrbye, 2012).

A number of studies have reported that clinicians involved in palliative care had neither more nor less stress and burnout than other health professionals (Vachon, 1995, 2008; Pereira et al., 2011). Some studies seem to indicate that palliative care clinicians have lower burnout levels (in all three dimensions), particularly when compared with physicians practising in other fields such as oncology (Ramirez et al., 1995; Schraub and Marx, 2004; Asai et al., 2006; Fanos, 2007). These results may derive, in part, from the self-selection of people with congruent personal and professional values who chose to work in palliative care and the support palliative care team members give to one another (Vachon, 1995; Pierce et al., 2007).

Consequences of burnout

Dissatisfaction and distress caused by burnout have significant costs for clinicians and their families, their patients, and the health-care settings in which they work. Burnout alters both the physician–patient relationship and the quality of care clinicians provide (West et al., 2006). High levels of burnout are associated with diminished empathy and compassion, lack of professionalism, and increased risk of making medical errors (West et al., 2006; Halbesleben et al., 2008; Sharp and Clancy, 2008; Ida et al., 2009). Clinicians who manifest burnout are more likely to endorse euthanasia or assisted suicide as appropriate end-of-life options (Portenoy et al., 1997). Given the potential human costs of medical mistakes, the emotional impact of actual or perceived errors can be devastating for clinicians. Burnout also appears to influence the degree of trust and confidence patients have in their treating clinicians and patients' satisfaction with their medical care (Halbesleben and Rathert, 2008).

In addition to these professional repercussions, burnout can have profound personal consequences for clinicians, including depression, substance abuse, intent to leave clinical practice, and even suicide (Vachon, 1995, 1999; Kuerer et al., 2007). Rates of psychiatric disturbances, including depressive symptoms, anxiety, and sleep disturbances (Grunfeld et al., 2000; Kash et al., 2000; Asai et al., 2006), in clinicians working in end-of-life care ranged from 12% in a study of palliative care physicians (Asai et al., 2006) to between one-quarter and one-third of oncologists in other studies (Grunfeld et al., 2000; Kash et al., 2000; Asai et al., 2006).

Factors mitigating burnout

Some researchers have focused on factors that promote a sense of well-being and which mitigate against the effects of stress. Among the factors identified were self-awareness, hardiness (resilience), promoting a sense of control, and good team function (Ablett and Jones, 2007).

Attitudes and values

Clinicians who strongly identify with the values central to palliative care are more likely to experience and to express feelings of energy, involvement, and efficacy which are essential for job engagement (Leiter, 2008; Leiter et al., 2009). Engaged palliative care clinicians often relate to their commitment to making the most out of life and out of relationships, they derive meaning from their contributions to the well-being of the patients and families they care for, they have realistic expectations as to what they can achieve, they are forgiving of themselves and of their colleagues when outcomes are less than optimal and they recognize that flexibility and compromise is often necessary in order to maintain coping.

Good team work

There is a substantial and growing body of evidence that well-functioning interdisciplinary team work characterized by shared philosophy of care, respectful interdisciplinary relationships, mutual trust and support, and strong culture of communication can mitigate the risk of burnout (Garman et al., 2002; Estryn-Behar et al., 2007; Bowers et al., 2011).

Resilience (hardiness) and coherence

The personality characteristic of hardiness or resilience is expressed as a sense of commitment, control, and readiness to meet and to cope with challenges (Sotile and Sotile, 2003; Nygren et al., 2005; Ablett and Jones, 2007; Swetz et al., 2009; Howe et al., 2012). Commitment refers to a sense of meaning and purpose in one's professional life; control refers not only to autonomy but to a feeling of empowerment to make a difference and to cope with challenges; and challenge relates to the ability to address new changes that, while not necessarily desired, are anticipated as an inevitable part of life. Resilience is related to a 'sense of coherence' which is a perception of one's life as being comprehensible (cognitively meaningful and predictable), manageable (personal resources sufficient to meet internal and external demands), and meaningful (life is emotionally meaningful and that problems are perceived as challenges rather than hindrances) (Antonovsky and Sagy, 1986; Nygren et al., 2005) (see Chapter 17.2).

Control (and training)

As described above, control is one of the elements contributing to resilience. A sense of competence, control, and pleasure in one's work were among the highest ranked coping mechanism of 584 caregivers to the critically ill, dying, and bereaved (Vachon, 1995). Competence and, more importantly, the perceived self-evaluation of competence of the clinician, are related to the adequacy of training. Training in palliative care, communication skills stress management, and conflict resolution reduces the likelihood of burnout (Fallowfield et al., 2002, 2003; Armstrong and Holland, 2004; Holland and Neimeyer, 2005; Jones, 2005; Bragard et al., 2006; Shanafelt and Dyrbye, 2012; Shanafelt et al., 2012).

A sense of control is also reflected in studies looking at sources of satisfaction from work in palliative care. Professional achievements such as successful engagement with patients and their relatives, helping dying people find meaning in suffering and death, and providing adequate comfort and support have all been identified as sources of personal reward derived from palliative care provision (Graham et al., 1996; DeLoach, 2003; Boston and Mount, 2006; Clark et al., 2007; Pierce et al., 2007; Slocum-Gori et al., 2013).

Use of wellness strategies

Multiple studies have demonstrated improved work satisfaction in clinicians who used wellness strategies in caring for themselves as they care for others (Shanafelt et al., 2005a, 2012; Balch and Copeland, 2007; Anewalt, 2009; Campbell, 2010) (see Box 4.16.2).

Box 4.16.2 Measures that may help prevent burnout and compassion fatigue

Personal wellness strategies

These include strategies that attend to personal, familial, emotional, and spiritual needs while attending to the needs and demands of patients. Suggestions for developing a good self-care plan that can minimize the impact of compassion fatigue include (Rourke, 2007):

1. Getting adequate sleep, good nutrition, and regular exercise (Jones, 2005; Wallace et al., 2009; Swetz et al., 2009; Newell and MacNeil, 2010).

2. Building relaxation into most daily activities including the regular use of tools such as meditation, deep breathing, visual imagery, and massage (Swetz et al., 2009; Wallace et al., 2009).

3. Engaging regularly in a non-work-related activity to rejuvenate and restore energy, commitment, and focus (Jones, 2005; Lovell et al., 2009; Swetz et al., 2009; Wallace et al., 2009).

4. Develop your supportive and enjoyable relationships with family and friends outside of work (Keidel, 2002).

5. Maintaining a good balance between work, family, and pleasurable activities to defuse work-related tensions (Lovell et al., 2009; Swetz et al., 2009; Wallace et al., 2009; Newell and MacNeil, 2010).

6. Monitor oneself for tendency to being over involved (Keidel, 2002).

7. Finding and allowing adequate personal time to grieve losses that come with losing a patient with whom one has a special bond (Wallace et al., 2009).

8. Self-awareness techniques including mindful communication (Jones, 2005; Shanafelt et al., 2005b; Harrison and Westwood, 2009; Rushton et al., 2009; Goodman and Schorling, 2012) and/or reflective writing (Bernardi et al., 2005, Fearon and Nicol, 2011, Meier et al., 2001, Coulehan and Granek, 2012, Wald et al., 2010).

9. Developing a specific set of coping skills, stress management, organization, time management, communication, and cognitive restructuring, to ease the challenges of day-to-day issues (Jones, 2005; Perry, 2008; Lovell et al., 2009; Newell and MacNeil, 2010).

10. Relying on psychotherapy or spiritual care, particularly for staff who are experiencing very strong emotional reactions to their work, staff who are strongly reminded of their own personal losses frequently, and those with no clear confidante in their daily lives (Holland and Neimeyer, 2005; Sinclair and Hamill, 2007; Newell and MacNeil, 2010).

11. Attending to one's spiritual needs and developing a philosophy of care that provides personal meaning and a sense of purpose in the delivery of palliative care (Holland and Neimeyer, 2005; Sinclair and Hamill, 2007; Swetz et al., 2009; Newell and MacNeil, 2010).

Professional development strategies

These approaches must recognize the realities of working in palliative care: many people die from their diseases and health-care providers are limited in their ability to relieve a patient's and family's suffering.

1. Remember who owns the problem: be interested in and challenged by your patient's physical, emotional and spiritual problems but don't make them your own.

2. Learning to handle conflict effectively (Jones, 2005).

3. Training in communication skills (Fallowfield et al., 2002; Fallowfield et al., 2003; Armstrong and Holland, 2004; Jones, 2005; Bragard et al., 2006; Shanafelt and Dyrbye, 2012; Shanafelt et al., 2012).

4. Maintaining a high level of clinical knowledge and familiarity with established clinical guidelines for management of common problems (Holland and Neimeyer, 2005; Rushton et al., 2009).

5. Engaging in peer consultation (most helpful if it occurs in a safe, confidential, and non-judgemental environment with conscious avoidance of catastrophization) (Perry, 2008; Swetz et al., 2009).

6. Developing assertiveness skills including learning to set limits, to say 'no', and to ask for what you need (Keidel, 2002).

7. Being clear and consistent with oneself and others about boundaries and personal limit-setting including taking vacations and limiting overtime and time on-call (Jones, 2005; Perry, 2008; Swetz et al., 2009; Newell and MacNeil, 2010) and maintaining a sustainable workload (Maslach et al., 2001; Jones, 2005; Kuerer et al., 2007; Maslach and Leiter, 2008).

8. Diversifying one's workload, so that not all professional time involves providing care to the most distressed patients. Examples include adding research, teaching, or other activities to round out clinical service (Quill and Williamson, 1990; Levine et al., 2005; Kuerer et al., 2007; Le Blanc et al., 2007).

9. Continuing educational activities (Robinson et al., 2004; Kuerer et al., 2007).

Box 4.16.2 Continued

10. Identifying the one or two scenarios that are most difficult and exhausting for a professional, and identifying and reviewing potential responses to use when these situations arise.

11. Finding and focusing on the positive features of one's own and one's patients' experiences (Jones, 2005; Perry, 2008; Swetz et al., 2009).

12. Connecting regularly with a respectful team of professionals that meets regularly and shares a common goal or mission (Jones, 2005; Sinclair and Hamill, 2007; Swetz et al., 2009).

13. Develop an approach/philosophy to dealing with death/end-of-life care (Jones, 2005; Shanafelt et al., 2005a).

Organizational strategies

The organization within which any palliative care provider works sets the stage for how stressful the work is, and for how effectively the provider is able to defuse that stress. It is essential that health-care organizations allocate adequate resources necessary to do the job well and provide structures for addressing compassion fatigue (Pisanti et al., 2011).

Organizations can be the focus for important interventions to prevent or reduce burnout and compassion fatigue. Some strategies that may move organizations closer to these goals include:

1. Providing adequate resources for the job, including regular and supportive supervision, continuing education opportunities, days off without undue hassle, appropriate benefits, and an overall positive work climate (Jones, 2005; Sinclair and Hamill, 2007; Newell and MacNeil, 2010; Pisanti et al., 2011).

2. Ensure schedules that accommodate work–life balance for providers as much as possible (Jones, 2005; Sinclair and Hamill, 2007; Perry, 2008; Swetz et al., 2009).

3. Providing clinical staff with physical settings that are comforting or soothing and offering meeting spaces that are appropriately furnished and private (Pisanti et al., 2011).

4. Encouraging and supporting choice and control (Shanafelt et al., 2006) and promoting fairness and justice in the workplace (Maslach et al., 2001; Maslach, 2003; Jones, 2005).

5. Appropriate recognition and reward (Maslach et al., 2001).

6. Developing a supportive work community (Maslach et al., 2001; Maslach and Leiter, 2008).

7. Adequate supervision and mentoring (Graham and Ramirez, 2002; Jones, 2005; Mackereth et al., 2005; Balch and Copeland, 2007).

8. Providing space for personal items that anchor clinicians to their lives outside of work (Pisanti et al., 2011).

9. Developing an atmosphere of respect for the work performed by palliative care clinicians (Jones, 2005; Pisanti et al., 2011).

10. Open acknowledgement, in routine and in education programmes, that compassion fatigue is an expected occupational hazard, not a weakness (Sinclair and Hamill, 2007; Newell and MacNeil, 2010).

11. Developing an interdisciplinary care team with an ethos of collaborative practice among professionals that values participation, fairness, freedom of expression, and interdependence (Jones, 2005; Sinclair and Hamill, 2007; Swetz et al., 2009).

12. Regular discussions of challenging cases, in which all team members, regardless of role, are encouraged to contribute, in an atmosphere that is safe supportive and which avoids catastrophization.

13. Mindfulness-based stress reduction for team (Cohen-Katz et al., 2004, 2005a, 2005b).

14. Meaning-centred intervention for team (Fillion et al., 2009).

Strategies particularly focused in improving self-awareness are discussed later in the section on 'Self-awareness (mindfulness) strategies'.

Spirituality and meaning

Studies of caregivers in end-of-life care have highlighted the importance of spirituality and meaning in preventing burnout (Holland and Neimeyer, 2005; Boston and Mount, 2006; Harrison and Westwood, 2009). Caregivers in oncology who rated themselves as being religious had a decreased risk of burnout (Kash et al., 2000). Huggard (2008) studied 230 New Zealand physicians and found an inverse correlation between burnout and spirituality.

Reducing burnout

Reducing burnout and promoting job engagement must include three dimensions: personal care, professional development, and infrastructural initiatives. Practical measures that may be used to reduce burnout and promote job engagement are outlined in Box 4.16.2. If distress persists despite use of these practices, and particularly if any objective impairment in functioning occurs, the clinician should seek psychiatric evaluation and treatment.

Administrators and clinical leaders have a major role in preventing or intervening in burnout (Medland et al., 2004; Estryn-Behar et al., 2007; Williams et al., 2007; Sprinks, 2012).

Clinical leaders have a responsibility to monitor staff conflicts and to promote positive staff relations through the use of support and discussion groups. Palliative care services must help prepare staff members to deal with the emotional needs of the patient and family through the development of counselling skills. Stress inoculation training may be useful for teaching appropriate coping skills (Admi, 1997; Medland et al., 2004). Workshops on job stress followed by small group discussions of concerned personnel may also be useful. One-to-one discussions to discuss mutual concerns between employees experiencing a conflict are sometimes necessary. If this is not comfortable for either party, an outside professional counsellor could be used (Keidel, 2002). These organizational interventions to reduce burnout can have additional flow-on benefits of increased staff retention and satisfaction, reduced absenteeism and staff conflicts, and improved patient and family satisfaction.

Compassion fatigue

Palliative care clinicians navigate situations of severe distress and they do this challenging work in the face of the intense emotions of the incurably ill patients and their families (Alkema et al., 2008). Many of the family members may demand time and attention that is simultaneously required to be directed towards helping the patient die peacefully and without pain or distress. Since most palliative care clinicians consider attentiveness to such distress to be part of their mandate, it is near impossible for them not be affected in some way by these interactions.

Compassion fatigue refers to the emotional impact of working with people involved in traumatic life events such as terminal illness; it has been referred to as the 'cost of caring', that comes from continuous compassion directed towards people in crisis (Booth, 1991). Some consider compassion fatigue to be a form of post-traumatic stress disorder (PTSD) in professional carers (Booth, 1991). Compassion fatigue is also known as secondary or vicarious traumatization (Tabor, 2011).

Clinicians may be more vulnerable to compassion fatigue in some situations than others. This is particularly true of the care of young people, be they patients or the children of patients (Robins et al., 2009), and when they are exhausted, stressed, or overworked. The intense relationships that often occur between palliative care providers and patients and their families can themselves be sources of compassion fatigue. Sometimes intense exposure to multiple deaths can lead to a feeling of 'grief overload' (Vachon, 1995).

The effects of compassion fatigue may endure or worsen over time, developing into serious reactions that compromise a health-care provider's ability to interact in positive and helpful ways with patients and families (Firth-Cozens, 2001)

Regarding the relationship between compassion fatigue and burnout, while compassion fatigue may be one of the factors contributing to burnout, it is important to appreciate one can have compassion fatigue whilst at the same time maintaining engagement and enthusiasm for one's work and with no sign of burnout (Booth, 1991; Keidel, 2002; Slocum-Gori et al., 2013).

Symptoms of compassion fatigue

Symptoms of compassion fatigue are similar to the three classic features of PTSD: hyperarousal, disturbed sleep, or outbursts of anger, and hypervigilance; avoidance, 'not wanting to go there again', and the desire to avoid thoughts, feelings, and conversations associated with the patient's pain and suffering (Wright, 2004). Compassion fatigue can have a profound impact on personal well-being and function and express itself across psychological, cognitive, and interpersonal domains (Box 4.16.3). Clinicians with compassion fatigue often have intrusive thoughts or dreams, and psychological or physiological distress in response

---

Box 4.16.3 Impact of compassion fatigue

Psychological

- Strong emotions (sadness, anger, guilt, worry)
- Intrusive thoughts or images/nightmares
- Feeling numb or frozen
- Avoiding the patient/family or situation
- Somatic complaints (gastrointestinal distress, headaches, fatigue)
- Anxiety or agitation
- Compulsive or addictive behaviours (drinking, smoking, shopping sprees)
- Feeling isolated or personally responsible, with no back-up
- Inability to make self-protective measures leading to maladaptive or harmful behaviours such as overworking, decision-making difficulties and a loss of sensitivity to one's own needs.

Cognitive

- Mistrust of others (family, patient, other staff)
- Increased personal vulnerability or lack of safety
- Belief that others aren't competent to handle the problem
- Increased or decreased sense of power or control
- Increased cynicism
- Increased sense of personal responsibility or blame
- Belief that others don't understand the work that you do.

Interpersonal

- Withdrawal from the larger treatment team
- Withdrawal from personal relationships (because people 'don't understand')
- Difficulty trusting others personally and professionally
- Over-identifying with the distress of others leading to skewed boundaries in relationships
- Detachment from emotional situations or experiences (including the patient/family)
- Becoming easily irritated with others.

Adapted from *Pediatric Clinics of North America*, Volume 54, Issue 5, Rourke, M. T., Compassion fatigue in pediatric palliative care providers, pp.631–644, Copyright © 2007, with permission from Elsevier, http://www.sciencedirect.com/science/journal/00313955.

to reminders of work with the dying (Valent, 2002; Showalter, 2010). They may manifest as either over-involvement or detachment and these can impact on clinicians' relationships with their patients, colleagues, and family members.

Among the complications of compassion fatigue are several syndromic behaviour patterns: splitting, the so-called saviour syndrome, and detachment.

Splitting

Splitting is form of good–bad polarization. It involves perceiving oneself or other members of the care team as entirely good and helpful, and others as entirely bad and extremely unhelpful. It produces intra-team conflicts and tensions that compromise team work and the cohesiveness of the care team. Additionally, caregivers may demonstrate splitting between their 'good patients' and their 'bad patients'.

The saviour (in contrast to helper) syndrome

The ultimate denial of the traumatic tragedy of terminal illness is to avoid the tragedy by rescuing the patient. Taking on the role of the saviour is one of the manifestations of compassion fatigue. It avoids the role of helping (which just feels too hard) by devoting energies to rescuing the situation. Among oncologists with compassion fatigue the saviour syndrome is often manifested as a 'counterphobic determination to treat'.

Becoming detached

Clinicians with compassion fatigue may gradually or abruptly withdraw as the emotional intensity increases. This occurs most commonly when clinicians are working alone or not being part of a supportive and collaborative team when providing end-of-life care.

Strategies to mitigate compassion fatigue

Empathic engagement between clinician and patient is at the heart of palliative care. It is hard to imagine a palliative care clinician who is not occasionally emotionally impacted by their work. The challenge is how to prevent these normal responses developing in strongly negative and destructive ways. The usual recommendation for mitigating compassion fatigue is 'good professional boundaries' (Anewalt, 2009; Hall, 2011). While professional boundaries are important, exclusive reliance on this as the main self-care strategy to prevent secondary traumatization may result in objectification, detachment, and reduced empathy. Hence, the need to consider other ways. As with burnout there has been increasing focus on factors that mitigate against the effects of compassion fatigue.

Exquisite empathy

Qualitative research on outstanding therapists who were thriving in their work with traumatized clients, including palliative care patients and their families, has identified a variety of protective practices that enhance caregivers' professional satisfaction and help prevent or mitigate compassion fatigue (Harrison and Westwood, 2009). In particular, trauma therapists who engaged in *exquisite empathy*, defined as 'highly present, sensitively attuned, well-boundaried, heartfelt empathic engagement', were 'invigorated rather than depleted by their intimate professional connections with traumatized clients' and protected against compassion fatigue and burnout (Harrison and Westwood, 2009).

This idea, which has also been referred to as bidirectionality (Katz, 2006), refutes the commonly held notion that being empathic to dying patients must lead to emotional depletion (Pearlman, 1995; Figley, 2002) and it challenges the characterization of empathy as 'emotional liability'.

The practice of exquisite empathy is facilitated by clinician self-awareness and mindful communication skills (discussed later) which were identified in another study as the most important factor in psychologists' functioning well in the face of personal and professional stressors (Coster and Schwebel, 1997).

Resilience (hardiness) and coherence

Personal and professional resilience predicate the capacity for positive outcomes from caring even in the most challenging of circumstances. These positive outcomes have been referred to as compassion satisfaction and post-traumatic growth.

Compassion satisfaction is pleasure derived from the work of helping others. Acknowledging the risks of work-related secondary exposure to trauma, Stamm (2002) identified compassion satisfaction as a possible factor that counterbalances the risks of compassion fatigue and suggested that this may partially account for the remarkable resiliency of the human spirit.

Post-traumatic growth (Tedeschi and Calhoun, 2004) is characterized by positive changes in interpersonal relationships, sense of self, and philosophy of life subsequent to direct experience of a traumatic event that shakes the foundation of an individual's worldview (Tedeschi and Calhoun, 2004). Post-traumatic growth is not uncommon and may occur concurrently with negative sequelae of trauma (Tedeschi and Calhoun, 2004). The term describes the phenomenon of clinician growth and inspiration that results from witnessing positive sequelae of other people's experiences of trauma. This may include the clinician's feelings that his or her own life has been enriched, deepened, or empowered by witnessing the patient's or family's post-traumatic growth (Harrison and Westwood, 2009; Splevins et al., 2010). When patients experience meaning and peacefulness in relation to their approaching death, this enriches the lives of the clinicians involved. This phenomenon appears similar to the 'healing connections' identified by Mount and colleagues (Mount et al., 2007).

Research has provided empirical evidence for the construct of vicarious post-traumatic growth (Linley et al., 2005; Harrison and Westwood, 2009). Exemplary therapists who were thriving in their work with traumatized clients experienced positive shifts in their sense of meaning or spirituality. Therapists enrolled in a study (Harrison and Westwood, 2009) described having gained an expanded worldview, even paradoxically feeling enriched, as a result of witnessing the sequelae of other people's experiences of trauma. Research on exemplary oncology nurses has focused on feelings of personal growth and development derived from moments of connection, making moments matter, and energizing moments with their patients and their families (Perry, 2008).

Grieving strategies

Approaches that facilitate grieving may be useful particularly for clinicians who are exposed to frequent and multiple deaths. Approaches that have been suggested include departmental memorial services, journaling, attending a funeral, or participating in a post-bereavement family visit (Vachon, 1998).

Use of mindfulness strategies

Mindfulness strategies, which will be described in greater detail later in the chapter, focus on enhancing intrapersonal and interpersonal self-awareness and can assist practitioners in becoming more attentive to the presence of stress, to their relationship with the sources of stress, and to their own personal capacity to to self-monitor and be less emotionally reactive in stressful situations.

Use of wellness strategies

Wellness approaches have been strongly advocated as a means to mitigate against compassion fatigue (Mulligan, 2004; Benson and Magraith, 2005; Aycock and Boyle, 2009; Slatten et al., 2011) (see Box 4.16.2).

Moral distress

Clinicians working in palliative care are confronted with many ethically challenging situations. Sometimes the chosen course of clinical action runs contrary to what individual clinicians would see as the most ethically appropriate approach and yet they are expected to go along with the committed action plan that they ethically disagree with (Weissman, 2009). This is the scenario that creates moral distress.

Moral distress is a stress reaction characterized by feelings of frustration, anger, and anxiety. It occurs when an individual has a conviction of what is ethically correct but is constrained from acting in accordance with their convictions and often expected to act against their convictions (Andre, 2002; Rushton, 2006). External constraints that contribute to moral distress include power imbalances between members of the health-care team (the doctor has decided), patient or family preferences, poor communication between team members, pressure to reduce costs, fear of legal action, lack of administrative support, or hospital policies that may conflict with patient care needs. Although the phenomenon was initially described in nurses it has been identified among nearly all health-care professionals, including physicians.

Sources of moral distress in palliative care

While research has identified common sources of moral distress (Kalvemark et al., 2004; Cohen and Erickson, 2006; Ferrell, 2006; Rushton, 2006; Schluter et al., 2008), not every clinician will experience distress when faced with these situations, and some clinicians will experience distress from other circumstances.

- *Clinical decisions*: continued life support even though it is not in the best interest of the patient; inappropriate use of health-care resources, overaggressive care, nihilistic care, requests for cardiopulmonary resuscitation by terminally ill patients or their family members, inadequate pain relief, sedation at the end of life.

- *Communication issues*: inadequate communication about end-of-life care between providers and patients and families, false hope given to patients and families.

- *Resources*: when the interests of the organization override the interests of a particular patient because of limited resources or when working is situations in which appropriate medications, equipment, or staff are not available to provide optimal care.

- *Lack of staff time*: such as the distress of professional staff caused by the proportion of time devoted to administrative tasks rather than attending to the physical and psychological needs of patients and their families.

- *Rules and regulations*: this occurs when there is a conflict between the regulations and what the clinicians regard as the best for the patient. Moral distress can arise in situations in which clinicians break rules or when they are constrained by the rules against their better judgement.

Consequences of moral distress

Moral distress can commonly produce feelings of frustration, anger, and anxiety and of having been devalued and marginalized. Moral distress can be devastating, leading to nightmares, headaches, and depression (Schluter et al., 2008). Affected staff often feel disenfranchised and may be reluctant to divulge their distress and feelings of impotence. This can contribute to feelings of isolation, which is an additional threat to their self-worth. The issue of isolation is further confounded by the fact that in any given situation, not all of the involved clinicians will disagree with morality of the approach taken.

Moral distress can certainly be a factor contributing to burnout and, among nurses, it has been identified as a major risk factor for leaving either a department or the field of nursing entirely (Ferrell, 2006; Repenshek, 2009; Piers et al., 2011).

Moral distress, and the feeling that one has seriously compromised oneself or allowed oneself to be compromised tend to linger and, especially if repeated frequently, can impact adversely on self-worth. This has been called 'moral residue' (Hardingham, 2004; Epstein and Hamric, 2009).

Management of moral distress

Approaches to the management of moral distress should be developed at both an organizational level and at an individual level.

Organizational

Palliative care and hospice services must provide support resources and structures to decrease moral distress including a forum for discussing ethically troubling situations experienced in the daily practice. The development of an institutional and/or departmental culture of moral sensibility and commitment is probably the most important step that can be undertaken to relive the burden of moral distress. Development of a strong moral culture and the provision of support structures for ethical discussions can help reduce moral distress and moral residue (Kalvemark et al., 2004). An open and interactive approach to moral conflicts can assist care providers to cope better with ethical conflicts that will always occur in their day-to-day practice. Teamwork is important since interdisciplinary issues, particularly a lack of opportunity to discuss and achieve wide consensus regarding ethically sensitive clinical decisions, often contributes to moral distress. This work can be facilitated by the development of an ethics infrastructure including the availability of ethics consultations (Schneiderman et al., 2000; Schneiderman, 2006; Pfafflin et al., 2009; Romano et al., 2009).

When similar problems tend to recur in a work setting, this often signals that there are issues in the workplace or organizational dynamic that may be contributing. Consequently, remedial approaches should focus on the work environment and organizational issues. All involved parties must engage together to evaluate the work environment or team dynamic factors that may be generating these dilemmas. Generating factors need to be evaluated to distinguish between those which are amenable to change and those which are not. Those which are amenable to change need to be targeted. The participation of a skilled ethics consultant in such situations has been shown to help resolve underlying structural issues that sometime contribute to moral distress (Schneiderman et al., 2000; Pfafflin et al., 2009).

Individual

Palliative care staff should be trained and encouraged to recognize moral distress in their professional lives and to discuss their concerns with their peers. Managing a situation of moral distress starts with a careful evaluation of one's own position and then of the constraining issues of the other involved stakeholders. A key question is whether the constraining factors are amenable to change.

Many sources of moral distress are caused by constraints that are potentially amenable to change; for instance, the orders of a doctor, the opinion of a consultant, a family member, or a religious advisor to a patient. When constraints are potentially amenable to change, clinicians are encouraged to articulate their concerns and to possibly relieve the constraints through discussion, negotiation of the issues, or persuasion. This approach requires moral courage (Gallagher, 2011). Situations when clinicians fail to act on their concerns in the face of potentially resolvable obstacles (moral cowardice) may contribute to reactive distress or feelings of guilt for not having spoken out (Jameton, 1993).

Some sources of moral distress are caused by constraints that are rigid and which are not amenable to change. Examples may include constraints caused by rationing of limited clinical resources, and patients who demand life-prolonging interventions on the basis of inflexible vitalist religious considerations. In these situations, the primary strategy relates to coping with the challenge of providing care and trying to understand the moral reasoning that has led other stakeholders to conclusion that vary with one's own. This requires personal flexibility and adaptability. Coping theory suggests that when the preferred ethical approach cannot be achieved, flexible people can maintain a sense of control by finding an alternative satisfying way to conceptualize the situation (Thompson, 2009). This is personally and ethically challenging and it requires a different form of moral courage that incorporates the ability to see the problem from the perspective of someone else rather than one's own to be able to function and care without feeling compromised or violated. There is indeed enhanced control in the 'capacity for choice', rather than reflex, as to how one sees the differing moral perspectives.

Clinicians need to develop an appreciation that there are different ways of reasoning in ethical dilemmas, a better understanding of their own process of ethical decision-making, and create a readiness to cope with situation when other critical stakeholders come to different conclusion to their own. Team and personal strategies need to be developed to cope with situations being generated by factors that cannot be changed. Coping and flexibility are vital skills and often there is more than one right way. Clinicians need to develop an understanding that circumstances may render their best moral option unworkable in prevailing circumstances and that sometimes the best we can do is a compromise. Learning to compromise, and the insight that compromise often comes from strength rather than weakness, is an important part of 'self-compassion'.

In the face of situations contributing to moral distress there is great healing wisdom in the Serenity Prayer: 'God grant me the serenity to accept the things I cannot change, the courage to change the things that I can, the wisdom to know the difference.' This approach, though soothing, can contribute to complacency. Betty Cherny (1932–2000) championed an inspirational version that challenges the reader to push the boundaries to render obstacles one considered fixed, as changeable: 'God grant me the serenity to accept the things I cannot change, the courage to change the things that I can, the wisdom to know the difference and the chutzpah [audacity in Yiddish] to push the boundaries.'

Self-awareness (mindfulness) strategies for prevention of burnout, compassion fatigue, and moral distress

Traditionally self-care strategies have emphasized the value of 'good professional boundaries' and 'effective self-care strategies outside the workplace.' These alone, however, can lead to emotional detachment by the clinician, leading to less job satisfaction, less patient-centred care, and less satisfied patients (Jackson et al., 2008).

Another approach to addressing loss of meaning and lack of control in life is developing greater self-awareness or mindfulness which includes four cardinal skills (Epstein et al., 2007):

1. The ability to notice and observe sensations, thoughts, and feelings even though they might be unpleasant

2. The ability to lower one's tendency to respond reactively to emotionally charged experiences

3. An enhanced ability to react with awareness and intention rather than being on reactive 'auto-pilot'

4. Focusing on experience, not the labels or judgements we apply to them (e.g. feeling an emotion rather than wondering if it is okay to feel that emotion).

It is proposed that by enhancing intrapersonal and interpersonal self-awareness practitioners can become more attentive to the presence of stress, to their relationship with the sources of stress, and to their own personal capacity to 'to self-monitor, to be less emotionally reactive in stressful situations, and to respond more skillfully to patient and family's needs' (Novack et al., 1999). This approach reduces burnout and compassion fatigue and it enhances the potential for job engagement and compassion satisfaction.

Kearney at al. have suggested that 'clinicians working in end of life care who are experiencing distress related to burnout, compassion fatigue or moral distress who use self-care strategies alone may feel as though they are drowning and barely able to come up for air, whereas self-care with self-awareness is like learning to breathe underwater' (Kearney et al., 2009).

There are a number of practical ways of enhancing self-awareness and mindfulness. These include initiatives such as participation in educational projects (Robinson et al., 2004; Le Blanc et al., 2007), and peer-support (Balint) groups (Rabinowitz et al., 1996; Benson and Magraith, 2005; Kjeldmand and Holmstrom, 2008; Bar-Sela et al., 2012). Two methods of enhancing self-awareness that have empirical data to support their effectiveness are mindful practice training (Epstein, 1999; Kabat-Zinn, 2003; Grossman et al., 2004; Shanafelt et al., 2005b; Krasner et al., 2009) and reflective writing (Frisina et al., 2004, Harris, 2006).

Mindful practice and mindful communication training

Mindful practice describes four qualities that are inherent in the behaviour of exemplary clinicians: *attentiveness* refers to the capacity to observe without making judgements that would otherwise distort or diminish one's capacity to understand. This involves monitoring one's own biases, thoughts, and emotions: observing the observer observing the observed. *Critical curiosity* refers to the ability to open up to possibilities, rather than premature closure and discarding new information or insights. *Informed flexibility* (sometimes referred to as having a 'beginner's mind') refers to the ability to be able to adopt a fresh perspective or to consider more than one perspective simultaneously rather than taking only a single fixed perspective on a problem. Finally *presence* which involves being there physically, mentally, and emotionally for patients, and accurately communicating an understanding of the patient's concerns and feelings back to the patient (empathy) (Epstein et al., 2007). This approach is predicated on the characteristics of mindfulness described earlier.

Mindful communication brings this approach to the situation of challenging communication encounters between clinicians and their patients (and family members of patients) and between professional colleagues in their professional deliberations and interdisciplinary discussions. The aim of mindful practice and communication training is to contribute to the ability of clinicians to respond to challenging situations with more flexibility, greater sensitivity, and less reactivity (Shapiro et al., 2007) and enhance their capacity to be more appreciative and forgiving of themselves (self-compassion) as well as to have greater empathy for others (Shapiro and Izett, 2008).

Researchers and educators from Rochester University School of Medicine, New York, United States, reported the results of an intensive course in 'mindful communication' which included a variety of self-awareness and body-awareness exercises, narratives about meaningful clinical experiences, appreciative interviews, didactic material, and discussion. The 70 participating physicians not only reported lower burnout and lower psychological distress, but also greater empathy and psychosocial orientation in care (Krasner et al., 2009; Beckman et al., 2012).

Strategies to teach mindful practice have been developed and initiated at a number of sites including the Stress Reduction

---

Box 4.16.4 Some suggested self-care and self-awareness practices in the workplace

- As you walk from your car to your workplace or through the corridors of your workplace, attend carefully to the sensation of contact between your feet and the ground.

- Set your watch or telephone alarm for midday each day. Use this as a prompt to perform some simple act of centring, for example, take four deep, slow breaths; think of a loved one; recite a favourite line of poetry or a prayer; imagine weights around your waist and the words 'ground, down'.

- Reward yourself after the completion of a task, for example, an early coffee break.

- Call a 'time out' (usually just a few minutes) as way of dealing with emotional flooding after a traumatic event; call a colleague saying, 'I need a walk' or take a break.

- Stop at a window in your workplace and notice something in nature; consciously give it your full attention for a few moments.

- Take half a minute of silence or take turns to choose and read a poem at the beginning of weekly interdisciplinary team meetings.

- Before going into the next patient's room, pause and bring your attention to the sensation of your breathing for two to five breaths.

- Take a snack before the end of clinic to prevent neuroglycopenia.

- Stay connected to the outside world during the day, for example, check in with loved ones.

- Multitask self-care, for example, dictate or meditate while using the treadmill in your office.

- Use the suggested 20 seconds of hand washing in creative ways, for example, pay attention to the sensation of the water on your skin and allow yourself to sink into this experience; make this an act of conscious receiving by acknowledging to yourself 'I am worthy of my own time'; or repeat a favourite line from a poem or prayer; or sing yourself 'Happy Birthday!'

- Don't be afraid to ask the question 'Is it time for a break?'

- Deliberately make connections during the day with colleagues and with patients, for example, use humour; look for something particular or unusual in the patient's room; or notice patient's birth date or age.

- Keep a notebook and write 'field notes' on traumatic or meaningful encounters and events; occasionally take time at interdisciplinary team meetings to share this material.

- Deliberately develop a 'role-shedding ritual' at the end of the day, for example, pay attention to putting away your stethoscope or hanging up your white coat; use the drive home from work deliberately, for example, take the longer, more interesting route; listen attentively to the news, music, or books-on-tape.

Text extracts reproduced permission from Kearney, M.K. et al, Self-care of physicians caring for patients at the end of life: "Being connected... a key to my survival", *Journal of American Medication Association* (JAMA), Volume 301, Issue 11, pp.1155-64, Copyright © 2009.

and Relaxation Program of the University of Massachusetts Medical Center (<http://www.umassmed.edu/cfm/index.aspx>) (Kabat-Zinn, 2003), the American Academy on Communication in Healthcare (<http://www.aachonline.org>), the Northwest Center for Physician Well Being (<http://www.tfme.org>), and the Mindful Practice Programs at the University of Rochester (Epstein et al., 2007). The Mindful Practice Program at the University of Rochester has published a curriculum which is also available online (Epstein et al., 2007).

Reflective writing

Writing in a reflective and emotionally expressive way is another form of self-care that enhances self-awareness. Physical and psychological benefits of expressive writing have been demonstrated in patients (Smyth et al., 1999; Stanton et al., 2002; Petrie et al., 2004; Cepeda et al., 2008; Morgan et al., 2008; O'Cleirigh et al., 2008) and this practice has been promoted as a tool to develop reflection and empathic engagement in clinicians (Charon, 2001; Brady et al., 2002).

In this approach, clinicians are encouraged to diarize challenging and/or rewarding clinical encounters, recording personal thoughts and along with the objective clinical data of the narrative (Pennebaker, 1997; DeSalvo, 1999; Charon, 2001; Spann, 2004). Narratives can be shared and explored in small group discussions or in one-on-one supervision or debriefing. The aims of the discussion are to facilitate a reflective/evaluative approach to understanding one's thoughts, thought processes, feelings, and responses. This approach aims to help foster better self-understanding, and the mindfulness skills described in the previous section.

Practising self-care

Although clinician self-care may happen through some of the formal practices and methods discussed earlier, it may also happen in countless informal ways as an everyday part of a physician's working life. Many experienced clinicians have evolved what are sometimes unique yet time-tested methods of self-care. A collection of suggested self-care and self-awareness practices in the workplace are listed in Box 4.16.4.

Conclusion: ongoing tasks

There remains abundant scope for research to address the prevention and management of burnout, compassion fatigue, and moral distress in palliative care. Specifically, there remains relatively little data on the frequency and specific nature and impact of compassion fatigue and moral distress among palliative care clinicians and the knowledge base regarding strategies for management remains largely anecdotal with only a very limited evidence base to inform practice beyond expert opinion. Researchers will be aided by the well-validated tools that are available to measure burnout (Maslach et al., 1996), compassion fatigue (Bride et al., 2007), and moral distress (Eizenberg et al., 2009). We look forward to being able to revise our next edition with additional knowledge you may have generated.

Online materials

Complete references for this chapter are available online at <http://www.oxfordmedicine.com>.

References

Ablett, J.R. and Jones, R.S. (2007). Resilience and well-being in palliative care staff: a qualitative study of hospice nurses' experience of work. *Psycho-Oncology*, 16, 733–740.

Andre, J. (2002). Moral distress in healthcare. *Bioethics Forum*, 18, 44–46.

Anewalt, P. (2009). Fired up or burned out? Understanding the importance of professional boundaries in home healthcare and hospice. *Home Healthcare Nurse*, 27, 590–597.

Antonovsky, H. and Sagy, S. (1986). The development of a sense of coherence and its impact on responses to stress situations. *Journal of Social Psychology*, 126, 213–225.

Arigoni, F., Bovier, P.A., Mermillod, B., Waltz, P., and Sappino, A.P. (2008). Prevalence of burnout among Swiss cancer clinicians, paediatricians and general practitioners: who are most at risk? *Supportive Care in Cancer*, 17, 75–81.

Armstrong, J. and Holland, J. (2004). Surviving the stresses of clinical oncology by improving communication. *Oncology*, 18, 363–368; discussion 373–375.

Aycock, N., and Boyle, D. (2009). Interventions to manage compassion fatigue in oncology nursing. *Clinical Journal of Oncology Nursing*, 13, 183–191.

Balch, C.M. and Copeland, E. (2007). Stress and burnout among surgical oncologists: a call for personal wellness and a supportive workplace environment. *Annals of Surgical Oncology*, 14, 3029–3032.

Beckman, H.B., Wendland, M., Mooney, C., *et al.* (2012). The impact of a program in mindful communication on primary care physicians. *Academic Medicine*, 87, 815–819.

Bernardi, M., Catania, G., and Marceca, F. (2005). [The world of nursing burnout. A literature review]. *Professioni Infermieristiche*, 58, 75–79.

Booth, E.W. (1991). Compassion fatigue. *Journal of the American Medical Association*, 266, 362.

Bragard, I., Razavi, D., Marchal, S., *et al.* (2006). Teaching communication and stress management skills to junior physicians dealing with cancer patients: a Belgian Interuniversity Curriculum. *Supportive Care in Cancer*, 14, 454–461.

Bride, B.E., Radey, M., and Figley, C.R. (2007). Measuring compassion fatigue. *Clinical Social Work Journal*, 35, 155–163.

Cohen-Katz, J., Wiley, S., Capuano, T., Baker, D.M., Deitrick, L., and Shapiro, S. (2005a). The effects of mindfulness-based stress reduction on nurse stress and burnout: a qualitative and quantitative study, part III. *Holistic Nursing Practice*, 19, 78–86.

Cohen-Katz, J., Wiley, S.D., Capuano, T., Baker, D.M., Kimmel, S., and Shapiro, S. (2005b). The effects of mindfulness-based stress reduction on nurse stress and burnout, Part II: A quantitative and qualitative study. *Holistic Nursing Practice*, 19, 26–35.

Cohen-Katz, J., Wiley, S.D., Capuano, T., Baker, D.M., and Shapiro, S. (2004). The effects of mindfulness-based stress reduction on nurse stress and burnout: a quantitative and qualitative study. *Holistic Nursing Practice*, 18, 302–308.

Cohen, J.S. and Erickson, J.M. (2006). Ethical dilemmas and moral distress in oncology nursing practice. *Clinical Journal of Oncology Nursing*, 10, 775–780.

Coulehan, J. and Granek, I.A. (2012). Commentary: 'I hope I'll continue to grow': rubrics and reflective writing in medical education. *Academic Medicine*, 87, 8–10.

Epstein, R.M. (1999). Mindful practice. *Journal of the American Medical Association*, 282, 833–839.

Epstein, R.M., Quill, T., Krasner, M., and McDonald, S. (2007). *A Curriculum in Mindful Practice for Students and Residents: Faculty Manual*. [Online] Available at: <http://www.urmc.rochester.edu/education/md/documents/MindfulPracticeFacilitatorManual_Final.pdf>.

Estryn-Behar, M., Van Der Heijden, B.I., Oginska, H., *et al.* (2007). The impact of social work environment, teamwork characteristics, burnout, and personal factors upon intent to leave among European nurses. *Medical Care*, 45, 939–950.

Fallowfield, L., Jenkins, V., Farewell, V., Saul, J., Duffy, A., and Eves, R. (2002). Efficacy of a Cancer Research UK communication skills training model for oncologists: a randomised controlled trial. *The Lancet*, 359, 650–656.

Fallowfield, L., Jenkins, V., Farewell, V., and Solis-Trapala, I. (2003). Enduring impact of communication skills training: results of a 12-month follow-up. *British Journal of Cancer*, 89, 1445–1449.

Fearon, C. and Nicol, M. (2011). Strategies to assist prevention of burnout in nursing staff. *Nursing Standard*, 26, 35–39.

Ferrell, B.R. (2006). Understanding the moral distress of nurses witnessing medically futile care. *Oncology Nursing Forum*, 33, 922–930.

Figley, C.R. (2002). Compassion fatigue: psychotherapists' chronic lack of self care. *Journal of Clinical Psychology*, 58, 1433–1441.

Goodman, M.J. and Schorling, J.B. (2012). A mindfulness course decreases burnout and improves well-being among healthcare providers. *International Journal of Psychiatry in Medicine*, 43, 119–128.

Graham, J. and Ramirez, A. (2002). Improving the working lives of cancer clinicians. *European Journal of Cancer Care*, 11, 188–192.

Graham, J., Ramirez, A.J., Cull, A., Finlay, I., Hoy, A., and Richards, M.A. (1996). Job stress and satisfaction among palliative physicians. *Palliative Medicine*, 10, 185–194.

Harrison, R.L. and Westwood, M.J. (2009). Preventing vicarious traumatization of mental health therapists: Identifying protective practices. *Psychotherapy*, 46, 203–219.

Holland, J.M. and Neimeyer, R.A. (2005). Reducing the risk of burnout in end-of-life care settings: the role of daily spiritual experiences and training. *Palliative & Supportive Care*, 3, 173–181.

Howe, A., Smajdor, A., and Stoeckl, A. (2012). Towards an understanding of resilience and its relevance to medical training. *Medical Education*, 46, 349–356.

Jones, S.H. (2005). A self-care plan for hospice workers. *American Journal of Hospice and Palliative Medicine*, 22, 125–128.

Kalvemark, S., Hoglund, A.T., Hansson, M.G., Westerholm, P., and Arnetz, B. (2004). Living with conflicts-ethical dilemmas and moral distress in the health care system. *Social Science & Medicine*, 58, 1075–1084.

Kearney, M.K., Weininger, R.B., Vachon, M.L., Harrison, R.L., and Mount, B.M. (2009). Self-care of physicians caring for patients at the end of life: 'Being connected . . . a key to my survival'. *Journal of the American Medical Association*, 301, 1155–1164, E1.

Keidel, G.C. (2002). Burnout and compassion fatigue among hospice caregivers. *American Journal of Hospice and Palliative Medicine*, 19, 200–205.

Krasner, M.S., Epstein, R.M., Beckman, H., *et al.* (2009). Association of an educational program in mindful communication with burnout, empathy, and attitudes among primary care physicians. *Journal of the American Medical Association*, 302, 1284–1293.

Kuerer, H.M., Eberlein, T.J., Pollock, R.E., *et al.* (2007). Career satisfaction, practice patterns and burnout among surgical oncologists: report on the quality of life of members of the Society of Surgical Oncology. *Annals of Surgical Oncology*, 14, 3043–3053.

Le Blanc, P.M., Hox, J.J., Schaufeli, W.B., Taris, T.W., and Peeters, M.C.W. (2007). Take care! The evaluation of a team-based burnout intervention program for oncology care providers. *Journal of Applied Psychology*, 92, 213–227.

Leiter, M.P., Frank, E., and Matheson, T.J. (2009). Demands, values, and burnout: relevance for physicians. *Canadian Family Physician*, 55, 1224–1225.e1–6.

Levine, R.B., Hebert, R.S., and Wright, S.M. (2005). Resident research and scholarly activity in internal medicine residency training programs. *Journal of General Internal Medicine*, 20, 155–159.

Lovell, B.L., Lee, R.T., and Frank, E. (2009). May I long experience the joy of healing: professional and personal wellbeing among physicians from a Canadian province. *BMC Family Practice*, 10, 18.

Mackereth, P.A., White, K., Cawthorn, A., and Lynch, B. (2005). Improving stressful working lives: complementary therapies, counselling and clinical supervision for staff. *European Journal of Oncology Nursing*, 9, 147–154.

Maslach, C. (2003). Job burnout: new directions in research and intervention. *Current Directions in Psychological Science*, 12, 189–192.

Maslach, C., Jackson, S.E., Leiter, M., Schaufeli, W.B., and Schwab, R.L. (1996). *The Maslach Burnout Inventory* (3rd ed.). Palo Alto, CA: Consulting Psychologists Press.

Maslach, C. and Leiter, M.P. (2008). Early predictors of job burnout and engagement. *Journal of Applied Psychology*, 93, 498–512.

Maslach, C., Schaufeli, W.B., and Leiter, M.P. (2001). Job burnout. *Annual Review of Psychology*, 52, 397–422.

Masterson-Allen, S., Mor, V., Laliberte, L., and Monteiro, L. (1985). Staff burnout in a hospice setting. *The Hospice Journal*, 1, 1–15.

Meier, D.E., Back, A.L., and Morrison, R.S. (2001). The inner life of physicians and care of the seriously ill. *Journal of the American Medical Association*, 286, 3007–3014.

Newell, J.M. and MacNeil, G.A. (2010). Professional burnout, vicarious trauma, secondary traumatic stress, and compassion fatigue: a review of theoretical terms, risk factors, and preventive methods for clinicians and researchers. *Best Practices in Mental Health*, 6, 57–68.

Payne, N. (2001). Occupational stressors and coping as determinants of burnout in female hospice nurses. *Journal of Advanced Nursing*, 33, 396–405.

Perry, B. (2008). Why exemplary oncology nurses seem to avoid compassion fatigue. *Canadian Oncology Nursing Journal*, 18, 87–99.

Pisanti, R., van der Doef, M., Maes, S., Lazzari, D., and Bertini, M. (2011). Job characteristics, organizational conditions, and distress/well-being among Italian and Dutch nurses: a cross-national comparison. *International Journal of Nursing Studies*, 48, 829–837.

Portenoy, R.K., Coyle, N., Kash, K.M., *et al.* (1997). Determinants of the willingness to endorse assisted suicide. A survey of physicians, nurses, and social workers. *Psychosomatics*, 38, 277–287.

Quill, T.E. and Williamson, P.R. (1990). Healthy approaches to physician stress. *Archives of Internal Medicine*, 150, 1857–1861.

Ramirez, A.J., Graham, J., Richards, M.A., Cull, A., and Gregory, W.M. (1996). Mental health of hospital consultants: the effects of stress and satisfaction at work. *The Lancet*, 347, 724–728.

Robinson, K., Sutton, S., von Gunten, C.F., *et al.* (2004). Assessment of the Education for Physicians on End-of-Life Care (EPEC) Project. *Journal of Palliative Medicine*, 7, 637–645.

Rokach, A. (2005). Caring for those who care for the dying: coping with the demands on palliative care workers. *Palliative & Supportive Care*, 3, 325–332.

Rourke, M.T. (2007). Compassion fatigue in pediatric palliative care providers. *Pediatric Clinics of North America*, 54, 631–644.

Rushton, C.H. (2006). Defining and addressing moral distress: tools for critical care nursing leaders. *AACN Advanced Critical Care*, 17, 161–168.

Rushton, C.H., Sellers, D.E., Heller, K.S., Spring, B., Dossey, B.M., and Halifax, J. (2009). Impact of a contemplative end-of-life training program: being with dying. *Palliative & Supportive Care*, 7, 405–414.

Schneiderman, L.J., Gilmer, T., and Teetzel, H.D. (2000). Impact of ethics consultations in the intensive care setting: a randomized, controlled trial. *Critical Care Medicine*, 28, 3920–3924.

Shanafelt, T., Chung, H., White, H., and Lyckholm, L. J. (2006). Shaping your career to maximize personal satisfaction in the practice of oncology. *Journal of Clinical Oncology*, 24, 4020–4026.

Shanafelt, T. and Dyrbye, L. (2012). Oncologist burnout: causes, consequences, and responses. *Journal of Clinical Oncology*, 30, 1235–1241.

Shanafelt, T.D., Oreskovich, M.R., Dyrbye, L.N., *et al.* (2012). Avoiding burnout: the personal health habits and wellness practices of US surgeons. *Annals of Surgery*, 255, 625–633.

Shanafelt, T.D., West, C., Zhao, X., *et al.* (2005b). Relationship between increased personal well-being and enhanced empathy among internal medicine residents. *Journal of General Internal Medicine*, 20, 559–564.

Showalter, S.E. (2010). Compassion fatigue: what is it? Why does it matter? Recognizing the symptoms, acknowledging the impact, developing the tools to prevent compassion fatigue, and strengthen the professional already suffering from the effects. *American Journal of Hospice and Palliative Medicine*, 27, 239–242.

Sinclair, H.A.H. and Hamill, C. (2007). Does vicarious traumatisation affect oncology nurses? A literature review. *European Journal of Oncology Nursing*, 11, 348–356.

Stamm, B.H. (2002). Measuring compassion satisfaction as well as fatigue: developmental history of the Compassion Satisfaction and Fatigue Test. In C.R. Figley (ed.) *Treating Compassion Fatigue*, pp. 107–119. New York: Brunner-Routledge.

Swetz, K.M., Harrington, S.E., Matsuyama, R.K., Shanafelt, T.D., and Lyckholm, L.J. (2009). Strategies for avoiding burnout in hospice and palliative medicine: peer advice for physicians on achieving longevity and fulfillment. *Journal of Palliative Medicine*, 12, 773–777.

Tedeschi, R.G. and Calhoun, L.G. (2004). Posttraumatic growth: conceptual foundations and empirical evidence. *Psychological Inquiry*, 15, 1–18.

Vachon, M.L. (1995). Staff stress in hospice/palliative care: a review. *Palliative Medicine*, 9, 91–122.

Vachon, M.L. (1998). Caring for the caregiver in oncology and palliative care. *Seminars in Oncology Nursing*, 14, 152–157.

Vachon, M.L. (1999). Reflections on the history of occupational stress in hospice/palliative care. *The Hospice Journal*, 14, 229–246.

Vachon, M.L.S. (2008). Oncology staff stress and related interventions. In J.C. Holland, W.S. Breitbart, P.B. Jacobsen, M.S. Lederberg, M.J. Loscalzo, and R. McCorkle (eds.) *Psycho-Oncology*, pp. 2111–2143. New York: Oxford University Press.

Wald, H.S., Reis, S.P., Monroe, A.D., and Borkan, J.M. (2010). 'The Loss of My Elderly Patient': Interactive reflective writing to support medical students' rites of passage. *Medical Teacher*, 32, e178–184.

Wallace, J.E., Lemaire, J.B., and Ghali, W.A. (2009). Physician wellness: a missing quality indicator. *The Lancet*, 374, 1714–1721.

Weissman, D.E. (2009). Moral distress in palliative care. *Journal of Palliative Medicine*, 12, 865–866.

Integrative oncology in palliative medicine

Gary Deng and Barrie R. Cassileth

Introduction to integrative oncology in palliative medicine

Patients under palliative care, facing poor prognoses and a heavy symptom burden, often seek health-care practices and agents outside of mainstream medicine (Hyodo et al., 2005; Molassiotis et al., 2005). Collectively these modalities often are termed 'complementary and alternative medicine' (CAM), to describe a diverse group of therapies that range from unproved alternative 'cures' offering false hope, to adjunctive complementary therapies that provide legitimate supportive care and that comprise integrative oncology. Although complementary therapies and alternative approaches are sometimes discussed under the umbrella of CAM, it is clinically and conceptually necessary to distinguish between the two because they are profoundly different in approach. The acronym is an easy but incorrect and counterproductive conflation of two unrelated approaches.

In the cancer setting, 'alternative' therapies generally are promoted for use instead of standard treatment, despite the fact that there are no viable 'alternatives' to mainstream cancer treatment. Alternative purveyors cater to people who have lost confidence in or grown antagonistic to mainstream medicine. In palliative care, these may be patients aware of their poor prognosis and limited therapeutic options, but unready to give up the hope of cure. Alternative therapies by definition are not supported by evidence. If they were backed by solid data, they would not be 'alternative', but used instead as viable treatments. Alternative regimens typically are costly and potentially harmful, either directly through physiological activity, or indirectly when patients forego legitimate cancer treatment in favour of 'alternatives'. Patients in palliative care are especially vulnerable to these schemes, as they often promise a cure even in advanced or end-stage disease.

Complementary therapies, conversely, are used to control pain and other symptoms, enhance physical, mental, and spiritual well-being, and optimize quality of life for patients and their families. These goals are shared by the World Health Organization, the American Cancer Society, and the Society for Integrative Oncology (World Health Organization, 2006; Deng et al., 2009; American Cancer Society, 2012). Complementary or integrative therapies ease the symptoms associated with cancer and treatment side effects. Unlike 'alternative therapies', they are never offered as substitutes for mainstream treatment, but rather as adjuncts to proper care. Complementary therapies address physical and emotional symptoms. Thus, they are palliative and especially helpful for both patients and family members during end-stage disease. Complementary therapies are evidence-based and rational, and have a highly favourable risk/benefit ratio. Currently the terms 'integrative medicine', 'integrative oncology', and 'complementary therapies' denote incorporating adjunctive therapies that play a vital supporting role in optimal care (Cassileth et al., 2005; Remen, 2008). Some institutions use the term 'complementary and integrative medicine' (CIM) in another effort to distinguish their work from the 'alternative therapies' that fall under the 'complementary and alternative medicine/CAM' umbrella. The distinction is essential, and patients and oncologists should be aware of this unfortunate terminology issue.

Complementary/integrative therapies are increasingly available not only directly to patients on a private or in-home basis, but also in some hospitals and clinics. Health-care professionals should steer patients away from harmful or useless alternative therapies while making helpful complementary therapies available to patients and increasing patient awareness of those services.

This chapter summarizes the state of integrative medicine and medical oncology in the current health-care system. We discuss helpful complementary therapies applicable to palliative medicine and also describe the unproven alternatives that are widely proffered to patients and families internationally. When both approaches have been conflated for research purposes, we use the acronym CAM but, to the extent possible in terms of available information, discuss each separately.

Complementary therapies in the current health-care system

No longer a collection of covert practices (Cassileth et al., 1984), new approaches became increasingly visible in the 1990s, driven by public fascination with unconventional therapies, a growing acceptance of therapies from other cultures, legislative and regulatory changes propelled by various interest groups, and publications documenting the benefits of complementary modalities in symptom control. A 2012 Google search of 'alternative therapy' yielded 25.5 million hits. It is a multibillion dollar business in the United States (Nahin et al., 2009) and of equivalent impact and importance throughout the developed world. The popularity of both legitimate and unproven methods also has affected every component of the health-care system and all specialties of medicine, including palliative care. It has left its mark on the thinking and practice of physicians and other health professionals, and has broadened patients' involvement and participation in their own care.

Prevalence

Prevalence rates concerning complementary and/or 'alternative' therapies ('CAM') internationally vary from less than 10% to more than 70% (Molassiotis et al., 2005; Barnes et al., 2008). The wide range is attributable primarily to variable interpretations and definitions of CAM. Some surveys use broad definitions that include lifestyle activities such as weight loss efforts, exercise, church attendance, and group counselling, while other surveys specify only the use of herbal products. Approximately 40% of adults use CAM therapies in the United States (Mao et al., 2011), with increasing use by cancer patients (Fouladbakhsh and Stommel, 2010) and a strong association among patients under palliative care (Hyodo et al., 2005; Molassiotis et al., 2005).

A consistent finding in cancer patient surveys is that users typically are younger, more educated, and more affluent, with the desire and ability to play an active role in their own care. Interestingly, however, some patients use products that lack sufficient information or fail to consult with their own health-care team (Hyodo et al., 2005). Many also tend to equate a lack of information about adverse effects with implied safety (Wood et al., 2003).

This dichotomy presents a key issue that must be recognized on the front lines of patient care: not only is the treatment of disease important, but so too are the myriad physical, emotional, psychosocial, and spiritual needs that arise as a result of serious illness. Patient and family attempts to 'do something more' reveal the unmet psychological and physical needs of these patients, which require attention and are not likely to resolve on their own.

The 1994 United States legislation known as the Dietary Supplement Health and Education Act allowed 'dietary supplements', including herbs, to be sold without US Food and Drug Administration review (US Food and Drug Administration, 2014). The sales of dietary and herbal supplements skyrocketed thereafter, despite media reports about safety concerns and questionable effectiveness and public confusion about the vast array of products. According to the Natural Products Association, annual sales of dietary supplements reached US$26.9 billion in 2009, including US$5 billion in sales and a 5% growth rate for herbs (Natural Products Association, 2012). The ever-expanding variety of both over-the-counter remedies and new age therapies, coupled with instant access to health-related information on the Internet are key contributors to this boom.

Public access to misinformation and quackery

CAM is an open and public issue today, discussed in the mass media and readily found on the Internet. Moreover, practitioners and product promoters widely advertise misinformation in all media. Product marketers produce infomercials, mass-mail newsletters and catalogues, and engage in multi-level marketing schemes, all with minimal to no regulatory oversight. Information available to the public varies widely in accuracy, and misinformation about health issues is widespread.

As early as 1999, the US Federal Trade Commission (FTC) announced that it had identified approximately 800 websites promoting and selling phony cures for cancer and other serious ailments in an estimated 15,000–17,000 health-related sites (FTC, 1999; Brann and Anderson, 2002). Because millions of such sites exist today, it is likely that those selling bogus treatments have increased accordingly. More recently, the FTC launched a campaign to address bogus cancer cures directly with consumers in attempts to stem this trend (FTC, 2008a, 2008b).

Recognition of legitimate therapies by mainstream medicine

Legitimate complementary therapies have been increasingly recognized and integrated as important adjuncts to mainstream care at many medical institutions. The research landscape experienced several shifts from commentaries in the 1970s expressing concerns about quackery, to surveys of patients' knowledge and use of unproven methods in the 1980s and 1990s, to reports of actual research results in the mid 1990s. In 1996–1997, the National Library of Medicine added many new related search terms to its medical subject headings (MeSH), and began to cover alternative medicine journals previously not reviewed for inclusion in MEDLINE®.

Studies over the last two decades strongly support the use of rational, non-invasive, and inexpensive evidence-based modalities. These include acupuncture, massage therapy, music, fitness/physical activity, nutrition and mind–body techniques, which take advantage of the reciprocal relationship between the mind and body. In addition, the application and insistence of rigorous evidence within the field of integrative oncology is well established. Comprehensive evidence-based guidelines are available from both the Society for Integrative Oncology and the American College of Chest Physicians (Cassileth et al., 2007; Deng et al., 2009). Other organizations have also been established for the cause of integrating complementary therapies with mainstream care, for example, the Consortium of Academic Health Centers for Integrative Medicine (a group of 50 institutions) whose goal is to advance the principles and practice of legitimate integrative health care within academic institutions.

Increased research funding also has played an important part both by expanding the body of evidence for some complementary therapies, while debunking other approaches. The National Center of Complementary and Alternative Medicine (NCCAM) and the National Cancer Institute (NCI) Office of Cancer Complementary and Alternative Medicine (OCCAM), both divisions of the National Institutes of Health (NIH), each oversees approximately $120 million in annual support of complementary and alternative related research. More than 2500 projects funded by NCCAM in the last decade yielded over 3000 peer-reviewed scientific articles (NCCAM, 2012).

A health insurance programme in western Washington state covered 13.7% of its enrolees in 2002 for CAM claims, including acupuncture, naturopathy, massage, and chiropractic (Lafferty et al., 2006), and more than 30 major insurers in the United States cover more than one method. Coverage varies by state, with some carriers requiring a prescription or supervision by a physician. Acupuncture, massage therapy, and other complementary services are variably covered by insurers. Socialized medical programmes tend to focus on providing a small number of therapies. For example, the most commonly offered British National Health Service modalities were counselling (82% of 142 centres), although counselling is not a complementary or alternative modality, reflexology (62%), aromatherapy (59%), reiki (43%), and massage (42%) (Egan et al., 2012).

Expanding insurance coverage for these therapies reflects consumer demand along with managed care efforts to control costs. CAM users often have chronic conditions and use more health-care resources. If these patients are helped by complementary therapies or steered towards less expensive treatment regimens, overall health-care costs may be reduced. Interventions such as pre-surgical hypnotherapy have already been shown to reduce institutional costs associated with inpatient procedures (Montgomery et al., 2007). Acupuncture for the treatment of chronic headaches was found to be more cost-effective than other interventions (Wonderling et al., 2004). Future efficacy research that includes cost-effectiveness evaluations will be instrumental in the further expansion of coverage for services that also demonstrate reduced or controlled costs.

Unproven 'alternative' therapies

Alternative practices are unregulated, expensive, unsubstantiated, and often discredited, but they are aggressively promoted as curative treatments. Susceptible patients often embrace the promise of cancer cures without the toxic effects of mainstream treatment. In addition to creating unnecessary financial expenditures and false hopes, the use of these therapies delay receipt of mainstream care, enabling disease progression and even resulting in death. Some 'alternatives' seem especially aimed at reaching vulnerable cancer patients. These 'therapies' include metabolic therapies, herbal and dietary supplement regimens, and 'vibrational or 'energy healing'.

Unproven biological approaches

Protocols and regimens in this category can involve ingestion, or rarely, injection of substances claimed to induce physiological changes that prevent and treat disease. The regimen could be a specified dietary plan, herbs, vitamins, or other constituents extracted from natural sources. The rationale may be stated as based on laboratory findings such as anti-tumour activity *in vitro* or in animal models, or traditional use such as herbal preparations from Traditional Chinese Medicine, naturopathy, or homeopathy.

In palliative care, unproven biological approaches tend to be adopted for one of two reasons. First, patients may try them in a final effort to treat end-stage disease and, even in the absence of clinical data, to leave no stone unturned. Second, patients may use them as supportive measures to 'strengthen the body', 'boost the immune system', or 'improve nutrition'.

Metabolic therapies

So-called metabolic therapies are practitioner-specific combinations of diet plus vitamins, minerals, enzymes, and 'detoxification'. One of the best known sites for metabolic therapy is the Gerson Institute, which licenses clinics in Mexico and Hungary. Treatment is based on the belief that toxic by-products of cancer cells accumulate in the liver, leading to liver failure and death. The Gerson therapy aims to counteract liver damage with a low-salt, high-potassium diet, coffee enemas, and a gallon of fruit and vegetable juice daily (Green, 1992). The clinic's use of liquefied raw calf liver injections were suspended following sepsis in several patients and one death (Centers for Disease Control and Prevention, 1981). There are numerous such clinics, with many variations on the theme, in Mexico as well as in the United States and Europe.

Box 4.17.1   Reputable online information sources

Complementary and alternative therapies

American Cancer Society: *Guidelines for Using Complementary and Alternative Methods* <http://www.cancer.org/Treatment/TreatmentsandSideEffects/ComplementaryandAlternativeMedicine/guidelines-for-using-complementary-and-alternative-methods>

Cochrane Summaries Database <http://summaries.cochrane.org/>

National Center for Complementary and Alternative Medicine (NCCAM) <http://www.nccam.nih.gov>

NCCAM *Time to Talk* Toolkit: *Ask Your Patients About Their Use of Complementary* Health Practices <http://nccam.nih.gov/timetotalk/forphysicians.htm>

National Cancer Institute (NCI) *PDQ® Cancer Information Summaries: Complementary and Alternative Medicine* <http://www.cancer.gov/cancertopics/pdq/cam>

Quackwatch *Guide to Quackery, Health Fraud, and Intelligent Decisions* <http://Quackwatch.org>

Society for Integrative Oncology <http://www.integrativeonc.org/>

Herbs and dietary supplements

Medline Plus <http://www.nlm.nih.gov/medlineplus/druginfo/herb_All.html>

Memorial Sloan-Kettering Cancer Center's *About Herbs, Botanicals & Other Products* <http://www.mskcc.org/aboutherbs>

NIH Office of Dietary Supplements <http://dietary-supplements.info.nih.gov>

United States Pharmacopeia (USP) *Dietary Supplement Standards* <http://www.usp.org/dietary-supplements/overview>

Patients may also explore elaborate dietary plans, detoxification regimens, mega-dose vitamin therapy, laetrile, essiac tea, iscador (mistletoe extract), immuno-augmentative therapy, ozone oxygen therapy, and many others. Some alternative practitioners 'diagnose' disease, sell their remedies, and remain unaccountable for their actions. Several online sources provide reliable information for patients and health-care professionals about such products and regimens (Box 4.17.1).

Dietary supplements

Another common marketing tactic is to highlight a 'magic bullet' ingredient for its superlative anticancer properties. This approach also capitalizes on perceptions that herbs and other products of plant or animal origin are 'natural' and 'safe', as opposed to standard treatments, which are associated with undesirable side effects.

A prominent example is shark cartilage, which garnered attention with the 1992 book, *Sharks Don't Get Cancer*, and a television special that displayed apparent remissions in patients treated with shark cartilage in Cuba. These supposed outcomes were strongly disputed by US oncologists. Advocates based their therapy on its putative antiangiogenic properties. Although shark cartilage was found to contain a substance with antiangiogenic activity *in vitro* (Lee and Langer, 1983), the active component appears to be a large molecule proteoglycan with a molecular weight of 10,000 Daltons (Liang and Wong 2000). Whether such large molecules can be absorbed in the digestive tract and reach the target tumour tissue at a sufficiently high local concentration is questionable. Clinical studies have yet to show survival benefit or improved quality of life in advanced cancer patients (Miller et al., 1998; Loprinzi et al., 2005) and the product was poorly tolerated due to its unpleasant taste.

Another example, 'caesium therapy', is based on the theory that an alkaline environment discourages tumour growth and that, by ingesting caesium chloride, one can alkalinize the body and kill cancer cells. In actuality, the activity of caesium chloride does not appear to be cancer-tissue specific. Excessive alkalization creates electrolyte and pH imbalances that disrupt normal cell functioning. Moreover, caesium therapy has resulted in life-threatening cardiac arrhythmia (Satoh and Zipes, 1998; Pinter et al., 2002).

Unscrupulous business practices colour many of these 'alternative offerings'. For example, a blanket promotion of 'coral calcium' as a cancer cure (Marcason 2003), was finally suspended by a governmental crackdown. Another popular and successful sales approach is multilevel marketing, with sales 'associates' motivated to sell the product while shielding the root promoter from liability arising from unsubstantiated claims. Often the results of the research on which 'alternative' therapies are based, if any, have not been evaluated for clinical relevance, or are exaggerated claims based on pseudoscience.

Herbs and other botanical products

Processed and marketed herbs may contain many different chemicals or even contaminants, most undocumented with unpredictable effects. The amount of purported active ingredients in botanical products also varies considerably across batches and manufacturers. Moreover, because these agents may have biological activity, their side effects and interactions with other drugs cannot be overlooked.

Even for reputable products, herbs and other botanicals for cancer patients may not be safe (Table 4.17.1). The harmful effects of the misuse of herbal remedies are documented (Lazarou et al., 1998), and herb–drug interactions may be underreported (Brulotte and Vohra, 2008). Moreover, botanicals can interfere with prescription medications through physiological mechanisms, including the induction or inhibition of drug-metabolizing enzymes such as cytochrome P450 (Frye et al., 2004) and transporters such as P-glycoprotein (Zhou et al., 2004). Herbs and supplements may increase bleeding when taken with anticoagulants, cause unwanted interactions with anaesthetics, enhance skin toxicity, and decrease the effects of radiation therapy. They also may stimulate the growth of hormone-sensitive cancers or decrease the effectiveness of chemotherapeutic agents.

More common adverse effects include allergic conditions such as hives, itchiness, swelling and bruising, and gastrointestinal symptoms such as nausea, vomiting, stomach upset, and constipation. Therefore, current opinion on the use of herbs and botanicals by cancer patients, especially before surgery or during chemotherapy and radiotherapy, is that such supplements should be avoided. The evidence regarding their safety is conflicting or absent (Wells et al., 1995; Prasad, 2004).

Biologically active natural substances have and will continue to serve as a rich resource for the development of legitimate therapeutic agents. Some of the most successful chemotherapeutic agents, including paclitaxel, topotecan, irinotecan, vincristine, and vinorelbine, were made from botanical compounds or their derivatives.

Other natural substances have shown promise in supportive care, such as carnitine for the treatment of cancer-related fatigue (Graziano et al., 2002; Cruciani et al., 2004) and glutamine to prevent taxane-induced neuropathy (Savarese et al., 2003; Stubblefield et al., 2005). Traumeel®, a proprietary blend, has been studied for chemotherapy-induced stomatitis (Oberbaum et al., 2001). Although promoted and sold as a homeopathic agent, it contains extracts from belladonna, arnica, St. John's wort, and echinacea, and should therefore be viewed as a botanical formulation. Other botanicals such as medicinal mushroom extracts are also under study for their potential to enhance immune function and reduce treatment toxicity (Lin et al., 2004; Deng et al., 2009). These agents should be used only under the supervision of oncology professionals who are familiar with their potential benefit and risks, taking into consideration the patient's medical condition and current medications. Any questionable agent should be used in a clinical trial setting with close monitoring of adverse events.

Vibrational medicine or energy field/healing therapies

Therapies in this category involve manipulation of a putative human energy field. This intervention may be provided by a 'healer', an individual believed to possess a special gift for energy healing. Popular over the centuries in less developed areas of the world (Cassileth et al., 1995), 'energy work' or 'vibrational medicine' has gained increasing public interest and acceptance in the United States, with some healers claiming the ability to cure cancer.

Purported energy field manipulation is also provided by devices that sell for hundreds of dollars, such as the 'BioResonance Therapy Device', which claims to detect electromagnetic emissions from a patient's cancer cells, modify them and send them back to the patient to correct cancer cell defects. Obviously, no one with a basic understanding of the pathogenesis and treatment of cancer would subscribe to such a theory (Ernst, 2004), but the manufacturers of these devices propagate the myth and sell the equipment internationally.

Although these practitioners may cause minor if any clinical difficulties when patients also receive mainstream care, many patients are firmly convinced of the healers' abilities, or of their effect on a patient's own ability to self-heal, and decline even to have tumours removed surgically in favour of the ministrations of energy therapy. Energy healing devices also tend to be costly.

Health literacy: the antidote for unproven 'alternatives'

A recent study estimated that 25% of adults have inadequate health literacy (Bains and Egede, 2011), without which patients cannot make correct choices. Health-care professionals must know how to obtain reliable information and to advise patients accordingly. Cancer patients and survivors especially should be alerted to the

Table 4.17.1 A sample of botanicals and supplements, their purported uses, and potentially serious adverse effects[a]

Botanical or supplement	Some common or purported uses	Potential adverse effects
Astragalus *Astragalus membranaceus*	Support/enhance immune system, colds and respiratory infections, chemotherapy side effects	◆ Decreased efficacy of immunosuppressants such as cyclophosphamide ◆ Increase risk of bone marrow or organ transplant rejection
DHEA Dehydroepiandrosterone	Alzheimer's disease, memory loss, osteoporosis, depression, cancer treatment	◆ Androgenic and oestrogenic effects ◆ Increased risk of some cancers ◆ May interfere with tamoxifen
Garlic *Allium sativum*	Cancer prevention or treatment, circulatory disorders, skin infections	◆ Interacts with CYP450 and P-gP substrates ◆ Antiplatelet effects, postoperative haemorrhage, increased bleeding risk with anticoagulants ◆ Unwanted interactions with anaesthetics ◆ May interfere with hypoglycaemic medications or ciclosporin with potential transplant rejection
Ginkgo *Ginkgo biloba*	Circulatory disorders, dementia, Alzheimer's disease, hearing loss, tinnitus	◆ Interacts with CYP450, MAOI, P-gP and UGT substrates ◆ Anticoagulant/antiplatelet effects; case reports of spontaneous bleeding ◆ Seizures in predisposed patients and when combined with antipsychotics including prochlorperazine (also an antiemetic)
Ginseng *Panax ginseng*	Cancer prevention/treatment, diabetes, immunostimulation, strength/stamina	◆ May stimulate the growth of hormone-sensitive cancers due to oestrogenic activity ◆ Interact with many drugs including imatinib (increased hepatotoxicity risk), insulin, and sulfonylureas (increased hypoglycaemic effects), anticoagulants (antagonizes effects), MAOIs (manic-like symptoms)
Green tea *Camellia sinensis*	Blood pressure and cholesterol; cancer prevention/treatment; heart disease; weight reduction	◆ Interacts with CYP450 and UGT substrates ◆ Inhibits bortezomib and irinotecan; may antagonize the effects of antiplatelets/anticoagulants ◆ Diuretic effects; nausea and GI upset
Maitake *Grifola frondosa*	Cancer prevention/treatment; diabetes, immunostimulation, weight loss	◆ May lower blood glucose level and have synergistic effects with hypoglycaemic medications ◆ May interact with warfarin
Saw palmetto *Serenoa repens*	BPH, prostate cancer, prostatitis	◆ Interacts with CYP450 and UGT substrates ◆ May have additive anticoagulant effects and prolong bleeding time; case reports of severe intraoperative haemorrhage, haematuria and coagulopathy, acute pancreatitis, and severe liver damage ◆ Self-treatment with saw palmetto for symptoms such as BPH could delay diagnosis and treatment of serious conditions including prostate cancer
Soy *Glycine max*	Menopausal symptoms, coughs, cancer prevention, cardiovascular disease	◆ May stimulate the growth of hormone-sensitive cancers due to oestrogenic activity ◆ May inhibit the actions of chemotherapy drugs including tamoxifen and aromatase inhibitors
St John's wort *Hypericum perforatum*	Depression, anxiety, mood and sleep disorders	◆ Can alter the metabolism of many drugs ◆ May cause photosensitivity or enhance skin toxicity of radiation therapy ◆ May reduce efficacy of chemotherapy ◆ Withdrawal symptoms have occurred with sudden stopping ◆ May cause serotonin syndrome with concomitant antidepressant use
Turmeric *Curcuma longa*	Cancer prevention, infections, inflammation	◆ Interacts with CYP450, P-gP and UGT substrates including cyclophosphamide, doxorubicin, and norfloxacin ◆ May increase risk of bleeding due to its antiplatelet properties

BPH, Benign prostatic hyperplasia; CYP450, cytochrome P450; GI, gastrointestinal; MAOI, monoamine oxidase inhibitors, P-gP, P-glycoprotein; UGT, uridine 5'-dip hospho-glucuronosyltransferase.

Botanicals have many characteristics and therefore the potential for multiple effects. For example, immunostimulants or herbs with oestrogenic effects may also have antioxidant or blood-thinning properties.

fact that special dietary regimens, herbal supplements, and other remedies are not viable substitutes for mainstream cancer treatment, and that they are not necessarily 'safe' simply because they are not pharmaceuticals or by virtue of their lack of scrutiny in the medical literature.

Patients should be alerted to avoid concurrent use of these products with prescription medications or when undergoing surgery, chemotherapy, or radiation therapy, while being directed to complementary therapies that can support and enhance mainstream care and patient satisfaction. Appropriate patient education could help to avoid most interactions and delays in receiving appropriate mainstream treatment and beneficial integrative services.

Medical institutions must continue to expand their outreach in this area. Of 41 NCI-designated comprehensive cancer centres, 12 (29%) had no functional websites containing information about complementary therapies (Brauer et al., 2010). The International Collaboration on Complementary Therapy Resources, which includes national complementary and alternative medicine centres in Australia, Denmark, Norway, the United Kingdom, and the United States, aims to explore effective ways of presenting information to health professionals, patients, and the general public (Pilkington et al., 2011).

Complementary therapies in palliative care

Patients with late-stage cancer and other major illnesses experience a wide range of symptoms and treatment-related toxicities. Problems experienced during treatment such as lymphoedema, neuropathic and other pain, nausea and vomiting, depression, and anxiety often persist for years or even decades. Pharmaceuticals can relieve some of these problems but can produce their own undesirable and difficult-to-manage side effects.

Complementary therapies such as mind–body techniques, massage therapy, acupuncture treatment, music therapy, and physical activity/fitness can help ameliorate many symptoms without additional adverse effects. Some therapies are a blend of several modalities. For example, yoga is a physical practice with strong breath training and mind–body components. Some fitness therapies incorporate specific music genres to elevate the exercise experience by engaging the mind and emotions as well as the body.

Mind–body techniques

The very existence of placebo effect, in which suggestions and expectancy can induce biological change, demonstrates the connection between mind and body. The potential to influence health with our minds is an appealing concept and an underutilized opportunity. Mind–body therapies in palliative care are geared to decrease distress and promote relaxation. They can also satisfy the spiritual needs of dying patients.

Hypnotherapy can be integrated into the various stages of palliative care patients' reactions—identified as initial crisis, transition, acceptance, and preparation for death (Marcus et al., 2003a, 2003b). Visualization and progressive relaxation also decrease pain and promote well-being (Walker et al., 1999). Hypnotherapy has been shown to reduce nausea and vomiting, procedural anxiety, and acute or chronic pain in children as well as adults (Gellert et al., 1993; Ladas et al., 2006; Montgomery et al., 2010).

A meta-analysis of 37 clinical trials conducted between 1966 and 2010 highlights the value of psychosocial interventions in pain management for patients with cancer (Sheinfeld Gorin et al., 2012). The effectiveness of meditation, biofeedback, and yoga in stress reduction to control a variety of physiological reactions also is well documented (National Institutes of Health 1996; Carlson et al., 2004; Cohen et al., 2004; Deng and Cassileth, 2005; Kim et al., 2011). Conclusions from a meta-analysis of 116 studies indicate that mind–body practices decrease anxiety, depression, and mood disturbance in cancer patients, and improve coping skills (Devine and Westlake, 1995).

Attending to patients' psychological health is a fundamental component of good palliative care. Support groups, good physician–patient relationships, and the emotional and instrumental help of family and friends are vital. However, the incorrect idea that patients can influence the course of their cancer through mental or emotional work is not substantiated and typically evokes feelings of guilt and inadequacy when the disease continues to advance despite the patient's best spiritual or mental efforts (Cassileth 1989; Gellert et al., 1993; Cunningham et al., 1998).

An important feature of mind–body therapies is the use of regular practice to produce and sustain benefit (Shapiro et al., 2003). The adoption of realistic expectations with respect to mind–body therapies while recognizing their value and potential is key.

Massage therapy

Massage therapy is a popular and important component of palliative care for symptom management during all stages of cancer treatment and survivorship. An important type of massage that is standard practice for patients who suffer from lymphoedema is manual lymph drainage in combination with compression bandaging (Poage et al., 2008). Other types of massage therapy employ a variety of techniques on soft tissues and joints to improve circulation, reduce tension and pain, and encourage relaxation.

Massage therapy helps reduce anxiety, pain (Cassileth and Vickers, 2004), depression (Krohn et al., 2011), and physical discomfort, and improves mood (Listing et al., 2009). In a randomized controlled trial of 380 patients with advanced cancer, six 30-minute massage sessions and simple-touch sessions over 2 weeks reduced pain and elevated mood. Massage was significantly superior to simple touch in improving both immediate pain and mood, but not for sustained pain, quality of life or analgesic use (Kutner et al., 2008). Reflexology, which includes gentle manipulation of the palms and feet, is highly valued by patients and helpful for those who are frail or uncomfortable with body massage (Stephenson et al., 2000). According to a multicenter randomized controlled trial, aromatherapy massage improved clinical anxiety and/or depression in cancer patients for up to 2 weeks post-intervention (Wilkinson et al., 2007). Reiki, a practice from Japan that uses light touch, also may be helpful in both non-ambulatory and outpatient settings (Birocco et al., 2012; Coakley and Barron, 2012). Massage therapy is generally safe when offered by credentialed practitioners, and those specifically trained to work with cancer patients (MSKCC Integrative Medicine Service, n.d. c, n.d. d) are especially likely to avoid any negative side effects, such as tissue trauma from excessive pressure.

Acupuncture

Acupuncture, an enduring integral component of Traditional Chinese Medicine, involves the insertion and stimulation of needles at selected points on the body to achieve a therapeutic effect (Fig. 4.17.1). Although based on the theory that needling regulates the flow of vital energy, neuroscience research suggests that acupuncture induces clinical response through modulation of the nervous system (Kaptchuk, 2002; Han, 2004). Acupuncture needles are filiform, sterile, single use, and very thin (32–40 gauge). They are regulated as medical devices in the United States. Acupuncture treatment is safe and causes minimal or no pain when performed by experienced, well-trained practitioners (MSKCC Integrative Medicine Service, n.d. a, n.d. b). Serious adverse events are extremely rare.

Acupuncture is well documented for the reduction of symptoms related to cancer and cancer treatment. Multiple well-designed studies also support its use to reduce chemotherapy-induced nausea and vomiting (Molassiotis et al., 2007), several types of pain (Pfister et al., 2010), and aromatase inhibitor-induced joint pain and stiffness (Crew et al., 2010). Acupuncture also was shown to be as effective as venlafaxine, the standard treatment for hot flushes in breast cancer patients (Walker et al., 2010). Early indications further suggest that acupuncture may decrease arm circumference in breast cancer patients with chronic lymphoedema (Cassileth et al., 2011) and alleviate dysphagia (Lu et al., 2010) in patients with head and neck cancer. Importantly, it has been shown effective for symptoms refractory to conventional care and often experienced by palliative care patients, including xerostomia (Pfister et al., 2010) and neuropathic pain (Alimi et al., 2003). Other concomitant conditions that may be experienced by patients with cancer have also been effectively improved with acupuncture, including osteoarthritis (Selfe and Taylor, 2008), migraine (Linde et al., 2009), and the relief of procedural anxiety (Wang et al., 2007, 2008).

Music therapy

Music can evoke deep-seated emotion and spiritual experience. A particular composition or genre may hold special meaning to an individual depending on his or her life experience. Music therapy can be receptive or participatory, and is provided by trained music therapists adept in dealing with the psychosocial as well as clinical issues faced by patients and family members. Music therapy is particularly effective in the palliative care setting. It offers a creative, lyrical, and symbolic means to address existential and spiritual needs, and is aesthetic and expressive. It brings form, order,

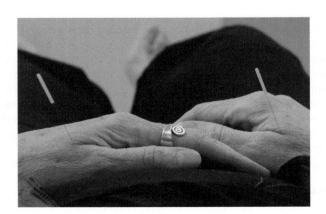

Fig. 4.17.1 Acupuncture.

comfort, and hope; transcends predicaments, space, and time; and affirms or re-establishes relationship with self, others, and the universe.

Many cancer centres in the United States and other countries offer music therapy programmes and studies have demonstrated its effectiveness in the oncology setting. A systematic review of 30 trials involving 1891 participants concluded that music therapy improves both psychological and physical outcomes in cancer patients by reducing anxiety and pain, and by improving mood and quality of life (Bradt et al., 2011). A randomized controlled trial of cancer patients undergoing autologous stem cell transplantation found that anxiety, depression, and total mood disturbance scores were significantly reduced in the music therapy group compared with standard-care controls (Cassileth et al., 2003). A perioperative music intervention suggests that music can reduce mean arterial pressure, anxiety, and pain among women undergoing mastectomy for breast cancer (Binns-Turner et al., 2011). In paediatric patients, music therapy-assisted procedures can reduce patient sedation, anxiety, and procedural time, and potentially prevent or reduce future negative associations (DeLoach Walworth, 2005).

Fitness/physical activity

An estimated 65% of all deaths worldwide currently are due to non-communicable chronic diseases such as cardiovascular disease, diabetes, and cancer. By 2030 that figure may exceed 75% (Blair et al., 2012). It is well known that physical inactivity affects mortality via risk factors such as obesity, diabetes, and hypertension. A growing body of literature also indicates that incorporating simple exercise regimens can improve survival in cancer patients.

In palliative care, fitness regimens can address many patient concerns including overall fitness, decreased mobility, breathing problems, difficulty relaxing, back and postural problems, and fear and anxiety (Selman et al., 2012). T'ai chi, a movement therapy derived from martial arts, can improve agility and reduce the risk of falls in frail and elderly patients (Faber et al., 2006; Lin et al., 2006). In a randomized controlled study of 256 elderly patients, a t'ai chi exercise programme resulted in significantly fewer falls, and fewer injurious falls when compared with a stretching control group. The risk for multiple falls in the t'ai chi group was 55% lower than that of the stretching control group. T'ai chi participants showed significant improvements in measures of functional balance, physical performance, and reduced fear of falling (Li et al., 2005). Yoga and yogic breathing also seem to improve persistent fatigue, sleep disturbance, anxiety, and mental quality of life (Dhruva et al., 2012; Bower et al., 2012), symptoms common among palliative care patients.

The issue of cancer cachexia is also of concern in the palliative phase (Fearon 2008). Multimodal approaches, including exercise, can stabilize and even improve nutritional status, function, and quality of life in patients with advanced cancer. A randomized controlled trial of physical exercise for 231 patients with advanced and progressive disease and a life expectancy of 3 months to 2 years found that physical exercise helped maintain physical functioning for at least a period of time (Oldervoll et al., 2011). For patients in palliative care, physical activity also can bring structure to everyday life and feelings of hope for the future (Gulde et al., 2011).

Other therapies

Other complementary therapies, such as spiritual care, counselling, and group support have been part of supportive, rehabilitative, and palliative care for decades. Many of these behavioural interventions fall in the grey area between mainstream treatment and complementary medicine. Animal-assisted therapy (pet therapy) is a low-tech, low-cost modality that can improve mood and provide meaning to hospitalized patients (Marcus, 2012). A randomized clinical trial underway is examining how animal-assisted therapy affects pain in cancer patients receiving pain and palliative care at the NIH Clinical Center (2012).

Art therapy is a behavioural modality that uses creative expression to help develop coping skills. Many cancer centres provide access to artistic expression on a recreational basis or guided by professional art therapists. A few reports have shown an association between art therapy and higher comfort levels of children with leukaemia undergoing painful procedures. Art as well as music therapy can also reduce stress and decrease anxiety in family caregivers. Although scientific study of art therapy is minimal, it is clear that many patients enjoy creative activity. That enjoyment per se is an important end in and of itself.

Summary

The public in general and palliative care patients in particular are interested in complementary and alternative therapies, which are diverse and have variable risk–benefit ratios. Alternative therapies are often marketed to palliative care patients, but are unproven or disproved, potentially harmful, and often fraudulent. In the context of palliative care, this can also present specific and critical issues with respect to optimal delivery or interference with needed mainstream treatment.

Hospitals and other research institutions recognize the appropriate role that complementary therapies bring by supporting mainstream treatments. An increasing body of evidence over the last two decades supports the use of acupuncture, massage therapy, music, mind–body therapies, and other complementary modalities to reduce physical and emotional symptoms. Recommended and non-invasive therapies with favourable risk–benefit profiles should be applied to bring symptom relief particularly when conventional treatments produce negative side effects.

In palliative care, complementary therapies also may reduce the level of opioids required for pain control. In providing patient-centred medical care, complementary therapies must be tailored to the needs and preferences of each patient. Economic concerns, patients' belief systems, and cultural backgrounds also influence selection of therapies.

At the same time, educating patients about cancer cure marketing schemes, avoiding unproven methods, and the potential dangers of using natural products that seem 'safe' will assist optimal patient care. In light of product quality control issues and potential interactions with prescription medications, it is important to access or refer patients and families to sources of reliable information about common herbs and dietary supplements, such as those listed in Box 4.17.1.

This dual approach to complementary modalities can help alleviate troubling symptoms, promote family involvement and patient self-care, improve patients' well-being, and enhance the physician–patient relationship.

References

Alimi, D., Rubino, C., Pichard-Leandri, E., Fermand-Brule, S., Dubreuil-Lemaire, M.L., and Hill, C. (2003). Analgesic effect of auricular acupuncture for cancer pain: a randomized, blinded, controlled trial. *Journal of Clinical Oncology*, 21, 4120–4126.

American Cancer Society (2012). *Cancer Facts & Figures 2012*. [Online] Available at: <http://www.cancer.org/Research/CancerFactsFigures/index>.

Bains, S.S. and Egede, L.E. (2011). Association of health literacy with complementary and alternative medicine use: a cross-sectional study in adult primary care patients. *BMC Complementary and Alternative Medicine*, 11, 138.

Barnes, P.M., Bloom, B., and Nahin, R.L. (2008). Complementary and alternative medicine use among adults and children: United States, 2007. *National Health Statistics Reports*, 12, 1–23.

Binns-Turner, P.G., Wilson, L.L., Pryor, E.R., Boyd, G.L., and Prickett, C.A. (2011). Perioperative music and its effects on anxiety, hemodynamics, and pain in women undergoing mastectomy. *AANA Journal*, 79, S21–27.

Birocco, N., Guillame, C., Storto, S., *et al.* (2012). The effects of reiki therapy on pain and anxiety in patients attending a day oncology and infusion services unit. *American Journal of Hospice and Palliative Care*, 29, 290–294.

Blair, S.N., Sallis, R.E., Hutber, A., and Archer, E. (2012). Exercise therapy—the public health message. *Scandinavian Journal of Medicine and Science in Sports*, 22(4), e24–28.

Bower, J.E., Garet, D., Sternlieb, B., *et al.* (2011). Yoga for persistent fatigue in breast cancer survivors: a randomized controlled trial. *Cancer*, 118, 3766–3775.

Bradt, J., Dileo, C., Grocke, D., and Magill, L. (2011). Music interventions for improving psychological and physical outcomes in cancer patients. *Cochrane Database of Systematic Reviews*, 8, CD006911

Brann, M. and Anderson, J.G. (2002). E-medicine and health care consumers: recognizing current problems and possible resolutions for a safer environment. *Health Care Analysis*, 10, 403–415.

Brauer, J.A., El Sehamy, A., Metz, J.M., and Mao, J.J. (2010). Complementary and alternative medicine and supportive care at leading cancer centers: a systematic analysis of websites. *Journal of Alternative and Complementary Medicine*, 16, 183–186.

Brulotte, J. and Vohra, S. (2008). Epidemiology of NHP-drug interactions: identification and evaluation. *Current Drug Metabolism*, 9, 1049–1054.

Carlson, L.E., Speca, M., Patel, K.D., and Goodey, E. (2004). Mindfulness-based stress reduction in relation to quality of life, mood, symptoms of stress and levels of cortisol, dehydroepiandrosterone sulfate (DHEAS) and melatonin in breast and prostate cancer outpatients. *Psychoneuroendocrinology*, 29, 448–474.

Cassileth, B., Deng, G., Vickers, A., and Yeung, K.S. (2005). *PDQ Integrative Oncology*. Hamilton: BC Decker.

Cassileth, B.R. (1989). The social implications of mind-body cancer research. *Cancer Investigation*, 7, 361–364.

Cassileth, B.R., Deng, G.E., Gomez, J.E., Johnstone, P.A., Kumar, N. and Vickers, A.J. (2007). Complementary therapies and integrative oncology in lung cancer: ACCP evidence-based clinical practice guidelines (2nd edition). *Chest*, 132, 340S–354S.

Cassileth, B.R., Lusk, E.J., Strouse, T.B. and Bodenheimer, B.J. (1984). Contemporary unorthodox treatments in cancer medicine. A study of patients, treatments, and practitioners. *Annals of Internal Medicine*, 101, 105–112.

Cassileth, B.R., Van Zee, K.J., Chan, Y., *et al.* (2011). A safety and efficacy pilot study of acupuncture for the treatment of chronic lymphoedema. *Acupuncture in Medicine*, 29, 170–172.

Cassileth, B.R. and Vickers, A.J. (2004). Massage therapy for symptom control: outcome study at a major cancer center. *Journal of Pain and Symptom Management*, 28, 244–249.

Cassileth, B.R., Vickers, A.J., and Magill, L.A. (2003). Music therapy for mood disturbance during hospitalization for autologous stem cell transplantation: a randomized controlled trial. *Cancer*, 98, 2723–2729.

Cassileth, B.R., Vlassov, V.V., and Chapman, C.C. (1995). Health care, medical practice, and medical ethics in Russia today. *Journal of the American Medical Association*, 273, 1569–1573.

Centers for Disease Control and Prevention (1981). Campylobacter sepsis associated with 'nutritional therapy'—California. *MMWR. Morbidity and Mortality Weekly Report*, 30, 294–295.

Coakley, A.B. and Barron, A.M. (2012). Energy therapies in oncology nursing. *Seminars in Oncology Nursing*, 28, 55–63.

Cohen, L., Warneke, C., Fouladi, R.T., Rodriguez, M.A., and Chaoul-Reich, A. (2004). Psychological adjustment and sleep quality in a randomized trial of the effects of a Tibetan yoga intervention in patients with lymphoma. *Cancer*, 100, 2253–2260.

Crew, K.D., Capodice, J.L., Greenlee, H., *et al.* (2010). Randomized, blinded, sham-controlled trial of acupuncture for the management of aromatase inhibitor-associated joint symptoms in women with early-stage breast cancer. *Journal of Clinical Oncology*, 28, 1154–1160.

Cruciani, R.A., Dvorkin, E., Homel, P., *et al.* (2004). L-carnitine supplementation for the treatment of fatigue and depressed mood in cancer patients with carnitine deficiency: a preliminary analysis. *Annals of the New York Academy of Sciences*, 1033, 168–176.

Cunningham, A.J., Edmonds, C.V., Jenkins, G.P., Pollack, H., Lockwood, G.A., and Warr, D. (1998). A randomized controlled trial of the effects of group psychological therapy on survival in women with metastatic breast cancer. *Psycho-Oncology*, 7, 508–517.

DeLoach Walworth, D. (2005). Procedural-support music therapy in the healthcare setting: a cost-effectiveness analysis. *Journal of Pediatric Nursing*, 20, 276–284.

Deng, G. and Cassileth, B.R. (2005). Integrative oncology: complementary therapies for pain, anxiety, and mood disturbance. *CA: A Cancer Journal for Clinicians*, 55, 109–116.

Deng, G., Lin, H., Seidman, A., *et al.* (2009). A phase I/II trial of a polysaccharide extract from Grifola frondosa (Maitake mushroom) in breast cancer patients: immunological effects. *Journal of Cancer Research and Clinical Oncology*, 135, 1215–1221.

Deng, G.E., Frenkel, M., Cohen, L., *et al.* (2009). Evidence-based clinical practice guidelines for integrative oncology: complementary therapies and botanicals. *Journal of the Society for Integrative Oncology*, 7, 85–120.

Devine, E.C. and Westlake, S.K. (1995). The effects of psychoeducational care provided to adults with cancer: meta-analysis of 116 studies. *Oncology Nursing Forum*, 22, 1369–1381.

Dhruva, A., Miaskowski, C., Abrams, D., *et al.* (2012). Yoga breathing for cancer chemotherapy-associated symptoms and quality of life: results of a pilot randomized controlled trial. *Journal of Alternative and Complementary Medicine*, 18, 473–479.

Egan, B., Gage, H., Hood, J., *et al.* (2012). Availability of complementary and alternative medicine for people with cancer in the British National Health Service: results of a national survey. *Complementary Therapies in Clinical Practice*, 18, 75–80.

Ernst, E. (2004). Bioresonance, a study of pseudo-scientific language. *Forsch Komplementarmed Klass Naturheilkd*, 11, 171–173.

Faber, M.J., Bosscher, R.J., Chin, A.P.M.J., and van Wieringen, P.C. (2006). Effects of exercise programs on falls and mobility in frail and pre-frail older adults: a multicenter randomized controlled trial. *Archives of Physical Medicine and Rehabilitation*, 87, 885–896.

Fearon, K.C. (2008). Cancer cachexia: developing multimodal therapy for a multidimensional problem. *European Journal of Cancer*, 44, 1124–1132.

Federal Trade Commission (1999). *FTC Sweep Stops Peddlers of Bogus Cancer Cures*. Available at: <http://www.ftc.gov/>

Federal Trade Commission (2008a). *Cure-ious? Ask*. Available at: <http://www.ftc.gov>.

Federal Trade Commission (2008b). *'Operation Cure.all' Targets Internet Health Fraud*. Available at: <http://www.ftc.gov>.

Fouladbakhsh, J.M. and Stommel, M. (2010). Gender, symptom experience, and use of complementary and alternative medicine practices among cancer survivors in the U.S. cancer population. *Oncology Nursing Forum*, 37, E7–E15.

Frye, R.F., Fitzgerald, S.M., Lagattuta, T.F., Hruska, M.W., and Egorin, M.J. (2004). Effect of St John's wort on imatinib mesylate pharmacokinetics. *Clinical Pharmacology and Therapeutics*, 76, 323–329.

Gellert, G.A., Maxwell, R.M., and Siegel, B.S. (1993). Survival of breast cancer patients receiving adjunctive psychosocial support therapy: a 10-year follow-up study. *Journal of Clinical Oncology*, 11, 66–69.

Graziano, F., Bisonni, R., Catalano, V., *et al.* (2002). Potential role of levocarnitine supplementation for the treatment of chemotherapy-induced fatigue in non-anaemic cancer patients. *British Journal of Cancer*, 86, 1854–1857.

Green, S. (1992). A critique of the rationale for cancer treatment with coffee enemas and diet. *Journal of the American Medical Association*, 268, 3224–3227.

Gulde, I., Oldervoll, L.M., and Martin, C. (2011). Palliative cancer patients' experience of physical activity. *Journal of Palliative Care*, 27, 296–302.

Han, J.S. (2004). Acupuncture and endorphins. *Neuroscience Letters*, 361, 258–261.

Hyodo, I., Amano, N., Eguchi, K., *et al.* (2005). Nationwide survey on complementary and alternative medicine in cancer patients in Japan. *Journal of Clinical Oncology*, 23, 2645–2654.

Kaptchuk, T.J. (2002). Acupuncture: theory, efficacy, and practice. *Annals of Internal Medicine*, 136, 374–383.

Kim, K.H., Yu, C.S., Yoon, Y.S., Yoon, S.N., Lim, S.B., and Kim, J.C. (2011). Effectiveness of biofeedback therapy in the treatment of anterior resection syndrome after rectal cancer surgery. *Diseases of the Colon and Rectum*, 54, 1107–1113.

Krohn, M., Listing, M., Tjahjono, G., *et al.* (2011). Depression, mood, stress, and Th1/Th2 immune balance in primary breast cancer patients undergoing classical massage therapy. *Supportive Care in Cancer*, 19, 1303–1311.

Kutner, J.S., Smith, M.C., Corbin, L., *et al.* (2008). Massage therapy versus simple touch to improve pain and mood in patients with advanced cancer: a randomized trial. *Annals of Internal Medicine*, 149, 369–379.

Ladas, E.J., Post-White, J., Hawks, R., and Taromina, K. (2006). Evidence for symptom management in the child with cancer. *Journal of Pediatric Hematology/Oncology*, 28, 601–615.

Lafferty, W.E., Tyree, P.T., Bellas, A.S., *et al.* (2006). Insurance coverage and subsequent utilization of complementary and alternative medicine providers. *American Journal of Managed Care*, 12, 397–404.

Lazarou, J., Pomeranz, B.H., and Corey, P.N. (1998). Incidence of adverse drug reactions in hospitalized patients: a meta-analysis of prospective studies. *Journal of the American Medical Association*, 279, 1200–1205.

Lee, A. and Langer, R. (1983). Shark cartilage contains inhibitors of tumor angiogenesis. *Science*, 221, 1185–1187.

Li, F., Harmer, P., Fisher, K.J., *et al.* (2005). Tai Chi and fall reductions in older adults: a randomized controlled trial. *Journals of Gerontology. Series A, Biological Sciences and Medical Sciences*, 60, 187–194.

Liang, J.H. and Wong, K.P. (2000). The characterization of angiogenesis inhibitor from shark cartilage. *Advances in Experimental Medicine and Biology*, 476, 209–223.

Lin, H., She, Y.H., Cassileth, B.R., Sirotnak, F., and Cunningham Rundles, S. (2004). Maitake beta-glucan MD-fraction enhances bone marrow colony formation and reduces doxorubicin toxicity in vitro. *International Immunopharmacology*, 4, 91–99.

Lin, M.R., Hwang, H.F., Wang, Y.W., Chang, S.H., and Wolf, S.L. (2006). Community-based tai chi and its effect on injurious falls, balance, gait, and fear of falling in older people. *Physical Therapy*, 86, 1189–1201.

Linde, K., Allais, G., Brinkhaus, B., Manheimer, E., Vickers, A., and White, A. R. (2009). Acupuncture for migraine prophylaxis. *Cochrane Database of Systematic Reviews*, 1, CD001218.

Listing, M., Reisshauer, A., Krohn, M., *et al.* (2009). Massage therapy reduces physical discomfort and improves mood disturbances in women with breast cancer. *Psycho-Oncology*, 18, 1290–1299.

Loprinzi, C.L., Levitt, R., Barton, D.L., *et al.* (2005). Evaluation of shark cartilage in patients with advanced cancer: a North Central Cancer Treatment Group trial. *Cancer*, 104, 176–182.

Lu, W., Posner, M.R., Wayne, P., Rosenthal, D.S., and Haddad, R.I. (2010). Acupuncture for dysphagia after chemoradiation therapy in head and neck cancer: a case series report. *Integrative Cancer Therapies*, 9, 284–290.

Mao, J.J., Palmer, C.S., Healy, K.E., Desai, K., and Amsterdam, J. (2011). Complementary and alternative medicine use among cancer survivors: a population-based study. *Journal of Cancer Survivorship*, 5, 8–17.

Marcason, W. (2003). What is the lowdown on coral calcium? *Journal of the American Dietetic Association*, 103, 1319.

Marcus, D.A. (2012). Complementary medicine in cancer care: adding a therapy dog to the team. *Current Pain and Headache Reports*, 16(4), 289–291.

Marcus, J., Elkins, G., and Mott, F. (2003a). The integration of hypnosis into a model of palliative care. *Integrative Cancer Therapies*, 2, 365–370.

Marcus, J., Elkins, G., and Mott, F. (2003b). A model of hypnotic intervention for palliative care. *Advances in Mind-Body Medicine*, 19, 24–27.

Miller, D.R., Anderson, G.T., Stark, J.J., Granick, J.L., and Richardson, D. (1998). Phase I/II trial of the safety and efficacy of shark cartilage in the treatment of advanced cancer. *Journal of Clinical Oncology*, 16, 3649–3655.

Molassiotis, A., Fernadez-Ortega, P., Pud, D., *et al.* (2005). Use of complementary and alternative medicine in cancer patients: a European survey. *Annals of Oncology*, 16, 655–663.

Molassiotis, A., Helin, A.M., Dabbour, R., and Hummerston, S. (2007). The effects of P6 acupressure in the prophylaxis of chemotherapy-related nausea and vomiting in breast cancer patients. *Complementary Therapies in Medicine*, 15, 3–12.

Montgomery, G.H., Bovbjerg, D.H., Schnur, J.B., *et al.* (2007). A randomized clinical trial of a brief hypnosis intervention to control side effects in breast surgery patients. *Journal of the National Cancer Institute*, 99, 1304–1312.

Montgomery, G.H., Hallquist, M.N., Schnur, J.B., David, D., Silverstein, J.H., and Bovbjerg, D.H. (2010). Mediators of a brief hypnosis intervention to control side effects in breast surgery patients: response expectancies and emotional distress. *Journal of Consulting and Clinical Psychology*, 78, 80–88.

MSKCC Integrative Medicine Service (n.d. a). *Acupuncture for the Cancer Patient.* [Online] Available at: <http://www.mskcc.org/cancer-care/integrative-medicine/professional-online-programs/acupuncture-patient>.

MSKCC Integrative Medicine Service (n.d. b). *Advanced Acupuncture for the Cancer Patient.* [Online] Available at: <http://www.mskcc.org/cancer-care/integrative-medicine/professional-online-programs/advanced-acupuncture-patient>.

MSKCC Integrative Medicine Service (n.d. c). *Medical Massage for the Cancer Patient I.* [Online] Available at: <http://www.mskcc.org/cancer-care/integrative-medicine/professional-online-programs/medical-massage-patient-i>.

MSKCC Integrative Medicine Service (n.d. d). *Medical Massage for the Cancer Patient II.* [Online] Available at: <http://www.mskcc.org/cancer-care/integrative-medicine/professional-online-programs/medical-massage-patient-ii>.

Nahin, R.L., Barnes, P.M., Stussman, B.J., and Bloom, B. (2009). Costs of complementary and alternative medicine (CAM) and frequency of visits to CAM practitioners: United States, 2007. *National Health Statistics Reports*, 18, 1–14

National Center for Complementary and Alternative Medicine (2011). *Budget Request for Fiscal Year 2011.* [Online] Available at: <http://nccam.nih.gov/about/offices/od/directortestimony/0410.htm>.

National Institutes of Health (1996). Integration of behavioral and relaxation approaches into the treatment of chronic pain and insomnia. NIH Technology Assessment Panel on Integration of Behavioral and Relaxation Approaches into the Treatment of Chronic Pain and Insomnia. *Journal of the American Medical Association*, 276, 313–318.

National Institutes of Health Clinical Center (2012). *Effects of Pet Therapy on Pain in Cancer Patients.* [Online] Available at: <http://clinicaltrials.gov/ct2/show/NCT00431639>.

Natural Products Association (2012). *Natural Products Association & Industry Facts.* [Online] Available at: <http://www.npainfo.org/>.

Oberbaum, M., Yaniv, I., Ben-Gal, Y., *et al.* (2001). A randomized, controlled clinical trial of the homeopathic medication TRAUMEEL S in the treatment of chemotherapy-induced stomatitis in children undergoing stem cell transplantation. *Cancer*, 92, 684–690.

Oldervoll, L.M., Loge, J.H., Lydersen, S., *et al.* (2011). Physical exercise for cancer patients with advanced disease: a randomized controlled trial. *The Oncologist*, 16, 1649–1657.

Pfister, D.G., Cassileth, B.R., Deng, G.E., *et al.* (2010). Acupuncture for pain and dysfunction after neck dissection: results of a randomized controlled trial. *Journal of Clinical Oncology*, 28, 2565–2570.

Pilkington, K., Gamst, A., Liu, I., Ostermann, T., Pinto, D., and Richardson, J. (2011). The International Collaboration on Complementary Therapy Resources (ICCR): working together to improve online CAM information. *Journal of Alternative and Complementary Medicine*, 17, 647–653.

Pinter, A., Dorian, P., and Newman, D. (2002). Cesium-induced torsades de pointes. *New England Journal of Medicine*, 346, 383–384.

Poage, E., Singer, M., Armer, J., Poundall, M., and Shellabarger, M.J. (2008). Demystifying lymphedema: development of the lymphedema putting evidence into practice card. *Clinical Journal of Oncology Nursing*, 12, 951–964.

Prasad, K.N. (2004). Multiple dietary antioxidants enhance the efficacy of standard and experimental cancer therapies and decrease their toxicity. *Integrative Cancer Therapies*, 3, 310–322.

Remen, R.N. (2008). Practicing a medicine of the whole person: an opportunity for healing. *Hematology/Oncology Clinics of North America*, 22, 767–773.

Satoh, T. and Zipes, D.P. (1998). Cesium-induced atrial tachycardia degenerating into atrial fibrillation in dogs: atrial torsades de pointes? *Journal of Cardiovascular Electrophysiology*, 9, 970–975.

Savarese, D.M., Savy, G., Vahdat, L., Wischmeyer, P.E., and Corey, B. (2003). Prevention of chemotherapy and radiation toxicity with glutamine. *Cancer Treatment Reviews*, 29, 501–513.

Selfe, T.K. and Taylor, A.G. (2008). Acupuncture and osteoarthritis of the knee: a review of randomized, controlled trials. *Family and Community Health*, 31, 247–254.

Selman, L.E., Williams, J., and Simms, V. (2012). A mixed-methods evaluation of complementary therapy services in palliative care: yoga and dance therapy. *European Journal of Cancer Care*, 21, 87–97.

Shapiro, S.L., Bootzin, R.R., Figueredo, A.J., Lopez, A.M., and Schwartz, G.E. (2003). The efficacy of mindfulness-based stress reduction in the treatment of sleep disturbance in women with breast cancer: an exploratory study. *Journal of Psychosomatic Research*, 54, 85–91.

Sheinfeld Gorin, S., Krebs, P., Badr, H., *et al.* (2012). Meta-analysis of psychosocial interventions to reduce pain in patients with cancer. *Journal of Clinical Oncology*, 30, 539–47.

Stephenson, N.L., Weinrich, S.P., and Tavakoli, A.S. (2000). The effects of foot reflexology on anxiety and pain in patients with breast and lung cancer. *Oncology Nursing Forum*, 27, 67–72.

Stubblefield, M.D., Vahdat, L.T., Balmaceda, C.M., Troxel, A.B., Hesdorffer, C.S., and Gooch, C. L. (2005). Glutamine as a neuroprotective agent in high-dose paclitaxel-induced peripheral neuropathy: a clinical and electrophysiologic study. *Clinical Oncology*, 17, 271–276.

US Food and Drug Administration (2014). *Dietary Supplements.* [Online] Available at: <http://www.fda.gov/Food/Dietarysupplements/default.htm>.

Walker, E.M., Rodriguez, A.I., Kohn, B., *et al.* (2010). Acupuncture versus venlafaxine for the management of vasomotor symptoms in patients with hormone receptor-positive breast cancer: a randomized controlled trial. *Journal of Clinical Oncology*, 28, 634–640.

Walker, L.G., Walker, M.B., Ogston, K., *et al.* (1999). Psychological, clinical and pathological effects of relaxation training and guided imagery during primary chemotherapy. *British Journal of Cancer*, 80, 262–268.

Wang, S.M., Escalera, S., Lin, E.C., Maranets, I., and Kain, Z.N. (2008). Extra-1 acupressure for children undergoing anesthesia. *Anesthesia and Analgesia*, 107, 811–816.

Wang, S.M., Punjala, M., Weiss, D., Anderson, K., and Kain, Z.N. (2007). Acupuncture as an adjunct for sedation during lithotripsy. *Journal of Alternative and Complementary Medicine*, 13, 241–246.

Wells, W.W., Rocque, P.A., Xu, D.P., Meyer, E.B., Charamella, L.J., and Dimitrov, N.V. (1995). Ascorbic acid and cell survival of adriamycin resistant and sensitive MCF-7 breast tumor cells. *Free Radical Biology and Medicine*, 18, 699–708.

Wilkinson, S.M., Love, S.B., Westcombe, A.M., *et al.* (2007). Effectiveness of aromatherapy massage in the management of anxiety and depression in patients with cancer: a multicenter randomized controlled trial. *Journal of Clinical Oncology*, 25, 532–539.

Wonderling, D., Vickers, A.J., Grieve, R., and McCarney, R. (2004). Cost effectiveness analysis of a randomised trial of acupuncture for chronic headache in primary care. *BMJ*, 328, 747.

Wood, M.J., Stewart, R. L., Merry, H., Johnstone, D.E., and Cox, J.L. (2003). Use of complementary and alternative medical therapies in patients with cardiovascular disease. *American Heart Journal*, 145, 806–812.

World Health Organization (2006). *Cancer Control: Knowledge into Action. WHO Guide for Effective Programmes. Palliative Care.* [Online] Available at: <http://www.who.int/>.

Zhou, S., Lim, L.Y., and Chowbay, B. (2004). Herbal modulation of P-glycoprotein. *Drug Metabolism Reviews*, 36, 57–104.

SECTION 5

Ethical issues

Human rights issues

Frank Brennan and Liz Gwyther

Introduction to human rights issues

The modern era has seen the articulation of a basic proposition: that palliative care should be viewed as a fundamental human right of all people. That proposition has been made in a context of, and in response to, clear inadequacies in the provision of palliative care around the world, absent or deficient national policies on pain and palliative care, restrictive opioid laws, and inadequate education of health professionals in all aspects of the care of people with life-limiting illnesses.

This chapter will examine:

1. the background of the concept

2. the fundamental argument and foundations of these rights in international human rights law

3. the content of the obligation

4. the response from the United Nations (UN) and the World Health Organization (WHO)

5. the counterarguments

6. current and future strategies in advancing palliative care by using a human rights discourse.

Background

Conscious of widespread deficits in the care of people throughout the world, the international pain and palliative care communities began, in recent years, to frame their advocacy in the language of rights. A series of declarations and statements emerged framing the provision of palliative care as a human right. These included the *Cape Town Declaration* (Mpanga-Sebuyira et al., 2003), the *Korea Declaration* (National Hospice and Palliative Care Associations, 2005), the *Joint Declaration of and Statement of Commitment to Pain Management and Palliative Care as Human Rights* (International Association for Hospice and Palliative Care (IAHPC) and the Worldwide Palliative Care Alliance (WPCA), 2008), the Panama Proclamation—*Proclamation of Pain Treatment and the Application of Palliative Care as Human Rights* (Latin American Federation of IASP Chapters and Foundation for the Treatment of Pain as a Human Right, 2008), the *Lisbon Challenge* (European Association of Palliative Care (EAPC), 2011) and the *Prague Charter* (EAPC, 2013).

These palliative care advocacy initiatives were concurrent to statements from within the international pain community. Indeed, as part of their response to the deficits around the world in pain management, clinicians, ethicists, and medical lawyers began, in the 1980s, to argue that pain management was a universal human right. To Michael Cousins, a past President of the International Association for the Study of Pain (IASP), 'the relief of severe unrelenting pain would come at the top of a list of basic human rights' (Cousins, 1999). These assertions were eventually followed by authoritative statements by multiple national and international pain associations articulating a right to pain management. Finally, the inaugural Global Day Against Pain in 2004 had as its theme 'Pain Relief: A Universal Human Right'. Subsequent international declarations, including the *Joint Declaration of and Statement of Commitment to Pain Management and Palliative Care as Human Rights* (IAHPC and WPCA, 2008), the *Proclamation of Pain Treatment and the Application of Palliative Care as Human Rights* (Latin American Federation of IASP Chapters and Foundation for the Treatment of Pain as a Human Right, 2008), the *Declaration of Montréal* (International Pain Summit of the IASP, 2011), the *WMA Resolution on the Access to Adequate Pain Treatment* (World Medical Association, 2011), and *The Morphine Manifesto* (Pallium India et al., 2012) have all endorsed this approach.

A summary of these statements and declarations appears in Box 5.1.1.

The foundation of these rights in human rights law

While admirable in rhetoric and potentially strong tools of advocacy, do these statements have any foundation in human rights law? That foundation rests on two pillars: the international conventions on drug control and the international right to health.

The international drug control conventions were promulgated for a dual purpose: to monitor and control the use of both licit and illicit controlled substances. The International Narcotics Control Board (INCB), the body established to oversee compliance with the conventions, stated the importance of ensuring 'adequate availability of narcotic drugs . . . for medical and scientific purposes while ensuring such drugs are not diverted for illicit purposes' (INCB, 2010, p. iii). The *Single Convention on Narcotic Drugs* (1961) expressly reminds and obliges signatory nations that the medical use of opioids is indispensable to the relief of pain and suffering (United Nations Conference for the Adoption of a Single Convention on Narcotic Drugs, 1961).

Several UN conventions articulate a right to the provision of health care. The central and most general statement of this is contained in the *International Covenant of Economic, Social and Cultural Rights* (ICESCR) (UN General Assembly, 1966,

Box 5.1.1 International statements articulating pain management and/or palliative care as human rights and their sponsoring organizations

Pain management

- Global Day Against Pain (2004)—IASP, EFIC, WHO.

- The Panama Proclamation—*Proclamation of Pain Treatment and the Application of Palliative Care as Human Rights* (2008)—Latin American Federation of IASP Chapters, Foundation for the Treatment of Pain as a Human Right.

- *Joint Declaration of and Statement of Commitment to Pain Management and Palliative Care as Human Rights* (2008)—IAHPC, WPCA.

- *Declaration of Montréal* (2011)—IASP.

- *WMA Resolution on the Access to Adequate Pain Treatment* (2011)—WMA.

- *The Morphine Manifesto* (2012)—Pallium India, IAHPC, PPSG, and 60 other organizations.

Palliative care

- *Cape Town Declaration* (2002)—African Palliative Care Educators.

- International Working Group (European School of Oncology) (2004).

- *Korea Declaration* (2005)—Second Global Summit of National Hospice and Palliative Care Associations.

- *Proclamation of Pain Treatment and the Application of Palliative Care as Human Rights* (2008)—Latin American Federation of IASP Chapters, Foundation for the Treatment of Pain as a Human Right.

- World Hospice Day (2008)—IAHPC.

- *Lisbon Challenge* (2011)—EAPC, IAHPC, HRW.

- *Prague Charter* (2013)—EAPC, IAHPC, WPCA, HRW.

EAPC, European Association of Palliative Care; EFIC, European Chapters of the IASP; HRW, Human Rights Watch; IAHPC, International Association of Hospice and Palliative Care; IASP, International Association for the Study of Pain; PPSG, Pain and Public Policy Studies Group, University of Wisconsin/WHO Collaborating Center for Pain Policy and Palliative Care; WPCA, Worldwide Palliative Care Alliance; WHO, World Health Organization.

Article 12). The right to health is articulated in several other conventions: Article 12, *Convention on the Elimination of All Forms of Discrimination Against Women* (UN General Assembly, 1979), Article 24, *Convention on the Rights of the Child* (UN General Assembly, 1989), Article 5(e), *International Convention on the Elimination of All Forms of Racial Discrimination* (UN General Assembly, 1965), and Article 25, *Universal Declaration of Human Rights* (UN General Assembly, 1948).

Given that pain management and palliative care fall within health care, the international right to health is a source of obligation on signatory governments in these areas. Other potential

sources of a human rights foundation to palliative care emerge from the international conventions:

1. Dignity. Each UN convention commences with a recognition of the 'the inherent dignity of the human person'. The attention to and the promotion of the dignity of individual patients is a central tenet of the practice of palliative care.

2. The right not to be subjected to inhuman or degrading treatment (UN General Assembly, 1976, Article 7). An example here would be a nation with laws prohibiting the availability of opioids for medical purposes.

3. The right to non-discrimination and equality (UN General Assembly, 1966, Preamble, Articles 2(2) and 3). The Committee overseeing the right to health in the ICESCR (UN General Assembly, 1966) stated that nations are obliged to respect the right to health and should not deny or limit equal access to all forms of health including palliative health services (Committee on Economic, Social and Cultural Rights (CESCR), 2000). An example would be a nation denying by law access to palliative care services to refugees or non-citizens. Arguably, an example of de facto discrimination would be a nation deliberately restricting the availability of opioids to a limited number of hospitals so that geographical distance and poverty means that only a small proportion of the population will realistically have access to these medications.

4. The right to seek, receive, and impart information (UN General Assembly, 1976, Article 19(2); CESCR, 2000, para. 12). An example would be a nation withholding information on analgesia or the nature and provision of palliative care.

5. Children. The *Convention on the Rights of the Child* contains a clear statement on the rights of all children and adolescents to the provision of health care (UN General Assembly, 1989). Significantly and expressly, the Committee overseeing the Convention identified States' responsibility to support the palliative care of children (Committee on the Rights of the Child, 2011). The Committee expressed concern that, in a particular country, most palliative care was provided by non-government organizations without sufficient financial support and recommended that the country establish adequate funding for these services (Committee on the Rights of the Child, 2011).

6. Older persons. The Committee overseeing the right to health in the ICESCR stated that State parties should uphold the right of elderly persons to the enjoyment of a satisfactory standard of physical and mental health (CESCR, 1995) and, in relation to older persons, to take a broad view of health including care of the terminally ill (CESCR, 1995).

The content of the obligation

Assuming that the right to pain management and palliative care exists under international human rights law, what obligations flow from that right? It is important to note that the rights articulated in the international conventions rest on individual nations, not on clinicians. Signatory countries are mandated to appear before that committee to outline their fulfilment of the rights enumerated in the covenant, including the right to health.

The content of the obligation on signatory countries in the provision of adequate pain management and palliative care can be gleaned from the Committee that oversees the ICESCR. In 2000, it issued a General Comment on the right to health (CESCR, 2000). In essence it stated that this right contained the following 'interrelated and essential elements': availability of health goods and services, accessibility of health services to all citizens, acceptability in terms of culture and religious beliefs, and quality in terms of skills and expertise. These foundation stones—availability, accessibility, acceptability, and quality—are useful points of reference in assessing the adequacy of any nation in the fulfilment of its obligations in the provision of palliative care.

The Committee went on to describe the 'core obligations' of all signatory nations, irrespective of resources. They included obligations to ensure access to health facilities, goods, and services on a non-discriminatory basis, to provide essential drugs, as defined by the WHO, and to adopt and implement a national public health strategy. Interpreting this Comment in the context of palliative care, this would oblige nations to ensure a universal access to services, the provision of basic medications for symptom control and terminal care, including analgesics, and the adoption and implementation of national pain and palliative care policies. In addition to the 'core obligations' the Committee also enumerated obligations 'of comparable priority'. These included health education, access to information, and the provision of appropriate training for health professionals. In the context of palliative care, a 'main health problem' in all countries, this would obligate governments to ensure the education of health professionals in the principles and practice of palliative care and, further, provide access to the general community to information regarding it.

Towards a transdisciplinary consensus on the content of the obligation

Do the obligations that derive from human rights law accord with recommendations articulated from other sources? And if so, is there a synergy between them? The first source is the WHO; the second is the international palliative care community itself. The WHO laid down minimum standards of palliative care expected of countries. Those standards included the adoption of national palliative care policies, ensuring the availability of essential medications, including morphine across all health-care settings and ensuring the education and training of health professionals. Those standards are consistent with the WHO 'Public Health Strategy for Palliative Care' (Sjernsward et al., 2007) and have been consistently replicated in the multiple statements and declarations by the principal international pain and palliative care representative bodies. Synthesizing these sources—the Committee overseeing the right to health care, the WHO, and the international palliative care community—a consensus begins to emerge. Whether as an obligation under international human rights law or as recommendations through the WHO and international palliative care bodies the content of that consensus includes the following:

1. The creation and implementation of national palliative care policies.

2. Equity of access to services, without discrimination.

3. Availability and affordability of critical medications, including opioids.

4. The provision of palliative care at all levels of care.

5. The integration of palliative care education at all levels of the learning continuum from informal caregivers to health professionals.

The response of the United Nations

Irrespective of the strength of the argument that the provision of palliative care constitutes a human right, it could only truly gain hold if the UN itself acknowledged its merit. The first and vital steps in that acknowledgement came in statements made by two UN Special Rapporteurs on human rights. In a statement made to the UN Human Rights Council in 2008, the Special Rapporteur on the Right to Health placed palliative care firmly within the obligations that derive from the international right to health:

> Many other right-to-health issues need urgent attention, such as palliative care . . . Every year millions suffer horrific, avoidable pain . . . Palliative care needs greater attention. (Hunt, 2008)

Similarly, the UN Special Rapporteur on Torture in his report to the Human Rights Council in 2009 stated 'the de facto denial of access to pain relief, if it causes pain and suffering, constitutes cruel, inhuman or degrading treatment or punishment' (UN Human Rights Council, 2009) and that everything should be done to overcome all obstacles—regulatory, educational, and attitudinal—to the provision of palliative care and access to appropriate medications such as opioids. A similar statement was made by the Rapporteur in a report to the UN Human Rights Council in 2013 (UN Human Rights Council, 2013). In addition, the two Rapporteurs made a joint statement to the Chairperson of the Commission on Narcotic Drugs in 2008. After reviewing the inadequacies of pain management and palliative care around the world, they stated that under international human right to health governments should provide essential medicines and that the lack of access to such medication, including for pain management, was a global human rights issue (Nowak and Grover, 2009).

That statement then proceeded to make clear, practical recommendations for all nations that they:

◆ Ensure that national drug laws reflect the legitimate medical needs of the population for the management of pain and suffering.

◆ Ensure that national laws and regulations do not unnecessarily prevent access to these medications.

◆ Ensure that national authorities and health ministries, in consultation with health-care providers, work to establish health-care systems that are capable of ensuring wide availability of controlled medicines

◆ Ensure appropriate education to health professionals on the medical use of all controlled medicines listed on the WHO Model List of Essential Medicines and on the legal requirements for prescribing and dispensing controlled medicines.

◆ Allocate sufficient funds and personnel to implement all the above stated objectives (Nowak and Grover, 2009).

These statements were a major breakthrough. They not only represent the most explicit linkage of human rights UN, but they also provide clinicians and advocates a clear statement of recommendations to present to the health ministries of individual countries.

The response of the World Health Organization

From its foundation, the WHO has promoted the universal right to health care (WHO 1946). The WHO has stated that under its Access to Controlled Medicines Programme (ACMP), access to WHO Essential Medicines is part of a nation's human rights obligations (WHO, 2011). Subsequent to the *Montréal Statement on the Human Right to Essential Medicines* (University of Montreal, 2005), the WHO requested the IAHPC prepare a list of Essential Medicines for Palliative Care (De Lima and Doyle, 2007).

In the modern era, the WHO has expressly linked the overall right to health care with certain aspects of care, including pain management and access to analgesia. They did so expressly in a major document: *Ensuring Balance in National Policies on Controlled Substances: Guidance for Availability and Accessibility of Controlled Medicines* (WHO, 2011). That document was followed shortly thereafter by a landmark collaboration between the WHO, the INCB, and the UN. They jointly released recommendations for nations to ensure they accurately report their opioid requirements for medical purposes to the INCB and a guide for nations on estimating those requirements (INCB et al., 2012).

The counterarguments

There are several counterarguments to the proposition that pain management and palliative care are basic human rights. The first is the nature of human rights themselves. For some nations the concept of individual human rights is contrary to a view of a collective view of society whereby the paramount obligation of a government is the collective welfare of the people and society rather than necessarily meeting the needs of an individual. A response to that argument in the context of palliative care would be, given that mortality is universal and that the caring for individuals with serious illness will come to most members of society at some point, the provision of adequate palliative care services fulfils both an individual-based view of society *and* a collective one.

The second is the danger of arguing in isolation. Any discussion about access to palliative care services must be predicated upon the fulfilment of many other interrelated needs of a person with a serious life-limiting illness—water, sanitation, warmth, bedding, and a habitable environment. It would be artificial to separate 'a right to palliative care' from a general right to health, housing, water, and sanitation—social determinants of health that are inadequate in many communities living in low socioeconomic conditions. That interconnectedness was made express by the General Comment on the right to health (CESCR, 2000). The other perspective that needs broadening is the sense of palliative care itself. Rather than sitting in isolation, the discipline of palliative care articulates well with broader public health approaches of promotive, preventative, curative, and rehabilitative health.

The third is misunderstanding. *That these rights demand perfection.* They do not. They simply ask of governments to pursue the fulfilment of these rights progressively. *That these rights are Western ideals and are unattainable in nations of limited resources.* Studies have clearly shown that the provision of palliative care services including palliative care education, policy development, and legislative reform to ensure availability of essential palliative care medications are neither expensive nor unsustainable. Indeed, the growth of palliative care services in resource-poor environments demonstrates their feasibility and the application of basic strategies can provide much benefit.

The final contrary argument is that the above discussion is largely confined to the direct obligations on governments, not individual clinicians. That is true. To examine the obligations of clinicians in any society one must look at both the professional responsibility of a health professional to a patient and the legal framework of the country. In terms of professional responsibility one could argue that there is a universal obligation on doctors to manage the pain of their patients. Certainly, the *Declaration of Montréal* (International Pain Summit of the IASP, 2011) sponsored by the IASP, included this obligation on health professionals. Indeed, there is a direct connection between obligations on national governments and clinicians. The lack of fulfilment by the former makes it impossible for the fulfilment by the latter. If the infrastructure of pain management—availability, accessibility, education—is absent then it is extremely difficult for doctors to adequately respond to the pain management needs of their patients. Beyond ethical obligations, obligations that may arise from a legal right emerge from the domestic laws of that country.

Employing a human rights discourse to advance palliative care—current and future strategies

> There are few things more elemental than pain, they tell us of the fundamental equality, the fundamental dignity that all of us should enjoy. (Longstaff, 2012)

The basic argument linking pain management, palliative care, and human rights has moved from advocacy and assertion to action. In numerous discussions, workshops, and submissions on the subject of pain management and palliative care, a foundation argument has been the universality of these issues and the responsibility of governments, morally and legally, to do better in providing adequate access to these services. Those arguments can be made significantly more robust where there is a clear foundation not only in evidence-based practice but also in human rights law. In addition to strengthening the argument, an approach based on human rights carries with it a coherent structure upon which to assess the performance of any individual nation in its provision of palliative care.

How can this approach be used practically? There are multiple points of possible application. A human rights perspective may be incorporated in:

1. A national pain/palliative care assessment. This would involve examining five critical issues:

   a. Does the nation have pain and palliative care policies?

   b. The national opioid laws. To what extent do they restrict the availability and accessibility of opioids?

   c. Does the nation report their annual opioid requirements for medical purposes to the International Control Board? If not, that is a critical threshold issue. If they do, are these estimates realistic and commensurate with need?

   d. Education. To what extent is the management of patients with life-limiting illnesses and the safe and appropriate use of opioids incorporated into the education of health professionals?

e. To what extent are palliative care services integrated across all levels of health care?

Each aspect of this assessment reflects the human rights obligations of individual countries as signatories to international human rights conventions as outlined earlier. An example of a national assessment was the report by Human Rights Watch (HRW) on paediatric pain management in Kenya (HRW, 2010).

2. Once a national assessment has been made, to employ a human rights argument to strengthen advocacy to national governments. In essence that argument would be that, in addition to any other imperative for government engagement and action, there are clear human rights obligations on governments in this area. An example is the Lisbon Challenge launched at the EAPC Congress in 2011 with four clear objectives of palliative care for the nations of Europe based on a human rights approach. If a nation is struggling to report accurate estimations of annual opioid use, to refer departments of health to guidelines that can assist them (INCB et al., 2012).

3. Advocacy and support of citizens in countries where a right to health care is entrenched in the national constitution. A good example is the Republic of South Africa where, pursuant to a constitutional right to health care, the Department of Health proclaimed the *Patients' Rights Charter* (South African Department of Health, 2007). That Charter included a right of all citizens to access to affordable and effective palliative care.

4. A point of collaboration between clinicians and human rights lawyers and advocates. Examples include collaborative workshops held in South Africa (2008) and the Ukraine (2009) organized by the Open Society Institute and in the Netherlands (2011) organized by the International Federation of Health and Human Rights Organisations.

5. As a basis of opioid law reform. An example of legislative reform is seen in Romania where the government, on advice from the Romanian Palliative Care Commission, changed restrictive and burdensome opioid legislation to legislation in line with international recommendations (Mosoiu et al., 2007). A critical catalyst of this work was the Pain and Policy Study Group (PPSG) at the University of Wisconsin, United States, which has an international expertise in the promotion of, and practicalities around, opioid law reform. The African Palliative Care Association has also influenced governments in Africa to reform opioid legislation through workshops focusing on accessibility of essential pain medications (Ddungu and Mugula, 2007).

6. Submissions to agencies within the UN, including the Committees that oversee the relevant international covenants.

In the modern world, the universality of mortality has not been met by a universality of response. For patients with life-limiting illnesses, there remains widely divergent access to palliative care services, availability and accessibility of analgesic medication, and training of health professionals in this area. A study in 2011 by the WPCA reported that, out of the world's 234 countries, only 136 (58%) have one or more hospice or palliative care services available to seriously ill people and their families and carers (WPCA, 2011). Many nations are either poorly engaged or simply unresponsive to these needs. An approach based on human rights has emerged in the interrelated disciplines of pain management and palliative care. That approach has a clear foundation in international human rights law. It has been acknowledged by the WHO, the World Medical Association, and from within the structure of the UN itself and remains an important agent for advocacy, change, and development.

It is clear that palliative care services worldwide are inadequate to meet the needs of patients with life-threatening and life-limiting illness and there is much work to be done to ensure that palliative care is accessible, available, and affordable to people needing this care. A human rights approach to facilitate development of these services provides a strong foundation plan for the implementation of palliative care services within countries.

Online materials

Complete references for this chapter are available online at <http://www.oxfordmedicine.com>.

References

African Palliative Care Association (APCA). Advocacy Workshop for Palliative Care in Africa, Report of workshop held in Accra, Ghana, May 2007. Kampala, Uganda. Acessible at http://www.apca.co.ug/advocacy/workshop/.htm.

Committee on Economic, Social and Cultural Rights (2000). *General Comment No. 14: The Right to the Highest Attainable Standard of Health* (Art. 12 of the Covenant), 11 August 2000, E/C.12/2000/4. New York: United Nations.

Cousins, M.J. (1999). Pain—the past, present and future of anesthesiology? The E.A. Rovenstine Memorial Lecture. *Anesthesiology*, 91, 538–551.

De Lima, L. and Doyle, D. (2007). The International Association of Hospice and Palliative Care list of essential medicines for palliative care. *Journal of Pain and Palliative Care Pharmacotherapy*, 21(3), 29–36.

European Association of Palliative Care (2011). *The Lisbon Challenge*. The 12th EAPC Congress, Lisbon Portugal, May 2011. [Online] Available at: <http://www.eapcnet.eu/Themes/Policy/Lisbonchallenge.aspx>.

European Association of Palliative Care (2013). *The Prague Charter*. [Online] Available at: <http://eapcnet.eu/Themes/Policy/PragueCharter.aspx>.

Hunt, P. (2008). *Statement by Paul Hunt, Special Rapporteur on the Right of Everyone to Highest Attainable Standard of Physical and Mental Health to the UN Human Rights Council*. [Online] Available at: <http://www.hospicecare.com/resources/painpallcarehr/docs/paulhuntoralremarks_hrcmarcch2008.pdf>.

International Association for Hospice and Palliative Care and the Worldwide Palliative Care Alliance (2008). *Joint Declaration and Statement of Commitment on Palliative care and Pain Treatment as Human Rights*. [Online] Available at: <http://www.hospicecare.com/resources/pain_pallcare_hr/docs/dsc.pdf>.

International Narcotics Control Board (2010). *Report of the International Narcotics Control Board on the Availability of Internationally Controlled Drugs: Ensuring Adequate Access for Medical and Scientific Purposes*. New York: United Nations.

International Pain Summit of the IASP (2011). Declaration of Montréal. *Journal of Pain and Palliative Care Pharmacotherapy*, 25(1), 29–31.

Latin American Federation of IASP Chapters and Foundation for the Treatment of Pain as a Human Right (2008). *Proclamation of Pain Treatment and the Application of Palliative Care as Human Rights*. [Online] Available at: <http://hospicecare.com/uploads/2011/8/panama_proclamation_pain_relief_as_a_human_right_english.pdf>.

Mpanga-Sbuyira, L., Mwangi-Powell, F., Pereira, J., and Spence, C. (2003). The Cape Town Palliative Care Declaration: home-grown solutions for Sub-Saharan Africa. *Journal of Palliative Medicine*, 6, 341–343.

National Hospice and Palliative Care Associations (2005). *The Korea Declaration*. Report of the second global summit of National Hospice and Palliative Care Associations, Seoul, Korea. [Online] Available at: <http://www.eolc-observatory.net/global/pdf/NHPCA_2.pdf>.

Nowak, M. and Grover, A. (2009). *Special Rapporteurs on Torture and the Right of Everyone to the Highest Attainable Standard of Physical and Mental Health*. Letter to Mr D. Best, Vice-Chairperson of the Commission on Narcotic Drugs, 10 December 2008. [Online] Available at: <http://www.hr.dp.org/files/wp-content/uploads/2009/12/SpecialRapporteursLettertoCND012009.pdf>.

Pallium India, International Association of Hospice and Palliative Care, and Pain and Policy Study Group, *et al.* (2012). *The Morphine Manifesto*. [Online] Available at: <http://www.palliumindia.org/manifesto>.

United Nations Conference for the Adoption of a Single Convention on Narcotic Drugs (1961). *Single Convention on Narcotic Drugs*. [Online] Available at: <http://www.incb.org/documents/Narcotic-Drugs/1961-Convention/convention_1961_en.pdf>.

United Nations General Assembly (1966). *International Covenant on Economic, Social and Cultural Rights*, 16 December 1966. New York: United Nations.

United Nations General Assembly (1989). *Convention on the Rights of the Child*, 20 November 1989. New York: United Nations.

UN Human Rights Council (2009). *Report of the Special Rapporteur on Torture and Other Cruel, Inhuman or Degrading Treatment or Punishment, Manfred Nowak*. 14 January 2009, A/HRC/10/44. New York: United Nations. Available at: <http://www.refworld.org/docid/498c211e2.html>.

UN Human Rights Council (2013). *Report of the Special Rapporteur on Torture and Other Cruel, Inhuman or Degrading Treatment or Punishment to the UN Human Rights Council*, 1 February 2013, A/HRC/22/53. New York: United Nations. Available at: <http://www.refworld.org/docid/51136ae62.html>.

University of Montreal (2005). *Montréal Statement on the Human Right to Essential Medicines*. Montreal: University of Montreal.

World Health Organization (2011). *Ensuring Balance in National Policies on Controlled Substances: Guidance for Availability and Accessibility of Controlled Medicines*. [Online] Available at: <http://www.atome-project.eu>.

World Medical Association (2011). *WMA Resolution on the Access to Adequate Pain Treatment. Adopted by the 62nd WMA General Assembly, Montevideo, Uruguay, October 2011*. [Online] Available at: <http://www.wma.net/en/30publications/10policies/p2>.

5.2

Confidentiality

Timothy W. Kirk

Introduction to confidentiality

This chapter offers an explanation of, and approach to, respecting confidentiality as an ethical obligation in the practice of hospice and palliative medicine. Understood in the context of coincident ethical obligations to maximize clinical benefit, avoid preventable harm, and restore moral agency, respecting confidentiality is embedded in the most basic philosophical precepts that define hospice and palliative care. *How* to respect confidentiality in everyday practice, however, can be a matter of unusual complexity. As such, following a brief conceptual framework, the chapter explores ways to employ the framework in the service of patients and families in clinical practice. While various regions and nationalities will have legal and regulatory requirements informing the definition and practice of respecting confidentiality, this chapter focuses instead on respecting confidentiality as an ethical value. Readers are encouraged to supplement the content of this chapter with the relevant requirements that apply in their practice location.

Agency, meaning, and interdisciplinary family-centred care: a brief philosophical context

Hospice and palliative care have a richly developed philosophical history, and it is only through that philosophy that the ethical significance of confidentiality can be fully articulated. Hospice care, in particular, is heavily informed by the clinical and philosophical work of Dame Cicely Saunders. Saunders was quite explicit in her writing that the defining feature of the hospice philosophy of care as she envisioned it was that it works with patients and families to restore and support the capacity of terminally ill persons to live meaningful lives. Indeed, while relief of symptom distress was an integral part of the hospice model Saunders established at St Christopher's Hospice in London, this relief was not an end in itself. Rather, it was a necessary condition employed, concomitantly with social and spiritual care, in the service of a more fundamental purpose: respecting the dignity of persons by allowing them to exercise their moral agency (Saunders, 1978; Kirk, 2014).

Restoring agency—the ability to intentionally express, live, and act upon the perception and creation of meaning—when possible, and respecting that agency in all cases, even when the capacity for restoration is minimal, are profoundly moral enterprises. By focusing on engaging patients at the level of their lived experience as persons, and not just their symptoms as bodies, hospice and palliative care clinicians acknowledge and affirm the value and dignity of patients and family members as human persons. It is

precisely this emphasis on restoring and respecting the agency of persons that led Saunders to construct hospice as a model of care that is interdisciplinary and family-centred.

Hospice and palliative care are interdisciplinary enterprises because assessing and addressing the multiple ways in which serious illness interrupts patients' lives require the coordinated intervention of multiple disciplines. Effective response to the vulnerability created by many serious illnesses requires a response more comprehensive and complex than can be delivered by a single discipline. And, because hospice and palliative care teams are restoring agency—and not just relieving symptom distress—the integrated work of expert medical and non-medical clinicians is necessary to mitigate the threats to personhood posed by serious and terminal illness.

Similarly, hospice and palliative care are family-centred care models because the professional care team recognizes that partnering with the support structures and meaningful relationships that patients have developed across their lifespans is often the most effective way to create and deliver a care plan that reduces levels of distress and suffering and empowers patients to recover and exercise their agency as moral persons.

Some (Randall and Downie, 1999) have argued that it is precisely this interdisciplinary, family-centred model of care that presents significant challenges to honouring ethical obligations related to maintaining confidentiality. However, this chapter presents an approach to understanding confidentiality as an instrumental value which gains its ethical significance through its connection to other, more fundamental ethical values of respecting persons, maximizing clinical benefit, and avoiding preventable harm.

Defining 'confidentiality'

Confidentiality is related to, but distinct from, privacy and secrecy. Privacy and secrecy focus on the phenomenon of disclosure. When we ask someone—whether a friend, colleague, or health-care provider—to keep a matter secret, we are asking them not to disclose the matter to others. Similarly, when we seek greater privacy in the form of closing window shades, closing doors, or planting trees along a property line, we are attempting to limit how much we disclose visually to others. *Why* we request secrecy or seek privacy is not germane to the nature of secrecy or privacy as phenomena.

Confidentiality, however, is more complex. While patients may be seeking privacy or secrecy when they request (or assume) confidentiality in health-care relationships, the very term itself points to the reason why: to establish or maintain confidence, or trust, in the relationship between patient and provider. In this way, confidentiality is primarily about the nature of therapeutic relationships, not about specific bits of information. That is, confidentiality is a *relational* value: its meaning and ethical significance arise only in the context of specific relationships.

Given the above, respecting confidentiality can be defined as follows: those practices and behaviours that serve to strengthen the trust and confidence between patients and their health-care providers, with special attention paid to the use of any and all information disclosed by, or obtained from, patients during their care experience.

Justifying a duty to maintain confidentiality

As noted by Thompson (1979), the *why* behind respecting confidentiality is often neglected in the literature, despite much ink being spilled on the legal and regulatory nuances of *how* to do so. Asking why confidentiality is important, however, yields an instructive response quite relevant to clinical practice.

The ethical duty to respect confidentiality is valuable because it generates and reflects other phenomena that are valued by professionals, patients, and families. As such, confidentiality is an instrumental, rather than an intrinsic, ethical value (see Fig. 5.2.1). That is, rather than being something we seek in itself, its value is rooted in its association with more fundamental ethical values in health care: respect for persons, avoiding preventable harm, and optimizing clinical outcomes (see Fig. 5.2.1). Each of these three values will be addressed in turn.

Respecting confidentiality respects persons insofar as it honours patients' discretion, protects their integrity, and exercises fidelity to promises made to them in the care relationship (see Fig. 5.2.2). Part of what it means to be a full moral person is that we have the right to exercise discretion over what aspects of ourselves to make public and what aspects of ourselves to keep private (Yeo and Moorhouse, 2010). Whether it is revealing certain parts of our bodies, certain facts about our identities, or certain pieces of our histories, what makes such matters 'personal' is precisely the fact that persons have discretion over when, in what conditions, and to whom they are revealed or hidden. Indeed, Cassell's (1982) influential model of suffering claims that suffering occurs when there is a threat—actual or perceived—to integrity of one's personhood. He defines such integrity as the way in which the different pieces of one's life fit together to form a whole person. One of those parts, according to Cassell, is one's 'secret life', the thoughts, hopes, fears, and history that we choose not to reveal to (or, to only reveal to carefully selected) others. In this model, violating confidentiality constitutes an affront to the personhood of patients by interrupting the integrity of their lives. Finally, if patients reveal personal information to health-care providers in the course of seeking care, then agreeing upon the terms of use for that information, and honouring such an agreement, is a way of respecting their personhood. This is especially so given that patients who seek the care of palliative care practitioners may be subject to increased vulnerability that accompanies the symptom and psychosocial distress attendant to serious or terminal illness. As such vulnerability creates a power imbalance between clinicians and patients, clinicians incur a fiduciary duty to safeguard the personhood of their patients. Honouring promises made by maintaining confidentiality exhibits fidelity to those promises. As promises are inherently moral acts made by and to persons, acting with fidelity honours patients' personhood.

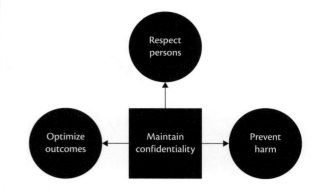

Fig. 5.2.1 The relationship between confidentiality and other core values in health care.

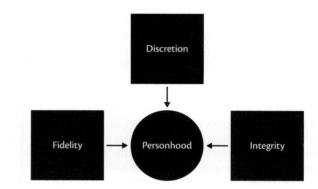

Fig. 5.2.2 Respecting confidentiality promotes three values essential for respecting a patient's personhood.

Respecting confidentiality facilitates beneficial clinical outcomes insofar as accurate diagnosis and treatment adherence are both linked to a patient's trust and confidence in her health-care providers (Hall et al., 2001; Graham et al., 2010). Simply stated, patients are more likely to adhere to the treatment recommendations of their health-care providers if they trust them. Respecting confidentiality generates trust. Similarly, as a successful diagnostic interview may require patients to disclose facts about their personal lives that they consider to be very private—facts about sexual behaviours, toileting patterns, illegal actions with health implications, etc.—the promise of confidentiality (and trust in the clinician to honour the promise) facilitates such disclosure. Failing to honour such a promise, or to adequately disclose the limits of confidentiality, constitutes a barrier to future disclosure. Whether via improved treatment adherence or truthful disclosure of relevant information, respecting confidentiality can improve outcomes (see Fig. 5.2.3).

Finally, respecting confidentiality can prevent avoidable harm (see Fig 5.2.4). Patients may choose which information to disclose to whom in what circumstances based on the perception of harm or benefit that accompanies such disclosure/nondisclosure. The ability to discern the degree to which such perceptions are accurate is often outside the scope of practice of hospice and palliative care clinicians. Knowing only a small part of each patient's story and life situation, failing to respect confidentiality by violating patients' requests to keep certain information private risks incurring precisely the harm they may have been avoiding by keeping such information private.

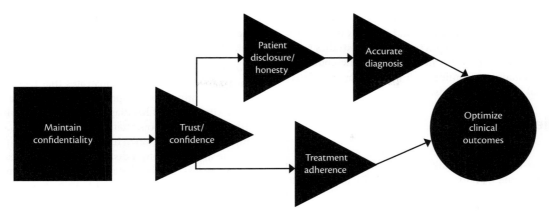

Fig. 5.2.3 The ways in which respecting confidentiality can optimize patient outcomes.

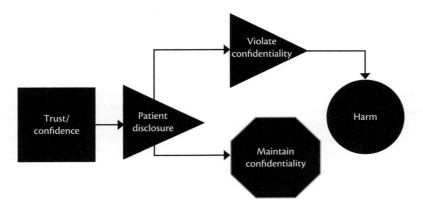

Fig. 5.2.4 The relationship between trust, disclosure, confidentiality, and patient harm.

Respecting confidentiality: the basics

Clinicians in hospice and palliative care can respect confidentiality in their relationships with patients and families by ensuring that three basic elements are a part of their practice.

1. *Establish and follow organizational practices that effectively respect confidentiality.* Effectively respecting confidentiality requires effort at the level of organizational policy, and cannot be accomplished only through the efforts of individual clinicians. Policies and procedures addressing disclosure, record-keeping, email/fax/phone communication, and compliance with regional and national law should be established and implemented, practices monitored, and needs reviewed regularly. Procedures surrounding hiring and termination of employees should address confidentiality. All employees—from senior management, to senior clinicians, to trainee clinicians, to administrative and clerical staff, to operations and janitorial staff—have an important role to play in respecting confidentiality and should be educated and incentivized accordingly.

2. *Be clear and explicit with patients and families about the principles and practices related to confidentiality in your practice environment.* Patients and their families should understand the scope and limits of confidentiality as they relate to each aspect of their care. As it is the trusting relationship with clinicians that confidentiality fosters, explanation and discussion of the nature and limits of confidentiality in the clinical encounter should be conducted by the primary clinicians involved in patients' care—not office staff or others outside of that relationship. This should connect the notion of confidentiality more directly with the clinical relationship in the minds of patients and families. Such discussions should address the following questions: who will have access to which information about patients? For what reasons? How will this be monitored? What information is considered 'confidential' and what is not considered so? How long does this confidentiality last? (Until the patient loses decision-making capacity? Until the patient's death? For a certain number of years following death?) What kind of information will need to be shared, under what conditions, regardless of a request for privacy, and with whom will it be shared?

3. *Immediately inform patients when breaches of confidentiality occur, and take action to mitigate the damages caused by such breaches.* Even in the presence of strong organizational policies and controls and in the practice of conscientious clinicians, breaches of confidentiality can occur. Quickly notifying patients of such breaches, and working with them to mitigate any short- and long-term harm arising from such breaches, fosters good will and is consistent with behaviours that maintain trust and confidence.

In sum, respecting confidentiality is intentionally engaging a set of behaviours that fosters the trust of patients and families in clinical relationships in a manner that maximizes beneficial clinical outcomes, avoids preventable harm, and respects the personhood of all parties involved. The following three case studies make use of this framework to identify ethical questions and courses of action that seek to maintain confidentiality while being attentive to multiple ethical and clinical goals.

Case studies and analysis

Case 1

Mr Q is a 67-year-old African American husband and father of three who lives at home with his wife in a small city in the southern United States. Diagnosed 4 years ago with stage IV breast cancer, he has received several courses of chemotherapy with adjuvant hormone therapy that have slowed, but not stopped, disease progression. Mr Q's illness experience has been especially difficult because, in addition to the significant distress of a cancer diagnosis and treatment, he has found the type of cancer—breast cancer—to be emasculating and humiliating. Believing it to be 'a lady's disease', he has not revealed his precise diagnosis to friends or family, speaking only generically of 'the cancer'.

Following a meeting with his oncology team, with whom Mr Q has an open and trusting relationship, he agreed to talk with a nurse about receiving home hospice care. Attracted to the possibility of dying in his own home, he enrolled in a hospice programme 3 months ago. Throughout the course of his illness, Mr Q has been adamant about making decisions independently, preferring not to involve his wife or children in any care discussion that might reveal the fact that his cancer is breast cancer. Indeed, his primary concern in beginning hospice care was that he would have to tell his diagnosis to clinicians outside of his closely trusted oncology team. It was only with his oncologist's ongoing reassurance that the hospice team would maintain the confidentiality of his diagnosis that he finally agreed to receive care.

As Mr Q progresses toward death, his wife's distress is increasing significantly. While social workers and spiritual caregivers are offering her support, she is upset that 'the man she has shared a bed with for 40 years will not tell me what is killing him'. Mr Q's children are also growing upset about the lack of disclosure, wondering if they are at risk for 'getting whatever he has' when they are older, and telling him that he is 'harming our future health' by not telling them his diagnosis. Mr Q remains firm in not discussing his diagnosis with his family, and is increasingly worried that the hospice team will not honour his wishes.

In weekly team meetings, hospice clinicians are expressing confusion and concern about what, and to whom, their most important ethical obligations are in this case. On the one hand, Mr Q is the dying patient, and some team members stress the importance of respecting his wishes—including not disclosing his diagnosis to his family. On the other hand, hospice care is family-centred care, and some team members emphasize the obligations they have to the family, questioning whether maintaining confidentiality for Mr Q is increasing the suffering of his family and, in turn, violating their obligations to support and care for family members.

Analysis of Case 1

1. *Respecting personhood.* Mr Q has been unambiguous about his desire to keep his diagnosis a secret from family and friends. Honouring his discretion about revealing personal information,

the integrity of his secret life, and the promises made to him at the time of admission to hospice care all support maintaining confidentiality and not disclosing his diagnosis to his family.

2. *Maximizing beneficial clinical outcomes.* Mr Q's history with his oncology team clearly demonstrates that trust and confidence in his care providers is important to him. Similarly, his concern about the impact of his diagnosis on his masculinity raises the risk for stoic behaviour that may make him reluctant to disclose important information to his current hospice care team—information about symptom distress that, he may fear, would make him seem less 'manly' if he reported it or requested intervention for relief (Robinson et al., 2001.). As such, respecting confidentiality by honouring his request not to disclose his diagnosis is important if the team wants to partner with Mr Q in effectively managing his symptoms. Similarly, an accurate assessment of his symptom profile—a process greatly aided by timely and accurate patient disclosure of symptom burden—will aid the team projecting his time until death. This, in turn, will be quite helpful in supporting Mr Q and his family as death nears.

3. *Preventing harm.* Mr Q perceives the diagnosis of breast cancer to be a threat to his identity as a husband, father, and man. The team does not agree with this perception. There may be an opportunity for a member of the team to work with him to challenge this perception, to educate him about the prevalence of breast cancer in men, and to distinguish the concept of 'breast' as an object of sexual pleasure/beauty or maternal nourishment from the concept of 'breast' as a type of fatty tissue that, in his case, is the primary site of disease. They could also offer to work with his family towards a shared understanding of this information.

In addressing the family's frustration/anxiety over (a) the perception that Mr Q's lack of disclosure reflects a lack of trust and (b) that his lack of disclosure may be withholding important information relevant to his children's future health, the team could work with Mr Q to do a thorough family health history related to the cancer. If there are not first-degree relatives in Mr Q's family who have breast cancer, they could counsel the family that Mr Q's condition does not suggest an elevated risk for contracting his illness, and do so without disclosing the precise diagnosis. If the family history does reveal the presence of breast cancer in first-degree relatives, the team can present this information, along with his children's concerns, to Mr Q and pursue ongoing persuasive efforts with the goal of supporting him in making the decision to tell his loved ones the diagnosis himself.

In sum, the three primary values implicated in maintaining confidentiality—respecting personhood, maximizing beneficial clinical outcomes, and preventing harm—are all best supported in this case by respecting the patient's request to not disclose his diagnosis to family members.

Case 2

Ms S is an 86-year-old Caucasian woman in a large teaching hospital in Sweden. Diagnosed 2 years ago with congestive heart failure, Ms S has declined rapidly in recent months. She is unable to walk her dog, Ludde, to the corner without becoming dyspnoeic, and has developed significant oedema that is no longer adequately responding to diuresis. She was admitted to hospital 4 days ago in respiratory distress, and has been transferred to the palliative care unit. Ms S's daughter, Marie, has been a constant presence at her side since hospitalization, leaving only once Ms S falls asleep in the evening and often arriving before she wakes in the morning.

On day five, Ms S encourages Marie to take some time away from the hospital to rest and check in on Ludde, who is being cared for by a neighbour. While her daughter is away, Ms S asks her primary nurse if she would be willing to witness a change in her last will and testament. In addition to Marie, Ms S has a son, Marc. Her current will leaves a modest estate split evenly between her two children. However, Marie has been so attentive during her hospitalization, and Marc so notably absent, Ms S now feels that an even split between the two may not be fair. 'After all,' she says, 'the end is near and I don't have much more time to make these changes. I may not even make it out of the hospital'. Ms S is adamant that no one, including Marie, be told of her desire to change the will.

The nurse is distraught. She has worked hard to establish a strong therapeutic relationship with Ms S and Marie. She is willing to be a witness for the document, but fears that not informing Marie (or, if he visits, Marc) might make them feel betrayed once they learn of the change. She does not want to be perceived by Marie or Marc as having colluded with Ms S behind their backs.

Analysis of Case 2

1. *Respecting personhood.* Ms S perceives, accurately, that the end of her life is very near. As such, her concern with the nature and content of her legacy with her family—in this case, her financial legacy—is an important expression of her personhood. Similarly, her desire to express her gratitude to her daughter, and express her feelings of loss and abandonment to her son, arise in the context of great vulnerability as she approaches the final transition of her life into death. Ms S surely has the right to discretion over to whom she leaves her estate, and how she does so. The role of a witness in this circumstance is simply to attest that Ms S had the decision-making capacity required to make an informed decision regarding her estate planning, and that she did so voluntarily. There are two distinct, though related, questions at play in this situation: (a) should the nurse serve as a signed witness to the document, and (b) should the nurse honour Ms S's request to not disclose the change in her estate plans?

    If the nurse agrees to witness the document, she should be very clear with Ms S about the terms of agreeing to do so. And, one of those terms should address whether or not, and for what reasons, the nurse also agrees to respect Ms S's request to not disclose that the document has been changed. In this case, the nurse would be agreeing or disagreeing to maintain confidentiality in her role as witness.

    Whether or not she agrees to witness the document, there is also the question of honouring Ms S's wishes to keep the fact that she is making changes to her estate planning confidential. If the nurse feels strongly that Ms S should discuss the changes with her family, she is free to explain that to the patient. However, as the patient waited until the daughter left the hospital to address the topic but openly discussed it with the nurse, this indicates that Ms S revealed her plan to the nurse under the implicit understanding that it would fall within the bounds of confidentiality. As such, maintaining that confidentiality also

maintains fidelity to the nurse's professional relationship with the patient.

2. *Maximizing beneficial clinical outcomes.* As noted in the discussion of Mr Q, effective symptom management and psychosocial support at the end of life requires the honest and timely disclosure of new or heightened symptom distress by the patient to the team. Building trust increases the likelihood of such disclosure, and respecting confidentiality contributes to that trust. For that reason, maintaining confidentiality is likely to maximize beneficial clinical outcomes for Ms S.

3. *Preventing harm.* It is not clear for what reasons Ms S wishes to keep the change in her estate plans confidential. If, however, one of the reasons has to do with Ms S's perception that disclosing the changes may result in harm to herself or her family, then exploring that perception of harm with the patient may be helpful for Ms S. Given the very brief relationship between the nurse and patient (less than a week), and absent robust evidence that the perception is inaccurate, the nurse should assume that Ms S knows the situation best and honour confidentiality to prevent the perceived harm from occurring, and the ensuing anxiety/distress on the part of Ms S that it may occur.

Case 3

Mr L is a 62-year-old patient who has amyotrophic lateral sclerosis. He lives at home with his partner, Robert, and is wheelchair dependent. As his symptoms progress, Mr L begins receiving visits from a home care nurse. Mr L has participated thoughtfully in advance care planning for himself, carefully documenting his refusal of ventilator support and artificial nutrition and hydration when he becomes unable to eat, drink, or breath on his own. Robert is supportive of Mr L's wishes and is active in his care.

At the end of an afternoon nursing visit, Robert and Mr L invite the nurse to stay for a cup of tea. During conversation, Mr L reveals that a veterinarian friend of his has given him some pentobarbital and that he plans to take it during the weekend and die with Robert at his side. When the nurse asks why, Mr L explains that he does not wish to continue to live as his function progressively declines, and that he is telling the nurse because he and Robert are both grateful for her support and care and wanted to 'say a proper goodbye'. When writing up her visit notes that evening, the nurse wonders whether or not to document the conversation, and realizes she may have a legal obligation to tell her supervisor that Mr L is 'suicidal'.

Analysis of Case 3

1. *Respecting personhood.* The question of whether or not Mr L is suicidal, and what ethical obligations arise from the answer to that question, is a complicated one. In patients who are terminally ill, there is an increasingly accepted distinction between (a) suicidal ideation and (b) the desire for hastened death (Breitbart et al., 2000). The latter is a common phenomenon (Arnold et al., 2004), and does not necessarily constitute a psychiatric emergency. Primary distinguishing features between the two include if, and how, the patient's desire is rational and voluntary (Bostwick and Cohen, 2009). We are not given enough information in this vignette to assess either, but such an assessment is important. If the patient's desire is rational and voluntary, it may be an important expression of his

personhood and maintaining confidentiality may be justified as a way to respect that personhood. If the patient's desire is not fully rational and voluntary, the patient's decision-making capacity—a crucial component of how personhood can be expressed—may be compromised, and intervention may be warranted, even if such intervention compromises confidentiality. In this case I would recommend that the nurse return to the patient's home to further explore the decision and the extent to which it is rational and voluntary. Such assessment will inform the extent to which the nurse has ethical obligations to the patient to keep his plans confidential or share them with her supervisor. (Note: the obligations discussed herein may be supplemented by legal and regulatory requirements specific to the nurse's care region.)

2. *Maximizing beneficial clinical outcomes.* Mr L's plans, and the circumstances in which they arise, reveal the ambiguity that can surround determining which clinical outcomes are 'beneficial', and for what reasons. Mr L has decided that death is a more beneficial outcome for him than continuing to live with his declining functional status. If such a decision is a rational and voluntary one resulting from careful consideration, there may be reason to accept Mr L's analysis even if it conflicts with regional practice norms or the nurse's own analysis. One complicating factor is the plan itself: ingestion of pentobarbital obtained from a veterinarian. The nurse does not know if Mr L has an adequate plan to result in a peaceful death, and cannot really confirm this without asking more questions about the source and dose of medication—questions that will further complicate her role in the process and, depending on her practice jurisdiction, may increase her exposure to criminal liability. As such, while a peaceful death may be beneficial to the patient based on his own analysis, the extent to which his current plan will bring about a peaceful death is not known.

3. *Preventing harm.* As with the determination of 'benefit', the case of Mr L also highlights the extent to which the definition of 'harm', and the relative weight of harms and benefits in ethical reasoning, is highly patient specific. Knowing the extent to which documenting the nurse's conversation with Mr L, or informing her supervisor of the same, affects the risk of harm for this patient requires not only consideration of what constitutes 'harm', but also consideration of what the likely outcomes are of documenting/informing about the conversation. If, for example, it would trigger a mandatory and involuntary psychiatric assessment, the nurse would have to weigh the perceived harm of undergoing such an assessment against the possibility of allowing Mr L to hasten his death—a calculation that would have to be informed by the extent to which the nurse has reason to believe Mr L's decision is, or is not, rational and voluntary. If, on the other hand, failing to document the conversation would, in turn, fail to instigate a more thorough review of the patient's history in which the district nursing supervisor would discover

a history of depression or compulsive harmful behaviour, the nurse would have to weigh the harm of violating Mr L's trust against the possible harm of missing information that could lead to a decision to intervene with more robust mental health support.

Conclusion

In each of the three cases discussed, the three-part model of an ethical duty to respect confidentiality—to respect personhood, to maximize beneficial clinical outcomes, and to avoid preventable harm—offers a useful framework to help guide clinicians in identifying questions and values to inform ethical decision-making about confidentiality. The framework does not change the reality that such ethical decision-making is fraught with difficulty and uncertainty. However, hospice and palliative care clinicians who use this framework will be well positioned to make clear and justified decisions on when and how to maintain confidentiality with their patients.

References

Arnold, E.M., Artin, K.A., Person, J.L., and Griffith, D.L. (2004). Consideration of hastening death among hospice patients and their families. *Journal of Pain and Symptom Management*, 27, 523–532.

Bostwick, J.M. and Cohen, L.M. (2009). Differentiating suicide from life-ending acts and end-of-life decisions: a model based on chronic kidney disease and dialysis. *Psychosomatics*, 50, 1–7.

Breitbart, W., Rosenfeld, B., Pessin, H., *et al.* (2000). Depression, hopelessness, and desire for hastened death in terminally ill cancer patients. *Journal of the American Medical Association*, 284, 2907–2911.

Cassell, E.J. (1982). The nature of suffering and the goals of medicine. *The New England Journal of Medicine*, 306, 639–645.

Graham, J.L., Gordiano, T.P., Grimes, R.M., Slomka, J., Ross, M., and Huang, L. (2010). Influence of trust on HIV diagnosis and care practices: a literature review. *Journal of the International Association of Physicians in AIDS Care*, 9, 346–352.

Hall, M.A., Dugan, E., Zheng, B., and Mishra, A.K. (2001). Trust in physicians and medical institutions: What is it, can it be measured, and does it matter? *The Milbank Quarterly*, 79, 613–639.

Kirk, T.W. (2014). Hospice care as a moral practice: exploring the philosophy and ethics of hospice care. In T.W. Kirk and B. Jennings (eds.) *Hospice Ethics*, pp. 35–56. New York: Oxford University Press.

Randall, F. and Downie, R. S. (1999). *Palliative Care Ethics: A Companion for All Specialties* (2nd ed.). Oxford: Oxford University Press.

Robinson, M.E., Riley, J.L., Myers, C.D., *et al.* (2001). Gender role expectations of pain: relationship to sex differences in pain. *The Journal of Pain*, 2, 251–257.

Saunders, C. (1978). The philosophy of terminal care. In C. Saunders (ed.) *The Management of Terminal Disease*, pp. 193–202. London: Edward Arnold.

Thompson, I.E. (1979). The nature of confidentiality. *Journal of Medical Ethics*, 5, 57–64.

Yeo, M. and Moorhouse, A. (2010). Confidentiality. In M. Yeo, A. Moorhouse, P. Kahn, and P. Rodney (eds.) *Concepts and Cases in Nursing Ethics* (3rd ed.), pp. 245–292. Peterborough, ON: Broadview Press.

Neuro-palliative care and disorders of consciousness

Joseph J. Fins and Barbara Pohl

Introduction: why palliative care and brain injury?

Whether one dates the origins of the palliative care movement to the hospice of the medieval pilgrimage or the advent of St Christopher's Hospice under Dame Cicely Saunders, a constant theme has been the care of patients on the margins, near death, often in pain, and likely abandoned in their distress (Fins, 2006a). This laudable history now continues with the proposition that palliative medicine expand the scope of its care to patients with disorders of consciousness, individuals with severe brain injury in the vegetative and minimally conscious states. Like more conventional beneficiaries of palliative care, these patients are also on the periphery of the acute care system. Recipients of brilliant care that saves their lives, these patients are often abandoned to an ill-equipped chronic care system that generally neglects their needs and those of their families.

These challenges are amplified because patients with disorders of consciousness generally cannot articulate their feelings or preferences and are prone to misdiagnosis. Some patients can experience pain, and perhaps suffer, even as they are unable to voice their discomfort. Families watch and wait and experience a vigil of either anticipatory grief or the pain of a slow bereavement, all in a context of care which is unable to meet these biopsychosocial needs.

This can be a difficult time for surrogates who are suddenly compelled to become decision-makers about conditions they likely know little about (Fins and Hersh, 2011). This places a tremendous burden on families and is an opportunity for engagement by skilled professionals, but too often there is no one available to comfort and provide informed counsel.

We envision this role as one that might be fulfilled by those who now provide palliative care, not because these patients will imminently die—although some certainly will—but rather because the profound burdens experienced by patients and families touched by brain injury are, in many ways, reminiscent of what the dying patient and family may experience. Thus, the skills gained in developing competence in palliative medicine could be readily transferrable to this new target population. When patients do die, palliative interventions can take hold. And when patients and families struggle to survive and adapt to a new reality, a palliative approach can help them recast their goals of care (Fins, 2006a) and make sense of an inalterably different life, much as a patient might grapple with the new knowledge of a terminal diagnosis.

The engagement of these patients will need to be orchestrated with care, lest it be communicated that they are being seen by palliative care specialists because they are dying. That would be the wrong message. Instead, the objective is to blend the skill-set that resides in palliative medicine with expertise in brain injury medicine that resides primarily in neuropsychology, rehabilitation medicine, and some sectors of neurology, thereby establishing the norms of *neuro*-palliative care. All of this would be in the service of a population which has historically been underserved and relegated to custodial care through benign neglect (Fins, 2003).

To that end, this chapter will define and describe the neuroscience of disorders of consciousness. We will consider emerging methods of diagnosis and treatment, including neuroimaging and neuroprosthetics, and address how the palliative care needs of patients and their surrogates might be better met. We will address questions of pain and suffering as they related to this cohort of patients. In addition, we will explore the ethical challenges of surrogate decision-making in light of neuroprosthetics that lead to re-emergent patient communication from patients who had previously been 'silenced' by their injury. We will explore how this variation on surrogate decision-making both enhances and complicates the informed consent process for both routine medical care and decisions to withhold and withdraw life-sustaining therapies. Finally, we will conclude with a systematic discussion of how the palliative medicine and hospice communities can better meet the needs of this vulnerable population by fostering links with both acute care and rehabilitative sectors.

Disorders of consciousness
Nosology and prognostication

Disorders of consciousness refer to severe brain injuries, which result in disturbances in arousal and awareness. A number of descriptive categories, which have characteristic, but somewhat overlapping, behavioural and neuroimaging stigmata, subsume these conditions. Generally, coma, the persistent and permanent vegetative states, and the minimally conscious state (MCS) fall under this broad classification (Laureys et al., 2004).

There are two conditions, which are often included under the rubric of disorders of consciousness, which should be distinguished from these conditions, namely brain death and the locked-in state (LIS). Brain death refers to whole-brain death involving both the brainstem and higher cortical function. The LIS is a disorder of motor output, but is often conflated with disorders of consciousness in error (Plum and Posner, 1972). Disorders of consciousness, in contrast, reflect composite disturbances of levels of arousal and awareness, that is, respectively, wakefulness or the 'readiness to respond to internal and external stimuli' (Bernat, 2009) and the ability to perceive aspects of the milieu and the self (Zemon et al., 1997).

In routine practice, and sometimes for polemical reasons (Fins and Plum 2004; Fins, 2006b) these categories are often conflated. When speaking with families of patients with disorders of consciousness, diagnostic clarity is important when invoking this nosology because each of these conditions has a particular time course and prognostic implications. Moreover, it is critical to appreciate that brain injury is dynamic and patients may start their disease trajectory in one state and evolve into another.

To track this trajectory, we will next define these brain states in more detail and suggest a means to convey prognostic information to expectant families as patients progress from initial stages of injury to later periods of recovery. Only as the course of the injury unfolds, can prognostic judgements reliably structure health-care decisions for patients with disorders of consciousness. As yet, no predictive model can fully account for the latent recovery of consciousness (Whyte et al., 2005; Katz et al., 2009). In the face of this knowledge deficit we suggest a method of *time de-limited prognostication* to structure clinical thinking and communication with surrogates (Banja and Fins, 2012). This method links clinical milestones, known to be associated with the process of recovery (The Multi-Society Task Force on PVS, 1994; Jennett 2002) with a longitudinal communication strategy to provide families with the information necessary to guide clinical care, both therapeutic and palliative (Fins 2007).

Coma

Coma may be the first clinical presentation of a severe brain injury or a complication or progression of an earlier insult. Patients do not exhibit wakefulness or respond to stimuli. It is an *eyes-closed* state of unresponsiveness, which represents dysfunction of the brainstem and higher cortical areas bihemispherically. Typically, they remain in this self-limited state for about 2 weeks, and can proceed in a variety of ways from brain death to full recovery (Schiff, 2009). If comatose patients do not devolve to brain death, or recover consciousness, they will progress to the vegetative state, either as a way station to higher levels of consciousness or to permanent unconsciousness as in the case of the permanent vegetative state.

Making a prediction regarding these variable outcomes depends on the history of the injury as well as the duration and time course of the comatose state. Comas from traumatic brain injury (TBI) have a far better prognosis than those following anoxia. Patients with a traumatic coma have a 50% chance of having an outcome at the level of the MCS or higher, while 77% of anoxic comas result in death or the vegetative state (Posner et al., 2007). The outcomes for anoxic coma with therapeutic hypothermia, as would follow cardiac arrest, is more favourable although precise data on outcomes are not yet available (Hypothermia after Cardiac Arrest Study Group, 2002; Scirica, 2013; Stevens and Sutter, 2013). Structural signs of herniation and loss of thalamic architecture are also associated with grave outcomes (Posner et al., 2007).

For the clinician, these distinctions in aetiology point to the importance of history taking in order to risk stratify outcomes. Overall the most important prognostic detail is how the patient was injured or became ill and distinguishing the aetiology as traumatic or anoxic, with vascular injuries being of intermediate severity. The exception to this general expectation is the emerging use of therapeutic hypothermia in the setting of cardiac arrest. This has a protective function that can be quite dramatic and cautions should be taken when prognosticating for recipients of this intervention.

Physicians may also be able to reliably formulate some expectations for recovery based on the length of time patients spend in the comatose state. Several studies indicate that while patients are in a coma, they exhibit neurological or electrophysiological signs that can reliably predict positive or negative moves to recovery (Posner et al., 2007). In most cases, an early versus late exit from coma portends a more favourable outcome, even if the patient only moves into the vegetative state, although a move to the vegetative state is less favourable than emergent consciousness. However, an early move to the vegetative state indicates recovery of brainstem function. The recovery of brainstem function defines the vegetative state.

Persistent and permanent vegetative states

Patients who do not recover consciousness after coma but recover brainstem activity, are vegetative, a state in which brainstem function is preserved but higher cortical functions are not. The vegetative state is a confounder for both clinicians and families alike. Unlike coma, it is an *eyes-open* state of unresponsiveness which can be both clinically confusing and ethically troubling. Clinically, the patient is in a state of what Jennet and Plum described as 'wakeful unresponsiveness', encapsulating both the physiological and ethical paradox of the condition (Jennett and Plum, 1972). Unlike comatose patients, patients in the *vegetative state* show signs of arousal but lack awareness. They will open their eyes in response to external stimuli, exhibit reflexive (but unintentional) movements and regain autonomic functions, such as respiratory or cardiac activity and sleep–wake cycles. None of these activities are purposeful and are basically autonomic functions.

This can be excruciatingly difficult for families. They become engaged with and generally ascribe awareness to individuals whose eyes are open. They can become optimistic about a patient's progress and think that their eyes-open state heralds a full recovery, only to become distressed when they are told that the patient is vegetative. Clinicians who consult with families need to appreciate how counter-intuitive the vegetative states can become for lay people and patiently help the surrogate understand this condition and its implication.

Most nosological schemes classify the vegetative state as *persistent* if it lasts for at least a month. It is considered *permanent* if it lasts for at least 3 months after an *anoxic* brain injury and for at least 12 months after a *traumatic* brain injury. Once the permanent vegetative state is reached, however, this neurological state is irreversible (Jennett, 2002). In addition, permanently vegetative patients have a mixed life expectancy. About 33% of patients in the permanent vegetative state die within a year of the injury (Jennett, 2002). Those patients who remain in the permanent vegetative state for more than a year typically do not die and can persist for many more years. Pulmonary and/ or urinary infections are frequent cause of death (Jennett 2002). In contrast, patients in the persistent vegetative state (PVS) have the potential to progress to the MCS (Giacino et al., 2009).

A patient's emergence from coma and move to the vegetative state does not necessarily mark a point where physicians can reliably make predictions of ultimate outcome. Most severely brain-injured patients will make this transition into the vegetative state, with it becoming the final outcome or a way-station to conscious recovery. The length of time that a patient remains in the vegetative state inversely correlates with the likelihood of further recovery. Based on a study done by the Multi Society Task Force for PVS, 52% of patients in the vegetative state for 1 month acquired consciousness a year after the initial injury while only 35% did so after being vegetative for 3 months. This contrasts with only 16% of patients regaining consciousness after 6 months in the vegetative state. A small number of cases move beyond the permanent vegetative state either to the MCS or to severe disability after these cut-offs, generally because they were misdiagnosed and had already reached the MCS by the 3-month or 1-year demarcations (The Multi-Society Task Force on PVS, 1994; Jennett, 2002).

Minimally conscious state and emergence from MCS

The MCS describes patients who have definitive evidence of consciousness demonstrating, by their behaviours, evidence of intention, attention, memory, and awareness of self, others or the environment. They may track objects in their visual field, say a word or phrase, or grasp a ball. But because of their state, they only do these actions intermittently and in an episodic fashion. If asked to perform the task, they will not reliably follow commands (Giacino et al., 2002). If a patient reaches the MCS, however, they have the potentiality to emerge and regain reliable functional communication (Giacino, 2005). At this juncture, we are unable to predict who in MCS will emerge and when or if it will happen. This is an area of active investigation (Schiff, 2010).

This prognostic uncertainty is highly problematic for surrogates who have to make decisions about quality of life and whether to maintain life-sustaining therapy. In the absence of prognostic clarity, care decisions can be difficult as possible trajectories are highly variable (Giacino, 2005). For some patients, MCS is a temporary bridge to further improvement and even emergence. For these patients, MCS is a transient state that will be overtaken by a higher functional status. However, other patients remain permanently in MCS, unable to reliably communicate but transiently exhibiting evidence of their consciousness. In the case of TBI, one study reported that 40% of MCS patients fully recovered 3 months after the initial insult and 50% a year after the initial insult (Lammi et al., 2005).

But it is even more confounding as the time spent in the MCS does not typically correspond to a positive or negative prognosis, as it does in the PVS (Schiff, 2005). In one highly publicized case, an MCS patient, regained functional communication after 19 years in what was thought at the time to have been the vegetative state. During that time, his parents observed behaviours that suggested he might have been aware, but their observations were ignored because they violated expectations and prevailing nosology. His emergence occurred in 2003, just 1 year after the Aspen Criteria describing MCS entered the lexicon (Fins and Schiff, 2003; Carey, 2006).

Once patients regain the ability to consistently and reliably communicate they are said to have emerged from MCS. This brain state is less ethically fraught than the MCS because the clinician has a direct resource to the thoughts and feelings of the patient, even as profound disability can persist. This vector of communication can help involve the patient in care decisions as we will discuss shortly.

Diagnostic assessment

As should be clear by now, the evaluation of patients with a disorder of consciousness is a dynamic process. Because brain states evolve over time, and sometimes do so with the assistance of drugs and devices, patients must be longitudinally evaluated (Fins, 2008b). Behavioural examinations, in skilled hands, are currently the standard way to diagnose patients and to track recovery. Most experts consider the Coma Recovery Scale-Revised (CRS-R) the most reliable way to make such assessments (Giacino et al., 2004). Unlike the more familiar Glasgow Coma and Outcome Scales (Teasdale and Jennett, 1974), CRS-R measures level of consciousness and is not wholly dependent on integrity of the motor system.

It is important to appreciate that behavioural signs do not always correlate with cognitive activity. Such misconstruals are an important source of error in assessing the related condition of the LIS where there is normal higher cortical function but absence of motor output through the brainstem. Although the LIS is technically not a disorder of consciousness, such patients can be mistaken as vegetative because of the paucity of behavioural signs offered by the LIS patient. These patients, however, are capable of communication using eye movements, and cranial nerves whose origins reside above the injured brainstem, as evocatively manifested in Bauby's memoir, *The Diving Bell and the Butterfly* (Bauby, 1997). Such patients can have misleadingly low scores on the conventional Glasgow scales because of their dependence on behavioural signs (Fins et al., 2007).

Increasingly, investigators are using functional neuroimaging to assess brain activity and delineate mechanisms of recovery (Laureys and Schiff, 2012). Methods like functional magnetic resonance imaging (fMRI) and positron emission tomography (PET) scans can provide information about metabolic activity and identify discordances between cognitive function and behavioural activity. Such results are most reliable when used in conjunction with the natural history and physical examination (Fins, 2008b) and need further validation within the research context (Laureys and Schiff, 2012).

At this juncture, the discordance between what physicians observe at the bedside and what they see using neuroimaging technology confounds the diagnostic process. Vegetative patients can have heterogeneous neuroimages (Schiff et al., 2002). A vegetative patient suffering an anoxic injury that impacts all parts of the brain will have significantly lower levels of metabolic activity as evinced by the PET scan. In contrast, in a vegetative patient with an injury to a particular structure like the thalamus, the fMRI will indicate the preservation of other portions of the cortex (Fins, 2011b).

Functional neuroimaging can lead to such provocative—and often confusing findings—but it can also help distinguish care needs by distinguishing the widely dispersed brain-wide neural networks of MCS from the non-integrated, even *dis*-integrated organization of the vegetative brain. This has clinical implications because the experience of pain, for example, requires an integrated pain network (Schnakers and Zasler, 2007). In a study done by Laureys et al., patients who were vegetative when given a noxious stimulus (nail-bed compression) only activated the primary sensory area, not the wider pain network as occurred in MCS patients. It is postulated that in the absence of such integration pain perception does not occur. Such first-order activations are necessary but not sufficient without engagement with higher level somatosensory and associative areas (Laureys et al., 2002; Fins, 2011b). Another study demonstrated the higher-order activation in MCS patients necessary for pain perception (Boly et al., 2005, 2008).

Medical management

Patients with disorders of consciousness have a number of complications with which palliative care practitioners must become familiar. Primarily, their medical issues relate to prolonged periods of immobility. These conditions, which are briefly outlined here, can be mitigated by appropriate exercise and rehabilitative programmes. (For a comprehensive discussion of the medical needs of this population of patients, please see Bell and Shenouda (2013).)

Such interventions are important because immobility can lead to deconditioning, catabolism and muscle wasting, osteopenia, and contractures, which can be quite painful. These can further limit mobility and may require tendon release. These orthopaedic problems may further compound any neurological complications of brain injury which might also lead to impaired mobility such as hemiparesis or spasticity.

From an infectious disease point of view, these patients are at risk for bedsores, which can occur because of poor skin turgor related to malnutrition and catabolism as well as immobility. This risk is heightened as well by decreased sensory input—due to cognitive impairment and/or decreased arousal—which may allow ulcers to progress without subjective complaint.

Patients with severe brain injury are also at risk for aspiration pneumonias, especially if they have a tracheostomy or require a feeding tube. The usual precautions about feeding (bed elevation) and about pulmonary toilet pertain to these patients as to others who are bed bound, although special care needs to be taken because their lower level of arousal make them less able to control and maintain secretions.

Patients also suffer from gastrointestinal problems such as poor motility, gastro-oesophageal reflux, and constipation (sometimes due to hypercalcaemia due to bone resorption, especially in younger patients). They may have a need to be fed via percutaneous endoscopic gastroscopy tubes because they are neither alert enough to eat by mouth, control secretions, nor masticate. They are also prone to catabolic weight loss or obesity depending upon their context of care.

These patients also *age in time* (Colantonio et al., 2004), and young people who are victims of brain injury in their 20s become prone to the illnesses of advanced age, heart disease, and diabetes at an accelerated pace because of immobility and associated deconditioning. This mix of circumstances—plus associated fluid fluxes like dehydration due to decreased thirst mechanisms or diabetes insipidus—may also increase episodes of orthostasis and the risk of venous thrombosis. This may require filter placement or anticoagulation treatment or prophylaxis, an intervention that needs to be done prudentially given any associated central nervous system risks related to brain injury.

Finally, because surrogates have decided to continue to care for these individuals into adult life, decisions will need to be made about routine health preventive measures, such as screening mammography and assessment of cardiovascular risk. There are no existing guidelines to provide direction for these decisions and it is best to have screening and therapeutic interventions harmonize with goals of care. Throughout, it is important to be cognizant of the burdens and benefits of any intervention and the epidemiology of the cohort, who as survivors of brain injury have an independent increased risk for premature death as compared to the general public (Ratcliff et al., 2005).

Neuro-palliative care

Chronic disorders of consciousness not only pose diagnostic and management challenges, they also present complex clinical and palliative issues across the continuum of care. Physicians cannot easily determine how to manage any symptoms or suffering or establish the priorities of care for patients unable to express their feelings and preferences. Families involved in making these difficult decisions may face significant emotional distress, perhaps already grieving the loss of the patient or suffering a slow bereavement.

Pain

Minimally conscious patients require interventions to ease their pain and suffering in an effort to promote an optimal quality of life. This aim, which is the central tenet of palliative care, has long been missing in the context of severe brain injury. Until recently, very few empirical studies explored the quality of life for these patients and most discussions centred on the family members' interpretation of their loved ones' behaviours (Phipps et al., 1997; Phipps and Whyte, 1999; Bullinger et al., 2002). Objective knowledge of this information is scarce because patients with impaired consciousness are unable to communicate their physical and psychological needs and others cannot easily discern what they are feeling or whether they suffer (Laureys and Boly, 2007).

A variety of different factors may cause pain in patients with disorders of consciousness. In the acute stage of the injury, fractures, abdominal wounds, and invasive procedures can all cause pain. Other physical complications that accompany the severe injury may also produce pain. Blood clots can form in arms or legs. Bedsores commonly result from poor maintenance practices. Seizures, hindering functional outcomes, often recur. Muscular contractions leading to painful twitches and jerks are likely. Some vegetative patients may exhibit symptoms in response to nociceptive stimuli which also require attention (Schnakers and Zasler, 2007; Zasler et al., 2007).

Ongoing behavioural assessments include motor response tests which can inform providers about whether these patients consciously experience pain. The CRS-R gives a high score to patients who reach towards the site of noxious stimuli, and therefore exhibit a localized response to pain. The localized response to pain indicates that patients have the potential for conscious perception of pain (Giacino et al., 2002). In contrast, responses such as frowns or shouts independent of connections to specific stimuli may not signify pain. Clinicians have misinterpreted these signs in some vegetative state patients who exhibit these behaviours, thus the critical importance of making the initial distinction between vegetative state and MCS (Bernat, 2009) as the same behaviour in different diagnostic contexts would have a differential significance.

It is important to note that there are no dedicated pain scales to assess MCS patients and this should be an area of investigation. Despite general acceptance of the CRS-R as the most reliable way to assess conscious perception, it is not intended to collect data about the level of pain or suffering. Palliative care providers will require a new behavioural scale that can evaluate pain in patients with disorders of consciousness. It may be possible to revise existing scales used to assess pain in patients who lack the ability to communicate, such as those with advanced dementia, infants, or intubated/sedated individuals (Schnakers and Zasler, 2007).

Similarly, there are currently no guidelines for how to manage pain in MCS patients. A simple clinical pearl will need to suffice: be attentive to the diagnosis and the potentiality for distress. Interestingly, clinical guidelines currently do not recommend the use of analgesics for vegetative state patients. Since physicians may misdiagnose as many as 40% of MCS patients as being in the vegetative state (Childs et al., 1993; The Multi-Society Task Force on PVS, 1994; Andrews et al., 1996; Wilson et al., 2007; Schnakers et al., 2009), clinicians should cautiously interpret this guideline. Practitioners should remain cognizant of the possibility of diagnostic error and appreciate that its consequence is unremitted pain which could be controlled *in a patient who is likely unable to ask for relief.*

Another key issue is the under-treatment of pain in MCS patients. Many clinicians conservatively administer analgesic to patients with impaired consciousness, sometimes leading to patients' 'agitation' often observed in the acute or rehabilitative facility (Zasler et al., 2007). To adequately manage pain, physicians must use their clinical judgement and assess autonomic findings as an indicator of potential distress (Fins, 2000).

Suffering

Pain management is further complicated by the fact that MCS patients are often conflated with ones who are vegetative (Fins and Plum, 2004), who as we have seen, neither experience pain nor suffering. Thus, the most critical step towards pain management is a proper diagnosis in order to identify who should be the subject of dedicated pain management. Clinicians must distinguish patients with MCS from the vegetative state because MCS patients are conscious and able to perceive pain, and potentially even suffer in the forward-looking definition offered by Eric Cassell (Cassell, 1991). Cassell distinguished somatic pain from suffering which he consider a threat to the *Ich*, the 'I' or the self. Correspondingly, MCS patients may be able to suffer given the isolation and the frustration of being unable to communicate if their motor output deficit far exceeds their cognitive impairment. This remains an unknown for many patients but a prudential ethic would call for good pain management and psychosocial support for the patient. At a minimum, it would preclude discussions about the patient *in the patient's presence* that assumed that the patient was not there and could not understand. Such 'casual' remarks have the potential for iatrogenesis.

Thus, in the absence of sophisticated assessment, it is difficult to evaluate the potential discordance between bedside behavioural activity and neural correlates. The clinician should assume that the MCS patient can understand what is being said, and exercise discretion with bedside conversation. Moreover, the skilled and compassionate practitioner should attempt to engage MCS patients in what may appear to be a unilateral conversation so as to assuage potential fear and feelings of isolation.

Patients persisting in the MCS may also require some psychological assistance as they remain conscious and may have an understanding of their situation, which is greater than their ability to demonstrate behaviourally. Without the ability to functionally communicate, it is impossible to know. This potential sense of isolation is plausible given evidence suggesting that MCS patients retain the ability to process language. In one study, MCS patients displayed large-scale network activation, which was similar to healthy controls, in response to spoken narratives (Schiff et al., 2005). This contrasts with vegetative patients who do not.

For patients who recover more significantly, supportive and psychotherapeutic measures may be indicated to assist individuals in grappling with their altered selves and diminished capabilities. These isolated losses can prove complex with patients having a self-identity but, for example, a lost temporal sense. That is, one could know who one was but not appreciate one's age and temporal context (Fins, in preparation; Windslade, 1998). Alternately, patients who recover from severe brain injury may recall a former capability that they no longer possess, prompting a sense of loss and depression (Meili, 1998; Osborn, 1998; Banja and Fins, 2007).

Goals of care: restoration of functional communication

In response to the threat of isolation is the neuro-palliative (Fins, 2005) care goal of restoring functional communication. The ability of MCS patients to process language in the absence of functional communication suggests that such patients could have greater awareness than is manifested behaviourally and thus potentially experience distress. No one knows what MCS patients are 'thinking' and if they could express themselves they would be out of that diagnostic frame. But if we adopt a prudential ethic, a clear palliative goal would be to promote communication whenever possible, maximizing the residual or dormant cognitive abilities of patients.

Families who have been interviewed express the restoration of functional communication as a primary goal of care and it is obvious why that would be so. At the most basic level, it would enable families and patients to re-establish vital ties and meaningful interactions. Once patients can communicate, they can engage in their treatment course, indicate their ability to feel pain, express psychological fears, or guide their end-of-life care decisions (Schiff et al., 2009).

There is a range of interventions that can facilitate communication. At its most basic level, it would be with the provision of a simple letter board, augmented potentially by a small cadre of pharmacological agents which are being studied to increase arousal and awareness (amantadine, zolpidem, and selective serotonin reuptake inhibitors). Drugs falling into three categories—psychostimulants, dopamine agonists, and tricyclic antidepressants—improve awareness, facilitate speech, and encourage new behaviours (Giacino et al., 2007). Zolpidem, paradoxically, leads to improvements in patients with impairments of consciousness, arousing them and increasing their interactive behaviours (Schiff and Plum, 2007; Whyte and Myers, 2009). A recent randomized controlled study in *The New England Journal of Medicine* demonstrated that amantadine increased the *rate* of recovery in patients with disorders of consciousness (Giacino et al., 2012). These relatively low-cost interventions, becoming the standard of care in the rehabilitation and neuropsychology communities (McNamee et al., 2012), should evolve as a standard neuro-palliative approach.

More involved interventions, also at the experimental level, include the use of what has been broadly termed neuroprosthetic devices (Fins, 2011a): deep brain stimulation (DBS) and neuro-imaging. In 2007, one of the authors was a co-investigator in a clinical trial describing the use of bilateral intralaminar nucleus thalamic DBS of a patient in MCS (Schiff et al., 2007). In *Nature*, we reported the case of 38-year-old man who had been in MCS for 6 years following an assault. Before DBS he could only intermittently respond to commands and was totally dependent upon tube feeds through his stomach. He was incapable of controlling his secretion and mastication. After the intervention, he was able to speak several words at a time and eat by mouth. Most critically, the device restored a degree of personal agency (Schiff et al., 2009). With the intervention he was able to communicate with his family, express preferences and emotions, and tell his caregivers that he was in pain, if they asked. While this remains an area of investigation and is ready for dissemination, the use of such neuromodulation technologies is likely to have a limited role for this population.

Neuroimaging methods are closer to clinical application and carry with them potential for neuro-palliative care. Over the past decade, functional neuroimaging has demonstrated the potential to use neuroimaging as a window on the brain and a communication vector for those who lack behavioural output (Owen et al., 2006; Schiff, 2006; Fins, 2008b). These methods have enabled patients to communicate without repairing the structural damage to the brain (Fins, 2009). Recent notable examples using fMRI have the patient 'imagining' that they are playing tennis or swimming or walking about their house and toggling these activations to yes/no questions (Monti et al., 2010; Bardin et al., 2012; Fins, 2012). Although the results are still primitive and the bandwidth of the communication channel is narrow, this is a promising area of research. The one caveat is how we interpret these *forme fruste* communications in light of prior wishes (Fins and Schiff, 2010). We will address this question in the next section.

Surrogate decision-making

One of the central ethical considerations in this neuro-palliative framework is the place of the MCS patients in relationships and in decision-making. This is a complex interaction because it involves surrogates and the patient, both how he or she was and how they are in present when medical choices have to be made. A key question is the valence given to prior wishes as against current claims and desires. This becomes apparent in a hypothetical DBS example, where the intervention improved communication as in the aforementioned study. The dynamic between the patient's former uninjured self and his current state comes to a fore when one considers whether such a patient can direct his or her medical care, much less assert a right to withhold or withdraw life-sustaining therapy. This determination will fundamentally hinge on a determination of decision-making capacity and awareness that the absence of communication via a prosthetic device may or may not preclude the presence of consciousness.

The re-entry of the patient's voice in the room, via assistive devices, presents a difficulty for surrogates who will need to weigh prior knowledge of the patient's choices, values, and expressed wishes against the cogency and reasonableness of what the patient is now saying. This mix of inputs from the past, the patient's present, and from the surrogate should be balanced together in the deliberative effort. Ultimately, a *mosaic* model of decision-making emerges which includes pieces from the patient and his past and the surrogate and her knowledge of the patient's values and current prospects.

Whatever the involvement of the patient, the burden of decision-making (for MCS patients) falls largely to families who must make choices amidst prognostic uncertainties. Clinicians should help families navigate the evolving trajectory of brain injury and help formulate temporally appropriate goals of care.

Right to care and right to die

Surrogates and clinicians must work together to respect the right to die and affirm the right to care (Fins, 2006b). Finding this balance amidst the general neglect of these patients, while advocating for care requires a balanced approach that recognizes the burdens associated with these conditions for patients and their families (Fins, 2003, 2010). Counselling about decisions to withhold or withdraw life-sustaining therapies can get overly focused on diagnostic and prognostic questions, often leading to an impasse.

In our view, it is better to identify goals of care and consider the feasibility of the patient reaching them. When articulated goals are elusive and likely not in reach, decisions to withhold or withdraw care may be more accepted. This functional approach to outcomes places the patient's condition into the context of a life narrative in a way that a simple diagnosis cannot (see Chapter 5.8).

Bereavement

Families caring for patients with disorders of consciousness face a significant burden; they must cope with severe emotional distress and be responsible for making health-care decisions amidst great prognostic uncertainty, and do so over the long haul. After their family member suffers a severe brain injury, they lose a psychological connection to their injured relative and often become socially isolated from family and friends. These losses may lead to what might be called a perpetual state of bereavement, heightening grief and distress when the patient actually passes. Some investigators liken their experience to caregivers of patients with dementia (Marwit and Kaye, 2006). Whether these factors lead to a complicated bereavement is a question for further study but our experience suggests that the mix of relief and sadness attending these loses make the recovery process for families more complex and nuanced and good candidates for follow-up support.

Expanding the mission of palliative care

Through our study of patients with disorders of consciousness and the experiences of their families we have come to appreciate that our systems of care neither accommodate the needs of this population vis-à-vis rehabilitation in the acute care setting, scientific advance in chronic care, nor palliation when it is most appropriate (Fins, 2003, 2005). All of this is in spite of the progress that has been made in this field (Fins, 2013). Curiously, this level of neglect has its origins in the evolution of the right to die in the vegetative state, observed in cases like Quinlan, Cruzan, and Schiavo

(Annas, 1996; Fins, 2009). In day-to-day practice, practitioners acculturated to modern notions of palliative care and medical ethics erroneously equate patients with brain injury with a dying patient: they see the loss of consciousness in brain injury as akin to that which occurs as a consequence of end-stage disease (Fins, 2007). This prematurely truncates care and precludes the potential of recovery, all in a misplaced exertion of palliative care.

So another rationale for expanding the mission of palliative care to this population is to help ensure that the application of this area of practice is not merely in the exercise of negative rights but rather a positive entitlement that brings comfort and relief to those patients and families who sought fuller recoveries but were left with chronic morbidity and mortality. Palliative medicine, properly exercised, can pre-empt its reflexive application to unconscious patients and more laudably apply its ministrations to a population that truly is in need. The main institutional features of palliative medicine—the use of interdisciplinary teams, the provision of care in a variety of settings, and its blending of comfort and curative interventions—have the potential to successfully coordinate care from the acute to chronic phases of severe brain injury. Such dedicated efforts can promote the integration of special neurorehabilitation programmes, which provide a variety of services that respond to the psychological, physical, and social aspects of the pathology (Bernat, 2009).

The reservoir of compassion, caring, and expertise that exists in the palliative care sector—in hospitals, hospice, and the community—is a ready resource for patients and families who will grapple with medically and psychologically complex conditions for decades in a state, as we have noted, that is often equated with perpetual bereavement. These families need biopsychosocial support, respite care, and counselling, much like families that are anticipating a death. And families of severely brain-injured patients also face a heightened prospect of mortality because of their loved one's condition and co-morbidities.

Because the acute care system has been so inhospitable to brain-injured patients after the initial heroic measures have been provided, policy needs to turn to alternative venues for optimal care. Although it is beyond the scope of this chapter, one might envision a collaborative dialogue between clinicians and institutions providing chronic care, rehabilitation, and palliation. Combining the best that each of these realms offer could lead to a care system that comprehensively and longitudinally meets the long-term care needs of this vulnerable population.

Online materials

Complete references for this chapter are available online at <http://www.oxfordmedicine.com>.

References

Bardin, J.C., Schiff, N.D., and Voss, H.U. (2012). Pattern classification of volitional functional magnetic resonance imaging responses in patients with severe brain injury. *Archives of Neurology*, 69, 176–181.

Fins, J.J. (2003). Constructing an ethical stereotaxy for severe brain injury: balancing risks, benefits, and access. *Nature Reviews Neuroscience*, 4, 323–327.

Fins, J.J. (2005). Clinical pragmatism and the care of brain damaged patients: toward a palliative neuroethics for disorders of consciousness. *Progress in Brain Research*, 150, 565–582.

Fins, J.J. (2006a). *A Palliative Ethic of Care: Clinical Wisdom at Life's End.* Sudbury, MA: Jones and Bartlett Publishers.

Fins, J.J. (2007). Ethics of clinical decision making and communication with surrogates. In J.B. Posner, C.B. Saper, N.D. Schiff, and F. Plum (eds.) *Plum and Posner's Diagnosis of Stupor and Coma* (4th ed.), pp. 376–380. New York: Oxford University Press.

Fins, J.J. (2010). Minds apart: severe brain injury, citizenship, and civil rights. *Law and Neuroscience: Current Legal Issues*, 13, 367–384.

Fins, J.J. (2011b). Neuroethics, neuroimaging, and disorders of consciousness: promise or peril? *Transactions of the American Clinical and Climatolology Association*, 122, 336–346.

Fins, J.J. (2013). Disorders of consciousness and disordered care: families, caregivers and narratives of necessity. *Archives of Physical Medicine and Rehabilitation*, 94(10), 1934–1939.

Fins, J.J. (in preparation). *Rights Come to Mind: Ethics and the Struggle for Consciousness.* New York: Cambridge University Press.

Fins, J.J. and Schiff, N. (2010). In the blink of the mind's eye. *The Hastings Center Report*, 40, 21–23.

Giacino, J., Childs, N., Cranford, R., *et al.* (2002). The minimally conscious state: definition and diagnostic criteria. *Neurology*, 58, 349–353.

Monti, M., Vanhaudenhuyse, A., Coleman, M., *et al.* (2010). Willful modulation of brain activity in disorders of consciousness. *The New England Journal of Medicine*, 362, 579–589.

Owen, A.M., Coleman, M.R., Boly, M., Davis, M.H., Laureys, S. and Pickard, J.D. (2006). Detecting awareness in the vegetative state. *Science*, 313, 1402.

Schiff, N.D., Giacino, J.T., Kalmar, K., *et al.* (2007). Behavioral improvements after thalamic stimulation after severe traumatic brain injury. *Nature*, 448, 600–603.

Schiff, N.D., Rodriguez-Moreno, D., Kamal, A., *et al.* (2005). fMRI reveals large-scale network activation in the minimally conscious state. *Neurology*, 64, 514–523.

5.4

Truth telling and consent

Linda L. Emanuel and Rebecca Johnson

Introduction to truth telling and consent

At the core of truth telling is a fairly new cultural value (Xue et al., 2011) that entails a revised role for 'healers' in society as well as care recipients (Cassell, 1985). Whereas in earlier times it was deemed helpful to shield people from the harsh reality of their conditions, clinicians practising palliative care in Western medicine today generally understand 'truth telling' as a legal and ethical professional responsibility. Persons with illness generally understand 'truth telling' as their right to information about their illness. This sea change in cultural values is reflected in the arts. Historically, cultural representations of the therapeutic relationship have emphasized physicians' dilemmas. For example, the tragic consequences of one-sided, professional honesty (Ibsen, 1984) and well-intentioned reticence (Narayan, 2006). More recently culture increasingly elects to profile individuals' illness dilemmas (Forster, 2010; Gurnah, 2011; Mankell, 2012).

This chapter focuses on the role of truth telling in the therapeutic relationship and the ways in which communications can maintain hopes and at the same time deliver information sufficient for informed consent. It outlines the evolution of standards for truth telling and consent and then presents practical approaches that can guide truth telling and informed consent. Finally, it concludes by considering these norms and some of their limitations from within a global cultural context.

History of truth telling

Truth telling in contemporary Western medicine has come to refer to the way in which information about the futility of treatment, a person's impending death, possible clinical pathways to death, and the possible impact of end-of-life decisions along those pathways should be communicated (Deschepper et al., 2008). Each person fears death in his or her own way (Yalom, 2008) and studies show that 'truth telling' around diagnosis or prognosis can be particularly difficult to communicate. For example, research shows that 'cancer' is a word which has the capacity to effect a blinding emotional reaction (Casarett et al., 2010; Nwankwo and Ezeome, 2011).

Research also suggests that communications which sustain hope along a disease trajectory are particularly effective in maintaining quality of life for individuals suffering from terminal or incurable diseases and their families (Clayton et al., 2008). However, these communications are sometimes difficult for clinicians. For example, some physicians are more comfortable talking about the disease or the technicalities of treatment than healing or choices that involve difficult decisions (Cassell, 1985; Deschepper et al., 2008). Importantly, many physicians and nurses are reluctant to communicate bad news (Gysels et al., 2004).

Approaches to medical truth telling in prognostic and diagnostic discussions differ around the globe. In Lebanon, China, Singapore, and Japan, for example, persons with cancer are often not told their diagnosis or their prognosis, whereas in the United States and United Kingdom, the American Medical Association and General Medical Council advocate truth telling and reject deception (Sokol, 2006). Studies in both these countries show that the gold standard is absolute truth about diagnosis and prognosis. Indeed, studies with families and persons with illness show that people appreciate honesty about their illness (Apatira et al., 2008). Preferred physician behaviours include being realistic, providing an opportunity for asking questions, and acknowledging the person as an individual while discussing the prognosis. However, it is less clear what each participant in the truth-telling interaction means by 'truth' and some studies show that preferences for information may change over time (Hagerty et al., 2004, 2005).

Hope is commonly equated with the potential for cure. Within the field of palliative care where cure is often a receding theme, hope still retains an important role. Observations in clinical practice suggest that when a future to hope for gets disturbed by difficult news, people move into a more fundamental emotional state in which dependence dominates and trust becomes more than usually essential. This response to disturbed hope underscores how powerful an emotional asset hope is (Hagerty et al., 2004, 2005; Eliott and Olver, 2006; Clayton et al., 2008; Kersten et al., 2012). In palliative care, the goal is to find something realistic to hope for and to tailor care towards that goal (Emanuel et al., 2007). For example, if a person says that he or she wants to attend a family life-cycle event, the care plan can focus on treatments which enable them to achieve this.

History of consent

Contemporary understandings of informed consent as a guiding ethical principle and practice within health-care settings have roots in the US and UK courts. Early English common law doctrine ensures that assault (the threat of bodily harm) and battery (the unlawful touching of another individual) are the key measures by which lawful behaviours are ascertained (Murray, 1990). Informed consent cases can be traced back to the early modern period of legal jurisdiction. Most cases present themselves in oppositional terms with the person with illness pitted against the physician, health-care team, and health-care provider. For example, a significant case in English medical law was *Slater v Baker and Stapleton* in 1767. Surgeons reset a femoral fracture without the person's consent and without giving sufficient prior warning. Custom dictated that physicians obtain consent to help patients 'take courage', and the judge ruled that failure to do so in this case was remiss (O'Shea, 2011).

Legal definitions of informed consent have evolved over the years. In the 1950s and 1960s, US courtroom debates focused on the question of medical judgement and how much a 'reasonable physician' might be expected to disclose. The normative assumption was that physicians knew how much to reveal about a medical procedure to patients and that professional bodies would provide guidelines. In the 1970s, a new formulation of person-orientated standards of care emerged, and the right to self-determined consent was enshrined in law (Bennett, 2000). Physicians were required to reveal as much information as a 'reasonable person' would wish to know. Informed consent was not just about protecting persons with illness from unwanted interference with their bodily integrity, it was also about enabling them to make informed choices about care (Appelbaum, et al., 1987).

The law of consent is now generally accepted as 'the vehicle by which the respect for personal autonomy' (MacLean, 1988) is translated into law. As a modern ethical formulation, informed consent can be seen as an attempt to codify and institutionalize a basic human right to self-determination of what happens to one's body (Bennett, 2000; Monagle, 1998). It has been argued that this is in part Western society's attempt to respond to some of the human rights violations which have occurred within medical practice and research. However, the relationship between consent and autonomy is not always as clear-cut as this implies. Autonomy can mean different things to different people in different contexts. For example, in geriatric palliative care autonomy for a person with illness may mean dignity in death. A person's definition of dignity may be strongly influenced by cultural or spiritual factors. For one person dignity in death may mean living for as long as possible and trying every curative treatment available (Johnson et al., 2005), to another it may mean relief from pain and suffering and no invasive end-of-life treatment (Deshpande et al., 2005).

Legal definitions of consent do not prescribe the type of interaction which should take place between a person, physician, health-care team, and families in order to ensure that consent is informed or articulate how it should be done. In fear of prosecution, many health-care providers have adopted a rigidly legalistic interpretation of informed consent, standardizing documentation and institutional review to deliver legal requirements. The danger of this approach is that communication about consent can become an 'empty ritual in which persons with illness are presented with complex information that they cannot readily understand and that has little impact on their decision making' (Grisso, 1998). Indeed, the legalistic approach seems a particularly poor match with the goals of palliative care where the person and his or her family is the 'unit of care' (McClement et al., 2007) within a complex and fluid system of health-care provision (Bowman, 2011).

Research has shown that single utilization of forms alone can result in limited person understanding of what they are consenting to (Tulksy, 2005). An alternative approach is the process model described by Appelbaum et al. (1987) where 'informed consent (is integrated) into the physician-person relationship as a facet of all stages of medical decision-making'. Constant communication around consent builds trust and services everyday norms of non-deception and non-coercion. Furthermore, persons and physicians build relationships of trust which can enable individuals to

exercise consent as 'a waiver (to) legitimate actions that (taken out of context) might otherwise be seen as breaches of rights and obligations towards them' (O'Neill, 2002). Take, for example, a person with illness who decides he or she wishes to die at home. Nursing staff know that the family carers will not be able to turn the person and that they may develop pressure ulcers. The health-care team holds a family meeting which includes the patient to discuss the benefits and barriers to a good death at home. The group decides that it is best for the individual to go home (Eisenberger and Zeleznik, 2004). This example suggests that there are diverse interpretations of autonomy as well as arguments for a non-autonomy rationale when seeking consent. It also suggests that continuing and sustained communication between professionals and the person with illness/family as 'unit of care' is essential for effective and considered consent (Appelbaum, 1987, Heinemann, et al. 2002).

A psychological perspective on consent

Any experience of significant illness is identity changing (Miller, 2010; Bowman et al., 2011). The shift from health to illness and self-confidence to constant watchfulness can be transformative, particularly for persons with illness living through long disease trajectories. Several conceptual approaches have been developed to facilitate understanding of these identity changes. For example, the concept of 'pre-morbid personality' notes that acknowledging one's illness entails '[entering] another way of being'. It notes that illness can impair or change a person's 'standard currency' (Bowman et al., 2011).

Taking in frame-altering news: a cognitively refractory state

Other conceptual models have facilitated predictions about how an emotional context will vary over time as a person processes illness-related losses (Emanuel et al., 2007). A first encounter with frame-altering news often leaves a person 'numb' and unable to absorb information. A key lesson from these models is that the decision-making behaviour of, say, a woman who gives consent for aggressive radiation treatment of breast cancer is unlikely to mirror the decision-making behaviour of the same woman who gives consent for transfer to hospice (Bowman et al., 2011). A different dynamic of contradictory feelings, experiences, family and health-care personnel, and motivations is likely to be in play at each stage of the illness (Covinsky, 1994, Mezey, 1997). Although in purely legal terms these identity changes don't matter (unless they affect the person's capacity to give consent), in practice they will affect the choices the individual makes (Bowman et al., 2011).

Adjusting to a new reality: an emotional and cognitive experimentation phase/creative adaptation

Recent scholarship has seen the emergence of a number of concepts and interventions relevant to the way individuals adjust to end-of-life losses at different stages of their illness journey (Munn et al., 2008). These include 'preparative waiting' around diagnosis (Giske, 2007); life review and emotional disclosure for persons with less than 6 months to live (Steinhauser et al., 2009); dignity therapy for terminally ill persons (McClement et al., 2007); and stages of change modelling for social workers preparing persons for end-of-life care planning and decision-making (Rizzo et al., 2010). Knight and Emanuel's reintegration model (Knight and

Emanuel, 2007) posits the idea that adjustment to losses are linked to a broader biopsychosocial context than hitherto acknowledged. As a person adjusts to illness, several cycles occur: comprehension (i.e. recognition of what has occurred), creative adaptation (i.e. experimentation with alternatives for living in the new circumstance), and reintegration (i.e. consolidation of a revised way of being). For example, take two individuals who have each had a leg amputated because of serious illness. Person one grieves for the loss of their mobility but seeks outside help to cope, and thinks of ways to continue to be mobile. Person two on the other hand does not accept the loss of his/her leg and does not adapt to the change. He/she refuses to leave his/her bed and dislikes having bed sheets changed because the amputation can be seen. This comparison illustrates how the reintegration model can help to 'place' the person in the trajectory of adjustment, and possibly thence guide approaches to foster optimal adjustment and functioning.

Reaching equilibrium; a mature state capable of durable decisions

Loss of function, body image, relationships, control, independence, dignity, and anxiety about death can occur at any time (Yalom, 2008). The literature on loss and grief tells us that loss is the condition of being deprived of something or someone (Kübler-Ross, 1969, Worden, 1991). Loss may be anticipated, real or perceived, primary or secondary. Grief is a personal and normal response to loss. It can be physical, (e.g. physiological capabilities, functions), psychological (e.g. emotions, cognitions, behaviours), social (e.g. role in relationships), or spiritual (beliefs, existential experiences). Mostly it is a complex combination of all these. The intensity of the response will vary according to the meaning of the loss to the person experiencing it (Yalom, 2008). Since all persons with illness and their families experience multiple losses associated with those illnesses, grieving can form a significant part of the end-of-life experience. Competence in helping those in care to adjust to losses is therefore a high priority for health-care professionals.

Working in clinical settings with different stages of adjustment

To be effective in end-of-life care, health-care teams must be able to recognize and anticipate grief (Kübler-Ross, 1969; Worden, 1991). Team members need to recognize individuals stuck in states of incomplete adjustment. Successful transitioning from one state to another takes time, reflection, regular communication, and an environment that offers hopeful alternatives to the state that has been lost. Team members should aim to anticipate grief reactions, providing basic supportive care to persons with illness and families and referring individuals to bereavement experts quickly when grief reactions become complicated. Observation in clinical practice suggests that active listening and unconditional support whilst acknowledging the unwanted reality can offer the best approaches. It also suggests that sources of help can feel like two-edged swords to persons who are having a hard time accepting the situation they are in. Worden and Rando advocate a process-orientated understanding of how people resolve grief (Worden, 1991; Rando, 1993). Their model offers guidance for identifying where individuals may be having difficulty in their trajectories of mourning.

Types of shared decision-making

Shared decision-making

In the last decade, as the therapeutic relationship has become more of a partnership (Joosten et al., 2008), shared decision-making has become a core imperative of person-centred care (Stacey et al., 2010). Conceptualizations of the nature of this partnership have identified an important common hallmark: 'that persons and providers have different but equally valuable perspectives and roles in the medical encounter' (Makoul and Clayman, 2006) when it comes to making decisions about treatment. Key questions for effective practice include how best to communicate these perspectives (Mok et al., 2010), which decision aids to use (Feldman-Stewart et al., 2006), who takes the lead and when, and what constitutes 'decision quality' (Joseph-Williams et al., 2010).

Current models of shared decision-making typically include the person with illness and one other health-care professional (Stacey et al., 2010) and can be plotted along a spectrum with paternalism at one end (i.e. physicians making the decisions) and informed choice at the other (i.e. where individuals make the decisions) (Makoul and Clayman, 2006). Some researchers suggest competencies for both clinician and persons with illness, while others argue that clinicians have the responsibility to elicit or respond to the views of the person with illness (Chwening et al., 2012). Self-help books urge individuals to proactively ask questions about diagnosis and prognosis (Lynn et al., 2011). At the same time, the evidence points to large variations in decision-making role preferences among and between persons with different disease trajectories (Tariman et al., 2010). A mismatch often exists between persons' stated preferences for and actually chosen roles. For example, while the majority of persons with cancer interviewed by Gaston and Mitchell expressed a wish for full information, only two-thirds wished to participate in active decision-making (Gaston and Mitchell, 2005). The nature of the decision and the stage of the therapeutic relationship can also influence a person's decision-making role preference (Chewning, 2012). All of these are important considerations, especially given that involvement in shared decision-making can improve the quality of end of life (Steinhauser et al., 2009).

Interprofessional and family perspectives on shared decision-making

A theory analysis of shared-decision-making models shows that although existing models identify the ways in which health-care professionals can work with persons with illness to achieve shared decisions, few discuss how the decision-making occurs 'with others involved beyond the person–practitioner dyad (e.g. family members, other professionals)' (Stacey et al., 2010). The person–practitioner dyad remains paramount in the literature and a core 'ethical unit' of shared decision-making.

An exception to this is family caregiving research, also referred to as family systems in nursing research, where there is a growing body of literature showing how the involvement of family in health-care decision-making can strengthen collaboration and trust between families and health-care teams (Anderson, 2000; Rempel, 2006). Family engagement reduces the risk of providing care which persons with illness and families don't want (Fineberg, 2005) and unnecessary and distressing hospital admissions among older persons (Ahearn, 2010). It can also impact positively on symptom management in non-verbal persons (Mentes et al., 2004), difficult invasive treatment choices (Deshpande et al., 2005), and the initiation of palliative care (Nolan, 2008). Wider dissemination of guidelines for palliative care in dementia, for example, has been linked to a decrease in the prescribing of antibiotics and increases in the use of analgesics with persons who are unable to verbally communicate their wishes and preferences (Volicer and Ganzini, 2003).

How to accomplish truth telling with good outcomes

In the determination to promote and improve communications around person-centred care, there is growing professional interest in matching different communication functions or behaviours to good outcomes (Back et al. 2009). The taxonomy illustrated in Fig. 5.4.1 suggests that six communication functions delivered at six stages along the cancer continuum can improve survival and health-related quality of life.

Epstein and Street suggest that a key task for researchers is to 'specify what [types of behaviours and interactions] will improve outcomes for a particular person at a given point in time on the continuum' (Epstein and Street, 2007). This is where many of the protocol-based guides designed for use by health-care professionals can be useful.

A stepwise guide

Stepwise protocols, for example, can help health-care teams to approach truth telling by structuring goals of care discussions with persons and their families. Protocols are essentially guidelines which can be adapted to local context and tailored for each individual transaction when required. SPIKES, the stepwise protocol recommended in the Education for Physicians in

End-of-Life Care (EPEC) project and widely used in other countries (Swaminath, 2008), is based on Buckman's protocol for communicating bad news (Buckman, 1992). SPIKES is a tool which respects the autonomy of the person and enables the clinician to determine how much 'truth' or information the individual wants to know and how he or she wants to receive it. Fig. 5.4.2 illustrates how a six-step SPIKES approach might be adapted to help the clinician determine the appropriate presentation of information for a person who has received a diagnosis of cancer and wants to talk about prognosis. Research suggests that older persons in particular expect physicians to initiate discussions around prognosis and so do many members of health-care teams (Adelman et al., 2000; Gutierrez, 2012).

Although stepwise approaches are useful tools when it comes to structuring sensitive communications and linking practice to legal frameworks, it is important to remember that to be successful they need to reflect the values, practices, and assumptions of the setting they are used within. For example, what happens when the prescribed norm is not the cultural norm for the person and family in question? The one-to-one communication model that SPIKES represents may not be an appropriate approach for a person who has never previously accessed health care, or who is non-verbal. It may be not applicable in cultural settings where families have traditionally shielded the person from prognosis (Chan, 2011). Furthermore, research shows that effective information sharing in end-of-life care depends on continuous ongoing communications that take into account a person's hope, despair, and regret.

How to accomplish informed consent

Informed consent is shorthand for two distinct duties in Westernized medicine. Firstly, the clinician's duty to obtain consent before treatment, and secondly the duty to ensure that the

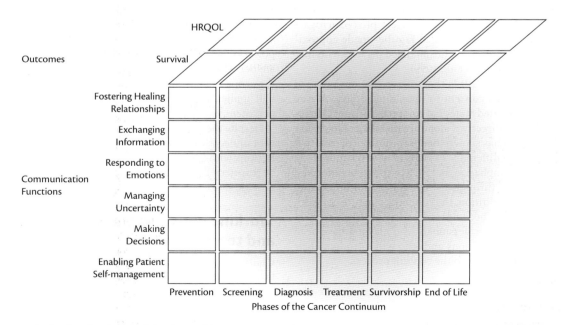

Fig. 5.4.1 Six communication functions in each of the phases of the cancer care continuum.
Reproduced from Epstein RM and Street RL, Jr., *Patient-Centered Communication in Cancer Care: Promoting Healing and Reducing Suffering*, National Cancer Institute, NIH Publication No. 07-6225, Bethesda, MD, USA, 2007.

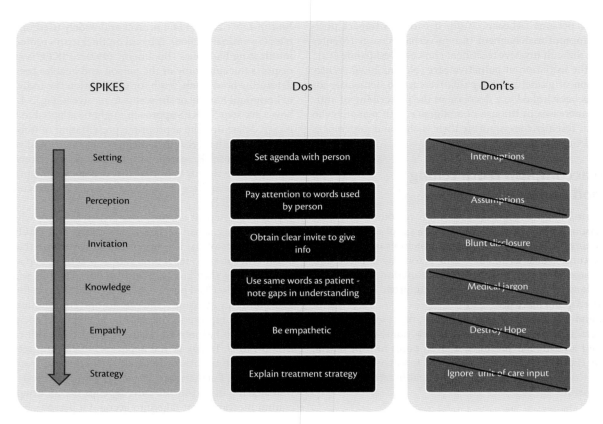

Fig. 5.4.2 SPIKES approach to breaking bad news.

Adapted with permission from M. Rinaldi and M. Potter at South West London & St George's Mental Health NHS Trust in, *Recovery is for All: Hope, Agency and Opportunity in Psychiatry. A Position Statement by Consultant Psychiatrists*, South London and Maudsley NHS Foundation Trust and South West London and St George's Mental Health NHS Trust, London, UK, Copyright © 2010. Contains data from Walter F. Bailea et al, SPIKES—A Six-Step Protocol for Delivering Bad News: Application to the Patient with Cancer, The Oncologist, Volume 5, Number 4, pp. 302-311, Copyright © 2000 by AlphaMed Press.

person has been properly informed about a treatment's risks and benefits (MacLean, 2013). A particular issue in end-of-life care is that many individuals are unable to make their own medical decisions and are increasingly being asked to elect proxy/surrogate decision-makers. One study showed that families made approximately 75% of medical decisions for hospitalized persons with life-threatening diseases (Hiltunen et al., 1999).

Advance care planning (ACP) is the process that has come to characterize true informed consent in the United States. A core outcome of ACP in the United States is a completed advance directive. Although advanced directives alone are insufficient to ensure successful ACP, research has shown that programmes of care that include ACP can make a difference to goals of care (Cantor et al., 2003). It is important to emphasize that ACP is a process. Informed consent is never achieved through a single act of communicating (Bowman et al., 2011). In addition, the systemized nature of health care means that as a person becomes sicker they are likely to meet more and more health-care professionals who may not have been privy to earlier consent discussions and who will introduce their own behaviours and attitudes into the consent process.

A stepwise guide

Analysis of the advanced care planning literature suggests five key elements to achieving informed consent. The steps are similar to those recommended for achieving truth telling: introduce the topic; engage in structured discussion; document the preferences

of the person with illness; review and update those preferences regularly; and apply the directives when needed. However, research has identified several deficiencies in ACP. Nursing home staff report that persons with illness do not understand the purpose of an advance directive with several thinking the directives appoint powers of attorney over their affairs (Moskop, 2004; Tulksy, 2005; Steiber-Roger, 2006). Other misunderstandings can arise around the scope of statutory document. For example, whether a living will applies if a persona has terminal conditions is in a coma or a persistent vegetative state (Gunter-Hunt, 2002).

Despite these drawbacks, ongoing ACP and discussion can prevent unnecessary admission to hospital and timely use of hospice. Persons with illness without ACPs or directives are more likely to be transferred to hospital for investigations and interventions that provide short-lived benefits (Moskop, 2004; Steiber-Roger, 2006).

Working with persons with illness, families, and team members

Continuous communication and information is essential for families to function and cope within what can be a bewildering health-care context. Most families have the capacity to share feelings of grief, open lines of communication, and eventually engage in collaborative decision-making. However, inconsistencies in information about a condition can fuel conflicts and disagreements between the person with illness and their family, between family members, and between family and health-care team members. Research also suggests that health-care team member attitudes to death and caring for dying persons can also be a significant factor in the provision of long-term care. For example, health-care team members who have completed an advance directive are more comfortable about discussing end-of-life planning with their patients than those who have no advance plan (Horgas et al., 2007; Guthell and Heyman, 2011).

As a life-threatening illness progresses, a person's family will have an increasingly important role to play, particularly in decisions about goals of care and treatment preferences. Some of the emerging roles for family or kin include emotional support for illness, advocacy for appropriate treatment for the individual, trusted confidantes about health-care issues, and surrogate decision-makers. These are not roles family members or the health-care teams caring for their loved ones are necessarily familiar or comfortable with. For example, research studies suggest that the desire to remain one's own person without becoming dependent on kin or family (children in particular) is particularly evident among older people growing old in America (Lamb, 2009). Comprehensive end-of-life care therefore requires that health-care teams know how to respond to family concerns and conflicts and how to help families and persons with illness reach informed consent.

Family systems

Family conferencing is a particular useful and well-evidenced tool that can promote communication around goals of care and ACP between the health-care team, person with illness, and family in a variety of health-care settings. For example, regularly scheduled nurse and clinician family meetings in intensive care units have the potential to maintain family health during chronic and terminal illness and enhance the care of the person with illness (Nelms and Eggenberger, 2010). Family meetings can also allow health-care teams to effectively acknowledge the suffering and vulnerability of families when a loved one is undergoing long-term care and offer families an opportunity for honest sensitive communication with health-care team members.

Alternative tools which have been successfully used in clinical family nursing practice to facilitate discussion around a person's individual and social network are genograms and ecomaps. Both are graphic portrayals of family structure and cultural, social, and spiritual relationships (Rempel et al., 2007). Wright and Leahey outline how health-care teams can conduct a 15-minute family interview that includes completing a genogram and ecomap (Wright and Leahey, 2009).

Cultural considerations

Culture is a vital factor for the clinician aiming to deliver person-centred health care. As clinical populations become increasingly diverse there is a growing premium on understanding and respecting cross-cultural difference and thus avoiding cultural stereotyping (Lasch, 2000). Research shows that the cultural factors which influence truth telling and consent around health care are complex. Age, gender, and ethnicity can all combine with spiritual beliefs, traditional family roles, and assumptions about the causes of an illness or stigma associated with treatments (e.g. opioids). Consequently, culture can

have a powerful influence on what clinicians and persons with illness are prepared to talk about, how they interpret one another's communications, and how they and their families make decisions.

Culture and truth telling

As noted at the beginning of this chapter, current ethical debates about truth telling and consent in Western medicine can be traced back to English common law and case law. Countries that share this tradition look to each other's jurisdictions for examples and precedents (Edwin, 2008). The outcome of several medical legal cases in Australia, Canada, Ghana, South Africa, and India, for example, all illustrate arguments which show that individual autonomy is fundamental to the rule of law and the basis for disclosure to persons with illness (Edwin, 2008). Truth telling is therefore grounded in a shared cultural value—respect for a person's autonomy and the 'right to know' (Xue et al., 2011). One result of this norm, as illustrated by this chapter, is that the research focus of much medical literature around truth telling is on how to divulge sensitive information (Xue et al., 2011) rather than whether to tell the truth.

Despite the links between culture and truth telling, a patient's desire for truth telling cannot be redacted down to cultural origins: 'neither cultural origin nor affiliation accurately predicts patient preferences regarding information transfer or decision making' (Cherny, 2012). Patients in both Western and non-Western cultures will exhibit considerable variation in their preferred style of disclosure of bad news or information. No one model will fit all. Indeed, data suggests that there is substantial heterogeneity of preferences that are not individually predicated by geography, culture, age, race, sex, religion, or educational level (Cherny, 2012).

Cultural approaches to screening bad news as a care function: some examples

National or minority cultures which emphasize family collectivism or familism can generate powerful arguments against the person's 'right to know' and for the family's right to a predominant role in therapeutic care and decision-making. In China and Asian countries which share similar cultures, philosophies of life and death, and laws and regulations, person autonomy is not a cultural 'norm'. Despite a legal mandate that physicians should tell the truth about a person's disease, family beliefs and norms of medical practice mean that 'truth telling' is not straightforward. The negative impact of learning that one has cancer, for example, is culturally well understood by many groups (Lasch, 2000; Rozario and DeRienzis, 2008; Xue et al., 2011) where familism is predominant. A cancer diagnosis is devastating for the whole family. The person's main source of financial and emotional support and care, particularly palliative care, will be their family. As a result many families adopt responsibility for the individual's therapy, protecting them against 'maleficence' (Chan, 2011). In practice this can mean families insisting that the person not be told 'the truth' about their disease (Chan, 2011), that particular family members be included or excluded from translation of negative news (Lasch, 2000), and that family caregivers may not seek information about help that they think the family should be able to deliver (Rozario and DeRienzis, 2008).

A practical guide

Clinicians can become more culturally sensitive and more effective in delivering person-centred palliative care. One approach is to purposefully ask patients about their individual preferences and act in accordance with their wishes (Cherny, 2012). Cherny, for example, recommends offering patients a range of options. These include: 'explain the results to me, explain the results to me with my family members, explain them first to my family and then to me, or tell the family first and let then them decide what I should be told'. The value of this approach is that it avoids cultural stereotyping, ensures authentic patient preferences are obtained, and reduces possible physician/family collusion. Other strategies include consulting with community organizations and community health advocates (Lasch, 2000) or engaging in cross-cultural discussion about truth telling and consent in the international arena (Xue et al., 2011).

Approaches to substandard norms of practice

The rights ethos is now firmly embedded in medical practice as is a culture of quality improvement (<http://www.medqic.org>; <http://www.ihi.org>; <http://www.capc.org>; <http://www.medicaring.org>). There are multiple measures and tools for determining a person's capacity to consent to treatment (Sturman, 2005), the effectiveness of risk communication and treatment decision-making (Edwards, 2003), the effectiveness of decision-making aids (Feldman-Stewart et al., 2006), and a person's regrets about decisions (Joseph-Williams et al., 2010). Despite these safeguards, no framework can predict all the factors which may influence treatment decisions and care near the end of life. As Lynn et al. argue 'in the care of very sick people, the error is not that we never provide good care, it is that we do not always provide good care' (Lynn, 2008). Research suggests that having the right people on a team which reflects and revises practice can be an effective way to improve palliative care and maintain high standards (Lynn, 2008; Hewison et al., 2009).

Conclusion

In Western medicine today, clinicians understand truth telling as a legal and ethical responsibility. Persons with illness understand truth as their right to be given the information in order to make informed decisions about end-of-life treatments and care.

Studies of person, family clinician, and caregiver experiences show that truth telling is difficult and distressing at all stages of a terminal illness for all involved. Delivering bad news goes against the grain; it challenges social norms and expectations about the role of physicians as healers. Communicated badly, without intimate knowledge of a person and their family's hopes, expectations, and wishes, 'truth' can have a devastating impact on quality of life and care.

In response, a rapidly increasing body of clinical practice guidelines and generic templates for ways to communicate around difficult topics are being created to assist health-care professionals and improve consumer confidence in decision-making. Analysis and development of more complex conceptual and theoretical models of the biopsychosocial experience of terminal illness is enabling verbal and non-verbal communication tools and approaches to be tailored to different person group typologies.

However, it would be dangerous to think that a cultural hiatus has been reached. The global research shows how familism has to be considered alongside autonomy. Recent cases relating to truth telling and consent in the media have been focused on the right to die rather than the right to know, suggesting that this may be the next legally inspired ethical debate to require professional standardization in the decade to come as populations get older.

Online materials

Additional online materials and complete references for this chapter are available online at <http://www.oxfordmedicine.com>.

References

Ahearn, D.J. , Jackson, T.B. and McIlmoyle, J. (2010) Improving end of life care for nursing home residents: an analysis of hospital mortality and readmission rates. *Postgraduate Medicine*, 86, 131–135.

Anderson, K. (2000). The family health system approach to family systems nursing. *Journal of Family Nursing*, 6, 103–119.

Appelbaum, P., Lidz, C., and Meisel, A. (1987). *Informed Consent: Legal Theory and Clinical Practice*. Oxford: Oxford University Press.

Back, A., Arnold, R., and Tulsky, J. (2009). *Mastering Communication with Seriously Ill Patients: Balancing Honesty with Empathy and Hope*. Cambridge: Cambridge University Press.

Bowman, D., Spicer, J., and Iqbal, R. (2011). *Informed Consent: A Primer for Clinical Practice*. Cambridge: Cambridge University Press.

Buckman, R. (1992). *How to Break Bad News: A Guide for Health Care Professionals*. London: Papermac.

Cantor, M. and Pearlman, R. (2003) Advanced Care Planning in Long Term Care Facilities, *Journal of American Medical Directors Association*, 4, 101–107.

Cassell, E. (1985). *The Healer's Art*. Cambridge, MA: MIT Press.

Chan, W.C.H. (2011). Being aware of the prognosis: how does it relate to palliative care patients anxiety and communication difficulty with family members in the Hong Kong Chinese context? *Journal of Palliative Medicine*, 14(9), 997–1003.

Chewning, B., Bylund, C., Shah, B., et al. (2012). Patient preferences for shared decisions: a systematic review. *Patient Education and Counseling*, 86, 9–18.

Clayton, J., Hancock, K., Parker, S., et al. (2008). Sustaining hope when communicating with terminally ill persons and their families: a systematic review. *Psycho-Oncology*, 17, 641–659.

Covinsky, K.E., Goldman, L., Cook, E.F., et al. (1994). The impact of serious illness on patients' families. Study to understand prognoses and preferences for outcomes and risks of treatment. *Journal of the American Medical Association*, 272, 1839–1844.

Deschepper, R., Bernheim, J., Vander Stichele, R., et al. (2008). Truth telling at the end of life: a pilot study on the perspectives of patients and professional caregivers. *Patient Education and Counseling*, 71, 52–56.

Deshpande, O., Carrington Reid, M., and Rao, A. (2005). Attitudes of Asian-Indian Hindus towards end of life care. *Journal of the American Geriatrics Society*, 53, 131–135.

Eliott, J.A. and Olver, I.N. (2006). Hope and hoping in the talk of dying cancer patients. *Social Science & Medicine*, 64, 138–149.

Emanuel, L.L., Bennett, K., and Richardson, V.E. (2007). The dying role. *Journal of Palliative Medicine*, 10(1), 159–168.

Emanuel, L.L., Danis, M., Pearlman, R.A., et al. (1995). Advance care planning as a process: structuring discussions in practice. *Journal of the American Geriatrics Society*, 43(4), 440–446.

Epstein, R. and Street, R. (2007). *Patient Centered Communication in Cancer Care: Promoting Healing, and Reducing Suffering*. Bethesda, MD: National Cancer Institute.

Gaston, C.M. and Mitchell, G. (2005). Information giving and decision-making in patients with advanced cancer: a systematic review. *Social Science & Medicine*, 61, 2252–2264.

Grisso T. and Appelbaum, P. (1998). *Assessing Competence to Consent to Treatment: A Guide for Physicians and Other Health Professionals*. Oxford: Oxford University Press.

Gunter-Hunt, G., Mahoney, J. and Sieger, C (2002). A Comparison of State Advance Directive Documents. *The Gerontologist*. 42(1). 51–60.

Guthell, I.A. and Heyman, J.C. (2011). A social work perspective: attitudes towards end-of-life planning. *Social Work in Health Care*, 50(10), 763–774.

Gutierrez, K.M. (2012). Prognostic communication of critical care nurses and physicians at end of life. *Dimensions of Critical Care Nursing*, 31(3), 170–182.

Gysels, M., Richardson, A., and Higginson, I.J. (2004). Communication training for health care professionals who care for patients with cancer: a systematic review of effectiveness. *Supportive Care in Cancer*, 12, 692–700.

Hagerty, R.G., Butow, P.N., Ellis, P.A., *et al.* (2004). Cancer patients' preferences for communication of prognosis in the metastatic setting. *Journal of Clinical Oncology*, 22, 1721–1730.

Hagerty, R.G., Butow, P.N., Ellis, P.A., *et al.* (2005). Communicating with realism and hope: incurable cancer patients' views of the disclosure of prognosis. *Journal of Clinical Oncology*, 23, 1278–1288.

Heinemann, G. and Zeiss, A. (2002). *Team Performance in Health Care: Assessment and Development*. New York: Kluwer Academic/Plenum Publishers.

Hiltunen, E.F., Medich, C., Chase, S., Peterson, L., and Forrow, L. (1999). Family decision-making for end of life treatment: the SUPPORT nurse narratives. Study to Understand Prognoses and Preferences for Outcomes and Risks of Treatments. *Journal of Clinical Ethics*, 10, 126–134.

Johnson, K., Elbert-Avila, K., and Tulksy, J. (2005). The influence of spiritual beliefs and practices on the treatment preferences of African Americans: a review of the literature. *Journal of the American Geriatrics Society*, 53, 711–719.

Joosten, E.A.G., DeFuentes-Merillas, L., de Weert, G.H., *et al.* (2008). Systematic review of the effects of shared decision-making on patient satisfaction, treatment adherence and health status. *Psychotherapy and Psychosomatics*, 77, 219–226.

Kersten, C., Cameron, M.G., and Oldenburg, M.D. (2012). Truth in hope and hope in truth. *Journal of Palliative Medicine*, 15(1), 128–129.

Knight, S. and Emanuel, L.L. (2007). Process of adjustment to end-of-life losses: a reintegration model. *Journal of Palliative Medicine*, 10(5), 1190–1198.

Kübler-Ross, E. (1969). *On Death and Dying*. London: Routledge.

Lamb, S. (2009). *Aging and the Indian diaspora: cosmopolitan families in India and abroad*. Bloomington: Indiana University Press.

Lasch, K. (2000). Culture, pain and culturally sensitive pain care. *Pain Management Nursing*, 1(3, Suppl. 1), 16–22.

Lynn, J., Schuster, J., Wilkinson, A., and Simon , L. (2008) *Improving Care for End of Life: A Sourcebook for Healthcare Managers and Physicians*. Oxford: Oxford University Press.

Lynn, J., Harrold, J., and Schuster, L. (2011). *Handbook for Mortals: Guidance for People Facing Serious Illness*. Oxford: Oxford University Press.

MacLean, A. (2013). *Autonomy, Informed Consent and Medical Law: A Relational Challenge*. Cambridge: Cambridge University Press.

MacLean, S. (1988). *First Do No Harm*. Farnham: Ashgate.

Makoul, G. and Clayman, M. (2006). An integrative model of shared decision-making in medical encounters. *Patient Education and Counseling*, 60, 301–312.

Mentes, J., Teer, J., and Cadogan, M. (2004). The pain experience of cognitively impaired nursing home residents: perceptions of family members and certified nursing assistants. *Pain Management Nursing*, 5(3), 118–125.

Mezey, M., Mitty, E., and Ramsey, G. (1997). Assessment of decision-making capacity: nurse's role. *Journal of Gerontological Nursing*, 23(3), 28–35.

Miller, J. (2010). *The Body in Question*. London: Random House.

Mok, E., Lau, K.-P., Lam, W.-M., *et al.* (2010). Health-care professionals' perspectives on hope in the palliative care setting. *Journal of Palliative Medicine*, 13(7), 877–883.

Moskop, J. (2004). Improving care at the end of life: how advance care planning can help. *Palliative and Supportive Care*, 2, 191–197.

Murillo, M. and Holland, J. (2004). Clinical practice guidelines for the management of psychosocial distress at the end of life. *Palliative and Supportive Care*, 2, 65–77.

Nelms, T. and Eggenberger, S. (2010). The essence of the family critical illness experience and nurse-family meetings. *Journal of Family Nursing*, 16(4), 462–486.

Nolan, M. *et al.* (2008) Family healthcare decision-making and self efficacy with patients with ALS at the end of life. *Palliative and Supportive Care*, 6, 273–280.

O'Neill, O. (2002). *Autonomy and Trust in Bioethics*. Cambridge: Cambridge University Press.

O'Shea, T. (2011). *Consent in History, Theory and Practice*. Essex Autonomy Project Green Paper Report. University of Essex: Essex Autonomy Project. [Online] Available at: <http://autonomy.essex.ac.uk/consent-in-history-theory-and-practice>.

Rando, T.A. (1984). *Grief, Dying and Death: Clinical Interventions for Caregivers*. Champaign, IL: Research Press.

Reinke, L., Shannon, S., Engelberg, R.A., *et al.* (2010). Supporting hope and prognostic information: nurses' perspectives on their role when persons have life limiting prognoses. *Journal of Pain and Symptom Management*, 39(6), 982–992.

Rempel, G. (2007). Interactive use of genograms and ecomaps in family caregiving research. *Journal of Family Nursing*, 13, 403–419.

Sokol, D. (2006). How the physician's nose has shortened over time: a historical review of the truth-telling debate in the physician-patient relationship. *Journal of the Royal Society of Medicine*, 99, 632–636.

Stacey, D., Legare, F. Pouliot, S., *et al.* (2010). Shared decision-making models to inform an interprofessional perspective on decision making: a theory analysis. *Patient Education and Counseling*, 80, 164–172.

Steiber-Roger, K. (2006). A literature review of palliative care, end of life and dementia. *Palliative and Supportive Care*, 4, 295–303.

Tariman, J., Berry, D.L., Cochrane, B., *et al.* (2010). Preferred and actual participation roles during health care decision-making in patients with cancer: a systematic review. *Journal of Oncology*, 21, 1145–1151.

Tulsky, J. (2005). Beyond advance directives: importance of communication skills at the end of life. *Journal of the American Medical Association*, 294(3), 359–364.

Volicer, L. and Ganzini, L. (2003). Health professionals' views on standards for decision-making capacity regarding refusal of medical treatment in mild Alzheimer's disease. *Journal of the American Geriatrics Society*, 51, 1270–1274.

Xue, D., Wheeler, J., and Abernethy, A. (2011). Cultural differences in truth telling to cancer persons: Chinese and American approaches to the disclosure of bad news. *Progress in Palliative Care*, 19(3), 125–131.

5.5

Ethics in paediatric palliative care

Richard D.W. Hain

Introduction: scope and function of medical ethics

A starting point for medical ethics is that there is potentially an imbalance of power between physician and patient that should be redressed by 'rules of engagement' setting out how a doctor should behave. That conception encompasses the idea of a moral obligation for persons to be fair to one another, and indicates that one requirement of fairness is that the strong should show special consideration to the weak. It is especially relevant to children needing palliative care, made multiply vulnerable by youth, small physical size, illness, and motor and cognitive impairment.

Ethical codes have elaborated on those basic ideas, through the Hippocratic Oath and principle of *primum non nocere* to the four-principles approach of Beauchamp and Childress (2009). The focus of medical ethics was how doctors should behave towards patients; the need for it also to account for a responsibility to society is recent.

The relationship between physician and child and family largely defines the *scope* of paediatric medical ethics. Its *function* can be expressed in several ways. From the perspective of child and family, it is an attempt to 'level the playing field' in relationship with the clinician. To society, it ensures doctors are not isolated from contemporary mores, including notions of how health-care money should be spent. From the perspective of the clinician, however, the task of medical ethics is analytical; to help resolve moral quandary and guide decision-making in patient management through an appeal to what is morally right, in clinical situations where rationality and medical competence alone do not provide a single clear answer.

This chapter sets out current approaches to ethics in paediatric palliative care, suggesting that none is completely satisfactory; a coherent, specifically paediatric account is needed.

Ethics in children: paradigms in practice

Two paradigms dominate contemporary ethical dialogue in children: rights-based arguments (United Nations General Assembly, 1989), and the 'four-principles' approach (Beauchamp and Childress, 2009). Rights-based claims are child specific (Goldhagen, 2003; Paul, 2007; Archard, 2010; Alderson, 2011; Streuli et al., 2011) but often not argued from an ethical premise. The four-principles approach flows from understandings of ethical theory, but is not designed for children. Each usefully informs

ethical discussions in children, though neither represents a complete account.

Rights

Rights-based dialogue provides a legalistic rather than ethical account of how a clinician should treat a child. Nevertheless, the idea that children have rights at all is a powerful and foundational ethical claim. Modern concepts of children's rights come largely from the United Nations (UN) Convention on the Rights of the Child (CRC) (UN General Assembly, 1989). The Convention is intended to give force to a child-focused legal agenda (Goldhagen, 2003); it does not provide any coherent ethical account of childhood or attempt a moral argument concerning the nature of rights. It invokes the earlier preamble of the UN Universal Declaration of Human Rights (UN General Assembly, 1948) in which rights were held to be self-evident, to apply to any human, and to be inherent in the individual. By applying this definition to children, the CRC insists there is no distinction between the moral values of child and adult. That is an important assertion. Children are often considered 'works in progress' whose moral value is as potential, rather than current, persons.

The CRC indicates that children are also distinct from adults in morally relevant ways. Their developmental nature imparts special value. It is their nature to be cared for in a family; society's responsibility to children is in supporting the family in caring for the child. These claims are in the preamble of the convention, identifying them as foundational.

As a matter of jural logic rights exist as the corollary of duties and must inevitably restrict the influence of states; even democracies (Hohfeld and Cook, 1978; Lazarev, 2005). That power concerns rights sceptics (Hafen and Hafen, 1995; Guggenheim, 2005). A lesser claim for rights (Alderson, 2011) as aspirational statements of moral intent, allows rights-based arguments more helpfully to inform an account of ethics in children.

Principlism

Thomas Beauchamp and James Childress (Beauchamp and Childress, 2009) famously articulated four principles: autonomy, beneficence, non-maleficence. and justice. Autonomy is the patient's own capacity to decide what medical treatment is done, beneficence is the responsibility of the clinician to do what is good for their patient, non-maleficence is the duty to avoid harm, and justice the responsibility of clinicians to participate in designing and maintaining a health-care system that is fair.

There may be no obvious way to resolve conflicts between the principles:

Following an uncomplicated pregnancy, a girl is born prematurely at 25 weeks' gestation. She weighs 695 g and is anatomically normal for post-conceptual age. She makes a respiratory gasp but clearly needs intubation and ventilation. Her parents request that 'everything' be done, but the neonatal paediatrician is reluctant to ventilate, knowing that majority of children born at this stage will suffer severe long-term cognitive and physical impairment, and that resuscitation of such children is expensive, not only in the immediately aftermath of the resuscitation, but in supporting the child medically and socially for decades afterwards.

Applying the four principles, it is possible to construct:

◆ An argument from respect for *autonomy* that the child should be resuscitated because her parents request it (either because they want it or because they think she would want it), or

◆ An argument from *beneficence* that she should be resuscitated because it will do her good, or

◆ An argument from *justice* that she should not be resuscitated because to do so would be unjustly consume resources in a world of finite health-care funding, or

◆ An argument from *non-maleficence* that she should not be resuscitated because to do so would do her harm.

This is not a shortcoming of the approach, but an illustration of the limitations of its scope. Principlism does not represent a single coherent ethical theory, but a practical heuristic for busy clinicians. The four principles represent a practical summary of complex philosophical deliberations, for use 'in the heat of battle', rather as a formulary summarizes practical prescribing but does not replace a sound knowledge of pharmacology.

In paediatric palliative care, however, there are important weaknesses in principlism as a result of the failure of some of the principles that lie behind it to account consistently for the nature of children. Autonomy is problematic in relation to children, accounts of beneficence and non-maleficence do not consistently distinguish between the interests of children and those of families, and establishing justice is complicated in a society composed mainly of adults. The status of the child in principlism is often unclear. Children ideally need a coherent ethical approach that is consistent with their nature as moral beings that are both distinct from, and have much in common with, adults.

The nature of children: special ethical considerations

Personhood and rationality

Personhood is often held to be a function of rationality, and the status of children in many ethical theories remains uncertain. Children probably rationalize differently from adults, but that is only determinative of rationality if the definition is limited to the way adults do it. Since even some non-human animals reason (Glackin, 2008), it seems unlikely that adult rationality is the only form of rationality there is among humans. In his book *Practical Ethics*, utilitarian philosopher Peter Singer (2011) asserts that infanticide is permissible. The infant, he says, lacks reason and

therefore awareness of self over time. Being killed cannot rob the infant of anything she can truly be said to possess. Given modern understandings of infant neurodevelopment (Gopnik, 2007; Bauer, 2008), Singer's claim is improbable. The idea that infants cannot reason is perhaps a contemporary parallel to earlier ideas that they cannot experience pain; a convenient and widely held belief about children that simplifies decision-making for adults but is ultimately untrue. Nevertheless, the moral status of children who are genuinely non-rational (such as those with severe cognitive impairment) presents paediatric clinical ethicists with a challenge.

Dependence and autonomy

Autonomy is often taken to mean freedom, in the sense of having no restrictions on actuating one's will. In practice, a child is multiply restricted in the influence he or she can exert. Many limitations are inherent to the nature of the child; children are physically small, and often lack verbal skills simply by virtue of their age. The child given less influence because she is unimportant inevitably becomes increasingly unimportant because she cannot exert influence, and lack of autonomy is self-perpetuating.

Properly understood, however, autonomy describes the freedom to decide for oneself which set of restrictions to acknowledge. That more realistic definition does not exclude children so clearly since children often manifest autonomy by allowing parents to make decisions on their behalf, seeing themselves in a reciprocal and balanced caring relationship with family members (Carnevale et al., 2008). Ambiguities in the nature of children's autonomy are particularly significant in palliative care. Cognitive impairment and severely restricted physical mobility are usual. Expectations that parental autonomy will be respected, as well as that of the child, interpose a layer of ethical complexity. Even caring parents may, rationally or otherwise, choose what is less than ideal for their children (Brierley et al., 2013). Disentangling what parents feel their child would want from what parents want for their child is morally relevant, but not always possible.

Limitations on understanding autonomy are relevant in considering the ethics of euthanasia and physician-assisted suicide legislation that extends into childhood or young adulthood. Adolescents may appear more autonomous than they are. A perfectly competent and rational adolescent may request euthanasia for reasons that have little to do with a considered desire to end life. The high frequency of risk-taking behaviour and suicide during adolescence (Self and Findley, 2010) illustrates that an actual desire to die is only one among many influences. Even if it is conceded that people who ask for it should be killed, it is not clear that it is possible, in practice, to distinguish clearly between an adolescent's request for death and (for example) a request for more attention, or a protest against parental restrictions. The assumption that there is always a straightforward relationship between what people say, and what they actually mean, is even less reliable in adolescents than it is in adults.

The concept of autonomy, then, is foundationally problematic in children. Autonomy requires some degree of control over one's own life. For all children, it is more limited than it is for adults, for various reasons of which some have no moral relevance. It is over-simplistic to suggest a child inherently lacks autonomy, and ethics therefore need account only for the wishes of parents. Nevertheless, a child is inherently in relationship with a family. To deny the importance of that relationship, and the authority it gives to parents to speak for their child, would be to deny something central to the ethical questions clinicians need to ask about children.

Interests: child versus family

Some sceptics of the concept of children's rights argue that it creates a separation between the interests of child and family that is spurious (Hafen and Hafen, 1995; Guggenheim, 2005). While that overstates the case, it is true that a child's moral deliberation normally occurs in a context in which family is extremely influential. The child will find it hard to articulate views of interests that differ from strongly expressed views of parents, potentially allowing coercion. Where differences are expressed, the medical team may need to arbitrate between them, or else privilege one over the other.

The concept of 'best interests' is especially problematic in children who are cognitively impaired. There are no objective measures of a good outcome. Survival probability is typically irrelevant, since death in childhood is expected. Other measures are subjective, requiring the child to be verbally and conceptually capable of articulating issues that relate to existential as well as physical components. In practice, this is difficult, and clinicians are often drawn instead to an account of ethics that allows us to regard a child's parents' interests as inseparable from those of the child. It is perhaps as a reaction to this problematic assumption that the modern children's rights movement has developed.

Relationality

It is important to individual families to know that a health-care system is fair, and to that extent, justice is appropriately considered one of the four medical ethical principles. In other respects, it appears out of place. Where autonomy, beneficence, and non-maleficence all relate primarily to decisions made in the context of a relationship between an individual child and an individual doctor, the principle of justice refers instead to 'states of affairs' (Smart and Williams, 1973). Typically, justice arguments are rooted in utilitarianism; that the ethically right decision depends on its impact on the whole community. While the other three principles focus on the needs of an individual patient, justice makes individuals subordinate to the needs of society.

A 3-year-old boy with an advanced metabolic degenerative condition was now felt by his paediatrician to be 'almost in a permanent vegetative state'. After a series of chest infections of increasing severity and frequency, his parents brought him to casualty with signs of another pneumonia, insisting that he should be ventilated again. The intensive care paediatrician saw the child in casualty and explained to the boy's parents that ventilation would not be offered, because it would mean their son occupying a bed that another child could use more effectively.

Few clinicians would disagree with the conclusion here that the child should not be ventilated. The ethical reasoning also appears sound. It is, however, cruel, unreasonable, and coercive to expect parents to sacrifice their child to the well-being of others

(American Academy of Pediatrics, 1996). Such an expectation flows from an ethical understanding that is hard to argue convincingly without ignoring the child's nature as a dependent being in the care of a family. Relationship has moral relevance in ethical deliberation around specific quandaries that is not easily accommodated by most forms of utilitarian consequentialism.

The relationship of physician and child is also of ethical relevance (Bartholome, 1985, 1996; Ramsey, 2002). In considering how to design a fair system of health care, it is a legitimate ethical starting point that all patients, real or hypothetical, are equally important. In the case described earlier, however, considering the impact on hypothetical 'other children' is outside the scope of this physician's relationship with this particular child.

Clinicians may need to make ethically relevant decisions in both modes. They will need to make some decisions in the context of their relationship with individual patients, and others in developing or maintaining fair systems. This is not inconsistent. It may even be ethically necessary; tension between the needs of the individual actual patient and those of hypothetical other patients is inevitable given limited health-care resources, and dialectic is integral to a consistent ethical approach, not antithetical to it.

Ethics in children: underlying theories

Deontology

Deontological arguments flow from an assumption that there is an absolute morality that is equally relevant to all people, in all situations, irrespective of the consequences. There at least three possible sources for an absolute moral code. One is the authority of God through religious scripture. Even in secular societies those codes are, it can be argued, authoritative at least to the extent that they are rational. Most scripture was, however, not designed primarily as an exposition of a consistent ethical code, and is often elliptical and/or subject to interpretation. Ethical accounts derived from religious understanding are rarely completely agreed, even among those who share that faith.

A second source of an absolute moral code might be the universe itself. Ancient and medieval understanding was that the universe was rationally ordered, and coherence with that rational order was the yardstick by which the rightness of behaviour should be measured. So, for example, the ethical rules by which children should live and by which parents should care for them both derive from the inherent nature of family.

A third authority might be that of pure reason. Kant (1785/2005) attempted to show that there were certain ethical premises that were beyond debate because for reasonable people they were logically inescapable. Some, he argued, were always true, irrespective of context (categorical imperatives) while others were contingent on the individual's prior beliefs about context (hypothetical imperative). Applying this to children is not straightforward; Kant considered the moral law to be co-extensive with rationality, and since he does not obviously consider children rational it is not clear in Kant whether a child has valid status as a moral being.

Consequentialism

In practice, the outcome of an ethical decision can be worse by obeying a rule than by breaking it. Consequentialists argue that this is an inherent weakness in 'rule-worship' itself, and that the only morally relevant aspect of an action is found in its consequences (Smart and Williams, 1973). Consequentialists differ about what outcomes should be measured. Libertarian consequentialists judge the moral 'rightness' of an action by the extent to which it contributes to freedom. In medical ethics, utilitarianism is the best-known form, and the most widely recognized outcome measure is the effect on 'the sum total of human happiness'.

Some important ambiguities restrict the usefulness of utilitarianism in practice. The sum total of happiness could relate to a great deal of happiness on the part of a few people, or moderate happiness on the part of many. The nature of happiness itself is not agreed, and may not be measurable. Evaluating happiness is particularly problematic in children needing palliative care, who are often non- or pre-verbal and cannot articulate feelings or preferences. A close correlation between happiness and observable function or cognitive ability is sometimes assumed (Shaw, 1977) but there is little reason or evidence to indicate that life quality is influenced in any readily predictable way by physical condition, or closeness to death.

Utilitarianism does not concern itself with the happiness of the individual, except insofar as it contributes to the sum total of human experience. A central principle is that the happiness of each individual person is equally important—or, perhaps more accurately, equally unimportant—to the agent making the ethical decision. A paradox in most forms of utilitarianism is that utilitarians can be concerned for the total happiness of society, while remaining indifferent to the happiness of all its individual members.

Finally, utilitarian consequentialism does not acknowledge any ethical relevance for intention. This again makes it problematic for most quandaries in medical ethics. A doctor trying to decide on a particular course of clinical action has to decide whether to do a particular act or not to do it. The quandary defines, and is defined by, the agent's intention. Utilitarianism does not provide a mechanism for that decision, because it claims that ethical 'rightness' depends on something entirely isolated from intention; that is, outcome. The physician cannot know the outcome at the time the decision needs to be made. She can only make a judgement on the basis of knowledge and prior experience. That informed judgement is what constitutes intention in the context of medical decision-making. The fact that utilitarianism cannot accommodate intention—still less complex intentions as in double effect—illustrates an important limitation of its scope.

Virtue ethics

Although deontology and consequentialism might appear to be opposites, they have two important things in common. Both are 'absolutist' approaches—they claim unlimited scope to provide moral values that are always and everywhere right. Both also ultimately elevate something abstract over real individual human beings. In the case of deontology, it is a concept of duty. In the case of utilitarian consequentialism, it is a concept of happiness or some other descriptor of persons. Since neither duty nor happiness can have any meaning independently of individual persons, neither deontology nor consequentialism can, on its own, provide an adequate account of medical ethics, which relates primarily, though not exclusively, to decisions in the context of relationships between individual persons.

In contrast, virtue ethics (Macintyre, 2007) has its roots in Aristotle's understanding that an action is right if it is done by a virtuous person for the right reason. Aristotle locates the quality of

virtue, not only in the ethical rightness of an act, but in the character of the moral agent whose act it is. Virtuous people, and ethically correct acts, are mutually defining in the same way that force and acceleration are mutually defining in Newton's second law of motion. One cannot argue from virtuous act to virtuous person; it is simply impossible for either to exist independently of the other.

An understanding of the 'virtuous doctor' emerges from the Hippocratic oath and underlies professionalism; that is, what constitutes good medical practice (General Medical Council, 2006). To be professional is to behave in a certain way that is, as a corollary, the way in which a professional behaves. Virtue ethics provides a coherent and consistent account of ethical behaviour that most other theories cannot, but it does not provide an obvious decision mechanism for resolving individual ethical quandaries. Virtue ethics can therefore shape expectations of professional behaviour from doctors, but may not in its own replace an analytical approach to clinical ethics.

Double effect and withholding of life-sustaining treatment in paediatric palliative care
Principle of double effect

A 9-year-old boy with severe cerebral palsy is admitted to the paediatric intensive care unit (PICU) with the latest in a series of severe chest infections. Each infection has been worse than the last, and on each admission it has become more difficult to wean him off the ventilator. Despite adequate and appropriate interventions, including ventilation and intravenous antibiotics, it seems likely that on this occasion it will not be possible for him to breathe independently of the ventilator. In discussion with his parents, a decision is made for 'compassionate extubation' (that is, extubation in anticipation that he will die). The child has not seemed to be in pain and has never received opioids, but 2 hours before extubation, the PICU physician prescribes the equivalent of 2 mg per kilogram of oral morphine as a single intravenous bolus. She is aware as she does so that three possible outcomes are analgesia, anaphylaxis, and abolition of respiratory effort at the time of extubation.

The principle of double effect (PDE) is an acknowledgement of the possibility that a clinician can foresee a range of outcomes from a single act, but intend only a subset of them. It is logically inescapable, and the basis on which good clinical decision-making is made in many specialties, including palliative medicine (Fohr, 1998). Despite its apparently self-evident nature, the PDE is considered by some simply to be a 'fudge factor' that allows physicians to feel comfortable making decisions at the end of life that, in reality, hasten or cause death. There are several reasons for this, of which this chapter will consider only two: it is sometimes misunderstood, and its self-evident first premise requires certain further qualifications that are not agreed. Those include, in particular, conceptions of proportionality, and the extent to which a single act can be defined within, and reliably distinguished from, a series of acts.

A common misunderstanding of the PDE is that it legitimizes equally all outcomes that are foreseen. In the earlier example, relief of pain is ethically permissible, while inducing apnoea is not.[1] It is sometimes thought that the PDE permits the overdose because the ethically problematic outcome is simply a secondary consequence of treating pain. The PDE does not allow this, however, for an important reason; the dose that is suggested is disproportionately high for the ethically permissible outcome. The dose required for pain in an opioid naïve child would be a tiny fraction of this (1 mg/24 hours). The dose suggested cannot be justified on the grounds of the permissible outcome.

The illustration shows that some element of proportionality must be shown between the act and its outcome in order to judge the intention. In palliative medicine, that proportionality can be considered in many ways. One is the reasonableness of the dose. Prescribing morphine analgesia is ethically justified only to the extent that the dose is appropriate for the degree of pain (Hain and Friedrichsdorf, 2012).

A second measure of proportionality is to consider 'directness' of the intention. Any action leads to a series of consequences that are increasingly remote from the agent's intention. It is not, as Glover humorously suggests (Glover, 1977, p. 89), a question of how long after the act its consequences manifest. The question of directness relates rather to the disposition of the agent; what result the physician expects from his or her action. Except to purist consequentialists, there is a morally relevant difference between intending A while recognizing that B is a consequence (that is, willing A but permitting B), and intending A and B equally. Temporal remoteness may be incidentally relevant, especially if it allows other agents to intervene to change the consequence as a result of their own intentions, but it is not of itself a measure of directness.

Proportionality can also be seen as a function of probability. Apnoea is likely at the dose suggested in the earlier example, but not inevitable. Pancuronium, however, guarantees it; a physician prescribing pancuronium during extubation intends apnoea and the PDE does not apply.[2] Conversely, anaphylaxis is a foreseen event for most drugs, but its rarity makes it obvious that a physician does not usually intend to cause death by prescribing it. Probability, as well as reasonableness and remoteness, are relevant to intention.

Problematically, the PDE demands that a single act can always be considered the sum of several smaller acts that are discrete. It is hard to find a valid basis for such analysis. The act of giving morphine could be said to begin with the injection, in choosing not to give naloxone to reverse it if apnoea occurs, or it could be considered inseparable from the overall act of caring for a dying child. According to utilitarian consequentialist understanding, the PDE is meaningless since it gives different ethical value to acts with the same outcome. Although utilitarians therefore dismiss the PDE as without moral meaning (Glover, 1977; Harris, 1985), it is equally rational to suggest that this is a further limitation of consequentialism in medical ethics.

The fact that application of the PDE in practice is not always straightforward does not, however, undermine its central thesis. It is a matter of everyday reality for paediatric palliative care physicians that it is possible to foresee consequences of an intervention that are not its aim. It is inconceivable, without re-evaluating the whole task of medical ethics, that the intention of the physician is not relevant. The ethical 'rightness' of an intervention with such multiple outcomes must rely on some concept of proportionality, measured as reasonableness of the dose, remoteness of the intention, or probability of a consequence.

Withholding and withdrawing life-sustaining treatment

The Royal College of Paediatrics and Child Health (RCPCH) (2004) in the United Kingdom recognizes several archetype situations in which medical treatment aimed at sustaining or saving life might be withheld. The guidelines represent a practical tool for considering the quandary, rather than a coherent ethical approach. Withholding and withdrawing are not the same decision, but if both serve the best interests of the child they are logically equivalent ethically.

Withholding or withdrawing treatment from *the child who is brain dead or in a permanent vegetative state* is permitted, not because the child is no longer of value, but because she no longer has interests and the residual interests are those of others, so that a beneficence argument need take only those into account. This situation therefore permits withdrawing or withholding, but it does not mandate it; for example, the family's interests may be best served by continuing. The justification for withdrawing in the *no chance situation* is not merely that the child cannot recover but, again, that the child's interests are best served by not prolonging treatment.

The same can be said of the *unbearable situation*. The term 'unbearable' is inherently subjective. There is an ethical duty on those caring for a child to explore with him what he feels about what is going on. That is not the same as securing the child's permission for treatment to be withdrawn. Although it is helpful if the child expresses a clear view, the *unbearable situation* does not preclude the possibility that carers will need to act as advocates, as well as proxies, for the child.

The *no purpose situation* appears to presuppose a provisional value for the child's life. What follows clarifies, however, that the purpose in question is that of treatment; that is, the benefit of that individual child. The *no purpose situation* is, again, a special example of beneficence, but unlike the *unbearable situation* it assumes the child cannot participate in the discussion. The responsibility of carers is therefore a little different; rather than giving a voice to his wishes, it is to make a wise and compassionate decision about what is best for the child.

Palliative care foundationally recognizes that death should sometimes be allowed to occur, even where it is technically possible to delay it. All the RCPCH 'situations' are best considered illustrations of the same principle of balancing burden and benefit, distinguished by what is at stake, whose interests are relevant, and the extent to which the child's own estimate of 'bearability' can be solicited. The only indisputably relevant ethical question in deciding whether treatment should be offered to or withheld from a child is whether the intervention is likely to do more good than it does harm to that individual child. That balance needs to take into account much more than the duration of life, including dimensions that are difficult to measure and/or are inherently subjective. A child's disability is relevant to the extent that it impacts on those dimensions.

Conclusion

This chapter has outlined some theories and paradigms in ethics of care at the end of life, and some special challenges of considering them in children's palliative care. Paediatric palliative care clinicians face all the moral ambiguities of their colleagues working with dying adults, and often have to turn for ethical guidance to sources that were not intended for that purpose. Of those, the most important currently are the four principles approach, and the UN CRC. The first was developed for adults and is often unsuitable for children, particularly because of its emphasis on autonomy. The second is a series of axiomatic rights claims that, while they make some important fundamental ethical claims about the nature of children, are not obviously justified philosophically. Neither on its own provides the kind of coherent account needed by those working in children's palliative care.

Because it does not accommodate the moral relevance of the relationship of clinician and child, the scope of utilitarian consequentialism (in its purest sense) in paediatric palliative care should be limited to development of fair systems, rather than to specific clinical decisions about individuals. Children are vulnerable to the misapplication of utilitarian ethics to individual patient quandaries because they are typically unable to express clearly what they want and their removal from the world, particularly as infants, does little to detract from the sum total of human happiness.

Many of the specific ethical quandaries faced by clinicians working with dying children have their counterparts in the adult specialty. It seems likely that, as it becomes technically possible to resuscitate children at ever earlier stages in fetal development, and to keep children alive but suffering for ever longer periods of time, it will also become increasingly important to be able to address those quandaries in a way that is specifically paediatric. To do so requires that we do more than extrapolate from existing accounts such as rights or principlism; paediatricians and bioethicists must develop an ethical account of childhood itself that is consistent, coherent, and complete.

Acknowledgement

The author is most grateful to Dr John Perry, Lecturer in Theological Ethics School of Divinity, University of St Andrews, for his comments on the manuscript.

Notes

1. Unless killing (active euthanasia) is considered a permissible outcome.
2. I am setting aside, for the purposes of this illustration, ethical arguments that support intentionally killing the child. Any ethical justification for giving pancuronium at the time of extubation flows from those arguments, rather than from the PDE.

Online materials

Complete references for this chapter are available online at <http://www.oxfordmedicine.com>.

References

American Academy of Pediatrics (1996). Ethics and the care of critically ill infants and children. American Academy of Pediatrics Committee on Bioethics. *Pediatrics*, 98, 149–152.

Beauchamp, T. and Childress, J. (2009). *Principles of Biomedical Ethics*. New York: Oxford University Press.

Carnevale, F.A., MacDonald, M.E., Bluebond-Langner, M., and McKeever, P. (2008). Using participant observation in pediatric health care settings: ethical challenges and solutions. *Journal of Child Health Care*, 12, 18–32.

Fohr, S.A. (1998). The double effect of pain medication: separating myth from reality. *Journal of Palliative Medicine*, 1, 315–328.

Royal College of Paediatrics and Child Health (2004). *Withholding or Withdrawing Life Sustaining Treatment in Children: A Framework for Practice*. London: RCPCH.

United Nations General Assembly (1989). *Convention on the Rights of the Child: Adopted and Opened for Signature, Ratification and Accession by General Assembly Resolution 44/25*. New York: United Nations.

5.6

Dignity and palliative end-of-life care

Harvey Max Chochinov, Susan E. McClement, and Maia S. Kredentser

Introduction to dignity and palliative end-of-life care

In recent years, the concept of dignity has garnered increased attention by health-care researchers and practitioners working across various disciplines. Despite this attention (Higginson and Hall, 2007) and debate regarding the overall usefulness of the concept (Macklin, 2004; Schroeder, 2008), there continue to be calls for more in-depth understanding of dignity and its applications to end-of-life care (Billings, 2008). Discussions of dignity remain pervasive, perhaps because health-care providers and patients alike understand that loss of dignity is particularly relevant in the face of declining health or heightened vulnerability. Indeed, the fear of losing one's dignity towards the end of life, and the implications of this, are very real, despite tensions regarding the use of the term.

These tensions are embedded within a highly politicized environment surrounding the notion of dignity at the end-of-life. 'Death with dignity' is often the rallying cry of supporters of assisted suicide and euthanasia (Death with Dignity, 2012). The hospice and palliative care movement, on the other hand, invokes notions of dignity with entirely different goals (Carstairs, 2010): those consistent with alleviating suffering and optimizing comfort to the very end of life. Given the complexities of the topic, the purpose of this chapter is to review issues pertaining to dignity, which are often faced by health-care providers in the context of end-of-life care, including definitions of dignity, discussion as to why dignity is important, and how it applies to clinical practice.

Defining dignity

The challenges of defining dignity are complex. The *Oxford Dictionary of English* describes dignity as, 'the quality of being worthy or honourable' ('Dignity', 2013). This definition appears to reflect Schroeder's (2008) *meritorious dignity*, a conceptualization stemming from Aristotle's idea that dignity is associated with virtue. This definition implies that one must deserve dignity, and in acting honourably, it may be achieved (Killmister, 2010). By contrast, the Kantian notion of dignity—commonly espoused in the context of health care, ethics, and human rights—purports that dignity is 'inalienable and normatively inviolable', a quality that all rational beings possess (Killmister, 2010, p. 160). Notions of dignity are often conflated with autonomy, and the seeming proximity of these two terms has led some to claim dignity as a 'useless concept' in medical ethics, no different from a basic respect for personhood and autonomy (Macklin, 2003). Yet, such claims are problematic in the sense that individuals who lack capacity for autonomous action or thought may consequently be seen as lacking dignity (McClement and Chochinov, 2006), which has particular implications in instances when illness and disability lay claim to personal or individual autonomy.

Efforts have been made to parse out the differences between dignity and autonomy. Pullman (2004) distinguishes between basic dignity and personal dignity. The former refers to the fundamental, intrinsic worth of all humans and is moralistic in nature, while the latter is a socially and individually referenced construction. This echoes work by Bechtel (2011), who distinguishes between inherent dignity—an irreducible and universal quality of all human beings—and non-inherent dignity—contingent on merit and social status. Inherent dignity, like Pullman's (2004) basic dignity and the concept invoked in documents such as the United Nations Universal Declaration of Human Rights (United Nations General Assembly, 1948), affirm dignity as inseparable from personhood and foundational to freedom and justice. Thus, in contrast to Macklin (2003) and others, inherent dignity is not synonymous with 'respect' but rather the justification for respect (Bechtel, 2011).

Self-respect, pride, poise, and self-esteem are all synonymous with dignity (Chapman, 1977). These multiple meanings and ambiguity led Levenson (2007) to describe dignity as a 'hurrah word—a term of general approval to which no one can object' (p. 8). *Dignity*, like the words *love* or *faith*, may seem intuitive, especially for professionals in health care who see helping as their primary goal (Chochinov, 2012). Others have suggested that they know dignity when they see it (Macklin, 2004). Perspectives such as these may contribute to the paucity of empirical work surrounding this topic, which has recently been placed under a more exacting, and in some instances empirical, lens.

Several organizations have formed to actively promote dignity in health care, and are beginning to offer helpful perspectives. In a comprehensive report by the UK organization Help the Aged, aimed at raising standards of care and behaviour in treating older people, Levenson (2007) describes dignity in a straightforward fashion; it is about how people feel when they are receiving care. Levenson outlines six guiding principles that underlie dignity in care, providing shape for how dignity manifests in a health setting: dignity in care is inseparable from the wider context of dignity as a whole; dignity is about treating people as individuals; dignity is not just about physical care but also psychosocial and spiritual care; dignity thrives in the context of equal power relationships; dignity must actively be promoted; and dignity is more than the sum of its parts. Within health care, dignity has been connected with how people perceive themselves as reflected through the attitudes and behaviour of others towards them (Chochinov, 2004). Such an explanation implies that how patients are treated by health-care providers has a significant impact on how they feel about themselves, which can profoundly influence their experience and satisfaction with health care.

Still others take an ontological approach to the meaning of dignity. Parse (2010) suggests four tenets of human dignity that emerge from a 'human becoming' perspective, wherein 'human dignity is an august presence, a noble bearing of inherent uniqueness' (p. 259). These tenets include reverence in terms of a deep respect for what it means to be human, and awe in terms of appreciating the wonders of humanity. Both betrayal (a violation of human trust) and shame (humiliation with dishonouring human worth), erode human dignity in the sense that they violate the core being of another person (Parse, 2010).

Relevance of dignity in end-of-life care

Much of the debate and confusion in the literature regarding the importance or utility of the term dignity pertains to its lack of definitional specificity (deRave, 1996; Street and Kissane, 2001). Progress in the field of palliative care in the twentieth century has seen increased attention to understanding dying in terms of dignity and autonomy of the person (Graham and Clark, 2008). Dignity has been identified as one of the five basic requirements in caring for dying patients (Geyman, 1983). A basic tenet of palliative care is to relieve suffering and improve quality of life by addressing physical, spiritual, and psychosocial issues affecting the patient and family (World Health Organization, 2012). Such care can readily be conceived of as enhancing dignity (McClement and Chochinov, 2006). Several researchers and clinicians have suggested that dignity should, in fact, be the central goal of palliative care, given the breath of issues and considerations it subsumes (Coppens, 1998). Recent work has also given voice to patients regarding their conceptualizations and experiences of dignity within the health-care system (Chochinov, 2004; Chochinov et al., 2005, 2006, 2009; Hack et al., 2004; McClement et al., 2004).

Continued discussions and research into the meaning, relevance, and importance of dignity is particularly salient, given the current climate surrounding assisted suicide and euthanasia. While dignity is seen as a fundamental aspect in palliative care (Geyman, 1983; Chochinov, 2006, 2007; World Health Organization, 2012), it is also invoked as the justification for death hastening practices. Organizations such as Death with Dignity National Centre, which promotes and defends assisted suicide, equate dignity with autonomy. Legislation passed in the US states of Oregon and Washington legalizing assisted suicide is coined the Death with Dignity Act. From this perspective, dignity is enhanced by patients exercising personal control over the exact timing and circumstances of their death (Death with Dignity, 2012).

Loss of dignity is indeed a central concern of patients requesting assisted suicide or euthanasia. In a study examining end-of-life decisions amongst patients with amyotrophic lateral sclerosis (ALS) in the Netherlands, Maessen and colleagues found significant differences between those who chose euthanasia or physician-assisted suicide (EAS), continuous deep sedation (CDS), or neither of those options. When informal caregivers were asked why the patient hastened their death, they reported the reasons as 'no chance of improvement', 'loss of dignity', 'being dependent', and 'fatigue'. These experiences were all significantly higher in patients choosing EAS compared to those who chose CDS or neither (Maessen et al., 2009). When asked why their patients had selected EAS, the most common reason cited by 57% of Dutch physicians was 'loss of dignity' (Van der Mass et al., 1991). In Washington state, physicians reported that 72% of their patients requesting hastened death were concerned about loss of dignity (Back et al., 1996).

Notably absent from much of the research surrounding concepts of dignity, suffering, and end-of-life choices are the voices of dying patients themselves (McClement and Chochinov, 2006). Karlsson and colleagues interviewed 66 dying cancer patients, inquiring about the nature of suffering with respect to euthanasia, a good death, and dignity. In this qualitative study, the general attitude of study participants toward euthanasia varied. Twenty-nine per cent of the sample were in favour of euthanasia, 20% opposed euthanasia, and the majority (51%) were undecided on the issue. Patients who feared intolerable suffering and were inclined to euthanasia discussed the complex nature of suffering, including meaninglessness, whereas those who felt euthanasia was unwanted or unnecessary felt that suffering could be overcome in various ways, often linking to their own experiences of ameliorated pain or supportive contact with health-care professionals (Karlsson et al., 2012).

Wilson and colleagues (2000) explored the personal attitudes of 70 terminally ill cancer patients receiving palliative care toward euthanasia and physician-assisted suicide. The study also examined specific end-of-life concerns identified in previous research exploring euthanasia and assisted suicide, including loss of dignity, sense of being a burden to others, and hopelessness. The majority of participants (73%) believed that EAS should be legalized. Reasons for this position included one's right to choose and the presence of pain. Moral and religious concerns were raised by those individuals who opposed such legalization. Eight of the patients interviewed (12%) who would have made a request for euthanasia at the time of the interview had greater loss of interest or pleasure in activities, felt more hopeless, and had a higher prevalence of depressive disorders compared to the rest of the sample. These findings underscore the salience of accessing patients' perspectives surrounding end-of-life choices, and the importance clinicians must assign to the psychological domains of care (see Chapter 5.7).

Personal experience: what dignity means for patients and providers

Increasingly, researchers are attending to patient and health-care provider experiences of dignity, providing a meaningful context to academic discourse. Participants in a multi-country, World Health Organization survey indicated that next to receiving prompt attention for medical issues, dignity was the most important aspect of non-clinical care (Valentine et al., 2008). Qualitative research by Jacobson has suggested that persons marginalized by poverty, illness, or both, are indeed very keen to discuss their views on and experiences with dignity in health care (Jacobson, 2009). Beach and colleagues found that the concept of autonomy (as gauged by involvement in treatment decisions) is culturally bound within Western ideologies. They reported that being treated with dignity, rather than only being involved in treatment decisions, resulted in greater treatment adherence for racial/ethnic minorities. Further, for patients from all backgrounds, being treated with dignity was significantly associated with receiving optimal preventative care, even when adjusted for involvement in treatment decisions (Beach et al., 2005).

Jacobson used grounded theory to describe patients' experiences of dignity violation within health care. In her interviews with experts in health and human rights and marginalized populations within the health-care system, several themes emerged. All participants reported experiences of rudeness, indifference, condescension, dismissal, disregard, dependence, objectification, restriction, labelling, contempt, discrimination, revulsion, deprivation, assault, and abjection as violations of dignity (Jacobson, 2009).

Explorations of how providers maintain patient dignity offers further insight into how dignity is constructed within health care. Lin and Tsai found that Taiwanese nurses ($N = 30$) maintain the dignity of their patients by showing them respect (100%), protecting privacy (93.3%), providing emotional support (40%), treating all patients in a similar fashion (13%), and maintaining patients' body image (13%) (Lin and Tsai, 2011). Dignity is seen as an essential component of nursing, suggesting that the nurse's role and how they experience the patient, often reveals more about what may be bothering them than a medical examination could (Castledine, 2006). In an observational study of nurse–patient interactions, Henderson and colleagues identified both physical and social environments that can enhance dignity, including maintenance of privacy during transfers and toileting, and treating patients in a courteous and age-appropriate manner (Henderson et al., 2009).

Chochinov and colleagues have been engaged in a programme of research seeking to better understand factors that enhance and erode dignity for terminally ill patients. In semi-structured interviews, they explored how patients with cancer perceived dignity. Using latent content analysis and constant comparative techniques, they identified three major categories that have a bearing on dignity-related issues, and generated an empirical model of dignity in the terminally ill (Chochinov et al., 2002b) (Table 5.6.1):

◆ *Illness-related concerns* that influence dignity derive, or are related to, the illness itself. These illness-mediated issues and their attendant themes and subthemes threaten or actually impinge a person's sense of dignity. For example, two themes within this category are 'level of independence' (the degree of reliance an individual has on others, influenced by cognitive acuity and functional capacity) and 'symptom distress' (the experience of discomfort or anguish related to the disease progression).

◆ *Dignity-conserving repertoire* includes a person's dignity-conserving perspectives, that is, a way of looking at one's situation that helps to promote dignity, and contains the subthemes of continuity of self, role preservation, generativity/legacy, maintenance of pride, hopefulness, autonomy/control,

Table 5.6.1 Model of dignity in the terminally ill. Summary of major categories, themes, and subthemes arising from qualitative work examining the construct of dignity from the perspective of the terminally ill

Illness-related concerns	Dignity-conserving repertoire	Social dignity inventory
Symptom distress	*Dignity-conserving perspectives*	*Social issues/ relationship dynamics affecting dignity*
Physical distress	Continuity of self	Privacy boundaries
Psychological distress	Role preservation	Social support
Medical uncertainty	Generativity/legacy	Burden to others
Death anxiety	Maintenance of pride	Aftermath concerns
	Hopefulness	
	Autonomy/control	
	Acceptance	
	Resilience/fighting spirit	
Level of independence	*Dignity-conserving practices*	
Cognitive acuity	Living in the moment	
Functional capacity	Maintaining normalcy	
	Seeking spiritual comfort	

Adapted from *The Lancet*, Volume 360, Issue 9350, Chochinov et al., Dignity in the terminally ill: a cross-sectional, cohort study, pp. 2026–2030, Copyright © 2002, with permission from Elsevier, http://www.sciencedirect.com/science/journal/01406736.

acceptance, and resilience/fighting spirit. Another facet of the dignity-conserving repertoire is dignity-conserving practices, that is, personal actions that can bolster or reinforce one's sense of dignity. These practices include living in the moment, maintaining normalcy, and seeking spiritual comfort.

◆ *Social dignity inventory* speaks to social concerns or relationship dynamics that enhance or detract from a patient's sense of dignity. Themes within this category include privacy boundaries, social support, care tenor, burden to others, and aftermath concerns.

The integration of these three categories forms the model of dignity in the terminally ill. Patients who experience difficulties with aspects of the social dignity inventory and/or illness-related concerns may experience an eroded sense of dignity. Yet, this can be moderated by their dignity-conserving repertoire. By invoking or utilizing resources contained within the dignity-conserving repertoire (i.e. feeling hopeful, maintaining normalcy, spiritual care), patients may be able to buffer dignity-associated challenges. The strength or integrity of those resources will determine the degree to which these assaults will erode or undermine individual sense of dignity. In this sense, the model is dynamic in that it incorporates aspects of dignity that are internal and external to the individual, and provides a framework for health-care providers to mitigate dignity-related distress (Chochinov et al., 2002b).

From patienthood to personhood: practical applications to enhance dignity

In an effort to better assess patients' distress at the end-of-life, Chochinov and colleagues created the Patient Dignity Inventory (PDI). Developed using the themes and subthemes of the model of dignity in the terminally ill, the PDI is a 25-item self-report

Table 5.6.2 The Patient Dignity Inventory

For each item, please indicate how much of a problem or concern these have been for you within the last few days	Not a problem	A slight problem	A problem	A major problem	An overwhelming problem
1. Not being able to carry out tasks associated with daily living (e.g. washing myself, getting dressed)	1	2	3	4	5
2. Not being able to attend to my bodily functions independently (e.g. needing assistance with toileting-related activities)	1	2	3	4	5
3. Experiencing physically distressing symptoms (such as pain, shortness of breath, nausea)	1	2	3	4	5
4. Feeling that how I look to others has changed significantly	1	2	3	4	5
5. Feeling depressed	1	2	3	4	5
6. Feeling anxious	1	2	3	4	5
7. Feeling uncertain about my health and health care	1	2	3	4	5
8. Worrying about my future	1	2	3	4	5
9. Not being able to think clearly	1	2	3	4	5
10. Not being able to continue with my usual routines	1	2	3	4	5
11. Feeling like I am no longer who I was	1	2	3	4	5
12. Not feeling worthwhile or valued	1	2	3	4	5
13. Not being able to carry out important roles (e.g. spouse, parent)	1	2	3	4	5
14. Feeling that life no longer has meaning or purpose	1	2	3	4	5
15. Feeling that I have not made a meaningful and/or lasting contribution in my life	1	2	3	4	5
16. Feeling that I have 'unfinished business' (e.g. things that I have yet to say or do, or that feel incomplete)	1	2	3	4	5
17. Concern that my spiritual life is not meaningful	1	2	3	4	5
18. Feeling that I am a burden to others	1	2	3	4	5
19. Feeling that I don't have control over my life	1	2	3	4	5
20. Feeling that my health and care needs have reduced my privacy	1	2	3	4	5
21. Not feeling supported by my community of friends and family	1	2	3	4	5
22. Not feeling supported by my health-care providers	1	2	3	4	5
23. Feeling like I am no longer able to mentally cope with challenges to my health	1	2	3	4	5
24. Not being able to accept the way things are	1	2	3	4	5
25. Not being treated with respect or understanding by others	1	2	3	4	5

measure (Table 5.6.2) that can be implemented to better understand the spectrum of patient dignity-related distress. The psychometric properties of the PDI have been examined, demonstrating robust internal consistency ($\alpha = 0.93$) and test–retest reliability ($r = 0.85$). Factor analysis revealed five factors, labelled *symptom distress, existential distress, dependency, peace of mind*, and *social support*. Concurrent validity was established with each factor showing significant correlations with other common measures of distress (Chochinov et al., 2008). This measure provides one way that dignity-related distress can be identified, measured, and possibly tracked in a range of care settings. Administration of the PDI to 253 patients receiving palliative care found that patients identified nearly six problems each. The most highly endorsed items included a combination of distressing physical symptoms,

functional limitations (not able to continue usual routines, not able to perform tasks of daily living, not able to carry out important roles), and existential concerns (no longer feeling like who I was) (Chochinov et al., 2009). These findings speak to the importance of conducting patient assessments that encompass more than physical symptom distress. The PDI may help clinicians identify and track the complex and diverse nature of distress in the terminally ill, hence paving the way toward effective, dignity-conserving, end-of-life care.

A recently completed study examined how psychosocial oncology professionals (N = 90) utilized the PDI as a clinical tool within their practice. In almost 80% of instances, the PDI was able to uncover one or more areas of distress previously unknown to the clinician. Thus, the PDI may enable more efficient and targeted psychosocial care amongst clients experiencing distress in the context of cancer (Chochinov et al., 2012b).

Dignity is profoundly influenced by the tone and texture of communication between the care provider and the patient; with acknowledgement of the patient as a whole person being paramount (Finset, 2010). Chochinov proposed an ABCD acronym for dignity-conserving care, rooted in the idea that how a patient views themselves is reflected in how they perceive they are seen by those providing care (Chochinov, 2002). This framework serves as a reminder to practitioners that their *Attitude, Behaviour, Compassion*, and *Dialogue* will markedly influence patient experience of dignity in care. Practical suggestions for implementing the ABCD framework are outlined in Table 5.6.3 (Chochinov, 2007).

Recognition for the importance of meaning and spiritual issues in palliative medicine (Puchalski et al., 2009) has seen the emergence of therapeutic interventions aimed at improving spiritual and psychological well-being at the end of life. Meaning-centred group psychotherapy has been shown to provide terminally ill patients with significant improvement in spiritual well-being and meaning, compared to patients participating in general supportive therapy (Breitbart et al., 2010). Breitbart and colleagues recently conducted a randomized controlled trial of individual meaning-centered psychotherapy (IMCP) with 120 patients who had stage III or IV cancer. Patients were assigned to receive either IMCP or a control treatment of therapeutic massage for 7 weeks, and were assessed on measures of spiritual well-being, quality of life, depression, anxiety, hopelessness, symptom burden, and symptom distress at baseline and 2 months post intervention. Patients in the ICMP condition showed significant improvement over the control group on measures of spiritual well-being (both sense of meaning and faith), quality of life, and symptom burden and distress (Breitbart et al., 2012).

Another approach coined dignity therapy consists of a brief psychotherapeutic intervention aimed at improving quality of life and reducing suffering for terminally ill patients and their families. The questions guiding dignity therapy are based on key themes and issues embedded within the model of dignity in the terminally ill. A trained professional guides the therapeutic encounter, helping the patient to elicit memories, hopes, and wishes for family members; life lessons they might wish to share; and legacy-related content they want to leave behind (Chochinov et al., 2011). Engagement in this process, along with affirmation from the dignity therapist, is meant to enhance a sense of meaning and purpose, sense of self, and overall sense of dignity. These sessions are recorded, transcribed verbatim, and then carefully edited into a readable narrative or *generativity document*. This document is returned to the patient, for any final editing and approval, for them to bequeath to friends and family of their choosing.

The effectiveness of dignity therapy has been demonstrated in various clinical trials. Chochinov and colleagues conducted a feasibility study of dignity therapy with terminally ill patients in Winnipeg, Canada and Perth, Australia. All patients who enrolled in palliative care in these cities and met eligibility requirements (less than 6 months to live, over age 18, English speaking, commitment to three to four contacts, no cognitive impairments, willing and able to provide verbal and written consent) were invited to participate. Over a 2-year timeframe, 100 patients—50 from each site—completed the study. Participants completed a broad range of tests to assess depression, anxiety, hopelessness, sense of dignity, suicidality, and sense of meaning and purpose, before and after completing the dignity therapy protocol. Ninety-one per cent of participants reported that they were satisfied or very satisfied with the intervention and 86% said it was helpful or very helpful. Patients also reported that the intervention helped their sense of purpose (68%) and meaning (67%). Just under half of participants indicated that dignity therapy increased their will to live (Chochinov et al., 2005).

A randomized controlled trial of dignity therapy provides further evidence for its application within palliative care. Data was collected between 2005 and 2011 at three study sites (Winnipeg, Canada; New York, United States; and Perth, Australia). Four hundred and forty-four participants aged 18 years and older with a life expectancy of less than 6 months who were receiving palliative care in a hospital or community setting were randomized to one of three study conditions: dignity therapy plus standard palliative care, client-centred care plus standard palliative care, and standard palliative care only. Participants in the dignity therapy condition received this intervention as described above. For client-centred care, participants engaged in supportive psychotherapy focused on present, rather than generativity-related, issues. Patients randomized to standard palliative care had access to all support services available within their site. The primary outcomes of the study were reductions in measures of distress, as measured by mean changes between baseline and post intervention. Standardized measures of psychosocial well-being, symptom distress, depression, anxiety, and hopelessness were used to assess these outcomes. The secondary outcomes were based on a post-intervention questionnaire capturing patient experiences regarding their participation in the study and the ways in which it was meaningful for them and their family.

Floor effects of initial distress resulted in non-significant differences between the study groups for the primary measures, such as depression, desire for death, and suicidality. However, dignity therapy outperformed the other study arms on the post-intervention questionnaire. Compared to client-centred therapy and standard palliative care, patients receiving dignity therapy were significantly more likely to report that the intervention was helpful, that it enhanced their sense of dignity, that it changed how their family saw or appreciated them, and that it would be helpful to their families (Chochinov et al., 2011).

Family members whose loved ones participated in dignity therapy have also been evaluated, to determine their perceptions of its impact on their deceased loved one, along with its influence on their bereavement experience. In a study of 100 patients who completed dignity therapy, 60 family members provided feedback on the experience approximately 1 year after the patient's death. Ninety-five per cent of family members whose loved ones received dignity therapy reporting it had helped the patient, and just over three-quarters indicated that the generativity document helped them during their grief and would be a source of comfort to them in the future (McClement et al., 2007).

Dignity therapy has been successfully delivered in various countries and languages, with minor adaptations for cultural differences (e.g. the notion of 'pride' did not resonate with Danish participants) (Houmann et al., 2010). It has also been implemented with geographically isolated patients using telemedicine (Passik

Table 5.6.3 Application of the dignity model to practice

Illness-related concerns	Directions for practice
Symptom distress	
Physical distress Psychological distress	Baseline and ongoing assessment of physical and psychological symptoms
Medical uncertainty	Provision of timely, relevant information about the illness and plan of care
Death anxiety	Exploration of concerns associated with illness progression
Level of independence	
Cognitive acuity	Baseline and ongoing assessment of cognitive functioning Vigilance in detection and treatment of delirium
Functional capacity	Baseline and ongoing assessment of ability to carry out activities of daily living Referrals to occupational and physiotherapy as appropriate Provision of supports needed to maintain independence (e.g. walker, raised toilet seat) Involvement in decision-making regarding plan of care, as desired by patient

Dignity-conserving repertoire	Directions for practice
Dignity-conserving perspectives	
Continuity of self	Communication with patient about those facets of life not affected by their disease Learn about the patient's biography, attending to those aspect of life that he or she values most
Role preservation	Exploration of roles important to the patient Facilitation of role enactment within limitations of patient's illness
Maintenance of pride	Discussion with patient about those aspects of their life that they are most proud of Professional demeanour in provision of care
Hopefulness	Talk with the patient about what is still possible, despite illness limitations Encourage redefining of goals and expectations
Autonomy/control	Assess patient's perceived level of control, and explore preference regarding level of involvement in care decisions and planning Where possible, provide choices
Generativity/legacy	Facilitate life review, or other activities that foster the sharing of memories that are meaningful to patient
Acceptance	Explore the impact of the illness for the patient Appreciate the dynamism of the process of responding to a life-threatening illness
Resilience/fighting spirit	Identify and promote patient participation in those interactions/activities that are most meaningful, given limited life expectancy
Dignity-conserving practices	
Living in the moment	Allow patient to participate in normal routines or take comfort in momentary distractions Identify things that can take the patient's mind off illness and provide comfort
Maintaining normalcy	Identify activities the patient still enjoys doing on a regular basis and enable them to participate in such activities where possible
Finding spiritual comfort	Inquire as to whether the patient is connected or would like to be connected with a spiritual or religious community Refer to a chaplain or spiritual leader and enable the patient to participate in the cultural/spiritual practices that are important to them

Social dignity inventory	Directions for practice
Privacy boundaries	Ask permission to examine a patient, use proper draping to respect modesty
Social support	Ask the patient who they are closest to and confide in Have liberal policies about visitation, rooming, and involve a wide support network
Care tenor	Ask the patient if any aspect of their care is undermining their dignity Treat the patient as worthy of honour, esteem, and respect
Burden to others	Inquire about whether the patient feels that they are a burden to others and encourage explicit discussions about these concerns with those they fear they are burdening
Aftermath concerns	Ask about the patient's concerns and encourage the settling of affairs, advance directives, making a will and funeral planning

et al., 2004). In addressing the floor effects of distress found in Chochinov et al.'s (2011) study, Julião and colleagues conducted a randomized controlled trial of dignity therapy with a Portuguese population experiencing high baseline levels of distress. Recruited from an inpatient palliative care unit, 29 patients received dignity therapy plus standard palliative care, while 31 control group patients received standard palliative care alone. Depression and anxiety, as measured by the Hospital Anxiety and Depression Scale (HADS—Portuguese version) (Pais-Ribeiro et al., 2007), were assessed at baseline (T1), day 4 (T2), day 15 (T3), and day 30 (T4). At baseline, compared to participants in the Chochinov et al. (2011) study, these participants had higher HADS-depression scores (12.9 versus 5.86) and HADS-anxiety scores (8.83 versus 5.22). For those in the dignity therapy condition, the intervention was conducted between baseline and T2.

Within the dignity therapy group, participants showed significant reductions from baseline in depression at T2 and T3, which plateaued by day T4; and significant reductions in anxiety at all three follow-ups. Within the standard palliative care group, depression ratings increased significantly between baseline and all three follow-up assessments, while no significant changes in anxiety were found. Compared to the standard palliative care group, patients in the dignity therapy group had significantly lower depression ratings at T2 and T3, and significantly lower anxiety ratings at T2, T3, and T4 (Julião et al., 2013).

The application of dignity therapy in community settings has also been explored, providing insights into the practical and logistical issues of offering this intervention. Montross and colleagues delivered dignity therapy to patients in a community-based hospice, with a psychologist trained in the protocol providing information about the service to members of the hospice team at meetings and rounds. This resulted in just over 100 referrals for dignity therapy, with 27 patients completing the full dignity therapy protocol (reasons for non-completion included cognitive/physical impairments impeding speech or comprehension, death before completion, patient declining participation, and patients lost to follow-up).

In terms of the logistics of providing the service, nearly three-quarters of referrals were from social workers. The average cost of a patients' transcript was US$55.94, and an average of 2993 words in length, with the therapist spending an average of 6.3 hours per patient in order to complete the dignity therapy document. Qualitative analysis of the themes of patients' documents revealed similarities to previous studies (Hack et al., 2010), including discussions of family, pride in their children/accomplishments, pleasure, and life experiences (Montross et al., 2011).

Dignity therapy has also been applied to participants who are not imminently dying. Avery and Baez recently published a case report in which a 61-year-old woman hospitalized for major depressive disorder participated in dignity therapy. She reported that dignity therapy had helped her feel more hopeful and improved her mood. That it can aid in improving depressive symptoms when distress is high (Julião et al., 2013), suggests that dignity therapy may facilitate feelings of increased purpose, meaning, and hopefulness in people with depression, and may also help their families (Avery and Baez, 2012). A recent feasibility study by Chochinov and colleagues has shown the benefits of dignity therapy for the frail elderly living in residential care. Dignity therapy was conducted with both cognitively intact residents and cognitively impaired residents by way of engaging family proxies.

While differing narrative themes emerged between the two groups, the majority of residents' family members and healthcare providers reported the intervention to be helpful to the patient. Further, family members felt the dignity therapy document would provide them comfort, and the majority of healthcare providers reported that the intervention changed how they saw and appreciated the resident and would be helpful in terms of how they provide care (Chochinov et al., 2012a). It thus appears that dignity therapy may have applications across a range of settings and a variety of patient populations. Moreover, the research on dignity therapy underscores the notion that knowing the patient as a person can improve care.

Future directions

Although more attention is being paid to notions of dignity, spirituality, and meaning at the end of life, further research is needed. While the term dignity is multifaceted and complex, its prominence in patient-centred care should spur inquiry across diverse context wherein notions of dignity are particularly salient, that is, the frail elderly, the chronically ill or disabled, those with major mental disorders, and patients encountering cognitively deterioration or impairment.

The notion of dignity in care and ways of affirming personhood also require further examination. These studies may broach cross-cultural comparisons of engaging dignity (Lee, 2010), and how cultural diversity impacts decision-making and experiences at the end-of-life for patients, families, and care providers. Longitudinal research, examining how patients experience dignity over the trajectory of their illness, would help inform dignity-based approaches that are sensitive to the needs and capacities based on disease imposed variables.

A central theme in palliative care is that the patient and the family constitute the unit of care; with the quality of life of family members directly impacted by the care the patient receives (McClement et al., 2007). Poor palliative care can complicate the grieving process and can leave family members with feelings of regret (Shiozaki et al., 2005; McClement et al., 2007), increasing bereavement-related health risks (Prigerson et al., 2009). Thus, researched aimed at better understanding family members' perspectives of dignity and how this impacts their experience of their loved one's illness would be beneficial.

Conclusion

The very nature of being a patient makes one vulnerable, wherein personal dignity may be in jeopardy (Jacobson, 2009). The violation of dignity at the end of life is a significant issue for patients and their families. Consistent with the goals of palliative medicine, dignity should be recognized as a key element of comprehensive care, with access to services—including optimal pain control, psychosocial, and spiritual support—posited as a fundamental human right (Breitbart, 2008). Understanding the multiple dimensions of dignity and how it is experienced in proximity to death, will contribute to a comprehensive and effective approach, which will improve care at the end of life.

Online materials

Complete references for this chapter are available online at <http://www.oxfordmedicine.com>.

References

Chochinov, H.M. (2002). Dignity conserving care: a new model for palliative care. *Journal of the American Medical Association*, 287, 2253–2260.

Chochinov, H.M. (2004). Dignity and the eye of the beholder. *Journal of Clinical Oncology*, 22, 1336–1340.

Chochinov, H.M. (2006). Dying, dignity, and new horizons in palliative end-of-life care. *CA: A Cancer Journal for Clinicians*, 56, 84–103.

Chochinov, H.M. (2007). Dignity and the essence of medicine: the A, B, C, and D of dignity conserving care. *BMJ*, 335, 184–187.

Chochinov, H.M. (2012). *Dignity Therapy: Final Words for Final Days*. New York: Oxford University Press.

Chochinov, H.M., Cann, B., Cullihall, K., *et al.* (2012a). Dignity therapy: a feasibility study of elders in long-term care. *Palliative and Supportive Care*, 10, 3–15.

Chochinov, H.M., Hack, T., Hassard, T., Kristjanson, L.J., McClement, S., and Harlos, M. (2002a). Dignity in the terminally ill: a cross-sectional, cohort study. *The Lancet*, 360, 2026–2030.

Chochinov, H.M., Hack, T., Hassard, T., Kristjanson, L.J., McClement, S., and Harlos, M. (2005). Dignity therapy: a novel psychotherapeutic intervention for patients near the end of life. *Journal of Clinical Oncology*, 23, 5520–5525.

Chochinov, H.M., Hack, T., McClement, S., Kristjanson, L., and Harlos, M. (2002b). Dignity in the terminally ill: a developing empirical model. *Social Science & Medicine*, 54, 433–443.

Chochinov, H.M., Hassard, T., McClement, S., *et al.* (2008). The patient dignity inventory: a novel way of measuring dignity-related distress in palliative care. *Journal of Pain and Symptom Management*, 36, 559–571.

Chochinov, H.M., Hassard, T., McClement, S., *et al.* (2009). The landscape of distress in the terminally ill. *Journal of Pain and Symptom Management*, 38, 641–649.

Chochinov, H.M., Krisjanson, L.J., Hack, T.F., Hassard, T., McClement, S., and Harlos, M. (2006). Dignity in the terminally ill: revisited. *Journal of Palliative Medicine*, 9, 666–672.

Chochinov, H.M., Kristjanson, L.J., Breitbart, W., *et al.* (2011). Effect of dignity therapy on distress and end-of-life experience in terminally ill patients: a randomised controlled trial. *The Lancet Oncology*, 12, 753–762.

Chochinov, H.M., McClement S.E., Hack, T.F., *et al.* (2012b). The Patient Dignity Inventory: applications in the oncology setting. *Journal of Palliative Medicine*, 15, 1–8.

Hack, T.F., Chochinov, H.M., Hassard, T., Kristjanson, L.J., McClement, S., and Harlos, M. (2004). Defining dignity in terminally ill cancer patients: a factor-analytic approach. *Psycho-Oncology*, 13, 700–708.

Hack, T.F., McClement, S.E., Chochinov, H.M., *et al.* (2010). Learning from dying patients during their final days: life reflections gleaned from dignity therapy. *Palliative Medicine*, 24, 715–723.

Julião, M., Barbosa, A., Oliviera, F., Nunes, B., and Vaz Carneiro, A. (2012). Efficacy of dignity therapy for depression and anxiety in terminally-ill patients: early results of a randomized controlled trial. *Palliative and Supportive Care*, 11(6), 481–489.

Levenson, R. (2007). *The Challenge of Dignity in Care: Upholding the Rights of the Individual*. London: Help the Aged.

McClement, S., Chochinov, H.M., Hack, T., Hassard, T., Kristjanson, L.J., and Harlos, M. (2007). Dignity therapy: family member perspectives. *Journal of Palliative Medicine*, 10, 1076–1082.

McClement, S., Chochinov, H.M., Hack, T., Kristjanson, L.J., and Harlos, M. (2004). Dignity conserving care: application of research findings to practice. *International Journal of Palliative Nursing*, 10, 173–179.

McClement, S.E. and Chochinov, H.M. (2006). Dignity in palliative care. In E. Bruera, I.J. Higginson, C. Ripamonti, and C. von Gunten (eds.) *Textbook of Palliative Medicine*, pp. 100–107. London: Hodder Arnold.

Montross, L., Winters, K.D., and Irwin, S.A. (2011). Dignity therapy implementation in a community-based hospice setting. *Journal of Palliative Medicine*, 14, 729–734.

Passik, S.D., Kirsh, K.L., Leibee, S., *et al.* (2004). A feasibility study of dignity psychotherapy delivered via telemedicine. *Palliative and Supportive Care*, 2, 149–155.

5.7

Euthanasia and palliative care

Lars Johan Materstvedt and Georg Bosshard

Introduction: definition of 'euthanasia'

The word euthanasia is a combination of the Greek *eu* = good, and *thanatos* = death. Literally and etymologically it therefore means 'good death'. In the modern setting, its meaning is much narrower; essentially how it is understood in the Netherlands.

The Netherlands is the only country in the world with a long history of practising euthanasia. Here, euthanasia dates back more than 40 years, to the court ruling in the Postma case in 1973, with subsequent de facto legalization through case law over the years, eventually followed by a law on euthanasia which entered into force in 2002 (Griffiths et al., 1998, 2008; Netherlands: Law on Euthanasia, 2002). In a scholarly article on the Dutch practice published in 2012, the authors observed that 'In the Netherlands, euthanasia is defined as the administering of lethal drugs by a physician with the explicit intention to end a patient's life on the patient's explicit request' (Onwuteaka-Philipsen et al., 2012). Dutch-American professor of sociology of law John Griffiths and colleagues shed the following light on the topic:

> 'Euthanasia' in the strict—and in the Dutch context the only proper—sense refers to the situation in which a doctor kills a person who is suffering 'unbearably' and 'hopelessly' at the latter's explicit request (usually by administering a lethal injection). . . . 'euthanasia' is in the Netherlands reserved for killing on request. (Griffiths et al., 1998, p. 17)

The Dutch medical association Koninklijke Nederlandsche Maatschappij tot bevordering der Geneeskunst, the KNMG, which is in favour of euthanasia, states that it takes place 'when a physician ends the life of a patient at his express request due to unbearable and lasting suffering. Euthanasia means that the physician administers a lethal substance to the patient' (KNMG, 2011).

A similar law to the Dutch one which took effect in 2002 was introduced in Belgium in the same year (Belgium: Law on Euthanasia, 2002). Here, euthanasia is 'defined as medical administration of life-ending drugs at the patient's explicit request' (Chambaere et al., 2011a). Subsequently, Luxembourg legalized euthanasia, in 2009 (Luxembourg: Law on Euthanasia, 2009), as did Québec, Canada, in 2014 (Québec: Law on Euthanasia, 2014).

The European Association for Palliative Care (EAPC; see <http://www.eapcnet.eu>), which is opposed to euthanasia, defines it in a way that is congruent with the conception in the BeNeLux countries; namely as 'a doctor intentionally killing a person by the administration of drugs, at that person's voluntary and competent request' (Materstvedt et al., 2003).

In concrete terms, euthanasia involves injecting the patient with two types of substances: barbiturates to induce coma, followed by neuromuscular blockers which cause respiratory muscle paralysis.

The consequent anoxia and cardiac arrest bring on immediate death.

Physician-assisted suicide (PAS): in contrast to in euthanasia, the doctor is not the final actor in PAS but instead provides medication for the patient to self-administer an overdose of barbiturates that suppresses respiration.

PAS is legal according to statute in the BeNeLux countries. It is also legal in four US states: Oregon, Washington, Montana, and Vermont (Oregon: Law on Physician-Assisted Suicide, 1997; Washington: Law on Physician-Assisted Suicide, 2009; Answers. USA.gov, 2013; CBSNEWS, 2013), and in Québec, Canada (Québec: Law on Euthanasia, 2014).

Assisted suicide: an act in which a lay person (i.e. someone who is not a *medical* professional) gives the drugs to the patient for self-administration. This practice is legally condoned in the penal code of Switzerland (Bosshard, 2008).

However, in all other jurisdictions that allow PAS (see earlier in this section), such *non*-physician assisted suicide is illegal.

Together, euthanasia, PAS, and assisted suicide comprise what is known as drug-induced 'assisted dying' (Bosshard and Materstvedt, 2011). Voluntary patient request is a key concept in the definition of all three.

Medicalized killing without request

Drugs are also used in the execution of what has been described as 'a life ending act without explicit patient request (LAWER)' (Chambaere et al., 2012).

Some regard such acts as falling within the category of assisted dying (Seale, 2009; Rady and Verheijde, 2010). It is our view that such non-requested ending of someone's life is by no means 'assistance'; it amounts to murder (Griffiths et al., 2008; Bosshard and Materstvedt, 2011; Materstvedt, 2012). There are two kinds of LAWER:

- *Non-voluntary medicalized killing*: this is a term used to describe induction of death in patients who lack decision-making competence—such as newborns and the senile demented, who concretely have no free will (Latin *voluntas*).

- *Involuntary medicalized killing*: such acts took place during and prior to the Second World War in what are often known as (the German) 'euthanasia clinics'. The name is misleading; in order to appropriately capture the true content of the practices in these institutions, they ought to be described as 'murder clinics' since the patient's life was taken against his or her will, regardless of the motivation for doing so—whether it be compassion, economic considerations, or other rationales (Materstvedt, 2003).

In a more recent example of involuntary medicalized killing, physician Wilfred van Oijen was convicted by the Dutch Supreme Court in 2002 of murdering one of his patients. Not only had this patient not requested a lethal injection, she had even made it clear that she did not want to die (Griffiths et al., 2008).

Assisted dying in practice

There exists a considerable amount of research data on legal assisted dying; however, we focus on selected findings pertinent to palliative care. We first and foremost report on the Netherlands, which has the most comprehensive evidence base on assisted dying by far (Youngner and Kimsma, 2012).

Frequency

Euthanasia is a much more common occurrence than PAS in the Netherlands. In 2005, for example, there were 2297 cases of euthanasia, compared to 113 cases of PAS (van der Heide et al., 2007). This yields a ratio of 20 to 1.

Age groups

Thirty-one per cent of the Dutch cases of assisted dying are found in the age group 40–59 years, while the majority (53%) are found in the 60–79 age bracket. In Belgium, the corresponding figures are 26% and 52%, respectively (Rurup et al., 2012).

Cancer predominant

The data on reported cases of assisted death in the Netherlands in 2010 show that general practitioners were involved in 92.5% of the cases, and that 83.1% of the diseased suffered from cancer, making it the predominant illness among those who were registered in the assisted dying statistics (Onwuteaka-Philipsen et al., 2012).

Relevance for palliative care

The fact that most patients who receive palliative care suffer from terminal cancer suggests that there is considerable overlap between this group and those who opt for assisted death. Hence, even if measured only by the numbers of patients involved, the issue of assisted dying is indeed relevant for palliative care.

Why patients request assisted death

The following findings can be listed:

- Over a 25-year period, pain became a significantly less important factor in patients' request for euthanasia in the Netherlands, whereas deterioration became more important (Marquet et al., 2003).

- Social, cultural, and existential issues such as loss of dignity and autonomy play a role in requests for assisted suicide in Switzerland (Fischer et al., 2009), and for PAS in Oregon. The 2013 annual report on Oregon's practice states that 'As in previous years, the three most frequently mentioned end-of-life concerns were: loss of autonomy (93.0%), decreasing ability to participate in activities that made life enjoyable (88.7%), and loss of dignity (73.2%)' (Oregon Public Health Division, 2014).

- Depression is another factor in these requests, according to a finding among terminally ill cancer patients in the Netherlands (van der Lee et al., 2005).

- Research in Oregon has similarly documented the impact of depression on decisions to request death (Ganzini et al., 2008).

- So-called tiredness of life has also been found to play a role, for example, in Switzerland. Weariness of life rather than a fatal or hopeless medical condition seems to be a more common reason among older members of the right-to-die organization Exit Deutsche Schweiz to request assisted suicide (Fischer et al., 2008).

What is a 'request'?

While much research has focused on requests for assisted dying, in clinical reality most patients' expression of a wish to die is not literally a plea for help to put an end to their life via drugs, but an expression of something else (Gudat et al., 2015). In particular, palliative care physicians and oncologists are familiar with this phenomenon from their clinical experience.

- This clinical knowledge has recently been scientifically confirmed in qualitative, semi-structured interviews with terminally ill inpatients at a palliative medicine unit in Norway about their attitudes and wishes regarding assisted dying (Johansen et al., 2005).

- It may be noted in this context that less than half of requests for assisted dying are granted by Dutch physicians (Onwuteaka-Philipsen et al., 2012).

Additionally, requests for euthanasia raise hugely difficult issues regarding patient autonomy and, at a deeper level, whether or not a person can know what are his or her best interests (Materstvedt, 2015).

How should palliative care deal with requests for assisted dying?

Various strategies for dealing with patients who request assisted dying are available. These include measures connected to all sorts of symptom treatment and psychosocial support.

The negative approach

Since all of these measures attempt to prevent premature death, they can be described as 'negative' responses. By contrast, the 'positive' or affirmative response is to comply with the request (Materstvedt, 2013a).

Because assisted dying is more or less universally prohibited, from the juridical point of view most palliative care providers are left with the option of pursuing the negative approach.

Where it *is* legal, however, or where it might be legalized in the foreseeable future, a real dilemma emerges. Should palliative care providers opt out of assisted dying, or should they be a part of the practice?

The World Health Organization stance

The World Health Organization (WHO) can offer guidance on this issue. According to its *Definition of Palliative Care*, such care 'affirms life and . . . intends neither to hasten or [sic] postpone death' and 'regards dying as a normal process' (WHO, 2014).

Death occurs as the culmination of a normal process when, for example, life-sustaining treatment (e.g. antibiotics) is withheld or withdrawn because contraindicated; that is, death is a normal occurrence when it is not artificially postponed or delayed in fatally ill patients. The patient is allowed to die of his underlying disease—of natural causes: the 'normal' way.

Accordingly, within palliative care a so-called non-treatment decision (NTD) (Griffiths et al., 2008; Chambaere et al., 2012), which is always combined with continued *palliative* treatment until death, is a matter of letting the patient die naturally. It does not hasten death (Materstvedt, 2013a).

By contrast, assisted dying does precisely that: it hastens death. It therefore follows from the WHO's palliative care ethics that palliative care providers should *not* participate in such procedures.

Belgium: offering euthanasia in a palliative care setting

Nevertheless, there is fundamental disagreement on this issue. In 2003, the Belgian Federatie Palliatieve Zorg Vlaanderen vzw (FPZV; see <http://www.palliatief.be>), published a statement, according to which there is no conflict between palliative care and euthanasia:

> Palliative care and euthanasia are neither alternatives nor opposites. When a doctor is prepared to accede to the euthanasia request of a patient who continues to find life unbearable despite the best treatment, then there is no gap between the palliative care given previously by the doctor and the euthanasia he applies now; on the contrary. In such a case, euthanasia forms part of the palliative care with which the doctor and the care team surround the patient and his or her nearest. (FPZV, 2003)

'Palliative care and euthanasia are neither alternatives nor opposites'

Findings on attitudes among Dutch doctors contradict on both accounts this claim. About one-third believed that euthanasia could be avoided by providing high-quality end-of-life care to terminally ill patients. Furthermore, this proportion remained relatively stable over the measured 11-year period (1990, 1995, and 2001) (Onwuteaka-Philipsen et al., 2003).

In another study, two-thirds of Dutch physicians disagree with the suggestion that adequate treatment of pain and terminal care make euthanasia redundant (Georges et al., 2006). But this position, too, reveals dualistic thinking: 'Palliative care is not the answer; euthanasia is.'

By moving from caring to killing, one abandons the dual commitment to treating symptoms and letting someone die of the disease. Euthanasia is therefore a totally different undertaking from palliative care. Accordingly, the claim that there is 'no gap' between the two is incorrect.

The FPZV continues:

> In view of the delicate, irreversible and radical nature of euthanasia, it is vitally important that euthanasia only be performed in cases where there is evidence of suffering 'which cannot be alleviated' (Art. 3, §1 Euthanasia Act), and a situation 'for which there is no other reasonable solution' (Art. 3, §2, 1° Euthanasia Act). (FPZV, 2003)

Suffering that 'cannot be alleviated'

This phrase is ambiguous; it is open to several interpretations. It might allude to the fact that palliative care does not always function optimally, and sometimes cannot be made to do so. Accordingly it is not always good enough in a very strict sense.

But it is wholly unrealistic to expect palliative care to make all patients completely free of all symptoms at all times, including pain, fatigue, cachexia, nausea, vomiting, dyspnoea, anxiety, depression, and delirium.

Additionally, how patients experience and cope with these symptoms is to a large extent a subjective matter.

Refractory symptoms

If, by contrast, symptoms have become *refractory*, 'despite the best treatment', as the FPZV puts it (see earlier quotation), the suffering can perhaps be said to be *objectively* unbearable. However, in a palliative care setting where patients are approaching the end of life, various degrees of palliative sedation can be offered to address such suffering, with terminal sedation as a last resort (Materstvedt and Bosshard, 2009). So even refractory suffering can be alleviated—or, perhaps more properly formulated in the case of terminal sedation, *erased* (Materstvedt, 2012, 2013b)—through reduction or complete removal of the ability to perceive symptoms.

Scope of suffering

Does the word 'suffering' in the above FPZV quotation refer exclusively to *medical* symptoms (be they somatic or psychiatric) of the kind mentioned earlier? Or does it also include broader issues such as loss of autonomy, loss of dignity, or tiredness of life?

As we have seen, these issues can be on a par with medical symptoms in terms of contributing to a patient's suffering. If this is indeed the case, it is even more unrealistic to expect palliative care to alleviate all suffering; especially suffering of such a very personal and subjective kind.

In this context, the findings of a qualitative study carried out in southern Switzerland are remarkable. The study involved 11 relatives of eight patients, looked after by a palliative care team, who had died by means of assisted suicide. It revealed that pain and symptom burden did not constitute the patients' key reasons for seeking assisted suicide. Instead, existential distress and fear of loss of control were the key determinants. The patients did not regard the provision of palliative care as an influential factor in their decision, according to the relatives (Gamondi et al., 2013).

No 'reasonable' alternative to euthanasia

Where does this leave the idea that euthanasia is a solution to a problem that cannot be solved in any other way? The FPZV refers to situations when there is 'no other reasonable solution' than euthanasia. The Belgian law in English translation uses the wording 'reasonable alternative' (Belgium: Law on Euthanasia, 2002); as does the Dutch law, stipulating that 'the attending physician must . . . have come to the conclusion, together with the patient, that there is no reasonable alternative in the light of the patient's situation' (Netherlands: Law on Euthanasia, 2002).

That there is no reasonable alternative to euthanasia, whatever the meaning of 'reasonable', does not imply that no alternative is available; it entails that the available alternative, namely treatment and/or psychosocial support, is rejected by the patient. Again, we can only conclude that palliative care and euthanasia are indeed alternatives.

'Medical futility' and the legal requirements of assisted dying

The Belgian law states in Chapter II, sect. 3, §1, that the patient must be: 'in a medically futile condition of constant and unbearable physical or mental suffering that can not be alleviated, resulting from a serious and incurable disorder caused by illness or accident' (Belgium: Law on Euthanasia, 2002).

Concept of futility

This concept is subject to much discussion and there are many interpretations of it. Non-resuscitation in the case of an old and severely demented patient when the likelihood of treatment having any effect on survival is less than 1% might be taken as an example of a decision based on a 'medically futile condition'.

Nevertheless, the fact remains that the 'inner life' of this patient is non-accessible to outsiders. For all we (can) know, he might be happy to go on living—despite the fact that to us his existence may look utterly miserable. Presuming that staying alive is a benefit or good in this and corresponding cases, one may ask if there ought to be such a thing as a right to futile treatment (Ackroyd, 2005).

It happens from time to time, although extremely rarely, that patients who have been judged to be beyond rescue in intensive care units—that is, whose chance of survival has been assessed as 0% (which makes them paradigmatic examples of medical futility)—do indeed recover and leave the hospital premises on their own two feet.

Another interpretation of futility is that it is present when treatment is of very limited usefulness weighed against the risks and/or side effects associated with it. For example, a terminally ill patient diagnosed with advanced pancreatic cancer can be given somewhat life-prolonging treatment. However, he may perceive the treatment as overly distressing, thus feeling that its limited advantages are outweighed by the disadvantages. Hence, the patient may decline further chemotherapy and accept only palliative care.

Criterion of medically 'futile' or 'hopeless' condition

What, then, is 'a medically futile condition' according to the Belgian euthanasia law: which interpretation would apply? The law contains no information that might help us answer this question. Also, we saw that the law's criterion of suffering that 'can not be alleviated' is a debatable premise.

Furthermore, why the law prescribes that the suffering must be 'constant' (a second translation is 'persistent' (Griffiths et al., 2008)) is not easy to understand. Does it mean that a patient whose suffering fluctuates may have his euthanasia request denied based on this fluctuation?

Another translation uses, in place of 'futile condition', the wording 'medically *hopeless situation* of persistent and unbearable . . .' (Griffiths et al., 2008; italics added by authors). In the Netherlands, the law stipulates that 'the attending physician must . . . be satisfied that the patient's suffering was unbearable, and that there was no prospect of improvement' (Netherlands: Law on Euthanasia, 2002).

'No prospect of improvement'

This formulation corresponds to the 'medically hopeless situation' wording of the Belgian law. Presuming that the translation 'medically futile condition' covers the same meaning, futility may then be understood as treatment that is unlikely to have any positive impact whatsoever.

However, both the treating physician and the second opinion physician (both laws require that a second doctor is consulted) might be wrong in their conclusion on this crucial issue.

What is more, beyond the strictly medical interpretation of 'improvement', even when there would be a standstill in this particular respect, the conception could be read in terms of *mental* improvement, for example, psychological or existential improvement. Thus it is not totally clear what the requirement actually entails.

'Unbearable' suffering

We noted above that perhaps some conditions are objectively in this category. But the laws quoted appear to be referring to suffering that is 'unbearable' according to the patient's subjective perspective. The physician needs, however, to comply.

This raises the question of how he, an 'outsider' who is not himself ill, can possibly be in a position to assess or vouch for the severity of the patient's subjectively perceived suffering.

No requirement of limited life expectancy

The Belgian law contains no restriction with regard to time left to live, and so chronic illness as well as psychiatric illness may provide legitimate grounds for assisted dying. In the Netherlands this has been the reality for many years (Griffiths et al. 1998, 2008).

And the Belgian law even includes suffering resulting from an 'accident' among the qualifying factors. Thus, a person who is paralysed from the neck down due to a car crash would in principle qualify for assisted dying.

Requirement of 'terminal' illness

The US states of Oregon and Washington, for example, are stricter on this point: the law requires that the patient be so-called terminally ill.

It should be noted, however, that 'terminally ill' is far from being a clear-cut concept. Nevertheless, it is defined in the following way in the Oregon Death with Dignity Act (the Washington act uses the exact same formulation): ' "Terminal disease" means an incurable and irreversible disease that has been medically confirmed and will, within reasonable medical judgment, produce death within six months' (Oregon: Law on Physician-Assisted Suicide, 1997). (It will be objected that it is impossible to accurately predict death within such a long time span.)

One may conclude from this that the two US laws, in contradistinction to the Dutch and Belgian ones, are discriminatory in that they 'reserve' assisted dying for particular patient groups and diseases. The same is true of the Québec law, which uses the expression 'an end-of-life patient' both with regard to PAS and euthanasia (Québec: Law on Euthanasia, 2014). How can this be legitimated?

PAS versus euthanasia

In explicitly prohibiting euthanasia, the two US laws also effectively ensure that any granted right to die does not apply to people who physically cannot, or who (for some reason or other) will not, or who psychologically cannot bring themselves to, commit suicide by swallowing or otherwise self-administering drugs.

The law in Oregon states that 'Nothing in ORS 127.800 to 127.897 shall be construed to authorize a physician or any other person to end a patient's life by lethal injection, mercy killing or active euthanasia' (Oregon: Law on Physician-Assisted Suicide, 1997). The wording of the Washington law is almost identical: 'Nothing in this chapter authorizes a physician or any other person to end a patient's life by lethal injection, mercy killing, or active euthanasia' (Washington: Law on Physician-Assisted Suicide, 2009).

The idea of 'palliative futility'

Regardless of what might be the meaning of 'medical futility', it has been claimed that similarly, 'there is also such a thing as palliative futility', implying 'the right of patients to decide that further conventional palliative care is futile and to request and obtain physician assisted death' within the palliative care unit (Bernheim et al., 2008).

It is true that palliative care may vary in quality and effectiveness, ranging from optimal across good and acceptable to poor. But it is never futile. Even in extreme cases of refractory suffering in the dying, palliative care can offer relief, as we pointed out above, through the option of terminal sedation.

The idea of palliative futility is therefore both clinically misplaced and conceptually incoherent (Materstvedt, 2013a). Accordingly, it should be discarded, and palliative care personnel should ignore it altogether.

A basic challenge for palliative care, and the model of 'integral' palliative care

Palliative care 'will enhance quality of life', states the WHO (2014). Obviously, if assisted dying is performed, it rules out such enhancement beyond the point of completing this procedure. But the task of enhancing the quality of life for terminally ill patients can be very demanding on the personnel involved in palliative care. According to Professor Franz Josef Illhardt, a fundamental challenge facing palliative caregivers is that they 'must know answers to the question: What makes a terminal and perhaps miserable life important and worth living for the dying person?' (Illhardt, 2001).

Faced with requests for assisted dying, finding answers to this question can be an even more difficult undertaking. And if assisted dying is practised within the walls of palliative care institutions, it might well prove a 'mission impossible' at times—for the very reason that the reality of the existing option may in itself cause particular patients to lose the will to live. This concern is sufficiently serious for many doctors and nurses to question or downright reject so-called integral palliative care.

Others think differently, believing this model to be a step in the right direction as practices evolve within palliative care, and as palliative care is increasingly institutionalized. Indeed, some even believe it to be *the* humane way to move forward in a civilized society.

In 2011, the EAPC published a report on palliative care development in countries with a euthanasia law (Chambaere et al., 2011b). The report highlighted that there has been substantial development in palliative care services in these countries, and that it was not possible to conclude that the development of palliative care had either been hindered or promoted by the legalization of elective death options.

By way of example, in Belgium, euthanasia or PAS seem not to be related to a lower use of palliative care, and often occur within the context of multidisciplinary care (van den Block et al., 2009). Some even claim that the domestic palliative care and euthanasia movements have reinforced one another in this country (Bernheim et al., 2008; Bernheim, 2011). However, that has been disputed (Gamester and van den Eynden, 2009). Whatever the truth of the matter, it is interesting to note that a Palliative care Act (as well as a Patients Rights Act) was passed simultaneously with the euthanasia law in 2002 (Bernheim and Mullie, 2010).

Table 5.7.1 lists some of the crucial arguments on either side of the important debate on the relationship between euthanasia and palliative care. A similar compilation appears in Materstvedt (2013a; see this article for an exposition of the various viewpoints).

The Swiss model of assisted suicide

Switzerland is known for its unique practice of assisted suicide involving lay people affiliated with right-to-die organizations. At first glance, this practice resembles the model of 'a suicide service outside clinical care' suggested by professor of palliative medicine Ilora Finlay and her colleagues (Finlay et al., 2005).

Role of the doctor

In the Swiss model, however, a medical doctor is involved in all cases of assisted suicide. He writes the lethal prescription—note that lethal injection upon request, that is, euthanasia, is prohibited in the penal code—and Swiss case law established in 1999 that a doctor can write such a prescription only on the basis of a clear diagnosis and indication, after personally having examined the patient, having checked his decisional capacity, and providing information on his prognosis and any existing treatment options (Bosshard, 2008).

Role of right-to-die organizations

Nevertheless, right-to-die organizations take responsibility for an important part of the assisted suicide process. The first step is often that the individual seeking to die contacts one of these organizations. If an applicant seems eligible in principle but his treating doctor is unwilling to participate, these organizations help the patient find a doctor who might be willing to assist.

Most importantly, right-to-die organization volunteers are present and provide counselling during the patient's self-administration of the lethal drug, that is, during the actual execution of the assisted suicide. They also give general support to the patient and his family (Ziegler and Bosshard, 2007).

Since Switzerland has no law on assisted suicide, there are no legal criteria for determining what patient groups may legitimately ask for such assistance. Hence the various right-to-die organizations operate according to their own rules. The common denominator for all of the organizations is that the patient must be competent. Beyond this basic requirement, their criteria for accepting an applicant for assisted suicide are as follows (Bosshard, 2008): 'hopeless prognosis or unbearable symptoms or unacceptable disabilities' (Exit; see also <http://www.exit.ch/en>); 'fatal disease or unendurable disability or uncontrollable pain' (Dignitas; see also <http://www.dignitas.ch>); or 'incurable disease with fatal prognosis or important disability or, and intolerable physical suffering, or incapacitating multimorbidity due to old age' (Exit A.D.M.D.; see also <http://www.exit-geneve.ch>).

Table 5.7.1 Combining palliative care and assisted dying

Arguments for	Arguments against
Assisted dying may be a part of palliative care	Assisted dying is not *palliative* care and by implication cannot be a part of it
The Belgian model of 'integral' palliative care has already been realized	That something is realizable does not necessarily make it desirable
Integral palliative care respects patient autonomy	The patient may not be capable of autonomous action
Assisted dying stops intolerable suffering at the end of life	Terminal sedation is an alternative procedure for stopping intolerable suffering
Patients may feel abandoned if they are denied access to assisted dying in palliative care institutions	Patients in wards offering 'integral' palliative care may lose the will to live and may also come to think that it is their duty to request assisted dying
Assisted dying and palliative care are neither alternatives nor antagonistic	Empirical research on the attitudes of Dutch doctors contradicts both claims
Palliative care needs a new ethical foundation that allows for assisted dying	The current, widely accepted WHO palliative care ethics rejects assisted dying
There is such a thing as 'palliative futility', which necessitates assisted dying	Palliative care is never futile, and the concept of 'palliative futility' is therefore both incoherent and clinically misplaced
In Belgium, the palliative care and assisted dying movements have reinforced one another	There is a danger that palliative care may become a neglected area in times of economic crises, with emphasis shifting to the less costly alternative of assisted dying
Doctors within palliative care are faced with decisions on life and death on a regular basis in the context of withholding or withdrawing life-sustaining treatment. Thus they are also the obvious and natural experts to carry out assisted dying	Withholding and withdrawing life-sustaining treatment (non-treatment decisions; NTDs) is not a matter of hastening death, but rather of not artificially prolonging life or postponing death. Such decisions are therefore fundamentally different from any decisions to hasten death through lethal injection or provision of lethal drugs for the patient to self-administer

Adapted from Materstvedt, L.J., Palliative care ethics: the problems of combining palliation and assisted dying, *Progress in Palliative Care*, Volume 21, Issue 3, pp. 158–64, Copyright © 2013, with permission from W. S. Maney & Son Ltd.

'Suicide tourism'

Also peculiar to the Swiss context is the phenomenon of 'suicide tourism', which means that patients travel from countries such as the United Kingdom and Germany to die (Bosshard 2008).

De-medicalizing assisted suicide

The Swiss practice is an instructive model in terms of showing what tasks and responsibilities can be dealt with without necessarily having to involve medical professionals. This division of tasks allows a certain distance between clinical practice and assisted suicide that may be perceived as helpful by many doctors.

The vast majority of cases of assisted suicide are carried out in the privacy of the patient's home. However, in recent years a number of nursing homes all over Switzerland, and a few hospitals in the French-speaking part of the country, have allowed assisted suicide to be performed on their premises (Pereira et al., 2008).

Statements on assisted dying by some palliative care organizations

Across the world, various palliative care organizations have published position statements on assisted dying.

We have seen that the Belgian FPZV is overtly supportive of elective death, however most such organizations oppose it, whereas some are neutral. The following is a selection that illustrates the spectre.

- *EAPC*: the EAPC's official position is that 'the provision of euthanasia and physician-assisted suicide should not be part of the responsibility of palliative care' (Materstvedt et al., 2003; Materstvedt, 2006, 2014; Payne, 2014).

- *The Australian and New Zealand Society of Palliative Medicine (ANZSPM)*: the ANZSPM is of a similar view, believing 'that the discipline of Palliative Medicine does not include the practice of euthanasia or assisted suicide' (ANZSPM, 2010).

- *The International Association for Hospice & Palliative Care (IAHPC)*: the IAHPC rejects assisted dying altogether in the short message that it 'believes that a plea for euthanasia is a plea for better care. There is no need or place for euthanasia in any form. The answer is the world-wide promotion and promulgation of the practice of Palliative Care' (IAHPC, 2012). They also stated 4 years earlier, in 2008, that 'assisted suicide and euthanasia should not be practiced in palliative care units' (IAHPC, 2008).

- *The Canadian Hospice Palliative Care Association (CHPCA)*: the CHPCA defends the right of those involved in palliative care not to contribute towards any hastening of death, stating that 'despite access to high quality end-of-life care, a small number of Canadians may still choose to have control over their own death . . . but we . . . have a choice not to participate or to be expected to assist in any efforts that intentionally hasten death' (CHPCA, 2010).

- *Canadian Society of Palliative Care Physicians (CSPCP)*: the position of the CSPCP is more conciliatory and is founded in membership opinion rather than ethical evaluation. They state: 'Based upon a membership survey, the Canadian Society of Palliative

Care Physicians strongly opposes the legalization of euthanasia and assisted suicide *at this time*, and most CSPCP members will not participate in euthanasia or assisted suicide' (CSPCP, 2012; italics added by authors). This position may be coined 'temporarily against', since by logical implication this means leaving the door open to legalizing assisted dying in the future.

◆ *The American Academy of Hospice and Palliative Medicine (AAHPM)*: the AAHPM 'takes a position of 'studied neutrality' on the subject of whether Physician-assisted Death should be legally regulated or prohibited, believing its members should instead continue to strive to find the proper response to those patients whose suffering becomes intolerable despite the best possible palliative care. Whether or not legalization occurs, AAHPM supports intense efforts to alleviate suffering and to reduce any perceived need for Physician-assisted Death' (AAHPM, 2007).

The future: palliative care on the 'slippery slope' towards euthanasia?

Against this background it is not easy to tell what the future holds for the relationship between assisted dying and palliative care. The picture is diverse. Will any of the organizations that have a somewhat unresolved attitude towards the topic today adopt a more accepting attitude towards combining palliative care and assisted dying?

Impact of new legislation

How will new legislation on assisted dying, if adopted by a particular country or state, impact on these views? Will some palliative care organizations abandon their long-standing resistance to assisted dying as a result of such legislation? And will we, as a consequence, be witnessing the realization, and hence the normalization, of the combination of palliative care and assisted dying?

Are we, in sum, going to see 'Palliative care on the "slippery slope" towards euthanasia?'—as asked in the title of a previous article by one of the present authors (Materstvedt, 2003). This issue has become all the more relevant with the very recent legalization of euthanasia in Québec, Canada, where the law requires that 'Every institution must adopt a policy with respect to end-of-life care', and that its annual 'report must also state, where applicable, the number of times . . . medical aid in dying were administered . . . *in the premises of a palliative care hospice* by a physician' (Québec: Law on Euthanasia, 2014; italics added by authors). In other words, the law explicitly paves the way for a practice akin to the Belgian 'integral' model (Bernheim et al., 2008; Materstvedt, 2013a). Accordingly, the Canadian organizations CHPCA and CSPCP, whose statements on assisted dying we quoted earlier, now face this reality.

Concluding remarks

For very many practitioners of palliative care the issue of assisted death is a potentially pressing one. They should therefore identify their own attitude towards it, and carefully think through the implications of this attitude. How do they justify their viewpoint? Would they or would they not be willing to participate in the practice?

Doctors' reluctance to participate in assisted dying: for clinicians, participating in assisted dying may prove to be a harder choice than abstaining. In a Dutch qualitative study of 22 primary care physicians, doctors described the emotional difficulties of performing euthanasia. One called euthanasia 'a rotten job'; another went as far as to depict himself as an 'executioner' (van Marwijk et al., 2007).

At the same time, doctors are becoming increasingly wary of being enlisted as experts in a field that extends far beyond medicine. There is often a presupposition in existing legislation and proposed bills that doctors' exclusive medical expertise can be utilized in the assisted dying process (Bosshard et al., 2008).

Doctors caught in the middle: doctors may also find themselves caught between society at large and professional concerns. On the one hand, a significant and growing proportion of the population in many Western countries seem to want assisted dying to be available as an option (Cohen et al., 2006). On the other hand, the overwhelming majority of medical organizations continue to view assisted dying as incompatible with the ethical codes of their profession (Bosshard et al., 2008).

From caring to killing?: but above all, the fact remains that moving from caring to killing is a big and fundamental step for palliative care personnel to take.

And for their patients, it is a matter of life and death—quite literally speaking.

Acknowledgement

The authors are grateful to Lise Utne, MA (English), for her thorough language editing of this chapter.

References

Ackroyd, R. (2005). Medically futile resuscitation: can it ever be justified? *European Journal of Palliative Care*, 12, 207–209.

American Academy of Hospice and Palliative Medicine (2007). *Position Statement on Physician-Assisted Death*. [Online] Available at: <http://www.aahpm.org/positions/default/suicide.html>.

Answers.USA.gov. (2013). *Assisted Suicide*. [Online] Available at: <http://answers.usa.gov/system/selfservice.controller?CONFIGURATION=1000&PARTITION_ID=1&CMD=VIEW_ARTICLE&USERTYPE=1&LANGUAGE=en&COUNTRY=US&ARTICLE_ID=11752>.

Australian and New Zealand Society of Palliative Medicine (2010). *Position Statement on Euthanasia*. [Online] Available at: <http://www.anzspm.org.au/c/anzspm?a=da&did=1005077>.

Belgium: Law on Euthanasia (2002). The Belgian Act on Euthanasia of May 28th 2002. *Ethical Perspectives*, 9(2–3), 182–188. [Online] Available at: <http://www.ethical-perspectives.be/viewpic.php?LAN=E&TABLE=EP&ID=59>.

Bernheim, J.L. (2011). Missed opportunity to advance debate on assisted dying. *BMJ*, 343, d4221.

Bernheim, J.L., Deschepper, R., Distelmans, W., Mullie, A., Bilsen, J., and Deliens, L. (2008). Development of palliative care and legalisation of euthanasia: antagonism or synergy? *BMJ*, 336, 864–867.

Bernheim, J.L. and Mullie, A. (2010). Euthanasia and palliative care in Belgium: legitimate concerns and unsubstantiated grievances. *Journal of Palliative Medicine*, 13, 798–799.

Bosshard, G. (2008). Switzerland. In J. Griffiths, H. Weyers, and M. Adams (eds.) *Euthanasia and Law in Europe*, pp. 463–482. Oxford: Hart Publishing.

Bosshard, G., Broeckaert, B., Clark, D., Materstvedt, L.J., Gordijn, B., and Müller-Busch, H.C. (2008). A role for doctors in assisted dying? An analysis of legal regulations and medical professional positions in six European countries. *Journal of Medical Ethics*, 34, 28–32.

Bosshard, G. and Materstvedt, L.J. (2011). Medical and societal issues in euthanasia and assisted suicide. In R. Chadwick, H. ten Have, and E.M. Meslin (eds.) *The SAGE Handbook of Health Care Ethics: Core and Emerging Issues*, pp. 205–221. London: SAGE Publications Ltd.

Canadian Hospice Palliative Care Association (2010). *Paper on Euthanasia, Assisted Suicide and Quality End-of-Life Care*. [Online] Available at: <http://www.chpca.net/media/7835/PAD_Issues_Paper_-_April_24_2010_-_Final.pdf>.

Canadian Society of Palliative Care Physicians (2012). *Position Statement: The Practice of Euthanasia and Assisted Suicide*. [Online] Available at: <http://www.cspcp.ca/english/Euthanasia%20pos%20state-FINAL4.pdf>.

CBSNEWS (2013). Vermont governor signs assisted-suicide bill. *CBSNEWS*, 20 May. [Online] Available at: <http://www.cbsnews.com/8301-201_162-57585348/vermont-governor-signs-assisted-suicide-bill/>.

Chambaere, K., Bilsen J., Cohen, J., Onwuteaka-Philipsen, B.D., Mortier, F., and Deliens, L. (2011a). Trends in medical end-of-life decision making in Flanders, Belgium 1998–2001–2007. *Medical Decision Making*, 31, 500–510.

Chambaere, K., Centeno, C., Hernández, E.A., *et al.* (2011b). *Palliative Care Development in Countries with a Euthanasia Law. Report for the Commission on Assisted Dying*. European Association for Palliative Care. [Online] Available at: <http://www.commissiononassisteddying.co.uk/wp-content/uploads/2011/10/EAPC-Briefing-Paper-Palliative-Care-in-Countries-with-a-Euthanasia-Law.pdf>.

Chambaere, K., Rietjens, J.A.C., Smets, T., *et al.* (2012). Age-based disparities in end-of-life decisions in Belgium: a population-based death certificate survey. *BMC Public Health*, 12, 447.

Cohen, J., Marcoux, I., Bilsen, J., Deboosere, P., van der Wal, G., and Deliens, L. (2006). Trends in acceptance of euthanasia among the general public in 12 European countries (1981–1999). *European Journal of Public Health*, 16, 663–669.

Federatie Palliatieve Zorg Vlaanderen vzw (2003). *Dealing with Euthanasia and Other Forms of Medically Assisted Death*. [Online] Available at: <http://www.consciencelaws.org/background/procedures/assist008-007.aspx>.

Finlay, I.G., Wheatley, V.J., and Izdebski, C. (2005). The House of Lords Select Committee on the Assisted Dying for the Terminally Ill Bill: implications for specialist palliative care. *Palliative Medicine*, 19, 444–453.

Fischer, S., Huber, C.A., Furter, M., *et al.* (2009). Reasons why people in Switzerland seek assisted suicide: the view of patients and physicians. *Swiss Medical Weekly*, 139, 333–338.

Fischer, S., Huber, C.A., Imhof, L., *et al.* (2008). Suicide assisted by two Swiss right-to-die organisations. *Journal of Medical Ethics*, 34, 810–814.

Gamester, N. and van den Eynden, B. (2009). The relationship between palliative care and legalized euthanasia in Belgium. *Journal of Palliative Medicine*, 12, 589–591.

Gamondi, C., Pott, M., and Payne, S. (2013). Families' experiences with patients who died after assisted suicide: a retrospective interview study in southern Switzerland. *Annals of Oncology*, 24, 1639–1644.

Ganzini, L., Goy, E.R., and Dobscha, S.K. (2008). Prevalence of depression and anxiety in patients requesting physicians' aid in dying: cross sectional survey. *BMJ*, 337, a1682.

Georges, J.J., Onwuteaka-Philipsen, B.D., van der Heide, A., van der Wal, G., and van der Maas, P.J. (2006). Physicians' opinions on palliative care and euthanasia in the Netherlands. *Journal of Palliative Medicine*, 9, 1137–1144.

Griffiths, J., Weyers, H., and Adams, M. (eds.) (2008). *Euthanasia and Law in Europe*. Oxford: Hart Publishing.

Griffiths, J., Weyers, H., and Bood, A. (eds.) (1998). *Euthanasia and Law in the Netherlands*. Amsterdam: Amsterdam University Press.

Illhardt, F.J. (2001). Scope and demarcation of palliative care. In H. ten Have and R. Janssens (eds.) *Palliative Care in Europe: Concepts and Policies*, pp. 109–116. Amsterdam: IOS Press.

International Association for Hospice & Palliative Care (2008/2012). *Homepage*. [Online] Available at: <http://hospicecare.com>.

Johansen, S., Hølen, J.C., Kaasa, S., Loge, J.H., and Materstvedt, L.J. (2005). Attitudes towards, and wishes for, euthanasia in advanced cancer patients at a palliative medicine unit. *Palliative Medicine*, 19, 454–460.

Koninklijke Nederlandsche Maatschappij tot bevordering der Geneeskunst (KNMG) (2011). *Position Paper: The Role of the Physician in the Voluntary Termination of Life*. [Online] Available at: <http://knmg.artsennet.nl/Publicaties/KNMGpublicatie/Position-paper-The-role-of-the-physician-in-the-voluntary-termination-of-life-2011.htm>.

Luxembourg: Law on Euthanasia (2009). [Online] Available at: <http://www.legilux.public.lu/leg/a/archives/2009/0046/a046.pdf>.

Marquet, R.L., Bartelds, A., Visser, G.J., Spreeuwenberg, P., and Peters, L. (2003). Twenty five years of requests for euthanasia and physician-assisted suicide in Dutch general practice: trend analysis. *BMJ*, 327, 201–202.

Materstvedt, L.J. (2003). Palliative care on the 'slippery slope' towards euthanasia? *Palliative Medicine*, 17, 387–392.

Materstvedt, L.J. (2006). The EAPC Ethics Task Force on Palliative Care and Euthanasia. *European Journal of Palliative Care*, 13, 69–71.

Materstvedt, L.J. (2012). Intention, procedure, outcome and personhood in palliative sedation and euthanasia. *BMJ Supportive & Palliative Care*, 2, 9–11.

Materstvedt, L.J. (2013a). Palliative care ethics: the problems of combining palliation and assisted dying. *Progress in Palliative Care*, 3, 158–164.

Materstvedt, L.J. (2013b). Erroneous assumptions about deep palliative sedation and euthanasia. *BMJ Supportive & Palliative Care*, 3(4), 458–459.

Materstvedt, L.J. (2014). Palliative care and euthanasia: what is the view of the EAPC? Editorial. *BMJ Supportive & Palliative Care*, 4(2), 124–125.

Materstvedt, L.J. (2015). Caring and killing in the clinic: the argument of self-determination. In C. Rehmann-Sutter, H. Gudat, and K. Ohnsorge (eds.) *The Patient's Wish to Die: Research, Ethics and Palliative Care*. Oxford: Oxford University Press.

Materstvedt, L.J. and Bosshard, G. (2009). Deep and continuous palliative sedation (terminal sedation): clinical-ethical and philosophical aspects. *The Lancet Oncology*, 10, 622–627.

Materstvedt, L.J., Clark, D., Ellershaw, J., *et al.* (2003). Euthanasia and physician-assisted suicide: a view from an EAPC Ethics Task Force. *Palliative Medicine*, 17, 97–101.

Netherlands: Law on Euthanasia (2002). *UK Parliament: Select Committee on Assisted Dying for the Terminally Ill Bill, Minutes of Evidence—Appendix*. [Online] Available at: <http://www.publications.parliament.uk/pa/ld200405/ldselect/ldasdy/86/4121603.htm>.

Onwuteaka-Philipsen, B.D., Brinkman-Stoppelenburg, A., Penning, C., de Jong-Krul, G.J., van Delden, J.J., and van der Heide, A. (2012). Trends in end-of-life practices before and after the enactment of the euthanasia law in the Netherlands from 1990 to 2010: a repeated cross-sectional survey. *The Lancet*, 380, 908–915.

Onwuteaka-Philipsen, B.D., van der Heide, A., Koper, D., *et al.* (2003). Euthanasia and other end-of-life decisions in the Netherlands in 1990, 1995, and 2001. *The Lancet*, 362, 395–399.

Oregon: Law on Physician-Assisted Suicide (1997). *Oregon Revised Statute*. [Online] Available at: <http://public.health.oregon.gov/providerpartnerresources/evaluationresearch/deathwithdignityact/Pages/ors.aspx>.

Oregon Public Health Division (2014). *Oregon's Death with Dignity Act Annual Report*. [Online] Available at: <http://public.health.oregon.gov/ProviderPartnerResources/EvaluationResearch/DeathwithDignityAct/Documents/year16.pdf>.

Payne, S. (2014). Response to the editorial 'Palliative care and euthanasia: what is the view of the EAPC?' *BMJ Supportive & Palliative Care*, 4(3), 226.

Pereira, J., Anwar, D., Pralong, G., Pralong, J., Mazzocato, C., and Bigler, J.M. (2008). Assisted suicide and euthanasia should not be practiced in palliative care units. *Journal of Palliative Medicine*, 11, 1074–1076.

Québec, Canada: Law on Euthanasia (2014). *Bill 52: An Act respecting end-of-life care.* [Online] Available at: <<http://www.scribd.com/doc/228378011/Quebec-s-Bill-52-Right-to-Die>.

Rady, M.Y. and Verheijde, J.L. (2010). Continuous deep sedation until death: palliation or physician-assisted death? *American Journal of Hospice & Palliative Medicine*, 27, 205–214.

Rehmann-Sutter, C., Gudat, H., and Ohnsorge, K. (eds.) (2015). The Patient's Wish to Die: Research, Ethics and Palliative Care. Oxford: Oxford University Press.

Rurup, M.L., Smets, T., Cohen, J., Bilsen, J., Onwuteaka-Philipsen, B.D., and Deliens, L. (2012). The first five years of euthanasia legislation in Belgium and the Netherlands: description and comparison of cases. *Palliative Medicine*, 26, 43–49.

Seale, C. (2009). Hastening death in end-of-life care: a survey of doctors. *Social Science & Medicine*, 69, 1659–1666.

Van den Block, L., Deschepper, R., Bilsen, J., Bossuyt, N., Van Casteren, V., and Deliens, L. (2009). Euthanasia and other end of life decisions and care provided in final three months of life: nationwide retrospective study in Belgium. *BMJ*, 339, b2772.

Van der Heide, A., Onwuteaka-Philipsen, B.D., Rurup, M.L., *et al.* (2007). End-of-life practices in the Netherlands under the Euthanasia Act. *The New England Journal of Medicine*, 56, 1957–1965.

Van der Lee, M.L., van der Bom, J.G., Swarte, N.B., Heintz, A.P., de Graeff, A., and van den Bout, J. (2005). Euthanasia and depression: a prospective cohort study among terminally ill cancer patients. *Journal of Clinical Oncology*, 23, 6607–6612.

Van Marwijk, H., Haverkate, I., van Royen, P., and The, A.-M. (2007). Impact of euthanasia on primary care physicians in the Netherlands. *Palliative Medicine*, 21, 609–614.

Washington: Law on Physician-Assisted Suicide (2009). *Washington Death with Dignity Act, Initiative 1000.* [Online] Available at: <http://www.doh.wa.gov/YouandYourFamily/IllnessandDisease/DeathwithDignityAct>.

World Health Organization (2014). *Definition of Palliative Care.* [Online] Available at: <http://www.who.int/cancer/palliative/definition/en/>.

Youngner, S.J. and Kimsma, G.K. (eds.) (2012) *Physician-Assisted Death in Perspective: Assessing the Dutch Experience.* Cambridge: Cambridge University Press.

Ziegler, S.J. and Bosshard, G. (2007). Role of non-governmental organisations in physician assisted suicide. *BMJ*, 334, 295–298.

Withholding and withdrawing life-sustaining treatment (including artificial nutrition and hydration)

Danielle N. Ko and Craig D. Blinderman

Introduction to withholding and withdrawing life-sustaining treatment

Although withholding medical treatment from the seriously ill is not new (Hippocrates et al., 1923), public debate over the appropriate use of life-sustaining treatment (LST) in seriously ill patients is at unprecedented levels, driven by multiple factors including advances in medical technology, an ageing population, ballooning health-care costs, the increased prevalence of life-threatening chronic disease, and more patients dying within health-care institutions.

LST is 'any treatment that serves to prolong life without reversing the underlying medical condition and includes but is not limited to cardiopulmonary resuscitation (CPR), mechanical ventilation, hemodialysis, left ventricular assist devices, antibiotics, as well as artificial nutrition and hydration' (Anonymous, 1992). *Withholding* LST is a deliberate decision not to initiate treatment aimed at prolonging life. *Withdrawing* LST involves removing a medical intervention without which life is not expected to continue due to the patient's underlying health status. Withholding/withdrawing LST is therefore performed with the expectation that the patient will die due to the natural progression of their underlying illness. This is in contrast to physician-assisted dying and euthanasia (see Chapter 5.6) which are acts intended to hasten death to prevent or alleviate patient suffering.

The primary goal of this chapter is to present a practical guide for clinicians who are faced with the prospect of withholding/withdrawing LST (as outlined in Box 5.8.1).

Consider the legal and ethical framework

Is withholding/withdrawing LST legal?

The legality of withholding/withdrawing LST differs between countries. In many countries (e.g. United States, United Kingdom, Germany, Japan, Netherlands, Taiwan, and Australia) withholding/withdrawing LST is legal, although each country tends to have different approaches for withholding/withdrawing LST (Mendelson and Jost, 2003). In contrast, within the developing world, withholding/withdrawing LST is either of uncertain legal status (e.g. China and Brazil) or illegal (e.g. Kenya, Turkey, and India) (Blank, 2011).

Even in those countries where withholding/withdrawing LST is legal, it has been shown that poor clinician knowledge of the law is associated with higher levels of legal defensiveness and consequently more aggressive and unjustified treatment at the end of life (McCrary et al., 1992; McCrary and Swanson, 1999; Meisel et al., 2000). It is therefore important that clinicians have a basic understanding of the relevant laws. Since a thorough review of the relevant laws around the world is beyond the scope of this chapter, readers are advised to familiarize themselves with the laws governing this clinical practice in their own jurisdiction. Nevertheless, we highlight here some of the general legal principles that one might need to consider, using the US legal framework as an example.

While there is no absolute right to die (*Vacco v Quill*, 1997; *Washington v Glucksberg*, 1997), US case and statutory law generally support the right of a person to refuse life-sustaining medical treatment. Prior to 1976, however, US courts were reluctant to allow patients to refuse treatment if this would result in their death. *In Re Quinlan* (1976), the first reported US 'end-of-life' case, the New Jersey Supreme Court recognized that the existing right to determine one's medical care included the right to refuse LST. Karen Quinlan had been in a persistent vegetative state (PVS) as a complication of drug and alcohol intoxication, and required respiratory support and artificial nutrition and hydration (ANH) to keep her alive. Quinlan's father, her legal guardian, requested that the ventilator be withdrawn. The Court ruled that there was a right to refuse medical care based on one's constitutional right to privacy—a right that is not expressly mentioned in the US constitution but is implied in a number of its amendments—and that this right could be exercised on behalf of a patient without decision-making capacity by her guardian.

In 1990, the US Supreme Court made its first decision on withdrawing LST in *Cruzan v Director, Missouri Department of Health* (1990). Nancy Cruzan was a young woman in a PVS following a

Box 5.8.1 Withholding and withdrawing life sustaining treatment—a practical approach to decision-making

We find that a systematic approach to withholding and withdrawing LST is important to ensure best clinical practice and optimal patient outcomes. When faced with a decision as to whether to withhold or withdraw LST from a seriously ill patient, the following approach is suggested:

1. Consider the legal and ethical framework for withholding/withdrawing LST

Is withholding/withdrawing LST legal in my jurisdiction?
What are the ethical principles/considerations relevant to a decision to withhold/withdraw LST?

2. Assess the consequences of utilizing or forgoing LST in this particular instance

What is the patient's current prognosis?
What are the current goals of care of the patient?
What are the likely outcomes of utilizing LST in this patient?

- What is the clinical evidence for utilizing LST in this context?
- Will it extend the patient's life? If so, for how long?
- How will the LST impact upon the patient's quality of life?
- What are the physical risks or complications likely to result from LST? How likely are these to occur?
- What are the emotional consequences of utilizing LST here?
- How will the LST impact upon specific goals of the patient? For example, LST may allow the patient to share a significant life event (e.g. seeing a child get married or a grandchild born) or to say goodbye to family.
- Will the LST facilitate other treatment aims? For instance, will it enable adequate time to treat a patient's underlying depression.
- How do these outcomes accord with the patient's known end-of-life values?

What are the likely outcomes of withholding/withdrawing LST in this patient?

- What is the expected clinical course if LST is withheld/withdrawn?
- How will withholding/withdrawing LST affect patient survival?
- What physical symptoms may occur? How can these be managed?
- What is the likely emotional impact of withholding/withdrawing LST on the patient? The caregiver(s)? The family?
- Will forgoing LST alleviate existing physical, emotional or existential distress?
- How do these outcomes accord with the patient's known end-of-life values?

3. Assess patient's decision-making capacity

Does the patient have capacity to make this particular decision at this particular time?

4. Make a decision regarding LST

We advocate using a shared decision-making model, in which the patient provides the expertise regarding his/her values and goals and the clinicians provide the expertise to determine whether utilizing LST will accord with the patient's values and help them to achieve their goals. In practice, we adopt the following approach:

(a) *If the patient has capacity, what is his preference regarding LST?* For patients who have not formed an opinion regarding LST, we should consider their health-care values and goals and make a recommendation as to whether the use of LST will honour those values and meet those goals.

(b) *If the patient lacks capacity, does the patient have an advance directive specifying his preference for LST? If not, is there a surrogate decision-maker who knows the patient's wishes or can use substituted judgement to decide on the patient's behalf?*

Taking this approach, we find that a consensus decision to utilize or forgo LST can be readily achieved in the vast majority of cases. However, sometimes disagreement/uncertainty regarding the best approach will remain. In this event, we suggest attempting to address the following questions:

Is the disagreement/uncertainty arising out of clinical uncertainty (e.g. uncertain prognosis, uncertain benefit?), an ethical dilemma (is this the right thing to do?), a legal issue (is what I am doing prohibited by law?) or a combination thereof?

- For clinical uncertainty, medical evidence, clinical experience and consultation with colleagues should be utilized.
- For ethical problems, consider the ethical principles of beneficence, non-maleficence, autonomy, justice, and the concepts of proportionality and quality of life as well as seeking the opinion of an ethics committee (if available).

Box 5.8.1 Continued

- ◆ For legal issues, obtain expert opinion regarding the laws governing withholding/withdrawing LST.

  Is the conflict within the team, between the team and the patient/family, or between the patient/family?

- ◆ For intra-team conflict, consider seeking advice from other senior physicians.

- ◆ For conflict between the team and the family/patient, is there a role for an ethics committee or is there a hospital policy that can provide guidance?

- ◆ For conflict between the family/patient, maintain focus on patient's goals. If the patient is competent, follow the patient's requests. Refer to social work/psychologists/chaplaincy if available for additional support.

5. If the decision to withhold/withdraw LST is made, make a treatment plan to actively manage resulting symptoms and provide support to patients/families and health-care providers

- ◆ A clear plan for the treatment of the patient's underlying symptoms should be in place given the expectation that the patient will become more symptomatic and die once LST is withheld/withdrawn.

- ◆ For patients, families and health-care providers, the decision to withhold or withdraw LST is emotionally charged. Good communication will significantly aid in alleviating some of the distress. Existential and spiritual issues may become more prominent as death is expected. Referrals to psychology, social work, and chaplaincy should be considered.

---

car accident. The hospital applied for a court order sanctioning the family's request to remove the feeding tube. The Missouri Supreme Court declined because of a lack of 'clear and convincing' evidence that this is what she would have wanted. On appeal, the US Supreme Court affirmed Missouri's right to require 'clear and convincing' evidence, but otherwise left it to individual states to set the evidentiary burden. The Court confirmed that both patients with and without decision-making capacity have a constitutional right to refuse medical care under the 14th amendment's Due Process Clause (that no person shall be deprived of life, liberty, or property, without due process of law). Shortly after the Cruzan case and its focus on patient preferences, the Patient Self Determination Act of 1990 was passed by the US Congress (Patient Self-Determination Act, 1990). This legislation requires that federally funded health-care institutions provide patients with information about their right to direct future medical care via written advance directives (ADs), which can be applied in the event of future incapacitation. By doing so, the Act forced health-care institutions to develop and outline policies regarding withholding/withdrawing of LST.

Withholding/withdrawing LST is *not* the same as physician-assisted suicide

Withholding/withdrawing LST is declining treatment that is artificially sustaining a person's life. In contrast, physician-assisted suicide (PAS) is the provision of means to end a life prematurely. In most countries where withholding/withdrawing LST is allowed, PAS is illegal. In *Washington v Glucksberg* (1997), the US Supreme Court held that while patients have the constitutional right to refuse medical treatment, individuals do not have a constitutional right to PAS (*Washington v Glucksberg*, 1997).

Withholding versus withdrawing LST

From a Western bioethical perspective, there is no moral reason to differentiate between withholding and withdrawing LST (President's Commission for the Study of Ethical Problems in Medicine and Biomedical and Behavioral Research, 1983;

Brock, 1997; Beauchamp and Childress, 2009). Notwithstanding this, withdrawing LST is an act of commission (as opposed to withholding LST which is an act of omission), and death usually follows more quickly than for withholding LST (Sprung et al., 2003). Consequently, withdrawing LST is frequently perceived to have direct causation in a patient's death. As a result, for many patients, family members, and clinicians withdrawal of LST carries a greater psychological burden (Solomon et al., 1993; Melltorp and Nilstun, 1997; Vincent, 1999; Dickenson, 2000). Moreover, for some orthodox religions, a distinction between withdrawal and withholding LST remains (Loike et al., 2010).

The common perception that withholding LST is morally more acceptable than withdrawing LST is further contributed to by the differential treatment the two acts are afforded in some legal jurisdictions. At a practical level, if only withholding treatment was allowed, time-limited trials of LST would not be acceptable and patients who chose LST would need to remain on those treatments until death.

What are the ethical considerations?

The ethical considerations around withholding/withdrawing LST have been the subject of considerable discussion. A summary of the important ethical principles that are relevant to withholding/withdrawing LST is outlined in the following sections. Since culture creates the context within which individuals comprehend the meaning of illness, suffering, and death, the moral considerations and the weight they carry are culturally determined (Vincent, 2001; Sprung et al., 2007b) and for any given patient, the most ethical option will depend on the individual circumstances of the case, and can only be determined by weighing all of the different principles.

General principles of modern bioethics

Beneficence, nonmaleficence, autonomy, and justice are the four guiding principles of modern bioethics (Beauchamp and Childress, 2009), and any decision to withhold/withdraw LST should carefully consider each of these.

Beneficence/non-maleficence

Dating back to the time of Hippocrates 2500 years ago, physicians have primarily acted to benefit their patients (beneficence) and refrained from causing harm (non-maleficence) (Will, 2011a). In modern medicine, where the ability to cure illness and extend life is widely celebrated, withholding/withdrawing LST can superficially be seen as running counter to the principle of beneficence. However, in those with serious advanced illness, clinicians need to be mindful that utilizing LST may not only be associated with significant physical harm (e.g. rib fractures frequently occur following chest compressions during resuscitation) but also be in violation of a patient's values and goals.

Autonomy

Autonomy is broadly defined as the human capacity for self-determination, that is, each person has the right to choose among the best alternatives according to a self-chosen plan (Kant and Gregor, 1998) and is derived from the basic moral obligation-respect for persons. Patient autonomy has a narrower definition, being the right of patients to make medical decisions and exert control over their medical care. Patient autonomy serves as the basis not only for informed consent to treatment but also for the right to refuse treatment (President's Commission for the Study of Ethical Problems in Medicine and Biomedical and Behavioral Research, 1982; Will, 2011b).

When considering withdrawing or withholding LST, the desire to uphold autonomy (or more aptly, patient preferences) may come into direct conflict with other ethical principles. For instance, patients and/or their families may request interventions that the physician considers harmful. In this regard, it is generally accepted that, while patients have the right to refuse medical treatments, they do not have the right to demand harmful and non-beneficial treatments (Luce, 1995; Brett and McCullough, 2012). Moreover, some authors have noted that an overemphasis and/or uncritical acceptance of patient autonomy risks putting unrealistic responsibility on patients and their families and may in fact compromise their ability for self-determination by forcing them to make decisions for which they lack the prerequisite knowledge and experience (Quill and Brody, 1996; Billings and Krakauer, 2011).

Justice

Given the finite nature of health-care resources, justice requires these resources be fairly allocated. Despite this, many clinicians feel that they should not have to bear in mind such considerations when determining whether to withhold/withdraw LST, since their duty of care is to the individual patient and not to society at large. In reality, however, resource allocation does limit the options one considers for seriously ill patients. For example, while there are often hospital policies regarding allocation of limited intensive care unit (ICU) beds, it is clinicians who make the final determination regarding who is allocated an ICU bed. This decision is inevitably made up of judgements regarding benefits and burdens to the individual patient but also must have regard for competing demands for a bed by other patients in the hospital at any given time.

Other ethical considerations

In addition to the general bioethical principles just outlined, an understanding of several other concepts is important when considering withdrawing/withholding LST.

Proportionality

Proportionality, a concept originating from the Catholic Church, supports the idea that LST should be forgone if it would cause more harm than benefit, and requires one to weigh the burdens and benefits of a particular treatment relative to the clinical situation and prognosis of a particular patient (Pence, 1995; Quill et al., 1997; Jansen and Sulmasy, 2002). For example, mechanical ventilation may be considered proportionate for a young, otherwise healthy adult, with a severe but reversible lung pathology/injury, but the same therapy may be disproportionate in a patient dying of metastatic cancer.

In a patient at the end of life there is a risk that LST may prolong the dying process and/or subject the patient to a quality of life that is unacceptable. In such cases where the burdens of the treatment outweigh any benefits, it has been argued that there is no ethical obligation to provide disproportionate treatment and that it is morally permissible to remove such treatments and focus exclusively on the patient's comfort even if this results in an earlier death (Shannon and Walter, 1993).

Extraordinary versus ordinary treatments

Previously, some ethicists and theologians advocated for a distinction between 'extraordinary' versus 'ordinary' treatments as a way to decide whether to withhold/withdraw LST, with foregoing of extraordinary treatment being more ethically justified. The extraordinary/ordinary distinction is no longer considered useful given it is unclear what aspect of a treatment (usualness, complexity, artificiality, availability, cost, etc.) would make it extraordinary or ordinary, and the concept has largely been replaced by considering proportionality, that is, benefits versus burdens instead (Beauchamp and Childress, 2009).

Futility

In everyday practice, futility is a concept that is frequently used as a justification to withhold/withdraw LST (Wilkinson and Savulescu, 2011). Indeed, some have argued that physicians should use futility to *unilaterally* decide to withhold/withdraw LST if such treatment will not change the patient's outcome (e.g. survival to discharge) (Schneiderman et al., 1990). Consistent with this notion, the Texas state legislature in 1999 passed legislation allowing health-care facilities to discontinue LST over patient and family objections, so long as the continuation of LST is deemed to be futile by the treating physicians and appropriate provisions are met (including an ethics committee review of the case) (Fine, 2009).

Despite this, we do not advocate the use of futility as a justification for withholding/withdrawing LST for the following reasons. First, there is no accepted definition of 'futile' treatment (Burns and Truog, 2007). Thus it is often unclear to a clinician what this actually means in practice (Solomon, 1993). For example, mechanical ventilation of a patient with multiorgan failure and end-stage cancer may enhance their respiratory function (and is therefore not futile from a physiological standpoint), but it is unlikely to have any significant impact on recovery (and is therefore futile in terms of achieving any improvement). Second, on a related note, what a clinician judges to be futile is inherently subjective and influenced by his own values (Truog et al., 1992; Ashby, 2011). For example, while a clinician may feel it is 'futile' to provide ongoing life support to a patient in a PVS, the family might feel quite differently, and there is no objective way to determine which of these value judgements is correct. Third, using futility as the basis for a unilateral decision to withhold/withdraw treatment enables clinicians to avoid having the difficult yet beneficial conversations that are frequently needed to bridge the gap between unrealistic family expectations and clinicians' prognosis.

Non-abandonment

Abandonment is when a physician withdraws from a therapeutic relationship without providing notice or reasonable alternative options for care. Withdrawing of LST is not a form of abandonment since the withdrawal of LST should always include a plan to continue care and provide intensive symptom management for the remainder of the patient's life. Especially around decisions to withhold LST, physicians should stress that the patient will not be abandoned and that every attempt will be made to ensure the patient's comfort. We should discourage clinicians from using the phrase 'withdrawing care' for the withdrawal of LST, as this gives an implicit message that we are no longer caring for the patient once we discontinue LST.

Double effect

The doctrine of double effect, originally formulated by Thomas Aquinas, applies to moral dilemmas in which it is impossible for a person to avoid all harmful actions and requires that (1) the nature of the act must be good or at least morally neutral; (2) the harmful effect must be foreseen but not intended; (3) the harmful effect must not be a way of producing the good effect; and (4) the good effect must outweigh the harmful effect (i.e. be proportionate). Thus, in the context of withdrawing LST, the doctrine of double effect has been used to justify the administration of high-dose opioids and sedatives for the purposes of pain and symptom relief during the withdrawal of mechanical ventilation, notwithstanding the unintended but foreseen risk of hastening the patient's death (Sulmasy and Pellegrino, 1999). The doctrine of double effect and its applicability to withholding/withdrawing LST was confirmed in the US Supreme Court decision of *Vacco v Quill* (1997).

Protection of vulnerable patients

Those at the end of life who often cannot speak for themselves require additional protections to make sure that their rights are not violated. The need to focus on patient values and protect the patient's best interests, when values cannot be discerned, is never stronger than when caring for the most vulnerable in society (children, elders, disabled, mentally incapacitated, minorities, prisoners, etc.). Members of cultural minorities with differing value structures and deep vitalist convictions also represent a group at significant risk of having their convictions dismissed by health care providers who do not ascribe the same value to survival (Burns and Truog, 2007).

Assess the consequences of utilizing or forgoing life-sustaining treatment

For any given clinical case, one of the primary tasks of a clinician is to consider the consequences (benefits and burdens) of either utilizing or forgoing LST. At the end of this chapter, we consider specific information pertaining to several common LSTs, including cardiopulmonary resuscitation (CPR), cardiac/circulatory support devices, haemodialysis, antibiotics, and ANH. In general,

however, we find the following questions helpful in determining the utility of any given LST.

What is the patient's current prognosis?

◆ How long are they likely to live?

◆ What is their expected quality of life?

What are the current goals of care of the patient?

What are the likely outcomes of utilizing LST in this patient?

◆ What is the clinical evidence for utilizing LST in this context?

◆ Will it extend the patient's life? If so, for how long?

◆ How will the LST impact upon the patient's quality of life?

◆ What are the physical risks or complications likely to result from LST? How likely are these to occur?

◆ What are the emotional consequences of utilizing LST here?

◆ How will the LST impact upon specific goals of the patient? For example, if it extends life, it might enable a patient to share a significant life event (e.g. seeing a child get married or a grandchild born) or to say goodbye to family.

◆ Will the LST facilitate other treatment aims? For instance, if it extends life, it might enable adequate time to treat a patient's underlying depression.

◆ How do these outcomes accord with the patient's known end-of-life values?

What are the likely outcomes of withholding/withdrawing LST in this patient?

◆ What is the expected clinical course if LST is withheld/withdrawn?

◆ How will withholding/withdrawing LST affect patient survival?

◆ What physical symptoms may occur? How can these be managed?

◆ What is the likely emotional impact of withholding/withdrawing LST on the patient? Their family? The caregivers?

◆ Will forgoing LST alleviate existing physical, emotional or existential distress?

◆ How do these outcomes accord with the patient's known end-of-life values?

Assess decision-making capacity

Decision-making capacity is defined as the cognitive ability to participate in making medical decisions. Strictly speaking, capacity is different from 'competence'. Competence is a legal determination made by the courts and relates to the presence or absence of global decision-making capacity. In contrast, health-care professionals determine capacity, which exists on a spectrum, or a sliding scale, rather than being strictly present or absent (President's Commission for the Study of Ethical Problems in Medicine and Biomedical and Behavioral Research, 1982; Drane, 1985). For example, a patient may have the capacity to make decisions about whether to have stitches for a wound, but may lack the sophisticated understanding to make decisions around withdrawing LST. In practice, the consequences that follow when a physician judges a person to lack capacity are often the same as a legal determination of incompetence. Indeed, in recent decades, competence and capacity have increasingly been used interchangeably in the legal, medical, and policy arenas.

At the end of life, cognitive failure and an associated lack of decision-making capacity is exceedingly common (due either to the disease itself, the treatments, or a combination thereof). In a recent study of almost 4000 adults who died, 42% were required to make important clinical decisions in their final days of life, but only 30% of those patients had sufficient capacity to do so (Silveira et al., 2010). Despite this, capacity assessments are frequently omitted under the mistaken assumption that sufficient capacity exists (Raymont et al., 2004; Sessums et al., 2011). And, even when an assessment is performed, clinicians repeatedly overestimate a patient's decision-making capacity (Fitten and Waite, 1990; Etchells et al., 1997; Marson et al., 1997; Sessums et al., 2011).

To help avoid such pitfalls, we advocate that a systematic capacity assessment be performed and documented in the medical record, whenever a decision to withhold/withdraw LST is being considered. To this end, we suggest a three-step approach. First, objective testing of cognition and reasoning should be performed (for instance, via the MacArthur Competence Assessment Tool (Dunn et al., 2006) or Aid to Capacity Evaluation (Etchells et al., 1999)). Second, clinicians should assess for the presence of depression, which will not only impair cognitive function but may also significantly bias patient preferences against LST (Ganzini et al., 1994; Hooper et al., 1996; Blank et al., 2001). If depression is suspected, discussion with family members regarding the patient's pre-morbid values and goals should be undertaken, and relevant treatment initiated if possible. Third, the following questions should be specifically addressed (Appelbaum, 2007):

1. Does the patient understand the relevant information? (e.g. *Can you tell me what you understand about your health problem and the treatments being offered?*)

2. Does the patient appreciate the medical consequences of the various treatment options? (e.g. *What do you believe will happen if you undergo this treatment and how will this likely impact your health?*)

3. Can the patient manipulate the information in a rational manner and state the reasons for making a particular decision? (e.g. *What makes treatment X better than treatment Y? Or why is not starting treatment Z better than starting treatment Z?*)

4. Can the patient communicate that choice? (e.g. *Can you tell me what your decision is?*)

Thus, the overarching question that a clinician should seek to address is not 'Does the patient have general decision-making capacity?' but rather 'Does the patient have capacity to make this particular decision at this particular time?' (Grisso and Appelbaum, 1998).

Make a decision regarding life-sustaining treatment

Up to this point, the necessary groundwork for making a decision regarding LST has been laid by assessing the legal and ethical context, the likely consequences of utilizing or forgoing LST, and the decision-making capacity of the patient. To proceed, we strongly advocate the adoption of a shared decision-making model where patients or their surrogates are encouraged to participate in selecting appropriate treatment options in accordance with the patient's values (Marshall and Bibby, 2011).

Shared decision-making: an introduction and some practical considerations

A shared decision-making model involves active dialogue and discussion between the clinician and the patient (and/or their families and surrogate), with specific roles for each (Charles et al., 1997; Frosch and Kaplan, 1999). The clinician (1) provides patients, their families and/or surrogates with information about the likely consequences of either utilizing or forgoing LST; (2) gains an understanding of the patient's values and goals; and (3) makes a recommendation, based not only on their own medical expertise and clinical experience but also their knowledge of the patient's values and goals and their assessment of whether utilizing LST will achieve those goals. Patients, families, and/or surrogates—with appropriate information regarding the likely consequences of LST and the clinician's recommendation—then make educated decisions that accord with the underlying values and goals of the patient. In this way, the shared decision-making model draws upon not only the clinician's expertise in LST but also the patient's, family's, and/or surrogate's expertise regarding the patient's values and goals (Elwyn et al., 2010; Health Foundation, 2010).

Ideally, clinicians will gain a good understanding of a patient's values and goals in the context of a long-term therapeutic relationship. However, in many areas the delivery of health care is often fragmented, such that patients are often cared for by providers who have no prior experience with them. In such instances, questions that may be helpful in eliciting a patient's values and health-care goals may include: *What is most important to you when you think about your health? What are you hoping for? What are your most important goals? What are your biggest fears about the future? Are there specific health states you would find unacceptable (for example, being a ventilator, dependent on others)?*

A shared decision-making model is a significant departure from how medicine is often practiced (Carlet et al., 2004; Cohen et al., 2005). Indeed, in some countries/cultures, it may be unacceptable to even discuss withholding or withdrawing of LST with a patient or base decisions on the patient's preferences and/or assessment of his/her quality of life (Thompson et al., 2004; Searight and Gafford, 2005). Nevertheless, we feel that a shared decision-making model is ideally suited to end-of-life care for several reasons. First, in the context of end-of-life decisions, data have shown that physicians are not only inaccurate in predicting what treatments their patients would want if they were seriously ill (Uhlmann et al., 1988) but also consistently underestimate a patient's quality of life (Uhlmann and Pearlman, 1991). The latter is exacerbated by the finding that ICU physicians and nurses place higher value on quality of life as opposed to quantity of life compared to patients and families (Sprung et al., 2007a). As a result, physicians are frequently biased toward withholding and withdrawing LST compared to their patients (Uhlmann and Pearlman, 1991). Second, a 2009 systematic review of 55 randomized controlled trials conducted over a 25-year period showed that patients involved in shared decision-making made clearer treatment decisions, were more likely to decline discretionary surgical intervention when compared to their doctors, and were no worse off in terms of health outcomes (O'Connor et al., 2009; Stacey et al., 2011). Third, what constitutes an acceptable quality of life for any given patient and how to weigh the benefits and burdens of treatment in this regard can only be truly known by that individual. It is therefore imperative that clinicians do not allow their own views on quality of life to unduly influence their assessment of whether it is appropriate to withhold/withdraw LST. Finally, on a related note, a decision regarding withholding/withdrawing LST will almost inevitably involve a judgement based upon values and goals and, while the physician remains the expert on the medical treatments, the patient is the only true expert on his/her values and goals. Understanding the patient's values and goals is therefore a crucial step in making an ethically sound recommendation and enabling patient autonomy.

It is important to note that we are not advocating leaving patients to make decisions on their own, which is a misunderstanding of patient autonomy and respect for persons. We have noticed that many practising physicians in the United States are less likely to make specific treatment recommendations. Instead they opt to present a range of treatment options without identifying which is best, ostensibly as a means of promoting patient choice and autonomy. However, such an approach actually withholds the expert opinion of the physician and not only risks causing harm to the patient but also places unreasonable and unwanted responsibility on patients and their families, especially in the context of end-of-life decision-making (Billings and Krakauer, 2011).

If a patient has decision-making capacity, determining their preference for LST is usually straightforward, although this may require extended discussion regarding the patient's health-care values and goals and how utilizing or forgoing LST will achieve those goals. Occasionally, even if a person has capacity, they may not wish to be involved in the decision-making process, due either to their personality, coping style, and/or cultural background (Azoulay et al., 2004; Searight and Gafford, 2005; Kelley et al., 2010). For instance, patients of some religious and cultural backgrounds will usually defer decision-making to family members or a religious authority (Kelley et al., 2010). Thus, it is important to ascertain the desire of each patient to participate in the decision-making process. Notwithstanding that, most patients still prefer to be informed that their condition is life threatening (Yun et al., 2010). Thus, even in cases where the patient does not want to play a major role in decision-making, it is essential to keep the person well informed of the basic information.

If a patient lacks capacity, determining their preference for LST is more complicated, but can usually be achieved via ADs and/or surrogate decision-makers as described next.

Advance directives

ADs are legal documents outlining preferences for end-of-life care and can take the form either of a document outlining one's goals, values, and preferences regarding end-of-life treatments (including a living will, instructional directive, and values history) or of a health-care proxy form (where one appoints a proxy to make health-care decisions if capacity is lost) (Gillick, 2004).

The clinical utility of ADs has been widely debated. On the one hand, ADs promote early discussion about death and dying, help to alleviate patients' anxiety about future decisions, guide decision-making when capacity is lost, and reduce stress, depression, and anxiety in surviving relatives (Detering et al., 2010).

On the other hand, ADs have major limitations. First, individuals find it very difficult to predict what they will want when they are seriously ill (Danis et al., 1994; Loewenstein, 2005; Ubel et al., 2005). Second, only a minority of patients have completed ADs (only 29% of US adults had ADs according to a 2005 survey) (Pew Research Center for the People and the Press, 2006). Third, even when an AD exists, they are often difficult to locate or too vague to be of any use (Gillick, 2010).

Allowing for these caveats, clinicians should at the very least inquire about the existence of an AD and follow the AD if it is applicable to the situation at hand. In many US states, patients' treatment preferences have been converted into medical orders (e.g. MOLST (Medical Orders for Life-Sustaining Treatment) and POLST (Physician Orders for Life-Sustaining Treatment)) that are portable and legally upheld throughout the state's health-care system, whether the patient is in hospital, a nursing home, or at home.

Surrogate decision-making

In the event of incapacity, current bioethical thinking favours the idea that in order to protect autonomy, physicians should liaise with a surrogate decision-maker who, ideally aided by ADs, can assist in determining the patient's goals, values, and preferences (Buchanan and Brock, 1989). At a practical level, this raises two questions.

First, who should be the surrogate? Ideally, the patient will have specified a proxy decision-maker via an AD. However, usually this is not the case, and it falls to the next of kin or else the person with the strongest genetic and/or emotional ties to the patient. Interestingly, studies of patients in the ICU have found that family members are frequently too emotionally distressed to make decisions regarding their loved ones (Pochard et al., 2001). Despite this, there is general academic agreement and support from many court decisions that close family members are in the best position to make decisions because they are most likely to know the patient's values and goals (President's Commission for the Study of Ethical Problems in Medicine and Biomedical and Behavioral Research, 1983).

Second, how should a surrogate decision-maker decide whether or not to forgo LST? In principle, surrogate decision-makers are supposed to use 'substituted judgement', that is, what the patient would have chosen. In some cases, this will be indicated in an AD or have been discussed previously with the patient. In the remaining cases, surrogate decision-makers should base the decision to withhold/withdraw LST on the patient's known values and goals or, if these are unknown, on what would generally be considered best for the patient (Pope, 2012). In reality however, achieving accurate substituted judgement is challenging (Emanuel and Emanuel, 1992). This was exemplified by one study which found that more than 30% of approximately 2600 surrogates incorrectly predicted patients' end-of-life treatment preferences, and that prior discussion regarding preferences between patients and their surrogates failed to improve the accuracy rate (Shalowitz et al., 2006).

Resolving conflict

Not surprisingly, there can be significant disagreement as to whether or not to withhold/withdraw LST. In such cases, trying to better understand the nature of the conflict can be very helpful. In particular, we usually try to address two key areas.

First, what is the nature of the conflict? For example, is there an ethical dilemma (e.g. is this the right thing to do?)? Is there legal uncertainty (e.g. is what I am doing prohibited by law?)? Or perhaps there is still clinical uncertainty (e.g. uncertain prognosis, uncertain benefit?)? Or a combination thereof? In answering the questions, clinicians will often be able to identify suitable strategies for moving forwards and obtaining resolution. For instance, where there are ethical problems, re-evaluating the relevant bioethical principles and/or consulting ethics committees can provide additional clarity. Where there are legal uncertainties, seeking proper legal counsel is important. And where there is clinical uncertainty, obtaining additional evidence from the literature and consulting with other colleagues can be helpful.

Second, where is the conflict arising? Is it within the treating team? Between the team and the patient/family? Or among the patient and their family? For conflicts within the treating team, an independent mediator can be helpful to draw out the relevant clinical issues and re-direct focus to achieving an outcome in best accordance with the patient's values and goals.

For conflict between the team and the patient/family, the role of good communication cannot be overstated. For example, studies in the ICU suggest that many families lack even a basic understanding of a patient's diagnosis, prognosis, and treatment options (Azoulay et al., 2000), and that better and more frequent communication is associated with greater consensus between families and medical teams regarding ICU treatment (Prendergast, 1997; Garros et al., 2003). Along similar lines, remembering that the emotional distress of families in ICU impairs their ability to make decisions on a patient's behalf (Pochard et al., 2001), addressing this distress either directly or with the support of social workers, psychologists, and/or nursing staff, can assist the therapeutic relationship and may also aid in resolving or avoiding conflict (McDonagh et al., 2004; Stapleton et al., 2006) as well as improve the mental health of surviving relatives (Lautrette et al., 2007). Adoption of mediation techniques such as the 'principled negotiation' approach (Fisher et al., 2011) can help to focus attention on common interests rather than individuals and emotions and may be a useful tool for resolving end-of-life conflicts (Burns and Truog, 2007). In addition, hospital ethics committees—if available—can be an invaluable resource to not only provide an opinion on valid ethical options but also help with conflict resolution (Schneiderman et al., 2003).

There sometimes remain cases that cannot be resolved despite good communication. For instance, some patients and families will want to 'do everything' to maintain life regardless of the quality of life or the chances of 'success', leaving clinicians in moral distress about providing inappropriate LST. If clinicians truly believe surrogates are making decisions that are harmful to a patient, an application to appoint a different surrogate decision-maker can be made to the courts. In the rare cases where there is in fact no real harm to the patient, one option that has been suggested is that care be continued and that the focus should be on finding additional ways to support the medical staff to minimize the damage to the morale of the treating team (Burns and Truog, 2007).

Finally, for conflicts between the patient and their families, it is important to maintain focus on the patient's goals and, again, support from colleagues in social work, psychology, and chaplaincy can be of tremendous assistance.

Withdrawing/withholding life-sustaining treatment

Once a decision to withhold/withdraw LST is made, it is important to make a clear treatment plan to manage the likelihood that the patient will become more symptomatic following the withdrawal/withholding of LST (Truog et al., 2008). The presence of interdisciplinary palliative care teams may help alleviate patient, family, and staff distress around the time of withholding or withdrawing LST. It is also important to carefully document the decision-making process, the consent of families and patients, the withdrawal process (if applicable), and the treatment of symptoms until death.

Before LST is withdrawn, clinicians should inform families of the expected signs of the dying process, including Cheyne–Stokes respiration, skin mottling, and increased secretions. Families should be given an approximation of how long the patient is expected to live but also advised of the possibility that death may not be as soon as expected. In the event there is prolonged time between withdrawal and death, opioids, sedatives and all medications should be administered in doses necessary for the patient's comfort. Attempts should also be made to avoid unnecessary interventions during this time, including monitoring devices, alarms, blood tests, intravenous fluids, and so on (Truog et al., 2008).

At the same time, it is important to provide psychosocial support not only to patients and their families but also clinicians. The decision to withhold or withdraw LST is emotionally charged for all involved, and existential and spiritual issues may become more prominent as death nears. Referrals to psychology, social work, and chaplaincy can be helpful where available and appropriate. Families should also be allowed adequate time with the patient to say their goodbyes. Ongoing support via bereavement services is valuable in aiding families after death and a forum or other professional services for clinicians to debrief may help to decrease burnout and distress amongst professional staff (Felton, 1998; Bar-Sela et al., 2012).

Notes on specific life-sustaining treatments

Here, we consider specific information pertaining to several common LSTs.

Cardiopulmonary resuscitation

Background

In 1960, Kouwenhoven and colleagues first described CPR as a medical intervention for cardiac arrest (Kouwenhoven et al., 1960). The success of this simple technique, originally used in the perioperative setting and in newly established coronary care units, was subsequently applied to anyone who suffered a cardiopulmonary arrest both in and outside the hospital. In 1973, the National Conference on Standards for CPR and Emergency Cardiac Care in the United States recommended universal use of CPR for sudden death. Today, presumed consent for CPR is still the norm in US hospitals and CPR is generally attempted whenever the heart stops.

Outcomes of CPR

The outcomes of CPR are generally quite poor. Unlike on TV where 67% of TV hospital patients who undergo CPR survive to discharge (Diem et al., 1996), in reality the success rate is considerably lower (15–18%) (Saklayen et al., 1995; Ehlenbach et al., 2009). Moreover, among high-risk patients, the prognosis is even more discouraging with survival to discharge rates of only 6–8% in those with hepatic insufficiency, haematological malignancy, metastatic cancer, or septicaemia (Larkin et al., 2010). Similarly, both advanced age and low pre-existing functioning are predictors of poor survival following CPR. For example, cancer patients with poor performance status at the time of admission (e.g. spending > 50% of time in bed) had only a 2.3% chance of surviving to discharge after receiving CPR (Vitelli et al., 1991). Indeed, the only cancer patients likely to survive to hospital discharge after CPR are those with good functional status who suffer an acute insult such as medication-induced cardiac toxicity (Faber-Langendoen, 1991). Thus, when cardiac arrest results directly or indirectly from advanced life-threatening illness, CPR is very unlikely to enable a patient to be discharged home.

Discussing code status

As clinicians and the public have become more aware of the poor outcomes associated with CPR—not to mention the likelihood of secondary chest pain and rib fractures—decisions not to attempt resuscitation using DNR (do not resuscitate) or AND (allow natural death) orders have become commonplace. Discussion of a patient's so-called 'code status' (i.e. whether or not to attempt CPR in the event of cardiac arrest) is therefore now quite common in places such as the United States, although most physicians lack adequate training in how to conduct such conversations (Anderson et al., 2011).

Like any LST, CPR is a medical intervention that requires a clinician to make a recommendation based on its likely outcomes and the patient's values and goals. We would therefore advise adopting the general approach we described earlier using a shared decision-making model to determine whether or not to utilize CPR. In actively dying patients or patients with significant co-morbid disease (e.g. multiorgan failure, metastatic cancer, advanced dementia), CPR is unlikely to prolong survival and should not be recommended (Blinderman et al., 2012).

Patient with a do not resuscitate/do not intubate (DNR/DNI) order requiring operative or sedative procedures

In some cases, suspension of DNR/DNI orders is appropriate. Ultimately, a decision will be made in light of a patient's values and health-care goals. For example, if a patient is planning to undergo a palliative procedure that would deliver good symptom relief, and expects post-operatively to have a reasonable quality of life and whose goal is prolongation of life and comfort, a suspension of the DNR/DNI order may be appropriate. In other cases, the patient or proxy decision-maker may prefer that no attempts to prolong life be made, even if the patient were to likely recover from an intraoperative cardiopulmonary arrest. In any case, the risks and benefits of the procedure should be made explicit with the patient or proxy decision-maker (American College of Surgeons, 1994) and a clear plan should be made with the responsible physician and the consulting interventionalist for the perioperative period.

Mechanical ventilation

Stopping mechanical ventilation is one of the most commonly performed withdrawals of LST. This issue is addressed in detail in Chapter 10.7.

Cardiac and circulatory support

Both continuous and intermittent inotrope therapy can provide symptomatic relief in patients at the end of life and may form part of a patient's hospice care plan (Stevenson, 2003; Lopez-Candales et al., 2004). Similar to other LSTs, the discontinuation or limitation of inotrope therapy should be considered when the therapy is no longer consistent with the values and goals of the patient, especially when continuation of inotropes seems only to be prolonging the dying process.

The deactivation or removal of cardiac and circulatory support devices, such as pacemakers, ventricular assist devices (VADs) and extracorporeal membrane oxygenation (ECMO), should be considered when such devices are no longer meeting the patient's goals, prolonging the dying process against the wishes of the patient, or when the benefits are outweighed by the burdens. The withdrawal of these devices is emotionally charged, since patients typically die shortly after the device is discontinued. Indeed, some describe these acts of withdrawal as 'justified killing' (Brock, 1992).

One scenario that is becoming increasingly common is the alert patient with a VAD or ECMO that has become a 'bridge to nowhere'. In such cases, the patient will usually have had a VAD or ECMO placed, as a bridge to future transplantation or to enable more time for clinicians to assess the patient's condition and prognosis and suitable treatment options, but subsequently become unsuitable candidates for either long-term device therapy (e.g. CentriMag®) or transplantation. Such patients thereby become confined to the critical care environment for the remainder of their lives and—although death will inevitably result from comorbid illness, an acquired nosocomial infection, or complications related to the device—discomfort about withdrawal of the device is inevitable as some of these patients appear 'well' and are not actively dying. Ultimately, the decision to discontinue the device rests with the patient and family, and withdrawal against patient or family objections should not be done (Abrams, et al., 2014). Ethical dilemmas encountered with the use of extracorporeal membrane oxygenation in adults. *Chest.* 145(4), 876–882). However, a disaster setting or serious epidemic that requires the availability of LST such as ECMO may change the ethical calculus in patients maintained on such therapies, but are not believed to survive to hospital discharge (Powell et al., 2008).

Haemodialysis

Interestingly, the withholding and withdrawing of haemodialysis frequently appears more acceptable to many people, since the patient is perceived to die more 'naturally'. Contrary to popular belief, death from uraemia is not symptom free but is often associated with symptoms such as pain, agitation, myoclonus/ muscle twitching, dyspnoea, pruritis, and nausea, particularly in the last 24 hours of life (Cohen et al., 2000; Murtagh et al., 2007a, 2007b; Kane et al., 2013). Appropriate symptom assessment and management must therefore be incorporated into the care plan in patients who decline or discontinue haemodialysis (Moss, 2000), and collaboration with renal specialists to ensure appropriate selection and dosing of medications is desirable. If severe agitation or delirium develops, neuroleptics and sedatives may be necessary. Discussions with the patients and their families regarding expected survival times post withdrawal of dialysis should occur: in patients with no renal function, average survival is 8–12 days (Sekkarie and Moss, 1998; Murtagh et al., 2007b).

Artificial nutrition and hydration

Patients with advanced disease (including dementia) often lose interest in food and drink, which frequently prompts the use of ANH. However, although effective in providing short-term support for acutely ill patients, ANH is unlikely to increase life expectancy in patients with advanced disease (Borum et al., 2000). In fact, ANH may actually add to suffering or even decrease life expectancy due to various complications such as line sepsis, aspiration pneumonia, diarrhoea, hypervolemia, as well as pressure ulcers, pain and local infection at the feeding tube site (Quill, 1989; Finucane et al., 1999; McClave and Chang, 2003; Casarett et al., 2005).

Despite the lack of strong evidence to support the use of ANH at the end of life, religious and cultural beliefs frequently support its use and oppose its withdrawal (Geppert et al., 2010). For example, according to Catholic, orthodox Jewish, and Islamic authorities, ANH has a special status and may not simply be removed in the same way. For example, ANH is considered basic humane care rather than medical treatment for devout Catholics (Pope John Paul II, 2004). That being said, one may be allowed to withhold or withdraw ANH if it is adjudged likely to cause more harm than benefit (Alsolamy, 2014). Similarly, for many cultures, food is believed to be necessary for the comfort of the patient, eliciting concerns that patients may be 'starving'. This issue needs to be approached with great care and sensitivity, and families can be reassured that once the patient no longer has the desire to eat the mechanism by which they feel hunger is no longer present and that the alleviation of thirst can be achieved by stopping anticholinergic medications, and providing good mouth care, ice chips, and sips of water (Burge, 1993; McCann et al., 1994).

Legally, US appellate courts have consistently found not only that ANH is a medical procedure that can be forgone in the same manner as other treatments but also that the cause of death is the disease that causes the inability to eat rather than the lack of nutrition itself (*Cruzan v. Director, Missouri Department of Health*, 1990). For example, in the highly publicized case of 'Terri' Schiavo, a woman who had been in a PVS for 8 years, her husband (and guardian) requested that ANH be withdrawn against the objections of her parents, and the Florida Supreme Court subsequently affirmed that her husband could exercise her right to discontinue treatments. After successive court appeals, the US Supreme Court refused to hear the case but reaffirmed the right to refuse medical treatments including ANH. Similarly, federal regulations and judiciary precedence in the US recognize that residents in long-term care facilities have the right to refuse all medical treatments including ANH (*Bouvia v Superior Court*, 1986; Department of Health and Human Services, 1989).

Antibiotics

Patients have a right to discontinue any and all medical treatments, including those that may be effective, like antibiotics for specific infections. The continuation or discontinuation of antibiotics is a highly contextualized medical decision at the end of life and antibiotics should not be withheld as a matter of policy from patients on hospice or those who wish to focus exclusively on comfort. In some cases, when the goal of care is to focus exclusively on comfort, starting or continuing antibiotics may assist in symptom relief (e.g. reduction of fevers from a bacterial infection) (White et al., 2003). On the other hand, discontinuation of antibiotics may be reasonable if the goal is no longer life prolongation, as antibiotics may prolong the dying process in patients with a terminal condition and acute infection.

Withdrawal/withholding of LST in the setting of severe neurological impairment

Patients with severe neurological injury may present a diagnostic dilemma that must be resolved if the withdrawal/withholding of LST is being considered. Specifically, clinicians should discriminate between patients in a PVS and those in a minimally conscious state (MCS), since management of the two is quite different. A patient in a PVS by definition lacks consciousness and therefore does not experience pain or dyspnoea and has no awareness of suffering. A MCS in contrast shows intermittent evidence of consciousness and offers the chance of further recovery. Despite these important differences, up to 40% of patients have been wrongly diagnosed as being in a PVS when in fact they have been in a MCS (Schnakers et al., 2009), highlighting the need to more accurately differentiate the two conditions (see Chapter 5.3).

In managing a patient in a PVS, the lack of consciousness is an important clinical factor that influences management. For example, if families perceive some behaviours as being signs of distress (e.g. reflexive coughing, posturing, secretions, tremors, respiratory patterns, and other physical signs), clinicians can gently and compassionately provide reassurance that the patient does not perceive these signs as distressful. Some have argued that for patients in a PVS, the focus of the clinician should turn to serving the best interests of the family rather than the patient who no longer has any true interests (Arras, 1991). In such cases, clinicians may therefore choose to treat upsetting physical signs not to alleviate suffering in the patient but to contain the family's distress.

In managing a patient in a MCS, it is important to optimize the conditions for neurological recovery and to attempt to communicate with them given the potential for awareness. Clinicians should also familiarize themselves with any special rules governing those in MCS. For example, in England and Wales, all decisions relating to the withdrawal or withholding of ANH in patients in MCS must be referred to the Court for a judicial ruling (*Airedale Hospital Trustees v Bland*, 1993; Mental Capacity Act 2005, 2005).

In patients where there is uncertainty about the neurological status of the patient, or the patient is found to have MCS, the same approach for non-neurologically injured patients should be employed when mechanical ventilation is withdrawn.

Conclusion

The appropriate use of LSTs in seriously ill patients is a controversial topic that continues to generate intense debate amongst private citizens as well as health-care professionals, bioethicists, lawyers, government, and religious institutions. Decisions to withhold/withdraw LST are difficult and will remain so. Ultimately, a clinician's approach to the issue of withdrawing and withholding LST will be influenced by many factors that shape the relationship between the patient and the physician/health-care system, and include the individual culture of the hospital/clinic in which a clinician works, the broader health-care system of a country and the historical developmental of that system, the availability of health-care resources, the ethical values and cultural norms dominant in that society, religious practices/beliefs, the legal system, as well as government policies.

Online materials

Complete references for this chapter are available online at <http://www.oxfordmedicine.com>.

References

Abrams, D.M., Prager, K., Blinderman, C.D., Burkart, K.M., Brodie, D. Ethical dilemmas encountered with the use of extracorporeal membrane oxygenation in adults. *Chest.* 2014 Apr;145(4):876–882.

Airedale Hospital Trustees v Bland (1993). UKHL 5 (4 February 1993).

Anonymous (1992). Decisions near the end of life. Council on Ethical and Judicial Affairs, American Medical Association. *Journal of the American Medical Association*, 267, 2229–2233.

Appelbaum, P.S. (2007). Clinical practice. Assessment of patients' competence to consent to treatment. *The New England Journal of Medicine*, 357, 1834–1840.

Arras, J.D. (1991). Beyond Cruzan: individual rights, family autonomy and the persistent vegetative state. *Journal of the American Geriatrics Society*, 39, 1018–1024.

Azoulay, E., Chevret, S., Leleu, G., *et al.* (2000). Half the families of intensive care unit patients experience inadequate communication with physicians. *Critical Care Medicine*, 28, 3044–3049.

Azoulay, E., Pochard, F., Chevret, S., *et al.* (2004). Half the family members of intensive care unit patients do not want to share in the decision-making process: a study in 78 French intensive care units. *Critical Care Medicine*, 32, 1832–1838.

Bar-Sela, G., Lulav-Grinwald, D., and Mitnik, I. (2012). 'Balint group' meetings for oncology residents as a tool to improve therapeutic communication skills and reduce burnout level. *Journal of Cancer Education*, 27, 786–789.

Beauchamp, T.L. and Childress, J.F. (2009). *Principles of Biomedical Ethics*. New York: Oxford University Press.

Blank, R.H. (2011). End-of-life decision making across cultures. *Journal of Law, Medicine & Ethics*, 39, 201–214.

Blinderman, C.D., Krakauer, E.L., and Solomon, M.Z. (2012). Time to revise the approach to determining cardiopulmonary resuscitation status. *Journal of the American Medical Association*, 307, 917–918.

Borum, M.L., Lynn, J., Zhong, Z., *et al.* (2000). The effect of nutritional supplementation on survival in seriously ill hospitalized adults: an evaluation of the SUPPORT data. Study to Understand Prognoses and Preferences for Outcomes and Risks of Treatments. *Journal of the American Geriatrics Society*, 48, S33–38.

Brett, A.S. and McCullough, L.B. (2012). Addressing requests by patients for nonbeneficial interventions. *Journal of the American Medical Association*, 307, 149–150.

Brock, D.W. (1992). Voluntary active euthanasia. *Hastings Center Report*, 22, 10–22.

Brock, D.W. (1997). Death and dying. In R.M. Veatch (ed.) *Medical Ethics* (2nd ed.), pp. 363–394. Sudbury, MA: Jones and Bartlett Publishers.

Burns, J.P. and Truog, R.D. (2007). Futility: a concept in evolution. *Chest*, 132, 1987–1993.

Casarett, D., Kapo, J., and Caplan, A. (2005). Appropriate use of artificial nutrition and hydration—fundamental principles and recommendations. *The New England Journal of Medicine*, 353, 2607–2612.

Charles, C., Gafni, A., and Whelan, T. (1997). Shared decision-making in the medical encounter: what does it mean? (or it takes at least two to tango). *Social Science & Medicine*, 44, 681–692.

Cohen, L.M., Germain, M., Poppel, D.M., Woods, A., and Kjellstrand, C.M. (2000). Dialysis discontinuation and palliative care. *American Journal of Kidney Diseases*, 36, 140–144.

Cohen, S., Sprung, C., Sjokvist, P., *et al.* (2005). Communication of end-of-life decisions in European intensive care units. *Intensive Care Medicine*, 31, 1215–1221.

Cruzan v. Director, Missouri Department of Health (1990). 497 U.S. 261.

Department of Health and Human Services (1989). Medicare and Medicaid: requirements for long term care facilities (comment to 42 CFR 483.10(b)(4)). *Federal Register*, 54, 5316–5321.

Drane, J.F. (1985). The many faces of competency. *Hastings Center Report*, 15, 17–21.

Dunn, L.B., Nowrangi, M.A., Palmer, B.W., Jeste, D.V., and Saks, E.R. (2006). Assessing decisional capacity for clinical research or treatment: a review of instruments. *American Journal of Psychiatry*, 163, 1323–1334.

Ehlenbach, W.J., Barnato, A.E., Curtis, J.R., *et al.* (2009). Epidemiologic study of in-hospital cardiopulmonary resuscitation in the elderly. *The New England Journal of Medicine*, 361, 22–31.

Etchells, E., Darzins, P., Silberfeld, M., *et al.* (1999). Assessment of patient capacity to consent to treatment. *Journal of General Internal Medicine*, 14, 27–34.

Faber-Langendoen, K. (1991). Resuscitation of patients with metastatic cancer. Is transient benefit still futile? *Archives of Internal Medicine*, 151, 235–239.

Felton, J.S. (1998). Burnout as a clinical entity—its importance in health care workers. *Occupational Medicine*, 48, 237–250.

Fine, R.L. (2009). Point: the Texas advance directives act effectively and ethically resolves disputes about medical futility. *Chest*, 136, 963–967.

Fitten, L.J. and Waite, M.S. (1990). Impact of medical hospitalization on treatment decision-making capacity in the elderly. *Archives of Internal Medicine*, 150, 1717–1721.

Gillick, M.R. (2004). Advance care planning. *The New England Journal of Medicine*, 350, 7–8.

Gillick, M.R. (2010). Reversing the code status of advance directives? *The New England Journal of Medicine*, 362, 1239–1240.

Grisso T. and Appelbaum, P. (1998). *Assessing Competence to Consent to Treatment: A Guide for Physicians and Other Health Professionals*. Oxford: Oxford University Press.

In re Quinlan. (1976). 70 N.J. 10, 355 A.2d 647 (NJ 1976)).

Kane, P.M., Vinen, K., and Murtagh, F.E. (2013). Palliative care for advanced renal disease: a summary of the evidence and future direction. *Palliative Medicine*, 27(9), 817–821.

Kant, I. and Gregor, M.J. (1998). *Groundwork of the Metaphysics of Morals*. Cambridge: Cambridge University Press.

Kelley, A.S., Wenger, N.S., and Sarkisian, C.A. (2010). Opiniones: end-of-life care preferences and planning of older Latinos. *Journal of the American Geriatrics Society*, 58, 1109–1116.

Kouwenhoven, W.B., Jude, J.R., and Knickerbocker, G.G. (1960). Closed-chest cardiac massage. *Journal of the American Medical Association*, 173, 1064–1067.

Larkin, G.L., Copes, W.S., Nathanson, B.H., and Kaye, W. (2010). Pre-resuscitation factors associated with mortality in 49,130 cases of in-hospital cardiac arrest: a report from the National Registry for Cardiopulmonary Resuscitation. *Resuscitation*, 81, 302–311.

Lautrette, A., Darmon, M., Megarbane, B., *et al.* (2007). A communication strategy and brochure for relatives of patients dying in the ICU. *The New England Journal of Medicine*, 356, 469–478.

Lopez-Candales, A.L., Carron, C., and Schwartz, J. (2004). Need for hospice and palliative care services in patients with end-stage heart failure treated with intermittent infusion of inotropes. *Clinical Cardiology*, 27, 23–28.

Luce, J.M. (1995). Physicians do not have a responsibility to provide futile or unreasonable care if a patient or family insists. *Critical Care Medicine*, 23, 760–766.

Marson, D.C., Mcinturff, B., Hawkins, L., Bartolucci, A., and Harrell, L.E. (1997). Consistency of physician judgments of capacity to consent in mild Alzheimer's disease. *Journal of the American Geriatrics Society*, 45, 453–457.

McCann, R.M., Hall, W.J., and Groth-Juncker, A. (1994). Comfort care for terminally ill patients. The appropriate use of nutrition and hydration. *Journal of the American Medical Association*, 272, 1263–1266.

McCrary, S.V. and Swanson, J.W. (1999). Physicians' legal defensiveness and knowledge of medical law: comparing Denmark and the USA. *Scandinavian Journal of Public Health*, 27, 18–21.

McCrary, S.V., Swanson, J.W., Perkins, H.S., and Winslade, W.J. (1992). Treatment decisions for terminally ill patients: physicians' legal defensiveness and knowledge of medical law. *Law, Medicine & Health Care*, 20, 364–376.

McDonagh, J.R., Elliott, T.B., Engelberg, R.A., *et al.* (2004). Family satisfaction with family conferences about end-of-life care in the intensive care unit: increased proportion of family speech is associated with increased satisfaction. *Critical Care Medicine*, 32, 1484–1488.

Mental Capacity Act 2005 (2005). London: The Stationery Office.

Murtagh, F.E., Addington-Hall, J.M., Edmonds, P.M., *et al.* (2007b). Symptoms in advanced renal disease: a cross-sectional survey of symptom prevalence in stage 5 chronic kidney disease managed without dialysis. *Journal of Palliative Medicine*, 10, 1266–1276.

Patient Self-Determination Act (1990). P.L. 101–508 (5 November 1990).

Pence, G.E. (1995). *Classic Cases in Medical Ethics: Accounts of Cases That Have Shaped Medical Ethics, with Philosophical, Legal, and Historical Backgrounds*. New York: McGraw-Hill.

Pew Research Center for the People and the Press. (2006). *More Americans Discussing and Planning End-Of-Life Treatment*. Washington, DC: Pew Research Center for the People and the Press.

Pochard, F., Azoulay, E., Chevret, S., *et al.* (2001). Symptoms of anxiety and depression in family members of intensive care unit patients: ethical hypothesis regarding decision-making capacity. *Critical Care Medicine*, 29, 1893–1897.

Prendergast, T.J. (1997). Resolving conflicts surrounding end-of-life care. *New Horizons*, 5, 62–71.

President's Commission for the Study of Ethical Problems in Medicine and Biomedical and Behavioral Research (1982). *Making Health Care Decisions: The Legal and Ethical Implications of Informed Consent in the Patient-Practitioner Relationship*. Washington, DC: President's Commission for the Study of Ethical Problems in Medicine and Biomedical and Behavioral Research.

President's Commission for the Study of Ethical Problems in Medicine and Biomedical and Behavioral Research (1983). *Deciding to Forego Life-Sustaining Treatment: A Report on the Ethical, Medical, and Legal Issues in Treatment Decisions*. Washington, DC: President's Commission for the Study of Ethical Problems in Medicine and Biomedical and Behavioral Research.

Quill, T.E., Lo, B., and Brock, D.W. (1997). Palliative options of last resort: a comparison of voluntarily stopping eating and drinking, terminal sedation, physician-assisted suicide, and voluntary active euthanasia. *Journal of the American Medical Association*, 278, 2099–2104.

Raymont, V., Bingley, W., Buchanan, A., *et al.* (2004). Prevalence of mental incapacity in medical inpatients and associated risk factors: cross-sectional study. *The Lancet*, 364, 1421–1427.

Saklayen, M., Liss, H., and Markert, R. (1995). In-hospital cardiopulmonary resuscitation. Survival in 1 hospital and literature review. *Medicine (Baltimore)*, 74, 163–175.

Schnakers, C., Vanhaudenhuyse, A., Giacino, J., *et al.* (2009). Diagnostic accuracy of the vegetative and minimally conscious state: clinical consensus versus standardized neurobehavioral assessment. *BMC Neurology*, 9, 35.

Schneiderman, L.J., Gilmer, T., Teetzel, H.D., *et al.* (2003). Effect of ethics consultations on nonbeneficial life-sustaining treatments in the intensive care setting: a randomized controlled trial. *Journal of the American Medical Association*, 290, 1166–1172.

Schneiderman, L.J., Jecker, N.S., and Jonsen, A.R. (1990). Medical futility: its meaning and ethical implications. *Annals of Internal Medicine*, 112, 949–954.

Searight, H.R. and Gafford, J. (2005). Cultural diversity at the end of life: issues and guidelines for family physicians. *American Family Physician*, 71, 515–522.

Sekkarie, M.A. and Moss, A.H. (1998). Withholding and withdrawing dialysis: the role of physician specialty and education and patient functional status. *American Journal of Kidney Diseases*, 31, 464–472.

Shalowitz, D.I., Garrett-Mayer, E., and Wendler, D. (2006). The accuracy of surrogate decision makers: a systematic review. *Archives of Internal Medicine*, 166, 493–497.

Shannon T.A. and Walter, J. (1993). The PVS patient and the foregoing/withdrawing of medical nutrition and hydration. In T.A. Shannon (ed.) *Bioethics: Basic Writings on the Key Ethical Questions that Surround the Major, Modern Biological Possibilities and Problems* (4th ed.), pp. 173–198. Mahwah, NJ: Paulist Press.

Silveira, M.J., Kim, S.Y., and Langa, K.M. (2010). Advance directives and outcomes of surrogate decision making before death. *The New England Journal of Medicine*, 362, 1211–1218.

Sprung, C.L., Carmel, S., Sjokvist, P., *et al.* (2007a). Attitudes of European physicians, nurses, patients, and families regarding end-of-life decisions: the ETHICATT study. *Intensive Care Medicine*, 33, 104–110.

Thompson, B.T., Cox, P.N., Antonelli, M., *et al.* (2004). Challenges in end-of-life care in the ICU: statement of the 5th International Consensus Conference in Critical Care: Brussels, Belgium, April 2003: executive summary. *Critical Care Medicine*, 32, 1781–1784.

Truog, R.D., Campbell, M.L., Curtis, J.R., *et al.* (2008). Recommendations for end-of-life care in the intensive care unit: a consensus statement by the American College [corrected] of Critical Care Medicine. *Critical Care Medicine*, 36, 953–963.

Uhlmann, R.F. and Pearlman, R.A. (1991). Perceived quality of life and preferences for life-sustaining treatment in older adults. *Archives of Internal Medicine*, 151, 495–497.

Uhlmann, R.F., Pearlman, R.A., and Cain, K.C. (1988). Physicians' and spouses' predictions of elderly patients' resuscitation preferences. *Journal of Gerontology*, 43, M115–121.

Vacco v Quill (1997). 521 U.S. 793.

Vitelli, C.E., Cooper, K., Rogatko, A., and Brennan, M. F. (1991). Cardiopulmonary resuscitation and the patient with cancer. *Journal of Clinical Oncology*, 9, 111–115.

Washington v Glucksberg (1997). 521 U.S. 702.

Yun, Y.H., Kwon, Y.C., Lee, M.K., *et al.* (2010). Experiences and attitudes of patients with terminal cancer and their family caregivers toward the disclosure of terminal illness. *Journal of Clinical Oncology*, 28, 1950–1957.

SECTION 6

Communication and palliative medicine

Communication with the patient and family

Thomas W. LeBlanc and James A. Tulsky

Introduction to communication with the patient and family

High-quality palliative medicine depends upon good communication, which can enhance the quality of care we provide while also improving patient and family satisfaction (Kaplan et al., 1989; Roter et al., 1995; Bertakis et al., 1991). Good communication fosters informed decision-making by improving the likelihood that patient choices remain consistent with individuals' stated goals, values, and preferences. This is particularly true at moments when patients and families face gut-wrenching dilemmas which require relatively sudden and difficult decisions to be made, often without sufficient certainty about the likely outcomes. Finally, by guiding terminally ill patients away from ineffective treatments towards care that is more likely to help them achieve realistic goals, good communication may also increase the delivery of high-value care (Wright et al., 2008).

Much of palliative medicine practice involves helping patients and families come to terms with serious illness and establish a care plan that reflects their goals. For example, in the United States, where 88% of hospitals with over 300 beds now have available specialist palliative care consult teams, a significant proportion of the work done by these services involves the management of difficult communication scenarios in critical care or advanced illness such as incurable cancer or end-stage heart failure (Center to Advance Palliative Care, 2012). Although symptom management is also key, communication is perhaps the most important and powerful skill that specialist palliative care clinicians bring to these cases. In fact, many palliative care clinicians believe that their specialist 'procedure' is the family meeting. Recognition of and investment in this unique skill set are important in the ongoing success and growth of palliative care as a medical specialty. Expansion of palliative care practice to the outpatient setting, where problems are no less difficult yet time constraints more prescient, further highlights the need for highly skilled communication.

While the benefits of good communication are significant, the reality can be difficult to achieve amidst the demands of daily clinical practice. In part, this difficulty stems from the enormous complexity of the clinical scenarios. For example, conflict is common within and between patients, families, and staff, and when tensions run high, communication is challenging regardless of one's skill level. In addition, clinical encounters may be further complicated by the recent disclosure of medical errors,

prior communication mistakes, or mistrust. Even in what appear to be the most routine settings challenges arise, as the skill set necessary to communicate well in clinical medicine is not necessarily intuitive, and may differ significantly from how clinicians approach communication in their personal lives.

Unfortunately, too few physicians have received adequate communication skills training and many experience low self-efficacy and avoid difficult discussions. A number of studies have documented that physicians can be taught to improve their communication skills, and such training needs to be widely disseminated (Fallowfield et al., 2002a; Back et al., 2007; Tulsky et al., 2011). Once learned, clinicians do best to assume a conscious daily practice utilizing proven communication techniques.

Difficult discussions are a reality of clinical palliative care practice. These conversations span from delivering bad news, to discussing prognosis, eliciting goals of care, identifying treatment options, and saying goodbye. They are made more challenging by high levels of emotion, cultural differences and the clinician's own prior history and attitudes. This chapter, using the available evidence, will present an outline of what comprises quality in communication and discuss the impact of communication on patient outcomes. Furthermore, we will describe what has been observed to occur in actual clinical practice, and conclude by presenting a framework with which to approach palliative care clinical encounters. We will offer concrete strategies and tips to best meet the needs of patients and families confronting serious illness.

What is 'good communication'?

As a start, all good clinical communication must meet the general criteria for 'patient-centeredness' (Institute of Medicine Committee on Quality of Health Care in America, 2001; Epstein et al., 2005; Epstein and Street, 2007). This framework includes four core components: (1) eliciting and understanding the patient's perspective, (2) understanding the patient's psychosocial context, (3) achieving a shared understanding of the problem and its appropriate treatment in the context of the patient's preferences and values, and (4) empowerment, by involving patients actively in decision-making. Patient-centred communication reflects the spirit and values inherent in palliative medicine.

Good communication, particularly in palliative medicine, must also account for the powerful role of affect, and most difficulties encountered are the result of inattention to this critical domain.

Affect refers to the feelings and emotions associated with the content of the conversation. Feelings such as anger, guilt, frustration, sadness, and fear modify our ability to hear, to communicate, and to make decisions. For example, after hearing bad news, most patients are so overwhelmed emotionally that they are unable to comprehend very much about the details of the illness or a treatment plan. Some studies have shown that emotion affects processing; people who are in negative moods may pay more attention to how messages are given than to the content of the messages (Bohner et al., 1994). Thus when patients are experiencing high levels of negative affect and caregivers do not ameliorate this affect, patients may be less likely to receive the health-care providers' messages. Unfortunately, in conversations between doctors and patients emotion is frequently not acknowledged and physicians miss opportunities to do so (Levinson et al., 2000; Pollak et al., 2007).

Physicians, as well as patients, experience many emotions as they care for people approaching the end of life. In addition to its effect on their own communication, physician affect plays an important role in patients' reactions to medical information. In one study, women were randomly assigned to view a video of an oncologist who was portrayed as either worried or not worried while presenting mammogram results. Those watching the 'worried' physician received less information, experienced higher anxiety levels, and perceived the situation as more severe compared with those watching the 'non-worried' physician (Shapiro et al., 1992).

When seriously ill patients and families are asked what is most important in their communication with physicians, several domains emerge (Wenrich et al., 2001). They want physicians to provide adequate information that is straightforward and understandable. They want clinicians to be receptive to when patients are ready to talk, and would like a balance between honesty and empathy. They want their doctors to elicit and respond to patient concerns, and they want them to attend to emotion. The overwhelming majority of patients with serious illness state that they want as much information as possible about symptoms, treatments, and side effects (Hagerty et al., 2004). However, that information is qualified, as 15–20% do not wish to discuss survival. And, among those that do want such information, they vary in when they want to hear it during the course of illness. Of note, giving more information to patients does not appear to increase anxiety, whereas greater encouragement of patient decision-making does increase stress (Gattellari et al., 2002). Patients overwhelmingly prefer an open-ended, empathic approach (Dowsett et al., 2000). They also prefer to maximize the quality of interactions, rather than the quantity thereof; when they are satisfied with the style and type of communication, patients tend to think that an encounter was longer than its actual duration (Cape, 2002).

Physicians are likely to be challenged trying to achieve a balance between being honest and straightforward and not being discouraging. Helpful approaches include leaving open the possibility that unexpected 'miracles' might happen (at least not disputing patient claims of such), discussing outcomes other than a cure that can offer patients hope and meaning, and helping patients prepare for the losses they may experience. Patients cope better when physicians emphasize what can be done, explore realistic goals, and discuss day-to-day living (Clayton et al., 2005). Although patients must receive adequate information to make informed choices,

they wish to receive that information in an emotionally supportive way (Parker et al., 2001).

Given the stress of decision-making, one might imagine that patients and families would welcome recommendations and, indeed, in a recent study of surrogate decision-makers for critically ill patients, 56% preferred a recommendation (White et al., 2009). However, given the large minority that feel otherwise and the great variability seen in communication preferences more generally, particularly from people from different cultures (Blackhall et al., 1995), we draw the conclusion that it is always prudent to ask patients and families about their communication preferences before entering into some of these sensitive topics.

Good communication in this patient population also includes techniques that allow for more accurate assessment of anxiety and depression and increased disclosure of patient concerns (Maguire et al., 1996; Fogarty et al., 1999). These include maintaining good eye contact, asking open-ended rather than closed-ended questions, focusing on the patient's concerns as well as the agenda for the visit, responding to the patient's affect, asking about the patient's life outside of their illness and the healthcare environment, attending to psychosocial concerns, and ensuring that non-verbal behaviour signifies attentiveness. In contrast, closed-ended or leading questions, focusing on physical aspects of illness, and offering of advice and premature reassurance inhibit patient disclosure of concerns (Maguire et al., 1996). Patients want to discuss emotional concerns but are frequently unwilling to bring them up spontaneously and may need to be prompted (Detmar et al., 2000).

Another quality of good communication is to 'ask before telling'. Patients often carry misperceptions or incomplete information obtained from the popular media, folklore, or friends and family. It is easier to deal with this information if it is discussed directly. Thus, it is usually helpful to ask patients about their understanding of their illness before educating them. Furthermore, one study of intensive care unit (ICU) family conferences observed that allowing families more opportunity to speak may improve family satisfaction (McDonagh et al., 2004).

Published literature also provides clear signals about factors associated with patient dissatisfaction, which further inform our approach here, and our working definition of 'good communication' in the setting of serious illness. These include a lack of warmth or friendliness, emotional distance, failure to consider patient concerns or expectations about the encounter, unclear explanations about a diagnosis or its cause, and the use of medical jargon (Korsch et al., 1968; Attree, 2001).

Finally, communication with family members includes some special considerations. Family members value being included in the decision-making process, and value open, honest communication (Tilden et al., 2001). In addition, they want assistance throughout this difficult time, whether via practical support at home, psychosocial support, or more concretely via medical equipment to facilitate daily caregiving. Providing compassionate support throughout the often foreign experience of caregiving is an important function of the palliative care team, and is facilitated by honest, open, empathic communication (Rabow et al., 2004). Family members also want honest information and disclosure. They have a dislike for the notion of 'false hope,' and feel that the avoidance of prognostic discussions and disclosure is an unacceptable way for clinicians to help them be hopeful (Apatira et al., 2008). They want to be listened to and feel heard, and there is an association between the proportion of time families speak and their rated satisfaction with clinical encounters in the intensive care setting, as well as a decreased perception of conflict (McDonagh et al., 2004). They also desire privacy, and hope to be contacted after a patient's death.

In summary, good communication in palliative medicine adopts a modern, patient-centred, biopsychosocial-spiritual framework, and focuses on eliciting patient concerns, identifying their agenda, providing complete information, but doing so in a way that allows patients and families to digest what they hear. It is respectful, empathic, inclusive, and efficient, seeks to elicit patients' goals and preferences, and to match these to an individualized plan of care. Finally, great attention is paid to the role of affect and difference, and each patient and family member is treated as a unique individual.

What are the outcomes of 'good communication?'

A growing literature describes the many benefits of good communication, particularly in the setting of palliative care and end of life. Discussions about end of life are associated with greater patient acknowledgment of terminal illness, preferences for comfort care over life extension, and receipt of less intensive, life-prolonging care and more palliative end-of-life care (Trice and Prigerson, 2009). Good communication is associated with significantly decreased anxiety in patients with cancer (Fogarty et al., 1999). Honest disclosure, along with the inclusion of sensitive yet pessimistic statements, is also associated with improved prognostic concordance between physicians and their patients (Robinson et al., 2008). Applied appropriately, good communication leads to a better matching of treatments with patients' preferences and goals.

Outside the setting of serious illness, patient perceptions of physician empathy are correlated with improved patient satisfaction and adherence to recommended treatments (Kim et al., 2004). A high-quality patient–doctor relationship is also linked with improved outcomes with regards to general health in the family practice setting (Sans-Corrales et al., 2006). And, in the psychiatric setting, an inclusive communication style that attends to patient beliefs and provides information about the recommended treatment is associated with improved satisfaction and better medication adherence (Bultman and Svarstad, 2000). Other specific styles of communication are known to be associated with good outcomes as well. For example, clinician statements associated with increased family satisfaction in the ICU setting include assurances that the patient will not be abandoned and will not suffer, and expressions of support of family decisions regardless of their nature (Stapleton et al., 2006). Finally, from a negative perspective, patients appear more likely to sue their physicians if they feel that they have failed to display empathy or to properly inform them about their diagnosis or recommended treatments (Levinson, 1994). Even in the event of undesirable outcome, patients and family members genuinely desire open, honest communication and disclosure, and the converse is more likely to lead to litigation (Forster et al., 2002). Overall, the published literature suggests that the quality of physician–patient communication significantly impacts health outcomes (Stewart, 1995).

Of note, good communication maps to several of the recently lauded beneficial outcomes of involving specialist palliative care practitioners in patient care. For example, in patients with advanced cancer, palliative care reduces re-hospitalizations, inappropriate ICU transfers, and chemotherapy in the last 30 days of life, while also increasing quality of life, quality of death, and possibly even length of life (Hearn and Higginson, 1998; Zhang et al., 2009; Temel et al., 2010, 2011). This reduction in the provision of unwanted, inappropriate, or unnecessary interventions is likely a result of good communication as defined above, wherein the matching of patient goals and values to a specific treatment plan results in appropriately aggressive care when warranted, but minimizes undesired or inappropriately aggressive care in the late stages of illness.

Current communication practice

Given what is known about what constitutes good communication and its powerful effects on patient care, it is natural to look to actual encounters and to see how close practising clinicians come to meeting these quality standards. Unfortunately, clinicians probably have an inflated perception of their communication ability. For example, in one study of trainee self-assessments about the quality of their communication in end-of-life situations, there was no significant correlation in their assessments with those of patients, family members, or instructors, suggesting poor self-awareness (Dickson et al., 2012). Evidence suggests that clinicians tend to avoid discussing negative prognostic information unless specifically requested, or they present it in an overly optimistic light (Lamont and Christakis, 2001; Daugherty and Hlubocky, 2008; Leydon, 2008). Furthermore, physicians appear to overestimate prognosis in general, with less accuracy as the length of the patient–doctor relationship increases, and also for those patients with cancer diagnoses (Christakis and Lamont, 2000; Glare et al., 2003). Other literature suggests that clinicians may believe they have conveyed key prognostic information effectively, while the patient still does not understand, or does not even recognize that a prognosis was rendered (Fried et al., 2003). This may, in part, be due to the commonplace use of medical jargon in communication, which is known to be poorly understood by many patients (Hadlow and Pitts, 1991; Lerner et al., 2000). Given these findings, not surprisingly, patients tend to rate physicians poorly with regards to issues of discussing prognosis and dying (Curtis et al., 2004). This well-intentioned omission is likely more harmful in the end, as it may impair the ability of patients and families to prepare for the end of life, to adapt their hopes and goals, and can even cause heightened fear or anxiety (Fallowfield et al., 2002b).

When surveyed after the death of a loved one, families sometimes report dissatisfaction with the quality of communication and care provided. For example, when the hospital is the place of death, bereaved family members tend to report insufficient contact with physicians, inadequate emotional support, and insufficient information about the dying process (Teno et al., 2004). In the intensive care setting, evidence suggests that at least half of families experience inadequate communication with physicians (Azoulay et al., 2000). Direct assessments of physician communication behaviour echo these family reports. Oncologists, for example, often seem to neglect patients' expressions of emotion, generally responding to empathic opportunities with terminating statements rather than exploring the emotional content in patients' statements (Pollak et al., 2007). Patient statements of difficult emotion may be rather subtle, and these cues are often missed by oncologists (Butow et al., 2002). Studies of physicians talking to patients about do-not-resuscitate orders or advance care planning have shown that they rarely adhere to the described standards for such conversations (Tulsky et al., 1995, 1998; Smith et al., 2006).

Physicians also tend to interrupt, and to redirect patients too early. In one study, physicians interrupted patients after an average of 23.1 seconds, and only 28% of patients were even allowed to complete their initial statement of concern. In addition, last-minute concerns were more common when patients were interrupted early; those who were not interrupted only used 6 more seconds of time (Marvel et al., 1999). The use of more open-ended, patient-centred communication methods is thus likely to improve the efficiency of the clinical encounter, by ensuring that patients' concerns are elicited upfront, thereby minimizing last-minute concerns while one's hand is on the doorknob at the end of a visit. In addition, rather than assessing patients' goals and preferences, and recommending a concordant plan of care, physicians tend to ask closed-ended questions about specific treatments, without adequate context.

The preponderance of the evidence from patient report and direct observation suggests that although physicians are well intentioned, the quality of their communication with patients, particularly in the setting of advanced illness, frequently does not meet the espoused quality standards. Although there are many reasons for this gap, the most likely explanation is that physicians are unprepared from their training to deal with complex communication challenges, particularly at the end of life. In a national survey of nearly 2000 students, house staff, and faculty, only 18% of students and residents reported receiving formal end-of-life care training, including communication skills training, and what they do receive is frequently inadequate (Sullivan et al., 2003).

Communication skills can be learned

Despite these difficult realities about current practice, we have learned over the last several decades that communication behaviours are readily measurable, teachable, and learnable. Good communication is ultimately the practice and performance of a series of discrete behaviours that can be observed and quantified. Practice leads to improvement. A number of studies have shown that communication skills teaching works and most educational programmes include the following elements. Learners must have the opportunity to first observe the behaviour done well, practise while being observed themselves (with either a real or simulated patient), and then receive feedback on their performance, ideally with the opportunity to try again with corrections.

One controlled trial of a communication intervention course to internal medicine residents led to significant improvements in delivering bad news (Alexander et al., 2006). Another targeted communication intervention for junior physicians in Australia improved participants perceptions of their skills, confidence, and the actual quality of their communication, as assessed via videotaped assessments before and after the intervention (Clayton et al., 2013). Courses for senior oncologists in the United Kingdom

resulted in improved communication confidence and positive behavioural changes, both initially and at 3 and 12 months, along with changes in attitudes towards patients' psychosocial needs (Fallowfield et al., 1998, 2002a, 2003). Tested in a randomized controlled trial, this intervention resulted in significant improvements in empathy, response to patient cues, and avoidance of leading questions (Fallowfield et al., 2002a). Similarly, a communication training course for oncology fellows, and more recently one to train faculty to teach communication skills, have resulted in improvements in oncologists' comfort level and skill with having difficult conversations, and teaching others to do so, respectively (Back et al., 2003b, 2009b).

Areas of uncertainty

Despite a growing and high-quality literature on effective doctor–patient communication, there remain several important areas of uncertainty. First, while it is clear that most patients and families value and desire communication that fits the 'patient-centred' model described earlier, a subset may explicitly reject central tenets of this framework. For example, not all patients wish to actively participate in decision-making (Blackhall et al., 1995). This may be a particularly important issue in cases of significant cultural difference. Sensitivity to the norms of particular cultural groups is thus an important part of effective communication in palliative care practice. In situations where shared decision-making is not desired, or is not a cultural norm, communicating within a patient-centred framework is likely to be at least ineffective, if not offensive. Assessing for this possibility upfront is important, and can be accomplished quite easily in many cases by asking an open-ended question such as, 'Some patients like to consider all the options before making a decision, whereas others prefer that their doctor makes a specific recommendation. Which of these styles appeals to you?'

Second, a minority of patients may prefer that physicians not engage with emotional issues and may not appreciate aspects of the recommended empathic communication style. As with most difficult communication scenarios, asking upfront and assessing preferences early usually goes a long way. For example, one might say: 'Some patients want their doctor to acknowledge and address the sometimes difficult emotional issues that go along with having an illness, while others prefer not to discuss these kinds of things with their physician. What's your preference about this?'

Third, in communication about serious illness, references to numbers and statistics often seem useful. Conveying information via numbers, however, is a difficult task (Apter et al., 2008). Just as many patients have low health literacy, many also have low numeracy, meaning they have difficulty fully understanding and contextualizing basic percentage estimates, fractions, and notions of risk. This issue may underlie the prevalence of misunderstanding one's prognosis in advanced cancer settings. While there is a growing literature on numeracy, including some recommendations about effective ways to present statistical information to patients, there remains much more to be studied.

Finally, the increasingly ubiquitous role of electronic health records poses a whole new set of challenges to clinician–patient communication. These include the challenge of maintaining a human connection with the patient while accessing and inputting data into a computer, as well as learning how to navigate electronic mail communications with patients in a way that ensures safety and leaves patients feeling cared for. Little data exists in this area and studies are just beginning to emerge.

Putting theory into practice: a communication skills overview

The data presented so far describes what high-quality communication for patients and families looks like and confirms that these are skills that can be taught. The rest of this chapter will focus on strategies and tips to put these skills into practice (Back et al., 2009a). While many models of communication have been proposed (Parle et al., 1997; Lo et al., 1999; Larson and Tobin, 2000; von Gunten et al., 2000), they have in common several principles. First, given that patients vary greatly in their desire for information and participation in decision-making, one should assess patients' preferences for communication as part of the medical encounter (Pfeifer et al., 2003; Hagerty et al., 2004). One cannot presume to 'intuit' patient's wants and needs, therefore one should ask. Second, information should be given using non-technical language and in brief, understandable chunks. This allows the physician to constantly reassess the patient's verbal or non-verbal reaction to the information, as well as their desire for more information. Third, while doctors focus on medical treatments and dying, patients focus on function and relationships. Therefore, treatments should be discussed within the framework of the patient's goals rather than in abstraction. Lastly, attention to the affective component of the conversation is as important as the cognitive aspects.

The 'SPIKES' protocol for delivering bad news, serves as an excellent overall framework for most difficult conversations (Baile et al., 2000). Each letter in the acronym denotes one component of this approach, including paying attention to Setting, assessing the patients Perception, providing an Invitation to the discussion, delivering Knowledge, offering Empathy, and Summarizing/strategizing (see Table 6.1.1) Paying attention to this overall schema, we offer specific strategies below.

Prepare in advance

A little effort spent on advance preparation can have a tremendous impact on the quality of the encounter. Whenever possible, important medical information, particularly bad or sad news, should be delivered during a scheduled meeting. This allows patients to prepare themselves for the type of information they will hear and to make sure that appropriate family members or friends are present. It also allows the physician to allocate the necessary time to the encounter and to come prepared with basic medical information and anticipate the most likely questions regarding treatment options, prognosis, and resources for support and guidance.

Part of the physician's preparation ought to include consideration of their own emotional state. When experiencing a strong emotion while interacting with a patient, one should ask oneself, 'Where is this coming from?'. Although it may be a result of what the physician brings to the encounter (e.g. one's own sense of mortality or how it makes one think of one's grandmother who died), it may also be a clue into what the patient is feeling. Thus, many doctors report feeling anxious when talking with a patient who has an anxiety disorder, or feeling overly sad when talking with a depressed patient. If the physician gets a sense that he or she is reflecting the patient's emotion it may help to ask the patient about this (e.g. 'I wonder if you're feeling sad?'). If the emotion is a result of the physician's reaction to the encounter, the next step is to discuss this with colleagues or confidants. In most cases, however, patients do not benefit from hearing such thoughts.

Whenever possible, communicate face-to-face

Telephones accentuate physical communication difficulties and there is no opportunity to employ the benefits of non-verbal communication. Given that over 50% of communication is non-verbal, both parties operate at a disadvantage if they cannot see each other. The physician should sit at eye level and within reach of the patient. If possible, one's pager or mobile phone should be turned off, or at least put on a quiet mode, and one should avoid interruptions. Finally, as many physicians are now compelled to interact

Table 6.1.1 Evidence-based communication strategies

Technique	Example	For further information
'I wish …'	'I wish the scan had turned out better for you'	Quill, T.E., Arnold, R.M., and Platt, F. (2001). 'I wish things were different': expressing wishes in response to loss, futility, and unrealistic hopes. *Annals of Internal Medicine*, 135, 551–555.
'Hope for the best …'	'I hope this treatment works well too. Let's also talk about other possible outcomes, to make sure we're prepared for anything'	Back, A.L., Arnold, R.M., and Quill, T.E. (2003a). Hope for the best, and prepare for the worst. *Annals of Internal Medicine*, 138, 439–443.
'Are you at peace?'	'Are you at peace?'	Steinhauser, K.E., Voils, C.I., Clipp, E.C., Bosworth, H.B., Christakis, N.A., and Tulsky, J.A. (2006). 'Are you at peace?': one item to probe spiritual concerns at the end of life. *Archives of Internal Medicine*, 166, 101–105.
'Ask–tell–ask'	Ask: 'What have the doctors told you about your illness?' Tell: Give the news Ask: 'I know this is a lot of information, and sometimes I don't do a very good job of explaining things. Tell me what you understand now about what we've been discussing'	Back, A.L., Arnold, R.M., Baile, W.F., Tulsky, J.A., and Fryer-Edwards, K. (2005). Approaching difficult communication tasks in oncology. *CA: A Cancer Journal for Clinicians*, 55, 164–177.
Praise	'You have been a truly remarkable advocate for your husband'	Back, A.L., Arnold, R.M., Baile, W.F., Edwards, K.A., and Tulsky, J.A. (2010). When praise is worth considering in a difficult conversation. *The Lancet*, 376, 866–867.

with electronic medical record systems during the office visit, they must be careful that accessing and inputting data do not compromise direct human interaction.

Use open-ended techniques

Patients and family members are more satisfied in encounters where they do much of the talking, so it is essential to develop the ability to communicate using open-ended prompts that solicit the required information from patients and family members while also not being inefficient in the face of time constraints. Rather than asking so-called closed-ended questions, which generally yield 'yes' or 'no' responses, or perhaps terminating, one-word responses, a more patient-centred communication strategy will utilize open-ended questions whenever possible. This might be as simple as to say, 'Tell me more about this back pain', rather than, 'Is it sharp, or dull?' The strategic use of open-ended framing of questions can improve patients' sense of being heard and listened to, and also improve the sense of connection patients have with their clinician.

Solicit the patient's agenda

The upfront solicitation of a patient's agenda may decrease the incidence of last-minute questions and requests at the end of a clinical encounter (Marvel et al., 1999). This is particularly important in the outpatient setting, where time pressures mandate effective, efficient communication. Here, a last-minute, unexpected 'doorknob question' or request can result in delays for subsequent patients' appointments, and also frustration on the part of both the clinician and the patient. Upfront efforts to ascertain the patient's agenda will allow one to negotiate a plan for the content of the visit within the constraints of the appointment time. Doing so can be relatively simple and straightforward, yet transformative with regards to time management. Consider asking the patient at the start of the visit, 'What were you hoping we could talk about today?' This should be followed by, 'Anything else?' This will elicit most patients' concerns, and minimize the chance of facing a 'doorknob question' later. Once these topics are out in the open, the clinician can thoughtfully propose an agenda and timeframe for each topic, also including other items which need to be discussed during the visit, such as a proposed radiographic test.

Ask permission

Physicians are not very good at predicting which patients want more and which patients want less information. Instead of assuming one should ask. For example, on a first visit one could say: 'I want to touch base with you about how you want me to handle information we get about your illness. Some patients want to know everything that is going on with their illness, the good and the bad. Other people do not want as much information and want me to speak more generally. And some would really prefer I do not discuss bad news with them but want me to discuss these issues with their family. Which kind of person do you think you are?' In addition, asking permission is an excellent way to gently move a conversation forward and engage a topic that may be threatening to a patient. For example, one might say, 'Would it be okay if we talked now about the latest tests and how your cancer is doing?'

Ask–tell–ask

The 'ask–tell–ask' framework is an excellent guide to any difficult conversation (Back et al., 2005). It operationalizes several core components of patient-centred communication, beginning with the first 'ask', which seeks to assess a patient's current knowledge, needs, or concerns. Starting an encounter in this manner, with an open-ended question that probes the issue from the patient's perspective, can be enormously illuminating regarding the appropriate next steps in the conversation. This technique thus often saves much time, energy, and difficulty, as it helps guide the conversation more naturally to wherever it needs to go, without as much input from the clinician's presumptions or agenda. After the 'tell,' which involves giving the news or information in small, digestible, sensitive, and non-technical language, one again 'asks' what the patient heard or understood. This 'teach-back' helps to gauge the efficacy of the conversation and information transfer, and again guides subsequent aspects of the discussion.

Empathize

Patients and family members appreciate and value clinician expressions of empathy. Unfortunately clinicians frequently miss opportunities to empathize in clinical practice, often responding with more cognitive 'terminating' statements, rather than exploring the emotional content of a patient's response (Robinson et al., 2008). Appropriate use of empathy can strengthen the patient–doctor relationship, and improve communication efficacy. Furthermore, non-verbal expressions of empathy (e.g. a concerned look, a touch on the hand) may demonstrate caring, yet also risk misinterpretation. Whenever possible, it is best to use clear verbal expressions of empathy. A popular acronym of commonly used empathic responses is known as 'NURSE' (see Table 6.1.2) (Smith, 2002). These five types of empathic statements (Name, Understand, Respect, Support, Explore) are not to be used at once, but rather represent a menu of options available to the clinician managing significant patient emotions.

Praise

The use of praise can be a particularly effective way to align oneself with a patient or family, and to encourage further productive discussions in the context of difficult clinical scenarios (Back et al., 2010). In the setting of a patient or family member who aggressively advocates for life-prolonging therapies that are unlikely to benefit the patient, it is not uncommon for clinicians to feel frustrated, and at odds with the very family they are trying to help. Rather than becoming frustrated, and expressing this frustration in the clinical encounter, however, the use of praise can help to create an alliance with family. One might say, 'You have been a truly remarkable advocate for your husband'. Judicial application of this technique sometimes marks the turning point in a difficult conversation.

Use 'wish statements'

'Wish statements' are a particularly powerful way to express empathy in the context of a difficult clinical encounter when bad news is involved (Quill et al., 2001). Expressing one's wish that the situation were different can align the clinician with the patient, while also helping to acknowledge and deliver the bad news itself. In the context of discussing an abnormal imaging result, for example, a

Table 6.1.2 Mnemonics for good communication[a]

	NURSE model for empathy		SPIKES method for giving bad news	
Name	'I imagine this must be upsetting' (naming the emotion)	**S**etting	Private room, silence pagers/phones, adequate time, key participants available
Understand	'I expect most people would feel that way in a situation like this'	**P**erception	'Tell me your understanding about the situation'
Respect	'I'm impressed with how well you've handled such a tough situation'	**I**nvitation	'Is it okay if we talk further about this?'
Support	'I'll be here to help you through this'	**K**nowledge	Give the news in short, digestible, clear, non-technical language, then be quiet and wait
Explore	'Tell me more about how you're feeling, and what this means for you'	**E**mpathy	Use NURSE or similar strategy to demonstrate empathy
		Summary/**S**trategy	'What kind of information would be helpful for you right now? 'Let's talk about the next steps ... '

[a] For further information see Schapira, L. (2008). Communication: what do patients want and need? *Journal of Oncology Practice*, 4(5), 249–253, Copyright © 2008.

patient might say, 'Does this mean my cancer is back?' Responding with a 'wish statement', as in, 'I wish things had turned out differently', acknowledges the bad news while aligning the clinician with the patient. This may lead to subsequent empathic opportunities, allowing one to further explore the important emotional issues relating to the bad news prior to discussing any medical or technical specifics.

'Hope for the best ... '

In situations where patients or families have unrealistic expectations for the future, it can be difficult to encourage discussion about less desirable outcomes. Sometimes clinicians also worry that doing so will crush a patient's hope, and lead to distrust. Patients and families, however, dislike the concept of 'false hope,' and generally want open, honest disclosure of even bad news (Apatira et al., 2008). One way to encourage exploration of the spectrum of outcomes while maintaining alignment with a patient's hopes is to use the 'hope for the best' phraseology (Back et al., 2003a). This allows the clinician to align with the patient's hopes, while also exploring other possibilities to ensure the patient is prepared in the event that things turn out differently. One might say, 'Let's hope for the best, while we also prepare for other possible outcomes'. This can be a less ominous way to explore goals and preferences for the future, when facing a likely poor prognosis.

'Are you at peace?'

Spiritual assessment is an important component of a comprehensive palliative care consultation, particularly in serious illness or end-of-life settings. Asking the simple question 'Are you at peace?' can be an effective way to screen for spiritual and psychosocial distress (Steinhauser et al., 2006). Without uncovering and addressing such distress, patients and families may be unable or unwilling to move forward with other important discussions and decision-making. This brief screening question can thus be transformative in moving discussions ahead in difficult clinical encounters, and in helping to expand a plan of care to include attention to important spiritual and psychosocial issues.

Use interpreters

Increasingly and in nearly all countries, clinicians encounter non-native language-speaking patients. One must absolutely employ the assistance of an interpreter in such settings. However, it is equally important to avoid using family members as interpreters. Not only does this run the risk of faulty translation or reinterpretation of the physician's statements, it also places family members into the uncomfortable position of being the physician's and patient's spokesperson (Forster et al., 2002). The common practice of using bilingual young children as translators is particularly problematic. Most hospitals and health-care facilities in regions with high numbers of immigrants employ professional translators or maintain lists of language skills among facility staff members.

Putting it all together

This chapter presents specific skills and even scripts that can improve communication efficacy and patient satisfaction. Translating this knowledge into practice, however, may prove difficult for many clinicians. Busy practitioners face increasing pressure to see more patients in less time, interact with more technology, and to meet new documentation requirements and quality monitoring standards. Adding the effort to be a high-quality empathic communicator can seem daunting, particularly if one presumes this will require even more time in an already overloaded schedule.

Contrary to popular belief, effective, empathic communication probably does not take any more time than communication that ignores emotional content, and may actually be more efficient (Fogarty et al., 1999; McDonagh et al., 2004; Kennifer et al., 2009). Proactively addressing patients' needs, setting an agenda for each visit, and ensuring that patients feel heard can actually be done relatively quickly, and can avoid time-consuming problems later.

High-quality empathic communication also depends upon the mindset of the health-care provider. When clinicians feel harried or disconnected in their practice of medicine, they are unable to focus meaningfully on the patient's concerns. 'Mindfulness' refers to the practice of being consciously present in everyday activities.

An intervention that helps clinicians achieve such mindful practice has been associated with less burnout and mood disturbance among primary care physicians, and at least a subjective sense of being more present with patients (Krasner et al., 2009). Finally, it is possible that conscious daily practice of empathic communication behaviours leads to longer-term improvements in communication skill (Fallowfield et al., 2003).

Conclusion

Communication in clinical practice is not intuitive, and requires conscious practice in order to achieve competency. This is especially true in the palliative care setting, where specialists are increasingly expected to help navigate difficult clinical situations, many of which involve communication challenges, or prior communication mistakes that complicate future encounters. Good communication can be deconstructed and conceptualized as a series of discrete behaviours. It is thus measurable, teachable, and learnable. Research shows that clinicians tend to overestimate their communication abilities, and that patients and families want better communication from the medical team, especially in settings of serious illness or at the end of life. They prefer open-ended, empathic communication and honest disclosure, even in the face of a bad prognosis. Family members expect to be listened to, and heard, to be involved in decision-making, and hope to be attended to even after the death of their loved one. As compassionate caregivers, palliative care specialists, and indeed all clinicians, we owe it to our patients and families to improve the quality of our communication, and to make this a conscious component and focus of our daily practice.

Online materials

Complete references for this chapter are available online at <http://www.oxfordmedicine.com>.

References

Azoulay, E., Chevret, S., Leleu, G., *et al.* (2000). Half the families of intensive care unit patients experience inadequate communication with physicians. *Critical Care Medicine*, 28, 3044–3049.

Back, A.L., Arnold, R.M., Baile, W.F., *et al.* (2007). Efficacy of communication skills training for giving bad news and discussing transitions to palliative care. *Archives of Internal Medicine*, 167, 453–460.

Back, A.L., Arnold, R.M., Baile, W.F., Edwards, K.A., and Tulsky, J.A. (2010). When praise is worth considering in a difficult conversation. *The Lancet*, 376, 866–867.

Back, A., Arnold, R.M., and Tulsky, J.A. (2009a). *Mastering Communication with Seriously Ill Patients: Balancing Honesty with Empathy and Hope*. Cambridge: Cambridge University Press.

Butow, P.N., Brown, R.F., Cogar, S., Tattersall, M.H., and Dunn, S.M. (2002). Oncologists' reactions to cancer patients' verbal cues. *Psycho-Oncology*, 11, 47–58.

Fallowfield, L., Jenkins, V., Farewell, V., Saul, J., Duffy, A., and Eves, R. (2002a). Efficacy of a Cancer Research UK communication skills training model for oncologists: a randomised controlled trial. *The Lancet*, 359, 650–656.

Fried, T.R., Bradley, E.H., and O'Leary, J. (2003). Prognosis communication in serious illness: perceptions of older patients, caregivers, and clinicians. *Journal of the American Geriatrics Society*, 51, 1398–1403.

Hagerty, R.G., Butow, P.N., Ellis, P.A., *et al.* (2004). Cancer patient preferences for communication of prognosis in the metastatic setting. *Journal of Clinical Oncology*, 22, 1721–1730.

Lamont, E.B. and Christakis, N.A. (2001). Prognostic disclosure to patients with cancer near the end of life. *Annals of Internal Medicine*, 134, 1096–1105.

Maguire, P., Faulkner, A., Booth, K., Elliott, C., and Hillier, V. (1996). Helping cancer patients disclose their concerns. *European Journal of Cancer*, 32A, 78–81.

Parker, P.A., Baile, W.F., De Moor, C., Lenzi, R., Kudelka, A.P., and Cohen, L. (2001). Breaking bad news about cancer: patients' preferences for communication. *Journal of Clinical Oncology*, 19, 2049–2056.

Pollak, K.I., Arnold, R.M., Jeffreys, A.S., *et al.* (2007). Oncologist communication about emotion during visits with patients with advanced cancer. *Journal of Clinical Oncology*, 25, 5748–5752.

Quill, T.E., Arnold, R.M., and Platt, F. (2001). 'I wish things were different': expressing wishes in response to loss, futility, and unrealistic hopes. *Annals of Internal Medicine*, 135, 551–555.

Tulsky, J.A., Arnold, R.M., Alexander, S.C., *et al.* (2011). Enhancing communication between oncologists and patients with a computer-based training program: a randomized trial. *Annals of Internal Medicine*, 155, 593–601.

Wright, A.A., Zhang, B., Ray, A., *et al.* (2008). Associations between end-of-life discussions, patient mental health, medical care near death, and caregiver bereavement adjustment. *Journal of the American Medical Association*, 300, 1665–1673.

6.2

Talking with families and children about the death of a parent

Mari Lloyd-Williams and Jackie Ellis

Introduction to discussing the death of a parent

Parental death is one of the most significant and stressful events children can encounter (Auman, 2007), one that could have a serious impact on adulthood. While no routine data is collected in the United Kingdom on this group, estimates suggests that over 24 000 children and young adults experience the death of a parent each year in the United Kingdom (Winston's Wish, n.d.). However, data may well reflect only those exhibiting some problem with their grief and may be underinflated (Thompson and Payne, 2000). A recent study (Parsons, 2011) found that 5% of young people have been bereaved of a parent by the time they are 16. For the majority of children, parents are the most significant people in their lives, so when one dies, life as the child knows it is disrupted and irrevocably changed. It is a time of suffering and confusion, both for the child and surviving parent. For diagnostic understanding, it is necessary that clinicians evaluate if the reaction is a part of 'normal life' or if it needs any type of specific intervention.

The parent's palliative stage of an illness exposes the child to significant levels of stress (Thastum et al., 2008; Kennedy and Lloyd-Williams, 2009a, 2009b) and yet there are limited resources available to this community of children (Lloyd-Williams et al., 1998; Dunning, 2006). Furthermore, these stress-related feelings are exacerbated because the non-bereaved community do not understand the loss or the associated pain which causes the bereaved to feel isolated and alone (Schultz, 2007).

Communication and information sharing are key factors in promoting children's coping strategies (Waskett, 1995; Christ, 2000; Rauch et al., 2003; Christ and Christ, 2006). Practitioners working in palliative care have a pivotal role in offering support to children and families and fundamental to this is their role in communicating with children and their families. While this chapter is not suggesting that all children experiencing or who have experienced the death of a parent are at risk of significant harm, they are, within the Children Act 1989 definition, 'children in need', although very rarely acknowledged as such.

Communicating with and sharing information with children is widely acknowledged as an important factor in supporting them when a parent is terminally ill or has died (Waskett, 1995; Christ, 2000; Rauch et al., 2003; Christ and Christ, 2006). Furthermore, communication within families about a parent's illness can act as a protective factor against children's distress (Kroll et al., 1998).

Research suggests that children's emotional well-being is adversely affected when a when a parent is terminally ill or has died (Christ and Christ, 2006). This anxiety is heightened when children are not provided with adequate information about their parent's illness (Beale et al., 2004).

This chapter discusses the key issues related to communicating and sharing information with families and children who have experienced parental death. Firstly, however, we briefly explore the literature that looks at the impact of early parental death. We then review the traditional theories of mourning and outline the dominant models of grief.

The impact of early parental death

A recent review (Akerman and Statham, 2011) on childhood bereavement following parental death reports that children that had lost a parent experience a wide range of emotional and behavioural symptoms often classified as 'non-specific disturbance'. The majority of children, however, do not experience serious problems (Haine et al. 2006). Even among children bereaved by parental suicide and cancer, most children reported low levels of psychological distress, suggesting a considerable degree of resilience (Ratnarajah and Schofield, 2007). This review also found that parents tend to report fewer symptoms and disorders in their children than children do themselves. The child often experiences an increase in anxiety with a focus on concerns about further loss, the safety of other family members, and fears around separation. Mild depression appears to be frequent, and can persist for at least a year (Akerman and Statham, 2011).

Akerman and Statham also found that psychiatric disorders are rare with only one in five bereaved children likely to manifest such disturbance at a level sufficient to justify referral to specialist services (Dowdney, 2000). This is most likely to take the form of depression or dysphoria (a combination of sadness and crying or irritability). Symptoms may include anxiety, depressive symptoms, fears, angry outbursts, and regression regarding developmental milestones. Across different types of potentially traumatic events, including bereavement, upward of 50% of people have been found to display resilience, suggesting that psychotherapeutic treatment should be reserved for those in genuine need (Bonanno and Mancini, 2008).

The evidence on children's bereavement outcomes is difficult to summarize and some findings contradict others (Ribbens McCarthy and Jessop, 2005). In part, this is because children experience bereavement in a wide range of circumstances and opposite effects can cancel each other out in large-scale quantitative studies (Ribbens McCarthy and Jessop, 2005). An 8-year-old child whose lone parent dies suddenly and who enters foster care will have a different experience from a 15-year-old whose parent's death is expected. Some children are more likely to experience bereavement; additionally, significant bereavement seems to bring greater risks to those who are already disadvantaged or have faced multiple losses (Ribbens McCarthy and Jessop, 2005).

Parsons (2011) found that there may be fewer longer-term effects for childhood bereavement and that children experiencing other forms of family disruption may suffer more extensive influences on their ability to negotiate successful transition to adult life. Many cumulative, interrelating risk and protective factors mediate or moderate children's experiences (Worden, 1996; Ribbens McCarthy and Jessop, 2005). These can be at the level of the child (such as their prior experiences of loss, their preferred coping style), their family and social relationships (including their prior and ongoing relationship with the person who has died), their wider environment and culture, and the circumstances of the death (including whether the child perceives this as traumatic) (Worden, 1996; Ribbens McCarthy and Jessop, 2005).

The family is a key context for bereaved children and young people. Studies consistently point to the importance of higher levels of caregiver warmth, coping styles, and lower levels of caregiver mental health problems, discipline, and communication in protecting against negative outcomes from the death of the parents (Worden, 1996; Lin et al., 2004; Ribbens McCarthy and Jessop, 2005; Haine et al., 2006; Luecken et al., 2009; Akerman and Statham, 2011).

Very few studies have explored the impact of bereavement in adult life, particularly in the United Kingdom. A recent study (Ellis, 2009; Ellis et al., 2013) employed qualitative methodologies and narrative analysis to explore the experiences of 33 individuals (seven men and 26 women) who had experienced the death of a parent before the age of 18, in order to better understand its perceived impact on adulthood. Ellis and colleagues found that while individual experiences of bereavement were unique, five common themes were identified across the narratives that impacted on the bereavement experience: (1) disruption and continuity, (2) recognition of loss, (3) family dynamics roles and responsibility and context, (4) the public world of bereavement, and (5) identity and aspects of personal growth. The findings are very important as they provide insight into the damage and effects on the individual in adulthood as a consequence of inappropriate or neglectful management.

Traditional theories of mourning

Much of the early evidence on the impact of early parental death is premised on traditional theories of mourning. Freud (1917/1957) developed the psychoanalytic theory of mourning based on his extensive research in this area. Until the 1960s, his theory had dominated clinical understanding, in the United States and the United Kingdom, of how children perceive and respond to the death of a parent (Saler and Skolnick, 1992). Freud explored the psychological process of mourning with individuals who had lost a parent through death and normalized the process of grief.

Freud (1917/1957) presented his theory of mourning in a paper entitled 'Mourning and Melancholia' in which he differentiated between healthy and unhealthy mourning. Freud's theory primarily focused on the individual process of mourning. He proposed that individuals develop attachment or love to significant others who are involved in satisfying their needs: the more important the person, the greater the attachment. Love is defined as the cathexis of libidinal (psychic) energy to the love object (the person). When the loved object is lost through death, the survivor's libidinal energy remains connected to the deceased through thoughts and memories. Freud argued that detaching or severing energy from the lost object is necessary. This process, which Freud referred to as hyper-cathexis, is achieved by reviewing all of the person's memories of the deceased. While Freud acknowledged that the process of letting go of the lost object is painful, he saw detachment as critical in order to free the ego so that it can invest in new relationships. Thus, psychoanalytic theory proposed that if hyper-cathexis did not occur, melancholia (i.e. lowered self-esteem caused by the unresolved ambivalence in the relationship with the deceased) or unhealthy mourning would result. Freud's theory referred to the adult experience, but succeeding generations of Freudian practitioners inferred that children and adolescents would be vulnerable to melancholia when a parent died because of their dependence on the parent and their developmental capacity for decathexis or 'grief work'.

Freud's understanding of loss and grief may be challenged because he worked from a psychiatric perspective and most of his theories were based on clinical experiences with depressed people and not on data from normal populations (Payne et al., 1999). Nevertheless, as Payne et al. point out, Freud's concept of grief work and the need to confront grief in order to gain detachment has had a powerful influence on both subsequent theory and clinical practice both in the United States and the United Kingdom.

Pollock (1961) extended Freud's theory of mourning. Pollock suggested that the main purpose of mourning is to facilitate the work of coming to terms with life without the deceased parent. According to Pollock, the process of mourning occurs in stages. The first stage is shock, which is followed by a period in which the work of mourning takes place. The final stage includes a separation reaction in which the presentation of the love object is restructured from present reality to that of memory.

Stages and phases models of grief

Bowlby (1961) originated the theory of attachment and this would seem to underpin the basis for understanding bereavement (Dent, 2005). Bowlby provides an explanation for the common human tendency to develop strong affectionate bonds. He views attachment as a reciprocal relationship that occurs as a result of long-term interactions, starting in infancy between a child and its caregivers. He suggests that grief is an instinctive universal response to separation.

Both Bowlby (1961) and Parkes (1972) were stage theorists. The stage model of grief is a linear progression in which the bereaved person moves through specific stages or phases of grief in order to reach the goal or stage of resolution. The first stage of grief involves denial, shock, and feelings of numbness. The second stage includes acute symptoms of grief such as intense emotional pain, social withdrawal, physical symptoms, and identification with the deceased. The final stage of grief includes a return to normal functioning and reintegration (entailing a letting go of the loved one). Success or resolution was determined by the extent to which the bereaved was able to give up his or her original attachment with the lost loved one (Wilcox-Rittgers, 1997). Many of the stage theorists such as Parkes (1986) proposed fluidity in this linear model whereby the bereaved may move back and forth between the stages of grieving before moving on to resolution. Kuber-Ross's (1969) stage model of the grief of terminally ill people is often applied to other loss situations such as bereavement.

In the stage model of grief the bereaved person is perceived as being relatively passive in terms of grieving (Holland, 2001). This theoretical perspective has become an established basis for professional training and self-help literature in the field of bereavement (Ribbens McCarthy, 2006). The stage-based model is criticized for having limited empirical evidence to support the existence of such stages in the grieving process (Shuchter and Ziscook, 1993). The early studies that informed these models have also been criticized, particularly for the dominance of young, white, middle-class widows (Payne et al., 1999) and for not accounting for diversity and individuality of reactions and for neglecting resourcefulness (Holland, 2001; Ribbens McCarthy, 2006).

Tasks models of grief

An alternative to stage models is the task model of grief whereby bereavement is seen as a series of tasks to work though rather than just being a series of stages through which the individual has to pass (Worden, 1982, 1991). Here the bereaved person plays an active rather than a passive role in the grieving process. Lindenmann (1944) developed the first task-based model of grief. He isolated three main tasks necessary for successful grief resolution. These tasks included (1) severing ties with the deceased, (2) adjusting to one's new environment without the deceased loved one, (3) and creating new bonds with others. Again, the task of breaking the emotional bonds was considered the ultimate goal of grief work.

Worden (1982) developed a task model of mourning which has been extremely influential and is widely used by those who work with bereaved people. In relation to parentally bereaved children, grief is seen as a set of tasks in terms of normal responses that children need to negotiate (Worden, 1996). Worden discusses the tasks as being: (1) to accept the reality of death, (2) to deal with the emotional impact of the loss, (3) to adjust to the environment in which the deceased is absent, and (4) to emotionally relocate the deceased. In the context of the lives of young people, this approach has been further elaborated by reference to what are theorized as the developmental tasks of adolescence, the aim being to achieve a 'healthy' rather than a 'pathological' outcome; that is, a medical model of grief (Ribbens McCarthy, 2006).

Fox (1988) identified the following tasks for children coping with grief or loss to work through: (1) understand and make sense out of what has happened; (2) identify, validate, and express strong reactions to the loss constructively; (3) commemorate the life that was lived; and (4) learn to go on living and loving. Fox also identified other factors which influence the process of bereavement in children such as their understanding of death, the type of loss, and subsequent life circumstances.

Tasks models have also been criticized for their failure to recognize individual differences and other relevant factors which may trigger upsurges of grief throughout the bereaved person's life (Rando, 1988).

Continuing bonds

An important development in grief theory has been provided by the work of Klass et al (1996), who challenged conventional thinking that the purpose of grieving was the reconstitution of an autonomous individual who could leave the deceased behind and form new attachments, in other words, 'break the bonds' with the deceased. Klass and his colleagues suggest that the purpose of grieving is instead to maintain a continuing bond with the deceased, compatible with other new and continuing relationships.

Dual process model

A more recent and significant advance in our understanding of grief work is the dual process model develop by Stroebe and Schut (1995, 1999). These authors suggest that avoiding grief may be both helpful and detrimental, depending on the circumstances. While previous models centred on loss, the dual process model recognizes that both expressing and controlling feelings are important and introduces a new concept: that of oscillation between coping behaviours.

Within this framework, grief is viewed as a dynamic process in which there is an alternation between focusing on the loss of the person who has died (loss orientation) and avoiding that focus (restoration orientation). The loss orientation encompasses grief work, while the restoration orientation involves dealing with secondary losses as a result of the death (Dent, 2005). For instance, a mother who loses her partner/spouse may have to deal with finances and house maintenance which previously her partner/spouse dealt with. Both the loss orientation and the restoration orientation are necessary for future adjustment, but the degree and emphasis on each approach will depend on the circumstances of the death, personality, gender, and cultural background of each person. The model also posits that by taking time off from the pain of grief, which can be overwhelming, a bereaved person may be more able to cope with their daily life and the secondary changes.

Such an approach is in line with recent discussion of the goal of 'coping' with bereavement rather than finding a resolution (Corr, 2000). Thompson (2002, p. 7) argues that this dual process model 'alerts us to the complex web of psychological, cultural and socio-political factors which interact to make the loss experience far more complex than traditional approaches would have us believe'. However, a potential problem with extending the adult model to children is that it assumes that their experiences of bereavement are similar (Holland, 2001).

Taking with families and children about death of a parent

Much of the communication literature emphasizes the importance of open and honest communication (Jordan, 1990; Broderick, 1993)—this is seen as the most essential element in grief resolution in a family. Anxiety in children is increased when information is available but no opportunities are provided to allow them to discuss the information (Beale et al., 2004). Providing clear, honest information prevents misunderstandings, which may lead to frightening fantasies and fears (Saldinger et al., 2004; Turner et al., 2007). Euphemisms and abstractions are not advisable. Telling a young child that the deceased is 'sleeping' could cause the child to fear going to bed (McGuinness, 2011).

The importance and value of age-appropriate, open, honest communication with the child is discussed in Rauch et al. (2003). This information also needs to be timely and in a language appropriate to the child's level of understanding which has been linked to their cognitive development, but it also reflects their experiences of death and dying (Slaughter, 2005). Such factors are acknowledged by more recent understanding of children's concept of learning which has emerged in cognitive developmental research and theorizing in recent years (Slaughter, 2005). This intuitive theory approach of cognitive development emphasizes the role of casual-explanatory models in organizing children's knowledge and driving learning about different domains of experience and recognizes the importance of conceptual change in children's learning (Carey, 1985; Wellman and Geelman, 1992; Gopnick and Meltzoff, 1997; Inagakie and Hatano, 2002).

One of the seminal works in this new tradition analysed the development of young children's conception of the biological world (Carey, 1985). From this perspective, an important factor influencing children's understanding of death is the child's personal experience with people and other living things that have died (Hunter and Smith, 2008). Intuitive theory challenges Piaget's (1976) very influential theory of cognitive development, based on the chronological age of the child. Piaget addressed the ways in which children's thought processes changed over time, regardless of the environment in which they grow. The Piagetian research documenting consistent stages of death established that children's understanding of death is closely tied to cognitive developmental maturation. Within this explanatory framework it is believed that very young children do not have the capacity to understand abstraction such as finality and irreversibility, an understanding that only emerges when the child is capable of operational thinking (Piaget, 1956). Children may in fact see death as reversible. As children grow older, they develop the capacity to understand the abstractions associated with death (Worden, 1996). From this perspective, the development of an understanding of death appears to be most strongly influenced by developing cognitive competency (Slaughter, 2005). Piaget saw these development stages as universal, homogenous, and stable across cultures.

Piaget's model has also been challenged by scholars such as Bluebird-Langer (1989). Bluebird-Langer describes how very young children who are terminally ill or life-threatened have a sophisticated understanding of death through their observation of how adults respond, knowledge of their own symptoms and treatment, and interactions with other dying children. Bluebird-Langer recognizes therefore that although the development of children's understanding of death has been linked to their cognitive development, it also appears to reflect their experience of death and dying.

Research would suggest that younger children are less likely to receive the same amount of information as older children (Christ and Christ, 2006). Beale et al. (2004) delineate that a reason why parents do not share information with their children is because of their belief that the children are not aware of what is happening within the family. This is an important factor in communication and information sharing; younger children are frequently not included because of the belief that they are too young to understand. However, children from a very young age will be acutely aware that something is different within their family life. While they may be unable to comprehend completely what is happening, they will know that things are different and without some age-appropriate explanations it is likely that their assumptive world (Parkes, 1972) will be thrown into confusion and fear. The information given to children also needs to be repeated over time (Worden, 1996). Worden asserts that the repetitive questions that children ask about a death are a way for them to grapple with the reality of the death as well as a test to ensure that the story has not changed.

A recent retrospective study (Ellis et al., 2013) of adults bereaved as children found that those who had not been given timely and accurate information not only felt confused and fearful, they also often felt let down and betrayed by their surviving parent (or surrogate parent). The perception was that this had implications in adulthood, as it often led to trust issues which in turn affected their relationships. According to Herman (1992) one of the most important factors that make childhood loss traumatic is the feeling of having been betrayed by trusted adults.

Children need information not only at the time of the physical death but also when a parent that was known to them in terms of 'mothering /fathering' is lost to them due to illness, as this experience was very distressing for informants as they felt bewildered and confused as they didn't understand what was happening (Ellis et al., 2013). Christ (2000) and Fearnley (2010) reported that regular medical updates about their parent's condition were helpful. In common with Worden (1996), Ellis et al. found that children who are not given accurate information make up a back story to fill in the gaps and this can be more frightening than what actually happened. Ellis et al. also found that while as a mature adult, respondents were able to reflect on their experience and appreciate that it may have been done with the best of intentions (i.e. protectionism), and/or associated with dominant beliefs about parenting at the time, it was still very difficult for them to come to terms with.

The recent cognitive development literature generates specific guidelines for talking about death with children, which acknowledges the importance of children's underlying folk biology to their capacity to conceptualize death. Slaughter states that even when adults provide explanations that appear to be clear and straightforward, such as 'he died because his heart gave out' or 'the doctors did all they could but her body was too weak to keep living' (2005, p. 184), such explanations may not be appropriate for young children if they presuppose a biological conceptualization of the human body. Slaughter goes on to say that even explanations that frame death in terms of a breakdown of the body, while concrete and unambiguous, are likely to be meaningless to a young child who does not recognize that death is characterized and ultimately caused by the cessation of bodily function.

However, the open expression of feelings highly valued in both psychodynamic and stage models of grief, can become destabilizing to a family's negotiated rules for shared emotional stability. Social development theory highlights that in the absence of social resources, such as economic security or social support, bereaved families are forced to rely on interpersonally negotiated emotional controls as strategies for stability. Interpersonal control strategies in response to overwhelming grief, such as interactions suppressing differences in shared experience or restricting destabilizing change, interfere with the individual and family capacity for open communication, cohesion, and mutual support and may narrow the capacity for flexible coping with future development challenges (Shapiro, 1994, 1996). Shapiro (2001) states that the greater the stressors and discontinuities and the fewer social supports there are, the more likely families will be to rely on interpersonal control strategies that limit their ability to adapt. Such families inhibit their growing children whose maturing cognitive capacities generate new questions about the death and its meaning from exploring the experience of the death and their images of the deceased family member in ways that enhance ongoing development (Shapiro, 1994; Silverman, 2000).

Research undertaken by MacPherson (2005) found that not sharing information and communicating with the children was directly related to the parents' ability to talk together about the illness. It was found that the dying parent influenced the decision whether the children were informed about the prognosis and the well parent followed their example. Fearnley (2010) refers to an interview with a specialist nurse who spoke at length about how in her opinion she had a significant role to facilitate those difficult conversations. She discussed how, by asking the parents questions about what their children knew of the situation and their understanding of it, new communication lines were opened and opportunities created for proactive supportive work to be undertaken. However, she also stressed that the initial discussions were 'very gentle to test out what the children may have been told' and to see what hesitations or beliefs the family may hold that prevented them from talking with their children. It would appear that these initial conversations are imperative so that the channels of communication can be opened.

In common with Hooghe et al. (2011), Ellis et al. (2013) suggest that if the negative consequences of bereavement are to be minimized, it is crucial that rather than unilaterally advocating the promotion of open communication, those working with bereaved families first discuss the complexities of communication with the family members, specifically those concerning talking and keeping silent, and explore the different meanings associated with sharing grief experiences with each other. Such an intervention may help the family as a unit, through interpersonal communication, to integrate experience and adapt to changes with few attempts to control thoughts and feelings in ways that impede shared development (Shapiro, 2008).

However, according to Fearnley (2010), the quality of information exchange is often dependent on the practitioner's professional background. Fearnley reported that a number of families in her study talked about how the focus of support from the nursing teams was medically orientated. Furthermore, it was noted that the nursing staff generally visited the family home during the day, when the children were at school, and therefore their issues were not discussed nor were they party to any information. Fearnley also found that when specialist social care staff were involved there was typically an increase in the amount of information provided to the children. This was provided directly through discussions and therapeutic sessions.

The emerging findings from this study also indicate that some qualified practitioners have difficulties using the words death, dying, and dead. This avoidance of the words and to supplement the conversations with euphemisms (which may lead to misunderstanding of information) were indicative of the individual's personal difficulties and how in general society has a death-denying attitude (Fearnley, 2010). Fearnley reflected about the choice of language and whether this was symptomatic of the notion that the subject is taboo within some cultures. Drawing on the evidence from her research, Fearnley suggests that there is a stigma attached to talking about death and dying and that practitioners find it difficult and embarrassing to discuss such topics. Fearnley asserts that this sequestration leads to a pattern of communicating that avoids any involvement of such unmentionable vocabulary. The metaphor of the elephant in the room is used to delineate how practitioners avoid such discussions and thereby miss opportunities to support children experiencing potentially the most traumatic event they have ever faced. Fearnley suggests that this is related to a lack of training for practitioners both as students and through continual professional development.

Conclusions

In this chapter we have explored the literature that looks at the impact of parental death. We have also outlined some of the dominant models of grief. Most suggest that bereaved people need to engage with their loss and work through it, so that life can be reordered and meaningful again. Worden's tasks of bereavement give a framework to guide the bereaved in their grief work, while the dual process model demonstrates the need to deal with secondary stresses as well as the primary loss, with time away from both. It is also important to recognize that the bereaved do not need to forget and leave the deceased behind, but can integrate them into their future lives by means of a continuing bond. An understanding of the different models of grief together with an understanding of the relationship between age, experience, and manifestations of grief in children are crucial for practitioners to provide effective support. An understanding the family dynamic is also of great importance for those working to enhance communication in identifying possible tensions between members and assessing how members may influence or be influenced by others, as well as understanding what the death means to each member. Each bereaved person is unique and will deal with a significant death in their own way; therefore there is no one right or wrong way to grieve. In many cases, the family is very often the prime provider of socialization, social control, and support. Certain factors either inhibit or enhance a family's grief. Families in which there are fragile relationships, secrets, and divergent beliefs may have more difficulty in adjusting; whereas families who have frequent contact, rituals, and a willingness for each member to share their feelings may find it easier. Those talking to families and children about the death of a parent need to acknowledge the complexities involved. They also need to acknowledge that a family's capacity to communicate and share information with their children is historically driven and mediated by the social, cultural, and economic context in which it resides. If families and children are to be supported at potentially the most traumatic time in their life, practitioners also need to ensure that they have the necessary skills, competencies, and confidence to engage with families in ways that enhance communication and information sharing.

Online materials

Complete references for this chapter are available online at <http://www.oxfordmedicine.com>.

References

Bowlby, J. (1961). Childhood mourning and its implications for psychiatry. *American Journal of Psychiatry*, 118, 481–498.

Carey, S. (1985). *Conceptual Change in Childhood*. Cambridge, MA: MIT Press.

Christ, G.H. (2000). Impact of development on children's mourning. *Cancer Practice*, 8, 72–81.

Christ, G.H. and Christ, A.E. (2006). Current approaches to helping children cope with a parent's terminal illness. *CA: A Cancer Journal for Clinicians*, 56, 197–212.

Ellis, J., Dowrick, C., and Lloyd-Williams, M. (2013). The long-term impact of early parental death: lessons from a narrative study. *Journal of the Royal Society of Medicine*, 106, 57–67.

Ellis, J.E. (2009). *An Exploration of the Impact of Early Parental Death on Adult Life: A Narrative Study*. PhD thesis, University of Liverpool.

Freud, S. (1957). Mourning and melancholia. In J. Strachey (ed.) *The Standard Edition of the Complete Psychological Works of Sigmond Freud*. London: Hogarth Press. (Original work published in 1917.)

Klass, D., Silverman, P.R., and Nickman, S.L. (1996). *Continuing Bonds: New Understandings of Grief*. Washington, DC: Taylor and Francis.

Kuber-Ross, E. (1969). *On Death and Dying*. New York: Macmillan.

Lindenmann, E. (1944). Symptomatology and management of acute grief. *American Journal of Psychiatry*, 101, 141–148.

Parsons, S. (2011). *Long-Term Impact of Childhood Bereavement: Preliminary Analysis of the 1970 British Cohort Study (BCS70)*. London: Childhood Wellbeing Research Centre.

Worden, J.W. (1996). *Children and Grief: When a Parent Dies*. New York: Guilford Press.

Communication between professionals

Jane deLima Thomas, Katie Fitzgerald Jones, Amanda Moment, and Janet L. Abrahm

Introduction to communication between professionals

Communication between health-care professionals is a core element of palliative care and is increasingly recognized as critical to health-care quality (National Healthcare Quality Report, 2011). The growing complexity of health-care delivery systems worldwide has led to a stronger emphasis on interprofessional communication, resulting in changes in health professional school curricula (McDonough and Bennett, 2006), institution accreditation requirements (Joint Commission Resources, 2009), and standards of interprofessional education (Interprofessional Education Collaborative Expert Panel, 2011). The importance of interprofessional collaboration was underscored in 2010 when the World Health Organization published its *Framework for Action on Interprofessional Education and Collaborative Practice*, emphasizing the need for more integrated and collaborative models of health-care training and delivery.

The focus on interprofessional communication comes, in part, as the result of the growing evidence about the practical consequences of communication successes and failures between health-care providers. The data show that failures in communication may lead to inferior palliative care, including medication errors, delays in treatment, wrong-site surgeries, higher patient mortality rates, longer hospital stays, and worse pain control and functional status (Mills et al., 2008; Martin et al., 2010). Poor communication may also lead to negative consequences for health-care professionals, including higher nursing turnover, negative feedback, and demoralization of colleagues (Health Professions Regulatory Network, 2008). Conversely, successful communication leads to better outcomes for patients and health-care teams including improved understanding by clinicians of patient care goals, improved team morale, higher staff retention, positive feedback from colleagues, and increased productivity (Health Professions Regulatory Network, 2008; Chang et al., 2009).

Palliative care clinicians are often in the position to facilitate communication among various members of the health-care team caring for a patient with a serious illness. First, a palliative care clinician's initial assessment includes an evaluation of the patient's overall clinical status and the roles of and relationships with the providers involved. Second, palliative care clinicians are often consulted for complex patients with difficult to manage symptoms and emotional suffering, leading to team distress, interpersonal conflict, ethical dilemmas, and lack of clarity about the plan of care. Third, most palliative care clinicians have had some communication skills training, and while their focus of care is patients and their families, many of the same communication techniques are effective with colleagues. Fourth, palliative care clinicians are accustomed to working in interdisciplinary teams (IDTs), where open, respectful communication is the expectation. As a result of these factors, palliative care clinicians can play a key role in pulling together the various providers and ensuring that their points of view are heard, misunderstandings are focu minimized, and a comprehensive plan of care is created that reflects input from all.

Principles of good interprofessional communication

Many clinicians believe that the ability to communicate well is innate, that is, that people are either born to be good communicators or they are not. Evidence, however, shows that communication skills are both teachable and learnable (Back et al., 2007; Krimshtein et al., 2011). This is especially encouraging since health-care professionals' communication skills do not improve reliably with experience alone (Wilkinson et al., 2008; Back et al., 2009a). Health-care providers that participate in communication skills training manifest changes in their behaviour that enhance communication (Reeves et al., 2008, Reeves, 2009), increased confidence as communicators (Back et al., 2007), improved assessment of interprofessional communication (Zwarenstein et al., 2007), and have increased patient satisfaction rates (Back et al., 2007). What's more, communication skills training has been shown to have an impact on participants' skill level even 5 years afterward (Roter and Hall, 2006). While the majority of interventions shown to improve communication in the health-care setting have been geared towards communication with patients, there is growing interest in designing interventions to improve interprofessional communication, too (Norgaard et al., 2012).

The guiding principles of good communication are familiar to many palliative care clinicians and are explored in more depth in Chapter 6.1. We summarize three key points here that are particularly important when considering interprofessional communication.

1. *Good communication begins by adopting an attitude of curiosity.* When starting from a position of curiosity, one is open to

the perspective, rationale, and motivation of the other parties involved (Stone et al., 2010). This attitude minimizes the risk of assuming one knows all the facts, leaping to conclusions prematurely, or alienating the other party. Curiosity relies on active listening (Back and Arnold, 2005): paying close attention, asking facilitating questions, and following up on verbal and non-verbal cues.

2. *Communication happens on many levels simultaneously.* The verbal communication exchanged is only one part of the conversation, which at deeper levels also includes underlying emotions and issues of self-identity for each participant (Stone et al., 2010). Good communicators, therefore, can attend to all of the elements of the conversation, even while maintaining self-awareness about their own communication styles, emotional reactions, and triggers for conflict (Back et al., 2009b).

3. *Good communication requires skill in managing conflict.* While conflict managed poorly can prove destructive to relationships and team function, conflict managed well can be productive and even necessary for healthy interaction between colleagues (Ezziane et al., 2012). Healthy conflict can serve to elucidate and contextualize points of disagreement, promote sharing of new ideas and perspectives, and enhance productivity (Lencioni, 2002; Ezziane et al., 2012).

While palliative care clinicians communicate with other professionals in a wide variety of ways, we have chosen to consider two major categories as prototypes: communication within palliative care IDTs and communication between palliative care consultants and other providers.

Communication within palliative care interdisciplinary teams

Given the complex symptoms, psychosocial issues, and important choices that arise for patients and families facing life-limiting illness, skilful communication among members of the palliative care IDT is essential (Blacker and Deveau 2010). Good communication is a result of—and contributes to—important team attributes. The first attribute that facilitates team communication is having mutual goals and a process for evaluating team function in pursuit of those goals (Dahlin, 2010). When a palliative care team creates shared objectives, usually aimed at the relief of suffering, clinicians become more collaborative and work towards group aspirations rather than individual goals (McPherson et al., 2001). These goals are re-evaluated regularly since they often shift in response to new initiatives, challenging cases, and evolving staff competencies (Lencioni, 2002). Additionally, members of a team that communicates well have a clear understanding of individual responsibilities and roles. Each member of the team should be able to articulate the specific skill and expertise he or she brings to patients and the team (Orchard et al., 2005) and how it differs from that of other team providers. When these areas of knowledge and skill are communicated and respected, the group can function with more cohesion and greater utilization of one another's skill sets (Hall, 2005). What's more, if collaboration is carried out effectively, the clinician's team identity trumps the clinician's discipline identity (e.g. nursing, social work, pharmacy, etc.) and team outcomes supersede those of the individual (Lencioni, 2002). Well-communicating teams also have standards for communication

among providers, including conflict negotiation (Lencioni, 2002). Interprofessional relationships are based on respectful communication, trust in one another's motives, and commitment to accountability when discord arises (Interprofessional Education Collaborative Expert Panel, 2011). A high-functioning palliative care team recognizes the importance of good communication in attaining these three attributes and actively work towards cultivating a culture that supports it.

Barriers to communication in palliative care IDTs

Even teams that acknowledge the importance of communication face many types of barriers that compromise it. First, there are practical and organizational issues such as staffing, geography, and caseloads. Since palliative care is a young and rapidly evolving field clinical teams are often in flux, with staffing models changing according to each institution's demand for palliative care services and the resources allocated to team development (Billings, 2008). Palliative care teams can have any number of part-time or full-time clinicians of different disciplines rotating on and off service, leading to significant communication challenges and variable team cohesion. Moreover, palliative care can be delivered to patients with a wide variety of underlying conditions, leading to geographic spread even within a single institution and creating another obstacle to good communication. Lastly, in rapidly growing programmes caseloads can exceed staffing, leaving little time for the team to ensure that lines of communication are maintained. Teams that have stressful caseloads can abandon interdisciplinary work (where providers work together) for multidisciplinary work (where providers 'divide and conquer') as they struggle to meet the clinical demands. The result is poorer communication and integration of each provider's skill sets and more working in parallel (Hall, 2005).

Second, there are barriers related to information value, hierarchy, and provider insight. In teams that emphasize biomedical information, non-medical providers can feel diminished (Wittenberg-Lyles, 2005). For example, if a social worker has to struggle to make his or her viewpoint heard, even when social or emotional distress is central to the patient's needs, the result can be feelings of disempowerment for the clinician and an incomplete plan of care for the patient. Also, the standard medical hierarchy may lead to barriers in interprofessional communication by causing team members to feel uncomfortable raising concerns (Irvine et al., 2002). For example a floor nurse may have concerns about the safety of a patient's discharge plan but feel unable to voice her worry to the physician who seems sure the patient is ready to go home. Lastly, clinicians can lack of insight about their own communication style and effectiveness. Physicians, in particular, tend to overestimate the efficacy of their communication with other team members (Mills et al., 2008; Chang et al., 2010).

Other hurdles to interdisciplinary communication relate to professional education and identity. Traditionally, skills are taught in 'professional silos' that can foster 'power, competition, and hierarchy not teamwork and collaboration' (Angelini, 2011, p. 175). This can result in limited understanding of or compassion for one another's professional perspectives, priorities, and education (Leipzig et al., 2002). For example, a nurse may view social workers more as 'friendly visitors' than as clinicians who work from a solid clinical or theoretical grounding. In addition to misunderstandings about one another's skill sets, palliative care IDT members can struggle with overlapping skills. IDT members share both 'ingroup membership (the IDT) and outgroup membership (occupational group)' (Wittenberg-Lyles et al., 2009, pp. 38–39) and clinicians can become protective of their disciplines and specific skill sets, leading to turf wars and interpersonal conflicts (Larson, 2003). For example, a palliative care nurse practitioner who enjoys exploring the psychosocial aspects of his patients' care might worry that the social worker's expertise will relegate him to medical management only.

Strategies for communication in palliative care IDTs

Given the barriers just described, palliative care IDTs must take a purposeful approach to maximize team communication and function. One strategy receiving increasing attention is the use of structured communication tools (Byres et al., 2009; Denver Health, 2012). For example, structured team rounds have been shown to encourage meaningful contributions from all providers involved in patient care (O'Leary et al., 2010) and to increase team satisfaction and interprofessional teamwork (Maeyama et al., 2003). Not surprisingly, team members' satisfaction increases based on the number of team members involved in the care meeting (Maeyama, 2003). Another example of structured communication is the model developed by Michael Leonard in 2002 called SBAR (Situation–Background–Assessment–Recommendation) (Institute for Health Care Improvement, n.d.). In this model, a clinician is encouraged to provide four categories of information when communicating a concern. The first is to describe the situation—the patient's name, location, and cause for concern: 'I am calling about Mrs X in room 14 who is having new episodes of apnoea.' The second is to give a one-line summary of the background: 'She is a 45-year-old woman with end-stage lung cancer who has required increasing doses of morphine in the last 48 hours.' The third is to provide an assessment of what is occurring: 'I believe that the change in her breathing indicates that she is close to death.' The fourth is to offer a recommendation based on that assessment: 'I think we should contact her husband to let him know that time might be short.' A standardized method like this creates a mutual language and process for conveying information no matter who is calling, the nature of the concern, or the level of urgency.

A second strategy to enhance IDT communication is to have designated forums for discussion and feedback. Difficult patient cases should be debriefed either in real time or soon after to help the team grieve, air misgivings, provide support, and assess team process (Salas et al., 2005; Salas et al., 2008). Any member of the team should be able to initiate this for a patient and have the team respond, with time and support from leadership. An example is to hold 'escalating patient care meetings' where the team convenes at the first signs of a difficult patient case to map out a plan, raise concerns, and involve appropriate clinicians. Additionally, team members should have opportunities to provide critical feedback to one another and their leaders by using 360-degree reviews or feedback tools (Lockyer, 2003; Massagli and Carline, 2007). Feedback must be separated from compensation or performance evaluations so that it remains constructive and not punitive (Lencioni, 2002). No matter the method, teams should have mechanisms for providing feedback to one another both in times of high stress and in times of relative calm (Salas et al., 2005; Salas et al., 2008).

A third strategy to maximize IDT communication is taken from the study of high-reliability organizations (HROs) such as

air-traffic control systems, nuclear power plants, and aircraft carriers. HROs deliberately create an organizational structure that flattens hierarchy by seeking input from front-line members and acknowledging expertise regardless of rank (O'Leary et al., 2012). In this manner each team member's contribution is sought and valued, leading to empowerment for every team member to participate and voice suggestions and concerns (Hempel et al.2012). If we imagine applying these principles to a palliative care IDT, we can consider a case where a palliative care patient dies suddenly in the hospital and in the ensuing confusion the patient's wife is not informed until she comes in to visit the patient. An HRO approach would include soliciting the perspective of all those involved, including the floor nurse, the administrative staff, the physician, the social worker, and so on. Protocols for notifying family members after the death of a loved one would then be studied and revised based on the input from all team members and communicated clearly back to all. With this approach the tendency to blame particular individuals, especially those in a lower position of power, is minimized, and team trust and communication is enhanced.

A fourth, closely related strategy to enhance IDT communication is to cultivate an open, no-fault culture in addressing medical errors (O'Daniel and Rosenstein, 2008). This requires a shift away from regarding medical errors as individuals' mistakes and instead viewing them as a reflection of systems problems (Berwick and Leape, 1999; Institute of Medicine 1999; Institute of Medicine Committee on Quality of Healthcare in America, 2001). A particular danger arises when organizations focus on correcting mistakes by initiating checklists and safety systems but don't recognize the more insidious problem that occurs when errors are identified through these mechanisms and people are afraid to speak up (Maxfield et al., 2005). In order to minimize this dynamic, organizations must tap into personal motivation and agency, that is, the belief that it is important to speak up and that one has the ability to do so. This is best achieved by interventions such as providing examples of non-threatening language to use when discussing mistakes; setting the expectation that each person is accountable for his or her own behaviour as well as that of colleagues; and encouraging providers to share their experiences of speaking up and empowering others to do the same. The effectiveness of these measures rests on the approach of team leaders, who must create an environment of 'psychological safety that fosters open reporting, active questioning, and frequent sharing' (Edmondson 2004, pp. ii8–ii9).

In this section about IDT communication, a number of themes emerge as important in maximizing good IDT communication and function. Table 6.3.1 integrates and expands on many of these points.

Communication in palliative care consultation

As with communication between members of the palliative care IDT, skilled communication is crucial between palliative care providers and other professionals. First, as noted in the introduction, palliative care clinicians are often consulted for difficult patient cases with complex medical, psychosocial, ethical, and emotional issues. Moreover, since palliative care addresses all of the biopsychosocial and spiritual domains of a patient's care, clinicians collaborate with a wide range of providers of different disciplines across many

Table 6.3.1 Effective interdisciplinary team communication

Characteristic	Description/examples
Team leadership	Facilitate problem-solving
	Create effective systems for conflict resolution
	Communicate performance expectations
	Clarify roles
Mutual performance monitoring	Debrief difficult cases
	Use peer assessment tools (e.g. 360-degree evaluations or multisource feedback)
Supportive teamwork behaviour	Anticipate, communicate, and respond to one another's needs
	Adjust workload distribution
	Accept shared responsibilities
Adaptability	Ability to modify processes as new information arrives
Shared mental model and team process	Acknowledge interdependence
	Agree on team goals and how they will be achieved
	Commit to reaching team goals
Closed-loop communication	Acknowledge information received
	Clarify requests
	Follow up on outcomes
Mutual trust	Discuss mistakes and accept feedback
	Practise constructive (not blaming) communication
Clear and respected boundaries	Communicate roles and responsibilities
	Acknowledge and communicate when boundaries are blurred or crossed
Comfort with conflict and error	Raise concerns freely and openly
	Recognize that conflict is inherent in healthy team process
Standardization of communication	Prioritize frequent face-to-face communication
	Use of structured models for interprofessional collaboration (e.g. team rounds, daily goals-of-care forms and checklists, joint visits)
	Participates in interprofessional education
Accountability	Examine and take responsibility for own actions and those of colleagues.

Source: data from O'Leary, K.J. et al., Interdisciplinary teamwork in hospitals: A review and practical recommendations for improvement, *Journal of Hospital Medicine*, Volume 7, Issue 4, pp. 48–54, Copyright © 2012; Angelini, D.J., Interdisciplinary and interprofessional education, *Journal of Perinatal Neonatal Nursing*, Volume 25, Issue 2, pp. 175–179, Copyright © 2011; Leonard, M., *Achieving safe and reliable healthcare*, Health Administration Press, Chicago, USA, Copyright © 2004; and Lencioni, P., *The Five Dysfunctions of a Team*, Jossey-Bass, San Francisco, USA, Copyright © 2002.

settings. Furthermore, and perhaps most important, there is huge variability from country to country in access to palliative care services, ranging from no hospice or palliative care presence in some countries to one provider per 158 million people in Pakistan to one provider per 43 000 per people in the UK (Wright et al., 2008). Even in a single country palliative care programmes can vary widely from institution to institution depending on the history, level of development, and make-up of the programme (Goldsmith

et al., 2008). Palliative care clinicians therefore meet varying levels of understanding and acceptance from other clinicians, and must often identify and overcome misperceptions even while trying to provide patient care.

Palliative care consultation rests on the same core principles as consultation by other specialists, including the fundamental importance of good communication. Consultants must remember that a basic principle of consultation etiquette is that the referring clinician is the consultant's primary customer, and not the patient (Goldman et al., 1983). A consultant's recommendations are conveyed to the referring clinician and the consultant does not have control over which—if any—recommendations will be followed (Meier and Beresford, 2007). Studies of physician compliance rates with consultants' recommendations, however, highlight the importance of good communication with referring clinicians, with communication skills comprising ten of the 11 proven factors that increase compliance (the exception being the severity of the illness) (Cohn, 2003):

◆ Response within 24 hours (Pupa et al., 1986)

◆ 5 or fewer recommendations (Sears and Charlson, 1983)

◆ Identification of critical recommendations (versus routine ones) (Pupa et al., 1986)

◆ Focus on central issues (Ballard et al., 1986)

◆ Specific, relevant recommendations (Horwitz et al., 1983)

◆ Definitive language (Klein et al., 1983)

◆ Specificity in drug dosage, route, frequency, duration (Horwitz et al., 1983)

◆ Frequent follow up including progress notes (Mackenzie et al., 1981)

◆ Direct verbal contact (Pupa et al., 1986)

◆ Therapeutic (versus diagnostic) recommendations (Ballard et al., 1986)

◆ Severity of illness (Sears and Charlson, 1983).

Reproduced with permission from Cohn SL, Macpherson DS. Overview of the principles of medical consultation and perioperative medicine. In: UpToDate, Post TW (Ed), UpToDate, Waltham, MA. (Accessed on 14th November 2014) Copyright © 2014 UpToDate, Inc. For more information visit www.uptodate.com.

Conversely, studies have also shown that if consultants do not follow these guidelines they will be more likely to receive poor feedback and fewer referrals (Goldman et al., 1983).

Communication challenges in palliative care consultation

While all specialist consultation requires effective communication, it can be argued that palliative care consultation carries particular complexity and requires even greater attention to communication. First, providers in other specialties are sometimes uncertain about what palliative care is and which patients might benefit from palliative care consultation (Shipman et al., 2008). Some referring clinicians worry that there is a 'palliative care agenda' to stop aggressive treatments or to encourage patients to sign on to hospice. One survey of 131 clinicians, for example, found there was widespread concern that palliative care consultants would prematurely discuss end-of-life issues, which led to significant barriers to consultation requests (Rodrigues et al., 2007). Other referring clinicians delay referral to palliative care due to worry that it would alarm patients and families (Smith et al., 2012). Yet other referring clinicians find the name 'palliative care' problematic and would more readily refer patients if the consultation were called 'supportive care' (Ferrell, 2005). In each case, the interaction between palliative care providers and referring clinicians requires thoughtful clarification from the beginning in order to identify concerns or misperceptions before proceeding with the consult.

Second, palliative care consultation usually happens at a time of high emotion, in the context of disease progression leading to considerable symptom burden, psychosocial distress, or a turning point in disease course requiring clarification of the goals of care. Clinicians caring for patients with advanced illness often experience strong emotions themselves, including helplessness, frustration, guilt, and grief (Meier et al., 2001). Palliative care consultants must be able to manage the emotions evoked by the situation, and then communicate clearly in the midst of the turbulence in order to facilitate team health and effectiveness and arrive at the best plan of care (Loscalzo, 2008).

Third, unlike consultants whose specialties are defined by organ system (e.g. cardiology) or disease (e.g. oncology), palliative care addresses the whole patient, including physical, emotional, social, and spiritual aspects. The role of consultant, where the focus of evaluation is limited by the scope of the request, can therefore seem restricting and sometimes lead to internal conflict for the consultant (Meier and Beresford, 2007). Examples include seeing a patient to help with advance care planning who has significant physical symptoms not part of the original consult request; seeing a patient who asks direct questions about topics expressly forbidden by the referrer to discuss; seeing a patient who confides goals or worries not known by the referrer; or seeing a patient whose management the consultant strongly disagrees with (Meier and Beresford, 2007). These situations can be particularly challenging for palliative care clinicians whose aim is to relieve total suffering for patients who may define their needs differently from the referring clinician.

Communication strategies in palliative care consultation

While there is no data supporting the use of a particular strategy in palliative care consultation, we draw from the evidence of medical consultation generally, on the opinions of experts in the field, and on our own clinical experience to recommend an approach that uses five core themes.

1. *Curiosity*: as noted earlier, starting from a position of curiosity leads a palliative care consultant to be non-judgemental and open to the perspective, rationale, and motivation of the other members of the team caring for the patient (Back and Arnold, 2005). Important questions include the following: 'What can we do to be helpful?' 'What do you think this patient or family understands about the disease or prognosis?' 'What have you chosen to talk about and why?' 'What is the current treatment plan and why?' 'What are your hopes and worries for this patient?'

2. *Humility*: when palliative care clinicians are brought into situations with high levels of suffering, the temptation can be to

assume that greater expertise would have prevented the distress. It is important to remember that (a) referring clinicians are acting in what they understand to be the best interests of their patients, (b) the clinician who has cared for a patient over time may have knowledge that the consultant does not have, and (c) certain cases will carry high levels of suffering even when the clinicians involved have considerable expertise (Meier and Beresford, 2007). Acknowledging other clinicians' efforts, expertise, and relationship with the patient can be helpful (Back and Arnold, 2005): 'It sounds like you have gone to great lengths to help this patient and family.' 'Could you explain to me what the risks and benefits of the various treatment options are in a case like this?' 'You have known this patient longer than I have so there may be things I'm missing.'

3. *Transparency*: transparency in a consultant's communication can be helpful in several ways (Back and Arnold, 2005). First, transparency about a consultant's viewpoint and prior experience can help other clinicians understand why the recommendations are being made and consider the rationale when deciding whether to take the recommended course of action. Additionally, transparency in thought processes helps show other clinicians what factors in palliative care are considered important, what assessments are made, and what outcomes are aimed for. Furthermore, a consultant's transparency about biases or areas of uncertainty models an attitude of openness, trust, and mutual respect. An example might be, 'We only have observational studies supporting this recommendation but my own experience is that it can be very helpful in patients like this.'

4. *Clarity*: it is crucial that a palliative care consultant have the ability to distil the many elements of a patient's care—medical data, psychosocial issues, team dynamics, etc.—and provide clear information to facilitate a common understanding of the issues. Ensuring clarity rests on the core principles of consultation outlined above, includes making a careful assessment of the reason and urgency for the consult; obtaining a thorough history from the medical record, patient, and family; keeping the consult recommendations and documentation brief and focused; using specific, definite language in the consult recommendations (e.g. medication dosing); contacting the referring clinician with recommendations; and making specific plans for follow-up, including leaving progress notes and signing off (Cohn, 2003).

5. *Judiciousness*: palliative care consultants must sometimes balance their desire to advocate for their patients with the need to preserve the relationship with the referring clinician and respect the boundaries of consultation etiquette (Weissman and von Gunten, 2012). Many factors can influence how strongly a consultant recommends a certain course of action, including the nature of the relationship between consultant and primary clinician, the risks and benefits of following one course of action or the other, the level of institutional support for palliative care, and the degree of suffering in the patient, family, or other clinicians (Weissman and von Gunten, 2012). Weissman notes that ultimately, palliative care clinicians will be most successful at consultations and collaboration if the provider requesting the consult or stakeholder trusts the consultant to make decisions that benefit the patient and family and preserve the authority of the referring clinician (Weissman, 2007, 2011).

Conclusion

As outlined in the chapter, interprofessional communication is crucial in palliative care, both within palliative care IDTs and between palliative care clinicians and others. Strategies to improve interprofessional communication in palliative care have been named throughout the chapter, but what are the next steps?

Efforts to improve interprofessional communication in health care are happening at many levels. One is the increasing emphasis on integrated care pathways (ICPs), defined as 'multidisciplinary tool[s] to improve the quality and efficacy of evidence based care and communication tool between professionals to manage and standardize the outcome of coordinated care' (Vanhaecht et al., 2006, p. 28). ICPs should if possible be evidence based and act as a guide on how to diagnose, treat, and follow-up the patients and the families. ICPs can also act as standardized communication tools showing promise in improving both clinical outcomes and communication between providers (Mahmoud et al., 2008). Another effort is the convening of expert consensus panels to set standards for interprofessional communication in specific disciplines, fields, or locations, which then can be used by clinicians, administrators, and educators designing clinical or educational programmes (Interprofessional Education Collaborative Expert Panel, 2011). A third effort is the increasing attention from regulatory bodies to tie measures of interprofessional communication to accreditation of clinical and educational institutions (Joint Commission Resources, 2009). A fourth is the development of government health-care policies emphasizing the importance of interprofessional communication and providing guidelines and structures (including funding) for its implementation (The Enhancing Interdisciplinary Collaboration in Primary Health Care Initiative, Nolte, J., 2006). A fifth is continued research to expand the evidence base on interprofessional communication, including outcomes for individuals, programmes, and institutions (Manser, 2009; Martin et al., 2010), as well as efficacy studies for interventions designed to improve it (Baker et al., 2008). A sixth and perhaps most notable effort, however, is the increasing focus on interprofessional education. Clinicians in training (Carpenter, 2009) as well as practising providers (McPherson et al., 2001) are participating in innovative interdisciplinavry educational initiatives, which have been variably studied but have demonstrated efficacy in improving collaborative practice and clinical outcomes (Reeves et al., 2008; Reeves 2009).

Palliative care can clearly benefit from the growing attention on interprofessional communication worldwide and the resulting development of these communication protocols, policies, and curricula. In fact, palliative care as a field is positioned to help lead the way, since clinicians are often experts in both communication and interdisciplinary practice. The task now is to be sure the field keeps current with the evolving scholarship on interprofessional communication and continues to contribute to and apply the emerging wisdom for the benefit of terminally ill patients and the providers who care for them.

Online materials

Complete references for this chapter are available online at <http://www.oxfordmedicine.com>.

References

Angelini, D.J. (2011). Interdisciplinary and interprofessional education. *Journal of Perinatal Neonatal Nursing*, 25(2), 175–179.

Back, A., Arnold, R.M., Baile, W.F., *et al.* (2007). Efficacy of communication skills training for giving bad news and discussing transitions to palliative care. *Archives of Internal Medicine*, 167, 453–460.

Berwick, D. and Leape, L. (1999). Reducing errors in medicine. *Quality in Health Care*, 8, 145–146.

Carpenter, J. (2009). Interprofessional education for medical and nursing students: evaluation of a programme. *Medical Education*, 29(4), 265–272.

Cohn, S. (2003). The role of medical consultant. *Medical Clinics of North America*, 87, 1–6.

Goldman, L., Lee, T., and Rudd, P. (1983). Ten commandments for effective consultations. *Archives of Internal Medicine*, 143, 1753–1755.

Horowitz, R., Henes, C., and Horwitz, S. (1983). Developing strategies for improving diagnostic and management efficacy or medical consultations. *Journal of Chronic Disease*, 36(2), 213–218.

Interprofessional Education Collaborative Expert Panel (2011). *Core Competencies for Interprofessional Collaborative Practice: Report of an Expert Panel*. Washington, DC: Interprofessional Education Collaborative. Available at: <http://www.aacn.nche.edu/education-resources/ipecreport.pdf>.

Joint Commission Resources (2009). *The Joint Commission Guide to Improving Staff Communication* (2nd ed.). Oakbrook Terrace, IL: Joint Commission Resources. Available at: <http://www.jcrinc.com/assets/1/14/GISC09_Sample_Pages1.pdf>.

Lencioni, P. (2002). *The Five Dysfunctions of a Team*. San Francisco, CA: Jossey- Bass.

McPherson, K., Headrick, L., and Moss, F. (2001). Working and learning together: good quality care depends on it, but how can we achieve it? *Quality in Health Care*, 70(30), 1–12.

Meier, D. and Beresford, L. (2007). Consultation etiquette challenges palliative care to be on its best behavior. *Journal of Palliative Medicine*, 10(1), 7–12.

Norgaard B., Kofoed P.E., Kyvik K.O., Ammentorp J. (2012). Communication skills training for health care professionals improves the adult orthopaedic patient's experience of quality of care. *Scand J Caring Sciences*, 26, 698–704.

Pupa, L., Conventry, J., Hanley, J., and Carpenter, J. (1986). Factors affecting compliance for general medicine consultants to non-internist. *American Journal of Medicine*, 81(3), 508–514.

Wittenberg-Lyles, E.M., Oliver, D.P., Demiris, G., and Regehr, K. (2009) Exploring interpersonal communication in hospice interdisciplinary team meetings. *Journal of Gerontological Nursing*, 35(7), 38–45.

World Health Organization (2010). *Framework for Action on Interprofessional Education and Collaborative Practice*. Geneva: World Health Organization. Available at: <http://www.who.int/hrh/resources/framework_action/en/index.html>.

Communications with the public, politicians, and the news media

Barry R. Ashpole

The communications environment

Two universal issues to have emerged in recent years continue to generate a great deal of attention in both the political and public arenas: (1) the future provision and delivery of health care and social services to the population at large; and (2) meeting the needs of the elderly, who are living longer, in greater numbers than in past generations, and with a corresponding increase in the incidence of chronic or long-term illness or disability. Running parallel is the trend in many countries away from institutionalized care to accommodate the preference expressed by many people to receive care and support in their own home in the event of illness or incapacity; the potential economic benefits of which have not escaped policymakers, presenting them with a persuasive argument that suggests a significant shift in the focus and scope of community care in the decades ahead. Against this backdrop is the increasing attention on all fronts given to the quality of care and support—or lack of—for those living with a terminal illness, both patients and their families or loved ones.

In assessing the prevailing communications environment, it is important not to lose sight of the growing evidence in the literature that the philosophy and principles of hospice and palliative care are gaining currency beyond meeting the immediate needs of those living with a shortened life expectancy. The holistic concepts of 'whole-person' care and managing 'total' pain are steadily working their way into family and hospital practice, long-term or extended care, and home care. This emerging trend has served to facilitate discussion about when, during the illness trajectory, should patients be referred to specialized end-of-life care. Almost from its earliest days, however, hospice and palliative care have been associated in the minds of many people—among them health professionals—with dying and death. This has created at times almost insurmountable barriers in the medical decision-making process and in conversations about life's last chapter.

Coverage of end-of-life issues in the news media has tended to be in the context of 'patient choice', which has done much to fuel the highly contentious public debates on assisted or facilitated death, medical futility, and on who has the 'final say' in the medical decision-making process. The protagonists in these debates focus on their respective interpretations of 'dying with dignity', which inevitably encompass the potential cost—both emotionally and financially—of sustaining life. This has resulted in a broad range of initiatives to promote advance care planning. Honouring the principle of patient autonomy and respecting patient wishes,

nonetheless, has become something of an ethical minefield. A residual effect has been the increased support given—ironically on *all* sides in the 'dying with dignity' debate—to the need to improve access to quality end-of-life care.

The communications environment in which to engage in an open dialogue with the public, politicians and policymakers, and the news media, suggests a far more proactive approach to communications than has hitherto been the norm.

The language of end-of-life care

There are differing points of view regarding language usage, particularly with patients, families, or lay people in general. This is not in reference to medical speak or terminology. Discussed here is how people are inclined to *interpret* language. As pointed out, 'hospice' and 'palliative care' are associated in the minds of many people with dying and death and, as a consequence, are taboo subjects or at least exceedingly difficult ones to broach. An important starting point in any dialogue, therefore, is to establish what a patient or family understands of the illness and what they want to know (or not know) in terms of, say, prognosis and likely scenarios as illness progresses—the 'what ifs'. From here, one can begin to gauge expectations with regard to end-of-life care, which can then lead into a discussion of hospice and palliative care. The challenge, however, can be compounded by modern language usage.

As individuals, we may go to extraordinary lengths in our day-to-day lives to avoid being the bearer of 'bad news' in almost any context. We consciously work, it often seems, in overdrive—to 'soften the blow', 'sugar-coat the message', to be 'politically correct' or 'culturally sensitive'. In doing so, we risk living much of our lives evading reality. As an example, 'openness' and 'transparency' have come to replace 'honesty' and 'truth', fundamental principles of hospice and palliative care. Also, is the 'conspiracy of silence' that so often prevails as death approaches—or, for that matter, whenever confronted with crises in our lives—nothing more than a manifestation of a life-long discomfort with the acceptance of the inevitable, of reality—or of truth itself? We live in a society that has, to a greater or lesser degree, devalued or inflated the meaning of words and, as individuals, we often manipulate their use and meaning to serve whatever our individual or collective ends might be. This begs the question: are we losing the ability or capacity to communicate effectively—or to hear what we need to hear—with empathy and without hurt or hurting?

An often overlooked and underappreciated 'component' of language is 'non-verbal' communication. People are not always conscious of how and what they communicate through their body language, facial expressions, or in their tone, no matter whether they are in a one-on-one situation or addressing a large audience or meeting with a small group of people.

Engaging in a dialogue with the public, politicians, and the news media

There is a direct correlation between the quality of care and the quality of communication. The quality of care for the terminally ill patient rests almost entirely on empathetic and meaningful two-way communication among or between all protagonists. It is essential to building a therapeutic relationship, facilitating informed decision-making, and effecting a positive change in the illness experience. The need is to transport this same mindset in reaching out to a far broader audience with the ultimate purpose of improving public understanding, advancing policy development, and building an informed news media. In other words, advocacy, which can be broadly defined as either taking a proactive stance (i.e. capital 'A' advocacy) or taking a reactive stance (i.e. small 'a' advocacy), in other words, acting 'after the fact'. Given the nature of the news media, 'yesterday's news' remains always 'yesterday's news', and opportunities for a meaningful response or redress fade—quickly.

The public

Patient choices tend to be at the forefront of public discussion on many aspects of health care. In the shadow of this discussion is the widespread concern in most countries over the needs of an ageing population. Added to this is the call to improve resource allocation to allow people to remain in their own homes and, if the option is available, to die there. The demands on informal or family caregivers has gained increasing attention also and added yet another dimension to the public discussion on meeting future demand for health-care and social services. Each of these issues should be considered 'avenues' to broaden discussion to encompass the provision and delivery of specialized end-of-life care.

Opportunities for community outreach come in many forms, particularly at the local or regional level, such as participating in public forums, speaking to special or public interest groups . . . and, of course, engaging the news media. Towards this end, a proven strategy has been to establish a pool of local experts, people who can speak with some authority on a given issue. Commonly referred to as a speaker's bureau, this can be an invaluable community resource (for the news media also).

Politicians

National ageing, home care or end-of-life care strategies are lacking in many, if not most, countries. For policymakers, each represents something of a political minefield and the real threat of political 'suicide'. A cautionary note: in countries where there is government funding or resource allocation for hospice or palliative care, there is an ever-present risk when speaking out on end-of-life issues of being seen to 'bite the hand that feeds you'. There can be negative consequences or repercussions if heard or seen to challenge or comment negatively on government action or inaction. This can present health-care professionals with both

an ethical and moral dilemma. Understandably, they are guarded in their expressions of concern or criticism, opting to err on the side of caution. This has the potential for neutralizing opposing points of view.

It is important to establish a dialogue with key politicians, at the local, regional, and national level. Policy may emanate at, say, the national, state, or provincial levels of government, but resource allocation may be a shared responsibility with other levels of government, for example, municipal. While politicians are the public face of government, it is important to identify and connect with those individuals who advise or counsel politicians on policy, who are involved in researching and gathering background information on a given issue or topic, and who can help navigate the political system—most importantly at the ministerial level.

The news media

The news media stands as one of the principal arbiters of social attitudes on a broad range of issues; its selection and interpretation shapes public opinion. With this in mind, there is an understandable and widespread scepticism or reluctance on the part of many health professionals to engage with journalists or reporters. It can be a risky business and also a mixed blessing. It is possible, nonetheless, if not imperative to take part in public discussion and, through the news media, give the general public a chance to make up its own mind from a broader set of arguments and different points of view. A prerequisite is to monitor the news media—much in the same way a health professional monitors the literature—to keep abreast of current thinking.

Engaging the news media is a formidable challenge, particularly since it is becoming increasingly more fragmented with each advance in technology. Gone are the days of only a few major news outlets. And, there is a notable change in the calibre of journalists who might be assigned to a 'health story'. Informed medical or policy writers, as examples, are not as commonplace as, say, a decade or two ago. There are, nonetheless, thoughtful elements in the news media, but a health professional may often be faced in an interview with a journalist with less than a general knowledge of the subject matter or issue in question. Brevity is invariably the requirement, most notably in the broadcast media where the ambiguous 'sound bite' seems the overriding order of the day. Inherent in this approach to news reporting is the probability of comments or information taken out of context.

A common technique used by news reporters is to ask a question, rapidly followed by two or three possible answers, in effect 'managing' the interview, for example:

> Why do you think government is not prepared to commit to funding additional free-standing hospices? Is it because it is relying too heavily on the community for financial support . . . or, that the economic case for hospice has yet to be made?

This can flummox the subject being interviewed, who is faced with responding, not to the initial question, but to one or both of the fabricated answers, which are more often than not purely speculative. Lost may be the opportunity for a more accurate or truthful—less provocative—response. Another technique is to ask a 'loaded' question:

> Is it true that as a consequence of government budget cuts, the hospital will reduce the number of desperately needed palliative care beds?

The response may indeed be a simple 'yes' (or, conceivably, 'no'), but the broadcasted or published news item might read:

> Physicians are critical of the government decision to close palliative care beds. Dr X said in an interview that the proposed budget cuts will mean reducing the desperately needed beds for dying patients.

With this in mind, it is critically important not to be diverted from the key points that need to be made. At the outset, stay focused, deliver the 'bottom line' first and then the background or rationale. Keep in mind also that there really is no such thing as 'off the record' and that the journalist you are talking with is not your 'best friend'. Respect that the journalist has a job to do, but do not relax your guard. The watchword should always be preparedness.

The Internet and social media should be considered in the same context as the more conventional print and broadcast news media, with added reservations. While they offer a means of reaching a far wider audience, the Internet and social media function with few conventions or 'rules of engagement'. They might be considered the ultimate in terms of opportunities for freedom of expression. In this technology-fixated age, the Internet and social media fit neatly Marshall McLuhan's theory of 'the medium is the message', by which the medium influences how the message is received. Much is contradictory, distorted or one-sided, emotionally charged, inaccurate, unsubstantiated, or unverifiable. The Internet and social media are something of a 'free for all' in the exchange of information and ideas. Proceed, therefore, with guarded optimism.

A preparedness plan

While the public, politicians, and the news media may be more than familiar, if not personally acquainted, with mainstream medicine, and health-care and social services in general, end-of-life care remains largely unfamiliar territory. For one, it demands dedicating time with a patient or family in a system where time is more often than not at a premium. An example of its complexity is the psychosocial aspects of hospice and palliative care in, say, an ethnically diverse or multicultural society. Dying and death is not something that lends itself easily to a 'tick box' or 'checklist' mentality. Therefore, no matter with whom you are trying to communicate, one needs to develop a preparedness plan for each and every encounter or opportunity.

There are a number of different approaches to formulating such a plan. One that serves the purpose of giving realistic and understandable guidance to effective, empathetic communications asks and answers five key questions: 'Who are we talking to?', 'Where are we now in their minds?', 'Where would we like to be?', 'How do we get there?', and 'How do we know we are right?'

Who are we talking to? (i.e. the 'target' audience)—the term 'target' is used only to characterize those people who are most likely to receive the intended message with sympathetic eyes or ears. Try to describe them demographically and psychographically. If you cannot with reasonable precision, research to find out who and what kind of people they are . . . and, in the case of politicians, what their position or stand is or has been on the issue or subject in question.

Where are we now in their minds? (i.e. perceptions)—this question should be answered in the language of the audience you are trying to reach. It is a summation of what you think the person or people you are trying to reach say or think about the issue you would like to address or discuss. Once again, it may be necessary to conduct research to answer this question with reasonable accuracy. A starting point at this stage of the process is to acknowledge a basic premise of communication: perception is fact.

Where would we like to be? (i.e. communications 'objective')—after your message has been heard or read, what response can realistically be expected from the communication?

How do we get there? (i.e. 'strategy')—if you think of the objective in terms of how you want your audience to respond, then the 'strategy' has to be what it is you say or do to create that response.

How do we know we are right? (i.e. 'support')—whenever possible support the answers to the first four questions. If you have done your homework before starting this exercise, you will constantly refer back to available information as the exercise progresses. If any answer is questionable supposition, decide that it should be checked out or researched. In any event, 'How do we know we are right?' is not a question you ask at the end of the exercise. It is one you ask all the way through: each answer to the four questions requires back-up support, a rationale. A reason why.

Conclusion

Engaging in a dialogue with the public, politicians, or the news media is challenging and requires careful consideration and planning. It demands dedicated time. It can indeed be a harrowing experience navigating the emotional and political terrain that is involved, but, ask yourself, who is better qualified to help shape both opinion and understanding, and policy development, with regard to end-of-life care?

SECTION 7

Assessment tools and Informatics

Palliative care needs assessment tools

Afaf Girgis and Amy Waller

Introduction to palliative care needs assessment tools

The delivery of appropriate and equitable care is a challenge facing many areas of health-care, including palliative care. The World Health Organization defines palliative care as 'an approach that improves the quality of life of patients and their families facing the problems associated with life-threatening illness, through the prevention and relief of suffering by means of early identification and impeccable assessment and treatment of pain and other problems, physical, psychological, and spiritual' (World Health Organization, 2013, p. 11). Issues surrounding when and how palliative care should be delivered, as well as to whom, are yet to be resolved. However, inherent in the World Health Organization definition of palliative care is the assessment of needs. In this chapter, we discuss the concept of needs assessment and consider strategies for assessing people's needs and experiences, with a focus on the tools developed specifically for this purpose. Finally, we reiterate the importance of needs assessment tools being implemented as part of routine care to facilitate the right care being offered to people at the time they most need it, by the people or service which is most appropriate to meet identified needs.

Measures to inform clinical care

Patient satisfaction with care, or the extent to which an individual's experience compares with his or her expectations, has been used widely as a proxy measure of disease-related morbidity. Despite its continued popularity, its value in facilitating the process of clinical care is arguably uncertain at best. There are few reports on the reliability of satisfaction surveys (Aharony and Strasser, 1993; Nabati et al., 1998; Bredart et al., 2001). For many decades, patient morbidity has also been studied through assessment of quality of life, or the ramifications of a disease on aspects of life experience (Gustafson, 1991; Lehr and Strosberg, 1991; Gustafson et al., 1993; Skeel, 1993; Akechi et al., 2011; Molassiotis et al., 2011). A wide range of validated measures are available to assess the physical and psychosocial impacts of a disease. More recently, distress has been advocated as the sixth vital sign, alongside temperature, respiration, heart rate, blood pressure, and pain (Bultz and Carlson, 2006; Holland and Bultz, 2007).

Needs assessment has become a more widely utilized measure informing clinical practice since the late 1990s, as it spans both quality of life and quality of care issues (Bonevski et al., 2000).

Richardson et al. (2007) argue that 'from a patient's perspective, the quality of supportive care can be considered to be the extent to which needs are addressed and met, and if they are to be addressed adequately, must first be identified' (Richardson et al., 2007). The relationship between patient needs and other measures, including quality of life and satisfaction, has been the topic of much debate and discussion in the literature (Asadi-Lari et al., 2004; Wen and Gustafson, 2004). There is some evidence demonstrating significant relationships between unmet needs and poor emotional health and dissatisfaction with health services. A recent study evaluating the ability of distress screening to uncover unmet need for psychosocial services in cancer patients concluded that direct assessment of unmet needs was a more efficient strategy for identifying specific need for services (van Scheppingen et al., 2011). Carlson et al. (2012) have argued for a more complementary model, in which screening for distress is augmented usefully by the assessment of meetable unmet needs, with further assessment and empirically supported treatments as needed. The question about 'meetable unmet needs' is clearly complex.

Needs assessment in palliative care

Not all patients for whom death is expected will need specialist palliative care (Palliative Care Australia, 2005a), but for those who do, non-referral, late referral, or crisis referral may affect adversely the quality of care they receive near the end of life. Many factors contribute to non- or late receipt of palliative care. A key factor has been a reliance on prognosis and patient symptoms as the main triggers for specialist palliative care referrals by both generalist and specialist practitioners (Johnson et al., 2008, 2011a, 2011b, 2011c). However, a reliance on prognosis is fraught with problems given evidence of high levels of inaccuracy (systematically optimistic) in doctors' prognoses for terminally ill patients (Glare et al., 2003; Gwilliam et al., 2013). A longer doctor–patient relationship appears to reduce prognostic accuracy further, rather than improve it. The growing and compelling evidence base against prognostication supports the position of international bodies, including Palliative Care Australia and the World Health Organization, which have long advocated for a move away from prognosis and diagnosis-based models to guide delivery of care, to recommending needs-based care (Palliative Care Australia, 2005b; World Health Organization, 2007).

Needs assessment in palliative care inevitably must be guided by the domains of palliative care. These have been well articulated by the World Health Organization as including pain, physical, psychological, social, cultural, and spiritual needs (World Health Organization, 2013); with a detailed overview of the domains of palliative care, as defined by the Canadian Hospice Palliative Care Association (2002), presented in Fig. 7.1.1.

Needs assessment tools have been developed and tested to assess palliative care and support needs across a variety of settings and diseases. Choosing the most appropriate tool depends on the purpose of the assessment, the target population, and the acceptability and psychometric qualities of the instrument.

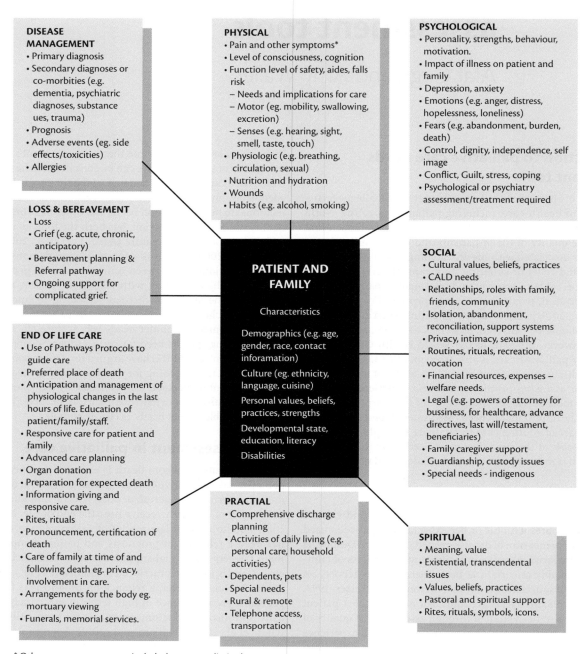

DISEASE MANAGEMENT
• Primary diagnosis
• Secondary diagnoses or co-morbities (e.g. dementia, psychiatric diagnoses, substance ues, trauma)
• Prognosis
• Adverse events (eg. side effects/toxicities)
• Allergies

LOSS & BEREAVEMENT
• Loss
• Grief (e.g. acute, chronic, anticipatory)
• Bereavement planning & Referral pathway
• Ongoing support for complicated grief.

END OF LIFE CARE
• Use of Pathways Protocols to guide care
• Preferred place of death
• Anticipation and management of physiological changes in the last hours of life. Education of patient/family/staff.
• Responsive care for patient and family
• Advanced care planning
• Organ donation
• Preparation for expected death
• Information giving and responsive care.
• Rites, rituals
• Pronouncement, certification of death
• Care of family at time of and following death eg. privacy, involvement in care.
• Arrangements for the body eg. mortuary viewing
• Funerals, memorial services.

PHYSICAL
• Pain and other symptoms*
• Level of consciousness, cognition
• Function level of safety, aides, falls risk
  – Needs and implications for care
  – Motor (eg. mobility, swallowing, excretion)
  – Senses (eg. hearing, sight, smell, taste, touch)
• Physiologic (e.g. breathing, circulation, sexual)
• Nutrition and hydration
• Wounds
• Habits (e.g. alcohol, smoking)

PATIENT AND FAMILY

Characteristics

Demographics (e.g. age, gender, race, contact inforamation)

Culture (eg. ethnicity, language, cuisine)

Personal values, beliefs, practices, strengths

Developmental state, education, literacy

Disabilities

PRACTIAL
• Comprehensive discharge planning
• Activities of daily living (e.g. personal care, household activities)
• Dependents, pets
• Special needs
• Rural & remote
• Telephone access, transportation

PSYCHOLOGICAL
• Personality, strengths, behaviour, motivation.
• Impact of illness on patient and family
• Depression, anxiety
• Emotions (e.g. anger, distress, hopelessness, loneliness)
• Fears (e.g. abandonment, burden, death)
• Control, dignity, independence, self image
• Conflict, Guilt, stress, coping
• Psychological or psychiatry assessment/treatment required

SOCIAL
• Cultural values, beliefs, practices
• CALD needs
• Relationships, roles with family, friends, community
• Isolation, abandonment, reconciliation, support systems
• Privacy, intimacy, sexuality
• Routines, rituals, recreation, vocation
• Financial resources, expenses – welfare needs.
• Legal (e.g. powers of attorney for bussiness, for healthcare, advance directives, last will/testament, beneficiaries)
• Family caregiver support
• Guardianship, custody issues
• Special needs - indigenous

SPIRITUAL
• Meaning, value
• Existential, transcendental issues
• Values, beliefs, practices
• Pastoral and spiritual support
• Rites, rituals, symbols, icons.

* Other common symptoms include, but are not limited to:
Cardio-respiratory: breathlessness, cough, edema, hiccups, apnea, agonal breathing patterns
Gastrointestinal: nausea, vomiting, constipation, obstipation, bowel obstruction, diarrhea, bloating, dysphagia, dyspepsia
Oral conditions: dry mouth, mucositis
Skin conditions: dry skin, nodules, pruritus, rashes
General: agitation, anorexia, cachexia, fatigue, weakness, bleeding, drowsiness, effusions (pleural, peritoneal), fever/chills, incontinence, insomnia, lymphoedema, myoclonus, odor, prolapse, sweats, syncope, vertigo

Fig. 7.1.1 A model to guide hospice palliative care: based on national principles and norms of practice.
Reproduced with permission from Ferris FD et al., *A Model to Guide Hospice Palliative Care*, Figure 7, p. 15, Canadian Hospice Palliative Care Association, Ottawa, Ontario, Canada, Copyright © 2002.

Selecting the most appropriate assessment tool requires a balance between obtaining the most accurate and comprehensive information possible, while minimizing the burden placed on the patient and clinician. Brief screening tools (1–14 items) (Mitchell, 2010) can provide a quick snapshot of the person's needs and may be most appropriate in busy clinical settings or if the patient has limited functioning. Ideally, this brief screening should be followed up by administering longer assessment tools to ascertain more comprehensive information on the range, severity, and complexity of any identified needs. The choice of assessment tool will be informed by the issues identified through the brief screening. For example, if a patient reports needs in only one domain of a brief tool (e.g. information needs), clinicians may consider using a unidimensional tool to explore that specific area of need in more detail. However, administration of a multidimensional tool which includes items assessing a range of need domains may be more informative when patients identify a number of domains of unmet need in the brief screening tool. For people with advanced disease or who are at the end of life, the mode of administration and participant burden are important considerations for health-care providers when selecting an assessment tool.

Many patients with advanced disease depend upon health-care providers for symptom assessment. However, research examining the extent of agreement between patient and provider symptom assessments (Nekolaichuk et al., 1999a; Laugsand et al., 2010) and patient psychosocial well-being (Newell et al., 1998; Jones et al., 2011a) suggests a need for caution in cases where a total reliance on health-care provider assessments is necessary. For example, a very large cross-sectional study of 1933 cancer patient–health-care provider dyads from 11 European countries revealed an under-estimating of symptoms by health professionals in one in ten cases, with patients with low Karnofsky Performance Status, high Mini Mental State-score, hospitalized, recently diagnosed, or undergoing opioid titration being at significantly increased risk of symptom underestimation by providers (Laugsand et al., 2010).

From a patient care perspective, patient-reported outcomes provide the highest level of accuracy of physical as well as psychosocial assessments (Sprangers and Aaronson, 1992; Nekolaichuk et al., 1999a, 1999b; Sneeuw et al., 2002; Tang and McCorkle, 2002). They may also be least burdensome in terms of financial costs and clinician time (Wen and Gustafson, 2004). The latter is a particularly important consideration for promoting needs-based care, with clinicians often reporting that time is a factor affecting the accurate and timely identification of needs (Pruyn et al., 2004; Waller et al., 2012b). However, the capabilities of the patient at the time of assessment and the clinical setting may necessarily become overriding factors in the choice of assessment mode (Wen and Gustafson, 2004). Caregivers and health professionals have been relied on for proxy assessments, with variable information about the severity and complexity of needs, in populations with advanced disease, where patients may have difficulty completing tools themselves due to the complexity and gravity of their symptoms (Carson et al., 2000). Tools which incorporate both patient and health-care provider input may provide the most detailed information to inform needs-based care.

The following section provides an overview of tools currently available for assessment of needs in a palliative care population, with more detailed information regarding each of these tools in Table 7.1.1. Some of these tools, such as the Palliative care Outcomes Scale (POS), the Needs at the End-of-Life Screening Tool (NEST), and the Sheffield Profile for Assessment and Referral to Care (SPARC-45) do not focus on a particular disease and have been validated in different patient groups. However, much of the work on development and validation of needs assessment tools has focused primarily on the palliative care needs of cancer patients, with fewer tools developed specifically for non-malignant conditions such as heart failure, chronic obstructive pulmonary disease (COPD), dementia, and HIV/AIDs.

Generic needs assessment tools for patients with any chronic disease

Only three generic measures were identified which are suitable for assessment of needs across a range of chronic diseases, two quite brief tools and one comprehensive assessment tool. One of the most established and well-validated tools for use across different patient groups is the POS (Hearn and Higginson, 1999; Bausewein et al., 2011). This 10-item measure assesses physical, practical, family, information, and psychological problems along with quality of life in the previous 3 days, with an additional item for open-ended patient comments. It includes both patient and clinician assessment components and has been used in a variety of clinical settings, including inpatient, home, hospice, and primary care. The POS has been implemented as an assessment tool in a mixture of palliative situations which include cancer, HIV/AIDS, COPD, dementia, heart failure, renal, and neurological populations. A recent systematic review highlights the studies validating or collecting data using the original and adapted versions of the POS, focusing on different patient groups, languages, and cultures (Bausewein et al., 2011).

The NEST is a 13-item measure identifying the subjective experiences and overall care of people at the end of life (Emanuel et al., 2000, 2001; Scandrett et al., 2010) and can be self-completed by the patient or by using a health professional interview. It assesses a wide range of domains of need including caregiver/family, physical, psychological, practical, spiritual, and social problems. Multiple strategies were used to provide evidence of content validity and adequate construct validity and internal consistency are reported. A recent study found that it is a feasible tool for assessing patient needs in the clinical setting (Scandrett et al., 2010); however, further evidence of reliability and responsiveness is needed.

The SPARC-45 (Ahmed et al., 2009) is a longer multidimensional assessment tool consisting of 45 items, developed to assess the palliative and supportive care needs of malignant and non-malignant conditions across general and specialist settings, prompting referrals to palliative care services where necessary. Like the NEST, content validity has been assessed, but there is limited information on other aspects of validity and on the reliability of the tool.

Tools specific to advanced cancer

Given the high representation of cancer patients in palliative populations, most of the published palliative care needs assessment tools have been developed and validated in cancer populations. These range from brief screening tools to longer self-report and interview measures.

The Three Levels of Need Questionnaire (3LNQ) (Johnsen et al., 2011), the Needs Assessment for Progressive Disease-Cancer (NAT: PD-C) (Waller et al., 2008, 2010, 2012a, 2012b) and the Screen for Palliative and End-of-Life Care Needs in the Emergency

Table 7.1.1 Summary of psychometric properties of palliative care needs assessment tools

Measure	Items and domains	Question format	Completion	Population	Psychometrics
Malignant and non-malignant conditions					
NEST Needs near the end-of-life scale	**13 items:** Financial, access to care, social connection, caregiving needs, psychological distress, spirituality, sense of purpose, patient–clinician relationship, clinician communication, personal acceptance	Assesses care needs of people at the end of life Scale ranges from 0 (no need) to 10 (highest need); higher scores indicate higher needs	Patient or health-care provider	Advanced cancer (Emanuel et al., 2000, 2001; Scandrett et al., 2010) Stroke, dementia, liver, renal, pulmonary (Grudzen et al., 2010)	Content validity Internal consistency Construct validity
POS Palliative Outcome Scale (see Bausewein et al. (2011) for a detailed overview))	**10 items:** Pain and other symptoms, patient anxiety, family anxiety, information, level support, life worth, self-worth, waste time, personal affairs Patients also asked open-ended item to identify main problem; staff asked additional performance status item	Assesses problems and quality of life over the last 3 days Scales range from 0 (no problem) to 4 (overwhelming problem); higher scores indicate more problems	Patient and health-care provider Time taken: 10 minutes	Cancer Dementia HIV/AIDS COPD Heart failure Kidney Neurological	Content validity Internal consistency Test–retest reliability Inter-rater reliability Construct validity Responsiveness Translations available
SPARC-45 Sheffield Profile for Assessment and Referral to Care	**45 items:** Communication/information, physical, psychological, religious and spiritual, independence and activity, family and social, treatment	Assesses level of need and desire for help in the last month Need scale ranges from 0 (not at all) to 3 (very much) Desire for help: scale scored as yes or no	Patient	Malignant and non-malignant Cancer (Ahmed et al., 2009; Wilcock et al., 2010) Stroke (Burton et al., 2010)	Validation manuscript in preparation
Malignant only—generic tools (all stages of disease)					
CaNDI Cancer Needs Distress Inventory	**39 items in 7 domains:** Depression, anxiety, emotional, social, health-care, practical, physical	Assess problem intensity and desire for help in past 2 weeks Intensity: scale ranges from 1 'not a problem', to 5 'very severe problem' Desire for help/discussion with health professionals: 'yes' or 'prefer not to'	Patient	Cancer (Lowery et al., 2012)	Content validity Construct validity Internal consistency Test–retest reliability Predictive validity
CARES-SF Cancer Rehabilitation Evaluation System Short Form	**38-57 items in 5 domains:** Physical, psychological, medical interaction, marital, sexual Also Global CARES score	Assesses physical and psychosocial issues affecting cancer patients; and in the clinical version, desire for help Scale ranges from 0 'does not apply to 4 'applies very much'	Patient (interview follow-up) Time taken: 11 minutes	Cancer (Schag et al., 1991; te Velde et al., 1996)	Content validity Internal consistency Test–retest reliability Construct validity Responsiveness
Palliative Care Screening Tool & NCCN Palliative Care Referral Criteria	**Screening tool 5 items:** Metastatic disease, functional status, serious complications, comorbidities, palliative problems **NCCN 24 items:** Physical, psychological, cognitive, treatment, communication, practical, family, spiritual, social	Identifies patients for whom specialist palliative care referral may be required **5 items:** score range from 0 to 13; higher scores indicate worse functioning; cut-off of 5 indicates need for referral **24 items:** NCCN criteria for referral	Health-care provider	Cancer (Glare et al., 2011)	Content validity

Instrument	Domains/items	Description	Respondent	Population (reference)	Psychometric properties
PCM Patient Care Monitor	**80 items in 6 domains:** General physical symptoms, treatment side effects, distress, despair, impaired performance, impaired ambulation. Also a QoL index (54 items)	Assesses symptoms on a scale ranging from 0 to 11; PCM distress score > 65 prompts further assessment by psychosocial	Patient	Cancer (Abernethy et al., 2010)	Content validity Internal consistency Test–retest reliability Concurrent validity
SCNS-SF34 Supportive Care Needs Survey Short Form	**34 items in 5 domains:** Psychological, physical, patient care and support, sexual and health system and information	Assesses level of need for help in the last month Scales range from 1 (no need/not applicable) to 5 (high need)	Patient time taken: 10 minutes	Cancer (Boyes et al., 2009; Schofield et al., 2012)	Content validity Internal consistency Construct validity Responsiveness
SCNS-ST9 Supportive Care Needs Survey Screening Tool	**9 items:** 2 psychological, 2 physical, 2 patient care and support, 1 sexual, and 2 information items	Assesses level of need for help in the last month Scales range from 1 (no need/not applicable) to 5 (high need)	Patient	Cancer (Girgis et al., 2011)	Content validity Construct validity Predictive validity
Malignant: advanced disease only					
3LNQ Three-Levels-of-Needs Questionnaire	**14 items (11 EORTC QLQ-C30 items + 3 additional):** Physical function, role function, social function, psychological (depression, worry), physical symptoms (pain, fatigue, nausea, dyspnoea, appetite), sexuality, feeling burden, loneliness	Assesses problem intensity, problem burden, and felt need in the past week Intensity and burden: scale ranges from 'not at all' to 'very much' Felt need: scale ranges from 'no need'/'met need'/'unmet need'	Patient	Advanced cancer (Johnsen et al., 2011)	Content validity Internal consistency
NA-ACP Needs Assessment of Advanced Cancer Patients	**132 items in 7 domains:** Daily living, physical symptom, psychological, social, spiritual, financial, medical communication & information	Assesses needs and desire for help in past 4 months Scale ranges from 1 (no need/not applicable) to 5 (high need); higher scores indicate higher needs	Patient Time taken: 76 minutes	Advanced cancer (Rainbird et al., 2005)	Content validity Internal consistency Test–retest reliability Construct validity
NAT: PD-C Needs Assessment for Progressive Disease—Cancer	**18 items in 3 domains:** Patient well-being, ability of caregiver/family to care for patients, caregiver/family well-being	Assesses the level of concern and actions taken to address concerns Level of concern ranges from 'none' to 'significant' Provider indicates action taken to manage concern ('directly managed', 'managed by team', or 'referral')	Health-care provider Time taken: 5–10 minutes	Advanced Cancer (Waller et al., 2008, 2010, 2012a, 2012b)	Content validity Inter-rater reliability Concurrent validity
PNPC Problems and Needs in Palliative Care	**132 items in 6 domains:** Physical/daily living, autonomy, psychological, social, spiritual, information, financial	Assesses problems and need for assistance using 2 questions for each item: (1) Is this a problem? (2) Do you want attention?	Patient	Advanced cancer (Osse et al., 2004)	Content validity Construct validity Internal consistency
PNPC-SF Problems and Needs in Palliative Care Short Form	**33 items in 6 domains:** Physical/daily living autonomy, psychological, social, spiritual, information, financial	Assesses problems and need for assistance using 2 questions for each item: (1) Is this a problem? (2) Do you want attention?	Patient Time taken: 5–10 minutes	Advanced cancer (Osse et al., 2007)	Content validity Construct validity Internal consistency

(continued)

Table 7.1.1 Continued

Measure	Items and domains	Question format	Completion	Population	Psychometrics
SISC Structured Interview of Symptoms and Concerns in Palliative Care	**13 items:** Pain, drowsiness, nausea, weakness, dyspnoea, loss control, loss dignity, burden, anxiety, depression, loss interest, hopelessness and desire death	Assesses common symptoms and concerns; scale ranges from 0 (none) to 6 (extreme) 3 and above as clinical cut-off	Health-care provider Time taken: 28–60 minutes	Advanced cancer (Wilson et al., 2004)	Inter-rater reliability Test–retest reliability Concurrent validity
SPEED Screen for Palliative and End-of-Life Care Needs in the Emergency Department	**13 items in 5 domains:** Social, therapeutic, physical, psychological, spiritual	Assesses the level of need Scale ranges from 0 (not at all) to 10 (a great deal); higher scores indicate higher needs	Health-care provider	Cancer patients in emergency department (Richards et al., 2011)	Content validity Construct validity
Malignant: specific tumour group or domain of need					
NA-ALCP Needs Assessment for Advanced Lung Cancer Patients	**38 items in 7 domains:** Daily living, physical symptom, psychological, social, spiritual, financial, medical communication & information	Assesses needs and desire for help in past 4 months. Scale ranges from 1 (no need/not applicable) to 5 (high need); higher scores indicate higher needs	Patient	Advanced lung cancer (Schofield et al., 2012)	Content validity Internal consistency Construct validity
PAQ Patient Autonomy Questionnaire	**9 items in 3 domains:** Dependency, losing control, limitation of activity	Assesses autonomy needs of cancer patients using 2 questions for each item: (1) Is this a problem? (2) Do you want attention?	Patient	Advanced cancer (Vernooij-Dassen et al., 2005)	Content validity Internal consistency Construct validity
Dementia					
EOLD (3 scales) End of Life in Dementia **SWC-EOLD** Satisfaction care **SM-EOLD** Symptoms **CAD-EOLD** Comfort	**SWC-EOLD 10 items:** Decision-making, communication with providers, understanding condition, medical and nursing care **SM-EOLD 9 items:** Physical (pain, shortness breath, skin); psychological (calm, depression, fear, anxiety, agitation, resistive to care) **CAD-EOLD 14 items:** Discomfort, pain, shortness breath, choking, gurgling, swallowing, fear, anxiety, crying, moaning, serenity, peace, calm	**SCW-EOLD** Assesses satisfaction in last 90 days of life ('strongly disagree' to 'agree'). Scores range from 10 to 40; higher scores indicate higher satisfaction **SM-EOLD** Assesses symptom frequency in last 90 days of life ('never' to 'once a month'). Scores range from 0 to 45; higher scores indicate better symptom control **CAD-EOLD** Assesses frequency in last 7 days life ('not at all' to 'a lot'). Scores range from 14 to 42; higher scores indicate better symptom control	Health-care provider	Dementia (Kiely et al., 2006, 2012; Volicer et al., 2001)	Internal consistency Content validity Construct validity Responsiveness
DCNA John Hopkins Dementia Care Needs Assessment	**86 items in 19 domains:** Safety, management cognitive and neurocognitive symptoms, medical comorbidities, daily activities, caregiver education and support	Assesses degree to which patients and caregiver needs are met Level need: 'unmet', 'partially met', 'met'	Health-care provider	Dementia	Unknown

Instrument	Items and domains	Description	Completed by	Condition (reference)	Psychometric properties
CANE Camberwell Assessment of Needs for the Elderly	**24 patient items and 2 caregiver items:** Daily living, self-care, physical, psychological, safety, social, financial, medications, behaviour, practical, patient and caregiver information, patient and caregiver distress	Assesses presence of need, level of help from family/friends and services and whether amount of help was adequate Scale ranges from 'no need', 'met/partially met need' 'unmet need' or 'not known'	Patient and health-care provider Time taken: 30 minutes	Dementia (initially developed for mentally ill elderly patients) (Reynolds et al., 2000)	Content validity Inter-rater reliability Test–retest reliability Construct validity Criterion validity
CareNap-D Care Needs Assessment pack for Dementia	**57 items in 7 domains:** Health and mobility, self-care and toileting, social interaction, thinking and memory, behaviour and mental state, house care, community living	Assesses intensity of need and for unmet needs the type action required Scale ranges from 'no need', 'unmet need', 'met need'	Health-care provider	Dementia (McWalter et al., 1998)	Content validity Inter-rater reliability Social validity
Heart failure					
NAT: PD-HF Needs Assessment Progressive Disease—Heart Failure	**18 items in 3 domains:** Patient well-being, ability of caregiver/family to care for patients, caregiver/family well-being	Assesses the level of concern and actions taken to address concerns Level of concern 'none' to 'significant' Provider indicates action to manage concern ('directly managed', 'managed team', 'referral')	Health-care provider Time taken: 5–10 minutes	Heart Failure (Waller et al., 2013)	Content validity Inter-rater reliability Concurrent validity
HFNAQ Heart Failure Needs Assessment Questionnaire	**30 items in 4 domains:** Physical (10 items), psychological (9 items), social(8 items), existential (3 items)	Assesses need for help in the last month Scale ranges from 1 (hardly ever) to 5 (always)	Patient Time taken: 10 minutes	Heart failure (Davidson et al., 2008)	Content validity Internal consistency Construct validity Concurrent validity Discriminant validity
Chronic obstructive pulmonary disease (COPD)					
CCQ Clinical COPD Questionnaire	**10 items in 3 domains:** Symptoms (4 items), functional state (4 items) and mental state (2 items)	Assesses symptom intensity during the past week Scale ranges from 0 (never/asymptomatic) to 6 (almost all of the time/extremely symptomatic)	Patient Time taken: 2 minutes	COPD (van der Molen et al., 2003; Jones et al., 2011)	Content validity Internal consistency Test–retest reliability Construct validity Responsiveness
CAT COPD Assessment Test	**8 items:** Cough, phlegm, chest tightness, breathlessness, activities, confidence in leaving home, sleep and energy	Assesses impact of symptoms on quality of life and well-being Scale ranges from 0 (I am very happy) to 5 (I am very sad)	Patient Time taken: 2 minutes	COPD (Tsiligianni et al., 2012)	Content validity Internal consistency Test–retest reliability Construct validity Responsiveness
SGRQ St George Respiratory Questionnaire	**50 items in 3 domains:** Symptoms (8 items), activity (16 items) and impact on daily life (26 items)	Assess frequency and severity of symptoms, limitation breathlessness on activities and disturbances of social and psychological functioning Scores range from 0 (no impairment) to 100 (maximum impairment)	Patient	COPD (Meguro et al., 2007)	Content validity Construct validity Internal consistency Test–retest validity Responsiveness

(continued)

Table 7.1.1 Continued

Measure	Items and domains	Question format	Completion	Population	Psychometrics
HIV/AIDS					
ECSQ Events in care Screening Questionnaire	**54 items in 9 domains:** Adherence to medical instructions, medical problems, specialty and inpatient care, preventative health-care and screening, sexual risk behaviour, family planning, psychological symptoms, substance use and life demands	Part 1 of Dynamics of Care assessment Assesses problems in last 3 months Scored as yes or no Dynamics of Care Assessment (interview) assesses need for additional information and whether provider has discussed each need identified	Health-care provider	HIV/AIDS (Patel et al., 2008)	Content validity Construct validity
HOPES HIV Overview if Problems Evaluation System	**106 items in 5 domains:** Physical, psychosocial, sexual functioning, medical interaction and partner relationship	Assesses quality of life and rehabilitation needs Scale ranges from 0 'does not apply' to 4 'applies very much'	Patient	HIV/AIDS (adapted from CARES) (Schag et al., 1992; De Boer et al., 1996)	Content validity Internal consistency Criterion validity Construct validity Responsiveness
MOS-HIV Medical Outcomes Study HIV Health Survey	**35 items in 10 domains:** Health perceptions, pain, physical, role, social and cognitive functioning, mental health, energy, health distress and quality of life	Assesses functional status and well-being Scores range from 0 to 100; higher scores indicate better health	Patient (also interview version) Time taken: 5 minutes	HIV/AIDS (Hughes et al., 1997; Wu et al., 1997; Revicki et al., 1998, Clayson et al., 2006)	Content validity Internal consistency Construct validity Responsiveness

Department (SPEED) (Richards et al., 2011) are all comparatively brief measures (13–18 items) for rapid needs assessment. The 3LNQ (Johnsen et al., 2011) assesses unmet need and desire for help in physical, social, psychological, and sexuality domains, through patients' self-rating of problem intensity, problem burden, and felt need. Preliminary evidence of content validity and internal consistency has been reported. Given its recent development, additional measures of reliability, construct validity or responsiveness are still needed. The NAT: PD-C was developed for completion by a range of health professionals in both generalist and specialist settings. It is the only identified multidimensional tool which assesses the needs of both the patient and caregiver/family concurrently. The reliability and content validity of the NAT: PD-C have been established in both a research and a clinical setting. Concurrent validity is available for some, but not all, subscales of the tool. The SPEED is a tool for health professional assessment of social, therapeutic, physical, psychological and spiritual palliative care needs, specifically for patients seen in the emergency department. It has been tested initially on people with metastatic disease, providing evidence for construct validity. Further work is needed to establish reliability and utility in non-cancer populations.

The Needs Assessment of Advanced Cancer Patients (NA-ACP) (Rainbird et al., 2005), Problems and Needs in Palliative Care (PNPC) (Osse et al., 2004), and Structured Interview of Symptoms and Concerns in Palliative Care (SISC) (Wilson et al., 2004) are longer measures administered by either self-report (NA-ACP, PNPC) or by interview (SSISC). The NA-ACP (Rainbird et al., 2005) is a 132-item multidimensional measure of needs that has undergone rigorous psychometric testing, including content and construct validity, internal consistency and test-retest reliability. The 132-item PNPC (Osse et al., 2004) also assessed the needs of people with advanced cancer across a range of domains, with adequate content and convergent validity as well as internal consistency. A 33-item shorter version of this tool is available, the PNPC-sv (Osse et al., 2007), which covers the same domains as the 132-item PNPC. The short completion time of 5–10 minutes increases the acceptability and clinical utility of this version. Whilst both the PNPC and NA-ACP are acceptable to patients, the time taken to complete these tools may make them less feasible for some palliative patients, particularly toward the end of life.

The SISC (Wilson et al., 2004) is an interview-style assessment covering 13 areas: pain, drowsiness, nausea, weakness, dyspnoea, loss of control, loss of dignity, burden, anxiety, depression, loss of interest, hopelessness, and desire for death. This tool may be useful as a follow-up assessment following initial screening, given the completion time ranging from 28 to 60 minutes.

As indicated in Table 7.1.1, varying levels of psychometric evidence are available for the tools targeting people with advanced cancer specifically. Content validity was established using literature reviews and reviews of existing measures (3LNQ, NAT: PD-C, NA-ACP, PNPC, PNPC-sv, SPEED, SISC) and clinical/expert options (NA-ACP, NAT: PD-C, PNPC, PNPC-sv, SPEED). Construct validity was established using factor analysis (NA-ACP) and correlations with other validated measures (NAT: PD-C, SPEED, PNPC, PNPC-sv). Evidence of inter-rater reliability (NAT: PD-C) and internal consistency (NA-ACP, PNPC, PNPC-sv) was available for some tools; however, all tools require further studies to establish test–retest reliability, predictive validity, and responsiveness.

Cancer-specific tools: across the illness trajectory

Needs assessment tools have been developed for use by cancer patients across the illness trajectory. The Palliative Care Screening Tool & NCCN Palliative Care Referral Criteria (Glare et al., 2011) can be used by health-care providers to identify patients for whom specialist palliative care referral may be required. The 34-item Supportive Care Needs Survey Short Form (SCNS-SF34) (Boyes et al., 2009), the Supportive Care Needs Survey Screening Tool (SCNS-ST9) (Girgis et al., 2012), the Patient Cancer Monitor (PCM) (Abernethy et al., 2010), the Cancer Rehabilitation Evaluation System Short Form (CARES) (Schag et al., 1991; te Velde et al., 1996), and the Cancer Needs Distress Inventory (CaNDI) (Lowery et al., 2012) are also suitable for patients along the cancer continuum and have undergone rigorous psychometric testing. Other tools such as the Needs Assessment for Advanced Lung Cancer Patients (NA-ACLP) (Schofield et al., 2012) and the Patient Autonomy Questionnaire (PAQ) (Vernooij-Dassen et al., 2005) may be useful for assessing particular tumour groups or domains of need.

Dementia

The assessment of needs in people with dementia can be complicated by the patient's limited cognitive functioning and loss of language skills (Schmid et al., 2012). The Camberwell Assessment of Need for the Elderly (CANE) is a structured interview that assesses 24 patient and two caregiver needs (Reynolds et al., 2000). It can be used for research and clinical purposes and performs well on psychometric criteria. Its advantage is that it enables patients, caregivers, and health-care providers to rate level of need, enabling a more comprehensive and accurate assessment of the patient situation. The Care Needs Assessment Pack for Dementia (CarenapD) (McWalter et al., 1998) is a software package assessing the needs of people with dementia living in the community and their carers. This package can be used by multidisciplinary health-care providers and combines patient and caregiver opinions regarding care needs. The End of Life in Dementia (EOLD) scale (Kiely et al., 2006, 2012) is comprised of three scales assessing satisfaction with care, symptoms, and comfort at the end of life. It is completed by the health-care provider and has demonstrated reliability, validity, and sensitivity to change over time. The Tayside Profile for Dementia Planning (Gordon et al., 1997) was developed for clinical use and can be administered as a questionnaire or interview. Unlike the other measures that utilize both patient and caregiver perspectives, the Tayside Profile for Dementia Planning assesses needs from the perspective of the caregiver only. It is also limited in the domains of need assessed (Schmid et al., 2012).

Heart failure

Fewer needs assessment tools are specific to people with heart failure. The Needs Assessment for Progressive Disease—Heart Failure (NAT: PD-HF) (Waller et al., 2013) was adapted from the NAT: PD-C, assessing multidimensional needs for both patients and carers. Preliminary evidence for inter-rater reliability, content and concurrent validity has been established in a clinical heart failure clinic. Similar to the cancer version of this tool, further work is needed to establish reliability, validity, and responsiveness. The Heart Failure Needs Assessment Questionnaire (HFNAQ) is a 30-item measure with adequate content validity, internal consistency, as well as concurrent and discriminant validity (Davidson et al., 2008). Heart failure-specific tools that have focused on assessment of health-related quality of life, rather than focusing on unmet needs, are the subject of a systematic review (Johansson et al., 2004). The most commonly used include the Minnesota Living with Heart Failure (MLwHF) tool, the Chronic Heart Failure Questionnaire (CHQ), and Quality of Life in Severe Heart Failure (QLQ-SHF) (Johansson et al., 2004).

Chronic obstructive pulmonary disease

The Clinical COPD questionnaire (CCQ) and the COPD Assessment Tool (CAT) are two brief tools that can be used to screen patients for physical symptoms, functional status, and emotional well-being (van der Molen et al., 2003; Jones et al., 2011b). These tools can be completed by the patient and take approximately 2 minutes. Both tools exhibit adequate reliability and validity but a recent study showed patients prefer the CCQ (Tsiligianni et al., 2012). The St George Respiratory Questionnaire (SGRQ), a longer patient-completed measure assessing severity of symptoms and limits on functioning, is used widely in people with respiratory problems. A COPD-specific version has been developed and validated in this population (Meguro et al., 2007).

HIV/AIDS

The Events in Care Screening Questionnaire (ECSQ) (Patel et al., 2008) is the first part of a larger interviewer-administered assessment (Dynamics of Care assessment). The ESCQ can be used as a stand-alone measure to assess needs and concerns, if patients want more information and if the health-care provider had discussed identified needs with the patient in the last 3 months. Construct validity and clinical utility was demonstrated in 628 HIV/AIDs patients. The ESCQ may be a valuable tool for use as an initial screen for patient needs in this population. Further work is needed to establish reliability and validity.

The HIV Overview of Problems Evaluation System (HOPES) (De Boer et al., 1996, Schag et al., 1992) scale was adapted from the cancer version (CARES) to assess the needs of people with HIV/AIDs. Items were derived from the CARES and by expert and clinical opinion, then piloted with 38 HIV patients. This 106-item tool has high internal consistency, convergent, divergent, and construct validity, and is responsive to changes in clinical status over time. While this measure is longer and may be potentially burdensome, the detailed approach allows the health-care provider to obtain more comprehensive information.

Many of the remaining tools available to assess needs in the HIV/AIDS population focus on health-related quality of life rather than unmet needs. Missoula–VITAS Quality of Life index (MVQOLI) (Byock and Merriman, 1998; Schwartz et al., 2005) was developed specifically for palliative care terminal patients. Items were initially identified from a review of the literature and informal interviews of hospice professionals, patients, and their families, then were pilot tested with patients. Convergent, divergent, and concurrent validity have been established; however, further work is needed to assess responsiveness. The tool allows respondents to rate the importance of each dimension and the patient-weighted dimensional sub-scores offer clinical utility.

The Medical Outcomes Study HIV Health Survey (MOS-HIV) is the most widely-used measure in HIV/AIDs (Hughes et al., 1997; Wu et al., 1997; Revicki et al., 1998). It has adequate reliability, validity, and responsiveness and has been tested in patients at all stages of disease. It has significant advantages including availability in numerous languages and 5-minute administration time via self-report or face-to-face and telephone interviews. However, it has been suggested that the MOS-HIV has limitations including possible ceiling effects associated with scoring; that it may be too general and some aspects of disease may not be assessed; and that it has not been extensively tested in some subgroups of patients (e.g. women, lower socioeconomic status, drug users). A systematic review of quality of life measures recommended the MOS-HIV and the Functional Assessment of HIV Infection (FAHI), but cautioned that these measures have limitations (Clayson et al., 2006).

Integrating needs assessment into routine clinical practice

For a needs-based model of palliative care to demonstrate systematic positive impacts on patient outcomes, it must inevitably involve more than needs assessment. Such a model needs to be well integrated into routine clinical practice, with key components including the following:

◆ Accessibility to people with a life-limiting illness, irrespective of their diagnosis.

◆ Assessment of unmet needs across the spectrum of palliative care domains (see Fig. 7.1.1), systematically and repeatedly to identify changes in needs over time.

◆ Clear care pathways for addressing identified needs by the most appropriate provider or service, including generalist and specialist care providers.

◆ Continuity of care across care settings through efficient communication strategies within and between these care settings.

◆ Training of staff to support the best quality generalist and specialist palliative care to patients and their families.

◆ Rigorous evaluation of outcomes to determine the physical and psychosocial impact on patients and carers of adopting a needs-based model of palliative care, as well as the economic costs and benefits to the health-care system.

Conclusion

◆ Most needs assessment tools have been developed for oncology patients, with validation and other psychometric testing largely being reported for this population. There are fewer tools for other patient groups.

◆ Brief tools, including the POS, NEST, NAT: PD-C, 3LNQ, and SPEED, may be more feasible in routine clinical practice with heavy patient throughput or for patients for whom longer measures may be too burdensome. Longer, more intensive tools can then be administered to provide more comprehensive information for health-care providers.

◆ Other disease-specific tools that have undergone rigorous psychometric testing include the CARES, CaNDI, and SCNS (across cancer trajectory); the NA-ACP (advanced cancer patients); EOLD and CANE (dementia); HFNAQ (heart failure); CCQ and CAT (COPD); and HOPES and MOS-HIV (HIV/AIDs).

- Tools such as the POS may be applied to various patient groups and provide information from patient and health-care provider perspectives.

- Further evidence of psychometric quality is needed, particularly test–retest reliability, predictive validity, responsiveness, and clinical utility of these tools.

- Integration of needs assessment into an overall needs-based model of palliative care will have the greatest likelihood of positive impacts on patients, carers, and health system outcomes.

References

Abernethy, A.P., Zafar, S.Y., Uronis, H., *et al.* (2010). Validation of the Patient Care Monitor (Version 2.0): a review of system assessment instrument for cancer patients. *Journal of Pain and Symptom Management*, 40, 545–558.

Aharony, L. and Strasser, S. (1993). Patient satisfaction: what we know about and what we still need to explore. *Medical Care Research and Review*, 50, 49–79.

Ahmed, N., Bestall, J.C., Payne, S.A., Noble, B., and Ahmedzai, S.H. (2009). The use of cognitive interviewing methodology in the design and testing of a screening tool for supportive and palliative care needs. *Supportive Care in Cancer*, 17, 665–673.

Akechi, T., Okuyama, T., Endo, C., *et al.* (2011). Patient's perceived need and psychological distress and/or quality of life in ambulatory breast cancer patients in Japan. *Psycho-Oncology*, 20, 497–505.

Asadi-Lari, M., Tamburini, M., and Gray, D. (2004). Patients' needs, satisfaction, and health related quality of life: towards a comprehensive model. *Health and Quality of Life Outcomes*, 2, 32.

Bausewein, C., Le Grice, C., Simon, S., and Higginson, I. (2011). The use of two common palliative outcome measures in clinical care and research: a systematic review of POS and STAS. *Palliative Medicine*, 25, 304–313.

Bonevski, B., Sanson-Fisher, R., Girgis, A., Burton, L., Cook, P., and Boyes, A. (2000). Evaluation of an instrument to assess the needs of patients with cancer. Supportive Care Review Group. *Cancer*, 88, 217–225.

Boyes, A., Girgis, A., and Lecathelinais, C. (2009). Brief assessment of adult cancer patients' perceived needs: development and validation of the 34-item Supportive Care Needs Survey (SCNS-SF34). *Journal of Evaluation in Clinical Practice*, 15, 602–606.

Bredart, A., Razavi, D., Robertson, C., *et al.* (2001). A comprehensive assessment of satisfaction with care: preliminary psychometric analysis in French, Polish, Swedish and Italian oncology patients. *Patient Education and Counseling*, 43, 243–252.

Bultz, B.D. and Carlson, L.E. (2006). Emotional distress: the sixth vital sign—future directions in cancer care. *Psycho-Oncology*, 15, 93–95.

Burton, C.R., Payne, S., Addington-Hall, J., and Jones, A. (2010). The palliative care needs of acute stroke patients: a prospective study of hospital admissions. *Age and Ageing*, 39, 554–559.

Byock, I.R. and Merriman, M.P. (1998). Measuring quality of life for patients with terminal illness: the Missoula-VITAS quality of life index. *Palliative Medicine*, 12, 231–244.

Carlson, L.E., Waller, A., and Mitchell, A.J. (2012). Screening for distress and unmet needs in patients with cancer: review and recommendations. *Journal of Clinical Oncology*, 30, 1160–1177.

Carson, M.G., Fitch, M.I., and Vachon, M.L. (2000). Measuring patient outcomes in palliative care: a reliability and validity study of the Support Team Assessment Schedule. *Palliative Medicine*, 14, 25–36.

Clayson, D.J., Wild, D.J., Quarterman, P., Duprat-Lomon, I., Kubin, M., and Coons, S.J. (2006). A comparative review of health-related quality-of-life measures for use in HIV/AIDS clinical trials. *Pharmacoeconomics*, 24, 751–765.

Davidson, P.M., Cockburn, J., and Newton, P.J. (2008). Unmet needs following hospitalization with heart failure: implications for clinical assessment and program planning. *Journal of Cardiovascular Nursing*, 23, 541–546.

De Boer, J.B., Sprangers, M.A., Aaronson, N.K., Lange, J.M., and Van Dam, F.S. (1996). A study of the reliability, validity and responsiveness of the HIV overview of problems evaluation system (HOPES) in assessing the quality of life of patients with AIDS and symptomatic HIV infection. *Quality of Life Research*, 5, 339–347.

Emanuel, L.L., Alpert, H.R., and Emanuel, E.E. (2001). Concise screening questions for clinical assessments of terminal care: the needs near the end-of-life care screening tool. *Journal of Palliative Medicine*, 4, 465–474.

Emanuel, L.L., Alpert, H.R., Baldwin, D.C., and Emanuel, E.J. (2000). What terminally ill patients care about: toward a validated construct of patients' perspectives. *Journal of Palliative Medicine*, 3, 419–431.

Ferris, F.D., Balfour, H.M., Bowen, K., *et al.* (2002). *A Model to Guide Hospice Palliative Care*. Ottawa: Canadian Hospice Palliative Care Association.

Girgis, A., Stojanovski, E., Boyes, A., King, M., and Lecathelinais, C. (2011). The next generation of the supportive care needs survey: a brief screening tool for administration in the clinical oncology setting. *Psycho-Oncology*, 2, 827–835.

Glare, P.A., Semple, D., Stabler, S.M., and Saltz, L.B. (2011). Palliative care in the outpatient oncology setting: evaluation of a practical set of referral criteria. *Journal of Oncology Practice*, 7, 366–370.

Glare, P., Virik, K., Jones, M., *et al.* (2003). A systematic review of physicians' survival predictions in terminally ill cancer patients. *BMJ*, 327, 195–198.

Gordon, D.S., Spicker, P., Ballinger, B.R., *et al.* (1997). A population needs assessment profile for dementia. *International Journal of Geriatric Psychiatry*, 12, 642–647.

Grudzen, C.R., Richardson, L.D., Morrison, M., Cho, E., and Morrison, R.S. (2010). Palliative care needs of seriously ill, older adults presenting to the emergency department. *Academic Emergency Medicine*, 17, 1253–1257.

Gustafson, D.H. (1991). Expanding on the role of patient as consumer. *QRB Quality Review Bulletin*, 17, 324–325.

Gustafson, D.H., Taylor, J.O., Thompson, S., and Chesney, P. (1993). Assessing the needs of breast cancer patients and their families. *Quality Management in Health Care*, 2, 6–17.

Gwilliam, B., Keeley, V., Todd, C., *et al.* (2013). Prognosticating in patients with advanced cancer—observational study comparing the accuracy of clinicians' and patients' estimates of survival. *Annals of Oncology*, 24, 482–488.

Hearn, J. and Higginson, I.J. (1999). Development and validation of a core outcome measure for palliative care: the palliative care outcome scale. Palliative Care Core Audit Project Advisory Group. *Quality in Health Care*, 8, 219–227.

Holland, J.C. and Bultz, B.D. (2007). The NCCN guideline for distress management: a case for making distress the sixth vital sign. *Journal of the National Comprehensive Cancer Network*, 5, 3–7.

Hughes, T.E., Kaplan, R.M., Coons, S.J., Draugalis, J.R., Johnson, J.A., and Patterson, T.L. (1997). Construct validities of the Quality of Well-Being Scale and the MOS-HIV-34 Health Survey for HIV-infected patients. *Medical Decision Making*, 17, 439–446.

Johansson, P., Agnebrink, M., Dahlstrom, U., and Brostrom, A. (2004). Measurement of health-related quality of life in chronic heart failure, from a nursing perspective-a review of the literature. *European Journal of Cardiovascular Nursing*, 3, 7–20.

Johnsen, A.T., Petersen, M.A., Pedersen, L., and Groenvold, M. (2011). Development and initial validation of the Three-Levels-of-Needs Questionnaire for self-assessment of palliative needs in patients with cancer. *Journal of Pain and Symptom Management*, 41, 1025–1039.

Johnson, C.E., Girgis, A., Paul, C.L., and Currow, D.C. (2008). Cancer specialists' palliative care referral practices and perceptions: results of a national survey. *Palliative Medicine*, 22, 51–57.

Johnson, C.E., Girgis, A., Paul, C.L., and Currow, D.C. (2011c). Palliative care referral practices and perceptions: the divide between metropolitan and non-metropolitan general practitioners. *Palliative and Supportive Care*, 9, 181–189.

Johnson, C., Girgis, A., Paul, C., Currow, D.C., Adams, J., and Aranda, S. (2011a). Australian palliative care providers' perceptions and experiences of the barriers and facilitators to palliative care provision. *Supportive Care in Cancer*, 19, 343–351.

Johnson, C., Paul, C., Girgis, A., Adams, J., and Currow, D.C. (2011b). Australian general practitioners' and oncology specialists' perceptions of barriers and facilitators of access to specialist palliative care services. *Journal of Palliative Medicine*, 14, 429–435.

Jones, J.M., McPherson, C.J., Zimmermann, C., Rodin, G., Le, L.W., and Cohen, S.R. (2011a). Assessing agreement between terminally ill cancer patients' reports of their quality of life and family caregiver and palliative care physician proxy ratings. *Journal of Pain and Symptom Management*, 42, 354–365.

Jones, P.W., Price, D., and van der Molen, T. (2011b). Role of clinical questionnaires in optimizing everyday care of chronic obstructive pulmonary disease. *International Journal of Chronic Obstructive Pulmonary Disease*, 6, 289–296.

Kiely, D.K., Shaffer, M.L., and Mitchell, S.L. (2012). Scales for the evaluation of end-of-life care in advanced dementia: sensitivity to change. *Alzheimer Disease and Associated Disorders*, 26, 358–363.

Kiely, D.K., Volicer, L., Teno, J., Jones, R.N., Prigerson, H.G., and Mitchell, S.L. (2006). The validity and reliability of scales for the evaluation of end-of-life care in advanced dementia. *Alzheimer Disease and Associated Disorders*, 20, 176–181.

Laugsand, E.A., Sprangers, M.A., Bjordal, K., Skorpen, F., Kaasa, S., and Klepstad, P. (2010). Health-care providers underestimate symptom intensities of cancer patients: a multicenter European study. *Health and Quality of Life Outcomes*, 8, 104.

Lehr, H. and Strosberg, M. (1991). Quality improvement in health-care: is the patient still left out? *QRB Quality Review Bulletin*, 17, 326–329.

Lowery, A.E., Greenberg, M.A., Foster, S.L., et al. (2012). Validation of a needs-based biopsychosocial distress instrument for cancer patients. *Psycho-Oncology*, 21, 1099–1106.

McWalter, G., Toner, H., McWalter, A., Eastwood, J., Marshall, M., and Turvey, T. (1998). A community needs assessment: the care needs assessment pack for dementia (CarenapD)—its development, reliability and validity. *International Journal of Geriatric Psychiatry*, 13, 16–22.

Meguro, M., Barley, E.A., Spencer, S., and Jones, P.W. (2007). Development and validation of an improved, COPD-specific version of the St. George Respiratory Questionnaire. *Chest*, 132, 456–463.

Mitchell, A.J. (2010). Short screening tools for cancer-related distress: a review and diagnostic validity meta-analysis. *Journal of the National Comprehensive Cancer Network*, 8, 487–494.

Molassiotis, A., Wilson, B., Blair, S., Howe, T., and Cavet, J. (2011). Unmet supportive care needs, psychological well-being and quality of life in patients living with multiple myeloma and their partners. *Psycho-Oncology*, 20, 88–97.

Nabati, L., Shea, N., McBride, L., Gavin, C., and Bauer, M.S. (1998). Adaptation of a simple patient satisfaction instrument to mental health: psychometric properties. *Psychiatry Research*, 77, 51–56.

Nekolaichuk, C.L., Bruera, E., Spachynski, K., Maceachern, T., Hanson, J., and Maguire, T.O. (1999a). A comparison of patient and proxy symptom assessments in advanced cancer patients. *Palliative Medicine*, 13, 311–323.

Nekolaichuk, C.L., Maguire, T.O., Suarez-Almazor, M., Rogers, W.T., and Bruera, E. (1999b). Assessing the reliability of patient, nurse, and family caregiver symptom ratings in hospitalized advanced cancer patients. *Journal of Clinical Oncology*, 17, 3621–3630.

Newell, S., Sanson-Fisher, R.W., Girgis, A., and Bonaventura, A. (1998). How well do medical oncologists' perceptions reflect their patients' reported physical and psychosocial problems? Data from a survey of five oncologists. *Cancer*, 83, 1640–1651.

Osse, B.H., Vernooij, M.J., Schade, E., and Grol, R.P. (2004). Towards a new clinical tool for needs assessment in the palliative care of cancer patients: the PNPC instrument. *Journal of Pain and Symptom Management*, 28, 329–341.

Osse, B.H., Vernooij-Dassen, M.J., Schade, E., and Grol, R.P. (2007). A practical instrument to explore patients' needs in palliative care: the Problems and Needs in Palliative Care questionnaire short version. *Palliative Medicine*, 21, 391–399.

Palliative Care Australia (2005a). *A Guide to Palliative Care Service Development: A Population Based Approach*. Canberra: Palliative Care Australia.

Palliative Care Australia (2005b). *Standards for Providing Quality Palliative Care for all Australians*. Canberra: Palliative Care Australia.

Patel, S., Weiss, E., Chhabra, R., et al. (2008). The Events in Care Screening Questionnaire (ECSQ): a new tool to identify needs and concerns of people with HIV/AIDS. *AIDS Patient Care STDS*, 22, 381–393.

Pruyn, J.F., Heule-Dieleman, H.A., Knegt, P.P., et al. (2004). On the enhancement of efficiency in care for cancer patients in outpatient clinics: an instrument to accelerate psychosocial screening and referral. *Patient Education and Counseling*, 53, 135–140.

Rainbird, K.J., Perkins, J.J., and Sanson-Fisher, R.W. (2005). The Needs Assessment for Advanced Cancer Patients (NA-ACP): a measure of the perceived needs of patients with advanced, incurable cancer. a study of validity, reliability and acceptability. *Psycho-Oncology*, 14, 297–306.

Revicki, D.A., Sorensen, S., and Wu, A.W. (1998). Reliability and validity of physical and mental health summary scores from the Medical Outcomes Study HIV Health Survey. *Medical Care*, 36, 126–137.

Reynolds, T., Thornicroft, G., Abas, M., et al. (2000). Camberwell Assessment of Need for the Elderly (CANE). Development, validity and reliability. *British Journal of Psychiatry*, 176, 444–452.

Richards, C.T., Gisondi, M.A., Chang, C.H., et al. (2011). Palliative care symptom assessment for patients with cancer in the emergency department: validation of the Screen for Palliative and End-of-life care needs in the Emergency Department instrument. *Journal of Palliative Medicine*, 14, 757–764.

Richardson, A., Medina, J., Brown, V., and Sitzia, J. (2007). Patients' needs assessment in cancer care: a review of assessment tools. *Supportive Care in Cancer*, 15, 1125–1144.

Scandrett, K.G., Reitschuler-Cross, E.B., Nelson, L., et al. (2010). Feasibility and effectiveness of the NEST13+ as a screening tool for advanced illness care needs. *Journal of Palliative Medicine*, 13, 161–169.

Schag, C.A., Ganz, P.A., and Heinrich, R.L. (1991). CAncer Rehabilitation Evaluation System—short form (CARES-SF). A cancer specific rehabilitation and quality of life instrument. *Cancer*, 68, 1406–1413.

Schag, C.A., Ganz, P.A., Kahn, B., and Petersen, L. (1992). Assessing the needs and quality of life of patients with HIV infection: development of the HIV Overview of Problems-Evaluation System (HOPES). *Quality of Life Research*, 1, 397–413.

Schmid, R., Eschen, A., Ruegger-Frey, B., and Martin, M. (2012). Instruments for comprehensive needs assessment in individuals with cognitive complaints, mild cognitive impairment or dementia: a systematic review. *International Journal of Geriatric Psychiatry*, 27, 329–341.

Schofield, P., Gough, K., Ugalde, A., et al. (2012). Validation of the needs assessment for advanced lung cancer patients (NA-ALCP). *Psycho-Oncology*, 21, 451–455.

Schwartz, C.E., Merriman, M.P., Reed, G., and Byock, I. (2005). Evaluation of the Missoula-VITAS Quality of Life Index—revised: research tool or clinical tool? *Journal of Palliative Medicine*, 8, 121–135.

Skeel, R.T. (1993). Quality of life dimensions that are most important to cancer patients. *Oncology (Williston Park)*, 7, 55–61.

Sneeuw, K.C., Sprangers, M.A., and Aaronson, N.K. (2002). The role of health-care providers and significant others in evaluating the quality of life of patients with chronic disease. *Journal of Clinical Epidemiology*, 55, 1130–1143.

Sprangers, M.A. and Aaronson, N.K. (1992). The role of health-care providers and significant others in evaluating the quality of life of patients with chronic disease: a review. *Journal of Clinical Epidemiology*, 45, 743–760.

Tang, S.T., and McCorkle, R. (2002). Use of family proxies in quality of life research for cancer patients at the end of life: a literature review. *Cancer Investigation*, 20, 1086–1104.

Te Velde, A., Sprangers, M.A., and Aaronson, N.K. (1996). Feasibility, psychometric performance, and stability across modes of administration of the CARES-SF. *Annals of Oncology*, 7, 381–390.

Tsiligianni, I.G., van der Molen, T., Moraitaki, D., *et al.* (2012). Assessing health status in COPD. A head-to-head comparison between the COPD assessment test (CAT) and the clinical COPD questionnaire (CCQ). *BMC Pulmonary Medicine*, 12, 20.

Van der Molen, T., Willemse, B.W., Schokker, S., ten Hacken, N.H., Postma, D.S., and Juniper, E.F. (2003). Development, validity and responsiveness of the Clinical COPD Questionnaire. *Health and Quality of Life Outcomes*, 1, 13.

Van Scheppingen, C., Schroevers, M.J., Smink, A., *et al.* (2011). Does screening for distress efficiently uncover meetable unmet needs in cancer patients? *Psycho-Oncology*, 20, 655–663.

Vernooij-Dassen, M.J., Osse, B.H., Schade, E., and Grol, R.P. (2005). Patient autonomy problems in palliative care: systematic development and evaluation of a questionnaire. *Journal of Pain and Symptom Management*, 30, 264–270.

Volicer, L., Hurley, A.C., and Blasi, Z.V. (2001). Scales for evaluation of end-of-life care in dementia. *Alzheimer Disease and Associated Disorders*, 15, 194–200.

Waller, A., Girgis, A., Currow, D., and Lecathelinais, C. (2008). Development of the palliative care needs assessment tool (PC-NAT) for use by multi-disciplinary health professionals. *Palliative Medicine*, 22, 956–964.

Waller, A., Girgis, A., Davidson, P.M., *et al.* (2013). Facilitating needs-based support and palliative care for people with chronic heart failure: preliminary evidence for the acceptability, inter-rater reliability, and validity of a needs assessment tool. *Journal of Pain and Symptom Management*, 45, 912–925.

Waller, A., Girgis, A., Johnson, C., *et al.* (2012a). Improving outcomes for people with progressive cancer: interrupted time series trial of a needs assessment intervention. *Journal of Pain and Symptom Management*, 43, 569–581.

Waller, A., Girgis, A., Johnson, C., *et al.* (2012b). Implications of a needs assessment intervention for people with progressive cancer: impact on clinical assessment, response and service utilisation. *Psycho-Oncology*, 21, 550–557.

Waller, A., Girgis, A., Lecathelinais, C., *et al.* (2010). Validity, reliability and clinical feasibility of a Needs Assessment Tool for people with progressive cancer. *Psycho-Oncology*, 19, 726–733.

Wen, K.Y., and Gustafson, D.H. (2004). Needs assessment for cancer patients and their families. *Health and Quality of Life Outcomes*, 2, 11.

Wilcock, A., Klezlova, R., Coombes, S., *et al.* (2010). Identifying supportive and palliative care needs in people with a recent diagnosis of thoracic cancer: acceptability of the SPARC questionnaire. *Thorax*, 65, 937–938.

Wilson, K.G., Graham, I.D., Viola, R.A., *et al.* (2004). Structured interview assessment of symptoms and concerns in palliative care. *Canadian Journal of Psychiatry*, 49, 350–358.

World Health Organization (2007). *Cancer Control: Knowledge into Action*. Geneva: WHO.

World Health Organization (2013). *WHO Definition of Palliative Care*. [Online] Available at: <http://www.who.int/cancer/palliative/definition/en/>.

Wu, A.W., Revicki, D.A., Jacobson, D., and Malitz, F.E. (1997). Evidence for reliability, validity and usefulness of the Medical Outcomes Study HIV Health Survey (MOS-HIV). *Quality of Life Research*, 6, 481–493.

The measurement of, and tools for, pain and other symptoms

Jane M. Ingham, Helen M. Moore,
Jane L. Phillips, and Russell K. Portenoy

Introduction to measurement tools for pain

For patients with advanced or incurable illnesses, the disease experience is inextricably linked to symptoms, and to the distress that symptoms produce. Symptom assessment is essential in developing and implementing a plan of care intended to reduce illness burden and suffering. The measurement of symptoms is both a key element in this assessment and the means by which therapeutic interventions can be tested in clinical research.

Symptoms are multidimensional and symptom measurement is complex. Addressing this complexity requires consideration of (1) symptom assessment and measurement principles, (2) the clinical and research applications of these principles, (3) measurement instruments for common symptoms, and (4) challenges in the application of symptom measures in palliative care settings.

Symptom assessment and measurement principles

Symptoms—a general definition

The study of symptoms has been hampered to some degree by a lack of consistency in terminology. According to the *Oxford Dictionary of English*, a symptom is 'a physical or mental feature which is regarded as indicating a condition of disease, particularly such a feature that is apparent to the patient' ('Symptom', 2013). Symptoms are inherently *subjective*. They are perceptions, and are usually conveyed by language. Symptom measurement attempts to quantify aspects of this perception in a manner that is valid and reliable.

Symptoms may be distinguished from *signs*, which are objective indicators of disease, and from pathological processes or diagnoses. Although neither symptoms nor signs are diagnoses, some symptoms are used clinically like diagnoses, as a guide to assessment or treatment. For example, 'confusion' is a symptom which, in the context of advanced illness, may imply the existence of cognitive impairment or delirium and lead promptly to a search for reversible causes. A comprehensive evaluation, seeking signs of cognitive disturbance, or change in level of consciousness, is needed, to establish the diagnosis of delirium. It is important to recognize that symptoms by themselves have a differential diagnosis, which may be explored by examination and review of objective data.

Specific symptom descriptors

While languages are enriched by the subtle differences in the meaning of words used to describe human perceptions, the measurement of these perceptions is made more challenging by these nuances. The complexity of measurement is compounded when the symptoms themselves are highly variable and the words used to label them, such as 'pain' or 'fatigue', have a plethora of meanings for patients and a wide range of implications. To address the complexity of pain, for example, the International Association for the Study of Pain (IASP) created a taxonomy that defines pain-related terms, characterizes various dimensions, and links these characterizations to specific diagnoses (IASP, 2011). This work has helped define the parameters of appropriate measurement strategies—what should be measured and how—in relation to varied painful conditions.

In contrast, there is no comparable framework for the meanings, dimensions, and linkages to diseases of other common symptoms, such as 'fatigue', 'confusion', and 'breathlessness'. Fatigue may be interpreted by some patients as sleepiness and by others as muscle weakness or exhaustion. The word 'confusion' may be used variably to refer to impaired concentration, disorganized thinking, forgetfulness, or even hallucinations. The variability of these meanings and the complexity of symptom linguistics are among the many factors that justify the need for formal validation of symptom measurement instruments. Validation determines whether a word or set of words to describe subjective experience has sufficient common meaning to allow accurate determination of characteristics such as presence/absence, intensity, and duration. Without a common meaning, there is the potential for instrument-to-instrument variation in the prevalence of seemingly identical symptoms (Bruera et al., 1991; Cella et al., 1993; Portenoy et al., 1994b; Chang et al., 2000a).

'Dyspnoea' illustrates this complexity. There is no consensus regarding the most appropriate definition for dyspnoea, but it is broadly accepted to be subjective, and hence a symptom. Affirming this view, the American Thoracic Society stresses that self-report is the appropriate means to assess dyspnoea and that dyspnoea is comprised of quantitatively distinct sensations that vary in intensity (American Thoracic Society, 1999). The symptom is not easily described by those who experience it, however. In a study of patients with dyspnoea, 8% answered 'no' to the statement 'I feel breathless' despite answering 'yes' for numerous other descriptors that are applied to dyspnoea (Elliott et al., 1991). Among healthy individuals, the descriptors applied to breathlessness appear to relate to various physiological mechanisms and not to any specific underlying pathophysiology or disease condition (Mahler et al., 1996). Clusters of descriptors have been found to associate with different diagnostic groups, suggesting that patients are describing qualitatively different experiences of breathlessness (Wilcock et al., 2002).

Another study found similar complexity in the variation across instruments when patients were asked to endorse similar symptoms. Intra-individual variation of about 10% was apparent in the prevalence of 'feeling sad' versus 'depression', and 'feeling nervous' versus 'anxiety' (Chang et al., 2000a). These differences could potentially relate to variation in the meaning of descriptors determined by culture, education, symptom experience (e.g. severity), or attributions specified by the instrument (such as assessment timeframe).

Subjectivity in assessment and measurement

Because symptoms are inherently subjective, patient self-report must be the primary source of information (Slevin et al., 1988; Kahn et al., 1992; Hinton, 1996; National Institutes of Health, 2011a; National Cancer Institute, 2013). This reliance on self-report to measure symptoms resonates well with a broad initiative—most notable in oncology—to validate and promote the use of so-called 'patient-reported outcomes' (PROs) as key metrics in clinical care. The emerging emphasis on PROs reflects increasing consumer demand for patient-centred care, ensuring that the voice of the patient is considered as the plan of care is elaborated.

The National Institutes of Health (NIH) in the United States has supported the development of a Patient-Reported Outcome Measurement Information System (PROMIS®), which aims 'to provide clinicians and researchers access to efficient, precise, valid, and responsive adult- and child-reported measures of health and well-being' (NIH, 2011b). The network advancing the PROMIS® system has developed item banks for measurement of major self-reported health domains that are affected by chronic illness. Item banks are collections of calibrated items from which short-form measures and computer-adaptive tests can be derived. As examples, this network has addressed fatigue, pain, physical function, and emotional distress (Garcia et al., 2007) for cancer clinical trials. The National Cancer Institute (NCI) in the United States has been particularly focused on an expanded role for PROs as outcomes in cancer trials (NIH, 2011a). In the United Kingdom, an example of these efforts is to be found in the Department of Primary Health Care Services, Health Service and Policy Research Group's work on patient-reported measures of outcome and experiences of health-care (PROMs and PREMs) (Department of Primary Care Health Sciences, 2013), and in the palliative care setting, the European Association on Palliative Care has a Task Force working actively on patient-reported outcome measurement (European Association for Palliative Care, 2012).

From a research perspective, direct measurement of PROs is supported by numerous studies that demonstrate poor correlation between observer and patient assessments (Slevin et al., 1988; Grossman et al., 1991; Kahn et al., 1992). There is a poor correlation, for example, between patients' visual analogue scale (VAS) scores for pain and those completed by their health-care providers, with some evidence that the poorest accuracy may be among patients with the most severe pain (Grossman et al., 1991). Another study that assessed concurrently patients and their spouse caregivers found that, although the spouse caregivers agreed with patients on objective measures with observable referents (e.g. ability to dress independently), they disagreed with subjective aspects of patient functioning (e.g. depression, fear of future, and confidence in treatment) (Clipp and George, 1992). Similarly, evidence from retrospective surveys completed by family members after the patient's death has suggested that assessment by family is better for symptoms that are more observable, such as vomiting (Hinton, 1996), than those that depend more on subjective indicators, such as psychological distress (McPherson and Addington-Hall, 2004) and the impact of events that occur during the dying process (Mularski et al., 2004).

Although the optimal approach to symptom assessment and measurement incorporates patient ratings, it may not be possible to obtain or interpret self-report. This can be the case, for example, in pre-verbal patients and those with cognitive impairment from delirium or dementia. In these groups, symptom measurement can only be done using proxy reports, or determination of pain-related behavioural or physiological changes. These data must be interpreted cautiously when used to quantify symptom distress and quality of life (QOL), particularly towards the end of life (Greer et al., 1986; Morris et al., 1986; Reuben and Mor, 1986; Mor, 1987; Mor and Masterson-Allen, 1990; Higginson and McCarthy, 1994; The Support Principal Investigators, 1995; Kutner et al., 2006). In clinical settings and in studies, the source of the data should always be acknowledged and the self-report and proxy data described separately, if both are acquired (Aaronson, 1990; Kutner et al., 2006).

Symptoms as measurable multidimensional experiences

The effective implementation of therapeutic strategies is contingent on comprehensive symptom assessment. Assessment involves a broad characterization of the nature of the symptom, including measurement of key dimensions (Tables 7.2.1 and 7.2.2) (Foley, 1993; Cherny and Portenoy, 1994; Sui et al., 1994; Ingham and Portenoy, 1996).

Symptom dimensions

Every symptom may be measured in terms of one or more specific dimensions (Dunlop, 1990; Portenoy and Hagen, 1990; Welch

Table 7.2.1 The measurable aspects of symptoms

Specific dimensions	Frequency
	Severity
	Distress
Symptom impact on specific factors	Other physical and psychological symptoms or diagnoses
	Function
	Family, social, financial, spiritual, and existential resources and concerns
Symptom impact on global constructs	Global symptom distress
	Health-related quality of life

Table 7.2.2 Clinical assessment with particular focus on symptom assessment

Assessment: eliciting medical history, examination, investigation review		Formulating a care plan

Identify presenting concerns	*Past history*
	Identification of other intercurrent conditions and previous illnesses and procedures
		Formulate a summary that identifies current:
		◆ Identified medical problems. This should include consideration of the following for each symptom:
		  • Inferred pathophysiology
		  • Relationship to other symptoms. Is symptom—same pathophysiology as other symptom/s, differing pathophysiology from other symptoms, triggering other symptoms, caused by treatment directed at other symptom/s
		◆ Identified psychosocial problems
		◆ Patient concerns, needs, priorities, and goals
		◆ Family/carer concerns, needs, priorities, and goals
		◆ Anticipated concerns

History of current illness Including therapeutic interventions, e.g. operative procedures, chemo- and radiotherapy. (The detail provided by the patient may serve to provide the clinician with some understanding of the patient's understanding of current extent of disease.)	*Family history* Identification of family illness history. This can also be an opportunity to address experiences relevant to current illness, e.g. carer roles etc. *Social history* Identification of social circumstances. If not addressed already, this can also be another opportunity to explore the impact of disease and symptoms on patient and family and factors that modulate global symptom distress, e.g. coping strategies and family supports	

History of each current symptom
Consider addressing:
◆ Chronology, frequency, other clinical characteristics, e.g. location, etc.
◆ Severity
◆ Degree of associated distress or burden
◆ Other factors that alleviate or modulate distress
◆ Impact of each symptom on any other symptoms
◆ Prior treatment modalities and their efficacy
◆ Impact on function
◆ Patient perception of aetiology
◆ Impact of the specific symptom (or constellation of symptoms) on QOL—physical condition, psychological status, social interactions
	Allergies, drug reactions, and medications
	If not addressed already, this can be an opportunity to ensure that the impact of medications on symptoms, barriers to use of medications, and concerns about medications are addressed
	
	Undertake physical examination
	In addition to a full examination in relation to medical problems, particular attention should be paid to identifying findings in physical examination that may relate to symptoms in terms of explaining their pathophysiology, and identifying consequences of symptoms and/or side effects of symptom treatments
		Formulate an appropriate strategy and 'next steps' in relation to:
		◆ Addressing current and anticipated medical and psycho-social problems, concerns, and needs within context of both patient priorities and goals and medical urgency. This should include addressing specific symptoms considering the role of:
		  • Additional diagnostic tests to assess each symptom's pathophysiology
		  • Therapeutic interventions to address cause of each symptom
		  • Therapeutic interventions to address distress related to each symptom
		◆ Informing patient/family/carers about new findings and, as needed, readdressing goals

Systems review Assessment of other symptoms that the patient may not have raised specifically	*Assess available laboratory and imaging data* In addition to identifying extent of disease, in relation to symptoms particular attention should be paid to identifying findings among data that may relate to symptoms in terms of explaining their pathophysiology, identifying consequences of symptoms and/or treatments, and problems that will be important to consider in developing a therapeutic plan	

et al., 1991; Portenoy et al., 1994a, 1994b; Chang et al., 2000b, 2000c; Collins et al., 2002). An early study of adult cancer patients noted that patients can separately measure the frequency, severity, and distress associated with 32 physical and psychological symptoms (Portenoy et al., 1994a). Some of the symptoms were reported to be frequent or severe, but not highly bothersome or distressing, suggesting that the mere report of a symptom does not imply that it is burdensome or in need of treatment. Similar variability in the characteristics of symptoms has been demonstrated in the paediatric setting (Collins et al., 2002).

The temporal dimension of symptoms

Although reference is commonly made to the temporal features of a symptom as if this was one important dimension, there are multiple aspects inherent in the change of symptoms over time. Measurement can focus on onset (abrupt or insidious), duration, trajectory (worsening or improving), and daily pattern

(continuous or intermittent). The occurrence of discrete episodes of worsening symptoms may be relevant as well.

The temporal features of a symptom also can focus on the change over time of other descriptors, such as severity or distress, or various types of symptom impact. Characteristics may change with progression or remission of the disease, or with evolution of perceptions related to the availability of treatment, psychosocial support or adaptation, or the impact of comorbid disorders or symptoms. A key descriptor such as severity may worsen, but associated dimensions, such as distress or impact on QOL, may stay the same or even improve.

Although longitudinal symptom measurement is challenging to accomplish, there is substantial value in doing so. Studies have shown that measurements of symptom distress, functional status and QOL may change dramatically in the months preceding death, but this occurs at different rates and at different points along the disease trajectory (Higginson et al., 2012; Hung et al.,

2013; Sutradhar et al., 2013). When changes in functional status are subtle, findings of changes in symptom distress may be more informative. Clinically, serial measurements and feedback to physicians have been reported to facilitate physician–patient communication and exert a positive impact on QOL and emotional functioning (Velikova et al., 2004). Research in this area is evolving but the overall clinical goal is to ensure the information gathered about symptoms can be applied at multiple points along the trajectory of a disease.

Symptom impact

The impact of symptoms may be described in relation to varied domains of functioning (such as family, social, financial, spiritual, and existential issues) or in terms of global constructs such as overall symptom distress or QOL (Dunlop, 1990; Welch et al., 1991; Portenoy et al., 1994a). Pain provides a useful example of this complexity in the measurement of symptom impact. Unrelieved pain may be associated with depressed or anxious mood, insomnia, anorexia, or interference in the ability to socialize, function physically, or work. Pain may reduce income or lead to role disruption in the family. Although challenging to do, instruments for the valid measurement of each of these domains could be combined to obtain a very broad understanding of the outcomes related to pain.

Given the complexity of multidimensional symptom measurement, the decision usually is made to focus on high-impact concerns. Instruments have been developed with this goal. Again using pain as an example, a commonly used measurement tool—the Brief Pain Inventory (BPI) —focuses on measures of pain severity (0–10 scales) and a validated subscale that assesses pain-related interference with function, mood, relationships, sleep, and enjoyment of life (Daut et al., 1983). The use of an instrument like the BPI (Daut et al., 1983) provides a simple approach to the measurement of multiple domains, but leaves the potential to assess other domains unfulfilled. The online version of this tool is available at: <http://www.mdanderson.org/education-and-research/departments-programs-and-labs/departments-and-divisions/symptom-research/symptom-assessment-tools/brief-pain-inventory.html>.

Symptoms and global constructs

Although the individual measurement of specific symptom dimensions can be highly informative, the value of global constructs to broadly characterize the experience of illness is clear. Fig. 7.2.1 illustrates the impact that a pathophysiological process and various modifying factors may have on the perception of symptom-associated distress and overall QOL. These global constructs can be measured with multidimensional QOL instruments (see Chapter 7.1) or more specific measurements of symptom distress. The multidimensional construct of QOL especially reflects the broad influence of many positive and negative factors on perceived well-being (Aaronson et al., 1988; Moinpour et al., 1989; Aaronson, 1990; Cella and Tulsky, 1990; Moinpour et al., 1990; Aaronson, 1991; Nayfield et al., 1992; Aaronson et al., 1993; Till, 1994).

Physical and psychological symptoms, or the distress that they cause, contribute to QOL, but may or may not be the predominant determinants of well-being (Levine et al., 1978; Derogatis et al., 1983; Reuben et al., 1988; Grosvenor et al., 1989; Brescia et al., 1990; Coyle et al., 1990; Dunlop, 1990; Dunphy and

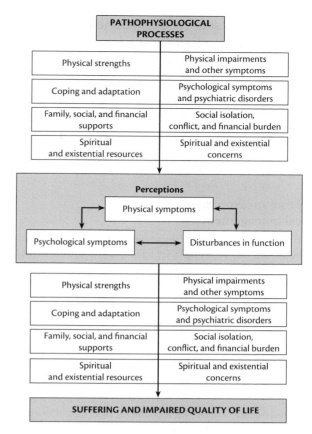

Fig. 7.2.1 Interactions among symptoms, suffering, and quality of life.

Amesbury, 1990; Ventafridda et al., 1990; Curtis et al., 1991; Fainsinger et al., 1991; Portenoy et al., 1994a; Chang et al., 2000c; Collins et al., 2002). A study of symptoms in cancer patients provided empirical evidence that information relating to the impact of symptoms on QOL was maximized by concurrent measurement of other factors, including 'symptom distress' and either frequency or intensity (Portenoy et al., 1994b). Of the three dimensions assessed, distress was the most informative. This observation, which was replicated in another study (Chang et al., 2000c), suggests that distress should be assessed if the goal of the evaluation is to clarify the interaction between symptoms and QOL.

Brief measures of symptom distress have been used as screening tools in clinical practice. The Distress Thermometer, for example, is a simple, self-report, pen and paper measure that asks patients to mark an 'X' on the 'thermometer' scale (0–10) that correlates with their level of distress in the previous week (National Comprehensive Cancer Network (NCCN), 2013b). Given that the score on this unidimensional scale has uncertain diagnostic accuracy, this, and other ultra-short methods, cannot be used alone to diagnose depression, anxiety, or distress in cancer patients (Mitchell, 2007; Thewes et al., 2009). That stated, such instruments may be considered as a first-stage screen to help rule out cases of depression (Mitchell, 2007). Also, the items on associated check lists can be used to identify and triage some 'realms' of concern.

Clinical and research applications of symptom assessment and measurement principles

Historically, symptom measurement has been used in clinical investigations to create primary or secondary treatment outcome variables. In recent decades, however, measurement has been brought more forcefully into clinical practice, where it has been shown to have a use as a part of the routine monitoring of patients (Grossman et al., 1991; Jacox et al., 1994a, 1994b; Foley, 1995; Bookbinder et al., 1996; Gordon et al., 2005).

Symptom measurement in routine clinical management

The clinical use of symptom measurement is evolving. Although it may be accomplished using brief hard-copy questionnaires, such as the Distress Thermometer (NCCN, 2013b) or the Edmonton Symptom Assessment Scale (Bruera et al., 1991), various types of computer-based methods have been developed and promise much greater flexibility in the future (Velikova et al., 1999; Taenzer et al., 2000; Carlson et al., 2001; Cull et al., 2001; Chang et al., 2002; Davis et al., 2007; Velikova et al., 2002; Abernethy et al., 2008, 2009; Mark et al., 2008; Wolpin et al., 2008).

A standardized approach using a validated symptom assessment instrument can serve to give the patient a voice and enable consistent symptom detection, assessment, and documentation. Ideally, assessment should be repeated at intervals. The challenge lies in selecting the right instrument for the patient population and integrating it into clinical practice. The simplest approach—routine screening with a brief instrument—may be best for large populations, notwithstanding the potential lack of diagnostic accuracy noted previously.

Another approach to systematic assessment focuses on single high-impact symptoms, such as pain and this symptom has been given particular attention in the cancer population (Foley, 1995). More broadly, systematic pain assessment has been shown to improve the understanding of health professionals of the pain status of individual hospitalized patients (Au et al., 1994; Gordon et al., 2002), and numerous guidelines now recommend the regular use of pain rating scales in all care settings (ambulatory care, community care, and acute care) (Jacox et al., 1994a; Gordon et al., 2005). In addition, educating people living with pain, and their caregivers, to use assessment tools at home has become a part of a self-management strategy to promote better pain management and continuity across care settings (Koller et al., 2012). An example of a tool for systematic recording of pain observations in the inpatient setting is the tool linked with the National Early Warning Score (NEWS) that has been devised by the Royal College of Physicians in the United Kingdom (Royal College of Physicians, 2012). This early warning score system and linked tool has been designed to trigger a clinical response to acute deterioration. The NEWS tool (Royal College of Physicians, 2012) has capacity to capture various observations such as temperature, pulse, and others, and a place for recording pain observations—indicating that pain should also be regularly recorded and responded to (Royal College of Physicians, 2012).

The experience with pain measurement has encouraged an expansion of routine assessment to the clinical measurement of other symptoms. Simple, face-valid, symptom screening tools developed to explore the spectrum of common physical and psychological symptoms in particular disease states can be helpful in the clinical setting where the screening measurement is complemented by a full clinical evaluation. Several measurement tools have been used routinely in palliative care units for some time (Bruera et al., 1991; Donnelly and Walsh, 1995). More recently, some investigators have explored the utility of symptom and QOL measures in the clinic setting using computer-based touchscreen methodology (Velikova et al., 1999; Taenzer et al., 2000; Carlson et al., 2001; Cull et al., 2001; Chang et al., 2002; Velikova et al., 2002; Davis et al., 2007; Abernethy et al., 2008, 2009). Evidence suggests the computer-based touchscreen methodology is valid, feasible, and acceptable to patients (Abernethy et al., 2008, 2009) and assuming confidentiality is ensured this may be a preferred approach for some patients, in contrast to paper questionnaires.

A number of organizations, including those that accredit hospitals, and national bodies such as the NCCN in the United States, have recommended the implementation of routine screening for pain, and potentially for distress and other symptoms (Holland, 1997; Payne, 1998; Mock et al., 2000; Scottish Intercollegiate Network, 2008; National Comprehensive Cancer Network, 2013a). There is now some evidence that improved outcomes can be achieved when routine symptom measures are augmented with clinical pathway implementation and access to expert consultation. A recent systematic review concluded that there is growing evidence in support of routine collection of symptom measures, as a means to achieve better, patient-centred care in cancer settings, particularly in relation to patient-provider communication and patient satisfaction, and to a lesser extent, in relation to the monitoring of treatment response and the detection of unrecognized problems. In contrast, to date, evidence is weak or non-existent in relation to the impact on changes to patient management and improved health outcomes; changes to patient health behaviour or the effectiveness of quality improvement of organizations; or the transparency, accountability, public reporting activities, and performance of the health-care system (Chen et al., 2013). All of these goals, as well as the goals of focusing staff attention on symptom assessment, reviewing the quality of patient care, and ascertaining the situation-specific barriers to symptom control, are important and warrant further investigation.

The emerging area of implementation and dissemination science will inevitably contribute to the future development of evidence based strategies by which recommendations for 'routine' symptom assessment can be implemented using an array of efficient, user-friendly (for both patients and clinicians), and valid methodologies, including face-to-face patient-physician interviews, pen and paper surveys, and/or computer-based methodology. At this time, and importantly, in implementing screening assessment strategies, clinicians should consider carefully how to optimize the integration of the screening strategy into clinical care. Response strategies should be identified, and consideration given to the development of plans for appropriate and timely response to identified levels of distress that can be feasibly implemented in the particular institution or health system (Seow et al., 2012; Cancer Quality Council of Ontario, 2014). Defined levels of distress for intervention may, for some symptoms, be defined by research-based evidence and for other symptoms, by expert input. As examples at the extreme level, an institution or health system should identify a response pathway for a pain report that suggests the presence of extreme pain and similarly, for a report of psychological distress that may indicate that a patient is at risk of self-harm. In addition to identifying 'alert' levels, in the clinical setting there is a need to develop institutionally-specific policies and procedures for responses. One approach is to align the responses to symptom distress with existing institutional risk management policies.

Symptom measurement in clinical research

Systematic symptom measurement can provide valid endpoints in clinical research, elucidating both the palliative potential of a treatment and its toxicity profile. Numerous factors must be considered when planning symptom-related research (Table 7.2.3). When observational studies or clinical trials seek detailed information about symptoms, face-valid symptom checklists are not preferred (Miller et al., 1981; Bruera et al., 1991; Burgess et al., 1993; Osoba, 1993; Donnelly and Walsh, 1995). Greater accuracy is achievable with validated measures that address more than one symptom dimension (McCorkle and Quint-Benoliel, 1983; De Haes et al., 1987; de Haes et al., 1990; Portenoy et al., 1994a, 1994b). When symptom related outcomes are secondary endpoints, as they are in most trials of cancer therapy, the use of simpler, standardized toxicity scales, such as those recommended by the World Health Organization and the NCI in the United States (Miller et al., 1981), may be sufficient. The challenge is to capture the relevant concerns as they evolve, using measures that are simple, and brief enough to limit participant burden and encourage compliance (Ingham et al., 1996).

When study aims include evaluation of a number of subjective endpoints, an investigator may decide to combine questionnaires, or alternatively, use a multidimensional measure such as the European Organization for the Research and Treatment of Cancer (EORTC), Quality of Life Questionnaire—Palliative (EORTC QLQ-C15-PAL) (Groenvold et al., 2006) or a short-form version of the EORTC's widely-used cancer-specific QOL measure (EORTC QLQ-C30) (Aaronson et al., 1993). Other instruments include the Functional Living Index-Cancer (FLIC) (Schipper et al., 1984; Morrow et al., 1992), the Functional Assessment of Cancer Therapy (FACT) System (Cella et al., 1993), the Cancer Rehabilitation Evaluation System (Ganz et al., 1992), the SF-36 of the Medical Outcome Study (Stewart et al.,

1988) and others. All of the validated, multidimensional measures of health-related QOL assess a selected group of prevalent symptoms, including pain, fatigue, and anxiety (Schipper et al., 1984; Ganz et al., 1992; Aaronson et al., 1993; Cella et al., 1993). Yet another approach is to use a core instrument with modules that target specific issues, disorders or treatments (Aaronson et al., 1988; Moinpour et al., 1989; Aaronson et al., 1993; Cella et al., 1993).

Although QOL information is important and may be sufficient for many purposes (Carlson et al., 2001; O'Brien et al., 2001; Chang et al., 2002; Millsopp et al., 2006), QOL instruments were not developed as symptom assessment instruments. Neither the prevalence rates nor the characteristics and dimensions of the diverse array of physical and psychological symptoms experienced by patients may be captured adequately by these instruments. Depending on the purpose of the assessment, the aims of the research, the anticipated outcomes and toxicities, and the resources of the investigator, other measures can be added to capture symptom-related information (Aaronson et al., 1988; Moinpour et al., 1989, Aaronson et al., 1993; Cella et al., 1993; Ingham et al., 1996). One way in which this can be accomplished is by the concurrent use of a QOL instrument and a symptom measurement tool.

The utility of a tailored approach to QOL and symptom assessment was demonstrated in a study that explored the importance of specific pain assessments during routine QOL evaluation (Ingham et al., 1996). After clinical observations suggested that the combination of paclitaxel and recombinant human granulocyte-colony stimulating factor for breast cancer was associated with frequent short-lived episodes of pain, supplemental pain measurements were included with QOL measures in a phase II trial. The 'tailored' assessment revealed a marked disparity between the pain data obtained during a routine QOL assessment performed at 3-week intervals and those acquired through the supplemental pain evaluation obtained twice weekly. Despite the interval assessment revealing a marked decline in median pain scores, the supplemental assessment demonstrated transient acute and severe pains in almost half the patients. Clearly, this was important to identify in order to provide information to patients and clinicians on expected transient concerns and management of side effects. Such a tailored approach to measurement may be important in anticipating side effects of treatments, clarifying the usefulness

Table 7.2.3 Methodological considerations for symptom measurement in research setting

Patient-related factors	Factors related to investigator goals and resources	Instrument-related factors
Patient's ability to provide consent and comprehend instruments:	*Study aims and method:*	*Validity and reliability:*
Age-related factors	Which symptoms and dimensions of symptoms need to be assessed?	Validity of instrument for assessment of symptom in general and in particular population
Cognitive state	When should symptoms be assessed?	
Cultural and language barriers	What methodological controls are needed?	Ability of instrument to assess the dimensions and impact of symptom
Patient's descriptors for symptom		
Presence of other symptoms		
Patient's willingness to participate in data collection:	*Data management and statistical analysis:*	*Clinical utility and appropriateness:*
Patient reluctance to participate in investigation or to report specific symptom	Available resources for data collection and analysis	Capacity of instrument to assess hypothesis
		Instrument complexity and respondent burden

of a therapy in symptom palliation, guiding clinical management at the time of treatment, and/or determining the time-dependent effects of therapy on well-being.

In contemplating measurement in any clinical research, consideration must not only be given to the utility of an instrument to measure a subjective effect, but also to whether a reasonable presumption can be made about the extent to which a change in the measured score reflects a 'clinically relevant' change in symptom severity or distress. Statistical significance, particularly in tests of group averages, may or may not indicate that the difference is meaningful in the clinical sense. For example, a clinical trial of an analgesic with a large sample size may show that the group receiving treatment 'A' had an average change in a pain score of 1.0 on a 0–10 scale, whereas the group that received treatment 'B' had an average change of 1.8. This difference may be statistically significant but clinically irrelevant. Moreover, this difference reflects average scores and may hide the fact that some patients had very large changes after a treatment, whereas some did not change at all.

Information about the responsiveness of a questionnaire to clinical changes and the minimal important difference (MID) in scores that depicts a clinically important change (Revicki et al., 2006) are very helpful in determining whether the differences observed during a study actually reflect a clinically meaningful event. There are a number of 'anchor-based' and 'distribution-based' methods to determine MID. Once a MID is determined, data from a trial can be subjected to a responder analysis, which can determine whether the proportion of experimental patients with a clinically meaningful change is statistically different than the proportion in a control group.

The MID may be derived empirically or reflect clinical impression. Analyses of data from a large pain study, for example, suggested that change scores of two or more on a 0–10 scale, or 30% or more on an analogue scale reflect clinically meaningful change (Farrar et al., 2000). Alternatively, it also is widely accepted on clinical grounds that the number of patients who achieve pain relief greater than 50% is a reasonable MID.

Other metrics also can be used to provide a clinical framework for the understanding of scores, or differences in scores, on symptom measures. A common approach is to use the number needed to treat (NNT), which gives the number of people you need to treat with the intervention (compared with the control) to prevent one event (The Cochrane Collaboration, 2002). The number of days on which symptoms reached a level of 'control' also can be employed (Zech et al., 1995). In pain research using the BPI (Daut et al., 1983), an analysis can be applied that first categorizes pain scores into 'mild', 'moderate', or 'severe', and then determines group differences in the proportion of patients who change from one category to another (Daut and Cleeland, 1982; Serlin et al., 1995; Cleeland et al., 1996; Paul et al., 2005).

Additional information about the clinical relevance of a change in symptom scores may be accessible by combining outcomes. In one study of a chemotherapeutic agent, for example, a combination of changes in three variables (reduction in pain by 50%, weight gain of 5%, and improvement in performance status of 20%) along with duration of improvement (4 weeks) was proposed a priori as an indicator of benefit (Rothenberg et al., 1996; Burris et al., 1997; Rothenberg et al., 1998).

Recent work has suggested that severity cut-off points may differ among different symptoms, at least when the object is to relate these cut-offs to physical functioning (Given et al., 2008). In this regard, systematic reviews may offer a method to assess the impact of symptom-related therapies by combining data through meta-analyses. Research has defined MIDs in six PROMIS®-Cancer scales in advanced-stage cancer patients and further work is underway to explore these in relation to other disease states. Of note, these MIDs are applicable to the total scores on 'instruments' made up of items from the PROMIS® item bank, rather than the scores related to specific symptom scales (Yost et al., 2011).

Another recent study provides an example of how investigators explored the MID using a 'well-being' anchor from the Edmonton Symptom Assessment Scale (ESAS) (Bedard et al., 2013). This study found that different changes were relevant for improvement and deterioration; a decrease of 1.2 and 1.1 units in pain and depression scales, respectively, reflected clinically relevant improvement, whereas an increase of at least 1.4, 1.8, 1.1, 1.1, and 1.4 units, respectively, were associated with deterioration in pain, tiredness, depression, anxiety, and appetite loss (Bedard et al., 2013). This work suggests that conclusions about the clinical relevance of changes in symptom scores are best grounded in empirical observations in appropriate clinical populations.

There continue to be many questions to be resolved through future studies. For example, is an improvement from 2 to 1 on an 11-point numeric scale (50% change) as clinically significant as a change from 9 to 4.5 (also a 50% change)? Can the clinical significance of a therapy be evaluated without controlling for side effects, and if not, how should these be measured and indexed? In the complex palliative care setting, how can the clinical relevance of a single symptom be explored fully when most patients experience multiple distressing symptoms concurrently? The latter concern has been raised in studies of symptom clusters that suggest important commonalities across symptoms (Walsh and Rybicki, 2006). If symptom cluster research ultimately demonstrates relevance to assessment, prognostication or treatment, the therapeutic targeting of clusters may have the potential to reduce polypharmacy, lessen drug side effects, and provide pharmacoeconomic benefits (Cheung et al., 2009).

Measurement instruments for common symptoms

Instrument selection for symptom measurement must be guided by an understanding of the goals of assessment and the practicality, applicability, and acceptability of the instrument in the particular patient population. Evidence that the instrument is valid and reliable for the purposes intended should be considered carefully. Concern about the potential burden imposed on patients, clinicians, and investigators, which may justify the use of simple and brief questionnaires, must be balanced against the scientific need to capture complex symptom-related concerns or QOL. If the information is salient and would not be assessed otherwise, the increased burden of the assessment itself may be warranted.

Instruments for the measurement of multiple symptoms

Simple, face-valid checklists may be used to determine the incidence or prevalence of multiple physical and psychological symptoms (Miller et al., 1981; Bruera et al., 1991; Fainsinger et al., 1991;

Donnelly and Walsh, 1995). This approach is limited, however, by the lack of instrument validation and the inability of such checklists to ascertain important dimensions of the symptom experience, such as intensity or distress.

Validated measures can supersede these simple checklists in many clinical situations and many types of studies. A systematic review identified 21 instruments that may be used to measure multiple symptoms in cancer patients (Kirkova et al., 2006). Those that are used commonly vary substantially in design and purpose (Table 7.2.4). Experience in the use of these instruments in non-cancer populations also varies, and the extent to which each has been validated externally or even field tested in other patient groups should be considered when selecting a specific instrument.

Edmonton Symptom Assessment System (ESAS) (Bruera et al., 1991). The ESAS has been used extensively in palliative care research. It evaluates intensity of nine common symptoms of cancer using VASs; a tenth symptom can be added. Patient ratings are preferred but there is extensive experience with proxy ratings. It also has been modified for use in the critically ill (Nelson et al., 2001). One study in an outpatient setting reported a completion rate of 60% for lung cancer patients and almost 40% for all other cancer patients (Dudgeon et al., 2012). Validation in a sample of patients with advanced cancer noted that test–retest validity was better at 2 days than 1 week, and the total score was most reflective of physical well-being (Chang et al., 2000a). This instrument's brevity and established utility in populations with advanced illness are advantageous. In addition, some clinicians have been exploring the use of revised versions of the ESAS (Watanabe et al., 2011).

Memorial Symptom Assessment Scale (MSAS) (Portenoy et al., 1994b). The MSAS is a validated, patient-rated measure that provides multidimensional information about a diverse group of common symptoms (Fig. 7.2.2). The original form characterizes 26 physical and six psychological symptoms in terms of intensity, frequency, and distress. A validated short-form (MSAS-SF), which evaluates these 32 symptoms in terms of a single dimension, has been translated into numerous languages and is widely used in studies of diverse populations (Chang et al., 2000c). A briefer version (the condensed MSAS or CMAS) that depicts 15 symptoms in terms of one dimension (Chang et al., 2004) and paediatric versions (Collins et al., 2002) also have been validated.

Although the MSAS provides ratings for individual symptoms, the tool generally is not used when the research question focuses on one or a small number of symptoms, as it might in an intervention trial. Rather, the MSAS, like other multi-symptom questionnaires, is more valuable as a means to determine the presence or absence of numerous symptoms concurrently and to measure symptom distress. All adult versions of the MSAS have a subscale that measures global symptom distress (Global Distress Index, or MSAS-GDI), and both the MSAS and the MSAS-SF have other subscales that describe physical symptom distress (MSAS-PHYS) and psychological symptom distress (MSAS-PSYCH), respectively. The MSAS-GDI, which is the average of the frequency of four prevalent psychological symptoms and the distress associated with six prevalent physical symptoms, may be the most meaningful clinically, because of its high correlation with measures of QOL and clinical status (Portenoy et al., 1994b).

MD Anderson Symptom Inventory (MDASI) (Cleeland et al., 2000). The MDASI evaluates the presence and severity of 13 core symptoms and has six items that rate the extent to which symptoms

interfere with various domains of function. It has been translated into many languages and several supplemental modules have been developed that contain items that augment the core items with disease-specific, disease-site-specific or treatment-specific use. The format of the MDASI is based on the BPI (Daut et al., 1983) and Brief Fatigue Inventory (Mendoza et al., 1999). Studies have demonstrated its utility when administered via interview or an interactive voice response system, and the core-plus-module approach may be advantageous when considering populations with specific symptoms that may be mild but distressing or significantly impacting on function. Examples include the MDASI-BT (brain tumour) (Armstrong et al., 2009) and MDASI-HN (head and neck) (Rosenthal et al., 2007).

Symptom Distress Scale (SDS) (McCorkle and Young, 1978; McCorkle and Quint-Benoliel, 1983). The SDS is a 10-item patient-rated scale that evaluates 10 symptoms, in terms of presence and intensity. The time frame of assessment is 1 day. Although the SDS provides only limited information about specific symptoms, it is a valid measure of global symptom distress. Some have recommended it as a screening instrument for cancer patients in the outpatient (Degner and Sloan, 1995) and community settings (Peruselli et al., 1992). Its potential utility has been suggested in one study of lung cancer patients, which found that the total symptom distress score was a significant predictor of survival (Kukall et al., 1986).

Rotterdam Symptom Checklist (RSCL) (de Haes et al., 1987, 1990). The RSCL is a validated, patient-rated measure that evaluates a spectrum of common symptoms in terms of distress. Thirty physical and psychological symptoms are included and an additional eight items define the impact of symptoms on physical activity and function. The total score assesses global symptom distress and there are subscales that measure physical and psychological symptom distress, respectively. The inability to assess dimensions other than distress, including intensity, and the lack of a general pain item, may be a disadvantage. A validated modified version with the addition of several key physical symptoms has improved its breadth and utility (Stein et al., 2003).

Instruments for the measurement of specific symptoms

Although numerous instruments have been validated for the assessment of some symptoms, such as pain, breathlessness, and depression, there are fewer for other prevalent symptoms, such as anorexia, dry mouth, or change in appearance. Many instruments have been validated in specific populations and may not be valid in others. For example, studies of dyspnoea measures have largely focused on populations with pulmonary or cardiac disease (Stark, 1988; Cockcroft et al., 1989; McCord and Cronin-Stubbs, 1992; Eakin et al., 1993; Mahler et al., 1996; Mahler and Harver, 2000; Mahler, 2006), and these instruments may or may not be valid and reliable when dyspnoea is a result of advanced cancer (Brown et al., 1986; Bruera et al., 1993; Roberts et al., 1993). Recognizing these concerns about generalizability across disease states, there is an emerging focus on the development of instruments for specific disorders (Chen et al., 2007). The development of disease-specific PROs reflects this trend.

To illustrate the range of options available and some of the practical issues that may be important in selecting an instrument, the following discussion focuses on measures for three common symptoms—pain, dyspnoea, and impaired cognition.

Table 7.2.4 Physical symptoms and dimensions of symptoms in selected symptom assessment instruments

Symptoms	ESAS (Bruera et al., 1991)	MDASI (Cleeland et al., 2000)	MSAS (Portenoy et al., 1994b)	MSAS-SF (Chang et al., 2000c)	RSCL (de Haes et al., 1990)	SDS (McCorkle and Young, 1978)	CAMPAS-R (Ewing et al., 2004)	Symptom Monitor (Hoekstra et al., 2004)
Pain	X	X	X	X		X	X	X
Low back pain					X			
Headaches					X			
Abdominal aches					X			
Insomnia						X		
Tiredness					X			
Activity	X							
Fatigue		X				X		X
Fatigue/tiredness							X	
Lack of energy			X	X	X			
Nausea	X	X	X	X	X	X	X	X
Depression	X							
Depressed mood					X			
Feeling sad		X	X	X				
Anxiety	X				X			
Feeling nervous/nervousness			X	X	X			
Feeling irritable/irritability			X	X	X			
Drowsiness/drowsy	X	X	X	X				
Appetite	X					X		X
Lack of appetite		X	X	X	X			
Well-being	X							
Shortness of breath	X	X	X	X	X			X
Breathlessness							X	
Disturbed sleep		X						
Difficulty sleeping			X	X	X			
Sleep								X
Dry mouth		X	X	X	X			
Mouth sores			X	X				
Vomiting		X	X	X	X		X	X
Distress		X						
Worrying			X	X	X			
Remembering		X						
Difficulty concentrating/concentration			X	X	X	X		
Numbness/tingling hands or feet		X	X	X	X			
Cough			X	X				X

(continued)

Table 7.2.4 Continued

	ESAS (Bruera et al., 1991)	MDASI (Cleeland et al., 2000)	MSAS (Portenoy et al., 1994b)	MSAS-SF (Chang et al., 2000c)	RSCL (de Haes et al., 1990)	SDS (McCorkle and Young, 1978)	CAMPAS-R (Ewing et al., 2004)	Symptom Monitor (Hoekstra et al., 2004)
Feeling bloated		.	X	X				
Problems with urination			X	X				
Diarrhoea			X	X	X			X
Sweats			X	X				
Problems with sexual interest or activity			X	X				
Decreased sexual interest					X			
Itching			X	X				
Dizziness			X	X	X			
Difficulty swallowing			X	X				
Change in the way food tastes			X	X				
Sore mouth/pain when swallowing					X			
Weight loss			X	X				
Hair loss			X	X	X			
Constipation			X	X	X		X	X
Swelling of arms or legs			X	X				
I don't look like myself			X	X				
Appearance						X		
Changes in skin			X	X				
Despairing about the future					X			
Sore muscles					X			
Acid indigestion					X			
Shivering					X			
Mood						X		
Bowel pattern						X		
Mobility						X		
Tension					X			
Burning/sore eyes					X			
Patient anxiety/feeling tense							X	
Patient depression/feeling low							X	
Carer anxiety/feeling tense							X	
Carer depression/feeling low							X	
Other (patient choice)	X		X	X			X	X

(continued)

Table 7.2.4 Continued

	ESAS (Bruera et al., 1991)	MDASI (Cleeland et al., 2000)	MSAS (Portenoy et al., 1994b)	MSAS-SF (Chang et al., 2000c)	RSCL (de Haes et al., 1990)	SDS (McCorkle and Young, 1978)	CAMPAS-R (Ewing et al., 2004)	Symptom Monitor (Hoekstra et al., 2004)
Dimensions of symptoms assessed in each candidate symptom assessment instrument								
Presence or absence	X	X	X	X	X	X	X	X
Severity	X	X	X		X	X	X	X
Frequency			X					
Associated distress/ how bothersome			X	X				X
Interference with function		X			X		X	

ESAS, Edmonton Symptom Assessment System; MSAS, Memorial Symptom Assessment Scale; MSAS-SF, Memorial Symptom Assessment Scale-Short Form; MDASI, MD Anderson Symptom Inventory; RSCL, Rotterdam Symptom Checklist, SDS, Symptom Distress Scale; CAMPAS-R, Cambridge Palliative Assessment Schedule.

Instruments for the assessment of pain

There are many validated instruments for the measurement of pain. Unidimensional scales measure the dimension, usually severity or relief, using a 10-cm line (VAS), numerals (e.g. 0–10), verbal categories (e.g. mild, moderate or severe), or various types of pictures (faces or other pictures). The Memorial Pain Assessment Card (MPAC) (Fishman et al., 1987) is a brief, validated measure that combines several unidimensional scales, including analogue scales to characterize pain intensity, pain relief, and mood, respectively, and an 8-point verbal rating scale (VRS) to further characterize pain intensity.

Multidimensional pain instruments include the McGill Pain Questionnaire (MPQ) (Melzack, 1975; Graham et al., 1980; Melzack, 1987) and the BPI (Daut et al., 1983). The BPI (Daut et al., 1983) has been translated into many languages, repeatedly validated, and used in many studies. It provides information about pain history, intensity, location, and quality (see Daut et al. 1983). It has numeric scales that define pain intensity 'in general', 'at its worst', 'at its least', and 'right now'. A percentage scale quantifies relief from current therapies and body figure allows localization of the pain. Seven questions evaluate the degree to which pain interferes with function, mood, and enjoyment of life.

The MPQ (Melzack, 1975; Graham et al., 1980; Melzack, 1987) evaluates the sensory, affective, and evaluative dimensions of pain, and provides global scores and subscale scores for each of these dimensions. The scores are derived from the adjectival pain descriptors selected by the patient. A 5-point verbal categorical scale characterizes the intensity of pain and a pain drawing localizes the pain. Additional information is collected about the impact of medications and other therapies. To date, the predominant application of the MPQ has been in the assessment of chronic, non-malignant pain and the utility of the subscale scores has not been demonstrated for pain associated with cancer or other medical illnesses (de Conno et al., 1994; Caraceni et al., 2005).

Although self-report is the 'gold standard' for the measurement of pain and other symptoms (Zwakhalen et al., 2006), difficulty exists even for some cognitively intact individuals when completing VASs (Stark et al., 1982; Ganz et al., 1988; Stark, 1988). Since cognitive impairment is prevalent in medically ill populations, this may interfere further with the completion of even unidimensional measures. Much work has been done to develop and validate pain measures that use behavioural indicators of intensity (Gagliese and Melzack, 1997; Gagliese, 2001), particularly for populations with dementia (Herr et al., 2010). For patients with milder cognitive impairment, the Resident's Verbal Brief Pain Inventory, a modification of the BPI (Daut et al., 1983), focuses on the physical and psychosocial elements of pain assessment and is useful, reliable, and valid (Gibson et al., 2004).

Instruments for the assessment of dyspnoea

Breathlessness is highly prevalent and may be associated with underlying disease, concomitant symptoms, psychological well-being and socio-demographic circumstances (Kamal et al., 2011). Like other symptoms, varied dimensions of breathlessness can be assessed (Dudgeon, 2003) and validated instruments are now available (Bausewein et al., 2007).

Unidimensional breathlessness measures include numerical rating scales (NRS) or VASs for the specific dimension under evaluation (e.g. intensity, unpleasantness, or distress), and the modified Borg Scale (Kendrick et al., 2000), which uses a combined numerical and categorical scale to rate the patient's perception of their dyspnoea in relation to a perceived level of exertion. The VAS has good within-subject reproducibility when applied repeatedly in a single session (O'Neill et al., 1986; de Torres et al., 2002), but less reproducibility when the same exercise task is repeated at longer intervals, such as 2 weeks (Wilson and Jones, 1989). Considerable between-subject variation has been demonstrated (Stark et al., 1983). The NRS is highly correlated with the VAS and can be easier for some patients to master (Gift and Narsavage, 1998). Both the NRS and modified Borg Scale have been validated for use over the phone (Bausewein et al., 2008).

The modified Borg Scale has been validated in healthy individuals and in patients with chronic pulmonary disease (Borg, 1982; Kendrick et al., 2000). Although developed to measure dyspnoea in relation to exertion, in addition it now is widely used to rate spontaneous breathlessness. Patients report that the language used in the modified Borg Scale adequately captures their experience of breathlessness (Kendrick et al., 2000) and the scores

MEMORIAL SYMPTOM ASSESSMENT SCALE

NAME: DATE:

SECTION 1:

INSTRUCTIONS: We have listed 24 symptoms below. Read each one carefully. If you have had the symptom during this past week, let us know how OFTEN you had it, how SEVERE it was usually and how much if DISTRESSED OR BOTHERED you by circling the appropriate number. If you DID NOT HAVE the symptom, make an "X" in the box marked DID NOT HAVE.

DURING THE PAST WEEK. Did you have any of the following symptoms?	DID NOT HAVE	IF YES How OFTEN did you have it?				IF YES How SEVERE was it usually?				IF YES How much did it DISTRESS or BOTHER you?				
		Rarely	Occasionally	Frequently	Almost Constantly	Slight	Moderate	Severe	Very Severe	Not At All	Alittle bit	Somewhat	Quite A Bit	Very Much
Difficulty concentrating		1	2	3	4	1	2	3	4	0	1	2	3	4
Pain		1	2	3	4	1	2	3	4	0	1	2	3	4
Lack of energy		1	2	3	4	1	2	3	4	0	1	2	3	4
Cough		1	2	3	4	1	2	3	4	0	1	2	3	4
Feeling nervous		1	2	3	4	1	2	3	4	0	1	2	3	4
Dry mouth		1	2	3	4	1	2	3	4	0	1	2	3	4
Nausea		1	2	3	4	1	2	3	4	0	1	2	3	4
Feeling drowsy		1	2	3	4	1	2	3	4	0	1	2	3	4
Numbness/tingling in hands/feat		1	2	3	4	1	2	3	4	0	1	2	3	4
Difficulty sleeping		1	2	3	4	1	2	3	4	0	1	2	3	4
Feeling bloated		1	2	3	4	1	2	3	4	0	1	2	3	4
Problem with urination		1	2	3	4	1	2	3	4	0	1	2	3	4

Continued on other side..........

DURING THE PAST WEEK. Did you have any of the following symptoms?	DID NOT HAVE	IF YES How OFTEN did you have it?				IF YES How SEVERE was it usually?				IF YES How much did it DISTRESS or BOTHER you?				
		Rarely	Occasionally	Frequently	Almost Constantly	Slight	Moderate	Severe	Very Severe	Not At All	Alittle bit	Somewhat	Quite A Bit	Very Much
Vomiting		1	2	3	4	1	2	3	4	0	1	2	3	4
Shortness of breath		1	2	3	4	1	2	3	4	0	1	2	3	4
Diarrhea		1	2	3	4	1	2	3	4	0	1	2	3	4
Feeling sad		1	2	3	4	1	2	3	4	0	1	2	3	4
Sweats		1	2	3	4	1	2	3	4	0	1	2	3	4
Worrying		1	2	3	4	1	2	3	4	0	1	2	3	4
Problems with sexual interest or activity		1	2	3	4	1	2	3	4	0	1	2	3	4
Itching		1	2	3	4	1	2	3	4	0	1	2	3	4
Lack of appetite		1	2	3	4	1	2	3	4	0	1	2	3	4
Dizzlness		1	2	3	4	1	2	3	4	0	1	2	3	4
Difficulty swallowing		1	2	3	4	1	2	3	4	0	1	2	3	4
Feeling irritable		1	2	3	4	1	2	3	4	0	1	2	3	4

Continued on other side..........

SECTION 2:

INSTRUCTIONS: We have listed 8 symptoms below. Read each one carefully. If you have had the symptom during this past week, let us know how SEVERE it was usually and how much if DISTRESSED OR BOTHERED you by circling the appropriate number. If you DID NOT HAVE the symptom, make an "X" in the box marked DID NOT HAVE.

DURING THE PAST WEEK. Did you have any of the following symptoms?	DID NOT HAVE	IF YES How SEVERE was it usually?				IF YES How SEVERE was it usually?			
		Rarely	Occasionally	Frequently	Almost Constantly	Slight	Moderate	Severe	Very Severe
Mouth sores		1	2	3	4	1	2	3	4
Change in the way food tastes		1	2	3	4	1	2	3	4
Weight loss		1	2	3	4	1	2	3	4
Hair loss		1	2	3	4	1	2	3	4
Constipation		1	2	3	4	1	2	3	4
Swelling of arms or legs		1	2	3	4	1	2	3	4
"I don't look like myself"		1	2	3	4	1	2	3	4
Changes in skin		1	2	3	4	1	2	3	4

** IF YOU HAD ANY OTHER SYMPTOMS DURING THE PAST WEEK, PLEASE LIST BELOW AND INDICATE HOW MUCH THE SYMPTOM HAS DISTRESSED OR BOTHERED YOU.

OTHER:	0	1	2	3	4
OTHER:	0	1	2	3	4
OTHER:	0	1	2	3	4

Fig. 7.2.2 Revised version of the Memorial Symptom Assessment Scale (Portenoy et al., 1994).

Reprinted from *European Journal of Cancer*, Volume 30A, Number 9, Portenoy, R. K., et al., The Memorial Symptom Assessment Scale: An instrument for the evaluation of symptom prevalence, characteristics and distress, pp. 1151–8, Copyright ©1994, with permission from Elsevier, http://www.sciencedirect.com/science/journal/09598049.

appear to be more reproducible than the VAS (Wilson and Jones, 1989). Ceiling effects can be a concern and there continues to be debate about the change needed to equate with 'clinical significance.' Expert opinion (Booth, 2006; Dorman et al., 2009) supports the available evidence (Ries, 2005; Oxberry et al., 2012; Johnson et al., 2013) suggesting that a change of 1 in the modified Borg Scale score or 10 mm in the VAS is the minimal clinically important difference in chronic breathlessness; a larger change in VAS may be needed to be clinically important in acute breathlessness (Karras et al., 2000; Ander et al., 2004).

Another unidimensional scale, the Medical Research Council Dyspnoea Scale (Medical Research Council Committee on the Aetiology of Chronic Bronchitis, 1960), assesses the consequences of breathlessness in relation to limitations on function. It is particularly useful if breathlessness is the only symptom experienced by the patient, but is too insensitive to detect subtle breathlessness changes following an intervention (Mahler, 2006).

Other scales developed to measure dyspnoea are multidimensional. A recent systematic review identified 33 instruments of this type (Bausewein et al., 2007). In selecting one of these instruments clinicians must give careful consideration to the goal of assessment.

The Cancer Dyspnoea Scale (CDS) rates effort, anxiety, and discomfort severity on 5-point Likert scales (Tanaka et al., 2000). It may capture the complex interaction between dyspnoea and anxiety (Smoller et al., 1996). The Chronic Respiratory Disease Questionnaire (CRQ) focuses on the population with chronic obstructive pulmonary disease and measures the impact of dyspnoea on QOL by examining concurrently breathlessness, fatigue, emotional function, and mastery over the disease (Guyatt et al., 1987). With regular use, the instrument requires 10–15 minutes to complete (Moran et al., 2001; Schunemann et al., 2005). Despite limitations in identifying treatment responsiveness for specific clinical interventions (Cullen and Rodak, 2002), instruments like the CRQ that quantify function and health-related QOL have great utility for documenting outcomes.

Dyspnoea also can be measured in terms of exercise tolerance. Several instruments have been validated in advanced disease, namely the Shuttle Walking Test (Booth and Adams, 2001), the Reading Numbers Aloud Test (Wilcock et al., 1999), and the Upper Limb Exercise Test (Wilcock et al., 2005). Unfortunately, the burdensome and time-consuming nature of these tests currently limits their applicability in the clinical setting (Bausewein et al., 2007).

Instruments for the assessment of impaired cognition

Cognitive impairment is a symptom if reported by the patient and a sign if noted by a clinician. Although some data suggest that most patients approach the end of life with cognitive capabilities retained (Seeman, 1992), surveys in populations with advanced cancer indicate a varying prevalence of impaired understanding and communication (Exton-Smith, 1961; Hinton, 1963; Witzel, 1975; Saunders, 1984; Fainsinger et al., 1991), which increases as death approaches (Morita et al., 2003). These findings support the clinical need to evaluate cognitive capability and when doing so, to determine whether patient self-report is possible.

Some assessment instruments have been developed to screen for impairment, or quantify its intensity or impact, and some have been developed to determine the likelihood that the cognitive impairment can be ascribed to a specific diagnosis, such as delirium, mild cognitive impairment (described as mild neurocognitive disorder in American Psychiatric Association's *Diagnostic and Statistical Manual of Mental Disorders*, fifth edition (DSM-5) (American Psychiatric Association, 2013), or dementia.

The most commonly used screening tests for cognitive impairment are the Mini Mental Status Examination (MMSE) (Folstein et al., 1975) and the Blessed Orientation-Memory-Concentration Test (Katzman et al., 1983). These tools are sensitive indicators of cognitive impairment (Bruera et al., 1992; Stiefel et al., 1992; Fainsinger et al., 1993), but are not specific for the diagnosis of delirium or dementia. The MMSE has some noted limitations, namely its length and administration time (approximately 10 minutes), poor sensitivity for frontal lobe dysfunction, and scoring influenced by culture and education levels (Anthony et al., 1982). A rapid cognitive screening approach for clinical practice involves the use of the Clock Drawing Test (CDT) with the Mini-Cognitive Assessment (Mini-Cog). The latter approach has been found to be helpful for detecting gross cognitive impairment, and has been demonstrated to compare well to longer cognitive impairment instruments (Borson et al., 1999; Borson et al., 2000; Ketelaars et al., 2013).

In addition, several instruments have been developed to address some of the MMSE limitations and are increasingly being used. The Rowland Universal Dementia Assessment Scale (RUDAS) is a multicultural cognitive assessment scale that aims to minimize the effects of cultural learning and language diversity (Rowland et al., 2006, Storey et al., 2004) and the Montreal Cognitive Assessment (MoCA) has been demonstrated to be superior to the MMSE at identifying mild cognitive impairment (Nasreddine et al., 2005; Dong et al., 2012; Markwick et al., 2012).

Some instruments aim to improve the detection of delirium, a highly distressing and prevalent condition in medically ill populations (Lipowski, 1987; Levkoff et al., 1992; Lawlor et al., 2000a; Breitbart et al., 2002a; Lam et al., 2003). Given the particularly high prevalence of delirium in inpatient palliative care populations, it has been suggested that routine screening ought to be considered to enable early identification of any reversible cause of the syndrome and to better manage distressing symptoms (Hosie et al., 2013). The DSM-5 (American Psychiatric Association, 2013) and a clinical interview remains the 'gold standard' for diagnosing delirium. Delirium screening or assessment instruments generally attempt to evaluate the key elements identified in this manual (Adamis et al., 2010). Of note, the recent edition has further modified the criteria for diagnosis of delirium (American Psychiatric Association, 2013). A recent review, prior to the publication of the DSM-5 (American Psychiatric Association, 2013), identified 11 instruments that had been developed (Wong et al., 2010), but at this time there is no consensus about the optimal approach for screening (Caraceni and Grassi, 2011). The various measures have been designed for different purposes (Adamis et al., 2010).

The Nursing Delirium Screening Scale (Nu-DESC) is a five-item observational screening tool that can be administered by nurses in the clinical setting in 1 minute. The Nu-DESC has been demonstrated to be psychometrically valid, with sensitivity and specificity similar to the Memorial Delirium Assessment Scale (MDAS) (Gaudreau et al., 2005).

The MDAS (Breitbart et al., 1997) is a widely used ten-item instrument that incorporates both diagnosis and measurement of symptom severity and takes approximately 10 minutes to be completed. It is based on criteria that are included in both the DSM-III-R (American Psychiatric Association, 1987) and the DSM-IV (American Psychiatric Association, 2000) and has been validated in palliative care and advanced cancer populations (Breitbart et al., 1997; Lawlor et al., 2000b). The MDAS is intended for repeated administration over a short time period and is useful for capturing short-term fluctuations in delirium (Breitbart et al., 2002b) and for determining delirium severity (Adamis et al., 2010). This instrument has now been translated into Italian and Japanese (Grassi et al., 2001; Matsuoka et al., 2001), and it has also been used for routine detection of symptoms in a French-speaking palliative care setting (Mancini et al., 2002).

The 16 item Delirium Rating Scale-Revised-98 (DRS-R-98) (Trzepacz et al., 2001), a more comprehensive version of the original Delirium Rating Scale (Trzepacz et al., 1988), also incorporates detection and severity ratings. It was developed based on the DSM-III-R (American Psychiatric Association, 1987) and has been demonstrated to be a useful instrument for diagnosing and rating delirium severity, and for use in longitudinal studies (Wong et al., 2010).

The Confusion Assessment Method (CAM) (Inouye et al., 1990) is a dichotomous scale that can be used by trained clinicians as a screening and diagnostic tool. It is brief, available in multiple languages (Adamis et al., 2010), and widely used in varied populations, including those with advanced illness (Ryan et al., 2009; Wong et al., 2010). It may not be possible to use it in those approaching the end of life (Gagnon et al., 2012) and a four-question version has been developed in an effort to broaden its applicability (Rao et al., 2011).

Challenges in the application of symptom measures in palliative care settings

There are numerous challenges to the systematic measurement of symptoms in both clinical and research settings. These challenges may be attributed to professionals and the systems within which they work, to patients, and to limitations in the instruments used to acquire data.

Professionals may have conceptual and attitudinal barriers to the use of health status measures in patient care and clinical trials (Deyo and Patrick, 1989). These barriers may be relatively more significant in populations with advanced illness. They include scepticism about the validity and importance of self-rated health measures, preferences for physiological and observable disease-related outcomes, and unfamiliarity of health-care providers with the scoring of measures. Knowledge and skills in symptom assessment also may be a problem in some settings (Donovan et al., 1987; Von Roenn et al., 1993). Professional education (Bourbonnais Fothergill et al., 2004) and the routine use of symptom measures in clinical practice (Foley, 1995) may be useful to address these concerns.

There is enormous variation in the health-care systems that provide care to patients with serious illness. Systems vary at every level—from national health services to protocols that guide care in individual units. The ability to measure symptoms systematically, incorporate screening or treatment algorithms, and facilitate quality improvement, is strongly influenced by numerous system-related facilitators and impediments. For example, the Canadian Cancer Quality Council of Ontario has reported that systematic symptom screening had been incorporated into all 14 regional cancer centres with a steady increase in use—from 51% of cancer patients using the screening tool in 2011 to 59% in 2013 (Cancer Quality Council of Ontario, 2014). That latter group has identified such screening as an important quality indicator. That stated, there is evidence to suggest that further work is needed to identify optimal strategies for systematizing responses to levels of distress, particularly when moderate to severe distress is identified (Seow et al., 2012). Quality improvement methods may be a useful avenue for the development of these approaches.

In some settings, system-related barriers may be addressed through adaptation of the electronic health record. Point-of-care evaluation, decision support, telehealth strategies, and other technological advances may drive improvement in symptom measurement and the management of symptom distress. These changes have begun in many developed countries and will continue to evolve wherever the technological and financial capacity exists.

If professional and system-related barriers to symptom assessment were eliminated, daunting challenges would remain, particularly in populations with serious illness. Patient self-report may be impaired by cognitive impairment or other medical problems associated with progressive illness, or by the highly prevalent symptom of fatigue (Coyle et al., 1990; Dunlop, 1990; Dunphy and Amesbury, 1990; McCarthy, 1990; Ventafridda et al., 1990; Curtis et al., 1991; Portenoy et al., 1994a). For example, one survey demonstrated that patients in a palliative care unit gradually reduced their compliance with twice-daily completion of the ESAS (Fainsinger et al., 1991) from 69% on the day of admission to 8% on the day of death.

Symptom distress or complexity also may be barriers. Severe distress may produce the paradox that those with greatest need of symptom management are least able to provide the information necessary for treatment. This problem highlights the importance of detailed clinical assessment in all instances, particularly in the very ill. The complexity of symptom measurement is evident in the common occurrence of multiple concurrent symptoms (Van Lancker et al., 2014). A study using the MSAS observed that the median number of symptoms per patient was 11.5 and the range was 0–25 (Portenoy et al., 1994a). Instruments that measure global symptom distress may be helpful when multiple symptoms contribute to illness burden but these measures may lack validation in populations other than those with cancer (McCorkle and Quint-Benoliel, 1983; Portenoy et al., 1994a, 1994b).

The realization that time is limited may be a factor in changing the priorities of patients or caregivers, and this shift also may become a challenge in symptom assessment (Perkins et al., 2007). The salience of these changing priorities is uncertain, however. Observational studies suggest that most patients with advanced illness are willing to provide information for research (Cleeland et al., 1994; Cunningham et al., 1995). Some studies indicate that most very ill patients will respond to questions about even highly sensitive topics (Townsend et al., 1990).

When instruments are used to evaluate the medically ill, each item should be considered in terms of its own potential to generate distress. The concern that patients may be relatively disinclined to respond to sensitive questions is especially pertinent to the measurement of some psychological symptoms. One group of investigators, for example, has described observations that some patients find it difficult to address issues such as suicidal ideation,

hopelessness, and emptiness in life, and can experience distress when queried about such items (Wilhelm et al., 2004). The group did not suggest that these important questions should be omitted from clinical assessment but did suggest the use of depression screening instruments that use less contentious questions within the tool, provided those questions can still identify depressed patients. A person to person clinical interaction is important for potentially distressing but nonetheless important questions. This is an important consideration when tools are being used in the absence of a clinician being in the patient's immediate vicinity to provide ongoing assessment and support.

These and other patient-related barriers to symptom measurement may be particularly challenging in several highly vulnerable subpopulations. In addition to those with cognitive impairment, populations of concern include children, minorities, and the imminently dying. Relatively few studies have evaluated symptom screening in sick children and there is no established approach (Dupuis et al., 2012). Validated verbal rating scales or observational scales provide the means to evaluate pain in children of any age (Jay and Elliott, 1984; LeBaron and Zelter, 1984; Elliott et al., 1987; Gauvain-Piquard et al., 1987; Jay et al., 1987; Katz et al., 1987; Kuttner et al., 1988; Manne et al., 1990; Karoly, 1991; Manne and Andersen, 1991; Matthews et al., 1993; Gaffney et al., 2003), and other scales have been developed for the assessment of chemotherapy-related nausea and vomiting (Zeltzer et al., 1988; Tyc et al., 1993). Paediatric versions of the MSAS have been validated (Collins et al., 2002; Hunt, 2006) and can provide information about multiple symptoms concurrently. The development and application of symptom measurement tools for diverse populations of children remain an area in need of further research.

Significant problems in symptom measurement also may be encountered in patients whose culture and language differ from the professionals involved in their care (Waxler-Morrison et al., 1990). Although some instruments have been shown to be reliable and valid across cultures and languages (Cleeland et al., 1988; Cleeland and Ryan, 1994; Grassi et al., 2001), translation and validation of other symptom measures is needed. In the clinical setting, health-care professionals may need to develop simple, face-valid symptom measures to overcome language barriers.

Although most patients will retain the ability to interact at a time very close to death (Seeman, 1992), evaluation of subjective reports may become impossible or very difficult due to cognitive impairment and other concerns (Exton-Smith, 1961; Hinton, 1963; Witzel, 1975; Saunders, 1984; Fainsinger et al., 1991). A transition from verbal rating scales to observational scales, and sometimes to proxy assessments may be necessary to provide data throughout the terminal phase. The validity of this approach, however, remains to be determined.

Yet another group of potential barriers to systematic measurement of symptoms in populations with advanced illness relate to the limitations of the available instruments. Although the increasing availability of validated symptom measures has been an important advance, valid measures are still lacking for some common symptoms, and many tools validated in one population have uncertain generalizability to others. With the exception of selected pain measures, symptom questionnaires have frequently not been tested for validity in patients with cognitive impairment or multiple symptoms (Stark, 1988).

Conclusion

Systematic symptom assessment is a foundation of clinical practice and research. Instruments for the measurement of symptoms have been developed and may facilitate this process. Quantification of symptoms may be able to improve symptom management and further the goal of enhanced QOL. Clinicians and investigators should become familiar with the instruments that are applicable in the population for whom they provide care, and develop methods for their use in routine clinical practice, the research environment, and the palliative care setting.

Acknowledgements

Professor Ingham and Professor Phillip's research work on this paper was undertaken, in part, with funding support from the Cancer Institute New South Wales Academic Chairs Program. The views expressed herein are those of the authors and are not necessarily those of the Cancer Institute NSW. The authors wish to acknowledge the work of Dr Paula Mohacsi, PhD, MBA, MSc (Ed Studies) RN in preparation of the manuscript.

Online materials

Complete references for this chapter are available online at <http://www.oxfordmedicine.com>.

References

Bruera, E., Kuehn, N., Miller, M.J., Selmser, P., and MacMillan, K. (1991). The Edmonton Symptom Assessment System (ESAS): a simple method for the assessment of palliative care patients. *Journal of Palliative Care*, 7, 6–9.

Chang, V.T., Hwang, S.S., Feuerman, M., Kasimis, B.S., and Thaler, H.T. (2000c). The Memorial Symptom Assessment Scale Short Form (MSAS-SF). *Cancer Investigation*, 89, 1162–1171.

Cleeland, C.S., Mendoza, T.R., Wang, X.S., *et al.* (2000). Assessing symptom distress in cancer patients: the M.D. Anderson Symptom Inventory. *Cancer*, 89, 1634–1646.

Daut, R.L., Cleeland, C.S., and Flanery, R.C. (1983). Development of the Wisconsin Brief Pain Questionnaire to assess pain in cancer and other diseases. *Pain*, 17, 197–210. The online version of this tool is available at: <http://www.mdanderson.org/education-and-research/departments-programs-and-labs/departments-and-divisions/symptom-research/symptom-assessment-tools/brief-pain-inventory.html>.

De Haes, J.C., Van Knippenberg, F.C., and Neijt, J.P. (1990). Measuring psychological and physical distress in cancer patients: structure and application of the Rotterdam Symptom Checklist. *British Journal of Cancer*, 62, 1034–1038.

Ewing, G., Todd, C., Rogers, M., Barclay, S., McCabe, J., and Martin, A. (2004). Validation of a symptom measure suitable for use among palliative care patients in the community: CAMPAS-R. *Journal of Pain and Symptom Management*, 27, 287–299.

Hoekstra, J., Bindels, P. J., Van Duijn, N.P., and Schade, E. (2004). The symptom monitor. A diary for monitoring physical symptoms for cancer patients in palliative care: feasibility, reliability and compliance. *Journal of Pain and Symptom Management*, 27, 24–35.

McCorkle, R. and Young, K. (1978). Development of a symptom distress scale. *Cancer Nursing*, 1, 373–378.

National Institutes of Health (2011b). *PROMIS Mission, Vision and Goals* [Online]. Available at: <http://www.nihpromis.org/about/missionvisiongoals>.

Portenoy, R.K., Thaler, H.T., Kornblith, A.B., *et al.* (1994b). The Memorial Symptom Assessment Scale: an instrument for the evaluation of symptom prevalence, characteristics and distress. *European Journal of Cancer*, 30A, 1326–1336.

Royal College of Physicians (2012). *National Early Warning Score (NEWS): Standardising the Assessment of Acute-Illness Severity in the NHS. Report of a Working Party*. London: RCP. NEWS tool available at: <http://www.rcplondon.ac.uk/sites/default/files/documents/news-observation-chart-with-explanatory-text.pdf>.

Symptom (2013). In *Oxford Dictionary of English* (3rd ed.) [Online] Available at: <http://oxforddictionaries.com/definition/english/symptom>.

7.3

Informatics and Literature Search

Jennifer J. Tieman and David C. Currow

Introduction to informatics and literature search

Technology has accelerated the ability of individuals and systems to capture, analyse, and distribute data and information. As a result, there is now an unprecedented capacity to access literature and evidence, to improve clinical decision-making and service delivery. Technology has also enabled the development of tools and resources that can enhance clinical care and patient involvement. However, the value of such applications rests upon the quality of the professional knowledge embedded in these applications. The knowledge to support such systems and applications is domain specific. In any field or discipline knowledge builds on, or reacts to, previous research and thought. Therefore, being able to find what has previously been published is critical. While availability and access to literature and evidence is a necessary prerequisite to use, there are still challenges for individuals and systems in retrieving relevant and good quality literature. Finding the right information is not as simple as typing a search term into a database. Indeed, searching for palliative care's literature and evidence is complex and time-consuming, given the way peer-reviewed literature is described and distributed within journals and bibliographic databases.

The role of health informatics

Technology is accelerating the rate at which data can be captured, organized, analysed, distributed, and accessed across the health system and these capabilities are transforming how health-care is conceived and delivered (Australian Health Ministers' Conference, 2008; Mattke et al., 2010; World Health Organization, 2011). This transformation reflects not only the possibilities afforded by technological innovations but the pressures being placed on the health system due to an ageing population, changing patterns of disease burdens, and increasing expectations of health consumers and involvement by health consumers in their care decision-making and management. Ready access to tools, information, and resources is not only driving change but raising expectations. Investment in health information technology (HIT) has been seen to offer many health system benefits, such as point-of-care clinical information, automated patient-record keeping, facilitated access to and exchange of patient data, enhanced coordination of care across settings and providers, and public health interventions for consumers use (Bennett and Glasgow, 2009; Jamal et al., 2009; Kreps and Neuhauser, 2010; Lobach et al., 2012).

Technology is not enough

It is, however, the quality and currency of the information and knowledge embedded in, and transmitted through, HIT that provides its clinical value. The importance of this concept can be seen in the emergence of the field of health informatics with its specific focus on the contribution of the information, rather than the characteristics of the technology alone (Hersch, 2009). This reinforces the importance of domain knowledge and its purpose in assisting professionals in their cognitive tasks and professional responsibilities. The potential links between evidence-based medicine and health informatics are highlighted by the capacity of HIT to make research evidence available to support clinical judgement and to help patients identify and articulate their preferences (Bloomrosen and Detmer, 2010). The definition of medical informatics in Haux's review of the development of this field as 'the systematic processing of data, information and knowledge in medicine and health-care' (Haux, 2010) again recognizes the significance of the knowledge base within HIT. Haux went on in this review to reflect on the forces that are shaping the field: the progress in information and communications technology; the expansion of the knowledge base for health and medicine; and changing expectations of the professions and the society.

For palliative medicine, health informatics and HIT could have many roles to play in supporting clinical decision-making and in enhancing care delivery. Indeed, HIT may be particularly valuable in this field, given palliative medicine is practised in hospices, in-patient wards, residential aged care facilities and other community settings, as well as patients' homes, and given that co-morbidities are common and care needs will change over time, in accordance with the underlying disease. HIT solutions may ease problems in managing a diffuse and multidisciplinary knowledge base and by supporting care within and across multiple settings.

There have already been a number of reviews of e-health and HIT initiatives within palliative care which show that HIT applications are feasible and can provide solutions to a range of practice issues in this field (Kidd et al., 2010; Corn et al., 2011; Demiris et al., 2011; Johnston, 2011; Oliver et al., 2012). There are also completed and in-progress trials and studies looking at diverse HIT applications within palliative care, ranging from community data collection (Abernethy et al., 2011) and palliative telemedicine in the home (Duursma et al., 2011), to symptom assessment in palliative radiotherapy using e-technology (Cox et al., 2011) and Internet-based self-help bereavement interventions (van der Houven et al., 2010). Such investigations ultimately could result in widely available HIT resources.

The challenge is to ensure that HIT resources reflect the best available evidence from research and practice (Banzi et al., 2010; Ketchum et al., 2011). Palliative medicine as a specialty, and palliative care as a discipline and area of professional practice, need to ensure that HIT applications and systems in this field incorporate what is known from palliative care's expanding research base and from the review of the specialty's current professional practice. Furthermore, HIT applications will need to be monitored, to ensure that they are updated or modified as new evidence emerges and the knowledge base changes.

The literature and evidence base for palliative care

Palliative medicine is a complex specialty drawing on many fields of expertise and academic interest to inform practice. It is a referral-based field of clinical care, not limited by the underlying disease or prognosis. Palliative care physicians can face specific challenges in their clinical practice relating to the changing nature of the knowledge and competencies needed in care delivery. Care is active but not curative in intent, addressing physical symptoms as well as psychosocial needs, and supporting both the patient and the family (World Health Organization, 2011). This reflects an expanding definition of palliative care from terminal care alone to a dynamic responsibility for supportive and palliative care across a time and disease continuum (Currow and Abernethy, 2005). Physicians, therefore, require a knowledge base that enables excellent symptom control as well as identifies emerging factors that could influence the course of the life-limiting illness or active co-morbid illnesses.

Engagement with knowledge and evidence is a critical component of such informed and current practice. However, the ability of palliative care physicians and palliative care as a discipline to use knowledge and evidence in practice depends on the ability to find, retrieve and assimilate this information. Hence, searching and accessing relevant material is a fundamental part of up-to-date and ethically responsible practice. However, finding relevant information can be a complex and time-consuming task yielding suboptimal results.

Size of the evidence base

The technicalities of evidence retrieval are heightened by a rapidly expanding biomedical literature. Each day over 1000 articles are indexed to the Medline database (Straus and Haynes, 2009), and each day reports of 75 clinical trials and 11 systematic reviews are published (Bastian et al., 2010). Such figures challenge the perception that clinicians have the time and ability to remain involved with, and informed by, the biomedical literature.

Concerns about the expanding literature base also apply to palliative care's literature. Research has shown that the absolute number of palliative and hospice care articles indexed on Medline increased in each 5-year period from 1970 to 2005, as did reports of palliative care clinical trials. Over the same time period, the proportion of indexed articles on Medline that were related to palliative and hospice care more than doubled. By 2005, 0.38% of all items indexed on Medline were relevant to palliative and hospice care (Tieman et al., 2008). A related bibliometric analysis not only confirmed that there was a substantial and increasing amount of palliative care literature, but calculated that keeping up to date with the published palliative care literature would mean that health professionals needed to read 19 articles every day (Tieman et al., 2009).

Diffuse nature of palliative care's interests

As a referral-based specialty, information needs in this context can be extensive. Doyle, in his review of the palliative medicine as a subspecialty, noted that the challenge for palliative medicine is:

> To espouse and demonstrate the principles of palliative care ('integral to all good clinical care') whilst at the same time developing the unique skill and knowledge base of specialist palliative care . . . This skill and knowledge base is a big challenge now that patients are being referred with every major pathology. (Doyle, 2005)

Understanding the commonalities and particular care needs of palliative care patients with different disease trajectories has been highlighted, as have the specific palliative care requirements of populations with diagnoses other than cancer. Potentially relevant literature that could inform the palliative care knowledge base will not necessarily be limited to studies in palliative care populations. In particular, it may be necessary to scan other specialist literature for studies of common symptoms and care issues in palliative care such as pain, breathlessness, fatigue, or depression which may be investigated by other medical specialties.

An analysis of the references contained in the 2010 edition of the *Oxford Textbook of Palliative Medicine* demonstrates this crossover in literature. Using a three-term search (palliative.tw. OR hospice.tw. OR terminal.tw.), retrieval rates for each chapter's references were calculated. There was a significant amount of variability between chapters in how many references were retrieved (range: 8–80%), with an overall retrieval of only 26% of the total reference dataset. Chapters which had the lowest rates of retrieval using the three-term search were those looking at the management of common symptoms and disorders, geriatric palliative medicine, issues in neoplastic disease, palliative medicine in non-malignant disease, and complementary therapies in palliative medicine. This suggests that these areas of palliative medicine are using literature that arises from other disciplines and medical specialties (Tieman, 2012).

The diffuse nature of palliative care's interests is likely to be compounded by the issue of scatter in the reporting of research. Hoffmann et al. have shown that the publication of trials and systematic reviews for specialty areas is not confined to specialist journals or even common generalist journals. This means that physicians are likely to miss relevant trials and reviews if they only read specialist journals. The authors noted in their article that:

> Scatter is also likely to be greater in specialties that typically concern patients with a wide variety of conditions. Examples include emergency medicine, primary care, palliative care, and allied health disciplines. (Hoffmann et al., 2012)

Scatter as an issue for palliative care has been reported. In 2005, 6983 palliative care related articles were published in 1985 different journals (Tieman et al., 2009). While most of these articles would not necessarily have been clinical trials or systematic reviews, such spread in palliative care publication suggests that a comprehensive review of the literature is challenging.

Not published, not indexed

Published indexed literature may represent only a portion of the knowledge materials that could be relevant to palliative care clinicians, educators, and researchers. Unpublished reports and documents that have not been indexed form an important part of the knowledge base. Limitations to, and idiosyncrasies of, indexing systems compound further potential losses to the retrieval of literature. Navigating both the formal and informal literature to acquire relevant and significant materials is an important issue for all fields, but may have specific resonance for palliative care, given the diffuse nature of this field.

Research from other fields has shown that material presented at conferences does not always lead to publication. Indeed, the conference conversion rate for biomedical presentations may be as low as 44% (Scherer et al., 2007). According to a 2010 *Heath Technology Assessment* report, positive studies are more likely to be published than negative studies and they are likely to be published more quickly (Song et al., 2010). One study has confirmed similar concerns for this discipline. It demonstrated multiple losses to the effective retrieval of published palliative care literature arising from non-publication of palliative care research, publication in non-indexed journals, and incomplete or idiosyncratic indexing of palliative care articles (Tieman et al., 2010).

Issues in searching the knowledge base

Where literature is held

The size of the literature database is only one source of difficulty in being able to retrieve literature effectively and evidence relevant to palliative care. Understanding where relevant literature is being held, the technical characteristics of individual databases, and the requirements of the different searching interfaces is also important. Each database has its own set of rules for citation referencing, storage, and retrieval, which adds to the complexity of effective searching. Various studies have reported on issues relating to database coverage and technical requirements of searching within different databases (Falagas et al., 2008; Wider and Boddy, 2009; Spreckelsen et al., 2011). Without detailed technical knowledge, seemingly sensible searching decisions can lead to loss of relevant literature. As an example, applying the '*humans*' limit to a search in PubMed will remove items that are not yet indexed or which will never be indexed under this database's rules. This will exclude automatically from retrievals some of the most recent literature that is awaiting indexing but which may already be published online (Sladek et al., 2010).

Unfortunately, not all of palliative care's literature is indexed on Medline. Highly relevant, unique literature is found on other databases including Embase, CINAHL, and PsycINFO. Depending on the specific information needs, this means that a searcher will have to interrogate multiple databases to ensure comprehensive coverage and, therefore, be familiar with the requirements and unique search interfaces of these repositories. Otherwise, the 40% of published palliative care items not indexed on Medline may not be retrieved (Tieman et al., 2009).

Physicians' technical skills in searching

The capacity to access a bibliographic database and construct a search should not be confused with creating an effective search. Information retrieval through searching requires technical expertise as well as content knowledge. The *PRESS: Peer Review of Electronic Search Strategies* report documents the complexities associated with expert searching and demonstrates the many simple errors that can affect retrieval (Sampson et al., 2008). Given that even expert searchers make errors, it is likely that health professionals without formal training will also make errors that will limit what they retrieve.

A recently completed study of palliative care clinicians' search constructions confirms that many clinicians struggled to create useful searches. The analysed searches were often rudimentary with nearly half of the clinical participants using only a single search term to try and retrieve *as many articles as possible that were relevant to palliative care*. The average retrieval in the study of a known set of relevant articles by the searchers was only 25%. Unnecessary limits, incorrect use of Boolean operators and inappropriate narrowing of searches were all common errors in the group (Tieman, 2012).

Although searching competence continues to be identified as an important component of evidence based practice, competence in this skill cannot be assumed. Problems with health professionals abilities in this field have been reported in various systematic reviews (Coumou and Meijman, 2006; Davies, 2007; Masters, 2008; Younger, 2010). There is increasing interest in interventions to support clinicians' use of clinical information retrieval systems, such as Medline. Although these interventions have shown some success in improving searching skills when using electronic bibliographic databases, the overall effectiveness of such training remains uncertain (McGowan et al., 2009; Gagnon et al., 2010).

Using Google

Given the many complexities of accessing and constructing searches in formal bibliographic databases, it is perhaps unsurprising that many health professionals use Google or Google Scholar as a search option. These search engines offer a simple and fast interface with a vast repository of content. However, a variety of concerns have been documented about their effectiveness. Such criticisms relate to a lack of advanced search features to enable the user any control over retrievals, insufficient and unclear indexing, uncertainty about coverage, and a lack of transparency about the embedded search algorithm (Falagas et al., 2008; Anders and Evans, 2010).

Similar concerns have also been raised about the use of Wikipedia as a source of a medical information (Clauson et al., 2008; Munger, 2009), particularly given its impact as a primary retrieval site by search engines (Laurent and Vickers, 2009).

Implications of ineffective searching

Poor searching can have many implications. If a health professional is seeking immediate clinical evidence to inform decision-making, ineffective retrieval may reduce the value of the clinical advice. For those who seek to maintain currency of their professional knowledge by monitoring emerging findings, inefficient retrieval may not only reduce their actual knowledge base, but may increase inappropriately the searcher's self-belief that their knowledge is current. Finally, the clinical authority of health and social guidance is put at risk, as errors in search strategies reduce the value of the retrieved results (Sampson et al., 2008).

Knowledge solutions in palliative care

Dealing with the information flood

Building a comprehensive knowledge base for palliative care practice and research remains an important priority for the discipline. Relying on health professionals to have the appropriate skills to retrieve needed knowledge from such a complex bibliographic environment may be an ineffective response to a fundamental problem. Straus and Haynes have argued that while research-based evidence is being generated at ever faster rates, much of this evidence is not readily available to the clinicians it is intended to support. They highlight a number of potential approaches to providing better infrastructure in the management of evidence-based knowledge, including better knowledge products and tools that are reliable, relevant, and readable, and more efficient search strategies (Straus and Haynes, 2009).

There is already a range of knowledge resources for palliative care, including specialist journals and journal subsets, web-based evidence repositories, and palliative care segments in major database repositories. Specialist journals such as *Palliative Medicine* and specialist database repositories, such as the pain, palliative and supportive care topic in the Cochrane Library, provide a focus for the publication of research work and its promulgation through the sector. Web resources such as the National End of Life Care Intelligence Network in the United Kingdom, National Hospice and Palliative Care Organization in the United States, the Canadian Virtual Hospice, and the Australian website CareSearch provide national and international access to high-quality evidence resources including guidelines, clinical guidance, and evidence summaries for palliative care specialists, other health professionals, and for palliative care patients and their families and carers. The CareSearch Review Collection provides details on systematic reviews and structured literature reviews relevant to palliative care, offering another approach to synthesized knowledge on palliative care issues. Table 7.3.1 outlines a range of web-based resources for palliative care. Such resources begin to address the need for better knowledge products and tools in this field.

To ensure that all research efforts are captured, academics, researchers, and clinicians involved in research projects need to be encouraged and supported in publishing their findings. This may be particularly important where the results are negative, to reduce publication bias. Clinical trials registration on one of the publicly available registers is an important step in preventing the loss of research. Grey literature repositories of project and research reports may also improve the comprehensiveness of evidence capture. There are some grey literature repositories that include palliative care content including Open Grey at <http://www.opengrey. eu/> and the New York Academy of Medicine's Grey Literature report at <http://www.nyam.org/library/online-resources/ grey-literature-report/>. The CareSearch website maintains a grey literature database of 'hard-to-find' Australian materials, including conference presentations, research reports, non-indexed Australian journal articles, and government and organizational reports. Such repositories may be especially important in finding information and evidence relating to the local factors that may influence the relevance or capacity to translate evidence to individual services or specific areas.

Role and contribution of search filters

Different strategies to deal with the searching issues for palliative care are being explored. Search filters represent a brokered informatics-based search solution. A search filter is an experimentally created and tested search strategy that is designed to find particular types of studies or articles dealing with a specific topic, in a particular database and remove material that does not meet these criteria. Effectively, a filter is an evidence-based search for relevant literature. Haynes and colleagues undertook the first work in this field constructing, testing, and validating scientifically a

Table 7.3.1 Major knowledge resources for palliative medicine available on the web

Name of knowledge resource	Specific resources available	Web address
Canadian Virtual Hospice ◆ Open access	Tools for practice	<http://www.virtualhospice.ca/en_US/Main+Site+Navigation/Home.aspx>
CareSearch ◆ Open access	Clinical practice CareSearch review collection Search filters and PubMed topic searches	<http://www.caresearch.com.au>
Cochrane Library ◆ May require registration	Pain, palliative and supportive care systematic reviews	<http://www.thecochranelibrary.com/view/0/index.html>
ESMO	Palliative Care Working Group Practice guidelines	<http://www.esmo.org/home.html>
European Association for Palliative Care ◆ Open-access resources and registered resources	Clinical and Care Specific groups	<http://www.eapcnet.eu/Home.aspx>
Medical College of Wisconsin	EPERC fast facts	<http://www.eperc.mcw.edu/EPERC/FastFactsandConcepts>
NHS Evidence ◆ Registration required	Palliative care subset National Institute of Health and Care Excellence pathways	<https://www.evidence.nhs.uk/>
NHS National End of Life Care Programme ◆ Open access and registered resources	Tools Care pathway Care setting Data and statistics	<http://www.endoflifecareforadults.nhs.uk/>
Shaare Zedek Cancer Pain and Palliative Care Reference Database ◆ Open access	narrow focus pain and palliative care reference library	<http://www.chernydatabase.org/>

Table 7.3.2 Palliative care search filter options: assisting searchers to automatically retrieve palliative care literature in Medline

Ovid Medline version[a]	PubMed version[b]	CareSearch version[c]
1 exp advance care planning/	advance care planning[mh] OR attitude to death[mh] OR bereavement[mh] OR terminal care[mh] OR hospices[mh] OR life support care[mh] OR palliative care[mh] OR terminally ill[mh] OR death[mh:noexp] OR palliat*[tw] OR hospice*[tw] OR terminal care[tw] OR 1049-9091[is] OR 1472-684X[is] OR 1357-6321[is] OR 1536-0539[is] OR 0825-8597[is] OR 1557-7740[is] OR 1552-4264[is] OR 1478-9523[is] OR 1477-030X[is] OR 0749-1565[is] OR 0742-969X[is] OR 1544-6794[is] OR 0941-4355[is] OR 1873-6513[is] OR 0145-7624[is] OR 1091-7683[is] OR 0030-2228[is] OR ((advance care plan*[tw] OR attitude to death[tw] OR bereavement[tw] OR terminal care[tw] OR life supportive care[tw] OR terminally ill[tw] OR palliat*[tw] OR hospice*[tw] OR 1049-9091[is] OR 1472-684X[is] OR 1357-6321[is] OR 1536-0539[is] OR 0825-8597[is] OR 1557-7740[is] OR 1552-4264[is] OR 1478-9523[is] OR 1477-030X[is] OR 0749-1565[is] OR 0742-969X[is] OR 1544-6794[is] OR 0941-4355[is] OR 1873-6513[is] OR 0145-7624[is] OR 1091-7683[is] OR 0030-2228[is]) NOT Medline[sb]) AND English[la]	Run Filter now
2 exp attitude to death/		
3 exp bereavement/		
4 death/		
5 hospices/		
6 life support care/		
7 Palliative care/		
8 exp terminal care/		
9 terminally ill/		
10 palliat$.af.		
11 hospice$.af.		
12 terminal care.af.		
13 OR/1-12		
14 journal of palliative care.jn.		
15 journal of palliative medicine.jn.		
16 hospice journal physical psychosocial & pastoral care of the dying.jn		
17 supportive care in cancer.jn.		
18 palliative medicine.jn.		
19 palliative & supportive care.jn.		
20 journal of supportive oncology.jn.		
21 journal of social work in end of life & palliative care.jn.		
22 journal of pain & symptom management.jn.		
23 journal of pain and palliative care pharmacotherapy.jn.		
24 international journal of palliative nursing.jn.		
25 death studies.jn.		
26 death education.jn.		
27 american journal of hospice care.jn.		
28 american journal of hospice & palliative care.jn.		
29 omega journal of death &dying.jn.		
30 OR/14-29		
31 13 OR 31		

Source: Data from [a] Sladek, R. and J. Tieman, Applying evidence in the real world: a case study in library and information practice, *Health Information & Libraries Journal*, Volume 25, Issue 4, pp. 295–301, Copyright © 2008 The authors; [b] Sladek, R., J. Tieman, et al., Development of a subject search filter to find information relevant to palliative care in the general medical literature, *Journal of the Medical Library Association*, Volume 94, Issue 4, pp. 394–401, Copyright © 2006; and [c] CareSearch, available from http://www.caresearch.com.au.

best performing Medline search strategy to retrieve literature with a particular research study design, using an approach more commonly used to test the performance of new diagnostic tests (Haynes and Wilczynski, 2004; Haynes et al., 2005). This enabled them to measure sensitivity, specificity, and accuracy to assess the performance of each individual search strategy. The resulting study design search filters have been utilized within the National Library of Medicine's PubMed website as the Clinical Queries filters.

Until recently search filter research has focused on methodological filters, that is, search filters designed to find research across any content or topic area but which all use the same study design. The last 5 years has seen increasing interest in developing content filters that look for literature on a particular topic, such as adverse events (Golder and Loke, 2009) or renal information (Iansavichus et al., 2010), regardless of the underlying study design. Importantly, a recent study has shown that the use of search filters improves the efficiency of physician searching (Shariff et al., 2012).

It is worth noting that one of the first content search filters developed in the world was a search filter for palliative care literature (Sladek et al., 2006; Sladek and Tieman, 2008). This search filter was developed using the approach applied by Haynes et al. of testing retrieval in a gold standard set of references identified by hand searching the general biomedical literature. The search filter for palliative care literature comprised nine MeSH terms and three textwords (Sladek et al., 2006). The inclusion of a subset of journals in the search filter followed subsequent research that that showed that not all articles from a set of specialist journals was captured by the search filter (Sladek and Tieman, 2008). The search construction of the current palliative care search filter for use in Ovid Medline can be seen in Table 7.3.2.

Making search filters useful: a PubMed option

A search filter is an extremely valuable health informatics tool as it provides a transparent and reproducible mechanism for identifying relevant literature within a particular bibliographic database, such as Ovid Medline. Developing or translating a search filter for use in a publicly available database that can be openly accessed through the web, increases dramatically its utility and reach. PubMed is an open access bibliographic database which contains over 19 million biomedical citations. Translating the Ovid Medline palliative care search filter for use in PubMed, means that web users can click on a hyperlink loading the search filter automatically to PubMed and initiating the retrieval of relevant citations. The PubMed translation of the palliative care search filter is detailed in Table 7.3.2.

By combining the palliative care search filter with expert searches on a range of care issues, such as dyspnoea or distress, it is possible to offer a technology-based solution to the problem of individuals' search competence. Visitors to the PubMed Palliative Care Filter page in the CareSearch website have immediate access to PubMed citations filtered by their relevance to palliative care and their specific topic interest. As the PubMed database is updated daily, by providing real-time links, the resulting search is always current. The utility of this searching solution has been enhanced by providing options to refine the search further by limiting to free full text or to randomized controlled trials and systematic reviews only.

The benefits associated with the provision of a PubMed version of the palliative care search filter work have been extended by the introduction of a Heart Failure Search Filter (Damarell et al., 2011) into the CareSearch website in 2010 and a Lung Cancer Search Filter in 2011. A Residential Aged Care Search Filter (Dicker and Hayman, 2014) and a Bereavement Search Filter (Tieman et al., in press) were developed and added to the CareSearch website in 2014.

The future of search

As technological capacities develop, different approaches to search and information retrieval will emerge, to assist in the issues of knowledge management highlighted by Straus and Haynes. There has been substantial work around the possibilities of natural text language analysis (Chung, 2009; Névéol et al., 2009). Another approach looks at the semantic web and semantic wikis, which marry information semantics (or meaning) with the dissemination platforms commonly being accessed by health professionals (Boulos, 2009; Kroeker, 2010). The value of federated searching across personalized web resources is also being explored. Word add-in technology may enable more efficiently tagged literature to be tracked by search engines such as Google (Fink et al., 2010).

There has also been some preliminary research into the role of social media functionalities such as Twitter*, Blogs*, and YouTube* (Fernandez-Luque et al., 2012; Gruzd et al., 2012).

The role of apps for phones in searching remains new territory. The Pew Internet Project has surveyed users and reported on the 'rise of the apps culture' (Purcell et al., 2010). There are already some iPhone apps that can be used to support searching and these applications are likely to grow in the coming years (Kubben, 2010).

Conclusion

HIT provides both a challenge and a solution for the management and activation of palliative care's knowledge base. New technologies are emerging that enable applications to be built that ultimately can enhance care delivery and service provision if taken up

systematically. However, the quality of these applications relies on the quality and currency of the domain knowledge that is embedded within them and distributed through them. The capacity to identify and retrieve palliative care's evidence base is, therefore more critical than ever. Searching, however, remains complex, given an expanding literature base and a diffuse and multidisciplinary set of information needs and information sources. Search strategies, such as the use of search filters that offer validated access to the literature, offer avenues to improve retrieval. Accessibility can also be enhanced by web-based availability to ensure immediate access.

Online materials

Complete references for this chapter are available online at <http://www.oxfordmedicine.com>.

References

Bastian, H., Glasziou, P., and Chalmers, I. (2010). Seventy-five trials and eleven systematic reviews a day: how will we ever keep up? *PLoS Medicine*, 7(9), e1000326.

Bennett, G. and Glasgow, R. (2009). The delivery of public health interventions via the internet: actualizing their potential. *Annual Review of Public Health*, 30, 273–292.

Bloomrosen, M. and Detmer, D. (2010). Informatics, evidence-based care, and research; implications for national policy: a report of an American Medical Informatics Association health policy conference. *Journal of the American Medical Informatics Association*, 17(2), 115–123.

Corn, M., Gustafson, D., Harris, L.M., Kutner, J.S., McFarren, A.E., and Shad, A.T. (2011). Survey of consumer informatics for palliation and hospice care. *American Journal of Preventive Medicine*, 40(5, Suppl. 2), S173–178.

Currow, D. and Abernethy, A. (2005). Quality palliative care: practitioners' needs for dynamic lifelong learning. *Journal of Pain and Symptom Management*, 29(4), 332–334.

Dicker, R. and Hayman, S. (2014). Online tool gives access to residential aged care research. *Australian Nursing and Midwifery Journal*, 21(7), 41–42.

Doyle, D. (2005). Palliative medicine: the first 18 years of a new sub-specialty of general medicine. *The Journal of the Royal College of Physicians of Edinburgh*, 35, 199–205.

Duursma, F., Schers, H., Vissers, K.C., and Hasselaar, J. (2011). Study protocol: optimization of complex palliative care at home via telemedicine. A cluster randomized controlled trial. *BMC Palliative Care*, 10, 13.

Falagas, M.E., Pitsouni, E.I., Malietzis, G.A., and Pappas, G. (2008). Comparison of PubMed, Scopus, Web of Science, and Google Scholar: strengths and weaknesses. *FASEB Journal*, 22(2), 338–342.

Fink, J., Fernicola, P., Chandran, R., *et al.* (2010). Word add-in for ontology recognition: semantic enrichment of scientific literature. *BMC Bioinformatics* 11(103).

Gagnon, M., Pluye, P., Desmartis, M., *et al.* (2010). A systematic review of interventions promoting clinical information retrieval technology (CIRT) adoption by healthcare professionals. *International Journal of Medical Informatics*, 79, 669–680.

Haux, R. (2010). Medical informatics: past, present, future. *International Journal of Medical Informatics*, 79, 599–610.

Hoffmann, T., Erueti, C., Thorning, S., and Glasziou, P. (2012). The scatter of research: cross sectional comparison of randomised trials and systematic reviews across specialties. *BMJ*, 344, e3223.

Iansavichus, A., Haynes, R., Shariff, S.Z., *et al.* (2010). Optimal search filters for renal information in EMBASE. *American Journal of Kidney Diseases*, 56(1), 14–22.

Kidd, L., Cayless, S., Johnston, B., and Wengstrom, Y. (2010). Telehealth in palliative care in the UK: a review of the evidence. *Journal of Telemedicine and Telecare*, 16(7), 394–402.

Laurent, M.R. and Vickers, T. (2009). Seeking health information online: does Wikipedia matter? *Journal of the American Medical Informatics Association*, 16(4), 471–479.

Lobach, D., Sanders, G.D., Bright, T.J., *et al.* (2012). *Enabling Health Care Decisionmaking Through Clinical Decision Support and Knowledge Management*. Evidence Report No. 203. Rockville, MD: Agency for Healthcare Research and Quality.

Névéol, A., Shooshan, S., Humphrey, S.M., Mork, J.G., and Aronson, A.R. (2009). A recent advance in the automatic indexing of the biomedical literature. *Journal of Biomedical Infomatics*, 42(5), 814.

Oliver, D.P., Demiris, G., Wittenberg-Lyles, E., Washington, K., Day, T., and Novak, H. (2012). A systematic review of the evidence base for telehospice. *Telemedicine Journal and e-Health*, 18(1), 38–47.

Purcell, K., Entner, R., and Henderson, N. (2010). *The Rise of Apps Culture*. Washington, DC: Pew Research Center.

Sampson, M., McGowan, J., Lefebvre, C., *et al.* (2008). *PRESS: Peer Review of Electronic Search Strategies*. Ottawa: Canadian Agency for Drugs and Technologies in Health.

Scherer, R., Langenberg, P., and von Elm, E. (2007). Full publication of results initially presented in abstracts. *Cochrane Database of Systematic Reviews*, 2, MR000005.

Shariff, S., Sontrop, J., Haynes, R.B., *et al.* (2012). Impact of PubMed search filters on the retrieval of evidence by physicians. *Canadian Medical Association Journal*, 184(3), E184–90.

Sladek, R. and Tieman, J. (2008). Applying evidence in the real world: a case study in library and information practice. *Health Information and Libraries Journal*, 25, 295–301.

Sladek, R., Tieman, J., Fazekas, B.S., Abernethy, A.P., and Currow, D.C. (2006). Development of a subject search filter to find information relevant to palliative care in the general medical literature. *Journal of the Medical Library Association*, 94(4), 394–401.

Song, F., Parekh, S., Hooper, L., *et al.* (2010). Dissemination and publication of research findings: an updated review of related biases. *Health Technology Assessment*, 14(8), iii, ix–xi, 1–193.

Straus, S. and Haynes, B. (2009). Managing evidence-based knowledge: the need for reliable, relevant and readable resources. *Canadian Medical Association Journal*, 180(9), 942–945.

Tieman, J., Abernethy, A., and Currow, D.C. (2010). Not published, not indexed: issues in generating and finding hospice and palliative care literature. *Journal of Palliative Medicine*, 13(6), 669–675.

Tieman, J., Sladek, R., and Currow, D. (2008). Changes in the quantity and level of evidence of palliative and hospice care literature: the last century. *Journal of Clinical Oncology*, 26, 5679–5683.

Tieman, J., Sladek, R., and Currow, D.C. (2009). Multiple sources: mapping the literature of palliative care. *Palliative Medicine*, 23(5), 425–431.

Tieman J (2012) Palliative Care Search Filter: Effectiveness Studies 2010-2011. Discipline of Palliative and Supportive Services, Flinders University: South Australia (Australia). 2012: Evaluation Report No 17

Tieman, J., Hayman, S., and Hall, C. (in press) Find me the evidence: connecting the practitioner with the evidence on bereavement care. *Death Studies*.

World Health Organization (2011). *Health Topics: eHealth*. [Online] Available at: <http://www.who.int/topics/ehealth/en/>.

Younger, P. (2010). Internet-based information-seeking behaviour amongst doctors and nurses: a short review of the literature. *Health Information and Libraries Journal*, 27, 2–10.

Validated assessment tools for psychological, spiritual, and family issues

Linda L. Emanuel, Richard A. Powell, George Handzo, Kelly Nichole Michelson, and Lara Dhingra

Introduction to validated assessment tools for psychological, spiritual, and family issues

Palliative care stands out among other medical disciplines for its foundational commitment to the inclusion of psychological, spiritual, and family issues, premised on founding pioneer Dame Cicely Saunders' assertion that 'total pain' involves suffering in the physical, psychological, spiritual, and social domains (Saunders, 1978).

Saunders further contended that suffering in one domain 'migrates' to others. For example, spiritual pain could be somatized or expressed by a person as physical pain. Indeed, research is beginning to identify some of the neurobiological mechanisms for physical expression of pain (García-Campayo et al., 2009; Borkum, 2010). Psychological distress has a reciprocal relationship with social distress, each produced by, and creating, distress in the other. Physical suffering may trigger psychological, spiritual, and social suffering. With the task of the palliative care team being to address suffering in all domains, occasionally resolution of one source will relieve suffering in other domains. Commonly, suffering adopts a life of its own in each domain and needs to be assessed and managed. For instance, an individual in distress who cannot eat due to oesophageal cancer may benefit greatly from palliative surgery. However, the impact of the experience on the individual's psychological and spiritual states, and their relationships with others, may take longer to resolve and entail anticipatory anxieties or concerns that the situation may recur and worsen in the future. If the individual undergoes palliative surgery successfully but these other domains are unaddressed, he/she remains incompletely managed.

Palliative care providers, therefore, should assess all domains competently and understand how suffering 'travels' from one realm to others. The provider must not only assess and address this multi-domain suffering, but measure how well the interventions applied have alleviated it. This applies to the patient and their family, who are considered a unit of care in palliative care, with the provider considering, first and foremost, the patient and then the family.

The patient may experience manifold challenges and losses, starting with the loss of their expectation of health. As each challenge and loss occurs, the patient must absorb the new situation, adapt to it, and reach a new equilibrium (Knight and Emanuel, 2007b). Confronted by serious and rapidly evolving illness, these losses can be overwhelming. Constant reassessment by the provider is essential, as is reconsideration of how to support comprehension, adaptation, and resolution in each of the physical, psychological, spiritual and social domains.

If this were not sufficiently complex, interactions between the patient and their circle of loved ones and community compound it. Understanding how the patient and family impact on one another's experience is a considerable but necessary challenge. Examples are myriad: a patient with depression due to pancreatic cancer transmits the burden of this depression to those who love them; a family unready to accept the terminal nature of their loved one's illness may complicate the patient's acceptance of their own condition and hinder the social tasks of dying that both sides need.

With these interacting dynamics, the provider is greatly assisted by practical assessment approaches and measures of relevant outcomes.

Assessment and measurement

Improving the quality of palliative care is now recognized as a high social priority. Advances in the field's development, however, are impeded by difficulties achieving reliable assessments and management of the 'total pain' domains that matter most in the discipline. These domains are often: (1) subjective, (2) of an impractically large scope, (3) reliant on interviews undertaken at a time when people may be too burdened or ill to answer multiple questions, and (4) difficult to study longitudinally due to the often contracted survival time of this population. Methods to enable measurement of patients' palliative care needs must be adapted to address these challenges. The availability of psychometrically sound and clinically relevant screening, diagnostic, and outcome evaluation tools that optimize patient evaluation, prognostication, and treatment selection, as well as patient satisfaction and quality of life, are essential to high-quality palliative care.

The following sections describe commonly used assessment and outcome measurement tools in a routine clinical setting—some of which are used, often erroneously, interchangeably. These can be employed in making general patient evaluations across multiple domains, as well as specifically addressing psychological, spiritual, and familial issues. We will discuss their development and, where it exists, validation.

Assessment

Comparing patient-reported symptoms following open-ended questioning versus a structured survey among 265 advanced disease patients in the United States, Homsi et al. (2006) reported that the median number of symptoms found using the latter was tenfold higher than those volunteered, with most non-volunteered symptoms being moderate or severe and distressing. Effective patient management is therefore based on active, systematic health assessments by providers. These evaluations may improve the accuracy of diagnostic and prognostic determinations and the development of individual treatment plans.

Given its holistic nature, palliative care assessment should include, but extend beyond, traditional medical assessments (Arseven et al., 2005). As suggested by the US-based National Consensus Project for Quality Palliative Care (2013), care plans should involve a comprehensive, timely assessment that is interdisciplinary, coordinated, and include: patient and family interviews; medical record review; discussion with other providers; physical examination and assessment; and relevant laboratory and/or diagnostic tests or procedures. Consultative evaluations should include the patient's current medical status, adequacy of diagnosis and treatment consistent with review of past history, diagnosis, and treatment, and past treatment responses.

Assessment includes documentation of disease status (diagnosis and prognosis); co-morbid medical and psychiatric disorders; physical and psychological symptoms; functional status; and social, cultural, spiritual, and future care planning concerns and preferences. Assessment of children must be conducted with sensitivity to their age and neurocognitive development stage. Patient and family expectations, goals of care and living, understanding of the disease and prognosis, and preferences for the type and site of care, should also be assessed and documented. Regular reassessment and updating are necessary.

Individual clinical assessment approaches have developed organically over time and are often not rigorous, systematic procedures using valid and reliable measurement tools to supplement skilled clinical interviewing. Such instruments exist in abundance, with a systematic literature review by Stiel et al. (2012) identifying 528 different tools (372 targeting patients) for use in palliative care research and clinical practice. Many are not well validated or designed for clinical use and it will likely always remain the case that the clinical interview and some intuitive assessment are essential. Nonetheless, validated instruments should have a role in the clinical setting. The following sections focus on a limited number that have been tested empirically and can facilitate a comprehensive bedside assessment.

Needs at the End-of-Life Screening Tool

The Needs at the End-of-Life Screening Tool (NEST) (Emanuel et al., 2001) is a general assessment tool that uses a holistic approach and 13 questions that are grouped into four thematic dimensions—corresponding, for mnemonic purposes, to each letter of NEST (Needs in the social domain, Existential matters, Symptom management needs, and Therapeutic relationship

matters)—to screen patients for needs of concern. The tool was developed using 15 focus groups and six in-depth interviews among patients, family caregivers, and professionals, followed by a survey of a nationally representative sample of 988 patients (650 at 4–6-month follow-up) with any terminal diagnosis of less than 6 months prognosis, except AIDS. The qualitative work identified areas of importance in end-of-life care, which were tested empirically using factor analysis of patients' survey responses. The tool was assessed further for its feasibility and effectiveness as a screening tool for advanced illness care needs among 451 cancer patients in tertiary care (Scandrett et al., 2010). An adaptation for use in the emergency ward setting is called SPEED (Screen for Palliative and End-of-life needs in the Emergency Department) (Richards et al., 2011).

Measurement

Measuring palliative care outcomes, and the totality of care provided, is an important mechanism by which high-quality health-care systems are developed and maintained (Pasman et al., 2009). Given that health-care costs are a substantial portion of public and private budgetary expenditures, the medical profession is obliged increasingly to generate quantifiable evidence demonstrating the effectiveness, efficacy, appropriateness, and acceptability of services. In some countries, the commissioning of health-care services is dependent upon evidence from patient-reported outcome measures (PROMs) (Bausewein et al., 2011a), where results of importance from the patient perspective play a critical role in care provision, audit, and research.

Outcome measurement

Care is focused on achieving positive clinical and satisfaction outcomes for patients and families by using quality services. Correspondingly, four types of health outcome measurement are patient-, carer-, staff-, and service-based (Jocham et al., 2009). Many measures are part of service assessment rather than direct patient care. However, PROMs can be used routinely in care, patient assessment, and as a continuing measure of progress such as effective pain management. Completed measures can be retained in the patient's medical record to help the clinician monitor change over time.

Identifying good outcome measures, however, is problematic. The utility of a measure is determined by its psychometric properties and how well it relates to its aim. A measure could be referred to as 'good' if it is shown to have validity (face, content, criterion, and construct), reliability (inter-rater, test–retest, and internal consistency), appropriateness and acceptability, responsiveness to change, and interpretable results (Bausewein et al., 2011b). Additionally, in the pressured, time-sensitive environment of the clinical setting, a measure should be easy and relatively quick to administer. These are the benchmarks against which the quality of a measure should be evaluated.

A small number of multidimensional palliative care outcome measures have been developed that meet at least some of the above criteria, including the Palliative care Outcomes Scale (POS).

Palliative care Outcomes Scale

The POS was developed in 1999, for use with patients with advanced disease, and to improve outcome measurement by evaluating essential palliative care components partly from the patients' perspectives (Hearn and Higginson, 1999). There are currently two versions of the original POS: one for patients to complete, the other for staff. The tool was developed initially across eight palliative care centres across England and Scotland (including inpatient, outpatient, day, home, and primary care settings) among 148 patients for the patient version, and 337 for the staff version. It has since been adapted and validated in multiple regions, from Europe (e.g. Bausewein et al., 2005), to Latin America (Eisenchlas et al., 2008), to Africa (Harding et al., 2010; Powell et al., 2007), and is being adapted for use among children (Downing et al., 2012).

The POS has ten items assessing physical symptoms, emotional, psychological, and spiritual needs and the provision of information and support, with one open question on main problems. Responses are rated on a 5-point Likert-type scale ranging from 0 ('No effect') to 4 ('Overwhelming').

Quality improvement

Quality improvement (QI) is a formal, systematic approach to performance analysis that seeks to measure the status quo and identify and implement ways to initiate improvements. Clinical audit can be the first step in the QI cycle; a method of reviewing existing clinical practice against agreed standards of care to identify areas for improvement, and re-evaluating those care practices after a designated period of time, to assess their outcome compared with baseline data.

Gould et al. (2007) reported a QI collaborative that was conducted to develop capacity among health-care providers in New York City to apply QI methodology—delivering 4-year-long implementation cycles with a total of 82 teams—to palliative care services. They found significant improvements in most team projects and substantial gains made in familiarity with continuous QI techniques and in building palliative care programmes and networks.

Measurements that have been developed for use in outcome assessments and QI exercises, and which focus on the particular health-care domains of the psychological, spiritual and familial, are discussed in the following sections.

Domain-specific tools

Psychological domain

Advanced medical illness and its treatment are associated with high rates of psychological distress in patients and families. The most common psychological problems occurring near the end of life include depression and anxiety (Mitchell et al., 2011). Rates vary widely across studies and are influenced by multiple factors, including the population assessed, the type and severity of disease, and the treatment setting (Mitchell et al., 2011). Depression ranges from 5.1% to 30.1% in populations with advanced illness, such as cancer, AIDS, chronic obstructive pulmonary disease, and congestive heart failure, and up to 15.4% for anxiety (Mitchell et al., 2011).

This section reviews validated screening tools for the assessment of general psychological distress, depression, and anxiety in populations with advanced illness, discussing multiple considerations for assessment and specific tools that may assist providers in timely and appropriate evaluation. For a review of tools that assess other common psychiatric problems—such as adjustment disorders (Akechi et al., 2006) and delirium (Breitbart et al.,

1997)—and family caregiver problems—including bereavement (Zisook et al., 1982) and complicated grief (BrintzenhofeSzoc et al., 1999)—readers may refer to Chapters 17.3, 17.4, 17.6, 17.7 and other published reviews (Stroebe et al., 2007; Thekkumpurath et al., 2008; Grover and Kate, 2012). For diagnosis and management, provide detailed overviews.

Studies show that untreated psychological distress undermines medical decision-making and treatment adherence, which can result in disability and high health-care usage (Colleoni et al., 2000; Prieto et al., 2002). Psychological distress may augment pain perception (Pincus et al., 2002), undermine symptom control (Spiegel and Giese-Davis, 2003), and impair quality of life (Skarstein et al., 2000; Stark et al., 2002). Patients commonly report a perceived loss of meaning or purpose in life, a decrease in engagement in valued activities, and a reduction in pleasure from the social environment (Parker et al., 2003; Hopko et al., 2008). This can impede the ability to cope with the emotional stress of preparing for death and separating from loved ones, and worsen distress in family members (Pessin et al., 2002). Despite effective interventions for psychological distress (Fawzy et al., 1990; Sheard and Maguire, 1999; Donker et al., 2009), it is under-diagnosed (Steinberg et al., 2009; Holland et al., 2010) and screening is rare in practice (Institute of Medicine Committee on Treatment of Posttraumatic Stress Disorder, 2008).

Psychological distress

In the past, one barrier has been the lack of validated tools for screening (Vodermaier et al., 2009). The US National Comprehensive Cancer Network (NCCN) has developed guidelines for regular screening and management (NCCN, 2013). The NCCN defines psychological distress as 'a multifactorial, unpleasant, emotional experience of a psychological (cognitive, behavioural, emotional), social, and/or spiritual nature that may interfere with the ability to cope effectively with cancer, its physical symptoms and its treatment' (NCCN, 2013). The detection of psychological distress often relies on physician assessment and patient-initiated reports; however, they are frequently discordant (Söllner et al., 2001). Consequently, the following tools can assist providers in more accurate identification.

When selecting an appropriate tool, important considerations include the psychometric properties, particularly sensitivity and specificity, treatment setting, and disease severity. Each tool has its own advantages and limitations. Ideally, validated cut-offs provide high sensitivity (i.e. identify all patients in need of support) and specificity (minimize false positives) (Vodermaier et al., 2009). For example, shorter measures are useful clinically (in terms of cost and time), but have fewer domains and, sometimes, limited specificity. In general, tools are classified as ultrashort (one to four items), short (five to 20 items), and long (21–50 items) (Vodermaier et al., 2009).

One ultrashort screening tool recommended by the NCCN is the Distress Thermometer (NCCN, 2013). A single item measures overall psychological distress in the past week on a 0–10 numeric rating scale, with an accompanying Problem List assessing five domains. It has high sensitivity and specificity with the Hospital Anxiety and Depression Scale (HADS) and the Center for Epidemiologic Studies of Depression Scale (CES-D) (Hurria et al., 2009) and good reliability (Hoffman et al., 2004). While a cut-off score of 4 or higher is meaningful (Hurria et al., 2009), scores of 7 or above may provide optimal sensitivity and specificity (Hegel et al., 2008).

Another ultrashort tool, the four-item Patient Health Questionnaire-4 (PHQ-4) (Kroenke et al., 2009) screens for anxiety and depression. Anxiety items include: 'Feeling nervous, anxious, or on edge' and 'Not being able to stop or control worrying', two diagnostic criteria for Generalized Anxiety Disorder in the *Diagnostic and Statistical Manual of Mental Disorders*, fourth edition, text revision (DSM-IV-TR). Depressive items include: 'Feeling down, depressed, or hopeless' and 'Little interest or pleasure in doing things'. Responses are rated on a 4-point Likert-type scale ('Not at all' to 'Nearly every day'), with total subscale scores ranging from 0 to 6; cut-offs of 3 or above are clinically significant (Mitchell et al., 2009; Kroenke et al., 2010), with 0–2 (normal), 3–5 (mild), 6–8 (moderate), and 9–12 (severe). Like other tools, it does not diagnose depression or anxiety. However, its predictive ability and reliability (Kroenke et al., 2009) and brevity are advantages.

The short Brief Profile of Mood States Total Mood Disturbance Score (Brief POMS TMDS) includes 11 items evaluating general distress in cancer patients (breast, pancreatic, gastric cancer, and myeloma) (Cella et al., 1987). It reduced the 58-item TMDS with one factor of general distress. Five mood factors include: tension-anxiety, depression-dejection, anger-hostility, fatigue, and confusion-bewilderment. Items are rated on a 5-point Likert-type scale ('Not at all' to 'Extremely'), with total scores ranging from 0 to 44. It is internally consistent and correlated with the long version. Criterion validity discriminates between pancreatic patients, who typically exhibit higher distress scores, and gastric cancer patients. Other strengths include brevity, sensitivity, and true assessment of psychological distress without the 'vigour' mood factor (i.e., measures physical well-being) (McNair et al., 1971; Cella et al. 1987).

Depression

Two widely-used, short screening tools for depression are the HADS (Zigmond and Snaith, 1983) and the CES-D (Radloff, 1977). Both are validated in palliative care populations (Le Fevre et al., 1999; Härter et al., 2006; Vodermaier et al., 2009).

The HADS includes two 14-item subscales measuring depressive and anxiety symptoms (HADS-D) (HADS-A). Items are rated on a 4-point Likert-type scale ('Not at all' to 'Very often'), with subscale scores ranging from 0 to 21 (Zigmond and Snaith, 1983). It is clinically relevant, responsive to treatment (Smarr et al., 2011), validated in multiple languages, including Spanish, Chinese, French, and Italian (Smarr et al., 2011), and reliable (Bjelland et al., 2002). However, the cut-offs vary, ranging from 8 to 22 (total score) and 5 to 11 (subscale scores) (Vodermaier et al., 2009). A cut-off of 8 or more provides optimal sensitivity and specificity (Bjelland et al., 2002), with probable major depression rated as: 8–10 (mild), 11–15 (moderate), and 16 or higher (severe) (Snaith and Zigmond, 1994).

The CES-D (Radloff, 1977) includes 20 items measuring depression and identifying individuals at risk of depression. It assesses mood and level of functioning in the past week, and rates symptom frequency across four domains: positive and negative affect, somatic and interpersonal problems. Items are rated on a 4-point Likert-type scale ('Rarely' to 'Most or all of the time'), with total scores ranging from 0 to 60. Internal consistency is good (Radloff, 1977). Cut-off scores greater than 16 suggest probable clinical depression (Katz et al., 2004), yielding a sensitivity of 100% and specificity of 85% in cancer patients (Katz et al., 2004). The increased false-positive risk is balanced by brevity, validation in multiple languages, and free use. Shorter five- and ten-item versions (Shrout and Yager, 1989; Irwin et al., 1999) have improved upon response wording.

Anxiety

While tools such as the HADS screen for depression and anxiety, several provide detailed anxiety assessments. The long State-Trait Anxiety Inventory (Spielberger et al., 1983) includes two 40-item subscales assessing State Anxiety (S-Anxiety) and Trait Anxiety (T-Anxiety). S-Anxiety measures current apprehension and tension on a 4-point Likert-type scale ('Not at all' to 'Very much'). T-Anxiety measures anxiety (i.e. discomfort or worry) during typical daily situations (responses range from 'Almost never' to 'Almost always'; Spielberger et al., 1994). Total subscale scores range from 20 to 80. Cut-off scores of 30 and below (no–low anxiety) or higher than 30 (moderate–high anxiety) (Glozman, 2004) and higher than 54 in geriatric populations have been suggested (Kvaal et al., 2005). Advantages include good reliability (Spielberger et al., 1983) and translation into multiple languages, but use requires purchase (Mind Garden, 2013).

The Beck Anxiety Inventory (Beck et al., 1988) includes 21 items assessing cognitive and somatic symptoms. Items are rated on a 4-point Likert-type scale ('Not at all' to 'Severely'), with total scores ranging from 0 to 63. A cut-off score greater than 10 provides high sensitivity and specificity (Hopko et al., 2008), with 0–9 (normal), mild to moderate (10–18), moderate to severe (19–29), and severe (30–63). While brief, easily administered, and validated in oncology populations (Hopko et al., 2008), specific drawbacks include the multitude of somatic symptoms, which can overlap with medical conditions (Julian et al., 2011). Although internally consistent (Fydrich et al. 1992), further validation in palliative populations is suggested (Vodermaier et al., 2009).

The extent of the family carer's burden and impact are becoming better understood and characterized. There are many potential stressors associated with caring, including managing psychological and physical needs, instrumental assistance with a range of practical and medical tasks, such as adherence to medical regimens and decision-making and providing seemingly constant vigilance. Qualitative data reveal common themes in subjective caregiver impact (Dellon et al., 2010; Braithwaite et al., 2011) and several questionnaires report both positive and negative consequences of caregiving (Glajchen et al., 2005). Although carers are often inadequately trained, under-supported, misunderstood, and distressed, there are also positive aspects of providing care to a family member, including satisfaction in caring for a loved one (Glajchen et al., 2012).

Spirituality domain

When confronted by suffering, distress, and mortality across the disease trajectory, patients may articulate spiritual concerns. Despite professional sensitivity regarding the investigation of patients' spiritual distress and the feasibility of addressing issues identified in the typically brief clinical encounter, the spiritual concerns of patients with a life-limiting illness can impact upon treatment choices (Balboni et al., 2013; Peteet and Balboni, 2013). However, research in the spiritual domain remains one of the least investigated in palliative and hospice care provision, in contrast to the physical-functional aspects.

Whilst instruments to assess religious/spiritual (R/S) issues within the discipline exist—with more being developed due to a growing appreciation of their need (for a more comprehensive list of existing R/S tools, see a review by Büssing (2012))—much of the work has three significant shortcomings: lack of a generally accepted conceptual definition of spirituality (Puchalski et al., 2009), resulting in confusion (la Cour and Götke, 2012); a paucity of tools validated in cross-cultural palliative care populations (Selman et al., 2011); and the dearth, or lack of reporting, of methodologically rigorous supportive validation studies per se, especially for clinical tools (Galek et al., 2011).

Three categories of formal assessment tool in the spiritual domain are screening, history taking, and assessment (Puchalski, 2010). These categories are aligned with normal medical practice and are the best current models for interdisciplinary spiritual care (Puchalski et al., 2009). For a fuller description of this model, see Chapter 4.5.

Spiritual screening

Spiritual screening questions are designed for insertion into routine assessment or screening processes to identify patients with significant spiritual needs. The widely used Distress Thermometer (NCCN, 2012)—a patient-rated tool whose specificity and sensitivity have been demonstrated among bone marrow transplant patients (Ransom et al., 2006) and among a heterogeneous mix of Swedish oncology patients (Thalén-Lindström et al., 2013)—includes 'spiritual/religious concerns' on its problem list. However, no research exists determining what this category means to patients, and therefore what it is measuring.

Some clinicians use the one-question screen 'Are you at peace?', with a 5-point Likert-type scale, that was evaluated by Steinhauser et al. (2006). Although the question was found to provide a brief gateway to assessing spiritual concerns, to date the screen has only been tested with patients with advanced, life-limiting illnesses such as stage IV cancer, congestive heart failure, or chronic obstructive pulmonary disease, despite research indicating such concerns can influence medical decision-making throughout the disease trajectory.

The only multi-question screening instrument supported by a published partial validation study was developed by Fitchett and Risk (2009). The brief screening protocol, subsequently named the Rush Religious Struggle Screening Protocol and used in a QI pilot project among oncology patients (Blanchard et al., 2012) and blood and marrow transplant patients (King et al., 2013), focuses on the identification of patients who may be experiencing R/S struggle—a well-researched concept that has been shown to be related to several significant health outcomes, including mortality (Pargament et al., 2004)—and patents who would like a visit from a chaplain. The triage method consists of three questions that can be administered by anyone on the health-care team without significant training, while the protocol for making referrals to a chaplain is simple and transparent. In a pilot study among non-chaplain health colleagues in an 18-bed, Chicago-based acute medical rehabilitation unit, the protocol identified 7% (n = 12) of patients possibly experiencing R/S struggle, with all but one of these confirmed in need following a chaplain assessment (Fitchett and Risk, 2009).

Spiritual history

Spiritual history questions are recommended for inclusion in the social history section of the routine history. The HOPE tool (sources of Hope, Organized religion, Personal spirituality, Effects on care) (Anandarajah and Hight, 2001), and the SPIRIT tool (Spiritual belief, Personal spirituality, Integration with community, Rituals, Implications for care, Terminal events planning) (Maugens, 1996) are often used.

However, the FICA (Faith, Importance, Community, and address in Care) spiritual history tool (Puchalski, 2006) is the only such instrument partly supported by a validation study (Borneman et al., 2010). Developed in a consensus expert-review process, and then modified based on anecdotal feedback from users, this tool is not intended to be used as a checklist, but rather as a guide to initiate dialogue with patients to explore deeper questions their relationship to spirituality, their spiritual beliefs, and their goals for spiritual health. One of the weaknesses of the limited validation conducted on the tool is the lack of heterogeneity in the R/S preferences of its sample, with over 70% declaring themselves Catholic or Protestant.

Spiritual assessment

Spiritual assessment is, 'A more extensive [in-depth, on-going] process of active listening to a patient's story as it unfolds in a relationship with a professional chaplain and summarizing the needs and resources that emerge in that process (see Chapters 4.5 and 17.1). The summary includes a spiritual care plan with expected outcomes which should be communicated to the rest of the treatment team' (Fitchett and Canada, 2010).

However, although intended, in North America and elsewhere, to guide the work of professional chaplains in detailed discussions with patients about their R/S strengths and issues and how they might affect their care, all existing spiritual assessment tools are unvalidated. Moreover, all require significant training to use and are best reserved for patients whose R/S concerns affect their coping and care planning significantly. Among these unvalidated instruments, the recommended include the following:

♦ The Guidelines for Pastoral Diagnosis, which provides a diagnostic taxonomy framed in theological language (Pruyser, 1976) across seven dimensions: awareness of the holy, providence, faith, grace or gratefulness, repentance, communion, and sense of vocation.

♦ The 7X7 model, developed in the mid 1980s, which uses a functional approach to assessment—concerned with how a person finds meaning and purpose in life and with the behaviour, emotions, relationships, and practices associated with that meaning and purpose. It assesses two broad thematic areas comprised of seven *holistic* (medical, psychological, family systems, psycho-social, ethnic, racial, and cultural, social issues and spiritual) and seven *spiritual* domains (beliefs and meaning, vocation and obligations, experience and emotions, courage and growth, rituals and practice, community, and authority and guidance) (Fitchett, 2002).

♦ Outcome Oriented Chaplaincy, described as, 'the operational paradigm for professional chaplaincy for the twenty-first century' (Peery, 2012, p. 346) that 'emphasizes achieving, describing, measuring, and improving outcomes that result from a chaplain's work' (Peery, 2012, p. 348). It includes an assessment template as part of an overall system for chaplaincy care based on the mnemonic 'Run In On A Prayer': Reason for Visit, Interventions, Outcomes, Assessment, and Plan.

Spiritual measurement

Like spiritual assessment tools, most spiritual measurement instruments are unvalidated. Two exceptions that have been used widely among physically ill populations are the Brief RCOPE and the Functional Assessment of Chronic Illness Therapy—Spiritual (FACIT-Sp).

The Brief RCOPE (Pargament et al., 2000) features 14 items across two scales: positive religious coping and negative religious coping, recognizing that religion can support or impede coping. It identifies spiritual adjustment; that is, the extent to which conflict, self-blame, or anger at God is present.

The tool was tested initially on a sample of 540 college students coping with a significant negative life event. They were predominantly white (93%), single (99%), female (69%), and Catholic (45%) or Protestant (41%). Factor analysis of the results produced factors largely consistent with the conceptualization and construction of the subscales. Subsequently confirmatory factor analysis of the RCOPE was undertaken in a second sample composed of 551 elderly hospital patients, and found to be moderately supportive of the initial factor structure. Studies have adjusted the tool for individuals with a Buddhist background (Phillips et al., 2009) and adapted the underlying coping concept for use in cancer patients (Zwingmann et al., 2006).

The tool can be very helpful to the clinician or researcher trying to identify patient use of religion in coping and contains a good deal of religious language. As such, it is more appropriate for populations with a theistic and Western, largely Christian, background (Pargament et al., 2011).

The FACIT-Sp (Peterman et al., 2002) focuses on spiritual well-being, another useful concept for clinicians, and is available in several variations aimed at specific populations, such as pain patients. Developed among cancer patients, and avoiding religious language, two subscales, measuring a sense of meaning and peace and the other assessing the role of faith in illness, were determined from the 12-item tool. A total score for spiritual well-being is produced. Based upon two studies, the tool has demonstrated good internal consistency and reliability, a significant association with quality of life, and convergent validity with five other measures of religion and spirituality in a sample of patients with mixed early-stage and metastatic cancer diagnoses. A subsequent study among 240 long-term (average of 10 years post-diagnosis) white, female survivors of cancer supported a three-factor model (meaning, peace, and faith) (Canada et al., 2008). However, this was later found to have less stability as a model across 8805 cancer survivors from a much more ethnically diverse sample, suggesting that items and their constructs might be understood differently across groups (Murphy et al., 2010). Consequently, because the variations of the scale are generally based on specific populations, users should determine whether the version they use is appropriate for their population.

Many of these measurement tools also have been used as spiritual screening tools, in part because of the dearth of validated tools designed explicitly for screening. However, clinicians are cautioned that even the varyingly validated tools have not been validated for clinical screening purposes. Additionally, since these are paper and pencil instruments, they are limited by the language

they use. For instance, several use references to 'God' or other higher powers which may be unhelpful to an increasing number of patients, such as in the United States, who perceive themselves as not religious (Pew Research Center's Forum on Religion and Public Life, 2012). Conversely, other instruments use no explicitly religious language, which may not resonate with patients who only express their R/S issues in such terms. Lastly, the terms 'spiritual risk', 'spiritual struggle', and 'spiritual pain' are not well defined or differentiated in the extant literature, although 'risk' is normally understood as a condition which renders the patient susceptible to 'pain' or 'struggle'. Clinicians and investigators should, therefore, be aware of possible ambiguity in the use of these terms.

Family domain

Support for the family is particularly important in palliative care. The needs of family members, many of whom contribute as carers, can shape the patient's experience and ultimately become the focus of bereavement care. Assessment of family members must address their role as carers as well as members of a larger family. While many tools exist, identifying appropriate tools and integrating them into routine clinical management or research is not standard, is poorly tested, and therefore problematic for practical implementation.

The types of caring roles family members adopt stem from diverse patient needs. Family carers can find themselves supporting a patient's physical, psychological, existential, and social needs. An abundant supply of carer burden scales and questionnaires exist that investigate the multidimensional impact on the carer's daily life and well-being. In a review of instruments related to carers in palliative care, the following categories were identified:

- satisfaction with service delivery
- psychiatric disorders
- quality of life
- needs
- grief and bereavement
- burden
- preparedness/competence
- family functioning
- a group of miscellaneous tools (Hudson et al., 2010).

A unitary comprehensive 'gold standard' assessment tool has not emerged, and is unlikely to do so. Although the diversity of existing instruments is potentially valuable—providing the clinician and researcher with choices based upon specific characteristics of a given disease site or caregiving burden domain of interest—the plethora of instruments carries the risk of 'confusing the marketplace' with a multitude of divergent questions, rating scales, and aggregated scores. Despite the wide availability of such instruments, few providers use them in routine practice.

Moreover, challenges exist to using assessment tools that evaluate the family itself and the specific roles of family members of a palliative care patient. There are varying contextual components that impact on the focus of assessment tools. For example, the relationship of a patient to his/her family and family structure can vary considerably depending on whether the patient is an infant, adolescent, adult, or elderly person. Similarly, assessing the family needs of a household with multiple young children differs from assessing those of a patient and their spouse, or adult child. Categories of existing family assessment tools based on their contextual focus include characteristics of the patient (e.g. spouse vs parent vs child); attention to the family as a unit versus members/caregivers within the family; disease categories, for example, patients with cancer versus those with Alzheimer's disease; location of patient, such as home versus at the hospital; and timing of illness, such as during chronic phases of illness versus end-of-life versus bereavement.

Few existing instruments that focus on families have been evaluated for their utility in guiding clinical practice. Rather, many have been developed based on a particular theoretical framework and validated in specific clinical settings (Neabel et al., 2000). How and when to use such tools clinically, and the mechanisms for implementing interventions based on their results, remain poorly established. While this area is clearly underdeveloped, the following sections discuss tools for assessing and measuring the family unit. (For a more comprehensive list of existing family assessment tools, see a review by Neabel et al. (2000) and of instruments related to family caregivers of palliative care patients by Hudson et al. (2010).)

Family assessment

The Needs Assessment Tool Progressive Disease (NAT-PD, nd) or the Needs Assessment Tool—Progressive Disease Cancer (NAT-PD-C, nd) is recommended by the Centre for Palliative Care's practice guidelines (Hudson et al., 2010) to assess carers' needs. These tools were developed by an expert consensus panel of 66 leaders and key stakeholders in palliative care, based on an extensive literature review. Initially, face and content validity, acceptability, and feasibility were confirmed by health-care professionals who viewed video-recorded, simulated consultations involving actors as patients (Waller et al., 2008). Further testing was undertaken in a clinical setting to determine the inter-rater reliability, validity, and feasibility of the tool (Waller et al., 2010). The impact of using this tool in the clinical setting was assessed for cancer patients and associated with significant reduction in health system, information, patient care, and support needs (Waller et al., 2012). These screening tools include six items to assess the ability of the carer/family to care for the patient across the physical, daily living, psychological, information, financial and legal, and family relationship domains as well as two items to assess the carer's well-being in relation to their own physical, psychological, and bereavement issues.

The Family Crisis Oriented Personal Evaluation Scales (F-COPES) is a 29-item self-report questionnaire intended to identify problem-solving and behavioural strategies used by families during crises (McCubbin et al., 1987). It measures five subscales related to acquiring social support, reframing, seeking spiritual support, mobilizing family to acquire and accept help, and passive appraisal. The tool can help health-care teams identify which families may need additional assistance with managing crises.

Family measurement

Like assessment tools, identifying measurement tools for carers and families requires consideration of the specific contextual components important to the families assessed and the area of interest. For example, some tools are developed specifically for use with cancer patients. Tools measuring the management of carer psychological distress differ from those addressing a family's ability to cope. Moreover, the questions of interest for the health-care teams and organizations will determine which tool to use and how to implement identified tools in the clinical setting. Measuring family needs consecutively over time may be necessary to determine the efficacy of the palliative care team in addressing them. Alternatively, it may be beneficial to measure carer bereavement following the death of their loved one, to consider whether palliative care services are providing long-term outcomes for family members. Needs assessment tools can be useful also for health-care organizations in determining resource allocation. Finally, many measures of families and carers have been developed and studied in non-palliative care settings, meriting a degree of caution if employed in palliative care situations.

Broad categories of relevance for measuring families and carers in palliative care include carer satisfaction with service delivery, carer quality of life, psychological impact, and bereavement. Many tools used to measure psychological domains for patients can also be used for carers.

The Quality of Life in Life-Threatening Illness—Family Carer Version (QOLLTI-F) is a 16-item tool measuring caregiver quality of life and includes the carer's perception of patients' conditions. There are seven subscales: environment, patient state, carer's own state, carer's outlook, quality of care, relationships, and financial worries. It was developed from qualitative research, asking carers what is important to their own quality of life, rather than focusing on the changes or burdens related to caring, with most domains responsive to change (Cohen et al., 2006). All items, the subscale scores and the total score (the mean of the seven subscale scores) have a scoring range from '0' to '10'; to ensure '0' always indicates the worst situation and '10' the best, item numbers 3, 4, 14, 15, and 16 must have their scores transposed.

The Family Appraisal of Caregiving Questionnaire for Palliative Care (FACQ-PC) is a 25-item tool that measures four theoretically derived domains: caregiver strain, positive caregiving appraisals, caregiver distress, and family well-being. Among 160 adult primary carers of a relative with cancer receiving home-based palliative care, it showed acceptable psychometric properties (internal consistency, factorial validity, and convergent and discriminant validity), can be used in clinical assessment, and has potential use in evaluating the effectiveness of palliative care (Cooper et al., 2006). However, one limitation is that the content validation process did not include carers, but rather a small group of professionals (n = 5).

Based upon the FAMCARE scale (Kristjanson, 1993), which was developed using qualitative research to identify indicators of family care satisfaction and their subsequent reduction using Q-sort study to the most salient, the FAMCARE-2 was developed among 497 carers from 29 Australian inpatient- and community-based palliative care services. FAMCARE-2 includes 17 items and is measured using a 5-point Likert-like scale (from 1 = 'Very satisfied', to 5 = 'Very dissatisfied') and an additional 'Not relevant to my situation' option.

What we don't know: assessments and measures yet to come

The tools available for the assessment and measurement of psychological, spiritual, and family care issues remain largely inadequate, both in terms of their psychometric validation and applicability in divergent diagnostic, ethnic and age groups, service delivery settings, and cultural contexts. As understanding of the nature of needs and care in the setting of serious illness deepens, we should expect improvements both in the tools available and how to integrate them into processes of care and QI.

Additional concepts need to be developed and integrated into mainstream palliative care. For instance, work exists on the nature of the state of peace that some attain near the end of life and that many aspire to (Emanuel et al., 2010). Yet, delineation of this state of peace as a construct that can be assessed, measured, and addressed has not developed to the point that tools are integrated into care delivery. Similarly, further understanding of what makes for resilience and successful adaptation are necessary if more patients are to achieve the best death possible for themselves, their families, and society (Knight and Emanuel, 2007a).

All this will be possible only if the culture of palliative care remains seriously committed to the inclusion of psychological, spiritual, and family care within palliative care. While the specialty may still be better at this than other medical disciplines, it is also the case that advances in the clinical sciences of physical symptoms have outpaced other areas. Approaches to address mental health are improving; information on anxiety, depression, delirium, and other psychological suffering encountered in palliative care is increasing, but still there is far to go. Similarly, counselling and psychotherapy for patients and families facing serious illness is a developing area, as are the economics at the household level of palliative care. However, to date there are limited data and clinical guidance available for either. Most striking of all is the sparse empirical knowledge of spiritual care in palliative care. Readers are advised to keep abreast of advances in all of these fields and participate in the culture of palliative care that insists on their importance. If patients are assessed for needs in these areas, and if care outcomes in these areas are measured, increased understanding and improvement will be possible.

Acknowledgements

Dr Dhingra wishes to thank Jack Chen, Huiyan Ye, and Anna Gordon for their assistance with literature reviews and references.

Online materials

Complete references for this chapter are available online at <http://www.oxfordmedicine.com>.

References

Balboni, T.A., Balboni, M., Enzinger, A.C., *et al.* (2013). Provision of spiritual support to patients with advanced cancer by religious communities and associations with medical care at the end of life. *JAMA Internal Medicine*, 173, 1109–1117.

Bausewein, C., Daveson, B., Benealia, H., Simon, S.T., and Higginson, I.J. (2011b). *Outcome Measurement in Palliative Care: The Essentials*. London: King's College London and PRISMA.

Borneman, T., Ferrell, B., and Puchalski, C. (2010). Evaluation of the FICA tool for spiritual assessment. *Journal of Pain and Symptom Management*, 20, 163–173.

Büssing, A. (2012). Measures. In M. Cobb, C.M. Puchalski, and B. Rumbold (eds.) *Oxford Textbook of Spirituality in Healthcare*, pp. 323–331. New York: Oxford University Press.

Glajchen, M., Kornblith, A., Homel, P., Fraidin, L., Mauskop, A., and Portenoy, R.K. (2005). Development of a brief assessment scale for caregivers of the medically ill. *Journal of Pain and Symptom Management*, 29, 245–254.

Hearn, J. and Higginson, I.J. (1999). Development and validation of a core outcome measure for palliative care: the palliative care outcome scale. Palliative Care Core Audit Project Advisory Group. *Quality in Health Care*, 8, 219–227.

Hudson, P.L., Trauer, T., Graham, S., *et al.* (2010). A systematic review of instruments related to family caregivers of palliative care patients. *Palliative Medicine*, 24, 656–668.

Neabel, B., Fothergill-Bourbonnais, F., and Dunning, J. (2000). Family assessment tools: a review of the literature from 1978–1997. *Heart and Lung*, 29, 196–209.

Richards, C.T., Gisondi, M.A., Chang, C.H., *et al.* Palliative care symptom assessment for patients with cancer in the emergency department: validation of the Screen for Palliative and End-of-life care needs in the Emergency Department instrument. *Journal of Palliative Medicine*, 14, 757–764.

Selman, L., Harding, R., Gysels, M., Speck, P., and Higinson, I.J. (2011). The measurement of spirituality in palliative care and the content of tools validated cross-culturally: a systematic review. *Journal of Pain and Symptom Management*, 41, 728–753.

Common symptoms and disorders

Common symptoms and disorders

Fatigue and asthenia

Sriram Yennurajalingam and Eduardo Bruera

Introduction to fatigue and asthenia

Fatigue is the most frequent and debilitating symptom in patients with advanced-stage cancer, with a prevalence of 60–90% in various studies (Stone et al., 2000; Cella et al., 2001; Servaes et al., 2002; Lawrence et al., 2004). In the palliative care setting, the frequency ranges from 48% to 78% (Stone et al., 2000; Lawrence et al., 2004; Teunissen et al., 2007). Fatigue adversely impacts the physical, functional, and psychological domains of quality of life, resulting in an inability to perform daily activities and affecting mood, social relationships, and work (Wilson and Cleary, 1995; Östlund et al., 2007; Teunissen et al., 2007; Beijer et al., 2008). It may influence patients' decision-making capabilities regarding future treatment and lead to the refusal of potentially curative treatment.

In the past, the term 'asthenia' was used to describe a subjective sensation of tiredness and the term 'fatigue' was used to describe a symptom of tiredness precipitated by effort. However, the terms are currently often used in the same context. In this chapter, we consider the two terms synonymous, and by convention, 'fatigue' is generally used.

Fatigue may include three major features:

1. Easy tiring and reduced capacity to maintain performance.

2. Generalized weakness, defined as the anticipatory sensation of difficulty in initiating a certain activity.

3. Mental fatigue, defined as the presence of impaired mental concentration, loss of memory, and emotional lability.

The National Comprehensive Cancer Network defined cancer-related fatigue as follows: 'Cancer-related fatigue is a distressing persistent, subjective sense of physical, emotional, and/ or cognitive tiredness or exhaustion related to cancer or cancer treatment that is not proportional to recent activity and interferes with usual functioning' (Berger et al., 2010).

Fatigue occurs as a result of both cancer and its treatment. The onset of fatigue may precede the diagnosis of cancer or it may occur at any stage in the course of the illness. It may first occur after or be exacerbated by chemotherapy, radiotherapy, or surgery, and may be present for prolonged periods after these treatments. In patients with advanced cancer, fatigue usually coexists with a number of other symptoms, including pain, anorexia, nausea, vomiting, dyspnoea, sleep disturbance, anxiety, and depression (Yennurajalingam et al., 2008).

In recent years, as the management of other symptoms (e.g. pain, dyspnoea, and nausea) has improved, there has been an increased awareness of the importance of recognizing fatigue as a symptom deserving of attention. The management of fatigue is confounded by a limited research base and a lack of data supporting an established therapeutic strategy.

Most of the evidence presented in this chapter relates to studies in cancer patients. However, similar principles can be applied to fatigue in patients with other end-stage diseases such as end-stage AIDS and cardiac conditions.

Pathophysiology

The basic mechanisms by which fatigue is caused are not well understood, and several possible underlying causes of fatigue exist in most patients. Occasionally, one predominant abnormality is present and appears to be the main contributor to the symptom; however, in most cases, several abnormalities and other symptoms are present that may contribute to the genesis of fatigue.

In patients with cancer, complex interactions occur between the tumour and host. Table 8.1.1 outlines mechanisms by which tumours have the potential to directly or indirectly produce fatigue in patients with advanced-stage cancer. Fig. 8.1.1 summarizes contributors to fatigue in cancer patients.

Tumours, host-derived factors, and cytokines

Tumours can produce various by-products, including lipolytic and proteolytic factors and cytokines capable of interfering with the host metabolism and causing fatigue. These factors are believed to also play a role in the development of cancer-related cachexia (Miller et al., 2008; Fearon et al., 2012). The relationship between cachexia and fatigue is discussed later in this chapter.

The evolving literature supports the current hypothesis that the presence of a tumour and/or cancer-related treatment such as radiotherapy and/or chemotherapy induces the dysregulation of pro-inflammatory cytokines such as tumour necrosis factor-alpha (TNF-α), interleukin (IL)-1, and IL-6 (Dantzer and Kelley, 2007; Miller et al., 2008; Seruga et al., 2008). Further, these cytokines have been implicated in the pathophysiology of fatigue by acting on multiple systems, including the brain (hypothalamic–pituitary–adrenal (HPA) axis, sleep, psychological, and dopaminergic alterations), muscles (reductions in mass and strength), immune system (cellular and humoral changes), and metabolism (Dantzer and Kelley, 2007; Seruga et al., 2008; Bower and Lamkin, 2013).

Rats and mice showed increased signs of fatigue when infection and other conditions associated with an increase in pro-inflammatory cytokines were present (Dantzer and Kelley, 2007; Burton et al., 2011). Drugs such as interferon-alpha, IL-2, and TNF-α have been associated with symptoms of fatigue, mood swings, sleep disturbance, and cognitive changes (Dantzer

Table 8.1.1 Mechanisms by which tumours may directly or indirectly cause fatigue

Direct effects	Induced host factors	Accompanying factors
Lipolytic factors	Interleukin-6	Psychological issues
Proteolytic factors	Interleukin-1	Anaemia
Tumour degradation products	Tumour necrosis factor	Cancer-related symptoms: pain, sleep disturbance, dyspnoea, drowsiness
Invasion of brain or pituitary gland by tumour or metastases		Cachexia, hypoxia, and infection; metabolic disorders; dehydration; neurological disorders; endocrine disorders; paraneoplastic syndromes

and Kelley, 2007; Miller et al., 2008; Raison et al., 2010). Cytokine-associated symptoms such as anorexia or cachexia, chronic nausea, fever, depression, pain, and sleep disorders may also contribute to fatigue (Miller et al., 2008).

The proinflammatory cytokines are further regulated by host-related factors such as genetic factors, immune factors, and HPA axis alterations. However, the lack of consensus on the definition of cancer-related fatigue (phenotype), challenges with the methodology used to measure these cytokines, the lack of a standard methodology used for measuring these cytokines, and the limited number of fatigue studies using animal models limit our understanding of the link between inflammation and cancer-related fatigue (Barsevick et al., 2010; Gilbertson-White et al., 2011).

Muscle abnormalities

Impaired muscle function may be one of the main underlying mechanisms of fatigue (Al-Majid and McCarthy, 2001). The fatigue-related muscular abnormalities may be related in part to known abnormalities in cytokine production, but the production of other fatigue-inducing substances by the tumour or the host has been postulated.

Muscle alterations in patients with tumours are well known. Cachexia leads to a loss of muscle and fat, which may partially

explain the relationship between cachexia and fatigue (Fearon et al., 2012; Gould et al., 2013). However, patients with tumours can have muscle abnormalities even in the presence of normal caloric intake and a constant body weight and lean body mass. The muscle tissues of cancer patients have been found to contain excessive amounts of lactate (Holroyde et al., 1979). It is unclear whether this lactate is part of the pathogenic mechanism of muscle weakness or a consequence of it. Atrophy of type II muscle fibres has been suggested to be a systemic effect of cancer, even in early or non-metastatic stages (Barron and Heffner, 1978). Tumour-free muscle from tumour-bearing animals shows alterations in the activity of various enzymes, the distribution of isoenzymes, and the synthesis and breakdown of myofibrillar and sarcoplasmic proteins (Fearon et al., 2012). Our group found impaired maximal strength, decreased relaxation velocity, and increased fatigue after electrical stimulation of the abductor pollicis muscle via the ulnar nerve in patients with breast cancer as compared with normal controls (Bruera et al., 1988).

Myopathies can also be caused by medications taken by cancer patients. Corticosteroids can cause loss of muscle mass, and cyclosporin has been implicated as a cause of mitochondrial myopathy (Schäcke et al., 2002).

Interestingly, a recent preliminary study comparing ten advanced-stage cancer patients and 12 healthy volunteers to determine the contribution of muscle fatigue to overall fatigue found no alteration in the muscle contractile property in advanced-stage cancer patients; therefore, the authors of the study suggested that the early motor task failure in cancer-related fatigue was primarily due to a central mechanism (Kisiel-Sajewicz et al., 2012). However, further studies are needed, as more recent studies targeting the fatigue mechanisms involving muscle found no correlation between muscle and fatigue. These studies included supplementation of adenosine triphosphate (Beijer et al., 2008) and L-carnitine (Cruciani et al., 2009).

Deconditioning

Prolonged bed rest and immobility lead to loss of muscle mass and reduced cardiac output. This deconditioning results in reduced endurance for exercise and activities of daily living and may be compounded by other muscle abnormalities in patients

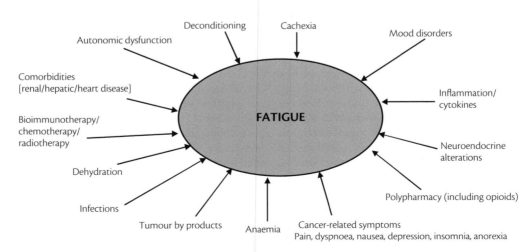

Fig. 8.1.1 Contributors to fatigue.

with cancer (Berger et al., 2010; Neil et al., 2013). Recent studies have found that endurance exercise training can reduce fatigue and improve physical performance in cancer patients undergoing chemotherapy, cancer survivors, and patients who have undergone bone marrow or autologous stem cell transplantation (Cramp and Byron-Daniel, 2012).

Overexertion

Overexertion is a frequent cause of fatigue in cancer and non-cancer patients (Siegel et al., 2012). It should also be considered in young cancer patients who are receiving aggressive antineoplastic treatment, such as radiotherapy and chemotherapy, and who are trying to maintain their social and professional activities. Research in sports medicine has shown that for prolonged endurance, it is important to provide muscles with adequate substrate (carbohydrate loading). Unfortunately, cancer patients frequently present with abnormalities in muscle metabolism that may not allow adequate use of this substrate (Fearon et al., 2012).

Central nervous system abnormalities

The mechanisms by which fatigue is perceived or induced in the central nervous system (CNS) are poorly understood. Primary or secondary tumours involving the CNS and leading to the invasion of brain tissue (particularly the pituitary gland, with resulting endocrine abnormalities) appear to be possible causes of fatigue in cancer patients.

Disturbed cognitive functioning may be caused by fatigue but may also contribute to fatigue. Brain tumours can cause cognitive dysfunction and other tumours, such as small cell lung cancers, can affect brain function by producing hormones or neurotransmitters (Ronnback and Hansson, 2004; Dantzer and Kelley, 2007; Schagen and Vardy, 2007). Antineoplastic treatments, such as chemotherapy and radiotherapy, and drugs used to treat complications of cancer, such as opioids and corticosteroids, can also affect the CNS (Wood et al., 2006). Research findings suggest that inflammatory cytokines play a role in mental fatigue (Ronnback and Hansson, 2004). However, much more research is needed to improve our understanding of the mechanisms by which fatigue is induced at the CNS level.

Other CNS mechanisms that have been proposed include (a) dysregulation of serotonin and/or its receptors in the brain due to cancer or cancer treatment; (b) circadian rhythm disruptions, which negatively impact arousal and sleep patterns (prior studies suggest that fatigue is positively correlated with decreased daytime activity and restless sleep at night); and (c) dysregulation of the hypothalamic–pituitary axis (Bower et al., 2005). However, there are no trials of patients with advanced-stage cancer to support the hypothesis that any of these CNS-mediated aetiologies is the primary mechanism of cancer-related fatigue (Servaes et al., 2002).

Relationship between fatigue and cachexia

Fatigue and cachexia coexist in the great majority of patients with advanced-stage cancer, and it is likely that malnutrition is a major contributor to fatigue. The loss of muscle mass resulting from progressive cachexia can cause profound weakness and fatigue. As previously discussed, even in the presence of normal protein and caloric intake and normal body weight, structural and biochemical muscle abnormalities are frequently found in cancer patients

(Lawrence et al., 2004; Tisdale, 2009; Barsevick et al., 2010). Similar abnormalities often are used to explain fatigue associated with chronic cardiac and respiratory disease (von Haehling et al., 2009; Briggs et al., 2012).

It is important to recognize, however, that profound fatigue can exist in the absence of significant weight loss. Fatigue is common in patients with breast cancer and lymphomas, which have a low prevalence of cachexia. In non-malignant conditions such as chronic fatigue syndrome and depression, profound fatigue is generally not associated with malnutrition. Our group found no correlation between fatigue and nutritional status or weight in a population of breast cancer patients (Bruera et al., 1989). However, severe malnutrition without fatigue can be observed in patients with anorexia nervosa and in some patient populations with solid tumours. Fig. 8.1.2 illustrates the potential relationship between cachexia and fatigue.

It has been proposed that anorexia and fatigue may be an expression of the major metabolic abnormalities that occur in cancer patients, rather than simply an expression of malnutrition per se (Seruga et al., 2008). This situation would be similar to the occurrence of a catabolic state owing to a viral infection or in the early postoperative period. In these conditions, patients experience anorexia and fatigue that are secondary to the metabolic abnormalities rather than being causes of those abnormalities. Some interventions used to treat cancer cachexia, such as corticosteroid agents, have been found to be effective in the management of fatigue. The mechanisms by which these agents ameliorate cachexia and fatigue, however, are not well understood. Current pharmacological interventions for cachexia are discussed elsewhere in this book.

Infection

Fatigue is frequently associated with infections, particularly those that are recurrent or protracted. It may occur as a prodrome, and it may outlast the infection by weeks or even months (Chrousos, 1995; Rovigatti, 2012). In patients with cancer, immunosuppression due to the cancer itself or to cancer treatment increases the risk of infection and its complications. Chronic infection and cancer induce the same mediators for cachexia, including inflammatory cytokines (Seruga et al., 2008; Bennett et al., 1998). It can be hypothesized that they share similar mediators for fatigue as well.

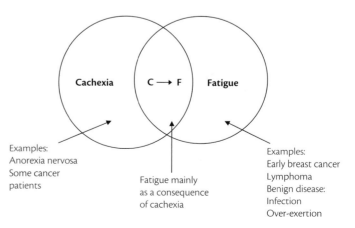

Fig. 8.1.2 Possible relationship between cachexia and fatigue.

Anaemia

Anaemia is prevalent in cancer patients (see Chapter 8.3). Common causes of anaemia in cancer patients are myelosuppression by chemotherapeutic agents, iron deficiency, bleeding, haemolysis, nutritional deficiencies, and anaemia owing to chronic disease (Grotto, 2008). Severe anaemia (haemoglobin < 8 g/dL) is known to be a cause of profound fatigue. In patients receiving chemotherapy, treating less severe anaemia has been shown to improve energy levels, activity levels, and quality of life. In a prospective, open-label study of epoetin-alpha in 2342 anaemic patients receiving chemotherapy, mean energy levels, activity levels, and quality of life were found to improve with increases in mean haemoglobin levels from approximately 9 g/dL to 11 g/dL (Glaspy et al., 1997; Demetri et al., 1998). The improvements were independent of tumour response and correlated with the increases in haemoglobin levels. Similar findings were reported in a study of 2289 patients receiving chemotherapy: increased haemoglobin was correlated with improvements in energy, activity, and quality of life (Demetri et al., 1998). Although these data suggest an association between anaemia and fatigue, there are limited studies that specifically assess this relationship in populations with advanced illness.

Autonomic dysfunction

Autonomic dysfunction is a common complication of advanced-stage cancer. This syndrome includes malnutrition, delayed gastric emptying, chronic nausea, anorexia, and poor performance status (Bruera et al., 1986; Walsh and Nelson, 2002). Postural hypotension has been documented in patients with a specific type of severe chronic fatigue syndrome (Newton et al., 2009). Autonomic dysfunction may contribute to fatigue as well as to orthostatic hypotension. The association between fatigue and autonomic dysfunction has not been established in cancer patients and should be investigated in future research (Strasser et al., 2006).

Psychological issues

Anxiety, depression, and psychological distress can all contribute to fatigue (Yennurajalingam et al., 2008). However, the nature of these relationships is unclear (Brown and Kroenke, 2009). While some depressive symptoms are frequent in cancer patients, only a minority of patients develop adjustment disorders and only a small percentage present with major depressive or anxiety disorders (Reeve et al., 2008; Rosenstein, 2011). The diagnosis of a major depressive episode in patients with advanced-stage cancer is difficult because the patients frequently present with neurovegetative and somatic symptoms that are part of the disease itself. The diagnosis of major depression thus should rely more on the presence of psychological and cognitive signs and symptoms in these patients than in those without advanced-stage cancer (Chochinov, 2001) (see Chapter 17.3).

Nevertheless, cancer patients presenting with an adjustment disorder or a major depressive disorder can have fatigue as one of the prevalent symptoms. One prospective cohort study of elderly patients with cancer found a significant association between the intensity of fatigue and psychological symptoms such as anxiety and depression (Respini et al., 2003). In a double-blind clinical trial of 94 women with breast cancer, depression was significantly reduced in the 44 patients receiving paroxetine compared to the 50 patients receiving placebo, indicating that a biologically active dose was used; however, the groups did not differ in regard to any measures of fatigue (Roscoe et al., 2005). Thus, the role of psychological factors, including anxiety and depression, in the development of fatigue among cancer patients needs further research.

Metabolic and endocrine disorders

Endocrine disorders (e.g. diabetes mellitus, Addison's disease, and hypothyroidism) and electrolyte disorders (e.g. hyponatremia, hypokalaemia, and hypercalcaemia) are possible causes of fatigue and in many instances have relatively simple and effective treatments.

Interest in hypogonadism as a cause of fatigue and loss of muscle mass has increased in recent years as a result of the prevalence of these symptoms in HIV-infected men. Testosterone deficiency results in the loss of muscle mass, fatigue, reduced libido, and reduced haemoglobin (Basaria et al., 2001). Androgen insufficiency in cancer patients can result from anorexia-cachexia syndrome (Burney et al., 2012). In addition, chemotherapy and radiotherapy can cause hypogonadism. Hormonal ablative therapy has been found to significantly increase the incidence of fatigue in patients with prostate cancer (Storey et al., 2012). In patients with testosterone insufficiency due to HIV disease and other causes, treatment with androgenic anabolic steroids, including testosterone and its derivatives, has been found to increase muscle mass (Grinspoon, 2005), improve energy and libido (Snyder et al., 2000), and increase haemoglobin levels (Snyder et al., 2000). Androgenic anabolic steroids are regularly used for the treatment of hypogonadism in HIV-infected men. A randomized, single-blind, placebo-controlled trial of testosterone replacement in 35 men with mild Leydig cell insufficiency after chemotherapy found that physical fatigue significantly improved in the testosterone-treated group and was associated with a borderline increase in physical activity (Howell et al., 2001). Other variables such as bone mineral density and body composition were not significantly altered. The effects of treating hypogonadism in cancer patients should be researched further.

Abnormalities of the HPA axis concerning corticotrophin-releasing factor have been postulated as another possible endocrine-related cause of fatigue (Tsigos and Chrousos, 2002; Silverman et al., 2010). Corticotrophin-releasing factor levels increase in situations of physical or emotional stress and thus may cause fatigue (Makino et al., 2002; Miller et al., 2008). In addition, the HPA axis is activated by stress; while hyperactivity in this system can lead to depression (Glaspy et al., 1997), reduced HPA activity also has been postulated as a possible cause of chronic fatigue syndrome (Papadopoulos and Cleare, 2012). The proinflammatory cytokines IL-1, IL-6, and TNF-α are central mediators of the inflammatory process that can result in the dysregulation of the HPA axis and the secretion of mediators that induce such symptoms as pain, fatigue, anxiety, and depression, leading to an impaired quality of life (Bruera et al., 1988; Servaes et al., 2002; Bower et al., 2005; Miller et al., 2008). Further research is needed to clarify the role of abnormalities of the HPA axis in the genesis of fatigue.

Paraneoplastic neurological syndromes

Paraneoplastic neurological syndromes are rare but are important to recognize, as many of these syndromes can precede the clinical

Table 8.1.2 Paraneoplastic neurological syndromes associated with fatigue

Syndrome	Characteristics
Progressive multifocal leucoencephalopathy	Leukaemia and lymphoma are the cancers in which this syndrome is most often found
Paraneoplastic encephalomyelitis	70% of cases occur in patients with lung cancer and 30% in patients with other cancers
Amyotrophic lateral sclerosis	
Subacute motor neuropathy	Proximal or distal, often asymmetric (e.g. after radiotherapy for lymphoma)
Subacute necrotic myelopathy	Mainly found in patients with lung cancer
Peripheral paraneoplastic neurological syndrome	Often precedes diagnosis of the primary tumour, similar to Guillain–Barré syndrome
Ascending acute polyneuropathy (Guillain–Barré syndrome)	Mainly found in patients with lymphoma
Neuromuscular paraneoplastic syndromes	
Dermatomyositis, polymyositis	Associated with malignancy in about 50% of cases (onset within 1 year)
Eaton–Lambert syndrome	Strongly associated with small cell lung cancer. Can precede detection of tumour by months. Improves with successful treatment
Myasthenia gravis	30% of cases occur in patients with thymoma, while most of the rest occur in those with lymphoma

Source: data from Warenius, H.M. (1989). Paraneoplastic neurological syndromes. In R. Tallis (ed.) *The Clinical Neurology of Old Age*, pp. 323–34. New York: John Wiley and Sons Ltd.

presentation of a malignancy. They may be partially reversible with primary treatment of the tumour. Table 8.1.2 summarizes some of the paraneoplastic neurological syndromes associated with fatigue (Darnell and Posner, 2006; Gandhi and Johnson, 2006).

Other cancer-related symptoms

Various correlative studies have shown that fatigue is associated with pain, psychological symptoms such as anxiety and depression, dyspnoea, sleep disturbances, anorexia, and constipation (Echteld et al., 2007; Okuyama et al., 2008; Yennurajalingam et al., 2008). However, the intensity of the individual symptoms in a given patient may determine the symptoms' ultimate contribution to the fatigue (Respini et al., 2003).

Side effects of cancer treatment

Treatments for both cancer and the symptoms and conditions caused by cancer can cause or aggravate fatigue. Worsening of fatigue is common during chemotherapy and radiotherapy (Wang et al., 2010). The mechanisms by which these treatment modalities cause fatigue are not fully understood. Radiotherapy can result in anaemia, diarrhoea, anorexia, and weight loss, and chemotherapy commonly causes anorexia, nausea, vomiting, and anaemia; all these events may contribute to fatigue. In addition, these treatments have secondary effects that may cause or exacerbate fatigue;

Box 8.1.1 Cancer therapies and medications that commonly contribute to fatigue

Cytotoxic therapeutic agents

Radiotherapy

Biological response modifiers (e.g. interferon)

Targeted therapy (tyrosine kinase inhibitors)

Opioids

Polypharmacy: hypnotics/anxiolytics, anticholinergics, antiepileptics, neuroleptics, opioids, alpha adrenergic blocking agents, diuretics, selective serotonin reuptake inhibitors and tricyclic antidepressants, and benzodiazepines

for instance, fatigue may be a consequence of chronic pain resulting from radiotherapy- or chemotherapy-induced immunosuppression that predisposes patients to infection. Such effects may persist long term. One study found that patients with breast cancer who had undergone adjuvant chemotherapy or autologous bone marrow transplantation appeared to experience fatigue for months to years after the completion of treatment (Cohen et al., 2012; Goldstein et al., 2012).

Biological response-modifying agents have also been implicated in fatigue; for instance, interferon-alpha was shown to cause fatigue in 70% of patients (Jones et al., 1998). In fact, fatigue is the most frequent dose-limiting side effect in patients receiving biological response-modifying treatments for cancer (Aparicio et al., 2011).

Opioids such as morphine have significant effects on the reticular system and are capable of inducing sedation, cognitive changes, and fatigue in some patients. In addition, anxiolytics, hypnotics, and other drugs may cause sedation and fatigue. Box 8.1.1 outlines cancer therapies and drugs that frequently contribute to fatigue in patients with cancer.

Genetics and cancer-related fatigue

There is preliminary evidence that various single nucleotide polymorphisms of proinflammatory cytokine genes (which affect the gene expression levels) are associated with cancer-related fatigue (Barsevick et al., 2010; Bower et al., 2011). Prior studies found overrepresentation of the IL-1B-511 CC alleles among cancer survivors with fatigue (Collado-Hidalgo et al., 2008; Jim et al., 2012). A study by Smith and Humphries found that homozygosity for both the variant C allele and the wild-type G allele of the IL-6-174 polymorphism was overrepresented in patients with fatigue (Collado-Hidalgo et al., 2008; Reyes-Gibby et al., 2008). Another recent study by Miaskowski et al. found a significant association between polymorphisms in the TNF-alpha and IL-6 genes and fatigue (Miaskowski et al., 2010).

In summary, evidence clearly shows that fatigue is a complex, subjective, multidimensional syndrome that can be attributed to multiple causes. It is particularly important to note that not only cancer but also cancer treatments, cancer-related symptoms (e.g. anorexia-cachexia, pain, sleep disturbances, drowsiness, anxiety, depression, cognitive dysfunction, and dyspnoea), metabolic causes, endocrine dysfunction (e.g. HPA axis dysfunction) cytokine dysregulation, and neuromuscular dysfunction may be among those causes, making a comprehensive assessment of paramount importance.

Assessment

Fatigue is one of the most common and complex symptoms in patients receiving palliative care. Due to the lack of consensus on the definition of fatigue and limited understanding of the exact causative mechanisms, its measurement can be challenging (Jean-Pierre et al., 2007; Minton and Stone, 2009; Mortimer et al., 2010; Seyidova-Khoshknabi et al., 2011). Hence there is no 'gold standard' tool that exists for the assessment of fatigue. Its multidimensional nature adds to the complexity of assessment.

The assessment of fatigue routinely should involve the evaluation of the severity of the fatigue; its onset, duration, and level of interference with everyday life; associated psychological or social problems; and possible underlying causes. Table 8.1.3 outlines some assessment tools for fatigue; several others also exist.

Subjective measures of fatigue are generally considered to be the most relevant in clinical practice and in clinical trials. Visual analogue scales, numerical scales, the Functional Assessment of Cancer Therapy–Fatigue (FACIT-F) (Cella et al., 1993), the Piper Fatigue Scale (Piper et al., 1998), and the Brief Fatigue Inventory (Mendoza et al., 1999) have all been validated and can be used in both pharmacological and non-pharmacological studies. In addition to these tools, there are validated functional assessments of fatigue in most frequently applied quality-of-life questionnaires, such as the European Organisation for Research and Treatment of Cancer QLQ-C30 (Knobel et al., 2003) and Functional Assessment of Cancer Therapy-G (Cella et al., 1993). However, there are studies indicating that the short scales within these instruments have certain limitations (Knobel, et al., 2003). The unidimensional scale is useful for the routine assessment of the severity of fatigue in clinical practice, but these tools may only predominantly assess the physical impact of fatigue and not its mental and emotional dimensions.

Multidimensional tools help us to understand various dimensions of fatigue, such as cognitive and emotional dimensions, in addition to the physical dimension. Tools that are multidimensional are generally preferred to those that are not because they give a broader picture of the problem and can highlight both general and specific management approaches that may benefit a specific patient. However, the trade-off is that it requires more time to administer the questionnaire. Examples of multidimensional tools used to assess fatigue include the Fatigue Questionnaire and Multidimensional Fatigue Inventory. For more details, see Chapter 7.1.

Table 8.1.3 Assessment approaches for fatigue

Functional capacity	Task-related fatigue
Treadmill performance (speed, duration)	Visual analogue/numerical rating scale
	Pearson and Byars Fatigue Feeling Checklist
Number of errors (pilot, driver)	
6-minute walk	
Performance status	**Subjective assessment tools**
Karnofsky Performance Status	Visual analogue/numerical rating scale
European Cooperative Oncology Group criteria	Functional Assessment of Cancer Therapy-Fatigue
Edmonton Functional Assessment Tool	Piper Fatigue Scale
	Brief Fatigue Inventory

Functional capacity tests attempt to objectively determine a patient's ability to perform a standard task, such as walking on a treadmill, riding a bicycle, or driving for a prolonged period (in a simulator). These tests are of very limited value in cancer care and research, as they are very difficult for patients with advanced-stage cancer to perform. A suitable alternative is measuring daily physical activity and fatigue by means of actigraphy (Berger et al., 2007). An actigraph can also be used to record and evaluate sleep quantity and quality, daytime activity levels, and napping. Roscoe et al. (2002) found that actigraph measurements significantly correlated with fatigue in patients with breast cancer. Conversely, Dimsdale and colleagues found no correlation between fatigue expression and actigraph measurements in healthy controls (Dimsdale et al., 2003). Task-related fatigue tests attempt to assess the fatigue induced by standard tasks. The 6-minute walk test, for example, is commonly used to assess physical function (ATS Committee on Proficiency Standards for Clinical Pulmonary Function Laboratories, 2002).

Assessment of performance status is the most commonly used measure of a patient's physical condition in oncology. Two popular tools, the Karnofsky Performance Status score (Karnofsky and Burchenal, 1949) and the European Cooperative Oncology Group score (Zubrod, 1960), rely on a physician's rating of the patient's functional capabilities after a regular medical consult. Another tool used in oncology, the Edmonton Functional Assessment Test (Kaasa et al., 1997), is administered by a physiotherapist and attempts to determine a patient's functional status in addition to identifying obstacles to clinical performance.

Assessment of fatigue also involves the assessment of possible underlying causes, including those factors shown in Fig. 8.1.1. A full assessment therefore involves a careful systems review and psychological assessment, a detailed physical examination, and blood tests that would detect anaemia and electrolyte or endocrine abnormalities. Multiple causes should be suspected in all patients, and the possible impact of various factors should be weighed according to their severity.

Screening for fatigue

Routine screening for fatigue using single-item screening for cancer-related fatigue has become more common in clinical practice as patients seldom report fatigue so as to avoid distracting the treating physician from the management of their disease.

Guidelines of the National Comprehensive Cancer Network Fatigue Practice Guidelines Panel (Berger et al., 2010) recommend that patients be screened for the presence and severity of fatigue at the time of their initial contact with a doctor and that ongoing assessments be made. The guidelines suggest that the screening data be used to designate the fatigue as mild, moderate, or severe (on a 0–10 numerical rating scale, with 1–3 considered mild, 4–6 moderate, and 7–10 severe). A patient diagnosed with mild fatigue would be re-evaluated on an ongoing basis, whereas patients diagnosed with moderate or severe fatigue would undergo more focused assessment and intervention. A recent study found that a fatigue score of 5 or more out of 10 indicated clinically significant fatigue (Butt et al., 2008).

Management

Because fatigue is complex, multifactorial, and multidimensional, it is crucial that an adequate therapeutic approach be used to identify

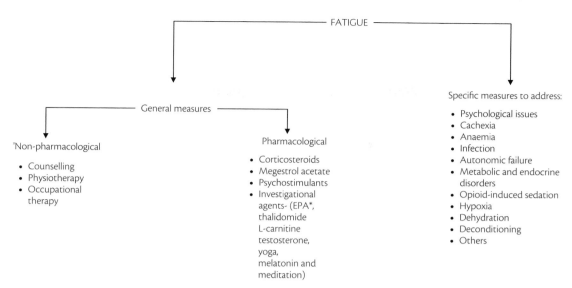

Fig. 8.1.3 Therapeutic approach to managing fatigue. * Eicosapentaenoic acid.

and prioritize the different underlying factors (Yennurajalingam and Bruera, 2007; Bruera and Yennurajalingam, 2010). Alterations in fatigue over time may demonstrate a relationship with a particular factor (e.g. fatigue may increase following an increase in tumour size, a change in medication, or a reduction in the haemoglobin concentration). This temporal pattern underscores the importance of continuous assessment and monitoring of symptoms and signs, even in palliative medicine. In planning a therapeutic approach, it is also important to answer the following questions:

1. Is fatigue a symptom of primary concern to this patient?

2. What are the major probable causes?

3. Are there therapeutic measures available that have a reasonable cost/benefit ratio?

An intervention may have the purpose of decreasing the intensity of fatigue, allowing the patient to express a maximal level of functioning with a stable level of fatigue, or both. In palliative care, the satisfactory treatment of a symptom such as fatigue does not mean that the symptom must be eliminated completely. Even minor improvements can be enough to shift fatigue downward on the patient's list of priorities.

In a given patient, it is often impossible to determine with certainty whether or not an identified problem is a major contributor to fatigue or simply coexists with the fatigue. Therefore, it is of great importance to measure the intensity of fatigue and the patient's performance status before and after treating any suspected contributing factor. For example, fatigue should be measured before and after correcting hypercalcaemia or treating anaemia. This can be done in a number of ways, including using a simple numerical scale (e.g. 0 = best, 10 = worst) or a visual analogue scale (e.g. 0 = best, 100 = worst imaginable) or using a patient-reported outcomes measure such as the Patient Reported Outcomes Measurement Information System from the National Institutes of Health (Yost et al., 2011). If the level of fatigue does not improve after correction of an underlying abnormality, it is clear that further treatment of that abnormality will not improve the fatigue in the future.

Fig. 8.1.3 outlines some general and specific measures that may be useful in the management of fatigue in patients with cancer. In many patients, no reversible causes will be identified. Several pharmacological and non-pharmacological approaches may be effective in these patients, however, including those that reduce energy expenditure or levels of fatigue. Specific treatments may also be used to address underlying abnormalities believed to contribute to the fatigue of an individual patient.

Non-pharmacological approaches

Of the various treatment strategies, exercise has the strongest empirical support in patients with early cancer and cancer survivors, with several recent meta-analyses concluding that physical activity has a moderate beneficial effect on cancer-related fatigue (Cramp and Byron-Daniel, 2012). There is also some support for psychological interventions, with a meta-analysis showing a small to moderate beneficial effect (standardized mean difference in the range of 0.10 to 0.30) (Yennurajalingam et al., 2008). The modest effect sizes in the psychological studies may be a result of the fact that many did not include a cancer-related fatigue-related aim or hypothesis (Jacobsen et al., 2007; Yennurajalingam et al., 2008). The few trials that explicitly focused on fatigue, providing education about fatigue and instruction in self-care, coping techniques, and activity management, were more effective than non-specific interventions (Jacobsen et al., 2007).

Physical activity or exercise

A recent Cochrane review confirmed the beneficial effects of exercise in the management of cancer-related fatigue (Cramp and Byron-Daniel, 2012). In a total of 56 studies in which 1461 participants received an exercise intervention and with 1187 control participants, exercise was seen to be statistically more effective than the control intervention (standardized mean difference, −0.27, 95% confidence interval (CI) −0.37 to −0.17). Both aerobic and resistance exercises, such as brisk walking, cycling, swimming, and weight lifting, are helpful; at least one 30-minute episode per day (at least 150 minutes per week) has been shown to reduce fatigue levels. The benefits of exercise for patients with fatigue were observed for interventions delivered during or after cancer therapy. In relation to diagnosis, they found that exercise benefits patients with fatigue and breast and prostate cancer but not those with haematological malignancies. In addition, they found that aerobic exercise significantly reduced fatigue but that resistance training and alternative forms of exercise failed to reach significance. Further research is necessary to determine the most effective type (aerobic vs resistance), frequency, duration, and intensity of exercise in palliative care patients.

There is limited evidence of beneficial effects of exercise in palliative care patients. In a recent randomized controlled study in advanced-stage cancer patients, 121 patients were referred to exercise and 110 were referred to usual care. After 8 weeks of a standardized 60-minute, twice-a-week intervention, no significant differences were found in the primary outcome of physical fatigue as assessed by a fatigue questionnaire. Statistically significant results were noted in the physical performance measures, including a shuttle walk test and a hand grip strength test; however, this study had a relatively lower adherence rate (69%) and a high dropout rate (36%) (Oldervoll et al., 2011).

Although no level 1 evidence exists on the efficacy of exercise, exercise should be prescribed for patients with advanced-stage cancer, if appropriate, as exercise may be beneficial to maintain muscle mass and physical strength, which are commonly affected due to cachexia related to progressive cancer (Oldervoll et al., 2011). Exercise may further be beneficial in improving outcomes, including maintaining independence, self-reported physical functioning, well-being, self-esteem, and energy (Segal et al., 2009).

Usually in cases of deconditioning, if appropriate, the physiotherapist can suggest suitable exercises and encourage increased activity, which may have beneficial effects from both physical and psychosocial perspectives. In addition, if the patient is immobile, a physiotherapist can perform passive movements that will help the patient maintain flexibility and decrease painful tendon retraction. Occupational therapists can allow patients to remain safe and increase their activity at home by providing such resources as ramps, wheelchairs and walkers, elevated toilets, safety devices for bathrooms, and hospital beds. In addition, these therapists can give patients and families useful tips that enhance mobility and help prevent further muscle atrophy, tendon retraction, and pressure ulcers.

Counselling

Patient education and cognitive behavioural therapy were found to improve fatigue in patients with advanced-stage cancer (Kwekkeboom et al., 2012). Counselling can be very useful for both patients and families. Patients frequently underestimate the side effect burden at the beginning of chemotherapy. In one study, only 8% of patients expected tiredness but 86% experienced it (Kirsh et al., 2001). This result suggests that many patients undergo treatment without sufficient information to develop realistic expectations about what that treatment entails.

Counselling and informing the patient of the possible causes of fatigue and the types of therapeutic options available may allow the patient the opportunity to develop realistic expectations. As the disease progresses, the patient will be required to adapt to further limitations in physical functioning and activity; similarly, the family will need to have realistic expectations for the patient.

Patients who are empowered by receiving correct and full information and by undergoing counselling, they may combat fatigue by:

1. adapting their activities of daily living by reducing the amount of housework they do or by enlisting the help of others to perform physical duties

2. spending more time in bed or, alternatively, exercising more (the latter if deconditioning is considered to be a contributor to the fatigue)

3. rearranging their schedules within the day, depending on their fatigue patterns

4. requesting changes in medications perceived to be causing a loss of energy

5. avoiding expending energy on unnecessary activities.

Acupuncture

Several studies have been conducted using acupuncture as an intervention for cancer-related fatigue (Garcia et al., 2013). Of these, a recent study by Malossitis et al. (2012) of patients with breast cancer shows the most promise. In this study, 75 patients were randomly assigned to usual care and 227 patients to acupuncture plus usual care. The difference in the mean General Fatigue score of the multidimensional fatigue inventory, which was the primary outcome, between those who received the intervention and those who did not was −3.11 (95% CI, −3.97 to −2.25; P < 0.001). The intervention also improved all other fatigue aspects measured by the Multidimensional Fatigue Inventory. The authors concluded that acupuncture is an effective intervention for managing the symptom of cancer-related fatigue and improving patients' quality of life (see Chapter 9.12).

Pharmacological treatments

In patients with fatigue of unknown origin and those for whom specific treatment is not available, several non-specific pharmacological interventions have been proposed. Corticosteroids, megestrol acetate, other anti-cachexia agents, and psychostimulant drugs are the most studied of these interventions. Unfortunately, there is a lack of compelling data to support any of these approaches other than very short term treatment with corticosteroids.

Corticosteroids

Studies have suggested that corticosteroids decrease fatigue in patients with advanced-stage cancer (Moertel et al., 1974; Bruera et al., 1985; Della Cuna et al., 1989; Peuckmann et al., 2010). The mechanism of action by which corticosteroids combat fatigue is unknown. The inhibition of tumour or tumour-induced substances, as well as central euphoriant effects, are potential mechanisms (Moertel et al., 1974). One potential mechanism of improvement of fatigue is by improvement of the physical symptoms commonly associated with cancer and treatment, such as pain, nausea, anorexia, dyspnoea, and drowsiness (Wilcox, 1984; Bruera et al., 1985; Yennurajalingam et al., 2012).

In a preliminary randomized, controlled, double-blind cross-over trial study of 31 patients with advanced-stage cancer, 32 mg/day of methylprednisolone was found to significantly improve subjective fatigue (P < 0.01), pain (P < 0.01), and appetite (P < 0.05) compared with the patients receiving placebo, with no significant differences in side effects between the methylprednisolone and the placebo groups (Bruera et al., 1985). In a recently concluded randomized, double-blind placebo-controlled study (Yennurajalingam et al., 2012) of 84 patients with advanced-stage cancer, an oral dosage of 8 mg/day of dexamethasone for 14 days was found to be more effective in relieving cancer-related fatigue than the placebo. The mean (standard deviation) improvement in the Functional Assessment of Cancer Therapy–Fatigue subscale at day 15 was significantly higher in the dexamethasone group than in the placebo group (9 (10.3) vs 3.1 (9.59), P = 0.008). However, the numbers of grade 3 and higher adverse effects did not significantly differ between dexamethasone and placebo groups at day 15 (17/62 vs 11/58, P = 0.14). Two other multicenter European trials have confirmed that corticosteroids can improve quality of life and reduce fatigue (Della Cuna et al., 1989; Tisdale, 2009).

Corticosteroid effects usually last only 2–4 weeks. In addition, corticosteroids can cause metabolic abnormalities and serious long-term toxic effects, including osteoporosis, myopathies, and increased risk of infections. Therefore, long-term treatment with corticosteroids should usually be avoided. In addition, the best types and doses of corticosteroids as a treatment for fatigue have not been established. Most studies have used doses equivalent to approximately 40 mg/day of prednisone.

Progestational agents

Preliminary studies involving terminally ill patients have demonstrated rapid (within 10 days) improvement in fatigue and general well-being in patients treated with megestrol acetate at a dose of 160–480 mg/day as compared to patients receiving the placebo, without any significant change in nutritional status (Bruera et al., 1998; De Conno et al., 1998). The mechanism of action by which progestational agents confer these benefits is unclear, although it is believed to be related to glucocorticoid or anabolic activity, as well as effects on cytokine release. A randomized controlled study showed that megestrol improves appetite and fatigue and has a better safety profile than corticosteroids. However a meta-analysis of four clinical studies of progestational agents showed no benefit of progestational agents compared with placebo for treating cancer-related fatigue (Minton et al., 2008).

Other agents of potential benefit in the management of cachexia

Other pharmacological agents that have potential benefit in the management of cachexia, such as thalidomide and omega-3 fatty acids, may also have a beneficial effect on fatigue. Thalidomide was found to preserve performance status in a randomized, double-blind, placebo-controlled study of 28 patients with advanced HIV and cachexia (Reyes-Terán et al., 1996). A pilot study of thalidomide (100 mg/day) in 37 evaluable cancer patients with cachexia found that the patients' sense of well-being had improved after 10 days of treatment (Bruera et al., 1999).

Aspirin and other non-steroidal anti-inflammatory agents have been investigated for the treatment of cancer-related symptoms, more specifically in the management of cachexia (Madeddu et al., 2012). There is evidence that these agents were associated not only with reduction of inflammatory markers associated with the cachexia but also with improvement of function and alleviation of quality of life (Madeddu et al., 2012). However, further studies are needed to determine whether treatment of these agents will result in clinically effective improvement of fatigue.

Psychostimulants

Clinical experience with cancer patients indicates that psychostimulants promote a sense of well-being, decrease fatigue, and alleviate depression. Methylphenidate, a presynaptic norepinephrine (noradrenaline) and dopamine reuptake inhibitor, is the most researched psychostimulant drug used in the treatment of fatigue and other symptoms such as depression and sedation in patients with advanced-stage cancer (Minton et al., 2008).

Methylphenidate has been used to manage opioid-induced sedation and depression in the palliative care setting (Bruera et al., 1992; Homsi et al., 2001; Minton et al., 2011; Kerr et al., 2012). A recent meta-analysis of psychostimulants (Minton et al., 2011) concluded that methylphenidate may be effective for fatigue based on the finding of trends towards benefits for the treatment of fatigue and a lack of a significant difference in side effects between methylphenidate and placebo. However, the authors suggested that perhaps larger trials may be able to detect a significant difference between methylphenidate and placebo. They observed that the under-powering of the studies due to small sample sizes could have resulted in the lack of statistically significant difference between the methylphenidate and placebo.

However, since the publication of the meta-analysis, larger studies using long-acting methylphenidate (Moraska et al., 2010) and short-acting methylphenidate for fatigue (Bruera, 2013; Bruera et al., 2013) have again failed to show any statistically significant benefit of methylphenidate as compared to placebo. On the basis of these findings and preliminary data showing some trends of benefit in fatigued patients with depression or anxiety, the authors concluded that future studies are needed to explore the benefits of psychostimulants in a subset of fatigued patients with a predominance of depressed mood or sedation (Bruera, 2013; Bruera et al., 2013).

Modafinil, whose mechanism of action is postulated to be via enhanced catecholaminergic signalling and decreased gamma aminobutyric acid release, primarily at the anterior hypothalamus, has also been shown to have benefits for the treatment of severe fatigue (Jean-Pierre et al., 2007) and impaired cognition (improved attention and psychomotor speed) (Lundorff et al., 2009). In a study in N-(2-chloroethyl)-N-ethyl-2-bromobenzylamine (DSP-4)-treated mice non-noradrenergic, dopamine-dependent adrenergic signalling was associated with the activation of the wake-promoting mechanism of modafinil (Cooper et al., 2009).

Modafinil is indicated in the treatment of excessive daytime sleepiness in patients with narcolepsy and conditions such as Parkinson's disease and obstructive sleep apnoea (Cooper et al., 2009). It appears to have less potential for abuse than amphetamines (Cooper et al., 2009). This agent also reduces fatigue in healthy individuals during sustained mental work and may have fewer side effects than D-amphetamine (Rammohan et al., 2002; Schwartz et al., 2003). A phase III randomized, placebo-controlled double-blind study of 631 cancer patients receiving chemotherapy showed significant benefit of modafinil treatment in a subset of cancer patients with severe fatigue greater or equal to 7/10 in a 0–10 scale (Jean-Pierre et al., 2007).

Modafinil's role in patients with advanced-stage cancer, however, has not been established, and in general, more research is needed to define the role of psychostimulants in the management of fatigue in patients with advanced-stage cancer.

Treatment/management of underlying factors

As previously discussed, fatigue is often multicausal and may appear as a consequence of other conditions, such as cachexia, infection, or anaemia (Yennurajalingam and Bruera, 2007). Any intervention capable of reversing an underlying contributor should alleviate fatigue. Thus, it is useful to consider all factors that may be contributing to fatigue in any given patient, with the aim of identifying and treating reversible causes. It is also important to remember that reversible causes, such as dehydration, metabolic disorders, or severe anaemia, may coexist with non-reversible causes.

Infection

As infections may cause fatigue, they should be treated appropriately. Factors leading to recurrent infections should be addressed where possible.

Anaemia

In patients with anaemia, determining the underlying cause is important, as it may influence the choice of treatment (see Chapter 8.3). Treatment may also be influenced by the speed at which the anaemia develops. Severe anaemia (haemoglobin < 8 g/dL) is usually treated with blood transfusion. A recent prospective study of 61 patients receiving care in a palliative care unit has shown that blood transfusions in patients with a haemoglobin level of < 8 g/dL improved the patients' fatigue, dyspnoea, and well-being for a period of 15 days; however, further studies are needed (Mercadante et al., 2009; Preston et al., 2012). As noted earlier, there is evidence that patients with less severe anaemia also benefit from increases in haemoglobin levels from the use of an erythropoietic-stimulating agent with chemotherapy (Demetri et al., 1998).

In a study of 4382 anaemic cancer patients receiving chemotherapy, improvement of haemoglobin of 2 g/dL or higher after treatment with an erythropoietic-stimulating agent was significantly associated with improvement of fatigue, with maximum benefit occurring when the patients' haemoglobin level improved to 12 g/dL (Crawford et al., 2002).

The main disadvantages of erythropoietic-stimulating agent include its cost, recent evidence that it may cause increased thrombotic events, suggestions that it may reduce survival times (Fishbane and Jhaveri, 2012), and the delay of 4–8 weeks until an increase of 1–2 g/dL in haemoglobin concentration, with resulting symptomatic improvement, can be observed. These disadvantages are particularly relevant in palliative care patients who have a short life expectancy.

Although treatment of anaemia has been shown to decrease fatigue in patients receiving chemotherapy, the correction of anaemia in patients with advanced-stage cancer at the end of life was found to have a limited impact on the intensity of fatigue (Stone et al., 2000; Munch et al., 2005). This is probably due to the fact that multiple factors contribute to fatigue in these patients, including cachexia, depression, pain, and deconditioning.

Autonomic failure

Autonomic failure in patients with diabetes and neurological disorders has been effectively managed by midodrine, a specific alpha

1-sympathomimetic agent (Low et al., 1997, Singer et al., 2006). Other measures that could be considered to treat such patients include (a) adjusting the dosages of medications that contribute to fatigue or ceasing polypharmacy so as to reduce drug interactions, (b) having the patient exercise, (c) increasing the patient's salt intake or considering mineralocorticoid (fludrocortisone), if indicated, and (d) having the patient avoid triggers of autonomic insufficiency, such as large morning meals, heat (including showers), alcohol intake, and motionless standing.

Psychological factors

Counselling should be considered for patients with adjustment disorders, depression, anxiety, and coping difficulties. Various randomized clinical trials have shown that supportive interventions (group and individual), such as education and stress management groups, coping strategies training, and behavioural interventions, can help cancer patients manage their fatigue (Homsi et al., 2001; Jacobsen et al., 2007). Patients with major depression should be treated with antidepressant medication. As in the general population, the choice of antidepressant in a patient with advanced-stage cancer will depend on other patient factors. Selective serotonin reuptake inhibitors are commonly used and have fewer side effects than tricyclic antidepressants. An alternative is to consider using a psychostimulant, such as methylphenidate or modafinil, to treat the depression. Psychostimulants have been found to be effective antidepressants and are also useful in the treatment of opioid-induced sedation (Parker and Brotchie, 2010). An advantage of psychostimulants is their rapid antidepressant effect, which is usually apparent within a few days. Disadvantages include their neurotoxic side effects and the risk that patients will develop tolerance or dependency.

Sleep disturbances

Daytime sleepiness and sleep disturbances have been reported to influence the cancer related fatigue (Berger and Mitchell, 2008; Liu et al, 2012) (see Chapter 8.6). Hence interventions treating sleep disturbances could improve fatigue. Berger et al., in a study of 219 women with breast cancer receiving chemotherapy, found that a 1-year four-component behavioural therapy (BT) sleep intervention (Individualized Sleep Promotion Plan) compared to healthy living control was associated with no significant improvement in fatigue as measured Piper Fatigue Scale; however, global sleep quality as measured by the Pittsburg Sleep Quality Index was improved in the BT group compared to the control (Berger et al., 2009). In a pilot study of 86 advanced-stage cancer patients, Kwekkeboom et al. found that patient-controlled cognitive behavioural intervention for 2 weeks resulted in improvement of pain, fatigue, and sleep disturbance cluster (P = 0.032) compared to patients on wait-list controlled condition (Kwekkeboom et al., 2012). Further studies are warranted, especially those targeting common underlying mechanisms such as inflammation (Liu et al., 2012).

Metabolic disorders

Metabolic disorders, such as hypercalcaemia, hyponatremia, hypomagnesaemia, and hypokalaemia, should be corrected where possible. Endocrine deficiencies, such as hypothyroidism and Addison's disease, require treatment with hormones. Hypogonadism affects two-thirds of men with advanced-stage cancer. Low testosterone in men with cancer is associated with fatigue, anorexia, depression, and insomnia. Testosterone replacement therapy can be considered for patients with hypogonadism. A preliminary placebo-controlled study in 26 evaluable patients with hypogonadic advanced-stage cancer (bioavailable testosterone levels of 70–270 ng/dL) showed a trend towards improvement in the fatigue scores after 4 weeks of treatment using intramuscular testosterone (Pulivarthi et al., 2012). Larger prospective studies are needed to look at the effects of testosterone replacement in cancer patients with fatigue and to determine which of these patients are most likely to benefit from treatment.

Dehydration and hypoxia should be managed as appropriate, and the treatment of underlying cardiac or respiratory conditions should be optimized.

Drug induced

The list of prescribed drugs should be monitored regularly to ensure that the fatigue is not an iatrogenic effect. Fatigue is a common complication of cancer-specific therapy including cytotoxic therapy, radiation therapy, hormonal therapy, surgery, and targeted therapy, and this adverse effect may be dose related.

Nutritional deficiencies

Studies have found that the micronutrient carnitine is frequently deficient in patients with advanced-stage cancer, and preliminary studies using escalating doses (250–3000 mg/day) of carnitine supplementation have shown improvements in fatigue. However, a recent randomized controlled study for the treatment of fatigue in 376 cancer patients showed that 2 g/day of L-carnitine did not significantly improve fatigue compared to a placebo (Cruciani et al., 2012).

Nutritional supplements

Various nutritional supplements such as *Ginseng quinquefolius* (American ginseng), *Paullinia cupana* (guarana), co-enzyme Q10, and L-carnitine, have been investigated in cancer patients to manage fatigue with various levels of success.

In a recently published randomized controlled study, Barton et al. found that American ginseng at a dose of 2000 mg daily over an 8-week period improved cancer fatigue significantly compared to placebo (Barton et al., 2013). Three hundred and sixty-four participants were enrolled from 40 institutions in United States. Changes from baseline in the general subscale of the Multidimensional Fatigue Symptom Inventory—Short Form were 14.4 (standard deviation (SD) = 27.1) in the ginseng arm versus 8.2 (SD = 24.8) in the placebo arm at 4 weeks (P = 0.07). A statistically significant difference was seen at 8 weeks with a change score of 20 (SD = 27) for the ginseng group and 10.3 (SD = 26.1) for the placebo group (P = 0.003). Greater benefit was reported in patients receiving active cancer treatment vs those who had completed treatment. Toxicities per self-report and Common Terminology Criteria for Adverse Events (CTCAE) grading did not differ statistically significantly between arms.

In another study by de Oliveira Campos and colleagues, patients with progressive fatigue after their first cycle of chemotherapy were randomized to receive either *Paullinia cupana* (guarana) 50 mg by mouth twice daily (32 patients) or placebo (43 patients) for 21 days (de Oliveira Campos, 2011). After a 7-day washout period, patients

were crossed over to the opposite experimental arm. All patients were evaluated on days 1, 21, and 49. Guarana significantly improved the Functional Assessment of Chronic Illness Therapy—Fatigue (FACIT-F) score compared to placebo on days 21 and 49 (P < 0.01). The Chalder Scale improved significantly on day 21 (P < 0.01) but not on day 49 (P = 0.27). Guarana did not produce any CTCAE grades 2, 3, or 4 toxicities and did not worsen sleep quality or cause anxiety or depression. Lesser and colleagues found that 300 mg coenzyme Q10 supplementation compared to placebo was not significantly associated with improvement of fatigue as measured by FACIT-F scores at the end 24 weeks (37.6 vs 37.6, P = 0.965) (Lesser et al., 2013). However, further studies are needed in palliative care population to determine the effectiveness and safety of standardized nutritional supplements in patients receiving palliative care.

Nutritional support (enteral and/or parenteral)

Studies in patients with advanced cancer suggest that there is limited evidence to suggest that artificial nutrition improves patient survival, performance status, quality of life, treatment toxicity, or psychological well-being. Further studies are needed to determine which subset of palliative patients would benefit from nutritional support so as to improve fatigue and quality of life (Chermesh et al., 2011; Dev et al., 2012).

Multimodal therapy

Symptomatic treatment of fatigue should be considered in cases in which fatigue is not effectively managed by treatment of reversible causes (Yennurajalingam and Bruera, 2007). In these cases, due to the multidimensional nature of fatigue, it is unlikely that fatigue can be effectively treated using a single intervention. A combination of pharmacological and non-pharmacological treatments should be considered on the basis of a predominant pathophysiological mechanism for a given patient (Bruera and Yennurajalingam, 2010). For example, a patient with a significant component of physical fatigue may benefit from a combination of dexamethasone and exercise tailored to the patient's needs. Similarly, various combinations of treatment that have shown preliminary beneficial effects on fatigue in patients with advanced-stage cancer should be considered on an individual basis. These may include interventions such as cognitive behavioural therapy, educational interventions, anti-inflammatory drugs, and exercise. However, further studies using sound research methodology are needed to investigate the efficacy of multimodal intervention in patients with fatigue.

Conclusion

Fatigue in cancer patients is now accepted as a symptom that should be studied in its own right. Unfortunately, few studies have addressed fatigue in palliative cancer populations. Consequently, most of the insight into the complexity of fatigue must be based upon extrapolation from studies performed with patients earlier in the disease trajectory. To improve treatment, we must gain a better understanding of the many aspects of fatigue. Thus, identifying the pathophysiological mechanisms that cause fatigue is important. Assessment and staging tools that are valid and reliable are needed to assist in clinical practice and research. Clinical syndromes of fatigue (cognitive, affective, and physical) also must be better characterized. The roles of nutritional interventions and commonly used agents, such as corticosteroids, also need to be more thoroughly investigated. The potential of agents such as eicosapentaenoic acid, thalidomide, and anabolic steroids must be explored in studies in which fatigue is a primary endpoint. Finally, the role of psychostimulants should be further researched, and the importance of counselling, rest, and exercise in cancer patients receiving palliative care should be clarified.

Online materials

Complete references for this chapter are available online at <http://www.oxfordmedicine.com>.

References

Barsevick, A., Frost, M., Zwinderman, A., Hall, P., and Halyard, M. (2010). I'm so tired: biological and genetic mechanisms of cancer-related fatigue. *Quality of Life Research*, 19, 1419–1427.

Barton, D.L., Liu, H., Dakhil, S.R., *et al.* (2013). Wisconsin Ginseng (Panax quinquefolius) to improve cancer-related fatigue: a randomized, double-blind trial, N07C2. *Journal of the National Cancer Institute*, 105, 1230–1238.

Berger, A.M., Abernethy, A.P., Atkinson, A., *et al.* (2010). Cancer-related fatigue. *Journal of the National Comprehensive Cancer Network*, 8, 904–931.

Kerr, C.W., Drake, J., Milch, R.A., *et al.* (2012). Effects of methylphenidate on fatigue and depression: a randomized, double-blind, placebo-controlled trial. *Journal of Pain and Symptom Management*, 43, 68–77.

Minton, O., Richardson, A., Sharpe, M., Hotopf, M., and Stone, P. (2008). A systematic review and meta-analysis of the pharmacological treatment of cancer-related fatigue. *Journal of the National Cancer Institute*, 100, 1155–1166.

Minton, O., Richardson, A., Sharpe, M., Hotopf, M., and Stone, P.C. (2011). Psychostimulants for the management of cancer-related fatigue: a systematic review and meta-analysis. *Journal of Pain and Symptom Management*, 41, 761–767.

Molassiotis, A., Bardy, J., Finnegan-John, J., *et al.* (2012). Acupuncture for cancer-related fatigue in patients with breast cancer: a pragmatic randomized controlled trial. *Journal of Clinical Oncology*, 30, 4470–4476.

Oldervoll, L.M., Loge, J.H., Lydersen, S., *et al.* (2011). Physical exercise for cancer patients with advanced disease: a randomized controlled trial. *The Oncologist*, 16, 1649–1657.

Yennurajalingam, S. and Bruera, E. (2007). Palliative management of fatigue at the close of life. *Journal of the American Medical Association*, 297, 295–304.

Yennurajalingam, S., Frisbee-Hume, S., Delgado-Guay, M.O., Bull, J., and Bruera, E. (2012). Dexamethasone (DM) for cancer-related fatigue: a double-blinded, randomized, placebo-controlled trial. *Journal of Clinical Oncology*, 31, 3076–3082.

8.2

Dyspnoea and other respiratory symptoms in palliative care

Kin-Sang Chan, Doris M.W. Tse, and Michael M.K. Sham

Introduction to dyspnoea and other respiratory symptoms in palliative care

A breath is a vital sign of a living creature. When one dies, one expires. A breath, however, serves more than physiological purposes. A sigh often carries unspeakable messages from the inner being. Hence a breath may be filled with physiological, psychological, and spiritual signals.

Breathing, an automatic activity which one undergoes hundreds of millions of cycles throughout one's life, is mostly effortless. Breathlessness serves as a warning signal in responding to the metabolic demand on a person. When the respiratory system is compromised by diseases, every breath may become laborious. Every day, millions of people throughout the world are distressed by breathlessness and other respiratory symptoms. Control of respiratory symptoms remains challenging towards the end of life.

Dyspnoea becomes an important factor predicting the will to live in the terminally ill while approaching death (Chochinov et al., 1999). Relieving distress related to respiratory symptoms is key to addressing suffering.

Definition of dyspnoea

The American Thoracic Society defines dyspnoea as 'a subjective experience of breathing discomfort that consists of qualitatively distinct sensations that vary in intensity' (American Thoracic Society, 1999).The experience is derived from interactions among physiological, psychological, social, and environmental factors, and may induce secondary physiological and behavioural responses. Dyspnoea per se can only be perceived by the person experiencing it. Perception entails conscious recognition and interpretation of sensory stimuli and their meaning (Parshall et al., 2012). Dyspnoea is a term we use for a symptom that patients often describe as breathlessness. In the following text, the two terms are used interchangeably.

Dyspnoea prevalence, pattern, and trajectory

Dyspnoea is common among patients with advanced cancers and non-cancer life-limiting illnesses. The prevalence of dyspnoea varies with the site of primary cancers and the stage of illness. In patients with primary lung cancers, the prevalence of dyspnoea reported ranges from 75% to 87% (Muers and Round, 1993; Smith et al., 2001). In a systematic review comparing the prevalence of 11 symptoms in patients with advanced cancer, AIDS, heart disease, chronic obstructive pulmonary disease (COPD), and renal disease, breathlessness was found in more than 50% of patients (Solano et al., 2006). Dyspnoea was prevalent among 10–70% of patients with cancer, 90–95% of patients with COPD, 60–88% of patients with heart disease, 11–62% of patients with AIDS, and 11–62% of patients with renal disease. In a cohort of 5682 palliative care patients, breathlessness increased from around 50% at 3 months before death to 65% at the time of death, with severe breathlessness increased from less than 10% to 26% at the two time points respectively. Absence of breathlessness between referral and death was only recorded in 11.4% of patients (Currow et al., 2010).

Two patterns of dyspnoea have been reported by cancer patients: the breakthrough-only dyspnoea in 61%, and constant dyspnoea in 39% of patients, among which 20% presented as breakthrough episodes (Reddy et al., 2009). The majority of patients with breakthrough episodes presented with fewer than five episodes daily, with each episode frequently lasting for less than 10 minutes. Simon et al. (2013b) observed two categories of breathlessness among patients with chronic heart failure, COPD, lung cancer, and motor neurone disease: episodic breathlessness that occurs in less than 24 hours (seconds, minutes, or hours) and continuous breathlessness lasting more than 24 hours (days to weeks or months or years). Episodic breathlessness could be triggered by exertion, emotion, or environment; or occur spontaneously without trigger. It could also occur independently or on top of continuous breathlessness. However, episodic breathlessness was only reported as a primary outcome in eight among 27 studies (Simon et al., 2013a).

Dyspnoea along the trajectory of life-limiting illnesses has been evaluated by several longitudinal studies. Bausewein et al. (2010) studied individual and summary trajectories of breathlessness of cancer and COPD patients at baseline and monthly over 6 months or until death. In people with COPD, breathlessness increased over time, on average by one Borg score over 6 months, while in people with cancer, breathlessness increased in the last month of life and towards death. Four breathlessness trajectory patterns have been identified: fluctuating, increasing, stable, and decreasing, with fluctuating breathlessness being most common in people with both severe COPD and advanced cancer (Bausewein et al., 2010).

In a cohort study of 5862 patients by Currow and colleagues, breathlessness as assessed at three time points before death (60–53 days, 30–23 days, and 7–0 days) was compared between cancer and non-cancer patients (heart failure, end-stage pulmonary disease, and no identifiable cardiopulmonary cause) (Currow et al., 2010). Patients with non-cancer diagnoses had significantly higher levels of breathlessness at all three time points, while cancer patients had less breathlessness initially but increased significantly at day 10 and day 3 before death. In another cohort of over 10,000 cancer patients, the trajectories of performance status and symptom scores during the last 6 months of life were evaluated (Seow et al., 2011). Breathlessness increased in severity over time, particularly in the month before death. With functional decline or towards the end of life, the intensity of dyspnoea progressively increased as Karnofsky Performance Status (KPS) score fell below 60 and peaked between KPS scores of 30 and 20 (Mercadante et al., 2000).

Qualities of dyspnoea and neurophysiology

There are at least three separate qualities of dyspnoea: air hunger or unsatisfied inspiration; work or effort; and tightness (Lansing et al., 2009; Parshall et al., 2012). This classification depends on different perceptual qualities with distinct afferent sources:

1. *Air hunger or unsatisfied inspiration*: this is the conscious perception of the urge to breathe. Patients describe this as 'I cannot get enough air', 'My breaths don't satisfy me', or 'I'm starving for air'. This sense of air hunger can be experimentally induced by hypercapnia, hypoxia, exercise, or acidosis, all leading to increase in respiratory drive. The signal comes from the motor drive of the respiratory centres in the brainstem, and is conveyed to the cerebral cortex as corollary discharge. When this is not matched by an adequate ventilatory response by feedback from afferent receptors throughout the respiratory system, individuals perceive air hunger or unsatisfied inspiration. Afferent information about the pulmonary ventilation achieved from mechanoreceptors in the lungs, airways, and chest wall can relieve or inhibit air hunger or unsatisfied inspiration. Air hunger is positively correlated with automatic drive to breathe (i.e. brainstem motor activity), and negatively correlated with the amount of ventilation.

2. *Work or effort*: this is an uncomfortable sense of respiratory work and effort. Patients describe this as 'It's an effort to breathe', or 'My breathing requires more work'. The perceptions of work and effort probably arise through some combinations of respiratory muscle afferents and perceived cortical motor command or 'corollary discharge' projecting to sensory areas. The sense of work or effort can be produced experimentally by external resistive or elastic load, volitional hyperpnoea, or by weakening of the respiratory muscles.

3. *Tightness*: tightness appears to be specific to bronchoconstriction. Patients describe this as 'My chest feels tight or constricted'. The sensation of tightness arises from pulmonary afferents through the stimulation of airway receptors.

Neuroimaging by positron emission tomography (PET) and functional magnetic resonance imaging (fMRI) has been employed recently for locating the activating areas during dyspnoea. The most consistent and the strongest area of activation is in the right anterior insula (Lansing et al., 2009; Parshall et al., 2012). Other activations can be seen in the left anterior insula, anterior cingulate, supplementary motor area, prefrontal cortex, cerebellum, and amygdala (Parshall et al., 2012). Dyspnoea is associated with activation of cortico-limbic structures, which overlap with that observed in pain (Lansing et al., 2009; Parshall et al., 2012). As demonstrated by fMRI, the unpleasantness of perceived dyspnoea is processed in the right insula and amygdala (von Leupoldt et al., 2008).

Similar to the pain model, it is postulated that dyspnoea consists of multiple dimensions, including the independent component of sensory dimension (sensory intensity and sensory quality), immediate affective stage which trigger immediate behaviour, and a stage of cognitive evaluative and emotional response which affects long-term behaviour (Lansing et al., 2009). Against the traditional neurochemical and neuromuscular model, a neuromatrix-gated model has been proposed to unify multiple factors by recognizing different inputs from afferents at receptor levels and inputs from different areas of the brain (Williams, 2011).

The impact of dyspnoea

Breathlessness correlates with survival and is a predictor of poor prognosis in cancer. In a systematic review of the value of symptom assessment to predict survival in people with advanced cancer, dyspnoea was evaluated in 35 studies involving 9155 patients (out of 44 studies included). Dyspnoea was correlated with survival in 22 studies in univariate analysis, and in ten studies in multivariate analysis. In 23 studies including 6806 patients in the symptom-oriented palliation stage, dyspnoea was also a predictor for survival in multivariate analysis in 30–50% of studies (Trajkovic-Vidakovic et al., 2012). Dyspnoea is one of six parameters used in the Palliative Prognostic Score that predicts 30-day survival of palliative care patients (Pirovano et al., 1999).

Dyspnoea also affects advanced cancer patients through individuals' symptom experience. Previous studies have shown that dyspnoea often brings panic, fear, anxiety, depression, hopelessness, sense of loss of control, and impending death to patients (Gysels et al., 2007). Dyspnoea affects daily and social functions, leading to dependence and loss of role. A more recent study on people with advanced cancer found that dyspnoea was closely associated with fatigue, pain, and depression on multivariate analysis, and interfering with general activities, mood, and enjoyment of life (Reddy et al., 2009). A qualitative study illustrated the meaning of breathlessness experience among patients with cancer, COPD, heart failure, and motor neurone disease (Gysels and Higginson, 2011). For people with cancer, breathlessness, apart from being a signal of cancer, is also a reminder of mortality, despite their optimism with treatment. In people with COPD, breathlessness is perceived as self-inflicted resulting from life-time smoking. People are alarmed by the debilitation caused by breathlessness often in the later stages of disease because of its insidious nature. For people with heart failure, breathlessness is associated with functional limitations and contributes to the negative effects of other symptoms. In people with motor neurone disease, breathlessness makes people realize that the illness affects mechanisms essential for living (Gysels and Higginson, 2011).

Under-recognition of dyspnoea by health-care workers adds to people's helplessness. Each person has to develop their own coping strategies (O'Driscoll et al., 1999).

Clinical assessment of dyspnoea

Clinical assessment of dyspnoea aims at identification of all underlying causes of dyspnoea and assessment of the distress and impact as experienced by patient so as to guide the management plan. The vehicles for assessment should include detailed history taking and physical examination, carefully selected investigations, and the use of dyspnoea measuring tools appropriate to the clinical context.

History taking

No objective test can replace a patient's own description of the symptom and its experience. Apart from information that helps in elucidating the underlying causes of dyspnoea, a good history from a dyspnoeic patient should include the quality of dyspnoea, its profile (episodic or constant), intensity, associated distress or affective states, impact on the patient's life, and concerns of the patients and caregivers (online Table 8.2.2).

Physical examination

Physical examination is important in evaluating the severity of the clinical situation and the possible underlying causes. Patients with severe dyspnoea may not be able to provide a history, appear exhausted, and have to sit up while breathing rapidly. In such circumstances, initial management plans rely on findings from physical examination and preliminary bedside tests. Warning signs calling for urgent review include the presence of stridor, marked tachypnoea (e.g. respiratory rate > 30 breaths per minute), tachycardia (e.g. heart rate > 130 per minute), marked respiratory distress, and altered level of consciousness (online Table 8.2.3).

Investigations

Investigations, when carefully selected, help to elucidate the underlying cause(s) of dyspnoea and guide the management plan for patients at different stages of illness. The choice of investigations depends on the balance of their benefits and burdens, treatment goals, and patients' preferences. First-line investigations include haemoglobin level, oxygen saturation by oximetry, and, if indicated chest radiograph. The intensity of dyspnoea correlates poorly with degree of hypoxaemia (Bruera et al., 2000) and lung function parameters (Heyse-Moore et al., 2000) and therefore these tests cannot substitute for a patient's own report of dyspnoea. Changes in the chest radiograph including shadows of lung parenchyma, pleura, airway, mediastinum, diaphragm, cardiac silhouette, and pulmonary vessels should be systematically observed.

Specialized investigations are less readily available in palliative care setting. Rarely are arterial blood gases indicated. Lung function tests with a flow volume loop are helpful to look for upper airway obstruction. Maximum inspiratory pressure or nasal sniff inspiratory pressure can detect inspiratory muscle weakness. Echocardiography and Doppler ultrasound may serve diagnostic or guide therapeutic procedures in pericardial or pleural effusion, heart failure, deep vein thrombosis, and pulmonary embolism. D-dimer is raised in cancer and has limited value for diagnosis of pulmonary embolism.

Third-line investigations should be considered in highly selected cases. Computed tomography (CT) may be valuable in delineating conditions including pulmonary embolism, major airway obstruction, superior vena cava obstruction, and lymphangitis carcinomatosis.

Measurement of dyspnoea

For the comprehensive assessment of dyspnoea as a multidimensional symptom, a dyspnoea measuring tool should reflect the subjective sensory experience of individual patients, provide objective measurement of dyspnoea, and serve as an effective means for communication to health-care workers. There are three domains of dyspnoea measurement as proposed by the American Thoracic Society in 2012 (Parshall et al., 2012). They are:

1. *Sensory-perceptual experience*: this includes ratings of symptom intensity, frequency, duration, and the sensory quality. Dyspnoea intensity can be assessed by a visual analogue scale, Borg scale, Likert-type ratings, or numerical rating scale (NRS). Dyspnoea is also among the symptoms assessed in validated multidimensional symptom assessment tools such as the Memorial Symptom Assessment Scale and Edmonton Symptom Assessment Scale. For the sensory quality, Simon and colleagues reported 15 dyspnoea descriptors used by breathless patients in eight clusters (rapid, exhalation, shallow, work, suffocating, hunger, tight, and heavy) (Simon et al., 1990). Simon et al. suggested the possible associations of dyspnoea descriptors with the specific conditions producing dyspnoea (Simon et al., 1990), but a subsequent study by Wilcock et al. (2002) failed to demonstrate the robustness of these descriptors in assisting diagnosis when applied to patients with cancer and cardiopulmonary diseases.

2. *Affective distress*: this may refer to the immediate distress (e.g. unpleasantness) or the cognitive-evaluated distress subsequent to appraisal of its meaning or consequences. Distress or unpleasantness may be rated as a single item as in the case for dyspnoea intensity. Scales with multiple items, such as the Cancer Dyspnoea Scale, assess emotional responses including anxiety (Tanaka et al., 2000).

3. *Symptom impact or burden*: this includes the effect of dyspnoea on behaviour, functions, quality of life (QOL), or health status. The Medical Research Council (MRC) scale provides unidimensional rating of disability (Mahler and Wells, 1988), while the Chronic Respiratory Disease Questionnaire (CRQ) is a multidimensional scale used for assessment of functional abilities (Guyatt et al., 1987). Various QOL scales have been validated for use in cancer or specific for lung cancer and in chronic lung diseases, for example, CRQ (Guyatt et al., 1987), EuroQol 5D (EuroQol Group, 1990), FACT-L (Cella et al., 1995), QLQ-C15-PAL (Groenvold et al., 2006), and QLQ-LC13 (Bergman et al., 1994).

Currently there are over 50 dyspnoea measurements scales readily available to readers (Parshall et al., 2012) covering various domains of dyspnoea and different diseases. However, a unified dyspnoea measurement tool for clinical use in palliative care setting is still lacking. One may consider combining rating of dyspnoea intensity with assessment of the impact of dyspnoea on a patient's QOL (Bausewein et al., 2008b), the NRS, Modified Borg Scale, CRQ-dyspnoea scale, Motor Neurone Disease Rating Scale (modelled on the CRQ), and Cancer Dyspnoea Scale appear most suitable for the palliative care setting (Dorman et al., 2007).

Elucidate the underlying causes of dyspnoea

Multiple underlying causes may coexist in a patient with dyspnoea. Causes of dyspnoea can be classified according to malignant, paramalignant, or non-malignant causes and cardiopulmonary causes versus systemic causes (Table 8.2.1).

Table 8.2.1 Causes of dyspnoea and management of potential treatable causes

Malignant and paramalignant causes	**Cardiopulmonary causes**	**Treatment**
	Lung cancer	Chemotherapy in selected patients
	Secondary to lung	Molecular targeted therapy for adenocarcinoma of lung with epidermal growth factor receptor mutation
	Pleural effusion	Repeated thoracentesis
		Chemical pleurodesis: talc 90% efficacious
		Thoracoscopic pleurodesis more effective than medical pleurodesis (Shaw and Agarwal, 2004)
		Indwelling pleural catheter (especially for trap lung) (Davies et al., 2012)
	Superior vena cava obstruction	Stents (95% have relief and faster) (Rowell and Gleeson, 2001)
		Chemotherapy and radiotherapy (60% in NSCLC)
		Trial of steroid, diuretics
	Pulmonary embolism	Low-molecular-weight heparin (more efficacious than warfarin)
	Pericardial effusion	Pericardiocentesis, catheter drainage, pericardial window, pericardiotomy
	Major airway obstruction	Radiotherapy, bronchial stent, endobronchial treatment- laser therapy, cryotherapy
		Trial of steroid
	Lymphangitis carcinomatosis	Trial of steroid
	Radiation-induced pneumonitis	Trial of steroid
	Drug-induced pneumonitis	Trial of steroid
	Chest infection	Antibiotics according to sensitivity
	Systemic causes	
	Cancer cachexia	Prevention of aspiration
	Ascites	Abdominal paracentesis
	Gross hepatomegaly	Prop up position
Non-malignant causes	**Cardiopulmonary causes**	**Treatment**
	COPD	Non-pharmacological therapy, breathing exercise
		Inhaled short acting bronchodilators, Inhaled long acting bronchodilators (beta$_2$ -agonist, anticholinergic), inhaled steroid, theophylline, phosphodiesterase-4 inhibitors
	Bronchiectasis	Airway clearance, antibiotics for infective exacerbation
	Interstitial pulmonary fibrosis	
	Congestive heart failure	Angiotensin converting enzyme inhibitors, beta-blockers/hydralazine + nitrate
		Angiotensin receptor blockers, spironolactone
		Digoxin, diuretics
	Arrhythmias	Anti-arrhythmic agents
	Systemic causes	
	Muscle weakness: motor neuron disease, muscular dystrophy	Non-invasive ventilation
	Anaemia	Blood transfusion, erythropoietin
	Acidosis	NaHCO$_3$
	Deconditioning	Exercise
	Respiratory panic attack	Anxiety management, benzodiazepines

Management of dyspnoea

The objectives of dyspnoea are to reduce its frequency and severity, minimize its psychological and spiritual distress, and maximize patients' function and QOL. To achieve these goals, identification of all of the underlying causes of dyspnoea are required, and use of specific or combinations of modalities of management may include the following:

1. Specific disease management

2. Non-pharmacological intervention

3. Pharmacological treatment

4. Palliative non- invasive ventilation

5. Palliative sedation.

Specific disease management

The underlying diseases causing dyspnoea, when reversible or modifiable, should be treated accordingly (Table 8.2.1). Among the diverse causes of dyspnoea, some have the propensity to present with acute, and even life-threatening dyspnoea, including tension pneumothorax, large pleural effusion, asthma attack, COPD exacerbation, fulminant chest infection, acute pulmonary oedema, arrhythmia, major airway obstruction, pulmonary embolism, cardiac tamponade, and metabolic acidosis. Clinicians may face the dilemma of having to decide on the extent of disease-specific and life-sustaining treatments in the presence of a life-limiting illness. Diagnosing the end of life in people with organ failure may be particularly difficult as the disease trajectory is fluctuating and less predictable.

Disease-modifying treatments are often applicable despite the progressive nature of cancer and other chronic debilitating diseases. Emergence of newer chemotherapeutic agents and targeted therapies such as tyrosine kinase inhibitors, monoclonal antibodies, and angiogenesis inhibitors have changed the landscape of cancer treatment with palliative intent, offering opportunity for life prolongation and symptom control. On the other hand, there is evidence that early palliative care integrated with standard oncology care for patients with metastatic non-small cell lung cancer (NSCLC) improves QOL (Temel et al., 2010). A randomized controlled trial (RCT) also showed that metastatic NSCLC patients assigned to early palliative care had a better QOL, less depressive symptoms, longer median survival, received less aggressive chemotherapy, and were more likely to be enrolled in hospice compared to patients receiving standard oncology care (Temel et al., 2010; Greer et al., 2012).

Disease-specific needs of patients with non-cancer diseases should also be recognized. Palliative care has been developing for patients with advanced COPD, chronic heart failure, end-stage renal failure, and neuromuscular and degenerative diseases. A collaborative model involving the palliative care team and other respective specialty teams should be considered to ensure access for patients to disease-specific treatments when indicated.

In both cancer and non-cancer diseases, the palliative care phase may go hand in hand with the disease-modifying phase. As disease progresses, symptom palliation will be more relevant than disease modification as the primary treatment goal. Dyspnoea-based care, such as the Breathlessness Intervention Service at Addenbrooke's Hospital, United Kingdom, has been established recently for management of dyspnoea caused by different diseases (Booth et al., 2011).

Non-pharmacological interventions

'Non-pharmacological interventions' is a broad term referring to any non-drug therapy and its scope for management of dyspnoea is developing. Non-pharmacological interventions for dyspnoea aim at improving the symptom experience and addressing the multidimensional needs of patients that are identified by comprehensive assessment (Booth et al., 2011). Non-pharmacological intervention may be delivered as a single component or as multiple components by health-care professionals including nurses, physiotherapists, occupational therapists, psychologists, and social workers in a multidisciplinary team.

The spectrum of non-pharmacological interventions varies from low-complexity interventions such as positioning to more sophisticated psychological interventions.

The effectiveness of non-pharmacological interventions for breathlessness in patients with advanced malignant and non-malignant diseases (mostly COPD) (Bausewein et al., 2008a), and patients with lung cancer (Rueda et al., 2011), has been reported in two Cochrane reviews. A further review of six systematic reviews of non-pharmacological interventions was recently published (Yates and Zhao, 2012). The following non-pharmacological interventions have been reviewed with different levels of evidence:

Interventions that are supported by good evidence

Breathing training (Bausewein et al., 2008a): as shallow breathing and dynamic hyperinflation increase breathlessness, the following breathing techniques may counteract this mechanism to improve breathing efficiency, including pursed-lipped breathing, diaphragmatic breathing, 'blow-as-you-go', positioning, and pacing technique. Two out of three studies in people with COPD showed positive outcomes. Activity pacing and energy conservation techniques are often taught together with breathing training, but this is less supported by evidence.

Walking aids (Bausewein et al., 2008a): wheeled-walker/rollators are helpful to relieve dyspnoea. Four out of seven studies in people with COPD showed positive results. Walking aids probably exert their effects on breathlessness by increasing the maximal voluntary ventilation as patients brace the arms on the walking aid and lean forward.

Neuromuscular electric stimulation (Bausewein et al., 2008a): muscle deconditioning and wasting can contribute to breathlessness. This modality is particularly useful for patients who are too weak to exercise. Increase in walking distance and decrease in dyspnoea have been reported by three trials performed in people with COPD.

Chest wall vibration (Bausewein et al., 2008a): modifies respiratory sensations by activation of muscle spindles in the intercostal muscles. In the studies of people with motor neurone disease and COPD, there was significant reduction in dyspnoea in four out of five studies.

Exercise (Koelwyn et al., 2012): has been shown to be effective for relieving dyspnoea in COPD but evidence for cancer is conflicting.

Interventions that are supported by some evidence

Handheld fan (Bausewein et al., 2008a): cool air has been shown to reduce the sensation of breathlessness in normal subjects. The effect of handheld fans was demonstrated by a randomized controlled crossover trial reported by Galbraith et al. (2010). Bausewein et al. compared the fan with a waistband but were unable to demonstrate any benefit over 2 months. However 50% of patients continued to use the fan compared to 20% who used the waistband.

Nurse follow-up programmes (Rueda et al., 2011): three trials on nursing intervention showed benefits in terms of symptom experience, emotional functioning, and performance status.

Acupuncture/ acupressure (Bausewein et al., 2008a): four studies were performed in people with COPD, one study in people with cancer and mixed patients respectively. The results are conflicting.

Interventions that require more evidence

Various interventions including relaxation, music, counselling support, counselling and support with breathing-relaxation training, case management, and psychotherapy are frequently practised (Bausewein et al., 2008a), but require more studies to confirm their effectiveness or the populations who will most benefit from them.

Pharmacological treatment

Unlike pain which has specific pain receptors which can be targeted by pain control treatments, the sensations of dyspnoea are mediated through multiple neurophysiological mechanisms. As the evidence supporting different pharmacological treatments in relieving dyspnoea are emerging, they can be grouped under three categories. A combined modalities approach involving several treatments has not yet been formally evaluated (Clemens et al., 2012).

1. Treatments with clear evidence: oxygen and opioids.

2. Treatments with some evidence: anxiolytics, nebulized furosemide, and Heliox.

3. Treatments with limited evidence: antidepressants, phenothiazines, indomethacin, and inhaled topical anaesthetics.

Pharmacological treatments with clear evidence

Oxygen therapy

Hypoxia triggers the sense of air hunger by stimulation of peripheral chemoreceptor. However, it has been shown that dyspnoea in the terminally ill does not correlate with the degree of hypoxaemia (Bruera et al., 2000). This can be explained by the multiple causes of dyspnoea in cancer. Oxygen therapy has been widely used in acute hypoxaemic conditions, while its long-term use in chronic hypoxaemic COPD to improve survival has been supported by studies. In palliative care settings, oxygen is mainly used for symptom relief of dyspnoea without fulfilling the criteria of long-term oxygen therapy, described by the term 'palliative oxygen therapy'. Palliative oxygen therapy has been studied in the following conditions:

Palliative oxygen for advanced cancer patients

Six RCTs were conducted to compare oxygen with air, with two trials on hypoxaemic patients, combined hypoxaemia, and non-hypoxaemic patients, and non-hypoxaemic patients respectively (Ben-Aharon et al., 2008). In studies on hypoxaemic patients, oxygen therapy was more effective than air in a single advanced-cancer patient by the N-of-1 RCT (Bruera et al., 1992) and in 12 hypoxaemic cancer patients (Bruera et al., 1993),

However, in a meta-analysis of the RCTs on combined hypoxaemia and non-hypoxaemic patients, oxygen was not superior to air in relieving dyspnoea (Uronis et al., 2008).

Palliative oxygen for non-hypoxaemic COPD

In a systematic review of 18 trials on people with COPD (N = 431), oxygen reduced dyspnoea with a standardized mean difference of -0.37 (95% confidence interval (CI) -0.50 to -0.24, $p < 0.00001$) (Uronis et al., 2011). The reviewers concluded that oxygen can relieve dyspnoea in mildly and non-hypoxaemic COPD patients, who otherwise would not fulfil the criteria for long-term oxygen therapy. Because of the significant heterogenicity among the studies reviewed, use of oxygen in COPD should be evaluated on an individual basis. In another RCT on 143 COPD patients without resting hypoxaemia, ambulatory oxygen, as compared with air, had no benefits in terms of dyspnoea relief, functional improvement, and QOL (Moore et al., 2011).

Palliative oxygen for patients with mixed diagnoses

Palliative oxygen has been evaluated in patients with mixed diagnoses but with no definite benefit proven. A 4-year consecutive cohort from a regional community palliative care service was reviewed to assess the effectiveness of home oxygen therapy on breathlessness (Currow et al., 2009). Out of the 5862 study population, 1239 patients (21.1%) were prescribed oxygen, and 413 patients had before and after data that could be evaluated, among which the majority had cancer (n = 270). There were no significant differences between the mean dyspnoea scores before and after 1 and 2 weeks of home oxygen. Among the 413 patients, about one-third had significant improvement in breathlessness (more than 20% improvement in mean dyspnoea scores), but demographic factors, baseline breathlessness or underlying causes of breathlessness failed to predict these responders.

In a well-designed RCT reported by Abernethy and colleagues, palliative oxygen was compared against room air in 239 patients with life-limiting illnesses. The majority were non-hypoxaemic with a mixed diagnosis of COPD and other lung diseases (73.6%), followed by primary and secondary lung cancer (15.9%) (Abernethy et al., 2010). These patients were non-hypoxaemic but suffered from refractory dyspnoea. Breathlessness and QOL as assessed twice a day at baseline and day 6 showed improvements in both arms, but with no significant difference between oxygen and room air. The authors concluded that oxygen provides no additional symptomatic benefit to room air for relief of refractory dyspnoea in non-hypoxaemic patients with life-limiting illnesses. The effect of air flow in decreasing dyspnoea may account for the effect in the control arm.

Palliative oxygen for patients with chronic heart failure

Three cross-over studies compared the use of oxygen inhalation to air inhalation in adults with stable chronic heart failure for dyspnoea management during exercise testing (Cranston et al., 2008). A systematic review conducted in 2008 failed to demonstrate a consistent beneficial effect of oxygen inhalation over air inhalation (Cranston et al., 2008). More updated studies in this area are lacking. Based on the observation that one-third of people with chronic heart failure have sleep-disordered breathing with intermittent hypoxaemia at night, the value of oxygen for nocturnal hypoxaemia associated with sleep disordered breathing deserves further evaluation.

Based on the above evidence and a systematic review (Davidson and Johnson, 2011), it is recommended that oxygen should only be prescribed to patients with hypoxaemia for its survival effect in COPD and possibly symptomatic benefits in other life-limiting illnesses especially if people are relatively hypoxaemic. For non-hypoxaemic patients with life-limiting illnesses, the effectiveness of palliative oxygen for relieving breathlessness is similar to air and there is no evidence to support its routine use.

Opioids for breathlessness

In a study on 17 COPD patients undergoing treadmill exercise, the level of endogenous opioids released demonstrates the role of opioids in modulating breathlessness (Mahler et al., 2009). The blood beta-endorphin levels increased threefold from rest to end-exercise. Patients received either blinded naloxone or normal saline intravenously before crossing over in a subsequent study. The peak ratings of breathlessness and regression slope of breathlessness as a function of oxygen consumption were significantly higher with naloxone than normal saline. The effectiveness of opioids in relieving dyspnoea has been studied among people with cancer, COPD, and chronic heart failure.

Opioids for breathlessness in cancer patients

There were six RCTs on the use of opioids in cancer patients (Ben-Aharon et al., 2008). Two studies, reported by Mazocatto et al. (1999) and Bruera et al. (1993), compared subcutaneous morphine with placebo, showed improvement of dyspnoea with subcutaneous injection of morphine. Another two studies reported by Davis et al. (1996) and Grimbert et al. (2004) comparing nebulized morphine with placebo showed no significant difference between nebulized morphine and placebo. One study by Bruera et al. (1993) compared subcutaneous morphine with nebulized morphine reported no significant difference between the two routes. Lastly, Allard et al. (1999) studied the morphine dose adjustments for breathlessness control in patients who previously treated with opioid and found no significant difference in dyspnoea with 25% or 50% increments of morphine dosage.

Opioids for breathlessness in COPD patients

A systematic review by Jennings and colleagues on the use of opioids in the management of dyspnoea identified nine placebo controlled studies of oral or parenteral opioids and nine studies of nebulized opioids (Jennings et al., 2002). All nine studies on systemic opioids and three out of nine nebulized opioid studies were recruited for meta-analysis. Seven systemic and two nebulized studies were COPD studies. The meta-analysis on the subgroup of COPD studies showed a highly significant result in reducing dyspnoea (p = 0.004) with a standardized mean difference of −0.26. The nebulized opioid group failed to show positive effect (p = 0.31).

The strongest evidence was shown by a double-blind controlled trial by Abernethy et al. with 48 opioid naïve breathless patients (Abernethy et al., 2003). The majority of patients (87.5%) had COPD, who were assigned to receive 20 mg once-daily oral sustained-release morphine or placebo for 4 days, followed by 4 days of cross over. Participants of the morphine arm reported significant improvement in dyspnoea scores and sleep.

Opioids for breathlessness in chronic heart failure patients

There were three RCTs with two yielding positive outcomes and the other recent study with a negative outcome. The first double-blind randomized study was performed in 11 men with chronic heart failure who received either dihydrocodeine or placebo as a single dose (Chua et al., 1997). There was a significant fall in hypoxic and hypercapnic chemosensitivities with dihydrocodeine 1 hour after administration when compared to placebo, together with significant improvement in exercise duration and reduction in dyspnoea.

Another double-blind, cross-over RCT was performed by Johnson in ten patients with chronic heart failure (New York Heart Association (NYHA) class III/IV) (Johnson et al., 2002). Oral morphine 5 mg four times daily was given for 4 days, followed by a 2-day wash out period and then crossed over. There was significant reduction in dyspnoea and five patients were on morphine for 1 year upon follow-up.

A larger-scale RCT on 39 people with chronic heart failure (NYHA class III/IV) was reported (Oxberry et al., 2011). Oral morphine, oral oxycodone, and placebo were given for 4 days each, followed by a 3-day washout and cross over. Breathlessness severity was reduced from baseline with all three interventions, with no statistically significant difference between the two active interventions and placebo. With these conflicting results, the role of opioids for relieving dyspnoea in chronic heart failure requires further study.

Opioids for breathlessness in interstitial lung disease and amyotrophic lateral sclerosis patients

The use of low-dose nebulized morphine (2.5 and 5.0 mg) for relieving dyspnoea in severe interstitial lung disease was not supported by a single RCT with six patients as reported by a Cochrane review (Polosa et al., 2002). A recent RCT reported the effectiveness of nebulized morphine on dyspnoea of mustard gas-exposed bronchiolitis obliterans (Shohrati et al., 2012). A case series reported the effectiveness of 2.5 mg diamorphine in 11 elderly opioid naïve patients with terminal stage of idiopathic pulmonary fibrosis. Follow-up treatment with oral diamorphine remained effective in reducing dyspnoea and no patient showed signs of respiratory depression (Allen et al., 2005).

Morphine was shown to be effective in reducing dyspnoea in a single-arm study of six patients with terminal amyotrophic lateral sclerosis (Clemens and Klaschik, 2008). A significant decrease was seen in both respiratory rate and the intensity of dyspnoea at 120 minutes after morphine administration with no significant respiratory depression.

Opioids for incident or episodic breathlessness

Few RCTs have been performed for episodic breathlessness. A double-blind, cross-over RCT was performed by Charles et al. comparing nebulized hydromorphone, systemic hydromorphone, and nebulized saline in 20 patients (Charles et al., 2008). There were significant improvements in breathlessness before and after each treatment but no difference among three treatments. Oral transmucosal fentanyl has been reported to provide rapid relief of breathlessness in small observational studies (Gauna et al., 2008).

Long-term use of opioids for dyspnoea, opioid safety, and acceptance of opioids

The dosage of opioid and its usage for the long term was reported by a phase II dose increment and pharmacovigilance study by Currow et al. (2011). Sustained-release morphine at a dose of 10 mg daily was administered to 83 opioid naïve patients with modified MRC dyspnoea scores of 3 or 4, and dosage was increased in non-responders by 10 mg each week to a maximum of 30 mg daily. The dominant underlying causes of dyspnoea were COPD (54%), cancer (29%), and interstitial lung disease (12%). Sixty-two per cent of participants derived more than 10% benefit. For every 1.6 people commenced on morphine for chronic refractory dyspnoea, one person responded. For every 4.6 people commencing the study, one stopped the medication due to side effects that all reversed with cessation. The dose of morphine was 10 mg daily for 70% of participants, and the benefit was maintained at 3 months in 33% of all patients. There were no episodes of respiratory depression or hospitalizations as a result of the sustained-release morphine. The authors concluded that sustained-release oral morphine 10 mg once daily is safe and effective for most people.

Clemens investigated the effects of opioids on ventilation in two studies. Morphine or hydromorphone were titrated according to dyspnoea intensity in 11 dyspnoeic patients excluding COPD. Opioids produced a significant decrease in dyspnoea intensity at 30 and 90 minutes, but no significant respiratory depression as demonstrated by changes in oxygen saturation and transcutaneous arterial pressure of carbon dioxide ($TcPaCO_2$) (Clemens and Klaschik, 2007). Another prospective, non-randomized study involving 27 patients (25 people with cancer and two with amyotrophic lateral sclerosis) compared opioid-naïve palliative care patients to patients pretreated with strong opioids. No higher risk of respiratory depression or increase in $TcPaCO_2$ was observed in opioid-naïve patients (Clemens et al., 2008). The results of opioid safety from these reports are consistent with the Cochrane review by Jennings and colleagues, which showed that among 11 studies which collected post-opioid blood gases and/or oxygen saturation, there was no report of any significant desaturation, increased $PaCO_2$, and no excess mortality (Jennings et al., 2002).

In a recent qualitative study on use of opioids for dyspnoea involving eight patients, 12 caregivers, and 27 physicians, patients reported a sense of calm and relief from severe dyspnoea and substantial improvement in their QOL (Rocker et al., 2012). Family caregivers felt that opioids helped patients to breathe more 'normally', were effective in relieving patients' anxiety and depression as well as caregivers' own stress, and adverse effects were not a key concern. While all patients and family caregivers preferred to continue opioids, most physicians were reluctant to prescribe opioids for refractory dyspnoea.

Clinical use of opioids

There is clear evidence to support the use of systemic opioids for the control of breathlessness in patients with advanced cancer and COPD without causing excessive respiratory depression. The opioids studied include morphine, diamorphine, and dihydrocodeine. There is limited evidence to support the use of nebulized opioids for controlling breathlessness. The evidence for using opioids for controlling breathlessness in chronic heart failure is conflicting and requires further study. The use of opioids for breathlessness in other life-limiting illnesses such as interstitial lung disease and motor neurone disease are based on anecdotal reports.

There is no universally agreed starting dosage of opioids for the control of breathlessness. Factors to be considered include renal function, hepatic function, severity of pre-existing type II respiratory failure, the patient's frailty, body size, and the availability of nursing monitoring. Sustained-release morphine 10 mg daily has

been most systematically studied. In patients who are already taking opioids for pain control, an increment of 25% of the baseline dosage is supported by one previous study (Allard et al., 1999). Episodic breathlessness can be addressed by morphine given on an 'as needed' basis. The use of fast-acting opioids such as oral transmucosal fentanyl requires further study. Communication with patients and families on the indication and adverse effects of opioids is important for an informed choice and to address myths and concerns.

Pharmacological treatments with some evidence

Anxiolytics

The routine use of benzodiazepines for relief of breathlessness in patients with advanced cancer and COPD has not been supported by the Cochrane review on seven studies and meta-analysis on six studies (Simon et al., 2010). However, there were reports of successful use of benzodiazepines for the control of breathlessness in people with cancer with or without anxiety. One study reported the effective use of subcutaneous midazolam as adjunct therapy to morphine in the alleviation of severe dyspnoea in people in the last hours or days of life (Navigante et al., 2006). These patients had anxiety level correlated with their degree of dyspnoea. In another study, 63 patients were randomized to either oral morphine (starting dose 3 mg) or oral midazolam (starting dose 2 mg) with stepwise titration according to level of dyspnoea in initial in-clinic phase for recent acute onset breathlessness while causes were being investigated. In the subsequent 5 days of ambulatory phase, midazolam was superior to morphine in controlling baseline and breakthrough dyspnoea (Navigante et al., 2010). In another prospective, non-randomized study among people with cancer with dyspnoea associated with anxiety, a combination of morphine with lorazepam was shown to be effective in decreasing respiratory rate and dyspnoea intensity, without causing respiratory depression (Clemens et al., 2008). There may be a role for benzodiazepines for dyspnoea that is associated with anxiety. While the role of benzodiazepines in relieving breathlessness requires further evaluation, benzodiazepines are widely used (Booth et al., 2008).

Inhaled furosemide

Multiple mechanisms are proposed for the effects of inhaled furosemide in relieving breathlessness, including enhanced pulmonary receptor activity, suppression of the pulmonary irritant activity and vasodilation (Newton et al., 2008). The role of inhaled furosemide for relieving breathlessness has been studied in healthy subjects, and in patients with asthma, COPD, and advanced cancer. A systematic review by Newton et al. included 42 studies, of which 39 studies were RCTs (34 studies in asthma, eight studies in healthy subjects, four studies recruited both healthy subjects and asthma, one study in COPD) (Newton et al., 2008). Studies performed in people with cancer included one open clinical trial and one case series. Recently, two more RCTs were reported, one on COPD (Jensen et al., 2008) and one on advanced cancer patients (Wilcock et al., 2008). Overall, three RCTs are relevant to palliative care: two performed in COPD and one in advanced cancer. Both the COPD studies performed by Ong et al. (2004) and Jensen et al. (2008) showed effectiveness of inhaled furosemide in decreasing breathlessness when compared to placebo (Jensen et al., 2008; Newton et al., 2008). One study showed significant bronchodilatation, and the other showed increase in exercise endurance. For people with advanced cancer, the study by Wilcock et al. showed no difference in breathlessness reduction or isometric arm exercise test in 15 patients (Wilcock et al., 2008). Inhaled furosemide may exert its effect on the airway and be useful in relieving dyspnoea due to airway diseases, but is not proven to be of benefit for breathlessness in cancer which involves multiple mechanisms.

Heliox

Helium has a low density and the potential of reducing the work of breathing and improving alveolar ventilation when nitrogen in air is replaced by helium. A systematic review has shown that Heliox can effectively improve exercise limitation, decrease the work of breathing, and reduce dyspnoea in people with lung cancer and COPD (Laude and Ahmedzai, 2007). In a phase II double-blind, randomized, cross-over, controlled study comparing Heliox28 (72%He/28%O_2) with oxygen-enriched air (72%N_2/28%O_2) on dyspnoea in lung cancer, Heliox28 was shown to be more effective than oxygen-enriched air in improving oxygen saturation, exercise capacity, and dyspnoea scores (Ahmedzai et al., 2004). Since there are individual variations in patients' responses to supplemental oxygen, breathing Heliox with supplemental oxygen may give additional benefits in patients who respond to supplemental oxygen alone. However, its cost and availability will continue to limit its use in clinical practice.

Pharmacological treatments with little evidence

Phenothiazines such as chlorpromazine, promethazine, and levomepromazine have been reported in small studies to provide relief of breathlessness in COPD patients with inconsistent results (Parshall et al., 2012). The management of depression is an important component in managing patients with chronic dyspnoea. However, the evidence of antidepressant in relieving dyspnoea is inadequate. Likewise there is insufficient evidence to support the use of indomethacin and inhaled topical anaesthetics to relief dyspnoea (Parshall et al., 2012).

Palliative non-invasive ventilation (NIV)

There are expanding roles of NIV as a form of palliative ventilatory support. The indication to use NIV for improving survival is well established in patients with acute COPD with type II respiratory failure, hypoxaemic cardiogenic pulmonary oedema, hypoxaemic respiratory failure in the immunocompromised host, and advanced neuromuscular disorders (Elliott, 2004). 'Palliative NIV' (Azoulay et al., 2011) has been used in do-not-intubate (DNI) patients, for dyspnoea palliation, and for prolonging life in terminally ill patients temporarily to meet patients' short-terms goals. In a 5-year follow-up of a 2-year cohort of 38 DNI patients who received NIV, 11 patients survived the hospital stay, four patients (10.5%) were still alive after 5 years (Bulow and Thorsager, 2009). NIV is widely delivered as a ceiling treatment for respiratory failure patients with a DNI order. In a survey on the use of NIV among DNI patients, 75% of physicians and respiratory therapists reported the use of NIV for DNI patients, with more in COPD or heart failure patients than in cancer patients (Sinuff et al., 2008).

Increasing numbers of people with severe respiratory compromise have been put on NIV in clinical practice. Four randomized controlled studies reported the use of NIV in relieving dyspnoea in acute exacerbation of COPD (Smith et al., 2012). One study yielded negative result, the other three studies showed relief of dyspnoea by NIV but only two studies reported statistically significant relief (Smith et al., 2012). In one RCT, NIV was more effective compared with oxygen in reducing dyspnoea and decreasing the doses of morphine needed in people with end-stage cancer (Nava et al., 2013).

NIV is recommended as a standard of care to be offered to people with motor neurone disease with respiratory insufficiency. In a recent survey on the practice of NIV for motor neurone disease among neurologists in the United Kingdom, 612 patients were referred for NIV over 12 months, and 72.5% were successfully established on NIV (O'Neill et al., 2012). Three-quarters of responding neurologists accessed palliative care service towards patients' end of life. A collaborative approach between respiratory team and palliative care team is essential. NIV is a labour intensive procedure that requires skilled respiratory care, and can be burdensome to patients and their families. In the advanced care planning process with patients and their families, patients' concerns, goals, and overall QOL can be addressed in a holistic manner. The goals of treatment, and the benefits and burdens of NIV, should be constantly reviewed with the option of withdrawal of NIV especially towards the end of life.

Palliative sedation for refractory dyspnoea

Palliative sedation is defined as 'the administration of non-opioid drugs to sedate a terminally ill patient to unconsciousness as an intervention of last resort to treat severe, refractory pain or other clinical symptoms that have not been relieved by aggressive, symptom-specific palliation' (National Ethics Committee and Veterans Health Administration, 2006) (see Chapter 18.2). Agitated delirium, dyspnoea, and pain were the most common indications for palliative sedation. Such sedation has been delivered in inpatient and community settings. In a systematic review on six studies, palliative sedation for people with advanced cancer in the home setting had an incidence of 5–36%, with a mean duration of 1–3.5 days and no association with hastened death.

Cough in palliative care

Prevalence of cough

Cough is prevalent in cancer and in COPD (Kvale, 2006; Chung and Pavord, 2008). Cough was present in 42.9% of general cancer patients at treatment initiation (Molassiotis et al., 2010b) and in more than 65% of lung cancer patients at the time of diagnosis (Kvale, 2006). Prevalence of chronic cough and sputum also increases with age and smoking, and cough is present in 70% of people with COPD (Chung and Pavord, 2008). Cough can cause physical complications including chest wall pain, fracture of ribs, urinary incontinence, sweating, exhaustion, and disturbance of sleep. Patients may also experience psychological impacts, social embarrassment, and isolation (Molassiotis et al., 2011).

Function of cough

Cough comprises of three phases: the inspiratory phase with lengthening of expiratory muscles; the compression phase whereby the glottis is closed with building up of the intrathoracic pressure; and the expiratory phase to expel air at high velocity together with dynamic compression of the airways, producing the characteristic sound of cough (Chang, 2006). Cough reflex protects the airway by clearing the inhaled materials, accumulated airway mucus secretion, and sputum. The efficiency of cough depends on the optimal function of the three phases of cough, mucus properties, and mucociliary clearance all of which may be affected in cancer or chronic lung diseases. Coughing effort is reduced in respiratory muscle weakness or mechanical disadvantage as in general debility, cachexia, steroid myopathy, gross ascites, or hepatomegaly, and neurological conditions affecting conscious level. Dynamic compression of the airway is affected by vocal cord paralysis, presence of tumour, and stent insertion. Changes in mucus properties occur in chronic inflammation or infection of the lungs and dehydration. In COPD, cystic fibrosis (CF) and chronic smokers, mucociliary action is impaired.

Regulation of cough

Cough reflex is modulated by vagal afferent pathways, including the rapidly adapting receptors (RARs) and the C fibres. The RARs are myelinated fibres activated by cigarette smoke, hypertonic saline, and other stimuli that evoke bronchoconstriction and obstruction (Chung and Pavord, 2008; Canning, 2011). The C fibres are non-myelinated fibres activated by capsaicin, bradykinin, protons (acid pH), but C-fibre dependent cough is prevented by anaesthesia. A new vagal afferent subtype distinct from RAR and C fibre, called the cough receptor, has been identified. Unlike C-fibre dependent cough, the cough receptor-dependent cough is not inhibited by general anaesthesia. It appears to be protective by evoking robust cough efforts in response to touch and acid (Canning, 2011).

The activation of these vagal afferents is dependent on expression of ion channels, the TRP vanilloid 1 (TRPV1) and TRP ankyrin 1 (TRPA1). Both are calcium-permeable, non-selective cationic channels belonging to the family of transient receptor potential (TRP) receptors. TRPV1 receptors are chemosensitive, activated by capsaicin, acid and endogenous inflammatory mediators. The TRPA1 receptors are not activated by capsaicin, but are sensitive to cold temperatures and activated by irritants present in air pollution, vehicle exhaust, cigarette smoke, and endogenous inflammatory mediators (Canning, 2011; Grace et al., 2012).

Afferent sensory nerves converge, interact, and synapse in the tract of the nucleus solitarius (NTS) in the brainstem before being transmitted to the cough centre, which coordinates the efferent cough response (Chung and Pavord, 2008; Canning, 2011). Upregulation and increased expression of TRPV1 are present in airway inflammation. Hypersensitivity and plasticity in brainstem and NTS plays a role in chronic cough. Higher cortical involvement is suggested by the phenomenon that the urge to cough can be voluntarily suppressed and placebo has a profound effect on cough.

Causes of cough in palliative care

Tumours are more likely to cause cough with involvement of airways than the lung parenchyma (Kvale, 2006). Cancer involvement of pleura, pericardium, mediastinum, pulmonary lymphatics, and blood vessels may cause cough, and airway hypersecretion is associated with chest infection or inflammation. People with advanced cancer are predisposed to swallowing problems and aspiration

due to various factors, and may present with cough on feeding or at night, aspiration pneumonitis, or pneumonia (Bolser, 2010) (online Box 8.2.1). Conditions with hypersecretion of mucus are associated with cough (see section on airway secretion).

Non-cancer causes of cough in life-limiting diseases include respiratory conditions like COPD, asthma, bronchiectasis, interstitial lung diseases, and non-respiratory conditions like upper airway cough syndrome (UACS) which comprises of a variety of allergic, vasomotor, infectious, and anatomical rhinosinus conditions and gastro-oesophageal reflux disease (GORD) (Chung and Pavord, 2008; De Blasio et al., 2011) (online Table 8.2.4). Cough is significantly more prevalent in smokers.

Assessment of cough in palliative care

Despite the prevalence of cough and its appearance with other symptoms such as dyspnoea, insomnia, and fatigue in symptom clusters (Chen et al., 2011; Molassiotis et al., 2011), cough assessment is under-represented in research. A validated tool for cough for systematic assessment in palliative care is lacking (Molassiotis et al., 2010a; Leconte et al., 2011; Yorke et al., 2012). The clinical approach in cough assessment aims at evaluation of the cough symptom and the possible underlying causes. History, physical examination, and chest radiograph remain the mainstay in elucidating the underlying causes of cough.

The characteristics of cough should be defined from history taking, including associated sputum production, precipitating factors such as smoking, irritants, drugs, feeding, posture, association with timing of the day, and other associated symptoms such as dyspnoea, insomnia, choking, or fatigue. History of previous cancer treatment, smoking, use of angiotensin-converting enzyme (ACE) inhibitors, and concomitant chronic cardiac and lung diseases should be obtained. Visual analogue scale or visual descriptive scale (VDS) may be used for assessing intensity of cough but there are no validation studies. Cough monitors serve to provide objective cough counts. Cough-specific quality of life (EuroQol) questionnaires have been validated for assessing the impact of cough, such as the Leicester Cough Questionnaire, Cough Quality of Life Questionnaire, Burden of Cough Questionnaire, and Lung Cancer Cough Questionnaire (Molassiotis et al., 2010a; Leconte et al., 2011). While cough-specific QOL scores correlated well with cough counts, the relationship between VDS or visual VAS with cough counts or QOL scores are inconsistent (Molassiotis et al., 2010a). A lung function test can help in diagnosis of asthma or COPD. Sputum culture can guide antimicrobial treatment in chest infections. Application of other investigations including a CT scan looking for major airway obstruction has to be carefully considered if it will affect the ultimate management of patient. In patients with suspected aspiration or who fail the bedside swallowing test, referral to a speech therapist for comprehensive assessment should be considered.

Management of cough in palliative care

Evidence for cough treatment in advanced cancer has been disappointing, and the approach to cough in palliative care and lung cancer is formulated based on expert consensus and limited evidence (Molassiotis et al., 2010a; Wee et al., 2012). There is also no evidence to support efficacy of nurse-led management (Yorke et al., 2012). Management of cough in cancer can be categorized to treatment for specific cancer and non-cancer causes, and modifying cough by enhancing clearance or suppressing cough.

Treatment for cancer related causes

Radiotherapy, chemotherapy, especially with gemcitabine, and endobronchial treatment may palliate cough due to tumours (Kvale, 2006). Thoracic radiotherapy is effective in relieving cough in around 50% of NSCLC, ranging from 20% to 80% (Kepka and Olszyna-Serementa, 2010; Reinfuss et al., 2011). The decision to deliver palliative radiotherapy involves consideration of tumour stage, pulmonary function, symptoms, the patient's performance status, and preference (Rodrigues et al., 2012). Data on cough relief by brachytherapy, laser, or photodynamic therapy are limited (Molassiotis et al., 2010b).

Steroids may be useful in reducing tumour-related oedema, airway obstruction, lymphangitis carcinomatosis, or radiotherapy- or chemotherapy-induced pneumonitis. A steroid trial may be recommended as an early step in the treatment pyramid for cough in lung cancer after considering disease-specific treatments (Molassiotis et al., 2010a).

Antimicrobial treatment is indicated for chest infections but its outcome may be poor in the presence of drug-resistant pathogens and frail patients especially near the end of life. In two recent surveys on antimicrobial prescription in people with advanced cancer near the end of life, empirical broad-spectrum antibiotics were given in 58.7% of patients in one study (Chun et al., 2010), while in another, about one-third of patients were prescribed more than one antibiotic (Abduh Al-Shaqi et al., 2012). There is a call for more careful consideration of antimicrobial use in these patients. Data on efficacy of antimicrobials in relieving cough from chest infection is limited, and in one study, physicians but not patients reported improvement in cough (Mirhosseini et al., 2006).

Treatment for non-cancer causes

ACE inhibitors should be discontinued and irritants of cough should be avoided if possible. When appropriate, considerations should be given to empirical treatment of the most common causes of cough, namely UACS, asthma, and GORD by a trial of first-generation antihistamine or decongestant, bronchodilators, and proton pump inhibitors respectively (Bolser, 2010; Wee et al., 2011). Steroids may be indicated for uncontrolled asthma, non-asthmatic eosinophilic bronchitis, and chronic interstitial lung disease. Antibiotics are indicated for infection precipitating exacerbations in chronic lung diseases.

Suppressing cough by antitussives

Cough suppression aims at symptomatic treatment in cases of dry cough or disturbing cough. Over-the-counter antitussives, often mixed with antihistamines or decongestants, have doubtful efficacy and adverse side effects such as sedation, nausea, and constipation, especially in children under the age of 2 (Ostroff et al., 2011).

Antitussives can be classified as centrally acting and peripherally acting. Most centrally acting antitussives are opioids that suppress cough primarily by the μ-opioid receptors in the central nervous system, while peripherally acting antitussives target the sensory afferents. Among the agents reviewed (Bolser, 2010; Molassiotis et al., 2010a; Wee et al., 2011), hydrocodone, dihydrocodeine, levodropropizine, benzonatate, and sodium cromoglycate have been specifically studied in cancer patients. Only

sodium cromoglycate has been evaluated in a double-blind, placebo controlled RCT.

Centrally acting antitussives

Slow-release morphine has been evaluated in a double-blind placebo-controlled study in patients with chronic persistent cough (Morice et al., 2007). Morphine sulphate given at 5–10 mg twice daily provided a significant improvement of 3.2 points over baseline on the Leicester Cough Questionnaire, and a rapid reduction by 40% in daily cough scores.

Hydrocodone is a codeine derivative with hydromorphone as one of the metabolites. Hydrocodone was studied in an uncontrolled phase II dose titration trial in 20 people with advanced cancer (Homsi et al., 2001). The median best response was a 70% reduction in cough frequency, achieved with a median hydrocodone dose of 10 mg/day. Hydrocodone may be given orally at 5–10 mg every 4–6 hours.

Codeine is a pro-drug that is metabolized by the liver to morphine, norcodeine, normorphine, and hydrocodone. Codeine has been regarded as the gold standard antitussive based on earlier reports, but a recent well-designed RCT did not find it more effective than placebo. Codeine is given at 10–20 mg orally every 4 hours as needed.

Dextromethorphan, a common over-the-counter antitussive, is a non-opioid with fewer side effects and more effect when compared with codeine in suppressing cough. It is administered orally as 10–20 mg every 4–6 hours. Dextromethorphan is metabolized in the liver by the cytochrome P450 isoform CYP2D6 and hence potential drug interaction should be noted.

Peripheral acting antitussives

Sodium cromoglycate, given at two puffs twice daily (total 40 micrograms/day), has been evaluated in a double-blind RCT involving 20 people with lung cancer. It significantly reduced cough when compared with placebo without serious side effects (Moroni et al., 1996). A trial of sodium cromoglycate is recommended by an expert group as a safe choice (Wee et al., 2011).

Levodropropizine, as reviewed for its efficacy for cough in cancer and chronic lung disease, was significantly more effective than placebo and equally effective as dihydrocodeine or moguisteine in reducing cough frequency and severity (Schildmann et al., 2011). Levodropropizine at 75 mg three times daily produces the same efficacy as dihydrocodeine 10 mg three times daily but is associated with less somnolence.

Benzonatate at doses of 100–200 mg three times daily has been reported to be useful for cancer cough in a case series (Doona and Walsh, 1998). The patient should be instructed not to chew the capsule to avoid any local anaesthetic effects in the oropharynx.

Moguisteine has been evaluated in a multicentre, double-blind, parallel group study involving 113 patients with chronic lung diseases and lung cancer (Barnabe et al., 1995). Moguisteine 100 mg three times daily, when compared with codeine 15 and 30 mg, three times daily, was as safe and as effective in suppressing cough (Aversa et al., 1993).

Gabapentin, as evaluated in a RCT for refractory chronic cough, significantly improved Leicester Cough Questionnaire scores as compared with placebo (between-group difference in LCQ score 1.80, 95% CI 0.56–3.04; p = 0.004; NNT of 3.58) (Ryan et al., 2012). Gabapentin is postulated to exert its effect on underlying central sensitization of the cough reflex.

Potential novel antitussives

Agents targeting the primary afferent nerves by inhibiting TRPV1 and TRPA1 have emerged as potential effective novel antitussive drugs. Several selective TRPV1 antagonists have been studied in phase I and phase II clinical trials (Grace et al., 2012).

Airway secretion

Mucociliary clearance (MCC) is a defence mechanism of the airway but may be overwhelmed by mucus hypersecretion. Secretory hyper-responsiveness is a feature of severe chronic lung diseases such as COPD and cancer due to underlying infection and inflammation. There is hypertrophy and hyperplasia of goblet cells and submucosal glands, associated with loss of ciliary function, destruction of surfactant layer, and alteration of mucus properties. Neutrophil-derived DNA and filamentous actin (F-actin), apoptotic cells, and bacteria contribute to purulence (Rogers, 2005). Cough clearance is more effective for higher-viscosity secretion while ciliary clearance is most effective with fairly low viscosity (Balsamo et al., 2010).

Excessive airway secretions can give rise to symptoms of cough, dyspnoea, or noisy breathing as seen in noisy breathing in the terminal phase of life. Mucus hypersecretion is also significantly associated with a more rapid decline in forced expiratory volume in 1 second and increased hospitalization of patients with COPD. Chronic cough and sputum in COPD are associated with poor outcomes (Rogers, 2005; Miravitlles, 2011).

Airway hypersecretion can be managed by treatment of underlying diseases, mucoactive agents, and non-pharmacological airway clearance techniques. Most experiences are derived from chronic lung diseases.

Mucoactive agents

Mucoactive agents act by increasing the ability to expectorate sputum and/or decrease mucus hypersecretion. Categories of mucoactive agents are shown in online Table 8.2.5, but they also overlap in their actions. Variable levels of evidence are provided by studies in people with severe chronic lung diseases (Rogers, 2005; Bhowmik et al., 2009; Bolser, 2010)

Nebulized saline is effective in CF in a dose-dependent manner (Jones and Wallis, 2003), and a lower concentration of 3% saline is safe in COPD (Miravitlles, 2011). Guaifenesin, though commonly available in various oral preparations, lacks an RCT to prove its effectiveness.

Carbocysteine is effective and safe in reducing exacerbations and improving QOL in Chinese COPD patients (Zheng et al., 2008). Beta-adrenergic agonists are used for improving mucus clearance by increasing ciliary activity, but studies give variable results (Rogers, 2005; Balsamo et al., 2010). Macrolides, acting as immuno-modulators of mucin gene expression, are used for hypersecretion, bronchorrhoea and CF. However, data in COPD patients are limited and safety of its long-term use awaits further studies (Martinez et al., 2008).

N-Acetylcysteine based on its mucolytic, antioxidant and anti-inflammatory properties, is a commonly used mucolytic in COPD. Doses used in various studies range from 400 mg/day to 1200 mg/day orally. However, the optimum dose and duration of its use remains to be defined. Mucolytics may produce a small reduction in acute exacerbations without significant adverse effects in COPD, but have little or no effect on lung function and the overall QOL (Poole et al., 2012). Dornase alfa, acting on polymerized DNA and F-actin network, is not effective for COPD but used for CF (Rogers, 2005; Balsamo et al., 2010).

Ambroxol 75 mg has been compared with placebo in an RCT on COPD. Post hoc analysis showed that subjects with more severe symptoms who were treated with ambroxol were more likely to be exacerbation-free through the study period (Malerba et al., 2004).

Airway clearance techniques

Airway clearance therapies (ACTs) include active cycle of breathing technique (ACBT), autogenic drainage, and forced expiration. Passive techniques include postural drainage and percussion. Studies of ACT in COPD have considerable methodological limitations with relatively small sample sizes (Osadnik et al., 2012). ACT use is safe but no significant long-term benefits on the number of exacerbations or hospitalizations, or any short-term beneficial effect on health-related QOL, has been reported (Malerba et al., 2004). A recent randomized controlled equivalence trial on the effectiveness of manual chest physiotherapy techniques on COPD also failed to show any additional benefit when compared with advice on chest clearance alone on QOL at 6 months after an exacerbation of COPD (Cross et al., 2012).

Bronchorrhoea

Bronchorrhoea is defined as production of more than 100 mL of watery sputum daily, well above the average of 25 mL (Lopez-Vidriero et al., 1975). Massive bronchorrhoea may occur in bronchioloalveolar carcinoma, metastatic cancer growing in a bronchioloalveolar pattern, chronic bronchitis, asthma, and bronchiectasis. The sputum in bronchorrhoea is typically mucoid, transparent, and topped by a thick frothy layer. Its property of increased viscosity on standing is distinguished from sputum production without bronchorrhoea and saliva (Lopez-Vidriero et al., 1975). Bronchorrhoea is associated with hypoxia, dyspnoea, exhaustion, chest pain, functional decline, and social limitation. Radiological features include diffuse consolidation, nodules, and solitary or localized lesions. These diagnoses have to be differentiated from pneumonia, pulmonary oedema, haemorrhage, and other lung infiltrates (Polo et al., 2001). Anecdotal reports of treatments include that of palliative radiotherapy, macrolides, anticholinergics, octreotide, steroids, inhaled indomethacin, and epidermal growth factor receptor tyrosine kinase inhibitor (Zylicz, 2010).

Noisy airway secretions in the last hours or day of life (death rattles)

Death rattles occur due to vibration of accumulated pharyngeal and pulmonary secretions in patients who are unconscious or semi-conscious and too weak to expectorate. Death rattles occur in 23–44% of terminal patients (Back et al., 2001; Morita et al., 2004; Wildiers and Menten, 2002), especially associated with lung cancer, pneumonia, and dysphagia. Very severe secretions occur in 4.5%. Death rattle is a strong predictor for death: 76% of patients died within 48h after onset in one study (Wildiers and Menten, 2002).

Previous studies on the use of hyoscine hydrobromide and glycopyrronium did not confirm the superiority of one over the other (Lawrey, 2005). A systematic review of interventions for noisy breathing at end of life in 2008 failed to identify evidence in supporting the superiority of any anticholinergic agent or non-pharmacological treatment over placebo in a RCT (Wee and Hillier, 2008). Recently, a randomized trial was conducted in 333 terminal patients assigned to 0.5 mg atropine, 20 mg hyoscine butylbromide, or 0.25 mg scopolamine. Results showed no significant difference in effectiveness or survival among the three drugs. The study was not designed to show that this made a difference to the natural history of noisy breathing. For the three drugs, death rattle became non-disturbing or disappeared after 1 hour in 42%, 42%, and 37% of cases, respectively, and further improved to 76%, 60%, and 68%, respectively at 24 hours before levelling off. Treatment appears to be more effective when started at lower initial rattle intensity (Wildiers et al., 2009).

Patients may be positioned on one side. Gentle oral suction may be considered when secretions are in the oropharynx but the distress associated should not be overlooked. Death rattle may have a negative impact on staff, and some doctors and nurses may feel obliged to intervene despite the absence of any evidence that the natural history of noisy breathing is changed by medications (Wee et al., 2008). However, family members of dying patients may not be universally distressed by death rattle (Wee et al., 2006). Individualized treatment is recommended, taking into consideration the potential distress experienced by caregivers.

Haemoptysis

The volume of expectorated blood is often used to define the severity of haemoptysis, but there is no agreed cut-off point (see also Chapter 8.7). Various subjective terms have been used, describing haemoptysis as massive, major, exsanguinating, or life-threatening (Sakr and Dutau, 2010). Massive haemoptysis has been defined as the expectoration of more than 300 mL of blood in a single episode of haemoptysis (Qiu et al., 2009). Massive haemoptysis has also been defined as haemoptysis of over 500 mL within 24 hours, haemoptysis needing volume resuscitation, or haemoptysis causing airway obstruction and asphyxia.

However, the amount of expectorated blood used by other authors to define massive haemoptysis ranged from 100 to 1000 mL/24 hours (Sakr and Dutau, 2010). In untreated massive haemoptysis, 80% of patients may die (Sirajuddin and Mohammed, 2008). In addition to the amount of bleeding, other determinants of morbidity and mortality from haemoptysis include the rate of bleeding, underlying cardiopulmonary conditions, and the patient's ability to maintain patent airways (Sakr and Dutau, 2010).

Causes of haemoptysis, differential diagnoses

The bronchial arterial supply and, to a lesser extent, the non-bronchial systemic arterial supply are responsible for the majority of cases of massive haemoptysis. In a minority, massive haemoptysis may also arise from pulmonary vessels (Sakr and Dutau, 2010). The cause of death is usually asphyxiation.

The causes of haemoptysis include pulmonary infections such as tuberculosis, lung abscess or invasive pulmonary fungal infection, neoplasms, pulmonary conditions such as bronchiectasis and CF, cardiovascular causes, vasculitis, trauma, drugs, coagulopathy, and platelet disorders (Sirajuddin and Mohammed, 2008;

Sakr and Dutau, 2010). Haemoptysis occurs in up to 60% of CF patients over 18 years of age (Efrati et al., 2008). There is a small risk of pulmonary haemorrhage in patients with NSCLC treated by bevacizumab, a humanized monoclonal antibody against vascular endothelial growth factor (Reck et al., 2012). Often, the precipitating factor for haemoptysis is concomitant pulmonary infection, especially with *Pseudomonas aeruginosa* as the causative agent (Efrati et al., 2008). However, the precipitating cause for haemoptysis cannot be found in 15–30% (Sirajuddin and Mohammed, 2008). Fatal haemoptysis could also result from diagnostic or therapeutic procedures, such as transbronchial lung biopsy, lung radiofrequency ablation, or endobronchial high-dose brachytherapy (Carvalho Hde et al., 2005).

Clinical approach

Initial management of haemoptysis includes airway protection and volume resuscitation. The patient should be placed in a lateral decubitus position, with the bleeding side down. A detailed history should then be taken with complete physical examination, followed by laboratory investigations. Differential diagnoses include epistaxis, bleeding from the mouth or pharynx, haematemesis, and false haemoptysis (aspiration of blood) (Andersen, 2006). Baseline investigations include complete blood count, renal and liver function tests, prothrombin time, and activated partial thromboplastin time.

Localization of the site and source of bleeding may define the best treatment for stopping the bleeding. Chest radiograph can identify the site of bleeding in 33–82% of cases of massive haemoptysis, in the form of a mass, pneumonia, atelectasis, or cavitary lesion. Diffuse alveolar haemorrhage typically appears as alveolar infiltrates on chest radiography (Sirajuddin and Mohammed, 2008). Bronchoscopy plays an important role in localization of the anatomical site of bleeding, isolation of the involved airway, control of bleeding and treatment of the underlying cause of haemoptysis. In massive, life-threatening haemoptysis, rigid bronchoscopy, rather than fibreoptic bronchoscopy, is more efficient in ensuring airway patency, and maintaining ventilation and clearance of secretions to improve visualization. A fibreoptic bronchoscope can still be useful, being introduced through the rigid scope to access the upper lobes and peripheral bronchi (Sakr and Dutau, 2010).

CT thorax is comparable to bronchoscopy for detecting the bleeding site, but much more efficient for determining the cause of bleeding (Sakr and Dutau, 2010), such as the presence of bronchiectasis (Efrati et al., 2008). This is because CT can show distal airways beyond the reach of the bronchoscope, and the lung parenchyma (Sirajuddin and Mohammed, 2008). CT-guided transcutaneous biopsy of pulmonary lesions can be used to confirm invasive pulmonary fungal infections (Qiu et al., 2009). Multi-detector CT angiography is useful in evaluation of the integrity of pulmonary, bronchial and non-bronchial systemic arteries. CT, however, may have a limitation in differentiating a blood clot from a tumour.

Management

Management depends on the quantity of bleeding, urgency, and the patient's basic health status. A majority of patients respond well to conservative medical therapy, with or without blood transfusion. The effectiveness of various treatments is only supported by case reports.

Where possible, treatment should be directed at the underlying causes of the haemoptysis, such as oncological treatment, antibiotic, antituberculosis or antifungal therapy, and correction of coagulopathy. In CF, this may be due to malabsorption of vitamin K and liver cirrhosis (Efrati et al., 2008). Drugs such as non-steroidal anti-inflammatory agents or anticoagulant should be withheld.

Systemic treatment includes oxygen, oral or intravenous tranexamic acid (Sakr and Dutau, 2010), aerosolized vasopressin in the dosage of 5 units of orthnithine-8-vasopressin for mild and moderate haemoptysis (Anwar et al., 2005) and recombinant activated factor VII for massive haemoptysis (Lau et al., 2009).

Endobronchial treatment can be applied through the bronchoscope, including cold saline, epinephrine (adrenaline), tranexamic acid, antidiuretic hormone derivatives, such as terlipressin and ornipressin, fibrinogen-thrombin combination, factor XIII, and aprotonin. Endobronchial tamponade could be achieved with balloon, stent (Brandes et al., 2008), spigot, oxidized regenerated cellulose mesh, or biocompatible glue. Endobronchial tumours could be treated with laser photocoagulation, argon plasma coagulation, or electrocautery (Sakr and Dutau, 2010).

Indications for bronchial arterial embolization (BAE) include failure of conservative treatment, massive haemoptysis, recurrent haemoptysis, and poor surgical risk (Sirajuddin and Mohammed, 2008). Immediate control of haemoptysis has been reported in 57–100% of patients (Sakr and Dutau, 2010). Common complications of BAE include chest pain, fever (Efrati et al., 2008), transient dysphagia, groin haematoma, dissection or perforation of arteries (Sakr and Dutau, 2010), and contrast nephropathy (Sirajuddin and Mohammed, 2008). The most dreaded complications are neurological deficits, which could be reduced by cannulation of the target vessel beyond the origin of spinal branches (Sakr and Dutau, 2010). The mortality rate is 7.1–18.2%, considerably less than that of emergency surgery (40%) (Sirajuddin and Mohammed, 2008).

Surgery is reserved for cases of technical failure of arteriography, or when the patient is not fit for transfer to radiological intervention (Sakr and Dutau, 2010). Surgery is also performed when BAE has failed, such as in conditions resistant to embolization, for example, thoracic vascular injury or bronchial adenoma. On the other hand, if the patient is unfit for surgery, BAE may be the only treatment option (Noe et al., 2011). Surgery is also performed as a definitive treatment, to prevent recurrence, as in aspergilloma (Sakr and Dutau, 2010). When the patient is unfit for surgery, percutaneous treatment such as radiofrequency ablation of lung cancer has been used to control severe haemoptysis (Baisi et al., 2010).

Management of fatal haemoptysis

If a patient is at risk of massive haemoptysis, it is essential to establish an action plan in anticipation (see Chapter 8.7). This is a very uncommon way to die. The patient and family need to be informed, psychologically prepared, with possible treatment options discussed. Within the hospital setting, an 'emergency box' with the necessary drugs and towels in the ward will facilitate timely intervention of such crisis. If a massive life-threatening haemoptysis occurs, sedation to relieve the distress should be given as soon as possible. Midazolam 2.5–5.0 mg can be given intravenously as

the subcutaneous route will not provide relief quickly enough. Morphine can also lessen the dyspnoea and distress. A dark towel to cover the patient and dark basin for collecting blood helps to reduce the visual impact. The psychological impact of a patient dying from massive haemoptysis is enormous. Support and attention should be given to the family and people who witness the event. Debriefing and support should be provided to team members after the event.

Online materials

Additional online materials and complete references for this chapter are available online at <http://www.oxfordmedicine.com>.

References

Abernethy, A.P., McDonald, C.F., Frith, P.A., et al. (2010). Effect of palliative oxygen versus room air in relief of breathlessness in patients with refractory dyspnoea: a double-blind, randomised controlled trial. *The Lancet*, 376, 784–793.

Andersen, P.E. (2006). Imaging and interventional radiological treatment of hemoptysis. *Acta Radiologica*, 47, 780–792.

Bausewein, C., Booth, S., Gysels, M., and Higginson, I. (2008a). Non-pharmacological interventions for breathlessness in advanced stages of malignant and non-malignant diseases. *Cochrane Database of Systematic Reviews*, CD005623.

Ben-Aharon, I., Gafter-Gvili, A., Paul, M., Leibovici, L., and Stemmer, S.M. (2008). Interventions for alleviating cancer-related dyspnea: a systematic review. *Journal of Clinical Oncology*, 26, 2396–2404.

Booth, S., Moffat, C., Farquhar, M., Higginson, I.J., and Burkin, J. (2011). Developing a breathlessness intervention service for patients with palliative and supportive care needs, irrespective of diagnosis. *Journal of Palliative Care*, 27, 28–36.

Chung, K.F. and Pavord, I.D. (2008). Prevalence, pathogenesis, and causes of chronic cough. *The Lancet*, 371, 1364–1374.

Currow, D.C., McDonald, C., Oaten, S., et al. (2011). Once-daily opioids for chronic dyspnea: a dose increment and pharmacovigilance study. *Journal of Pain and Symptom Management*, 42, 388–399.

Currow, D.C., Smith, J., Davidson, P.M., Newton, P.J., Agar, M.R., and Abernethy, A.P. (2010). Do the trajectories of dyspnea differ in prevalence and intensity by diagnosis at the end of life? A consecutive cohort study. *Journal of Pain and Symptom Management*, 39, 680–690.

Jennings, A.L., Davies, A.N., Higgins, J.P., Gibbs, J.S., and Broadley, K.E. (2002). A systematic review of the use of opioids in the management of dyspnoea. *Thorax*, 57, 939–944.

Kvale, P.A. (2006). Chronic cough due to lung tumors: ACCP evidence-based clinical practice guidelines. *Chest*, 129, 147S–153S.

Molassiotis, A., Bailey, C., Caress, A., Brunton, L., and Smith, J. (2010a). Interventions for cough in cancer. *Cochrane Database of Systematic Reviews*, 9, CD007881.

Parshall, M.B., Schwartzstein, R.M., Adams, L., et al. (2012). An official American Thoracic Society statement: update on the mechanisms, assessment, and management of dyspnea. *American Journal of Respiratory and Critical Care Medicine*, 185, 435–452.

Sakr, L. and Dutau, H. (2010). Massive hemoptysis: an update on the role of bronchoscopy in diagnosis and management. *Respiration*, 80, 38–58.

Sirajuddin, A. and Mohammed, T.L. (2008). A 44-year-old man with hemoptysis: a review of pertinent imaging studies and radiographic interventions. *Cleveland Clinic Journal of Medicine*, 75, 601–607.

Wee, B. and Hillier, R. (2008). Interventions for noisy breathing in patients near to death. *Cochrane Database of Systematic Reviews*, 1, CD005177.

Anaemia, cytopenias, and thrombosis in palliative medicine

Nancy Y. Zhu and Cynthia Wu

Anaemia and cytopenias

Introduction to anaemia and cytopenias

The illnesses, malignant or benign, that bring patients to a palliative care setting are often complicated by haematological problems such as anaemia, bone marrow failure, disseminated intravascular coagulopathy, and thrombosis. Supportive therapy for these problems can provide gratifying relief of symptoms and improvement in overall quality of life. This chapter emphasizes a practical approach to assessment and therapy intended to maximize quality of life.

Anaemia

Anaemia is present in 77% of men and 68% of women receiving palliative care (Dunn et al., 2003). Typical symptoms associated with a sudden drop in haemoglobin as seen with acute blood loss include tachycardia, orthostatic hypotension, and dyspnoea. If the onset of anaemia is more gradual, compensatory mechanisms can help lessen these symptoms by increasing the cardiac output, increasing plasma volume and shifting the haemoglobin dissociation curve.

Patients can often remain symptom free if mild to moderate anaemia evolves gradually. More commonly, however, a diminished overall well-being is seen manifesting as fatigue, decreased exercise capacity, and decreased appetite. Some patients can also complain of dizziness, headache, syncope, tinnitus, vertigo, and impaired cognitive function. Patients with underlying cardiac disease are more susceptible to anaemic symptoms as they are unable to compensate as readily (Mercadante et al., 2000).

Determining the cause of anaemia in the palliative care setting can be challenging, since the aetiology is often multifactorial. Disease-related causes include bone marrow infiltration, blood loss, haemolysis, and anaemia of chronic disease. Cancer-related treatment can also result in anaemia such as myelosuppression from chemotherapy and treatment-related myelodysplastic syndrome. Concomitant factors such as folate deficiency from malnutrition and gastrointestinal resections can also contribute to anaemia (Mercadante et al., 2000).

Anaemia of chronic disease

Anaemia of chronic disease (ACD) is a hypoproliferative anaemia caused by an immunological reaction to the presence of inflammation and malignancy. It results from the release of multiple cytokines from T cells and monocytes including interferon-gamma (INFγ), tumour necrosis factor α (TNFα), interleukin (IL)-1, IL-6, and IL-10. These cytokines stimulate the uptake into and storage of iron in macrophages and monocytes while also preventing the export of iron out of these cells. Hepcidin, a hepatic peptide stimulated by IL-6 and lipopolysaccharide, contributes to the retention of iron within the reticuloendothelial system. This results in a paradoxical situation of iron-deficient erythropoiesis occurring in a marrow replete with iron. Simultaneously, the cytokines also suppress the ability of the kidneys to produce erythropoietin, enhance red blood cell membrane damage, and prevent the differentiation and proliferation of red cell progenitors in the marrow. Together, erythropoiesis is reduced resulting in anaemia (Weiss and Goodnough, 2005).

The diagnosis of ACD is often based on the exclusion of other forms of anaemia but should always be considered in the palliative care setting. It is present in almost 50% of men and over 70% of women (Dunn et al., 2003). The anaemia is typically normocytic, normochromic, and is usually mild to moderate (80–95 g/L). The reticulocyte count will be low, reflecting a reduced marrow output. Serum iron studies can be helpful in differentiating ACD from iron-deficiency anaemia. Serum iron, total iron binding capacity (transferrin), and iron saturation are all low in ACD while total iron binding capacity is elevated in iron deficiency. Serum ferritin is a reflection of total body iron storage, and since iron stores within the reticuloendothelial system is abundant, ferritin is normal or elevated in ACD (Weiss and Goodnough, 2005).

Acute and chronic haemorrhage

Acute and chronic blood loss is common in a palliative patient, especially in gastrointestinal, head and neck, respiratory, uterine, and urinary cancers. Bulky sarcomas, hepatomas, melanomas, and ovarian cancers can bleed into the malignant masses as well (Mercadante et al., 2000). Even the loss of a few millilitres of blood a day can result in iron deficiency over time. In the early stage of iron deficiency, iron stores are low resulting in a reduced ferritin but normal serum iron, iron saturation, and haemoglobin levels. As iron deficiency worsens, serum iron and iron saturation falls but the haemoglobin is preserved. Anaemia is the end result of severe iron deficiency with the presence of microcytic hypochromic red blood cells. Abnormally shaped cells like target cells and pencil cells are seen as the severity of the iron deficiency advances (Beutler, 2010). In most cases, the chronic blood loss is obvious from the presence of blood in bodily fluids, but occasionally tests for occult blood or endoscopic examination is necessary to determine the presence and site of the bleeding.

The first step in management of haemorrhage is to control the bleeding lesion if practical (see Chapter 8.7). This may be accomplished surgically, endoscopically, or by radiation of the bleeding lesion (Videtic, 2013). Iron supplementation should be started concomitantly if iron deficiency is present. Treatment can be provided either orally in the form of simple iron salts or parentally as iron–carbohydrate complex. The oral route is preferred as parenteral iron is associated with more severe adverse effects. The dosage for adults should provide 150–200 mg of elemental iron a day. This is ideally taken orally in three or four separate doses 1 hour before meals. Mild gastrointestinal side effects like nausea, heartburn, constipation, or diarrhoea are common. For these patients, changing to another form of iron or reducing the dose initially can be helpful (Beutler, 2010).

Parenteral iron is useful for patients who are intolerant of oral iron, have intestinal malabsorption issues, or may be losing iron more quickly than can be replaced with oral supplementation. The total dose required can be calculated by this formula:

$$\text{Dose of iron (mg)} = \text{whole-blood haemoglobin deficit (g/dL)} \times \text{body weight (lb)}$$

Iron sucrose contains 20 mg of elemental iron per millilitre and is recommended by the manufacturer to be administered at a maximum of 100 mg three times weekly. However, it has been safely given to chronic kidney disease patients at doses of 500 mg over 3 hours on 2 consecutive days. Typical adverse effects include hypotension, cramps, nausea, headache, vomiting, and diarrhoea (Beutler, 2010).

Iron dextran contains 50 mg of elemental iron per millilitre and is recommended by the manufacturer to be administered at a maximum of 100 mg per dose preceded by a 0.5 mL test dose. Larger doses are frequently used and considered safe with an increase in minor adverse effects. Iron dextran can result in a severe anaphylactic reaction occurring in less than 1% of patients. It is not dose dependent so can occur within the first few millilitres of the infusion. Typical presentation includes difficulty breathing, a choking sensation, becoming sweaty and anxious, nausea, and vomiting within the first few minutes of starting the iron dextran infusion. The infusion should be stopped immediately, resuscitation initiated, and epinephrine (adrenaline) be readily available. For patients with severe anaemia, transfusions may be necessary to help boost their haemoglobin. As each millilitre of blood contains 1 mg of elemental iron, blood transfusions will also help boost iron stores as well. Transfusion therapy is discussed later in this chapter in 'Transfusions in the palliative care setting' (Beutler, 2010).

Nutritional deficiencies

Cancer cachexia is seen in about half of all cancer patients, characterized by anorexia and loss of adipose tissue and skeletal muscle mass (Suzuki et al., 2013), leading to progressive nutritional deficiency (Segura, et al., 2005). The incidence of vitamin B_{12} deficiency was similar to that of the general elderly population at 7% but low serum folic acid level was significantly increased at 22%. Folic acid levels have been found to be an insensitive marker of occult folate deficiency, especially in those with weight loss. For

example, 58% of patients with major weight loss in the palliative care setting have been found to have features of megaloblastic anaemia with a normal folate level (Dunn et al., 2003).

Folic acid is critical in the metabolism and DNA synthesis of all cells, especially cells that are highly proliferative including haematological cells. Fruits and vegetables are rich in folic acid and the recommended dietary intake for an adult is 0.4 mg. When folic acid intake is reduced to less than 5 micrograms, megaloblastic anaemia ensues in approximately 4 months. Folic acid is absorbed in the duodenum and proximal jejunum so patients with intestinal resections or masses involving this area are at high risk of developing megaloblastic anaemia.

Megaloblastic anaemia results in enlarged megaloblastic bone marrow precursor cells and consequently enlarged red blood cells increasing the red cell volume. Hypersegmented neutrophils with the presence of more than the usual three to five nuclei lobes are classically described in megaloblastic anaemia. All cell lines can be affected resulting in anaemia, thrombocytopenia, and/or neutropenia.

Dietary supplementation can be given orally, usually at a dose of 1 to 5 mg/day. Typically 1 mg a day is adequate to correct anaemia even if malabsorption is present (Green, 2010).

Bone marrow infiltration

While anaemia from metastatic cancer is most commonly related to anaemia of chronic disease, iron deficiency, or other nutritional deficiencies, bone marrow infiltration from metastatic disease can occur. All malignancies can metastasize to the marrow, but the most common are from the lung, breast, and prostate. While not common, the classic clinical picture is that of a leucoerythroblastic blood picture with the presence of immature nucleated red cells, myeloid white cell precursors, and teardrop-shaped red cells. A bone marrow biopsy can help to confirm the diagnosis but since the majority of metastatic malignancies with marrow involvement are incurable, it is oftentimes not clinically necessary (Agarwal and Prchal, 2010).

Mild to moderate marrow infiltration is often times asymptomatic with minimal blood count changes. With more significant marrow involvement, anaemia can be more severe and accompanied by an elevated white blood cell count. Platelets can be low, normal, or elevated. Treatment is focused at managing the underlying disease and symptom control.

Patients with haematological malignancies (Franchini et al., 2013) and bone marrow failure disorders like myelodysplastic syndrome (Foran and Shammo, 2012) have diseased marrows that are unable to produce adequate blood cells, often resulting in pancytopenia. While thrombocytopenia can result in easy bruising, it is unlikely to result in spontaneous bleeding at a platelet count of more than 20×10^9 or in fatal intracranial haemorrhage at a platelet count of more than 5×10^9 (Franchini et al., 2013).

Neutropenia

Neutropenia in the palliative setting is most commonly due to bone marrow failure from myelosuppressive chemotherapy, disease infiltration of the bone marrow, or from intrinsic bone marrow failure. The definition of neutropenia is defined as an absolute neutrophil count (ANC) less than 1500 cells/microlitre with severe neutropenia being ANC less than 500 cells/microlitre. Patients with neutropenia are at high risk of developing severe bacterial and fungal infections. The Infectious Diseases Society of America defines fevers in neutropenic patients as a single oral temperature of greater than 38.3° Celsius or a sustained temperature of greater than 38.0° Celsius for more than 1 hour (Freifeld et al., 2011).

Patients at highest risk of severe febrile neutropenia are those with ANC less than 500 cells/microlitre for more than 7 days. Those with active comorbidities or significant hepatic or renal dysfunction are also considered to be high risk of severe bacterial infections.

Patients with prolonged neutropenia with ANC less than or equal to 100 cells/microlitre for more than 7 days should be considered for fluoroquinolone prophylaxis with levofloxacin or ciprofloxacin. In patients with fevers and neutropenia, the decision about management is dependent on the patient's values and disease stage. If life prolongation is deemed appropriate, then a discussion about the extent of investigation and management should be discussed on a per case basis.

Standard investigations for febrile neutropenia include complete blood cell (CBC) count with differential leucocyte count and platelet count, serum electrolytes, hepatic enzymes, total bilirubin, and creatinine. At least two sets of blood cultures are recommended, one from each lumen of a central venous catheter and one from a peripheral vein. Cultures from other sites should be taken as appropriate and a chest radiograph should be performed if respiratory findings are present.

High-risk patients with febrile neutropenia should be hospitalized for intravenous empiric antibiotic therapy with an anti-pseudomonal beta-lactam agent such as cefepime, meropenem, imipenem–cilastatin, or piperacillin–tazobactam. Vancomycin should be added for empiric treatment of suspected catheter-related infection, skin or soft-tissue infection, pneumonia, or haemodynamic instability. If fevers persist or new infectious symptoms develop, additional investigations and alterations in the antimicrobials may be necessary. Management should be guided by clinical microbiological data derived from investigations undertaken. Treatment is generally continued until neutrophil recovery (ANC ≥500 cells/microlitre) plus whatever duration is appropriate for the site of infection and organism identified. For patients without neutrophil recovery, antimicrobials should be continued until all signs and symptoms of a documented infection have resolved.

While hematopoietic growth factors such as granulocyte colony-stimulating factor (G-CSF) are frequently used to prevent infections associated with chemotherapy-related neutropenia, it is generally not used to prophylactically raise neutrophil counts in the palliative population. In addition, G-CSF is not recommended for routine use as adjuncts to antimicrobials in febrile neutropenia either. While the days of neutropenia, duration of fever, and length of hospital stay have been minimally reduced in some trials, no survival benefit has been seen.

Disseminated intravascular coagulopathy

Disseminated intravascular coagulopathy (DIC) results from an overproduction of procoagulants, which overwhelms the anticoagulant mechanism resulting in a systemic generation of intravascular microthrombi. Two-thirds of DIC cases are a result of underlying severe infection or malignancy (Levi and Seligsohn, 2010). The incidence of DIC in solid tumours is 7% but is much higher in acute leukaemia, up to 15–20%, which can increase further with chemotherapy treatment. Patients with acute promyelocytic leukaemia have a very high risk of DIC with more than 90% diagnosed at some point in the course of the disease (Levi, 2009). The risk of DIC increases with advanced age, more advanced stages of cancer, and the use of chemotherapy or anti-oestrogen therapy. Triggers for DIC include sepsis, immobilization, and liver metastases (Levi, 2013).

The production of intravascular microthrombi results in multiorgan failure, while the consumption of platelets, fibrinogen, and other coagulation factors increases bleeding. Hence, this results in a contradictory increased risk of both bleeding and clotting. Solid organ tumours are more prone to thrombosis while leukaemia patients are more prone to bleeding. Mucocutaneous bleeding is classic with cutaneous purpura, haemorrhagic bullae, oral and intestinal mucosal bleeding, and bleeding from intravenous sites. Other sites including intracranial haemorrhage, pulmonary haemorrhage, and haemorrhagic necrosis of the adrenals can also be seen. Ischaemic organ failure from microthrombi classically results in renal insufficiency, liver failure, intestinal ischaemia, cutaneous focal necrosis, acral gangrene, and respiratory failure. With severe DIC, cardiovascular shock can ensue (Levi and Seligsohn, 2010).

While DIC from infection and acute leukaemia typically presents very acutely, solid-organ cancer-related DIC can be more subacute and less fulminant with a more chronic presentation (Levi, 2009).

Laboratory findings classically reveal thrombocytopenia and prolonged prothrombin time/international normalized ratio (INR) or activated partial thromboplastin time and a suppressed fibrinogen level. Since fibrinogen acts as an acute-phase reactant and is elevated in the presence of infection or malignancy, it can remain within normal range despite an active DIC process. The most important diagnostic tool is to maintain a high clinical suspicion for DIC in patients with bleeding or clotting symptoms (Levi, 2013).

As the mainstay of treatment for DIC is supportive care while treating the underlying disease, its management becomes very difficult in palliative patients with incurable cancer. Prognosis is poor with a high mortality rate, especially with more severe DIC. Mortality rates range from 31% to 86% depending on the severity of DIC (Levi, 2013).

Supportive care of DIC in palliative cancer patients involve cardiovascular support and replacement of coagulation factors by using blood products. Cryoprecipitate contains large quantities of fibrinogen and factor VIII while fresh-frozen plasma helps replace the remaining coagulation factors. Platelet transfusions are sometimes necessary as well. In patients with clotting as the main presentation, anticoagulation should be initiated cautiously as the risk of bleeding is high (Levi, 2013).

Transfusions in the palliative care setting

The most common indication for blood transfusion in the setting of advanced cancer is fatigue and dyspnoea. Unfortunately, data regarding the relationship between fatigue and dyspnoea and the presence of anaemia remains controversial. In addition, there are currently no randomized controlled trials assessing the effectiveness of blood transfusions in this population. A Cochrane review found a subjective improvement in fatigue and dyspnoea at a rate of 31% to 70% with red blood cell transfusions (Preston et al., 2012).

Blood products are scarce and costly and hence use in the terminally ill evokes ethical discussions involving the principles of autonomy, beneficence, nonmaleficence, and justice. There are currently no guidelines on transfusions for palliative care patients, and each case should be assessed on an individual basis (Smith et al., 2013).

Red cell transfusion rapidly improves tissue oxygenation in the presence of anaemia or acute blood loss. Unfortunately, there is no evidence regarding red cell transfusions in the palliative population. Among non-palliative care patients, a Cochrane review comparing restrictive to liberal transfusion strategies did not find any adverse health outcomes and concluded that in patients without acute coronary artery disease, red cell transfusions is generally not necessary until haemoglobin levels approach 70–80 g/L as long as there is no evidence of bleeding (Carson et al., 2012).

Thrombocytopenia in the palliative setting is most commonly seen in patients with haematological malignancy and bone marrow failure. They can also be seen in advanced liver disease and splenomegaly. Platelet transfusions are scarcer and have a shorter duration of effect in raising the platelet count. They are generally indicated in patients with thrombocytopenia and active bleeding. Extrapolating from surgical patients, a platelet count above 50,000/microlitre should be adequate for bleeding control. Prophylactic platelet transfusions are considered for patients with platelet count less than 10,000/microlitre as they are at higher risk of severe spontaneous bleeding (Kaufman, 2013).

Blood cell transfusions like red cells and platelets have associated with it potential adverse events including transmission of blood-borne viral, bacterial, parasitic, and prion infections as well as transfusion reactions. With improved blood donor screening and blood testing strategies, the associated risks of receiving a transfusion-transmitted infection can been significantly reduced (Katz and Menitove, 2013).

Transfusion reactions range from frequent to rare, and from mild to severe (see Table 8.3.1). The most common are febrile reactions and mild allergic reactions. Febrile non-haemolytic transfusion reactions are likely related to cytokines released in response to antibody–leucocyte or antibody–platelet interactions. Fevers usually respond to antipyretics such as acetaminophen, which does not have the anti-platelet effect of aspirin and non-steroidal anti-inflammatory drugs. Prophylactic antipyretics are not necessary unless there is a history of febrile reactions. Rigor can be ameliorated with a small dose of meperidine, which can stop the symptom almost immediately. In patients with persistent febrile or allergic reactions despite premedication, hydrocortisone 1–2 hours before a transfusion can be used. Leucoreduction of blood products if available can significantly reduce the frequency of febrile reactions as well (Choate et al., 2013).

Mild allergic transfusion reactions are believed to be a result of plasma proteins in the blood products to which the patient has formed antibodies. They are quite common, occurring in approximately 1% of all transfusions. At the onset of pruritus and hives, the transfusion should be stopped and a dose of 25–50 mg of diphenhydramine given. Once the rash improves and the patient fells well without signs of fever, chills, or vasomotor instability, transfusion of the same unit can be re-initiated. In patients with frequent mild allergic transfusion reactions, pre-medication with diphenhydramine can be utilized (Choate et al., 2013).

Table 8.3.1 Types of acute transfusion reactions

Type of reaction	Presentation
Acute intravascular haemolytic	Fever, chills, dyspnoea, hypotension, tachycardia, flushing, vomiting, back pain, haemoglobinuria, haemoglobinaemia, shock
Acute extravascular haemolytic	Fever, indirect hyperbilirubinaemia, post-transfusion haematocrit increment lower than expected
Febrile non-haemolytic	Fever, chills
Allergic (mild)	Urticaria, pruritus, rash
Anaphylactic	Dyspnoea, bronchospasm, hypotension, tachycardia, shock
Transfusion-associated circulatory overload (TACO)	Dyspnoea, tachycardia, hypertension, headache, jugular venous distension
Septic	Fever, chills, hypotension, tachycardia, vomiting, shock
Transfusion-related acute lung injury (TRALI)	Dyspnoea, decreased oxygen saturation, fever, hypotension

Source: data from Choate, J. D. et al., Transfusion Reactions to Blood and Cell Therapy Products, in R. Hoffman et al. (Eds.), *Hematology: Basic Principles and Practice*, Sixth Edition, Elsevier Saunders, Philadelphia, USA, Copyright © 2013.

Transfusion-associated circulatory overload (TACO) results from excess fluid accumulation in the lungs. Transfused blood products rapidly increase a patient's intravascular volume and can exceed the ability of the cardiovascular system to compensate. Patients with pre-existing cardiovascular disease are especially at risk, and transfusing at a rapid rate in the absence of acute haemorrhage is an additional risk factor. Reducing the rate of transfusion in those at risk for fluid overload and the administration of diuretics before a transfusion can be preventative (Choate et al., 2013).

Acute intravascular haemolytic transfusion reactions are a result of the acute haemolysis of ABO incompatible red blood cells in a patient with the corresponding antibody. The reactions are very rapid, occurring within minutes after initiating the transfusion. The transfusion needs to be stopped immediately, cardiorespiratory support initiated, and a crystalloid solution infused to maintain a good urine output (Choate et al., 2013).

Erythropoietin-stimulating agents

Erythropoietin is a hormone naturally produced by the kidney and is an essential growth factor for red cell progenitors in the bone marrow. It is traditionally used to manage anaemia associated with advanced renal disease (Marks et al., 2013) but has become increasingly common in cancer-related anaemia as well. The use of erythropoietin-stimulating agents (ESAs) like epoetin and darbepoetin in patients on myelosuppressive chemotherapy has been shown to reduce the need for red cell transfusions, but can also increase the risk of hypertension, thromboembolic events, and death. There is some suggestion that ESAs may improve quality of life but the data is not definitive. Also controversial is whether ESAs worsen tumour control (Tonia et al., 2012).

The American Society of Hematology/American Society of Clinical Oncology 2010 guideline recommends that ESAs be considered in patients undergoing myelosuppressive chemotherapy who have a haemoglobin level less than 100 g/L and cautions against ESA use under any other circumstances of cancer-related anaemia. They also recommend using the lowest ESA dose possible and targeting a haemoglobin level to avoid transfusions. If no response is seen after 6–8 weeks, the ESAs should be discontinued (Rizzo et al., 2010).

Venous thrombosis

Introduction to venous thrombosis

Venous thromboembolism (VTE) is a category of disease comprised of deep vein thrombosis (DVT) and pulmonary embolism (PE). Although venous thrombosis can occur in any site, the vast majority of what we know is focused on lower extremity DVT and PE. VTE is associated with significant morbidity and mortality. The link between cancer and thrombosis has long been established and was first described by French internist Armand Trousseau in 1865. Cancer patients experience a higher rate of VTE (Blom et al., 2006). It is estimated that one in 1000 adults per year develop VTE in the general population. About 15% of patients with cancer develop symptomatic VTE, 15–20% of patients with VTE have cancer, and about 10% of patients presenting with idiopathic VTE will develop cancer within a year (Lee, 2004). Cancer is also associated with both a higher rate of anticoagulant failure and a two- to sixfold higher rate of major bleeding (Palareti et al., 2000; Prandoni et al., 2002). Cancer patients with thrombosis also have a shortened life expectancy (Sorensen et al., 2000; Chew et al., 2006).

The pathophysiology of thrombosis in cancer is often complex and multifactorial but can be generally thought of in a simple framework developed in 1856 by the German physician Rudolf Virchow. Together, venous stasis, endothelial injury, and hypercoagulability are now commonly known as Virchow's triad. Large lymphadenopathy or tumours causing local compression, paralysis from spinal cord compression, and hospitalization from complications of cancer can contribute to venous stasis. Many chemotherapeutic agents, surgical interventions, and central venous access can contribute to endothelial injury. Cancer causes various procoagulant changes in the blood, including, for example, an increase in circulating levels of tissue factor, and thrombogenicity often depends on tumour type and stage (Otten et al., 2004; Lee et al., 2006).

VTE continues to be a significant problem throughout a cancer patient's care, from pre-diagnosis to diagnosis to treatment to palliation and death. Older studies carried out in a time when autopsies were done more frequently estimate that up to 50% of patients with cancer have VTE at the time of death. Despite recognizing this link between cancer and thrombosis, there is a paucity of data in the palliative care setting and there still remains the question of how aggressively we should try and prevent, diagnose, and treat thrombosis in the end stages of life.

Goals of VTE treatment

To help answer this question, it is important to understand what treatment of VTE accomplishes for patients. The initial phase is targeted at decreasing symptoms (leg swelling and pain, chest pain, shortness of breath), preventing clot extension, preventing embolic events, preventing early recurrence, and decreasing upfront mortality. Longer-term treatment is targeted at decreasing the risk of recurrent VTE and mitigating post-thrombotic symptoms (Lee, 2004). In most patients, the risk of haemorrhage is outweighed by the thromboembolic risk in the first few weeks to months after a new VTE is diagnosed and, in the absence of major contraindications, prompt investigations and initiation of treatment is usually recommended. Duration of treatment hinges on the fine balance between thrombotic complications and haemorrhagic complications, both of which can change over time (Noble et al., 2008).

Complications of VTE treatment

Treatment of VTE is based largely on anticoagulant therapy. Although new oral anticoagulant agents are being developed, none have currently been studied in the cancer or palliative setting. At present, the mainstay of treatment consists of administering a fast acting agent such as intravenous (IV) unfractionated heparin (UFH) or subcutaneous (SC) low-molecular-weight heparin (LMWH). This is frequently followed by initiation of oral warfarin therapy to target an INR of 2–3 for ongoing maintenance therapy. An overlap of about 5–7 days is required between the parenteral and oral medications as there is a delay in the onset of anticoagulant effect of warfarin.

More recent data has supported the ongoing use of LMWH rather than warfarin in cancer patients, particularly in those receiving active chemotherapy (Lee et al., 2005). Prophylactic anticoagulants for VTE prevention is mostly comprised of low-dose SC UFH or LMWH. All anticoagulants are associated with a risk of major or fatal haemorrhage. IV or SC modalities are additionally cumbersome for patients and may cause discomfort and decrease quality of life. Other considerations for those undergoing anticoagulant therapy include the need for continued monitoring of laboratory parameters including potentially INR, CBC count (to look for thrombocytopenia), and liver and kidney function tests.

Goals of palliative care

The line between active treatment and palliation can often be unclear. Palliative care is targeted at symptom control, maintaining quality of life and psychosocial supports, and decreasing suffering. In the treatment and prevention of VTE, there are many overlapping features. Although anticoagulant therapy is in part used to decrease mortality, much is also used to decrease clot burden and improve symptoms (McLean et al., 2010). Investigation for VTE will often require a hospital visit and potential need for admission. Administration of anticoagulant therapy, as described earlier, is associated with its own challenges (Soto-Cardenas et al., 2008; McLean et al., 2010). Given this, it is prudent to individually tailor treatment plans and care plans for different patients. For example, for a patient who is palliative but still ambulatory and living independently at home, it is very reasonable to consider investigation for and treatment of newly diagnosed VTE, or prophylactic anticoagulation in case of temporary immobilization, as controlling the complications of VTE can help maintain their state of independence.

At the extreme of life, a terminally ill patient who is bedridden and approaching death may benefit more from symptom control only, regardless of aetiology, rather than being subjected to hospital transport for further investigation, uncomfortable administration of medications with frequent monitoring, and potentially the need for further intervention if complications such as bleeding occur (Tran, 2010).

Conclusions

Haematological complications are common and significant issues in cancer patients and those who eventually require palliative care. The complications of investigation and treatment make devising care decisions for such patients a challenging process. Frank and open discussions with each patient regarding the overall goals of care can help guide management. It is important to remember that a patient's status and thus these very goals will change over time and constant re-evaluation is essential. This will help shape plans that avoid unnecessary testing and intervention, as well as avoid depriving a patient of the compassionate care needed in the end of life.

Online materials

Complete references for this chapter are available online at <http://www.oxfordmedicine.com>.

References

Carson, J.L., Carless, P.A., and Hebert, P.C. (2012). Transfusion thresholds and other strategies for guiding allogeneic red blood cell transfusion. *Cochrane Database of Systematic Reviews*, 4, CD002042.

Choate, J.D., Maitta, R.W., Tormey, C.A., Wu, Y., and Snyder, E.L. (2013). Transfusion reactions to blood and cell therapy products. In R. Hoffman, E.J. Benz Jr, L. Silberstein, H.E. Heslop, J.I. Weitz, and J. Anastasi (eds.) *Hematology: Basic Principles and Practice* (6th ed.), pp. 1727–1737. Philadelphia, PA: Elsevier Saunders.

Chew, H., Wun, T., Harvey, D., Zhou, H. and White, R.H. (2006). Incidence of venous thromboembolism and its effect on survival among patients with common cancers. *Archives of Internal Medicine*, 16, 458–464.

Dunn, A., Carter, J., and Carter, H. (2003). Anemia at the end of life: prevalence, significance, and causes in patients receiving palliative care. *Journal of Pain and Symptom Management*, 26, 1132–1139.

Franchini, M., Frattini, F., Crestani, S., and Bonfanti, C. (2013). Bleeding complications in patients with hematologic malignancies. *Seminars in Thrombosis and Hemostasis*, 39, 94–100.

Freifeld, A. G., Bow, E. J., Sepkowitz, K. A., *et al.* (2011). Clinical practice guidelines for the use of antimicrobial agents in neutropenic patients with cancer: 2010 update by the Infectious Diseases Society of America. *Clinical Infectious Diseases*, 52 (4), pp. e56–e93.

Lee, A.Y.Y. (2004). Management of thrombosis in cancer: primary prevention and secondary prophylaxis. *British Journal of Haematology*, 128, 291–302.

Lee, A.Y.Y., Levine, M.N., Butler, G., *et al.* (2006). Incidence, risk factors, and outcomes of catheter-related thrombosis in adult patients with cancer. *Journal of Clinical Oncology*, 24(9), 1404–1408.

Levi, M. (2009). Disseminated intravascular coagulation in cancer patients. *Best Practice & Research Clinical Haematology*, 22(1), 129–136.

McLean, S., Ryan, K., and O'Donnell, J.S. (2010). Primary thromboprophylaxis in the palliative care setting: a qualitative systematic review. *Palliative Medicine*, 24(4), 386–395.

Mercadante, S., Gebbia, S., Marrazzo, A., and Filosto, S. (2000). Anaemia in cancer: pathophysiology and treatment. *Cancer Treatment Reviews*, 26, 303–311.

Preston, N.J., Hurlow, A., Brine, J., and Bennett, M.I. (2012). Blood transfusions for anaemia in patients with advanced cancer. *The Cochrane Database of Systematic Reviews*, 2, CD009007.

Rizzo, J.D., Brouwers, M., Hurley, P., *et al.* (2010). American Society of Hematology/American Society of Clinical Oncology clinical practice guideline update on the use of epoetin and darbepoietin in adult patients with cancer. *Blood*, 116(20), 4045–4059.

Smith, L.B., Cooling, L., and Davenport, R. (2013). How do I allocate blood products at the end of life? An ethical analysis with suggested guidelines. *Transfusion*, 53, 696–700.

Weiss, G. and Goodnough, L.T. (2005). Anemia of chronic disease. *The New England Journal of Medicine*, 352(10), 1011–1023.

Genitourinary aspects of palliative care

Olivia T. Lee, Jennifer N. Wu, Frederick J. Meyers, and Christopher P. Evans

Introduction to genitourinary aspects of palliative care

Patients receiving palliative care often face problems related to the genitourinary system, whether their primary disease is of urologic origin or not. Factors contributing to common genitourinary pathology in this setting include advanced and metastatic malignancy, chronic illness, neurodegenerative disease, prior radiation, chemotherapy, or surgery (Doherty and O'Sullivan, 2004; Wu et al., 2011) In particular, this chapter will focus on urinary tract obstruction (upper and lower tract obstruction), intractable bleeding, fistulae, and bladder-associated pain. Management of each process should take into account the patient's symptom severity, performance status, and life expectancy. Treatment options must weigh the benefits of a particular modality against the risks of intervention, with the goal of reducing suffering and improving quality of life. Common genitourinary surgical interventions in the palliative care setting are summarized in Table 8.4.1.

Lower urinary tract obstruction

Lower urinary tract obstruction in the palliative care setting can be due to benign or malignant disease. Primary urologic causes include benign prostatic hyperplasia (BPH), invasive prostate or bladder cancer, urethral stricture, or bladder neck contracture. Non-urologic causes include invasive gynaecological or colorectal malignancies. Symptoms of outlet obstruction include urinary retention, suprapubic pain, frequency, urgency, dysuria, and urinary tract infection. Untreated severe bladder outlet obstruction leads to bladder dysfunction, bladder stones, and kidney injury.

In the work-up of bladder outlet obstruction, a proper history will guide diagnosis and treatment. Prior radical prostatectomy would suggest bladder neck contracture, while prostate radiation therapy (brachytherapy or external beam radiotherapy) suggests urethral stricture. Prior endourologic procedures (transurethral resection of prostate (TURP), bladder tumour, direct vision internal urethrotomy (DVIU), urethral dilation) could suggest urethral stricture disease or BPH recurrence. In women, it is pertinent to know if there is a history of bladder suspension surgery or mid urethral slings. A neurologic history is important to rule out neurogenic causes of urinary retention, such as pelvic plexus injuries (pelvic trauma, abdomino-perineal resection, or low anterior resection) or systemic neurologic disease such as multiple sclerosis, Parkinson's disease, or multiple systems atrophy.

In severe bladder outlet obstruction, physical examination may reveal abdominal or suprapubic distension and tenderness. A digital rectal examination is appropriate to evaluate BPH, invasive and recurrent prostate cancer, or rectal masses. In women, a pelvic examination could reveal a vaginal, uterine, or adnexal mass. A urinalysis and urine culture will detect infection or microscopic haematuria. Performing a bladder scan to determine a post-void residual volume allows one to assess incomplete emptying and the amount of retention. A post-void residual volume greater than 90–100 mL is concerning for outlet obstruction. Formal urodynamic studies will provide more accurate information about bladder pressure, capacity, compliance, and risks of upper tract injury. Renal ultrasound may detect hydronephrosis and parenchymal thinning if obstruction is severe. Further imaging with computed tomography (CT) or magnetic resonance imaging (MRI) can aid in diagnosis of a pelvic or abdominal disease process or evaluate progression of a known disease. If one suspects concomitant neurogenic bladder dysfunction with outlet obstruction, urodynamic testing will help in deciphering the primary cause for incomplete emptying. Cystoscopy would aid in diagnosing a bladder mass or prostatic invasion. Prior to performing invasive diagnostic procedures, however, one must assess the utility of each in its role in guiding palliation of symptoms. For example, if a man has progression of known prostate cancer and evidence of incomplete emptying with a large volume post-void residual, then one could forego additional studies and proceed with catheter drainage. Lastly, in the setting of bladder outlet obstruction, one should rule out constipation or faecal impaction causing obstruction, as it is common in the palliative care population and is possible to treat.

Management of bladder outlet obstruction varies from pharmacologic therapy to catheterization (urethral or suprapubic), endoscopy, or major open surgery. Each approach depends on the source and aetiology of the obstruction. In the case of BPH, patients who have lower urinary tract symptoms that include frequency, urgency, weakened force of stream, sensation of incomplete emptying, dysuria, and evidence of retained urine, one would start an alpha-blocker, a 5-alpha reductase inhibitor, or both to improve emptying. The 5-alpha reductase inhibitors have minimal benefit improving obstruction from prostate cancer. In an acute episode of complete urinary retention, an indwelling urethral catheter or

Table 8.4.1 Palliative urologic procedures

Procedure	Indication	Anaesthesia
Suprapubic catheterization	Bladder outlet obstruction	General or spinal anaesthesia
Ureteral stents	Ureteral stricture	General anaesthesia
	Malignant extrinsic compression	
	Retroperitoneal fibrosis	
Percutaneous nephrostomy tube placement with or without ureteral occlusion	Ureteral obstruction or fistula	Conscious sedation or general anaesthesia
	Bladder haemorrhage	
Intravesical instillation of formalin	Intractable haemorrhagic cystitis	General anaesthesia
Transurethral resection of prostate (TURP)	Bladder outlet obstruction from BPH or invasive prostate cancer	General or spinal anaesthesia
Direct vision internal urethrotomy (DVIU)	Urethral stricture	General or spinal anaesthesia
Cystourethroscopy, transurethral resection of bladder tumour (TURBT), fulguration, clot evacuation	Bleeding from bladder tumour	General or spinal anaesthesia
Urethral stent placement	Urethral stricture, non-healing urethra	General or spinal anaesthesia
Selective angioembolization	Intractable haemorrhage or urovascular fistula	Conscious sedation or general anaesthesia
Diverting ileal conduit	Pelvic malignancy obstructing bladder	General anaesthesia
Palliative cystectomy/palliative cystoprostatectomy	Intractable bleeding	General anaesthesia
	Invasive pelvic malignancy obstructing urine	
	Chronic bladder pain	
Palliative nephrectomy	Bleeding	General anaesthesia
	Pain from mass	
	Recurrent infection	
Fistula repair	Uroenteric or urovaginal/uterine fistulae	General anaesthesia

suprapubic catheter is required, followed by close monitoring of serum electrolytes and water losses due to post-obstructive diuresis. While post-obstructive diuresis (defined as > 200 cc/hour urine output) is most often self-limiting, in the patient who is unable to replace water losses enterally either due to altered mental status or physical barriers, support with isotonic intravenous fluids is required. After the acute episode of urinary retention, the goal is to transition the indwelling catheter to clean intermittent catheterization (CIC) if the patient is physically and mentally able and willing.

If patients continue to suffer from outlet symptoms despite medications or cannot tolerate catheter diversion, then surgical approaches should be considered. The common surgical intervention for BPH is TURP. For invasive prostate cancer, a 'channel TURP' is appropriate, in which a more limited resection is performed to avoid incontinence. If prior prostate radiation with external beam or brachytherapy was performed, endoscopic treatment with TURP or DVIU risks urinary incontinence and tissue non-healing and therefore should be carefully considered.

For urethral stricture disease, conservative measures include urethral dilation and indwelling urethral catheter or diversion using a suprapubic catheter. Endoscopic options include DVIU or placement of urethral stents. The role of urethral stents is limited to the bulbar urethra and remains controversial due to the high complication rate of urethral ingrowth, stent migration, encrustation, infection, and irritative voiding symptoms (De Vocht et al., 2003). Primary anastomotic or substitution urethroplasty should

have no role in the palliative care setting as urethral reconstruction is very involved and often requires multistage repair in a patient population with potentially compromised wound healing. Surgical treatment should be reserved for select patients who can tolerate an intervention and have a prognostic time course that would benefit from surgery. It is important to note that recurrence of obstruction is not uncommon, for cancer regrowth or stricture disease. Furthermore, complications from invasive procedures such as bladder or urethral injury, problematic bleeding, and electrolyte disturbances can occur. Thus, a thorough discussion must be held with the patient and family before proceeding and should only be considered if a patient cannot be managed with an indwelling urethral catheter, intermittent catheterization, routine urethral dilation, or suprapubic catheterization. In the setting of invasive pelvic masses that compress or invade the bladder outlet, pelvic irradiation or palliative surgery with urinary diversion using a bowel segment conduit with or without cystectomy/pelvic exenteration may be appropriate.

Urinary catheters and catheter-associated urinary tract infections

In choosing catheter type and technique, infection risk and the patient's functional capacity are important considerations (Cespedes and Gerboc, 2012; Niel-Weise et al., 2012). An indwelling urethral catheter is the most common method of relieving bladder outlet obstruction. When used chronically, however, indwelling catheters cause recurrent urinary infections, urethral erosion, and irritative bladder symptoms. If given the choice, CIC is preferred over an indwelling urethral catheter; however, it requires patient compliance, mental capacity and physical dexterity, or it requires attentive nursing staff. If CIC is not a viable option, then indwelling suprapubic catheter is an alternative to urethral catheters. Suprapubic catheters reduce the risks of infection, urethral erosion, periurethral abscess, epididymitis, and urethral trauma (National Institute for Health and Clinical Excellence, 2003; Cottenden, 2009). It does, however, require surgery to place a suprapubic catheter and in the process, carries the risk of an anaesthetic, and injuring surrounding structures such as bowel. Again, a global assessment of the patient's clinical and psychosocial situation is necessary to decide whether a urethral catheter, intermittent catheterization, or suprapubic catheter will serve the patient best, while avoiding unnecessary risk.

The major risk of chronic indwelling catheters is urinary infection (Schaeffer and Schaeffer, 2012). Catheter-associated bacteriuria risk increases by 10% for each indwelling catheter day. This is in contrast to a 1–3% risk for each sterile or CIC (Warren et al., 1999). Note that asymptomatic bacteriuria associated with chronic catheters does not need treatment and routine urine culture is not necessary in patients with chronic catheters. Only symptomatic catheter-associated urinary tract infections (CAUTIs) require treatment with appropriate antibiotics. Symptoms such as fever, urgency, frequency, dysuria, and urine culture with at least 10^5 colony-forming units of no greater than two species of organisms warrant an infectious work-up (Centers for Disease Control and Prevention, 2012). Proper sterile technique with catheter placement and routine 3–4-week exchanges of indwelling catheters and clean technique for intermittent catheterization should be followed. In patients who develop recurrent, symptomatic CAUTIs, low-dose prophylactic antibiotics may be appropriate (Petronella et al., 2012). For patients who have problematic encrustation due to a chronic catheter, consider more frequent exchange of catheters or genitournary irrigation using sterile saline or neomycin-polymyxin solution daily or twice daily, as needed.

Selection of catheter material is also important in the setting of chronic indwelling catheters, as infection, encrustation, allergy, and comfort vary. Among them, latex rubber and silicone are the most common materials. Silicone catheters (100% or silicone coated) are preferable for long-term use because they reduce the risk of encrustation and 100% silicone catheters are safe for patients who have latex allergy (Jahn et al., 2007; Cottenden, 2009; Gould et al., 2010). Silicone-coated latex catheters are softer than 100% silicone catheters and cause less discomfort. Silver alloy-coated and antibiotic-impregnated catheters are also available and have been found to reduce the risk of catheter-associated bacteria only in the short term (1-week) duration of use (Schumm and Lam, 2008; Tenke et al., 2008). In the long term (> 14 days), the silver alloy- or antibiotic-impregnated catheters have not shown benefit in reducing infection (Geng et al., 2012). Similarly, nitrofurazone impregnated catheters were found to reduce *Escherichia coli* and *Enterococcus faecalis* adherence to catheters; however, this effect was lost beyond 5 and 3 days of incubation, respectively (Desai et al., 2010).

Upper urinary tract obstruction

Upper tract obstruction involves the renal collecting system and ureters. Intraluminal sources of obstruction include masses (transitional cell carcinoma, fibroepithelial polyps), stricture, or stones. Extraluminal sources include pelvic or retroperitoneal malignancy, fibrosis, or prior radiation. Patients may present with flank pain, nausea, or vomiting. If untreated, ureteral obstruction can cause loss of unilateral or bilateral renal function, end-stage renal disease, pyelonephritis, or urosepsis.

If ureteral obstruction is suspected, preliminary studies should include urinalysis, renal ultrasound, and serum creatinine or an estimated glomerular filtration rate. If hydronephrosis is present and the source is known (i.e. progressive retroperitoneal or pelvic mass), then further diagnostic tests may not be necessary, and percutaneous nephrostomy tube can be placed to relieve obstructive pain and renal insufficiency. If the source is unclear and if a ureteral stent is considered, then additional imaging with CT urogram will help characterize the location and source of the ureteral obstruction. Further, nuclear renal function studies may be considered only if it will help guide treatment.

In the acute setting of obstructive uropathy, the patient's and family's wishes in regard to relief of obstructive pain and improvement of renal function must be addressed. If the patient and family wish to accept renal failure, then symptom relief with analgesics may be sufficient for palliation. In order to treat obstructive nephropathy, endoscopic procedures with a nephrostomy tube placed percutaneously or a ureteral stent placed transurethrally are common approaches. Benefits of a nephrostomy tube include sparing the patient an anaesthetic by having an interventional radiologist place it under conscious sedation and diverting the urine proximal to the source of obstruction. These tubes and stents require exchange every 3 months or calcifications and encrustation can become problematic. The placement risks include bleeding in patients with coagulopathy, vascular injury, perinephric hematoma, discomfort, and social stigma associated with an external drainage bag.

Ureteral stents also alleviate obstruction but have a higher failure rate due to inability to traverse the site of blockage, and if successful, external malignant compression leads to eventual obstruction despite a ureteral stent (Docimo and Dewolf, 1989; Chung et al., 2004; Kamiyama et al., 2011). Metallic stents have shown success in keeping ureters patent in the setting of malignant compression (Borin et al., 2006; Liatsikos et al., 2010). If a ureteral stent fails, then a percutaneous nephrostomy tube is required (Gasparini et al., 1991; Wilson et al., 2005; Allen et al., 2010). Stent placement requires a patient that is fit for general anaesthesia routinely every 3–4 months for exchanges and is associated with the risks of genitourinary trauma, bleeding, urinary extravasation, and infection. Ureteral stents are appealing because they are internal and not visible; however, patients and families should be counselled on the effects of colicky pain, frequency, dysuria, and pelvic pressure. Alternatives to urinary diversion in the face of malignant extrinsic obstruction include reducing the obstructive mass with appropriate chemotherapy, radiation, or debulking surgery.

Benign causes of ureteral obstruction, including stones, stricture, or retroperitoneal fibrosis can be managed similarly with ureteral stents or nephrostomy tubes. Attempts to definitively treat the source of obstruction in such scenarios will depend on the patient's competing comorbidities, life expectancy, and ability to tolerate the risks associated with intervention. In the case of obstructing ureteral stones, one could discuss treatment with shockwave lithotripsy or ureteroscopy and laser lithotripsy. In the case of stricture, balloon dilation or laser endoureterotomy are reasonable options (Banner and Pollack, 1984). Ureterectomy and further reconstruction (i.e. ureteroneocystostomy, ureteroureterostomy) has an unlikely role in this setting due to the invasive nature and risk involved. Similarly, ureterolysis for retroperitoneal fibrosis is unlikely.

Intractable haematuria

Intractable haematuria in the palliative care patient can be difficult to control and may be life-threatening (see also Chapter 8.7). Depending on the source of bleeding, symptoms can be painful or painless, accompanied by lower urinary tract symptoms, clot retention, or infection. If untreated, patients will continue to have anaemia requiring frequent transfusions, clot retention, and secondary obstructive uropathy, and eventually haemorrhagic shock and death. Risk factors in this population include bleeding diatheses due to impaired synthetic function, anticoagulant medication, and poor wound-healing ability. Management depends on the aetiology and location within the upper or lower urinary tract (Garber and Wein, 1989).

For upper urinary tract bleeding involving the kidneys or ureters, sources include renal cell carcinoma, urothelial carcinoma, arteriovenous malformation, angiomyolipoma, haemorrhagic cysts, or metastatic disease. While rare, upper urinary tract communications with nearby vessels (ureterovascular, pyelovascular, and renovascular fistulae) can cause brisk bleeding and require quick intervention with transfusion, and angioembolization. Ureterovascular fistulae, although rare, occur with risk factors that are more common in the palliative care population, such as chronic ureteral stents, vascular stents, significant atherosclerosis, arterial aneurysms, or history of radiation. Renovascular or pyelovascular fistulae are usually iatrogenic after percutaneous kidney surgery (i.e. percutaneous nephrolithotomy). The clinician must have a high level of suspicion in order to detect this pathology, as presentation and diagnostic studies can be elusive.

General work-up of gross haematuria includes cystourethroscopy and upper urinary tract imaging with a CT urogram or retrograde pyelography. If the bleeding source is localized to a lesion in the collecting system, then ureteroscopy and endoscopic fulguration with or without excision is a reasonable approach. If bleeding recurs despite endoscopic treatment or if the source of bleeding is not amenable to endoscopic fulguration, then selective arterial embolization is recommended. In the setting of life-threatening haemorrhage, haemodynamic stabilization and blood transfusion should be followed quickly by angiography with selective arterial embolization. Any anticoagulants should be held until bleeding is controlled. Surgical exploration to control bleeding is an option if endovascular embolization is not possible. For bleeding renal masses that cannot be managed endoscopically or endovascularly, palliative nephrectomy or nephroureterectomy could be considered in very select patients.

For ureterovascular fistulae, control of the communicating vessel can be achieved by endovascular stenting, open reconstruction, embolizing, or ligating with or without arterial bypass (Rovner, 2012). Consideration must be taken for infection due to urine contamination, and treated as needed. Control of the urinary tract can be achieved via urinary diversion, least invasive of which would be placement of a nephrostomy tube with ureteral coiling. More involved and less feasible in this population includes open reconstruction to perform a uretero-ureterostomy, transuretero-ureterostomy, or cutaneous ureterostomy.

Lower urinary tract sources of haematuria include bladder tumour (urothelial or non-urothelial origin), haemorrhagic cystitis secondary to chemotherapy (cyclophosphamide and ifosfamide) or radiation, bleeding prostatic varices, or urethral trauma. First, anticoagulant medications should be held if possible, coagulopathies should be corrected, and blood transfusion should be performed in anaemic patients.

Initial management includes hand irrigation and continuous saline bladder irrigation with a large-calibre Foley catheter. For prostatic bleeding, gentle Foley catheter traction can help tamponade the source. Medical management with 5-alpha reductase (finasteride) or androgen deprivation can reduce prostatic bleeding in the long term (Sieber et al., 1998). Persistent prostatic or bladder bleeding refractory to conservative measures will require operative intervention to fulgurate sites of bleeding, resect bladder or prostatic tumour, and evacuate clots.

For persistent bladder bleeding from malignancy, radiation, or cyclophosphamide-induced haemorrhagic cystitis, epsilon aminocaproic acid (Amicar®) may be used in intravenous, oral, or intravesical form, to aid in clot formation (Stefanini et al., 1990). Patients on Amicar® should be monitored for rhabdomyolysis, a rare but serious adverse event reported in the literature. Those patients who are on therapy for greater than 24 hours should have routine tests for myoglobinuria, myoglobinaemia, creatine kinase, lactate dehydrogenase, aspartate aminotransferase, decreased muscle strength, and myalgia (Seymour and Rubinger, 1997). If bleeding is ongoing, then bladder irrigation with 1–2% alum (potassium or ammonium aluminium sulphate) or 1% silver nitrate can be effective (Goel et al., 1985). If renal insufficiency is present or bladder lesions allow a significant amount of alum to enter the vascular system, then serum aluminium levels should be monitored. Patients can typically tolerate these intravesical treatments and anaesthesia is not usually required.

For haematuria refractory to the above-mentioned agents, formalin instillation is very effective but carries a high toxicity risk, including severe lower urinary tract symptoms, incontinence, small capacity bladder, fibrosis, and perforation (Donahue and Frank, 1989; Ghahestani and Shakhssalim, 2009). Formalin at 2.5–4% concentration is instilled passively until half the bladder capacity is reached and then left in for 20–30 minutes. Then the bladder is irrigated continuously with normal saline. Since this procedure is very painful, general or regional anaesthesia is required. Prior to formalin instillation, vesicoureteral reflux must first be ruled out with an intraoperative cystogram. If reflux is present, balloon catheters should be inserted into the lower ureters and the patient placed in reverse Trendelenburg position to prevent formalin reflux and subsequent upper tract damage (Sarnak et al., 1999). The effect of intravesical instillations can be maximized with urinary diversion (percutaneous nephrostomy tubes and ureteral occlusion) in order to minimize the effects of urokinase, a clot inhibitor present in urine (Sneiders and Pryor, 1993; Zagoria et al., 1993; Russo, 2000).

An alternative to intravesical agents in the treatment of haematuria from a malignant source includes radiation therapy. In one study, up to 59% of patients with advanced bladder cancer had resolution of haematuria and 73% had pain reduction after

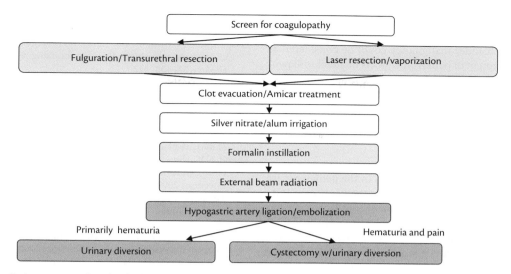

Fig. 8.4.1 Simplified palliative treatment algorithm for bleeding and pain of bladder origin, including malignant and benign conditions. All of the treatment steps are not required. Some treatments will be bypassed depending on the severity of the symptoms.
Reprinted from *The Journal of Urology*, Volume 174, Issue 4, Part 1, Joon-Ha Ok et al., Medical and Surgical Palliative Care Of Patients with Urological Malignancies, pp. 1177–1182, Copyright © 2005 American Urological Association, Inc., with permission from Elsevier, http://www.sciencedirect.com/science/journal/00225347.

treatment (Srinivasan et al., 1994). In another study, complete palliation of locally advanced bladder cancer was found in 43% of patients (Salminen, 1992). Although bladder and bowel complications are possible, radiation therapy is generally well tolerated. Chemotherapy has not been as well studied for palliation of pain or bleeding in advanced bladder cancer.

If conservative methods fail, embolization or surgical ligation of hypogastric arteries may be required. Palliative cystectomy with urinary diversion such as an ileal conduit should only be considered if all other options have failed or are not feasible, as it is the most invasive treatment associated with the greatest morbidity. The various treatments and recommended algorithm for intractable haematuria are depicted in Fig. 8.4.1.

Urinary tract fistulae

Risk factors that contribute to vesicoenteric and vesicovaginal fistulae (VVF) are common to the palliative care patient, such as advanced malignancy, prior pelvic surgery, radiation, poor nutrition, poor wound-healing ability, and infection (Rovner, 2012). Common causes specific to vesicoenteric fistulae are colon malignancies, diverticulitis, and Crohn's disease. Similarly, gynaecologic malignancies and pelvic inflammatory disease contribute to VVF. Symptoms of fistulae involving the urinary tract include pneumaturia, urinary tract infection, suprapubic pain, and incontinence. Faecaluria, diarrhoea, and tenesmus are associated with vesicoenteric fistulae. Vaginal leakage can be significant in VVF. Untreated, these symptoms lead to rash, skin breakdown, ulcers, chronic infection, and sepsis.

Diagnostic studies include pelvic examination, urinalysis, contrast imaging with a CT cystogram, CT urogram (to detect ureterovaginal or ureteroenteric fistula), CT scan with rectal contrast, or MRI. Endoscopy with cystoscopy and colonoscopy may also help confirm the diagnosis. Goals of palliative management of urinary fistulas include symptom management and containment of urinary leakage. Spontaneous closure is rare. These goals can be

achieved conservatively with diversion of urine using a Foley or suprapubic catheter or bilateral nephrostomy tubes with or without permanent ureteral occlusion (Gupta et al., 2009). Surgical diversion with an ileal conduit or formal fistula repair are more involved and only appropriate in select patients. For vesicoenteric fistulas, a diverting colostomy or the use of rectal stents may temporize symptoms (Harford et al., 2008). Depending on the severity of the fistulae, conservative measures may or may not alleviate symptoms.

Pelvic and bladder pain

Pelvic and bladder pain can cause significant distress with symptoms of suprapubic pressure, urgency, or dysuria. The aetiology of bladder and pelvic pain will dictate the treatment approach. Diagnostic work-up includes drawing a urinalysis and culture, pelvic exam, imaging with X-ray and ultrasound to evaluate for obstructing urolithiasis or bladder stones. A CT scan or MRI is indicated to better identify abdominal or pelvic masses. Cystoscopy can be performed to identify an intravesical mass, bladder stone, or fistula. If the patient has a known malignancy as the source of pelvic pain, extensive work-up may be unnecessary.

Invasive pelvic masses cause pain due to the loss of bladder capacity and compliance, leading to high filling pressure, urgency, frequency, incontinence, and infection. Extrinsic compression on the bladder can cause similar lower urinary tract symptoms. Initial treatment includes placement of a urethral catheter to facilitate drainage. Ongoing bladder pressure and spasms despite drainage could be treated with analgesics, antimuscarinic medication, or belladonna and opium suppository. Urinary diversion with nephrostomy tubes could further alleviate symptoms of voiding dysfunction; however, it *may not* address pain from mass effect.

Neuropathic pain caused by mass compression onto the lumbosacral plexus can be treated medically with analgesics, antidepressants, or antiepileptics (Jaeckle et al., 1985; Rigor, 2000).

Radiation, chemotherapy, or surgery is appropriate in very select patients, to reduce the size of the mass. Transurethral resection of invasive prostatic or bladder malignancy could be considered as well. Alternative treatment of pain from cystitis includes oral pentosan polysulphate sodium (Elmiron®). Intravesical agents include dimethyl sulphoxide, heparin, and hyaluronic acid, which have variable success. Management of haematuria related to radiation cystitis is addressed earlier in this chapter.

Conclusion

Genitourinary problems are not uncommon in the palliative care setting and can become more severe as a patient's disease state progresses. Diagnostic tests and management approaches need to be tailored to each patient's clinical and social situation. Selection of tests and treatment modalities should be based on using the least invasive means to achieve the most relief in suffering. Some genitourinary conditions in this setting are potentially fatal, such as urinary tract haemorrhage and renal failure, and in the acute or subacute setting, require re-evaluation of the end-of-life goals and wishes of the patient and family.

Online materials

Complete references for this chapter are available online at <http://www.oxfordmedicine.com>.

References

Borin, J.F., Melamud, O., and Clayman, R.V. (2006). Initial experience with full-length metal stent to relieve malignant ureteral obstruction. *Journal of Endourology*, 20, 300–304.

Centers for Disease Control and Prevention (2012). Catheter-associated urinary tract infection (CAUTI) event. In *National Healthcare Safety Network, Device-Associated Module*. Atlanta, GA: Center for Disease Control and Prevention.

Chung, S.Y., Stein, R.J., Landsittel, D., *et al.* (2004). 15-year experience with the management of extrinsic ureteral obstruction with indwelling ureteral stents. *Journal of Urology*, 172, 592–595.

Docimo, S.G. and Dewolf, W.C. (1989). High failure rate of indwelling ureteral stents in patients with extrinsic obstruction: experience at 2 institutions. *Journal of Urology*, 142, 277–279.

Doherty, A.P. and O'Sullivan, J.M. (2004). Symptom control in urological malignancy. In G.P. Dunn and A.G. Johnson (eds.) *Surgical Palliative Care*, pp. 186–210. Oxford: Oxford University Press.

Donahue, L.A. and Frank, I.N. (1989). Intravesical formalin for hemorrhagic cystitis: analysis of therapy. *Journal of Urology*, 141, 809–812.

Garber, B.B. and Wein, A.J. (1989). Common urologic bleeding problems part I & II. *AUA Update Series*, Lesson 34.

Gasparini, M., Carroll, P., and Stoller, M. (1991). Palliative percutaneous and endoscopic urinary diversion for malignant ureteral obstruction. *Urology*, 38, 408–412.

Ghahestani, S.M. and Shakhssalim, N. (2009). Palliative treatment of intractable hematuria in context of advanced bladder cancer: a systematic review. *Urology Journal*, 6, 149–156.

Goel, A.K., Rao, M.S., Bhagwat, A.G., Vaidyanathan, S., Goswami, A.K., and Sen, T.K. (1985). Intravesical irrigation with alum for the control of massive bladder hemorrhage. *Journal of Urology*, 133, 956–957.

Gould, C.V., Umscheid, C.A., Agarwal, R.K., Kuntz, G., and Pegues, D.A. (2010). Guideline for prevention of catheter-associated urinary tract infections 2009. *Infection Control and Hospital Epidemiology*, 31, 319–326.

Jaeckle, K.A., Young, D.F., and Foley, K.M. (1985). The natural history of lumbosacral plexopathy in cancer. *Neurology*, 35, 8–15.

Jahn, P., Preuss, M., Kernig, A., Seifert-Huhmer, A., and Langer, G. (2007). Types of indwelling urinary catheters for long-term bladder drainage in adults. *Cochrane Database of Systematic Reviews*, 3, CD004997.

National Institute for Health and Clinical Excellence (2003). *Infection Control: Prevention of Healthcare-Associated Infections in Primary and Community Care*. London: National Institute for Health and Clinical Excellence.

Niel-Weise, B.S., Van Den Broek, P.J., Da Silva, E.M., and Silva, L.A. (2012). Urinary catheter policies for long-term bladder drainage. *Cochrane Database of Systematic Reviews*, 8, CD004201.

Petronella, P., Scorzelli, M., Fiore, A., *et al.* (2012). Antibiotic prophylaxis in catheter-associated urinary infections. *New Microbiologica*, 35, 191–198.

Rigor, B.M. Sr. (2000). Pelvic cancer pain. *Journal of Surgical Oncology*, 75, 280–300.

Rovner, E.S. (2012). Urinary tract fistulae. In A.J. Wein (ed.) *Campbell-Walsh Urology* (10th ed.), pp. 415–421. Philadelphia, PA: Elsevier Saunders.

Schaeffer, A.J. and Schaeffer, E.M. (2012). Infections of the urinary tract. In A.J. Wein (ed.) *Campbell-Walsh Urology* (10th ed.), pp. 257–326. Philadelphia, PA: Elsevier Saunders.

Schumm, K. and Lam, T.B. (2008). Types of urethral catheters for management of short-term voiding problems in hospitalized adults: a short version Cochrane review. *Neurourology and Urodynamics*, 27, 738–746.

Seymour, B.D. and Rubinger, M. (1997). Rhabdomyolysis induced by epsilon-aminocaproic acid. *Annals of Pharmacotherapy*, 31, 56–58.

Sneiders, A. and Pryor, J.L. (1993). Percutaneous nephrostomy drainage in the treatment of severe hemorrhagic cystitis. *Journal of Urology*, 150, 966–967.

Wu, J.N., Meyers, F.J., and Evans, C.P. (2011). Palliative care in urology. *Surgical Clinics of North America*, 91, 429–444.

Zagoria, R.J., Hodge, R.G., Dyer, R.B., and Routh, W.D. (1993). Percutaneous nephrostomy for treatment of intractable hemorrhagic cystitis. *Journal of Urology*, 149, 1449–1451.

8.5

Oral care

Andrew N. Davies

Introduction to oral care

Epidemiology

Oral symptoms are common in patients with advanced cancer (see below) (Davies and Epstein, 2010). Most patients have at least one symptom, and many patients have several symptoms. Oral symptoms are also common relative to other symptoms in patients with advanced cancer (Davies and Epstein, 2010). Indeed, xerostomia (dry mouth) is consistently ranked as one of the five most common symptoms in this group of patients.

Investigators have found disparities between the recorded prevalence of certain oral symptoms and the true prevalence of these oral symptoms in patients with advanced cancer (Shah and Davies, 2001). These disparities probably relate to service-related factors (e.g. inadequate oral assessment procedures), professional-related factors (e.g. perception that these symptoms are unimportant), and patient-related factors (e.g. perception that other symptoms are more important).

Oral problems are also common in other groups of patients with life-limiting illnesses (and more generally in patients with chronic illness) (Davies and Finlay, 2005). For example, the reported prevalence of oral problems in a study of patients with Parkinson's disease was as follows: xerostomia—55%; loose dentures—31%; sore gums—23%; ulcers—17%; bleeding gums—12%, burning sensation—10%; loose teeth—8%; sore teeth—5% (Clifford and Finnerty, 1995). Similarly, the reported prevalence of oral problems in a study of patients with multiple sclerosis was as follows: orofacial paraesthesia—37%; orofacial pain—30%; taste disturbance—23%; orofacial muscle spasm/palsy—17%; difficulty chewing—8% (Fabiano, 1983).

Aetiology

Oral problems may be related to:

- Direct ('anatomical') effect of the primary disease
- Indirect ('physiological') effect of the primary disease
- Treatment of the primary disease
- Direct/indirect effect of a coexisting disease
- Treatment of the coexisting disease
- Combinations of the above factors.

One of the most important causes of oral problems is the indirect ('physiological') effects of the primary disease. Thus, patients often develop physical problems (e.g. fatigue), which impedes their ability to undertake oral hygiene measures. Moreover, patients often develop psychological problems (e.g. depression), which further affects their ability/motivation to undertake oral hygiene measures (Friedlander and Mahler, 2001).

Clinical features

Oral problems are a significant direct cause of morbidity in palliative care patients. Table 8.5.1 shows the severity of oral symptoms, whilst Table 8.5.2 shows the distress caused by oral symptoms, in an advanced cancer population (Davies, 2000b). Moreover, oral problems can lead to a more generalized deterioration in a patient's physical state, and also in their psychological state (Rydholm and Strang, 2002). Oral problems are also an indirect cause of mortality in palliative care patients (i.e. oral colonization/infection leading to systemic infection) (Mandel, 2004).

Assessment

The assessment of oral problems is essentially similar to the assessment of other medical problems. It involves taking a history, performing an examination, and the use of appropriate investigations (Birnbaum and Dunne, 2000). Many of the oral assessment tools that are used in palliative care are not validated for use in this clinical setting (and indeed are not appropriate for use in this clinical setting) (Davies, 2005).

A wide range of investigations are used in everyday clinical practice (Birnbaum and Dunne, 2000), but only some of these investigations will be relevant in patients with advanced cancer (e.g. microbiological testing). The decision to perform an investigation will depend on the nature of the problem (important or not), the nature of the investigation (invasive or not), the likely outcome of the investigation (management altered or not), and the condition/prognosis of the patient (Davies, 2005).

Management: general principles

The successful management of oral problems involves adequate assessment, appropriate treatment, and adequate re-assessment. The aims of assessment are to determine the nature of the problem, and factors that may influence the choice of treatment: inadequate assessment may result in the use of ineffective or inappropriate interventions. The aims of re-assessment are to determine the response to the treatment (i.e. efficacy of treatment, tolerability of treatment): inadequate re-assessment may result in the continued use of ineffective or inappropriate interventions (and ongoing morbidity from the oral problem).

The treatment of oral problems may involve definitive management of the problem ('cure'), symptomatic management of the

Table 8.5.1 Severity of oral symptoms in patients with advanced cancer (Davies, 2000)

Symptom (N = 120)	'Slight'	'Moderate'	'Severe'	'Very severe'
Dry mouth (n = 93)	14%	37%	33%	16%
Mouth discomfort (n = 55)	40%	29%	22%	9%
Change in the way food tastes (n = 53)	30%	45%	19%	6%
Difficulty speaking (n = 37)	40%	30%	19%	11%
Difficulty swallowing (n = 28)	46%	29%	14%	11%
Difficulty chewing (n = 27)	41%	41%	11%	7%
Mouth sores (n = 17)	59%	35%	6%	0%

Reproduced from Davies, A.N., *An investigation into the relationship between salivary gland hypofunction and oral health problems in patients with advanced cancer* (Dissertation), Kings College, University of London, UK, Copyright © 2000, with permission of the author.

Table 8.5.2 Distress caused by oral symptoms in patients with advanced cancer (Davies, 2000)

Symptom (N = 120)	'Not at all'	'A little bit'	'Somewhat'	'Quite a bit'	'Very much'
Dry mouth (n = 93)	16%	21%	23%	26%	14%
Mouth discomfort (n = 55)	16%	31%	18%	26%	9%
Change in the way food tastes (n = 53)	17%	32%	23%	21%	7%
Difficulty speaking (n = 37)	3%	32%	24%	22%	19%
Difficulty swallowing (n = 28)	11%	28%	36%	14%	11%
Difficulty chewing (n = 27)	11%	44%	15%	30%	0%
Mouth sores (n = 17)	18%	35%	18%	29%	0%

Reproduced from Davies, A.N., *An investigation into the relationship between salivary gland hypofunction and oral health problems in patients with advanced cancer* (Dissertation), Kings College, University of London, UK, Copyright © 2000, with permission of the author.

problem ('palliation'), management of the cause of the problem, and/or management of the complications of the problem. Whilst there may be a range of options for management in everyday practice, there may be fewer options for management in patients with advanced cancer. The decision to undertake a treatment depends on a number of factors, including the nature of the problem, the nature of the treatment, the availability of the treatment, the general health/condition of the patient, and, particularly, the wishes of the patient.

In some cases the most appropriate treatment for a patient with advanced cancer is the same treatment that would be given to a patient with early cancer (or no cancer). Thus, intensive treatment of the oral problem often results in the best palliation of the oral problem. It is not justified to withhold treatment on the grounds that the patient has advanced cancer. However, it may be justified to amend treatment (when appropriate). For example, the standard treatment for a poorly fitting denture involves fabrication of a new denture. However, in patients with a poor performance status, an alternative treatment for a poorly fitting denture would involve re-lining of the old denture (Walls, 2005).

Management: multidisciplinary working

Oral care/problems should be the concern of all clinical members of the core palliative care multidisciplinary team (MDT). Dental professionals are important members of the extended palliative care MDT (i.e. dentists, dental hygienists). They have a number of key roles, including (a) training of other members of the MDT, (b) management of specific oral problems (e.g. dental caries), and (c) management of complex oral problems (in combination with other members of the MDT). Many dental procedures can be performed in the home or hospice setting, although such 'domiciliary dentistry' requires specialized skills and appropriate equipment (Walls, 2005).

Other members of the MDT team will, of course, have a major role in the management of certain oral problems (e.g. speech and language therapists, dieticians).

Management: evidence-based practice

Oral care in palliative care is frequently based on historical anecdote, rather than on available research evidence. Hence, many patients continue to receive relatively ineffective treatments for their oral problems (e.g. ice cubes for xerostomia), whilst some patients continue to receive entirely inappropriate treatments for their oral problems (e.g. vitamin C tablets for 'dirty mouth'). However, there is a wealth of evidence for the efficacy of various interventions in the non-palliative care population, and increasingly in the palliative care population (Davies and Finlay, 2005; Davies and Epstein, 2010).

Oral hygiene

Maintenance of good oral hygiene is important for the maintenance of good quality of life in patients with cancer and other life-limiting illnesses (Sweeney and Davies, 2010).

Dental care

Toothbrushing

The single most important oral hygiene measure is toothbrushing, which should be undertaken at least twice daily (Sweeney and Davies, 2010).

A wide range of toothbrushes is available, including powered ('electric') toothbrushes. It is recommended that a small-headed brush, which has soft-to-medium texture bristles is used. 'Ultra-soft' toothbrushes can be used for patients whose mouths are sore; such toothbrushes include baby brushes and specialist brushes, for example, TePe® Special Care toothbrush. Powered toothbrushes with a rotation-oscillation action appear to be better at removing dental plaque than manual toothbrushes (and other types of powered toothbrushes) (Robinson et al., 2005).

The recommended life span of a toothbrush is about 3 months, but it should be replaced sooner if the filaments of the brush become softened and/or misshapen. (At this stage the brush is no longer effective at removing dental plaque). Toothbrushes should be replaced sooner if the patient is immunosuppressed or receiving chemotherapy. Furthermore, toothbrushes should be immediately replaced if the patient has experienced any type of oral infection.

Patients should use toothpaste containing at least 1000 ppm fluoride. Most toothpaste contains a foaming agent, which may prove problematic for those patients who have difficulty swallowing (and who are at risk of aspiration). In these cases, a non-foaming alternative should be used (e.g. Biotene® toothpaste, chlorhexidine gel). If patients cannot tolerate the use of toothpaste (due to oral discomfort), then they can simply use water during toothbrushing.

Interdental cleaning

Interdental aids are designed to remove dental plaque from the areas between teeth that cannot be reached by a toothbrush. Ideally, some form of interdental cleaning should be used on a daily basis (Sweeney and Davies, 2010), although this may not be achievable or appropriate for some patients. The types of cleaning aids available include dental floss, dental tape, wood sticks, and interdental brushes.

Chemical plaque control

For some patients, mechanical control of dental plaque is extremely difficult because of their level of debilitation and/or the presence of oral pathology. In such cases chemical control of dental plaque may be considered for maintenance of oral hygiene (Sweeney and Davies, 2010).

Currently the most effective anti-plaque agent is chlorhexidine (Jones, 1997). The chlorhexidine molecule has a positive charge at either end, and binds readily to negatively charged sites on the dental enamel pellicle, mucosal cells, and bacterial cells. Chlorhexidine is slowly released from such surfaces, so maintaining its antimicrobial activity (a property known as substantivity).

Chlorhexidine is used most commonly as a 0.12–0.2 % mouthwash (10–15 mL twice a day), although it is also available as a 1% gel and a 0.2% spray in certain countries. Indeed, there are no indications for using chlorhexidine more than twice a day (see earlier). It is important to realize that chlorhexidine will not remove established dental plaque—this must be physically removed by a dentist or dental hygienist.

The most common side effect associated with long-term use of chlorhexidine is staining of the teeth and the dorsal surface of the tongue. The tooth staining can easily be removed by a dentist or dental hygienist. Other problems include the taste of the mouthwash, and the alcohol content of some mouthwashes (which may cause mucosal discomfort). These problems may be overcome by diluting the mouthwash with up to an equivalent volume of water (Axelsson and Lindhe, 1987).

Denture care

Denture hygiene must be carried out regularly and should be incorporated into a daily oral care routine (Sweeney and Davies, 2010). It should is done at least once per day (preferably at night). All dentures must be cleaned outside the mouth, and the soft tissues of the mouth cleaned separately (see below).

The denture should first be held under running water to remove debris, and then be brushed thoroughly with a large toothbrush, denture brush, or personal nailbrush to dislodge any remaining debris or plaque. Commercial products are available for cleaning dentures, but soap and water, or water on its own, is usually satisfactory. Ordinary toothpaste should not be used, because they are quite abrasive and may damage the polished surface of the denture. The denture should be rinsed well before placing it back in the patient's mouth.

Dentures should ideally be rinsed under running water after every meal, and the lining of the mouth checked for food debris before re-inserting the dentures. Calculus ('tartar') may form on the smooth surfaces of a denture as a result of deposition of calcium from the saliva. Calculus may irritate/damage the underlying oral mucosa, and should be professionally removed as soon as it is noticed.

In order to maintain a healthy oral mucosa, it is advisable to leave dentures out of the mouth overnight. Plastic dentures should be soaked in a dilute solution of sodium hypochlorite (1 part Milton® sterilizing fluid to 80 parts water). This allows disinfection of the denture, and reduces the likelihood of denture stomatitis. Dentures with metal parts should be soaked in chlorhexidine (0.12–0.2% solution), since sodium hypochlorite can potentially damage the metal parts.

Care of the oral mucosa

The oral mucosa should be cleaned three to four times per day, ideally after each meal (Sweeney and Davies, 2010). For those patients who are able, rinsing the mouth with water is adequate to remove any debris. For those who are unable to rinse, the mucosa should be cleaned mechanically with a water-moistened gauze or foam stick.

Salivary gland dysfunction

Xerostomia is 'the subjective sensation of dryness of the mouth', whilst salivary gland hypofunction is 'any objectively demonstrable reduction in either whole and/or individual gland flow rates' (Davies, 2010a). Salivary gland dysfunction (SGD) has been defined as 'any alteration in the qualitative or quantitative output of saliva caused by an increase (hyperfunction) or decrease (hypofunction) in salivary output', although SGD is more often used as an umbrella term to describe patients with xerostomia and/or salivary gland hypofunction (Davies, 2010a).

Epidemiology

The prevalence of xerostomia is 22–26% in the general population (Davies, 2010a), whereas the prevalence of xerostomia is 78–82% in patients with advanced cancer (Davies et al., 2001; Tranmer et al., 2003). Similarly, the prevalence of salivary gland hypofunction has been reported to be 82–83% in patients with advanced cancer (Chaushu et al., 2000; Davies et al., 2002b). SGD is common in patients with other life-limiting conditions, and indeed in patients with many chronic conditions (Davies and Finlay, 2006)

Aetiology

There are numerous causes of SGD in the oncology population, with the most common cause being drug treatment (Davies et al., 2001). SGD is a side effect of many of the drugs used in day-to-day practice, including many of the drugs used in supportive and palliative care (e.g. analgesics, antiemetics) (Sreebny and Schwartz, 1997). Other causes of SGD include: (a) cancer related, for example, tumour infiltration, paraneoplastic syndrome; (b) cancer treatment-related, for example, radiotherapy, graft-versus-host disease; and (c) other causes, for example, dehydration, malnutrition, anxiety, and depression (Davies, 2010a).

Xerostomia is usually the result of a decrease in the volume of saliva secreted (i.e. salivary gland hypofunction). However, xerostomia may also result from a change in the composition of the saliva secreted.

Clinical features

The clinical features of SGD are very variable, and reflect the differing functions of saliva (Davies, 2010a). SGD is associated with a number of oral problems, but is also associated with more generalized problems. Indeed, SGD is associated with a significant negative impact on quality of life (Rydholm and Strang, 2002):

◆ General problems—oral discomfort, lip discomfort, cracking of lips

◆ Eating-related problems—anorexia, taste disturbance, difficulty chewing, difficulty swallowing, decreased intake of nutrition

◆ Speech-related problems—difficulty speaking

◆ Oral hygiene—poor oral hygiene, halitosis

◆ Oral infections—oral candidosis, dental caries, periodontal disease, salivary gland infections

◆ Systemic infections—secondary to oral infection (e.g. pneumonia, septicaemia)

◆ Dental/denture prosthesis problems—dental erosion (leading to dental sensitivity/trauma to oral mucosa)

◆ Psychosocial problems—embarrassment, anxiety, depression, social isolation

◆ Miscellaneous problems—sleep disturbance, difficulty using oral transmucosal medication (i.e. sublingual/buccal medication), oesophagitis, urinary frequency (secondary to increased intake of fluid).

It is important to emphasize that there may be a discrepancy between the symptoms experienced by patients and the signs identified by health-care professionals. The classic signs of salivary gland hypofunction include dryness of the oral mucosa, dryness of the lips, absence of a pool of saliva in the floor of the mouth, fissuring of the oral mucosa (especially of the tongue), and cracking of the lips. However, patients with xerostomia, and some patients with salivary gland hypofunction, may have no obvious abnormalities on examination.

Assessment

A wide range of investigations may be employed in the management of SGD in the general population (Davies, 2010a). Some of these investigations are used to diagnose SGD (e.g. measurement of salivary flow rates), whilst other investigations are used to determine the cause of the SGD (e.g. detection of auto-antibodies). However, most of these investigations are not indicated in the assessment of SGD in the oncology population. Indeed, a diagnosis of SGD can invariably be made on the basis of routine clinical skills, that is, taking a history and performing an examination (Navazesh et al., 1992).

Management

SGD is a heterogeneous condition, and so requires individualized management (Davies, 2010a). The management of SGD depends on a variety of different factors, including the aetiology/pathophysiology of the SGD, the clinical features of the SGD, the general condition of the patient, the dental status of the patient, the treatment preferences of the patient, the availability of specific interventions, and the affordability of specific interventions. The management of SGD involves a number of different strategies, including (a) treatment of the cause of SGD, (b) symptomatic treatment of SGD, and (c) the treatment of the complications of SGD.

The symptomatic treatment of SGD involves the use of saliva stimulants (agents that promote saliva secretion) and saliva substitutes (agents that replace missing saliva) (Davies, 2010a). There are good reasons for prescribing saliva stimulants rather than saliva substitutes. Thus, saliva stimulants increase the secretion of 'normal' saliva, and so will ameliorate xerostomia and the other clinical features of SGD. In contrast, saliva substitutes, which are very different from normal saliva (i.e. physically, chemically), will usually only ameliorate xerostomia. Moreover, in studies that have compared saliva stimulants with saliva substitutes, patients have generally expressed a preference for the saliva stimulants (Bjornstrom et al., 1990; Stewart et al., 1998). Nevertheless, some patients do not respond to treatment with saliva stimulants, and so will require treatment with saliva substitutes (e.g. some patients with radiation-induced SGD).

Saliva stimulants

Chewing gum

Chewing gum increases salivary flow by two mechanisms; approximately 85% of the increase is related to stimulation of chemoreceptors within the oral cavity (i.e. taste effect), whilst approximately 15% of the increase is related to stimulation of mechanoreceptors in and around the oral cavity (i.e. chewing effect).

Chewing gum has been reported to be effective in the management of xerostomia in various groups of patients, including advanced cancer patients with drug-induced SGD (Davies, 2000a). Moreover, chewing gum has been reported to be more effective than organic acids and artificial saliva in studies involving mixed groups of patients with SGD (Bjornstrom et al., 1990; Stewart et al., 1998). Patients with SGD should use 'sugar-free' chewing gum, and patients with dental prostheses should use 'low-tack' (less sticky) chewing gum.

Chewing gum is generally well tolerated. However, side effects can occur, and may be related to (a) chewing, for example, jaw discomfort, headache; (b) inappropriate ingestion, for example, respiratory tract obstruction, gastrointestinal obstruction; (c) non-allergic reactions to additives, for example, oral discomfort, flatulence; and (d) allergic reactions to additives, for example, stomatitis, perioral dermatitis. Chewing gum is an acceptable form of treatment for most patients, including most elderly patients (Davies, 2000a).

Organic acids

Various organic acids have been used as saliva stimulants, including ascorbic acid (vitamin C), citric acid (the acid in citrus fruits), and malic acid (the acid in apples and pears). Organic acids increase salivary flow through stimulation of chemoreceptors within the oral cavity.

Ascorbic acid has been reported to be relatively ineffective in a study involving a mixed group of patients with SGD (Bjornstrom et al., 1990). Thus, only 33% of the patients rated ascorbic acid as either 'good' or 'very good', and only 23% of patients wanted to continue with it after the study.

Studies suggest that citric acid can provide symptomatic improvement for some groups of patients with SGD, although not patients with radiation-induced SGD. However, in the study by Stewart et al., only 24% patients expressed a preference for the citric acid product, compared with 46% for the chewing gum and 30% for the artificial saliva (Stewart et al., 1998).

Malic acid has been reported to be relatively more effective in a study involving a mixed group of patients with SGD (Bjornstrom et al., 1990). Thus, 51% of the patients rated malic acid as either 'good' or 'very good', and 44% of patients wanted to continue with it after the study.

The use of organic acids is associated with the development of oral discomfort. Thus, organic acids should not be used in patients with dry mucosae, cracked mucosae, stomatitis, and/or mucositis. Moreover, the use of organic acids may be associated with the exacerbation of certain pH-related complications of SGD (i.e. demineralization of the teeth, dental caries, oral candidosis). Thus, organic acids should not be used in patients with teeth, and should be used with caution in patients with dental prostheses.

Parasympathomimetic drugs

Parasympathomimetic drugs stimulate the part of the autonomic nervous system responsible for the secretion of saliva from the salivary glands. The parasympathomimetic drugs include choline esters (e.g. pilocarpine, cevimeline) that have a direct effect, and cholinesterase inhibitors (e.g. distigmine, pyridostigmine) that have an indirect effect by inhibiting the metabolism of endogenous acetylcholine.

Pilocarpine has been reported to be effective in the management of SGD due to salivary gland disease (e.g. Sjögren's syndrome), drug treatment (Davies et al., 1998), radiotherapy (Davies and Shorthose, 2007), and graft-versus-host disease. Indeed, it has been reported to be more effective than artificial saliva in the management of SGD secondary to drug treatment (Davies et al., 1998), and radiotherapy (Davies and Singer, 1994).

The side effects of pilocarpine are usually related to generalized parasympathetic stimulation, and include sweating, headache, urinary frequency, and vasodilatation. The incidence of side effects is dose related, that is, the higher the dose of pilocarpine, the higher the incidence of side effects. A systematic review found that few (6%) patients with radiotherapy-related SGD discontinue

pilocarpine due to side effects at the standard dose of 5 mg three times daily (Davies and Shorthose, 2007).

The other choline esters that have been used in clinical practice include bethanechol, carbacholine, and cevimeline (Davies, 2010a). Bethanechol has been reported to be effective in the management of drug-induced SGD, and of radiotherapy-induced SGD. Similarly, cevimeline has been reported to be effective in the management of Sjögren's syndrome, radiotherapy-induced SGD, and graft-versus-host disease. The cholinesterase inhibitors that have been used in practice include distigmine and pyridostigmine (Davies, 2010a).

Acupuncture

Acupuncture has been reported to be useful in the management of SGD secondary to benign salivary gland disease, drug treatment, and radiotherapy, Nevertheless, a recent systematic review concluded that (at present) 'there is no evidence for the efficacy of acupuncture in the management of xerostomia', and stated that 'there is a need for future high quality randomized controlled trials' (Jedel, 2005).

Saliva substitutes

Water

Patients often use water to treat dryness of the mouth. However, in studies, patients have reported that water is less effective than 'artificial saliva'. Moreover, in one study, patients reported that the mean duration of improvement of dryness of the mouth was only 12 minutes (range 4–29 minutes) (Olsson and Axell, 1991).

In spite of this, many patients choose to use water rather than other saliva substitutes. The reasons for this phenomenon include familiarity, efficacy (moderate), tolerability, availability, and affordability. The use of water is not associated with side effects per se, although polydipsia is inevitably associated with polyuria (and nocturia).

It should be noted that there is no scientific rationale, and indeed no research evidence, to support the use of chilled or frozen water (i.e. ice chips, ice cubes).

'Artificial saliva'

It is common practice for health-care professionals to prescribe 'artificial saliva' for the treatment of SGD. A number of commercial products have been developed, which differ in formulation (e.g. spray, gel, lozenge), lubricant (e.g. carboxymethylcellulose, hydroxyethylcellulose, mucin), and additives (e.g. flavourings, fluoride, antimicrobial factors).

The 'ideal' artificial saliva should be easy to use, pleasant to use, effective, and well tolerated (Davies, 2010a). Moreover, it should have a neutral pH (to prevent demineralization of the teeth), and contain fluoride (to enhance remineralization of the teeth). Unfortunately, some commercial products have an acidic pH, and these should definitely not be prescribed in dentate patients, and should probably not be prescribed in any patient with SGD.

It should be noted that most of these commercial products have not been formally tested in any group of patients with SGD. However, there are positive studies in the literature involving patients with advanced cancer of a specific mucin-based artificial saliva (Sweeney et al., 1997; Davies et al., 1998; Davies, 2000a).

Artificial saliva is generally well tolerated, although some patients report local problems (e.g. oral irritation, taste disturbance), whilst some patients even report systemic problems (e.g. nausea, diarrhoea). The duration of effect of artificial saliva is invariably short, which necessitates the repeated use of these products during the day and night. Indeed, the short duration of effect is one of the main reasons why patients do not continue to use artificial saliva. In an attempt to overcome this problem, a number of investigators have developed intra-oral artificial saliva reservoirs. Reservoirs can be incorporated into new (purpose-built) dental prostheses, or into existing (standard) dental prostheses. Moreover, reservoirs can be incorporated into bite guards that may be worn throughout the day, or simply at night-time.

Sialorrhoea

Sialorrhoea has been defined as 'an excessive secretion of saliva' (Davies, 2010b). Sialorrhoea is not synonymous with drooling, although patients with sialorrhoea may also experience drooling. The symptomatic management of sialorrhoea is similar to the symptomatic management of drooling (see 'Drooling') (Davies, 2010b).

Drooling

Drooling has been defined as 'abnormal spillage of saliva from the mouth on to the lips, chin and clothing' (Davies, 2010b). Drooling is usually not related to sialorrhoea, but is related to difficulty in retaining saliva within the mouth (secondary to facial weakness/deformity) and/or removing saliva from the mouth (secondary to dysphagia). Indeed, many patients with drooling have salivary gland hypofunction rather than sialorrhoea. The symptomatic management of drooling includes anticholinergic drugs (e.g. oral or nebulized glycopyrronium bromide, transdermal or nebulized hyoscine hydrobromide), botulinum toxin A, parasympathetic nerve ablation, and salivary gland duct relocation (Davies, 2010b).

Tenacious saliva

The strategies used to manage tenacious saliva include treatment of any SGD (see earlier), treatment of any dehydration (and encouragement of drinking), oral rinsing (e.g. soda water, sodium bicarbonate), humidification, and dietary manipulation (e.g. avoidance of milk, avoidance of caffeine) (British Columbia Cancer Agency, n.d.). Other strategies have been reported to be effective in patients with non-malignant diseases, include drinking of fruit juices (e.g. dark grape, pineapple) (Anonymous, 2000), and treatment with beta blockers (Newall et al., 1996).

Taste disturbance

Taste disturbance occurs as a result of a reduction in taste sensation (hypogeusia), an absence of taste sensation (ageusia), or a distortion of normal taste sensation (dysgeusia) (Ripamonti and Fulfaro, 2010). The prevalence of taste disturbance has been reported to be 44–50% in patients with advanced cancer (Shorthose and Davies, 2003; Tranmer et al., 2003). Taste disturbance is relatively common in patients with cancers of the head and neck region, and extremely common in patients that have received radiotherapy to the head and neck region.

There are a variety of different causes of taste disturbance in patients with cancer (Ripamonti and Fulfaro 2010): (a) cancer

related, for example, damage to taste buds, damage cranial nerves, damage to central nervous system (CNS); (b) cancer treatment related, for example, local surgery, local radiotherapy, systemic chemotherapy; (c) oral problems, for example, SGD, poor oral hygiene, oral infections; (d) neurological problems, for example, damage cranial nerves, damage to CNS; (e) metabolic problems, for example, malnutrition, zinc deficiency, renal dysfunction; (e) miscellaneous, for example, ageing, menopause, drug treatment.

Patients may complain of a single taste problem (e.g. ageusia for all foods), or a combination of taste problems (e.g. hypogeusia for some foods, dysgeusia for other foods). For example, in a study involving patients with advanced cancer and taste disturbance, 40% reported ageusia, 31% reported hypogeusia, and 53% reported dysgeusia (Davies and Kaur, 1998). Patients with dysgeusia may report a variety of different sensations, but invariably report that food tastes unpleasant. Taste disturbance can lead to other physical, psychological, and social problems, which, in turn, can lead to a further deterioration in quality of life (Rydholm and Strang, 2002; Hutton et al., 2007). For, example, impairment of taste may be associated with anorexia, decreased nutritional intake, and weight loss.

The assessment of taste disturbance involves taking a history, performing an examination, and undertaking appropriate investigations. However, it is usually not necessary to undertake an objective assessment of the taste disturbance (i.e. measure taste acuity). The management of taste disturbance involves treatment of the underlying cause, dietary intervention, zinc therapy, and/or other (anecdotal) therapies (Ripamonti and Fulfaro 2010). In some cases it may be possible to treat the underlying cause of the taste disturbance, for example, SGD. Indeed, studies have shown that saliva stimulants improve both the xerostomia, and the associated taste disturbance (Davies and Singer, 1994). Nevertheless, in many cases, it is not possible to identify and/or treat the underlying cause of the taste disturbance.

Dietary intervention involves (a) utilization of foods that taste 'good'; (b) avoidance of foods that taste 'bad'; (c) enhancing the taste of the food (using salt, sugar, and other flavourings); and (d) addressing the presentation, smell, consistency and temperature of the food (Twycross and Lack, 1986; Komurcu et al., 2001). Ideally, a dietician should review all patients with taste disturbance, since dietary intervention requires an individualized approach. Studies of zinc therapy in various patient groups have produced conflicting results (Ripamonti and Fulfaro, 2010). Thus, it may be that zinc is effective for some, but not all, causes of taste disturbance. Oral zinc supplements are generally well tolerated, although they can cause dyspepsia, and abdominal pain. Hence, it seems reasonable to offer patients with taste disturbance a trial of an oral zinc supplement (in the absence of other treatment options).

Oral infections

Oral infections are common in patients with advanced cancer. A number of studies have assessed oral candidosis in this group of patients (see 'Oral candidosis' section), and there appears to be an association between the presence of oral candidosis and poor performance status (Davies et al., 2006, 2008). In contrast, few studies have assessed other oral infections in this group of patients. Nevertheless, dental caries has been reported in 20–35%

of patients (Aldred et al., 1991; Jobbins et al., 1992), and gingivitis in 36% of patients (Gordon et al., 1985). Oral herpes simplex virus infections are also relatively common in patients with advanced cancer (Sweeney and Bagg, 2000).

Oral candidosis

A variety of different fungi have been reported to cause oral infections. However, *Candida* species are responsible for almost all oral fungal infections. This chapter will confine itself to a discussion of infection caused by *Candida* and related species, that is, oral candidosis.

Epidemiology

Certain *Candida* species are considered to be commensal organisms within the oral cavity. Indeed, the median reported prevalence of oral yeast carriage in the general population is 34%. Oral yeast carriage is very common in patients with advanced cancer, with a reported prevalence of between 47% and 87% (Davies et al., 2002a). Similarly, oral candidosis is very common in patients with advanced cancer, with a reported prevalence of between 8% and 83% (Davies et al., 2008).

Aetiology

Candida albicans is the most common species isolated from the oral cavity, although other species are being increasingly isolated from the oral cavity for example, *C. glabrata*, and *C. dubliniensis* (Finlay and Davies, 2005). The main explanation for the increasing frequency of non-*C. albicans* species is the increasing use of antifungal drugs. The main consequence of the increasing frequency of non-*C. albicans* species is the increasing occurrence of antifungal drug resistance.

Candida species are relatively non-pathogenic organisms. Hence, oral candidosis usually occurs as a result of changes in host and/or intraoral factors. Oral candidosis is very common in immunocompromised patients. It is widely believed that systemic corticosteroids cause oral candidosis. However, most studies involving patients with advanced cancer have failed to identify such an association (Finlay and Davies, 2005). Moreover, a review of the literature concluded that, 'the relationship between systemic steroid therapy and oral candidal carriage or infection is not clear' (Samaranayake, 1990). Similarly, it is widely believed that systemic antibiotics cause oral candidosis. However, studies involving patients with advanced cancer have again failed to identify such an association (Finlay and Davies, 2005). Moreover, a review of the literature concluded that, 'the relationship between antibiotic therapy and candidosis is far from unequivocally proven' (Odds, 1979). However, there is a strong association between oral candidosis and the use of topical antibiotics and topical corticosteroids. Oral candidosis is very common in patients with SGD, and common in patients with a denture, particularly an upper denture (Finlay and Davies, 2005).

Clinical features

Oral candidosis can present in different clinical forms, with several forms sometimes being found in one patient. Patients with oral candidosis may, or may not, have oral symptoms. Moreover, these symptoms may be due to the infection, or the underlying cause of the infection (e.g. SGD). Indeed, many patients continue to have oral symptoms, even after they have been treated for oral candidosis (Finlay, 1986).

Pseudomembranous candidosis is the most common type of oral candidosis (Finlay and Davies, 2005). It is generally asymptomatic. Pseudomembranous candidosis is characterized by the presence of off-white spots/plaques on the buccal mucosa, or elsewhere in the oral cavity: the lesions can be easily removed. Erythematous candidosis is relatively common. Patients often complain of localized discomfort/pain. Erythematous candidosis usually involves the tongue or the buccal mucosa, and presents as an area of inflamed (reddened) mucosa.

Denture stomatitis is a very common type of oral candidosis in patients with dentures (Finlay and Davies, 2005). It is generally asymptomatic, although some patients complain of palatal discomfort. Denture stomatitis is characterized by varying degrees of inflammation of the hard palate: the lesion may consist of patchy inflammation, confluent inflammation, and/or areas of hyperplasia. Angular cheilitis is relatively common, particularly in edentulous patients. Patients often complain of localized discomfort, and the lesions may 'weep' or bleed. Angular cheilitis invariably involves both angles of the mouth, and presents as cracking/inflammation of the mucosa and skin. (The lesions may be covered with a crust/clot.) Denture stomatitis is often associated with angular cheilitis.

The other types of oral candidosis are relatively uncommon (e.g. median rhomboid glossitis) (Finlay and Davies, 2005). Oesophageal candidosis is a frequent complication of oral candidosis (Samonis et al., 1998). The clinical features of oesophageal candidosis include odynophagia (pain on swallowing), and dysphagia (difficulty swallowing). The diagnosis can be confirmed by performing an oesophagoscopy, or a barium swallow. The appearance on barium swallow is typical, with 'fluffy', punched-out lesions along the length of the oesophagus. Candidaemia/systemic candidosis are less frequent complications of oral candidosis.

Assessment

A diagnosis of oral candidosis should be based on a combination of clinical features and microbiological investigations (Finlay and Davies, 2005).

The clinical features of oral candidosis are relatively non-specific. For example, white patches on the oral mucosa (akin to pseudomembranous candidosis) can also occur in bacterial infections (Tyldesley et al., 1977). Similarly, erythematous patches on the oral mucosa (akin to erythematous candidosis) can also occur in a number of other conditions, for example, chemotherapy-induced mucositis.

As discussed above, it is common to isolate yeasts from the mouths of patients. Thus, a diagnosis of oral candidosis should only be made if there is heavy growth from targeted microbiological swabs. (A light growth would indicate oral yeast carriage, rather than oral candidosis.) Other microbiological tests are warranted if a patient suffers from persistent/recurrent oral candidosis (e.g. species typing, sensitivity testing).

Management

The management of oral candidosis involves:

♦ Treatment of the infection

♦ Treatment of the cause of the infection

♦ Symptom management.

A variety of different topical and systemic treatments are available for treating oral candidosis (Table 8.5.3 and 8.5.4) (Pappas et al., 2009; Anonymous, 2012). A recent Cochrane systematic review concluded that drugs absorbed from the gastrointestinal tract appeared to be more effective than drugs not absorbed from the gastrointestinal tract (Worthington et al., 2010). It should be noted, however, that the evidence for the effectiveness of individual antifungal drugs in treating cancer patients is somewhat limited (Worthington et al., 2010).

The choice of treatment depends on a number of factors (Finlay and Davies, 2005):

1. Extent of disease: topical agents are appropriate for treating localized disease, whilst systemic agents are more appropriate for treating multifocal/generalized disease.

2. Immunocompetence: systemic agents are more appropriate for treating immunosuppressed patients than topical agents.

3. Drug resistance: resistance to the polyenes is uncommon, although resistance to the azoles is becoming increasingly common.

4. Concomitant disease: the azoles have a number of relative/absolute contraindications, which may limit their usage.

5. Concomitant drug treatment: the azoles have a number of drug interactions, which may limit their usage.

6. Patient preference for medication.

7. Patient adherence with medication: topical agents are associated with greater non adherence than systemic agents.

8. Availability/affordability of different treatments.

In view of the problem of antifungal drug resistance, it is recommended that antifungal drugs, particularly azoles, should usually only be prescribed for microbiologically proven cases of oral candidosis. Furthermore, antifungal drug should be prescribed for short periods, since longer courses promote the development of resistance (White et al., 1998). However, 'single-dose' treatments are invariably ineffective in the management of oral candidosis (as opposed to vaginal candidosis). Similarly, antifungal drug should be prescribed in high doses, since lower doses also promote the development of resistance (White et al., 1998).

Many patients suffer with recurrent episodes of oral candidosis. The reason for this phenomenon is that although the infection is adequately treated, the underlying cause of the infection is not treated. For example, patients with oral candidosis secondary to SGD will usually respond to antifungal drugs, but will often relapse on withdrawal of the antifungal drugs. However, studies have shown that treatment of SGD significantly reduces the subsequent prevalence of oral candidosis (Rhodus et al., 1998).

The successful management of denture stomatitis and/or angular cheilitis depends on a combination of antifungal drug treatment, and disinfection of the denture (see earlier) (Finlay and Davies, 2005). Moreover, maintenance of denture hygiene is essential to prevent recurrence of these infections.

Denture-related problems

Denture-related problems are again common in patients with advanced cancer. The reported prevalence of subjective problems is 45–86% (Gordon et al., 1985; Aldred et al., 1991; Jobbins et al., 1992), and of objective problems is 57–83%, in published studies of

Table 8.5.3 Topical antifungal agents for managing oral candidosis (i.e. localized infections in non-immunosuppressed patients)

Drug group	Drug	Recommended regimen	Comments
Polyene group	Nystatin	1–5 mL suspension (100,000 U/mL) four times a day or 1–2 pastilles (200,000 U/pastille) four times a day 7–14-day course: continue drug for 48 hours after lesions resolved	Drug needs to be kept in contact with lesions. (Larger volumes of suspension may be used with diffuse lesions.) Suitable for treating pseudomembranous candidosis. Chlorhexidine may inactivate nystatin—it is advisable not to use chlorhexidine immediately before/after using nystatin. Resistance uncommon
	Amphotericin B	1 lozenge (10 mg) four times a day or 1 mL suspension (100 mg/mL) four times a day 10–15-day course	Drug needs to be kept in contact with lesions. Resistance uncommon
Azole group (imidazoles)	Miconazole	5–10 mL oral gel (20 mg/g) four times a day or 1 mucoadhesive buccal tablet (50 mg) once a day 7–14-day course: continue drug for 48 hours after lesions resolved	Drug needs to be kept in contact with lesions. Some systemic effect. (Smaller volumes of gel may be used with localized lesions). Suitable for treating pseudomembranous candidosis, denture stomatitis and angular cheilitis. Miconazole is also active against staphylococci, which may be present in some cases of angular cheilitis
	Clotrimazole	1 troche (10 mg) five times a day 7–14-day course	Drug needs to be kept in contact with lesions. Some systemic effect. Suitable for treating pseudomembranous candidosis
Other topical agents	Chlorhexidine		Mainly used as an adjunctive agent
	Gentian violet		Successfully used to treat oral candidosis in HIV patients
	Tea tree oil		Successfully used to treat oral candidosis in HIV patients

Table 8.5.4 Systemic antifungal agents available to treat oral candidosis (i.e. generalized infections in non-immunosuppressed patients, persistent/recurrent infections in non-immunosuppressed patients, infections in immunosuppressed patients)

Drug group	Drug	Recommended regimen	Comments
Azole group (tiazoles)	Fluconazole	50–200 mg once a day (capsule/oral suspension) 7–14-day course	Considered first-line systemic treatment Inhibits cytochrome P450 leading to certain drug interactions Resistance becoming a problem
	Itraconazole	100–200 mg per day (capsule/oral liquid) 7–14-day course	Indicated for fluconazole resistant/refractory disease Not recommended for routine use in patients with/at risk of cardiac failure Capsule absorption dependent on low pH within stomach Inhibits cytochrome P450 leading to certain drug interactions Resistance becoming a problem
	Posoconazole		Option for managing refractory disease
	Voriconazole		Option for managing refractory disease

patients with advanced cancer (Gordon et al., 1985; Aldred et al., 1991; Jobbins et al., 1992). Most problems relate to poor fitting of the dentures (e.g. oral discomfort, oral ulceration, food getting stuck under denture). Denture-related fungal infections are also common in patients with advanced cancer (i.e. denture stomatitis, angular cheilitis). The reported prevalence of denture stomatitis is 12.5%, of angular cheilitis is 5%, and of combined denture stomatitis and angular cheilitis is 3.5% in a published study of patients with advanced cancer (Davies et al., 2006).

Oral care in terminal phase

Oral care often takes prominence during the terminal phase of the illness. Indeed, oral care is a major component of so-called integrated care pathways ('care of the dying' pathways). However, the oral care protocols in these pathways are not evidence based, and are reported to produce somewhat disappointing outcomes (Fowell et al., 2002).

Certain authors recommend 1–2-hourly oral care patients in the terminal phase (Anonymous, 1996). This is very obtrusive for patients (and families), and very time consuming for health-care professionals. Some patients may require this frequency of care, although many patients require much less frequent care, to maintain oral comfort. Thus, the frequency of oral care should be determined on an individual basis, rather than on the basis of a protocol.

Oral care is often delegated to families in the terminal phases. Some family members relish this task, whilst others find it difficult and/or distressing. It is important, if appropriate, that families are given the opportunity to provide oral care. Equally, it is important that families are not coerced into providing oral care. Furthermore, health-care professionals must provide adequate instructions, and ongoing support and supervision, for families that do undertake this task.

One of the most common problems amongst unconscious patients is the presence of a desiccated oral mucosa. Family members (and health-care professionals) often perceive this as a source of discomfort, although this is unlikely to be the case in an unconscious patient. Oral care protocols often recommend the regular application of water. However, this strategy is largely ineffective, since the water rapidly dissipates as a result of swallowing and/or evaporation. A more effective intervention involves the regular application of a suitable water-based moisturizing gel (e.g. K-Y® jelly, Oral Balance® gel).

The philosophy of care in the terminal phase should be the maintenance of patient comfort (Sweeney, 2005). It is relatively easy to determine the merits of oral care in conscious patients. Thus, health-care professionals should always ask patients about their experiences of oral care, that is, whether the oral care makes them feel better, whether the oral care causes any problems. Nevertheless, it is much less easy to determine the merits of oral care in unconscious patients. However, if an intervention causes or appears to cause distress, then that intervention should be discontinued.

Online materials

Complete references for this chapter are available online at <http://www.oxfordmedicine.com>.

References

Aldred, M.J., Addy, M., Bagg, J., and Finlay, I. (1991). Oral health in the terminally ill: a cross-sectional pilot survey. *Special Care in Dentistry*, 11, 59–62.

Bjornstrom, M., Axell, T., and Birkhed, D. (1990). Comparison between saliva stimulants and saliva substitutes in patients with symptoms related to dry mouth. A multi-centre study. *Swedish Dental Journal*, 14, 153–161.

Chaushu, G., Bercovici, M., Dori, S., *et al.* (2000). Salivary flow and its relation with oral symptoms in terminally ill patients. *Cancer*, 88, 984–987.

Clifford, T. and Finnerty, J. (1995). The dental awareness and needs of a Parkinson's disease population. *Gerodontology*, 12, 99–103.

Davies, A. and Finlay, I. (2005). *Oral Care in Advanced Disease*. Oxford: Oxford University Press.

Davies, A.N. (2000a). A comparison of artificial saliva and chewing gum in the management of xerostomia in patients with advanced cancer. *Palliative Medicine*, 14, 197–203.

Davies, A.N. (2000b). *An Investigation into the Relationship Between Salivary Gland Hypofunction and Oral Health Problems in Patients with Advanced Cancer*. [Dissertation]. London: Kings College, University of London.

Davies, A.N., Brailsford, S., Broadley, K., and Beighton, D. (2002a). Oral yeast carriage in patients with advanced carriage. *Oral Microbiology and Immunology*, 17, 79–84.

Davies, A.N., Brailsford, S.R., and Beighton, D. (2006). Oral candidosis in patients with advanced cancer. *Oral Oncology*, 42, 698–702.

Davies, A.N., Brailsford, S.R., Beighton, D., Shorthose, K., and Stevens, V.C. (2008). Oral candidosis in community-based patients with advanced cancer. *Journal of Pain and Symptom Management*, 35, 508–514.

Davies, A.N., Broadley, K., and Beighton, D. (2001). Xerostomia in patients with advanced cancer. *Journal of Pain and Symptom Management*, 22, 820–825.

Davies, A.N., Broadley, K., and Beighton, D. (2002b). Salivary gland hypofunction in patients with advanced cancer. *Oral Oncology*, 38, 680–685.

Davies, A.N., Daniels, C., Pugh, R., and Sharma, K. (1998). A comparison of artificial saliva and pilocarpine in the management of xerostomia in patients with advanced cancer. *Palliative Medicine*, 12, 105–111.

Davies, A.N. and Epstein, J.B. (2010). *Oral Complications of Cancer and its Management*. Oxford: Oxford University Press.

Davies, A.N. and Kaur, K. (1998). Taste problems in patients with advanced cancer. *Palliative Medicine*, 12, 482–483.

Davies, A.N. and Shorthose, K. (2007). Parasympathomimetic drugs for the treatment of salivary gland dysfunction due to radiotherapy. *Cochrane Database of Systematic Reviews*, 3, CD003782.

Davies, A.N. and Singer, J. (1994). A comparison of artificial saliva and pilocarpine in radiation-induced xerostomia. *Journal of Laryngology and Otology*, 108, 663–665.

Fabiano, J.A. (1983). Orofacial involvement in multiple sclerosis. *Special Care in Dentistry*, 3, 61–64.

Finlay, I.G. (1986). Oral symptoms and candida in the terminally ill. *British Medical Journal*, 292, 592–593.

Gordon, S.R., Berkey, D.B., and Call, R.L. (1985). Dental need among hospice patients in Colorado: a pilot study. *Gerodontics*, 1, 125–129.

Jobbins, J., Bagg, J., Finlay, I.G., Addy, M., and Newcombe, R.G. (1992). Oral and dental disease in terminally ill cancer patients. *BMJ*, 304, 1612.

Odds, F.C. (1979). Factors that predispose the host to candidosis. In F.C. Odds (ed.) *Candida and Candidosis*, pp. 82–85. Leicester: Leicester University Press.

Olsson, H. and Axell, T. (1991). Objective and subjective efficacy of saliva substitutes containing mucin and carboxymethylcellulose. *Scandinavian Journal of Dental Research*, 99, 316–319.

Rydholm, M. and Strang, P. (2002). Physical and psychosocial impact of xerostomia in palliative cancer care: a qualitative interview study. *International Journal of Palliative Nursing*, 8, 318–323.

Samaranayake, L.P. (1990). Host factors and oral candidosis. In L.P. Samaranayake, and T.W. MacFarlane (eds.) *Oral Candidosis*, pp. 66–103. London: Wright.

Shah, S. and Davies, A.N. (2001). Symptom prevalence in palliative care. *Palliative Medicine*, 17, 805–806.

Shorthose, K. and Davies, A. (2003). Symptom prevalence in palliative care. *Palliative Medicine*, 17, 723–724.

Sreebny, L.M. and Schwartz, S.S. (1997). A reference guide to drugs and dry mouth—2nd edition. *Gerodontology*, 14, 33–47.

Stewart, C.M., Jones, A.C., Bates, R.E., Sandow, P., Pink, F., and Stillwell, J. (1998). Comparison between saliva stimulants and a saliva substitute in patients with xerostomia and hyposalivation. *Special Care in Dentistry*, 18, 142–148.

Sweeney, M.P., Bagg, J., Baxter, W.P., and Aitchison, T.C. (1997). Clinical trial of a mucin-containing oral spray for treatment of xerostomia in hospice patients. *Palliative Medicine*, 11, 225–232.

Tranmer, J.E., Heyland, D., Dudgeon, D., Groll, D., Squires-Graham, M., and Coulson, K. (2003). Measuring the symptom experience of seriously ill cancer and noncancer hospitalized patients near the end of life with the Memorial Symptom Assessment Scale. *Journal of Pain and Symptom Management*, 25, 420–429.

Worthington, H.V., Clarkson, J.E., Khalid, T., Meyer, S., and McCabe, M. (2010). Interventions for treating oral candidiasis for patients with cancer receiving treatment. *Cochrane Database of Systematic Reviews*, 7, CD001972.

Sleep disorders

Kyriaki Mystakidou, Irene Panagiotou, Efi Parpa, and Eleni Tsilika

Introduction to sleep disorders

Sleep disturbances can present independently or concomitantly with other medical and/or psychiatric disorders, such as chronic pain and depression. Insomnia is the most prevalent sleep disorder and can become a persistent problem for patients with serious or life-threatening illnesses. The burden of chronic sleep disturbances is heavy for patients, caregivers, and health-care providers and its impact can affect physical, psychological, occupational, and economic well-being (Morin and Benca, 2012). Assessment and management of sleep disorders is necessary when treating chronically ill patients.

Sleep physiology

Sleep is a state that shows alternating patterns of neural activity controlled by homeostatic and circadian mechanisms interacting in complex ways. The sleep–wake cycle is a highly regulated process that involves two distinct types of sleep: (1) rapid eye movement (REM) sleep, which is the active phase of sleep defined by faster electroencephalography (EEG) activity, rapid horizontal eye movements seen on electrooculography, vital sign instability, and occurrence of skeletal muscle hypotonia, as well as dreams; and (2) non-REM sleep (Kryger et al., 2000).

The major characteristics of normal sleep architecture include the generalized slowing of EEG activity that characterizes the transition from drowsiness to light sleep (stage one), the emergence of sleep spindles and K-complex waveforms that accompany the onset of deeper sleep (stage two), and the desynchronized slow (delta) waves of slow-wave sleep (SWS) (stages three and four) (Kryger et al., 2000). Sleep occurs in a circadian pattern, with most deep sleep (SWS, delta sleep) occurring during the first half of the night, and the most REM sleep occurring during the second half of the night. During an average night, individuals experience five cycles of non-REM and REM sleep that last for approximately 70–90 minutes each. Sleep normally progresses slowly from stage one to stage four of non-REM sleep. Periods of non-REM sleep constitute approximately 80% of total sleep time and non-REM reaches its greatest depth during SWS. After a period of SWS, the individual enters an episode of REM sleep, followed by re-progression through stages one to four of non-REM sleep (Kryger et al., 2000). Sleep architecture varies widely from person to person in terms of the amount of time spent in each sleep stage, the number of cycles, and the amount of interruption by waking. There are individuals who, because of their circadian rhythm patterns and chronotype, prefer early bed times and wake times and there are those who prefer later bed times and wake times.

Sleep is generated by two opposing processes that interact together to strengthen sleep: the homeostatic drive for sleep and the circadian system that regulates wakefulness (Borbely and Achermann, 1999;Kryger et al., 2000). The homeostatic drive for sleep involves mutually inhibitory interactions between sleep- and arousal-promoting systems and increases with the length of time that an individual has been awake. Non-REM sleep and SWS appear to be primarily controlled by this homeostatic process.

The circadian system plays an important role in the control of the timing of sleep onset, the timing of sleep offset, and the distribution of REM sleep. The circadian system is known as the wake-promoting system because it determines the timing of sleep propensity and wakefulness (Borbely and Achermann, 1999). Individuals who sleep in phase with their circadian rhythm obtain a better quality of sleep, with minimal time to fall asleep and fewer awakenings, than those who sleep outside of their circadian chronotype (i.e. shift workers, jet-lagged pilots and airline attendants). The central pacemaker of the circadian system for all physiological processes (including the modulation of sleep and wakefulness) is located in the suprachiasmatic nucleus of the hypothalamus. Retinal light input synchronizes the pacemaker to the external light–dark cycle via a direct retinal hypothalamic tract. A complicated neural pathway links the suprachiasmatic nucleus to the pineal gland, where melatonin is secreted in a circadian pattern with onset of the secretion in the early evening, peak levels occurring in the middle of the night, and very low or non-existent melatonin levels during the day. In the mammalian circadian system, melatonin serves as a chemical messenger of the circadian pacemaker. Central melatonin receptors are concentrated primarily in the suprachiasmatic nucleus, where melatonin functions in a feedback loop (Borbely and Achermann, 1999).

Prevalence of sleep disorders

The reported prevalence of sleep disturbances depends on the definitions used and the underlying pathology (Roth, 2007). A general consensus has emerged from population-based studies that approximately 30% of adults report one or more of the symptoms of insomnia: difficulty initiating sleep, difficulty maintaining sleep, waking up too early, and, in some cases, non-restorative or poor quality sleep (Roth, 2007). Rates of insomnia with associated daytime dysfunction in attendees of general medical practices range from 10% to as high as 34% (Sateia and D' Nowell, 2004). This high prevalence of chronic insomnia is supplemented by an additional 25% to 35% who experience transient or occasional insomnia (Sateia and D' Nowell, 2004; Morin and Benca, 2012). It has been estimated that approximately 6–10% of adults meet the criteria for an insomnia disorder (Sateia and D' Nowell, 2004; Morin and Benca, 2012).

Given the prevalence of sleep problems, it is remarkable that sleep disturbance is seldom considered to be a primary cause of patients' distress. Often, it is perceived to be important only in the context of other symptoms. Clinicians caring for patients with serious illness should have a stronger foundation in at least those disorders for which medically ill patients often seek care—insomnia, excessive daytime sleepiness, obstructive sleep apnoea syndrome, and restless legs syndrome.

Classification of sleep disorders

Sleep disorders are classified according to the International Classification of Sleep Disorders of the American Sleep Disorders Association (Freedom, 2011). This system categorizes sleep disorders into two large categories: primary sleep disorders, such as dysomnias and parasomnias (Kryger et al., 2000; Morin and Benca, 2012), and secondary sleep disorders due to medical or psychiatric conditions (Borbely and Achermann, 1999).

Primary insomnia and hypersomnia, narcolepsy, breathing-related sleep disorders such as sleep apnoea, and circadian rhythm sleep disorders are all classified in the dysomnia category. These disorders may disturb sleep quality, quantity, or timing of nocturnal sleep, or may cause excessive daytime sleepiness. Parasomnias are unusual experiences or behaviours that occur during sleep; they include sleep terror disorder and sleepwalking, as well as nightmare disorder (Freedom, 2011).

This classification is largely based on phenomenology. Although research may ultimately identify measurable physiological disturbances that allow classification based on test results, diagnosis now relies mainly on patient reports. This may pose diagnostic challenges, particularly given the heterogeneity that exists in medically ill populations. These challenges are exemplified by several of the more common disorders, such as insomnia, excessive daytime sleepiness, and circadian rhythm sleep disorders.

Insomnia

In clinical practice, insomnia can be defined as the patient's subjective report of difficulty initiating or maintaining sleep, despite adequate opportunity and circumstance to sleep. The predominant complaint is dissatisfaction with sleep quality or quantity. Additional components may include early awakening and interrupted or non-restorative sleep, along with nightmares (Sateia and D' Nowell, 2004; Roth, 2007; Morin and Benca, 2012). Daytime tiredness or poor functioning; fatigue or malaise; naps during daytime; disturbances in concentration, memory, and mood; tension headaches; or gastrointestinal symptoms, along with impairment of quality of life, represent additional criteria for the diagnosis of acute and chronic insomnia (Morin and Benca, 2012).

Acute or adjustment insomnia is often associated with life events or unscheduled sleep changes, usually remits when the precipitating event has subsided, and lasts no more than 3 months. The criteria for chronic insomnia, which may be primary or secondary to a medical and/or psychiatric condition, includes sleep disturbance for at least 3 nights/week that persists for more than 3 months, although night-to-night variability in sleep is often reported and there may be an occasional good night sleep intertwined with periods of disrupted sleep (Sateia and D' Nowell, 2004; Morin and Benca, 2012).

Excessive daytime sleepiness

Excessive daytime sleepiness is a common symptom, particularly among patients with serious medical illness. It may be secondary to neurological dysfunction caused by the disease itself, to a disease-modifying or symptomatic treatment, or to a factor unrelated to the disease or its treatment. For example, excessive daytime sleepiness may result from cancer involvement of brain or leptomeninges, or as a result of chemotherapy or cranial radiotherapy (Davidson et al., 2002; (Phillips et al., 2012). Because sleepiness renders patients 'calmer', caregivers (including medical staff) do not always identify sleepiness as a problem. While some degree of sedation during the day may be beneficial for the terminally ill patient, excessive somnolence can potentially be quite disabling and compromise physical functioning and social interactions of patients, which might be extremely important even in the final weeks of life (Regestein, 1977).

Patients with primary or secondary forms of insomnia may experience excessive daytime sleepiness. In this situation, patients or their families may report recurrent episodes of drowsiness or involuntary dozing that arise mainly in sedentary situations (Sateia and D' Nowell, 2004). This phenomenon, which should not be confused with fatigue or tiredness, is very common among patients receiving palliative care services. Paradoxically, some patients with primary insomnia report excessive daytime sleepiness but demonstrate findings indicative of normal or even increased daytime alertness (Bonnet and Arand, 1996). As a result, subjects with primary insomnia who additionally manifest convincing evidence of excessive daytime sleepiness should be assessed for other potential causes of sleepiness, such as sleep apnoea or periodic limb movement (Regestein, 1977).

Circadian rhythm sleep disorders

Maintenance of a normal sleep pattern is dependent on adherence to a well-established schedule of sleep and wakefulness. Patients with serious illnesses are particularly prone to disturbances of the sleep–wake schedule: when night sleep has been poor, there is an inclination to delay the hour of rising and/or to engage in lengthy daytime naps. Disorders of the circadian sleep rhythm, such as complete disappearance of the normal sleep pattern, delayed sleep, and advanced sleep phase syndromes, all may occur in these patients (Dagan, 2002).

The delayed sleep phase syndrome consists of a problematic sleep onset, with further delay in rising and increased napping. With difficulty in falling asleep until the early morning hours, sleeping till the early afternoon may occur and further promote the vicious cycle of problematic sleep onset during bedtime (Dagan, 2002). In other cases, fatigue and sedation associated with major medical illness may result in advancement of the normal sleep–wake schedule, resulting in early morning awakening (advanced sleep phase syndrome). The disappearance of the normal circadian rhythm results in a pattern of multiple shorter sleep periods, which are interspersed with wakefulness throughout the 24-hour cycle (Dagan, 2002). As a result, the patient is able to sleep at other times, but unable to sleep at the desired time.

Causes of primary sleep disorders

Primary sleep disorders presumably result from varied neurological diseases, and given the variation in presentation, there are likely to be multiple pathophysiological processes that initiate or sustain these disturbances. An increased vulnerability to sleep disturbances has been associated with a positive family history of insomnia and, possibly, genetic factors, such as the presence of the short allele of the serotonin transporter gene (Morin and Benca, 2012). A rare and fatal familiar insomnia is autosomal dominant and characterized by severe autonomic disturbances, hallucinations, dementia, and severe progressive insomnia (Montagna et al., 1994).

Some primary sleep disturbances are thought to be a disorder of hyperarousal; this may be experienced throughout the entire day and manifests as hypervigilance during the day and difficulty in initiating and maintaining sleep during the night (Roth, 2007). This state has been demonstrated through measurements of the whole-body metabolic rate, heart rate variability, neuroendocrine measures, and functional neuroimaging. For example, a pattern of hyperarousal in patients with primary sleep disorders was shown by raised body temperature, increased 24-hour metabolic rate, heart rate, and electromyographic activity (Bonnet and Arand, 2012). Hypothalamic–pituitary–adrenal axis dysfunction has been confirmed through plasma and urinary measures of norepinephrine (noradrenaline), cortisol, and adrenocorticotropic hormone—all of which appear to have higher levels in subjects with primary sleep disturbances (Bonnet and Arand, 2012).

Using quantitative electroencephalogram analysis, subjects with primary sleep disturbance also have been shown to have an increase in beta and gamma frequencies at sleep onset and during non-REM sleep; these are thought to be associated with increased cognitive activity, as well as greater cerebral glucose metabolism during waking and non-REM sleep states (Nofzinger et al., 2004). In imaging studies, reduced grey matter volume in the left orbitofrontal cortex and hippocampus also has been reported (Altena et al., 2010).

Secondary sleep disorders and contributing factors

Sleep disorders have been associated with a very large number of potential causes. One or more of these may be the main driver for disturbed sleep, or may contribute to another primary cause. Patients with serious medical illnesses often have more than one. In those with advanced cancer, for example, sleep disturbance may be related to neoplastic involvement of the central nervous system, various treatments for the cancer, or to symptoms such as pain, nausea or constipation (Regestein, 1977; Katz and McHorney, 1998; Davidson et al., 2002; Roth, 2007; Palesh et al., 2010; Phillips et al., 2012). Advanced illness also may be associated with other conditions, such as nutritional deficiency, respiratory disorders, or nocturia, which are strongly linked to sleep disturbances (Regestein, 1977; Crisp, 1980).

Many specific medical conditions, such as chronic pain, hypertension, pulmonary and/or heart diseases, and prostatism, have been associated with sleep disturbances (Regestein, 1977; Crisp, 1980; Katz and McHorney, 1998). Substance abuse also may contribute, as can any cause of delirium, a movement disorder, or any primary disease of the central nervous system (Regestein, 1977; Crisp, 1980; Katz and McHorney, 1998). Delirium is especially common among terminally ill patients (Regestein, 1977; Crisp, 1980; Katz and McHorney, 1998) and is associated with a distorted sleep–wake cycle: wakefulness during daytime is typically reduced, while night-time brings increased alertness and agitation (Dagan, 2002). As a result, the circadian rhythm is severely reversed or disrupted. Sleep deprivation itself may also predispose to the development of delirium.

Dementia also is associated with sleep disruption. Sleep studies of dementia patients reveal increased sleep latencies, lighter sleep, reduced REM sleep, and increased awakening after sleep (Klink et al., 1992; Katz and McHorney, 1998).

Sleep-disordered breathing is a particularly common cause of disturbed sleep and can be an important comorbidity in populations with life-limiting illnesses. Central sleep apnoea is the absence of airflow for more than 10 seconds with an absence of ventilatory effort. Obstructive sleep apnoea is associated with continued ventilatory effort. One review noted that 29–67% of older adults with insomnia had obstructive sleep apnoea, with the apnoea–hypopnea index greater than five (Luyster et al., 2010). Obstructive sleep apnoea is associated primarily with heavy snoring and excessive daytime sleepiness although some patients report frequent nocturnal wakening, morning headaches, choking or gasping, nocturia, and fatigue (Regestein, 1977; Crisp, 1980; Chilcott and Shapiro, 1996; Morin and Benca, 2012). The syndrome is associated with obesity, male sex, older age, short neck, and redundant pharyngeal tissues.

Patients with serious illnesses also can develop periodic limb movement in sleep (Regestein, 1977; Katz and McHorney, 1998). This disorder consists of repetitive stereotyped leg and/or arm movements which occur at intervals of 20–40 seconds, typically in clusters throughout the night. It can be secondary to sedative-hypnotic withdrawal, tricyclic medication, anaemia, uraemia, leukaemia, diabetes mellitus, or peripheral neuropathy. In some cases, it might also be associated with restless legs syndrome (Regestein, 1977; Katz and McHorney, 1998), which interferes with sleep onset. This syndrome is characterized by an uncomfortable sensation, localized to the lower legs, producing an urge to move the lower extremities. The sensation is usually worst at night and is relieved by movement. As a result, both disorders can lead to great difficulty falling and staying asleep (Morin and Benca, 2012).

Environmental factors and/or poor sleep hygiene, such as a sleeping environment not conducive to sleep, snoring, and/or restless bed partner, also have been included among the psychophysiological conditions that precipitate insomnia or predispose to it (Crisp, 1980; Klink et al., 1992; Chilcott and Shapiro, 1996; Katz and McHorney, 1998). Hospital admission, for example, has been associated with marked sleep disruption (Klink et al., 1992; Katz and McHorney, 1998). The more common complaints include difficulty falling asleep, frequent awakenings, somnolence, and poor sleep quality (Klink et al., 1992; Katz and McHorney, 1998).

Although an increasing rate of insomnia has been noted in older people, debate exists as to whether increasing age is associated with sleep disturbances (Ohayon et al., 2001). Investigators suggest that progressive inactivity, dissatisfaction with social life, and presence of comorbid illnesses (both physical and psychological) can induce insomnia in older people (Sateia et al., 2000; Ohayon et al., 2001). Insomnia also is more common in women, and in individuals who are less educated or are unemployed, separated, or divorced (Sateia et al., 2000). In chronically ill non-cancer patients, age and gender were the most clearly identified demographic factors associated with insomnia, with an increased prevalence in women and older adults (Roth, 2007; Morin and Benca, 2012). On the contrary, younger age increases the risk of sleep disturbances in the cancer population.

Common psychiatric disorders and sleep disturbance

Numerous psychosocial and psychiatric conditions have been linked to sleep disturbance. An anxiety-prone personality with hyperarousability, unrealistic sleep expectations, incorrect perceptions about sleep difficulties, as well as misconceptions about causes of insomnia, represent common perpetuating factors (Chilcott and Shapiro, 1996; Weissman et al., 1997; Katz and McHorney, 1998; Ohayon et al., 2001). Psychiatric disorders linked to the onset and persistence of a life-threatening illness may lead to disturbances of sleep (Pasacreta and Pickett, 1998; Verhaak et al., 1998; Bower, 2008; Du-Quiton et al., 2010; Ewertz and Jensen, 2011). Negative cognitions, such as uncertainty about the disease and its treatment, fear of death, and concerns about disease progression and diminished quality of life, can contribute (Bailey et al., 2007; Mishel et al., 2009). Although the linkages between specific psychiatric disorders and sleep disturbances are complex, their elucidation may lead to innovative insomnia treatments focused on psychological and/or pharmacological interventions (Van't Spijker et al., 1997).

Moderate to severe depression is common in medical illness, occurring for example in 25–50% of cancer patients, and insomnia may be considered an important diagnostic marker for depression in populations with serious illness (Palliative Care Notes, 2000). Indeed, the most robust correlate of insomnia in cancer patients is depressed mood (Davidson et al., 2002) and 90% or more of depressed patients experience abnormal sleep patterns. Supporting the salience of this relationship is evidence linking depression to disturbances in the continuity of sleep, decreased latency to the first REM sleep period, and diminished SWS (stages three and four) (Reynolds, 1987). These associations underscore the importance of assessing mood in patients with sleep disorders and sleep in those with mood disorders.

This relationship between insomnia and depression is not simple, however. Uncertainty exists regarding the use of a somatic symptom, like sleep, in establishing the diagnosis of depression, since such symptoms may be a result of the illness. There also is no specific evidence regarding the efficacy of antidepressant medications in the treatment of insomnia associated with depression in the terminally ill.

Sleep disturbances also are associated with anxiety. In one study, 63% of cancer patients with anxiety had insomnia, the multifactorial causes of which included nightmares (Palliative Care Notes, 2000). Many situational factors can drive anxieties, including fear of illness progression, forthcoming procedures, or family or financial distress. For terminally ill patients, sleep-associated anxiety may be related to a fear of death.

The subjective experience of anxiety may occur with over-activation of stress response systems, notably the hypothalamic–pituitary–adrenal axis; this phenomenon is associated with insomnia (Roth, 2007). Some have argued that chronic activation of these physiological systems may explain why insomnia is an independent risk factor for medical conditions such as coronary artery disease (Mallon et al., 2002).

Chronic pain and sleep disturbance

Chronic pain also is highly associated with disturbed sleep (Klink et al., 1992; Verhaak et al., 1998; Roehrs et al., 2006; Kundermann and Lautenbacher, 2007). It is estimated that 50–90% of patients with chronic pain report poor sleep quality (Menefee et al., 2000; Lavigne et al., 2005; Breivik et al., 2006). The sleep disturbances that may accompany pain include difficulty falling and staying asleep, lack of restful sleep, frequent awakening, and daytime somnolence (Klink et al., 1992; Menefee et al., 2000; Okura et al,. 2008). Chronic pain from musculoskeletal diseases has been found to affect sleep architecture (Mahowald et al., 1989; Branco et al., 1994), abnormalities in REM sleep architecture have been noted in patients with fibromyalgia (Branco et al., 1994), and decreased SWS and increased alpha sleep changes have been associated with both fibromyalgia and rheumatoid arthritis (Mahowald et al., 1989; Branco et al., 1994).

Pain and sleep disorders also can have a reciprocal relationship. Just as poorly controlled pain can disrupt sleep, chronic sleep deprivation may increase pain (Smith and Perlis, 2004; Lavigne et al., 2005; Roehrs et al., 2006). Indeed, it has been reported that sleep quality can predict the levels of pain the following day and that the number of hours of sleep reported the previous night represents a highly significant predictor of pain during the next day (Edwards et al., 2008). It has been suggested that the relationship is so close that even healthy subjects can suffer from hyperalgesia due to sleep deprivation (Roehrs et al., 2006; Kundermann and Lautenbacher, 2007). If untreated, the conjunction of these two processes can have drastic consequences; the combination of high pain intensity and insomnia has been shown to increase the already-doubled suicide risk found in patients suffering from chronic pain (Smith and Perlis, 2004).

Opioid therapy and sleep disturbance

Opioids have a variety of effects on sleep and can cause sleep disturbances even in the absence of pain (Lydic and Baghdoyan, 2007). It has been shown that increased opioid medication during the day can represent a significant predictor of poor sleep during the following night and a night of poor sleep can be followed by higher levels of opioid intake the following day (Mystakidou et al., 2011). These phenomena have not been directly linked to the sedative effects of these drugs, to which tolerance usually develops (Benyamin et al., 2008). If sedation is severe or persistent, however, it can disrupt daytime arousal and lead secondarily to sleep problems. Opioid-induced daytime somnolence may be manageable with opioid dose reduction, opioid rotation, or the use of a psychostimulant (Mystakidou et al., 2011).

Opioids also are associated with sleep-disordered breathing (Mahowald et al., 1989; Lydic and Baghdoyan, 2007; Panagiotou and Mystakidou, 2012). Both central and obstructive sleep apnoea have been associated with chronic opioid treatment (Walker et al., 2007; Webster et al., 2008; Walker and Farney, 2009; Luyster et al., 2010; Mystakidou et al., 2011; Panagiotou and Mystakidou, 2012).

Sleep disturbances in the palliative care setting

Sleep disorders in the cancer population

As noted, cancer patients may experience sleep disturbances as a direct effect of the neoplasm; as a consequence of cancer surgery, chemotherapy, and/or radiation therapy (Davidson et al., 2002; Phillips et al., 2012); or as a correlate of pain or other symptoms, related disorders such as delirium, treatment with opioids or other medications, or varied psychological or psychiatric conditions (Davidson et al., 2002; Palesh et al., 2010). Sleep and fatigue have been reported as important components of a symptom cluster in cancer and a longitudinal study suggested that fatigue in breast cancer patients undergoing chemotherapy was significantly associated with subjective reports of poor sleep and objective measures of daytime sleepiness (Liu et al., 2012).

The prevalence and characteristics of sleep disturbances vary within the cancer population. Breast and lung cancer patients have the highest rates of sleep disturbances and insomnia symptoms are more likely to be reported by younger patients (Davidson et al., 2002; Palesh et al., 2010). There are no reported sex differences (Palesh et al., 2010). Phillips et al. (2012) reported that poorer overall sleep in cancer patients was predicted by less education, more medical comorbidities, and previous radiotherapy, while depression and fatigue were significantly related to problematic sleep.

The few studies that have recorded objective data from cancer patients with sleep disturbances suggest a complex relationship between subjective events and neural processes. For example, there is evidence that self-report of sleep duration and latency correlates poorly with polysomnographic or actigraphic sleep data (Roscoe et al., 2011; Liu et al., 2012). The relationship between self-reported sleep disturbance and cancer-related fatigue was not confirmed in actigraphic studies (Roscoe et al., 2011; Liu et al., 2012), and sleep architecture was not affected by cancer treatment. Another study found no relationship between fatigue and insomnia in men with prostate cancer (Savard et al., 2004).

Insomnia also is a serious concern among cancer survivors, including children and adolescents (Kaleyias et al., 2012). Children with brain tumours have the highest prevalence of long-term morbidities. The most prevalent sleep disorders included insomnia, excessive daytime fatigue and sleepiness, as well as restless legs syndrome.

Sleep disorders in other chronic diseases

Sleep disorders are common other serious or life-threatening illnesses. In populations with HIV/AIDS, fatigue, daytime sleepiness, and difficulties initiating and maintaining sleep have been reported (Norman et al., 1990; Moeller et al., 1991). The severity of sleep disturbance and associated daytime dysfunction is correlated with progression of the disease (Moeller et al., 1991). The presence of depression, anxiety, and cerebral involvement, particularly in HIV-dementia complex (Norman et al., 1990), is likely to have major impact on the sleep of these patients. Sleep disturbances may represent early changes in the central nervous system associated with the infection or an adaptation to bolster immune response (Norman et al., 1990). Studies have shown that sleep alterations of asymptomatic HIV-infected males include increased SWS in the second half of the night, while, on the contrary, a decreased percentage of SWS has been reported in patients with diagnosed cerebral disease (Norman et al., 1990). Sleep disturbances have also been described in association with treatment for HIV infection (Moeller et al., 1991).

Patients with chronic obstructive pulmonary disease have been traditionally reported as poor sleepers. Severe daytime hypoxia and/or hypercapnia, as well as dyspnoea, chronic cough, and sadness/anxiety may play an important role in the increased prevalence of sleep disturbances (Budhiraja et al., 2012; McSharry et al., 2012). Insomnia, shorter sleep time, increased light sleep with multiple arousals, lower sleep efficiency, and increased daytime sleepiness have all been reported (Budhiraja et al., 2012; McSharry et al., 2012). Furthermore, altered sleep architecture with decreased REM sleep was found as a criterion of impaired sleep efficiency (McSharry et al., 2012). These abnormalities were reported separate and distinct from the obstructive sleep apnoea syndrome, which can impose an additional significant burden in such patient cohort.

Liver diseases also have been associated with sleep disturbances (De Cruz et al., 2012). Relatively high rates of insomnia, daytime sleepiness, daytime napping, and nocturnal awakenings occur in patients with cirrhosis, even in the absence of hepatic encephalopathy. Derangements in sleep patterns include circadian rhythms disorders, restless leg syndrome, and a progressive decrease in total wake time, with an increase in total SWS and REM (De Cruz et al., 2012). Patients with primary biliary cirrhosis suffer from profound fatigue and excessive daytime somnolence, resulting in poor night sleep. Sleep disruption in hepatitis C is mainly due to neurological disturbances involving both the peripheral and central nervous system, comorbid psychiatric disorders (both mood disorders and psychosis), and fatigue due to interferon therapy. Polysomnographic studies confirm decrease in SWS and sleep efficiency, and an increase in REM latency, stage two sleep, and awakenings after sleep onset (De Cruz et al., 2012). Patients with Wilson's disease may experience disorders of REM sleep, reduced total sleep time, and hypersomnia; several cases with significant increases in REM-related disturbances (cataplexy and sleep paralysis) have been reported (De Cruz et al., 2012). A dysfunctional suprachiasmatic nucleus has been suggested to contribute to a circadian rhythm disturbance in patients with Wilson's disease, and some patients have a dopaminergic deficit that leads to secondary Parkinsonism, which itself may be associated with REM sleep disturbances, especially REM behaviour disorder (De Cruz et al., 2012). Degenerative brain diseases, such as Alzheimer's disease, also can produce chronic insomnia and related disturbances of the sleep–wake cycle (Morin and Benca, 2012).

Diagnosis and evaluation of sleep disorders

Clinical assessment

The diagnosis of sleep disturbances requires a comprehensive history (Sateia and D'Nowell, 2004; Morin and Benca, 2012). In view of the high prevalence and substantial morbidities in palliative care setting, patients should routinely be evaluated for sleep problems. Evaluation includes careful analysis of the sleep–wake cycle and identification of all sleep-related symptoms, as follows:

◆ Identify the type of primary complaint (dysomnia, parasomnia) by evaluating difficulty initiating/maintaining sleep, early awakening, non-restorative sleep, and daytime consequences.

◆ Characterize the complaint by assessing its onset, severity, course, and duration (e.g. gradual or abrupt, frequency, and intensity).

◆ Document the sleep–wake cycle by noting sleep schedule, naps, activities, medications, pre-sleep activities, wake-up time and time out of bed, and regularity of schedules.

◆ Document cognitions such as negative expectations (e.g. 'I will never get to sleep'), distortions (e.g. 'Should I stay in bed and rest if I cannot sleep?') and catastrophization (e.g., 'If I cannot sleep I cannot work', 'I cannot function'; 'My life is falling apart').

◆ Evaluate daytime function, as well as the patient's particular sleep requirements; patients may be short/average/long sleepers, and the absence of daytime consequences suggests clinical insignificance or short sleepers.

◆ Identify possible precipitants, perpetuating factors, and causative factors, and record ameliorating or exacerbating factors, including substance use (medications, alcohol or other drugs, caffeine, and nicotine).

◆ Identify medical and neuropsychiatric (personal/family) history, along with other sleep-related symptoms.

◆ Assess previous treatments response and attitudes.

◆ Complement the information from the history with data from a sleep log or diary, if possible; this should cover at least 2 weeks.

Findings from a physical examination and laboratory data also may be important in establishing the significance of factors that could cause or contribute to a sleep disorder. Objective sleep studies, including polysomnography or actigraphy, may be helpful in selected cases. Polysomnography is considered the 'gold standard' and generally is not indicated for the routine assessment of insomnia (Sateia and D' Nowell, 2004; Morin and Benca, 2012). Nonetheless, it may provide definitive information in cases of suspected sleep apnoea or sleep-related movement disorders, when violent or potentially self-injurious behaviour occurs during sleep, or when patients are treatment resistant (Littner et al., 2003). Actigraphy is an indirect measure of the sleep–wake cycle, which is inferred by means of movement recording. It, too, can be a helpful adjunct in some patients, although it is not indicated in clinical practice (Littner et al., 2003).

Questionnaires

'Sleep quality' includes quantitative aspects (such as sleep duration, sleep latency, and number of arousals) and subjective aspects (such as 'depth' or 'restfulness' of sleep) (Beck et al., 2004). Self-report measures, including sleep diaries, sleep logs, and questionnaires, have been developed to aid the assessment of these features (Davidson et al., 2001).

Daily sleep diaries can record timing of retiring and rising, sleep onset latency, number and duration of awakenings, time and duration of naps, use of hypnotic medications, and overall ratings of feeling rested and sleep quality. Sleep logs can be used to give a day-to-day account of sleep activities 24 hours per day over a period of time (Davidson et al., 2001).

Other types of self-report questionnaires also have been developed. The Pittsburgh Sleep Quality Index (PSQI) represents one of the most useful (Beck et al., 2004; Mystakidou et al., 2007, 2009).

It may be used as a simple screening measure to identify cases and controls, or 'good' and 'bad' sleepers. It is self-administered and collects data on multiple facets of sleep quality. It takes only 5–10 minutes to complete, and has a possible range of 0–21 points. The Global Sleep Quality Index (GSQI) is obtained from the sum of seven components: subjective sleep quality, sleep latency, sleep duration (hours of actual sleep at night), habitual sleep efficiency, sleep disturbances, use of sleeping medication, and daytime dysfunction (Beck et al., 2004). A higher score indicates poorer sleep quality. Studies suggest that a cut-off score of equal or more than 5 can be used to identify poor sleepers (Beck et al., 2004).

Other self-report instruments used to measure the perceived severity of sleep problems include the Insomnia Severity Index (Morin, 1993; Savard et al., 2005) and the Epworth Sleepiness Scale (ESS) (Johns, 1991). The latter tool is widely used and is a subjective measure of daytime sleepiness. It is brief and self-administered, and asks the subject to rate his or her likelihood of sleeping in eight specific situations that are commonly encountered in daily life. The items are each scored on a 0–3-point scale, which are added to give an overall total score of 0–24. The results represent the subjects' average sleep propensity across these situations of daily life. Higher scores indicate more sleepiness. An ESS score of 2–10 is considered 'normal' and more than 10 is indicative of pathological sleepiness (Johns, 1991).

Another important tool for the clinical assessment of sleep disturbances is the Medical Outcomes Study (MOS) Sleep Scale (Sprintzer and Hays, 2003). This scale quantifies the effects of sleep problems on individuals. It uses 12 questions to assess the effects of sleep problems through several individual dimensions of sleep including sleep disturbance, snoring, sleep adequacy, headache, somnolence, and respiratory impairments with sleep. Similar to the PSQI, it allows calculation of a 'global sleep problems index'. It is scored from 0 to 100; for sleep adequacy, a high score indicates better sleep ('more adequate'), and for the remaining parameters, a high score indicates more pathology (Sprintzer and Hays, 2003).

Treatment of sleep disorders

When sleep disorders are secondary to medical and/or psychiatric conditions, or are exacerbated by these factors, treatment directed at the cause should be undertaken if possible. Symptomatic drug therapy may be needed concurrently, typically with a sedative-hypnotic or an antidepressant. Factors that affect drug choice may include nature of insomnia symptoms, the medical and psychological status of the patient, age, and response to previous treatments. Once treatment is begun, continuous re-evaluation is warranted to determine efficacy and complications, and to adjust dosage or type of medication accordingly. If possible, drug therapy should be used on an intermittent basis, rather than continuously, with the theoretical appeal of preserving effectiveness over time (Schuman and Attarian, 2012).

According to recent guidelines, the treatment of insomnia should be initiated with either a short-acting or intermediate-acting benzodiazepine-receptor agonist or with ramelteon, unless the patient has a depressive disorder, in which case a sedating antidepressant should be used (Morin and Benca, 2012; Schuman and Attarian, 2012) (Table 8.6.1). An antidepressant also should be considered if the first-line drug is ineffective. A benzodiazepine with a longer half-life may be chosen if the hypnotic's duration of

Table 8.6.1 Pharmacotherapy of sleep disturbances

Drug name	Dose (mg) [dose recommended in elderly and medically ill (mg)]	Metabolism	Half-life (hours) and peak plasma concentration (hours after administration)	Adverse effects
Benzodiazepine hypnotic drugs (benzodiazepine receptor agonists)				
Alprazolam	0.5–1	Hepatic via CYP3A4	11.2	Abnormal coordination, depression, drowsiness
Diazepam	5–10	Hepatic	20–50	Agitation, amnesia, anxiety, ataxia, confusion, depression, drowsiness, dizziness
Estazolam	1–2 [0.5]	Hepatic	10–24, 2	As for diazepam
Flurazepam	15–30 [15]	Hepatic	47–100, 2	As for estazolam
Quazepam	7.5–15 [7.5]	Hepatic	25–41, 1.5	As for estazolam
Temazepam	7.5–30 [7.5]	Hepatic	6–16, 1	As for estazolam
Triazolam	0.25–0.50 [0.125–0.250]	Hepatic	1.5–5.5, 2	As for estazolam
Non-benzodiazepine hypnotic drugs (benzodiazepine receptor agonists)				
Zaleplon	10–20 [5–10]	Extensive, primarily via aldehyde oxidase	1, 1	Chest pain, peripheral oedema, amnesia, anxiety, depersonalization, depression, gastrointestinal symptoms
Zolpidem	5–10 [5]	Hepatic, primarily via CY3A4	2.5–2.8, 1.6	Dizziness, headache, somnolence
Zopiclone	3.75–7.5 [7.5]	Extensively hepatic	5–7, > 2	Palpitations, agitation, anterograde amnesia, asthenia, gastrointestinal symptoms
Antidepressant drugs				
Amitriptyline	25–100 [20]	Hepatic to nortriptyline (active)	9–27, 4–8	Restlessness, dizziness, insomnia, sedation, fatigue, anxiety, impaired cognitive function, blurred vision, dry mouth, arrhythmias, orthostatic hypotension
Mirtazapine	15–45 [7.5–15]	Extensively hepatic via CYP1A2, CYP2C9, CYP2D6, CYP3A4, and via demethylation and hydroxylation	20–40, 2	Somnolence, constipation, xerostomia, increased appetite, weight gain
Doxepin	75–100 [25–50]	Hepatic	8–24, 2–3	As for amitriptyline
Trazodone	150–400 [150]	Hepatic	7, 1	As for amitriptyline
Non-prescription medications				
Melatonin	0.5–6	–		No known toxicity or serious side effects
Alternative agents				
Ramelteon	8 (30 min before bedtime)	Extensive first-pass effect; oxidative metabolism primarily through CYP1A2 and to a lesser extent through CYP2C and CYP3A4		Central nervous system depression, reproductive hormonal regulation disturbances

(continued)

Table 8.6.1 Continued

Drug name	Dose (mg) [dose recommended in elderly and medically ill (mg)]	Metabolism	Half-life (hours) and peak plasma concentration (hours after administration)	Adverse effects
Anticonvulsants				
Gabapentin	300–600 [300]	Hepatic, renal	5–7, 2–4	Drowsiness, dizziness, ataxia, tremor, diplopia, nystagmus, myalgia, peripheral oedema
Clonazepam	0.25–0.50 [0.25]	Hepatic	30–40, 1–4	Drowsiness, dizziness, ataxia, nervousness
Tiagabine	4–8 [4]	Hepatic	7–9, 0–75	Drowsiness, dizziness, ataxia, tremor, new onset of seizures in patients without epilepsy, asthenia, gastrointestinal disturbances
Antipsychotics				
Olanzapine	5–10, 5	Hepatic	21–54, 6	Drowsiness, dizziness, ataxia, tremor, extrapyramidal symptoms, new-onset diabetes mellitus
Quetiapine	25–200, 25	Hepatic	6, 15	As for olanzapine

effect is insufficient. Although evidence of efficacy for sleep disturbances is lacking, other drugs are considered in refractory cases or when a specific disorder is identified. For example, a neuroleptic may be appropriate when sleep disruption occurs in association with an organic brain syndrome.

Benzodiazepine receptor agonists

Zolpidem, zaleplon, and zopiclone are currently the medications of choice in the treatment of short-term or transient insomnia. Although their use in chronic insomnia remains unclear due to uncertainty about long-term effectiveness, they are used for various types of chronic insomnia (Sateia and D' Nowell, 2004). These drugs reduce sleep latency and wake time after sleep onset. Side effects are usually minimal. There is a very small chance of abuse, dependence, and tolerance, and no withdrawal or rebound insomnia is observed after long-term use (Schuman and Attarian, 2012).

Although generally considered safe, the use of the benzodiazepine receptor agonists in populations with advanced illness must be undertaken cautiously. The rate of drug metabolism may be significantly slower in medically ill and geriatric patients, predisposing to greater drug accumulation and daytime carry-over effects. Studies suggest that the use of sedative-hypnotics in the elderly is associated with increased risk of falls, hip fracture due to motor incoordination, and cognitive impairment (Sateia and D' Nowell, 2004). Perhaps the most common undesirable side effects are those of daytime sedation, nocturnal confusion, and performance decrement (Sateia and D' Nowell, 2004).

Other sleep medications

Sedative antidepressants have also assumed an important role in the treatment of chronic insomnia and non-restorative sleep (Sateia and D' Nowell, 2004). The tricyclic compounds, amitriptyline and doxepin, can be administered at lower dosages than those typically required for the treatment of major depression (Schuman and Attarian, 2012). Although usually safe with cautious dosing,

the risk of toxicity related to excessive sedation, orthostatic hypotension, cardiotoxicity, and anticholinergic effects (including delirium from central effects) must be recognized (Sateia and D' Nowell, 2004). In some countries, mirtazapine and trazodone are used for their potential effects on sleep. Clinicians must always have in mind that the metabolism of antidepressants may be substantially slower in chronically medically ill patients and the elderly.

Melatonin is a hormone produced by the pineal gland that contributes to reinforcement of circadian and seasonal rhythms (Morin and Benca, 2012). It has received widespread attention for treating chronic insomnia and other sleep disorders, particularly sleep–wake cycle disturbances, Recent evidence suggests that it can be used in elderly patients, since melatonin is normally reduced as part of ageing. Ramelteon, a melatonin receptor agonist, reduces latency to sleep, but does not increase total sleep time; it has been reported that it might help promote circadian rhythm entrainment at lower doses (Morin and Benca, 2012; Schuman and Attarian, 2012).

Other drugs are sometimes tried when insomnia has been refractory to routine therapies. Antihistamines used as sleep-inducing agents include diphenhydramine and doxylamine succinate. An herbal preparation, valerian, has been shown to bind to gamma-aminobutyric acid type A receptors and to improve subjective improvement in sleep quality without improvement in quantitative measures (Morin and Benca, 2012). Some anticonvulsants, such as tiagabine hydrochloride and pregabalin, have been reported to increase SWS, as well as to decrease wakefulness after sleep onset and decrease sleep latency (Morin and Benca, 2012). Pregabalin has been reported to decrease insomnia and anxiety in patients with comorbid generalized anxiety and insomnia (Montgomery et al., 2009), and to reduce insomnia and pain in patients with fibromyalgia (Russell et al., 2009). Finally, atypical antipsychotics, quetiapine and olanzapine in particular, are occasionally used for insomnia, particularly if there are associated signs of organicity (Morin and Benca, 2012). All of these drugs must be used very cautiously in the medically ill due to concerns about daytime sedation, dizziness, cognitive impairment, and falls (Morin and Benca, 2012).

Non-pharmacological interventions

The management of sleep disorders in the medically ill should aim to improve the quality and quantity of sleep, mitigate the impact of contributing comorbid disorders, and improve quality of life (Schutte-Rodin et al., 2008; National Cancer Institute, 2010). From this perspective, cognitive and behavioural therapies may have advantages for some patients (Lindley et al., 1998; Smith et al., 2005; Irwin et al., 2006; Page et al., 2006; Kozachik and Bandeen-Roche 2008; Harsora and Kessman, 2009; Harvey, 2010). Some studies suggest that a large majority of patients with chronic diseases can benefit from cognitive behavioural therapy (CBT) (Belanger et al., 2006), notwithstanding the potential for limited effectiveness in some populations, such as the elderly (Irwin et al., 2006).

CBT is an integration of cognitive therapy and behavioural modification techniques. In the 1950s, Skinner, Pavlov, and Wolpe developed behaviour therapy from learning theories derived from their experiments in classical conditioning, operant conditioning, and desensitization. Behavioural therapy focuses on observable behaviours that can be modified in the present; the patient gradually is taught to replace maladaptive learned responses with healthier behaviours, through positive, and negative reinforcement (O'Donohue and Krasner, 1995; Belanger et al., 2006). The advantages of behavioural therapy for sleep disorders is the durability and the lack of dependency or rebound insomnia; the disadvantages are that the technique requires regular practice and the effect may take 2 weeks or longer to appear (Morin et al., 1999).

Cognitive therapy, which was initially developed in the 1960s by Beck, helps patients to evaluate and change negative thoughts or cognitive distortions, a process known as cognitive restructuring (Belanger et al., 2006). Patients can be educated to identify dysfunctional beliefs related to sleep or the consequences of insomnia, interventions that aim to reduce anticipatory anxiety (fear of insomnia). They also may learn specific techniques to reduce symptoms and enhance self-efficacy.

CBT is goal-oriented and requires active participation by the patient (Belanger et al., 2006; Reeve and Bailes, 2010). It is predicated on an understanding of insomnia as a problem that has transitioned from acute to chronic as a result, at least in part, of maladaptive compensatory strategies and behavioural contingencies separate from medical or psychiatric causes (Buysse et al., 1994). To address these issues, patients who are able to participate in this therapy can be taught specific cognitive and behavioural strategies to improve sleep hygiene, correct misconceptions about sleep, and manage symptoms and distress (Turner and Asher, 1979; Smith et al., 2005).

In CBT, patients may learn specific techniques, such as relaxation training, guided imagery, diaphragmatic breathing, meditation, autogenic training, and biofeedback (McCurry et al., 2007). Hypnosis can reduce the frequency and severity of hot flashes and may also improve sleep quality in breast cancer patients. (Becker, 1993; Elkins et al., 2008; Jensen et al., 2012). Relaxation training, usually progressive relaxation, is probably the most frequently employed technique, and is based on procedures developed by Jacobson in the early twentieth century (Jacobson, 1938; McCurry et al., 2007). The approach involves progressively tensing and then relaxing each muscle group while concentrating on and contrasting sensations of tension and relaxation.

Studies suggest that CBT may improve time to fall asleep and nocturnal wake time, as well as inducing other benefits, such as improved pain management and reduced anxiety (Smith et al., 2005; Espie et al., 2008). Compared to the control group, a group of 30 cancer patients with chronic sleep-onset insomnia who underwent three sessions of progressive muscle relaxation training, with instructions to practise twice per day for 9 days, achieved a significant, 83-minute differential reduction in latency to sleep onset, which was maintained at a 3-month follow-up (Cannici et al., 1983). In another study, 12 cancer patients benefited from stimulus control, relaxation techniques, sleep hygiene, and cognitive approaches to decrease worry and emotional arousal during pre-sleep intervals (Schutte-Rodin et al., 2008). Stimulus control in this model was based on the principles of classical conditioning and attempted to associate the bed with sleep in an effort to re-associate the bedroom with a rapid onset of sleep and to establish a set wake-up time that stabilises the sleep–wake rhythm. Patients experienced significant improvements by the end of treatment, as well as a post-treatment reduction in fatigue, improvement in role functioning, and a trend towards improvement in depressive symptom severity (Davidson et al., 2001).

When a few CBT strategies are combined and focused specifically on the management of sleep disturbance, they may be termed cognitive behaviour therapy for insomnia (CBT-I) (Smith and Neubauer, 2003). Studies of CBT-I for primary insomnia have demonstrated large effect sizes on a variety of sleep parameters. Benefits of brief CBT-I, including improved sleep parameters and reduced medication use, have continued for follow-up periods up to 2 years after treatment completion (Smith et al., 2005). Studies of CBT-I in medically ill populations indicate similar benefits (Simeit et al., 2004; Espie et al., 2008; Woodward, 2011). Some authors, however, note that patients' access to CBT-I practitioners is limited and cost often is prohibitive (Espie, 2009; Savard et al., 2010).

Future work

Many challenges remain in characterizing and treating sleep disorders in populations with medical illness. Future research must expand our knowledge about the biological dimensions, as well as the behavioural aspects of these disorders. Awareness of accurate diagnosis of sleep disturbances and of effective treatment strategies using both pharmacological and non-pharmacological approaches should be developed.

Online materials

Complete references for this chapter are available online at <http://www.oxfordmedicine.com>.

References

Bailey, D.E., Wallace, M., Jr, and Mishel, M.H. (2007). Watching, waiting and uncertainty in prostate cancer. *Journal of Clinical Nursing*, 16(4), 734–741.

Beck, S., Schwartz, A.L., Towsley, G., Dudley, W., and Barsevick, A. (2004). Psychometric evaluation of the Pittsburgh Sleep Quality Index. *Journal of Pain and Symptom Management*, 27, 140–148.

Benyamin, R., Trescot, A.M., Datta, S., *et al.* (2008). Opioid complications and side effects. *Pain Physician*, 2(Suppl.), S105–S120.

Bonnet, M.H. and Arand, D.L. (1996). Metabolic rate and the restorative function of sleep. *Physiology & Behavior*, 59(4–5), 777–782.

Budhiraja, R., Parthasarty, S., Budhiraja, P., Habib, M.P., Wendel, C., and Quan, S.F. (2012). Insomnia in patients with COPD. *Sleep*, 35, 369–375.

Cannici, J., Malcolm, R., and Peek, L.A. (1983). Treatment of insomnia in cancer patients using muscle relaxation training. *Journal of Behavior Therapy and Experimental Psychiatry*, 14, 251–256.

Dagan, Y. (2002). Circadian rhythm sleep disorders (CRSD). *Sleep Medicine Reviews*, 6, 45–54.

Davidson, J.R., MacLean, A.W., Brundage, M.D., and Schulze, K. (2002). Sleep disturbance in cancer patients. *Social Science & Medicine*, 54, 1309–1321.

De Cruz, S., Espiritu, J.R.D., Zeidler, M., and Wang, T. (2012). Sleep disorders in chronic liver disease. *Seminars in Respiratory and Critical Care Medicine*, 33, 26–35.

Espie, C.A., Fleming, L., Cassidy, J., *et al.* (2008). Randomized controlled clinical effectiveness trial of cognitive behavior therapy compared with treatment as usual for persistent insomnia in patients with cancer. *Journal of Clinical Oncology*, 26, 4651–4658.

Freedom, T. (2011). Classification of sleep disorders. *Disease-a-Month*, 57, 323–327.

Harsora, P. and Kessmann, J. (2009). Nonpharmacologic management of chronic insomnia. *American Family Physician*, 79(2), 125–130,131–132.

Jacobson, E. (1938). *You Can Sleep Well*. New York: McGraw-Hill.

Jensen, M.P., Gralow, J.R., Braden, A., Gertz, K.J., Fan, J.R., and Syrjala, K.L. (2012). Hypnosis for symptom management in women with breast cancer: a pilot study. *International Journal of Clinical and Experimental Hypnosis*, 60(2), 135–159.

Katz, D.A. and McHorney, C.A. (1998). Clinical correlates of insomnia in patients with chronic illness. *Archives of Internal Medicine*, 158, 1099–1107.

Klink, M., Quan, S., Kaltenborn, W., and Lobowitz, M. (1992). Risk factors associated with complaints of insomnia in a general adult population. *Archives of Internal Medicine*, 152, 1634–1637.

Lavigne, G.L., McMillan, D., and Zucconi, M. (2005). Pain and sleep. In M.H. Kryger, T. Roth, and W.C. Dement (eds.) *Principles and Practice of Sleep Medicine* (4th ed.), pp. 1246–1255. Philadelphia, PA: Elsevier Saunders.

Littner, M., Hirshkowitz, M., Kramer, M., *et al.* (2003). For the American Academy of Sleep Medicine Standards of Practice Committee. Practice parameters for using polysomnography to evaluate insomnia: an update. *Sleep*, 26, 754–760.

Liu, L., Rissling, M., Natarajan, L., *et al.* (2012). The longitudinal relationship between fatigue and sleep in breast cancer patients undergoing chemotherapy. *Sleep*, 35, 237–245.

Luyster, F.S., Buysse, D.J., and Strollo, P.J., Jr. (2010). Comorbid insomnia and obstructive sleep apnoea: challenges for clinical practice and research. *Journal of Clinical Sleep Medicine*, 6, 196–204.

Menefee, L.A., Cohen, M.J., Anderson, W.R., *et al.* (2000). Sleep disturbance and non-malignant chronic pain: a comprehensive review of the literature. *Pain Medicine*, 1, 156–172.

Morin, C.M. (1993). *Insomnia: Psychological Assessment and Management*. New York: The Guilford Press.

Morin, C.M., Colecchi, C., Stone, J., and Sood, R.M. (1999). Behavioral and pharmacological therapies for late-life insomnia: a randomized controlled trial. *Journal of the American Medical Association*, 281, 991–999.

Morin, M.M. and Benca, R. (2012). Chronic insomnia. *The Lancet*, 379, 1129–1141.

Montgomery, S.A., Herman, B.K., Schweizer, E., and Mandel, F.S. (2009). The efficacy of pregabalin and benzodiazepines in generalized anxiety disorder presenting with high levels of insomnia. *International Clinical Psychopharmacology*, 24, 214–222.

Mystakidou, K., Clark, J., Fischer, J., Lam, A., Pappert, K., and Richarz, U. (2011). Treatment of chronic pain by long acting opioids and their effect on sleep. *Pain Practice*, 3, 282–289.

Mystakidou, K., Parpa, E., Tsilika, E., Gennatas, C., Galanos, A., and Vlahos, L. (2009). How is sleep quality affected by the psychological and symptom distress of advanced cancer patients? *Palliative Medicine*, 23, 46–53.

Mystakidou, K., Parpa, E., Tsilika, E., *et al.* (2007). Sleep quality in advanced cancer patients. *Journal of Psychosomatic Research*, 62, 527–533.

O'Donohue, W. and Krasner, L. (1995). Theories in behavior therapy: philosophical and historical contexts. In W. O'Donohue and L. Krasner (eds.) *Theories of Behavior Therapy: Exploring Behavior Change*, pp. 1–22. Washington, DC: American Psychological Association.

Palesh, O.G., Roscoe, J.A., Mustian, K.M., *et al.* (2010). Prevalence, demographics, and psychological associations of sleep disruption in patients with cancer: University of Rochester Cancer Center-Community Clinical Oncology Program. *Journal of Clinical Oncology*, 28, 292–298.

Panagiotou, I. and Mystakidou, K. (2012). Non-analgesic effects of opioids: opioids' effects on sleep (including sleep apnoea). *Current Pharmaceutical Design*, 18(37), 6025–6033.

Phillips, K.M., Heather, J.S., Donovan, K.A., Pinder-Schenck, M.C., and Jacobsen, P.B. (2012). Characteristics and correlates of sleep disturbances in cancer patients. *Supportive Care in Cancer*, 20, 357–365.

Reeve, K. and Bailes, B. (2010). Insomnia in adults: etiology and management. *Journal for Nurse Practitioners*, 6, 53–60.

Regestein, Q.R. (1977) Sleep disorders in the medically ill. In A. Stoudemire and B.S. Fogel (eds.) *Principles of Medical Psychiatry*, pp. 186–191. Orlando, FL: Grune and Stratton.

Roth, T. (2007). Insomnia: definition, prevalence, aetiology and consequences. *Journal of Clinical Sleep Medicine*, 3, 7–10

Sateia, M.J., Doghramji, K., Hauri, P.J., and Morin, C.M. (2000). Evaluation of chronic insomnia: an American Academy of Sleep Medicine Review. *Sleep*, 23, 243–308.

Schuman, C.C. and Attarian, H.P. (2012). Integrating sleep management into clinical practice. *Journal of Clinical Psychology in Medical Settings*, 19, 65–76.

Schutte-Rodin, S., Broch, L., Buysse, D., Dorsey, C., and Sateia, M. (2008). Clinical guideline for the evaluation and management of chronic insomnia in adults. *Journal of Clinical Sleep Medicine*, 4, 487–504.

Simeit, R., Deck, R., and Conta-Marx, B. (2004). Sleep management training for cancer patients with insomnia. *Supportive Care in Cancer*, 12, 176–183.

Smith, M.T., Huang M.I., and Manber, R. (2005). Cognitive behavior therapy for chronic insomnia occurring within the context of medical and psychiatric disorders. *Clinical Psychology Review*, 25, 559–592.

Smith, M.T. and Neubauer, D.N. (2003). Cognitive behavior therapy for chronic insomnia. *Clinical Cornerstone*, 5, 28–40.

Turner, R.M. and Asher, L.M. (1979). Controlled comparison of progressive relaxation, stimulus control, and paradoxical intention therapies for insomnia. *Journal of Consulting and Clinical Psychology*, 47(3), 500–508.

Walker, J.M. and Farney, R.J. (2009). Are opioids associated with sleep apnea? A review of the evidence. *Current Pain and Headache Reports*, 13, 120–126.

The management of bleeding in palliative care

Jose Pereira and Jennifer Brodeur

Introduction to the management of bleeding in palliative care

Bleeding is one of the more distressing symptoms experienced by patients with advanced life-threatening illnesses. It may be the presenting symptom that prompts patients to seek medical attention (Moreno-Otero et al., 1987; Jellema et al., 2010), or the harbinger of disease recurrence and progression. Bleeding is associated with a poorer prognosis in some cancers, such as gastric cancers (Prommer, 2005), and the cause of death in others (Stalfelt et al., 2003; Rimmer et al., 2012). For some patients it is the principal symptom, overshadowing others (Stalfelt et al., 2003).

Frequency of bleeding

The prevalence and incidence of bleeding in patients with progressive, life-limiting illnesses vary depending on the disease and the illness trajectory. In a study of patients with lung cancer, bloody sputum was present at the time of diagnosis in 17% of patients, varying across cancer cell types (Buccheri and Ferrigno, 2004). Throughout the illness, haemoptysis occurs in a quarter to a third of lung cancer patients (Chute et al., 1985; Hopwood and Stephens, 1995) and 3% experience catastrophic terminal haemoptysis (Prommer, 2005). About 10% of patients with renal cancer present with haematuria at the time of diagnosis (Schips et al., 2003). Bleeding occurs in 5–15% of patients with hepatocellular cancer (Zhu et al., 1996; Okuda, 1997).

While most cases of upper gastrointestinal bleeds in patients with cancer are due to gastritis and ulcerative disease, up to 27% are caused by tumour invasion (Shivshanker et al., 1983).

In a study of patients with advanced cancer cared for by a home-based palliative team until death, 2.5% experienced gastrointestinal bleeding (melena or haematemesis) (Mercadante et al., 2000). In patients with acute myeloid leukaemia, bleeding occurred in 44% of cases in the last week of life; cerebral haemorrhage was listed as the cause of death in 9.4% (Stalfelt et al., 2003).

Bleeding also occurs in terminally ill patients with non-cancer diagnoses. Variceal haemorrhage, for example, occurs in 25–35% of patients with cirrhosis (Burroughs, 1993; Sharara and Rockey, 2001). Recent studies have noted a reduced rate of rebleeding in these patients, from 47% in 1980 to 13% in 2000 (Carbonell et al., 2004). There have also been improvements in survival after variceal bleeding (Carbonell et al., 2004).

Causes of bleeding

The causes of bleeding in patients with advanced disease are varied and may sometimes have several aetiologies or aggravating factors in any given patient (DeLoughery, 2009). Gagnon and colleagues proposed three major categories of causes: (1) anatomical (or local), (2) generalized (e.g. coagulation dyscrasias), or (3) a mixed (local and generalized) (Gagnon et al., 1998). Prommer proposes a more detailed classification of six causal categories (Prommer, 2005): (1) cancer invasion and destruction, (2) treatment-related causes, (3) thrombocytopenia/marrow failure, (4) nutritional deficits, (5) drugs, and (6) coagulation disturbances.

The primary tumour may invade tissues, including small and large vessels. Metastatic lesions and the granulation tissue within a malignant wound are often friable and hypervascular, increasing the risk for bleeding. Reduced fibroblast activity and ongoing thrombosis of larger vessels in infected and malignant wounds may render the granulation less resilient to trauma. Minor trauma, such as removal of dressings, may trigger bleeding. Some cancers such as renal cell carcinoma, choriocarcinoma, and melanoma are particularly vascular. In head and neck cancer, the walls of blood vessels may be weakened by exposure to saliva and prior radiation or surgery.

Chemotherapy and/or radiotherapy treatments may affect haemostatic mechanisms and damage mucosae, resulting in bleeding (Peterson and Cariello, 2004; Takemoto et al., 2012). Mucositis of the upper gastrointestinal tract is a frequent complication in patients receiving fractionated radiotherapy with or without concomitant chemotherapy for head and neck cancer and lung cancer (Trotti et al., 2003). Incidence of severe mucositis of the entire gastrointestinal tract can be as high as 75% in patients undergoing hematopoietic stem-cell transplantation (Peterson et al., 2009). Bone marrow transplantation and severe graft-versus-host disease are associated with the risk of haemorrhagic complications (Pihusch, 2004).

Treatment-related causes of bleeding include thrombocytopenia secondary to myelosuppressive chemotherapy such as imatinib mesylate (Croom and Perry, 2003), microangiopathic haemolytic anaemia syndrome associated with agents such as mitomycin (Rosen, 1992), haemorrhagic cystitis secondary to drugs such as cyclophosphamide and ifosfamide, and angiogenesis inhibition with agents such as bevacizumab (Kilickap et al., 2003; Hapani et al., 2010). Post-radiotherapy telangiectasia can cause bleeding following treatments of bladder, cervix, and prostate cancer.

Solid tumours with extensive bone metastases, leukaemias, and lymphomas may cause marrow failure by invading the marrow, resulting in thrombocytopenia (Prommer, 2005). Some cancers, such as prostate cancer, can also cause thrombocytopenia due to disseminated intravascular coagulopathy (DIC). Mucin-producing carcinomas of the prostate, pancreas, lung, breast, ovary, and gastrointestinal tract are associated with increased risk for DIC, as are acute leukaemias (Bick et al., 1996). The increased risk for bleeding in prostate cancer has also been attributed to increased fibrinolysis, preventing healing of the vascular endothelium (Kohli et al., 2003). Thrombocytopenia could occur due to immune-related mechanisms as well as sequestration, from advanced liver disease and associated splenomegaly.

Patients with very advanced disease suffer from a variety of nutritional deficits that could cause or aggravate bleeding. These include deficits of vitamin B_{12}, folate (Stefanini, 1999), zinc (Dunn et al., 2003), and vitamin K (Harrington et al., 2008).

Non-steroidal anti-inflammatory medications may interfere with platelet function or cause gastrointestinal ulceration. The use of anticoagulant medication, particularly warfarin, has been associated with excess bleeding in patients at the end of life Johnson, 1997). A number of commonly used drugs occasionally cause thrombocytopenia. These include trimethoprim-sulfamethoxazole, cimetidine and ranitidine, acetaminophen (paracetamol), carbamazepine, and heparin-related drugs.

Not all episodes of bleeding in patients with advanced cancer are related to the cancer or its treatments. Although rarer, bleeding may be caused by conditions such as idiopathic thrombocytopenic purpura and Goodpasture's syndrome.

Clinical presentation

The clinical presentation of bleeding in the palliative care setting is variable. It may be visible, as in haemoptysis or hematemesis, or invisible, as in cerebral haemorrhaging (Mandybur, 1977) or rupture of a liver mass (Zhu et al., 1996; Akriviadis, 1997). Volumes may vary, from low-grade oozing from a malignant wound to massive and catastrophic in the case of a ruptured carotid artery (Recka et al., 2012). Bleeding may be continuous or intermittent. Bleeding may be localized or from multiple sites as in the case of systemic coagulopathies.

Some patients present with small prodromal bleeding occurring several hours or days before the rupture of a larger artery (Harris and Noble, 2009) referred to as 'sentinel' or 'herald' bleeds. It is prudent to consider most initial presentations of bleeding as sentinel bleeds. This is particularly true of haemoptysis or bleeding from a malignant neck wound (Fernando et al., 1998).

Catastrophic, terminal haemorrhaging warrants special attention because of its dramatic clinical presentation and the profound distress it causes to patients, families, and caregivers (Harris and Noble, 2009). The rapid sequence of events gives little time to support and comfort the patient. Harris and Noble define it as 'a major haemorrhage, from an artery, which is likely to result in death within a period of time that may be as short as minutes, because of the rapid internal or external loss of circulating blood volume' (Harris and Noble, 2009).

Back defined it as major arterial haemorrhage with loss of more than 1.5 L of blood in 30 seconds which will inevitably cause death in minutes (Back, 2001). Prommer defines massive

haemoptysis as expectoration of at least 100–600 mL of blood in 24 hours (Prommer, 2005). Fernando et al. used the presence of one or more of the following criteria to define major haemoptysis: (Fernando et al., 1998) bleeding 200 mL or more per 24 hours; bronchial blood loss that caused haemodynamic or respiratory compromise; or bleeding that resulted in a haematocrit of less than 0.30 (< 30%).The terms 'massive' or 'catastrophic' are sometimes preferred over the term 'terminal' haemorrhage because not all large bleeds result in death. Harris and Noble propose that any major bleed should be managed in the same way as there is no way of knowing which will be terminal events (Harris and Noble 2009). The mortality rates of massive haemoptysis may be as high as 60–100% in patients with bronchogenic carcinoma (Fernando et al., 1998; Kvale et al., 2003).

Carotid blow-out (CBO), a complication that has a high mortality rate, usually occurs proximal to the carotid bifurcation and is commonly associated with soft tissue necrosis in the neck (55%) and mucocutaneous fistulas (40%) (Citardi et al., 1995; Powitzky et al., 2010) (see Chapter 14.5). Citardi and colleagues suggested that CBO is a syndrome with three distinct clinical entities (Citardi et al., 1995): (1) 'threatened' CBO (when the artery is clinically exposed or there is radiological evidence of carotid invasion), (2) 'impending' CBO (a herald bleed has settled spontaneously or with treatment), and (3) 'acute' CBO (rupture with profuse bleeding). All three presentations require urgent attention (Harris and Noble, 2009) as even the smallest of bleeds should be taken seriously (Fortunato and Ridge, 1995).

Patients at risk for bleeding

Factors that place cancer patients at increased risk for bleeding have been proposed (Prommer 2005; Harris and Noble, 2009) (see Table 8.7.1). It is important to initiate pre-emptive treatments when possible and to prepare caregivers.

Table 8.7.1 Risk factors for bleeding in cancer patients

Overall risk factors for bleeding in cancer patients (Prommer, 2005)	Risk factors for terminal haemorrhaging in head and neck cancers (Harris and Noble, 2009)
◆ Thrombocytopenia <20,000/μL	◆ Radical neck dissection
◆ Large head and neck cancers	◆ High-dose radiotherapy
◆ Large centrally located lung cancers	◆ Postoperative healing problems
◆ Refractory acute and chronic leukaemias	◆ Visible arterial pulsation
◆ Myelodysplasia	◆ Pharyngocutaneous fistula
◆ Sever liver disease and metastatic liver disease	◆ Fungating tumours with artery invasion
◆ Hepatocellular carcinoma	◆ Direct observation during surgery or imaging (e.g. magnetic resonance imaging) of artery wall invasion
◆ Oral anticoagulants	◆ Sentinel bleed
◆ High-dose radiation therapy	

Column 1 adapted with permission from Prommer, E., Management of bleeding in the terminally ill patient, *Hematology*, Volume 10, Number 3, pp. 167–175, Copyright © W. S. Maney and Son Ltd 2005, Column 2, data from Harris, D. G. and Noble, S. I., Management of terminal hemorrhage in patients with advanced cancer: a systematic literature review, *Journal of Pain and Symptom Management*, Volume 38, Number 6, pp. 913–927, Copyright © 2009 U.S. Cancer Pain Relief Committee. Published by Elsevier Inc. All rights reserved.

Impact on patients, families, and care providers

Except for in malignant wounds (Goode, 2004; Lo et al., 2008; Alexander, 2009) there are few studies that explore the meaning that patients associate with bleeding and its psychological impact (Maida et al., 2009). In addition to morbidity and mortality, bleeding may also result in increased used of emergency services. In a large Canadian study of cancer patients who visited an emergency department at the end of life, about 2% did so because of gastrointestinal bleeding or haematuria (Barbera et al., 2010).

Management plan

General

Communication and clarifying goals of care

The management plan should be individualized; several factors need to be considered. These include the patient's life expectancy, performance status, quality of life, previous therapies, acuteness of situation, likelihood of reversing or controlling the underlying cause of the bleeding, access to interventions such as interventional radiology, and patient preferences. A newly diagnosed patient with good performance status will be managed differently from a patient at the end of life with a poor performance status.

Establishing goals of care is important, particularly in patients at risk for a major bleed. The discussion should be consistent with a patient's information needs and preferences and the care plan should, amongst others, be compatible with the patient's wishes (Prommer, 2005).

Whether the patient, family, and caregivers should be informed of the risk of terminal haemorrhage poses an ethical dilemma. Arguments for and against full disclosure to patients exist (Frawley and Begley, 2006b; Harris and Noble, 2009). An individualized approach is recommended; finding a balance between information needs against the potential psychological impact of full disclosure (Frawley and Begley, 2006a). Some suggest that, although patients need not be universally informed about the risk, families and caregivers should be made aware so as to prepare them for what could be a very distressing event (Gagnon et al., 1998; Pereira and Phan, 2004). Unprepared caregivers may panic, calling emergency services that are required to institute resuscitative measures. The implications of asking a caregiver and family member to administer prefilled syringes of sedatives in the event of a massive bleed should be considered (Harris and Noble, 2009).

History and physical examination

A comprehensive history and examination is required. The goals of the clinical assessment are to establish the scope of the problem, identify patients at risk and in the setting of active bleeding, identify underlying causes and aggravating factors, and assess its impact on the patient and family.

Current and recent medications as well as past medical history should be reviewed. The benefits versus burden of continuing prophylactic anticoagulation treatments or medications that may be causing or aggravating bleeding need to be assessed. In addition to assessing the location, pattern, and severity of bleeding, the physical examination may also provide valuable clues as to its origin; the presence of multiple sites of bleeding, for example, points to systemic problems.

Investigations

Investigations are warranted in some situations, especially if a patient is not at the end of life. A full blood count and basic coagulation blood work-up may be useful, including the international normalized ratio (INR), activated partial thromboplastin time, platelet count, and fibrinogen level. Coagulation defects vary across different problems (DeLoughery, 2009). Procedures such as endoscopy and angiography may be required in select cases to identify and treat the source of bleeding. Magnetic resonance imaging may be useful when exploring CBO risk in a patient with a fungating neck wound

Prevention

Strategies to prevent or reduce the risk of bleeding should be implemented where possible. Bleeding from ulcerated wounds can be minimized by using non-adherent dressings, maintaining a moist wound bed, and gently irrigating rather than swabbing. Dry dressings should be avoided. Pre-emptive treatments, such as endovascular stents in the case of large neck tumours, may be considered in very select cases. A randomized placebo controlled trial of preventative topical rectal beclometasone dipropionate found a significantly reduced risk of rectal bleeding in patients receiving radiation for prostate cancer (Fuccio et al., 2011). Beta blockers may play a role in preventing bleeding from high-risk oesophageal varices in end-stage liver disease; endoscopic prophylactic sclerotherapy is not recommended in these cases (The Veterans Affairs Cooperative Variceal Sclerotherapy Group, 1991; Pagliaro et al., 1992).

Treatment options

A number of treatment modalities are available. These can be divided into (a) general measures, (b) local measures (see Box 8.7.1), and (c) systemic measures. The decision to select one or the other is dependent on a number of factors. In addition to goals of care, functional status, co-morbidity, and patient preference, they include aetiology of the bleed, availability of the modality, benefit versus burden, and cost. Unfortunately studies in the palliative care setting comparing various modalities and approaches are generally lacking and guidelines are largely based on case reports and expert opinion (Regnard and Makin, 1992; Harris and Noble, 2009).

General measures

General supportive measures include, in addition to proactive planning, the use of dark towels and staying with and comforting the patient in the case of a massive bleed (Harris and Noble, 2009; Harris et al., 2011). General resuscitative measures, including aggressive fluid replacement or blood products, are generally inappropriate in patients with very advanced disease but may be appropriate alongside interventional measures to stop bleeding in some patients.

Management: local modalities

Compression, compression dressings, and packing

Pressure, using surgical gauze and dressings, is the simplest form of haemostasis, particularly in emergency situations. For minimal bleeding, compressive dressings generally suffice (Recka et al.,

---

Box 8.7.1 Local and systemic modalities

Local modalities[a]

◆ **Compression dressings and packing**
◆ Topical haemostatic agents:
  • **Absorbable agents: gelatin foams, oxidized cellulose, microfibrillar collagen**
  • Biologic agents (*limited usefulness in palliative care*): topical thrombin, fibrin sealants, platelet sealants
  • Alginates
  • **Astringents, sclerosing and vasoconstrictor agents**: silver nitrate, alum solutions, sucralfate, formalin, acetone, epinephrine (adrenaline), topical cocaine, zinc chloride, oxymetazoline
  • Synthetic agents: cyanoacrylates, glutaraldehyde cross-linked albumin
  • Haemostatic dressings: fibrin dressing, chitin/chitosan dressings, mineral zeolite dressings
  • Other: tranexamic acid, steroids
◆ **Radiation therapy**
◆ **Embolization and balloon tamponade**
◆ **Endoscopy**: ligation, sclerosing agent, cauterization, balloon tamponade, thrombin/fibrinogen application
◆ **Surgery**: vessel ligation, resection

Systemic modalities[a]

◆ **Antifibrinolytic agents**
◆ Somatostatin analogues (octreotide)
◆ Vasopressin analogues (desmopressin/DDAVP)
◆ **Vitamin K**
◆ Blood/plasma products:
  • Platelets
  • Fresh frozen plasma
  • Cryoprecipitate
◆ Recombinant coagulation factors (VIIa, VIII, IX)
◆ Hyperbaric oxygen therapy
◆ Other modalities: pentosanpolysulphate, melatonin, thalidomide

[a] First-line modalities in bold.

2012). With the exception of alginate dressings, most compressive dressings are not inherently haemostatic (Terrill et al., 2003).

Packing, with saline-soaked dressings, surgical swabs, or special haemostatic dressings, is useful for bleeding from accessible hollow organs such as the nose, rectum, and vagina. Haemostatic or vasoconstrictor agents, such as silver nitrate, cocaine, and/or epinephrine (adrenaline) may be added to the dressings. Vaginal bleeding, for example, has been controlled with packs soaked with formaldehyde or acetone (Patsner, 1993; Fletcher et al., 2002). If possible, the frequency of dressings should be reduced and non-adherent dressings used.

Compression can also be achieved with inflatable balloons. Specially designed catheters with inflatable balloons may be used to control severe posterior nasal bleeding. In emergent cases, urinary catheters have been used. Such measures are temporary since prolonged pressure may cause tissue necrosis.

Topical haemostatic agents

A large number of topical agents are available (see Box 8.7.1). They differ in constitution, mechanisms of action, indication, packaging, and price. Many, such as the absorbable agents and biologic agents, were designed for intraoperative control of minor bleeding during vascular, cardiac, oral, and reconstructive surgery when other conventional methods are ineffective (Achneck et al., 2010). They are often used for one-time applications. A large number of products are available, from powders, sponges, pads, and ribbons, to dual-syringe systems. Their costs vary; some such as topical thrombin and fibrin sealants are prohibitively expensive for multiple applications.

Absorbable products

Absorbable products are amongst the least expensive of the surgical haemostatic products and are easy to apply (Achneck et al., 2010). Gelatin foams can be applied as a sponge, powder, or film (Achneck et al., 2010). The powder is mixed with a sterile saline solution and applied as a paste. Sponges can be applied either dry or saturated with sterile saline or topical thrombin solutions. Unlike oxidized cellulose, the pH of gelatin foams is neutral; so they can be combined with thrombin to provide a physical matrix for fibrin deposition and clotting to be initiated. These products are usually fully absorbed approximately 4–6 weeks following application, except in the nose and nasal pharynx where it liquefies within 2–5 days. Occasionally, gelatin can swell to twice its size and may lead to compressive complications when used in confined spaces or near nerves.

Oxidized regenerated cellulose products are available as sponges and pads and have been used in the palliative setting (Lagman et al., 2002). They are more pliable than the gelatin foams. They should be applied dry, and tend to expand and dissolve in 2–6 weeks.

Microfibrillar collagen is available in sponge and powder forms. The mesh form may be cut to size and conforms well to irregular surfaces. The preparations can be stored at room temperature and are ready to use out of the box. Platelets adhere to the fibres and are activated, resulting in platelet aggregation and thrombus formation (Wagner et al., 1996). It is therefore less effective in patients with severe thrombocytopenia but effective in heparinized patients. It appears to be useful in large areas of parenchymal bleeding (Chapman et al., 2002).

Biologic agents

Thrombin forms the basis of a fibrin clot by promoting the conversion of fibrinogen to fibrin. It requires the presence of fibrinogen. Bovine plasma-derived products are associated with the development of antibodies to thrombin and other clotting factors, while products derived from pooled human plasma cause fewer immunological complications. A recombinant product is now available (Chapman et al., 2007). The bovine and recombinant products require reconstitution in sterile isotonic saline solution, while the human-derived product is 'ready to use'. The human-derived product is available in small vials with syringe and spray applicators. An epistaxis kit is also available. Thrombin may be applied either directly to the bleeding site or soaked in gelatin sponge.

Thrombin vials are for single use only and require frozen storage and thawing before application. They cannot be refrozen.

Fibrin sealants are made of two components: thrombin and fibrinogen (Kanaoka et al., 2001; Mankad and Codispoti, 2001). They are applied with a dual-syringe delivery system that mixes the two components as it is applied (Achneck et al., 2010). The components interact to form a stable fibrin clot. In contrast to passive haemostatic agents such as collagen, alginate, and cellulose products that promote the patient's own blood clotting mechanism, fibrin sealants coagulate independently from patient blood and are therefore useful even in patients with severe coagulopathy. They are derived from pooled or autologous human plasma or bovine plasma and may cause immunological reactions; less so with human-only derived. They are available in 2 mL and 5 mL single dosing syringes and are very costly and need to be thawed prior to usage. Fibrin sealant, instilled via bronchoscopy, has been used to control massive haemoptysis (Pandya et al., 2011).

Platelet sealant is a thrombin/collagen suspension which works in combination with the patient's own plasma to form a fibrin/collagen clot. It is resorbed in 30 days and is intended to be left *in situ*. It is not very practical in the palliative care setting as it requires centrifugation of the patient's own plasma and significant pre-application processing.

Alginates

Alginate dressings are readily available for minor bleeds, particularly oozing from malignant wounds. They are fibre dressings containing alginic acids (mannuronic and guluronic) which are extracted from seaweed species and are available as pads or ribbons (Timmons, 2009). Alginates are best used on wounds with a large amount of exudate; but are not useful in large-volume bleeds. The fibrous dressings form a gel when in contact with wound exudate; the calcium alginate in the dressing forms sodium alginate and calcium ions which in turn support the normal clotting process. The gel prevents the wound from drying out and assists in autolytic debridement. This function precludes alginates from being used in dry or low exuding wounds, as they may adhere to the wound bed.

Alginates require a secondary cover dressing such as a bio-occlusive thin film, hydrogel sheet, or gauze to keep them in place. They can absorb up to 20 times their weight in fluid. Alginates can be rinsed away with saline irrigation, so removal of the dressing does not interfere with healing granulation tissue. Some alginates contain a silver compound which provides antimicrobial protection. Wounds are generally irrigated with sterile saline when the dressings are removed so as to remove the fibres.

Alginates are also useful for deep, undermined wounds as the risk of infection or tissue inflammation is reduced if they are left *in situ*. Alginates are usually changed every 12–48 hours, but in some cases may be left in place for up to 7 days. Wounds with lots of exudates may require more frequent dressing changes (Grocott, 1998).

Astringents, sclerosing, and vasoconstrictor agents

Astringents induce chemical cauterization and are best used to control minor to moderate bleeds. The two most commonly used astringents are silver nitrate and aluminium-based solutions. Silver nitrate acts as a strong oxidizing agent, causing tissue coagulation (Hanif et al., 2003). Silver nitrate, fused with potassium nitrate on the end of thin wooden applicators, has been extensively used in the management of epistaxis. The ends of the sticks are gently applied with minimal pressure to the vessel. It is relatively inexpensive and requires minimal technical skill to apply.

Silver nitrate, in a concentration of 0.5–1% and instilled for 10–20 minutes, has been used to manage bladder bleeding (Jerkins et al., 1986); ureteral stenosis, however, is a potential complication (Vijan et al., 1988).

Intravesical alum bladder irrigations have been described in the management of bladder-related haematuria, with response rates of 66–100% (Ostroff and Chenault, 1982; Arrizabalaga et al., 1987; Octavio and Buizza, 1989). A recommended regimen consists of using a 1% alum solution, dissolving 50 g of alum in 5 L sterile water and irrigating the bladder at 250–300 mL per hour (Choong et al., 2000). Alum (either aluminium ammonium sulphate or aluminium potassium sulphate) causes the precipitation of protein in the interstitial tissue spaces, resulting in decreased capillary permeability, vasoconstriction, constriction of the interstitial spaces, and hardening of the capillary endothelium. The treatment duration is usually 3–4 days, but can be extended up to 1 week. It is generally safe and well tolerated. It should be avoided in patients with renal impairment or very large bladder tumours as aluminium encephalopathy and death have been described in these patients (Murphy et al., 1992; Shoskes et al., 1992). Ureteral fibrosis has been reported.

Sucralfate has a cytoprotective action derived from the production of prostaglandins and promotion of epithelial cell proliferation (Prommer, 2005). Sucralfate enemas (usually 20 mL of 10% sucralfate suspension), applied twice a day until bleeding stopped, successfully controlled bleeding from radiation proctitis (Cotti et al., 2003; Chun et al., 2004). Sucralfate can be mixed with K-Y® Jelly forming a paste for direct application to bleeding sites, including malignant wounds (Regnard 1991; Thomas et al., 1998). A preparation made up of a 1 g tablet of sucralfate, crushed and mixed into 5 mL of water-soluble gel for twice-daily application, has been suggested for malignant wounds (Woodruff 1993).

Topical formalin, usually in concentrations of 4–5%, has been used to control haemorrhaging from radiation proctitis (Biswal et al., 1995b; Roche et al.,1996; Saclarides et al., 1996; Parikh et al., 2003), rectal cancer (Zbar et al., 2005), bladder lesions (Donahue and Frank, 1989; Vicente et al., 1990; Redman and Kletzel, 1994; Fu et al., 1998; Sarnak et al., 1999), vaginal/cervix tumours (Yegappan et al., 1998), and cutaneous ulcers (Adebamowo, 2000). Formalin controls bleeding by fixing tissue, causing the cross-linkage of tissue proteins. Coagulation of tissue also occurs (Parikh et al., 2003). In rectal bleeding it is applied as an irrigation or soaked in gauze. In a case series, topical formalin controlled bleeding in 89% of patients (Cotti et al., 2003). In another series, haemorrhagic proctitis was controlled with 500 mL of a 4% formalin solution instilled in the rectum in 50 mL aliquots (Saclarides et al., 1996). Treatments were done under local, regional, or general anaesthesia. Endoscopy-aided insertion of cotton pledgets soaked in 5% formalin has been used to control bleeding from multiple foci in the bladder (Choong et al., 2000). Intravesicular formalin instillation is done with solutions of 1%, 4%, or 10% for a period of between 5 and 30 minutes (Ghahestani and Shakhssalim, 2009; Guven et al., 2011). Despite good response rates, formalin is associated with severe adverse effects, including spasms, kidney failure, retroperitoneal fibrosis, incontinence, reduced bladder capacities, and even death (Braam et al., 1986).

Acetone-soaked packs may control vaginal bleeding from recurrent pelvic malignancy, particularly in patients who have previously undergone radiotherapy or when embolic techniques are not available (Patsner, 1993).

Vasoconstrictors such as cocaine and epinephrine have been used to control epistaxis (Katz et al., 1990; Chrisman, 2010). Cocaine can be applied to cotton pledgets and packed into the nasopharynx (Kothari et al., 2001); 4 mL of a 4% solution is used. Prostaglandins E_2 and F_2 have been used to control intractable haemorrhagic cystitis but bladder spasms may limit their utility. Epinephrine can also be used but liberal use can lead to necrosis and neurological and cardiac complications. Oxymetazoline is a local vasoconstrictor that works via stimulation of alpha-adrenergic receptors. It has been used to achieve haemostasis perioperatively in nasal surgery (Krempl and Noorily, 1995). Oxymetazoline spray combined with non-occlusive dressing helped to control bleeding in a malignant neck wound (Recka et al., 2012). Successful use of aerosolized vasopressin to stop mild to moderate haemoptysis has been reported in a small series in palliative care (Anwar et al., 2005).

Synthetic agents

A number of synthetic haemostatic agents are used as glues or mechanical sealants intraoperatively, including vascular, oncological (Carmignani et al., 2006; Chen et al., 2009), and cosmetic surgery. They include polyethylene glycol hydrogels, cyanoacrylates, and glutaraldehyde cross-linked albumin. Cyanoacrylates are synthetic resin glues that provide haemostasis by forming polymers when in contact with a basic medium such as blood or water. Lal and colleagues reported successful use of cyanoacrylate glue in a case of intractable bleeding from locally advanced duodenal cancer (Lal et al., 2009). Cyanoacrylate sclerotherapy by endoscopy has been used to stop bleeding of cholecystojejunostomy varices in a patient with pancreatic cancer (Hsu et al., 2010).

Haemostatic dressings

Haemostatic dressings and granules were developed to control ballistic injuries in battlefield injuries (Holcomb et al., 1998; Achneck et al., 2010). To date, there have been no reports of their use in the palliative care settings. The agents include chitin (a polysaccharide with haemostatic properties that is found in arthropod skeletons), chitosan (a deacetylated form of chitin) (Wedmore et al., 2006; Brown et al., 2009), zeolite agents (Neuffer et al., 2004; Rhee et al., 2008; Achneck et al., 2010), and kaolin-containing products (Kheirabadi et al., 2009).

Other haemostatic agents

Topical application of zinc chloride-containing paste (Mohs' paste) achieved haemostasis in bleeding from malignant wounds in five patients with breast cancer (Kakimoto et al., 2010). Local application of antifibrinolytic agents has been reported as has intravesicular instillation of E-aminocaproic acid (Lakhani et al., 1999). Tranexamic acid can also be applied topically to cancer in the rectum, bladder, and pleura (5 g in 50 mL of water, instilled once or twice a day). Tranexamic acid tablets (500 mg) have been crushed and dissolved in 5 mL of normal saline, soaked in gauze, and applied to skin wounds for 10 minutes (Twycross and Wilcock 2014b). It has also been used to control haemothoraces (De Boer et al., 1991), rectal bleeding (McElligott et al., 1991), and bleeding from oral lesions.

Steroid suppositories or enemas have been used in bleeding caused by radiation-induced proctitis (Takemoto et al., 2012). Carboplast (prostaglandin $F_{2\alpha}$) intravesical instillation (at doses of 0.4 mg/dL to 1 mg/dL four times a day alternating with continuous saline bladder irrigation for 2 hours over 4–5 days) has been reported in several case series; with a success rate of up to 54% (Levine and Kranc, 1990; Levine and Jarrard, 1993; Miller et al., 1994; Ippoliti et al., 1995; Laszlo et al., 1995). Bladder spasm is the most common side effect.

Radiation therapy

Radiation therapy (RT) is a very useful modality. RT appears to cause erosion of the surface of blood vessels, leading to formation of thromboses and capillary necroses (Lee et al., 2009). Benefits have been reported in patients with cancers of the lung (Medical Research Council Lung Cancer Working Party, 1992; Brundage et al., 1996; Fernando et al., 1998; Harris and Noble, 2009), uterus and cervix (Halle et al., 1986; Biswal et al., 1995a), ovary (Tinger et al., 2001), bladder (Srinivasan et al., 1994), rectum (Taylor et al., 1987; Hoskin et al., 2004), stomach (Myint, 2000; Tey et al., 2007), haemoptysis from metastatic thyroid cancer (Ulger et al., 2006), sarcoma metastatic to the vagina (Park et al., 2005), and prostate (Thurairaja et al., 2008; Din et al., 2009). Response rates ranging from 45% to 100% across a variety of cancers have been reported (Cihoric et al., 2012). RT was used to control intractable bleeding from a hypervascular mandibular metastasis in a patient with hepatocellular carcinoma (Huang et al., 2007) (see Chapter 12.3).

The reduction of haemoptysis by palliative RT in non-small cell lung cancer has been demonstrated in randomized trials using varying fractions (Bleehen et al., 1992; Langendijk et al., 2000). Response rates vary but are generally high with up to 75% or more of patients responding. Single or hypofractionated doses appear as effective and safe, with minimal toxicity, as multiple fractions in the management of haemoptysis.

Endoluminal brachytherapy is an option for managing bleeding in patients who are not eligible for more aggressive treatment (Klopp et al., 2006; Ozkok et al., 2008). Allison et al., reported the combined use of high-dose rate brachytherapy and flexible metallic stenting for palliation of haemoptysis and shortness of breath due to bronchial obstruction (Allison et al., 2004); haemoptysis resolved within 1 week of therapy.

Positive results have also been reported for the use of RT in the management of refractory haemorrhaging from carcinoma of the uterine cervix. In a small study, six out of 20 patients had a complete response and 12 had a partial response; improvements were noted within 24–48 hours after completing treatment (Biswal, et al., 1995a). In another study, treatment with single fractions of 10 Gy were successful in almost all patients with uterine and cervical cancer (Onsrud et al., 2001).

External beam RT has been shown to control cases of haematuria in patients with advanced bladder cancer. Initial response rates of 60–81% have been reported using single or hypofractionated regimens (Srinivasan et al., 1994; Duchesne et al., 2000; Din et al., 2009). Following intra-urethral brachytherapy, haematuria resolved in 19 of the 23 patients with intractable bleeding from advanced prostate cancer (Thurairaja et al., 2008). Haemostasis usually occurs within a few days. The role of RT for managing bleeding from inoperable renal carcinoma is unclear.

Palliative RT, either alone in varying fractions or in combination with chemotherapy, has shown benefits in controlling bleeding from gastric cancer, with response rates of 51–73% (Tey et al., 2007; Kim et al., 2008; Lee et al., 2009; Asakura et al., 2011). Rebleeding appears to occur in approximately half of the patients who responded. Lee et al. (2009) have suggested the following criteria for palliative radiotherapy to control bleeding in patients with gastric cancer: (a) Eastern Cooperative Oncology Group performance status score 3 or better, (b) expected survival duration of more than a few months, (c) failure or contraindication of other treatment modalities, and (d) oozing cancer bleeding accompanied by intractable pain. Endoscopic confirmation of cancer-related bleeding is suggested to avoid unnecessary RT for bleeding from benign causes, particularly bleeding in the gastrointestinal and urogenital tracts.

The role of RT to control bleeding malignant wounds has not been adequately explored. RT is often not an option in patients presenting with bleeding malignant neck wounds as most cases would have already received maximum doses.

Endoscopy

Endoscopy provides access to bleeding in the upper and lower gastrointestinal (Loftus et al., 1994; Savides and Jensen, 2000), bronchial, and genito-urinary tracts (Kimmey, 2004). It allows the operator to visualize the source of bleeding, take a tissue biopsy if required, and initiate definitive treatment. Once visualized, several options are available (Savides and Jensen, 2000): (a) cauterization or coagulation with electrocautery, heat probes, laser, argon plasma coagulation, or cryotherapy; (b) balloon tamponade; (c) ligation using endoclips or banding; (d) injection of a vasoconstrictor or sclerosing agents such as epinephrine, ethanol (Loscos et al., 1993), or cyanoacrylate; (e) application of haemostatic agents; or (f) instillation of agents for irrigation (Conlan and Hurvitz, 1980). The choice of method varies amongst endoscopists (Tang et al., 2009).

Cauterization can be done with electrocoagulation heat probes, cryotherapy probes, laser, or argon plasma coagulation. Heat probes require direct contact between the probe and the tissue. Neodymium:yttrium aluminium garnet (Nd:YAG) laser allows cauterization of the vessel and, in select cases, vaporization of cancerous tissue (Birnbaum and Mercer, 1990; von Ditfurth et al., 1990). In argon plasma coagulation (APC) (Akhtar et al., 2000; Reichle et al., 2000), a jet of ionized argon gas (plasma) is directed through a probe that is passed through the endoscope. The argon gas is then ionized by a high-voltage discharge and an electrical current is conducted through the jet onto the lesion, thereby coagulating it. There is no physical contact between the probe and the tissue. High-volume bleeds may make visualization difficult (Mathus-Vliegen and Tytgat, 1990; Lee et al., 2009). APC has been used in palliative surgeries of patients with head and neck cancers (Hauser et al., 2002).

Endoscopy has been used at various levels of the gastrointestinal tract, including the oesophagus and stomach (Suzuki et al., 1989; Gupta and Fleischer, 1993; Loscos et al., 1993; Savides et al., 1996; Akhtar et al., 2000), duodenum (Loftus et al., 1994), and rectosigmoid colon (Schrock, 1989; Birnbaum and Mercer, 1990; von Ditfurth et al., 1990; Schulze and Lyng 1994; Chun et al., 2004; Kimmey, 2004). Bipolar probe cauterization has been used to treat radiation-induced rectal bleeding (Chun et al., 2004).

Endoscopic haemostasis of gastric bleeding has provided temporary relief prior to elective surgical palliation for advanced gastric cancer (Cook et al., 1992; Loftus et al., 1994; Savides et al., 1996). Endoscopic sclerotherapy with cyanoacrylate was used to control cholecystojejunostomy variceal bleeding in a patient with pancreatic head cancer (Hsu et al., 2010). In a case series, APC was successful in reducing or halting rectal bleeding related to radiotherapy for prostate cancer (Takemoto et al., 2012).

Endoscopy has been used to control haemoptysis (Freitag, 1993; Knott-Craig et al., 1993; Patel et al., 1994; Kato et al., 1996; D'Amico et al., 2003; Tuller et al., 2004). Kaaragac et al. successfully used neodymium:yttrium aluminum perovskite (Nd:YAP) laser repetitively over the course of the illness of two patients (Karaagac et al., 2005). Balloon catheters may be used as temporary measures (24–48 hours) before proceeding with more definitive treatments such as radiotherapy (Freitag, 1993). Bronchoscopy has been used to instil a variety of agents around or into the lesion, including cold saline, epinephrine solution, antidiuretic hormone derivatives such as ornipressin (Tuller et al., 2004), or thrombin/fibrinogen (Patel et al., 1994; de Gracia et al., 2003). Successful use of fibrin sealant applied via bronchoscopy was reported in a warfarin anticoagulated patient who had presented with massive haemoptysis that did not respond to irrigation with cold saline and epinephrine (Pandya et al., 2011). Definitive treatment with coil embolization via angiography followed.

Cystoscopy-aided laser or argon beam coagulation (Quinlan et al., 1992) of bleeding lesions in the bladder is now considered standard second-line treatment if bladder irrigation and clot evacuation through a three-way catheter is unsuccessful (Choong et al., 2000; Guven et al., 2011). As previously described, a number of agents have been instilled into the bladder for irrigation (including alum, silver nitrate, formalin, e-aminocaproic acid, phenol, prostaglandin F_2/carboplast) or injected around or into the bleeding tissue, including fibrin sealants (Ouwenga et al., 2004; Tirindelli et al., 2009) and cyanacrylate glue (Carmignani et al., 2006). Access to the bladder is through cystoscopy or cystostomy (Baronciani et al., 1995). Continuous bladder irrigation with saline solution can aid in preventing further clotting.

Embolization

Percutaneous transcatheter arterial embolization (TAE) involves the intravascular deposition of haemostatic material to produce permanent or temporary vessel occlusion (Angle et al., 2010). It has been used in many different vascular territories, including bronchial, coeliac, superior and inferior mesenteric, renal, hypogastric, and carotid territories. The potential role of TAE in palliative care has been described (Broadley et al., 1995).

Access to the vessel is usually under local anaesthesia through a femoral or axillary approach. The interventional radiologist performs an arteriogram to identify the vessel responsible for the bleeding and then threads a smaller catheter as close to the site of bleeding as possible—referred to as 'superselection'. The choice of material employed for embolization depends on the size of the vessel and the desired duration of occlusion.

Materials used in embolization include coils, microspheres, gelatin sponge (Gelfoam®) and haemostatic agents such as ethanol, sodium tetradecyl sulfate, cyanoacrylate, and polyvinyl alcohol (Angle et al., 2010). In the case of coils, occlusion occurs as a result of coil-induced thrombosis rather than mechanical occlusion of the lumen. The thrombogenic effect primarily results from the addition of silk or synthetic fibres. Microcoils can be particularly useful when superselective coil embolization is required. Microspheres are biocompatible, hydrophilic, non-resorbable particles produced from an acrylic polymer and impregnated with porcine gelatin or starch. Microspheres are available in different sizes and are supplied in apyrogenic sterile sodium chloride solution. Gelfoam® is usually absorbed completely, with little tissue reaction, and the vessel recanalizes within a few weeks. Some patients develop postembolization syndrome which is usually transient and is characterized by nausea, vomiting, pain, and fever due to tissue necrosis (Pisco et al., 1989).

Bronchial artery embolization plays a pivotal role in management of massive haemoptysis (Mal et al., 1999; White, 1999; Pandya et al., 2011). Shigemura et al. reported reduced morbidity and mortality in patients with massive haemoptysis with an embolization technique compared to a surgical approach (Shigemura et al., 2009). In a study by Fernando and colleagues, embolization of the bronchial artery gave an initial success rate of 85% (Fernando et al., 1998). However, there was a significant rate of recurrent bleeding (50%). Poyanli et al. described a large series of 140 patients treated with bronchial artery embolization; most had tuberculosis and only four had cancer (Poyanli et al., 2007). Embolization was successful in all but two of the patients immediately post intervention. Two of the patients, both with cancer, experienced fatal bleeds a month after the procedure.

TAE has been used extensively in managing severe bladder or pelvic haemorrhaging (Pisco et al., 1989; Gine et al., 2003; De et al., 2005; Palandri et al., 2005; El-Assmy and Mohsen, 2007; Ghahestani and Shakhssalim, 2009; Delgal et al., 2010; Liguori et al., 2010; Guven et al., 2011). Success rates of 70–100% have been reported. Selective internal iliac embolization is being replaced by superselective embolization of bladder arteries, which is associated with fewer side effects (gluteal pain, claudication, or tissue necrosis and pain) and has a lower recurrence rate.

Endovascular management of head and neck bleeding was initially done with endovascular balloon occlusion of the bleeding vessel (Citardi et al., 1995). This has been replaced with embolization; newer techniques are showing reductions in vascular complications and improvements in survival and quality of life (Morrissey et al., 1997; Chaloupka et al., 1999; Levy et al., 2002; Broomfield et al., 2006; Rimmer et al., 2012). More recently, endovascular stent repair of carotid rupture has been described (Cohen and Rad, 2004; Hoppe et al., 2008). Successful stent grafting in combination with coil embolization has been reported in a patient with impending carotid rupture secondary to head and neck cancer (Bates and Shamsham, 2003). Chang et al. reported the use of endovascular therapy in patients with CBO syndrome; self-expandable stent grafts or insertions of balloons, coils, or acrylic adhesives were used (Chang et al., 2008). Rebleeding occurred in a small number of these patients. Chen and colleagues used a variety of methods (Gelfoam® sponge, coils, microcoils, or combinations of these) to manage carotid bleeding following RT or chemotherapy for head and neck tumours (Chen et al., 2010).

Some authors advocate stents only as an interim measure while more definitive management is planned. Potential complications include infections or extrusion or occlusion of the stent, with subsequent cerebrovascular accident (Simental et al., 2003). Carotid artery rupture is also a risk (Kwok et al., 2001). All things

considered, the benefits appear to outweigh the risks (Rimmer et al., 2012).

TAE of the adrenal artery has been reported for controlling gastroduodenal bleeding (Eckstein et al., 1984; Loffroy and Guiu, 2009), and massive retroperitoneal adrenal haemorrhage secondary to lung cancer metastasis (Ambika et al., 2009). Selective intra-arterial terlipressin infusion stopped acute lower gastrointestinal haemorrhage in a patient with abdominal lung cancer mestastases (Favalli et al., 2004). In a retrospective case series of 85 patients undergoing preoperative embolization of tumours or vascular lesions of the head and neck or embolization for refractory tumour bleeding and epistaxis, embolization was achieved in 83.5% of patients (Zahringer et al., 2005). Transhepatic arterioembolization was used to control bleeding in five patients with bleeding from oesophageal varices or direct invasion of the duodenum, transverse colon, or stomach from inoperable hepatocellular cancer (Srivastava et al., 2000) and four patients with spontaneous rupture of hepatocellular carcinoma (Recordare et al., 2002).

Surgery

Palliative surgery to stop severe haemorrhaging may be appropriate in select cases. Surgery may range from ligation of a vessel, to fulguration and excision of tissue (Baum et al., 1993). Cystectomies have been successfully performed to control massive intractable bladder haemorrhaging (Choong et al., 2000; Ghahestani and Shakhssalim, 2009; Guven et al., 2011). Laparoscopic cystoprostatectomy and mini-laparotomy ileal conduit diversion were successfully performed in one patient with radiation-induced haemorrhagic cystitis following treatment for prostate cancer (Alkan et al., 2006). Schneider and colleagues performed a segmental duodenal resection with side-to-side duodenojejunostomy in a patient with occult gastrointestinal bleeding due to metastatic endometrial cancer (Schneider et al., 2005). Witz et al. reported three patients with head and neck cancers whose carotid arteries were successfully ligated following acute or imminent carotid artery rupture (Witz et al., 2002). Ligation of a vessel was successful in some patients who presented with bleeding from radiation proctitis (Yegappan et al., 1998). Pulmonary resections to manage massive haemoptysis may be considered in very exceptional situations (Gourin and Garzon, 1974; Jewkes et al., 1983).

Management: systemic modalities

Antifibrinolytic agents

Antifibrinolytic drugs can be useful to control bleeding in patients who are unable to get definitive haemostatic treatment such as irradiation in a previously irradiated field, or patients who are too frail for invasive procedures such as embolization (Prommer, 2005). They are synthetic drugs that stabilize clots by blocking the binding sites of plasminogen, thereby inhibiting the conversion of plasminogen into plasmin. This results in decreased lysis of fibrin clots.

Tranexamic acid (TA) and epsilon aminocaproic acid (EACA) are the two most commonly used antifibrinolytic agents and can be administered orally or intravenously; TA is more potent than EACA *in vitro* and is also a weak direct inhibitor of plasmin.

Antifibrinolytic drugs have been used successfully in a variety of oncological and non-oncological settings (Biggs et al., 1976; Chandra, 1978) to assist in controlling bleeding in thrombocytopenic patients (Garewal and Durie, 1985; Kalmadi et al., 2006), DIC (Cooper et al., 1992), lung cancer (Kaufman and Wise, 1993), mesothelioma (De Boer et al., 1991), gastric cancer (Roberts et al., 2010), and leukaemia (Avvisati et al., 1989; Shpilberg et al., 1995).

In the palliative care setting, Dean and Tuffin found that cessation of bleeding occurred in 14 out of 16 cancer patients treated with TA for a variety of bleeding problems, including haematuria, haemoptysis, and bleeding from fungating tumours and the rectum (Dean and Tuffin, 1997). The average time until significant improvement in bleeding was 2 days and for complete cessation was 4 days.

Doses of tranexamic acid were 1.5 g followed by 1 g three times a day. Aminocaproic acid was dosed at a 5 g load followed by 1 g four times a day. Treatment was continued for another 7 days after the bleeding stopped. Others have recommended similar doses (Twycross and Wilcock, 2014a). If ineffective after 3 days, the dose of TA can be increased to 1.5–2 g three times a day, with a maximum dose of 2 g four times a day. The suggested intravenous dose of TA is 10 mg/kg over 5–10 minutes. The intravenous route is generally reserved for patients who are unable to swallow oral medications. Treatment can be restarted if bleeding resumes. For EACA, a stat dose of 5 g orally (or 4–5 g intravenously in 250 mL of 0.9% saline for 8 hours or until the bleeding stops) is recommended, followed by daily doses of 5–30 g orally or intravenously in divided doses at 4–6-hour intervals, with a maximum daily dose of 30 g per day orally or intravenously (Twycross and Wilcock, 2014a).

The most common adverse effects are gastrointestinal (nausea, vomiting, and diarrhoea), occurring in about 25% of cases. Adverse effects appear to be dose dependent and thromboembolism is uncommon (Hashimoto et al., 1994). EACA and TA are excreted mainly unchanged in the urine. Doses therefore need to be reduced in renal impairment. It is generally recommended that these drugs not be used in DIC. Caution is advised in the case of haematuria as there is a risk of clot formation causing ureteric obstruction or urinary retention (Twycross and Wilcock, 2014a).

In patients with thrombocytopenic haemorrhage, 66% achieved a complete response and 17% a partial response with EACA treatment (Kalmadi et al., 2006). The median initial dose was 4 g per day and the median dose during the whole course of treatment was 6 g per day (range, 2–24 g per day). Aminocaproic acid was successfully used to manage upper gastrointestinal bleeding in a patient with metastatic gastric cancer who wished to avoid invasive procedures (Roberts et al., 2010) Benefits have also been reported with TA in managing bleeding during treatment of acute myeloid leukaemia (Shpilberg et al., 1995).

Somatostatin analogues (octreotide)

Octreotide, an analogue of somatostatin, has been used to manage upper gastrointestinal bleeds, including peptic ulcers, and oesophageal varices (Lin et al., 1995; D'Amico et al., 2003). It has also been used perioperatively to reduce bleeding in pancreatic cancer resections (Halloran et al., 2002). Somatostatin reduces splanchnic flow and pressure by causing venous dilatation, thereby reducing portal pressure and portal venous flow. A starting dose of 50–100 micrograms subcutaneously or intravenously twice daily is recommended (Lamberts et al., 1996). The dose may be titrated, up to 600 micrograms per day if needed. An alternative regimen of

a bolus of 50 micrograms given intravenously or subcutaneously, followed by a continuous subcutaneous or intravenous infusion of 50 micrograms/hour for 48 hours, has been suggested (Burroughs et al., 1990). Few side effects are reported at low doses but nausea, abdominal discomfort, and diarrhoea may occur with doses greater than 100 micrograms/hour.

Vasopressin analogues

Vasopressin is a posterior pituitary hormone that causes splanchnic arteriolar constriction and reduction in portal pressure (Octavio and Buizza, 1989). The vasopressin analogue 1-desamino-8-D-arginine vasopressin (desmopressin, DDAVP) is the treatment of choice for patients with von Willebrand disease and mild haemophilia A. The compound has also proved useful for the treatment of patients with other inherited or acquired haemostasis disorders. It has been used in the management of variceal bleeding related to portal hypertension (Gross et al., 2001; D'Amico et al., 2003).

In cancer care, a small pilot study evaluated the use of vasopressin for the management of bleeding in patients with various haematological malignancies and thrombocytopenia (Castaman et al., 1997). All the patients responded to a single infusion of desmopressin (0.4 micrograms/kg) diluted in 100 mL of isotonic saline and infused over 30 minutes; no toxicities were reported. Vasopressin therapy, given in doses of 0.1–0.4 mg by continuous infusion, stopped bleeding in about half of patients with stomach cancer (Prommer 2005). Terlipressin (triglycyl lysine-vasopressin), a long-acting vasopressin analogue, was used to control acute, severe lower gastrointestinal bleeding in a patient with gastric metastases from a lung primary (Favalli et al., 2004). Selective angiography was used to administer the drug into the middle colic artery.

Aerosolized vasopressin has been reported in the management of mild to moderate recurrent haemoptysis in palliative patients (Anwar et al., 2005). Five units (1 mL) of ornithine-8-vasopressin, diluted in 1 or 2 mL of physiological saline solution and administered in aerosol, as needed, was used.

Vitamin K

Vitamin K (phytonadione) is fat soluble and is necessary for the hepatic production of a number of clotting factors, including factors II (prothrombin), VII, IX, and X. Liver disease, decreased intake, small bowel disease or resection, and biliary obstruction can lead to deficiencies in these factors. Vitamin K is indicated in the management of bleeding from oral anticoagulants, liver disease, and DIC.

Oral administration of vitamin K is the preferred route (Whitling et al., 1998). Although its onset of action is slower than the intravenous route, it is more reliable than the intravenous and subcutaneous routes. Serious allergic reactions are more frequent with intravenous administration (Riegert-Johnson and Volcheck, 2002); 1.9% of patients (Shields et al., 2001). The onset of action of the intravenous route is as soon as 4 hours. Intravenous administration should be slow, not exceeding 1 mg per minute. Oral vitamin K lowers INR levels more rapidly than subcutaneous vitamin K in patients with excessive oral anticoagulation (Crowther et al., 2002). For most situations, the oral route will result in reliable results with an onset of action within 12 hours (Whitling et al., 1998).

A number of regimens have been recommended for managing INR levels. For non-bleeding patients with elevated INRs less than 5, warfarin can simply be omitted or the dose lowered. A study comparing 2.5 mg oral vitamin K versus omission alone in 30 asymptomatic patients with INR levels of 6–10 found that treatment with oral vitamin K (accompanied by holding further warfarin dosing) reduced the time to achieve a normal INR by a day (Patel et al., 2000). Other studies found similar results (Fondevila et al., 2001).

For INRs in the 5–10 range, the next doses of warfarin should be held and 1–2.5 mg of vitamin K given orally (DeLoughery, 2009). For INRs greater than 10, 2.5–5 mg of vitamin K should be given with the expectation that the INR will be lowered in 24–48 hours (DeLoughery, 2009).

If the patient requires rapid full reversal because of bleeding or the need for surgery when the INR is high, intravenous vitamin K and fresh frozen plasma (FFP) should be considered (DeLoughery, 2009). Note that one unit of plasma raises, on average, coagulation factors by only 5% therefore large doses (15 mg/kg or 4–5 units) must be given. In the case of intracranial haemorrhage occurring in patients taking warfarin, 10 mg of vitamin K may be given slowly intravenously alongside FFP (Aguilar et al., 2007). Recombinant factor VIIa may be effective in reversing warfarin-induced bleeding in these cases (Aguilar et al., 2007).

Blood and plasma products

Platelets

There appears to be lack of consensus on when to transfuse platelets in patients with advanced disease. Some guidelines suggest prophylactic transfusions triggered by predefined platelet counts (usually $10–20 \times 10^9$/L). Others recommend platelets transfusions only when bleeding occurs or when there are additional risk factors (Schiffer et al., 2001; British Society for Haematology, 2003). Not all thrombocytopenic patients require or benefit from platelet transfusion and the decision to administer transfusion is not based solely on the platelet count but should be individualized for specific clinical settings and patient circumstances (Wandt et al., 2005).

Salacz and colleagues reviewed the management of thrombocytopenia in bone marrow failure (Salacz et al., 2007). They recommend considering prophylaxis with aminocaproic acid (500–1000 mg four times a day) in high-risk patients. If a prophylactic transfusion strategy is appropriate, a platelet count should be taken. If the count is 10×10^9/L or lower, continue with regularly scheduled platelet counts; initially weekly and then up to 3 weeks apart if the patient remains asymptomatic. Consider a platelet transfusion if platelet levels are 5×10^9/L or lower. A higher threshold can be considered if there are coexistent conditions such as coagulopathy or a recent episode of bleeding. If bleeding occurs with counts less than or equal to 10×10^9/L, consider therapeutic transfusions of platelets. If platelet counts are consistently greater than 10×10^9/L, then the patient should be followed clinically without scheduled platelet counts.

Platelet transfusion is rarely needed in patients with increased platelet destruction such as autoimmune or drug-associated immune thrombocytopenia, and is relatively contraindicated in patients with thrombotic thrombocytopenic purpura because of concerns about the risk of precipitating thromboses (Schiffer et al.,

2001). Many patients with chronic, stable, severe thrombocytopenia can be observed without prophylactic transfusion, reserving transfusions for episodes of haemorrhage or during time of active chemotherapy.

A recent Cochrane review concluded that there is no evidence that a prophylactic platelet transfusion policy prevents bleeding; but the review was unable to make a final recommendation regarding prophylactic transfusion versus therapeutic treatment (Estcourt et al, 2012). Risk factors that would sway towards considering prophylactic transfusions when the count was below 10×10^9/L may include sepsis, concurrent antibiotic use, or other haematological disorders.

Although guidelines may vary, it is generally accepted that a count of greater than 50×10^9 /L (or 50,000/μL) is sufficient for most invasive procedures and surgeries. Platelet counts of greater than 100×10^9 /L (> 100,000/μL) are recommended for ophthalmic and neurosurgery. Higher transfusion thresholds may be appropriate for patients with platelet dysfunction.

Transfused platelets have a short life span and will need to be re-dosed within 3–4 days if given for prophylaxis. Suboptimal increases can be seen due to non-immune destruction or immune refractoriness. Clinicians should suspect immune-mediated refractoriness to platelet transfusions if post-transfusion increases are minimal. This can be confirmed by screening for the presence of lymphocytotoxic (anti-HLA) antibodies. Patients with autoimmune destruction of platelets, such as ITP, may not receive therapeutic benefit from prophylactic transfusion, but may however benefit from therapeutic transfusions.

Severe thrombocytopenia presents many difficult management choices at the end of life and may pose an ethical dilemma in some situations. The use of platelet transfusions in this patient population presents complex issues; platelets are logistically more difficult to transfuse than red cells and carry risks including acute febrile episodes, alloimmunization, and infection. Platelet transfusion in the setting of advanced cancer should be on a case-by-case basis with the aim of controlling symptoms. The short half-life of platelets limits the usefulness of platelet transfusions in patients with end-stage disease. Moreover, the half-life decreases as the platelet count drops. Indications for the transfusion of platelets in patients with advanced haematological malignancies have been recommended (Lassauniere et al., 1996) and include (a) continuous bleeding of the mouth and gums, (b) overt haemorrhage (gastrointestinal tract, gynaecological, urinary), (c) extensive and painful hematoma, (d) recent disturbed vision (in the setting of thrombocytopenia), (e) severe and recent headache (in the setting of thrombocytopenia), (f) severe anaemia (and thrombocytopenia). Detailed reviews of the management of blood dyscrasias in patients with cancer (DeLoughery, 2009) and terminally ill patients with haematological malignancies (Salacz et al., 2007; Gertz 2009) are reported elsewhere.

Fresh frozen plasma

Generally, haemostasis can be achieved when the activity of coagulation factors is at least 25–30% of normal, assuming the absence of inhibitors (including heparin) and the presence of adequate fibrinogen levels (> 100 mg/dL) (Prommer, 2005). FFP contains all the plasma clotting factors and is the most commonly used plasma product to correct severe clotting factor deficiencies in urgent situations, particularly coagulopathies that are attributable to multiple clotting factor deficiency states as in liver disease, DIC, or warfarin anticoagulation. It is used to prevent bleeding prior to an urgent invasive procedure (e.g. thoracentesis) in patients requiring replacement of multiple coagulation factors, including patients over-coagulated with warfarin. Usually, there is an increase of at least 1.5 times the normal prothrombin time or partial thromboplastin time, or an INR of 1.6 or above before clinically important factor deficiency exists. This corresponds to factor levels lower than 30% of normal.

The volume of each unit is usually 200–250 mL. A dose of about 15 mL/kg (10–20 mL/kg) of FFP is usually recommended and translates to about 4 units (about 800 mL). (American Society of Anesthesiologists Task Force, 1996). This is expected to increase factor levels by 20–30% and fibrinogen levels by about 1 g/L. Volume overload may be a risk in some patients. The frequency of the transfusion depends on the half-life of the deficient factor(s). However, coagulation screening tests may be poor predictors of coagulation factor levels.

Reversal of warfarin anticoagulation with plasma is indicated only if significant bleeding or risk is present. Often it will require recurrent transfusion to maintain normal factor levels. Otherwise, reversal can be achieved by giving vitamin K or holding warfarin 2–3 days prior to a planned procedure. Recombinant or factor VIII concentrates should be used to replace factor VIII. FFP should not be used for haemophilia B (factor IX) deficiency unless factor IX concentrate is not available.

Cryoprecipitate

Cryoprecipitate is a concentrated blood component made by thawing FFP between 1°C and 6°C. Each unit (usually 10–15 mL) contains a minimum of 80 IU of factor VIII (stabilizes fibrin) and at least 150 mg of fibrinogen, in addition to significant amounts of von Willebrand factor (promotes platelet adhesion), factor XIII, and fibronectin. It is primarily used to treat patients bleeding as a result of reduced levels of fibrinogen activity (functional defects or deficiency in amount). Better treatments are now available for von Willebrand disease, haemophilia A and B, and factor XIII deficiency.

Cryoprecipitate is indicated in association with bleeding or prior to an invasive procedure when the following are present: (a) hypofibrinogenaemia due to reduced synthesis (severe liver disease), consumption (e.g. DIC), dilution following massive transfusions, or inherited deficiency; (b) von Willebrand disease when desmopressin (DDAVP) is ineffective or contraindicated and von Willebrand factor-containing concentrates are not immediately available; (c) haemophilia A when factor VIII concentrate is not immediately available; (d) factor XIII deficiency; and (e) uraemia with bleeding if the patient is unresponsive to other treatments such as dialysis, and DDAVP. For fibrinogen replacement, 2 units of cryoprecipitate per 10 kg of body weight generally raise fibrinogen concentration by 100 mg/dL, except in cases of DIC or continued bleeding with massive transfusion. Treatment should therefore be based on clinical status with a goal of achieving and maintaining a fibrinogen concentration of 100 mg/dL.

Recombinant coagulation factors (VIIa, VIII, IX)

Several recombinant factors are now available, including recombinant factors VIII, IX and VIIa.

Recombinant factor VIIa (rFVIIa) is currently approved for use in haemophilia patients with inhibitors. It has apparent value in a variety of other situations, including massive bleeding resulting from massive trauma and bleeding from liver disease (Kenet et al., 1999; Roberts et al., 2004; Dutton et al., 2011), but its role in these settings is controversial. Recombinant factor VIIa has been reported to have value in a variety of disorders involving thrombocytopenia (Goodnough, 2004) and/or platelet dysfunction, including benefit for patients who are refractory to platelet transfusions (Vidarsson and Onundarson, 2000). A recent meta-analysis concluded that treatment with high doses of rFVIIa in off-label indications may significantly increase the risk of arterial but not venous thromboembolic events, especially among the elderly (Levi et al., 2010). A multicenter, placebo controlled trial of rFVIIa in cirrhotic patients with gastrointestinal haemorrhage failed to show a beneficial effect of rFVIIa over standard therapy (Bosch et al., 2004). However, post hoc analysis showed a subpopulation in which it could be useful, namely Child–Pugh B and C cirrhotic patients.

Hyperbaric oxygen therapy

Hyperbaric oxygen is thought to promote granulation tissue and neovascularization and to cause vasoconstriction, which decreases haemorrhaging. Case series have reported response rates of up to 85% from hyperbaric oxygen therapy for patients with bleeding from radiation- or chemotherapy-induced cystitis (Schoenrock and Cianci, 1986; Weiss et al., 1994; Bevers et al., 1995; Del Pizzo et al., 1998; Corman et al., 2003; Bratsas et al., 2004). The downside of this treatment is that it requires multiple treatments (up to 20 sessions), each lasting 90 minutes. Contraindications include active cancer, active viral infection, pneumothorax, treatment with doxorubicin or cisplatin, and ear reconstruction.

Other modalities (pentosanpolysulphate, melatonin, thalidomide)

Oral sodium pentosanpolysulphate has been reported in a small case series to control chronic haematuria secondary to pelvic irradiation (Parsons, 1986; Toren and Norman, 2005). The therapy consisted of 100 mg of oral sodium pentosanpolysulphate three times per day; the average time to control bleeding was 4–7 weeks of therapy. Precisely how sodium pentosanpolysulphate controls haematuria is unknown, but it is postulated to increase the natural defence of the bladder–urine interface by coating the lining of the bladder. Oral sodium pentosanpolysulphate has no detectable anticoagulant activity, is safe, and not toxic

Recent pilot studies suggest that melatonin (MLT) may ameliorate thrombocytopenia in patients being treated for cancer (Lissoni et al., 1995; Lissoni et al., 1999). Similar benefits have been reported in cases with refractory idiopathic thrombocytopenic purpura (Todisco and Rossi, 2002; Todisco et al., 2003). Recommended dosage is 20 mg/day (orally) during the dark period of the day. One study suggested a greater decrease in the frequency of thrombocytopenia and lymphocytopenia in patients treated with MLT than in those who received supportive care alone (Lissoni, 2002).

Thalidomide, given its antiangiogenic properties, has been reported in a palliative patient who experienced severe upper gastrointestinal bleeding secondary to gastric cancer (Lambert and Ward, 2009). Bleeding settled within 1 week of starting 300 mg of thalidomide nocte.

Specific clinical scenarios in palliative care

Management of terminal haemorrhaging

The options for managing terminal haemorrhage can be divided into three categories (Harris and Noble, 2009): (1) general supportive measures such as the use of dark towels and staying with and comforting the patient; (2) general resuscitative measures such as fluid replacement; and (3) specific measures to stop the bleeding such as wound packing, haemostatic agents, haemostatic radiotherapy, and interventional radiology.

Sedative medications to alleviate patient distress and provide comfort are often recommended (MacMillan and Struthers, 1987; Regnard and Makin, 1992; Fortunato and Ridge, 1995; Gagnon et al., 1998; Oneschuk, 1998; Prommer, 2005; Frawley and Begley, 2006a). It is important to note that the intent is to relieve distress and not to hasten death. Midazolam is the most frequently recommended drug because of its rapid onset and short duration of action (Oneschuk, 1998). The commonly recommended routes are intravenous or subcutaneously, at doses of between 2.5 and 10 mg. Some guidelines suggest a repeat dose within 5–10 minutes if necessary. The intramuscular route has been suggested but bioavailability of this route may be compromised by peripheral circulation shutdown during hypovolemic shock

Harris and colleagues recently explored the utility of crisis medication in the management of terminal haemorrhage by interviewing 11 nurses who had managed such events (Harris et al., 2011). Participants reported crisis medication (such as midazolam) to have little role in many cases. Terminal haemorrhage often occurred rapidly, with the majority of patients dying before medications could be administered. Many events had not been predicted and so anticipatory prescribing of crisis medications did not always occur. A focus on accessing crisis medicines was done to the detriment of staying with and supporting the patient and using dark-coloured towels, which were reported to be the most useful measures. The researchers stressed that crisis medications, although generally not useful, may be of benefit in some situations, specifically those in which bleeding occurs over several hours.

Harris and Noble (2009) and Regnard and Makin (1992) have published guidelines in this area.

Bleeding oesophageal varices

Current therapies and recommendations for the management of oesophageal and gastric variceal haemorrhage from advanced liver disease are published elsewhere (Garcia-Tsao et al., 2007). A meta-analysis recommends pharmacological management (vasopressin, nitroglycerin, terlipressin, somatostatin, or octreotide) over endoscopic sclerotherapy as first-line treatment of variceal bleeding (D'Amico et al., 2003). The use of beta blockers is not recommended during acute episodes of bleeding.

When endoscopy is used, variceal ligation appears to be generally preferred over sclerotherapy (Garcia-Pagan and Bosch, 2005; Garcia-Tsao et al., 2007). A meta-analysis showed superiority of endoscopic (sclerotherapy or variceal ligation) plus pharmacological (octreotide, somatostatin, vapreotide) therapy over endoscopic therapy alone (Banares et al., 2002). Despite urgent endoscopic and/or pharmacological therapy, variceal bleeding cannot be controlled or recurs early in about 10–20% of patients (Banares et al., 2002). Shunt therapy, either shunt surgery or transjugular intrahepatic portosystemic shunt (TIPS), has proven clinical efficacy as salvage therapy for patients who fail to respond to endoscopic or pharmacological therapy (Sanyal et al., 1996).

Balloon tamponade is effective in controlling bleeding temporarily with immediate control of haemorrhage in over 80% of patients (Avgerinos and Armonis, 1994). However, its use is associated with potentially lethal complications such as aspiration and necrosis and perforation of the oesophagus. Therefore, it should be restricted to patients with uncontrollable bleeding for whom a more definitive therapy such as TIPS is planned within 24 hours.

Haemorrhagic bladder

Three reviews of the topic provide a comprehensive review of the management of intractable bladder haemorrhaging in cancer care (Choong et al., 2000; Ghahestani and Shakhssalim, 2009; Guven et al., 2011) (see also Chapter 8.4). They highlight considerable variation in practices and recommendations.

Ghahestani and Shakhssalim propose alum instillations or radiotherapy, after irrigation and evacuation of blood clots, as first-line options. In the case of a sloughing tumour as aetiology, internal iliac artery embolization is a second-line option, while hyperbaric oxygenation and embolization or transurethral fulguration are second-line options in the case of radiation cystitis. Formalin, because of significant adverse effects, is relegated to a last-resort option. Guven et al. also suggest intravesical irrigation with alum, EACA or silver nitrate as first-line options, followed by hyperbaric oxygen in the case of haemorrhagic cystitis or radiation cystitis and arterial embolization, with formalin irrigations and surgery as last-resort options (Guven et al., 2011).

Guven et al. suggest that the first step in the treatment of haemorrhagic cystitis should be directed towards making sure that the bladder does not become overly distended. Bladder outlet obstruction from clots can lead to urosepsis, bladder rupture, and renal failure. Clot evacuation can be performed at the bedside by carefully placing a large, stiff-walled haematuria catheter. After clot evacuation, if haematuria persists, a three-way catheter can be inserted and continuous bladder irrigation with saline can be started. All clots must be removed before continuous irrigation is started to avoid over distention and bladder rupture. The patient should be vigorously hydrated using oral and/or intravenous fluids to keep clots from reforming. If clot evacuation is unsuccessful with this approach, the patient should undergo cystoscopy with clot evacuation and consideration of treatments previously described, including fulguration and instillation/injection of agents.

A variety of approaches have been reported. These include instillation of astringents and other agents (including alum, silver nitrate, formalin, prostaglandin F_2, EACA, phenol), intravesical hydrostatic pressure treatment with fluid instillation or compression balloons (but there is a risk for bladder rupture) (Antonsen et al., 1986; Choong et al., 2000), hyperbaric oxygen therapy, transarterial embolization, and surgery as last-resort options (ranging from percutaneous nephrostomy diversion (Pomer et al., 1983; Sneiders and Pryor, 1993) to cystectomy (Zebic et al., 2005; Fergany et al., 2009).

Last-resort options include urinary diversion (prevents urine urokinase from coming into contact with the fragile haemorrhagic mucosa) and radical cystectomy (Zebic et al., 2005; Alkan et al., 2006).

Malignant wounds

Slow capillary oozing is common in malignant wounds. The use of sucralfate paste or an alginate often suffices (Thomas et al., 1998; Emflorgo, 2014). For heavier bleeding, haemostatic surgical dressings will provide rapid haemostasis and can be left on the wound and covered with an appropriate dressing. A number of other options are available and these are described above and elsewhere (Grocott, 2000; McDonald and Lesage, 2006).

Conclusion

Bleeding in the palliative care setting may have a variety of causes and clinical presentations. It is often complicated by a number of co-morbidities and underlying pathologies. It is often very distressing to patients, families, and caregivers. A large number of treatment modalities, local and systemic, are available to address bleeding and massive haemorrhages. The large majority of evidence in support of these modalities, however, is based on case reports, case series, and expert opinion, with only a small number of large randomized studies. Selecting between the different modalities is therefore seldom guided by comparative studies between the modalities. A number of factors need to be considered when selecting between modalities and the overall care approach. These include patient prognosis and expected survival, access to modalities, quality of life, functional status, and ultimately goals of care and patient wishes.

Online materials

Complete references for this chapter are available online at <http://www.oxfordmedicine.com>.

References

Achneck, H.E., Sileshi, B., Jamiolkowski, R.M., Albala, D.M., Shapiro, M.L., and Lawson, J.H. (2010). A comprehensive review of topical hemostatic agents: efficacy and recommendations for use. *Annals of Surgery*, 251(2), 217–228.

Anwar, D., Schaad, N., and Mazzocato, C. (2005). Aerosolized vasopressin is a safe and effective treatment for mild to moderate recurrent hemoptysis in palliative care patients. *Journal of Pain and Symptom Management*, 29(5), 427–429.

Dean, A. and Tuffin, P. (1997). Fibrinolytic inhibitors for cancer-associated bleeding problems. *Journal of Pain and Symptom Management*, 13(1), 20–24.

Gagnon, B., Mancini, I., Pereira, J., and Bruera, E. 1998). Palliative management of bleeding events in advanced cancer patients. *Journal of Palliative Care*, 14(4), 50–54.

Grocott, P. (2000). The palliative management of fungating malignant wounds. *Journal of Wound Care*, 9(1), 4–9.

Harris, D.G., Finlay, I.G., Flowers, S., and Noble, S.I. (2011). The use of crisis medication in the management of terminal haemorrhage due to incurable cancer: a qualitative study. *Palliative Medicine*, 25(7), 691–700.

Harris, D.G. and Noble, S.I. (2009). Management of terminal hemorrhage in patients with advanced cancer: a systematic literature review. *Journal of Pain and Symptom Management*, 38(6), 913–927.

Kakimoto, M., Tokita, H., Okamura, T., and Yoshino, K. (2010). A chemical hemostatic technique for bleeding from malignant wounds. *Journal of Palliative Medicine*, 13(1), 11–13.

Lagman, R., Walsh, D., and Day, K. (2002). Oxidized cellulose dressings for persistent bleeding from a superficial malignant tumor. *American Journal of Hospice and Palliative Medicine*, 19(6), 417–418.

Maida, V., Ennis, M., Kuziemsky, C., and Trozzolo, L. (2009). Symptoms associated with malignant wounds: a prospective case series. *Journal of Pain and Symptom Management*, 37(2), 206–211.

McDonald, A. and Lesage, P. (2006). Palliative management of pressure ulcers and malignant wounds in patients with advanced illness. *Journal of Palliative Medicine*, 9(2), 285–295.

Mercadante, S., Barresi, L., Casuccio, A., and Fulfaro, F. (2000). Gastrointestinal bleeding in advanced cancer patients. *Journal of Pain and Symptom Management*, 19(3), 160–162.

Pereira, J. and Phan, T. (2004). Management of bleeding in patients with advanced cancer. *Oncologist*, 9(5), 561–570.

Prommer, E. (2005). Management of bleeding in the terminally ill patient. *Hematology*, 10(3), 167–175.

Regnard, C. and Makin, W. (1992). Management of bleeding in advanced cancer—a flow diagram. *Palliative Medicine*, 6(1), 74–78.

Sexual dysfunction: discussing patient sexuality and intimacy in palliative care

Amanda Hordern

Introduction to sexual dysfunction

Experiencing a life-limiting illness has the potential to radically transform every aspect of a person's life, including how they feel about themselves, their body, and their sense of self within intimate and sexual relationships. For many terminally ill people, intimate and sexual moments are a vital aspect of their life, providing a sense of connectedness and assisting the person to explore and find meaning to living, dying, and death (Rothenberg and Dupras, 2010). Entering the palliative phase of any disease frequently results in a reappraisal of life priorities and relationships in the remainder of life. This has the potential to directly impact the manner in which a person connects at the deepest level with a significant other, at a time when chronic and debilitating illness may precipitate a longing for intimate touch and communication. Sexual expression through all of life, but particularly during end-of-life phases, provides a vital form of communication, reassurance, tenderness, and validation of self when grappling with the vulnerability of changing health and wellness (Lemieux et al., 2004; Shell, 2008; Redelman, 2010; Gianotten and Hordern, 2011; Vitrano et al., 2011). Gianotten challenges health professionals to consider that sexual and intimate moments provide a welcome respite and distraction from all that is going as death approaches (Gianotten, 2007). Yet few health professionals view patients in their care as sexual beings and if they do, they struggle to know what and how to raise the topic of sexuality and intimacy within their clinical roles (Hordern and Street, 2007a, 2007b; Gianotten and Hordern, 2011). The following chapter will:

- define patient sexuality and intimacy in the context of palliative care

- explore the impact of natural ageing and treatment for cancer and chronic illnesses

- provide an introduction to opening communication and providing practical strategies to support the patient through intimate and sexual changes.

What is sexuality and intimacy?

Sexuality and intimacy are lived experiences that mean different things to different people, at different stages of their lives. There has been a reassuring shift in recent cancer and palliative care literature from a traditional, medicalized, and functional focus on patient sexuality, where the emphasis has remained on rates of penetration and orgasmic responses, strength of erections, libido, and menopausal status (Schover, 2005; Miles et al., 2007; Potter, 2007; Ochsenkuhn et al., 2011) to a more person-centred definition of sexuality, where psychological aspects of sexual identity have been described more extensively (Manne et al., 2007; Manne and Badr, 2009; Manne et al., 2010; Cleary and Hegarty, 2011). A particularly poignant definition is 'sexuality is the process of giving and receiving sexual pleasure and is closely connected to a sense of being. Sexuality is a feeling of belonging, of being accepted by another, and the conviction that we are worthy to live and enjoy life' (Shell, 2008).

Intimacy has been defined as the 'sharing of identity, closeness, and reciprocal rapport' (Mercadante et al., 2010), where the emphasis is usually on emotional closeness and intimate communication rather than sexual function. When viewed in this context, a patient's sexuality and intimacy have the potential to be altered and redefined, at every stage of life-limiting illness.

Health benefits of sexual and intimate expression

Sexuality and intimacy can reduce emotional distress, anxiety, stress, and depression (Redeleman, 2010) and improve psychosocial responses to living with a cancer diagnosis (Sadovsky et al., 2010). Gianotten and Hordern (2011) outline a comprehensive list of the benefits including the following:

- Pain-relieving effects of sexual expression that is enjoyable.

- A distraction from the day-to-day challenges.

- Evidence to support a heightened pain threshold. Muscle relaxation following sexual stimulation and orgasm can reduce muscular tension for many hours, having a positive effect on inducing sleep. The same authors discuss the release of oxytocin after skin contact, body massage and sexual intercourse which has been associated with increased levels of trust and intimacy between couples as well as lower anxiety and fewer depressive symptoms.

The impact of a life-limiting illness on a person's sexual and intimate world

Despite increasing emphasis on patient sexuality in the general cancer and cancer survivorship literature, patient and carer sexuality in the context of palliative care has only recently been receiving attention (Lemieux et al., 2004; Hordern, 2008; Anderson, 2009; Gianotten and Hordern, 2011).

Lemieux et al. (2004) conducted seminal work exploring the patient's perspective of sexuality in palliative care and highlighted that sexuality remained an important aspect of patients' lives even until the last weeks and days of the person's life. Nine out of the ten participants interviewed for this study reiterated the importance of being given an opportunity to discuss intimate and sexual changes with a health professional, yet only one had been given the opportunity. Lemieux suggested that the focus of sexuality changed from an emphasis on intercourse before the disease, to an emphasis on longing to be touched through hand, body, kissing, hugging, and 'meaningful' eye contact as the disease advanced. These findings support the earlier work of Anath and colleagues (2003) who used a cross-sectional, survey to find that sexual function was more affected in palliative care patients than in the other control group of patients from a general practice clinic.

Rothenberg and Dupras (2010) used the Kübler-Ross five-stage of death theory to explore the impact of impending death on the sexual and intimate world of palliative care patients. Drawing upon qualitative data obtained through a small number of clinical interviews, this discussion paper illuminates the range of sexual issues emerging for people during the final phases of their lives. Case studies were used to highlight how the phases of denial, anger, bargaining, depression, and acceptance all impacted sexual and intimate expression. This work revealed the relationship between health professionals validating the topic by opening a discussion and dying patients being able to actively shape their final intimate and sexual connections, enabling patients to find meaning in their last weeks and days.

As difficult and rare as it is to quantify sexuality and intimacy in the face of advanced disease, Vitrano et al. (2011) explored the attitudes and feelings of people with advanced cancer to sexual and intimate practices before and after their diagnosis. Of the 65 male and female respondents, most respondents (86%) felt it was important to be offered the opportunity to discuss changes to sexuality with trained professionals and half (47%) of the respondents felt sexuality was very important for psychological well-being.

While the study did not explore the rate of discussions patients had with their health-care professionals, it was interesting to note that 60% of the patients in this study did not feel less attractive than prior to their diagnosis; however, only 30% respondents felt satisfied with their sexual activity compared to 67% feeling satisfied with their sexual activity prior to the diagnosis. Whilst the reasons for these findings were not explicated in the study, one could assume that if people facing these issues were provided with an opportunity to explore the challenges, and receive practical and evidence-based solutions, then satisfaction rates may have increased.

Assessing the need

Drawing upon findings from research into cancer and sexuality, it becomes apparent that even when a cancer diagnosis directly impacts body parts traditionally associated with sexual expression, such as breasts, prostate, and genital organs, patients are rarely given an opportunity to engage in meaningful discussions with health professionals about how to cope with these changes. A study highlighted this when a sexual well-being for people with breast cancer survey was conducted by Ussher et al. (2011). Out of 2210 respondents, 1956 women (88.5%) reported changes to their sexual well-being, including emotional consequences, physical changes, changes to self and femininity, and reconciliation of self to changes. By contrast, only 25% of respondents had discussed sexual well-being with a health professional, despite high levels of distress associated with sexual changes. Furthermore, over half of the sample of 1907 participants who responded to the question 'Have you obtained information about breast cancer and sexual well-being?' said no (n = 1117). These results reveal a gulf between patient expectation and experience, with unmet needs emerging from an area of cancer care that is well resourced (breast cancer) and could raise the profile of sexuality. The likelihood of these findings being far more exaggerated in cancer and palliative care areas which have not received the same research focus as breast cancer would be highly likely. This has been confirmed by Low et al. (2009), who stated that sexuality is ill-defined and under-reported in people experiencing head and neck cancer. In a qualitative study exploring the effects of lung cancer on physical and emotional intimacy for 13 married couples, most patients and spouses perceived sexuality and intimacy were still important to them since the lung cancer diagnosis yet very few respondents had discussed this with a health professional (Tessler Lindau et al., 2011).

The partner's perspective

The partners' perspectives of experiencing end-of-life issues have rarely been described in the palliative care literature. An Australian study has shed light on the intimate and sexual disruptions experienced by carers who are partners of people with cancer (Gilbert et al., 2010). When Gilbert and colleagues interviewed 20 participants who were partners across a range of cancer types, stages, and age groups, they found that all partners reported a decrease in levels of sexual expression and frequency of intercourse. The authors highlighted the experience of some partners who were unable to negotiate other forms of intimacy when penetration was no longer an option. They also described a group of participants who managed to successfully 'renegotiate' their sexual experiences of sex, drawing on mutual masturbation, self-masturbation, manual stimulation, oral sex, use of massage and vibrators as alternate forms of sexual expression, bringing couples closer together (Gilbert et al., 2010). This study also highlighted the importance of couple communication, where poorer communication decreased both relationship and sexual satisfaction. When couples found it difficult to communicate about their own sexual needs and concerns, a cycle increasing distance occurred between the partners causing isolation, fear, and distress. Due to the lack of research into the impact of sexuality and intimacy on the partner in non-cancer-related areas of palliative care, one can assume that these findings are transferable to other life-limiting diseases.

Health professionals can play an important role in assisting both the patient and their partner to communicate about the impact of advanced disease on intimacy and sexuality (Cort et al., 2004; Manne and Badr, 2009; Street et al., 2009; Manne et al., 2010).

Barriers and challenges of discussing patient sexuality in the clinical setting

Despite the integral role human sexuality and intimacy plays across a person's entire life, patient sexuality and intimate needs are rarely addressed in clinical care, let alone in the cancer and palliative care setting (Manne et al., 2010; Ussher et al., 2011).The challenges faced by health-care professionals who 'don't know where to begin' in raising the topic of patient sexuality have been discussed throughout the literature. Hordern and Street (2007b, 2007d) explored issues of intimacy and sexuality in cancer and palliative care, through a lens of reflexivity, enabling them to critically examine the structures, rules, and ideas that traditionally shape and influence patients' and health professionals' interactions. This was done through in-depth interviews with 32 health professionals representing a multidisciplinary team, a critical review of the literature, and a contextual analysis of 33 national and international cancer and palliative care clinical practice guidelines. The majority of health professionals did not see their patients as sexual beings, avoiding the topic, feeling vulnerable to the reactions of patients and colleagues, and rarely taking the risk of venturing into such a taboo topic with patients in their care. If sexuality were ever raised, it was done from the safety of a medicalized perspective, where sexuality could be reduced to measuring erectile function, menopausal status, or levels of libido and the emphasis on the communication remained at the level of 'fighting the cancer' (Hordern and Street, 2007b). Unchecked assumptions about the patient's sexuality were frequently made on the patient's behalf, based on the person's age, gender, stage of disease, culture, and partnership status (Hordern and Street, 2007c).

The same researchers also interviewed 50 patients across a range of ages, cancer types, and stages (who were increasingly armed with information downloaded from the Internet). People wanted to play an active role in decision-making. The patients wanted information and support about how to live with and manage the side effects of treatment that was impacting their sexual and intimate worlds, how others cope, and the choices they could make to regain sexual confidence until the end of life. Hordern and Street suggested that these mismatched expectations between patient and health professionals could be overcome by health professionals reflecting upon and recognizing the personal and professional influences that shape their beliefs about patient sexuality and checking their assumptions with the patients in their care (Hordern and Street, 2007b, 2007d).With the dearth of research into the area of communicating about patient sexuality in the non-cancer palliative care context, one can assume that the key barriers and challenges in the communication process are transferable to other advanced and terminal disease states.

Whose role is it to raise the topic?

Although patients' sexuality has been recognized as an important aspect impacting quality of life in clinical practice guidelines for psychosocial care of people with cancer (National Cancer Institute / National Breast and Ovarian Cancer Centre) and in National Consensus Project for Quality Palliative Care (2004), little guidance has been offered on best practice approaches to discussing patient sexuality and intimacy in clinical care. Cagle and Bolte (2009) propose that multidisciplinary teams are required to delegate a team member who will address issues of intimacy and sexuality, taking an advocacy role in ensuring patient-centred sexuality discussions occur. These authors suggest social workers are well equipped to conduct discussions and take on patient-centred roles within teams. Similarly, de Vocht et al. (2011) proposes that a team approach with clearly defined roles and referral pathways for different team members is required to ensure patient sexuality is on the agenda. These authors propose that all team members have a responsibility to be 'spotters' for identifying sexuality and intimacy issues in the palliative care context, and that designated 'skilled companions' within the team take on the more in-depth advocacy and coordinated method of patient-centred communication about these issues as they emerge. De Vocht et al. (2011) propose that the skilled companions are primarily well-educated nurses who show an interest in this area of health care. Other authors suggest that that as long as the communication is patient-centred, well documented, and that the patient feels well supported with information and practical strategies, then the type of health professional providing this level of communication is irrelevant (Hordern and Street, 2007a; Woodhouse and Baldwin, 2008; Hawkins et al., 2009). Cort et al. emphasize that it is the openness of the health professional committed to incorporating patient sexuality and intimacy into routine health care that results in growing confidence in the required communication skills to achieve this. Health professionals do not require specialist training in sexuality to achieve patient-centred outcomes and patients want links to their regular team rather than to a separate sexual counsellor (Cort et al., 2004). Hordern et al. (2009) propose that a brief communication skills training model for clinicians has the potential to reduce perceived barriers and increase confidence and frequency of discussing the topic of sexuality in the clinical setting.

Normal ageing processes for women

Irrespective of health and disease status, men and women experience changes to sexual function as a result of natural ageing processes. For example, in natural menopause the vaginal tissue becomes drier, thinner, and more fragile. There is a reduced amount of natural lubrication and a shortening in the length and width of the vagina (Hickey et al., 2008). There are also physical changes to the labia, which shrink in size, exposing the clitoris, so that some of the sensitivity and involuntary contractions after orgasm are altered (Gianotten, 2007). Experiencing pain related to a dry vagina and a decrease in the intensity and speed of a sexual response may result in a loss of libido. The frequency of these symptoms varies among women and is less marked with regular intercourse (Quinn, 2007). Women also may experience mood changes, night sweats, fatigue, and changes to their body shape as they age (Hickey et al., 2008). These issues do not equate to women becoming asexual but do raise challenges for older women who may choose to embark on new relationships or to explore their sexual identity from a non-reproductive focus.

Normal ageing processes for men

As a man experiences physiological changes related to ageing, he is more likely to increase the time required to achieve an erection. Changes may include the erection being less rigid for extended periods without ejaculation and the amount of seminal fluid decreases

(Corona et al., 2010). A man's orgasmic strength and pleasure may also lessen throughout the ageing process (Gianotten, 2007; Corona et al., 2010), and older men may experience a decrease in the size and firmness of the testes and a change in testicular elevation (Shell and Smith, 1994). Erectile dysfunction has also been attributed to many common drugs including some medications for hypertension or depression, interferon-based therapies, excessive alcohol consumption, and cigarette smoking (Corona et al., 2010).

With so many predisposing factors relating to erectile dysfunction, it is important for health professionals to assess accurately and differentiate between physical and psychological causes of erectile dysfunction and loss of libido. With adequate support and information, many men who are unable to experience an erection are able to explore more flexible forms of intimacy with a partner such as massage, hugging, oral sex, and sexual responses to fantasies produced without physical touch (Gilbert et al., 2010). Therefore it is important to emphasize to men that they do not need an erection to experience orgasm, ejaculate, or feel intimately and sexually connected to their partner.

Impact of cancer treatment and chronic illness on sexuality

Facing advanced cancer, living extended periods with chronic and debilitating disease and entering the palliative phase of illness inevitably brings a range of physical and emotional responses to the person, and their carers, and families. People frequently say they are 'on an emotional and physical roller coaster ride' as they face changes that have the potential to transform how they view themselves as a man or a woman. Many medical conditions such as cancer, hyper- and hypo-tension, diabetes, renal failure, depression, stroke, multiple sclerosis, and Parkinson's disease have all been associated with changes to sexual function in men and women (Wylie and Kenney, 2010). Irrespective of age or partnership status, chronic illness, fatigue, depression, anxiety, surgery, living with uncertainty, or just feeling unwell, can cause a person to look at their body differently and make them more sensitive to the reactions of partners, other family members, and friends. When these issues are combined with fatigue, dyspnoea, incontinence, disfigurement, pain, nausea and vomiting, weight changes, fluid retention, xerostomia, and other forms of alteration to body image, it is difficult to overstate the enormity of the impact on a person's overall body image and confidence (Hordern, 2012).

Understanding the impact of previous cancer treatment on a person's sexuality can provide a deeper understanding and insight into the complex loss, change, and grief associated with a person's altered sexuality and intimacy in the palliative care setting. Even when non-genital or non-sexual areas of a person's body have been affected by surgery or disease, a person's intimate and sexual world has the potential to be altered. Catheters, colostomy bags, subcutaneous medicines, syringe drivers, intravenous poles, and enteral feeding tubes can become intrusive to intimate moments such as holding hands, cuddling, and kissing. For highly detailed information about the sexual ramifications of a broad range of cancer types and treatment see Sadovsky et al. (2010).

Impact of chemotherapy

Treatment-induced infertility may result from chemotherapy, radiotherapy, and hormone treatment (Su et al., 2008; Stovall and McGee, 2010). The effects of chemotherapy on reproductive capacity depend on the age, sex, and chemotherapy regimen (treatment dose, cycles, and time between treatments). The impact of radiotherapy on fertility is determined by the location and size of the radiation field, the total dose, and dose intensity. Thus the residual effect of therapy on the reproductive capacity of both men and women is complex and individually determined, ranging from little or no effects to prolonged and permanent sterility (Otkay and Meirow, 2007). It is important that options for preserving fertility are routinely discussed with patients prior to commencement of fertility compromising treatment and due to the complexity and individual variation it is advised that these discussions take place with reproductive specialists (Su et al., 2008; Stovall and McGee, 2010).

Women are often anxious and seek practical advice on managing the symptoms of treatment induced menopause such as vaginal dryness, atrophy, reduced libido, and hot flushes (Leyden Wiggens and Dizon, 2008). In premature menopause, the vaginal mucosa will remain thin and fragile and therefore easily irritated by intercourse, resulting in dyspareunia. Dyspareunia combined with treatment-induced vaginal dryness can inevitably lead women to avoid sexual intimacy of any type, for fear it will lead to painful intercourse and moderate to severe vaginal discomfort for women (Su et al., 2008; Stovall and McGee, 2010). This also has the potential to impact the quality of life for women in day-to-day activities like wearing jeans, sitting in trousers for long periods of time, and experiencing routine medical examinations. Experiencing these vaginal symptoms for extended periods can become debilitating to women, irrespective of age, disease, or relationship status. For practical advice on managing these side effects, refer to the 'Vaginal moisturizers, lubricants, and topical oestrogen' section later in this chapter.

Chemotherapy can also reduce circulating androgens. In both men and menstruating women, androgens act in the body to promote sexual desire and arousability (Hickey et al., 2008) so that men and women may experience changes in mood, energy, and libido as a result of their treatment. Hormonal manipulation, particularly in treatment for metastatic prostate and breast cancer, can also reduce circulating androgens (Couper, 2007; Hickey et al., 2008). Patients claim that these physical and psychological symptoms may persist for months or years after completion of treatment yet there is a paucity of literature around the length of time that people may experience reduced libido and arousal and evidence-based approaches to managing these side effects of treatment (Ochsenkuhn et al., 2011).

Safe sex while undergoing chemotherapy

Cytotoxic waste can be excreted through any blood and body fluid during chemotherapy, hence the need for partner protection in the first 48 hours after completion of the chemotherapy (Cancer Council Victoria, 2012a). Surprisingly little research has been done in this area of partner protection after cytotoxic therapy; however, general advice can be offered to people undergoing chemotherapy (including oral regimens) to wear a condom for sexual intercourse or use a dental dam for oral sex (Schover, 2008). Dental dams are approximately A4-sized latex that can be purchased from sex shops (not dentists!), in a variety of colours and flavours and protect the partner's mouth from sexually transmitted infections and cytotoxic irritation. Similarly a condom or a dental dam should be used to cover sex toys like vibrators and dildos which require washing after each use.

Side effects of radiotherapy

Radiotherapy and women

Sexuality can also be affected by radiotherapy—side effects of treatment include fatigue, nausea, diarrhoea, and skin reactions. All have the potential to affect the way people feel about themselves. Pelvic and intracavity radiation can result in vaginal tissue becoming thinner, ulcerated, and scarred, making sexual intercourse very painful. Vascular damage to the pelvic or vaginal areas results in a reduced blood flow to the area, often leading to the vagina being less lubricated and less dilated (Quinn, 2007). In severe cases, the scarring and vaginal atrophy can be so marked that the vagina shortens and shrinks in width, making it difficult or impossible for the woman to have sexual intercourse. During treatment a woman can be encouraged to have sexual intercourse, or use a vaginal vibrator or dilator three or four times a week to reduce the chances of her vagina shrinking (Quinn, 2007).

Radiotherapy and men

Radiotherapy to the testes and total body irradiation in men as part of stem cell transplant can also result in men becoming permanently infertile (Stovall and McGee, 2010). Vascular insufficiency caused by pelvic or testicular irradiation may result in erectile dysfunction (Shell and Smith, 1994). A spinal cord lesion may affect the nerve centres that control erectile function and neurologic erectile dysfunction can be induced by damage to the prostatic nerve plexus during radical pelvic surgery. Erectile dysfunction rates for both radiotherapy and surgery (including robotic) after prostate cancer are similar, despite the belief that some prostate treatment is more successful than others (Barry et al., 2012; Cooperberg et al., 2012). More research is required to determine whether the long-term benefits of high-frequency ultrasound will reduce incidence or severity of erectile dysfunction experienced by men as a result of their cancer treatment (Barry et al., 2012; Cooperberg et al., 2012).

Myths and misconceptions

Many myths and misconceptions exist about being 'radioactive' following radiotherapy. Couples fear having sexual intercourse during radiotherapy for fear of transmitting radiation from one person to the other. Other people ask if it is safe to cuddle and kiss, hold beloved grandchildren, or even sit in the same car or lie in the same bed while having radiotherapy. It is important for health professionals to explain to patients and carers that external beam radiation does not leave the body radioactive; nor do radiation implants once they are removed from the body (Cancer Council Victoria, 2012b). While temporary internal radiation implants are in place, guidelines recommend that patients avoid all close contact with people, especially children under 18 years of age and pregnant women. Visitors are advised to sit approximately 2 metres from the bed and remain in the hospital room only 30 minutes each day (American Cancer Society, 2011). Once the temporary implant is removed, sexual and intimate contact is considered safe for the partner. People with permanent implants (using lower radiation) are advised to avoid close contact with people for the first few days while the radiation is most active and then to use condoms for several days post procedure (American Cancer Society, 2011; Cancer Council Victoria, 2012b).

Addressing the sexual and intimate needs of hidden communities in palliative care

Heterosexual norms

People who deviate from heterosexual norms of society (Rondahl et al., 2006), young adolescents, and the elderly all share some form of discrimination when it comes to health professionals avoiding or failing to discuss patient sexuality in a palliative care context (Redelman, 2010). Same-sex, bisexual, transsexual, and transgender populations enter a health-care system that not only fails to view patients as sexual beings, but does little to encourage open and honest discussions about the impact a life-limiting diagnosis may have on minority groups who are often hidden from view and feel too vulnerable to have a voice, in a system where homophobia and heterosexism is prevalent (Rondahl et al., 2006; Hyde, 2007). Added to that, any attempt to explore the impact a cancer diagnosis or chronic illness has on intimate and sexual relationships is almost always considered and discussed through the lens of a heterosexual health system (Hordern and Street, 2007b, 2997c), where dominant heterosexual assumptions hinder free expressions of sexuality for all minority groups (De Santis and Vasquez, 2010; Redelman, 2010). Non-heterosexual relationships can vary from heterosexual relationships in terms of communication, conflict negotiation, and connectedness (Gilbert et al., 2009) so that discrimination against non-heterosexual minority groups can result in profound loss of identity and isolation (Hordern and Currow, 2003). The resultant grief, pain, and suffering become deep sadness, particularly in the face of a life-limiting illness (Redelman, 2010). Health professionals play a vital role in recognizing not only the assumptions they bring to practice but also the structures and influences which can positively or negatively impact and shape a person's ability to embrace intimacy and sexuality. Irrespective of the sexual orientation of the clinician, this must be part of practice so that sexuality is viewed as 'life affirming way of achieving intimacy and human contact' (Gilbert et al., 2009, p. 537).

Young adolescents

Similarly, the unique sexual and intimate needs of adolescents and young adults who face end-of-life issues have been largely ignored (Zebrack, 2011). For example, what has been identified is that when a person experiences a cancer diagnosis as an adolescent or young adult it has direct ramifications on their ability to develop a positive self-esteem, body image, sexual identity, reproductive capacity, communication with peers, and confidence associated with entering the dating world. Parental and health-care dependency, confronting mortality at such a young age, and experiencing late effects and ongoing palliative care issues make this another priority area for health professionals to increase their understanding of, and willingness to, communicate about patient sexuality and intimacy (Schover, 1997; Thaler DeMers, 2001).

Single people facing chronic illness

Similarly, the impact of experiencing life-limiting illness as a single person and for those entering new relationships, irrespective of how poor the prognosis, is another area that requires attention in the palliative care arena. Issues such as a desire to seek or engage in a new sexual relationship are challenging for patients who are in a palliative phase of their disease. Lack of confidence can be compounded by changes to body image, scars, leaking orifices and odours (Lawton, 1998, 2000), fears of being rejected, and lack of uninterrupted time and energy (Shell, 2008). Yet remarkably, the majority of palliative care clinicians can vividly recall patients who have formalized relationships with wedding ceremonies around a hospice bed, or participated in symbolic ceremonies that recognized and validated significant relationships involving a patient with very advanced disease and their (relatively new) partner.

Ageist assumptions

Similar discrimination is felt by the elderly whose sexual identity is written off and discounted as soon as they age (Hordern and Street, 2007b, 2007d; Shell, 2008). It has been refreshing to note that researchers, particularly from the fields of palliative care have been embracing opportunities to explore how people engage in many forms of sexuality as a form of intimate expression and communication, particularly when grappling with cognitive, physical, and life-limiting changes associated with ageing (Cort et al., 2004; Mercadante et al., 2010). Discussing sexuality late in the course of a life-limiting disease could be perceived as distasteful, an enduring taboo, or breaching social norms. Yet sexual expression can also be life affirming, an antidote for pain and misery, and provide a deep connection to another—which is important to most of humankind irrespective of the age, sexual orientation or disability (Gianotten, 2007; Cagle and Bolte, 2009; Gianotten and Hordern, 2011). When illness is incurable, there are social rules and norms about what is acceptable pre- and post-death and each individual has a unique opportunity to seek comfort in a relationship or shying away from such new adventures, depending on the individual need (Cort et al., 2004; Rothenberg and Dupra, 2010; Ussher et al., 2011).

Similarly, opening communication about life and new relationships after the death of a partner warrants discussion as part of regular palliative care follow-up (Cort et al., 2004). Complex and varying emotions are enmeshed in the phases of loss and grief post death of a partner and while some shy away from new relationships, others seek comfort from the sexual release and physical contact of a new lover (Gianotten, 2007). Social etiquette and cultural 'rules' vary about the length of time required after the death of a partner before pursuing new intimate and sexual experiences (Cort et al., 2004). Importantly however, a study has found that couples who communicated more frequently about how the man would cope physically and emotionally after a wife's death to cancer resulted in less guilt and potentially better psychological health 6 months after the death than men who did not have such discussions with their wives (Miao Jonasson et al., 2011). Although the authors do not make the link, one could suggest that reduced feelings of guilt and better psychological health would be more conclusive to better sexual and intimate health after death and bereavement of the partner.

Not surprisingly, patients frequently report that even though they feel it is a health professional's responsibility to raise the topic, health professionals rarely do (Hawkins et al., 2009). Discussions about the impact of an advanced life-limiting illness on intimate and sexual aspects of a person's life and the provision of information relating to physical, psychological, and relationship changes after a diagnosis, remain an unmet need (Stead et al., 2001, 2007; Canada et al., 2005; Ussher et al., 2011).

Opening the communication

If sexuality and intimacy are raised as an important and valid part of patient assessment in the palliative care setting, practical solutions to many issues can be offered to the patient and their partners, so that treasured moments of meaningful and intimate connections can occur until the moment of death. Unless the topic is raised by a health professional, people are likely to suffer in silence, as sexual and intimate relationships decline. Offering opportunities to discuss intimate and sexual ramifications of a life-limiting illness demonstrates that a health professional regards this as a legitimate and important topic that is open for discussion along the whole illness trajectory (Katz, 2009; Sadovsky et al., 2010).

Recognizing the barriers and assumptions in health professional communication

Few health professionals feel comfortable or confident raising the topic of patient sexuality in palliative care settings (Hordern and Street, 2007b, 2007d), yet people affected by progressive life-limiting illnesses often search for ways to deal with altered self-perception and body image, negotiating relationships with partners or the desire for practical ways to adjust to living with sexual and intimate changes after alterations to health. In general terms, the majority of patients search for how other people cope in similar situations, what is 'normal', and ways to adapt to many of the side effects of treatment that impact upon their sexual and intimate world (Hordern and Street, 2007b, 2007c).

Health professionals' attitudes and barriers that prevent conversations about patient intimacy and sexuality include:

◆ lack of time

◆ the belief that the patient is too ill or not interested in sex

◆ belief that disfigured bodies are not sexually attractive

◆ fear of opening a 'Pandora's box'

◆ transgressing medico-legal boundaries

◆ the presence of third parties at the consult (Sunquist and Yee 2003).

Barriers to discussions about patient sexuality in the context of cancer may also arise because health professionals believe their conversations may be construed as disrespectful and inappropriate by the patient, where gender, age, disease, partnership status, culture, socioeconomic factors, and religion all contribute to health professionals' avoidance of the topic (Sunquist and Yee, 2003; Hordern and Street, 2007d).

Health professionals often worry about what their patients or colleagues would think of them if they raised the topic of sexuality and intimacy in the clinical setting, particularly when they have little sexual experience themselves or struggle to communicate about such difficult topics in their personal lives (Hordern and Street, 2007a, 2007b, 2007c, 2007d). Reflecting on personal definitions of sexuality and intimacy and how this may impact on feelings of discomfort, embarrassment, or awkwardness when raising the topic of patient sexuality is a good starting place.

Recognizing one's own comfort zone is vital for effective, open, and patient-centred communication, and this will improve with practice and experience. Validating the importance of the topic, ensuring confidentiality, and moving from a less sensitive to more sensitive topics are all vital elements in open communication about sexuality. Few patients will actually bring up the subject of sexuality unless the health professional caring for them provides permission by raising the topic as part of routine health assessment. Conversation starters may be as follows:

◆ Many people who have undergone this kind of treatment tell me they experience sexual or intimate changes. How has this been for you?

◆ How has your sexual confidence changed since . . . ?

◆ How has all of this made you feel about yourself as a man/a woman?

◆ How do you think this treatment has affected the way you feel about yourself or your relationship with your partner?

◆ Now let's focus on the more intimate changes you may have experienced since this all began.

◆ It is also important for me to support you through the personal side of this management plan. Let's spend some time exploring some of the sexual and intimate issues you may have been facing . . .

◆ Sometimes a person's body image changes with this illness . . .

Health professionals who continue to feel uncomfortable about discussing sexuality with patients should, with the patient's permission, arrange referral to another health professional and document this in the patient's history. With adequate information, support, and training, health professionals can become aware of their assumptions and barriers, and increase their confidence and frequency in discussing sexuality and intimacy with patients in their care (Hordern et al., 2009).

Dispelling myths and clarifying beliefs

Health professionals often make assumptions about a person's knowledge and understanding of human anatomy and how their body works, without checking baseline knowledge and beliefs. This may result in the patient or their partner failing to really understand the whole conversation (Katz, 2005). Furthermore, many people subscribe to the myths that sexual activity can spread the cancer to the partner, or that any sexual activity can cause cancer (Katz, 2005), make the cancer or life-limiting disease worse, or negate the benefits of treatment. It is not uncommon for patients to express beliefs that past actions such as extramarital affairs, abortions, illegitimate children, and other 'sins of the past' have contributed to their ill health (Kishore et al., 2007).

Strategies for helping people help themselves

Patients want practical strategies and approaches to engaging in sensual body touch, communicating more openly about sex with their partners that will result in increasing expressions of affection, and more sensual aspects of intimacy (Canada et al., 2005). Validating sexuality and intimacy in the context of palliative care legitimizes the notion that sexuality can be impacted but not destroyed by life-limiting illness and people need permission to divert attention and energy to their body image, rather than solely focusing on the illness (Shell, 2008). Discussing the extensive range of vaginal moisturizers and lubricants that are available is a helpful way to support men and women through managing the side effects of natural ageing processes and reducing side effects of medical treatments.

Vaginal moisturizers, lubricants, and topical oestrogen

Differentiating lubricants from vaginal moisturizers and topical oestrogen is a good place to begin the conversation as there are important differences in their formulas and instructions for use (Leyden Wiggens and Dizon, 2008; Carter et al., 2011). Vaginal moisturizers are a helpful way to optimize hydration of the vaginal mucosa and relieve some of the symptoms associated with atrophy, yet little clinical research has been published in this area. Replens® (<http://www.replens.com.au/>) is an example of a vaginal moisturizer containing purified water, glycerine, mineral oil, hydrogenated palm oil, and sorbic acid, and in two small studies has been shown to offer a non-hormonal alternative for the management of vaginal dryness and irritation, as well as providing vaginal comfort when used three times a week to daily use (Leyden Wiggens and Dizon, 2008; Carter et al., 2011).

Regular use of lubrication to the genital areas can promote awareness of new erotic zones, changes in foreplay patterns, and validation that exploring intimacy, sensuality, and sexuality (no matter what stage of illness) is good for the mind and body. Lubricants can also prevent genital irritation, abrasions, and vaginal tears (Carter et al., 2011). Water- or silicon-based lubricants that are oestrogen free (for oestrogen-dependent cancers) and do not contain perfumes or colourings can be purchased at a pharmacy and suit many people. Both silicon- and water-based lubricants can be broken down with warm soapy water, and generally, silicon-based lubricants last longer but may be more expensive. However, some water-based lubricants do contain glycerine, increasing the risk of yeast infections (such as *Candida albicans*) as do oil-based lubricants. There are many options available and it is advisable to encourage patients to try different options until they find one that suits them. It is best to instruct patients to apply the lubrication to their genital areas and to their partner's (if applicable) prior to any manual caressing, intercourse, or use of vibrators.

Vaginal oestrogen

Lowered oestrogen levels as a result of natural ageing or treatment-induced menopause, is associated with vaginal pain and dryness, which has the potential to negatively impact sexual function and enjoyment (Carter et al., 2011). Topical or systemic oestrogen therapy is an effective treatment for managing vaginal symptoms; however, the whole issue of hormone replacement therapy is complex and controversial. Carter et al. (2011) provide a comprehensive review of benefits, risks, and knowledge to date, as do Hickey et al. (2008).

Managing a range of common side effects

Many of the palliative care population experience dyspnoea, pain, degenerative muscle weakness, fatigue, nausea and vomiting, incontinence, and xerostomia, all of which have the potential to negatively impact sexual function and confidence. Table 8.8.1 provides some practical approaches to managing these symptoms, to enhance sexual and intimate expression (Shell, 2008).

Table 8.8.1 Approaches to managing physical issues impacting sexual function

Pain	◆ Pain management—as pain negatively impacts libido and sexual performance
	◆ Dyspareunia due to vaginal dryness from radiation therapy, chemotherapy, or hormone therapy. Vaginal moisturizer Replens® (<http://www.replens.com.au/>), lubricating products such Pjur® water-based/silicon-based products (<http://www.pjur.com/>), and SYLK® (<http://www.sylk.co.uk/>) may be helpful
Dyspnoea	◆ Medical assessment and management of the dyspnoea
	◆ Practical measures include a well-ventilated room with fan and comfortable bed (consider water bed)
	◆ Encourage patient to explore gentle intimacy with partner (gentle hugging, hand holding, soft caressing, or light massage with oils or creams). Use water bed to conserve energy
	◆ During sex, control shortness of breath with pursed-lip breathing. Take extra pillows and covers off the bed to create open sensation. Avoid long kisses on the mouth to take away fear of 'not getting enough air'. Avoid positions that restrict breathing or put pressure on the chest (Shell, 2008)
Fatigue and weakness	◆ Set aside a time of the day when patient feels most energy and encourage them to set the scene; phone on answer machine, nap first, ensure privacy and light candles, play music, burn oils to create intimate atmosphere with self or partner
	◆ Explore different positions to conserve energy. A warm bath together, lying on side, explore oral and mutual masturbation options for self and/or partner
	◆ Avoid extreme temperature, heavy meals, and alcohol
Nausea and vomiting	◆ Medical assessment and antiemetic regimen
	◆ Avoid use of oils, perfumes, and deodorants
	◆ Explore gentle sensuality as above
Xerostomia	◆ Education on regular oral hygiene
	◆ Artificial saliva (consider Moi-Stir® <http://www.kingswood-labs.com/>, Optimoist® spray, Saliva Substitute® liquid and Xero–Lube® Artificial Saliva sodium-free spray
	◆ Saliva stimulants: over-the-counter (OTC) saliva stimulants include Natrol Dry Mouth Relief® lozenges may be dissolved in the mouth three times daily
	◆ Pilocarpine tablets: Salagen® stimulates the salivary glands to produce saliva
Incontinence	◆ Encourage use of bath and shower as places for foreplay and post-coital relaxation
	◆ Utilize shower chair, disabled baths, fluffy towels over an incontinent sheet for intimate foreplay and sexual contact

Source: data from *Seminars in Oncology Nursing*, Volume 24, Issue 2, Sexual issues in the palliative care population, pp. 131–134, Copyright © 2008 Elsevier Inc. All rights reserved.

Providing privacy in the clinical setting

Many situations arise in the clinical setting through lack of privacy, which is created at an architectural level in most institutions. How can we offer people the privacy they have had throughout their lives when there are no locks on doors, only a flimsy curtain shields semi-private rooms, and only single beds are provided? There is also a general acceptance that health professionals have the right to 'barge' into any room at any time of day or night to 'attend' to a patient, irrespective of whether the door is closed or a visitor is present.

Placing 'do not disturb' signs on patients' doors when people request some privacy, knocking before entry, and announcing arrival prior to sweeping back curtains all create a respectful environment. Some palliative care organizations have ensured there is at least one double bed in the setting, which patients and their partners can use, to create intimate and private shared moments. Incorporating the topic of patient sexuality and intimacy into the routine assessment of patients entering the clinical setting invites an open discussion about what needs to be put into place to ensure privacy and respect for intimate and sexual expression up until the moment of death. Partners may wish to bathe the patient or to have the opportunity to shower or bathe together. Couples may find comfort knowing they can intimately hold one another in bed, nap, or sleep together with the certainty that they will not be disturbed by health professionals for negotiated periods of time through the day. If designated sensuality areas (private rooms with double beds, massage oils, access to music, satin sheets, boas, etc.) are actively promoted by health professionals, inpatients will feel they legitimately have an opportunity to be intimate with themselves or their partner for as long as they are able or desire. Similarly, community-based palliative care can encourage the hiring of double hospital beds and embrace intimate sensual moments to legitimize the need for people to remain connected with others until they die.

Having realistic expectations

When people have faced considerable changes to their physical and emotional health it is common for them to fear any form of intimacy that will be painful or 'may make things worse'. Patients frequently wonder: 'Is my partner still attracted to me?' 'Will everything be able to work as it did?' 'How can I bear to look at my body?' 'How do other people cope with these changes?' 'Will I ever feel interested in sex again?' 'Will I ever find a new partner after all I have been through and all that lies ahead?' Relearning to love a changed body, have sexual confidence, and explore new techniques and expressions of intimacy that suit the stage of the disease require changes to ways of expressing intimacy, past foreplay patterns, or sexual positions, and takes time. Advise patients and their partners that first attempts may be disappointing but that with time and patience, people can relearn the feeling of sexual pleasure and intimate connection until they die.

Coping with physical disfigurement

Some people are happy to be naked with their partner despite physical disfigurement. Others are not. Some women wear soft lacy camisoles or night wear to conceal the scars of surgery. Others use the power of fantasy to imagine themselves as 'whole' people with two breasts or without a syringe driver or colostomy bag. Many men have spoken about the confidence they feel in taking the time to dress up for sex, with vests and cummerbunds to conceal scars and altered body parts. Granting patients permission to explore these options is usually the most crucial step in the communication process and having access to a private room as an inpatient offers a remarkable step forward in acknowledging the intimate and sexual needs of the palliative care community.

Setting the scene

Encouraging patients to set a 'date' with themselves and or their partner validates the importance of promoting intimacy and sexuality throughout all phases of care. Creating a relaxed and comfortable environment to explore sensual and intimate moments can be achieved by encouraging patients to block out times of the day when they experience energy, allowing the phone to divert to an answering machine, setting the scene with candles, soft lighting, and favourite music. Encouraging patients to dress up into clothing that makes them feel more sensually confident, showering or bathing alone or with a partner, using soft fluffy towels on the bedding to absorb any incontinence, and exploring their body to find out what feels satisfying, are the type of practical strategies patients often search for. Taking the pressure off intercourse and encouraging people to rebuild intimate and sensual enjoyment takes time, practise, and a willingness to try new things.

Pelvic floor muscle control and self-stimulation

There is increasing evidence that teaching muscle awareness and control can enhance sexual function, increase blood flow to the clitoris and penile area, and enhance sexual arousal in men and women (Carter et al. 2011). Self-stimulation using masturbation is not only viewed by sex therapists as a normal activity, it is used as a form of therapy for the majority of sexual changes that arise from chronic illness and significant life changes. Making this an 'okay' topic by suggesting to people that they may like to 'have a try yourself', can set the scene for undisturbed sexual and intimate exploration after physical and emotional changes arising from illness. If individuals no longer know what and how they like to be touched, it would be difficult for them to convey this to a partner and this type of sensual self-exploration may give them the confidence to review and potentially alter previous sexual patterns and habits. Along with pelvic floor awareness, self-stimulation using lubrication with digital or oral exploration, with or without a vibrator, can enhance sexual response rates, increase arousal, confidence, and have broader health benefits (Cass, 2004; Gianotten and Hordern, 2011).

Conclusion

In conclusion, the more comfortable you feel about your own sexuality the more likely you will be to respond to and address issues relating to the sexual and intimate worlds of patients in your care. If you have given patients permission to discuss their sexuality with you there is a good chance that they will bring up issues when they feel ready to address them. Every person has a different comfort zone, and recognizing the barriers and assumptions brought to clinical practice is a good place to begin. Raising the topic, validating sexual and intimate changes in the context of palliative care, and offering practical strategies have the potential to legitimize intimate and sexual expression until the moment of death.

Online materials

Complete references for this chapter are available online at <http://www.oxfordmedicine.com>.

References

Anath, H., Jones, L., King, M., and Tookman, A. (2003). The impact of cancer on sexual function: a controlled study. *Palliative Medicine*, 17, 202–205.

Cagle, J. and Bolte, S. (2009). Sexuality and life-threatening illness: implications for social work and palliative care. *Health & Social Work*, 34(3), 223–233.

Carter, J., Goldfrank, D., and Schover, L.R. (2011). Simple strategies for vaginal health promotion in cancer survivors. *Journal of Sexual Medicine*, 8(2), 549–559.

Cass, V. (2004). *The Elusive Orgasm*. Bentley, WA: Brightfire Press.

Cort, E., Monroe, B., and Oliviere, D. (2004). Couples in palliative care. *Sexual and Relationship Therapy*, 19(3), 337–354.

De Vocht, H., Hordern, A., Notter, J., and van de Wiel, H. (2011). Stepped skills: a team approach towards communicating about intimacy in cancer and palliative care. *Australian Medical Journal*, 4(11), 610–619.

Gianotten, W. (2007). Sexuality in the palliative-terminal phase of cancer. *Sexologies*, 16, 299–303.

Gianotten, W. and Hordern, A. (2011). Sexual health in the terminally ill. In J.P. Mulhall, L. Incrocci, I. Goldstein, and R. Rosen (eds.) *Cancer and Sexual Health*, pp. 577–587. New York: Springer.

Gilbert, E., Ussher, J., and Hawkins, Y. (2009). Accounts of disruptions to sexuality following cancer from the perspective of informal carers who are partners of a person with cancer. *Health: An Interdisciplinary Journal*, 13(5), 523–541.

Gilbert, E., Ussher, J., and Perz, J. (2010). Renegotiating sexuality and intimacy in the context of cancer: the experience of carers. *Archives of Sexual Behavior*, 39, 998–1009.

Hawkins, Y., Ussher, J., Gilbert, E., *et al.* (2009). Changes in sexuality and intimacy after the diagnosis and treatment of cancer. *Cancer Nursing*, 32(4), 271–280.

Hickey, M., Saunders, C., Partridge, A., Santoro, N., Joffe, H., and Stearns, V. (2008). Practical guidelines for assessing and managing menopausal symptoms after breast cancer. *Annals of Oncology*, 19, 1669–1680.

Hordern, A. (2008). Intimacy and sexuality after cancer: a critical review of the literature. *Cancer Nursing*, 31(2), E9–E 17.

Hordern, A. (2012). Sexuality and intimacy in palliative care. In M. O'Connor, S. Lee, and S. Aranda (eds.) *Palliative Care Nursing: A Guide to Practice*, pp. 236–254. Melbourne: Ausmed Publications.

Hordern, A. and Currow, D. (2003). A patient-centred approach to sexuality in the face of life-limiting illness. *The Medical Journal of Australia*, 179(6), s8–s11.

Hordern, A., Grainger, M., Hegarty, S., *et al.* (2009). Discussing sexuality in the clinical setting: The impact of a brief training program for oncology health professionals to enhance communication about sexuality. *Asia-Pacific Journal of Clinical Oncology*, 5, 270–277.

Hordern, A. and Street, A. (2007a). Communicating about patient sexuality and intimacy after cancer: mismatched expectations and unmet needs. *Medical Journal Australia*, 186(5), 224–227.

Hordern, A. and Street, A. (2007b). Constructions of sexuality and intimacy after cancer: patient and health professional perspectives. *Social Science & Medicine*, 64(8), 1704–1718.

Hordern, A. and Street, A. (2007c). Issues of intimacy and sexuality in the face of cancer: the patient perspective. *Cancer Nursing*, 30(6), E11–E 18.

Hordern, A. and Street, A. (2007d). Let's talk about sex: risky business for cancer and palliative care clinicians. *Contemporary Nurse*, 27(1), 49–60.

Katz, A. (2009). Interventions for sexuality after pelvic radiation therapy and gynecological cancer. *The Cancer Journal*, 15(1), 45–47

Kishore, J., Ahmed, I., Kaur, R., and Mohanta, P. (2007). Beliefs and perceptions about cancer among patients attending a radiotherapy OPD in Delhi India. *Asia Pacific Journal of Cancer Prevention*, 8, 155–158.

Lemieux, L., Kaiser, S., Pereira, J., and Meadows, L.M. (2004). Sexuality in palliative care: patient perspectives. *Palliative Medicine*, 18, 630–637.

Leyden Wiggens, D. and Dizon, D. (2008). Dyspareunia and vaginal dryness after breast cancer treatment . *Sexual Reproduction and Menopause*, 6(3), 18–22.

Low, C., Fullarton, M., Parkinson, E., O'Brien, K., Jackson, S., Lowe, D., and Rogers, S. (2009). Issues of intimacy and sexual dysfunction following major head and neck treatment. *Oral Oncology*, 45(10), 898–903.

Manne, S. and Badr, H. (2009). Intimacy processes and psychological distress among couples coping with head and neck or lung cancer. *Psycho-Oncology*, 18(7), 735–746.

Mercadante, S., Vitrano, V., and Catania, V. (2010). Sexual issues in early and late stage cancer: a review. *Supportive Care in Cancer*, 18, 659–665.

Miao Jonasson, J., Hauksdottir, A., Nemes, S., *et al.* (2011). Couples' communication before the wife's death to cancer and the widower's feelings of guilt or regret after the loss—a population-based investigation. *European Journal Cancer*, 47(10), 1564–1570.

Otkay, K. and Meirow, D. (2007). Planning for fertility preservation before cancer treatment. *Sexuality, Reproduction & Menopause*, 5(1), 17–22.

Redelman, M. (2010). Is there a place for sexuality in the holistic care of patients in the palliative care phase of life? *American Journal of Hospice and Palliative Medicine*, 25(5), 366–371.

Rothenberg, M. and Dupras, A. (2010). Sexuality of individuals in the end of life stage. *Sexologies*, 19, 147–152.

Sadovsky, R., Basson, R., Krychman, M., *et al.* (2010). Cancer and sexual problems. *Journal of Sexual Medicine*, 7(1 Pt2), 349–373.

Schover, L. (2005). Sexuality and fertility after cancer. *American Society of Haematology*, 2005, 523–527.

Shell, J.A. (2008). Sexual issues in the palliative care population. *Seminars in Oncology Nursing*, 24(2), 131–134.

Shell, J.A. and Smith, C.K. (1994). Sexuality and the older person with cancer. *Oncology Nursing Forum*, 21(3), 553–558.

Sunquist, K. and Yee, L. (2003). Sexuality and body image after cancer. *Australian Family Physician*, 32(1/2), 19–22.

Tessler Lindau, S., Surawska, H., Paice, J., and Baron, S.R. (2011). Communication about sexuality and intimacy in couples affected by lung cancer and their clinical-care providers. *Psycho-Oncology*, 20, 179–185.

Vitrano, V., Catania, V., and Mercadante, S. (2011). Sexuality in patients with advanced cancer: a prospective study in a population admitted to an acute pain relief and palliative care unit. *American Journal of Hospice and Palliative Care*, 28(3), 198–202.

Woodhouse, J. and Baldwin, M. (2008). Dealing sensitively with sexuality in the palliative care context. *British Journal of Community Nursing*, 13(1), 20–25.

Zebrack, B. (2011). Psychological, social and behavioral issues for young adults with cancer. *Cancer*, 117(10 Suppl.), 2280–2294.

SECTION 9

Common symptoms and disorders: pain

Principles of drug therapy: focus on opioids

Ruth Branford, Emily Wighton, and Joy Ross

Introduction to principles of drug therapy: focus on opioids

An understanding of the principles of clinical pharmacology is essential to enable clinicians to prescribe drugs safely and effectively. When prescribing any drug the intention is to gain a therapeutic effect (e.g. the use of opioids to reduce pain), while avoiding harm (e.g. opioid-induced drowsiness). All drugs have the potential to cause side effects, many of which are predictable from knowledge of clinical pharmacology.

Patients with serious or life-threatening illness present challenges to the safe and effective use of medications. Patient-related factors, such as age, gender, and co-morbidities, may influence the choice of drug, starting dose, and route of administration. Most patients receive multiple drugs and clinicians must always be mindful of the risk of drug–drug interactions. Given the risks of polypharmacy in those with advanced illness, options for concurrent non-drug therapy always should be considered. This is certainly important in the case of pain, for which a holistic approach, one that acknowledges that pharmacotherapy is only one strategy among many that may yield favourable outcomes, is often best.

Opioids and other drugs that have the potential for misuse or abuse, addiction, or drug diversion (see Chapter 9.5) are commonly used in palliative care, and these drugs are regulated to a greater or lesser extent in every country. Prescribers may need to make adjustments based on the wider social context implicated in these regulations, and impact of taking medications that may be inconsistently available or arduous to prescribe. In some countries, excessive regulation impedes patient access, particularly in community settings. Clinicians may need to consider whether therapy can be more effectively provided in different care settings (e.g. hospital versus community) or when using specific drugs or formulations, or rates of titration and monitoring. Inclusion of a drug, such as codeine or morphine, on the World Health Organization (WHO) Model List of Essential Medicines (WHO, 2013) increases the likelihood of availability, but does not mean unrestricted access in every country (Junger et al., 2013). Indeed, opioid drugs exemplify the international variation in access that characterizes many types of drugs; some provide their populations with a large number of different opioids and opioid formulations, whereas others fail to ensure access to any. The WHO continues to seek to improve international access to controlled drugs, in particular opioids.

With increasing health-care costs, groups of clinical, pharmacy, and finance professionals are working to promote cost-effective and safer prescribing. In the United Kingdom, efficacy and cost-effectiveness of drugs are assessed at a national level by the National Centre for Health and Care Excellence (NICE). Consideration of cost-effectiveness is now an integral part of the rationale for appropriate prescribing.

Guidelines and formularies

Clinical guidelines are recommendations, based on appraisal of the best available evidence. When evidence is limited or absent, expert opinion is necessary to guide and support best practice. For example, most of the evidence-based guidelines for opioid use in palliative care that have been developed by the European Association of Palliative Care are based on weak evidence (Caraceni et al., 2012). In addition to the development of guidelines by professional societies, national guidances (e.g. NICE (2012) or Scottish Intercollegiate Guidelines Network (2008)) have been developed to help inform local, regional, or hospital-specific practices in a manner that considers local variation in resources and practice. A working knowledge of both international guidelines and national guidances is essential.

Formularies are also a useful resource to guide the prescribing and dispensing of medicines. Many provide detailed information about formulations and doses of drugs. If a formulary is promoted or required in practice, it is important to consider the target audience and the context for any recommendations provided. In palliative care, the most widely recognized formulary is the *Palliative Care Formulary* (Palliativedrugs.com, 2012). This is regularly updated and includes advice about the many drugs that are used off-licence in the palliative care setting. Other generic formularies, such as the *British National Formulary* (BNF), include a much wider selection of medications (Joint Formulary Committee, 2014). The choice of drugs in local or regional formularies is often restricted due to budget constraints.

Efficacy, effectiveness, and cost-effectiveness

Evidence-based medicine (EBM) is centred on the judicious use of current best evidence about the risks and benefits of interventions to inform clinical decision-making. The principles of EBM are discussed in detail in Chapter 19.2. It is important to recognize that the evidence provided by clinical trials evaluates the efficacy of an intervention, such as an opioid, in an ideal/controlled setting. Strict inclusion and exclusion criteria are applied and an enriched or selected sample may be studied, with structured and often short-term follow-up. Conducting high-quality clinical trials in the palliative care setting is especially challenging (Kaasa et al., 2006) and the evidence used to inform prescribing in patients with advanced illness typically originates from studies of relatively healthier populations.

Effectiveness should be distinguished from efficacy. Effectiveness refers to the benefits and burdens of a drug in the wider context, at a population level and as part of everyday practice. Information about efficacy is needed to identify substances that have the potential for clinical benefit; information about effectiveness provides more relevant and actionable information about the likelihood and extent of the therapeutic effect in a given patient.

Cost-effectiveness refers to a comparison of effectiveness for a target indication against cost, that is, the ratio of effectiveness to cost. Clearly, it is more efficient to use the cheaper of two drugs that are equally effective and safe, and this information often informs local guidance.

Therapeutic benefit and risk

From the clinical perspective, the expectation of benefit must be compared to the expectation of risk to determine whether treatment or a change in treatment is justified. Although it can be difficult to estimate the balance between the potential risks and benefits of a particular treatment in an individual case, it is necessary to do so before action is taken.

The likelihood of benefit or risk in the individual is informed by an understanding of likely outcomes in the population overall. Two broad measures that can be useful as part of this assessment are number needed to treat (NNT) and number needed to harm (NNH). The NNT estimates the number of patients that would need to be given a treatment for one of them to achieve a desired outcome (e.g. 50% pain relief). The NNH is calculated for adverse effects in a similar way. Although these measures have been criticized because they are derived from controlled clinical trials data, they nevertheless provide a useful point of comparison among drugs (Christensen and Kristiansen, 2006).

The cut-offs in pain relief or severity of an adverse effect used to calculate the NNT and NNH, respectively, are accepted by convention. In fact, perceived benefit or risk may be strongly influenced by individual variation or therapeutic context. For example, patients with severe pain may feel that a 30% or smaller reduction in pain relief is clinically meaningful. In addition, some patients may be willing to tolerate mild/moderate side effects to achieve a small improvement in pain control if this translates into improved function or quality of life. Knowledge of the patient's drug history in terms of previous success or failures of treatment will also guide choice of drug in prescribing. Prescribers also must always check individual patient factors, such as renal function and known allergies, to further inform assessment of risk/harm and potential for drug interactions.

Information about side effects of a drug must continue to be gathered after the drug is licensed. This is particularly important when a drug is used in the palliative care context, which is usually characterized by patients with advanced illness and the use of multiple drugs adapted for off-licence indications. In these situations, the use of a drug may be associated with a side effect liability quite different than that expected based on clinical trials information.

Principles of clinical pharmacology

Clinical pharmacology is broadly divided into pharmacokinetics ('what the body does to the drug') and pharmacodynamics ('what the drug does to the body'). In palliative medicine, drugs are not often used to cure or modify underlying disease but are predominantly focused on improving symptoms. They often are administered with the intent to continue treatment until death. Knowledge of pharmacokinetic variation, between patients and across time as disease worsens, combined with an understanding of the basic modes of drug action, underpins the logical selection and use of the most appropriate treatment.

Pharmacokinetics

Pharmacokinetics encompasses the *a*bsorption, *d*istribution, *m*etabolism, and *e*xcretion of drugs (ADME). Detailed descriptions of each of these processes are available in pharmacology textbooks. To some extent, inter-individual variation in kinetics is genetically determined. Each process also is influenced by many other factors, however, and in the the palliative care setting, these also contribute to large inter-individual variation and the potential for significant changes across time (Box 9.1.1).

Box 9.1.1 Factors affecting pharmacokinetics

- Age. Both pharmacokinetic and pharmacodynamic factors change at the extremes of age. Metabolism and volume of distribution are often reduced in the elderly leading to increased free drug concentrations in the plasma. Hepatic blood flow may have declined by 40–50% by age 75, with reduced clearance of opioids. Increased central nervous system sensitivity to opioid effects is also found in the elderly.

- Hepatic disease has unpredictable effects. Although there may be little clinical consequence, severe hepatic failure with coexisting encephalopathy can lead to a marked increase in sensitivity to drug effects. Reduction in plasma protein concentration, which occurs with liver failure, will also have an effect on plasma concentrations of free unbound drug.

- Renal failure has a significant impact on drug response. Some of this effect is due to changes in the concentrations of parent drug and metabolites. Some is related to pharmacodynamic changes apparent when drug effects compound the uraemic state. Drugs with active, renally-cleared metabolites, for example, morphine, tend to be more problematic because of metabolite accumulation.

- Obesity results in a larger volume of distribution and prolonged elimination $t_{1/2}$.

- Hypothermia, hyperthermia, hypotension, and hypovolaemia may also result in variable absorption, distribution and metabolism of opioids.

Absorption

At the cellular level, absorption occurs across lipid cell membranes and is a passive process along a concentration gradient. For most drugs, this process takes place in the small intestine. As long as the drug is in solution, has a degree of lipid solubility, and there is sufficient surface area and time for diffusion in the small bowel, then problems should not arise.

A reduced rate of absorption may occur if there is delayed emptying of the stomach. This might arise as part of a pathological process or pharmacological agents that slow gastric motility, such as anticholinergic drugs or opioid analgesics.

Many drugs are now formulated as modified-release preparations, which need to remain in the small bowel for a specified period to achieve the expected absorption profile. In patients with either increased or decreased gastrointestinal transit time, there is a risk that the expected time–action relationship may not materialize. In either case, the prolonged duration or extent of therapeutic effects may be lost.

Bioavailability

Absorption and bioavailability are not the same. The bioavailability of a drug is the percentage of administered drug that gains access unchanged to the systemic circulation. Bioavailability is of most clinical relevance after oral administration. Extensive first-pass hepatic metabolism results in relatively low bioavailability and/or large inter-individual variability for some drugs. For example, the bioavailability of oral morphine is just 35% on average and the range is 15–64%, whereas oxycodone has a bioavailability of 75% and range of 60–87%. The difference in bioavailability complicates the challenge of safe dose selection when changing between oral and parenteral routes and is one of the main reasons that dose titration is essential to identify an effective opioid dose.

Bioavailability can be altered by disease processes that affect hepatic function, or by exposure to drugs that either induce or inhibit enzymes of the cytochrome P450 (CYP450) system. In patients with chronic liver disease, for example, blood may be 'shunted' from portal to systemic vessels; this bypasses hepatic enzymes, reduces the first-pass effect, and increases bioavailability. These changes in hepatic function may have a profound effect on drug levels after oral administration but relatively little effect when the drug is given parenterally.

Distribution

The volume of distribution (V_d) is a theoretical volume in which the total amount of drug would need to be uniformly distributed to achieve the blood concentration. For very lipophilic drugs which are taken up into fat stores or muscle, such as fentanyl, the volume may be many times body size.

The V_d is important as a determinant of half-life ($t_{1/2}$) and is also of theoretical importance in the calculation of the loading dose of a drug where one is needed. Changes caused by disease, such as cachexia or renal failure, may shift a drug's concentration–time relationships. Other related processes with potentially profound effects on drug kinetics or dynamics also may occur as a result of alteration in body composition or physicochemical environment. For example, all opioids are weak bases and dissociate into free-base and ionized fractions when dissolved in solution. The ionized form is active at the receptor site, whereas the free-base form is more lipid soluble. The relative proportions of ionized and unionized drug are dependent on pH and pK_a, and may change with the effects of disease.

All opioids also bind to plasma proteins, such as albumin and glycoproteins, in varying degrees. Opioid molecules which are unbound and unionized are capable of diffusing to the site of action, the proportion of which is known as the diffusible fraction. The concentration of the diffusible fraction and other factors such as lipid solubility determine the speed of onset of the drug. The diffusible fraction of a drug may change with hypoalbuminaemia associated with advanced illness.

A high lipid solubility facilitates diffusion across the blood–brain barrier into the brain and therefore is associated with a rapid onset of action. However this view is simplistic in that it is the ionized form that is active at opioid receptor. Speed of onset is therefore better represented as a complex function of both lipid solubility and percentage of the drug that ionized at physiological pH. Morphine has a high diffusible fraction but low lipid solubility which results in a slow onset of action. Alfentanil, however, has both a high diffusible fraction and a higher lipid solubility, which together explain the more rapid onset of action. Baseline values for both drugs may shift with varied disease-related factors that alter V_d, protein binding or the proportion of the ionized form of the drug.

Metabolism

Drug biotransformation takes place mainly in the liver and contributes both to the rate of elimination of a drug and its bioavailability. The rate at which metabolism proceeds usually determines the clearance; however, where removal is particularly rapid (high extraction ratio) the rate of delivery of drug to the liver rather than the rate of metabolism, may determine clearance (flow-dependent kinetics). For such drugs, if liver blood flow is markedly reduced, drug accumulation will result.

The biochemical processes of drug metabolism are complex. Two phases of metabolism are usually described. Phase I reactions involve oxidation, reduction, hydrolysis, hydration, dethioacetylation, and isomerization. Of these reactions, oxidation catalysed by members the CYP450 superfamily of enzymes are the most important and best characterized. Phase II reactions usually involves conjugation; this may take the form of glucuronidation, glycosylation, sulphation, methylation, acetylation, or conjugation with glutathione or certain amino acids. All of the reactions involve the production of products which are more water-soluble and amenable to excretion by the kidney. In some circumstances, phase II reactions may take place without a prior phase I reaction. When phase I reactions do occur, they may prepare the drug molecule for a phase II reaction by producing or uncovering a chemically reactive group, which then forms the substrate for a phase II reaction.

Most opioid metabolism, both phase I and II reactions, occurs in the liver. Hydrophilic metabolites are predominantly excreted renally, although a small amount may be excreted in the bile or unchanged in the urine. Opioid metabolites may be active and contribute to both the overall analgesic and side effect profile (Smith, 2011). Metabolism of individual opioids is shown in Table 9.1.1.

Elimination

The two major organs of elimination are the liver and kidneys, both of which are susceptible to pharmacological and pathophysiological sources of variability. Clearance is defined as the volume

Table 9.1.1 Properties of commonly used opioids in palliative medicine

Drug	pK$_a$	Oral bioavailability (%)	Lipophilicity	Protein binding (%)	Volume of distribution	Metabolic enzymes	Active metabolites	Excreted unchanged in urine (%)	Half-life
Morphine	7.9	15–64	+	30	3–5 L/kg	UGT2B7	M6G (A) M3G (CNS+)	10	1.7–3 hours
Codeine	8.2	60–90	+	20	3–4 L/kg	UGT2B7 CYP2D6	Morphine (A)	0	2–4 hours
Diamorphine	7.6	–	++	–	70 L	Esterases	Morphine (A)	Minimal	2–3 minutes
Hydromorphone	8.2	50	+	<10	295 L	UGT2B7 UGT1A3	H3G (I) H6G (A)	6	2–3 hours
Tramadol	9.4	70–90	+	20	2.6–2.9 L/kg	CYP3A4 CYP2D6	M1	90	6 hours
Buprenorphine	8.4	15	+++	96	430 L	CYP3A4 UGT1A1/1A3	–	Minimal	*Complicated by enterohepatic recirculation
Meperidine (pethidine)	8.5	–	++	60–80	3–5 L/kg	CYP3A4 CYP2B6 CYP2C19	Norpethidine (A, CNS+)	5	3–6 hours
Oxycodone	8.5	60–87	+	45	2–3 L/kg	CYP3A4 CYP2D6	Oxymorphone (A)	< 10	3–4 hours
Methadone	8.3	60–90	++	60–90	3–6 L/kg	CYP3A4 CYP2B6 (CYP2D6,2C9,2C19,1A2)	–	15–60	15–20 hours (13–47)
Fentanyl	8.4	–	+++	90	3–8 L/kg	CYP3A4	–	< 7	2–7 hours
Alfentanil	6.5	–	++	90	0.4–1 L/kg	CYP3A4	–	Minimal	1–2 hours

Enzymes: CYP, cytochrome P450, UGT, UDP-glucuronosyltransferase. *Metabolites*: M3G, morphine-3-glucuronide, M6G, morphine-6-glucuronide H3G, Hydromorphone-3-glucuronide, H6G, Hydromorphone-6-glucuronide, M1, O-desmethyl tramadol. *Active metabolites*: A, analgesically active, CNS+, CNS excitability.

Source data from: Medicines and Healthcare Products Regulatory Agency (MHRA), available from <http://www.mhra.gov.uk>; Drugs.com, <http://www.drugs.com>, Copyright © 2000–2014 Drugs.com. All rights reserved.; Twycross R. WA (ed), *Palliative Care Formulary 4+*, Palliativedrugs.com Ltd, Copyright © 2012; Rook EJ et al., Pharmacokinetics and pharmacokinetic variability of heroin and its metabolites: Review of the literature, *Current Clinical Pharmacology*, Volume 1, Issue 1, pp. 109–18, Copyright © 2006; and Ashley C et al. (ed), *The Renal Drug Handbook*, Third Edition, Radcliffe Publishing, Oxford, UK, Copyright ©2008.

of blood which is completely cleared of the drug in a unit of time and reflects the efficiency of the elimination process. It is usually measured in mL/minute or L/hour. It is a major determinant of $t_{1/2}$ and of the steady-state drug concentration.

Half-life

This is perhaps the most well-known and commonly used pharmacokinetic parameter. The elimination half-life ($t_{1/2}$) is a measure of the time taken for half the drug in the body to be removed and generally correlates closely with duration of action. After repeated dosing is initiated, or the dose of an existing regimen is changed, five to six half-lives are required to approach steady-state concentration, irrespective of the route of administration or dosing interval. Drugs with a long $t_{1/2}$ accumulate for a relatively prolonged period of time, and as a result, the concentration may surpass the effective therapeutic range and build up to toxic levels. In the clinical setting, this accumulation has largely been a problem during methadone therapy. Methadone is exceptionally complex because its slow elimination phase is highly variable (beta $t_{1/2}$, 15–60 hours) and preceded by a rapid distribution phase ($t_{1/2}$, 2–3 hours); the overall half-life is relatively long (> 20 hours).

Steady-state plasma concentration

The aim of any dosing regimen in an individual patient is to achieve a concentration of drug in the blood that is high enough to give the intended effect without producing side effects. This concentration can never be completely steady as peaks will occur at the point of maximum drug absorption after administration, and troughs will occur immediately before each dose (Fig. 9.1.1). The degree of swing between peak and trough concentrations is determined by the drug's elimination $t_{1/2}$ and the frequency of drug administration.

Time to reach steady-state plasma concentration

The time taken for a drug to reach steady-state plasma concentration is dependent on the half-life. As noted, five to six half-lives are required to approach steady-state drug concentration if the same dose of drug is given at a constant time interval; four $t_{1/2}$ yields approximately 95% of this concentration. This applies only to drug where elimination is governed by 'first-order' kinetics. Fortunately, this comprises the vast majority of drugs, including opioids. Phenytoin is a notable exception, which involves both 'first-' and 'zero-order' processes.

The $t_{1/2}$ of morphine is 2–4 hours. Therefore, when morphine is administered every 4 hours, steady state will be 95% achieved

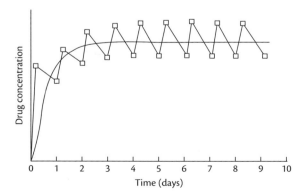

Fig. 9.1.1 Steady-state plasma concentration of a short-acting drug showing peaks and troughs after each dose.

after approximately 16 hours. Titration of the dose on a daily basis ensures that dose changes are occurring at steady state. In contrast, the methadone requires approximately 4–7 days, and occasionally much longer, to achieve steady state. Taking this into consideration a loading dose of methadone is often used followed by a period of cautious titration (after a number of days) to minimize the risk of toxicity.

Pharmacodynamics

Drugs produce their effects on the body by binding with receptors, modifying enzyme processes, or by direct chemical or physical actions. Opioids exert their influence by interacting with opioid receptors (primarily the mu opioid receptor).

Receptors

Receptors are specialized proteins within the cell membrane which are integral for communication between the cell and the outside world. They are highly specific for certain ligands, such as specific hormones, cytokines and/or drugs.

Opioid receptors

Opioid receptors were originally classified by pharmacological activity and later by molecular sequencing (Pasternak, 2004). There are three types of classical opioid receptor: μ (mu) or MOR, κ (kappa) or KOR, and δ (delta) or DOR. Another opioid-like receptor has been identified named the nociceptin or orphanin FQ peptide receptor or NOR (Mollereau et al., 1994).

The three classical receptors are activated differentially by the endogenous opioids (encephalins, endorphins, and dynorphins) (Table 9.1.2). Exogenous opioids, such as morphine, act primarily at the MOR. Different opioids may show differential binding to sites on the MOR and may also bind to other opioid or non-opioid receptors (Pasternak and Pan, 2011).

The opioid receptors belong to the superfamily of G protein-coupled receptors. Each consists of an extracellular N-terminus, seven transmembrane helices, three extra and intracellular loops, and an intracellular C-terminus. Each receptor type is coded for by a different gene (Meng et al., 1993; Knapp et al., 1994; Wang et al., 1994). The three receptors share a high degree of homology with most variation found in the extracellular loops and N-terminal domains (Minami and Satoh, 1995). The extracellular loops are particularly important as they determine ligand binding. Opioid receptors are widely, yet differentially, distributed in both central and peripheral nervous systems (Table 9.1.2) (Minami and Satoh, 1995).

The μ-opioid receptor. The μ-opioid receptor is clinically the most important of the family is, as it is responsible for the inhibition of nociceptive pathways and is exploited by all exogenous opioids. Knockout studies in mice show that the MOR is essential for morphine-induced analgesia (Matthes et al., 1996). Many of the unwanted effects of opioids are also related to activity at this receptor (Table 9.1.2). The MOR is expressed on central and peripheral neurons, and the latter are up-regulated in response to inflammatory stimuli. Peripherally, MOR are found pre- and post-synaptically. For example, approximately 70% of MOR receptors in the dorsal horn are expressed on the primary afferent terminations (presynaptic), where they modulate afferent transmission (Stein et al., 2003). At a cellular level, μ-opioid receptor activation results in an overall inhibitory effect (Box 9.1.2).

Table 9.1.2 Classical opioid receptor genes, distribution, endogenous ligands, and function

Receptor	Gene	Expression*	Endogenous ligand	Function
Mu (μ) MOR	OPRM1	Central nervous system: ◆ Brain including cerebral cortex, thalamus, hypothalamus, striatum, amygdala, periaqueductal grey. ◆ Spinal cord, pre- and postsynaptic neurons Peripheral nervous system Immune cells	◆ Beta-endorphin ◆ Encephalins ◆ Endomorphins	◆ Analgesia ◆ Respiratory depression ◆ Reduced GI motility ◆ Miosis ◆ Euphoria ◆ Sedation ◆ Physical dependence
Kappa (κ) KOR	OPRK1	Central nervous system: ◆ Brain including cerebral cortex, thalamus, hypothalamus, striatum, periaqueductal grey ◆ Spinal cord Peripheral nervous system	◆ Dynorphins	◆ Analgesia ◆ Miosis ◆ Dysphoria ◆ Hallucinations ◆ Sedation
Delta (δ) DOR	OPRD1	Central nervous system: ◆ Brain including cerebral cortex, striatum, olfactory bulb Peripheral nervous system	◆ Encephalins ◆ Beta-endorphin	◆ Analgesia ◆ Respiratory depression ◆ Reduced gastrointestinal motility ◆ Tolerance ◆ Mood regulation

Source: data from Peckys D, and Landwehrmeyer GB, Expression of mu, kappa, and delta opioid receptor messenger RNA in the human CNS: A 33P *in situ* hybridization study, *Neuroscience*, Volume 88, Issue 4, pp. 1093–135, Copyright © 1999; Stein C et al., Attacking pain at its source: new perspectives on opioids. National Medicine, Volume 9, Issue 8, pp. 1003–8, Copyright © 2003; and Borner C et al, Comparative analysis of mu-opioid receptor expression in immune and neuronal cells, *Journal of Neuroimmunology*, Volume 18, Issue 1–2, pp. 56–63, Copyright © 2007.

Box 9.1.2 Downstream consequences of μ-opioid receptor activation

◆ Inhibition of adenylyl cyclase

◆ Increased opening of potassium channels (hyperpolarization of post-synaptic neurons, reduced synaptic transmission)

◆ Inhibition of calcium channels (decreases pre-synaptic neurotransmitter release).

δ- and κ-opioid receptors. δ- and κ-opioid receptors also are involved in the modulation of pain. Knock-out studies in mice show that KOR may influence chemical visceral pain and thermal nociception (Simonin et al., 1998). Studies with selective opioid antagonists suggest that oxycodone analgesia depends on binding to the KOR receptor (Smith et al., 2001); other studies indicate that oxycodone is more like morphine and exerts its analgesic effects through MOR activation (Kalso et al., 1990; Chen et al., 1991; Yoburn et al., 1995). Pharmacological studies also suggest a role for KOR in mediating the dysphoric and sedative effects of opioids (Mark, 1990).

Combination opioid receptor knockout studies suggest that DOR plays a role in modulating mechanical and inflammatory pain (Martin et al., 2003). δ-opioid receptor knock-out mice also do not exhibit analgesic tolerance to morphine (Nitsche et al., 2002).

G-protein-coupled receptors, including MOR, KOR and DOR, have been shown to form different configurations, including homo- and hetero-dimers and oligomers, with unique internalization and activation pathways. Dimerization modulates receptor pharmacology and this process could present targets for novel interventions (Milligan, 2005). The development of MOR-DOR heteromers exemplifies this potential. There is evidence that there is an increased abundance of MOR–DOR heteromers in chronic pain and/or chronic exposure to morphine, and that ligand binding to DOR in the context of MOR-DOR is not associated with the development of opioid tolerance, in contrast to ligand binding to DOR alone. MOR-DOR may represent a new pharmacological target with the potential induce analgesia without tolerance (Costantino et al., 2012).

Modulation of opioid responses

Genetic polymorphism caused by alternative splicing of mRNA has been shown to give rise to various human MOR receptor subtypes. Much of the variation is found in the intracellular C-terminal domain and includes the creation of potential phosphorylation sites (Pasternak and Pan, 2011). These receptor subtypes have differential expression patterns and demonstrate activation profiles that vary among the various MOR agonists; they are likely to explain some of the clinical variation in opioid response (Pasternak, 2004). Genetic polymorphism also may be involved individual variation in pain responses. For example, the minor T allele of *OPRM1* rs563649 is associated with higher expression levels of the MOR-1K isoform and also with high pain sensitivity (Shabalina et al., 2009).

Other cellular adaptations are likely to be involved in the varied responses to chronic opioid exposure, such as variation in the development of tolerance (Ferguson, 2001; Bailey and Connor, 2005). Chronic morphine exposure leads to little change in MOR expression but does seem to produce changes in the non-neuronal population of glial cells, with increased activation provoking central sensitization (Watkins et al., 2005).

Although it is widely accepted that clinically relevant pharmacological tolerance to opioid analgesic effects is not an issue for the majority of patients with cancer-related pain, it is difficult to assess analgesic tolerance clinically (Chang et al., 2007). There does not appear to be a simple correlation between exposure to opioids and induction of analgesic tolerance. A process of adaptation occurs, which is likely to depend on diverse factors, but this process cannot be fully explained on the basis of current knowledge of cellular mechanisms.

Agonists, agonist–antagonists, and antagonists

Based on their interactions with receptors, opioid compounds can be divided into agonist, agonist–antagonist, and antagonist classes (Table 9.1.3). Most opioids used in the clinical setting are full agonist drugs. Opioid antagonists, such as naloxone and naltrexone, bind to MOR and produce no agonist activity. Agonist-antagonist drugs include a group of mixed agonist–antagonists, which are agonists at one or more opioid receptor subtypes and antagonists at others, and partial agonists. The mixed agonist–antagonists, such as pentazocine, are seldom used in the management of patients with advanced illness. Buprenorphine is a partial agonist that is being used more as an analgesic with the advent of a transdermal delivery system. Buprenorphine is believed to have a ceiling effect at doses of 8–16 mg/day (Walsh and Eissenberg, 2003). However as the recommended analgesic doses are much lower than the ceiling dose (equivalent to up to 3–4 mg/day, or 2 × 70-microgram/hour patches), buprenorphine typically is used with doses in the linear part of the dose-response curve and clinically performs as a full agonist during the management of pain. At the higher doses used to treat heroin addiction, the partial agonist effect may be encountered (Greenwald et al., 2003).

Efficacy, potency, and relative potency

Efficacy is defined by the maximal response induced by administration of the active agent. In practice, this is determined by the degree of analgesia produced following dose escalation through a range limited by the development of adverse effects. Potency, in contrast, reflects the dose–response relationship and is typically defined by the intensity of a specified effect, such as analgesia, associated with a specific dose. Potency is influenced by pharmacokinetic factors (i.e. how much of the drug enters the body's systemic circulation and then reaches the receptors) and by affinity to drug receptors.

Clinically, the utility of potency measurements is created by comparing drugs using relative potency ratios, or the ratio of doses required to produce the same analgesic effect. The relative potency of each of the commonly used opioids is based upon a comparison with 10 mg of oral morphine. Data from single-and repeated-dose studies in patients with acute or chronic pain have been used to develop 'equianalgesic' or dose conversion tables. The term 'equianalgesic' is however misleading as there is wide inter-individual differences in response to different opioids and such tables should be used only as a guide when switching between opioids (Riley et al., 2006). In particular, care should be exercised when switching from one opioid to another as part of the management of opioid toxicity. In this situation, conservative conversions should be used followed by individual titration. Opioid switching is discussed in detail in Chapter 9.4.

The clinical utility of an opioid therapy is determined by a favourable balance between analgesic efficacy and side effects. Many variables may influence whether a dose exists that yields this balance. These include intensity of pain; prior opioid exposure in terms of drug, duration, and dose (and the degree of cross-tolerance that this confers); age; route of administration; level of consciousness and metabolic abnormalities; and genetic polymorphism in the expression of relevant enzymes or receptors (Droney et al., 2012).

Opioid combination therapy. The clinical use of combinations of different opioids is increasing with the aims to (a) improve analgesia, (b) reduce side effects, and (c) limit the development of opioid tolerance. The rationale behind this practice is to utilize

Table 9.1.3 Table of opioid receptor agonists and antagonists

Receptor effect	Description	Examples
Agonists	An agonist is a drug that has affinity for and binds to cell receptors to induce changes in the cell that stimulate physiological activity The agonist opioid drugs have no clinically relevant ceiling effect to analgesia	Morphine Diamorphine Oxycodone Pethidine Hydromorphone Methadone Fentanyl Tramadol
Partial agonist	A partial agonist has low intrinsic activity (efficacy) so that its dose–response curve exhibits a ceiling effect at less than the maximum effect produced by a full agonist	Buprenorphine
Antagonist	Antagonist drugs have no intrinsic pharmacological action but can interfere with the action of an agonist Competitive antagonists bind to the same receptor and compete for receptor sites, whereas non-competitive antagonists block the effects of the agonist in some other way	Naloxone Naltrexone
Mixed agonist–antagonist	The mixed agonist–antagonist drugs produce agonist effects at one receptor and antagonist effects at another	Pentazocine Butorphanol Nalbuphine

the inherent differences in the pharmacodynamic and pharmacokinetic properties of this group of drugs to maximize potential benefit and minimize adverse effects (Fallon and Laird, 2011). Hypotheses of the pharmacodynamic mechanisms include splice variation in opioid receptors, the receptor activation versus endocytosis (RAVE) theory, and the formation of opioid receptor homo- and heterodimers which results in changes to G-protein signalling cascades (Davis et al., 2005).

In animal studies, there is some evidence of analgesic synergism between methadone and other μ-agonist opioids (Bolan et al., 2002). In addition two small retrospective case series of patients with uncontrolled cancer-related pain have reported that low dose methadone in combination with existing opioid improved analgesia (McKenna and Nicholson, 2011; Haughey et al., 2012).

A combination product of oxycodone with morphine in a fixed-dose ratio 3:2 is currently being evaluated in clinical trials (MoxDuo®). It has been trialled in phase II and phase III studies for the management of acute postoperative pain and results suggest that there may be a difference in side effect profile when compared with the individual opioids (Webster et al., 2010; Richards et al., 2011; Webster, 2012). There are currently no trials published in the chronic pain or cancer pain setting.

Further research into the use of opioid combinations in warranted. The potential benefits from this strategy must be weighed against other factors, such as poor patient compliance, confusion over dosing, and prescriber dosing errors, along with potentially unanticipated increased side effects.

Drugs which alter enzyme activity or have a direct chemical or physical action

Some drugs exert effects by affecting enzyme processes, rather than by binding to receptors. Many act by inhibition of enzyme actions. For example, non-steroidal anti-inflammatory drugs block the effect of the enzyme cyclooxygenase and thereby interfere with the synthesis of prostaglandins and exert anti-inflammatory activity.

Other drugs produce intended effects through a direct chemical or physical action. Antacids are an example of drugs with a direct chemical action; they are bases which neutralize gastric acid. Drugs with a physical mode of action include the bulk laxatives, such as ispaghula husk.

Drug interaction

Patients with palliative care needs may already be receiving drugs for a variety of conditions. Some may still be beneficial but others may no longer contribute to improving prognosis or symptoms. Rationalization of the therapeutic regimen always should be considered. If further drugs to relieve symptoms are added, this adds to the potential for drug interaction. Interaction is adverse if it causes therapeutic failure or toxicity from any one drug. Remembering all the possible drug interactions is virtually impossible, but knowledge of the underlying mechanisms of drug interaction can put the prescriber on guard together with frequent consultation with prescribing information is important.

Adverse drug reactions

An adverse drug reaction can be defined as an unwanted or harmful reaction experienced following administration of a drug, or combination of drugs, under normal conditions of use that is suspected of being related to the drug. For example opioids act via the μ-opioid receptor to slow gut transit and cause constipation.

Box 9.1.3 Opioid side effects listed by system

Gastrointestinal system
- Nausea
- Constipation
- Dry mouth
- Vomiting
- Ileus

Nervous system
- Somnolence
- Confusion
- Myoclonus
- Abnormal dreams
- Hallucinations
- Hyperalgesia

Genitourinary system
- Urinary retention

Respiratory system
- Cough decreased
- Respiratory depression

Skin
- Hyperhidrosis
- Pruritus

Endocrine
- Hypogonadism
- Immunosuppression

Opioid-related side effects are summarized in Box 9.1.3 and can be transient or persistent. Chapter 9.4 describes in more detail the principles of opioid switching which can reduce individual adverse drug reactions.

Opioid analgesics are one of the drugs most frequently associated with adverse drug events. A study of 3695 inpatient adverse drug reactions found that 16% were attributable to opioids (Davies et al., 2009). Risk of opioid drug reactions increases in older patients, in those with underlying cardiac or respiratory disease, and when co-prescribed with other sedative medications such as benzodiazepines (Bernard and Bruera, 2000).

Pharmacokinetic drug interaction

Pharmacokinetic interaction arises through alterations in the rate and extent of absorption and changes in metabolism (both pre-systemic and elimination), distribution, and renal excretion. The clinical impact of theoretical interactions can be difficult to predict.

Drugs such as metoclopramide and anticholinergics, which alter the rate of gastric emptying, may affect the speed of absorption of other agents. Some drugs bind others in the gastrointestinal tract and affect their bioavailability. For example, care is necessary if antacid preparations, iron salts, or cholestyramine are used concurrently with certain drugs.

Drug interactions resulting from changes in the rate of metabolism by the liver will result both in changes of bioavailability for those drugs with a significant first-pass effect, and decreased clearance. Steady-state concentrations of drug may be profoundly affected.

A number of drugs (particularly phenobarbital, carbamazepine, phenytoin and rifampicin) are capable of inducing the cytochrome P450 and glucuronidase enzymes in the liver. There are a myriad of substrates for this interaction, including methadone, warfarin, corticosteroids, and anticonvulsant drugs. Increased pre-systemic metabolism may result in the need to increased doses to achieve therapeutic levels. Conversely some drugs may inhibit CYP enzymes, individually or as an entire superfamily (Table 9.1.4). Certain foodstuffs may also induce or inhibit hepatic enzyme systems; for example, grapefruit contains furanocoumarins which inhibit CYP3A (Hanley et al., 2011).

The most important drug interactions in the kidney involve competition between agents for active tubular secretion. Active tubular secretion is used by organic acids, and the most frequent interactions are caused by the loop diuretics and some non-steroidal anti-inflammatory drugs. Although renal excretion of some drugs is pH dependent, in general this has minor implications in normal therapeutics. There are a few exceptions, however; for example, methadone's renal clearance is considerably enhanced by concurrent use of urinary acidifiers such as acetazolamide (Bellward et al., 1977).

Pharmacodynamic drug interaction

Some drug–drug interactions occur at a receptor level. For example, buprenorphine is a partial agonist and morphine is a full agonist, and morphine-induced analgesia may be reversed or limited by competition at the receptor level if buprenorphine is added.

Drug formulations and route of administration

The preferred route of administration for many drugs including opioids is oral. Oral formulations of opioids include immediate-release (IR) syrups, tablets or capsules, and modified-release (MR) tablets or capsules. MR formulations slowly release the drug into the gut, allowing treatment once or twice daily depending on the formulation (e.g. morphine, oxycodone). Care must be taken in prescribing, such that the correct formulation is dispensed, and when more than one formulation is given (e.g. IR and MR) the patient understands how and when to use each preparation.

Opioid drugs can also be given by other routes, including, transdermal, transmucosal (sublingual, buccal, nasal, rectal), and parenteral by injection either intravenously or more commonly subcutaneously. Fentanyl and buprenorphine products have been formulated for the transmucosal and transdermal routes. In addition specialist pain services may use epidural or intrathecal opioids in the palliative setting where appropriate. Prescriptions of these drugs should specify the exact formulation, as formulations differ in systemic availability and may not be interchangeable.

Immediate and modified-release formulations

IR preparations are absorbed in the stomach or proximal small bowel, so that absorption is complete within a few hours on ingestion. For example, IR morphine and oxycodone reach peak effects within 1 hour. Modified- or sustained-release formulations allow a drug to be released over 12–24 hours, resulting in a smoother concentration profile of the drug in the blood, extended duration of action, and reduction in tablet burden for the patient.

Transmucosal preparations

Drugs that are absorbed through the buccal, nasal, or rectal mucosa avoid first-pass metabolism in the liver by uptake into veins that drain directly into the systemic circulation. This results in higher bioavailability and often a faster onset of action when compared to the oral route. IR transmucosal fentanyl products may be useful in treatment of breakthrough/incident pain. The rapid speed of onset of action (approximately 10 minutes) and short duration of action ($\geq$ 1 hour) may sometimes be more suited to the temporal characteristics of breakthrough/incident pain than conventional IR opioid (Twycross et al., 2012; Davies et al., 2013). There does not, however, appear to be a meaningful relationship between background opioid dose and the effective dose of transmucosal fentanyl, and therefore, titration is essential (Zeppetella, 2011).

Transdermal preparations

Some lipid-soluble drugs are well absorbed through the skin, and their transdermal delivery via 'patches' allows controlled release over many hours or days. Opioid examples include fentanyl and buprenorphine. Different formulations have been developed and are not interchangeable and preparations may last for 3–7 days depending on drug/formulation. Clinical trials suggest good patient satisfaction with this mode of delivery. Care must be taken, given the wide variability in drug absorption, especially in cachexic or pyrexial patients (Heiskanen et al., 2009).

Parenteral preparations for subcutaneous, intravenous, and intrathecal delivery

The preferred parenteral route of administration in palliative patients is subcutaneous and opioids may be given as stat injections or as a continuous subcutaneous infusion. When continuous subcutaneous infusions are used and multiple drugs combined, care must be taken to ensure drug interactions are avoided, as precipitation of one drug in solution will clearly limit therapeutic effect (e.g. cyclizine and oxycodone are not compatible) (Dickman et al., 2002).

Combination formulations in oral therapy

Combination products are attractive and may aid compliance by reducing tablet burden. To be effective, the frequency of administration of the two drugs should be the same. Combination products to not allow for titration of one drug without the other, and this may be a concern with some combinations. For example, concerns have been raised regarding combinations of opioid analgesics with paracetamol because of the need to limit titration of the paracetamol and risk of liver damage in overdose.

The patient's use of a drug: compliance and adherence

Compliance or adherence is the extent to which a patient follows a prescribed drug regimen. It is important that decisions regarding treatment are jointly made by the prescriber and patient. Allowing adequate time to explain principles and goals of therapy, expected benefit and possible side effects, and plans for review and follow-up is essential. In addition, exploration of patient

Table 9.1.4 Potential for drug interactions involving the cytochrome P450 enzyme system

Inhibitors –	CYP1A2	CYP2B6	CYP2C8	CYP2C9	CYP2C19	CYP2D6	CYP2E1	CYP3A4
	Amiodarone	Clopidogrel	Amiodarone	Amiodarone	Celecoxib	Amiodarone	Alcohol (acute use)	Amiodarone
	Ciprofloxacin	Paroxetine	Fluconazole	Fluconazole	Esomeprazole	Celecoxib	Disulfram	Bicalutamide
	Diclofenac	Sertraline	Ibuprofen	Ibuprofen	Fluconazole	Duloxetine		Clarithromycin
	Fluvoxamine		Omeprazole	Metronidazole	Fluoxetine	Fluoxetine		Diclofenac
			Pantoprazole	Miconazole	Lansoprazole	Haloperidol		Diltiazem
			Quinine	Omeprazole	Modafinil	Levomepromazine		Erythromycin
			Trimethoprim	Pantoprazole	Omeprazole	Methadone		Fluconazole (high dose)
				Quinine	Rabeprazole	Paroxetine		Grapefruit juice
					Sertraline	Quinine		Haloperidol
						Sertraline		Imatinib
								Itraconazole
								Verapamil

Substrates	CYP1A2	CYP2B6	CYP2C8	CYP2C9	CYP2C19	CYP2D6	CYP2E1	CYP3A4	CYP3A4
	Amitriptyline	Diclofenac	Diclofenac	Amitriptyline	Amitriptyline	Amitriptyline	Domperidone	Alfentanil	Metronidazole
	Domperidone	Ketamine	Ibuprofen	Celecoxib	Citalopram	Codeine	Paracetamol	Amitriptyline	Midazolam
	Duloxetine	Methadone	Naproxen	Diclofenac	Clopidogrel	Duloxetine	Theophylline	Carbamazepine	Mirtazapine
	Flutamide		Omeprazole	Fluoxetine	Diazepam	Fluoxetine		Citalopram	Modafinil
	Haloperidol		Repaglinide	Gliclazide	Diclofenac	Haloperidol		Clonazepam	Omeprazole
	Methadone		Rosiglitazone	Glimepiride	Esomeprazole	Methadone		Dexamethasone	Ondansetron
	Mirtazapine		Tamoxifen	Glipizide	Ibuprofen	Methylphenidate		Diazepam	Oxycodone
	Naproxen			Ibuprofen	Lansoprazole	Metoclopramide		Domperidone	Pantoprazole
	Olanzapine			Ketamine	Methadone	Mirtazapine		Esomeprazole	Quinine
	Ondansetron			Methadone	Naproxen	Omeprazole		Etoricoxib	Rabeprazole
	Paracetamol			Metronidazole	Omeprazole	Ondansetron		Exemestane	Reboxetine
	Ropinirole			Naproxen	Pantoprazole	Oxycodone		Fentanyl	Risperidone
	Theophylline			Omeprazole	Phenobarbital	Paroxetine		Finasteride	Sertraline
	Warfarin			Tamoxifen	Rabeprazole	Promethazine		Granisetron	Simvastatin
				Warfarin	Sertraline	Risperidone		Haloperidol	Tamoxifen
					Warfarin	Sertraline		Ketamine	Trazodone
						Tamoxifen		Medroxyprogesterone	Venlafaxine
						Tramadol		Methadone	Zopiclone
						Trazodone		Methylphenidate	
						Venlafaxine			

Inducers +	CYP1A2	CYP2B6	CYP2C8	CYP2C9	CYP2C19	CYP2D6	CYP2E1	CYP3A4
	Carbamazepine	Carbamazepine	Carbamazepine	Carbamazepine	Carbamazepine		Alcohol (chronic use)	Carbamazepine
	Phenobarbital	Modafinil	Phenobarbital	Phenobarbital	Phenobarbital		Phenobarbital	Dexamethasone
	Rifampicin	Phenobarbital	Rifampicin	Rifampicin				Modafinil
	Tobacco	Rifampicin						Phenobarbital
								Phenytoin
								Rifampicin
								St John's wort

Adapted with permission from Andrew Dickman, *Drugs in Palliative Care*, Second Edition, Oxford University Press, Oxford UK, Copyright © 2012 Andrew Dickman by permission of Oxford University press.

(and family) concerns regarding addiction, tolerance, side effects, or fear that treatment implies the final stages of life are essential when using opioids for patients with advanced illness (NICE, 2012). The proactive management or prevention of side effects, for example, provision of laxatives for opioid-induced constipation, can improve compliance. In general, more complex regimens with high frequency of administration and/or multiple drugs reduce compliance.

Pharmacogenomics

Pharmacogenomics is the study of how genetic variation influences response to drugs. It is the cornerstone of personalized medicine, which aims to tailor treatment to the individual to maximize efficacy and minimize adverse reactions. Two techniques have been used to study pharmacogenomics: the candidate gene approach and genome-wide association. The candidate gene approach targets single nucleotide polymorphisms (SNPs) in genes already known to be important in pharmacokinetic (e.g. drug metabolizing enzymes, drug transporters) and pharmacodynamic (e.g. receptors, ion channels, enzymes) pathways. Genome-wide association studies cast a much wider net examining millions of SNPs across the entire genome at a time and may therefore provide new biological insights into mechanisms (Wilke et al., 2008).

In recent years, the field of pharmacogenomics has exploded to provide a wealth of information to inform personalized prescribing across the medical specialties. In oncology, response to certain chemotherapy agents can now be predicted, for example, variation in *UGT1A1* is associated with severe neutropenia from irinotecan (Innocenti et al., 2004). In cardiology, response to warfarin, statins, and clopidogrel have all been associated with genetic factors (Johnson and Cavallari, 2013). In HIV medicine, screening programmes have been used to reduce the risk of hypersensitivity reactions to abacavir by testing for *HLA B*5701*, which is associated with the condition (Mallal et al., 2008). Work continues on how this knowledge may best be translated into clinical practice (Johnson et al., 2012).

Opioid pharmacogenomics

Study of the CYP enzyme 2D6 (*CYP2D6*) gene has provided perhaps the best examples of how pharmacokinetics and ultimately opioid response is linked to genetic variation. CYP2D6 is involved in the metabolism of several opioids including codeine, tramadol, and oxycodone. Over 70 *CYP2D6* alleles have been described which directly affect the final protein; these include SNPs, deletions, insertions, and copy number variation (Leandro-Garcia et al., 2009). The sum functional effect of this variation has been classified into four main phenotypes: poor, intermediate, extensive, and ultrarapid metabolizers.

Codeine is partially (10%) metabolized to morphine by CYP2D6 (Lotsch, 2005). Approximately 10% of Caucasians are poor metabolizers and experience little analgesia from codeine (Sindrup et al., 1990; Persson et al., 1995). Conversely 3% of Caucasians are ultrarapid metabolizers and have a higher incidence of codeine-related adverse reactions (Kirchheiner et al., 2007). There have been case reports of fatal neonatal opioid toxicity in children breastfed by mothers who are ultrarapid metabolizers following ingestion of codeine (Madadi et al., 2007). The CYP2D6 phenotype has also been suggested to affect response to tramadol and oxycodone by altering ratios of the parent opioid to the more active metabolites (Samer et al., 2003, 2010b), although the clinical relevance of this is debated (Gronlund et al., 2010; Samer et al., 2010a, 2010b; Andreassen et al., 2012).

Pharmacodynamic candidate gene studies in palliative care patients suggest that opioid receptor SNPs, for example, *OPRM1* A118G, influence patients' requirements for opioids (Klepstad et al., 2004; Campa et al., 2008; Walter and Lotsch, 2009). Individual pain susceptibility also influences analgesic response, and therefore, many more candidate genes from pain signalling and modulatory pathways, for example, *COMT* (Rakvag et al., 2005; Rakvag et al., 2008), also may be important in opioid responsiveness.

Pain experience and opioid response are complex traits and therefore influenced by a myriad of gene–gene and gene–environment interactions. Recently, genetic association studies have begun to explore interactions between variants from more than one gene. This has thus far been limited to two candidate SNPs at a time (Reyes-Gibby et al., 2007; Campa et al., 2008). The concept of gene–gene/environment interactions or epistasis provides a huge challenge for the future of opioid pharmacogenetics, both practical and analytical. Further work needs to be done to unpick the complexities behind opioid response to be able to develop a useful predictive tool to inform clinical practice.

Online materials

Complete references for this chapter are available online at <http://www.oxfordmedicine.com>.

References

Ashley, C. and Currie, A. (2008). *The Renal Drug Handbook* (3rd ed.). Oxford: Radcliffe Publishing.

Bernard, S.A. and Bruera, E. 2000. Drug interactions in palliative care. *Journal of Clinical Oncology*, 18, 1780–1799.

Borner, C., Stumm, R., Hollt, V., and Kraus, J. (2007). Comparative analysis of mu-opioid receptor expression in immune and neuronal cells. *Journal of Neuroimmunology*, 188(1–2), 56–63.

Caraceni, A., Hanks, G., Kaasa, S., *et al.* (2012). Use of opioid analgesics in the treatment of cancer pain: evidence-based recommendations from the EAPC. *The Lancet Oncology*, 13, e58–e68.

Dickman A. (2012). *Drugs in Palliative Care* (2nd ed.). Oxford: Oxford University Press.

Dickman A., Littlewood, C., and Varga J. (2002). *The Syringe Driver: Continuous Subcutaneous Infusions in Palliative Care*. Oxford: Oxford University Press.

Droney, J., Riley, J., and Ross, J. (2012). Opioid genetics in the context of opioid switching. *Current Opinion in Supportive and Palliative Care*, 6, 10–16.

Fallon, M. T. and Laird, B. J. (2011). A systematic review of combination step III opioid therapy in cancer pain: an EPCRC opioid guideline project. *Palliative Medicine*, 25, 597–603.

Joint Formulary Committee (2014). *British National Formulary* (68th ed.). London: BMJ Group and Pharmaceutical Press.

Junger, S., Brearley, S., Payne, S., *et al.* (2013). Consensus building on access to controlled medicines: a four-stage Delphi consensus procedure. *Journal of Pain and Symptom Management*, 46(6), 897–910.

Minami, M. and Satoh, M. (1995). Molecular biology of the opioid receptors: structures, functions and distributions. *Neuroscience Research*, 23, 121–145.

National Institute of Health and Clinical Excellence (2012). *Opioids in Palliative Care: Safe and Effective Prescribing of Strong Opioids for Pain in Palliative Care of adults* CG140. London: NICE.

Palliativedrugs.com (2012). *Palliative Care Formulary 4+*. [Online] Available at: http://www.palliativedrugs.com>.

Pasternak, G.W. (2004). Multiple opiate receptors: deja vu all over again. *Neuropharmacology*, 47(Suppl. 1), 312–323.

Peckys, D. and Landwehrmeyer, G.B. (1999). Expression of mu, kappa, and delta opioid receptor messenger RNA in the human CNS: a 33P in situ hybridization study. *Neuroscience*, 88(4), 1093–1135.

Rook, E.J., Huitema, A.D., Van Den Brink, W., Van Ree, J.M., and Beijnen, J.H. (2006). Pharmacokinetics and pharmacokinetic variability of heroin and its metabolites: review of the literature. *Current Clinical Pharmacology*, 1(1), 109–118.

Shabalina, S.A., Zaykin, D.V., Gris, P., *et al.* (2009). Expansion of the human mu-opioid receptor gene architecture: novel functional variants. *Human Molecular Genetics*, 18(6), 1037–1051.

Smith, H.S. (2011). The metabolism of opioid agents and the clinical impact of their active metabolites. *Clinical Journal of Pain*, 27, 824–838.

Stein, C., Schafer, M., and Machelska, H. (2003). Attacking pain at its source: new perspectives on opioids. *Nature Medicine*, 9(8), 1003–1008.

Walter, C. and Lotsch, J. (2009). Meta-analysis of the relevance of the OPRM1 118A>G genetic variant for pain treatment. *Pain*, 146, 270–275.

Zeppetella, G. (2011). Opioids for the management of breakthrough cancer pain in adults: a systematic review undertaken as part of an EPCRC opioid guidelines project. *Palliative Medicine*, 25, 516–524.

9.2

Pathophysiology of pain in cancer and other terminal illnesses

Richard M. Gordon-Williams and Anthony H. Dickenson

Introduction to pathophysiology of pain in terminal illness

Acute pain involves a series of excitatory events at peripheral and central levels that faithfully transmit signals about noxious events, leading to clinical reports of pain that usually have an overt relationship to identifiable peripheral damage, lesion, or abnormality. In contrast, clinically important chronic pains have altered neurophysiological and pharmacological substrates at many levels, from the periphery to the central nervous system (CNS), and the relationship between noxious phenomena and the level of pain experienced can become altered. Clinically, pain may be present, or unexpectedly severe, in the absence of an explanatory peripheral process. Plasticity, the ability of the nervous system to alter in response to injury-evoked dysfunction, leads to changes that can be observed throughout the pathways involved in the perception of pain.

Exploitation of continually developing pharmacological, anatomical, molecular, and genomic techniques is providing a basis for understanding the molecular and cellular mechanisms that contribute to the pain associated with varied pathophysiologies. Some chronic pains arise from persistent damage to tissue, such as that from arthritis, whereas others arise in the absence of these changes. Plasticity may alter pain responses in all these cases, but may be particularly notable with chronic neuropathic pains, which can arise from injury, a lesion, or a disease to either the peripheral or central nervous somatosensory systems.

Patients with cancer may develop injury to somatic or visceral tissues, or damage to neural structures. The aetiology may be related to the tumour itself, to various antineoplastic therapies, or to comorbid disorders. Cancer pain, therefore, often has a mix of mechanisms. Some mechanisms are broadly characterized as nociceptive, and some of these are inflammatory. Others are neuropathic. This complexity, which is shared by other types of advanced illnesses, such as HIV/AIDS, can complicate treatment but also offer more treatment options—a double-edged sword.

Recent animal studies are shedding light on some of the specific mechanisms underlying cancer pain. Importantly, whereas nociceptive pain results from activation of sensory afferents, neuropathic pain originates from damage to nerves and may prominently feature disturbances in ion channels. Thus, treatments aimed at the peripheral mechanisms are different for these two types of pain.

Plasticity in the nervous system in response to injury may lead to characteristic symptoms that contribute to the pain experience. These include expanded receptive fields, increased amplitude of response to a given stimulus (hyperalgesia), pain elicited by normally innocuous stimuli (allodynia), and spontaneous pain in the absence of external stimuli. Sensory deficits can also exist in neuropathic pain. In addition, as pain persists, affective and emotional responses must be considered along with the sensory aspects of the stimulus. It is clear that, although the sensory and psychological aspects of pain are separable, the neural pathways that contribute to these aspects of pain are interlinked. Furthermore, at both peripheral and central sites, there are mechanisms that can amplify and prolong the painful stimulus so that the pain becomes greater—this can result in severe pain in the presence of relatively minor peripheral pathology. This chapter considers these signalling systems and changes therein in the context of pain in cancer.

Anatomy of pain

Primary afferents and inputs to the dorsal horn

The dorsal horn receives sensory information from somatosensory receptors in the periphery via primary afferents. The area of the dorsal horn in which these primary afferents terminate is determined by the type of primary afferent and, therefore, the nature of the information that they carry. Different sensory inputs are carried by fibres of different thickness, from thick myelinated to thin and unmyelinated. Due to the differing degrees of myelination, these different groups exhibit differing conduction velocities at which they transmit a stimulus. The largest of the afferent sensory fibres, with thick myelin sheaths, are the $A\beta$ fibres that carry information from muscle and tendons; these are the fastest conducting. A subset of thickly myelinated fibres carries mostly information from cutaneous mechanoreceptors; these usually do not transmit nociceptive signals. Neurons that carry nociceptive information include the thinly myelinated $A\delta$ nociceptors and the thin unmyelinated C fibres. The latter two types of fibres are therefore pivotal in detection of potentially harmful stimuli in the external environment.

$A\delta$ and C fibres terminate primarily in the superficial laminae of the dorsal horn, namely lamina I, which is an area intrinsically important in pain processing due to its large output to supraspinal areas. The large majority of neurons found within lamina I are nociceptive-specific; these neurons have small receptive fields and respond to only noxious pinch and/or heat stimulation. This region also contains a smaller population of polymodal neurons that are also cold responsive (Andrew and Craig, 2002; Craig and Andrew, 2002) and also a small population of so-called wide dynamic range (WDR) neurons that code throughout innocuous and noxious stimulus intensities (Seagrove et al., 2004). Finally, other neurons that respond purely to itch-inducing stimuli or to non-noxious heat have been noted (Light et al., 1993; Andrew and Craig, 2001).

Lamina I neurons have been shown to project to areas in the brain, such as the periaqueductal grey (PAG), lateral parabrachial nucleus, thalamus, nucleus tractus solitarius, and the medullary reticular formation (Todd, 2002). A large number of projection neurons from lamina I express the receptor for substance P, which is also known as neurokinin 1 (Todd et al., 2000). This group of neurons is the origin of a spinobulbospinal loop that ascends from the cord to the brain and then drives descending controls back to the cord; in this way the circuit can control dorsal horn excitability from higher centres (Bannister et al., 2009).

Deep dorsal horn neurons are mostly WDR neurons and consequently have larger receptive fields than the neuronal populations of the superficial dorsal horn (SDH). Projections from the deep dorsal horn neurons have been shown to be mainly to the reticular nuclei (Raboisson et al., 1996) and to the thalamus in the spinothalamic pathways. These nuclei of the brain have good connections with areas concerned with primary somatosensory cortex and therefore discriminatory perception of pain.

Acute pain

Peripheral sensitization

Peripheral receptors and channels involved in transduction of nociceptive stimuli in the periphery (see Fig. 9.2.1). The diagram depicts a C fibre and a polymodal nociceptor comprising numerous receptors and channels activated by voltage changes (voltage-gated ion channels) or chemical mediators of pain. The latter mediators include adenosine (acting at P2Y), bradykinin (B2), prostaglandin (endoprostinoid receptor (EP)), noradrenaline (β2), protons (acid sensing ion channel (ASIC)/TRPV1), heat/capsaicin (TRPV1), adenosine triphosphate (ATP) (P2X), and nerve growth factor (NGF) (trkA/p75). The precise molecular identity of a mechanoreceptor is still unclear.

In order to sense the external environment, it is necessary to convert peripheral stimuli into signals that can be carried by nerves to the CNS, a process known as transduction. There are a number of transduction molecules on the peripheral neuron that allow detection of a wide range of both exogenous and endogenous stimuli. While the full pharmacology and physiology of each of these peripheral sensory transducers falls outside the scope of this chapter, Table 9.2.1 illustrates a number of mechanisms through which a peripheral neuron can sense the peripheral environment. Needless to say, the actions of these transducers have a large part to play in pathological states where tissue and nerves are damaged, including cancer pain.

Transduction molecules seem to be highly preserved throughout evolution, with homology found throughout non-mammalian and mammalian species. This suggests the huge importance of an animal's ability to sense its surroundings (Caterina and Julius, 2001). Peripheral tissue damage and subsequent local inflammation can cause the release of a wide variety of chemical factors that are able to sensitize primary afferent fibres. Pro-inflammatory compounds also can be released by nerve endings themselves in a process known as neurogenic inflammation.

Neurogenic inflammation is one of the mechanisms of peripheral sensitization and can further amplify the peripheral response of nociceptors. Peripheral terminations of nociceptors may arborize over a large area. Activation of peripheral afferents may cause neuromodulator release from nearby peripheral branches into peripheral tissues. These include factors such as substance P, neuropeptide Y, calcitonin gene-related peptide (CGRP), ATP, and glutamate. These compounds may act on peripheral blood vessels, mast cells, and sympathetic nerve fibres, leading to an increase

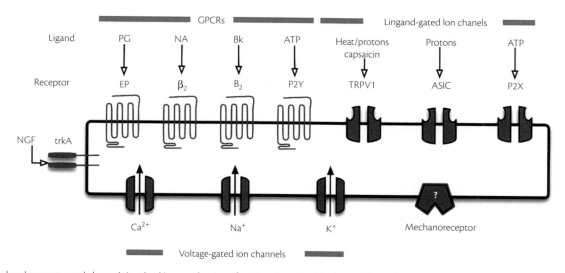

Fig. 9.2.1 Peripheral receptors and channels involved in transduction of nociceptive stimuli in the periphery. The diagram depicts a C fibre where the polymodal nociceptor is comprised of numerous receptors, channels activated by voltage changes (voltage-gated ion channels) or chemical mediators of pain. Adenosine (acting at P2Y), bradykinin (B2), prostaglandin (endoprostinoid receptor, EP), noradrenaline (β2), protons (acid sensing ion channel, ASIC/TRPV1), heat/capsaicin (TRPV1), ATP (P2X), NGF (trkA/p75). The precise molecular identity of a mechanoreceptor is still unclear.

Table 9.2.1 Algogenic ligands: their origins and their cognate receptors

Ligand	Origin	Receptor
H+	Tissue damage, macrophages	ASIC, TRPV1
Bradykinin	Macrophages, mast cells	B2/B1 (TRPV1)
Histamine	Mast cells	H1
Prostaglandins	Mast cells, fibroblasts	EP
Nerve growth factor	Macrophage, fibroblasts	TrkA
ATP	Platelets, sympathetic terminals	P2X3
Adenosine	Tissue damage	A1/A2
5-HT	Platelets, mast cells	5-HTr
IL-1	Macrophage	IL-1r
Heat	Exogenous, inflammation	TRPV
Cold		TRPM8

in vasodilation, vascular permeability, and therefore plasma extravasation, causing erythema and oedema. Serotonin, bradykinin, glutamate, NGF, and other cytokines in the inflammatory infiltrate can cause further activation of primary afferent fibres and help propagate nociception when tissue is damaged and the production of these molecules is promoted.

Peripheral sensitization also involves change in ion channels. TRPV1 is a ligand-gated ion channel that is responsive to noxious heat and capsaicin, the pungent component of chilli peppers (Caterina and Julius, 2001). This channel is able to drive a neural response when exposed to noxious heat in the normal physiological setting. When inflammation occurs, however, a decrease in local tissue acidity can potentiate the channel's response so that it is active at temperatures nearer body temperature (Caterina and Julius, 2001). This is a good example of how inflammation may cause a lowering of the nociceptive threshold in peripheral fibres and how hyperalgesia can result. A hugely intriguing point of note is that a receptor for noxious mechanical transduction, a much more obvious clinical issue, has yet to be fully elucidated. As mechanical allodynia presents such a large problem in the clinic, a cognate receptor for mechanical noxious stimuli may be of great therapeutic benefit.

Ion channels

There is very strong evidence pointing to the key role of ion channels in the production of electrical activity within sensory nerves and altered function of these channels after nerve damage (Suzuki et al., 2002). This evidence ranges from preclinical studies, the actions of drugs used in patients, and the discovery of familial pain disorders. Ion channels are important in the occurrence of altered transduction and disordered neural activity in damaged and intact fibres when neuropathy occurs.

The opening of sodium channels depolarizes neurons and generates the action potential. Injury to peripheral nerve can alter the normal arrangement of these channels along the length of a nerve. This is particularly notable in the development of neuromas after axons have been injured. Neuromas are associated with 'ectopic' electrical activity, which results from the accumulation of sodium channels at this site of injury. There also are many reports of altered distribution and levels of these channels in adjacent nerves, not just the damaged ones. Some inherited pain disorders arise from genetic mutations that either increase or decrease the functioning of a specific sodium channel subtype known as Nav 1.7 (Yang et al., 2004; Cox et al., 2006). Less dramatic polymorphisms in this channel impact on the level of pain experienced in several groups of pain patients. The latter observation suggests that inherited variations in channel function might be behind some of the variability in pain within patient groups (Reimann et al., 2010). Blockers of the channels Nav1.7 and Nav1.8, the major pain-related channels, have been described but have yet to reach the clinic. Thus, treatments presently use non-selective blockers, such as lidocaine and some anticonvulsants (e.g. carbamazepine, which is approved for the treatment of trigeminal neuralgia (Suzuki et al., 2002).

Central sensitization

While peripheral mechanisms play a large role in development of pain states, a large amount of interest has been generated in the CNS's abilities to amplify the inputs it receives from the peripheral nervous system and therefore cause an increased perception of pain. The mechanisms are multiple and complex, and again, involve changes in ion channel functioning. At spinal levels, upregulation and enhancement of transmitter release occurs via calcium channels. The drugs gabapentin and pregabalin modulate the function of these channels and, in this way, reduce transmitter release and excessive hyperexcitability.

One mechanism at the spinal level that has relevance to pain perception is called 'wind up'. 'Winding up' of neuronal responses is made possible by the physiological properties of the N-methyl-D-aspartate (NMDA) receptor (Seagrove et al., 2004). The NMDA receptor is a ligand-gated ion channel whose central pore is, under normal neuronal activity, blocked by a magnesium ion. Due to this, the NMDA receptor plays little part in normal neuronal activity. However, after prolonged peripheral C-fibre nociceptive drive, increased presynaptic release of neurotransmitters, such as glutamate and substance P, causes depolarization of the postsynaptic neurons via their actions on the α-amino-3-hydroxy-5-methyl-4-isoxazole propionic acid (AMPA) and neurokinin 1(NK1) receptors, respectively (Bannister et al., 2009). This membrane depolarization allows the release of the magnesium ion blocking the pore of the NMDA receptor, and calcium to flow through the pore, further increasing postsynaptic excitability. The influx of calcium through the NMDA receptor allows short-term changes, such as phosphorylation of AMPA and NMDA receptors in the postsynaptic membrane. All these events lead to the potentiation of postsynaptic response. NMDA receptor blockers, such as ketamine and MK-801, have been shown to be effective in the reduction of neuronal actions and pain behaviours in animal models of acute and chronic pain, as well as in human acute and chronic pain states. However, due to the widespread nature and important role that the NMDA receptor plays in many other physiological systems, NMDA blockers may cause unacceptable neurological side effects, resulting in a limited utility in the clinic.

Pathophysiology of chronic cancer pain
Aetiology

Pain is prevalent in populations with active cancer or other serious or life-threatening illnesses. As noted, cancer pain may be due directly to the tumour (tissue or nerve destruction) or may occur as a result of cancer therapy (e.g. chemotherapy-induced neuropathic pain). Bone is a common site of metastatic disease, exceeded only by lung and liver (Tubiana-Hulin, 1991), and bone pain is the most common cause of pain among patients with active cancer. Metastatic disease in bone occurs in 64–80% of those with solid tumours (Mercadante et al., 1997), and cancer-induced bone pain affects 28% of hospice inpatients, 34% of those patients in cancer pain clinics (Banning et al., 1991), and 45% of advanced cancer patients followed at home (Mercadante et al., 1997). This epidemiology highlights the need to find better drug therapies to combat pain in the clinical setting and recent progress in understanding bone pain illustrates the potential of translational research that links discoveries in the laboratory with potentially useful clinical treatments.

Animal models of cancer-induced bone pain

Until recent years, advances in the treatment of malignant bone pain were hindered by the lack of knowledge of the basic mechanisms of disease (Fig. 9.2.2). Original attempts at modelling this pathology involved administering a systemic bolus injection of metastatic tumour cells. This, however, led to systemically unwell animals, from which it was hard to draw conclusions about underlying mechanisms specific to pain rather than those related to systemic cancer (Kostenuik et al., 1993; Sasaki et al., 1998). As a consequence of these recognized deficiencies in earlier models, a number of novel approaches were developed to elucidate the mechanisms of cancer-induced bone pain. These new models rely on injecting a bolus of a variety of different tumour cells into either the long bones or the calcaneum of rodents. In general,

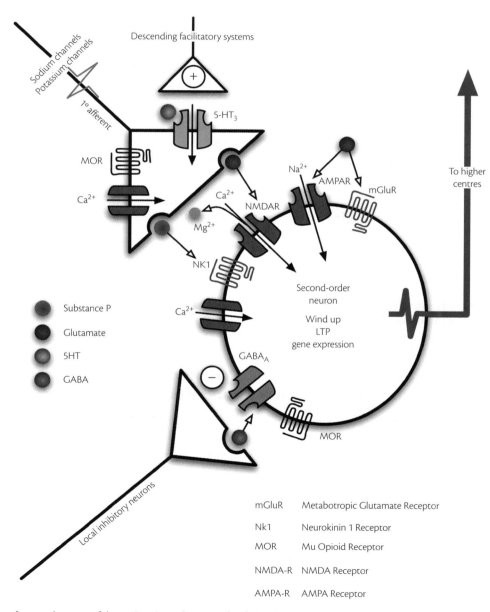

Fig. 9.2.2 Pharmacology of a central synapse of the nociceptive pathway. For details see text.

this leads to the progressive and reliable development of pain-like behaviours to either mechanical or thermal stimuli in the post-operative period. This model has been used to explore a number of pharmacological, genetic and anatomical manipulations. As a result, some basic mechanisms have now been uncovered.

Pain arising from tumour within the bone

Originally, evidence supporting innervation of tumours was limited, and therefore the precise peripheral mechanisms underlying bone pain were of great debate (see also Chapter 13.2). While there were suspect players implicated in the generation of this particular pain state, such as primary afferents, interactions in the bone/cancer microenvironment, tumour-associated macrophages and others, none had substantial support. The information was insufficient to determine whether bone pain was related to neural mechanisms, to inflammation, or to other processes. Indeed, to this day the question remains: 'Is bone cancer pain one of neuropathic or inflammatory origin?' Answering this question will involve dissecting apart the various mechanisms implicated thus far.

Structure and innervation of bone

Bone is not simply a framework to support and protect the body's internal organs. It is an active tissue and plays key roles as a reservoir for calcium and phosphate and as a source of blood cells from the bone marrow. Its mechanical characteristics permit movements via actions of the muscles. The multitude of functions carried out by bone is reflected in its complex physiology and innervation.

Structure of bone

There are two main types of bone which differ in structure and density: cortical bone and trabecular bone. Cortical bone is the dense outer layer of all bones, representing nearly 80% of all skeletal mass; it has a high resistance to torsion and bending forces. The periosteum forms the fibrous sheath surrounding the outer surface of cortical bone. Trabecular bone is found in the epiphyseal regions of long bones and constitutes a large proportion of the bone tissue of the ribs, spine, and skull. Paradoxically, this tissue type represents 20% of the skeletal mass, yet 80% of its surface area. Trabecular bone has a much less dense, woven appearance, created by interspersed trabeculae (plates) and bars of bone adjacent to red marrow cavities. For these reasons, it has more of an elastic characteristic compared with cortical bone. The cavities are connected through canaliculi, through which they receive their blood supply. Trabecular bone undergoes a greater amount of constitutive remodelling compared with the dense cortical bone and therefore bone pathology is often largely evident in bone of this type.

The remodelling of bone is reliant on an equilibrium of two main cell groups (Blair, 1998; Mackie, 2003): osteoclasts and osteoblasts. Osteoblasts are derived from primitive mesenchymal cells and are responsible for bone formation through the secretion of an array of extracellular matrix proteins (type I collagen, proteoglycans). Once osteoblasts have finished their function, they either apoptose or terminally differentiate into osteocytes, which remain viable surrounded by the bone matrix. Osteoblasts also have the interesting role of interacting with osteoclast progenitors and therefore regulate osteoclast activity.

Osteoclasts are derived from the monocyte-macrophage lineage and are the primary bone resorption cells. They are of great interest in bone pathologies such as osteoporosis and cancer-related bone pain. While a specialized cell for bone degradation may seem counterintuitive, it permits regulation of extracellular calcium and periodic bone repair, as well as remodelling in response to mechanical loads (Blair, 1998). An acidic extracellular microenvironment is highly important for an osteoclast to function properly as it is involved in the predominant mechanism through which osteoclasts degrade the base mineral hydroxyapatite. High expression of the vacuolar-(v) type electrogenic ATP-H+ channel is found along the ruffled border of the resorptive surface of an osteoclast, permitting the required development of an acidic environment of around pH 4.0–4.5 (Blair, 1998).

Mechanisms of cancer-induced bone pain

Innervation of bone

Even though it has been shown since the 1500s that nerve fibres are present in mineralized bone and the marrow cavity, tracing along the paths of blood vessels, the consensus of thought had been that pain arising from bone was principally the result of dense periosteal innervations (Mundy, 2002; Foley, 2004). While the periosteum is the most densely innervated structure, the bone marrow space receives the highest number of sensory and sympathetic fibres (Mantyh et al., 2002). Mineralized bone also receives a high volume of sympathetic and sensory fibres, more so than that of the densely innervated periosteum. All of the bone marrow, mineralized bone, and the periosteum receive both myelinated and unmyelinated sensory afferent fibres, as well as sympathetic fibres. Interestingly, of these small diameter unmyelinated fibres (presumably C-fibre population), only the CGRP trkA expressing peptidergic neurons are found to innervate bone and not the non-peptidergic IB4 labelled populations.

The theory that pain arising from bone metastases is only the result of structural weakness leading to mechanical distortion of the periosteum by innocuous stressors did not explain pain arising from bone with little or no radiographic evidence of periosteum involvement. Models of cancer-induced bone pain have now highlighted a number of other mechanisms that may be important both in peripheral and central sites.

Peripheral mechanisms of cancer-induced bone pain

Factors released in the periphery

Changes in the periphery have been shown to cause peripheral sensitization of the primary nociceptive afferents, and this peripheral sensitization can, in turn, drive central changes and hyperexcitability. When considering a tumour seeded within a bone, it is important to recognize that this includes not only cancer cells but also an inflammatory infiltrate, including macrophages, neutrophils, and T-lymphocytes (Mantyh et al., 2002). The immune-mediated response to the tumour leads to the release of a plethora of factors, such as cytokines, interleukins (ILs), chemokines, prostanoids, growth factors, and endothelins (Suzuki and Yamada, 1994; Safieh-Garabedian et al., 1995).

Peripheral nociceptors have an array of receptors that respond to these algogenic agents in the periphery. These factors are therefore able to sensitize and/or directly excite nociceptive fibres by acting on these peripheral receptors and lowering their threshold for activation. Pharmacological manipulation of these factors in a murine model of cancer-induced bone pain has shown promise in reducing measures of pain behaviour. Antagonism of endothelins, tumour necrosis factor alpha (TNFα), and bradykinin, all reduced pain behaviours (Baamonde et al., 2004; Wacnik et al., 2005), and endothelin antagonism also reduced central neurochemical markers that have been associated with the development of cancer-induced bone pain (Sorkin et al., 1997). As previously stated, the peptidergic CGRP-expressing neurons are the exclusive group of unmyelinated neurons that innervate the bone (Davar, 2001). This group of neurons express the receptor for NGF, namely trkA/p75. Macrophages, tumour cells, and other immune cells associated with the tumour mass have been previously shown to express NGF (Vega et al., 2003). The use of a NGF sequestering antibody attenuated both early and late phases of pain in the murine model of cancer-induced bone pain (Halvorson et al., 2005; Sevcik et al., 2005b) and reduced central markers of this pain state. Due to the exclusivity of trkA expressing peptidergic neurons in the bone, antagonism of this fibre type means that there can be no compensatory mechanisms in a differing fibre type.

Most importantly, as a tumour grows, there is a progressive increase in the innervation of the tissue, driven by NGF that is secreted by tumour-associated stromal cells. This pathological sprouting leads to a hyper-innervation of bone. Since almost all of the fibres express the receptor for NGF, sequestration of NGF has been shown to block both the reorganization of the sensory fibres and the associated nociceptive responses seen in models of cancer pain (Jimenez-Andrade et al., 2010).

Recently, emphasis has turned to ATP, which is present within all cells and is a purine that is algogenic and will be released into local tissues by damage. ATP has long been recognized as a local pain mediator and it is now clear that the P2X2/3 receptors are activated at peripheral and central levels in a model of cancer-induced bone pain. The data suggest that ATP may increase the activation of the central terminals of sensory afferents and so enhance spinal hyperexcitability (Kaan et al., 2010). Another receptor for ATP is the P2X7 receptor and this has been implicated in a number of animal pain models and also as a contributor to pain levels in postoperative and osteoarthritis patients. However, in a bone cancer model, deletion of the receptor had no effects on the pain behaviour, again reiterating the point that cancer pain is different from other pain conditions (Hansen et al., 2011).

The osteoclast and acidosis

With an uncertain relationship between bone destruction and pain, a number of other mechanisms for the generation of this pain state have been studied, one of which involves the activation of osteoclasts. Osteolytic tumours have been widely studied in the animal literature and have been shown to involve the recruitment of osteoclasts within the bone, leading to bone resorption. Primary tumours in bone (i.e. osteosarcoma) and secondary tumours in bone (i.e. metastatic spread from primary lung, breast, or prostate tumours) each have a profile of effects on the remodelling of bone. While some have a mainly osteolytic profile (i.e. osteosarcoma) others have a predominately osteoblastic profile (i.e. prostate carcinoma). However, in both osteolytic and osteoblastic tumours abnormal osteoclast regulation has been proposed as

both a mechanism through which tumours destroy bone and a process that generates pain in cancer patients.

Cancer-induced bone destruction has been shown to be osteoclast-mediated, and, in a proportion of cases, dependent on the receptor activator of nuclear factor kappa B (RANK)/RANK ligand (RANKL) regulatory axis. In the non-pathological situation, osteoblast and osteoclast activity are in equilibrium so that normal bone remodelling can occur (Wacnik et al., 2005). In the presence of the growth factor colony stimulating factor-1 (CSF-1), osteoblasts expressing RANKL bind to RANK on local osteoclasts and osteoclast progenitor cells to stimulate bone resorption. This in turn stimulates nearby osteoblast activity and local bone formation (Boyle et al., 2003). It has been shown that metastatic cancer cells release a number of factors that may disrupt this axis, among the most important of which is parathyroid-hormone-related peptide (PTHrP). Metastatic breast cancer in bone has a higher expression of PTHrP than metastases in soft tissue (Powell et al., 1991). In light of this, it is apparent that PTHrP causes up-regulation of RANKL on osteoblast cells, which causes terminal differentiation of osteoclast progenitor cells (Guise, 2000). Activated T lymphocytes in the immune infiltrate of the tumour mass may also express RANKL and cause further osteoclast activation (Kong et al., 1999).

Given the importance of the RANK/RANKL regulatory axis, it is unsurprising that osteoprotegerin, the soluble ligand of RANKL, has shown efficacy in preventing cancer-induced bone destruction in animal models of osteolytic skeletal destruction (Clohisy et al., 1995). Additionally, osteoprotegerin attenuates development of pain behaviours in a murine model of osteolytic sarcoma bone pain (Honore et al., 2000). As mentioned previously, osteoclasts rely on an acidic extracellular microenvironment at the osteoclast/bone interface to facilitate resorption (Delaisse and Vaes, 1992). Moreover, increased osteoclast activation leads to a decreased extracellular pH. CGRP fibres that innervate the marrow or mineralized bone express ASIC (Safieh-Garabedian et al., 1995), as well as TRPV1 (Tominaga et al., 1998). Both of these channels are either sensitized or excited by protons and therefore likely to cause nociceptive transmission due to a decrease in extracellular pH. The increase in osteoclast actions may not be solely responsible for the decrease in extracellular pH, as tumours themselves lower the extracellular pH in order to assist invasion into surrounding tissues (Stubbs et al., 2000).

Both TRPV1 antagonism and TRPV1 knock-out in murine models of bone-cancer pain show attenuation of pain behaviours (Ghilardi et al., 2005). However, in these models, both osteoclast inhibition and TRPV1 antagonism does not completely attenuate all facets of the pain behaviours seen, even in light of the fact that osteoprotegerin almost completely prevented bone destruction and osteoclast activation (Guise, 2000; Kaan et al., 2010). This suggests that while osteoclast-induced acidosis and structural weakening may play an important role in the development of malignant bone pain, it is not the sole mechanism through which this pain is generated.

Structural damage to the bone and damage to nerves

Increased osteoclast activity in this setting may also cause structural weakness. Mechanical stress upon the periosteum and its distension due to tumour burden may well result in peripheral fibre activation and the sensation of pain (Mach et al., 2002). It would be expected that the tumour growing within bone would damage the distal processes of nerves within the bone marrow, mineralized bone, and the periosteum. Studies in animal models suggest that this is indeed the case. A marker for neuronal cell injury ATF-3, which is up-regulated in the dorsal root ganglion in peripheral neuropathic pain models, is also found to be up-regulated in models of malignant bone pain. Of interest is that gabapentin, a drug that has been shown to be efficacious in models of neuropathic pain, has also been shown to be of benefit in models of cancer-induced bone pain (Sevcik, 2004; Donovan-Rodriguez et al., 2005). This suggests that nerve injury may play a role in the development of bone cancer pain. Mechanisms underlying neuropathic pain will be discussed in greater depth later in this chapter.

Central mechanisms of cancer-induced bone pain

It is also clear that the CNS undergoes changes that aid the maintenance of this pain state. The early murine models of cancer-induced bone pain involving confinement of tumour (NCTC 2472 sarcoma cells) within the femur established the neurochemical 'fingerprint' of cancer-induced bone pain. Confinement of tumour to within the bone not only leads to development of postoperative behavioural signs of pain, but increased osteoclastic bone destruction in the periphery (Schwei et al., 1999). However, of greater interest in this murine model of malignant pain were the immunohistochemical studies showing a number of central cellular and neurochemical changes in the segments of the spinal cord relating to the peripheral input. The spinal cord segments that receive afferent input from tumour-laden femur showed a massive astrocyte hypertrophy and elevation of the pro-hyperalgesic peptide dynorphin (Schwei et al., 1999). These changes were seen exclusively in the side of the spinal cord ipsilateral to the affected limb and not on the contralateral side. Glia, a family of which astrocytes are a member, are in the normal situation quiescent. Upon becoming activated, glia release a myriad of pro-inflammatory cytokines, including IL-1, TNF, IL-6, reactive oxygen species, nitric oxide, prostaglandins, excitatory amino acids, and ATP (Watkins and Maier, 2003). This in turn can cause enhanced second-order neuron excitability within the dorsal horn and further exaggerate primary afferent neurotransmitter release. It has also been demonstrated in murine models that normally non-noxious palpation of the affected femur not only produced nocifensive behaviour but an increase in substance P receptor internalization and an increase in c-Fos expression in lamina I neurons of the dorsal horn (Schwei et al., 1999).

These findings provide a weight of evidence showing that primary afferent fibres are sensitized following tumour growth in the periphery. This astrocyctosis, increased dynorphin expression, increased substance P internalization, and increased c-Fos expression has been shown in models of inflammatory and/or neuropathic pain. While substance P levels in primary afferent neurons have been shown to increase in inflammatory models and decrease in neuropathic models, levels remain unchanged in cancer-induced bone pain states. However, the coexistence of all these features in cancer-induced bone pain provides evidence that this is a unique pain state that may have mechanisms similar to inflammation and neuropathy (Schwei et al., 1999). Furthermore, this may well be the basis of reasoning behind why conventional

treatments have failed thus far in the battle with malignant bone pain and further highlights the need for unique pharmacotherapy (Fig. 9.2.3).

By recording second-order neurons in the dorsal horn of the spinal cord using in vivo electrophysiology, we can gain an idea of the supra-threshold response to peripheral stimuli that cannot be ascertained using behavioural techniques (Urch et al., 2003; Donovan-Rodriguez et al., 2005). Neurons can be characterized, based on their responses to mechanical, thermal, and electrically evoked stimuli. The SDH is predominantly populated with nociceptive specific (NS) neurons, which respond to nociceptive stimuli. These cells are distinguished from WDR neurons, which respond to a wide range of both noxious and innocuous stimuli (Seagrove, 2004). Establishment of cancer-induced bone pain changes the ratio of WDR:NS neurons in the SDH from the 26% WDR:74% NS in a sham animal to 47% WDR to 53% in the pathological setting (Stubbs et al., 2000). The phenotype shift seen in the superficial dorsal horn was also paralleled by the development of superficial and deep dorsal horn neuronal hyperexcitability to mechanical, thermal, and electrical stimuli, further suggesting ongoing central sensitization. Furthermore, these lamina I neurons that become hyperexcitable after cancer-induced bone pain now show a *de novo* or increased responsivity in the innocuous range (Stubbs et al., 2000). Thus pain selective neurons can now be activated by innocuous stimuli. This may allow the limbic areas of the brain, concerned with affective/emotional aspects of pain, to have an influence via the parabrachial pathways, and also increase the effects of low-threshold stimuli. Plausibly, this may result in affective areas of the brain now being dominated by painful messages and so relate to the distress and co-morbidities such as fear, anxiety, mood changes and sleep disorders caused by pain.

This hyperexcitability in lamina I also plays a role in further maintaining neuronal dorsal horn hyperexcitability through descending facilitations. Spinal events are not only controlled by afferent input but also by descending controls from higher centres (Bannister et al., 2009). Higher-order cognitive and emotional processes such as anxiety, mood, and attention can influence perceived pain. Such phenomena are enabled by the convergence of somatic and limbic systems into such descending modulatory systems. Areas in the midbrain and brainstem, such as the PAG and the rostroventral medial medulla (RVM), are key structures in the descending modulatory repertoire (Bannister et al., 2009). Such a system is important as it provides neural networks by which cognitive and emotional states can influence pain processing at the level of the spinal cord (Suzuki et al., 2004; Bannister et al., 2009). In short, these circuits allow the brain to exert some control over spinal pain events. Recent animal studies suggest that in addition to inhibitory systems, there are important descending facilitations that can be engaged by external and internal processes, and act to enhance intrinsic spinal mechanisms of pain. Lamina I neurons expressing the substance P receptor NK1 form the origin of a spinobulbospinal loop, which relays through the RVM (Todd, 2002; Bannister et al., 2009). The RVM has been highlighted as a key area involved with descending facilitations which are thought to be mediated through the 5-hydroxytryptamine type 3 (5-HT$_3$) receptor. Blockade of spinal 5-HT$_3$ receptors with intrathecal ondansetron reduces the mechanical and thermal evoked responses of superficial and deep dorsal horn neurons (Bannister et al., 2009). This suggests that descending facilitations are indeed

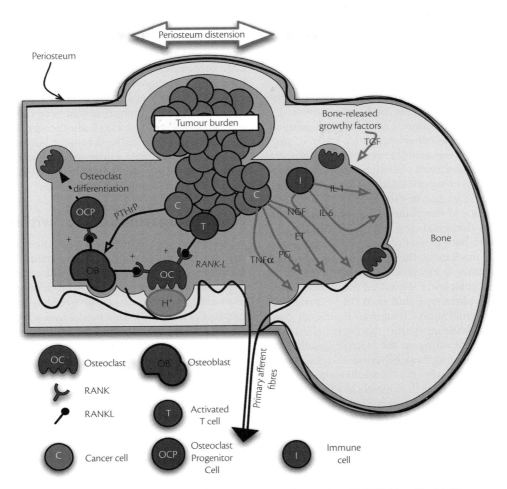

Fig. 9.2.3 A summary of the peripheral mechanisms of cancer-induced bone pain. Increased expression of RANKL (ligand for RANK, receptor activator of nuclear κ B—activator of osteoclast progenitor cells, OCP), on osteoblasts (due to interaction with tumour cells via PTHrP) and activated T cells in the tumour mass causes increased activation of osteoclasts. An increasingly acidic extracellular environment may activate/sensitize peripheral neurons, by activating TRPV1/ASIC on the peripheral neuron (see Fig. 9.2.1). This in conjunction factors release from tumour cells, bone matrix, and tumour-associated immune cells that are known to sensitize primary afferents acting at their cognate receptors (see text) on primary afferent neurons innervating the bone. Disease progression may lead to further bone destruction and a swelling of the periosteum leading to activation of periosteal nerve fibres and the transmission of noxious stimuli.

important in amplifying nociceptive transmission from the dorsal horn to higher centres (Suzuki et al., 2004; Bannister et al., 2009).

Mechanisms of cancer-induced bone pain related to treatment

Current therapies give researchers a great insight into the possible mechanisms underlying cancer pain. Opioids are the mainstay of treatment of severe malignant pain in the clinic (Mercadante et al 1997). However, while the benefits to be gained from opioid therapy are obvious, opioid treatment is associated with a large number of side effects, such as nausea, vomiting, constipation, sedation, and delirium. At the high doses sometimes required to relieve persistent cancer pain, these side effects become even more problematic to control and, in some cases, may be the reason for inadequate analgesia. In line with clinical evidence, opioids are effective in reducing pain-like behaviours in a number of animal models of cancer-induced bone pain.

Early data from murine models suggest that higher doses of morphine were required to attenuate cancer-induced bone pain

than those needed in inflammatory pain, and this point was used to further highlight the mechanistic differences between these two pain states (Luger et al., 2002). The relatively low efficacy of acute morphine has since been further validated (Mercadante et al., 1997; Vermeirsch et al., 2004); however, a situation that more closely mimicked the clinical paradigm was sought. A bi-daily injection schedule over 5 days after the establishment of the pain state has been shown to be highly effective in reducing behavioural signs of cancer-induced bone pain (Urch et al., 2005). This regimen also was found to be more efficacious than a single acute dose (Sevcik et al., 2004). However, even in light of this, behavioural measurements taken pre and post the final morphine administration, at peak disease progression, indicated a significantly reduced analgesia between consecutive morphine administrations. This is not to say that the analgesia provided by morphine completely wore off between doses. Behavioural signs of pain were still, 12 hours after the last dose, significantly reduced from that of the vehicle-treated animals and no different from that of the acutely treated group. However this may help to explain the requirement for escalated doses of opioids to treat severe cancer-induced bone pain.

Chronic, but not acute, gabapentin administration also has been shown to be effective in these models (Donovan-Rodriguez et al., 2005; Peters et al., 2005). Gabapentin acts by binding to the calcium channel accessory subunit α2δ. This implies a role of α2δ in the pathology underlying this pain state. Yet looking at the response of neurons in chronic morphine and chronic gabapentin regimens highlights two differing mechanisms involved in cancer-related bone pain. While chronic morphine and gabapentin administration both lead to behavioural attenuation of pain, chronic morphine treatment was unable to completely reset dorsal horn excitability and the associated phenotype shift towards the WDR neuronal population in superficial dorsal horn (Urch et al., 2005). The bias of superficial neurons toward the WDR phenotype, even in the presence of morphine analgesia, suggests that low-threshold inputs to the spinal cord may still access areas of the brain concerned with both pain affect and perception. This is a possible physiological mechanism through which breakthrough pain may remain refractory to morphine analgesia in the clinic. In contrast, gabapentin completely attenuated dorsal horn excitability and reversed the phenotype shift of WDR:NS ratio back towards that seen in a normal animal (Donovan-Rodriguez et al., 2005). This suggests that while morphine may cause behavioural attenuation of pain, it is not acting on the mechanisms that are intricately involved in producing those behavioural signs. On the other hand, gabapentin is able to inhibit the mechanisms that lead to cancer-induced bone pain rather than merely blocking sensory inputs as seen with morphine. Upon the termination of gabapentin treatment, pain behaviours and dorsal horn excitability returned to their hyperexcitable 'pathological' state, implicating neuronal physiological mechanisms rather than anatomical changes to be key in development of cancer-induced bone pain.

Peripheral opioids may also have a role to play in the management of malignant cancer pain. In support of this potential is evidence showing that loperamide, the peripheral mu opioid receptor agonist, is able to attenuate thermal hyperalgesia in a murine model of cancer-induced bone pain (Menendez et al., 2003).

Non-steroidal anti-inflammatory drugs (NSAIDs) are the first step on the World Health Organization's (WHO) ladder for the use of analgesics for the relief of cancer pain. Although NSAIDs are still used as an analgesic additive even after increased pain severity (Mercadante et al., 1997), the clinical data supporting their efficacy is limited (Urch, 2004). NSAIDs inhibit the cyclooxygenase (COX) enzyme and therefore attenuate the synthesis of prostaglandins from arachidonic acid. This ultimately prevents sensitization or activation of primary afferents by prostaglandins produced locally by tumour cells and/or the immune response. Inhibition of the COX-2 enzyme, the local inducible form of COX, using three different COX-2 selective inhibitors in a rat and murine models of cancer-induced bone pain has been shown to be effective in ameliorating behavioural pain signs. In both these studies, chronic COX-2 inhibition has been shown to be better at attenuating pain-like signs than a single acute dose. Chronic administration reduced tumour burden and bone destruction (Sabino et al., 2002; Fox et al., 2004), suggesting that COX-2 inhibition may be acting at multiple sites rather than at a single point in a pathway.

Bisphosphonates are used widely in the clinical setting and prevent bone resorption by osteoclast inhibition. Bisphosphonates were able to reduce pain scores, as well as bone and sensory nerve destruction, in both rat and mouse models of cancer-induced bone pain (Sevcik et al., 2004; Walker et al., 2002). However, tumour burden was found to not be affected, with both tumour burden and tumour necrosis increasing (Sevcik et al., 2004). Bisphosphonates, therefore, may have a role to play in reducing bone pain in malignancy, especially if combined with other analgesics (Mercadante et al., 1997).

Radiotherapy of tumours within bone causes analgesia but the mechanism is still unclear. Radiotherapy in the murine model of bone cancer pain reduced tumour burden by more than 75% (Goblirsch et al., 2005). However, it did not affect the osteoclast density, suggesting that radiotherapy causes analgesia via direct mechanisms on tumour cells themselves.

Pain arising from tumour within soft tissues

While pain arising from bone is a common clinical problem, pain arising from soft tissue can also be painful. The pathophysiology in this pain state, however, is still not clear. A novel model of pancreatic cancer pain has been developed to elucidate the relationship between disease progression and pain development (Lindsay et al., 2005). This model uses a transgenic mouse that develops pancreatic cancer and shows changes similar to that seen in the human condition. These include tumour growth, increased innervation, macrophage infiltration, weight loss, and pain. More significantly, pain was only evident at a point at which cancer progression was highly advanced. Sensory innervation has now been quantified and models such as these will hopefully provide mechanistic insights in to the development of pancreatic cancer pain in the future.

Neuropathic pain

The International Association for the Study of Pain (IASP) defines neuropathic pain as 'pain initiated or caused by a primary lesion or dysfunction in the nervous system'. This may not be a complete definition of neuropathic pain, and the definition is changing to be 'a lesion or disease' affecting the 'sensory nervous system' (Treede et al., 2008). These definitions hint at broad mechanisms. After nerve injury occurs, there are large-scale changes that occur within the peripheral and central nervous systems. This nerve plasticity has been heavily scrutinized and some of these plastic changes have been proposed as possible important mechanisms for the generation of pain in neuropathic states.

Mechanisms of cytotoxic neuropathy

Neuropathic pain may arise in the palliative care setting for a multitude of reasons. Nerve damage is known to occur as a result of tumour compressing a nerve, surgical resection, radiotherapy, and chemotherapy. Numerous pre-clinical animal models have been developed in an effort to elucidate the basic mechanisms involved in the generation and maintenance of neuropathic pain. These include models of peripheral nerve injury (common in traumatic neuropathic pain) and chemotherapy-induced neuropathic pain. Peripheral lesions to nerves are obvious, and therefore many models of traumatic peripheral nerve injury exist. Consequently, a multitude of mechanisms have been implicated in painful peripheral nerve lesions. It would be wrong to believe that mechanisms of peripheral nerve injury are the same whether caused by chemical injury, constriction, or by the surgeon's scalpel. It is for these reasons that the pharmacotherapy of different types of neuropathic pain should differ. One only has to look at the different responsiveness of trigeminal neuralgia and other neuropathic pain syndromes to drugs such as carbamazepine to see that mechanisms underlying these neuropathies must differ. Iatrogenic neuropathic pain caused by various drug treatments is well recognized. Theoretically, it should be of no surprise that chemotherapeutic agents and antiretrovirals, compounds which broadly act through inhibiting cellular processes, may have neuropathic side effects.

The chemotherapy agents vincristine and paclitaxel and the nucleoside reverse transcriptase inhibitors (NRTIs) such as dideoxycytidine have a well-established history of causing painful neuropathy (Berger et al., 1993; Forsyth et al., 1997), with the incidence of painful neuropathies in paclitaxel-treated patients suggested to be around 22% (Forsyth et al., 1997). Paclitaxel binds to microtubules and promotes hyperpolymerization. This interferes with the mitotic spindle formation and promotes cellular arrest in the metaphase-anaphase transition, and consequently apoptosis (Jordan et al., 1996; Yvon et al., 1999). As the precise mechanism of paclitaxel-induced neuropathy is still not clear, it has been assumed that the binding of paclitaxel to microtubules of neurons, which consequently prevents anterograde and reterograde axonal transport, could lead to a neuropathic state. However, these proposed mechanisms of both tumour apoptosis and neuropathy have been questioned, and the precise mechanisms are still not clear (Komiya and Tashiro, 1988; Fan, 1999). Another chemotherapeutic agent, vincristine, is said to act via a similar mechanism, inhibiting normal polymerization of β-tubulin, leading to abnormal spindle function. Early studies showed that epineural injection of paclitaxel caused oedema and axonal degeneration (Roytta and Raine, 1986) along with interference of axonal transport and microtubule anomalies. However, a number of sources have doubted the theory that axonal degeneration and microtubule anomalies occur, citing the unusually high concentrations of paclitaxel in the epineural injections responsible for the local axonal reactions (Polomano and Bennett, 2001). These local epineural injections allowed paclitaxel to bypass the liver, so that any metabolites usually involved in the development of pathology would not be present.

Mitochondria have now been shown to play an important role in the establishment of some pain states, especially chemotherapy and NRTI-induced neuropathic pain. Change in mitochondrial function has been shown to be involved in the pathogenesis of neurodegenerative diseases; however, this has not previously been widely studied in pain. In patients, neuropathies solely due to disarray in mitochondrial function have been shown to have an increased incidence of developing pain (Finsterer, 2004).

These mitochondrial effects may be relevant to the mechanisms described recently in models of chemotherapy-induced neuropathic pain that are more akin to the clinical scenario. Low-dose systemic injections of paclitaxel produced mechanical hypersensitivity, yet even at the stage of peak pain-like behaviours, there were no signs of axonal degeneration, markedly altered microtubules, or impairment of axonal transport (Flatters and Bennett, 2006). However, abnormal mitochondria in C fibres and myelinated axons were noted and this was suggested to be the cause of paclitaxel's actions. In this model, it was proposed that paclitaxel's binding to mitochondria caused opening of the mitochondria permeability transition pore, causing calcium ion influx into the cytosol. This mitochondrial calcium efflux has been suggested to be both the cause of mitochondrial swelling as well as of primary afferent excitability and pain behaviour (Flatters and Bennett, 2006). The T-type calcium channel blocker ethosuximide, α2δ calcium channel subunit ligand, gabapentin, and calcium chelators, all block neuropathic pain behaviours caused by chemotherapeutic agents (Flatters and Bennett, 2004; Xiao et al., 2006).

Mitochondrial damage is also the proposed mechanism for the neuropathy seen after treatment with NRTIs for HIV/AIDs (Joseph et al., 2004; Joseph and Levine, 2006). The mitochondrial electron transport chain and its end product, ATP, have also been a suggested pathological player in the development of neuropathic pain due to both chemotherapy and antiretroviral treatment; however, the downstream targets in the pathological setting are still to be elucidated (Joseph and Levine, 2006). It has also been noted that both paclitaxel- and vincristine-evoked painful peripheral neuropathies show a loss of innervation of the epidermal sensory fibres as well as the Langerhans cells, the skin's resident immune cells. Whether this is a causal or merely consequential finding is yet to be shown (Siau et al., 2006).

Pain associated with HIV infection

Iatrogenic neuropathic pain due to treatment with NRTIs is not the only cause of neuropathic pain in HIV/AIDS patients. Around 10–15% of all HIV-1 infected patients have a symptomatic distal polyneuropathy (Verma, 2001), a proportion of which experience pain as a result. It has been shown that direct infection of neurons by HIV has a negligible incidence rate and it is for this reason that the attention of researchers turned to the neuroimmune system. An envelope protein of HIV-1, gp120 has been widely shown to produce hindpaw hypersensitivity to thermal and mechanical stimuli when injected into the intrathecal space (Milligan et al., 2001), as well as directly to the sciatic nerve of the rat (Herzberg, and Sagen, 2001). Astrocytes and microglia have been shown to bind to the virus epitope gp120, which in turn causes their activation. Milligan et al. showed that attenuating glial activation ameliorates the development of behavioural hypersensitivity of animals once exposed to gp120 (Milligan et al., 2001). In this study, the response of microglia and astrocytes to gp120 was blocked. As mentioned previously, activation of glia in the spinal cord by exogenous factors, such as gp120, causes the transcription and release of factors such as prostaglandins, excitatory amino acids, IL-1, and IL-6 as well as inducing nitric oxide synthetase expression in glial cells (Kreutzberg, 1996; Kong et al., 1996). The release of these factors from glia in the dorsal horn may well be able to directly excite local sensory neurons and propagate the sensation of pain, even without the presence of a peripheral pathology. The development of spinal sensitization has been put forward as an explanation for why pains in HIV-1 infected patients commonly present without obvious peripheral pathologies and are vague and diffuse in nature (Breitbart et al., 1996; Hewitt et al., 1997).

Mechanisms underlying the generation of pain in neuropathy

Many changes in the periphery have been implicated in the development of neuropathic pain, but none have been more heavily studied than the role of ion channel dysregulation on peripheral nerves. Normally, tactile stimulation of sensory nerve terminals in the skin, viscera, or bone leads to the propagation of an action potential and sensory signalling. However, after nerve injury, many peripheral nerves display ectopic discharge, which may lead to an increased barrage of nociceptive signalling onto dorsal horn transmission neurons without a peripheral stimulus. Electrophysiologically, neuronal responses of second-order deep dorsal horn neurons are heightened after nerve injury in rodent models, with an increase in receptive field size and an increased response to natural stimuli applied to the hindpaw. This goes hand in hand with increased spontaneous activity and hyperexcitability of these neurons.

Changes in the sodium channel populations on peripheral nerves and their subsequent aberrant activity have been of great interest due to their key role in setting neuronal excitability and therefore the development of pain states (Suzuki et al., 2002; Cox et al., 2006; Cummins et al., 2007). Expression of sets of sodium channels on the peripheral neurons shows plasticity after nerve injury. The mRNA of NaV1.3, a usually embryonic TTX-sensitive current, has been found to increase after axotomy and this may play a role in the generation of ectopic activity in peripheral nerve fibres. The sensory neuron specific sodium channel, NaV1.8 is also thought to play a key role in the generation of abnormal sensory signalling following nerve injury. NaV1.8 protein is markedly decreased in the dorsal root ganglion of predominantly small fibres after nerve injury. This is paralleled by an increase in immunoreactivity of the channel in the distal axons and nerve terminals, representing a redistribution of the channel to the distal sites of the neuron, where it may take part in the development of hyperexcitability and increased nociceptive transmission. Both in humans and animals, sodium channel accumulation has been shown to occur around the neuroma formed at the site of the nerve lesion. This has long been the pharmacological basis for the use of drugs such as carbamazepine, lamotrigine, and local anaesthetics in patients with neuropathic pain. After nerve injury, demyelination and abnormal trafficking of sodium channels occurs along the membrane of injured nerves and maybe in the uninjured neighbours. This may lower the threshold for activation and induce ectopic activity in the peripheral nerve. This contributes to the development of central sensitization and amplification of peripheral events, possibly leading to the allodynia and hyperalgesia seen in patients (see Suzuki et al., 2002; Cox et al., 2006).

Voltage-gated calcium channels (VGCCs) may also play a large hand in the increased peripheral nociceptive drive in neuropathic pain. VGCCs play a key role in permitting neurotransmitter release from the presynaptic terminal and, therefore, the postsynaptic propagation of the sensory signal. As with sodium channels, there are a large number of calcium channels that play a role in neuronal excitability. Activation of calcium channels by peripheral electrical events causes the inward flow of calcium and allows neurotransmitter vesicle exocytosis and thus postsynaptic depolarization. However, VGCCs not only have presynaptic actions but also act at the postsynaptic site, allowing activation of postsynaptic second messenger cascades. This may lead to altered gene expression, protein synthesis, and therefore long-term plastic changes. Long-term potentiation of dorsal horn neurons, caused by repetitive afferent stimulation, may be of importance in maintaining exaggerated neuronal responses for long periods after increased peripheral drive has subsided (Rygh et al., 2006).

Specific targeting of these VGCCs and their accessory subunits seems to be beneficial in the treatment of neuropathic pain, with novel drugs acting at these sites now available. Gabapentin and its newer analogue pregabalin have shown benefit to patients with neuropathic pain. Their target is thought to be the α2δ accessory subunit of calcium channels. Gabapentin has been shown to be effective in reducing neuronal responses in a model of neuropathic pain (Suzuki et al., 2005). However, gabapentin's inability to reduce neuronal responses in normal animals highlights a clear state dependency of gabapentin's action and implicates a role for the α2δ subunit in neuropathic pain pathology. The α2δ subunit has been shown to up-regulate after nerve injury and this correlates not only with the development of behavioural allodynia in these animals but also with gabapentin's behavioural antiallodynic efficacy (Luo et al., 2001). Gabapentin's actions have now been characterized in many differing animal models of neuropathic pain including a model of chemotheraputic paclitaxel-induced neuropathic pain (Xiao et al., 2006).

Another target for the treatment of neuropathic pain is the N-type calcium channel. It was shown that blockade of the N-type calcium channel with ω-conotoxin-GIVA reduced dorsal horn neuronal responses in animals with neuropathic pain and that the release of substance P and CGRP from primary afferents was N-type dependent (Matthews and Dickenson, 2001). An analogue of ω-conotoxin-GIVA, ziconotide, has now been developed and is now licensed for the treatment of neuropathic pain.

In addition to spinal changes, higher brain centres are able to facilitate dorsal horn neuronal activity. An ascending descending facilitatory pathway seems to play a critical role in chronic pain states, such as neuropathic pain. Superficial dorsal horn NK1 neurons project to higher brainstem nuclei, such as the parabrachial nucleus, which receives connections from amygdala and hypothalamus and may explain the ability of emotion to affect pain processing (Bannister et al., 2009). Along with the affective implications, these brainstem nuclei form a part of a spinal-bulbo-spinal loop, which through the RVM, can facilitate dorsal horn neuronal responses. Ablation of these NK1-expressing projection neurons, using a saporin toxin conjugated to substance P, is able to attenuate dorsal horn neuronal responses to stimuli evoked in the periphery (Suzuki et al., 2005). Using an antagonist of the excitatory 5-HT$_3$ receptor, it is clear that these descending facilitations are in the large part serotonergic acting at the 5-HT$_3$ receptor in the spinal cord. These descending facilitations contribute to maintaining central sensitization in pathological pain states and may well aid the development of tactile allodynia seen in patients with chronic pain. The analgesia produced by tricyclic antidepressants and serotonin-norepinephrine reuptake inhibitors are no doubt due to interactions with these descending controls, which are altered in many pain states, including cancer pain (Dickenson and Ghandehari, 2007; Bannister et al., 2009).

Astonishingly, gabapentin's actions in reducing neuronal responses in nerve-ligated animals were blocked by both the ablation of these superficial projection neurons and by the application of ondansetron (Suzuki et al., 2005). However, the activation of the 5-HT$_3$ receptor allowed gabapentin to reduce neuronal responses in normal animals, suggesting that this supraspinal loop needs to be in place for gabapentin's action to be unmasked.

Conclusion

Any advances in the understanding and treatment of pain in cancer and other terminal illnesses will need to be based on a better understanding of pain mechanisms, so that existing therapies can be used with greater efficacy. Further knowledge of these mechanisms is a basis for the development of future therapeutic approaches based on controlling the pathophysiology, as well as the pain itself.

This chapter illustrates how important advances in understanding the pathophysiology of pain have been made in recent years and provide a basis for improvements in the treatment of the pain, distress, and co-morbidities. Tumour growing in the periphery elicits a series of changes that run from peripheral tissue and nerve, causes profound changes in spinal cord function, and in the final experience of pain, involves complex circuits in the brain that link pain with affective function.

Acknowledgements

The authors acknowledge funding from the Wellcome Trust London Pain Consortium.

Online materials

Complete references for this chapter are available online at <http://www.oxfordmedicine.com>.

References

Bannister, K., Bee, L.A., and Dickenson, A.H. (2009). Preclinical and early clinical investigations related to monoaminergic pain modulation. *Neurotherapeutics*, 6(4), 703–712.

Blair, H.C. (1998). How the osteoclast degrades bone. *Bioessays*, 20(10), 837–846.

Breitbart, W., McDonald, M.V., Rosenfeld, B., *et al.* (1996). Pain in ambulatory AIDS patients. I: pain characteristics and medical correlates. *Pain*, 68(2–3), 315–321.

Caterina, M.J. and Julius, D. (2001). The vanilloid receptor: a molecular gateway to the pain pathway. *Annual Review of Neuroscience*, 24, 487–517.

Dickenson and Ghandehari. (2007). Anti-convulsants and anti-depressants. *Handbook of Experimental Pharmacology*, 177, 145–177.

Donovan-Rodriguez, T., Dickenson, A.H., and Urch, C.E. (2005). Gabapentin normalizes spinal neuronal responses that correlate with behavior in a rat model of cancer-induced bone pain. *Anesthesiology*, 102(1), 132–140.

Flatters, S.J. and Bennett, G.J. (2006). Studies of peripheral sensory nerves in paclitaxel-induced painful peripheral neuropathy: evidence for mitochondrial dysfunction. *Pain*, 122(3), 245–257.

Foley, K.M. (2004). Treatment of cancer-related pain. *Journal of the National Cancer Institute, Monographs*, 32, 103–104.

Forsyth, P.A., Balmaceda, C., Peterson, K., *et al.* (1997). Prospective study of paclitaxel-induced peripheral neuropathy with quantitative sensory testing. *Journal of Neurooncology*, 35(1), 47–53.

Ghilardi, J.R., Rohrich, H., Lindsay, T.H., *et al.* (2005). Selective blockade of the capsaicin receptor TRPV1 attenuates bone cancer pain. *Journal of Neuroscience*, 25(12), 3126–3131.

Hansen, R.R., Nielsen, C.K., Nasser, A., *et al.* (2011). P2X7 receptor-deficient mice are susceptible to bone cancer pain. *Pain*, 152(8), 1766–1776.

Hewitt, D.J., McDonald, M., Portenoy, R.K., *et al.* (1997). Pain syndromes and etiologies in ambulatory AIDS patients. *Pain*, 70(2–3), 117–123.

Jimenez-Andrade, J.M., Bloom, A.P., Stake, J.I., *et al.* (2010). Pathological sprouting of adult nociceptors in chronic prostate cancer-induced bone pain. *Journal of Neuroscience*, 30(44), 14649–14656.

Joseph, E.K., Chen, X., Khasar, S.G., *et al.* (2004). Novel mechanism of enhanced nociception in a model of AIDS therapy-induced painful peripheral neuropathy in the rat. *Pain*, 107(1–2), 147–158.

Kaan, T.K., Yip, P.K., Patel, S., *et al.* (2010). Systemic blockade of P2X3 and P2X2/3 receptors attenuates bone cancer pain behaviour in rats. *Brain*, 133(9), 2549–2564.

Lindsay, T.H., Jonas, B.M., Sevcik, M.A., *et al.* (2005). Pancreatic cancer pain and its correlation with changes in tumor vasculature, macrophage infiltration, neuronal innervation, body weight and disease progression. *Pain*, 119(1–3), 233–246.

Luger, N.M., Sabino, M.A., Schwei, M.J., *et al.* (2002). Efficacy of systemic morphine suggests a fundamental difference in the mechanisms that generate bone cancer vs inflammatory pain. *Pain*, 99(3), 397–406.

Luo, Z.D., Chaplan, S.R., Higuera, E.S., *et al.* (2001). Upregulation of dorsal root ganglion (alpha)2(delta) calcium channel subunit and its correlation with allodynia in spinal nerve-injured rats. *Journal of Neuroscience*, 21(6), 1868–1875.

Mantyh, P.W., Clohisy, D.R., Koltzenburg, M., *et al.* (2002). Molecular mechanisms of cancer pain. *Nature Reviews Cancer*, 2(3), 201–209.

Milligan, E.D., O'Connor, K.A., Nguyen, K.T., *et al.* (2001). Intrathecal HIV-1 envelope glycoprotein gp120 induces enhanced pain states mediated by spinal cord proinflammatory cytokines. *Journal of Neuroscience*, 21(8), 2808–2819.

Peters, C.M., Ghilardi, J.R., Keyser, C.P., *et al.* (2005). Tumor-induced injury of primary afferent sensory nerve fibers in bone cancer pain. *Experimental Neurology*, 193(1), 85–100.

Polomano, R.C. and Bennett, G.J. (2001). Chemotherapy-evoked painful peripheral neuropathy. *Pain in Medicine*, 2(1), 8–14.

Reimann, F., Cox, J.J., Belfer, I., Diatchenko, L., and Zaykin, D.V. (2010). Pain perception is altered by a nucleotide polymorphism in SCN9A. *Proceedings of the National Academy of Sciences of the United States of America*, 16, 107(11), 5148–5153.

Schwei, M.J., Honore, P., Rogers, S.D., *et al.* (1999). Neurochemical and cellular reorganization of the spinal cord in a murine model of bone cancer pain. *Journal of Neuroscience*, 19(24), 10886–10897.

Seagrove, L.C.1, Suzuki, R., and Dickenson A.H. (2004). Electrophysiological characterisations of rat lamina I dorsal horn neurones and the involvement of excitatory amino acid receptors. *Pain*, 108(1–2), 76–87.

Sevcik, M.A., Luger, N.M., Mach, D.B., *et al.* (2004). Bone cancer pain: the effects of the bisphosphonate alendronate on pain, skeletal remodeling, tumor growth and tumor necrosis. *Pain*, 111(1–2), 169–180.

Siau, C., Xiao, W., and Bennett, G.J. (2006). Paclitaxel- and vincristine-evoked painful peripheral neuropathies: loss of epidermal innervation and activation of Langerhans cells. *Experimental Neurology*, 201(2), 507–514.

Sorkin, L.S., Xiao, W.H., Wagner, R., *et al.* (1997). Tumour necrosis factor-alpha induces ectopic activity in nociceptive primary afferent fibres. *Neuroscience*, 81(1), 255–262.

Stubbs, M., McSheehy, P.M., Griffiths, J.R., and Bashford, C.L. (2000). Causes and consequences of tumour acidity and implications for treatment. *Molecular Medicine Today*, 6(1), 15–19.

Suzuki, R., Matthews, E.A., and Dickenson, A.H. (2002). Neurobiology of neuropathic pain: mode of action of anticonvulsants. *European Journal of Pain*, 6, 51–60.

Suzuki, R., Rahman, W., Rygh, L.J., *et al.* (2005). Spinal-supraspinal serotonergic circuits regulating neuropathic pain and its treatment with gabapentin. *Pain*, 117(3), 292–303.

Treede, R.D., Jensen, T.S., Campbell, J.N., *et al.* (2008). Neuropathic pain: redefinition and a grading system for clinical and research purposes. *Neurology*, 70, 1630–1635.

Urch, C.E., Donovan-Rodriguez, T., and Dickenson, A.H. (2003). Alterations in dorsal horn neurones in a rat model of cancer-induced bone pain. *Pain*, 106(3), 347–356.

Urch, C.E., Donovan-Rodriguez, T., Gordon-Williams, R., *et al.* (2005). Efficacy of chronic morphine in a rat model of cancer-induced bone pain: behavior and in dorsal horn pathophysiology. *Journal of Pain*, 6(12), 837–845.

Verma, A. (2001). Epidemiology and clinical features of HIV-1 associated neuropathies. *Journal of the Peripheral Nervous System*, 6(1), 8–13.

Vermeirsch, H., Nuydens, R.M., Salmon, P.L., *et al.* (2004). Bone cancer pain model in mice: evaluation of pain behavior, bone destruction and morphine sensitivity. *Pharmacology, Biochemistry, and Behavior*, 79(2), 243–251.

Watkins, L.R. and Maier, S.F. (2003). Glia: a novel drug discovery target for clinical pain. *Nature Reviews Drug Discovery*, 2(12), 973–985.

Xiao, W., Boroujerdi, A., Bennett, G.J., *et al.* (2006). Chemotherapy-evoked painful peripheral neuropathy: analgesic effects of gabapentin and effects on expression of the alpha-2-delta type-1 calcium channel subunit. *Neuroscience*, 144, 714–720.

Definition and assessment of chronic pain in advanced disease

Clare Rayment and Michael I. Bennett

Background to chronic pain in advanced disease

Definition of chronic pain in advanced disease

The International Association for the Study of Pain (IASP, 2011) defines pain as an 'unpleasant sensory and emotional experience associated with actual or potential tissue damage, or described in terms of such damage'. Chronic pain is defined as 'pain which persists beyond the usual course of healing or is associated with chronic pathological illness which causes continuous pain or pain which recurs at intervals for months of years' (Bonica, 1990). Pain is always subjective, corresponding to what the patient describes. This point, which is emphasized by the IASP, underscores the observation that correlation between observed behaviour and patient reports of pain may be poor as individual response to pain varies considerably. All pain-related behaviour, including verbal report, is influenced by its perceived meaning, and an individual's culture, ethnicity, and mood (Cleeland et al., 1996; Twycross, 1997). Verbal report is the simplest to interpret clinically, but other behaviours are relevant to a broader understanding of the pain. In those patients unable to communicate effectively, such as infants or those who are cognitively impaired, changes in behaviour may be the key clinical finding.

The concept of 'total pain' acknowledges the physical, psychological, social, and spiritual influence on a patient's perception of pain, and the multidimensional effects it has on a person's life (Saunders, 1967; Portenoy and Lesage, 1999; Zaza and Baine, 2002; Foley, 2004; Ferreira et al., 2008; Portenoy, 2011). Without attention to all these areas, pain relief is unlikely to be optimal (Saunders, 1967).

Defining the likely pathophysiology of the pain is an essential part of the broader understanding which may help enable appropriate treatment. Nociceptive pain is defined as 'pain that arises from actual or threatened damage to non-neural tissue and is due to the activation of nociceptors' (IASP, 2011). In contrast, neuropathic pain is defined by the Neuropathic Pain Special Interest Group (NeuPSIG) of the IASP as 'pain caused by a lesion or disease of the somatosensory nervous system'. It is often then further classified as peripheral or central and by anatomical site and disease. Both these terms are descriptions of pain, not diagnoses.

Breakthrough pain is the term most widely used to describe variations in quality, intensity, and timing of pain on a background of stable pain control (Haugen et al., 2010). It can be predictable, unpredictable, spontaneous, or evoked with the same quality or a different quality to the baseline pain (Portenoy et al., 2006; Hagen et al., 2008). Patients with uncontrolled breakthrough pain are more likely to have a poorer quality of life and be depressed (Portenoy et al., 1999).

Pathophysiology and aetiology of pain in advanced disease

Pain occurs in more than 50% of patients with advanced disease, and although the 'analgesic ladder' approach to treatment promulgated by the World Health Organization is both accepted as the mainstay therapy and widely disseminated, pain is undertreated (Solano et al., 2006; van den Beuken-van Everdingen et al., 2007a; DeAndrea et al., 2008; Breivik et al., 2009). Unrelieved pain interferes with daily functioning and quality of life. It may have multiple negative effects, interfering with sleep, activity, and interaction with others, and causing psychological and existential distress (Sheinfeld et al., 2012).

Most of the empirical evidence about pain in advanced disease has been related to patients with cancer, but a review by Solano et al. (2006) shows that pain is a common feature of advanced disease in all patients regardless of the underlying pathology. Prevalence of pain in cancer patients was 35–96%, in those with heart disease, 41–77%, AIDS, 63–80%, chronic obstructive pulmonary disease (COPD), 34–77%, and renal disease, 47–50% (Solano et al., 2006). However, what is not clear is whether this pain is a result of the underlying advanced disease or associated co-morbidities. For example, a patient with COPD may have severe back pain but this may be due to osteoporotic fractures as a result of long-term steroid use.

In cancer patients, pain is more common as the disease progresses. A systematic review of 52 articles focusing on patients with cancer found that the prevalence was 64–74% in those with advanced disease, 59% of those on anti-cancer treatment, and 33% in those that had been cured of their cancer (Hearn and Higginson, 2003; van den Beuken-van Everdingen et al., 2007b). These findings are similar to those in a recent European Pain in Cancer survey of over 5000 patients in 11 European countries, which showed an overall pain prevalence of 72% of patients with cancer in the community (Breivik et al., 2009). Prevalence rates of pain associated with different types of cancer vary in the literature, but overall rates all remain over 50%. Breivik et al. (2009) found that the highest prevalence rates, of over 85%, were associated with cancers of the pancreas, bone, brain, lymphoma, lung, and head and neck.

Although confirming that pain is an extremely common symptom among diverse populations with serious illness, the specific prevalence rates must be interpreted with caution. Pain is heterogeneous and prevalence rates are affected by the setting of the patient, such as a specialist pain or a general respiratory clinic.

Pain prevalence may be related to aetiology. Pain may be due to a direct effect of underlying advanced disease or its treatment; an indirect effect of the disease, such as pressure sores from immobility; or a disorder unrelated to the primary disease, such as osteoarthritis. One survey observed that 76% of patients with cancer have pain directly related to the cancer, 11% have pain related to cancer treatment, 5% have pain due to an indirect effect, and 8% have pain due to unrelated conditions (Grond et al., 1996).

A study of patients with chronic cancer pain observed that somatic pains were more common (71%) than either neuropathic (39%) or visceral (34%) pains (Caraceni and Portenoy, 1999). Many patients experience both nociceptive and neuropathic pain, and the origin of pain must be considered when interpreting prevalence rates. In neuropathic cancer pain, for example, although the majority of pains are caused by cancer (64%), a significantly higher proportion is caused by cancer treatment (20%) in comparison with all cancer patients (Bennett et al., 2012).

The pathophysiology of pain affects its impact on patients and treatment. Patients with neuropathic pain have been shown to have greater pain intensity, a worse quality of life, and a greater negative impact on their daily living than patients with nociceptive pain (Torrance et al., 2006; Smith et al., 2007; Bouhassira et al., 2008). Similarly, those with neuropathic cancer pain have been shown to have a worse quality of life, poorer performance status, and a need for both higher opioid doses and a longer time to achieve pain control than those with nociceptive pain (Fainsinger et al., 2010; Rayment et al., 2013).

Further clouding interpretation of prevalence figures is the observation that patients often report more than one pain (Twycross and Fairfield, 1982). For example, a systematic review found that, on average, patients with cancer have two pains, 20% of which are neuropathic in origin; these patients with multiple types of pain contribute to a 40% prevalence rate for neuropathic pain overall (Bennett et al., 2012).

Finally, pain prevalence must be interpreted in light of severity and other factors. Pain severity varies, but as a minimum, more than one-third of patients with cancer pain grade their pain as either moderate or severe (van den Beuken-van Everdingen et al., 2007b; deAndrea et al., 2008). In hospitalized patients with cancer, patients reported a pain score of 3.7 on a 0–10 numerical rating scale for average pain; two-thirds of patients reported that their worst pain was higher than 5 (Klepstad et al., 2002; Yates et al., 2002). In the community, 93% of those patients who experienced cancer pain at least several times a month rated the severity as moderate to severe, 44% described it as severe, and 3% regarded it as the worst pain imaginable (Breivik et al., 2009).

Like pain itself, under-treatment has many influencing factors. Discrepancies between patient and physician rating of pain severity are one such predictor (deAndrea et al., 2008). Under-treatment also is more likely when patients have a better performance status

or are in the early stages of their diseases, findings that may suggest a reluctance to believe that those with early disease can have severe pain or an increased likelihood that those with advanced disease are managed by specialists (deAndrea et al., 2008).

It is not clear if older age has an effect on pain management. Evidence from the cancer population suggests that there are no differences in pain intensity but older people may require less or more analgesia than the younger population, perhaps due to altered physiology (Vigano et al., 1998; Mercadante and Arcuri, 2007; Hall et al., 2003; Mercadante et al., 2006; van den Beuken-van Everdingen et al., 2007b; Bennett et al., 2009). Older patients also do not have more adverse effects or more need for opioid switching (Mercadante et al., 2006). However, they may have different attitudes towards opioids and therefore may be more reluctant to use these drugs (Yeager et al., 1997; Closs et al., 2009). Gender does not alter pain prevalence rates, but education level and ethnicity may (van den Beuken-van Everdingen et al., 2007b; deAndrea et al., 2008).

Characterizing the pain complaint

Assessing a patient's pain should be a continual process supported by communication between patient, carer, and clinician. The aims are to characterize the complaint, correctly identify the underlying pathophysiology, and determine the effect of pain on the patient's life. All of this information informs the management plan. Without this focus on a comprehensive assessment, pain treatment becomes less targeted and less effective.

A history and clinical examination are vital for pain assessment and radiological and laboratory tests may be indicated. Inadequate pain control is most often due to a poor history and examination (Grossman et al., 1992; Von Roenn et al., 1993). Establishing the effect of pain on the person's quality of life and activities of daily living, recording previous effects of analgesic treatments, and exploring the patient's goals and expectations are crucial in being able to effectively treat all aspects of pain's impact on the person. Creating a trusting, open relationship encourages communication and allows patients to be involved in the management of their pain. Concerns generated by the experience of fear, such as worry about cancer progression or about the risks of addiction or tolerance to opioids, may affect the information given to the clinician.

The clinical history of pain

The acronym SOCRATES is useful in prompting systematic assessment of pain characteristics: *S*ite, *O*nset, *C*haracter, *R*adiation, *A*ssociated factors, *T*iming, *E*xacerbating/relieving factors, and *S*everity (Box 9.3.1). As previously mentioned, patients often report more than one pain and it is important to ascertain a pain history for each pain a patient reports, as its cause and therefore treatment may vary. Answers to these questions provide clues as to the likely underlying cause. For example, a patient who describes unpredictable severe shooting and stabbing pains in both toes and feet, with no radiation, may well be describing a peripheral neuropathic pain perhaps related to previous chemotherapy. In contrast, a patient describing severe shooting and stabbing pains radiating down both legs to their feet, which is worse on movement, may be describing impending cauda equina/spinal cord compression. Management of these two syndromes is substantially different

Box 9.3.1 SOCRATES acronym for pain assessment

Site
Onset
Character
Radiation
Associated factors
Timing
Exacerbating/relieving factors
Severity.

Box 9.3.2 Patient's description of neuropathic pain

As far as I can remember, my pain started during the second week of the radiotherapy and chemotherapy. In total I had six chemotherapy and 30 radiotherapy sessions over a 6-week period. I found the radiotherapy was the most painful. Not during treatment—it was the aftereffects. The headache seemed to get worse on a daily basis.

Trying to explain the pain is difficult. It is like hundreds of needles inside my head. I ended up trying to relate it to other pain I have suffered over my lifetime. For instance, ear infection at its worst, very bad migraine, tonsillitis. If you could imagine all this pain in one blast it is about right, maybe even worse. At this time of my life I was lucky if I managed to have an hour or two of undisturbed sleep. Now 10 months down the line, I am finding it much easier to cope as my nerve ends are healing. The medication as a pain patch has definitely been a great help with the nerve pain.

and requires physicians' knowledge of the underlying disease and likely prognosis.

The pain assessment also must clarify the history of the underlying disease process, including previous treatments and current status. This information informs both treatment selection and prognostication. Similarly, a history of other symptoms is needed to both predict the impact of pain therapy and assist in the development of a broader plan of care for symptom control.

For those patients who are cognitively impaired it can be harder to ascertain symptoms and there must be increased reliance on non-verbal cues, as well as proxy reports from families and other carers who can highlight abnormal behaviours. A recent Norwegian cluster randomized controlled trial of patients in nursing homes with moderate to severe Alzheimer's dementia and significant behavioural disturbances showed significant benefit in agitation in patients who received analgesia, the vast majority receiving just regular paracetamol (Husebo et al., 2011).

Character

English, which can express the thoughts of Hamlet and the tragedy of Lear, has no words for the shiver and the headache. . . . The merest schoolgirl, when she falls in love, has Shakespeare or Keats to speak her mind for her; but let a sufferer try to describe a pain in his head to a doctor and language at once runs dry. (Virginia Woolf, *On Being Ill*)

Although patients often find it difficult to articulate the character of their pains, it is important to elicit descriptors as a step in diagnosing the underlying pathophysiology. Nociceptive pain is divided into somatic pain, which arises from injury to the soft tissues and bone, and visceral pain, which arises from injury to internal organs. Somatic pain is usually well localized and described as aching, sharp, or throbbing. In contrast, visceral pain due to obstruction of a hollow viscus is poorly localized and can be described as gnawing or cramping; injury to other tissues, such deep fascia, or organs such as the heart, may be described as pressure or a deep pain. Visceral pain is commonly referred, such as shoulder tip pain from diaphragmatic irritation. Patients often find visceral pain harder to describe than somatic pain (Bennett et al., 2005; Osta and Bruera, 2008).

Neuropathic pain is often described as numb or burning with sharp, shooting pains on movement. Patients may describe spontaneous pains in the absence of any stimuli or evoked pains such as allodynia (painful response to a non-painful stimulus), hyperalgesia (increased painful response to a painful stimulus), and hyperpathia (delayed and prolonged response to painful stimulus). Due to cancer's natural history, neuropathic pain can

evolve as masses increase in size; over time, many patients with tumour-related neuropathic pain experience the emergence of deep aching related to the underlying lesion. See Box 9.3.2 for an example of a patient's description of neuropathic pain from head and neck cancer.

Neurological signs may precede pain and reflect the distribution and severity of nerve injury (Twycross, 1995). Sensory changes, weakness, and altered tendon reflexes can localize the site of injury and help clarify the aetiology of the pain.

However, distinguishing between neuropathic and nociceptive pain on the basis of pain descriptors alone is not easy. A study in non-cancer patients found that while patients with peripheral neuropathic pain reported more descriptors such as hot, cold, sensitive, itchy, and significantly less dull and deep than those with nociceptive pain, they still used nociceptive descriptors, although to a lesser extent (Dworkin et al., 2007). A study in lung cancer patients found that several words traditionally thought to describe neuropathic pain such as burning, shooting, tingling, and cold did not distinguish between the two pains (Wilkie et al., 2001).

As noted, individual pains also can have more than one mechanism. A patient describing pain from a vertebral metastasis that is compressing a nerve root is likely to describe features of both nociceptive and neuropathic pain. This would be classified as mixed pain or a more useful term to aid management may be whether the pain is more or less neuropathic in nature (Bennett et al., 2006).

Associated features

Pain is associated with many features that may be clinically important or predict treatment response. For example, interference is the extent to which pain has affected aspects of a patient's life. It is important to analyse because the extent to which pain interferes in various functional domains may enable better classification of its cause or predict those patients who are likely to have a poor response to management and a longer time to pain control. Although pain interference is strongly related to pain intensity at a group level (Serlin et al., 1995), there are significant inter-individual differences. In addition there are differences in reported levels of pain-related interference between patients with and without advanced medical illness: at any level of pain intensity, those without advanced illness report greater interference (Fayers et al., 2011).

Other associated features also are important. A recent longitudinal study by Knudsen et al. (2012) confirmed that pain intensity, incident pain, and younger patients predicted more complex pain and longer time to achieve pain control. In an international multicentre study, Fainsinger et al. (2010) showed that these three domains and psychological distress and neuropathic pain were associated with a longer time to pain control. Those with addictive behaviours, a history of drug or alcohol abuse, did not take longer to reach stable pain control but required higher opioid doses. Alcoholism is a major predictor of rapid escalation of opioids and opioid-related neurotoxicity (Bruera et al., 1995).

In addition, sleep disturbance, lack of social support, and concerns over finances and family all affect the impact pain has on the patient. Given this complexity, the treatment of pain with analgesics alone is unlikely to optimize outcomes. Working within a multiprofessional team to target and help each domain while expertly providing analgesics is more likely to result in better pain management for the patient.

Severity

It is important to assess the severity of pain, as the greater its severity the more impact it has on daily functioning and quality of life (Serlin et al., 1995). Various pain measurement tools can be applied to this task, ranging from simple unidimensional scales such as the visual analogue scale (VAS), to more complex pain questionnaires (see following sections). For some patients, facial scales may be more useful in establishing the severity of pain.

In the clinical setting, pain severity usually is measured by asking patients to rate their pains on a 0–10 scale or as mild, moderate, or severe. The response to this question may provide enough information to help initiate appropriate treatment, as well as its urgency. It may also help to establish the underlying cause of the pain; for example, severe pain on movement may support a diagnosis of a fracture, whereas mild pain may suggest osteoarthritis. Ongoing assessment of pain severity enables evaluation of interventions, and monitoring of variation over hours or days can help establish factors which worsen or ease the pain. All this information may be useful when there is a large team caring for the patient (Twycross, 1995).

Pain measurement scales

Intensity 0–10

Visual, categorical numerical, and categorical verbal rating scales are validated and used as tools to measure intensity of pain (Caraceni et al., 2002; Hjermstad et al., 2011) (see also Chapter 7.2). The VAS is a 10 cm line labelled at each end with the minimum or maximum extremes of what is being measured. In measuring pain, these anchors often are 'no pain' and 'pain as bad as you can imagine'. Patients indicate their pain severity on the line. Categorical numerical scales ask the patient to rate their pain on an 11-point numeric scale (e.g. '0 to 10, where 0 is no pain and 10 is pain as bad as you can imagine') or on a 5-point numeric scale (e.g., a 0–4 scale with the same anchors), and categorical verbal scales provide verbal descriptors, such as none, mild, moderate,

or severe. They are reliable and can be used clinically and in research. Expert consensus recommended an 11-point numerical rating scale with 'no pain' and 'pain as bad as you can imagine' as anchors for the assessment of chronic pain including cancer pain (Dworkin et al., 2005; Kaasa et al., 2011).

Brief Pain Inventory

The Brief Pain Inventory (BPI) (Daut et al., 1983; Cleeland and Rayn, 1994) has long (15 minutes) and short versions; either a health-care professional or patient can complete it. The short version assesses pain severity from four frames of reference—'pain right now', 'pain at its best', 'pain at its worst', and 'pain on average'—and also measures pain relief using a VAS. A pain schematic shows the localization of pain, and pain interference during the last 24 hours is determined in terms of various domains, for example, general activity, mood, walking ability, normal work, relations with other people, sleep, mood, and enjoyment of life. The longer version of the BPI also records information about medical history, has pain descriptors, and asks about interference with daily activities in the last month and last week. The BPI has been translated and validated in many languages. The short form has been recommended for cancer pain assessment (Caraceni et al., 2002).

McGill Pain Questionnaire

The McGill Pain Questionnaire (MPQ) is another self-report tool validated in cancer patients. It assesses intensity, quality, temporal pattern, relieving and exacerbating factors, and site of pain. Intensity is assessed on a categorical verbal rating scale, which uses the descriptors mild, discomforting, distressing, horrible, and excruciating (Melzack, 1987). It has been validated in the cancer pain population (Graham et al., 1980; Dudgeon et al., 1993).

Neuropathic pain screening tools

Various neuropathic screening tools exist (Bennett et al., 2007). The Leeds Assessment of Neuropathic Signs and Symptoms has five self-report pain items and two clinical examination items (Bennett 2001). PainDETECT is another self-report questionnaire consisting of seven questions related to the quality of the pain, a body map, and two further questions on radiation and timing (Freynhagen et al., 2006). The Douleur Neuropathique en 4 questions or DN4 has seven symptom and three clinical examination questions (Bouhassira et al., 2005), while the Neuropathic Pain Questionnaire has ten questions on sensation and two on affect (Krause and Backonja, 2003). All have been validated in populations without cancer and emerging evidence suggests that for screening tools in cancer populations these tools may be less reliable or require adapting (Rayment et al., 2013).

Alberta Breakthrough Pain Assessment Tool

The Alberta Breakthrough Pain Assessment Tool was developed for use in clinical studies. There are 15 patient answered questions and questions on aetiology, pathophysiology, medications, and descriptions of the pain for the health-care professional.

Clinical examination

Clinical examination is essential to ensure accurate diagnosis of the pathophysiology of pain. It not only aids accurate diagnosis but also allows for assessment of comorbidities and the patient's overall physical state. This information is essential when considering management strategies.

A neurological examination often provides valuable information and is essential if neuropathic pain is suspected. The recent IASP guidelines for neuropathic pain underline the importance of clinical examination for an accurate diagnosis (Haanpää et al., 2011), and the recent NeuPSIG guidance (Haanpää et al., 2011) proposed a four-criterion grading system for non-cancer neuropathic pain highlighting the importance of examination in this subgroup. This guidance indicates that the examination of the patient with presumed neuropathic pain should demonstrate that the pain is neuroanatomically plausible and the patient has a history suggestive of a relevant lesion or disease of the central somatosensory or peripheral nervous system. With these criteria, neuropathic pain may be considered possible if there is at least one confirmatory bedside measurement, and probable if there is at least one confirmatory test. If all four of these criteria are met, then neuropathic pain may be considered definite.

Confirmatory imaging will help in the assessment of pain if there is doubt as to its cause or if it may lead to further directed treatment, such as radiotherapy (Twycross, 1995). Analgesia should not be withheld while a diagnosis is being obtained. Plain radiography and bone scintigraphy may help in determining the appropriateness of radiotherapy or orthopaedic intervention. Computed tomography and magnetic resonance imaging help determine the causes of intrathoracic or intra-abdominal and pelvic pain, and nerve conduction studies may help localize the lesion.

Assessing pain in context of a palliative plan of care

Patients with advanced disease face many challenges. Pain is often only one symptom of an illness that may have been associated with many losses—normality, independence, health, and the future. The significance of pain varies among individuals; a patient with peripheral neuropathic pain due to diabetes may be very distressed but a patient with ischaemic heart disease may believe chest pain means they are dying. It is still common for people to believe that severe pain is unavoidable in advancing illness, especially cancer, and this may place extra suffering on patients. It therefore is a clinical imperative to understand a patient's understanding of the cause of their pain, and their concerns about management and what may happen in the future. This inevitably needs to be done with consideration for other symptoms. Other factors are important to help predict response to treatment. For example, organ failure, cachexia, and age affect pharmacokinetics and response to treatment, and should be considered within any management plan.

It is essential when considering a management plan to consider both the potential benefits and burdens. Performance status and likely prognosis may alter what treatment is offered. For example, a patient with pain from a femoral fracture due to metastatic disease who has been gradually deteriorating for many months, was bed bound before the fracture and is anorectic, cachectic, and fatigued with a prognosis of days will not benefit from radiotherapy, while a patient with a similar pain due to a femoral fracture who was walking and independent prior to the fracture, and has a prognosis of many months, should be considered for both orthopaedic and oncological intervention.

Explanation of the cause of pain and its management needs to be made not only to the patients but to any carers/family that the patient identifies as helping in their day-to-day life. Their understanding may be crucial in designing and implementing management. Consideration also needs to be made as to whether initial assessment and management is better done in an inpatient unit or on an outpatient basis.

Continuing assessment of pain and its response to management is vital in ensuring that patients get the treatment they deserve. Clinicians working within a multidisciplinary team with expertise in nursing, social work, physiotherapy, occupational therapy, spiritual care, and complementary therapies ensure a holistic assessment is made of a patient's pain and a holistic management plan is implemented.

Online materials

Complete references for this chapter are available online at <http://www.oxfordmedicine.com>.

References

Bennett, M. (2001). The LANSS Pain Scale; the Leeds Assessment of Neuropathic Symptoms and Signs. *Pain*, 92(1–2), 147–157.

Bennett, M.I., Attal, N., Backonja, M.M., *et al.* (2007). Using screening tools to identify neuropathic pain. *Pain*, 127(3), 199–203.

Bennett, M.I., Rayment, C., Hjermstad, M., Aass, N., Caraceni, A., and Kaasa, S. (2012). Prevalence and aetiology of neuropathic pain in cancer patients: a systematic review. *Pain*, 153, 359–365.

Bonica, J.J. (1990). Definitions and taxonomy of pain. In J.J. Bonica (ed.) *The Management of Pain*, pp. 18–27. Philadelphia, PA: Lea and Febiger.

Bouhassira, D., Attal, N., Alchaar, H., *et al.* (2005). Comparison of pain syndromes associated with nervous or somatic lesions and development of a new neuropathic pain diagnostic questionnaire (DN4). *Pain*, 114(1–2), 29–36.

Bouhassira, D., Lanteri-Minet, M., Attal, N., Laurent, B., and Touboul, C. (2008). Prevalence of chronic pain with neuropathic characteristics in the general population. *Pain*, 136(3), 380–387.

Breivik, H., Cherny, N., Collett, B., *et al.* (2009). Cancer-related pain: a pan-European survey of prevalence, treatment, and patient attitudes. *Annals of Oncology*, 20(8), 1420–1433.

Bruera, E., Schoeller, T., Wenk, R., *et al.* (1995). A prospective multicentre assessment of the Edmonton staging system for cancer pain. *Journal of Pain and Symptom Management*, 10(5), 348–355.

Caraceni, A., Cherny, N., Fainsinger, R., *et al.* (2002). Pain measurement tools and methods in clinical research in palliative care: recommendations of an Expert Working Group of the European Association of Palliative Care. *Journal of Pain and Symptom Management*, 23(3), 239–255.

Caraceni, A. and Portenoy, R. (1999). An international survey of cancer pain characteristics and syndromes. IASP task force on cancer pain. International association for the study of pain. *Pain*, 82(3), 263–274.

Cleeland, C.S. and Rayn, K.M. (1994). Pain assessment: global use of the Brief Pain Inventory. *Annals of the Academy of Medicine*, 32, 129–138.

Deandrea, S., Montanari, M., Moja, L., and Apolone, G. (2008). Prevalence of under treatment in cancer pain. A review of published literature. *Annals of Oncology*, 19, 1985–1991.

Fainsinger, R.L., Nekolaichuk, C., Lawlor, P., *et al.* (2010). An international multicentre validation study of a pain classification system for cancer patients. *European Journal of Cancer*, 45, 2896–2904.

Fayers, P.M., Hjermstad, M.J., Klepstad, P. *et al.*, on behalf of the European Palliative Care Research Collaboration (EPCRC) (2011). The dimensionality of pain: palliative care and chronic pain patients differ in their reports of pain intensity and pain interference. *Pain*, 152, 1608–1620.

Freynhagen, R., Baron, R., Gockel, U., and Tolle, T.R. (2006). painDE-TECT: a screening questionnaire to identify neuropathic components in patients with back pain. *Current Medical Research Opinion*, 22(10), 1911–1920.

Grond, S., Zech, D., Diefenbach, C., Radbruch, L., and Lehmann, K.A. (1996). Assessment of cancer pain: a prospective evaluation in 2266 cancer patients referred to a pain service. *Pain*, 64, 107–114.

Haanpää, M., Attal, N., Backonja, M., *et al.* (2011). NeuPSIG guidelines on neuropathic pain assessment. *Pain*, 152(1), 14–27.

Hjermstad, M.J., Fayers, P.M., Haugen, D.F., *et al.* (2011). Studies comparing numerical rating scales, verbal rating scales, and visual analogue scales for assessment of pain intensity in adults: a systematic literature review. *Journal of Pain and Symptom Management*, 41(6), 1073–1093.

Husebo, B.S., Ballard, C., Sandvik, R., Nilsen, O.B., and Aarsland, D. (2011). Efficacy of treating pain to reduce behavioural disturbances in residents of nursing homes with dementia: cluster randomised clinical trial. *BMJ*, 343, d4065.

International Association for the Study of Pain (2011). *IASP Taxonomy*. [Online] Available at: <http://www.iasp-pain.org/Content/NavigationMenu/GeneralResourceLinks/PainDefinitions/default.htm>.

Kaasa, S., Apolone, G., Kelpstad, P., *et al.* (2011). Expert conference on cancer pain assessment and classification, the need for international consensus: working proposals on international standards. *BMJ Supportive and Palliative Care*, 1, 281–287.

Mercadante, S. and Arcuri, E. (2007). Pharmacological management of cancer pain in the elderly. *Drugs & Aging*, 24(9), 761–776.

Portenoy, R.L. (2011). Treatment of cancer pain. *The Lancet*, 377(9784), 2236–2247.

Rayment, C.S., Bennett, M.I., Aass, N., Hjermstad, M.J., and Kaasa, S. (2013). Neuropathic cancer pain: prevalence, severity, analgesics, and impact from the European Palliative Care Research Collaborative Computerised Symptom Assessment study (EPCRC-CSA). *Palliative Medicine*, 27, 8, 714–721.

Solano, J.P., Gomes, B., and Higginson, I.J. (2006). A comparison of symptom prevalence in far advanced cancer, AIDS, heart disease, COPD and renal disease. *Journal of Pain and Symptom Management*, 31(1), 58–69.

Smith, B.H., Torrance, N., Bennett, M.I., and Lee, A. (2007). Health and quality of life associated with chronic pain of predominantly neuropathic origin in the community. *Clinical Journal of Pain*, 23(2), 143–149.

Torrance, N., Smith, B.H., Bennett, M.I., and Lee, A. (2006). The epidemiology of chronic pain of predominantly neuropathic origin. Results from a general population survey. *Journal of Pain*, 7(4), 281–289.

Twycross, R. (1995). *Pain Relief in Advanced Cancer*. Singapore: Longman Singapore Publishers Ltd.

Van den Beuken-van Everdingen, M.H.J., de Rijke, J.M., Kessels, A.G., Schouten, H.C., van Kleef, M., Patijn, J. (2007a). Prevalence of pain in patients with cancer: a systematic review of the past 40 years. *Annals of Oncology*, 18, 1437–1449.

Van den Beuken-van Everdingen, M.H.J., de Rijke, J.M., Kessels, A.G., Schouten, H.C., van Kleef, M., and Patijn, J. (2007b). High prevalence of pain in patients with cancer in a large population-based study in The Netherlands. *Pain*, 132, 312–320.

Wilkie, D.J., Huang, H.Y., Reilly, N., and Cain, K.C. (2001). Nociceptive and neuropathic pain in patients with lung cancer: a comparison of pain quality descriptors. *Journal of Pain and Symptom Management*, 22(5), 899–910.

Woolf, V. (1930). *On Being Ill*. London: The Hogarth Press.

Opioid therapy: optimizing analgesic outcomes

Marie T. Fallon and Nathan I. Cherny

Introduction to opioid therapy

Treatment with analgesic drugs is the mainstay of cancer pain management (World Health Organization (WHO), 1996; Portenoy and Lesage, 1999). Although concurrent use of other approaches and interventions may be appropriate in many patients, and necessary in some, analgesic drugs are needed in almost every case. Drugs whose primary clinical action is the relief of pain are conventionally classified on the basis of their activity at opioid receptors as either opioid or non-opioid analgesics. A third class, adjuvant analgesics, are drugs with other primary indications that can be effective analgesics in specific circumstances. The major group of drugs used in cancer pain management is the opioid analgesics.

During the last 30 years, there has been a dramatic increase in our knowledge of the sites and mechanism of action of the opioids. The development of analytical methods has also been of great importance in facilitating pharmacokinetic studies of the disposition and fate of opioids in patients. More recently, advances in genomic research have indicated the potential importance of pharmacogenetic factors in the response to opioid analgesics (Lötsch et al., 2002a, 2009). These studies have begun to offer us a better understanding of some of the sources of variation between individuals in their response to opioids and to suggest ways of minimizing some of their adverse effects. Although there are gaps in our knowledge of opioid pharmacology, the rational and appropriate use of these drugs is based on their clinical pharmacological properties demonstrated in well-controlled clinical trials. However, in order to reflect the dramatic increase in pre-clinical opioid research in recent years, this chapter has been divided into two; a pre-clinical and a clinical section.

Terminology

In this chapter and throughout this textbook, we have adopted the following conventions in terminology:

Opiate is a specific term that is used to describe drugs derived from the juice of the opium poppy. For example, morphine is an opiate but methadone (a completely synthetic drug) is not (Hughes and Kosterlitz 1983).

Opioid is a general term that includes naturally occurring, semi-synthetic, and synthetic drugs which produce their effects by combining with opioid receptors and are stereospecifically antagonized by naloxone. In this context we refer to opioid agonists, opioid antagonists, opioid peptides, and opioid receptors.

Narcotic is commonly used to describe morphine-like drugs and other drugs of abuse. The term is derived from the Greek *narke*, meaning numbness or torpor. Since this is an imprecise and pejorative term that is not useful in a pharmacological context, its use with reference to opioids is discouraged. The term narcotic is not used in this book.

Section 1: pre-clinical pharmacology

Opioid receptors

Opioid receptors were originally classified by pharmacological activity in animal preparations and later, by molecular sequence. The three main receptors were classified as μ (mu) or OP3, κ (kappa) or OP1, and δ (delta) or OP2. Another opioid-like receptor has been identified; it is termed the nociceptin orphanin FQ peptide receptor. Receptor nomenclature has changed several times in the last few years; the current International Union of Pharmacology (IUPHAR) classification is MOP (mu), KOP (kappa), DOP (delta), and NOP for the nociceptin orphanin FQ peptide receptor (Table 9.4.1).

The formerly identified sigma receptor is not a true opioid receptor and is not included in the opioid receptor group. Opioid receptors are widely distributed in both central and peripheral nervous systems. One of the characteristics of DNA and RNA is known as sequencing and this can be an indicator of normal biological processes, pathogenic processes, and/or response to a therapeutic or other interventions (see Box 9.4.1 for definitions of key terms in the discipline of pharmacogenomics and pharmacogenetics).

The mu, delta, and kappa receptors are very similar, sharing over 70% sequence homology, whilst the orphan receptor shares only 50% sequence homology (Pasternak 2001). Extensive pre-mRNA splicing gives rise to numerous splice-variants also known as receptor subtypes. The mu receptor gene has been shown to have 25 different splice variants in mice, eight in rats, and 11 in humans. These splice variants are controlled by diverse promoters. It has been demonstrated that different splice variants exhibit differences in agonist-induced G-protein activation, adenylyl cyclase activity, and receptor internalization or endocytosis. In addition, some differences can lead to modification of phosphorylation, membrane translation, scaffolding protein binding, and G-protein binding (Reisine and Pasternak, 1996). The potential activation and destination of the receptor is changed by such modifications. The different effects of currently available opioids are dependent on complex interactions at various receptors

Table 9.4.1 Classification of opioid receptors

Receptor	Molecular classification	Endogenous ligand	Site
Mu	OP3	Beta-endorphin, leu-and met-encephalin; endomorphins	Peripheral inflammation; pre- and postsynaptic neurons in spinal cord, periaqueductal grey, nucleus raphe magnus, thalamus, cortex
Kappa	OP1	Dynorphins	Spinal cord, supraspinal, hypothalamus
Delta	OP2	Encephalins, beta-endorphin	Olfactory centres, motor integration areas in cortex, limited distribution in nociception areas
Orphan	ORL-1 (opioid-like receptor)	Nociceptin	Spinal cord

Source: Data from UpToDate.

and they function as neurotransmitters, neuromodulators, and neurohormones.

The three families of endogenous opioid peptides are well characterized. They are the endorphins, encephalins, and dynorphines, which have binding affinities to all the receptors. Each family originates from a different gene, their precursors being pro-opiomelanocortin, proencephalin and prodynorphin. The endogenous tetrapeptide endomorphins 1 and 2 do not have an identified precursor; however, they are potent agonists acting very specifically at the mu receptor and they play a role in modulating inflammatory pain. Peripherally they interact extensively with immune cells, primarily in inflammatory states, when beta-endorphin-containing cells as well as signalling molecules (vascular P-selectin and intercellular adhesion molecule-I) which stimulate these cells, are up-regulated (Martin et al., 1976).

The receptor family

The mu opioid receptor

This is clinically the most important of all the receptor families. It is the main opioid receptor responsible for inhibition of nociceptive pathways, and is exploited by all exogenous opioids (Pasternak 1993). Many of the unwanted effects of opioids are also related to activity at this receptor.

Expression

The mu receptor is expressed on central and peripheral neurons, although in the latter it is only activated in response to inflammatory stimuli. Peripherally, mu receptors are found pre- and postsynaptically, for example, in the dorsal horn; approximately 70% are expressed on the primary afferent terminations (presynaptic) modulating afferent transmission (Sindrup et al., 1991). Mu receptors are present on C and A delta fibres, the sympathetic nervous system, and immune cells. Centrally, they are expressed widely including the cerebral cortex, the amygdala, and the periaqueductal grey. In the periaqueductal grey, the presence of mu receptors on inhibitory neurons seems to lead to disinhibition of descending pathways resulting in excitation, as opposed to the more usual result of inhibition of neural transmission.

The relative contribution of each binding site to the overall analgesic effects of systemic opioids has not been investigated. We do understand from both the pre-clinical and clinical paradigm of inflammatory pain, that the pain state itself is highly likely to have a major role in the pattern of binding. The receptor undergoes pre- and post-transcriptional splicing and alteration, leading to a huge variation in the activation state of the receptor (Pasternak 2001).

The delta receptor

Evidence suggests that other opioid endogenous ligands and receptors are linked to analgesic response and to mu receptor activation. It is interesting that deletion of the delta receptor gene and pre-proencephalins inhibits the development of morphine tolerance, but not withdrawal, in mice (Inturrisi et al., 1983). On the other hand, the potency of mu agonists can be increased by the co-administration of a delta agonist, and such co-administration can induce a translocation of delta receptors to the cell surface. This pre-clinical information is of interest in relation to methadone, which has strong delta, as well as mu, activity.

The kappa receptor

Kappa receptors are also involved in pain, in particular, in response to inflammation (peripherally); however, activation is associated clinically with a number of unpleasant side effects, such as nausea and vomiting and dysphoria. The latter have limited their clinical development for pain of gastrointestinal aetiology, which is often associated with inflammation.

The ORL-1 receptor

The ORL-1 receptor was identified because of its homology with classical opioid receptor types. Its natural ligand is 'nociceptin' or 'orphanin'. There is a suggestion that centrally ORL-1 agonists appear to antagonize mu opioids but this is not yet clearly elucidated. The ORL-1 receptor is involved in modulation of a range of biological functions including the stress response, movement, memory, cardiovascular, and renal mechanisms (Pasternak 2001).

Opioid receptors: structure and function

The opioid receptors belong to the superfamily of seven transmembrane-spanning G protein-coupled receptors (GPCRs). The three major opioid receptors (mu, delta, and kappa) originate from different genes. Each of the transcribed receptor proteins consists of an extracellular N-terminus, seven transmembrane helices, three extra- and intracellular loops, and an intracellular C-terminus characteristic of GPCRs.

The opioid receptor belongs to the rhodopsin family of GPCR (Christensen, 1993; Raynor et al., 1995; Heiskanen et al., 1998). The extracellular regions are involved in opioid binding and intracellular domains interact with G proteins. GPCRs were originally thought to function as monomers in a 1:1 stochiometric ratio with downstream heterotrimeric G proteins (Traynor, 1996). Their primary function is to transmit extracellular stimuli to intracellular signals. Opioid receptors are transduced by the Gi/Go proteins which are relatively resistant to tolerance or desensitization. Transport proteins, metabolizing enzymes, opioid receptors, and

Box 9.4.1 Terminology in pharmacogenomics

Genomic biomarker

Definition

A genomic biomarker is defined as:

A measurable DNA or RNA characteristic that is an indicator of normal biologic processes, pathogenic processes, and/or response to therapeutic or other intervention.

Additional information

1. The definition for a genomic biomarker is not limited to human samples.

2. A genomic biomarker could, for example, reflect:

   - the expression of a gene
   - the function of a gene
   - the regulation of a gene.

3. A genomic biomarker can consist of one or more deoxyribonucleic acid (DNA) or ribonucleic acid (RNA) characteristics.

4. The definition for a genomic biomarker does not include the measurement and characterization of proteins or low-molecular-weight metabolites.

5. DNA characteristics include, but are not limited to

   - single nucleotide polymorphisms (SNPs)
   - variability of short sequence repeats
   - DNA modification, for example, methylation
   - insertions
   - deletions
   - copy number variation
   - cytogenic rearrangements, for example, translocations, duplications, deletions, or inversions

7. RNA characteristics include, but are not limited to:

   - RNA sequence
   - RNA expression levels
   - RNA processing, for example, splicing and editing
   - microRNA levels.

Pharmacogenomics and pharmacogenetics

Definitions

Pharmacogenomics

Pharmacogenomics (PGx) is defined as:

The investigation of variations of DNA and RNA characteristics as related to drug response.

Pharmacogenetics

Pharmacogenetics (PGt) is a subset of pharmacogenomics and is defined as:

The influence of variations in DNA sequence on drug response.

Additional information

1. PGx and PGt are applied to activities such as drug discovery, drug development, and clinical practice.

2. Drug response includes drug disposition (pharmacokinetics (PK)) and drug effect (pharmacodynamics (PD)).

3. The term drug should be considered synonymous with investigational (medicinal) product, medicinal product, and pharmaceutical product (including vaccines and other biological products)

4. The definition of PGx and PGt does not include other disciplines such as proteomics and metabonomics.

Box 9.4.2 Factors influencing opioid effectiveness

- Absorption
- Distribution
- Metabolism
- Excretion
- Intrinsic efficacy at receptors:
  - transport proteins
  - metabolizing enzymes
  - opioid receptors
  - second messenger molecules.

---

second messenger molecules are central to the effect of opioids (Box 9.4.2). At a cellular level, mu receptor activation has an overall inhibitory effect via:

- inhibition of adenylyl cyclase
- increased opening of potassium channels (hyperpolarization of postsynaptic neurons, reduced synaptic transmission) and
- inhibition of calcium channels (decreases presynaptic neurotransmitter release).

Opioid receptors and the accompanying G proteins interact with a vast array of other intracellular proteins that are responsible for trafficking receptors to the cell membrane, anchoring, and scaffolding proteins. This combination of events alters the response of the receptor to a ligand. GPCRs, including mu, kappa, and delta receptors, have been shown to form different configurations including dimers, homo-, and hetero-oligomers, which have relevance in internalization and activation pathways (Hennessy and Spiers, 2007). This is discussed further in the section on receptor activation versus endocytosis (RAVE). Dimerization modulates receptor pharmacology and this process could present targets for novel interventions (Pasternak, 2001).

Modulation of opioid responses

There are multiple cellular adaptations in response to chronic opioid exposure, which may lead to tolerance (Inturrisi et al., 1983). Tolerance to exogenous opioids is relatively easy to produce in animal studies, where repeated doses of a given opioid rapidly lead to loss of efficacy in response to noxious stimuli. Cellular processes which occur in response to chronic ligand binding to mu receptors include diminution of spare opioid receptors, decreased receptor density, altered coupling, activation and phosphorylation of G proteins, and alteration of downstream pathways (Heiskanen et al., 1998).

It has been reported that chronic exposure to mu or delta agonists induces and up-regulates the pro-excitatory peptides, calcitonin-gene-related peptide (CGRP), substance P, and protein kinase C (responsible for phosphorylation). There is some evidence that the N-methyl-D-aspartate receptor (NMDA) or neurokinin 1 (NK1) receptors may play a role in acute tolerance. Interactions with the orphanin (NOP) receptor may also be important. The effect of these adaptations is to lead to a pro-excitatory state and an attenuation of the inhibitory effects of opioid activation (WHO, 1986; Johnson 1997).

Endogenous peptides such as neuropeptide FF, cholecystokinin, nociception, and dynorphin exhibit anti-opioid actions, which in turn modulate the physiological action and outcome of opioid agonists. Chronic morphine exposure leads to little change in mu receptor expression. There are interesting changes in the non-neuronal population of glial cells, with increased activation in response to chronic morphine exposure (Christensen 1993). Glia have come under increased scrutiny in many pain states. Although previously glia were considered an inert, supporting structure, there is increasing evidence of a key role, particularly in central sensitization where glia may modulate chronic opioid analgesia.

It is widely accepted that clinically relevant pharmacological tolerance to opioid analgesic effects is not relevant for the majority of patients with cancer-related pain. It is however difficult to assess analgesic tolerance clinically (Johnson 1997). There does not appear to be a simple correlation between exposure to opioids and induction of analgesic tolerance. A process of adaptation occurs which is highly likely to depend on many factors which do not necessarily relate easily to current knowledge of cellular processes.

Receptor activation versus endocytosis

The use of more than one opioid or partial opioid substitutions (or rotations) has been reported to reduce agitated terminal delirium, opioid tolerance, and dose escalation (WHO 1986; Ventafridda et al., 1987; Takeda, 1990). The potential benefits have been explained on the basis of RAVE. This is discussed here only to give the reader a complete picture of the evolving theories around opioid function. Potent opioids that activate but do not internalize or recycle the receptor are said to have a high RAVE value. Opioids which cause receptor endocytosis curtail opioid signalling. Paradoxically, sustained opioid signalling causes adenylyl cyclase superactivation and counter-opioid responses (Inturrisi et al., 1983; Walker et al., 1988; Goisis et al., 1989; Schug et al., 1990; Zech et al., 1995; Mercadante 1999).

The opioid receptor binding site is different for each opioid. The number of receptors needed to be activated in order to suppress adenylyl cyclase (a hallmark for analgesia) differs significantly between major opioid receptors. This difference is not related to receptor density or to the amount of intracellular G protein (Raynor et al., 1995). Opioid alkaloids (morphine, methadone, fentanyl) bind within the core of the transmembrane portion of the receptor, whereas large peptidyl ligands bind to the extracellular loops (Inturrisi et al., 1983; McQuay and Moore, 1997; Kalso et al., 1998).

A single receptor has the ability to activate multiple G protein heterotrimers independent of receptor density. Receptor conformation changes as a result of opioid binding and subsequently determines the efficacy of receptor activation and G-protein interactions. Opioid receptors naturally oscillate between active and inactive states. Full agonists stabilize the receptor in an active conformation; partial agonists favour receptor conformation between fully active and inactive states. Opioid antagonists stabilize the receptor in an inactive conformation and prevent G protein activation. Antagonists can become opioid agonists when mutations occur within the fourth membrane helix (TM4) which influences receptor conformation and G protein interactions. The efficiency by which an opioid activates the receptor is dependent on the conformation that allows G proteins to interact with certain transmembrane helices (TM1 and TM7) and the C-terminus (Raynor et al., 1995).

Opioid receptor conformational changes trigger conformational changes in the alpha subunit of G proteins (G alpha) that dissociate GDP from the alpha subunit of the G protein complex and promotes GTP binding to the G alpha subunit. The other component of the G protein (G beta-gamma) is released for downstream signalling. Receptor signalling is curtailed by regulators of G-protein signalling (RGS) and certain kinases (Jadad and Browman, 1995; Heiskanen et al., 1998). G-protein activation inhibits cyclic AMP production by adenylyl cyclase, and also initiates counter-opioid responses and receptor desensitization through the activation of G protein-coupled receptor kinase (GRK) as well as other protein kinases such as protein kinases A and C and mitogen-activated protein kinase (MAPK) (Benedetti et al., 2000; Cleary, 2000; Walsh, 2000).

GPCR activity is balanced by molecular signals that govern receptor desensitization and resensitization. Mechanisms by which receptors are desensitized involve GRK, RGS, kinases, and receptor endocytosis. Receptor desensitization, which is the diminution of receptor responsiveness to agonist activation over time, also represents an important mechanism which limits opioid tolerance. Desensitization prevents acute and chronic overstimulation (or, in the case of opioids, over inhibition) by agonists (Ventafridda et al., 1987). Receptor mechanisms that paradoxically reduce signalling (GRK) are responsible for resensitization by directing receptor trafficking into endocytosis and resensitization (Ventafridda et al., 1987). These acute desensitization processes may be a protective mechanism whereby cells adapt to avoid physiological tolerance by attenuating receptor response to a new sustainable level.

Endocytosis or internalization

G-protein activation (partially G beta-gamma subunits) activates GRK-2 which phosphorylates the C-terminus of the opioid receptor, as well as the second (TM2) and third transmembrane helices (TM3) (Ventafridda et al., 1987). Beta arrestin binds to the phosphorylated receptor, which then binds to clathrin pits within the membrane. Dynamin, a type of GTPase, causes fission of the membrane which results in the formation of small phosphorylase-rich endosomes (Walker et al., 1988; Agency for Health Care Policy and Research: Cancer Pain Management Panel, 1994; Heiskanen et al., 1998; Cleary, 2000; Hanks et al., 2001). The receptor is dephosphorylated within the endosome and returned resensitized to the membrane surface (or catabolized in the process of down-regulation) (Ventafridda et al., 1987). The degree of endocytosis is highly variable and depends on the opioid. Peptides and lipophilic alkaloid opioids (methadone and fentanyl) readily induce receptor endocytosis and recycling (Kristiansen, 2004). Clinically, both methadone and fentanyl have higher opioid intrinsic efficacy, and in some animal models reduced adenylyl cyclase superactivation associated with opioid tolerance (Schug et al., 1990; Agency for Health Care Policy and Research: Cancer Pain Management Panel, 1994; Sindrup and Brosen, 1995; Poulsen et al., 1996; McQuay and Moore, 1997; Mercadante, 1999). Morphine, on the other hand, is believed to activate MAPK resulting in opioid receptor phosphorylation and prevents internalization.

Genetic modulation of the response to opioid analgesics

Pharmacogenomics is currently an intensely studied area of medicine to which great hope and expectations are attached (Takeda, 1990). Research investigating the relationship between the genetic variability among individuals and susceptibility to disease, clinical symptoms or treatment responses has been growing exponentially.

There is considerable variability in response to opioid analgesics in clinical practice and in the balance of wanted and unwanted in individual patients. Pharmacogenetic factors are believed to play important roles in this variability. Possible candidates are polymorphisms in drug metabolizing enzymes, drug transporters, opioid receptors, or in the structures involved in the perception and processing of nociceptive information (Walker et al., 1988), all of which may result in the modulation of the pharmacokinetic or pharmacodynamic effects of opioid analgesics.

Candidate genetic polymorphisms are, of course, only identified on the basis of our current understanding of opioid analgesic mechanisms. Despite sufficient possible candidates with potential importance for pain therapy, evidence for a modulation of the effects of analgesics is only available for a few genes (Table 9.4.2). A variety of polymorphisms have been shown to be important for pain perception and processing and early work suggested that the mu-1 opioid receptor (*OPRM-1*) gene polymorphisms may relate to opioid dose requirements and side effects (de Crean et al., 1996). The numerous subtypes related to spice variants and alleles of the *OPRM-1* gene which result in genetic variations, helps explain the large intra-individual and inter-individual variation in response to the different mu agonist opioids (Pasternak, 2014). More than 100 polymorphisms have been identified in the human mu-opioid receptor gene alone, and some of these variants, such as the A118G nucleotide substitution, have been shown to alter the binding affinities of different opioids (Lötsch et al., 2002b; Beyer et al., 2004) and to effect analgesic outcomes (Chou et al., 2006; Hayashida et al., 2008; Zhang et al., 2010).

Identification of such polymorphisms in an individual patient would currently not provide an immediate individual therapeutic benefit. Benefit will only be obtained when pharmacogenetic testing provides a basis for individual drug selection or dosing. There are also polymorphisms which affect the plasma concentrations of analgesics but while this does not necessarily have any direct clinical implications as yet, the knowledge on the highly variable degree of codeine metabolism has influenced clinical prescribing in many countries (Lötsch, 2009).

Potential clinical applications

The substantial developments in the understanding of genetic polymorphisms, study of mutations affecting opioid receptors, activation, ligand response, and pain processing are of great interest, but as yet do not have direct clinical applications. The implications for clinical practice are that all known active pharmacogenetic variants would need to be tested.

One of the great challenges in translating pre-clinical and early clinical evidence to the clinic, especially concerning genetic modulation, is the undisputed complexity involved in pain perception in individual patients on the background of a heterogenous spectrum of pain syndromes along with environmental and behavioural factors. Improved, more robust clinical phenotyping is necessary in all genetic studies to allow better understanding and meaningful interpretation of any findings. Researchers and clinicians need to agree on well-defined, measurable end points and, of course, agree on how we will measure such end points (see also Chapter 19.1).

Table 9.4.2 Evidence for statistically significant pharmacogenetic modulation of the therapeutic effects of analgesic drugs and their consequences. The clinical significance of these effects has not been established

Gene	Frequency of affected subjects (%)	Affected analgesics (positive available evidence)
OPRM1 (mu opioid receptor)	17.2	Morphine (Goisis et al., 1989)
		M6G (Barnes and Goodwin, 1983; Rowell et al., 1983; Moore et al., 1997; Lötsch et al., 2002)
COMT (catechol-O-methyl transferase)	46.2	Morphine (Crome et al., 1984; Barnes et al., 1985)
	Protective to opioid central side effects	
MC1R (melanocortin-1 receptor)	2 (Inturrisi et al., 1982)	Morphine (Inturrisi et al., 1982)
	4.5	M6G (Inturrisi et al., 1982)
	4.3	Pentazocine (Beaver, 1984)
	3 (Inturrisi et al., 1982)	
CYP2D6 (cytochrome P450 2D6)	2 (Schug et al., 1990)	Codeine (Perrier and Gibaldi, 1972; Rosenberg et al., 1993; Lötsch et al., 2009)
	20.7 (Schug et al., 1990)	
	2 (Schug et al., 1990)	Tramadol (Zech et al., 1995)
	0.9 (Schug et al., 1990)	Codeine (McQuay and Moore, 1997; Mercadante 1999)
	0.1 (Schug et al., 1990)	
	0 (Schug et al., 1990)	
	2 (Schug et al., 1990)	
P-glycoprotein	47.6	Morphine (Kalso et al., 1998)
ABCB1 (adenosine triphosphate-binding cassette subfamily B member 1)	Protective to opioid central side effects	Morphine (Crome et al., 1984)
ABCB1 is also known as MDR-1 (multidrug resistance-1 gene)		

Opioid structure

The structures of opioid analgesics are diverse, although for most opioids it is usually the laevorotatory (*levo*)- stereoisomer that is the active compound. The structures of some of the common agents are shown. Those in current use include phenanthrenes (e.g. morphine), phenylpiperidines (e.g. fentanyl), and diphenylpropylamines (e.g. methadone). Structural modification affects agonist activity and alters physicochemical properties such as lipid solubility. Tertiary nitrogen is necessary for activity, separated from a quaternary carbon by an ethylene chain. Chemical modifications that produce quaternary nitrogen significantly reduce potency, due to decreased central nervous system (CNS) penetration. If the methyl group on the nitrogen is changed, antagonism of analgesia can be produced.

Other important positions for activity and metabolism, as seen on the morphine molecule, include the C-3 phenol group (the distance of this from the nitrogen affects activity) and the C-6 alcohol group. Potency may be increased by hydroxylation of the C-3 phenol; oxidation of C-6 (e.g. hydromorphone); double acetylation at C-3 and C-6 (e.g. diamorphine); hydroxylation of C-14 and reducing the double bond at C-7/8. Further additions at the C-3 OH group reduce activity. A short chain alkyl substitution is found in mixed agonist–antagonists, hydroxylation, or bromination of C-14 produces full antagonists, and removal or substitution of the methyl group reduces agonist activity (Hanks et al., 2001).

Pharmacokinetics and physicochemical properties

Knowledge of the specific physicochemical properties and pharmacokinetics of individual agents is important in determining the optimal route of drug delivery in order to achieve an effective receptor site concentration for an appropriate duration of action.

All opioids are weak bases. The relative proportion of free and ionized fractions is dependent on plasma pH and the pK_a of the particular opioid. The amount of opioid diffusing to the site of action (diffusible fraction) is dependent on lipid solubility, concentration gradient, and degree of binding. Plasma protein concentrations of albumin and acid glycoprotein as well as tissue binding determine the availability of the unbound, unionized fraction. This diffusible fraction moves into tissue sites in the brain and elsewhere; the amount reaching receptors is dependant not only on lipophilicity, but also the amount of non-specific tissue binding (e.g. CNS lipids).

The ionized, protonated form is active at the receptor site. This has important implications for speed and duration of activity. For example, morphine is relatively hydrophilic and penetrates the blood-brain barrier slowly. However, a large mass of any given dose eventually reaches the receptor site due to low levels of non-specific tissue-binding. This effect-site equilibration time ($t_{1/2}$keo) is measured by assessing the effect of opioids on the electroencephalogram. The offset time may also be prolonged with resultant longer duration of action than would be expected from the plasma $t_{1/2}$. Most opioids have a very steep dose–response curve. Therefore, if the dose is near the minimum effective analgesic concentration, very small fluctuations in plasma or effect-site concentrations can lead to large changes in the level of analgesia (Agency for Health Care Policy and Research: Cancer Pain Management Panel,1994).

Opioids tend to have a large volume of distribution (V_d) because of their high lipid solubility. A consequence of this can be that redistribution, particularly after a bolus dose or short infusion,

Table 9.4.3 Metabolism and excretion of some opioids

Drug	Metabolism	Faeces	Urine
Morphine	Glucuonidation Sulphation N-dealkylation	Trace	90% in 24 h (10% morphine; 70% glucuronides; 10% 3-sulphate; 1% normorphine; 3% normorphine glucuronide)
Codeine	O-demethylation Glucuronidation	Trace	86% in 24 h (5–10% codeine; 60% codeine glucuronide; 5–15% morphine (mainly conjugated); trace normorphine)
Diamorphine	O-deacetylation Glucuronidation	Trace	80% in 24 h (5–7% morphine; 90% morphine glucuronides; 1% 6-acetylmorphine; 0.1% diamorphine)
Buprenorphine	Glucuronidation N-dealkylation	70%. Mainly unchanged	2–13% in 7 days. Mainly N-dealkylbuprenorphine (and glucuronide), buprenorphine-3-glucuronide
Meperidine (pethidine)	N-demethylation Hydrolysis	No evidence of excretion	70% in 24 h (10% meperidine; 10% normeperidine; 20% mepridinic acid; 16% meperidinic acid glucuronide; 8% normeperidinic acid; 10% normeperidinic acid glucuronide; plus small amounts of other metabolites)
Methadone	N-dealkylation	30%	60% in 24 h (33% methadone; 43% EDDP; 10% EMDP plus small amounts of other metabolites)
Fentanyl	N-dealkylation Hydroxylation	9%	70% in 4 days (5–25% fentanyl; 50% 4-N-(N-proprionylanilino-piperidine) plus other metabolites)

can have significant effects on plasma concentrations. In addition, first-pass effects in the lung can remove significant amounts of drug from the circulation, reducing the initial peak plasma concentration. However, the drug re-enters the plasma several minutes later. Plasma concentrations of opioids such as fentanyl can be affected by this. Other lipophilic amines such as lidocaine and propranolol can be affected similarly and may reduce pulmonary uptake of co-administered opioids.

After prolonged infusion, significant sequestration in fat stores and other body tissues can occur for highly lipid soluble opioids. This is reflected in the 'context-sensitive $t_{1/2}$', that is, the time taken for the plasma concentration to fall by 50% after the infusion has stopped. The context-sensitive $t_{1/2}$ is increased after prolonged infusion for most opioids. For example, the elimination $t_{1/2}$ for fentanyl after bolus administration is 3–5 hours, but increases to 7–12 hours after prolonged infusion.

Most opioid metabolism occurs in the liver (phase I and II reactions) with the hydrophilic metabolites predominantly excreted renally, although a small amount may be excreted in the bile or unchanged in the urine. As a result, hepatic blood flow is one of the major determinants of plasma clearance. Metabolism of individual drugs is shown in Table 9.4.3. Enterohepatic re-circulation may occur when water-soluble metabolites excreted in the gut may be metabolized by gut flora to the parent opioid and then re-absorbed. Lipid soluble opioids may diffuse into the stomach, become ionized due to the low pH and then re-absorbed in the small intestine; this results in a secondary peak in plasma concentrations.

A summary of physicochemical and pharmacokinetic properties of some opioids is shown in Table 9.4.4. Metabolism (including production of active metabolites), distribution between different tissues, and elimination, all interact within individual subjects to produce clinically important actions at receptor sites. The physicochemical and pharmacokinetic properties of opioids can change when used for chronic pain relief.

Factors affecting pharmacokinetics include:

◆ *Age*. Age is important due to both pharmacokinetic and pharmacodynamic factors. Metabolism and volume of distribution are often reduced in the elderly, leading to increased free drug concentrations in the plasma. Hepatic blood flow may have declined by 40–50% by age 75, with reduced clearance of opioids. Increased CNS sensitivity to opioid effects is also found in the elderly.

◆ *Hepatic disease* has unpredictable effects, although there may be little clinical difference unless there is coexisting encephalopathy. Reductions in plasma protein concentrations will also have effects on plasma concentrations of free unbound drug.

◆ *Renal failure* may have significant effects for opioids with renally excreted active metabolites such as morphine and diamorphine.

◆ *Obesity* will result in a larger volume of distribution and prolonged elimination $t_{1/2}$.

◆ *Hypothermia, hypotension and hypovolaemia* may also result in variable absorption and altered distribution and metabolism of opioids.

Agonists, antagonists, potency, and efficacy

Based on their interactions with the various receptor subtypes, opioid compounds can be divided into agonist, agonist–antagonist, and antagonist classes (Table 9.4.5).

Agonists

An agonist is a drug that has affinity for and binds to cell receptors to induce changes in the cell that stimulate physiological activity. The agonist opioid drugs have no clinically relevant ceiling effect to analgesia. As the dose is raised, analgesic effects increase in a log linear function, until either analgesia is achieved or dose-limiting adverse effects supervene. Efficacy is defined by the maximal response induced by administration of the active agent. In practice, this is determined by the degree of analgesia produced following dose escalation through a range limited by the development of adverse effects. Potency, in contrast, reflects the dose–response relationship. Potency is influenced by pharmacokinetic factors (i.e. how much of the drug enters the body's systemic circulation and then reaches the receptors) and by affinity to drug receptors.

Table 9.4.4 Pharmacokinetic and physiochemical properties of some opioids

Opioid	pK_a	Protein binding (%)	Octanol: water partition coefficient	Terminal $t_{1/2}$(h)	Clearance (mL/kg/min)	Volume of distribution L/kg	Duration of action (h)
Morphine	7.9	30	6	1.7–3.0	15–20	3–5	3–5
Oxycodone	8.5	45	0.7	3–4	13	2–3	2–4
Codeine	8.2	20	0.6	2–4	9–13	2.5–3.5	4–6
Meperidine	8.5	70	39	3–5	8–18	3–5	2–4
Fentanyl	8.4	90	813	2–4	10–20	3–5	1–1.5
Alfentanil	6.5	91	128	1–2	4–9	0.4–1	0.25–0.4
Remifentanil	7.3	70	18	0.1–0.2	40–60	0.3–0.4	2–5 min
Methadone	8.3	90	26–57	15–20	2	5	4–8

Table 9.4.5 Classification of opioids for pain management

Opioid type	Medications	Notes about therapy
Pure agonists	Codeine[a] Hydrocodone Dihydrocodeine Morphine Hydromorphone Fentanyl Oxycodone Oxymorphone Levorphanol Methadone Meperidine	Mainstay of therapy in many countries for moderate to severe cancer pain No clinically relevant ceiling effect to analgesia; as dose is raised, analgesic effects increase until analgesia is achieved or dose-limiting side effects supervene Meperidine and propoxyphene are not preferred due to potential effects of toxic metabolites Methadone must be used with caution; only clinicians who are knowledgeable about the risks posed by long and variable $t_{1/2}$, unpredictable potency, and potential for QTc prolongation should use this drug without guidance

Agonists–antagonists	Partial agonists:
	  buprenorphine
	Mixed agonist–antagonists:
	  butorphanol
	  dezocine
	  nalbuphine
	  pentazocine
		Agonists–antagonists include mu-receptor agonists with lower intrinsic efficacy (partial agonists) and drugs that have agonist effects at one opioid receptor and antagonist effects at another (mixed agonist–antagonists)
		Most were developed to be less attractive to individuals with the disease of addiction; this characteristic does not rationalize widespread use for cancer pain
		All have a ceiling effect for analgesia
		All have the potential to induce acute abstinence in patients with physical dependency to agonist opioids
		Some (pentazocine and butorphanol) have a high risk of psychotomimetic side effects.
		Buprenorphine is available in a transdermal patch and may be of use in relatively opioid-naïve cancer patients

Pure antagonists	Alvimopan Methylnaltrexone Naloxone Naltrexone Nalmefene	Compete with endogenous and exogenous opioids at mu-receptor sites. Administered for prevention or reversal of opioid effects Alvimopan and methylnaltrexone have been developed specifically to treat opioid-induced bowel dysfunction
Mixed mechanism drugs	Tramadol Tapentadol	Centrally acting analgesics that have agonist actions at the mu-receptor and block reuptake of monoamines

[a] With a greater understanding of the variable handling of codeine and larger number of step 3 opioid options, codeine use is declining in many countries.

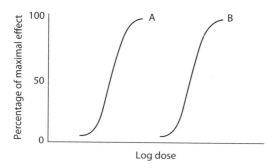

Fig. 9.4.1 Dose-response curves for two full opioid agonists (A and B) similar in efficacy but different in potency (A is more potent than B).

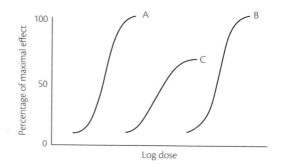

Fig. 9.4.2 Dose–response curves for two full opioid agonists (A and B) and a partial opioid agonist C.

The concepts of efficacy and potency are illustrated in Fig. 9.4.1, which shows the dose–response curves for two drugs A and B. If the logarithm of dose is plotted against response an agonist will produce an S-shaped or sigmoid curve. The efficacy of the two drugs, defined by maximum response is the same. Drug A produces the same response as B but at a lower dose, and therefore is described as more potent.

Antagonist

Antagonist drugs have no intrinsic pharmacological action but can interfere with the action of an agonist. Competitive antagonists bind to the same receptor and compete for receptor sites, whereas non-competitive antagonists block the effects of the agonist in some other way.

Opioid antagonists

Naloxone (short acting) and naltrexone (long acting) are opioid antagonists and block mu, delta, and kappa receptors equally. They are generally only used to reverse respiratory depression associated with opioid overdose as they will also reverse analgesia. Recently, however, combined opioid and peripherally acting antagonist preparations such as oxycodone/naltrexone have been made available for the prevention/management of opioid-induced constipation.

Agonist–antagonist

The agonist–antagonist analgesics can, in turn, be subdivided into the mixed agonist–antagonists and the partial agonists, a distinction also based on specific patterns of drug–receptor interaction. Both the partial agonist and agonist–antagonist drugs have a ceiling effect for analgesia, and although they produce analgesia in the opioid-naive patient, in theory they can precipitate withdrawal in patients who are physically dependent on morphine-like drugs. For these reasons, they have been considered generally to have a limited role in the management of patients with cancer pain.

Mixed agonist–antagonists

The mixed agonist–antagonist drugs produce agonist effects at one receptor and antagonist effects at another. Pentazocine is the prototype agonist–antagonist: it has agonist effects at kappa receptors and weak mu antagonist actions. Thus, in addition to analgesia, pentazocine may produce kappa-mediated psychotomimetic effects not seen with full or partial mu agonists. When a mixed agonist–antagonist is administered together with an agonist, the antagonist effect at the mu receptor can generate an acute withdrawal syndrome.

Partial agonists

A partial agonist has low intrinsic activity (efficacy) so that its dose–response curve exhibits a ceiling effect at less than the maximum effect produced by a full agonist. Buprenorphine is the main example of a partial agonist opioid. Increasing the dose of such a drug above its ceiling does not result in any further increase in response. This phenomenon is illustrated in Fig. 9.4.2 in which C is a partial agonist. C is more potent than B (in the lower part of the curve it will produce the same response at a lower dose), but is less effective than both A and B because of its ceiling effect.

When a partial agonist is administered together with an agonist, displacement of the agonist can cause a net reduction in pharmacological action which may be sufficient to generate an acute withdrawal syndrome. Whilst this is a theoretical possibility with morphine and buprenorphine, no such interaction has been reported. Similarly, it has been suggested that the effects of morphine may be blocked in a patient switched from buprenorphine, because of the prolonged action of buprenorphine and the assumption that it will 'antagonize' the effect of morphine. This has been one of the reasons why buprenorphine has not been used in cancer pain management. However, the recent development of a transdermal formulation of buprenorphine may encourage its use in chronic cancer pain (and chronic non-cancer pain). An analgesic ceiling with buprenorphine is only reached at doses of 8–16 mg or more in 24 hours (Sindrup and Brosen, 1995). When used in usual recommended doses (for example, two patches of 70 micrograms/h of transdermal buprenorphine, equivalent to 3–4 mg per 24 hours) buprenorphine can be considered a full mu agonist since at these doses its effect will lie on the linear part of the dose–response curve.

Mixed mechanism drugs

Tramadol and tapentadol are both centrally acting analgesics whose mechanism of action depends on both mu agonism and monoamine (serotonin and norephinephrine (noradrenaline)) reuptake inhibition. There is no evidence that tramadol is superior to pure mu agonists for cancer pain (Wilder-Smith et al., 1994; Leppert, 2009). It is used widely in some countries as an alternative step 2 approach. Tapentadol is a relatively new drug with little evidence for use in cancer pain (Mercadante et al., 2013). The monoaminergic mechanism results in a ceiling dose with both of these drugs

Relative potency and equianalgesic doses

Relative potency is the ratio of the doses of two analgesics required to produce the same analgesic effect. By convention, the relative potency of each of the commonly used opioids is based upon a comparison with 10 mg of parenteral morphine. Data from single- and repeated-dose studies in patients with acute or chronic pain have been used to develop an equianalgesic dose table (Table 9.4.6) that provides guidelines for dose selection when the drug or route of administration is changed. The information contained in the equianalgesic dose table does not represent standard doses, nor is it intended as an absolute guideline for dose selection. Many variables may influence the appropriate dose for an individual patient, including intensity of pain, prior opioid exposure in terms of drug, duration, and dose (and the degree of cross-tolerance that this confers), age, route of administration, level of consciousness, metabolic abnormalities (see following paragraphs), and genetic polymorphism in the expression of relevant enzymes or receptors. In particular, care should be exercised when switching from opioid to another as part of the management of opioid toxicity. In this situation highly conservative conversions should be used.

Dose–response relationship

As noted earlier, there is no ceiling to the analgesic effects of full agonist opioids. As the dose is raised, analgesic effects increase as a log linear function. In practice, the appearance of adverse effects, including confusion, sedation, nausea, vomiting, or respiratory depression, imposes a limit on the useful dose of an opioid agonist. Thus the efficacy of any particular drug in an individual patient will be determined by the degree of analgesia produced following dose escalation to intolerable and unmanageable side effects.

Section II: clinical aspects of opioid analgesia

The role of opioids in the management of cancer pain

Analgesic therapy with opioids, non-opioids, and adjuvant analgesics is developed for the individual patient through a process of continuous evaluation so that a favourable balance between pain relief and adverse pharmacological effects is maintained.

The analgesic ladder

An expert committee convened by the Cancer and Palliative Care Unit of the WHO proposed a structured approach to drug selection for cancer pain, which has become known as the 'WHO analgesic ladder' (Poulsen et al., 1996; WHO, 1996). When combined with appropriate dosing guidelines, this approach is capable of providing adequate relief to 70–90% of patients (Sawe et al., 1981a; Hoskin et al., 1989; De Conno et al., 1991; Kopp, 2000; Benyhe, 1994; St Charles et al., 1997; Innes et al., 1998). Emphasizing that the intensity of pain, rather than its specific aetiology, should be the prime consideration in analgesic selection, the approach advocates three basic steps (Fig. 9.4.3). This strategy should be integrated with non-pharmacological methods of cancer pain control including, radiotherapy, chemotherapy, hormone therapy, surgery, anaesthetic interventions, physiotherapy, and psychological/cognitive approaches:

◆ Patients with mild cancer-related pain should be treated with a non-opioid analgesic, which should be combined with adjuvant drugs if a specific indication for these exists. For example, a patient with mild to moderate arm pain caused by radiation-induced brachial plexopathy may benefit when a tricyclic antidepressant is added to paracetamol (acetaminophen) (Sawe et al., 1983; Gourlay et al., 1991).

◆ Patients who are relatively non-tolerant and present with moderate pain, or who fail to achieve adequate relief after a trial of a non-opioid analgesic, may be treated with an opioid conventionally used for mild to moderate pain (formerly known as a 'weak' opioid). This treatment is typically accomplished using a combination product containing a non-opioid (e.g. aspirin or paracetamol) and an opioid (such as codeine or oxycodone). This combination can also be coadministered with an adjuvant analgesic. The doses of these combination products can be increased until the maximum dose of the non-opioid analgesic is attained (e.g. 4000–6000 mg paracetamol); beyond this dose, the opioid contained in the combination product could be increased as a single agent, or the patient could be switched to an opioid conventionally used in step 3.

◆ Patients who present with severe pain, or who fail to achieve adequate relief following appropriate administration of drugs on the second step of the analgesic ladder, should receive an opioid conventionally used for moderate to severe pain (formerly known as a 'strong' opioid). This group includes morphine, diamorphine, fentanyl, oxycodone, phenazocine, hydromorphone, methadone, levorphanol, and oxymorphone. There is no inherent superiority of one opioid over another and treatment is individualized (Caraceni et al., 2012). These drugs may also be combined with a non-opioid analgesic or an adjuvant drug. Clearly, the boundary between opioids used in the second and third steps of the analgesic ladder is somewhat artificial since low doses of morphine or other opioids for severe pain can be less effective than high doses of codeine or propoxyphene.

According to these guidelines, a trial of opioid therapy should be given to all patients with pain of moderate or greater severity.

The evidence of the long-term efficacy of this approach and the evidence base underlying its recommendations has been the subject of criticism (Persson et al., 1992). However, this approach has been fundamental to improving cancer pain control on a worldwide basis. In recent years, application of the WHO ladder has been evolving in some countries towards omitting the second step. This is for several reasons:

1. Improved understanding of problems associated with the metabolism of codeine (Lötsch 2009)

2. A wider range of step 3 opioids and use of these drugs at a low dose instead of traditional step 2 opioids (Shimomura et al., 1971; Osborne et al., 1986; Pasternak et al., 1987; Paul et al., 1989; Caraceni, 2012).

3. An evolving suspicion that using a low dose of a step 3 opioid will be a more efficient way of controlling pain than starting at step 2 and moving upwards to a different drug. An international randomized controlled trial of the traditional three-step approach versus a two-step approach is underway (UK Clinical Research Network : Portfolio Database, n.d.).

Despite these reservations, the guiding principle that analgesic selection should be primarily determined by the severity of the pain remains sound, and continues to be widely endorsed (Paul et al., 1989; Osborne et al., 1992; Radbruch et al., 1996).

Opioid analgesics

The division of opioid agonists into 'weak' or 'strong' opioids, which was incorporated into the original analgesic ladder

Table 9.4.6 Opioid analgesics (pure mu agonists) used for the treatment of chronic pain

Morphine-like agonists	Equi-analgesic doses[a]	$t_{1/2}$ (h)	Peak effect (h)	Duration (h)	Toxicity	Comments	Oral bioavailability (%)	Active metabolites
Morphine	10 SC	2–3	0.5–1	3–6	Constipation, nausea, sedation most common; respiratory depression rare in cancer patients	Standard comparison for opioids; multiple routes available	20–30	M6G
	20–60 PO[b]	2–3	1.5–2	4–7				
Sustained-release morphine	20–60 PO[b]	2–3	3–4	8–12		Twice daily administration	20–30	M6G
Sustained-release morphine	20–60 PO[b]	2–3	4–6	24		Once-a-day morphine approved in some countries	20–30	M6G
Hydromorphone	1.5 SC	2–3	0.5–1	3–4	Same as morphine	Used for multiple routes	35–80	No
	7.5 PO	2–3	1–2	3–4				
Oxycodone	20–30	2–3	1	3–6	Same as morphine	Combined with aspirin or paracetamol (acetaminophen), for moderate pain in USA; available orally without non-opioid for severe pain	60–90	Oxymorphone
Sustained-release oxycodone	20–30	2–3	3–4	8–12				Oxymorphone
Oxymorphone	1 SC	—	0.5–1	3–6	Same as morphine	No oral formulation		Glucuronides
	10 PR	—	1.5–3	4–6				
Pethidine (meperidine)	75 SC	2–3	0.5–1	3–4	Same as morphine + CNS excitation; contraindicated in those on MAOIss	Not used for cancer pain due to toxicity in higher doses and short $t_{1/2}$	30–60	Norpethidine
Diamorphine	5 SC	0.5	0.5–1	4–5	Same as morphine	Analgesic action due to metabolites, predominantly morphine; only available in some countries		Morphine
Levorphanol	2 SC	12–16	0.5–1	4–6	Same as morphine	With long $t_{1/2}$ accumulation occurs after beginning or increasing dose		No
	4 PO							
Methadone[c]	10 SC	12– >150	0.5–1.5	4–8	Same as morphine	Risk of delayed toxicity due to accumulation; useful to start dosing on PRN schedule	60–90	No
	20 PO (see text)							
Codeine	200 PO	2–3	1.5–2	3–6	Same as morphine	Usually combined with non-opioid	60–90	Morphine

(continued)

Table 9.4.6 Continued

Morphine-like agonists	Equi-analgesic doses[a]	$t_{1/2}$ (h)	Peak effect (h)	Duration (h)	Toxicity	Comments	Oral bioavailability (%)	Active metabolites
Propoxyphene HCl (dextropropoxyphene)	—	12	1.5–2	3–6	Same as morphine plus seizures with overdose	Toxic metabolite accumulates but not significant at doses used clinically; usually combined with non-opioid	40	Norpropoxyphene
Propoxyphene napsylate (dextropropoxyphene)	—	12	1.5–2	3–6	Same as hydrochloride	Same as hydrochloride	40	Norpropoxyphene
Hydrocodone	—	2–4	0.5–1	3–4	Same as morphine	Only available combined with paracetamol; only available in some countries		Hydromorphone
Dihydrocodeine	—	2–4	0.5–1	3–4	Same as morphine	Only available combined with aspirin or paracetamol in some countries	20	Morphine
Fentanyl	—	3–12	—	—	Same as morphine	Can be administered as a continuous IV or SC infusion; based on clinical experience, 100 micrograms/h is roughly equianalgesic to morphine 4 mg/h IV	25/buccal <2/oral	No
Fentanyl transdermal system	—	13–22	—	48–72	Same as morphine	Based on clinical experience 100 micrograms/h is roughly equianalgesic to morphine 4 mg/h; recent study indicates a ratio of oral morphine: transdermal fentanyl of 100: 1	90/transdermal	No

[a] Dose that provides analgesia equivalent to 10 mg IM morphine. These ratios are only guidelines when switching drugs or routes of administration.

[b] Extensive survey data suggest that the relative potency of IM: PO or SC: PO morphine of 1: 6 changes to 1: 2–3 with chronic dosing.

[c] When switching from another opioid to methadone, the potency of methadone is much greater than indicated in this table.

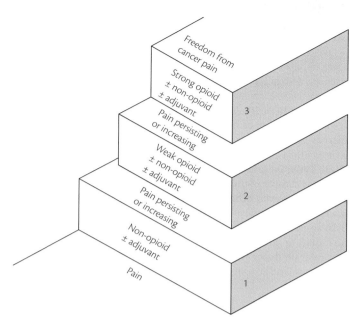

Fig. 9.4.3 The WHO three-step analgesic ladder.
Reproduced with permission from the World Health Organization, *WHO's cancer pain ladder for adults,* Copyright © WHO 2014, available from http://www.who.int/cancer/palliative/painladder/en/.

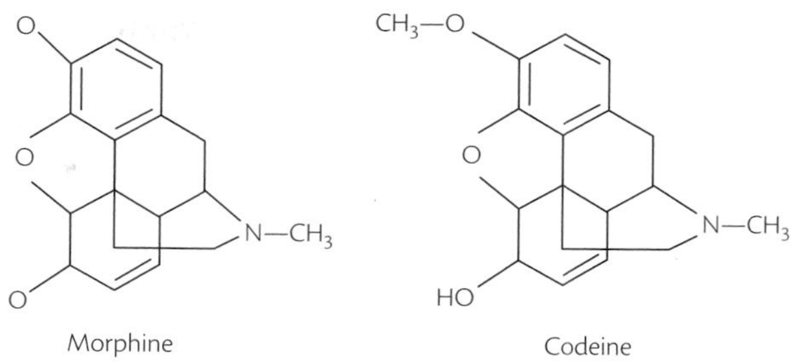

Fig. 9.4.4 The chemical structures of morphine and codeine.

proposed by the WHO, was not based on fundamental differences in their pharmacology, but rather reflected the customary manner in which these drugs were used. In this chapter, we will refer to opioids for mild to moderate pain and opioids for moderate to severe pain rather than 'weak' or 'strong' opioids. This terminology is now incorporated into the current version of the WHO analgesic ladder.

Opioids for mild to moderate pain

Codeine

Codeine (methylmorphine) is a naturally occurring opium alkaloid used as an analgesic, antitussive, and antidiarrhoeal agent (Fig. 9.4.4). Codeine is much less potent than morphine and produces its analgesic effects in part by binding to mu opioid receptors but with low affinity and, in part through biotransformation to morphine by cytochrome P450 (CYP) 2D6 (sparteine oxygenase) which exhibits genetic polymorphism. Approximately 7% of Caucasians lack CYP2D6 activity (poor metabolizers) due to inheritance of two non-functional alleles and in these individuals codeine has a diminished analgesic effect (Portenoy et al., 1991, 1992).

Codeine phosphate is absorbed well from the gastrointestinal tract, but oral bioavailability varies considerably between individuals (from 12% to 84% in one study (Vree and Verwey-van Wissen, 1992). The main metabolite is codeine-6-glucuronide, with much smaller amounts of norcodeine, morphine, and morphine 3- and 6-glucuronides also being produced (de Crean et al., 1996). The usual oral dose of codeine is 30–60 mg and its duration of action is 4–6 hours.

Codeine is not generally given as a single agent when used orally as an analgesic, but is usually combined with a non-opioid and recent systematic reviews confirm that the combination of codeine

and paracetamol is more effective than paracetamol alone (Peat et al., 1991; Penson et al., 2000a). A sustained-release formulation of codeine is available in some countries. When changing from regular administration of a codeine/non-opioid combination to morphine, patients receiving a total daily dose of 240–360 mg codeine are usually started on 60 mg morphine daily.

Dihydrocodeine

Dihydrocodeine is a semisynthetic analogue of codeine that is used as an analgesic, antitussive, and antidiarrhoeal agent. When administered by mouth, dihydrocodeine is equianalgesic to codeine. However, when administered parenterally, it is approximately twice as potent as codeine. This may be explained by the consistently poorer bioavailability of dihydrocodeine (20%), which probably results from hepatic pre-systemic metabolism (Moore et al., 1997).

The usual starting dose is 30 mg every 4–6 hours (by mouth), and this may be increased to 60 mg. However, dihydrocodeine appears to have a narrower therapeutic index than codeine, with a high incidence of adverse effects at the 60 mg dose. A controlled-release formulation of dihydrocodeine is available in several countries.

There have been a number of reports of severe toxicity associated with dihydrocodeine in patients with impaired renal function (Smith et al., 1990; Hanks 1991). The mechanism is not clear because of the limited data available on the pharmacokinetics of this drug, although it seems most likely that the cause is accumulation of active glucuronide metabolites, as occurs with morphine.

There is confusion about the relative analgesic potency of dihydrocodeine. It seems reasonable to assume that oral dihydrocodeine is roughly equipotent to oral codeine, and to use a similar conversion ratio when changing to morphine.

Dextropropoxyphene

Propoxyphene is a synthetic derivative of methadone, and its dextrorotatory stereoisomer dextropropoxyphene is responsible for its analgesic activity. Dextropropoxyphene is a mu agonist with low receptor affinity similar to that of codeine. It is readily absorbed from the gastrointestinal tract with peak serum levels about 2 hours after administration. The mean elimination $t_{1/2}$ is about 12 hours, with steady state levels being reached after 3–4 days of regular administration every 6–8 hours. The $t_{1/2}$ may be very long (over 50 hours) in elderly patients (Rowell et al., 1983).

Dextropropoxyphene undergoes extensive first-pass metabolism. Its principal metabolite is norpropoxyphene, which is active but penetrates the brain to a much lesser extent and has much weaker opioid effects. Norpropoxyphene has a longer $t_{1/2}$ (about 23 hours) than dextropropoxyphene itself and accumulates in plasma (Barnes and Goodwin 1983). Norpropoxyphene accumulation is associated with excitatory effects, including tremulousness and seizures.

The analgesic efficacy and relative potency of dextropropoxyphene have been questioned. This is in part because single-dose studies comparing aspirin, paracetamol, and non-steroidal anti-inflammatory drugs (NSAIDs), including ibuprofen 400 mg, mefenamic acid 250 mg, and fenoprofen 50 mg, have shown dextropropoxyphene to be a less effective analgesic (Barnes et al., 1985). A more recent systematic review found that paracetamol alone is as effective as the combination of paracetamol with dextropropoxyphene though the studies included were again all single-dose studies (Crome et al., 1984). Single-dose studies may be misleading, as is the case with single-dose studies of oral morphine.

The extensive first-pass metabolism of dextropropoxyphene is dose-dependent such that the systemic availability of the drug increases with increasing oral doses (Perrier and Gibaldi, 1972). Thus, with regular administration, there is enhanced bioavailability and some degree of accumulation because of the long elimination half-lives of the parent drug and its main metabolite. Both dextropropoxyphene and norpropoxyphene reach plasma concentrations in the steady state which are five to seven times greater than those found after the first dose. There is, therefore, a pharmacokinetic basis for believing that repeated doses of dextropropoxyphene are likely to be more effective than single doses. The usual starting dose of morphine for patients receiving dextropropoxyphene–paracetamol combinations every 4–6 hours (representing 260–390 mg of dextropropoxyphene daily) is 60 mg per day.

For a long time, a combination of dextropropoxyphene and paracetamol was the most commonly prescribed analgesic in the United Kingdom and some Scandinavian countries, but it received much adverse publicity because of its lethal effects in overdose and fears about its addiction potential. Part of this concern was stimulated by its very widespread use. In addition to usual opioid adverse effects, propoxyphene may rarely induce a hepatotoxic reaction (Beaver 1984), cardiac conduction disorder (Li Wan Po and Zhang, 1997), and potentially dangerous drug interactions have been reported when propoxyphene has been administered along with carbamazepine (Perrier and Gibaldi, 1972), warfarin (Perrier and Gibaldi, 1972), or alcohol (Hantson et al., 1995). Currently, however, there is insufficient evidence to conclude that dextropropoxyphene is inherently more toxic than codeine or other opioids of similar efficacy, nor is there evidence that one is more effective than another. In the United Kingdom, dextropropoxyphene in combination with paracetamol has been removed from the general prescribing list because of an association with fatal drug overdose; however, dextropropoxyphene remains available in several countries.

Oxycodone

Oxycodone is a semi-synthetic congener of morphine, which has been on the market for 80 years but until relatively recently was only available in formulations which effectively circumscribed its use. In the United States, it has been prescribed in low-dose combination products with a non-opioid for oral administration (usually 5 mg of oxycodone with either aspirin or paracetamol) and has traditionally been used as a step 2 analgesic. Historically, it had only been used as a rectal suppository in the United Kingdom,

and had been widely used by mouth as a first line step 2 and 3 opioid in Scandinavia (Pippenger 1987).

Over the past 20 years, oxycodone has been produced as a single agent in new oral formulations, both normal release and sustained release, which has substantially improved the convenience of administration. In many countries sustained-release oxycodone is available in 5, 10, 20, 40, and 80 mg formulations with a corresponding range of normal-release formulations. Oxycodone is increasingly used as a step 3 opioid, though the low-dose formulations allow its use at step 2 also (Savarese et al., 1986; Poulain et al., 1988; Gourlay et al., 1997). Oxycodone probably provides the best example of the overlap in efficacy between opioids at steps 2 and 3; however, other opioids now also fulfil this role (see following paragraphs).

In some countries, it is available in a combination slow-release formulation with naloxone in a 2:1 ratio. There is evidence that at moderate doses this formulation is associated with a reduced prevalence and severity of constipation (Ahmedzai et al., 2012).

Tramadol

Tramadol is a centrally acting analgesic which possesses opioid agonist properties and may also activate monoaminergic spinal inhibition of pain (Justice and Kline 1988). It has modest affinity with mu opioid receptors, with weak affinity to delta and kappa receptors, and its analgesic effect is reversed by naloxone. Unlike other opioids, it also inhibits the uptake of noradrenaline and serotonin, and in an animal model systemically administered yohimbine or ritanserin blocks tramadol-induced analgesia, suggesting that this effect contributes significantly to the drug's analgesic action (Justice and Kline, 1988; Leppert 2009).

Tramadol can be administered orally, rectally, intravenously, subcutaneously, or intramuscularly. In many countries, it is available in both normal- and sustained-release formulations. Parenterally, 50–150 mg of tramadol is equianalgesic to 5–15 mg morphine (Whittington 1984). There are insufficient data for a reliable assessment of its oral-to-parenteral relative analgesic potency and estimates range from 1:4 to 1:10 (Kaiko et al., 1981; Ripamonti et al., 1997).

Oral tramadol has demonstrated efficacy in the management of chronic cancer pain of moderate severity (Kaiko et al., 1981; Davis and Walsh 2001). Few patients with severe pain are adequately managed by tramadol (Grochow et al., 1989; Ripamonti et al., 1997; Davis and Walsh 2001). Tramadol has a similar side effect profile to morphine, but may cause less constipation and respiratory depression at equianalgesic doses.

A systematic review demonstrates a lack of evidence to support the routine use of tramadol as a step 2 analgesic in cancer pain (Tassinari et al., 2011).

Tapentadol

Several mechanisms can be proposed to explain an apparent synergistic analgesic action between mu-opioid and α2-adrenergic receptor agonists. Combining both effects in a single molecule eliminates the potential for drug–drug interactions inherent in multiple drug therapy. Tapentadol is the first approved centrally acting analgesic having both mu-opioid receptor agonist and noradrenaline (norepinephrine) reuptake inhibition activity with minimal serotonin reuptake inhibition. This dual mode of action is of interest, however cancer pain studies with tapentadol are awaited. Having limited protein binding, no active metabolites and no significant microsomal enzyme induction or inhibition, tapentadol has a limited potential for drug–drug interactions. Clinical trial evidence in acute and chronic non-cancer pain and neuropathic pain seems to support an opioid-sparing effect that reduces some of the typical opioid-related adverse effects (Hatrick and Rozek 2011; Riemsma et al., 2011).

While rapidly absorbed, the oral bioavailability of tapentadol under fasting conditions is only 32% due to an extensive first-pass effect (Tzschentke et al., 2006; LabelDataPlus, 2011). Only 20% of the drug is bound to plasma protein. Its $t_{1/2}$ of 4.9 hours permits achievement of steady-state concentrations at 25–30 hours when tapentadol is administered orally every 6 hours (Tzschentke et al., 2006, 2007). Extensive metabolism, primarily by the uridine diphosphate-glucuronosyltransferase (UGT) enzymes UGT1A9 and UGT2B7, results in renal elimination of inactive glucuronide or sulphate conjugates, with tapentadol-0-glucuronide being the major metabolite (Tzschentke et al., 2007; Kneip et al., 2008). Tapentadol follows first-order elimination kinetics over a wide range of conditions. Moderate hepatic dysfunction, however, warrants dose reduction (Xu et al., 2010; LabelDataPlus, 2011). Tapentadol is not recommended and should not be given to patients with severe hepatic dysfunction.

Since tapentadol is a noradrenaline reuptake inhibitor, it is contraindicated in patients receiving monoamine oxidase inhibitors (MAOIs) within the previous 14 days. Despite minimal serotonergic effect, theoretically a serotonin syndrome might be precipitated by concomitant use with serotonin noradrenaline reuptake inhibitor (SNRI), selective serotonin reuptake inhibitor (SSRI), TCA, MAOI, or serotonin 5-HT$_{IB/ID}$ receptor agonist (triptan) medications (LabelDataPlus, 2011).

The second step of the analgesic ladder

As previously described, by convention, formulations combining aspirin or paracetamol with a low dose of codeine, oxycodone, or propoxyphene have been recommended for pain of moderate intensity (step 2 of the analgesic ladder). This recommendation was pragmatic rather than evidence based. It reflected the concern that in many parts of the world it would be unacceptable to use morphine or other potent opioids for moderate pain.

The most frequently employed step 2 analgesics in cancer pain are combination preparations containing 300–500 mg paracetamol with 30 mg codeine, 32.5 mg dextropropoxyphene, or 5 mg oxycodone. The combination of dextropropoxyphene with paracetamol has been withdrawn in the United Kingdom and other parts of the world because of its lethal effects in overdose, and is much less used generally. Codeine plus paracetamol is still used in combination at step 2. As already discussed, the use of codeine is however evolving and is now used less frequently.

Studies comparing single doses of opioid/non-opioid combinations with various NSAIDs in postoperative pain have shown advantages for the latter in terms of greater efficacy and fewer adverse effects (Sawe et al., 1981b; Mercadante et al., 1996; Mathew and Storey, 1999). Chronic use of NSAIDs may negate any advantage in terms of unwanted effects, although at present there are no comparative data for chronic cancer pain. NSAIDs are increasingly employed as step 2 analgesics.

Given the limitations of the conventional approach many clinicians now use a variety of single agent opioid agonists, some

previously designated as 'step 3' opioids, in an appropriate dose, for moderate pain. Over recent years, sustained-release formulations of oxycodone, tramadol, and morphine in dose formulations appropriate for pain of moderate severity have become widely available and are now often used in this setting. This practice is supported by evidence of efficacy (Poulain et al., 1988; Bruera et al., 1991; Davis and Walsh, 2001).

The partial agonist opioid buprenorphine also may be used in this setting since it has recently become available in a transdermal formulation. A low-dose formulation of transdermal fentanyl (12 micrograms/hour) is designed for use in patients who may be opioid naive. More clinical trial data are required to clarify some of the issues surrounding these trends in opioid prescribing.

Opioids for moderate to severe pain

Morphine

Morphine is a potent mu-agonist drug that was first introduced into clinical use almost 200 years ago. It is the main naturally occurring alkaloid of opium derived from the poppy *Papaver somniferum* and is available for therapeutic use as the sulphate, hydrochloride, and tartrate. Recent evidence suggests that biosynthetic pathways for morphine exist in animal and human tissues such as liver, blood, and brain (Kalso et al., 1991). Its chemical structure is shown in Fig. 9.4.5. The WHO has placed oral morphine on the Essential Drug List, and preparations are available for oral, rectal, parenteral, and intraspinal administration.

Bioavailability

Morphine is available in four oral formulations: an elixir, a normal-release tablet, a modified-release tablet or capsule (of which there are now several preparations using different sustained-release mechanisms), and sustained-release suspensions. Absorption of morphine after oral administration occurs predominantly in the alkaline medium of the upper small bowel (morphine is a weak base) and is more or less complete. After oral administration, extensive pre-systemic elimination of the drug occurs predominantly in the liver. In healthy volunteers and cancer patients, the average bioavailability for oral morphine is 20–30% (Szeto et al., 1977; Umans and Inturrisi, 1982; Eisendrath et al., 1987). Like all other pharmacokinetic parameters, bioavailability demonstrates marked inter-individual variability. In patients with normal renal function the plasma $t_{1/2}$ (2–3 hours) is somewhat shorter than the duration of analgesia (4–6 hours). The pharmacokinetics remain linear with repetitive administration, and there does not appear to be autoinduction of biotransformation even following large chronic doses (Glare and Walsh, 1993). Rectal morphine bioavailability is similar to the oral route.

Morphine is relatively hydrophilic and, when administered epidurally or intrathecally, it is not rapidly absorbed into the systemic circulation. This results in a long $t_{1/2}$ in cerebrospinal fluid (90–120 minutes) and extensive rostral redistribution (Heiskanen and Kalso, 1997).

Morphine metabolism

About 90% of morphine is converted into metabolites (Fig. 9.4.5), principally the glucuronide conjugates morphine-3-glucuronide (M3G) and morphine-6-glucuronide (M6G); minor metabolites include codeine, normorphine, and morphine ethereal sulphate. The liver appears to be the predominant site of metabolism in humans, although in animal models extrahepatic metabolism

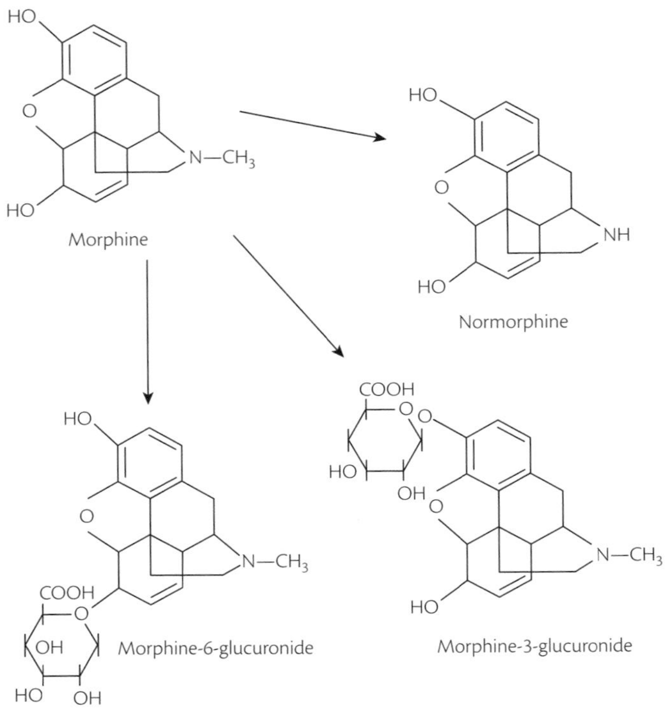

Fig. 9.4.5 The metabolites of morphine.

has been demonstrated in the small bowel and the proximal renal tubule of rodents. These sites may become important where liver function is impaired. M3G is the major metabolite and in recent years there has been some controversy about its possible role as an opioid antagonist or in mediating some of the adverse effects of morphine.

Morphine-6-glucuronide

M6G binds to opioid receptors (Hanks and Hawkins, 2000) and produces potent opioid effects in animals (Houde 1986; Agency for Health Care Policy and Research: Acute Pain Management Panel, 1992; Sarhill et al., 2001) and humans (Brose et al., 1991; Moulin et al., 1991; Agency for Health Care Policy and Research: Acute Pain Management Panel, 1992; Hays et al., 1994). M6G excretion by the kidney is directly related to creatinine clearance (Raffa et al., 1992); its elimination $t_{1/2}$ is 2–3 hours in patients with normal renal function (similar to that of morphine) but becomes progressively longer with deteriorating function, resulting in significant accumulation (Raffa et al., 1992). In patients with impaired renal function, M6G may accumulate in blood and cerebrospinal fluid (Lee et al., 1993), and high concentrations of this metabolite have been associated with toxicity (Moulin et al., 1991, Dixon et al., 1983). These data warrant caution when administering morphine to patients with renal impairment. Patients who are receiving regular morphine and develop acute renal failure in a previously stable situation (e.g. a rapidly developing obstructive uropathy in a patient with pelvic malignancy) may develop a sudden onset of signs and symptoms of opioid toxicity, necessitating temporary withdrawal of the morphine and subsequent dose reduction, and/or less frequent administration.

M6G is thought to be a potent analgesic and studies in acute postoperative pain are currently ongoing. There are some, albeit limited, data to suggest that M6G has fewer side effects than morphine (van Dorp et al., 2008).

Morphine-3-glucuronide

For many years, it has been assumed that M3G is inert as is the case with most glucuronide metabolites (Wilder Smith et al., 1994). Behavioural studies in rodents, however, suggested that M3G produces a functional antagonism of the analgesic effects of morphine and its active metabolite M6G (Kaiko et al., 1996; Salzman et al., 1999). There is also some evidence in animal models that M3G may be responsible for the CNS excitatory adverse effects seen with morphine, such as myoclonus (Eddy and Lee, 1959; Wilder Smith et al., 1994).

It is now clear that M3G does not bind to opioid receptors. Data from electrophysiological animal models indicate no evidence of an antagonistic effect of M3G (Grond et al., 1999) and recent studies in human volunteers indicate that M3G appears to be devoid of significant activity (Moulin et al., 1988; Rogers, 1991a). In particular, there is no evidence of functional antagonism of morphine or M6G in humans and overall it seems that M3G plays no significant role in the pharmacodynamics of morphine.

Oral to parenteral relative potency

Single-dose studies of morphine in postoperative cancer patients demonstrated an oral-to-intramuscular potency ratio of 1:6 (Petzke et al., 2001). However, empirical clinical practice using chronically administered oral morphine in cancer patients has generated a different ratio of 1:3 or 1:2 (Hess et al., 1972; Mather, 1983). The reason for the discrepancy between relative potency estimates derived from single-dose versus chronic dosing studies is probably associated with both methodology (Radbruch et al., 1996) and the pharmacokinetics and pharmacodynamics of M6G (McEvoy et al., 1996). It is possible that M6G accumulation relative to morphine may be greater with oral than with parenteral administration; this would lead to an increase in the relative potency of the orally administered drug when given on a chronic basis.

The important principle for clinical practice is that there is a difference in relative analgesic potency when the route of administration is changed, and that adjustment of dose is necessary in order to achieve an equivalent effect and to avoid either underdosing or toxicity. The usual practice when converting from oral morphine to subcutaneous morphine (or diamorphine) is to divide the oral dose by two or three (Osborne et al., 1986).

Parenteral morphine

The inorganic salts of morphine (morphine sulphate and morphine hydrochloride) have limited solubility. Standard formulations are available up to 20 mg/mL, and morphine can be constituted from lyophilized power up to 50 mg/mL. Morphine tartrate is substantially more soluble and, in some countries, is formulated in a concentration of 80 mg/mL.

Sustained-release morphine preparations

The development of modified-release morphine preparations has had a major impact on clinical practice. These preparations, which are usually administered on a 12-hour schedule, provide a much more convenient means of administering oral morphine (St Charles et al., 1997). Several preparations are available worldwide with a range of dose formulations (10, 15, 30, 60, 100, and 200 mg depending on the country), allowing considerable flexibility in their use. Some preparations allow once-daily administration and sustained-release suspensions are also available (Innes et al., 1998).

In contrast with morphine solution or normal-release tablets, where peak plasma concentrations are achieved within the first hour followed by a rapid decline and an elimination $t_{1/2}$ of 2–4 hours, sustained-release morphine typically achieves peak plasma concentrations 3–6 hours after administration, the peak is attenuated, and plasma concentrations are sustained over a 12- or 24-hour period (Portenoy et al., 1993; Jeal and Benfield, 1997; Megens et al., 1998). The type and incidence of adverse effects with sustained-release morphine and normal-release oral morphine appear to be similar with the currently available formulations.

Although some clinicians advocate the use of sustained-release morphine when initiating morphine therapy in cancer patients, a normal-release preparation is generally recommended in the dose titration period (Caraceni et al., 2012).

Initial dose titration using sustained-release morphine is difficult because of the delay in achieving peak plasma concentrations, the attenuation of peak concentrations, and the long duration of action. In this situation, dose finding is performed more efficiently with a short-acting morphine preparation. Once the effective dose is identified using a normal-release formulation, this may be changed to a sustained-release preparation using a milligram-to-milligram conversion. For the same reasons, sustained-release morphine is not appropriate for the treatment of acute pain or 'breakthrough' pain (BTP). A normal-release morphine preparation should be provided to patients stabilized on sustained-release morphine to be used 'as required' for BTP.

Diamorphine (heroin)

Diamorphine (diacetylmorphine) is a semi-synthetic analogue of morphine and has a long tradition of use for cancer pain in the United Kingdom. It is only available for legal medicinal use in the United Kingdom and Canada.

Following oral administration of diamorphine, only morphine can be measured in the patient's blood. The use of oral diamorphine is an inefficient way of delivering morphine to the systemic circulation. There is no good basis to believe that there is any difference between these two drugs when given by mouth. Sublingual administration of diamorphine has been advocated by some but, as discussed below, this route is not appropriate for either morphine or diamorphine because of poor absorption. It has been thought that diamorphine does not itself bind to the mu opioid receptor but must be biotransformed to 6-acetylmorphine and morphine to produce its analgesic effect (Kopp, 2000). However, recent studies with mor-knockout mice seem to indicate that it does not produce its effects through mu receptor binding and may have effects at other receptors (Benyhe, 1994). This may explain some of the pharmacodynamic differences between morphine and diamorphine when given parenterally.

Since diamorphine is more soluble and lipophilic than morphine, it does have some advantages for parenteral administration. When administered by subcutaneous or intramuscular injection, diamorphine is approximately twice as potent as morphine. There are also differences between diamorphine and morphine administered by intravenous injection: diamorphine has a marginally quicker onset of action, produces greater sedation, and possibly less vomiting (Sawe et al., 1981a). This may be explained by different receptor binding. The greater solubility of diamorphine (shared also with hydromorphone and morphine tartrate)

is of particular advantage for patients who require large doses of subcutaneous opioids.

Methadone

Methadone is a synthetic opioid with an oral-to-parenteral potency ratio of 1:2 and an oral bioavailability greater than 85%. In single-dose studies, methadone is only marginally more potent than morphine; however, with repeated administration it is several times more potent. Methadone has a very long plasma $t_{1/2}$, averaging approximately 24 hours (with a range from 12 to over 150 hours) (Hoskin et al., 1989; Gourlay et al., 1991). Whereas most patients can be well controlled on 8–12-hour dosing, some patients require dosing at a 4–8-hour interval to maintain analgesic effects (Sawe et al., 1983). Methadone may be a useful alternative to morphine, but its safe administration requires knowledge of its pharmacology and experience of its use.

After treatment is initiated or the dose is increased, plasma concentration rises over a prolonged period, and this may be associated with a delayed onset of side effects. Consequently, patients must be followed closely until there is reasonable certainty that a steady state plasma concentration has been approached (approximately 1 week). Serious adverse effects can be avoided if the initial period of dosing is accomplished with 'as needed' administration (Max et al., 1985). When steady state has been achieved, scheduled dose frequency should be determined by the duration of analgesia following each dose (Paul et al., 1989).

Oral and parenteral preparations of methadone are available. Subcutaneous infusion is possible (Shimomura et al., 1971) but caution is required since local skin toxicity may be a problem (Pasternak et al., 1987).

The equianalgesic dose ratio of morphine to methadone has been a matter of confusion and controversy. Data from cross-over studies with morphine and methadone and hydromorphone and methadone indicate that methadone is much more potent than previously described in literature, and that the ratio correlates with the total opioid dose administered before switching to methadone (Osborne et al., 1986). Among patients receiving oral equivalent doses of morphine (< 90mg/daily), the ratio is 4:1, a ratio of 8:1 for patients receiving 90–300 mg/day and for patients receiving greater than 300 mg morphine/day, a ratio of 12:1 should be used (Benitez-Rosario et al., 2009; Chatham et al., 2013).

Pethidine (meperidine)

Pethidine is a synthetic opioid with agonist effects similar to those of morphine but a profile of potential adverse effects that limits its utility as an analgesic for chronic cancer pain. Intramuscular pethidine 75 mg is equivalent to 10 mg of intramuscular morphine. Pethidine has an oral bioavailability of 40–60%, and its oral-to-parenteral potency ratio is 1:4. It is more lipophilic than morphine, and produces a faster onset and shorter duration of analgesia of 2–3 hours.

Pethidine is *N*-demethylated to norpethidine, which is an active metabolite that is twice as potent as a convulsant and half as potent as an analgesic compared with its parent compound. Accumulation of norpethidine after repetitive dosing of pethidine can result in central nervous system excitability characterized by subtle mood effects, tremors, multifocal myoclonus, and occasionally, seizures (Osborne et al., 1992; Portenoy et al., 1992). Naloxone does not reverse pethidine-induced seizures, and it is possible that its administration to patients receiving pethidine chronically could precipitate seizures by blocking the depressant action of pethidine and allowing the convulsant activity of norpethidine to become manifest (Portenoy et al., 1991). If naloxone is necessary in this situation, it should be diluted and slowly titrated while appropriate seizure precautions are taken.

Selective toxicity of pethidine can also occur following administration to patients receiving monoamine oxidase inhibitors. This combination may produce a syndrome characterized by hyperpyrexia, muscle rigidity, and seizures which may occasionally be fatal (D'Honneur et al., 1994). The pathophysiology of this syndrome is related to excess availability of serotonin at the 5-HT$_{1A}$-receptor in the central nervous system.

Although accumulation of norpethidine is most likely to affect patients with overt renal disease, toxicity is sometimes observed in patients with normal renal function. These potential adverse effects contraindicate pethidine for the management of chronic cancer pain. Given the availability of alternative drugs that lack these toxicities, its use in acute pain management is also not recommended (Lehmann and Zech, 1992).

Hydromorphone

Hydromorphone is another morphine congener. It is about five times more potent than morphine and can be administered by the oral, rectal, parenteral, and intraspinal routes. Its oral bioavailability varies from 35% to 80% (Peat et al., 1991). Its $t_{1/2}$ is 1.5–3 hours and it has a short duration of action. Although it is largely excreted unchanged by the kidney, it is partially metabolized in the liver to a 3-glucuronide, which is excreted by the kidneys (Peat et al., 1991; Penson et al., 2000a).

Its solubility, the availability of a high-concentration preparation (10 mg/mL), and high bioavailability by the subcutaneous route (78%) make it particularly suitable for subcutaneous infusion (Penson et al., 2000b). In the United States, it is routinely available in oral, rectal, and injectable formulations, and a sustained-release oral formulation (Hanks 1991).

For patients who require very high opioid doses via the subcutaneous route, hydromorphone can be constituted in concentrations of up to 50 mg/mL from lyophilized powder. It has also been administered via the epidural and intrathecal routes to manage acute and chronic pain. In fact for newer intrathecal pump devices, hydromorphone rather than diamorphine should be used because of device interactions with the latter. Hydromorphone is hydrophilic and, when administered via the epidural route, its pharmacokinetic profile, including its long $t_{1/2}$ and extensive rostral distribution in cerebrospinal fluid, is similar to that of morphine (Smith et al., 1990).

The equianalgesic ratio of parenteral morphine to hydromorphone has been a matter of controversy. There is evidence that potency ratios for hydromorphone are not bidirectional. An equianalgesic ratio of 7:1 is quoted when switching from morphine to hydromorphone but ratios of 4:1–8:1 are reported when switching in the other direction. The reported oral equianalgesic ratio for morphine to hydromorphone is 7.5:1, so when converting from oral to subcutaneous hydromorphone, the dose should be divided by two, presuming an oral to parenteral potency ratio for morphine of 1:2 (Gong et al., 1992).

Although some studies suggest a more favourable side effect profile than morphine, there is conflicting evidence. It is highly likely, as with all opioids, that it will depend on the individual patient. Systematic reviews of hydromorphone in cancer pain did not find any significant differences between hydromorphone and oxycodone for acute and chronic pain (Yaksh and Harty, 1987) and place it clearly as an alternative to morphine with no inferiority nor superiority (Pigni et al., 2011).

Levorphanol

Levorphanol is a morphine congener with a long $t_{1/2}$ (12–16 hours) (Labella et al., 1979). It shares a number of pharmacological properties with methadone. It is five times more potent than morphine and has an oral-to-parenteral potency ratio of 1:2 (Hewett et al., 1993). Like methadone, the discrepancy between plasma $t_{1/2}$ (12–16 hours) and duration of analgesia (4–6 hours) may predispose to drug accumulation following the initiation of therapy or dose escalation. Although dose titration needs to be done carefully in the opioid-naive patient, problems with drug accumulation appear to be less than those produced by methadone.

In the United States, levorphanol is generally used as a second-line agent in patients with chronic pain who cannot tolerate morphine. The possibility that this drug may be particularly useful in morphine-tolerant patients has been proposed on the basis of its affinity for kappa and delta receptors that are presumably not involved in morphine analgesia (Penson et al., 2001). It seems also to have NMDA antagonist activity. It is no longer available in the United Kingdom or Canada.

It has been suggested that because of the unique properties of levorphanol, it may prove useful to re-evaluate this drug in clinical studies (McNulty, 2007; Prommer, 2007).

Oxycodone

As previously described, oxycodone is a synthetic morphine congener that has a high oral bioavailability (60–90%) and an analgesic potency 30–50% greater than morphine (Houde et al., 1965; Hanks et al., 1987). Since the development of sustained-release formulations in doses suitable for severe pain, it is now widely used for this indication. The sustained-release formulation is available in a wide range of dose formulations (5, 10, 20, 40, and 80 mg) (Hanks and Hawkins, 2000) and has a duration of action of 8–12 hours. The sustained-release formulation achieves effective therapeutic levels within an hour (Kaiko, 1996) and appears to be suitable for dose titration (Salzman et al., 1999).

Oxycodone pectinate is available in the United Kingdom as a 30 mg rectal suppository which has a delayed absorption and prolonged duration of effect (Kaiko, 1986).

There has been confusion about the relative efficacy of oxycodone. It had been viewed primarily as a 'step 2' opioid because it had for long been available in low dose in combination products with non-opioid analgesics. It seems clear that the relative potency of oxycodone has been underestimated in early clinical studies in which it appeared to be less potent than morphine. Subsequent studies indicate that it is more potent, in a ratio of about 1.5:1 (Bruera et al., 1998).

There remains uncertainty also about the role of its active metabolite oxymorphone which accounts for 10% of its metabolites, in mediating the effects of oxycodone. However, current evidence suggests that the metabolites of oxycodone including oxymorphone do not contribute significantly to its pharmacological effects (Hanks, 1989).

A recent systematic review of oxycodone in cancer pain concluded that there is no evidence of a significant difference in analgesia or adverse effects between oxycodone and morphine or hydromorphone (King et al., 2011).

Oxymorphone

Oxymorphone is a lipophilic congener of morphine formerly available as a rectal formulation. It is now available in the United States in oral normal- and sustained-release preparations. It has a predictable dose response and linear pharmacokinetics. The injectable formulation is ten times more potent than morphine (Forman et al., 1993). The plasma $t_{1/2}$ of oxymorphone is 1.2–2 hours, and its duration of action is 3–5 hours. It is less likely to produce histamine release than morphine (Savarese et al., 1986), and may be particularly useful for patients who develop itch in response to other opioids (Poulain et al., 1988). It is not metabolized through CYP3A4 or CXP2D6 which is useful for avoiding drug–drug interactions.

A pilot of the effectiveness and safety of oral extended-release oxymorphone for the treatment of cancer pain, reported favourably. Patients stabilized on CR morphine or CR oxycodone were safely and rapidly converted to a lower milligram dose of oxymorphone ER that provided adequate pain relief with similar tolerability (Sloan et al., 2005; Slatkin et al., 2010).

Oxymorphone is currently not available in the United Kingdom.

Fentanyl

Fentanyl is a semi-synthetic opioid and is a highly selective mu agonist (Gourlay et al., 1997) that is about 80 times as potent as parenteral morphine in the non-tolerant acute pain patient. It is also extremely lipophilic and is extensively taken up into fatty tissue (Inturrisi et al., 1984). Its elimination $t_{1/2}$ ranges from 3 to 12 hours and is influenced by the duration of prior administration and the extent of fat sequestration. Fentanyl has been used mainly as an intravenous anaesthetic agent and continues to be used parenterally as a pre-medication for painful procedures and in continuous infusions. When used intravenously, fentanyl has a very short duration of action of 0.5–1 hours. This is related to the rapid re-distribution of the drug into body tissues rather than to hepatic and renal elimination (Pasternak and Standifer, 1995). The development of a transdermal system and an oral transmucosal formulation has broadened the clinical utility of fentanyl for the management of cancer pain.

Transdermal fentanyl

The low molecular weight and high lipid solubility of fentanyl facilitate absorption through the skin and a transdermal formulation that delivers 12.5, 25, 50, 75, or 100 micrograms/hour is widely available (Kaiko et al., 1981; Ripamonti et al., 1997; Davis and Walsh, 2001). Modern formulations incorporate the fentanyl in the adhesive matrix. The drug is released at a nearly constant amount per unit time along a concentration gradient from the patch to the skin. After application of the transdermal system, serum fentanyl concentration increases gradually, usually levelling off after 12–24 hours, and then remaining stable for a time before declining slowly. When the patch is removed, serum concentration falls 50% in approximately 17 hours (range 13–22 hours) (Grouchow et al., 1989). The slow onset of effect after application and an equally slow decline in effect after removal are consistent with the development of a subcutaneous depot of drug that maintains the plasma concentration. There is significant interindividual variability in fentanyl bioavailability by this route

and dose titration is necessary (Grouchow et al., 1989). The dosing interval for each system is usually 72 hours, but interindividual pharmacokinetic variability is large and some patients require a dosing interval of 48 hours (Sawe et al., 1981b; Gibbs, 2009; Yang et al., 2010).

Familiarity with the kinetics of the transdermal system is essential for optimal use. Since there is a delay of 8–12 hours in achieving effective analgesia after initial application of the patch, it is necessary to provide alternative analgesia for this initial period. It is prudent to apply the patch in the early hours of the day so that the patient can be observed as blood levels rise over the ensuing 12 hours to minimize the risk of overdosing during sleep. Significant concentrations of fentanyl can remain in the plasma for up to 24 hours after removal of the patch because of delayed release from tissue and subcutaneous depots. Neither age nor patch location appears to affect fentanyl absorption from the transdermal system (Davis and Walsh, 2001). There is a potential for temperature-dependent increases in fentanyl release from the system associated with increased skin permeability in patients with fever, who should be monitored for opioid side effects. Patients should also avoid exposing the patch to direct external heat.

Empirically, the indications for the transdermal route include intolerance of oral medication, poor compliance with oral medication, and occasionally the desire to provide a trial of fentanyl to patients who have reacted unfavourably to other opioids. However, there are a number of limitations. The delay in onset of analgesia and in the establishment of steady state blood levels require the liberal use of an alternative short-acting opioid (usually morphine) for breakthrough pain during the early treatment period. Because of its 3-day duration of action, transdermal fentanyl is generally unsuitable for patients with unstable pain, and if a patient's pain goes out of control management may be complicated because of the delay in re-establishing steady state. If dose reductions are required or discontinuation is indicated, the continuing absorption following patch removal must be taken into account. Poor patch adhesion may be a problem in some patients. Set against these considerations are the advantages in terms of convenience and compliance and there is high patient acceptability of this mode of administration. Additionally there are experimental and clinical data to suggest that transdermal fentanyl is associated with less constipation than morphine (Mercadante et al., 1996).

Empirical observations suggest that a 100-microgram/hour fentanyl patch is approximately equianalgesic to 2–4 mg/hour of intravenous morphine (or equivalent). The relative potency ratio that is applicable when converting patients from oral morphine to transdermal fentanyl has been the subject of some controversy, but the dosing recommendations of the manufacturer seem provide a reasonable guideline. The patch should be placed in an area where skin movement is limited, such as the upper anterior chest wall or either side of the midline on the back, preferably the lower back. Studies have shown that all areas of skin absorb the drug at roughly the same rate (Davis and Walsh, 2001). Since the adhesive strips on these patches are less than optimal, securing the patch with non-irritant tape is often necessary.

Transdermal fentanyl currently recommended for patients whose opioid requirements are stable (Caraceni et al., 2012) and in general it is likely to be a second-line choice. However, for suitable patients it works well and they like it (Mathew and Storey, 1999).

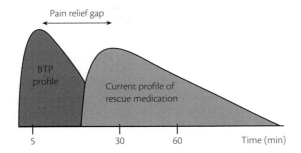

Fig. 9.4.6 Pain relief gap.

Oral transmucosal fentanyl citrate (OTFC)

An oral transmucosal formulation of fentanyl (which incorporates the drug in a hardened lozenge on a stick) that is absorbed across the buccal mucosa, has been available in many countries since the 1990s for the management of BTP. The lozenge is rubbed gently against the inside of the cheek until it has dissolved. The formulation is rapidly absorbed and achieves blood levels and time to peak effect that are comparable to parenterally administered fentanyl. Indeed, the time to onset of analgesia is 5–10 minutes (Eisendrath et al., 1987; Bruera et al., 1991; Szeto et al., 1997; Ripamonti et al., 1998), and studies in cancer patients suggest that it can provide rapid and very effective relief of BTP in well-chosen patients Formulations incorporating 200, 400, 600, 800, and 1600 micrograms are available. The most common adverse effects associated with this formulation are somnolence, nausea, and dizziness. One interesting observation which has emerged from the clinical trials and clinical use is that the successful dose of OTFC cannot be predicted and is not directly related to the daily dose of regular opioids being received for background pain.

OTFC was followed by a variety of other fentanyl preparations for BTP which are discussed below.

The oral immediate-release opioids have an extensive first-pass effect and are hydrophilic in nature, which slows the onset of analgesia to approximately 30 minutes and more. By the time these agents reach their peak of effect the pain has usually already resolved, unless of course the BTP is of longer duration (Fig. 9.4.6).

Rapid-onset oral fentanyl preparations

These are given either by the buccal or the sublingual route with the primary rationale being that the oral mucosa is very permeable. Although the oral mucosa is constantly washed by saliva which may disturb placement of devices like adhesive discs, its higher permeability could produce rapid onset of action and makes this an appropriate route for drugs administered for the management of BTP. Various formulations exist including fentanyl buccal tablets (FBT), OTFC as described above, and sublingual fentanyl citrate oral disintegrating tablet (ODT).

A Cochrane review examined opioids for the management of breakthrough (episodic) pain in cancer patients (Zeppetella and Ribeiro, 2006). As is the case with the methodology employed in Cochrane reviews, results were limited to randomized studies resulting in only four trials meeting the inclusion criteria (Christie et al., 1998; Farrar et al., 1998; Portenoy et al., 1999b; Coluzzi et al., 2001). All four studies involved OTFC and this was shown to be superior to placebo, normal-release morphine, and previously used rescue medications. A mixed treatment analysis

has also been conducted which demonstrated that FBT, ODT, and OTFC are more efficacious than oral morphine for breakthrough cancer pain (Jandhyala et al., 2013).

Rapid-onset nasal fentanyl preparations

The other main route of administering fentanyl is nasally. The nasal preparations are either unmodified fentanyl which results in a high, early peak or fentanyl in a pectin which also results in an early peak but the peak is attenuated due to the pectin delivery system. The unmodified fentanyl spray, intranasal fentanyl spray (INFS), has been shown to provide clinically relevant reductions in pain intensity and superior efficacy to OTFC (Kress et al., 2009; Mercadante et al., 2009). The pectin-based preparation fentanyl pectin nasal spray (FPNS) has also been shown to be superior to placebo and morphine in breakthrough pain (Taylor et al., 2010; Fallon et al., 2011).

Other drugs

Drugs such as phenazocine, dextromoramide, and dipipanone are now largely obsolete in chronic pain management.

Agonist–antagonist opioid analgesics

The agonist–antagonist opioid analgesics are a heterogeneous group of drugs with moderate-to-strong analgesic activity, comparable with that of the agonist opioids such as codeine and morphine. The group includes drugs which act as an agonist or partial agonist at one receptor and as an antagonist at another (pentazocine, dezocine, butorphanol, nalbuphine)—'the mixed agonist–antagonists'—and drugs acting as a partial agonist at a single receptor (buprenorphine). These two groups of drugs can be also classified as nalorphine- or morphine-like. Meptazinol fits neither classification and occupies a separate category. The place of this group of drugs in chronic cancer pain has been limited (Brose et al., 1991). However, the recent development of a transdermal formulation of buprenorphine may allow its more widespread use in both chronic cancer and non-cancer pain.

Mixed agonist–antagonist analgesics

The agonist–antagonists produce analgesia in the opioid-naive patient but may precipitate withdrawal in patients who are physically dependent on morphine-like drugs. Therefore, when used for chronic pain, they should be tried before repeated administration of a morphine-like agonist drug.

Pentazocine, butorphanol, and nalbuphine are mu antagonists and kappa agonists or partial agonists. All three drugs are strong analgesics when given by injection: pentazocine is one-sixth to one-third as potent as morphine, nalbuphine is roughly equipotent with morphine, and butorphanol is 3.5–7 times as potent. The duration of analgesia is similar to that of morphine (3–4 hours). Oral pentazocine is closer in analgesic efficacy to aspirin and paracetamol than the weaker opioid analgesics, such as codeine. Neither nalbuphine nor butorphanol is available as an oral formulation, and butorphanol is no longer available in any form in the United Kingdom.

At usual therapeutic doses, nalbuphine and butorphanol have respiratory depressant effects equivalent to that of morphine (although the duration of such effects may be longer with butorphanol). Unlike morphine, there appears to be a ceiling to both the respiratory depression and the analgesic action.

All three drugs have a lower abuse potential than the agonist opioid analgesics such as morphine. However, all have been subject to abuse and misuse, and pentazocine (but not the others) is subject to controlled drug restrictions. In North America, the oral preparation of pentazocine is marketed in combination with naloxone (but is available without naloxone elsewhere).

Meptazinol is a synthetic hexahydroazepine derivative with opioid agonist and antagonist properties, but is unlike either the nalorphine-type agonist–antagonists or buprenorphine. Meptazinol has central cholinergic properties which may account at least in part for its analgesic effects. Receptor-binding studies show it to be a specific mu1 agonist. Meptazinol is one-tenth as potent as morphine by intramuscular injection and has a duration of action of about 4 hours. Some studies have shown adverse effects to be more frequent than with morphine, although respiratory depression and constipation appear to be less.

In therapeutic doses, the mixed agonists–antagonists may produce certain self-limiting psychotomimetic effects in some patients; pentazocine is the most common drug associated with these effects. These drugs play a very limited role in the management of chronic cancer pain because the incidence and severity of the psychotomimetic effects increase with dose escalation, and nalbuphine and butorphanol are only available for parenteral use.

A transnasal formulation of butorphanol is now on the market in the United States, but there is no reported experience of its use in the management of chronic cancer pain.

Partial agonist analgesics

Buprenorphine is a semi-synthetic derivative of thebaine and chemically closely related to the strong agonist etorphine. Buprenorphine is a true partial agonist at the mu receptor and exhibits a ceiling effect in dose response curves in various animal models. In some, a bell-shaped curve is seen, indicating that at doses above a certain level the pharmacological effect actually decreases with increasing dose (Collins et al., 1996). Buprenorphine has until recently only been available by injection or for sublingual administration. A dose of 0.4 mg sublingually gives similar analgesia to 0.2–0.3 mg intramuscularly, with an onset of analgesia within 30–60 minutes of administration and a duration of 6–9 hours (Lawlor et al., 1997). In contrast, if taken orally, buprenorphine is a poor analgesic due to extensive pre-systemic elimination (Dixon et al., 1983). The long duration of analgesia with buprenorphine may be related to its affinity for the mu-opioid receptor and an unusually slow dissociation constant for the drug–receptor complex.

Buprenorphine has been in clinical use for more than 30 years and has been evaluated in a variety of acute pain models. Direct single dose comparisons with other analgesics such as morphine is complicated by its long duration of action, but results from a number of studies in postoperative pain suggest that single doses of 0.3 mg buprenorphine parenterally or 0.4 mg sublingually give equivalent analgesia to 10–15 mg intramuscular morphine. A ceiling effect for analgesia in humans has not been clearly demonstrated.

Buprenorphine produces typical opioid adverse effects. Overall the available data (which are limited) suggest that the incidence of common adverse effects compared with morphine is similar. Naloxone appears to be relatively ineffective in reversing opioid effects due to buprenorphine (Wallenstein et al., 1986). Clinical experience does not necessarily agree with this. Buprenorphine was introduced in high-dose sublingual tablet formulations in 1999 for the management of drug dependence. This potential use of the drug has long been recognized (Moulin et al., 1988) and it has been suggested that there is less overdose risk compared with other opioids (Kalso and Vainio, 1990).

Buprenorphine is available in a patch for transdermal administration. The drug is incorporated in a polymer adhesive matrix which controls the release of the drug by diffusion. There are two preparations; one lasting 4 days and the other 7. Three patch sizes of the 4-day preparation are available delivering 35, 52.5, and 70 mg buprenorphine per hour. Therapeutic plasma concentrations are achieved within 11–21 hours and steady state between the second and third applications of the patch. The 7-day patch also comes in three sizes, delivering 5, 10, and 20 mg buprenorphine per hour. At usual clinical doses of 3–4 mg per 24 hours buprenorphine functions as a pure mu agonist.

Transdermal buprenorphine has been licensed for use in both cancer pain and non-cancer pain. The lack of renal excretion (majority excreted unchanged in stool) makes this of potential use in renal dysfunction.

Principles of opioid administration

The effective clinical use of opioid drugs requires familiarity with the different drugs available, routes of administration, dosing guidelines, and potential adverse effects.

Indications

A trial of opioid therapy should be given to all patients with pain of moderate or greater severity, irrespective of the underlying pathophysiological mechanism. As discussed in Chapter 13.3, the suggestion that some forms of pain, such as neuropathic pain, are intrinsically refractory to opioid analgesia has been refuted by several studies that demonstrate that pain mechanisms do not accurately predict analgesic outcome from opioid therapy (Poyhia et al., 1993). Given the variability of response, all opioid trials in the clinical setting should include dose titration until adequate analgesia occurs or intolerable adverse effects supervene. This approach will identify those responders who can gain substantial clinical benefit from opioid therapy.

Patients whose pain is not easily controlled with an opioid analgesic because of troublesome adverse effects may benefit from alternative strategies and these are discussed below.

Drug selection

The factors that influence opioid selection include pain intensity, pharmacokinetic considerations and available formulations, previous adverse effects, and the presence of coexisting disease.

Pain intensity

Patients who present with severe pain are usually treated with a 'step 3' opioid (morphine, hydromorphone, oxycodone, oxymorphone, fentanyl, methadone, or levorphanol). Patients with moderate pain are conventionally treated with a combination product containing paracetamol or aspirin plus a conventional step 2 opioid (codeine, dihydrocodeine, hydrocodone, oxycodone (low dose), and propoxyphene), although increasingly, low dose of a step 3 opioid is used instead of a step 2 opioid.

Pharmacokinetic considerations and type of formulation

Any of the available agonist opioids can be selected for the opioid-naive patient without major organ failure. Short-$t_{1/2}$ opioids (morphine, hydromorphone, oxycodone, or oxymorphone) are generally favoured because they are easier to titrate than the long-$t_{1/2}$ drugs, which require a longer period to approach steady state plasma concentrations. Among the short-$t_{1/2}$ opioids, the range of available formulations often influences specific drug selection. For ambulatory patients who are able to tolerate oral opioids, morphine sulphate is generally preferred since it has a short $t_{1/2}$ and is easy to titrate in its normal-release form; it is also available as sustained-release preparations that allow 12- and 24-hour dosing intervals. The long-$t_{1/2}$ opioids methadone and levorphanol are not usually considered for first-line therapy because they can be difficult to titrate and present challenging management problems if delayed toxicity develops as plasma concentrations gradually rise following dose increments. For the reasons previously described, the use of pethidine, dextromoramide, and dipipanone for the management of cancer pain is discouraged.

When the oral route of opioid administration is contraindicated, the available routes of administration may become an important consideration in opioid selection. Fentanyl and buprenorphine are available for administration by the transdermal route. Although most of the full agonist drugs are well absorbed by subcutaneous infusion, some (like morphine tartrate, hydromorphone, and diamorphine) are more suitable by virtue of their high solubility and low irritability. Methadone and fentanyl may produce significant local irritation when administered by the subcutaneous route. For cultural and aesthetic reasons, the subcutaneous route is often preferred to rectal administration. Subcutaneous infusion may be also preferable in patients at the end of life because it is less disruptive than using intermittent analgesic suppositories when nursing a sick patient.

Response to previous trials of opioid therapy

It is always important to review the response to previous trials of opioid therapy. If the current opioid is well tolerated, it is usually continued unless difficulties in dose titration occur or the required dose cannot be administered conventionally. If dose-limiting side effects develop, a trial of an alternative opioid should be considered as discussed in the section on adverse effects.

Coexisting disease

Pharmacokinetic studies of pethidine, pentazocine, and propoxyphene have revealed that liver disease may decrease the clearance and increase the bioavailability and half-lives of these drugs (Kaiko et al., 1996; Salzman et al., 1999). These changes may result in above-normal plasma concentrations. Mild or moderate hepatic impairment has only a minor impact on morphine clearance (Eddy and Lee, 1959); however, advanced disease may be associated with reduced elimination (Hermens et al., 1985).

Patients with renal impairment may accumulate the active metabolites of propoxyphene (norpropoxyphene), pethidine (norpethidine), and morphine (M6G). Particular caution is required in the administration of these drugs to such patients (Hess et al., 1972; Mather, 1983; Yeadon and Kitchen, 1988; Rogers, 1991a; Raffa et al., 1992). Until more data are available, it may be wise to assume that other opioids with active metabolites may produce similar problems of toxicity in patients with impaired renal function. On this basis buprenorphine, fentanyl and alfentanil show potential advantages in renal impairment.

Morphine has been the standard step 3 opioid analgesic against which others are measured and is the most widely available in a variety of oral formulations (De Conno et al., 1991). It has limitations; the systemic availability of morphine by the oral route is poor (20–30%) and this contributes to the sometimes unpredictable onset of action and great interindividual variability in dose requirements and response. Active metabolites may contribute to toxicity particularly in patients with renal impairment (Mather, 1983). Sometimes the pain does not respond well or completely to morphine, notably neuropathic pain. However, none of the alternatives to morphine has so far demonstrated advantages which would make it preferable in routine use as the first-line oral opioid for cancer pain. Morphine remains the standard but for reasons of familiarity, availability and cost. A recent systematic review identified that there is no superiority of any of the commonly used opioids for moderate to severe pain over another (Caraceni, 2012). Early pilot work by Reid and Hanks comparing standard three-step approach with morphine versus a two-step approach with oxycodone indicates that such a two-step approach may be superior in terms of time to effective pain relief with all the associated secondary gains (Reid, 2007).

Routes of administration

Opioids should be administered by the least invasive and safest route capable of providing adequate analgesia. In a survey of patients with advanced cancer, more than half required two or more routes of administration prior to death, and almost a quarter required three or more (Lehmann and Zech, 1992).

Oral administration

The oral route of opioid administration remains the most important and appropriate in routine practice. Orally administered drugs have a slower onset of action, a delayed peak time, and a longer duration of effect compared with parenterally administered drugs. The time to peak effect depends on the drug and the nature of the formulation. For most normal-release oral formulations, peak effect is typically achieved within 60 minutes. The oral route of drug administration is inappropriate for patients who have impaired swallowing or gastrointestinal obstruction, and for some patients who require a rapid onset of analgesia. For patients who require very high doses, the inability to prescribe a manageable oral opioid regimen may be an indication for the use of a non-oral route.

When given orally, the opioids differ substantially with respect to their relative analgesic potency compared with parenteral administration. To some extent, this reflects differences in pre-systemic metabolism, that is, the degree to which they are inactivated as they are absorbed from the gastrointestinal tract and pass through the liver into the systemic circulation. As indicated in Box 9.4.2, morphine, diamorphine, pethidine, hydromorphone, and oxymorphone have ratios of oral to parenteral potency ranging from 1:3 to 1:12. Methadone, levorphanol, and oxycodone are subject to less pre-systemic elimination and also demonstrate a lower oral-to-parenteral potency ratio of at least 1:2. Failure to recognize these differences may result in a substantial reduction in analgesia when a change from parenteral to oral administration is attempted without upward titration of the dose, or toxic effects when changing in the opposite direction.

Rectal administration

The rectal route is a non-invasive alternative to parenteral routes for patients unable to use oral opioids. Rectal suppositories containing morphine, hydromorphone, oxymorphone, and oxycodone are available. The pharmacokinetics and bioavailability of drugs given rectally may differ from that of oral administration because of delayed or limited absorption and partial bypassing of pre-systemic hepatic metabolism. In practice, however, the potency of opioids administered rectally is approximately equal to that achieved by oral dosing (Varvel et al., 1989). In contrast with morphine, rectal oxycodone appears to have a delayed absorption and prolonged duration of action.

For many patients, the rectal route is not used because it is more convenient to convert directly to a subcutaneous infusion of opioid using a portable syringe driver or similar device.

Parenteral administration

Bolus injections via parenteral routes of administration are considered for patients who have impaired swallowing or gastrointestinal obstruction, those who require a rapid onset of analgesia, and those who require very high doses that cannot be conveniently administered by other methods. Repeated parenteral bolus injections, which can be delivered by the intravenous, intramuscular, or subcutaneous routes, may be complicated by the occurrence of untoward 'bolus' effects (toxicity at peak concentration and/or pain breakthrough at the trough). Intravenous bolus provides the most rapid onset; the time to peak effect correlates with the lipid solubility of the opioid, ranging from 2 to 5 minutes for methadone and from 10 to 15 minutes for morphine.

Although repeated intramuscular injections are commonplace in some countries, they are painful and offer no pharmacokinetic advantage, and their use is not recommended (Lehmann and Zech, 1992; Caraceni et al., 2012). Repeated bolus doses, if required, can be accomplished without frequent skin punctures by using an indwelling intravenous or subcutaneous infusion device. To deliver repeated subcutaneous injections, a 25–27 gauge 'butterfly' can be left under the skin for up to a week (Southam, 1995). The discomfort associated with this technique is partially related to the volume to be injected; it can be minimized by the use of concentrated formulations.

Continuous infusions

Continuous infusions avoid the problems associated with the 'bolus effect' and can be administered intravenously or subcutaneously (Portenoy et al., 1993; Jeal and Benfield, 1997). Continuous subcutaneous infusion using a portable battery-operated syringe driver or other similar device was originally devised to administer infusions of desferrioxamine to patients with thalassemia, but was subsequently used to deliver diamorphine to patients with advanced cancer who were unable to take oral drugs (Megens et al., 1998). This technique is now well established in palliative care and is used to administer analgesics, antiemetics, anxiolytic sedatives, and dexamethasone.

Ambulatory infusion devices vary in complexity, cost, and ability to provide patient-controlled 'rescue doses' as an adjunct to a continuous basal infusion. A variety of devices have been employed, all designed to be lightweight and portable, and in one case, disposable. Opioids suitable for continuous subcutaneous infusion must be soluble, well absorbed and non-irritant. Extensive experience has been reported with morphine, diamorphine, hydromorphone, fentanyl, and oxymorphone (Portenoy et al., 1993; Haazen et al., 1999; Penson et al., 2000b). Methadone (Pasternak et al., 1987) and fentanyl appear to be relative irritants and are best avoided by this route.

Studies suggest that dosing with subcutaneous administration can proceed in a manner identical to continuous intravenous infusion: a postoperative study comparing patients who received an identical dose of morphine by either intravenous or subcutaneous infusion found no difference in blood levels (Payne et al., 1998), and a controlled study of hydromorphone calculated a bioavailability of 78% for the subcutaneous route and observed that analgesic outcome was identical during intravenous or subcutaneous infusion. To maintain the comfort of an infusion site, the subcutaneous infusion rate should not exceed 5 mL/hour. Subcutaneous infusion has become the first choice when parenteral analgesia is required in palliative care patients.

Continuous intravenous infusion may be the most appropriate way of delivering an opioid for patients with a pre-existing implanted central line, when there is a need for infusion of a large volume of solution, or when using methadone. If continuous intravenous infusion must be continued on a long-term basis, a permanent central venous port is recommended.

Continuous infusions of drug combinations may be indicated when pain is accompanied by nausea, anxiety, or agitation. In such cases an antiemetic, neuroleptic, or anxiolytic may be combined with an opioid provided that it is non-irritant, miscible, and stable in combined solution. As noted later in the text, a variety of different combinations of drugs are commonly given by continuous infusion (Fine et al., 1991). However, the stability/compatibility of many of these combinations is not known. The compatibility of drug combinations is dependent on a number of factors, including the types of drugs, the concentrations of drugs, the diluent and temperature, and ultraviolet light. A database of compatible drug combinations is now available on the Internet (http://www.palliativedrugs.com). Generally infusions should contain as few drugs as possible, preferably no more than three. The absence of precipitation within a drug mixture is not synonymous with compatibility between the drugs in that mixture (Farrar et al., 1998).

Epidural, intrathecal, and intraventricular administration

The discovery of opioid receptors in the dorsal horn of the spinal cord led to the development of intraspinal opioid delivery techniques. In general, they provide a longer duration of analgesia at doses lower than required by systemic administration. The delivery of low opioid doses near the sites of action in the spinal cord may decrease supraspinally mediated adverse effects (see Chapter 13.2).

Opioid selection for intraspinal delivery is influenced by several factors. Hydrophilic drugs, such as morphine and hydromorphone, have a prolonged $t_{1/2}$ in cerebrospinal fluid and significant rostral redistribution (Christie et al., 1998). Lipophilic opioids, such as fentanyl and sufentanil, have less rostral redistribution and therefore fewer prolonged adverse effects if these become a problem.

The addition of local anaesthetic such as bupivacaine to an epidural or intrathecal opioid has been demonstrated to improve analgesia without increasing toxicity (Faull et al., 1994; Egan et al., 2000). Unlike in acute postoperative pain, where a large volume of low concentration local anaesthetic is used, in chronic cancer pain, a small volume of high concentration of local anaesthetic is preferred and can be mixed with an appropriate dose of a small volume of opioid.

The initial conversion of opioid dose from systemic subcutaneous diamorphine or morphine is:

- epidural—1/10 of systemic dose
- intrathecal—1/10 of epidural dose.

Thus, if a patient were on 100 mg of subcutaneous morphine or diamorphine/day, the equivalent epidural dose would be 10 mg, and the equivalent intrathecal dose would be 1 mg/day.

The initial solution used for epidural infusion is usually:

- 9 mL 0.5% bupivacaine
- 150 micrograms clonidine
- morphine or diamorphine dose according to individual patient requirements (as calculated above). This gives a total volume of 10 mL infused over 24 hours.

The initial solution used for intrathecal infusion is normally around 1/10 of the above, that is:

- 1 mL 0.5% bupivacaine
- 15 micrograms clonidine
- morphine or diamorphine according to individual patient requirements.

Hydromorphone is sometimes preferred to morphine for use in programmable intrathecal pumps because of incompatibility between some of the commonly-used devices and morphine.

There are no clinical studies comparing the intrathecal and epidural routes in cancer pain. The epidural route is sometimes preferred because the techniques to accomplish long-term administration are simpler. A combined analysis of adverse effects observed in numerous trials of epidural or intrathecal administration suggests that the risks associated with these techniques are similar. The potential morbidity associated with these procedures emphasizes the need for a well-trained clinician and long-term monitoring for individual patients.

Limited experience suggests that the administration of an opioid into the cerebral ventricles can provide long-term analgesia in selected patients. This technique has been used for patients with upper-body or head pain or with severe diffuse pain. Schedules have included both intermittent injection via an Ommaya reservoir and continual infusion using an implanted pump.

The indication for the spinal routes of administration of opioid analgesics in palliative care patients is discussed in more detail in Chapter 13.2.

Other routes and modes of administration

Transdermal

As previously described, fentanyl and buprenorphine are available in a transdermal formulation and their use is discussed above.

Sublingual

Sublingual absorption could potentially occur with any opioid, but bioavailability is very poor with drugs that are not highly lipophilic (Rance, 1979; Hoskin and Hanks, 1991). A sublingual preparation of buprenorphine is available in some countries, although not in the United States. Anecdotally, sublingual morphine has also been reported to be effective; given the poor sublingual absorption of this drug, this efficacy may be related in part to swallowing of the dose. Methadone is well absorbed sublingually. Sublingual administration has been discussed earlier.

Topical

There are several case series and one very small randomized controlled trial that examine the role of topical morphine for local analgesia. The small amount of existing evidence seems to point to a role in some situations, for example, cutaneous ulcers or tumour with cutaneous inflammation. Doses of 10–40 mg of morphine are used in simple gel, saline soaks, or local anaesthetic gel (Bullingham et al., 1981, 1983; Gal, 1989). Randomized controlled trials in non-malignant cutaneous pain, for example, burns or photodynamic therapy, have been negative.

Changing the route of administration

As described earlier, when changing from the oral to parenteral routes, or vice versa, an adjustment in dose is required to avoid either toxic effects or a reduction in analgesia. The ratios of oral to parenteral relative potency given in Table 9.4.5 are estimates and should not be taken as precise figures but used as guidelines to achieve a roughly equianalgesic effect. There is considerable variation between patients, and upward or downward adjustment may then be required for individual patients.

The slower onset of analgesia after oral administration often requires some adaptation on the part of a patient who is accustomed to the more rapid onset seen after parenteral opioid. In some patients, the problems associated with switching from the parenteral to the oral route of opioid administration may need to be minimized by slowly reducing the parenteral dose and increasing the oral dose over a 2–3-day period.

Usually, no dose adjustment is required when patients are switched from the subcutaneous to the intravenous route or vice versa.

Scheduling opioid administration

'Around-the-clock' dosing

To provide the patient with continuous relief by preventing the pain from recurring, patients with continuous or frequent pain are usually scheduled for 'around-the-clock' dosing. However, clinical vigilance is required in patients with no previous opioid exposure and those administered drugs with long half-lives. With methadone, for example, delayed toxicity may develop as plasma concentration rises slowly towards steady-state levels.

Rescue doses

All patients who receive an around-the-clock opioid regimen should also be offered a 'rescue dose', that is, a supplemental dose given on an as-needed basis to treat pain that breaks through the regular schedule (De Conno et al., 1991). The integration of scheduled dosing with rescue doses provides a method for safe and rational stepwise dose escalation and is applicable to all routes of opioid administration. The rescue drug is typically identical to that administered on a continuous basis, with the exception of transdermal fentanyl and methadone; the use of an alternative short-$t_{1/2}$ opioid is recommended for the rescue dose when these drugs are used. The frequency with which the rescue dose can be administered depends on the time to peak effect for the drug and the route of administration. Oral rescue doses can be offered up to every 60–90 minutes, and parenteral rescue doses can be offered up to every 15–30 minutes.

Clinical experience suggests that the size of the rescue dose should usually be equivalent to one-sixth of the 24-hour baseline dose, that is, the same as the 4-hourly dose of opioid. The magnitude of the rescue dose should be individualized and some patients with low baseline pain but severe exacerbations may require rescue doses that are substantially larger. As discussed in this chapter, in the setting of clinical trials where rescue doses are individualized, the effective doses rarely turn out to be one-sixth of the 24-hour dose.

Scheduling with sustained-release formulations

Sustained-release formulations can reduce the inconvenience associated with around-the-clock administration. These formulations should not be used for rapid titration of the dose in patients with severe pain. Sustained-release oral morphine sulphate and oxycodone, and transdermal fentanyl are now widely used, and sustained-release formulations of codeine, tramadol, and hydromorphone have been introduced in various countries.

A normal-release formulation of a short-$t_{1/2}$ opioid (usually the same drug) is often used as the rescue medication. Sustained- and normal-release formulations of oral morphine are dose equivalent; switching from one to the other is done on a milligram-for-milligram basis after the daily dose requirement is identified using a normal-release formulation.

As-needed dosing

In some limited situations, an as-needed dosing regimen alone can be recommended. This type of dosing provides additional safety during the initiation of opioid therapy in the opioid-naive patient, particularly when rapid dose escalation is needed or a long-$t_{1/2}$ drug is administered. This technique is strongly recommended when starting methadone therapy, and for patients with acute renal failure.

Patient-controlled analgesia

Patient-controlled analgesia is a technique of parenteral drug administration in which the patient controls a pump that delivers bolus doses of an analgesic according to parameters set by the physician. Use of a patient-controlled analgesia device allows the patient to titrate the opioid dose carefully to his or her individual analgesic needs. Long-term patient-controlled analgesia in cancer patients is accomplished via subcutaneous or intravenous routes using an ambulatory infusion device (Mello and Mendelson, 1980). The more technologically advanced of these devices have programmable variables, including infusion rate, rescue dose, and lock-out interval. The option for bolus dosing is typically used in conjunction with continuous opioid infusion.

Dose selection and adjustment

Initial dose selection

A patient with severe pain that is not controlled with a step 2 opioid– non-opioid combination in full dose should begin one of the opioid agonists at a dose equivalent to 10 mg oral morphine sulphate every 4 hours.

Dose titration

Inadequate pain relief should be addressed by gradual escalation of the opioid dose until adequate analgesia is reported or intolerable side effects (that cannot be managed by simple interventions) supervene. Because analgesic response to opioids increases linearly with the logarithm of the dose, dose escalations of less than 30–50% are not likely to improve analgesia significantly. Clinical experience indicates that a dose increment of this order of magnitude is safe and is large enough to observe a meaningful change in effects.

In most cases, gradual dose escalation identifies a favourable balance between analgesia and side effects which remains stable for a prolonged period. While doses can become extremely large during this process, the absolute dose is immaterial as long as the balance between analgesia and side effects remains favourable.

In a retrospective study of 100 patients with advanced cancer, the average daily opioid requirement was equivalent to 400–600 mg of intramuscular morphine, but approximately 10% of patients required more than 2000 mg and one patient required over 30 000 mg every 24 hours. Other centres have generally reported lower doses; a median dose of 60 mg/day in one centre and 120 mg/day in another (Hammersley et al., 1995).

A simple method of dose titration using oral morphine is to prescribe a dose of immediate-release morphine every 4 hours and the same dose for rescue for BTP (De Conno et al., 1991). The rescue dose can be given as often as required (e.g. every hour) and the total dose of morphine can be reviewed daily. The regular dose can then be adjusted according to how many rescue doses have been given.

Rate of dose titration

The severity of the pain should determine the rate of dose titration. Patients with very severe pain can be managed by repeated parenteral dosing every 15–30 minutes until pain is partially relieved when an oral dosing regimen should be started.

Tolerance

Patients vary greatly in the opioid dose required to manage their pain. The need for escalating doses is a complex phenomenon. Most patients reach a dose that remains constant for prolonged periods. When the need for dose escalation arises, any of a variety of distinct processes may be involved. Clinical experience suggests that true pharmacological tolerance is a much less common reason than disease progression or increasing psychological distress. Changes in the pharmacokinetics of an analgesic drug could also be implicated.

True pharmacological tolerance probably involves changes at the receptor level, and in this situation continued drug administration itself induces an attenuation of effect. Clinically, tolerance to the non-analgesic effects of opioids appears to occur commonly albeit at varying rates for different effects. For example, tolerance to respiratory depression, somnolence, and nausea generally develops rapidly, whereas tolerance to opioid-induced constipation develops very slowly, if at all. Tolerance to these opioid side effects is not a clinical problem, and indeed is a desirable outcome that allows effective dose titration to proceed.

From the clinical perspective, the concern is that tolerance to the analgesic effect of the drug will develop and that this will necessitate rapid dose escalation which may continue until the drug is no longer useful. Induction of true analgesic tolerance which could compromise the utility of treatment can only be said to occur if a patient manifests a need for increasing opioid doses in the absence of other factors (e.g. progressive disease) that would be capable of explaining the increase in pain. Extensive clinical experience suggests that most patients who require an escalation in dose to manage increasing pain have demonstrable progression of disease. With the emergence of our understanding of opioid-induced hyperalgesia (OIH), both generalized pain and/or appearance of features of central wind-up should be assessed very carefully.

This conclusion has two important implications: concern about tolerance should not impede the use of opioids early in the course of the disease, and worsening pain in a patient receiving a stable dose of opioid should not be attributed to tolerance but taken as presumptive evidence of disease progression or, less commonly, increasing psychological distress.

Determination of an equianalgesic dose

The overriding clinical issue with an opioid switch is that it is nearly always done because a problem exists. Assessment of appropriate dose conversion is critical when switching a patient from one opioid to another. The most common reason for a switch is an unacceptable side effect profile often also associated with uncontrolled pain. It is clear that any deterioration in either side effects and/or pain control is disastrous for the patient, therefore a switch needs to find the right balance. In practice this means a very conservative equianalgesic conversion should be made (no more than 75% of the equianalgesic dose and clearly less in the case of drugs such as methadone) and appropriate breakthrough analgesia prescribed in a clear and practical way to prevent any distress due to underdosing. Failure to do this can lead to the development of opioid toxicity or worsening of existing opioid toxicity.

Management of opioid adverse effects

Successful opioid therapy requires that the benefits of analgesia clearly outweigh treatment-related adverse effects. This requires understanding of adverse opioid effects and the strategies used to prevent and manage them are essential skills for all involved in cancer pain management. The adverse effects that are frequently observed in patients receiving oral morphine and other opioids are summarized in Table 9.4.7. The most common are sedation, constipation, and nausea and vomiting, but there are other adverse effects including confusion, hallucinations, nightmares, urinary retention, multifocal myoclonus, dizziness, and dysphoria. The mechanisms that underlie these adverse effects, even the most common, are only partly understood and, as discussed earlier, appear to depend upon a number of factors including age, extent of disease and organ dysfunction, concurrent administration of certain drugs, prior opioid exposure, and the route of drug administration. Studies comparing the adverse effects of one opioid analgesic with another in this population are lacking. Similarly, controlled studies comparing the adverse effects produced by the same opioid given by various routes of administration are also lacking.

As a general rule, caution is required when using opioids in patients in acute pain with impaired ventilation, bronchial asthma, or raised intracranial pressure; the same caveats do not usually limit dose titration in chronic cancer pain management.

Factors predictive of opioid adverse effects

Drug-related

Overall, there is very little reproducible evidence suggesting that any one opioid agonist has a substantially better adverse

Table 9.4.7 Common opioid-induced adverse effects

Gastrointestinal	Nausea
	Vomiting
	Constipation
Autonomic	Xerostomia
	Urinary retention
	Postural hypotension
Central nervous system	Drowsiness
	Cognitive impairment
	Hallucinations
	Delirium
	Respiratory depression
	Myoclonus
	Seizure disorder
	Hyperalgesia
Cutaneous	Itch
	Sweating

effect profile than any other. Pethidine is not recommended in the management of chronic cancer pain because of concerns regarding its side effect profile (Kaiko et al., 1983). Data from controlled studies indicate that the transdermal administration of fentanyl is associated with a lesser incidence of constipation than oral morphine (Donner et al., 1996; Ahmedzai and Brooks, 1997; Payne et al., 1998; van Seventer et al., 2003) or codeine (Mystakidou et al., 2005).

Route-related

There is very limited evidence to suggest differences in adverse effects associated with specific routes of systemic administration. Compared to oral morphine administration, small studies have demonstrated less nausea and vomiting with rectal (Babul et al., 1998) and subcutaneous administration (McDonald et al., 1991). Four studies comparing transdermal fentanyl to oral morphine demonstrated less constipation among the patients receiving transdermal fentanyl. It is not clear as to whether this is a route or drug related effect (Ahmedzai and Brooks, 1987; Donner et al., 1996; Payne et al., 1998; van Seventer et al., 2003).

Patient-related

For reasons that are not well explained, there is striking interindividual variability in the sensitivity to adverse effects from morphine and other opioid drugs. Genetic variability clearly affects the sensitivity to opioids (Somogyi et al., 2007) and it is reasonable to assume that the genetic background plays a similar important role in sensitivity to adverse effects and the pre-clinical evidence for this is discussed in the first part of this chapter (Stamer et al., 2005).

Some of this variability is related to co-morbidity. Ageing is associated with altered pharmacokinetics particularly characterized by diminished clearance and volume of distribution. This has been well evaluated for morphine (Baillie et al., 1989) and fentanyl (Bentley et al., 1982; Holdsworth et al., 1994). In a study of morphine use in the management of chronic cancer pain in the elderly, overall elderly patients required lower doses than their younger counterparts without exhibiting an enhanced risk for opioid induced adverse effects (Rapin, 1989). In patients with impaired renal function there is delayed clearance of an active metabolite of morphine, M6G (Osborne et al., 1993). Anecdotally, high concentrations of M6G have been associated with toxicity (Osborne et al., 1986; Hagen et al., 1991; Sjogren et al., 1993), however in a prospective study of patients with opioid-induced delirium or myoclonus no relationship to renal function was observed (Tiseo et al., 1995).

Other patient-related factors that may enhance the risk of adverse effects include the co-administration of drugs which may have cumulative toxicity, especially sedation or other concurrent co-morbidity (Table 9.4.8).

Opioid initiation and dose escalation

Among adverse effects there is substantial variability in their dose response. A dose response relationship is most commonly evident with regards to the central nervous system adverse effects of sedation, cognitive impairment, hallucinations, myoclonus and respiratory depression. Even among these, however, there is very substantial interindividual variability to many of these effects. Additionally, as tolerance develops to some effects, the spectrum of adverse effects varies with prolonged use. Commonly, patients who have had prolonged opioid exposure have a lesser tendency to develop sedation or respiratory depression, and the predominant central nervous system effects become the neuroexcitatory ones of delirium and myoclonus.

Gastrointestinal adverse effects generally have a weaker dose response relationship. Some, like nausea and vomiting, are common with the initiation of therapy but are subsequently unpredictable with resolution among some patients and persistence among others. Constipation is virtually universal and it demonstrates a very weak dose relationship.

Some adverse effects appear transiently after starting an opioid or after dose escalation and spontaneously abate. This phenomenon has been well demonstrated in a prospective study on the effect of morphine dose escalation on cognitive performance (Bruera et al., 1989). This study demonstrated that opioid induced cognitive impairment commonly improved after 7 days. This phenomenon, though often described, has not been formally studied in regards to other adverse effects and needs to be repeated in relation to cognitive performance in a larger population.

Differential diagnosis

Adverse changes in patient well-being among patients taking opioids are not always caused by the opioid. Adverse effects must be differentiated from other causes of co morbidity that may develop in the treated patient and from drug interactions. Common causes of co-morbidity that may mimic opioid induced adverse effects are presented in Table 9.4.8.

Indeed, the appearance of a new adverse change in patient well-being that occurs in the setting of stable opioid dosing is rarely caused by the opioid, and an alternate explanation should be vigorously sought. Since polypharmacy is common among patients with advanced cancer, it is essential to scrutinize medication records and patient report of medication administration to evaluate for possible drug interactions or some other drug-related explanation for the reported symptoms.

Table 9.4.8 Co-morbidity that may mimic opioid induced adverse effects

Cause		Adverse effects
Central nervous system	Cerebral metastases	Drowsiness, cognitive impairment, nausea, vomiting
	Leptomeningeal metastases	Drowsiness, cognitive impairment, nausea, vomiting
	Cerebrovascular event	Drowsiness, cognitive impairment
	Extradural haemorrhage	Drowsiness, cognitive impairment
Metabolic	Dehydration	Drowsiness, cognitive impairment
	Hypercalcaemia	Drowsiness, cognitive impairment, nausea, vomiting
	Hyponatremia	Drowsiness, cognitive impairment
	Renal failure	Drowsiness, cognitive impairment, nausea, vomiting, myoclonus
	Liver failure	Drowsiness, cognitive impairment, nausea, vomiting, myoclonus
	Hypoxemia	Drowsiness, cognitive impairment
Sepsis/infection		Drowsiness, cognitive impairment, nausea, vomiting
Mechanical	Bowel obstruction	Nausea, vomiting
Iatrogenic	Tricyclics	Drowsiness, cognitive impairment, constipation
	Benzodiazepines	Drowsiness, cognitive impairment
	Antibiotics	Nausea and vomiting
	Vinca alkaloids	Constipation
	Flutamide	Constipation
	Steroids	Agitated delirium
	Non-steroidal anti-inflammatory drugs	Nausea, drowsiness
	Chemotherapy	Nausea, vomiting, drowsiness, cognitive impairment
	Radiotherapy	Nausea, vomiting, drowsiness

Overview of the alternative approaches to treating opioid adverse effects

In general, four different approaches to the management of opioid adverse effects have been described:

1. Dose reduction of systemic opioid
2. Specific therapy to reduce the adverse effect
3. Opioid switching
4. Change route of administration

Dose reduction of systemic opioid

Reducing the dose of administered opioid usually results in a reduction in dose related adverse effects. When patients have well-controlled pain, gradual reduction in the opioid dose will often result in the resolution of dose related adverse effects whilst preserving adequate pain relief (Fallon and O'Neill, 1997).

When opioid doses cannot be reduced without the loss of pain control, reduction in dose must be accompanied by the addition of an accompanying synergist approach. Extensive experience has been reported with four accompanying approaches:

1. *The addition of a non-opioid co-analgesic.* The analgesia achieved from non-opioid co-analgesics is additive and often synergistic with that achieved by opioids. This is supported from a number of prospective studies (Nabal et al., 2012).

2. *The addition of an adjuvant analgesic that is appropriate to the pain syndrome and mechanism* (see Chapter 13.1). Adjuvant analgesics (see following) may be combined with primary analgesics to improve the outcome for patients who cannot otherwise attain an acceptable balance between relief and side effects (Lussier et al., 2004; Mitra and Jones, 2012). There is great inter-individual variability in the response to all adjuvant analgesics and, for most, the likelihood of benefit is limited. Furthermore, many of the adjuvant analgesics have the potential to cause side effects which may be additive to the opioid induced adverse effects that are already problematic (Bennett, 2011). In evaluating the utility of an adjuvant agent in a particular patient setting, one must consider the likelihood of benefit, the risk of adverse effects, the ease of administration and patient convenience.

3. *The application of a therapy targeting the cause of the pain.* Specific antitumour therapies, such as radiotherapy, chemotherapy, or surgery targeting the cause of cancer related pain can provide substantial relief and thus reduce the need for opioid analgesia. Radiotherapy is of proven benefit in the treatment of painful bone metastases, (Lutz et al., 2011) epidural neoplasm (Souchon et al., 2010; Holt et al., 2012) and headache due to cerebral metastases (Pease et al., 2005; Akhtar et al., 2012; Kong et al., 2012). In other settings there is a lack of well-established supportive data, and the use of radiotherapy is largely anecdotal (Lutz et al., 2010, 2012). Despite a paucity of evidence concerning the specific analgesic benefits of chemotherapy (Bang et al., 2005; von Gruenigen et al., 2006; Dahele et al., 2007), there is a strong clinical impression that tumour shrinkage is generally associated with relief of pain. Although there are some reports of analgesic value even in the absence of significant tumour shrinkage (Patt et al., 1985; Thatcher et al., 1995; Rothenberg 1996), the likelihood of a favourable effect on pain is generally related to the likelihood of tumour response (Bang et al., 2005; von Gruenigen et al., 2006; Dahele et al., 2007). Surgery may have a role in the relief of symptoms caused by specific problems, such as obstruction of a hollow viscus (Sartori et al., 2010; Dalal et al., 2011; Dolan 2011; Kolomainen and Barton, 2011), unstable bony structures (Ogilvie et al., 2008; Utzschneider et al., 2011), and compression of neural tissues (Dy et al., 2008; Eleraky et al., 2010; Quraishi et al., 2010).

4. *The application of a regional anaesthetic or neuroablative intervention* (see Chapter 13.2). The results of the WHO 'analgesic ladder' validation studies suggest that 10–30% of patients with cancer pain do not achieve a satisfactory balance between relief and side effects using systemic pharmacotherapy alone without unacceptable drug toxicity (Takeda, 1985; Ventafridda et al., 1987; Goisis et al., 1989; Schug et al., 1990; Grond et al., 1991).

Anaesthetic and neurosurgical techniques may reduce or eliminate the requirement for systemically administered opioids to achieve adequate analgesia. In general, regional analgesic techniques such as intraspinal opioid and local anaesthetic administration or intrapleural local anaesthetic administration are usually considered first because they can achieve this end without compromising neurological integrity. Neurodestructive procedures, however, are valuable in a small subset of patients; and some of these procedures, such as coeliac plexus blockade in patients with pancreatic cancer, may have a favourable enough risk: benefit ratio that early treatment is warranted.

Symptomatic management of the adverse effect

Symptomatic drugs used to prevent or control opioid adverse effects are commonly employed. Most of these approaches are based on cumulative anecdotal experience. With few exceptions, the literature describing these approaches is anecdotal or 'expert opinion'. Very few studies have prospectively evaluated efficacy and no studies have evaluated the toxicity of these approaches over long term. In general, this approach involves the addition of a new medication, adding to medication burden and with the associated risks of adverse effects or drug interaction.

Opioid rotation

Opioid rotation refers to an approach to reduce opioid side effects by switching to an alternative opioid (Quigley, 2004; Mercadante and Bruera, 2006; Vadalouca et al., 2008; Fine and Portenoy, 2009; Vissers et al., 2010).

Improvements in cognitive impairment, sedation, hallucinations, nausea, vomiting and myoclonus are commonly reported. This approach requires familiarity with a range of opioid agonists and with the use of equianalgesic tables to convert doses when switching between opioids. While this approach has the practical advantage of minimizing polypharmacy, outcomes are variable and unpredictable. When switching between opioids, even with prudent use of equianalgesic tables, patients are at risk for under or over dosing by virtue of individual sensitivities.

The biological basis for the observed intra-individual variability in sensitivity to opioid analgesia and adverse effects

The biological basis for the observed intra-individual variability in sensitivity to opioid analgesia and adverse effects is multifactorial (Ross et al., 2006) and is related to pharmacogenetics (Kadiev et al., 2008). The pharmacokinetic and pharmacodynamic differences among the opioids and the spectrum of proteins involved in determining response create great potential for response variability.

Heterogeneity of opioid metabolism

Different opioids have different metabolic and excretion pathways. Of the processes of metabolism and excretion, some are genetically determined and some reflect phenotypic changes particularly with regard to renal and hepatic function. The genetic factors influencing metabolism play an important role in analgesia for some opioids and similar phenomena may contribute to variability in adverse effect sensitivity (Stamer and Stuber, 2007; Kadiev et al., 2008; Kleine–Brueggeney et al., 2010).

Genetic influences of receptor function

The potential for genetic influences on opioid effects and tolerability is vast and understanding of this very complex system remains rudimentary (Stamer et al., 2005). Still several important findings have contributed to the understanding of differences in opioid effects:

1. Genetic factors influencing opioid receptors: The mu-opioid receptor is a GPCR the signalling of which results in inhibition of neuronal transmission of painful stimuli by a complex sequence of events. Pre-clinical studies show that opioids can act on different receptors or subtype receptors and, individual receptor profiles may influence the analgesia as well as the side effects (Pasternak, 2005). More than 100 polymorphisms have been identified in the human mu-opioid receptor gene alone, and some of these variants, such as the A118G nucleotide substitution, have been shown to alter the binding affinities of different opioids (Lötsch et al., 2002b; Beyer et al., 2004) and to effect analgesic outcomes (Chou et al., 2006; Hayashida et al., 2008; Zhang et al., 2010). Furthermore other factors involved in the processes of GPCR such as desensitization, endocytosis, and down-regulation may further add to the potential for variability (Kristiansen, 2004).

2. Control of opioid receptor gene expression: There are some data to suggest that differences in signal transfer function that controls the expression of the mu-opioid receptor gene may impact on opioid responsiveness (Ross et al., 2005). Research continues to examine other transcription factors that may be important in influencing response to different opioids.

Genetic factors influencing drug transport

The membrane-bound drug transporter P-glycoprotein influences drug absorption and drug excretion as well as transport of drugs in and out of the CNS across the blood–brain barrier (Hennessy and Spiers, 2007). Furthermore the P-glycoprotein modulation of opioid CNS levels varies substantially between different opioids (Dagenais et al., 2004). To add to the potential heterogeneity of responses, these critical transporter proteins are encoded by the multidrug resistance gene *MDR-1*, which has multiple genetic variations, some of which are associated with differences in P-glycoprotein expression or function (Hoffmeyer et al., 2000).

Switching route of systemic administration

Limited data indicate that some adverse side effects among patients receiving oral morphine can be relieved by switching the route of admission to the subcutaneous route. In one small study this phenomenon was reported for nausea and vomiting (McDonald et al., 1991), in another there was less constipation, drowsiness, and nausea (Drexel et al., 1989).

Initial management of the patient receiving opioids who presents with adverse effects

Among patients receiving opioid analgesic therapy there are two key steps in the initial management of adverse effects. Firstly, the clinician must distinguish morphine adverse effects from co-morbidity or drug interactions. This step requires careful evaluation of the patient for factors outlined in Table 9.4.8. If present, these factors should be redressed. Metabolic disorders, dehydration, or sepsis should be treated; non-essential drugs that may be producing an adverse interaction should be discontinued. Symptomatic measures may be required until an effect is observed.

Secondly, if indeed it seems that this is a true adverse effect of the opioid, consideration should be given to reducing the opioid dose. If the patient has good pain control, reduce morphine dose by 25%.

Adverse drug interactions

In patients with advanced cancer side effects due to drug combinations are common. The potential for additive side effects and serious toxicity from drug combinations must be recognized. The sedative effect of an opioid may add to that produced by numerous other centrally-acting drugs, such as anxiolytics, neuroleptics, and antidepressants (Bennett 2011). Likewise, drugs with anticholinergic effects probably worsen the constipatory effects of opioids. As noted previously, a severe adverse reaction, including excitation, hyperpyrexia, convulsions, and death, has been reported after the administration of pethidine (meperidine) to patients treated with a monoamine oxidase inhibitor (Browne and Linter 1987).

Gastrointestinal side effects

The gastrointestinal adverse effects of opioids are common. In general they are characterized by having a weak dose–response relationship.

Constipation

All opioids cause constipation and tolerance to this effect is not observed over time. Importantly, the dose–response relationship to this effect is very flat and the severity does not appear to be strongly dose related. There are some data to indicate that the severity is less severe with fentanyl and, possibly, methadone (Pappagallo, 2001; Staats et al., 2004). The likelihood of opioid-induced constipation is so great that laxative medications should be prescribed prophylactically to most patients (Ahmedzai and Boland, 2010). In general, bulking laxatives are discouraged. There is some evidence from randomized controlled trials, supported by consensus, that the oral laxatives lactulose, polyethylene gycol/electrolyte solutions and senna are probably of similar efficacy in people with opioid-induced constipation and that the polyethylene glycol/electrolyte solutions may have a better adverse effect profile than the other oral laxatives (Ahmedzai and Boland, 2010).

Methylnaltrexone, a quaternary derivative of naltrexone that does not cross the blood–brain barrier in humans, is a potentially important product recently licensed in Europe. It antagonizes only peripherally located opioid receptors while sparing centrally mediated analgesic effects of opioid pain medications. There is evidence of very predictable effectiveness after administration by either oral or parenteral routes of administration with most patients achieving defecation within 90 minutes of administration (Ahmedzai and Boland 2010; Candy et al., 2011; Licup and Baumrucker, 2011).

In many countries, an oral prolonged-release preparation containing oxycodone and naloxone in a ratio of 2 to 1, is available. Efficacy in preventing and or managing opioid related constipation is based on the fact that oral naloxone binds to gut opioid receptors with a greater affinity than oxycodone, however, naloxone that undergoes metabolism in the liver where it is rendered inactive, while oxycodone passes through the liver unchanged. The preparation is administered 12-hourly. A randomized controlled trial demonstrated that prolonged release oxycodone and naloxone combination provides superior bowel function in cancer pain patients, compared with prolonged release oxycodone alone, without compromising analgesic efficacy or safety (Ahmedzai et al., 2012).

Nausea and vomiting

Opioids may produce nausea and vomiting through both central and peripheral mechanisms. These drugs stimulate the medullary chemoreceptor trigger zone, increase vestibular sensitivity and have effects on the gastrointestinal tract (including increased gastric antral tone, diminished motility and delayed gastric emptying). With the initiation of opioid therapy, patients should be informed that nausea may occur. Routine prophylactic administration of an antiemetic is not necessary, except in patients with a history of severe opioid-induced nausea and vomiting, but patients should have access to an antiemetic at the start of therapy if the need for one arises. Nausea and vomiting that persists more than a few days is likely to be a chronic problem. No antiemetic has proven superiority over another and, indeed, there is little supportive evidence for any specific agent (Laugsand et al., 2011).

Additionally, there is also limited evidence supporting use of transdermal scopolamine (Ferris et al., 1991). A 'first principle' approach is usually adopted using metoclopramide or haloperidol. Persistent nausea and vomiting often necessitates opioid switching.

Central nervous system side effects

The CNS side effects of opioids are generally dose related. The specific pattern of CNS adverse effects is influenced by individual patient factors, duration of opioid exposure, and dose.

Sedation

Initiation of opioid therapy or significant dose escalation commonly induces sedation that persists until tolerance to this effect develops, usually in days to weeks. It is useful to forewarn patients of this potential, and thereby reduce anxiety and encourage avoidance of activities, such as driving, that may be dangerous if sedation occurs (Vainio et al., 1995). Some patients have a persistent problem with sedation, particularly if other confounding factors exist. These factors include the use of other sedating drugs or coexistent diseases such as dementia, metabolic encephalopathy, or brain metastases. Limited evidence supports the potential efficacy of amphetamines and amphetamine-like agents such as dextroamphetamine, methylphenidate, donepezil, and modafinil in the treatment of opioid-induced sedation (Reissig and Rybarczyk, 2005; Stone and Minton, 2011).

Treatment with methylphenidate or dextroamphetamine is typically begun at 2.5–5 mg in the morning, which is repeated at midday if necessary to maintain effects until evening. Doses are then increased gradually if needed. Few patients require more than 40 mg per day in divided doses. This approach is relatively contraindicated among patients with cardiac arrhythmias, agitated delirium, paranoid personality and past amphetamine abuse.

Confusion and delirium

Mild cognitive impairment is common following the initiation of opioid therapy or increase in dose. Similar to sedation, however, pure opioid-induced encephalopathy appears to be transient in most patients, persisting from days to a week or two (Banning and Sjogren, 1990; Vainio et al., 1995). Although persistent confusion attributable to opioid alone occurs (Gaudreau et al., 2007), the aetiology of persistent delirium is often related to the combined effect of the opioid and other contributing factors, including electrolyte disorders, neoplastic involvement of central nervous

---

> **Box 9.4.3** A stepwise approach to the management of confusion and delirium
>
> 1. Discontinue non-essential centrally acting medications.
> 2. If analgesia is satisfactory, reduce opioid dose by 25%.
> 3. Exclude sepsis or metabolic derangement.
> 4. Exclude CNS involvement by tumour.
> 5. If delirium persists, consider:
>   - trial of neuroleptic (e.g. haloperidol)
>   - change to an alternative opioid drug
>   - a change in opioid route to the intraspinal route (± local anaesthetic)
>   - a trial of other anaesthetic or neurosurgical options.

system, sepsis, vital organ failure and hypoxaemia (Centeno et al., 2004; Gaudreau et al., 2007).

A stepwise approach to management (Box 9.4.3) often culminates in a trial of a neuroleptic drug or opioid rotation. Among the neuroleptic agents, haloperidol in low doses (0.5–1.0 mg PO or 0.25–0.5 mg IV or IM) is most commonly recommended because of its efficacy and low incidence of cardiovascular and anticholinergic effects. As an alternative strategy, there is limited anecdotal experience with the use of acetylcholinesterase inhibitors; initiated with IV physostigmine, and then maintained with oral donepezil (Slatkin and Rhiner, 2004).

Respiratory depression

When sedation is used as a clinical indicator of CNS toxicity and appropriate steps are taken, respiratory depression is rare. When, however, it does occur it is always accompanied by other signs of CNS depression, including sedation and mental clouding (Dahan 2007). Respiratory compromise accompanied by tachypnoea and anxiety is never a primary opioid event. With repeated opioid administration, tolerance appears to develop rapidly to the respiratory depressant effects of the opioid drugs, consequently clinically important respiratory depression is a very rare event in the cancer patient whose opioid dose has been titrated against pain.

The ability to tolerate high doses of opioids is also related to the stimulus-related effect of pain on respiration in a manner that is balanced against the depressant opioid effect. Opioid-induced respiratory depression can occur however, if pain is suddenly eliminated (such as may occur following neurolytic procedures) and the opioid dose is not reduced (Wells et al., 1984).

Careful observation is the best method for monitoring sedation level and respiratory status. The University of Wisconsin Hospital and Clinics Sedation Assessment Scale (Gordon et al., 2000) is a very useful aid to assessment, particularly in the sleeping patient.

When respiratory depression occurs in patients on chronic opioid therapy, administration of the specific opioid antagonist, naloxone, usually improves ventilation (Dahan et al., 2010). This is true even if the primary cause of the respiratory event was not the opioid itself, but rather, an intercurrent cardiac or pulmonary process. A response to naloxone, therefore, should not be taken as proof that the event was due to the opioid alone and an evaluation for these other processes should ensue.

Naloxone can precipitate a severe abstinence syndrome and should be administered only if strongly indicated. If the patient is bradypnoeic but readily arousable, and the peak plasma level of the last opioid dose has already been reached, the opioid should be withheld and the patient monitored until improved. If severe hypoventilation occurs (regardless of the associated factors that may be contributing to respiratory compromise), or the patient is bradypnoeic and unarousable, naloxone should be administered. To reduce the risk of severe withdrawal following a period of opioid administration, dilute naloxone (1:10) should be used in doses titrated to respiratory rate and level of consciousness. In the comatose patient, it may be prudent to place an endotracheal tube to prevent aspiration following administration of naloxone.

Multifocus myoclonus

All opioid analgesics can produce myoclonus. Mild and infrequent myoclonus is common. In occasional patients, however, myoclonus can be distressing or contribute to breakthrough pain that occurs with the involuntary movement. If the dose cannot be reduced due to persistent pain, consideration should be given to either switching to an alternative opioid (Stone and Minton, 2011) or to symptomatic treatment with a benzodiazepine (particularly clonazepam or midazolam), dantrolene, or an anticonvulsant such as gabapentin (Mercadante et al., 2001; Stone and Minton, 2011).

Endocrine effects

Hypogonadism

Chronic opioid therapy may often cause endocrine dysfunction mainly in the form of hypo function of the pituitary–gonadal axis with sexual disturbance and menstrual irregularities. Chronic opioid therapy has an inhibitory effect on the hypothalamic–pituitary axis (Katz and Mazer, 2009; Elliott et al., 2011). It interferes with the release (including its pulsatile nature) of gonadotropin-releasing hormone, resulting in lower peak values of luteinizing hormone and follicle-stimulating hormone and an inhibitory effect of the opioids on the hypothalamic–pituitary levels with secondary effects on oestradiol and testosterone levels. Clinical manifestations may include fatigue, muscle wasting, erectile dysfunction, reduced libido, vaginal dryness, and menstrual abnormalities. More subtle symptoms such as hot flushes and anxiety may occur, rarely with changes in pubic hair distribution and breast size. This may require hormone replacement therapy (Aloisi et al., 2011; Blick et al., 2012; McWilliams et al., 2014).

Adrenal hormones

Chronic use of exogenous opioids has been found in several studies to decrease adrenocorticotropic hormone (ACTH) and cortisol levels and cortisol responses to adrenocorticotropin challenges. Opioids also affect the circadian rhythms of cortisol secretion, resulting in persistently raised levels of ACTH and cortisol and eventually blunting the stress response (Katz and Mazer, 2009; Elliott et al., 2011).

Obesity and diabetes

Chronic opioid use is associated with weight gain, hyperglycaemia, and worsening diabetes. This may be a central action via the sympathetic nervous system and impaired insulin secretion (Katz and Mazer, 2009; Elliott et al., 2011).

Immune effects

No clinical data exist on the effects of opioids on the immune system, when used for chronic cancer pain, however, a significant amount of pre-clinical data exist. Some theoretical differences between opioid classes have been suggested, however, clinical studies are needed to understand if this is a clinically relevant issue (Bortsov et al., 2012).

Other effects

Urinary retention

Opioid analgesics increase smooth muscle tone and can occasionally cause bladder spasm or urinary retention (due to an increase in sphincter tone). This is an infrequent problem that is usually observed in elderly male patients. Tolerance can develop rapidly but catheterization may be necessary to manage transient problems.

Opioid-induced hyperalgesia

The phenomenon of OIH may occur, whereby there is a paradoxical increase in pain with increasing or high doses of opioids. It is important to recognize when OIH occurs, in order to manage it correctly. Chronic opioid use may result in tolerance, when a higher dose is required to achieve the same degree of analgesia (with a right shift in a standard dose–response curve). In contrast, when OIH occurs, an increase in opioid dose results in an increase in pain (see Fig. 9.4.7) (Colvin and Fallon, 2010).

Laboratory studies of OIH in both acute and chronic models show a number of changes in pain processing, due to opioid administration. There are some variations, dependent on what model is used, but the underlying mechanisms may include central sensitization involving the glutaminergic system (Haugan et al., 2008; Zhao and Joo, 2008; Minville et al., 2010; Hutchinson et al., 2011; Wang et al., 2012); activation of glial cells via opioid binding to toll-like receptors, inducing a central neuroinflammatory response (Hutchinson et al., 2011; Wang et al., 2012); or alterations in the balance between anti-nociceptive and facilitatory descending systems (Vera-Portocarrero et al. 2007; Xie et al., 2005) and spinal alpha-2 receptors (Milne et al.. 2013). Improved understanding of the mechanisms that lead to OIH should allow us to develop more effective targeted therapies to treat it.

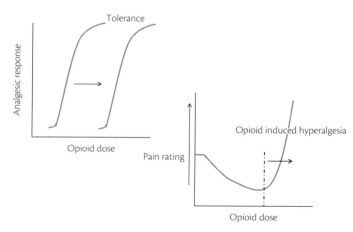

Fig. 9.4.7 Common adverse effects of opioid medication.

There has been much debate about the clinical relevance of OIH, but the evidence from basic science studies, human volunteer studies, and emerging clinical evidence indicate that it is a real clinical phenomenon, although an area where more research is urgently needed (Angst and Clark, 2006; Eisenberg et al.. 2010; Brush, 2012). A recent systematic review of OIH in the acute setting found 27 studies that were suitable to include in a meta-analysis, with a total of 1494 patients, where those patients who had received high dose intraoperative opioids compared to lower doses, had a significant increase in postoperative pain (Fletcher and Martinez, 2014). Many of the studies of chronic opioid use have been of patients on methadone for substance misuse, with some evidence of increased pain sensitivity (Doverty et al., 2001). This has been confirmed in chronic non-malignant pain, where reduced effectiveness of descending inhibitory pathways may contribute to OIH (Baron and McDonald, 2006; Ram et al., 2008).

Management of OIH may include gradual reduction in opioid doses and assessing the analgesic effect, which should improve, as the dose is decreased. Alternatively, opioid rotation may be useful: this may be due to genetic variation in opioid response, or due to differential binding at opioid receptor subtypes (Quigley, 2004; Jensen et al., 2009). For example, there is interest in developing novel dual-action opioids, with high binding affinity to mu and delta receptors, where there is early evidence of reduced OIH and other adverse effects (Dietis et al., 2009; Parenti et al., 2013; Podolsky et al., 2013). Other management strategies may include the use of NMDA receptors, such as ketamine, alpha-2 agonists, and in the future, agents that modify TRP receptors, or glial cell activity (Ramasubbu and Gupta, 2011; Mion and Villevieille, 2013).

There are no evidence-based therapeutic algorithms for this scenario. Commonly recommended strategies include dose reduction of the causative agent and/or substitution of the causative agent with another opioid. Naloxone does not reverse this effect. Anecdotal suggestions include, as above, a NMDA receptor antagonist such as ketamine, non-opioid co analgesics, spinal opioids, and hydration.

Opioids and driving

The ability to continue driving is very important to maintaining the quality of life of many patients with advanced cancer. Many assume that they must stop driving whilst taking regular potent opioid analgesics, but this is not necessarily so. The usual advice to patients is that they should not drive or engage in other skilled activities such as operating machinery when they first start on morphine or a similar opioid, or when they increase the dose. However, once the initial sedative effects have resolved and both the patient and physician are confident that cognitive and psychomotor performance is no longer impaired, driving and other similar activities may restart.

This advice is based to a large extent on empirical experience and there have been few objective data to substantiate it. However, recent studies confirm, perhaps surprisingly, that morphine produces little measurable impairment of cognitive and psychomotor function, particularly in patients receiving continuous treatment with stable doses (Vainio et al., 1995; Fishbain et al., 2003; Byas-Smith et al., 2005). In one study, which used a battery of performance tests designed specifically to assess functions related to driving ability, chronic morphine use was associated with slower reaction times, more mistakes, and a slowing in ability to process visual information and perform motor sequences, but these changes were not statistically significant compared with a control group of cancer patients not taking morphine (Vainio et al., 1995). These data support the clinical impression that stable doses of morphine are unlikely to cause substantial impairment of the psychomotor skills required for driving, and allow us to continue to advise patients to this effect.

Patients, however, must be reminded of the responsibility of critical self-examination of their fitness to drive on a moment-by-moment basis before and during operating a motor vehicle and should desist if they are aware of any impairment of concentration or alertness (Brandman, 2005; Kress and Kraft, 2005). Clearly a physician has a duty of care to society and if he feels a patient should not drive, has to report this to the relevant driving authority, if the patient continues to drive.

'Allergy' and intolerance to morphine

Morphine and other opioids cause histamine release, and this is said to contribute to asthma or urticaria in allergic patients (Hermens et al., 1985; Warner et al., 1991; Katcher and Walsh, 1999). There is no published information on the incidence of this phenomenon and, in our experience, it is very uncommon (Woodall et al., 2008).

However, it is not uncommon for patients to claim that they are 'allergic' to morphine. This usually means that they have had a bad experience with the drug but, on investigation, what they describe are its common side effects. There is no doubt that most patients experience some adverse effects when they first start regular morphine treatment. Most commonly this is sedation, nausea, and, less often, vomiting. All patients must be warned about this and appropriate measures must be taken, as described above. If patients are not warned and experience unpleasant adverse effects they will be discouraged from continuing with the drug, and if they do not understand what is going on they may assume they that are 'allergic' to it.

Opioid misuses and addiction

Opioid misuse is a generic term for the intentional or unintentional use of a prescribed medication other than as directed (see Chapter 9.5). Misuse can include a patient taking more pain medicine than prescribed to control otherwise inadequately controlled pain as well as criminal, abusive and addictive behaviours.

Abuse refers to the intentional self-administration of a medication for non-medical purpose or the use of an illegal drug.

Addiction is a primary, chronic disease defined by one or more of the following behaviours: impaired control over drug use, compulsive use, continued use despite harm, and craving.

Addiction and substance abuse are social and medical problems of pandemic proportions which are associated with major social and human costs. Commonly, opioid drugs are the preferred substances of abuse. This association, combined with the principle of non-maleficence is the basis for concern regarding risk of addiction caused by the medical use of opioids. In recent years, the relationship between the medical use of opioids and the risk of addiction has been the focus of policy makers, medical sociologists, and pain clinicians.

Overall, this body of research has demonstrated (1) the risk of developing addictive behaviours or substance abuse as a consequence of the medical use of opioids in a palliative care setting is low (Passik et al., 2000; Hojsted and Sjogren, 2007; Minozzi et al., 2013); (2) patient, family members, members of the health-care professions, and regulators commonly overestimate the risk of addiction; (3) patient, family members, members of the health-care professions, and regulators often confuse physical dependence and addiction; and (4) together, these concerns contribute substantially to physician reluctance to prescribe opioids and patient reluctance to use them (Goldberg, 2010).

Sadly, in the United States there is now clear evidence of an increasing problem of diversion of prescribed opioids (Epstein et al., 2007; Joranson and Gilson, 2007) as well as substance abuse and addiction among patients with chronic pain syndromes (Hojsted and Sjogren, 2007). This has generated much public discussion and anxiety about prudent opioid use and underscores the need for vigilance in patient evaluation and selection, the storage of opioid medications and the disposal of unused drugs, and used opioid patches.

To understand these phenomena as they relate to opioid treatment of cancer pain, it is useful first to present a concept that might be called 'therapeutic dependence'. Patients who require a specific drug therapy to control a symptom or disease process are clearly dependent on the therapeutic efficacy of the drugs in question. Examples of this 'therapeutic dependence' include the requirements of patients with congestive cardiac failure for cardiotonic and diuretic medication or the reliance of type 1 diabetics on insulin therapy. In these patients, undermedication or withdrawal of treatment would result in serious untoward consequences. Patients with chronic cancer pain have an analogous relationship to their analgesic therapy. This relationship may or may not be associated with the development of physical dependence, but is virtually never associated with addiction.

Psychological dependence and 'addiction'

The properties of the opioid analgesics that are most likely to lead to their being misused are effects mediated in the CNS. The term addiction refers to a psychological and behavioural syndrome characterized by a continued craving for an opioid drug to achieve a psychic effect (psychological dependence) and associated aberrant drug-related behaviours, such as compulsive drug-seeking, unsanctioned use or dose escalation, and use despite harm to self or others. Addiction should be suspected if patients demonstrate compulsive use, loss of control over drug use, and continuing use despite harm. The term addiction should not be used when physical dependence is meant.

There is a common perception that opioid use, for any reason, is associated with a high risk of iatrogenic psychological dependence and that it is best avoided or minimized. Many health-care professionals and laypersons fail to distinguish between patients with substance abuse disorder and psychologically well patients with pain, and consequently overestimate the risk of iatrogenic addiction. This skews evaluation of the therapeutic index of opioids, and impacts adversely on the likelihood of a clinician to prescribe opioids and on the patient's compliance with an opioid prescription.

Physical dependence

Physical dependence is the term used to describe the phenomenon of withdrawal when an opioid is abruptly discontinued or an opioid antagonist is administered (Jasinski, 1981). The severity of withdrawal is a function of the dose and duration of administration of the opioid just discontinued (i.e. the patient's prior opioid exposure). The administration of an opioid antagonist to a physically dependent individual produces an immediate precipitation of the withdrawal syndrome. Patients who have received repeated doses of a morphine-like agonist to the point where they are physically dependent may experience an opioid withdrawal reaction when given a mixed agonist–antagonist. It can be shown that prior exposure to a morphine-like drug greatly increases a patient's sensitivity to the antagonist component of a mixed agonist–antagonist. Therefore, when used for chronic pain, the mixed agonist–antagonists should be tried before prolonged administration of a morphine-like agonist is initiated.

The abrupt discontinuation of an opioid analgesic in a patient with significant prior opioid experience will result in signs and symptoms characteristic of the opioid withdrawal or abstinence syndrome (Rogers, 1991b). The onset of withdrawal is characterized by the patient's report of feelings of anxiety, nervousness and irritability, and alternating chills and hot flushes. A prominent withdrawal sign is 'wetness' including salivation, lacrimation, rhinorrhoea, sneezing, and sweating, as well as gooseflesh. At the peak intensity of withdrawal patients may experience nausea and vomiting, abdominal cramps, insomnia, and, rarely, multifocal myoclonus. The time course of the withdrawal syndrome is a function of the elimination $t_{1/2}$ of the opioid on which the patient has become dependent. Abstinence symptoms generally appear within 6–12 hours and reach a peak at 24–72 hours following cessation of a short-$t_{1/2}$ drug such as morphine, while onset may be delayed for 36–48 hours with methadone, which has a long $t_{1/2}$. Therefore, it is important to emphasize that, even in a patient in whom pain has been completely relieved by a procedure (e.g. a cordotomy), it is necessary to decrease the opioid dose slowly to prevent withdrawal.

Experience indicates that the usual daily dose required to prevent withdrawal is equal to 75% of the previous daily dose. Following this rule of thumb, doses can be gradually titrated down until the drug is discontinued.

'Pseudoaddiction'

Some cancer patients who continue to experience unrelieved pain manifest intense concern about opioid availability and drug-seeking behaviour that is reminiscent of addiction but ceases once pain is relieved, often through opioid dose escalation. This behaviour has been termed 'pseudoaddiction' (Weissman and Haddox, 1989). Pain relief usually produced by dose escalation eliminates this aberrant behaviour and distinguishes the patient from the true addict. Misunderstanding of this phenomenon may lead the clinician inappropriately to stigmatize the patient with the label 'addict', which may compromise care and erode the doctor–patient relationship.

For the treating clinician, differentiating pseudoaddiction from abuse or addiction can be challenging. Evaluation requires a complete pain assessment and review the recent analgesic history: is this a pain syndrome that typically responds to opioids? Is the current opioid dose, route and schedule appropriate? If so, has a reasonable attempt at dose escalation been made? Is there any past medical history to suggest a substance abuse disorder? Complete a comprehensive addiction assessment if such a disorder is suspected

(Weissman, 2005). Ultimately, the diagnosis can only be made retrospectively, that is, pseudoaddiction improves with the provision of adequate analgesia, including opioids. In contrast, behaviours associated with a substance abuse disorder will not change.

This concept has been criticized, arguing that it is difficult to empirically demonstrate and that it can only be diagnosed ex post facto, that is, it can only be recognized when pain is adequately relieved and the pseudoaddictive behaviours disappear (Bell and Salmon, 2009).

Screening for abuse risk or abuse

Whereas opioids analgesic therapy is a safe and effective treatment for pain in many, for some it carries risk of abuse and addiction. Patients with severe chronic pain and high risk of opioid misuse should not necessarily be denied opioid therapy but should be identified and managed with a modified treatment plan and be followed under closer supervision than those patients with lower risk estimates (Hojsted and Sjogren, 2006).

Especially in the United States, authorities have been advocating the use of a screening evaluation for risk of misuse and addiction before patients are commenced on chronic opioids therapy. Although no screening tests have been developed to screen for opioid misuse specifically in cancer or palliative care patients the *Screener and Opioid Assessment for Pain Patients* (SOAPP) appears to be the best validated tool. The SOAPP predicts risk potential for aberrant drug behaviour via a 14-item self-report. Items included in the SOAPP cluster into categories of antisocial behaviour, substance abuse history, doctor/patient relationship, medication-related behaviours, and psychiatric and neurobiological need for medicine. Responses are based on a 5-point Likert scale (possible score range 0–56). Using 7 as a cut-off, this test had a sensitivity of 91%, specificity of 69%, positive predictive value of 71% and negative predictive value of 90% to predict future likelihood of aberrant drug behaviour (Butler et al., 2004). It is important to note that while a score of 7 maximizes this test's sensitivity, that is, identifies most patients with a risk of opioid misuse, it will also result in a large number of false positive tests given the lower specificity at this cut-off. In a study of 48 chronic pain patients, the sensitivity of predicting aberrant behaviour using SOAPP (73%) was very close to the sensitivity of a trained psychologist's clinical interview (77%) (Akbik et al., 2006). More recently a 24 item, revised version SOAPP-R has been developed with greater reliability (Butler et al., 2008).

Current Opioid Misuse Measure (COMM) is a 17-item, self-report questionnaire to assist clinicians identify whether a patient, currently on long-term opioid therapy may be exhibiting aberrant behaviours associated with misuse of opioid analgesics. Since the COMM examines current behaviour, it is ideal for helping clinicians to monitor patients during the course of therapy (Butler et al., 2007). In validation studies among patients with chronic pain, a COMM score of 13 had a sensitivity of 77% and a specificity of 77% for identifying patients with prescription drug use disorder (Meltzer et al., 2011).

Management of cancer pain in patients with a history of drug abuse

Patients with a history of abuse of opioid analgesics may develop cancer and severe pain (Starr et al., 2010; Kircher et al., 2011). It is important to distinguish between the patient with a previous history of abuse and one who is currently abusing or who is in the company of active abusers. In general, a multidisciplinary team approach is recommended for the management of at-risk patients. Mental-health professionals who specialize in addiction therapy may be instrumental in helping palliative care team members develop strategies for management and treatment compliance (see Chapters 4.13 and 9.5).

Conclusion

This opioid chapter reinforces that we have to remain grounded in individual patient assessment and tailored prescribing, with the background knowledge that complex disease and genomic dynamics make the patient phenotype. The ultimate response to analgesia is complex, but can be managed in an optimal way.

The consensus that opioid-based pharmacotherapy remains the mainstay of chronic cancer pain management, drives a consensus to best practice and a clinically relevant research agenda.

Online materials

Complete references for this chapter are available online at <http://www.oxfordmedicine.com>.

References

Baron, M.J. and McDonald, P.W. (2006). Significant pain reduction in chronic pain patients after detoxification from high-dose opioids. *Journal of Opioid Management*, 2, 277–282.

Bennett, M.I. (2011). Effectiveness of antiepileptic or andidepressant drugs when added to opioids for cancer pain: systematic review. *Palliative Medicine*, 25(5) 553–559.

Caraceni, A., Hanks, G., Kaasa, S., et al. for EPCRC Collaborative on behalf of EAPC (2012). Evidence-based guidelines for the use of opioid analgesics in the treatment of cancer pain: the 2011 EAPC recommendations. *The Lancet Oncology*, 13, e58–e68.

Colvin, L.A. and Fallon, M.T. (2010). Opioid-induced hyperalgesia—a clinical challenge. *British Journal of Anaesthesia*, 104, 125–127.

Dahan, A., Aarts, L., and Smith, T.W. (2010). Incidence, reversal, and prevention of opioid-induced respiratory depression. *Anesthesiology*, 112, 226–238.

Dy, S.M., Asch, S.M., Naeim, A., Sanati, H., Walling, A., and Lorenz, K.A. (2008). Evidence-based standards for cancer pain management. *Journal of Clinical Oncology*, 26, 3879–3885.

Elliott, J.A., Horton, E., and Fibuch, E.E. (2011). The endocrine effects of long-term oral opioid therapy: a case report and review of the literature. *Journal of Opioid Management*, 7, 145–154.

Epstein, R.H., Gratch, D.M., and Grunwald, Z. (2007). Development of a scheduled drug diversion surveillance system based on an analysis of atypical drug transactions. *Anesthesia and Analgesia*, 105(4), 1053–1060.

Fine, P.G. and Portenoy, R.K. (2009). Establishing 'best practices' for opioid rotation: conclusions of an expert panel. *Journal of Pain and Symptom Management*, 38, 418–425.

Fishbain, D.A., Cutler, R.B., Rosomoff, H.L., and Rosomoff, R.S. (2003). Are opioid-dependent/tolerant patients impaired in driving-related skills? A structured evidence-based review. *Journal of Pain and Symptom Management*, 25, 559–577.

Jandhyala, R., Fullarton, J.R., and Bennett, M. (2013), Efficacy of rapid-onset oral fentanyl formulations vs oral morphine for cancer-related breakthrough pain: a meta-analysis of comparative trials. *Journal of Pain and Symptom Management*, 46(4), 573–580.

Joranson, D.E. and Gilson, A.M. (2007). A much-needed window on opioid diversion. *Pain Medicine*, 8(2), 128–129.

King, S.J., Reid, C., Forbes, K., and Hanks, G. (2011). A systematic review of oxycodone in the management of cancer pain. *Palliative Medicine*, 25(5), 454–470.

Kircher, S., Zacny, J., Apfelbaum, S.M., *et al.* (2011). Understanding and treating opioid addiction in a patient with cancer pain. *Journal of Pain*, 12, 1025–1031.

Laugsand, E.A., Kaasa, S., and Klepstad, P. (2011). Management of opioid-induced nausea and vomiting in cancer patients: systematic review and evidence-based recommendations. *Palliative Medicine*, 25, 442–453.

Licup, N. and Baumrucker, S.J. (2011). Methylnaltrexone: treatment for opioid-induced constipation. *American Journal of Hospice and Palliative Medicine*, 28, 59–61.

Nabal, M., Librada, S., Redondo, M.J., Pigni, A., Brunelli, C., and Caraceni, A. (2012). The role of paracetamol and nonsteroidal anti-inflammatory drugs in addition to WHO Step III opioids in the control of pain in advanced cancer. A systematic review of the literature. *Palliative Medicine*, 26, 305–312.

Pigni, A., Brunelli, C., and Caraceni, A. (2011). The role of hydromorphone in cancer pain treatment: a systematic review. *Palliative Medicine*, 25(5), 471–477.

Podolsky, A.T., Sandweiss, A., Hu, J., *et al.* (2013). Novel fentanyl-based dual mu-/-opioid agonists for the treatment of acute and chronic pain. *Life Sciences*, 93, 1010–1016.

Ramasubbu, C. and Gupta, A. (2011). Pharmacological treatment of opioid-induced hyperalgesia: a review of the evidence. *Journal of Pain & Palliative Care Pharmacotherapy*, 25, 219–230

Stone, P. and Minton, O. (2011). European Palliative Care Research collaborative pain guidelines. Central side-effects management: what is the evidence to support best practice in the management of sedation, cognitive impairment and myoclonus? *Palliative Medicine*, 25, 431–441.

Vissers, K.C., Besse, K., Hans, G., Devulder, J., and Morlion, B. (2010). Opioid rotation in the management of chronic pain: where is the evidence? *Pain Practice*, 10, 85–93.

Opioid therapy: managing risks of abuse, addiction, and diversion

Julie R. Price, Alric D. Hawkins, and Steven D. Passik

Introduction to opioid therapy

Over the past decade, an emerging societal health issue has been the troubling increase in prescription drug abuse in the United States (National Center on Addiction and Substance Abuse of Columbia University, 2005). Given the complex and chronic medical problems that are seen in the palliative care setting, there is an increasing need for awareness of this issue, in addition to the potential for diversion of medications to others for illicit use. Traditionally, patients with substance use problems have been considered a homogenous group, but there exists a wide array of patients ranging from those with frank dependency to others with self-escalation of their medication doses without their prescribers' knowledge. Regardless of where patients may lie on the spectrum of substance-related problems, awareness of the existence of such issues is an important component to establishing an appropriate treatment plan.

However, simple awareness is only the first step in management, as these patients create a quandary for well-intentioned providers, who must balance the potential for abuse of prescribed opioids with the need to provide appropriate analgesia for patients in the palliative care setting. Nevertheless, these patients can be treated safely and effectively while addressing both of these issues.

Prevalence

Substance use in the United States is not uncommon with approximately half of the population between the ages of 15 and 24 having previously used illicit substances, while another 6–15% has met criteria for a substance use disorder (Regier et al., 1990; Colliver and Kopstein, 1991; Groerer and Brodsky, 1992; Warner et al., 1995; Kessler et al., 2005a, 2005b). Reports in the European Union from 2013 cite up to 38% of the population having a 'disorder of the brain', which includes substance use disorders. This number does include issues of alcohol and tobacco dependence as well, accounting for some of the increased prevalence rates (Effertz and Mann, 2012). Perhaps even more alarming is the increasing misuse of prescription drugs, which increased approximately 94% between 1992 and 2003 (National Center on Addiction and Substance Abuse of Columbia University, 2005). The combination of this high prevalence of use and its association with conditions such as HIV/AIDS, hepatic cirrhosis, and certain cancers (Wells et al., 1989; Blot, 1992; Thun et al., 1997; Smith-Warner et al., 1998; Room et al., 2005) means that issues surrounding substance

misuse will arise in the palliative care setting, and will require increasing attention. Clinicians must be aware of the difficulties that may arise with the use of potentially abusable medications with patients who have an active or past problem with substance misuse and the potential difficulties this may cause in providing the patient with optimal care for management of their illness.

The problem of increasing prescription drug misuse is more than a complication of treatment, as it is contributing to a health care crisis where, in the United States, for the year of 2002 alone, it was implicated in approximately 30% of drug-related emergency-room deaths and at least 23% of emergency-room visits (National Center on Addiction and Substance Abuse of Columbia University, 2005). More concerning is that approximately one-third of abusers were new users with a growth of 225% in new opioid abusers between the years of 1992 and 2003. Additionally, during the same time period, there was a 150% increase in the abuse of tranquilizers, a 127% increase in the abuse of sedatives, and a 171% increase in the abuse of stimulants (National Center on Addiction and Substance Abuse of Columbia University, 2005). Given this rapid growth in the general population, new questions have to be raised about the prevalence of problematic use among those seen in the palliative care setting.

Fortunately, it appears that the prevalence of use amongst patients with cancer in tertiary care centres appears to be less than the frequency seen in society and general medical populations (Derogatis et al., 1983; Regier et al., 1984; Burton et al., 1991; Colliver and Kopstein, 1991; Groerer and Brodsky, 1992). For example, less than 1% of psychiatric consultations were requested for substance abuse concerns at Memorial Sloan Kettering Cancer Center (MSKCC) in a 6-month period in 2005 with only 3% of those patients eventually receiving a substance abuse diagnosis (Yu, 2005). A 1983 study by the Psychiatric Collaborative Oncology Group, found substance use conditions in less than 5% of 215 patients with cancer in the ambulatory care setting of several tertiary care hospitals based on structured clinical interviews (Derogatis et al., 1983). When compared to other settings, including emergency departments, general medical care providers, and society, this prevalence is fairly low (Derogatis et al., 1983; Regier et al., 1984; Burton et al., 1991; Colliver and Kopstein, 1991; Groerer and Brodsky, 1992).

However, this data must be considered carefully, due to the potential of bias, as prevalence has been found to be higher in other settings (Bruera et al., 1995). Potential contributors to lower than expected prevalence, include potential under-reporting and underrepresentation of groups, who may have a higher likelihood of substance misuse, due to potential barriers and access to care. Ultimately, more studies are needed to sort out the true prevalence, but until then, there should remain some index of suspicion for substance use issues so that they can be adequately addressed.

Abuse, dependence, and the terminology of substance misuse

The terminology used in describing the phenomena associated with substance misuse is often problematic, given the widespread misuse amongst members of both the medical community and lay public. Nevertheless, it is imperative that this nomenclature become more standardized and be utilized appropriately in order to facilitate communication between providers and with patients. The American Psychiatric Association (2000) has outlined their criteria for substance abuse and dependence, in the *Diagnostic and Statistical Manual of Mental Disorders* (4th edition, text revision) (DSM-IV-TR), but these can be problematic when applied in the context of medical illness. One major difficulty is inconsistent use or relevant terminology, which interferes with communication between care providers. What will follow is a discussion of the relative terminology.

Tolerance

Tolerance is defined as a need for increasing doses of a medication to facilitate an effect (Martin and Jasinski, 1969; Dole, 1972). This phenomenon has been observed in a variety of opioid effects including its analgesic effects, as demonstrated in animal models (Ling et al., 1989), as well as respiratory depression and cognitive impairment (Bruera et al., 1989). Although it is often considered negative, there is limited data to support that it creates problems in the medical setting (Foley, 1991; Portenoy, 1994a). In fact, it appears that most patients can be maintained on stable doses of their medications with tolerance being primarily a side effect of the medication. It appears the increasing needs for analgesia when using opioids is more related to progression of the underlying illness (Twycross, 1974; Kanner and Foley, 1981; Chapman and Hill, 1989; Zenz et al., 1992; Aronoff, 2000; McCarberg and Barkin, 2001; Meuser et al., 2001). Moreover, clinical practice does not reliably support the notion that tolerance is a harbinger of substance dependence.

Dependence

The notion of dependence has to be considered in the context of physical dependence and the much broader substance dependence. Substance dependence, as described in the DSM, is a syndrome that requires maladaptive substance use with drug-seeking behaviour and physical indicators of use including withdrawal and tolerance (American Psychiatric Association, 2000). This is to be considered differently from physical dependence which indicates the presence of withdrawal alone with cessation of use or administration of an antagonist (Martin and Jasinski, 1969; Dole, 1972; Redmond and Krystal, 1984). Although there is some overlap, with previous speculations that physical dependence drives some of the drug-seeking behaviour associated with substance dependence (Wikler, 1980), these are completely separate entities. Physical dependence is a physiological phenomenon which may not occur

in patients taking opioids for pain relief. This is confirmed by animal studies, which have demonstrated that drug-taking behaviour can occur without physical dependence (Dai et al., 1989), and in the clinical treatment of non-malignant pain where patients who have physical dependence are able to discontinue without developing problematic substance use behaviours (Halpern and Robinson, 1985). Clinically, this is an important concept to understand in order to avoid the stigmatization of patients and inappropriate management. This stigmatization is particularly typified in the use of terms such as addiction, which has a pejorative meaning to the general public. This ill-defined term may include both components of problem drug use behaviours as well as physical dependence, and when misused may place patients in danger of having their pain undertreated by well-intentioned clinicians. In general, the label of 'addict' should rarely be used, especially when describing a patient who only has the potential for developing a withdrawal syndrome with substance discontinuation and has no maladaptive behaviours associated with their exposure to the addictive substance.

Substance abuse and dependence

Substance abuse and dependence are the terms designated in the DSM-IV-TR for problematic substance use (American Psychiatric Association, 2000), and should be utilized when discussing these issues. A key component of these designations is the idea of maladaptive behaviours associated with use that occur outside typical societal/cultural norms. However, it is important to recognize that defining normative behaviour is problematic, as evidenced by a survey of pain clinicians which demonstrated significant individual differences when defining the behaviours that were most problematic when ranking aberrant drug-taking behaviours (Passik et al., 2002). Furthermore, normative behaviours will also vary based on the circumstances under which they occur, such as in the chronic pain and medical conditions seen in palliative care.

As a result, problem drug-related behaviours are poorly defined in medically ill populations, which limit appropriate assessment. Furthermore, what defines problem behaviour may differ between provider and the patient, which could impair formation of an appropriate treatment alliance. This was demonstrated in a 2000 pilot study at MSKCC, where inpatients with cancer condoned behaviours typically considered as misuse, when it was done in the context of symptom management, while women, who were inpatients with complications of HIV frequently engaged in behaviours that would commonly be labelled as misuse (Passik et al., 2000). Further complicating the use of these terms in medically ill patients is the lack of clarity with regards to which symptoms should be attributed to the substance use and which should be attributed to the underlying illness, such as the declining physical status of the patient being due to the underlying medical illness and/or their substance dependence. For example, a patient may become less engaged with those around him/her, which may be more related to the progression of their illness than deterioration in social functioning related to their ongoing substance use. Given these and other issues, it can be seen that the use of these terms in medically ill populations are limited.

Aberrant drug-related behaviour

A concise definition of substance dependence was previously proposed by Rinaldi et al., who described it as a 'compulsive use of a substance resulting in physical, psychological, or social harm to the user and continued use despite that harm' (Rinaldi et al., 1988). However, it could be argued that this definition is not sufficient to help in clinical decision-making. An attempt to develop a model that was more clinically useful has lent itself to the concept of 'aberrant drug-related behaviour'. The importance of this concept is that it moves away from defining and classifying the significance of behaviours that can be associated with misuse, and making it more clinically useful by defining it as an indication to assess patients for problematic substance use. Thus, in practice, a patient who presents with aberrant drug-related behaviours should be viewed as having a symptom of a potentially larger problem for which a differential should be constructed in order to fully address and provide an opportunity to manage a variety of issues that may be negatively impacting the patient's treatment including an underlying psychiatric illness or poor adaptive coping with the stressors of having a chronic medical illness.

At the core of this concept is the idea that aberrant substance use can represent more than a dependency syndrome. For example, a patient may ask aggressively for escalating drug dosage, which may be related to an intense desire to have adequate analgesia as opposed to representing true substance abuse or dependence (also known as pseudoaddiction). This, and other signs of distress, may appear to be aberrant drug-related behaviour and, if misdiagnosed, could produce a missed opportunity to help relieve patient suffering.

In using this model, the degree of aberrancy should be noted. Examples include:

- Mildly aberrant:
  - requests for specific pain medication
  - aggressive complaints about the need for medication
  - using drugs prescribed for a friend or family member
  - frequent prescription losses
  - hoarding drugs
- More highly aberrant:
  - forging prescriptions
  - obtaining drugs from non-medical source
  - sale of prescription drugs
  - crushing sustained-release tablets for snorting or injecting (Passik et al., 2002).

Less aberrant behaviours are more likely to represent patient distress whereas more aberrant behaviour is more consistent with problem substance use. However, it should be remembered that no specific behaviour should be viewed as pathognomonic for problem drug use and further exploration of any such behaviours should be undertaken if they are present. Examples include:

- a patient who is forging prescriptions in the context of borderline personality disorder due to their fears of abandonment instead of drug misuse
- a patient who self-medicates their underlying psychiatric illness, such as depression or anxiety
- a patient who misuses their medication due to confusion about their regimen in the context of cognitive deficits such as delirium or an underlying dementia.

In each of these examples, targets for treatment can be easily identified and would not preclude further prescribing of needed pain medications to the specific patient.

Empirical studies using the aberrant drug taking concept

The use of this model appears to have some support based on a few small studies (Dunbar and Katz, 1996; Compton et al., 1998; Passik et al., 2000) and appears to be a clinically useful tool, although larger empirical studies are needed. Dunbar and Katz (1996) examined 20 patients, with varying substance histories, who were being followed on chronic opioid therapy for 1 year. Ultimately, when compared to patients who abused their regimen, they found patients who did not abuse their opioid medications (11 of the 20 patients) were more likely to have abused alcohol alone or had a remote history of polysubstance use, were in community treatment programmes, and had strong psychosocial support. The patients who abused their regimen typically acquired opioids from more than one provider, increased their dose without permission, and made multiple phone calls or unscheduled visits to the clinic.

In another study, Compton et al. (1998) studied a group of patients who were referred to a multidisciplinary pain programme due to aberrant drug-taking behaviours. They examined these patients for a psychiatric diagnosis of substance dependence and found that those who met the criteria were more likely to have experienced a loss of control, increased their dose without permission, and received pain medications from multiple sources, compared to those without a psychiatric diagnosis.

Passik et al. (2000) examined patients with both cancer and AIDS for self-reported measures of attitudes and behaviours with regard to aberrant drug use. They found patients were not opposed either to themselves or others engaging in aberrant drug-taking behaviours if pain and other symptom management were not optimal. In addition, they found that the worry about developing substance dependence was greater than the actual risk.

These studies provide some insight into identifying potential behaviours that may be most concerning with regard to development of substance dependence syndromes with potentially abusable drugs. This is important to consider because of the potential to ascribe aberrant behaviours to substance dependence based on anecdotal evidence instead of following a more evidence-based approach. As a result, patients may be labelled inappropriately with dependence, which may jeopardize their ongoing management. Furthermore, it may lead to a missed opportunity to address the underlying needs or issues that resulted in the observed behaviour. For example, Passik et al. (2000) found that patients who had used anxiety medications that were intended for a friend appeared to have been doing so in an effort to manage undertreated anxiety instead of representing a true dependence syndrome.

Risk of substance abuse and dependence in the medically ill

Due to the growing prescription drug abuse problem in the United States, awareness has increased, which appears to have inappropriately raised the concern of both clinicians and patients with regard to the potential for developing opioid dependency when being treated for cancer pain. Contrary to this, is the increasing concern in the palliative care community that patients are being undertreated. This is based on available data that indicates the development of a significant substance abuse issue in patients being treated for cancer pain with opioids, with no previous substance abuse history, is a rare occurrence (Health and Public Policy Committee, 1983; Ventafridda et al., 1985, 1990; Walker et al., 1988; Jorgensen et al., 1990; Moulin and Foley 1990; Schug et al., 1990, 1992; World Health Organization, 1990; Ad Hoc Committee on Cancer Pain, 1992; American Pain Society, 1992; Agency for Health Care Policy and Research, 1994; Zech et al., 1995).

Considering this issue raises questions regarding the potential risks and benefits for chronic opioid treatment in patients with non-malignant pain (Zenz et al., 1992; Portenoy, 1994b), which has traditionally been considered negative, especially when considering that a large group of patients who have drug dependence issues began abusing substances after receiving prescribed opioids (Kolb, 1925; Pescor, 1939; Rayport, 1954). In one survey, Caucasian participants with substance dependence had a previous history of medical opioid prescriptions at a rate of approximately 27% compared to only 1.2% of their African American counterparts (Rayport, 1954). This may represent a differential effect that has yet to be identified or may reflect ongoing disparities in the adequate treatment of pain in African American patients.

However, these estimates are flawed, as they do not represent a sample of medically ill patients requiring opioid therapy with no known drug abuse history. One study, which included almost 12 000 inpatients that received opioids while hospitalized, only demonstrated four cases of substance abuse or dependence issues following discharge (Porter and Jick, 1980). In a series including more than 10 000 burn patients without a history of drug abuse, no cases were identified of patients who subsequently developed new substance use disorders. Another study of patients with chronic headaches demonstrated similarly low numbers of patients who developed substance misuse concerns (Medina and Diamond, 1977). Although this does not directly support the safety of long-term opioid therapy in chronic pain patients, it seems promising with regard to their safety potential.

The other component in the ultimate development of substance use issues is potential heritability or a predisposition for developing such a disorder. Evidence now exists that supports the idea of inheritance of predispositions for substance use (Grove et al., 1990), so patients with a genetic loading for these disorders along with exposure to opioids would be expected to have a higher rate of developing a substance use disorder. However, the data currently does not support the concept that patients are likely to develop these issues when treated with drugs that have abuse potential for appropriate medical indications if they have no personal history of substance use or psychopathology, no family history of substance abuse/dependence, and/or no membership in a subculture that fosters abuse (Grove et al., 1990; Zenz et al., 1992; Gardner-Nix, 1996; Aronoff, 2000; McCarberg and Barkin 2001; Meuser et al., 2001; Potter et al., 2004).

Risk in patients with current or remote drug abuse histories

The available information about the risk of exacerbating remote or active substance abuse/dependence issues in medically ill patients who require prescriptions for substances of abuse is inadequate.

There are small reports which seem to support safety in such prescribing in patients, especially when the substance use issues are remote (Macaluso et al., 1988; Gonzales and Coyle, 1992; Dunbar and Katz, 1996). This is further supported by a study of patients, who had AIDS-related pain, who were able to be treated effectively with morphine (Kaplan et al., 2000). Ultimately, this issue needs further investigation and caution should be exercised in these patients with close follow-up and attention to aberrant behaviours.

Clinical management

The presence of aberrant drug use amongst patients with advanced illness represents a major impediment to appropriate care, regardless of the context in which it occurs. In order to maximize patient outcomes and to prescribe needed medications both safely and fairly, the clinician should work to develop appropriate controls and monitoring within their clinical practice.

Multidisciplinary approach

Multidisciplinary teams in the palliative care setting can be an important tool in optimizing treatment for patients with substance use disorders. A structured approach can minimize impediments to treatment for both the patient and the prescriber, who can develop a variety of emotions while treating these patients that may inadvertently affect the quality of pain-related care that is being offered. Teams would ideally include a psychologist, who is trained in addictions, along with adequate nursing and social work support to address the complex needs that patients often have.

Assessment

Once a member of the treatment team becomes concerned about the potential for aberrant substance use, then the other team members should be notified in order to begin a multidisciplinary intervention (Lundberg and Passik, 1997). Due to safety concerns that may arise, a physician should be involved early in the process in order to rule out life-threatening issues such as respiratory depression due to intoxication and/or life-threatening withdrawal symptoms. Once immediate safety has been assured, then an organized assessment should be conducted where information is gathered concerning the nature and extent of the problematic substance use in a non-judgemental and empathetic manner.

One technique to accomplish this is by conducting a graduated interview that proceeds from open-ended and broad questioning to more specific details about substance use, which will allow for a positive rapport to develop and potentially minimize the patients denial of his/her use. In this same manner, information should be gathered about co-occurring psychiatric disorders including anxiety, mood, and personality disorders, which are often co-morbid (Regier et al., 1990; Penick et al., 1994; Grant et al., 2004). Once this information has been gathered a more comprehensive treatment plan can be developed that will allow for the patient's need to be most effectively met.

Pre-screening patients

Much of recent research has been done on developing screening tools that allow for appropriate risk stratification of patients who will require a treatment plan that includes chronic opioid prescribing. An important component of risk stratification is to be non-judgemental and to be mindful that aberrant substance use occurs on a spectrum that differs between recreational users and those requiring chronic pain treatment with opioids (Kirsh and Passik, 2008) (see Fig. 9.5.1). No assessment tool can diagnose substance misuse disorders alone, and some clinical acumen will need to be applied in order to identify the issues that may be leading to non-adherence.

Assessments tools are available for the purpose of identifying patients who may have problem substance use. A tool, called the Screener and Opioid Assessment for Patients with Pain (SOAPP) is a 24-item self-administered screen, which was validated in patients with chronic non-malignant pain (Butler et al., 2004). A shorter, five-item self-report tool, called the Opioid Risk Tool (ORT) was demonstrated in 2005 to be effective in identifying patients who would later develop aberrant substance use (Webster and Webster, 2005), although it is susceptible to deception. A study by Moore et al. demonstrated that a semi-structured clinical interview had the highest sensitivity alone (0.77), but this was increased to 0.90 when combined with the SOAPP (Moore et al., 2009). However, this study was done on patients primarily with chronic pain and its effectiveness in medically ill patients is unclear.

The four As for ongoing monitoring

Analgesia, Activities of daily living, Adverse side effects, and Aberrant drug-taking behaviours have been labelled the 'Four A's' of necessary monitoring for patients with chronic pain on opioids (Passik and Weinreb, 2000). Utilizing these four domains is useful in treatment planning and clinical decision-making. A checklist tool (Passik et al., 2004) has been developed:

- *Analgesia:* document and monitor patient's pain, using scales such as a 0–10 pain rating scale. Although listed as the first 'A,' analgesia is not necessarily to be considered the most important outcome of pain management. An alternate view is how much relief it takes for a patient to feel that their life is meaningfully changed so they can work toward the attainment of their own zgoals.

- *Activities of daily living:* monitor patient's typical level of daily activities and psychosocial functioning to observe increases over time. The second 'A' concerning activities of daily living refers to quality of life issues and functionality. It is necessary that patients understand that they must comply with all of their recommended treatment options so that they are better able to return to work, avocation, and social activities.

- *Adverse effects:* strive for the highest analgesia with the most benign side effect profile. Patients must also be made aware of the adverse side effects inherent in the treatment of their pain condition with opioids and other medications. Side effects must be aggressively managed so that sedation and other side effects do not overshadow the potential benefits of drug therapy. The most common side effects of opioid analgesics include constipation, sedation, nausea, vomiting, and dry mouth.

- *Aberrant behaviours:* be aware of aberrant behaviours suggestive of drug use, such as multiple 'lost' prescriptions or unauthorized dosing escalations. Patients must be educated through agreements, or other means, about the parameters of acceptable drug taking. Even an overall good outcome in every other domain might not constitute satisfactory treatment if the patient is non-adherent with the contract in concerning ways. Dispensing pain medicine in a highly structured fashion may become necessary for some patients who are in violation or constantly on the fringes of inappropriate drug taking behaviours.

Development of a treatment plan—general considerations

A treatment plan with clear goals will need to be individualized for each patient in an effort to curtail and manage aberrant drug-related behaviours. The ultimate overall goal is for 'harm reduction' as poor coping and dealing with chronic illness may interfere with adequate management (Passik et al., 1998). The key elements of this approach are:

1. Approach the patient with empathetic listening and attempt to understand their distress.

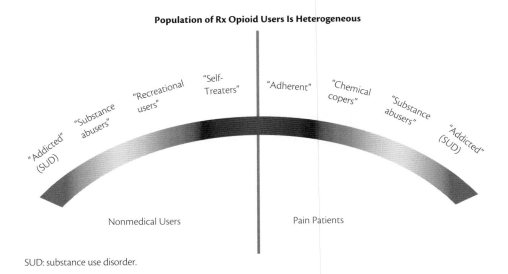

Population of Rx Opioid Users Is Heterogeneous

"Addicted" (SUD)   "Substance abusers"   "Recreational users"   "Self-Treaters"   "Adherent"   "Chemical copers"   "Substance abusers"   "Addicted" (SUD)

Nonmedical Users   Pain Patients

SUD: substance use disorder.

Fig. 9.5.1 The spectrum of adherence for pain patients versus the spectrum of illicit use by nonmedical users.
From Kirsh KL and Passik SD, The interface between pain and drug abuse the evolution of strategies to optimize pain management while minimizing drug abuse, *Experimental and Clinical Psychopharmacology*, Volume 16, Issue 5, pp. 400–404, Copyright © 2008 American Psychological Association. Reprinted with permission.

2. Utilize non-opioid interventions as part of management, but not as a substitute.

3. Utilize the patient's history of aberrant use in determining dosing and choice of medication that will offer the best outcome.

4. Frequent reassessment of the adequacy of pain and symptom control.

Urine toxicology screening

Non-adherence to treatment planning and aberrant substance use pose a variety of issues that could negatively impact prognosis. Due to this, it is imperative that appropriate monitoring be undertaken. The most useful and often easily obtained form of monitoring is the urine toxicology screening. However, one chart review in 2000 at a tertiary care centre showed that these screens were not often used by providers (Passik et al., 2000) and when used often demonstrated problems that decreased their effectiveness.

One of the difficulties in the use of urine toxicology screenings is a non-standardized approach, where clinicians make their decisions on who to test based on their own assessment of who they feel is at risk. However, this is not a reliable practice and could potentially miss problem behaviours, which would have been readily identified with testing. This unreliability was tested by Bronstein et al. (2011) who asked clinicians to identify patients who they felt were most at risk for aberrant drug use. They found that clinicians missed a significant group of patients who had no identifiable risk factors, but were able to identify patients more reliably when assessment tools were used.

Given that clinicians are not reliable in assessing those patients who do not have recognizable risk factors or problem behaviours, it is of great importance that drug screens be performed in a standardized and reliable way and performed on a randomized basis to minimize the ability of patients to predict testing in an effort to deceive screening.

The patient with advanced disease

The management of patients with advanced medical illness is a difficult task at baseline, but aberrant substance use can negatively impact efforts to offer appropriate palliative care. Ultimately the palliative care team and other treatment providers must work together to minimize risk, which may be as simple as a reduction in use, which could have a positive effect on the patient (Passik and Theobald, 2000). Box 9.5.1, lists some interventions that could be utilized in managing risk. These include screening tools for monitoring a variety of conditions, prescription monitoring programmes, which provides information on adherence to providers (Passik, 2009), and the previously mentioned urine drug screens. It is also important to remind patients to control their prescriptions carefully as studies have shown that prescription opioids are commonly diverted to family and friends for non-medical use (Passik, 2009). A final safety guard is opioid formulations and delivery strategies that minimize the potential for misuse, such as physical barriers.

Outpatient management

Outpatient management can be done safely and effectively. An important step to ensure a structure for appropriate management is to have the patient agree to a written treatment contract that is a mutually agreed upon document that establishes the boundaries

---

> **Box 9.5.1** Screening for substance abuse and treatment recommendations
>
> **Assessment guidelines**
>
> - Use a graduated interview approach beginning with broad questions about substances such as nicotine or caffeine and becoming more specific.
> - Assess for comorbid psychiatric disorders, such as anxiety, mood, and personality disorders.
> - Consider diagnostic instruments, such as the Screener and Opioid Assessment for Patients with Pain (Butler et al., 2004).
>
> **Treatment recommendations**
>
> *General*
>
> - Listen and accept the patient's report of distress.
> - Use behavioural and non-opioid interventions for pain when possible.
> - Consider drugs with slower onset and longer duration (e.g., transdermal fentanyl and modified-release opioids). Note that higher doses may be needed for adequate pain control in patients with a history of abuse or dependence.
> - Frequently assess adequacy of symptom and pain control.
>
> *Outpatients*
>
> - Limit amount of drug dispensed per prescription.
> - Make refills contingent on clinic attendance.
> - Consider urine toxicology screenings to assess usage.
> - Involve family members and friends in the treatment plan.
>
> *Inpatients*
>
> - Consider placing the patient in a private room near the nurses' station.
> - Consider daily urine collection.
>
> Source: data from Butler SF, et al. Validation of a screener and opioid assessment measure for patients with chronic pain, *PAIN*, Volume 112, Issue 1, pp.65–75, Copyright © 2004 International Association for the Study of Pain. Published by Elsevier B.V. All rights reserved.

---

of treatment. This may include such issues as frequency of urine drug screens, expectations in obtaining refills, expectations for outpatient substance abuse treatment, contingency plans for problem drug use, and expectations for the involvement of family and friends.

Inpatient management

In the inpatient setting, issues of misuse still remain a problem as patients may develop a variety of issues in regards to their substance use. This includes withdrawal syndromes, which may only become apparent after the patient no longer has access to the amount of medication they take at home. Aberrant substance use within the inpatient hospitalization can also be problematic and in extreme cases, visitors may need to be restricted and/or searched upon their arrival along with the patient's belonging. However, remain cognizant of the negative feelings that this may elicit from patients who may view this as an invasion of privacy. The goal of maintaining safety should be communicated to the patient and, when possible, the patient should be included in the process in order to facilitate a more positive working relationship. Clinicians should also be aware of intravenous access in patients with a known history of intravenous drug use and of the potential for patients to leave the floor to purchase illicit substances. The patient should be monitored carefully for both safety and adequate pain management with an individual plan that is designed to meet his/her needs.

Conclusion

Aberrant drug-related behaviour is a complex phenomenon that can occur in the chronic medically ill patient and needs to be approached in a manner that allows for recognition of the biological, chemical, psychological, and social aspects of it. The spectrum of behaviours that fall within this category is broad and, unfortunately, not well defined in terms of outcome, management, and potential difficulties. Nevertheless, we must continue to approach patients with these issues in an empathic manner, with the ultimate goal of safely managing their pain, while addressing other issues that are leading to their distress and perpetuating their aberrant drug use.

Online materials

Additional online materials and complete references for this chapter are available online at <http://www.oxfordmedicine.com>.

References

Blot, W.J. (1992). Alcohol and cancer. *Cancer Research*, 52, S2119–S2123.

Burton, R.W., Lyons, J.S., Devens, M., *et al.* (1991). Psychiatric consults for psychoactive substance disorders in the general hospital. *General Hospital Psychiatry*, 13, 83.

Colliver, J.D. and Kopstein, A.N. (1991). Trends in cocaine abuse reflected in emergency room episodes reported to DAWN. *Public Health Reports*, 106, 59–68.

Derogatis, L.R., Morrow, G.R., Fetting, J., *et al.* (1983). The prevalence of psychiatric disorders among cancer patients. *Journal of the American Medical Association*, 249, 751.

Groerer, J. and Brodsky, M. (1992). The incidence of illicit drug use in the United States, 1962–1989. *British Journal of Addiction*, 87, 1345.

Kessler, R.C., Berglund, P., Demler, O., *et al.* (2005a). Lifetime prevalence and age-of-onset distributions of DSM-IV Disorders in the National comorbidity survey replication. *Archives of General Psychiatry*, 62, 593–602.

Kessler, R.C., Chui, W.T., Demler, O., *et al.* (2005b). Prevalence, severity, and comorbidity of 12-month DSM-IV disorders in the National comorbidity survey replication. *Archives of General Psychiatry*, 62, 617–627.

National Center on Addiction and Substance Abuse of Columbia University (2005). *Under the Counter: The Diversion and Abuse of Controlled Prescription Drugs in the U.S.* New York: National Center on Addiction and Substance Abuse of Columbia University.

Regier, D.A., Farmer, M.E., Rae, D.S., *et al.* (1990). Comorbidity of mental disorders with alcohol and other drug abuse. *Journal of the American Medical Association*, 264, 2511–2518.

Room, R., Babor, T., and Rehm, J. (2005). Alcohol and public health. *The Lancet*, 365, 519–530.

Smith-Warner, S.A., Spiegelman, D., Yaun, S., *et al.* (1998). Alcohol and breast cancer in women: a pooled analysis of cohort studies. *Journal of the American Medical Association*, 279, 535–540.

Thun, M.J., Peto, R., Lopez, A.D., *et al.* (1997). Alcohol consumption and mortality among middle-aged and elderly U.S. adults. *The New England Journal of Medicine*, 337, 1705–1714.

Warner, L.A., Kessler, R.C., Hughes, M., *et al.* (1995). Prevalence and correlates of drug use and dependence in the United States. Results from the National Comorbidity Survey. *Archives of General Psychiatry*, 52, 219–229.

Wells, K.B., Golding, J.M., and Burnam, M.A. (1989). Chronic medical conditions in a sample of the general population with anxiety, affective, and substance use disorders. *American Journal of Psychiatry*, 146, 1440.

Yu, DK. (2005). Review of Memorial Sloan-Kettering Counselling Center Database (Unpublished manuscript).

9.6

Non-opioid analgesics

Per Sjøgren, Frank Elsner, and Stein Kaasa

Introduction to non-opioid analgesics

Non-opioid analgesics encompass the non-steroidal anti-inflammatory drugs (NSAIDs) and paracetamol (acetaminophen). All these drugs have analgesic and antipyretic properties. The NSAIDs include acetylsalicylic acid (ASA, aspirin), dipyrone (metamizole), and numerous other drugs in diverse classes. The advantages of non-opioid analgesics include their wide availability, familiarity to patients, effectiveness for milder pain conditions, ease of administration, additive analgesia when combined with other analgesics, and relatively low cost. The disadvantages include a ceiling effect for pain relief and the risk of side effects, including the potential for serious gastrointestinal (GI), renal, and cardiovascular toxicity (NSAIDs), and hepatotoxicity (paracetamol).

Non-opioid analgesics are widely used to manage mildto-moderate pain. In most Western societies, patients use over-the-counter formulations to treat pain related to headache and musculoskeletal ailments. In palliative medicine, they represent the first step of the analgesic ladder when used alone, or with adjuvant drugs, for mild pain and are an important supplement to opioids and adjuvant drugs at higher steps of the ladder (World Health Organization, 1996). The NSAIDs seem to be particularly useful in inflammatory pain and specific conditions such as bone pain. Paracetamol has limited anti-inflammatory effects, but is safer than the NSAIDs for long-term use. Dipyrone (metamizole) is used in some countries to treat pain, but has been removed from the market in others because of an association with life-threatening agranulocytosis.

Anti-inflammatory mechanisms

NSAIDs and paracetamol inhibit the production of prostaglandins (PGs). PGs are lipid-soluble molecules that are produced by enzymatic breakdown of arachidonic acid, which is itself produced from cell-membrane phospholipids. PGs are not stored in the body, but are produced constitutively as mediators of physiological effects in many tissues, or induced as part of the inflammatory cascade in in response to various noxious stimuli. Only 44 years ago, Vane postulated that inhibition of PG synthesis was the main effect of analgesics such as ASA (Vane, 1971). Subsequently, this led to the development of different types of drugs aiming at inhibiting the synthesis of PGs. A large number of NSAIDs were designed, and after the discovery of different isoforms of cyclooxygenase (COX), more selective COX-inhibitors became the focus of NSAID development. The selective COX-2 NSAIDs (coxibs) are the latest group to emerge from these activities.

The two isoforms of COX that have been best characterized are COX-1 and COX-2 (Fig. 9.6.1). COX-1 is largely a constitutive enzyme that produces PGs in many tissues. These PGs protect gastric mucosa, maintain normal kidney function, and promote platelet aggregation. Most COX-2 is induced as part of the complex processes that lead to inflammation, fever, and pain. All NSAIDs inhibit both COX-1 and COX-2, but there is a large variation in the relative effects on the two isozymes. Compared to conventional 'non-selective COX-1/COX-2' NSAIDs, coxibs inhibit COX-2 to a much greater extent.

The potential positive effects produced when NSAIDs inhibit PG synthesis include reduced inflammation and less pain. Serious adverse effects are possible, however, if the normal physiological effects of the PGs are disrupted (Abramson et al., 1985; McCormack, 1994; Richardson and Emery, 1995). Managing the latter risk is key to the use of these drugs in palliative care. The therapeutic benefit of the NSAIDs may be compromised if those PGs that are involved in nociception and inflammation cannot be reduced sufficiently, or adverse effects on normal physiology related to PG inhibition outweigh the therapeutic effects.

The tissue release of PGs is complex and is mediated by many types of noxious stimuli, and also by the actions of other substances like bradykinin and cytokines. The latter compounds induce nociception themselves and stimulate the synthesis of PGs and other mediators involved in nociception, such as substance P and calcitonin gene-related peptide (Burke et al., 2006).

Some of the functions affected by PGs also are mediated by leukotrienes. Leukotrienes are responsible for and involved in anaphylactic reactions, broncho-constriction, and chemotaxis, as well as vascular permeability and inflammation (Burke et al., 2006). PG synthesis inhibitors, such as NSAIDs and ASA, do not inhibit the production of leukotrienes, which to some extent may explain the limited efficacy of NSAIDs and ASA when treating pain of inflammatory origin.

The specific mechanisms underlying the beneficial antipyretic and analgesic actions of NSAIDs are not fully understood. Mediators of the inflammatory process—especially the cytokines—induce the production of COX-2 within hours. The induction of COX-2 does not only take place in injured tissues, but also in the central nervous system (CNS). In the CNS, high concentrations of COX-2 cause increasing concentrations of PGs, which, in turn, induce central sensitization and consequently more pain (Baba et al., 2001; Samad et al., 2001). However, under normal physiological conditions, COX-2 is found only at very low concentrations in the body, including brain tissue (Breder et al., 1995; Seibert et al., 1997). In animal studies, endothelial cells

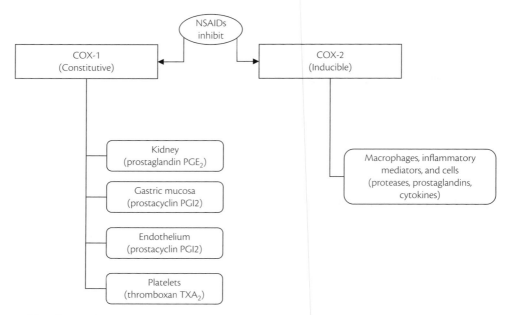

Fig. 9.6.1 Simple diagram of the influence of NSAIDs on prostaglandin synthesis.

express COX-2 mRNA in response to systemic interleukin-1 beta and the resulting production of PGs in the hypothalamus area may play an important role in producing fever (Cao et al., 1996).

In addition to COX-1 and COX-2, a COX-3 has been proposed as a variation expressed by the *COX-1* gene (Chandrasekharan et al., 2002). The existence of COX-3 in the CNS of humans has been controversial, and discussions regarding COX variants and their impact on antipyretic and analgesic effects are ongoing (Warner and Mitchell, 2002; Kis et al., 2003, 2004; Snipes et al., 2005).

COX-1 is constitutive, which means that it exists and acts continuously in many different tissues (Fig. 9.6.1). In gastric epithelial cells, COX-1 predominates and is responsible for the production of the protective PGI_2 (prostacyclin). Multiple actions of PGI_2 are involved in the protection of gastric mucosa: maintenance of mucosal blood flow, mucus production, secretion of bicarbonate, and also a positive influence on epithelial cell regeneration in order to provide a well-protected gastric mucosa. Thus, the inhibition of the production of PGI_2 by NSAIDs can upset this protective equilibrium (Scarpignato, 1995).

COX-1 is also responsible for the synthesis of PGE_2, which in addition to vasodilatation during inflammatory processes counteracts vasoconstriction in the kidneys. Under normal physiological conditions, the PG synthesis activity in the kidney is low and its role in modifying renal blood flow (RBF) is not of major importance (Ruilope et al., 1986). However, if RBF is critically lowered, glomerular filtration rate (GFR) may be partly restored by vasodilatatory effects of PGE_2. If PGE_2 production is reduced due to the use of NSAIDs, volume depletion of different aetiologies may aggravate the reduction of RBF. Moreover, inhibition of PGs may also result in a higher extracellular concentration of electrolytes such as sodium, which may cause water retention and oedema. In 10–25% of the patients treated with NSAIDs, sodium retention can be found (Burke et al., 2006).

There is growing evidence that nephrotoxicity is not only related to the influence of COX-1, but also to COX-2 activity. COX-2 is also constitutively expressed in the kidney and is regulated in

relation to changes in intravascular volume. Metabolites of COX-2 have also been discussed in the regulation of sodium excretion and renin release and the maintenance of RBF (Harris, 2006).

COX inhibition by NSAIDs also reduces platelet aggregation. Thromboxane A_2 (TXA_2) and PGI_2 are produced in platelets. PGI_2 prevents aggregation of platelets, but does not influence endothelial adherence, whereas TXA_2 is mainly responsible for coagulation. NSAIDs temporarily inhibit platelet aggregation by decreasing TXA_2 synthesis via incomplete and reversible inactivation of COX-1. The antithrombotic action of ASA is mainly due to inhibition of TXA_2-mediated platelet aggregation related to a complete and irreversible inactivation of COX-1 in platelets by acetylation of the enzyme (Patrono et al., 2004).

In an effort to minimize side-effects such as GI complications, renal impairment, and increased cardiovascular risk, efforts have been made to develop NSAIDs that selectively suppress the inducible form of COX, that is, COX-2, and also reduce the action of microsomal prostaglandin E_2 synthase (mPGES-1)-derived PGE_2. The coxibs have these effects. PGES-1 was identified as the most important PGE_2 synthase and its inhibition may lead to a relevant reduction of inflammation, fever, and pain in animal models. However, even if mPGES-1 seems to be a paramount target for inhibition resulting in a therapeutic use for any diseases related to inflammation and cancer, current knowledge about its role in clinical settings is limited (Koeberle and Werz, 2009).

NSAID-induced reduction in prostaglandin formation could potentially have other therapeutic effects, but supporting data are yet very limited. Epidemiological surveys of users and non-users of NSAIDs and ASA have shown that NSAIDs may alter the development and growth of malignancies. Clinical trials in patients with familial adenomatosis polyposis have shown the efficacy of NSAIDs in reducing the number as well as the size of colorectal polyps. However, a primary preventive effect has not yet been demonstrated. NSAIDs are also supposed to have a preventive and growth inhibitory effect in extracolonic epithelial malignancies. Pre-clinical studies show promising results with combination treatments of either chemotherapy or radiotherapy with NSAIDs. These NSAID effects in cancer cells may be mediated not only by COX enzymes, but also by interactions with downstream effectors of inflammation (Meric et al., 2006).

NSAIDS also have been proposed to be effective in the treatment of cancer-induced cachexia. The effect can be explained through the 'cytokine pathway' in the development of cachexia. Consequently, the blocking effect of NSAIDS on cytokines may slow down the development of cancer cachexia.

In general, the inhibition of cyclooxygenase isoforms is the main mechanism of the non-opioid analgesics, especially the NSAIDs. However, there are several other effects of non-opioid analgesics beyond COX inhibition, and these too may ultimately be shown to be important in the analgesic and anti-inflammatory effects. Interactions with cholinergic, monoaminergic, and endocannabinoid systems may be responsible for anti-inflammatory effects, as well as for the reduction of pain and fever; they also may be responsible for some adverse effects (Hamza and Dionne 2009).

The pharmacology of NSAIDs

Absorption, distribution, metabolism, and excretion

Most NSAIDs are administered orally, and absorption takes place mainly in the upper GI tract; stomach mucosa may also absorb a substantial proportion of the dose, especially at low pH. If administered as suppositories, most of the NSAID crosses the mucosal membrane easily. Recommended maximum doses and pharmacokinetic data of widely used NSAIDs are shown in Table 9.6.1.

With oral administration, effects usually begin within 30 minutes and peak effects, which mirror maximum concentration, occur within 120 minutes. The rate at which effects decline depends on the half-life of each NSAID.

There is evidence that topical administration of NSAIDs can be an effective way of treating pain in special indications. The pharmacology of topical-applied NSAIDs is not well understood (Mason et al., 2004).

Several NSAIDs, such as ketorolac and ibuprofen, are available in injectable formulations, which may be administered intravenously or intramuscularly. There are only a few publications which compare possible advantages and disadvantages of the parenteral and oral routes (Tramer et al., 1998).

All systemically administered NSAIDs are highly protein-bound. Plasma protein binding ranges from 90% to 99%. NSAIDs are predominantly metabolized in the liver by conjugation to sulphate and glucuronide compounds. Hepatic metabolism, which is by the cytochrome P450 system, is subject to many sources of individual variation, including genomic factors and the influence of other drugs. There may be circadian differences as well, but the potential clinical relevance of this phenomenon remains unclear (Burke et al., 2006). Conjugation of NSAIDs in other tissues of the body occurs, but accounts for a small and insignificant percentage of the metabolism.

Most of the NSAIDs are rapidly distributed in all tissues of the body. The more lipid-soluble a NSAID is, the more it will distribute into the CNS. However, the very high plasma protein binding will retain most of the drug within the plasma compartment (Burke et al., 2006).

NSAIDs are eliminated in the urine in free and conjugated forms. The relative amounts of free and conjugated compounds are highly dependent on urinary pH. Higher pH favours more acidic forms of elimination products. A small percentage of the drug can be found in the bile as well, which indicates that excretion also takes place via the intestines into the faeces (Burke et al., 2006).

Table 9.6.1 Choice of oral NSAIDs

NSAID	Pharmacokinetics		Dosage
Ibuprofen	◆ Peak Cp	◆ 15–30 min	400–800 mg 3–4 times/day
	◆ Protein binding	◆ 99%	
	◆ Half-life	◆ 2–4 h	
Diclofenac	◆ Peak Cp	◆ 2–3 h	50–75 mg 3 times/day
	◆ Protein binding	◆ 99%	
	◆ Half-life	◆ 1–2 h	
Naproxen	◆ Peak Cp	◆ 1 h	500 mg twice/day
	◆ Protein binding	◆ 99%	
	◆ Half-life	◆ 14 h	
Flurbiprofen	◆ Peak Cp	◆ 1–2 h	200–300 mg/day Resp. 100 mg 3 times/day
	◆ Protein binding	◆ 99%	
	◆ Half-life	◆ 6 h	
Indomethacin	◆ Peak Cp	◆ 1–2 h	25 mg 2–3 times/day
	◆ Protein binding	◆ 90%	
	◆ Half-life	◆ 2.5h	
Meloxicam	◆ Peak Cp	◆ 5–10 h	7.5–15 mg once/day
	◆ Protein binding	◆ 99%	
	◆ Half-life	◆ 24 h	
COX-2-inhibitors			
Celecoxib	◆ Peak Cp	◆ 2–4 h	200–400 mg twice/day
	◆ Protein binding	◆ 97%	
	◆ Half-life	◆ 6–12 h	
Etoricoxib	◆ Peak Cp	◆ 1 h	60–120 mg once/day
	◆ Protein binding	◆ 92%	
	◆ Half-life	◆ 20–26 h	

Cp, plasma concentration.

Clinical efficacy of NSAIDs alone and in combination with opioids

Although data from populations with musculoskeletal pain or pain due to inflammatory disorders suggest that NSAIDs are likely to be efficacious in the treatment of pain associated with cancer and other advanced medical illnesses, the evidence of efficacy is very limited. A useful measure of relative efficacy is the number needed to treat (NNT), which can be calculated from data aggregated through systematic reviews. The NNT is the number of patients who need to be treated before one patient benefits at a specified level—such as 30% or 50% pain relief for a specified period of time—when compared to placebo. A systematic review of NSAID efficacy in cancer pain, alone or in combination with opioids, was unable to provide a NNT for the analysed studies because few studies reported the percentage of responders as dichotomous data (McNicol et al., 2005). Based on limited data, the authors cautiously concluded that NSAIDs seem to be more effective than placebo for cancer-related pain. The evidence is not adequate to determine comparative efficacy or safety across NSAIDs, and the relative efficacy of NSAIDs in different cancer-related pain mechanisms cannot be established. There are no data specific to other severe illness. Given the short duration of studies, the long-term safety of NSAIDs for cancer pain also has not been established.

Side effects and toxicity of NSAIDs

NSAIDs administered alone or in combination with other analgesics should be used carefully. Potential adverse effects must be weighed carefully against potential advantages on a case-by-case basis, especially during chronic use. Given the broad role that PGs have in modifying physiological mechanisms, potential adverse effects vary widely.

Gastrointestinal effects

The most common adverse effects associated with the intake of NSAIDs occur in the GI tract (Table 9.6.2). The effects vary from symptoms without evident end-organ injury, such as nausea, pyrosis, pain, or bloating, to more serious problems, such as gastric and/or intestinal erosions followed by ulcerations. Erosions or ulceration, which can be observed in up to 30% of NSAIDs users, produce a range of associated symptoms of varying severity, and haemorrhage may range from harmless to life-threatening. Ulcers are often asymptomatic until haemorrhage occurs. Compared to non-users, patients who receive long-term treatment with a non-selective COX-1/COX-2 NSAID have an approximate fivefold higher risk of peptic ulcer disease and a fourfold higher risk of upper GI bleeding.

Patients receiving COX-2 selective inhibitors have significantly lower risk of GI toxicity than those receiving a non-selective COX inhibitor (Lanas, 2010). Although COX-1 inhibition is not the only mechanism involved in NSAID-induced GI toxicity, a systematic review of randomized controlled trials has shown that COX-2 selective inhibitors produced significantly fewer gastroduodenal ulcers and clinically important ulcer complications than non-selective NSAIDs (Rostom et al., 2007). Whether the outcome included bleeding events, symptomatic ulcers, or both, the GI risks with coxibs was consistently about half of that with traditional NSAIDs. However, there is evidence, both from this systematic review and from large controlled trials such as CLASS (Silverstein et al., 2000) and SUCCESS-1 (Singh et al., 2006), that this safety advantage is reduced in patients receiving concomitant low-dose ASA treatment. For example, in the SUCCESS-1 study, the risk of ulcer complications in patients receiving naproxen or diclofenac was significantly higher than in those receiving the COX-2 selective inhibitor celecoxib in the absence of ASA; in contrast, there was no significant difference in risk between the two groups of ASA users (Singh et al., 2006). A recent meta-analysis of all available trials including patients taking low-dose ASA combined with either non-selective NSAIDs or COX-2 selective inhibitors indicates a 28% reduction of GI risk in patients taking the combination of ASA + COX-2 (Rostom et al., 2009).

Celecoxib is the only COX-2 inhibitor currently available in the United States. Rofecoxib and valdecoxib were marketed but were withdrawn in 2004 and 2005, respectively, because of concern related to prothrombotic effects and other toxicities associated with long-term use.

The past decade has seen major advances in the prevention and management of ulcer complications, such as a decrease in the prevalence of *Helicobacter pylori* infection and improved treatment of acute ulcer bleeding. Recent evidence suggests that these developments have been reflected in a change in the pattern of NSAID-related GI complications seen in clinical practice (Lanas et al., 2009). Thus, while the incidence of complications involving the upper GI tract has decreased steadily during the last decade, perforations and bleeding in the lower GI tract have increased. Such findings suggest that, whereas attention has traditionally focused on NSAID-related complications in the stomach or duodenum, a broader perspective regarding the potential adverse effects of NSAIDs in the GI tract as a whole is needed.

Although there is a connection between NSAID use and lower GI haemorrhage, the evidence of NSAID-associated risk of lower GI bleeding is weaker than the evidence of upper GI bleeding. A systematic literature review reported that mucosal breaks or small intestinal injuries were present in up to 71% of NSAID users, and that up to 88% of patients with lower GI bleeding were NSAID users (Laine et al., 2006); the odds ratios (ORs) for upper GI and lower GI bleeding or perforation associated ranged from 1.9 to 18.4 and from 2.5 to 8.1, respectively. The risk of such problems was lower in patients receiving COX-2 selective inhibitors than in those receiving non-selective COX-1/COX-2 inhibitors (Laine et al., 2006).

The risk of GI toxicity varies among the non-selective COX inhibitors as well. Ibuprofen seems to be the least harmful drug in terms of the risk of upper GI bleeding. In comparison to non-users of NSAIDs, patients taking coxibs seem to have a low relative risk of GI bleeding followed by ibuprofen and diclofenac. A medium risk seems to be present for flurbiprofen, indomethacin, and naproxen, and a high risk has been proposed for ASA and ketorolac (Hernandez and Rodriguez 2000).

The risk of GI toxicity also varies with many other factors. The duration of the use of NSAIDs seem to be weakly associated with the risk of developing GI bleeding, whereas the incidence of haemorrhage is highly associated with high doses (Hawkins and Hanks, 2000). Specific characteristics and comorbidities also strongly influence the likelihood of adverse GI effects. Risk is related to age above 65 years; *Helicobacter pylori* infection; peptic ulceration within the last year; simultaneous intake of corticosteroids, low-dose ASA, and/or anticoagulants; far-advanced disease; cardiovascular disease, renal and hepatic impairment, and diabetes mellitus; smoking; and excessive alcohol use (Hernandez and Rodriguez, 2000).

Due to the high risks of GI side effects of traditional NSAIDs in frail patients, the use of gastroprotective strategies prevails, although the evidence is still limited. Proton pump inhibitors (PPIs) and misoprostol both reduce the incidence of gastric and duodenal ulcers, as well as recurrence in patients receiving traditional NSAIDs. Although misoprostol is slightly more effective in preventing gastric ulcers, PPIs are better tolerated, as misoprostol often causes diarrhoea (Rostom et al., 2002; Dubois et al., 2004). Patients at increased risk of GI complications should receive either a non-selective NSAID with an appropriate gastroprotective agent, such as a PPI, or a COX-2 selective inhibitor alone. These two strategies were compared in a randomized, double-blind trial involving 287 arthritis patients who received either diclofenac plus omeprazole, or celecoxib, 200 mg twice daily, for 6 months

Table 9.6.2 Side effects of NSAIDs in general

Where	What
◆ Gastrointestinal tract	◆ Pain
	◆ Nausea
	◆ Gastric erosion: ulceration
	◆ Bleeding
	◆ Perforation
◆ Kidney	◆ Water and sodium retention
	◆ Oedema
	◆ Hyperkalaemia
	◆ Decreased effectiveness of:
	• antihypertensive agents
	• diuretics
◆ Central nervous system	◆ Dizziness
	◆ Headache
	◆ Confusion
	◆ Vertigo
	◆ Depression
◆ Platelet function	◆ Inhibition of activation
	◆ Increased risk of haemorrhage
◆ Special areas of hypersensitivity	◆ Rhinitis
	◆ Bronchial asthma
	◆ Urticaria
	◆ Flushing
	◆ Hypotension
	◆ Shock

(Chan et al., 2002). The risk of recurrent ulcer bleeding did not differ significantly in the two groups. More recently, the combined use of a COX-2 selective inhibitor and a PPI to prevent recurrent ulcer bleeding in high-risk patients was studied. In this randomized, double-blind trial, 441 patients with upper GI bleeding received celecoxib, 200 mg twice daily, alone or in combination with esomeprazole, 20 mg twice daily, for 12 months (Chan et al., 2007). The incidence of recurrent bleeding within 12 months was significantly lower with combination therapy than with celecoxib alone, and there were no differences in discontinuation rate or the incidence of adverse events between the two groups.

Nephrotoxicity and hypertension

Non-selective NSAIDs inhibit both constitutive COX-1 and inducible COX-2, the rate-limiting enzymes involved in the production of PGs and thromboxane. In addition to their role in inflammation and pain, PGs are important mediators of vascular tone, salt and water balance, and renin release. PGE_2 is a mediator of sodium reabsorption in the distal renal tubule and acts as a counter-regulatory factor under conditions of increased sodium reabsorption by limiting salt and water reabsorption (Whelton, 2000). PGI_2 and PGE_2 increase potassium secretion, primarily by stimulating the secretion of renin and activating the renin–angiotensin system, which leads to increased aldosterone secretion. These vasodilatory PGs also increase RBF and GFR under conditions associated with decreased actual or effective

circulating volume, resulting in greater tubular flow and secretion of potassium. In healthy hydrated individuals, renal PGs do not play a major role in sodium and water homeostasis (Whelton, 2002). Under conditions of decreased renal perfusion, however, the production of renal PGs serves as an important compensatory mechanism. Numerous conditions are associated with a decrease in renal perfusion, including dehydration, blood loss, congestive heart failure, cirrhosis, diuretic use, and restricted sodium intake. Under these conditions, non-selective NSAIDs may produce adverse effects, including a decrease in GFR. Conversely, in conditions of high salt intake and/or volume expansion, non-selective NSAIDs may induce salt retention, which may elevate blood pressure or make pre-existing hypertension worse.

These effects produced by the non-selective COX-1/COX-2 inhibitors also occur with the selective COX-2 inhibitors. Both types of NSAIDs can cause acute renal failure and hypertension (Cheng and Harris, 2004) during short-term or long-term use. All these drugs are especially likely to reinforce renal impairment in patients with pre-existing renal insufficiency. Patients with chronic kidney diseases, like those with heart failure, cirrhosis, dehydration, or any other co-morbidity causing activation of the sympatho-adrenergic and/or renin–angiotensin system, depend very much on a normal PG status for maintaining adequate function of the kidneys. Because the production of PGE_2 and PGI_2 depends on the activity of COX-2 (Qi et al., 2002), there is no difference in this risk between the non-selective COX inhibitors and the selective COX-2 drugs. Long-term treatment with either non-selective COX-1/COX-2 inhibitors or the selective COX-2 inhibitors also may significantly increase the risk of developing and maintaining renal failure, as may the use of NSAIDs with a long half-life (Henry et al., 1997).

Renal papillary necrosis induced by the non-selective COX-1/COX-2 inhibitors is well recognized and case reports also have described this complication with the selective COX-2 inhibitors (Whelton, 1999; Akhund et al., 2003). Recently, tubulointerstitial injury has been reported with COX-2 inhibitors (Ortiz et al., 2005). The vascular supply within the renal papillae is dependent on local renal PG production. Clinical conditions resulting in volume depletion or decreased RBF in association with NSAID ingestion may lead to elevated concentrations of NSAIDs and their metabolites within the papillae, which inhibit the vasodilatatory effect of the PGs and lead to renal papillary necrosis.

Congestive heart failure, coronary heart disease, and thrombosis

Congestive heart failure also may result from treatment with NSAIDs, particularly in medically frail and elderly patients. Patients admitted to the hospital diagnosed with congestive heart failure had a higher prevalence (17%) of recent NSAID use than patients admitted with other diagnoses (12%) (Page and Henry, 2000; Merlo et al., 2001). The risk of congestive heart failure increased with an additional history of heart disease

As mentioned earlier, TXA_2 is a potent vasoconstrictor and promotes platelet aggregation. TXA_2 is induced by the activity of COX-1 and, in effect, acts as a prothrombotic agent. On the other hand, PGI_2 causes vasodilatation, and thereby inhibits the aggregation of platelets. Selective inhibition of COX-2 increases the relative activity of TXA_2, which subsequently may facilitate the formation of thromboses. The literature relating to the risk of prothrombotic complications from NSAIDs, including myocardial infarction and stroke, is complicated, but supports the conclusion that all NSAIDs—including non-selective COX-1/COX-2 inhibitors and selective COX-2 inhibitors—could pose a risk of these complications as a result of their effects on COX-2. There appears to be important variation across drugs, however. In patients with coronary heart disease, a reduction of COX-2 activity produced by treatment with selective COX-2 inhibitors increase the risks for acute cardiovascular events such as strokes, thromboses, and myocardial infarction (Fitzgerald, 2004; Bresalier et al., 2005; McGettigan and Henry, 2006). However, some studies do not observe these outcomes during treatment with celecoxib (McGettigan and Henry, 2006). A meta-analysis of randomized trials including coxibs and non-selective NSAIDs taken for more than 4 weeks showed that coxibs and high-dose regimens of ibuprofen and diclofenac were associated with a moderate increase in the risk of vascular events (defined as myocardial infarction, stroke, or vascular death) (Kearney et al., 2006). However, high-dose naproxen was not associated with such events. Another recent systematic review confirmed that the relative risk of myocardial infarction varied with the individual NSAIDs. An increased risk was observed for diclofenac and rofecoxib; the latter drug had a dose–response trend, with risk higher for doses greater than 25 mg/day (78%) than for lower doses (18%) (Hernandez-Diaz et al., 2006). Rofecoxib was withdrawn from the market in September 2004.

Notwithstanding the limitations in the literature, it is clinically prudent to include prothrombotic cardiovascular risk as among the potential adverse effects produced by both the selective COX-2 inhibitors (Flavahan, 2007) and the non-selective COX-1/COX-2 inhibitors (Kearney et al., 2006; Warner and Mitchell, 2008). The 'imbalance' theory alluded to previously offer a reasonable explanation: any NSAID that reduces COX-2-dependent PGI_2 in endothelium without a commensurate effect on COX-1-dependent TXA_2 in platelets will predispose to a prothrombotic state by increasing the relative activity of TXA_2. All NSAIDs may be prothrombotic because all have an inhibitory effect on COX-2 (Cheng et al., 2002).

Contraindications and drug interactions

Given the risk profile of the NSAIDs there are important relative contraindications to their use in palliative care. Treatment should be undertaken cautiously, if at all, in patients at high risk for GI haemorrhage, or those who would be unlikely to cope with bleeding should it occur. The former group includes those with a haemorrhage within the last year, a history of peptic ulcer disease or NSAID-induced gastroduodenopathy in the past, advanced age, severe medical frailty, or concurrent treatment with a corticosteroid.

Patients with clinically significant renal insufficiency usually are considered to have too high a risk for NSAID therapy, and patients with liver disease and those predisposed to adverse cardiovascular outcomes should be considered to have a relative contraindication. The latter group includes those with a history of symptomatic atherothrombotic disease in the past (myocardial infarction, angina, stroke, transient ischaemic attacks, or symptomatic peripheral vascular disease) and those with significant risk factors, such as a history of poorly controlled hypertension, hyperlipidaemia, or smoking. Patients with a history of

NSAID-induced asthma or a documented allergic reaction to any NSAID also should not generally be offered NSAID therapy. When the European Agency for the Evaluation of Medicinal Products reviewed a recent addition to the coxibs available in Europe, etoricoxib, it noted that the drug is contraindicated in cases of hypertension, severe hepatic dysfunction, inflammatory bowel disease, and congestive heart failure (European Medicines Agency, 2008).

NSAIDs also are associated with drug–drug interactions that may be particularly important in the medically ill. For example, they may reduce renal function during concomitant lithium, methotrexate, and amino-glycoside therapy, which can give rise to increased plasma concentrations. High plasma protein binding of NSAIDs can increase the concentration of free, active drug in some cases, such as phenytoin, and lead to unanticipated toxicity as a result. Patients who have a coagulopathy or are receiving anticoagulant therapy should be considered to have a strong relative contraindication to NSAID therapy. NSAIDs also may attenuate the metabolism of warfarin and thus increase its effect.

One should take into consideration that most of the studies of patients with advanced disease and short life expectancy typically involve small numbers of patients. Therefore, the studies investigating side effects are probably underestimating the frequency of such symptoms and signs. As a general rule in old and/or frail patients, polypharmacy should be limited if possible. Indications for the use of all drugs should be carefully considered by evaluating the probability of beneficial effects versus the probability of side effects. These considerations seem to be of utmost importance when using NSAIDS.

Topical NSAIDs

Topical NSAIDs, which may be applied via a rub-on solution, gel, or adhesive skin patch, offer obvious theoretical advantages by minimizing the systemic complications of these drugs. They have a relatively low bioavailability compared with oral NSAIDs and this may account for their favourable safety profile. Topical patches provide a fixed constant dose and local action. Gel formulations can be used on parts of the body that are not easily accessible by a patch, such as the fingers. Side effects tend to be localized to the site of application, such as itching and rashes.

Topical NSAIDs have been recommended for use in osteoarthritis (National Institute for Health and Clinical Excellence, 2010). After topical application, therapeutic levels of NSAIDs can be demonstrated in synovial fluid, muscles, and fasciae, and this finding suggests that they may have their pharmacological effects on both intra- and extra-articular structures. Although it is assumed that their mechanism of action is similar to that of oral NSAIDs, the topical drugs produce a maximal plasma NSAID concentration of only 15% of that achieved following oral administration of a similar dose (Lin et al., 2004). There have been no studies of topical NSAID therapy in palliative care and their efficacy for localized pain associated with non-musculoskeletal causes is unknown. The potential role of topical NSAIDs needs to be explored in palliative care.

Acetylsalicylic acid

ASA and its derivatives are the prototypes of NSAIDs and have been known since ancient times. In the mid-eighteenth century,

Edward Stone, an English clergyman, wrote the first scientific description of the effects of willow bark.

ASA covalently and irreversibly inhibits both COX-1 and COX-2. This is an important feature of ASA, as the duration of the effects are related to the turnover rate of COX in the different tissues. Platelets are particularly susceptible to ASA-mediated irreversible inhibition of COX, because they have limited capacity for protein synthesis and thus cannot regenerate COX enzymes. This means, that a single and small dose of ASA will inhibit the COX enzymes for the lifetime of the platelets (Patrono et al., 2004).

The prevalent use of low-dose ASA for cardioprotection must be considered when NSAIDs are administered for pain. The combination of a non-selective COX-1/COX-2 inhibitor and low-dose ASA increases the risk of GI toxicity. The combination of a selective COX-2 inhibitor and low-dose ASA reduces the relative benefit of the coxib on GI risk, particularly if treatment lasts more than 6 months. Some NSAIDs, such as ibuprofen, may attenuate the antithrombotic effects of ASA and reduce its cardioprotective effects. Because the latter interaction would be less likely to occur if the NSAID is taken after (perhaps 2 or more hours) the dose of ASA, patients should be instructed to do so. Paracetamol has no adverse interaction with low-dose ASA therapy (Gaziano and Gibson, 2006).

The results of systematic reviews of single-dose studies confirm ASA's efficacy as an analgesic. Analysis of the analgesic dose–response tells us that higher doses give more analgesia, and comparing ASA with paracetamol the analgesia produced by the two drugs are very similar. One gram of ASA gives the same analgesia as 1 g of paracetamol (Gaziano and Gibson, 2006; McQuay and Moore, 2007). Furthermore, significant benefit of ASA over placebo was shown for ASA 600–650 mg, 1000 mg, and 1200 mg, with NNT values for at least 50% pain relief of 4.4, 4.0, and 2.4, respectively. However, in single-dose studies even low doses of ASA 600/650 mg produced significantly more gastric irritation and drowsiness than placebo (Edwards et al., 1999). The GI side effects of ASA are the main reason for the limited use of ASA in palliative care.

Paracetamol (acetaminophen)

Paracetamol (acetaminophen; N-acetyl-p-aminophenol) is one of the most commonly used analgesic and antipyretic drugs worldwide, and it is widely available by prescription and over the counter. Paracetamol, a so-called coal-tar analgesic, was discovered by accident as an active metabolite of phenacetin. The site of action seems to be in the brain; however, the mechanism of action is still poorly understood. In a double-blind, placebo-controlled study in healthy volunteers, Piletta and colleagues obtained some evidence for a central analgesic action of paracetamol. Application of a transcutaneous electrical stimulus to the sural nerve caused a flexion reflex and a subjective sensation of pain. In contrast to ASA, paracetamol raised the threshold to both types of pain, indicating an analgesic action both at the spinal cord level and in higher centres (Piletta et al., 1991).

Although there is considerable overlap in the actions of paracetamol, NSAIDS, and ASA regarding inhibition of COX, in vitro studies show that paracetamol is not a highly potent inhibitor of COX-1 and COX-2 (Ouellet and Percival, 2001). As mentioned earlier, a third form of COX has been proposed, which has been referred to as COX-3 (Ayoub et al., 2006). However, cloning studies have failed to confirm the existence of COX-3 in humans and the search for a convincing mechanistic explanation of the therapeutic activity of paracetamol continues (Qin et al., 2005).

Paracetamol also possesses antipyretic activity and the brain is likely to be the site of its antipyretic effects. The antipyretic activity of the compound resides in its aminobenzene structure and the effect seems to be caused by inhibition of COX-2 or a variant of this enzyme (Simmons, 2003). Because of the association between ASA and Reye's syndrome in children, paracetamol is the antipyretic drug of choice in children, and when used in recommended doses, has few side effects, and is remarkably well tolerated.

Pharmacokinetics and metabolism

Paracetamol is commercially available in a considerable number of products, both alone and in combination with other drugs. It can be administered orally as tablets (conventional, sustained release, effervescent), capsules, powders, and elixirs, and can be given rectally as suppositories. Paracetamol is rapidly and almost completely absorbed from the GI tract. Gastric emptying rate rather than the diffusion across the intestinal mucosa is the rate-limiting step in paracetamol absorption after oral administration. Therefore, any drug, disease, or other condition that alters the rate of gastric emptying will influence the rate of absorption. Although paracetamol is rapidly absorbed from the GI tract, it is incompletely available to the systemic circulation due to hepatic first-pass metabolism accounting for a 10% loss in therapeutic doses. Intestinal metabolism also contributes to decreased bioavailability (Tone et al., 1990). In adults, the bioavailability of paracetamol after administration of suppositories is approximately 60% (Beck et al., 2000). After oral administration of therapeutic doses, the concentration in plasma reaches a peak in 30–60 minutes, and the half-life in plasma is about 2 hours. Paracetamol is relatively uniformly distributed throughout most body fluids (Prescott 1996). The proportion of paracetamol bound to plasma proteins is small and varies from 5% to 20% (Milligan et al., 1994). Biotransformation takes place primarily in the liver and the oxidative reactions via the cytochrome P450 system are followed by conjugation. After therapeutic doses, 90–100% of the drug may be recovered in urine within the first day, primarily after hepatic conjugation with glucuronic acid (about 60%), sulphuric acid (about 35%), or cysteine (about 3%); small amounts of hydroxylated and deacetylated metabolites also have been detected (Steventon et al., 1996).

Pharmacodynamics

The lack of dichotomous data in randomized trials, and a lack of trials in medically ill populations, largely precludes calculation of a NNT for paracetamol use in patients with serious illness. Studies also have not evaluated long-term efficacy. Nonetheless, evidence suggests the use of non-opioids alone is superior to placebo for mild pain in cancer and medical illness, at least during short-term treatment (McNicol et al., 2005).

The efficacy of paracetamol compared to NSAIDS has not been thoroughly investigated (Ventafridda et al., 1990) and the combination of paracetamol and NSAIDS has not been investigated in cancer-related pain. Most studies have assessed paracetamol in combination with other analgesics, and these studies do not give any information on the analgesic effect that paracetamol provides on its own (Carlson et al., 1990; Chary et al., 1994). Only one randomized, double-blind, placebo controlled study indicated that the addition of paracetamol to ongoing oral opioid therapy improved pain relief and general well-being in cancer patients (Stockler et al., 2004).

Side effects and toxicity

At therapeutic doses of paracetamol, side effects are rare, and the clinical advantage during long-term treatment is that the side effects are less severe than with the NSAIDS. Allergic reactions have been described, and during long-term treatment chronic headache may occur (Meskunas et al., 2006). Toxicity from paracetamol usually is due to either accidental or deliberate overdose. A small proportion of paracetamol undergoes P450-mediated N-hydroxylation to form N-acetyl-benzoquinoneimine, a highly reactive intermediate metabolite. This metabolite normally reacts with sulfhydryl groups in glutathione. At large doses of paracetamol (usually considered in those without liver disease to be a single dose > 10 g), the metabolite is formed in sufficient amounts to deplete liver cells completely of glutathione, which seems to trigger hepatotoxicity and a prolonged rise in liver-derived transaminase and alkaline phosphatase levels in the serum. Intervention to sustain hepatic glutathione is an effective treatment for paracetamol overdose and administration of N-acetyl-L-cysteine, which replenishes glutathione stores, remains the treatment of choice (Josephy, 2005).

Dipyrone (metamizole)

Dipyrone is a popular medicine for pain relief in many countries and is used to treat postoperative pain, colic pain, cancer pain and migraine. In other countries (e.g. United States, United Kingdom, and Japan), however, the drug has been removed from the market, or not approved, due to concerns about serious adverse effects. Although the data are insufficient to draw any conclusions about the influence of dose or route of administration, dipyrone has been associated with potentially life-threatening blood disorders, such as agranulocytosis.

A single 500 mg oral dose of dipyrone provides at least 50% pain relief to adults with moderate or severe postoperative pain, with efficacy similar to ibuprofen 400 mg. A single 2.5 g intravenous dose is equivalent to 100 mg intravenous tramadol for at least 50% pain relief. In efficacy studies, no serious events or adverse event withdrawals were reported (Edwards et al., 2010). A small controlled trial indicated that dipyrone adds significantly to the analgesic effect of morphine in patients with cancer-related pain (Duarte et al., 2007).

Conclusions and recommendations

NSAIDs have important risks and should be used cautiously in the medically ill. There are many factors that increase the risk of GI, renal, or cardiovascular toxicity, and populations with serious or life-threatening illness are likely to have one or more of these factors. Caution must be exercised in elderly or medically frail patients and those with significant disorders affecting liver or kidney. Risk factors for GI haemorrhage, such as peptic ulcer disease or *Helicobacter pylori* infection, and risk factors for cardiovascular disease, such as prior coronary artery disease, uncontrolled

hypertension, diabetes, and others, present relative contraindications to the long-term use of NSAIDs. The risk of these drugs increases when the potential for pharmacokinetic or pharmacodynamic drug–drug interactions occur, and co-treatment with corticosteroids, low-dose ASA, or anticoagulants, for example, should further increase caution in the use of these drugs.

Patients at high risk for adverse effects during long-term oral NSAID therapy should be considered for other strategies, such as paracetamol, topical NSAIDs, adjuvant analgesics, and opioids. When treatment with NSAIDs is indicated and effective, it is strongly recommended to use the lowest effective dose for the shortest period of time, and to combine the treatment with a gastroprotective agent (usually a PPI; misoprostol and higher-dose H_2 antagonists are alternatives). Unless otherwise contraindicated for other reasons, a COX-2-inhibitor, such as celecoxib, should be strongly considered. Patients with advanced illnesses are often at high risk and either lowest effective dose of an NSAID combined with PPI or the lowest effective dose of a coxib should be considered.

Cardiovascular risks are associated with COX-2 inhibition, and consequently, are concerns during treatment with all NSAIDs. Although the data are inconclusive, there do appear to be important drug-selective effects; naproxen, for example, may pose a lesser risk than other NSAIDs, and some studies suggest a low risk for celecoxib. Both relatively higher doses and longer treatment durations seem to increase the cardiovascular risks. Based on current evidence, patients at high cardiovascular risk should be treated with either naproxen (plus PPI) or celecoxib, and the use of the lowest effective dose for the shortest possible duration of time is recommended.

Generally, the efficacy and side effects of NSAIDs should be monitored and evaluated during long-term treatment. If effectiveness is doubtful, the drug should be discontinued.

Future trends

There remains a need for a substantial increase in the number of high-quality trials of non-opioid analgesics in patients with serious or life-threatening illnesses, such as cancer. Studies that specifically address the question of whether addition of a non-opioid to an opioid analgesic regimen actually increases efficacy and/or reduces side effects are required. In addition, the safety and efficacy of chronic use of non-selective COX-1/COX-2 inhibitors versus the coxibs needs to be established. Emerging questions about the selective COX-2 inhibitors, such as their potential anti-angiogenic properties, remain unanswered (Steinbach et al., 2000). Translation of emerging preclinical insights into distinct mechanisms for pain of different aetiologies (e.g. bone metastases) would be another step towards more rational pharmacotherapy (Davar, 2002).

Due to the potential for adverse effects encountered during NSAID therapy, combined with a very economically lucrative market, this is an area of continuing major investment in research. The COX-inhibiting nitric oxide donors (CINODs) are a new class of agents designed for the treatment of pain and inflammation. CINODs have a multi-pathway mechanism of action that involves COX-inhibition and nitric oxide donation. The anti-inflammatory and analgesic effects of COX-inhibition are reinforced through inhibition of caspase-1 regulated cytokine production, while nitric oxide donation provides multi-organ protection. The CINODs are devoid of hypertensive effects in animal models and their mechanism of action suggests that they may not cause oedema. CINODs also have other renal-sparing effects, being better tolerated than NSAIDs in models of kidney failure. CINODs have been shown to prevent platelet activation *in vitro* and exhibit antithrombotic activity *in vivo*. In animal models of ischaemia/reperfusion treatment with CINODs results in improved recovery of heart contractility and reduced left ventricular end-diastolic pressure, in contrast to the effects of NSAIDs and ASA. Naproxcinod has been the first, and so far the only, CINOD investigated in clinical trials. These studies have shown a slight improvement in GI tolerability in comparison to naproxen in surrogate endpoints (number of gastric and duodenal ulcers) and a significant reduction in the risk of destabilization of blood pressure control in patients with osteoarthosis taking antihypertensive medications in comparison to either naproxen and rofecoxib (Baerwald et al., 2010; White et al., 2011). The lack of outcome studies, however, has precluded the approval of naproxcinod by the US Food and Drug Administration.

NSAIDs that release H_2S as a mechanism may have greater GI and cardiovascular safety, and are being investigated in preclinical models. Both naproxen and diclofenac hybrids have been reported to cause less GI injury than parent NSAIDs. These novel chemical entities exert a variety of beneficial effects in rodent models of cardiovascular and metabolic disorders through a mechanism that might involve the release of H_2S and/or by exerting antioxidant effects. The beneficial role these mechanisms in clinical settings await a proof-of-concept study (Fiorucci and Distrutti, 2011).

The short-term use and benefits of topical NSAIDs have been reflected in guidelines for the treatment of osteoarthritis. The evidence with regards to efficacy of these drugs is predominantly limited to the osteoarthritis and rheumatoid arthritis populations (National Institute for Health and Clinical Excellence, 2010). Their efficacy needs to be further investigated in chronic cancer pain conditions of musculoskeletal origin.

Online materials

Complete references for this chapter are available online at <http://www.oxfordmedicine.com>.

References

Ayoub, S.S., Colville-Nash, P.R., Willoughby, D.A. *et al.* (2006). The involvement of a cyclooxygenase 1 gene-derived protein in the antinociceptive action of paracetamol in mice. *European Journal of Pharmacology*, 538(1–3), 57–65.

Baerwald, C., Verdecchia, P., Duquesroix, B., *et al* (2010). Efficacy, safety, and effects on blood pressure of naproxcinod 750 mg twice daily compared with placebo and naproxen 500 mg twice daily in patients with osteoarthritis of the hip: a randomized, double-blind, parallel-group, multicenter study. *Arthritis & Rheumatism*, 62(12), 3635–44.

Bresalier, R.S., Sandler, R.S., Quan, H., *et al.* (2005). Cardiovascular events associated with rofecoxib in a colorectal adenoma chemoprevention trial. *The New England Journal of Medicine*, 352(11), 1092–102.

Chan, F.K.L., Wong, V.W.S., Suen, B.Y., *et al.* (2007). Combination of a cyclo-oxygenase-2 inhibitor and a proton-pump inhibitor for prevention of recurrent ulcer bleeding in patients at very high risk: a double-blind, randomised trial. *The Lancet*, 369, 1621–1626.

Chandrasekharan, N.V., Dai, H., Roos, K.L. *et al.* (2002). COX-3, a cyclooxygenase-1 variant inhibited by acetaminophen and other analgesic/antipyretic drugs: cloning, structure, and expression. *Proceedings of the National Academy of Sciences of the United States of America*, 99(21), 13926–13931.

Cheng, H.F. and Harris, R.C. (2004). Cyclooxygenases, the kidney, and hypertension. *Hypertension*, 43(3), 525–530.

Cheng, Y., Austin, S.C., Rocca, B., *et al.* (2002). Role of prostacyclin in the cardiovascular response to thromboxane A2. *Science*, 296, 539–541.

Duarte Souza, J.F., Lajolo, P.P., Pinczowski, H., and del Giglio, A (2007). Adjunct dipyrone in association with oral morphine for cancer-related pain: the sooner the better. *Supportive Care in Cancer*, 15(11), 1319–1323.

Dubois, R.W., Melmed, G.Y., Henning, J.M. *et al.* (2004). Risk of upper gastrointestinal injury and events in patients treated with cyclooxygenase (COX)-1/COX-2 nonsteroidal antiinflammatory drugs (NSAIDs), COX-2 selective NSAIDs, and gastroprotective cotherapy: an appraisal of the literature. *Journal of Clinical Rheumatology*, 10(4), 178–189.

Edwards, J., Meseguer, F., Faura, C., *et al.* (2010). Single dose dipyrone for acute postoperative pain. *Cochrane Database of Systematic Reviews*, 8, CD003227.

European Medicines Agency (2008). *Etoricoxib*. [Online] Available at: <http://www.ema.europa.eu/ema/index.jsp?curl=pages/medicines/human/referrals/Etoricoxib/human_referral_000104.jsp>.

Fiorucci, S. and Distrutti, E. (2011). COXIBs, CINODs and H2S-releasing NSAIDs: current perspectives in the development of safer non steroidal anti-inflammatory drugs. *Current Medicinal Chemistry*, 18(23), 3494–3505.

Fitzgerald, G.A. (2004). Coxibs and cardiovascular disease. *The New England Journal of Medicine*, 351(17), 1709–1711.

Flavahan, N.A. (2007). Balancing prostanoid activity in the human vascular system. *Trends in Pharmacological Sciences*, 28, 106–110.

Gaziano, J.M. and Gibson, C.M. (2006). Potential for drug-drug interactions in patients taking analgesics for mild-to-moderate pain and low-dose aspirin for cardioprotection. *American Journal of Cardiology*, 97(9A), 23–29.

Hamza, M. and Dionne, R.A. (2009). Mechanisms of non-opioid analgesics beyond cyclooxygenase enzyme inhibition. *Current Molecular Pharmacology*, 2(1), 1–14.

Harris, R.C. (2006). COX-2 and the kidney. *Journal of Cardiovascular Pharmacology*, 47(Suppl. 1), S37–S42.

Josephy, P.D. (2005). The molecular toxicology of acetaminophen. *Drug Metabolism Reviews*, 37, 581–594.

Kearney, P.M., Baigent, C., Godwin, J., *et al.* (2006). Do selective cyclo-oxygenase-2 inhibitors and traditional non-steroidal anti-inflammatory drugs increase the risk of atherothrombosis? Meta-analysis of randomised trials. *BMJ*, 332(7553), 1302–1308.

Kis, B., Snipes, A., Bari, F., *et al.* (2004). Regional distribution of cyclooxygenase-3 mRNA in the rat central nervous system. *Brain Research Molecular Brain Research*, 126(1), 78–80.

Koeberle, A. and Werz, O. (2009). Inhibitors of the microsomal prostaglandin E2 synthase-1 as alternative to non steroidal anti-inflammatory drugs (NSAIDs)—a critical review. *Current Medicinal Chemistry*, 16 (30), 1–23.

Lanas, A. (2010). A review of the gastrointestinal safety data—a gastroenterologist's perspective. *Rheumatology*, 49(Suppl. 2), ii3–10.

Lanas, A., Garcia-Rodríguez, L.A., Polo-Tomás, M., *et al.* (2009). Time trends and impact of upper and lower gastrointestinal bleeding and perforation in clinical practice. *American Journal of Gastroenterology*, 104, 1633–1641.

Laine, L., Smith, R., Min, K., Chen, C., and Dubois, R.W. (2006). Systematic review: the lower gastrointestinal adverse effects of non-steroidal anti-inflammatory drugs. *Alimentary Pharmacology and Therapeutics*, 24, 751–767.

Mason, L., Moore, R.A., Edwards, J.E., *et al.* (2004). Topical NSAIDs for chronic musculoskeletal pain: systematic review and meta-analysis. *BMC Musculoskeletal Disorders*, 5, 28.

McGettigan, P. and Henry, D. (2006). Cardiovascular risk and inhibition of cyclooxygenase: a systematic review of the observational studies of selective and nonselective inhibitors of cyclooxygenase 2. *Journal of the American Medical Association*, 296(13), 1633–1644.

McNicol, E., Strassels, S.A., Goudas, L., *et al*. (2005). NSAIDS or paracetamol, alone or combined with opioids, for cancer pain. *Cochrane Database of Systematic Reviews*, 1, CD005180.

McQuay, H.J. and Moore, R.A. (2007). Dose-response in direct comparisons of different doses of aspirin, ibuprofen and paracetamol (acetaminophen) in analgesic studies. *British Journal of Clinical Pharmacology*, 63(3), 271–278.

Meric, J.B., Rottey, S., Olaussen, K., *et al*. (2006). Cyclooxygenase-2 as a target for anticancer drug development. *Critical Reviews in Oncology/Hematology*, 59(1), 51–64.

Meskunas, C.A., Tepper, S.J., Rapoport, A.M., *et al*. (2006). Medications associated with probable medication overuse headache reported in a tertiary care headache center over a 15-year period. *Headache*, 46(5), 766–772.

National Institute for Health and Clinical Excellence (2010). *Osteoarthritis: The Care and Management of Osteoarthritis in adults*. NICE Clinical Guideline 59. London: NICE. Available at: <http://www.nice.org.uk/nicemedia/pdf/CG59NICEguideline.pdf>.

Ortiz, M., Mon, C., Fernandez, M.J., *et al*. (2005). Tubulointerstitial nephritis associated with treatment with selective Cox-2 inhibitors, celecoxib and rofecoxib. *Nefrologia*, 25, 39–43.

Patrono, C., Coller, B., FitzGerald, G.A., *et al*. (2004). Platelet-active drugs: the relationships among dose, effectiveness, and side effects: the Seventh ACCP Conference on Antithrombotic and Thrombolytic Therapy. *Chest*, 126(3 Suppl.), 234S–264S.

Rostom, A., Muir, K., Dubé, C., *et al*. (2007). Gastrointestinal safety of cyclooxygenase-2 inhibitors: a Cochrane Collaboration systematic review. *Clinical Gastroenterology and Hepatology*, 5, 818–828.

Rostom, A., Muir, K., Dube, C., *et al*. (2009). Prevention of NSAID-related upper gastrointestinal toxicity: a meta-analysis of traditional NSAIDs with gastroprotection and COX-2 inhibitors. *Drug, Healthcare and Patient Safety*, 1, 1–25.

Samad, T.A., Moore, K.A., Sapirstein, A., *et al*. (2001). Interleukin-1beta-mediated induction of Cox-2 in the CNS contributes to inflammatory pain hypersensitivity. *Nature*, 410(6827), 471–475.

Singh, G., Fort, J.G., Goldstein, J.L., *et al*. (2006). Celecoxib versus naproxen and diclofenac in osteoarthritis patients: SUCCESS-1 study. *American Journal of Medicine*, 119, 255–266.

Snipes, J.A., Kis, B., Shelness, G.S., *et al*. (2005). Cloning and characterization of cyclooxygenase-1b (putative cyclooxygenase-3) in rat. *Journal of Pharmacology and Experimental Therapeutics*, 313(2), 668–676.

Stockler, M., Vardy, J., Pillai, A. *et al*. (2004). Acetaminophen (paracetamol) improves pain and well-being in people with advanced cancer already receiving a strong opioid regimen: a randomized, double-blind, placebo-controlled cross-over trial. *Journal of Clinical Oncology*, 22(16), 3389–3394.

Vane, J.R. (1971). Inhibition of prostaglandin synthesis as a mechanism of action for aspirin-like drugs. *Nature New Biology*, 231(25), 232–235.

Warner, T.D. and Mitchell, J.A. (2008) COX-2 selectivity alone does not define the cardiovascular risks associated with non-steroidal antiinflammatory drugs. *The Lancet*, 371, 270–273.

Warner, T.D. and Mitchell, J.A. (2002). Cyclooxygenase-3 (COX-3): filling in the gaps toward a COX continuum? *Proceedings of the National Academy of Sciences of the United States of America*, 99(21), 13371–13373.

White, W.B., Schnitzer, T.J., Bakris, G.L., *et al*. (2011). Effects of naproxcinod on blood pressure in patients with osteoarthritis. *American Journal of Cardiology*, 107(9), 1338–1345.

World Health Organization (1996). *Cancer Pain Relief: With a Guide to Opioid Availability*. Geneva: World Health Organization.

Adjuvant analgesics

David Lussier and Russell K. Portenoy

Introduction to adjuvant analgesics

The term 'adjuvant analgesic' has been defined as any drug that has a primary indication other than pain, but is analgesic in some painful conditions. As drugs in this category have begun to be used in the treatment of diverse chronic pain disorders, the term itself, and its definition, have become outmoded. There are now drugs in this category that are approved in many countries as primary analgesics for selected pain disorders. The evolution of this group of non-traditional drugs has been rapid and a strongly positive development in the search for a more effective pharmacological armamentarium for chronic pain.

In the palliative care literature, the term 'adjuvant analgesic' also is often used synonymously with 'co-analgesic'. These labels refer to drugs that may be administered with a primary analgesic, usually an opioid, to enhance pain relief, treat pain that is refractory to the analgesic, or allow reduction of the analgesic dose for the purpose of limiting side effects. In this context, adjuvant analgesics should be distinguished from other adjuvant drugs that are co-administered with analgesics for the specific purposes of treating side effects produced by the analgesic or managing symptoms other than pain. In the latter sense, laxatives and antiemetics are adjuvant drugs.

Given this imprecise terminology and the expanding use of adjuvant analgesics as non-traditional primary analgesics, it is important to understand the pharmacology of these drugs and their therapeutic role in varied patient populations. In this way, the use of the adjuvant analgesics can be optimized, both as 'add-on' therapy to an opioid regimen and as distinct, primary therapy in those painful disorders that are likely to demonstrate a good response.

General considerations

Several principles guide the administration of all adjuvant analgesics. These emphasize the importance of a comprehensive patient assessment and a broad foundation in analgesic pharmacotherapy.

Comprehensive assessment

The selection of a drug and optimal dosing regimen depends on a systematic assessment of the patient. This assessment requires a careful history and review of records, physical examination, and appropriate laboratory and imaging studies (Box 9.7.1).

The need for systematic assessment continues during the course of therapy. Over time, changes in pain, side effects, or any of the broader quality of life concerns may impel a shift in therapeutic strategy. The use of adjuvant analgesics in the management of pain may be a 'labour intensive' endeavour, which requires frequent contact with the patient to ensure continuous, appropriate administration of the drug.

Positioning of treatment

Adjuvant analgesics are, as a group, less reliable analgesics than opioids. This characteristic may be determined by a smaller proportion of treated patients who respond adequately, a higher likelihood of troublesome side effects, or a slower onset of analgesic effect for most drugs (perhaps due to the need to initiate therapy at low doses to avoid side effects). For example, in contrast to survey data that demonstrate a favourable outcome within days for 70–90% of cancer patients who receive opioid therapy (Schug et al., 1990; Grond et al., 1999) studies of the tricyclic antidepressants show that these drugs require treatment for weeks to obtain optimal results and offer 50%, or greater, relief to fewer than 50% of patients with neuropathic pain (Max et al., 1987; Kishore-Kumar et al., 1990).

This observation suggests that most patients with moderate or severe pain related to serious medical illness who have no relative contraindications to opioid therapy should not receive an adjuvant analgesic until opioid therapy has been optimized. Although some clinicians attempt to improve patient response by initiating therapy with an opioid and an adjuvant analgesic concurrently, this approach increases the risk of additive toxicity. Unless another indication for an earlier trial exists (e.g. a comorbidity that may also respond to the drug, a history of problems with opioids, or a type of pain that may be particularly responsive to a specific adjuvant), the safest and most efficient approach usually involves the addition of an adjuvant analgesic to an opioid regimen that is yielding inadequate analgesia despite dose escalation to limiting side effects. In the absence of data from comparative clinical trials, the decision to use an adjuvant analgesic drug instead of an alternative therapy, such as a trial of spinally administered opioids or a nerve block, is usually a matter of clinical judgement.

The selection of a specific adjuvant analgesic may be suggested by the characteristics of the pain (see 'Pharmacological characteristics') or, in some instances, by the existence of another symptom concurrent with pain that may be amenable to a non-analgesic effect of the drug. In many situations, multiple options exist and priorities for therapeutic trials must also be developed on the basis of a comprehensive assessment of the patient and best clinical judgement.

Pharmacological characteristics

Safe and effective prescribing requires familiarity with a drug's actions, approved indications, unapproved indications accepted in medical practice, likely side effects and potential serious adverse effects, usual time–action relationship, pharmacokinetics, specific dosing guidelines for pain, and interactions with other drugs. Very few of the adjuvant analgesics have been studied in populations with serious illness and this information is usually extrapolated from other patient populations.

Caution is appropriate when prescribing to the medically ill. Low initial doses and gradual dose escalation may avoid early side effects and identify dose-dependent analgesic effects that can be explored to optimize the balance between pain relief and adverse effects. The use of low initial doses and dose titration may delay the onset of analgesia, however, and patients must be forewarned of this possibility to improve adherence with the therapy.

Interindividual and intraindividual variability

There is great variability in the response to all adjuvant analgesics. The inability to reliably predict the outcome of therapy underscores the potential utility of sequential trials of adjuvant analgesics. The process of sequential drug trials, like the use of low initial doses and dose titration, should be explained to the patient at the start of therapy to enhance adherence and reduce the distress that may occur as treatments fail.

Risks and benefits of polypharmacy

The potential for additive side effects and unpredictable adverse effects must be anticipated by the practitioner whenever an adjuvant is added to an existing drug regimen. The decision to add, or continue, a therapy must be based on a careful assessment of outcomes and a clear understanding of the goals of care. If a treatment yields demonstrable benefit without serious risk, and without cumulative side effects that otherwise impair function or quality of life, there is ample justification for continuing. Additional pain relief at the price of somnolence or mental clouding is not acceptable for patients whose goals include restoration of function, but may be completely appropriate for those who seek comfort as the only goal.

The risks of additive toxicity from polypharmacy derive from both pharmacokinetic and pharmacodynamic changes. For example, the addition of a tricyclic antidepressant to a morphine regimen may produce somnolence due to an increase in morphine plasma concentration or a pharmacodynamic interaction independent of changes in drug concentration.

Adjuvant analgesics

The adjuvant analgesics comprise an extraordinarily diverse group of drug classes (Box 9.7.2). A generally useful, broad classification distinguishes those that may be considered non-specific, multipurpose analgesics from those used for more specific indications. A review of the evidence supporting the analgesic efficacy of agents in each class provides the foundation for the development of clinical guidelines.

Multipurpose analgesics

The data supporting the analgesic efficacy of some drug classes derive from numerous studies of very diverse syndromes. The range of positive outcomes for these drugs suggests that they can

Table 9.7.1 Multipurpose adjuvant analgesics

Class	Examples
Antidepressants:	
Tricyclic antidepressants	Amitriptyline, nortriptyline, desipramine, doxepin, imipramine
Serotonin/norepinephrine reuptake inhibitors	Venlafaxine, duloxetine, milnacipran
Selective serotonin reuptake inhibitors	Paroxetine, citalopram, escitalopram
Others	Bupropion
Alpha-2-adrenergic agonists	Clonidine
	Tizanidine
Corticosteroids	Dexamethasone, prednisone, methylprednisolone

be considered multipurpose analgesics, fundamentally similar in this respect to the opioid and non-opioid analgesics (Table 9.7.1).

Antidepressant drugs

The analgesic efficacy of antidepressant drugs has been shown in diverse types of chronic pain (Table 9.7.2).

In the palliative care setting, antidepressants can be used to improve pain control when a favourable balance between analgesia and side effects cannot be attained with an opioid, or to treat comorbid depression or anxiety. Along with the gabapentinoids (see below), specific antidepressants are usually considered first-line medications for the treatment of neuropathic pain (Dworkin et al., 2007). However, very few clinical trials have evaluated analgesic efficacy of antidepressants for cancer-related pain, and none have been approved by the US Food and Drug Administration for this use. Recommendations for their use in this setting are therefore derived from observational studies, clinical experience or shown efficacy for pain of a non-malignant origin.

Anecdotal observations suggest that there is substantial variability in the analgesic response to the different antidepressants. Failure of a drug due to inefficacy, therefore, might reasonably be followed by a trial of an alternative drug. There are no guidelines for drug selection during these sequential trials and the process usually proceeds by trial and error. In those patients with refractory pain that has responded in part to one antidepressant, combination antidepressant therapy using drugs in different classes is sometimes considered, as it is for treatment-refractory depression. The latter option is based on anecdotal observation and usually involves the combination of a tricyclic and a serotonin-norepinephrine reuptake inhibitor (SNRI), or bupropion (see later).

Given evidence of dose-dependent analgesic effects, at least for the tricyclic antidepressants, it is reasonable to continue upward dose titration beyond the usual analgesic doses in patients who

Table 9.7.2 Antidepressants

Drug	Starting dose	Usual effective dose[a]	Precautions and contraindications	Selected potential drug interactions	Commonly reported adverse effects
Tricyclics					
Amitriptyline Nortriptyline Desipramine	10–25 mg HS	50–150 mg HS	Caution in elderly and medically ill, patients with cardiovascular disorders, urinary hesitancy or seizure history. Contraindicated with narrow angle glaucoma, recent MI	Caution with MAOIs, SSRIs, anticholinergic agents, antiarrhythmics, clonidine, lithium, and tramadol. Combination with beta blockers or agents which prolong QTc interval may increase risk for cardiac arrhythmia	Sedation, confusion, orthostatic hypotension, heart block, weight gain, tachycardia, seizure, arrhythmia, anticholinergic effects (e.g. dry mouth, blurred vision, urinary retention, constipation)
Noradrenaline and serotonin reuptake inhibitors (NSRIs)					
Duloxetine	20 mg bid or 30 mg qd[b]	60 mg qd	Caution in patients with hypertension (for venlafaxine) or seizure disorders	Venlafaxine: increased risk of serotonin syndrome with MAOIs, TCAs, bupropion, SSRIs, buspirone, sibutramine, ritonivir	Nausea, headache, somnolence, tremor, nervousness, hypertension, dry mouth, diaphoresis, constipation, sexual dysfunction.
Milnacipran	25 mg bid	100 mg bid	Should be tapered down progressively when discontinued. Rapid discontinuation may lead to agitation, anxiety, insomnia		
Venlafaxine XR	37.5 mg qd	150–300 mg qd	Dose should be reduced by 25% in mild-moderate renal impairment and by 50% in dialysis patients		Duloxetine: dizziness, fatigue
Noradrenaline and dopamine reuptake inhibitor					
Bupropion	75 mg qd	75–150 mg bid–tid	Contraindicated with seizure disorder, anorexia/bulimia, use of MAOI within 14 days	Toxicity of bupropion is increased by levodopa and amantadine. Seizure risk increased with agents that lower the seizure threshold	Agitation, tremor, insomnia, nausea, decreased appetite, weight loss, headache, dry mouth, somnolence, hypertension, tachycardia

[a] These doses are the ones shown analgesic in RCTs, or suggested by clinical experience, if the patient responds to that drug; if there is no response with that dose, the medication can be titrated up to the maximum tolerated or recommended dose.

[b] In United States, duloxetine is available in 20-mg dosing, whereas the lowest dose is 30 mg in other countries.

fail to achieve benefit and have no limiting side effects. This course is clearly justified in patients with a coexistent depression, but should be considered even in patients without evidence of this disorder. There is currently no justification for increasing doses beyond the levels associated with antidepressant effects.

A favourable analgesic effect is usually observed within a week after achieving an effective dosing level and, in some patients, maximal effect appears to evolve over days or weeks thereafter. This delay, combined with the many days required to increase the dose to a therapeutic level, may result in a prolonged period during which patients experience unsatisfactory effects from the therapy, and sometimes experience uncomfortable side effects. To reduce non-adherence, the patient should be well informed about this potential.

Tricyclic antidepressants

There is evidence that the tricyclic compounds have analgesic efficacy in a variety of chronic pain syndromes (Dworkin et al., 2007). The evidence is stronger for the tertiary amine compounds, mainly amitriptyline. The secondary amines, desipramine and nortriptyline, are often preferred, however, because of a lower toxicity than the tertiary amines.

Although evidence is limited to a few partially controlled trials (Walsh, 1986; Ventafridda et al., 1987) and one randomized controlled trial with amitriptyline (Mishra et al., 2012), tricyclics are actually the only antidepressants for which there is some evidence of analgesic potential in the cancer population. Use of tricyclic antidepressants is often limited by their frequent association with adverse effects. Although they can be minimized by starting with a very low dose and titrating up slowly, adverse effects, especially mental clouding, often limit the use of tricyclics in this population.

SNRIs

SNRIs are the only antidepressants, along with the tricyclics, for which there is clear evidence of analgesic efficacy, with pain relief reported in several types of neuropathic pain, as well as in fibromyalgia.

In patients with breast cancer, venlafaxine prevented the development of chronic post-mastectomy pain when started the night before surgery and administered for 2 weeks (Reuben et al., 2004). A randomized trial also showed that venlafaxine, administered for 2 weeks during chemotherapy, reduced acute neurosensory symptoms and chronic oxaliplatin neurotoxicity (Durand et al., 2012). The analgesic efficacy of duloxetine and milnacipran has been established in several conditions and in the United States and several other countries, these drugs have been approved for the treatment of fibromyalgia and varied types of neuropathic pain.

Evidence has also started to accumulate for an analgesic effect of duloxetine in cancer-related neuropathic pain. In an open label study of 39 patients with colon cancer and chronic oxaliplatin-induced peripheral neuropathy, 63.3% of those who could tolerate duloxetine experienced improvement of their pain (Yang et al., 2012). Similar results were observed in a retrospective case series of patients who could not tolerate pregabalin (Matsuoka et al., 2012). A recent randomized controlled trial found that duloxetine significantly reduced pain associated with chemotherapy-induced peripheral neuropathy (Smith et al., 2013).

SSRIs

Although there is limited evidence that some selective serotonin reuptake inhibitors (SSRIs)—paroxetine, citalopram, and escitalopram—may have analgesic efficacy (Lee and Chen, 2010), drugs in this class appear to be less analgesic than other antidepressants. They are therefore not preferred when pain is the primary indication.

Others

Bupropion provided substantial pain relief in a randomized study of patients with neuropathic pain (Semenchuk et al., 2001). Although this finding has not been replicated, bupropion has favourable characteristics that may support a trial for pain. It has a low risk of somnolence and sexual dysfunction, side effects that may be limiting with other antidepressants. Anecdotally, patients may report increased energy that appears to be unrelated to mood effects, which has led to empirical use for fatigue. Bupropion should be considered as a potential treatment for pain in selected patients, especially those who are sedated, fatigued, or apathetic.

Whereas mirtazapine was shown to improve sleep, anxiety and depression in cancer patients diagnosed with depression, it did not improve pain (Cankurtaran et al., 2008).

Corticosteroids

Numerous studies have suggested that corticosteroids may improve appetite, nausea, malaise, and overall quality of life in populations with advanced illness (Tannock et al., 1989; Farr, 1990). Although concern about toxicity has generally limited the primary analgesic use of these drugs to those with short life expectancies, there is a substantial anecdotal experience with both short-term and long-term administration for a variety of clinical problems, including pain.

Data from controlled trials and clinical series support the classification of corticosteroids as multipurpose analgesics. Analgesic efficacy has been suggested in diverse types of cancer pain, including bone pain, neuropathic pain from infiltration or compression of neural structures, headache due to increased intracranial pressure, arthralgia, and pain due to obstruction of a hollow viscus (e.g. bowel or ureter) (Tannock et al., 1989; Fainsinger et al., 1994). Patients who present with these pain syndromes commonly have other symptoms that could potentially be improved by steroid therapy, such as nausea or malaise, and corticosteroid therapy may be considered earlier if primarily indicated by these other symptoms.

The relative risks and benefits of the various corticosteroids are unknown. In the United States, dexamethasone is usually selected, a choice that gains theoretical support from the relatively low mineralocorticoid effects of this drug. Prednisone and methylprednisolone have also been used.

On the basis of clinical experience, corticosteroids are usually administered either in a high-dose regimen or a low-dose regimen. A high-dose regimen (empirically ranging from an initial dose of dexamethasone of 20–100 mg followed initially by 32–96 mg per day in four divided doses, which is usually tapered concurrent with the initiation of other analgesic approaches) has been used for patients who experience an acute episode of very severe pain that cannot be promptly reduced with opioids, such as that associated with a rapidly worsening malignant plexopathy. The higher range of this regimen has been widely used in the setting of emerging spinal cord or cauda equina signs related to epidural metastasis and may also be appropriate when treating other oncological emergencies, such as superior vena cava syndrome.

A low-dose corticosteroid regimen (e.g. dexamethasone 1–2 mg once or twice daily) has been used for patients with advanced medical illness who continue to have pain despite optimal dosing of opioid drugs. Although a randomized controlled study of low-dose oral dexamethasone (8 mg daily) combined with an opioid failed to show any benefit on pain or most other symptoms in a sample of patients with far advanced illness, (Mercadante et al., 2007) gastrointestinal side effects of the opioid were diminished and the drug produced short-lasting improvement of weakness, drowsiness and well-being. In most cases, long-term therapy is planned when a low-dose regimen is initiated.

Well-recognized adverse effects are associated with short-term and long-term administration of corticosteroids, and with the withdrawal of these drugs following chronic use. The risk of serious toxicity increases with the dose of the drug, the duration of therapy, and predisposing factors associated with the medical condition of the patient. These risks are balanced by the need for enhanced comfort. Repeated assessments are required to ensure that benefits occur and are sustained. Ineffective regimens should be tapered and discontinued, and in all cases, the lowest dose that yields the desired results should be sought.

Alpha-2 adrenergic agonists

Reports suggest that clonidine can be analgesic in diverse pain syndromes, including cancer pain (Eisenach et al., 1995; Tumber and Fitzgibbon, 1998). A controlled trial of transdermal clonidine in diabetic painful polyneuropathy demonstrated that fewer than one-quarter of patients are potential responders, but that those who do respond can experience analgesia that is both substantial and sustained (Byas-Smith et al., 1995). A 14-day epidural infusion of clonidine (30 micrograms/hour) in cancer patients reduced pain in 45% of patients, compared to 21% with placebo, but did not reduce opioid consumption (Eisenach et al., 1995); neuropathic pain responded relatively well (56% vs only 5% with placebo). The most common adverse effects associated with systemic or epidural clonidine administration have been somnolence, hypotension (usually orthostatic), and dry mouth.

Tizanidine is another centrally acting alpha-2 agonist and is commercially available in the United States as an antispasticity agent (Nance et al., 1994). Although the evidence of analgesic efficacy is limited to a few open-label studies in myofascial pain syndrome, the mechanism of this drug and a favourable clinical experience has supported its use as a multipurpose analgesic. The most frequent side effects are somnolence and dry mouth. This drug has less affinity for the alpha-1 adrenergic receptor and therefore produces hypotension less often than clonidine.

Given limited experience with the adrenergic agonists in those with advanced illness, trials of these drugs are usually considered after other adjuvant analgesics, such as the antidepressants and anticonvulsants, have failed.

Neuroleptics

In the palliative care setting, neuroleptics are used commonly in the management of delirium or nausea. A systematic review suggested that the second-generation 'atypical neuroleptics' may have analgesic properties (Fishbain et al., 2004). According to a case series, olanzapine could decrease opioid-unresponsive cancer pain by potentiating the effect of opioids, thereby allowing a significant decrease of the opioid dose (Khojainova et al., 2002).

Nonetheless, there is relatively little evidence of analgesic activity for most neuroleptic compounds and their role as adjuvant analgesics is limited by this lack of definitive data and the potential for adverse effects (Fishbain et al., 2004). They should therefore only be considered for pain when treatment with many other drugs has proved unsuccessful, or there is concomitant delirium or nausea.

Adjuvant analgesics used for neuropathic pain

Although neuropathic pain may be relatively less responsive to opioid drugs than other pains (Portenoy et al., 1990; Mercadante et al., 1992; Cherny et al., 1994), combination therapy with an opioid and adjuvant analgesics can yield analgesic outcomes in cancer-related neuropathic pain that mirror those obtained during treatment of nociceptive or mixed pain syndromes (Grond et al., 1999). One survey found that absent and mild pain can be obtained in 53.2% and 41.9% of patients, respectively, after 6 months (Mishra et al., 2008).

Guidelines for the management of neuropathic pain recommend selected antidepressants (tricyclics and SNRIs) and the gabapentinoid anticonvulsants as the first-line drugs (Table 9.7.3). In the context of advanced illness, a corticosteroid also may be first-line drug. Drugs in many other classes are tried in refractory cases, despite limited data.

Anticonvulsant drugs

The analgesic potential of anticonvulsant drugs has been recognized for decades for the management of neuropathic pains. The older drugs, such as phenytoin and carbamazepine, are now complemented by a rapidly increasing number of newer agents (Table 9.7.4).

There is evidence that the gabapentinoids—gabapentin and pregabalin—are analgesic in diverse neuropathic pains (Caraceni et al., 2004; Mishra et al., 2012). Given good tolerability and no known drug–drug interactions, they are first-line agents for the

Table 9.7.3 Adjuvant analgesics used for neuropathic pain

Class	Examples
Antidepressants	See Table 9.7.1
Anticonvulsants	Gabapentin, pregabalin, topiramate, carbamazepine, phenytoin, valproate, oxcarbazepine, lamotrigine, levetiracetam
Topical agents	Capsaicin, lidocaine patch, EMLA[*]
Oral sodium channel blockers	Mexiletine, tocainide, flecainide
Alpha-2 adrenergic agonists	Clonidine, tizanidine
N-methyl-D-aspartate receptor antagonists	Dextromethorphan, ketamine
GABA agonists	Baclofen
Cannabinoids	Tetrahydrocanninol (THC), nabilone, THC:cannabidiol mixture
Miscellaneous	Calcitonin

Table 9.7.4 Anticonvulsants

Drug	Starting dose	Usual effective dose	Precautions and contraindications[a]	Selected potential drug interactions[b]	Commonly reported adverse effects
Gabapentin	100–300 mg daily; titrate by 100–300 mg every 1–3 days to an effective dose	300–1200 mg tid	Decrease dose in patients with renal dysfunction (avoid in severe renal dysfunction). Rapid discontinuation may result in headache, nausea, insomnia, and diarrhoea.	None	Sedation, dizziness, tremor, peripheral oedema, weight gain, nausea, headache
Pregabalin	25–75 mg qd–bid	150–300 mg bid			
Lamotrigine	25 mg qd; titrate by 25 mg every 7 days to an effective dose	100–200 mg bid	Black box warning: severe and potentially life threatening skin rashes have been reported	May increase carbamazepine levels	Headache, dizziness, ataxia, somnolence, tremor, nausea, diarrhoea, blurred vision, insomnia
Carbamazepine	100–200 mg qd–bid	300–800 mg bid	Contraindicated in bone marrow depression, or within 14 days of MAOI use. Caution in patients with cardiac disease, hepatic or renal dysfunction. Potentially fatal blood dyscrasias have been reported; monitor CBC, platelets, renal and liver function, and serum sodium. Potentially fatal severe dermatologic reactions (e.g. Stevens–Johnson syndromes) are rare	May decrease levels of drugs metabolized by CYP3A4	Somnolence, dizziness, blurred vision, headache, confusion, speech and memory difficulties, cardiovascular abnormalities (e.g. arrhythmia, bradycardia, hypertension, AV block), rash, SIADH, nausea, urinary retention, hematologic abnormalities (e.g. aplastic anaemia, bone marrow suppression, thrombocytopenia), increased liver enzymes, hepatic failure
Oxcarbazepine	150 mg qd; titrate by 150–300 mg every 3–5 days to an effective dose	150–600 mg bid	Clinically significant hyponatremia can develop: monitor serum sodium at baseline, during the first 3 months and periodically	May decrease levels/effects of CYP3A4 substrates and increase levels/effects of CYP2C19 substrates	Dizziness, somnolence, headache, ataxia, nausea, tremor, diplopia, nystagmus
Topiramate	25–50 mg qd; titrate by 25 mg every 5–7 days to an effective dose	100–400 mg bid	May significantly decrease serum bicarbonate; monitor serum bicarbonate at baseline and periodically. Often poorly tolerated: high rate of withdrawal due to adverse effects	Administration with anticholinergics may increase risk of hyperthermia and oligohydrosis	Somnolence, dizziness, ataxia, psychomotor slowing, speech and memory difficulties, decreased serum bicarbonate, metabolic acidosis, nausea, paraesthesia, tremor, abnormal vision, nystagmus, diplopia, weight loss, nephrolithiasis, secondary angle closure glaucoma
Lacosamide	50 mg bid	200–400 mg bid	—	—	Dizziness, fatigue, nausea/vomiting
Levetiracetam	250–500 mg bid	500–1500 mg bid		None	Somnolence, dizziness
Zonisamide	100 mg qd	100–300 mg bid	Use in patients with severe sulfonamide allergy is contraindicated; potentially fatal sulfonamide reactions (including Stevens–Johnson syndrome and toxic epidermal necrolysis) are rare. Use cautiously in patients with renal or hepatic dysfunction	CYP3A4 inhibitors may increase zonisamide levels/effects	Somnolence, dizziness, headache, confusion, ataxia, insomnia, tremor, nausea, weight loss, diplopia, nystagmus

[a] Avoid abrupt withdrawal of any anticonvulsant as this may increase the risk for seizure. Although the actual incidence of seizure following abrupt withdrawal of anticonvulsants in patients without seizure disorders, is unknown to discontinue over 1–2 weeks.

[b] CNS depressants (e.g. alcohol, benzodiazepines, barbiturates, opioids) may increase the CNS side effects of all anticonvulsants.

treatment of neuropathic pain of diverse aetiologies (Dworkin et al., 2007). Gabapentin is the most commonly used adjuvant analgesic in cancer patients with neuropathic pain and on palliative care units (Oneschuk and al-Shahri, 2003).

Although one controlled study of gabapentin failed to demonstrate any benefit in chemotherapy-induced peripheral neuropathy (Rao et al., 2007), others have been positive (Keskinbora et al., 2007; Rao et al., 2007). Another study found that low-dose gabapentin (200 mg twice daily) and imipramine (10 mg twice daily) produced good pain control with fewer adverse effects than high-dose gabapentin alone (Arai et al., 2010) and yet another demonstrated that treatment with oral gabapentin and local anaesthetics in the wound decreased acute and chronic pain after breast surgery for cancer (Fassoulaki et al., 2005). Controlled trials have similarly confirmed that pregabalin is analgesic in neuropathic pain (Sabatowski et al., 2004), including neuropathic cancer pain (Saif et al., 2010; Mishra et al., 2012), and also is analgesic in non-neuropathic conditions such as fibromyalgia (Crofford et al., 2005) and irritable bowel syndrome (Houghton et al., 2007). The onset of analgesic activity is faster with pregabalin (significant difference in pain on second day) than with gabapentin (Sabatowski et al., 2004).

A recent systematic review found insufficient evidence to conclude that other anticonvulsants have analgesic efficacy (Wiffen et al., 2013). It acknowledged, however, that decades of experience provided support for some agents and called for more research to assess effectiveness in clinical practice. Carbamazepine has been used for many years and is approved in the United States for trigeminal neuralgia. This drug raises concern about adverse effects, particularly leucopenia, and has been largely supplanted by others, including oxcarbazepine, which is a metabolite of carbamazepine and is better tolerated. A small, randomized open-label study has suggested that oxcarbazepine might significantly decrease the risk of oxaliplatin-induced painful neuropathy (31.2 vs 75%) (Argyriou et al., 2006). Both topiramate and lamotrigine are used empirically for refractory neuropathic pain; although case reports suggested possible efficacy for neuropathic cancer pain (Devulder, 2000) and chemotherapy-induced peripheral neuropathy (Durand et al., 2005), a randomized controlled crossover trial failed to show any pain relief with lamotrigine for the latter condition (Rao et al., 2008). Although some observational data supported the potential for analgesic effects from levetiracetam, recent controlled trials have yielded negative results (Holbech et al., 2011). Zonisamide has been shown to be effective in one randomized controlled trial of painful diabetic neuropathy (Atli and Dogra, 2005) and further evaluation of this drug is warranted. Similarly, recent studies of the newest anticonvulsant, lacosamide, suggest potential for analgesic effects in some situations (Wiffen et al., 2013). There is very scarce evidence related to other anticonvulsants, such as tiagabine and felbamate, and despite a large clinical experience, similarly limited data about several older drugs such as clonazepam, valproate, and phenytoin.

In sum, the first-line drugs for neuropathic pain remain the gabapentinoids followed by the analgesic antidepressants (the order may be reversed when the patient is depressed), in addition to the corticosteroids. Those who do not respond to any of the several drugs in these two classes may be considered for empirical trials of other anticonvulsants, notwithstanding the lack of evidence, or trials of one or more of the drugs described below. Drug selection is by trial and error. The preferred anticonvulsant drugs based on limited evidence, safety considerations and experience are usually considered to be oxcarbazepine, topiramate, lamotrigine, lacosamide and zonisamide; clonazepam may be considered as well, particularly when there is comorbid anxiety. The older anticonvulsants (carbamazepine, valproate, and phenytoin) usually are considered if access to other drugs is limited or patients have been highly refractory to treatment

Oral and parenteral sodium channel blockers

Several sodium channel blockers possess analgesic activity, including some anticonvulsants and anaesthetics/anti-arrhythmics. Although studies suggest that these drugs may be multipurpose analgesics, a large clinical experience has focused on their use for neuropathic pain. While controlled trials have demonstrated efficacy of a brief intravenous infusion of lignocaine (lidocaine) for diverse types of non-malignant neuropathic pain, several studies in neuropathic cancer pain have yielded negative results (Bruera et al., 1992; Chong et al., 1997).

Prolonged relief of pain following a brief intravenous infusion of a local anaesthetic is nevertheless possible. On the basis of clinical experience, a trial of a brief local anaesthetic infusion is sometimes implemented in patients with severe neuropathic pain that has not responded promptly to an opioid and requires immediate relief. Repeated infusions with escalating doses can be performed over a period of hours and may be a useful approach to the acute management of severe neuropathic pain even in those with advanced illness. If pain recurs, long-term subcutaneous administration of lignocaine also has been used anecdotally to yield sustained relief of refractory neuropathic pain in cancer patients (Brose and Cousins, 1991).

Oral formulations of sodium channel blockers (mexiletine, flecainide) are available and long-term systemic therapy can be accomplished simply using these drugs. A survey of cancer patients suggested that flecainide can be effective in the treatment of pain due to tumour infiltration of nerves (Dunlop et al., 1989). One study showed that the response to an intravenous infusion of lidocaine is a good predictor of the response to oral mexiletine treatment (Galer et al., 1996). It may therefore be useful to consider a brief infusion as a means to guide the selection of an oral therapy after trials of anticonvulsants and antidepressants have proved unhelpful.

N-methyl-D-aspartate receptor blockers

Excitatory amino acids, such as glutamate and aspartate, are released by primary afferent neurons in response to noxious stimuli and are important in the central processing of the pain-related information. Interactions at the *N*-methyl-D-aspartate (NMDA) receptor are involved in the development of central nervous system changes that may underlie chronic pain and modulate opioid mechanisms—specifically tolerance (Mao et al., 1995). Preclinical studies have established that the NMDA receptor is involved in the sensitization of central neurons following injury and the development of the 'wind-up' phenomenon, a change in the response of central neurones that has been associated with neuropathic pain (Dickenson and Sullivan, 1987).

Although there is evidence that antagonists at the NMDA receptor may be multipurpose analgesics, which could potentially ameliorate acute pain (Weinbroum et al., 2003) and diverse types

Table 9.7.5 NMDA antagonists

Drug	Starting dose	Usual effective dose	Precautions and contraindications	Selected potential drug interactions	Commonly reported adverse effects
Ketamine	Different intravenous or SC regimen, e.g. continuous infusion (0.05–1.5 mg/kg/h), IV boluses (0.25–0.5 mg/kg), IV 'burst' doses (100–500 mg/kg/d × 2-3 days) or oral doses (0.2–0.5 mg/kg bid–tid)	Unclear	Contraindicated with hypertension, heart failure, angina, aneurysms, cerebral trauma, recent myocardial infarct Caution with psychotic disorders, thyrotoxicosis, tachycardia, seizures	Increased levels/effects with CYP3A4 inhibitors	Hypertension, tachycardia, tremor, nystagmus, diplopia, airway resistance, myocardial depression, hallucinations, vivid dreams, tonic–clonic movements
Dextromethorphan	15–20 mg tid	Unclear		Increased levels/effects with CYP2D6 inhibitors	Dizziness, nausea, vomiting, confusion, hallucination, respiratory depression

of chronic pain (Graven-Nielsen et al., 2000), the most intense interest has focused on their role as new therapies for neuropathic pain. At the present time, there are four commercially available drugs in the United States that have primary effects at the NMDA receptor and have been explored as potential analgesics: ketamine, dextromethorphan, memantine, and amantadine (Table 9.7.5).

There is some evidence that ketamine is analgesic for non-malignant neuropathic pain (Schwartzman et al., 2009), and despite the negative results of a recent large and well controlled clinical trial evaluating subcutaneous ketamine infusion in cancer patients, (Hardy et al., 2012) a recent systematic review concluded that there is sufficient evidence to support the use of this drug in treatment-refractory cancer pain (Hardy et al., 2012). The drug can be used orally, as well as parenterally (Lauretti et al., 1999).

The side effect profile of ketamine can be daunting, particularly in the medically frail. Concurrent treatment with a benzodiazepine or a neuroleptic commonly is used to blunt or prevent these adverse effects. These side effects are unlikely to be problematic when low subanaesthetic doses are used. In the palliative care setting, ketamine may be a valuable strategy for severe refractory pain, particularly neuropathic pain, for pain emergencies and for pain that occurs in the context of a decision to offer sedation.

Evidence in favour of analgesic efficacy for the other commercially available NMDA receptor antagonists is very limited. One trial suggested that the antitussive dextromethorphan is analgesic in non-malignant neuropathic pain (Weinbroum et al., 2003), but a randomized trial of a mixture of morphine and dextromethorphan failed to show better analgesia than morphine alone (Galer et al., 2005). There is very little evidence on analgesic efficacy of memantine or amantadine.

The D-isomer of the opioid methadone also blocks the NMDA receptor (Davis and Inturrisi, 1999). In most countries, methadone is commercially available as a racemate containing 50% of the D-isomer. The contribution of this non-opioid molecule to the analgesia produced by methadone is uncertain, but the greater-than-anticipated potency of methadone in patients who undergo a switch to this drug from another mu agonist suggests that it can play a clinically important role. There are no data, however, to support the conclusion that methadone is better than other opioids for the treatment of neuropathic pain.

Cannabinoids

There are several cannabinoids now available and others in development. Clinical trials have established the analgesic efficacy of some of these drugs. Nabiximols, a cannabinoid oromucosal spray formulation primarily comprising delta (9)-tetrahydrocannabinol (THC) and cannabidiol, is approved in some countries for spasticity related to multiple sclerosis and opioid-refractory cancer pain. A recent large randomized graded-dose trial in cancer patients with persistent pain despite opioid treatment showed that the overall proportion of patients reporting analgesia was greater for nabiximols than placebo in the low-dose and medium-dose groups, but not the high-dose group (Portenoy et al., 2012). Other studies have demonstrated positive results in pain due to multiple sclerosis, cancer, peripheral nerve lesions, and rheumatoid arthritis (Rog et al., 2005; Russo et al., 2007).

The oral synthetic cannabinoid nabilone has been shown to be analgesic in spasticity-related pain from chronic upper motor neuron syndrome (Wissel et al., 2006) and fibromyalgia (Skrabek et al., 2008). An observational study of nabilone in patients with advanced cancer suggested significant benefit for pain and other symptoms (Maida et al., 2008).

The most common side effects associated with the cannabinoids are dizziness, somnolence, and dry mouth. An older study of THC for cancer pain noted a narrow therapeutic window and a relatively low efficacy, comparable to codeine at conventional doses (Noyes et al., 1976). Studies of the plant extracts suggest that better outcomes occur with drugs that include a combination of cannabinoid compounds. Additional studies will provide new agents for clinical use and hopefully clarify the relative benefits and burdens.

The existing data suggest that the newer cannabinoid drugs, such as the oromucosal spray containing THC and cannabidiol, ultimately will be characterized as multipurpose analgesics, potentially appropriate for a trial in the medically ill whenever pain is refractory to opioid therapy. At this point, however, both experience and available agents are limited, and most of the data in relation to this class has been collected in neuropathic pain populations. A trial of a commercially available cannabinoid usually is considered only in those patients who are refractory to opioids and other appropriate adjuvant analgesics; most of these patients will have neuropathic pain. Nabilone should be started at 0.5–1 mg at night and titrated up to 3 mg twice daily, or higher if tolerated. THC usually is started at a dose of 2.5 mg once or twice daily, and titrated. The oromucosal spray containing THC and cannabinol has been initiated with an 'as needed' schedule and effectively titrated by the patient to an effective dose.

Baclofen

Baclofen, an agonist at the gamma-aminobutyric acid type B (GABA$_B$) receptor, is efficacious in trigeminal neuralgia (Fromm et al., 1984). Intrathecal baclofen also is very effective in relieving pain related to spasticity. Although there have been a few observations that suggest a broader analgesic potential for systemically administered baclofen, the data are too limited to recommend a trial for non-neuropathic pain.

Topical analgesics

Topical therapies have the potential to deliver low doses of analgesic compounds directly to a site responsible for pain. There is a potential for benefit with a very low risk of systemic toxicity. Topical analgesics are used for many types of focal pain and commercially available agents include capsaicin preparations, formulations of aspirin or non-steroidal anti-inflammatory drugs (NSAIDs), creams, and patches containing local anaesthetics, and preparations containing tricyclic preparations. Other formulations compounded by pharmacies may include opioids, selected anticonvulsants, or other drugs.

Capsaicin is the naturally occurring constituent of the chili pepper that produces its pungent taste. When applied topically, it inhibits polymodal primary afferent nociceptive neurons by binding to the transient receptor potential vanilloid type 1 (TRPV1) receptor, and inhibiting the release of substance P and other compounds. The presumed analgesic mode of action is depletion of substance P from the terminals of afferent C-fibres, which occurs with regular use. Low-dose topical capsaicin (0.1%) has been demonstrated to be effective in both painful mononeuropathies and polyneuropathies, including peripheral painful mononeuropathies following cancer surgery (post-mastectomy, post-thoracotomy, post-amputation) (Fromm et al., 1984). A controlled trial in HIV-associated painful peripheral neuropathy, however, failed to show any analgesic effect (Paice et al., 2000). A high-dose capsaicin patch (8%), which is applied for only an hour and is available in some countries, has shown efficacy in post-herpetic neuralgia and HIV-associated painful peripheral neuropathy, with a duration of effect in responders that can last several months (Baranidharan et al., 2013).

Topical formulations of NSAIDs (e.g. diclofenac, aspirin) are widely available and used to treat common musculoskeletal pains, such as sprains and strains. The use of these creams, fluids, and patches to manage focal pains in those with serious illness is empirical; given the potential for some systemic absorption, they should not be given to patients with strong contraindications to systemic NSAID therapy, such as renal insufficiency.

There is ample evidence that topical local anaesthetics are analgesic. Given the observation that the lidocaine 5% patch may reduce pain and allodynia from diverse types of neuropathic pain and some presentations of osteoarthritis, a trial of this formulation can be considered for all patients with relatively small areas of pain unrelated to local skin injury. Topical local anaesthetic creams and gels also are available. A commercially available mixture of local anaesthetics, which contains a 1:1 mixture of prilocaine and lignocaine, is capable of penetrating the skin and producing a dense local cutaneous anaesthesia; this product, known as eutectic mixture of local anaesthetics (EMLA®), is widely used to prevent the pain of needle puncture or incision, as well as pain from debridement of leg ulcers. Although there is a very remote risk of toxicity from systemic absorption of a topical local anaesthetic, careful monitoring is needed if the anaesthetic is applied repeatedly to mucous membranes or open wounds.

Topical administration of tricyclic antidepressants sometimes is considered for focal neuropathic pain, despite conflicting data. There are favourable clinical observations pertaining to topical amitriptyline 2% cream, given alone or in combination with ketamine 1%, for the treatment of neuropathic pain (Lynch et al., 2005b), but randomized trials have not confirmed the efficacy of topical amitriptyline (Lynch et al., 2005a; Ho et al., 2008).

Compounded topical preparations also are used, based mostly on anecdotal observations. A topical gel made of amitriptyline, ketamine, and baclofen lessened tingling, cramping, and shooting/burning pain in patients with chemotherapy-induced peripheral neuropathy, without any systemic toxicity (Barton et al., 2011).

A topical gel of amitriptyline, ketamine, and lidocaine, used three times daily during radiation therapy and up to 2 weeks after, appeared to help pain caused by radiation skin reaction (Uzaraga et al., 2012).

Adjuvant analgesics used for bone pain

Radiation therapy is usually considered when bone pain is focal and poorly controlled with an opioid, or is associated with a lesion that appears prone to fracture on radiographic examination. Anecdotally, multifocal bone pain has been observed to benefit from treatment with a NSAID or a corticosteroid. Other adjuvant analgesics that are potentially useful in this setting include calcitonin, bisphosphonate compounds, gallium nitrate, and selected radiopharmaceuticals (Table 9.7.6). There have been no comparative trials of these adjuvant analgesics for bone pain and the selection of one over another is usually based on convenience, patient preference, and the clinical setting.

Calcitonin and bisphosphonates

Although evidence of its analgesic efficacy is mostly limited to case studies, clinical experience suggests that calcitonin may relieve pain from bone metastases (Hindley et al., 1982; Szanto et al., 1992; Mystakidou et al., 1999).

While calcitonin was most commonly administered intranasally, which was very convenient since less invasive, the intranasal formulation has recently been withdrawn from the European and Canadian markets because of poor evidence of analgesic efficacy and possible increased cancer risk when used on a long-term basis to treat osteoporosis (Overman et al., 2013). The only remaining route of administration is therefore subcutaneously, usually administered daily. Continuous subcutaneous administration also has been described (Mystakidou et al., 1999).

There is much more evidence that the bisphosphonates are analgesic for metastatic bone pain and one of these drugs typically is used first. The bisphosphonates are analogues of inorganic pyrophosphate and inhibit osteoclast activity. Studies have demonstrated that pamidronate is analgesic in breast cancer

Table 9.7.6 Adjuvant analgesics for cancer-related bone pain

Drug	Starting dose	Usual effective dose	Precautions and contraindications	Selected potential drug interactions	Commonly reported adverse effects
Corticosteroids	c.f. above text				
Calcitonin	100 IU SC daily	Dose can be progressively increased up to 200 IU SC daily	SC administration should be preceded by skin testing with 1 IU SC to screen for hypersensitivity, especially in patients with a history of allergy to salmon or seafood	None	Nausea/vomiting
Bisphosphonates					
Pamidronate	30 mg SC q 4 weeks	60–90 mg SC q 4 weeks, can increase up to 120 mg if well tolerated and not effective	Renal function should be checked prior to initiation and monitored during course of therapy		Renal toxicity
Zoledronic acid	4 mg IV in 15 minutes, q 3 weeks				Acute-phase (flu-like) reactions, usually transient and well controlled with acetaminophen and NSAIDs
Ibandronate	6 mg IV in 1–2 h, q 3–4 weeks or 50 mg po qd		Adherence to dosing instructions decrease risk of GI toxicity		Gastrointestinal toxicity, only with oral administration
					Osteonecrosis of the jaw (worrisome but uncommon)

(Hortobagyi et al., 1996) and multiple myeloma (Berenson et al., 1996); zoledronic acid decreases bone pain from breast, prostate, and lung metastases, and multiple myeloma (Vogel et al., 2004; Wardley et al., 2005); and ibandronate reduces pain and analgesic use in patients with breast cancer (Body et al., 2004; Mancini et al., 2004; Pecherstorfer et al., 2006). Ibandronate was shown to be helpful in opioid-resistant bone pain (Mancini et al., 2004) and to be safe for up to 4 years of use (Pecherstorfer et al., 2006). The bisphosphonates also reduce other skeletal morbidity, including pathological fractures, need for bone radiation or surgery, spinal cord compression, and hypercalcaemia (Berenson et al., 1996; Hortobagyi et al., 1996; Rosen et al., 2003).

Radiopharmaceuticals

Radionuclides that are absorbed at areas of high bone turnover have been evaluated as potential therapies for metastatic bone disease. Strontium chloride-89, rhenium-186 hydroxyethylene diphosphonic acid, and samarium-153 ethylene-diaminetetramethylene phosphonic acid have been most promising thus far. The data suggest that treatment with a radiopharmaceutical yields meaningful pain relief in approximately 80% of patients, 10% of whom attain complete relief (Robinson et al., 1995). Initial clinical response occurs in 7–21 days and peak response may be delayed for a month or more. Approximately 5–10% of patients experience a transitory pain flare immediately after treatment. The usual duration of benefit is 3–6 months, after which retreatment may regain a favourable effect. Following treatment, clinically significant leucopenia or thrombocytopenia peak a few weeks after treatment and occurs to a clinically significant degree in approximately 10% and 33% of patients, respectively. Bone marrow effects usually wane by 12 weeks after treatment. Given the effects on bone marrow and delayed onset, treatment with a radiopharmaceutical should not be considered in patients awaiting cytotoxic chemotherapy and those with a life expectancy of greater than 3 months. This delay also implies that treatment should not be considered as the sole approach for patients with severe pain.

Adjuvant analgesics used for bowel obstruction

The management of symptoms associated with malignant bowel obstruction may be challenging. If surgical decompression is not feasible, the need to control pain and other obstructive symptoms, including distension, nausea, and vomiting, becomes paramount. The use of opioids may be problematic due to dose-limiting toxicity (including gastrointestinal toxicity) or the intensity of breakthrough pains. Anecdotal reports suggest that anticholinergic drugs, the somatostatin analogue octreotide, and corticosteroids may be useful adjuvant analgesics in this setting. The use of these drugs may also ameliorate non-painful symptoms and minimize the number of patients who must be considered for chronic drainage using nasogastric or percutaneous catheters.

Anticholinergic drugs

Anticholinergic drugs theoretically relieve the symptoms of bowel obstruction by reducing propulsive and non-propulsive gut motility and decreasing intraluminal secretions. Some patients appear to benefit from the administration of hyoscine (scopolamine) (Baines et al., 1985).

In some countries, hyoscine is only commercially available as the hydrobromide salt, which readily crosses the blood–brain barrier. Although this formulation can be delivered via a transdermal system, which simplifies treatment in patients with bowel obstruction, it is likely to be associated with a relatively higher incidence of central nervous system side effects, such as somnolence and confusion, than an anticholinergic drug with less penetration through the blood–brain barrier. Hyoscine butylbromide, which is less likely to pass the blood–brain barrier due to low lipid solubility, can be effective for obstructive symptoms, including pain (Ripamonti et al., 2000). Glycopyrrolate has a pharmacological profile similar to hyoscine butylbromide, but has not been systematically evaluated in a population with symptomatic bowel obstruction.

Octreotide

The somatostatin analogue octreotide inhibits the secretion of gastric, pancreatic, and intestinal secretions and reduces gastrointestinal motility. These effects probably underlie the analgesic effects that have been reported in case series of symptomatic treatment of bowel obstruction (Ripamonti et al., 2000). The benefits of this drug may occur more rapidly than hyoscine (Mercadante et al., 2000).

Octreotide has also been used to manage severe diarrhoea due to enterocolic fistula, high output jejunostomies or ileostomies, or secretory tumours of the gastrointestinal tract. A newer long-acting formulation, administered intramuscularly once monthly, can provide sustained reduction of bowel obstruction symptoms (Massacesi et al., 2006).

Octreotide has a good safety profile but is expensive. In some settings, however, the cost may be balanced by an excellent clinical response or the avoidance of the costs involved in the use of a gastrointestinal drainage procedure.

Corticosteroids

As discussed previously, the symptoms associated with bowel obstruction may improve with corticosteroid therapy. The mode of action is unclear and the most effective drug, dose, and dosing regimen are unknown. A broad range of doses have been described anecdotally. For example dexamethasone has been used for this indication in a dose range of 8–60 mg/day (Fainsinger et al., 1994) and methylprednisolone has been administered in a dose range of 30–50 mg/day (Farr, 1990). The potential for complications during long-term therapy, including an increased risk of bowel perforation, may limit this approach to patients with short life expectancies.

Adjuvant analgesics used for musculoskeletal pain

Although pains that originate from injury to muscle or connective tissue are prevalent in the medically ill, there has been no systematic evaluation of analgesic therapies for this problem. In the management of acute traumatic sprains or strains in the non-medically ill, non-opioid and opioid analgesics are commonly supplemented by treatment with so-called muscle relaxant drugs or benzodiazepines. The role of the latter drugs for opioid-refractory musculoskeletal pains in populations with advanced medical illness remains ill defined.

Muscle relaxants

The so-called muscle relaxants include drugs in a variety of classes, all of which are marketed for the treatment of acute musculoskeletal pain. In the United States, this group includes drugs that are also administered as antihistamines (e.g. orphenadrine), tricyclic compounds structurally similar to the tricyclic antidepressants (e.g. cyclobenzaprine), and other types of drugs (e.g. carisoprodol, chlorzoxazone, metaxalone, and methocarbamol).

The efficacy of the muscle relaxant drugs in common musculoskeletal pains has been established in placebo-controlled studies (Bercel, 1977; Gold, 1978).

Some studies have demonstrated analgesic effects that are superior to either aspirin or acetaminophen, and others have shown that the combination of a muscle relaxant and one of the latter drugs provides better analgesia than does aspirin or acetaminophen alone. There have been no controlled comparative trials or studies that have directly compared the efficacy and side effect profiles of these drugs with either NSAIDs or opioids.

Although muscle relaxant drugs can relieve musculoskeletal pains, these effects may not be specific and do not depend on relaxation of skeletal muscle. The label 'muscle relaxant' notwithstanding, there is actually no evidence that these drugs relax skeletal muscle in the clinical setting. They should not be administered in the mistaken belief that they relieve muscle spasm. If muscle spasm is believed to be related to the pain, it may be justifiable to consider a trial of a drug with established effect on skeletal muscle, such as diazepam or another benzodiazepine, the alpha-2 adrenergic agonist tizanidine, or the $GABA_B$ agonist baclofen.

Conclusions

Although the use of adjuvant analgesics in palliative care remains largely guided by anecdotal experience, controlled clinical trials have begun to provide a scientific rationale for many therapies. Future investigations of nociceptive processes and pain pathophysiology will undoubtedly lead to the development of novel drugs. For example, the adjuvant analgesics may one day include drugs that modulate peripheral nociceptive processes, such a substance P or bradykinin antagonists, or drugs that alter central processing by interacting with gangliosides or second messenger systems activated by excitatory amino acids. Although opioid drugs continue to be the major approach to the treatment of pain in the palliative care setting, adjuvant analgesics offer opportunities for improved outcomes in the substantial group of patients who cannot attain an acceptable balance between pain relief and side effects.

Online materials

Complete references for this chapter are available online at <http://www.oxfordmedicine.com>.

References

Bredlau, A.L., Thakur, R., Korones, D.N., and Dworkin, R.H. (2013). Ketamine for pain in adults and children with cancer: a systematic review and synthesis of the literature. *Pain Medicine*, 14(10), 1505–1517.

Caraceni, A., Zecca, E., Bonezzi, C., et al. (2004). Gabapentin for neuropathic cancer pain: a randomized controlled trial from the Gabapentin Cancer Pain Study Group. *Journal of Clinical Oncology*, 22, 2909–2917.

Dworkin, R.H., O'Connor, A.B., Backonja, M., et al. (2007). Pharmacologic management of neuropathic pain: evidence-based recommendations. *Pain*, 132, 237–251.

Hardy, J., Quinn, S., Fazekas, B., et al. (2012). Randomized, double-blind, placebo-controlled study to assess the efficacy and toxicity of subcutaneous ketamine in the management of cancer pain. *Journal of Clinical Oncology*, 30(29), 3611–3617.

Hortobagyi, G.N., Theriault, R.L., Porter, L., et al. (1996). Efficacy of pamidronate in reducing skeletal complications in patients with breast cancer and lytic bone metastases. *The New England Journal of Medicine* 335, 1785–1791.

Lee, Y.C. and Chen, P.P. (2010). A review of SSRIs and SNRIs in neuropathic pain. *Expert Opinion on Pharmacotherapy*, 16, 2813–2825.

Russo, E.B., Guy, G.W., and Robson, P.J. (2007). Cannabis, pain, and sleep: lessons from therapeutic clinical trials of Sativex, a cannabis-based medicine. *Chemistry & Biodiversity*, 4, 1729–1743.

Sabatowski, R., Gálvez, R., Cherry, D.A., *et al.* (2004). Pregabalin reduces pain and improves sleep and mood disturbances in patients with post-herpetic neuralgia: results of a randomised, placebo-controlled clinical trial. *Pain*, 109, 26–35.

Smith, E.M., Pang, H., Cirrincione, C., *et al.* (2013). Effect of duloxetine on pain, function, and quality of life among patients with chemotherapy-induced painful peripheral neuropathy: a randomized clinical trial. *Journal of the American Medical Association*, 309, 1359–1367.

Wiffen, P.J., Derry, S., Moore, R.A., *et al.* (2013). Antiepileptic drugs for neuropathic pain and fibromyalgia—an overview of Cochrane reviews. *Cochrane Database of Systematic Reviews*, 11, CD010567.

Interventional approaches for chronic pain

Robert A. Swarm, Menelaos Karanikolas, Lesley K. Rao, and Michael J. Cousins

Introduction to interventional approaches for chronic pain

Severe, uncontrolled pain remains common in populations with serious or life-threatening illness. Despite the availability of oral opioid therapy in most developed countries, an estimated 10–30% of people with advanced cancer have inadequate pain control (Hoskin 2006). Published guidelines endorse the view that these patients should be considered for procedural, or so-called interventional, pain therapies (Ripamonti et al., 2012; National Comprehensive Cancer Network, 2013). These therapies are best used within a multimodal strategy for symptom management, including appropriate systemic pharmacological, non-pharmacological, and psychosocial therapies.

Generally accepted indications for interventional pain therapies include (a) uncontrolled pain despite systemic analgesics and (b) unacceptable systemic analgesic adverse effects. In practice, if pain is not adequately controlled with systemic analgesics, doses are increased until pain is controlled or dose-limiting adverse effects occur; therefore, analgesic adverse effects are common indications for procedural pain therapies. Procedural pain therapies potentially improve pain control and/or allow opioid dose reduction.

Disease and patient characteristics that limit the effectiveness of systemic opioid analgesics should be recognized as factors that also increase the likelihood that procedural pain therapies will be needed. These characteristics include neuropathic pain, somatic pain that is sharp and severe, and pain that fluctuates markedly. Some patients are poorly responsive because of adverse effects that cannot be adequately controlled. Opioids may cause sedation, constipation, pruritus, urinary dysfunction, or neuroendocrine abnormalities (Katz and Mazer, 2009). Research in the future may indicate other risks, such as opioid-related immune suppression (Odunayo et al., 2010) and proliferative effects (Lennon et al., 2012). Some patients develop aberrant patterns of drug use or addiction (Ballantyne and LaForge, 2007). Finally, a reluctance to use high-dose systemic opioid therapy may be justified by concerns related to facilitation of pain transmission (or opioid-induced hyperalgesia) (Ossipov et al., 2005; Angst and Clark, 2006). Although the importance of the latter phenomenon is uncertain, it occurs in humans (Chu et al., 2008), and anecdotally,

may compromise some high-dose systemic or spinal therapies (De Conno et al., 1991; Bruera and Pereira, 1998); management approaches have included interventional pain therapies (Carr and Cousins, 2009; Deer et al., 2012c), opioid rotation, and adjuvant drugs such as systemic lignocaine (lidocaine) (Tremont-Lukats et al., 2005) or ketamine infusions (Mercadante et al., 2000).

There are numerous interventional pain therapies. In populations with advanced illness, these techniques may be used to address acute pain, perioperative pain, exacerbations of chronic pain, and pain from diagnostic or therapeutic procedures, as well as chronic pain.

Injection therapies

Peripheral injections for muscular and arthritic pain

Trigger point injections

Myofascial pain syndromes (MPS) are common, can involve any muscle, and can be the primary problem, or a secondary manifestation of underlying pathology, such as infection, intervertebral disc disease, vertebral compression fracture, or bone metastasis. MPS diagnosis requires thorough physical examination for muscular 'trigger points' (TPs). A TP is a hyperirritable nodule in skeletal muscle that may be palpable, is painful on compression, and can cause characteristic referred pain and/or autonomic phenomena (Simons et al., 1999). Physical therapy alone may suffice, but many patients benefit from local anaesthetic TP injections. Other therapies comprise both interventional (e.g. dry needling, acupuncture, pulse radiofrequency, botulinum toxin (BTX) injection) and non-interventional (e.g. spray and stretch) approaches.

Intra-articular injections

Arthritis and joint-related pain are common in populations with advanced illness. Corticosteroids are most commonly used for intra-articular injections, although data comparing various agents are limited (Bliddal et al., 2006). Possible complications include infection, bleeding, nerve injury, or joint destruction.

Botulinum toxin injection

BTX is a potent neuroparalytic agent produced by the bacterium *Clostridium botulinum*. It irreversibly inhibits acetylcholine release at the neuromuscular junction, thereby causing localized chemodenervation at the target organ (e.g. muscle, glands), with minimal systemic adverse effects. More relevant to pain, BTX-A also may block peripheral sensitization and indirectly reduce central sensitization (Aoki, 2005).

In addition to its use in spasticity and movement disorders, BTX is used as an analgesic in migraine, interstitial cystitis, and chronic myofascial pain (Foster et al., 2001; Gobel et al., 2001). Evidence in the latter condition is inconclusive (Soares et al., 2012), but it is generally safe and well tolerated, and may be repeated. When effective, its effects usually become evident approximately 1 week after injection; benefit lasts 3–4 months and then fades. Repeated administration may lead to diminishing benefit due to the development of neutralizing antibodies. To limit this, an interval of at least 12 weeks between injections is recommended, and if positive effects are lost, they may be regained by using an alternative formulation. There are at least four commercially available BTX-A preparations, one BTX-B preparation, and recent report of a BTX-F preparation.

Regional administration of agents that modify neural transmission

Peripheral nerve blocks and catheters

Regional local anaesthetic neural blockade is best used for pain in the distribution of a peripheral nerve or plexus. It is most frequently used perioperatively and also is applied to the treatment of acute pain caused by tumour, pathological fractures, and/or ischaemia. Occasional patients with chronic pain are candidates for repeated or continuous local anaesthetic blockade, which may be facilitated by placement of a catheter near the peripheral nerve (Vranken et al., 2001; Okell and Brooks, 2009). Almost any somatic nerve can be blocked and ultrasound techniques have been developed to improve the accuracy of needle or catheter placement (Hadzic, 2012). Long-term catheters may be complicated by infection, local anaesthetic toxicity, catheter displacement, or technical difficulties such as catheter knotting. With good care and strict attention to sterility, however, peripheral nerve catheters can be maintained for several weeks.

Spinal corticosteroid injection techniques

Although efficacy data are inconclusive, broad experience suggests that selected patients with neck, back, and/or spinal radicular pain unrelated to serious illness may benefit from translaminar (Abram, 1999), transforaminal (Riew et al., 2000), or caudal epidural steroid injections. These and related injection techniques may be used to treat comorbid spinal pain or radiculopathy in populations with advanced illness. Despite limited data suggesting efficacy, subarachnoid steroid injection for intractable pain remains controversial because of concern about neurotoxicity, and should be considered experimental.

Neural destructive techniques: neurolytic blockade, surgical techniques

Chemical neurolysis: alcohol and phenol

Phenol and ethyl alcohol (ethanol) are the agents most frequently used for neurolytic blocks (Burton et al., 2009). Phenol has both local anaesthetic and neurolytic effects, resulting in nearly painless injection. Excessive doses or accidental intravascular phenol injection may cause convulsions, central nervous system depression, or cardiovascular collapse. In contrast, ethanol has few significant adverse effects from systemic absorption but may cause pain on injection. There are few comparative data for choosing a neurolytic agent.

Radiofrequency (RF) techniques: RF ablation and pulsed RF treatment

RF neurotomy is the destruction of neural tissue with heat generated by a high-frequency electrical current (Niemisto et al., 2003). Conventional (thermal) RF, which creates a thermal lesion at the tip of the wire probe, has been used to denervate painful spinal facet joints, ablate trigeminal or dorsal root ganglia, and lesion thoracic or lumbar sympathetic ganglia. RF is rarely used to lesion somatic nerves supplying the skin due to risk of generating neuropathic pain.

In contrast to thermal RF, pulsed radiofrequency (PRF) applies radiofrequency current in short, high-voltage bursts. The time between bursts allows heat to dissipate. Although sufficient heat to damage tissue may occur, the mechanism by which PRF yields pain relief is not clearly understood, and is thought to involve a neuromodulatory effect rather than neurodestruction. The relatively non-destructive nature and good safety profile of PRF make it attractive for treating pain, but its role in pain management remains unclear (Gofeld et al., 2012). The technique may be useful in cases where conventional RF has limited indications, such as peripheral neuropathies, arthrogenic pain, painful trigger points, and modulation of dorsal root ganglion (Chua et al., 2011). There is no published experience in the treatment of pain related to serious illness.

Sympathetic nervous system block

Sympathetic blockade, with local anaesthetic or neurolytic solutions, can be used for a variety of pain problems, including neuropathic, ischaemic, and/or visceral pain, complex regional pain syndrome (CRPS), and pain from other acute processes (e.g. renal colic, or ischaemic crises in Raynaud's disease or obliterative arteriopathies) (Breivik and Cousins, 2009). Local anaesthetic sympathetic block has been used to predict response to sympathetic neurolysis, but response to local anaesthetic blockade should be interpreted with caution because of the analgesic effect of absorbed (systemic) local anaesthetic and/or placebo response.

In advanced malignancy, neurolytic sympathetic blocks are used for abdominal (coeliac plexus block), pelvic (superior hypogastric plexus block), and perineal (ganglion impar block) pain of visceral origin (Table 9.8.1). These blocks are generally done with fluoroscopic or computed tomography (CT) imaging to guide needle placement; ultrasound guidance may also be an option (Bhatnagar et al., 2012). Although patients with mixed somatic (from tumour invasion of somatic structures) and visceral pain may experience incomplete relief, even partial relief from sympathetic blockade may allow reduction in opioid doses and fewer side effects as a result.

Coeliac plexus/splanchnic nerve block

Neurolytic coeliac plexus block (NCPB) and or neurolytic splanchnic block are used for upper abdominal pain from unresectable pancreatic or other upper abdominal malignancies (Burton et al., 2009). NCPB produces good to excellent relief in 85–90%

Table 9.8.1 Neurolytic sympathetic blockade by location and clinical indication

Location	Clinical use	Results
Stellate ganglion block[a]	Angina, inoperable coronary artery disease Upper extremity pain: ◆ complex regional pain syndrome ◆ peripheral vascular disease ◆ Raynaud's disease ◆ brachial plexus infiltration by tumour ◆ herpes zoster ◆ phantom pain	Rarely indicated[a] Upper thoracic (T2–3) paravertebral sympathectomy (surgical or radiofrequency ablation) is the preferred technique of cervicothoracic sympathectomy when needed
Coeliac plexus block[b]	Visceral pain from: ◆ pancreatic cancer ◆ other upper abdominal tumours	Partial to complete pain relief in 90% of patients alive after 3 months. Results similar for pancreatic cancer and other abdominal malignancies (Eisenberg et al., 1995)
Lumbar sympathetic block[b]	Kidney pain (including 'phantom kidney pain') Intractable lower extremity pain: ◆ inoperable peripheral vascular disease ◆ chronic painful leg ulceration ◆ complex regional pain syndrome ◆ phantom pain ◆ herpes zoster ◆ diabetic neuropathy Testicular pain	Variable, depending on pain condition Peripheral vascular disease: 50–80% of patients experience partial or complete relief of pain at rest (Breivik and Cousins, 2009)
Superior hypogastric plexus block[b]	Pelvic visceral pain from gynaecological, colorectal, or genitourinary cancer	Long-lasting relief in 70% of patients with positive response to diagnostic block (Burton et al., 2009)
Ganglion impar block[b]	Intractable perineal pain	Case series suggest efficacy but little data available (Burton et al., 2009)

[a] Neurolysis of the stellate ganglion is controversial, due to risk of complications. In some cases, persistent relief can be achieved from a series of local anaesthetic blocks (Breivik and Cousins 2009).

[b] Some clinicians do a local anaesthetic block before proceeding with neurolytic block to assess the effect of neurolysis.

of patients and pain relief persisting until death in 70–90% of responders (Eisenberg et al., 1995). A recent Cochrane review concluded that NCPB reduces opioid consumption and side effects (Arcidiacono et al., 2011). Given a favourable risk:benefit ratio, this approach is widely accepted as the next step for patients with pain due to upper abdominal malignancy that fails to respond promptly to systemic opioid therapy. Although NCPB was associated with longer survival in patients with significant preoperative pain (Staats et al., 2002), a subsequent study failed to confirm a survival benefit (Wong et al., 2004).

Both NCPB and neurolytic splanchnic block may be accomplished percutaneously, typically under fluoroscopic control, or by endoscopic ultrasound-guided transoesophageal injection. Extant data are not sufficient to determine whether any of these procedures is better than any other (Arcidiacono et al., 2011). Outpatient treatment is possible, but frail patients or those living far away may be best served by overnight observation. Immediately following the procedure, many patients have diarrhoea and/or orthostatic hypotension, which are typically transient; patients may rarely need oral ephedrine (30 mg three times daily) for orthostatic hypotension or an oral opioid for diarrhoea. Major catastrophic complications are rare: a survey of 2730 patients reported four cases of paraplegia (incidence 1:683)

(Davies, 1993). It is postulated that paraplegia after NCPB is due to ischaemic spinal cord injury from injury or spasm of the artery of Adamkiewicz. Other rare complications include aortic dissection, generalized seizures, and circulatory arrest (Burton et al., 2009). It is unclear if complication risk is affected by the technique or imaging used. Paralysis has even been reported after open, intraoperative NCPB (Abdalla and Schell, 1999).

Lumbar sympathetic block

Intractable lower extremity ischaemic pain due to inoperable peripheral vascular disease is the most common indication for neurolytic lumbar sympathetic block (NLSB). In such settings, NLSB appears to increase cutaneous blood flow, reduce rest pain, and enhance healing of chronic ischaemic ulceration (Breivik and Cousins, 2009). NLSB may also reduce neuropathic lower extremity pain, especially in CRPS. Less common indications are visceral pain from lower abdominal or pelvic structures, such as renal pain, testicular pain, and tenesmus. Serious complications from NLSB are rare when radiographic imaging is used. Lumbar sympathectomy done by NLSB or surgery has comparable results: most peripheral vascular disease patients experience partial or complete relief of pain at rest, and mean duration of effect is approximately 6 months. Compared to surgical sympathectomy,

NLSB is less invasive; has lower morbidity, mortality, and cost; and can be repeated.

Neuraxial neurolysis: spinal neurolytic injection techniques

The aim of neuraxial neurolysis is to produce a chemical posterior rhizotomy, interrupting pain signal transmission. Although use is decreasing, clinical experience supports the approach in selected patients with advanced cancer. Subarachnoid neurolysis should be restricted to patients with advanced malignancy and pain limited to a few dermatomes (Candido and Stevens, 2003), for example, perineal pain in patients with colostomy and permanent bladder catheter or in those with relatively localized (unilateral) chest wall or trunk pain (Burton et al., 2009). Pain relief may last for 6–12 months, with a rate of reported complications between 1% and 14%, which is acceptable to some patients. The approach also is considered for non-ambulatory, incontinent patients with severe lower-extremity spasticity that has not responded to systemic medications or spinal baclofen (Jarrett et al., 2002). Very rarely, extreme cases of lower-body and/or lower-extremity pain in bedbound, terminally ill patients with significant nerve root or spinal cord tumour involvement is managed with chemical cordectomy at the upper-lumbar or lower-thoracic dermatomal level (Burton et al., 2009).

Spinal analgesics: epidural and subarachnoid

Administration of analgesic drugs into either the epidural or subarachnoid (or intrathecal) space is the most common interventional pain therapy for patients with advanced malignancy whose pain cannot be controlled with systemic analgesics (Carr

and Cousins, 2009). These approaches allow one or more drugs to be delivered close to relevant spinal receptors (see Fig. 9.8.1) and will provide some patients with analgesia that could not be obtained with systemic therapies, and others with comparable analgesia but fewer side effects. A randomized controlled trial that compared an implantable subarachnoid drug delivery system to best medical management in patients with advanced cancer found that the spinal analgesic approach reduced pain and analgesic-related adverse effects, and perhaps increased 6-month survival (Smith et al., 2002). Spinal analgesics are included in widely accepted guidelines for the management of cancer pain that is poorly responsive to systemic analgesics (Ripamonti et al., 2012; National Comprehensive Cancer Network, 2013).

Morphine is the most frequently used spinal analgesic for chronic pain, but other opioids (hydromorphone, fentanyl, and sufentanil) are also used. When spinal opioid monotherapy is ineffective, opioids can be combined with other analgesics, most commonly local anaesthetics (bupivacaine, ropivacaine) and/or clonidine. Best practices for these and other drug combinations are outlined in the 2012 Polyanalgesic Consensus Conference report (Deer et al., 2012c). In the United States, morphine (epidural and subarachnoid), clonidine (epidural), baclofen (subarachnoid), and ziconotide (subarachnoid) are the only drugs approved for chronic spinal administration, and other drugs are used off-label. Due to concern about neurotoxicity, and the safety of compounded 'custom' preparations, great caution is needed when considering analgesics not approved for spinal administration, including non-standard drug preparations, concentrations, doses, or multiple-drug combinations of approved analgesics (Deer et al., 2012c).

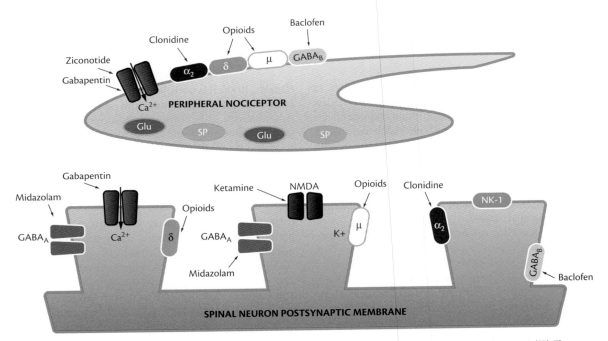

Fig. 9.8.1 Presynaptic primary afferent neurons (peripheral nociceptor) release neurotransmitters such as glutamate (Glu) and substance P (SP). These neurotransmitters stimulate secondary neurons in the dorsal horn (spinal neuron post synaptic membrane), sending pain signals to the brain. Inhibition of ion channel permeability decreases neurotransmitter release and decreases responsiveness of dorsal horn neurons to reduce transmission of noxious stimuli to the brain. Activation of inhibitory receptors (μ and δ opioid; GABA (γ-aminobutyric acid); $α_2$-adrenergic) also is a means by which pain transmission may be modulated. The drugs shown reduce pain transmission, and are believed to be active at the sites indicated (arrows). Some agents exert their effect presynaptically, others act on postsynaptic receptors, and many act on both.

Spinal opioid administration

Spinal administration delivers opioid close to the opioid receptors within the dorsal horns of the spinal grey matter, where they reside on both presynaptic (peripheral afferent nociceptor) and post-synaptic (second-order spinal neuron) nerve terminals. Opioid binding inhibits synaptic transmission between primary afferent nociceptors and second-order spinal neurons, and reduces the firing of the second-order neurons. Following spinal administration, cerebrospinal fluid (CSF) opioid concentrations are far in excess of plasma concentrations, and the time course of analgesia correlates with CSF opioid concentration rather than with plasma concentrations (Carr and Cousins, 2009).

Adverse effects of spinal opioids

Most common spinal opioid adverse effects are those of opioid therapy in general. The incidence of these effects is not high when spinal opioids are used in patients with advanced illness because these patients usually have developed opioid tolerance during prior systemic administration. When adverse effects occur, they are often self-limiting or can be successfully managed by dose adjustment. While the opioid dose is being adjusted, adverse effects due to excess opioid may be managed with small naloxone doses, often without reducing opioid analgesia. In this setting, naloxone is best administered as an intravenous loading dose, given in 40-microgram increments, followed by intravenous infusion (approximately 1–5 micrograms/kg/hour) titrated to effect. Constipation is a problem to which tolerance may not develop; therefore, it should be anticipated and managed.

Although respiratory depression from spinal opioid therapy is uncommon, it can occur at initiation of treatment or with subsequent spinal catheter or pump adjustments (Scherens et al., 2006; Deer et al., 2012b). Occasionally, delayed respiratory depression (onset 3–20 hours) occurs, presumably as a result of cephalad opioid migration within the CSF (Carr and Cousins, 2009). These risks require that opioid dosing adjustments be made cautiously. Other, more common adverse effects, such as endocrine abnormalities, sweating, and peripheral oedema, are associated with both systemic and spinal chronic opioid therapy (Katz and Mazer, 2009). In one study of spinal opioid for non-malignant pain (Winkelmuller and Winkelmuller, 1996), most male and all female patients developed hypogonadotropic hypogonadism, and other endocrine abnormalities were also common. Peripheral oedema associated with chronic spinal opioid, related to opioid antidiuretic effect, is usually managed with diuretics, but may require opioid rotation or change to non-opioid analgesics (Deer et al., 2012c). Analgesic tolerance and likely associated hyperalgesia also may accompany chronic systemic or spinal opioid administration (Angst and Clark 2006; Chu et al., 2008). Very high doses of either systemic or spinal opioid may cause an opioid-induced toxicity syndrome, potentially including delirium, myoclonus, and hyperalgesia (De Conno et al., 1991). The best way to avoid these effects is to limit opioid dose by optimizing non-opioid analgesics, and non-pharmacologic therapies; more severe toxicity may be managed with opioid rotation.

Non-opioid spinal analgesics

When spinal opioids do not provide adequate analgesia, addition of a local anaesthetic may help (Carr and Cousins, 2009; Deer et al., 2012c). Bupivacaine is most commonly used, whereas lignocaine (lidocaine) and tetracaine are generally avoided due to concern for neurotoxicity. Local anaesthetics may both decrease nociceptive input and reduce sensitization of spinal cord neurons. Blockade of pain transmission without loss of sensory or motor function is usually possible, and may be more readily obtained with epidural than with subarachnoid use. Subarachnoid local anaesthetic requires low (less than 20–30 mg bupivacaine per day) and carefully adjusted doses. Refractory pain in non-ambulatory terminally ill patients sometimes is managed with high-dose subarachnoid local anaesthetic (> 48 mg bupivacaine per day), which produces spinal anaesthesia, with dense sensory and motor block.

Clonidine, an α_2-adrenergic agonist, is well accepted as a spinal analgesic and typically is administered along with an opioid and/or local anaesthetic. Analgesic efficacy was demonstrated in randomized controlled trials that evaluated effects in cancer pain (Eisenach et al., 1995) and spinal cord injury pain (Siddall et al., 2000). Adverse effects, including hypotension, bradycardia, and sedation, are dose related and generally manageable. However, a case report of spinal cord damage after 3 years of uneventful subarachnoid clonidine-bupivacaine administration (Perren et al., 2004) is a reminder that there are few safety data on long-term administration of custom compounded combination spinal analgesic solutions.

Chronic subarachnoid baclofen infusion via an implanted pump is useful for severe spasticity in patients unresponsive to, or intolerant of, oral baclofen. There also may be some efficacy as a co-analgesic for CRPS, musculoskeletal pain related to spasticity, and neuropathic pain (Deer et al., 2012c). Spinal administration, which results in significantly higher CSF concentrations than oral administration (despite doses 100–1000 times lower), is generally well tolerated and no significant neurotoxicity has been identified.

Ziconotide, a synthetic analogue of an omega-conotoxin derived from the marine snail *Conus magus*, produces analgesia by blocking N-type calcium channels in the superficial dorsal horn of the spinal cord. Subarachnoid dosing starts from 0.5 to 1.5 micrograms/day and is slowly titrated to an average dose of 7 micrograms/day. There is a narrow therapeutic window as a result of neuropsychiatric adverse events, including depression (perhaps with increased risk of suicide), cognitive impairment, hallucinations and depressed level of consciousness; rare adverse effects include creatine kinase level elevation and meningitis (perhaps due to infusion device contamination). Because of its narrow therapeutic window, ziconotide is rarely used as a single agent, but has been combined with morphine to improve intractable pain (Deer et al., 2012c), with documented efficacy in advanced cancer pain (Alicino et al., 2012).

Indications for spinal analgesics in palliative care

Spinal analgesics are used to manage chronic cancer pain (Carr and Cousins, 2009; Deer et al., 2011) and non-cancer pain in populations with serious illness. Limited life expectancy should not deter consideration of this approach, but is a factor in selecting among spinal administration systems. Spinal opioids work best for deep, constant somatic pain, whereas other types of pain (e.g. cutaneous, intermittent somatic such as pathologic fracture, intermittent visceral from intestinal obstruction, and coexistent cancer and non-cancer pain) are variably responsive. Neuropathic pain may respond but often requires trials of drug combinations, including clonidine, local anaesthetic, or ziconotide). Patients with extreme opioid tolerance are unlikely to have good pain control with spinal opioid alone, and will likely require coadministration of non-opioid spinal analgesic(s). In general, a spinal analgesic trial through a temporary catheter is recommended before permanent spinal delivery system implantation.

Contraindications to spinal analgesic therapy are similar to those for any regional anaesthetic technique, with additional concerns due to chronicity of spinal analgesia. Coagulopathy increases risk and anticoagulation therapy should be withheld before implementing therapy. Specific recommendations vary depending on the anticoagulant and the indication for its use; consensus statements by anaesthesiology professional societies are a useful guide (Gogarten et al., 2010; Horlocker et al., 2010). Septicaemia is an important contraindication due to the risk of spinal delivery system infection, and local infection is a contraindication if a site free of infection cannot be found for spinal catheter system implantation. Immunosuppression is generally only a relative contraindication for implantable devices. Ongoing chemotherapy or radiation therapy is not a contraindication to spinal analgesic therapy, and radiation therapy is a concern only if the portal includes a surgical site. In the latter situation, a simple percutaneous spinal catheter may be used until the effects of radiation are clear; percutaneous spinal catheters have been utilized for prolonged periods with appropriate sterile technique (Nitescu et al., 1995; Aprili et al., 2009).

Spinal metastasis is not a contraindication for spinal therapy. To avoid trauma to a friable tumour mass or neural injury caused by needle or catheter placement into a stenotic spinal canal, catheters should be inserted away from metastases, under fluoroscopy. If CSF circulation may be impeded by an expanding tumour, the catheter should be placed cephalad to the lesion.

Technical considerations and complications in spinal drug administration

The system used to deliver intraspinal drug may be as simple as a 'low-tech', percutaneous catheter for intermittent injection or as sophisticated as a totally implanted high-tech infusion pump system. No single system is appropriate for all cases, and any system can result in complications, such as infection, catheter dislodgement, or other failures (Table 9.8.2) (Aprili et al., 2009; Carr and Cousins, 2009). Before initiating long-term spinal analgesia, adequate medical, nursing and social support to assist with maintenance of the specific system and address any complications should be confirmed.

'High-tech' implantable pump systems have long battery life, need refills at regular intervals (typically 1–2 months), and may have capacity for patient-activated bolus dose administration, in addition to continuous infusion (Brogan and Winter, 2011). They are generally reserved for patients with a life expectancy of at least a few months, because of high start-up costs. Because they have small medication-reservoir volume (20–50 mL), the use of commercially available (dilute) bupivacaine and/or clonidine preparations is impractical and custom-compounded solutions are needed (Deer et al., 2012c). Compounds pose a risk of contamination and infection, or potential overdose if high-concentration solution is inadvertently injected into the subcutaneous tissue surrounding the pump ('pocket fill') or into the spinal catheter injection port (allowing direct access to the spinal fluid) (Deer et

al., 2012b). Pump refill, accomplished by placing a needle through the skin into the pump refill port, is usually technically straightforward, but may be associated with devastating drug overdose if the refill solution is not correctly injected into the refill port; therefore, refills require physician or skilled nursing personnel.

'Low-tech' spinal infusion systems usually consist of an epidural or subarachnoid catheter connected to an implanted or externalized injection port (Carr and Cousins, 2009). Spinal analgesics are then administered by intermittent injection or external pump. Advantages of subarachnoid analgesia are efficiency and potency, which may translate into improved analgesia with lower drug cost. Therapy requires adequate skilled nursing assistance and/or physician evaluation. Percutaneous catheters or implanted injection port systems with or without external infusion pumps may be managed by some patients and/or family members, but still require periodic nursing support. It is possible to initiate and maintain percutaneous subarachnoid analgesia at home for terminally ill, homebound patients, if physician home visits can be arranged (Mercadante 1994).

Infection (meningitis, epidural abscess, or encephalitis) may occur with any delivery system but is more of a concern with the 'low-tech' spinal infusion systems (Aprili et al., 2009). Experience has shown that the risk is low if aseptic technique during placement is followed by careful maintenance and medication administration. Risk is further reduced by use of bacterial filters (0.2 micrometres) and a sterile technique that strictly minimizes changing external infusion pump reservoirs and tubing (Nitescu et al., 1995; Aprili et al., 2009). Infections are usually superficial, localized to skin at the catheter insertion or implantation site. Cultures of any drainage can guide antibiotic therapy. Epidural abscess and meningitis are rare, but must be treated aggressively because they may cause permanent neurological deficit or death. Although an epidural system usually is removed as part of epidural abscess management, the catheter may temporarily serve as a drainage conduit from the epidural space. Antibiotics may be delivered via the epidural catheter (Du Pen, 1999), but if infection does not rapidly improve, the catheter should be removed. Meningitis associated with subarachnoid catheter systems should be treated with intravenous antibiotics, but treatment may also include antibiotics delivered via the subarachnoid system (only antibiotics suitable for subarachnoid administration, such as vancomycin, should be administered through the spinal catheter). If the infection does not rapidly clear with antibiotics, the subarachnoid catheter system should be removed (Mercadante, 1999). In end-of-life care, attempts to contain the infection without removal of the system may be appropriate.

Any spinal catheter system may malfunction. Malfunction typically is signalled by abrupt or gradual worsening of pain (which may be difficult to distinguish from disease progression) or the development of withdrawal. Infusion device function can be evaluated using epidurography or myelography to verify catheter location and patency, and plain radiographs to help confirm the structural integrity of the spinal system.

The efficacy of epidural infusion also may be compromised by epidural fibrosis, that is, formation of scar tissue around the catheter within the epidural space (Cherry and Gourlay, 1992). Epidural fibrosis is a variable process and may develop as early as 2 weeks after epidural catheter placement. It limits analgesic solution spread, resulting in pain on injection and/or loss of analgesic

Table 9.8.2 Evaluation and management of spinal catheter complications

Catheter system	Symptoms	Complication	Prevention	Evaluation	Management
Epidural	Back pain Paraesthesias on injection Loss of analgesic effect No signs of infection	Epidural fibrosis (Cherry and Gourlay, 1992)	Unknown	Epidurography	Replace epidural or insert subarachnoid catheter
	Back and extremity pain Weakness Sensory abnormalities Fever, Leucocytosis	Epidural infection or abscess	Sterile technique, bacterial filters (Du Pen, 1999)	Catheter aspirate for Gram stain, culture; spine MRI	Catheter aspiration for decompression Intravenous antibiotics Remove catheter
Epidural or subarachnoid	Loss of analgesic effect Opioid withdrawal	Catheter dislodgement or disconnection	Implanted rather than percutaneous system; subarachnoid catheter anchored to fascia	Plain radiographs with contrast injection via catheter	Revise or replace catheter
		Pump malfunction	Pump maintenance; utilize low volume and low battery alarm	Pump analysis; technical support from manufacturer	Revise or replace pump
	Erythema, tenderness at catheter insertion point or incision site	Infection at catheter insertion site	Sterile technique Catheter care	Culture: catheter exit site catheter aspirate	Antibiotics Local site care Remove catheter system if no rapid improvement
Subarachnoid	Meningeal irritation: severe headache, cervical stiffness, photophobia, fever	Meningitis	Sterile technique Bacterial filters for pump refill or on percutaneous catheters	Catheter aspirate (CSF) for cell count, Gram stain, glucose, culture	Systemic (and possibly subarachnoid) antibiotics Remove catheter system if no rapid improvement
	Spinal cord compression: paraesthesias, weakness	Subarachnoid granuloma	Unknown Avoid excessive doses, concentrations of spinal opioid	Spine imaging: MRI or CT myelogram	Discontinue spinal analgesics Surgical consultation if significant sensory or motor deficits present

effect. Management requires repositioning the epidural catheter or replacing it with a subarachnoid catheter.

Although scarring around subarachnoid catheters rarely occurs, these systems may be complicated by catheter-tip granuloma formation. These lesions are rare, may develop slowly over several weeks, and can present with loss of pain control, sensory abnormality, or weakness progressing to paralysis. Most granulomas occur with chronic opioid administration and may be related to activation of opioid receptors on inflammatory cells. Consideration should be given to evaluating for catheter-tip granuloma whenever a patient reports worsening pain control, or the new onset of back pain, radicular pain, or sensory or motor abnormalities. Spine magnetic resonance imaging (MRI) is the preferred imaging technique (patients with spinal pumps can undergo MRI), but CT myelography is a good alternative. Surgical resection of a granuloma is only indicated if significant neurologic deficit is present. Otherwise, discontinuation of spinal analgesics may be followed by shrinkage of the granuloma and symptomatic improvement. Careful monitoring is required to ensure that improvement occurs (Deer et al., 2012a, 2012d).

Patients with worsening pain as a result of a technical problem or complication often require systemic analgesics to relieve pain and prevent opioid withdrawal. Subarachnoid morphine doses are approximately 10% of epidural doses, and 1% of systemic

(parenteral) doses, but these estimations are just starting points, and must be used cautiously in order to prevent significant under or over-dosing. Lignocaine (lidocaine), 50–100 mg/hour, or ketamine 10–20 mg/hour, by intravenous or subcutaneous infusion, may temporarily control intractable pain unresponsive to opioids (Tremont-Lukats et al., 2005). If intravenous ketamine is utilized, a benzodiazepine should be administered also to control possible dysphoric hallucinations.

Neurosurgical interventions for intractable pain: intracerebroventricular opioid and neuro-destructive interventions

Catheter techniques are rarely used for opioid administration directly into the cerebral ventricles (Raffa and Pergolizzi, 2012). Data suggest that intracerebroventricular opioid is a reasonable option for intractable pain (usually cancer related) in the following settings: inadequate analgesia through conventional techniques, inaccessible spinal epidural and subarachnoid spaces, known obstruction of spinal CSF circulation, and/or intractable head and neck pain. A Cochrane review (Ballantyne and Carwood, 2005) concluded on the basis of case series that intracerebroventricular opioid may have efficacy similar to spinal analgesics, with a lower incidence of complications, but no comparative studies are available.

In recent years, with increasing use of systemic and spinal analgesics, there has been a reduction in use of destructive neurosurgical procedures for control of intractable pain. Nonetheless, these techniques are potentially valuable in selected pain syndromes (Raslan and Burchiel, 2010). These procedures most commonly target the spinal cord, but may target the brainstem or brain. Percutaneous, image-guided ablation techniques potentially limit the need for open surgical interventions. Spinothalamic cordotomy, the most common, is best used for intractable unilateral somatic pain in the lower body (or at least below the level of the neck) (Raslan et al., 2011). Rarely, midline myelotomy (for midline visceral pain) and dorsal root entry zone lesioning (for localized neuropathic pain such as brachial plexopathy) are considered (Romanelli et al., 2004). Neurosurgical procedures to disrupt pathways involved in emotional processing (e.g. cingulotomy) are very rarely utilized.

Miscellaneous techniques for pain control

Vertebroplasty and kyphoplasty

Vertebral compression fractures are an important cause of pain and morbidity in patients with serious illnesses and can be caused by metastatic cancer, multiple myeloma, or bone loss after radiotherapy, hormonal treatment, steroids, and poor overall medical status (Aghayev et al., 2011) (see also Chapter 12.5). Osteoporotic vertebral compression fractures not only are painful, but increase mortality (Bliuc et al., 2009). Percutaneous vertebroplasty and kyphoplasty are similar minimally invasive procedures, in which a fractured vertebra is stabilized by injection of polymethylmethacrylate bone cement into the vertebral body via large-bore needles (Burton et al., 2005; Nairn et al., 2011). Both procedures provide good to excellent pain relief to 80–90% of people with painful vertebral compression fractures due to osteoporosis, and 50–60% of those with painful neoplastic vertebral fractures. In vertebroplasty, bone cement is injected through needles into the interstices of the vertebral body marrow space. Kyphoplasty includes inflation of a high-pressure balloon in the vertebral body to create a cavity, which is subsequently filled with bone cement. The balloon expansion may partially restore vertebral height, but the degree of height restoration may be modest and is of unclear significance. There are no comparative studies between these techniques. A randomized, controlled trial comparing kyphoplasty with non-interventional, conservative management strongly favoured kyphoplasty in terms of pain, disability, quality of life, and decreased analgesic use (Berenson et al., 2011). Rapid pain relief from percutaneous vertebroplasty or kyphoplasty may improve patient tolerance of needed antitumor therapies, such as positioning for radiation therapy (Aghayev et al., 2011).

Both vertebroplasty and kyphoplasty requires neuraxial imaging (MRI or CT) to evaluate vertebral anatomy, with attention to possible extension of bone fragments or tumour into the spinal canal. MRI is especially useful for detecting acute vertebral compression fractures because vertebral marrow oedema (indicating acute fracture) is readily identified. Bone scintigraphy is less useful because it will identify increased activity at a fracture site for up to 2 years, long after the fracture may have spontaneously stabilized.

Absolute contraindications for vertebral augmentation are spinal cord compression with clinical myelopathy, overt spinal instability

(i.e. subluxation), and osteomyelitis. Relative contraindications include posterior vertebral defects, epidural tumour spread, and cervical fractures. The overall complication rate for these procedures is low, but cement extrusion into the spinal canal can result in neural compromise, and cement venous embolism can cause pulmonary embolism (Burton et al., 2005; Nairn et al., 2011).

Spinal cord stimulation

Spinal cord stimulation (SCS) is a minimally invasive and readily reversible approach to neuropathic and nociceptive pain, most frequently used for post-laminectomy syndrome and CRPS (for detailed discussion see Chapter 9.9). It can be efficacious for intractable angina (Yu et al., 2004), peripheral neuropathic pain (e.g. diabetic or chemotherapy-induced neuropathy), abdominal visceral pain (Tiede et al., 2006), and ischaemic pain from peripheral vascular disease (Ubbink and Vermeulen, 2013). Its analgesic mechanism has not been fully elucidated.

SCS involves placing stimulating electrode arrays in the epidural space overlying the posterior aspect of the spinal cord. Current is delivered by an internal, battery-powered pulse generator. SCS stimulation paraesthesias are generally perceived as warm, soothing sensations associated with pain relief. A trial using temporary leads can help determine patient response prior to permanent placement. As many as 50–60% of patients who undergo a SCS trial experience meaningful pain relief (defined as reduction of pain by at least 50%). Although some stimulator systems have limited MRI compatibility, most are not MRI compatible; therefore, compatibility must be determined from the manufacturer for each specific stimulator and MRI study.

Palliative sedation: management of intractable pain when all else fails

Despite advances in palliative care, a few patients still experience distressing end-of-life symptoms, including pain or delirium (Maltoni et al., 2012). To address intractable pain and suffering, 'anaesthetic' rather than 'analgesic' interventions may be considered. Palliative sedation is a medical intervention, clearly different than euthanasia, and accepted guidelines for proper use have been proposed (Cherny and Radbruch, 2009). Appropriate use requires a clinician to distinguish symptoms that are merely difficult to control from symptoms that are truly refractory to standard treatments, including interventional pain therapies. This distinction will protect patients with refractory symptoms from futile interventions, and avoid unnecessary sedation in patients with difficult but controllable symptoms (Cherny and Radbruch, 2009). Obtaining 'second opinion' from a pain specialist or multidisciplinary palliative care team, may help determine if effective symptom management therapies are yet available. For detailed discussion of this issue see Chapter 18.2.

Conclusion

There have been important advances in the therapies used to control pain in populations with serious illness. In developed countries, systemic opioid and adjuvant analgesics are widely available and are used with increasing sophistication and improved effect, although cost and other barriers (Fisch et al., 2012) continue to limit analgesic access. Unfortunately, poor access to analgesics in developing nations often denies people their fundamental human right to pain treatment (Cousins and Lynch, 2011). Across the globe, there is increasing scrutiny on health-care institutions and providers, which is intended to encourage the delivery of patient-centred care that efficiently and effectively improves outcomes, including quality of life. In addition to assured access to systemic analgesics, the availability of selected interventional pain therapies should be viewed as a goal to optimize pain management.

The need for access to interventional pain therapies has become more certain with increasing recognition that opioid analgesia has significant limitations. For many patients, systemic opioids cannot provide satisfactory analgesia with acceptable side effects, and poor outcomes combined with emerging concerns about adverse effects such as neuroendocrine and sleep disturbances underscore the need to evaluate and manage risk when opioids are used. Interventional pain therapies are key components of this strategy and are now incorporated into best practices for cancer pain management (Ripamonti et al., 2012; National Comprehensive Cancer Network 2013). These therapies, especially spinal analgesics, NCPB, and vertebroplasty, have become essential components of palliative care, to control pain that cannot be safely and effectively managed with systemic analgesics. Most patients now suffering from uncontrolled pain need not await clinical application of new developments but could benefit from well-coordinated and consistent application of available techniques, including interventional pain management therapies.

Online materials

Complete references for this chapter are available online at <http://www.oxfordmedicine.com>.

References

Abdalla, E.K. and Schell, S.R. (1999). Paraplegia following intraoperative celiac plexus injection. *Journal of Gastrointestinal Surgery*, 3, 668–671.

Abram, S.E. (1999). Treatment of lumbosacral radiculopathy with epidural steroids. *Anesthesiology*, 91, 1937–1941.

Aghayev, K., Papanastassiou, I.D., and Vrionis, F. (2011). Role of vertebral augmentation procedures in the management of vertebral compression fractures in cancer patients. *Current Opinion in Supportive & Palliative Care*, 5, 222–226.

Alicino, I., Giglio, M., Manca, F., Bruno, F., and Puntillo, F. (2012). Intrathecal combination of ziconotide and morphine for refractory cancer pain: a rapidly acting and effective choice. *Pain*, 153, 245–249.

Angst, M.S. and Clark, J.D. (2006). Opioid-induced hyperalgesia: a qualitative systematic review. *Anesthesiology*, 104, 570–587.

Aoki, K.R. (2005). Review of a proposed mechanism for the antinociceptive action of botulinum toxin type A. *Neurotoxicology*, 26, 785–793.

Aprili, D., Bandschapp, O., Rochlitz, C., Urwyler, A., and Ruppen, W. (2009). Serious complications associated with external intrathecal catheters used in cancer pain patients: a systematic review and meta-analysis. *Anesthesiology*, 111, 1346–1355.

Ballantyne, J.C. and LaForge, K.S. (2007). Opioid dependence and addiction during opioid treatment of chronic pain. *Pain*, 129, 235–255.

Bliddal, H., Terslev, L., Qvistgaard, E., *et al.* (2006). A randomized, controlled study of a single intra-articular injection of etanercept or glucocorticosteroids in patients with rheumatoid arthritis. *Scandinavian Journal of Rheumatoloty*, 35, 341–345.

Bliuc, D., Nguyen, N.D., Milch, V.E., Nguyen, T.V., Eisman, J.A., and Center, J.R. (2009). Mortality risk associated with low-trauma osteoporotic fracture and subsequent fracture in men and women. *Journal of the American Medical Association*, 301, 513–521.

Brogan, S.E. and Winter, N.B. (2011). Patient-controlled intrathecal analgesia for the management of breakthrough cancer pain: a retrospective review and commentary. *Pain Medicine*, 12, 1758–1768.

Bruera, E. and Pereira, J. (1998). Recent developments in palliative cancer care. *Acta Oncologica*, 37, 749–757.

Candido, K. and Stevens, R.A. (2003). Intrathecal neurolytic blocks for the relief of cancer pain. Best Practice & Research. *Clinical Anaesthesiology*, 17, 407–428.

Carr, D.B. and Cousins, M.J. (2009). Spinal route of analgesia: opioids and future options for spinal analgesic chemotherapy. In M.J. Cousins, P.O. Bridenbaugh, D.B. Carr, and T.T. Horlocker (eds.) Cousins and Bridenbaugh's Neural Blockade in Clinical Anesthesia and Pain Medicine (4th ed.), pp. 886–947. Philadelphia, PA: Liippincott Williams & Wilkins.

Cherry, D.A. and Gourlay, G.K. (1992). CT contrast evidence of injectate encapsulation after long-term epidural administration. *Pain*, 49, 369–371.

De Conno, F., Caraceni, A., Martini, C., Spoldi, E., Salvetti, M., and Ventafridda, V. (1991). Hyperalgesia and myoclonus with intrathecal infusion of high-dose morphine. *Pain*, 47, 337–339.

Deer, T.R., Smith, H.S., Burton, A.W., et al. (2011). Comprehensive consensus based guidelines on intrathecal drug delivery systems in the treatment of pain caused by cancer pain. *Pain Physician*, 14, E283–E312.

Du Pen S. (1999). Complications of neuraxial infusion in cancer patients. *Oncology (Williston Park)*, 13(5 Suppl 2), 45–51.

Eisenach, J.C., DuPen, S., Dubois, M., Miguel, R., and Allin, D. (1995). Epidural clonidine analgesia for intractable cancer pain. *The Epidural Clonidine Study Group. Pain*, 61, 391–399.

Foster, L., Clapp, L., Erickson, M., and Jabbari, B. (2001). Botulinum toxin A and chronic low back pain: a randomized, double-blind study. *Neurology*, 56, 1290–1293.

Gobel, H., Heinze, A., Heinze-Kuhn, K., and Jost, W.H. (2001). Evidence-based medicine: botulinum toxin A in migraine and tension-type headache. *Journal of Neurology*, 248 Suppl 1, 34–38.

Gofeld, M., Restrepo-Garces, C.E., Theodore, B.R., and Faclier, G. (2012). Pulsed Radiofrequency of Suprascapular Nerve for Chronic Shoulder Pain: A Randomized Double-Blind Active Placebo-Controlled Study. *Pain Practice*, 13, 96–103.

Hadzic, A. (ed.) (2012). Hadzic's Peripheral Nerve Blocks and Anatomy for Ultrasound-Guided Regional Anesthesia, 2nd ed. (New York: McGraw-Hill Professional).

Jarrett, L., Nandi, P., and Thompson, A.J. (2002). Managing severe lower limb spasticity in multiple sclerosis: does intrathecal phenol have a role? *Journal of Neurology, Neurosurgery, and Psychiatry*, 73, 705–709.

Mercadante, S. (1994). Intrathecal morphine and bupivacaine in advanced cancer pain patients implanted at home. *Journal of Pain and Symptom Management*, 9, 201–207.

Mercadante, S. (1999). Problems of long-term spinal opioid treatment in advanced cancer patients. *Pain*, 79, 1–13.

Mercadante, S., Arcuri, E., Tirelli, W., and Casuccio, A. (2000). Analgesic effect of intravenous ketamine in cancer patients on morphine therapy: a randomized, controlled, double-blind, crossover, double-dose study. *Journal of Pain and Symptom Management*, 20, 246–252.

Nitescu, P., Sjoberg, M., Appelgren, L., and Curelaru, I. (1995). Complications of intrathecal opioids and bupivacaine in the treatment of "refractory" cancer pain. *Clinical Journal of Pain*, 11, 45–62.

Okell, R.W. and Brooks, N.C. (2009). Persistent pain relief following interscalene analgesia for cancer pain. *Anaesthesia*, 64, 225–226.

Ossipov, M.H., Lai, J., King, T., Vanderah, T.W., and Porreca, F. (2005). Underlying mechanisms of pronociceptive consequences of prolonged morphine exposure. *Biopolymers*, 80, 319–324.

Perren, F., Buchser, E., Chedel, D., Hirt, L., Maeder, P., and Vingerhoets, F. (2004). Spinal cord lesion after long-term intrathecal clonidine and bupivacaine treatment for the management of intractable pain. *Pain*, 109, 189–194.

Raffa, R.B. and Pergolizzi, J.V., Jr. (2012). Intracerebroventricular opioids for intractable pain. *British Journal of Clinical Pharmacology*, 74, 34–41.

Raslan, A.M., Cetas, J.S., McCartney, S., and Burchiel, K.J. (2011). Destructive procedures for control of cancer pain: the case for cordotomy. *Journal of Neurosurgery*, 114, 155–170.

Riew, K.D., Yin, Y., Gilula, L., et al. (2000). The effect of nerve-root injections on the need for operative treatment of lumbar radicular pain. A prospective, randomized, controlled, double-blind study. *Journal of Bone and Joint Surgery (American)*, 82-A, 1589–1593.

Romanelli, P., Esposito, V., and Adler, J. (2004). Ablative procedures for chronic pain. *Neurosurgery Clinics of North America*, 15, 335–342.

Scherens, A., Kagel, T., Zenz, M., and Maier, C. (2006). Long-term respiratory depression induced by intrathecal morphine treatment for chronic neuropathic pain. *Anesthesiology*, 105, 431–433.

Simons, D.G., Travell, J.G., and Simons, L.S. (1999). Travell & Simons' Myofascial Pain and Dysfunction: The Trigger Point Manual, 2nd ed. (Philadelphia: Lippincott Williams & Wilkins).

Soares, A., Andriolo, R.B., Atallah, A.N., and da Silva, E.M. (2012). Botulinum toxin for myofascial pain syndromes in adults. *Cochrane Database of Systemic Reviews*, Issue 4. Article No. CD007533.

Staats, P.S., Hekmat, H., Sauter, P., and Lillemoe, K. (2002). The effects of alcohol celiac plexus block, pain, and mood on longevity in patients with unresectable pancreatic cancer: A double-blinded, randomized, placebo-controlled study. *Pain Medicine*, 2, 28–34.

Tiede, J.M., Ghazi, S.M., Lamer, T.J., and Obray, J.B. (2006). The use of spinal cord stimulation in refractory abdominal visceral pain: case reports and literature review. *Pain Practice*, 6, 197–202.

Tremont-Lukats, I.W., Challapalli, V., McNicol, E.D., Lau, J., and Carr, D.B. (2005). Systemic administration of local anesthetics to relieve neuropathic pain: a systematic review and meta-analysis. *Anesthesia and Analgesia*, 101, 1738–1749.

Vranken, J.H., van der Vegt, M.H., Zuurmond, W.W., Pijl, A.J., and Dzoljic, M. (2001). Continuous brachial plexus block at the cervical level using a posterior approach in the management of neuropathic cancer pain. *Regional Anesthesia and Pain Medicine*, 26, 572–575.

Winkelmuller, M. and Winkelmuller, W. (1996). Long-term effects of continuous intrathecal opioid treatment in chronic pain of nonmalignant etiology. *Journal of Neurosurgery*, 85, 458–467.

Wong, G.Y., Schroeder, D.R., Carns, P.E., et al. (2004). Effect of neurolytic celiac plexus block on pain relief, quality of life, and survival in patients with unresectable pancreatic cancer: a randomized controlled trial. *Journal of the American Medical Association*, 291, 1092–1099.

Yu, W., Maru, F., Edner, M., Hellstrom, K., Kahan, T., and Persson, H. (2004). Spinal cord stimulation for refractory angina pectoris: a retrospective analysis of efficacy and cost-benefit. *Coronary Artery Disease*, 15, 31–37.

Neurostimulation in pain management

Joy Hao, Rae Lynne Kinler, Eliezer Soto, Helena Knotkova, and Ricardo A. Cruciani

Introduction to neurostimulation in pain management

Pain is highly prevalent and exerts a huge toll on individuals, families and society. A 2011 review conducted by the US Institute of Medicine exemplifies the scope of the problem. It found that 100 million American adults have chronic pain and estimated the annual cost burden to society at US$560–635 billion plus US$100 billion spent by the federal government (Institute of Medicine of the National Academies, 2011). Pain prevalence is likely to rise in most countries as age-related chronic illnesses increase and the long-term effects of HIV/AIDS evolve. Both health systems and individual health professionals face enormous challenges in providing safe and effective care for diverse populations with chronic pain.

Pain is a major factor in the burden associated with serious or life-threatening illnesses, and both the prevalence and the adverse consequences increase in advanced illness. Most studies have focused on populations with cancer and have determined that the prevalence of pain associated with varied solid tumours is 39–50% (Deandrea et al., 2014). The adverse effects of unrelieved pain on physical functioning, mood, coping and adaptation, and caregiver distress justify the widely-held view that pain management is a moral imperative in the clinical management of patients with advanced illness.

There is a strong international consensus that the first-line treatment for pain associated with serious or life-threatening illnesses is opioid therapy. Although broad experience with opioid therapy indicates that it is usually safe and effective, patients may not be able to access optimal therapy or may be unable to obtain satisfactory relief even when treatment is available. Indeed, some studies indicate a relatively high rate of inadequate pain relief (Nekolaichuk et al., 2013), the reasons for which are likely to be multifactorial and variable across settings.

Both non-opioid pharmacological therapies and non-pharmacological interventions are needed to optimize analgesic outcomes. If opioid therapy does not yield a favourable balance between analgesia and side effects, the patient should be considered to be poorly responsive to the current regimen and an alternative strategy should be selected. There are many options. Some, such as opioid rotation, the use of non-opioid or adjuvant analgesics, and varied interventions like neural blockade and neuraxial analgesia, are considered routinely.

Neurostimulation is another important strategy for pain. The term includes an array of interventions that involve precisely targeted stimulation of peripheral nerve, spinal cord, or the brain (Table 9.9.1). Some of these treatments, such as transcutaneous electrical nerve stimulation (TENS) and spinal cord stimulation (SCS), have been available for decades. Others, such as peripheral nerve stimulation (PNS) and transcranial stimulation techniques, have emerged more recently as viable options in pain management. Neurostimulation techniques are seldom used in the management of pain related to serious illness. A better understanding of the available treatments and the emergence of newer technologies, may increase access and use in the future.

Neurostimulation techniques

The treatments categorized as neurostimulation techniques are highly variable. They target different tissues with different stimulation modalities and use varied technologies to accomplish intended effects.

Transcutaneous electrical nerve stimulation

TENS is a non-invasive technique that uses electrodes on the skin to deliver electrical stimulation to peripheral nerves. The site selected for stimulation usually is in the region of the painful site, but may be at a distance, usually along the course of the peripheral nerves innervating the site (Atamaz et al., 2012). The approach is sometimes considered a rehabilitative modality comparable to heat, cold, vibration, or ultrasound; when used in this way, it may be directed by physical therapists as part of a programme intended to reduce symptoms and improve function. In some countries, however, TENS units may be acquired by patients for home use and applied primarily for the purpose of pain management.

TENS was developed after publication of the gate control theory, which suggested that stimulation of large-diameter, non-nociceptive primary afferent nerves may be able to modulate pain due to interactions with nociceptive pathways in the spinal cord (Johnson et al., 1991; Sluka and Walsh, 2003). Later studies demonstrated that stimulation of nerves can produce dose-dependent (80 Hz vs 30 Hz) segmental inhibition of

Table 9.9.1 Neurostimulation techniques

Strategy	Type of stimulation	Complexity and burden	Mechanism
Spinal cord stimulation (SCS)	Implantation of electrodes in the epidural space at the level of the posterior columns of the spinal cord	Invasive; outpatient surgical procedure; mid level of burden to patients	Modulation of pain signals at the level of the spinal cord and central modulation of the pain response
Transcutaneous electrical stimulation (TENS)	Electrodes are placed at the level of the painful region and stimulate the underlying area	Non-invasive; low level of burden to patients	Based on the 'gate theory' by Melzack and Wolf in which vibration closes the gate for pain information at the spinal cord level; also evidence for supraspinal mechanisms
Peripheral nerve stimulation (PNS)	Implantation of electrodes in the subcutaneous tissue over the peripheral nerve that innervates the affected area	Invasive; outpatient surgical procedure; intermediate level of burden to patients	Impulse interruption by collision; gate control within the spinal cord or supraspinal locations; inhibition of neuroma spontaneous activity
Transcranial direct current stimulation (tDCS)	Placement of electrodes on the scalp and forehead creating an electrical field between the two electrodes	Non-invasive; minimal burden to patients	Subthreshold modulation of neuronal resting membrane potential with subsequent changes of N-methyl-D-aspartate receptor
Transcranial magnetic stimulation (TMS)	Magnet placed on the scalp and stimulate the underlying brain tissue	Non-invasive; delivery can be painful; low burden to patients.	Modulation of brain neuronal excitability under the magnet and connections to other parts of the brain
Deep brain stimulation (DBS)	Leads placed in deep brain structures	Invasive; inpatient surgical intervention; high level of burden to patients	Modulates the activities of certain brain areas like the hypothalamus, thalamus, periaqueductal grey area
Motor cortex stimulation (MCS)	Grid placed on the motor cortex	Invasive; inpatient procedure; high level of burden to patients	Modulates the activity of the underlying cortex and connections to other brain areas

pressure-pain thresholds mediated by second-order neurons in the dorsal horn of the spinal cord (Chen and Johnson, 2009). Adenosine pathways are responsible, at least in part, for the TENS analgesia, as caffeine and adenosine antagonists can block the effect (Marchand and Charest, 1995). In addition, the endogenous opioid peptides, encephalins and dynorphins, may play a role and may actually mediate differential responses to low versus high TENS frequencies. Specifically, low-frequency TENS stimulation causes met-encephalin release (Han et al., 1991), implicating mu opioid receptors, and high-frequency TENS induces dynorphin A release that activates delta receptors (Kalra et al., 2001) at supraspinal and spinal levels (Sluka et al., 1999; Leonard et al., 2010).

The extent to which the effects of TENS is influenced by the placement of electrodes in the dermatome affected by injury has suggested the possibility that the effects of TENS in the spinal cord may be augmented or modified by more direct actions on peripheral nerves (Walsh et al., 1998). TENS can ameliorate chronic pain when applied to a region innervated by a specific peripheral nerve territory (Gersh et al., 1980; Engholm and Leffler, 2010) and TENS application to dermatomes can increases local pain threshold (Bjordal et al., 2007) and reduce postoperative pain (Chen et al., 1998; Yeh et al., 2010). The potential efficacy of TENS placed at traditional acupuncture points also suggests the importance of peripheral localization of the electrical stimulation (Ng and Hui-Chan, 2007, 2009).

The clinical use of TENS is largely based on favourable anecdotal experience. There have been few high-quality studies capable of determining safety and efficacy in different patient populations. Of the 43 studies in a recent systematic review of TENS treatment

for cancer pain, only two were randomized controlled trials (RCTs), 16 were non-randomized, 19 were educational articles, five were on non-cancer related pain, and one was on acute pain (Robb et al., 2009).

The two RCTs were too small to account for variability in settings and patients characteristics, and were considered yield inconclusive results. One of these studies randomly assigned 49 breast cancer patients with thoracic pain due to mastectomy to receive TENS, sham TENS, or transcutaneous spinal electro-analgesia (TSE) (Robb et al., 2007). Treatment for 3 weeks at the intensity recommended by the manufacturers produced no difference among the three arms in terms of the primary outcomes (pain intensity, anxiety, mood, and function); there was, however, less pain interference in the patients randomized to the TENS arm, and at study end, twice as many TENS than TSE patients decided to continue treatment. The second RCT randomized 15 cancer patients with advanced illness to sham, acupuncture-like TENS, or no treatment and found that 30-minute treatment periods for 5 consecutive days produced no difference in pain intensity among the groups (Gadsby et al., 1997).

A systematic review of TENS in patients with advanced illness who were receiving palliative care also noted that conclusions about efficacy are not possible given the limited data available (Pan et al., 2000). Most published experience is in the form of case series (Loh and Gulati 2013). More research is needed to determine whether TENS is efficacious and safe for pain associated with cancer or other serious illnesses.

The ability of TENS to increase blood flow at the site of high-frequency stimulation has raised concerns about the safety of TENS in patients with pain caused by tumour masses.

Theoretically, the application of TENS near a tumour could increase angiogenesis or tumour spread. Although recent studies indicate that the elevated blood flow at the TENS stimulation site is the result of increased muscle activity, and that high-frequency or low-frequency TENS below motor threshold has no clinically significant effect on blood flow in tumours (Cooperman et al., 1975; Cata et al., 2004), the limited data on safety may justify caution in the use of high-frequency TENS in those with metastatic disease.

Peripheral nerve stimulation

PNS for the management of pain is a strategy that became available in 1970s but has received more attention since the 1990s when more sophisticated leads and stimulators were developed (Verrills et al., 2009). Patients receiving PNS undergo implantation of one or more percutaneous leads adjacent to the peripheral nerves innervating a painful region (Long et al., 1981; Hassenbusch et al., 1996; Johnson and Burchiel, 2004). Nerve dissection is not required and the risk of nerve injury is minimal. Although the literature in support of this approach is mostly characterized by retrospective reviews and case series, the potential for this technology may be significant.

PNS has been utilized for a variety of pain syndromes, including occipital neuralgia, headache, and regional pains in the abdominal, pelvic, axial low back, and cervical regions. In a typical report, PNS was used to address pain in the distribution of sensory nerves that was part of a failed back surgery syndrome; all six patients experienced improvement in pain scores, decreased the utilization of pain medications, and experienced an improvement in function (Paicius et al., 2007). There have been no confirmatory controlled trials and no published experience in populations with serious medical illnesses.

Recently, a variation of PNS has been introduced, which is known as 'PNS cross- talk' (PNSCT). By creating an electrical circuit between leads, a larger area can be covered than would be possible using conventional PNS (Burgher et al., 2012). PNSCT has been proposed as an alternative to treat chronic regional and axial pain in patients refractory to conventional therapy (Falco et al., 2009). Controlled trials are needed to evaluate whether this approach is better than PNS and could be applied to the treatment of chronic pain in the medically ill.

Spinal cord stimulation

SCS is achieved by applying an electrical current to a specific area of the spinal cord (Shealy et al., 1967). Stimulation is accomplished using electrodes placed in the epidural space that deliver a current to the underlying posterior columns. Patient who are candidates for this therapy typically undergo an initial trial using percutaneous leads to determine whether stimulation can be provided to the painful area, and if so, whether it is associated with meaningful analgesia (Ghoname et al., 1999). Those who report benefit are offered subcutaneous implantation of the entire system, which includes the electrodes, connecting wires, and a radiofrequency transmitter. The system is equipped with an alarm that alerts when the batteries need to be replaced; newer systems are rechargeable.

The mode of action of SCS has not been elucidated, but like TENS and PNS, the approach was developed based on predictions developed from the gate control theory (Melzack and Wall, 1965). Specifically, stimulation of large-diameter afferents in the posterior columns may be able to segmentally inhibit transmission of impulses originating in small diameter nociceptive afferents. Ongoing research also suggests that SCS may inhibit transmission in the spinothalamic tract through the activation of central descending inhibitory mechanisms, influencing sympathetic efferent neurons, and releasing various inhibitory neurotransmitters (Oakley and Prager, 2002).

Stancak et al. tested patients with failed back surgery syndrome to determine the area of the central nervous system (CNS) where SCS has its effect. Functional magnetic resonance imaging (fMRI) technology showed that during SCS, there was a signal increase in the somatosensory cortex, primary motor cortex, and insula of the leg area and vicinity, while there was a concomitant signal decrease in the primary motor cortex corresponding to the shoulder. Applying a standardized suprathreshold heat stimulus to the lower leg of study subjects produced increases in the secondary somatosensory cortex, insula, thalamus, and cingulate cortex. During simultaneous spinal cord and painful heat stimulations, the left and right temporal poles and the ipsilateral cerebellar cortex were activated more strongly compared with the sum of the activations of the separate stimulations, suggesting modulation of pain-related activation by ongoing SCS.

In another study of SCS mechanisms, Nihashi and colleagues utilized fluorodeoxyglucose (FDG) positron emission tomography (PET) scanning to study metabolic/glucose uptake information in seven patients with complex regional pain syndrome (CRPS) and 13 controls (Nihashi et al., 2004). They found an increase of FDG metabolism in the left thalamus, secondary somatosensory cortex, anterior cingulate cortex, bilateral insula, dorsolateral prefrontal cortex, and bilateral superior temporal gyrus in the six patients where SCS was effective (defined by > 50% pain reduction). However, FDG uptake decreased in the posterior cingulate cortex.

Most reports of SCS have described case series of patients with neuropathic pains, such as radiculopathies, arachnoiditis (De La Porte and Siegfried, 1983), phantom limb pain, CRPS (Taylor 2006; Taylor et al., 2006), deafferentation syndromes (Sanchez-Ledesma et al., 1989), non-specific neuropathic pain (Kumar et al., 2008), brachial and lumbosacral plexopathies, and post-herpetic neuralgia (Tasker, 1998). Positive effects also were reported in 18 patients with visceral syndromes, such as interstitial cystitis, chronic abdominal pain, chronic pancreatitis, mediastinal pain (Guttman et al., 2009), and intractable angina (Kemler et al., 2000).

A systematic review of the literature on the use of SCS in cancer patients identified only four trials, all of them small observational or retrospective studies (Lihua et al., 2013). In one study, three of 11 patients reported greater than 50% analgesia and underwent implantation (Meglio et al., 1989). Another study of 14 lung cancer patients who underwent SCS implantation for the treatment of chest pain after surgical or radiological interventions noted a mean 71% decline in opioid use after implantation and a reduction in mean visual analogue score from 7.43 at baseline to 3.07 after 1 month and 2.07 after 12 months (Yakovlev et al., 2010). A survey of 15 patients with intractable, cancer-related, low back pain observed similar benefits after SCS implantation (Yakovlev and Resch, 2011).

A retrospective study of 454 patients undergoing SCS implantation for a variety of pain diagnoses observed that 71% of the patients reported partial to complete pain relief, 58% decreased analgesic use, and 11% stopped using analgesics completely

(Shimoji et al., 1993). Fifty-two of these patients had cancer-related pain, and 45 also experienced greater than 50% pain reduction. These retrospective data, like the case series, cannot confirm efficacy or establish the benefits of SCS relative to other treatments used for refractory pain. Nonetheless, the observational data are promising and suggest that a trial of SCS should be considered in patients who have pain related to serious illness that has not responded to conventional pharmacological management.

Central nervous system stimulation

Widespread use of neuroimaging techniques such as fMRI has shown that patients with chronic pain syndromes develop changes in the brain. For example, imaging shows changes in the excitability and/or somatotopic organization within specific cortical and subcortical regions, including structures generally considered to be part of a pain processing network or 'pain matrix' (e.g. areas of the motor and somatosensory cortices and parts of the thalamus) (Cohen et al., 1991; Elbert et al., 1994; Flor 2003). The observation that modulation of these neuroplastic changes may be accompanied by pain relief (Pleger et al., 2005; Birbaumer et al., 1997) has provided a physiological justification for trials of CNS neurostimulation for the treatment of chronic pain.

Both non-invasive and invasive techniques of neuromodulation have been studied in different types of chronic pain syndromes. Results have been promising and suggest that CNS neurostimulation could play a role in the treatment of pain related to serious medical illness.

Transcranial direct current stimulation

Transcranial direct current stimulation (tDCS) is a non-invasive technique that applies low-intensity direct current to the scalp (Nitsche and Paulus, 2000). The current penetrates the brain and modulates neuronal excitability by altering the firing rate of individual neurons. There are two modalities depending on current direction: anodal (excitatory) tDCS increases cortical excitability and cathodal (inhibitory) tDCS decreases excitability (Nitsche and Paulus, 2001).

Studies have shown that the analgesic effect of tDCS may be elicited by the application of anodal tDCS over the primary motor cortex (Fregni et al., 2006a, 2006b) or cathodal tDCS over the somatosensory cortex (Antal et al., 2008, Knotkova et al., 2009). Two randomized, sham-controlled studies showed that anodal stimulation improved pain in patients with fibromyalgia (Fregni et al., 2006b; Roizenblatt et al., 2007), and another sham-controlled trial showed promising results of tDCS for the treatment of central pain in patients with traumatic spinal cord injury (Fregni et al., 2006a). A case study suggested that cathodal tDCS over the somatosensory cortex also may be able to relieve chronic neuropathic pain (Knotkova et al., 2009).

Two recent sham-controlled studies evaluated the analgesic efficacy of tDCS for the treatment of chronic migraine headache: Antal et al. found that cathodal tDCS applied to the visual cortex resulted in a significant reduction in pain intensity when compared with the sham group (Antal et al., 2011), and Dasilva et al. showed that anodal tDCS applied over the primary motor cortex resulted in a delayed reduction in pain intensity four months after stimulation (Dasilva et al., 2012). Furthermore, tDCS was successfully applied in two patients with trigeminal neuralgia and neuropathic facial pain due to surgical disturbance

of the trigeminal nerve, resulting in greater than 50% reduction in pain scores and decreased use of pain medications (Knotkova 2009). A small observational study suggests that tDCS may be useful for the treatment of cancer pain (Silva et al., 2007).

Both studies and clinical experience with tDCS suggest that the analgesic properties are cumulative and that the duration of the analgesic effect outlasts the stimulation but is transitory. Pain usually returns to prestimulation levels. Independent investigators have shown greater pain relief with tDCS over 5 consecutive days as compared to a single session, and demonstrated a time course of the analgesic response that can outlast the last stimulation session by over 9 weeks (Fregni et al., 2006a, 2006b; Roizenblatt et al., 2007). However, the duration of the effect varies greatly from patient to patient, and predictions on the magnitude of the response and duration of the effect cannot be made based solely on the underlying pain syndrome, concomitant medications (opioids or adjuvants), co-morbidities like depression or anxiety, or other patient characteristics (e.g. age and gender). Indeed, a recent negative study in a group of patients with painful spinal cord injury suggested that time since the injury may affect the magnitude of the analgesic response (Wrigley et al., 2013).

TDCS may yield benefits for symptoms other than pain. One study showed that tDCS treatment in patients with fibromyalgia increased sleep efficiency by 11.8% and decreased arousal by 35% (Roizenblatt et al., 2007). Others have shown improvement in quality of life and a decrease in the use of pain medications (Fregni et al., 2006a, 2006b).

In summary, tDCS has been shown to be effective in relieving pain in a variety of chronic pain syndromes, with potential secondary benefits in sleep, quality of life, and use in pain medications. It is relatively inexpensive, easy to implement, and can be portable so that patients can be educated to self-administer the stimulation at home. These characteristics suggest that tDCS could play a useful role in the treatment of pain in populations with serious medical illness. Studies are needed to confirm these positive outcomes in medically ill populations.

Transcranial magnetic stimulation

Like tDCS, transcranial magnetic stimulation (TMS) is a non-invasive technique applied directly on the scalp. This technology entails the generation of a powerful magnetic field perpendicular to the brain cortex. This field induces the formation of electrical currents that are parallel to the cortex (similar to tDCS) and can modulate the neuronal excitability in underlying brain structures. The electrical field is relatively restricted in space due to the conical shape of the magnetic field, and as a result, TMS can produce more selective regional neuromodulation than tDCS.

TMS can be delivered as a single stimulation (sTMS) or a train of repetitive stimulations (rTMS). It was first explored for the treatment of pain in 1995 and numerous studies since then have been conducted to test various parameters of frequency, duration and width of the wave. The range of frequencies that have been tested is wide and is divided into high- and low-frequency stimulation based on efficacy.

In general, studies involving patients with various types of neuropathic pain suggest that high-frequency rTMS is more effective in eliciting long-lasting pain relief than low-frequency rTMS. For instance, André-Obadia et al. performed a double-blind study comparing the analgesic effect of a single session of

1 Hz and 20 Hz rTMS with sham stimulation in 14 patients with treatment-resistant neuropathic pain, including trigeminal, central post-stroke, and peripheral brachial plexus neuropathic pain. Although pain relief was achieved immediately after stimulation with both, the analgesic effect was maintained 1 week after stimulation in the 20 Hz group only (André-Obadia et al., 2006). Another sham-controlled study of 48 patients with trigeminal neuralgia or post-stroke pain syndrome reported that 20 Hz rTMS yielded significantly greater improvement in pain after five consecutive daily sessions of stimulation; the positive effect persisted for 2 weeks after treatment, suggesting that repeated rTMS sessions also can result in long-lasting pain relief (Khedr et al., 2005).

Other studies suggest that the outcome of TMS is influenced by the cause and location of the pain, and the somatotropic area where stimulation is applied. Lefaucher et al. conducted a study in 60 patients with intractable pain secondary to a variety of causes, including thalamic stroke, brainstem stroke, spinal cord lesion, brachial plexus lesion, and trigeminal nerve lesion. The overall pain reduction was significantly greater in rTMS as compared to sham stimulation, but rTMS was less effective in patients with brainstem stroke than with other lesions. The best results were obtained in patients with facial pain, rather than those with pain in the upper or lower limbs (Lefaucheur et al., 2004). In a later study, the same authors evaluated the relationship between the cortical stimulation site and pain site in 36 patients with chronic neuropathic pain located on the face or the hand. Interestingly, patients with facial pain experienced significantly better analgesic effects after stimulation to the hand rather than to the face. Similarly, patients with hand pain had greater pain relief after stimulation to the face rather than to the hand. The authors concluded that rTMS was the most effective for pain relief when stimulation was applied to an area adjacent to the cortical representation of the painful zone rather than to the motor cortical area corresponding to the painful zone itself (Lefaucheur et al., 2006).

Recent research in volunteers also has suggested that targets for rTMS treatment of pain may include brain regions that process pain perception, such as prefrontal cortex (Martin et al., 2013).

Some studies suggest that there are limitations in the use of rTMS in pain management. A randomized double-blind, sham-controlled, crossover study of patients with painful diabetic polyneuropathy demonstrated only a transient and modest improvement in pain scores following ten daily 5 Hz rTMS (500 pulses/session) of primary motor cortex (M1) (Hosomi et al., 2013). However, it has been proposed that a modification of the magnet (H-coil) would result in better stimulation of areas that otherwise are not easily accessible, like the lower limbs in diabetic neuropathy, hence achieving better pain relief (Onesti et al., 2013).

TMS may be efficacious in the treatment of headache. One evaluated sTMS as an abortive strategy for migraine and observed that pain relief occurred in 69% of the patients in the sTMS group as compared to 48% in the sham-controlled group (Mohammad et al., 2008). The second did not find a difference between the treatment and placebo groups (Clarke et al., 2006). Lipton et al. conducted a large multicenter, double-blind, sham-controlled study to evaluate the efficacy of a portable, self-administered sTMS device for the treatment of acute migraine, and found that 39% of the patients treated with sTMS were pain-free at 2 hours post-treatment, as compared to 22% of the sham controlled group (Lipton et al., 2010).

Four studies have evaluated the efficacy of rTMS for the treatment of frequent migraines. A small randomized study (Brighina et al., 2004) and an observational study Misra et al., 2012) suggested benefit, but this was not confirmed in two placebo-controlled studies (Teepker et al., 2010; Conforto et al., 2012).

There have been no studies of TMS in populations with acute or chronic pain related to serious illnesses. Extant data suggests that the strategy can be efficacious in some types of neuropathic pain and acute headache. Studies have shown that high-frequency stimulation is more effective in achieving long lasting pain relief than low-frequency stimulation, and that the outcome of TMS is influenced by the origin and location of the pain, and the somatotropic area where stimulation is applied. The best results have been obtained with facial pain, and when applied to an area adjacent to the cortical representation of the painful zone rather than to the motor cortical area corresponding to the painful zone itself. Like tDCS, TMS may prove to be a feasible, non-invasive alternative to pharmacological therapy for the treatment of refractory chronic pain.

Deep brain stimulation

Deep brain stimulation (DBS) is an invasive neurostimulatory technique that involves stereotactic implantation of electrodes directly into subcortical areas. It was first used for the treatment of chronic pain in the 1950s by placing electrodes in the hypothalamus (Pool et al., 1956), but later on, other brain areas were also considered to be good targets, including the thalamic nuclei and adjacent structures (Hosobuchi et al., 1973), subthalamic nucleus (Marques et al., 2013), the internal capsule (Adams et al., 1974; Hosobuchi et al., 1975), anterior cingulate cortex (Pereira et al., 2013), and the periventricular and periaqueductal grey area (Richardson and Akil, 1977a, 1977b). The analgesic mechanism of action of DBS for chronic pain is unclear and still debated, but the evidence favours modulation of brain activity (Kringelbach et al., 2007, Montgomery and Baker, 2000; McIntyre et al., 2004) over synaptic depression, synaptic inhibition (Dostrovsky et al., 2000), or depolarization blockade (Beurrier et al., 2001). DBS has been successfully used for the management of facial and head pain such as post-herpetic trigeminal neuralgia (Green et al., 2003), anaesthesia dolorosa (Green and Owen et al., 2006), multiple sclerosis (Hamani et al., 2006), genital pain, brachial plexus injuries, and malignancy (Nandi et al., 2003).

Although the recommendation of DBS for the management of headaches should be made with caution due to the limited evidence of its efficacy, there are reports of successful use of DBS for the management of cluster headaches. Leone et al. published the first case report of DBS in which a single patient with cluster headache underwent stereotactic implantation of an electrode in the posterior ipsilateral hypothalamic grey matter. The headaches stopped after 48 hours of stimulation, and the patient remained pain-free 13 months after implantation (Leone et al., 2001). Since then, multiple studies have been published evaluating the efficacy of DBS for the treatment of cluster headaches, most of which are case series. The largest study was a prospective, open-label study which included 16 patients, 13 of whom reported improvement in pain with DBS, and ten achieved a persistently pain-free state at 23 months' follow-up (Leone et al., 2006). The underlying mechanism seems to involve down-regulation of the increased regional blood flow in the posterior hypothalamus that occurs during an acute attack, as seen with both PET and fMRI techniques (May et al., 2006).

Kringelbach et al. published a case series comparing DBS with other invasive techniques for the management of chronic pain. Approximately 70% of the 65 patients who underwent DBS in the thalamus and/or periventricular or periaqueductal grey (PVG/PAG) experienced pain relief after 1 week post-implantation, and pain relief persisted more than 1 year in 60% of these patients (Nandi et al., 2002). Another study found very good efficacy of DBS for stroke patients complaining of burning hyperaesthesia (Owen et al., 2006) but less efficacy in patients with stroke overall.

Although the advent of the non-invasive CNS neurostimulation approaches may supplant DBS for pain, rare patients with severe treatment-refractory neuropathic pain still may be considered for a trial of invasive brain stimulation. Patient selection for DBS should be done by an experienced team, including a mental health professional experienced with this type of evaluations (Saint-Cyr and Trepanier, 2000; Lang et al., 2006). Medical contraindications to DBS include ventriculomegaly large enough to impede direct electrode passage to the surgical target (Kringelbach et al., 2010) and uncorrectable coagulopathy. The current recommendation is to utilize DBS as the last resort for patients who do not respond to standard of care.

Although the use of DBS is limited to a highly selected group of patients, the number of DBS implantations is greater than that for other invasive strategies such as motor cortex stimulation (MCS). According to a recent report, at least 1300 patients have been implanted with electrodes for DBS for the treatment of chronic neuropathic pain conditions (Kringelback et al., 2007), while only 400 patients have been implanted with motor cortex stimulators during a comparable period (Brown et al., 2003). The goal is to improve patient selection and thus outcomes. One intriguing possibility is the use of autonomic measures as potential objective markers, as shown by stroke patients' subjective preference for PVG/PAG stimulation over ventral posterolateral nucleus/ventral posteromedial nucleus, and correlations between analgesic efficacy and cardiovascular effects or burning hyperaesthesia (Green and Wang et al., 2006).

There are several types of complications that can occur as a result of the electrode implantation for DBS, including complications related to surgical procedures, complications due to the implanted devices, and side effects that result from the stimulation itself (Hariz 2002). According to Beric et al., 6.5% of the implantations can result in device-related complications, including infections, electrode fracture or dislocation, and hardware failure (Beric et al., 2001). Infrequent life-threatening complications can also occur and include intracranial haemorrhage (Benabid et al., 1996), haematoma, and paralysis (Beric et al., 2001). In addition, other complications like perioperative haemorrhage, occurred in 2.3% of patients undergoing DBS implantation (Beric et al., 2001). Stimulation-related side effects are the most frequently encountered problems in DBS. The symptom tends to correlate with the anatomical structure being stimulated (Hariz 2002), and can include paraesthesias, dysarthria, dyskinesia, gait disturbances, imbalance, confusion, depression, inappropriate laughter (Krack et al., 2001), and mood or personality changes (Bejjani et al., 2002).

Motor cortex stimulation

MCS is another invasive neurostimulation method, in which electrodes are surgically implanted in the epidural space to deliver an electric current to the motor cortex. This strategy requires the assistance of neuronavigation, most commonly fMRI or somatosensory evoked potentials, to localize the motor cortex. During the neurosurgical procedure, a lead with four electrodes is positioned above the dura and under the periosteum so that all four contacts are over the precentral gyrus of the motor cortex (Rasche et al., 2006). To verify the positioning of the electrodes, a suprathreshold stimulus is delivered that produces a contralateral motor response in the absence of concomitant sensory sensations (Brown and Barbaro, 2003). After the operation, a trial is performed to determine the best electrode combination and stimulation parameters that elicit the maximum response without significant side effects. A variety of settings have been proposed, but the most commonly utilized are an intensity of 2–3 V (range 0.5–9.5 V), with a frequency of 25–50 Hz (range 15–130 Hz), and a pulse width of 200 microseconds (range 60–450 microseconds). The stimulation can be tailored to the individual patient's needs by programming alternating cycles of stimulation with periods of no stimulation.

As noted, experience with MCS is far more limited than experience with DBS, and there have been no published trials of MCS in medically ill patients (Nguyen et al., 1998; Cioni and Megglio, 2007; Friedland et al., 2007; Arle and Shils, 2008; Lima and Fregni, 2008). Favourable case reports (Nguyen et al., 2000; Esfahani et al., 2011) are now supplemented by a few clinical trials suggesting positive outcomes from this approach. A randomized trial of MCS in 16 patients with chronic neuropathic pain following peripheral nerve lesions reported that 60% of patients had satisfactory levels of pain relief after 1 year (Lefaucheur et al., 2009).

The potential role of MCS is ill-defined. If non-invasive neurostimulation strategies are available, they will likely be tried first. If an invasive CNS neurostimulation treatment is considered for refractory chronic pain associated with serious illness, the choice between DBS and MCS is likely to revolve around the experience of the clinician.

Conclusions

Stimulation of the peripheral or central nervous systems for the management of chronic pain has been done for many years and the results have been mixed. Over the years, technology has improved and the delivery of current has become more sophisticated, allowing stimulation of discrete areas with a variety of intensities and frequencies that can be tailored to the underlying condition. The most efficacious parameters, stimulation targets, and devices have evolved with the improvement in technology, but selection of the proper stimulation strategy and patient population continues to be based on limited data and clinical experience. Studies are needed to confirm efficacy and illuminate those factors that predict a high likelihood of a favourable response. Further research also may reveal additional innovations, such as the potential utility of combinations of stimulations (e.g. SCS and DBS) (Chodakiewitz et al., 2013).

Online materials

Complete references for this chapter are available online at <http://www.oxfordmedicine.com>.

References

Adams, J.E., Hosobuchi, Y., and Fields, H.L. (1974). Stimulation of internal capsule for relief of chronic pain. *Journal of Neurosurgery*, 41(6), 740–744.

Brown, J.A. and Barbaro, N.M. (2003). Motor cortex stimulation for central and neuropathic pain: current status. *Pain*, 104, 431–435.

Chen, C.C. and Johnson, M.I. (2009). An investigation into the hypoalgesic effects of high- and low-frequency transcutaneous electrical nerve stimulation (TENS) on experimentally induced blunt pressure pain in healthy human participants. *Journal of Pain*, 11(1), 53–61.

Clarke, B.M., Upton, A.R., Kamath, M.V., *et al.* (2006) Transcranial magnetic stimulation for migraine: clinical effects. *Journal of Headache & Pain*, 7(5), 341–346.

Cohen, L.G., Bandinelli, S., Findley, T.W., and Hallett, M. (1991). Motor reorganization after upper limb amputation in man. *Brain*, 114, 615–627.

Hosomi, K., Shimokawa, T., Ikoma, K., *et al.* (2013). Daily repetitive transcranial magnetic stimulation of primary motor cortex for neuropathic pain: a randomized, multicenter, double-blind, crossover, sham-controlled trial. *Pain*, 154(7), 1065–1072.

Knotkova, H., Homel, P., and Cruciani, R.A. (2009). Cathodal tDCS over the somatosensory cortex relieved chronic neuropathic pain in a patient with complex regional pain syndrome (CRPS/RSD). *Journal of Pain Management*, 2(3), 365–368.

Lefaucheur, J.P., Drouot, X., Cunin, P., *et al.* (2009). Motor cortex stimulation for the treatment of refractory peripheral neuropathic pain. *Brain*, 132(6), 1463–1471.

Melzack, R. and Wall, P.D. (1965). Pain mechanisms: a new theory. *Science*, 150(3699), 971–979.

Ng, S.S. and Hui-Chan, C.W. (2007). Transcutaneous electrical nerve stimulation combined with task-related training improves lower limb functions in subjects with chronic stroke. *Stroke*, 38(11), 2953–2959.

Nitsche, M.A. and Paulus, W. (2001). Sustained excitability elevations induced by transcranial DC motor cortex stimulation in humans. *Neurology*, 57, 1899–1901.

Pleger, B., Tegenthoff, M., Ragert, P., *et al.* (2005). Sensorimotor returning in complex regional pain syndrome parallels pain reduction. *Annals of Neurology*, 57, 425–429.

Sanchez-Ledesma, M.J., Garcia-March, G., Diaz-Cascajo, P., Gomez-Moreta, J., and Broseta, J. (1989). Spinal cord stimulation in deafferentation pain. *Stereotactic & Functional Neurosurgery*, 53(1), 40–45.

Taylor, R.S. (2006). Spinal cord stimulation in complex regional pain syndrome and refractory neuropathic back and leg pain/failed back surgery syndrome: results of a systematic review and meta-analysis. *Journal of Pain and Symptom Management*, 31, S13–S19.

Yakovlev, A.E., Resch, B.E., and Karasev, S.A. (2010). Treatment of cancer-related chest wall pain using spinal cord stimulation. *American Journal of Hospice and Palliative Medicine*, 27 (8), 552–556.

Rehabilitation medicine approaches to pain management

Andrea L. Cheville and Jeffrey R. Basford

Introduction to rehabilitation medicine approaches to pain management

Pain is a frequent but poorly controlled aspect of cancer and other medical conditions which may, in part, stem from the clinician's lack of understanding of its severity or impact. However, even with the best of care, our current approaches are associated with poorly tolerated side effects and frequently fall far short of complete control. All pain is limiting, but bone pain from metastatic disease is particularly problematic in that it is provoked by movement or weight bearing and has profound effects on an individual's mobility, activities, and independence.

Rehabilitation medicine, with its focus on optimizing patient function irrespective of their symptom burden or impairments, has developed strategies that may reduce pain in general, but are particularly targeted to movement-related pain. For the most part, these approaches serve as adjuncts to, rather than replacements for, conventional analgesic approaches. Some may have a limited evidence base and most have not been validated in the palliative setting. Nevertheless, common sense and extensive experience argue persuasively for their clinical effectiveness. In addition, with few exceptions, they are patient controlled and largely free of side effects.

These approaches can be grouped into four general categories: (1) modulating nociception, (2) stabilizing and unloading painful musculoskeletal structures, (3) influencing pain perception, and (4) alleviating musculotendinous pain. This latter section is included since 'benign' pain related to the overloading or maladaptive use of muscles and connective tissues occurs with sarcopenia in the late stages of many diseases. This chapter will review each of these categories in detail and offer examples to illustrate their clinical application. It will be noted that the majority are focused on minimizing pain during periods of mobility and the performance of activities of daily living (ADLs).

Modulation of afferent nociceptive activity

Rehabilitation uses two approaches to modulate the input of nociceptive signals into the central nervous system (CNS). The first, the use of heat and cold, is traditionally associated with rehabilitation medicine and still has a role. The second, rather than trying to block the input of painful stimuli, uses benign afferent sensory input to reduce nociceptive activity. This approach, introduced and named by Melzack and Wall in the 1960s has been termed the 'gate theory of pain' (Melzack and Wall, 1965). The concept has been challenged but not disproved or seriously debunked even though the precise neural pathways and biochemical reactions continue to be studied.

Heat and cold

Heat and cold have powerful effects on the body. Metabolic and enzymatic processes may be markedly accelerated or slowed by temperature elevations of only a few degrees with changes of 3–7°C capable of altering nerve conduction, blood flow, and collagen extensibility (Knight, 1985; Guyton, 1986; Denys, 1991; Lehmann et al., 1966). Effects can be local or systemic: immersions of the body at robust but tolerable temperatures can alter core temperatures by 0.3–0.4°C with local effects being more pronounced (Doering et al., 1999). Ice massage over the knee can reduce intra-articular temperatures by as much as 6°C (Oosterveld and Rasker, 1994), and agents such as hot paraffin and diathermy can markedly raise local skin and intra-articular temperatures (Oosterveld and Rasker, 1994). Although the heating agents differ, most gain their effects by inducing analgesia, hyperaemia, or reducing muscle tone. Cold, while reducing perfusion, is also used for its analgesic and tone reduction capabilities.

Heat and cold have clear effects on a variety of physiological processes. As such, their main use has been primarily for the control of pain. Use is typically focused on the musculoskeletal system where there is support for its benefits as an adjunct to exercise (Brosseau et al., 2002; Lin, 2003; French et al., 2006; Chou et al., 2007).

Electrical stimulation

Electrical stimulation is used for a variety of indications that range from moving and strengthening limbs to analgesia and even the healing of soft tissue injuries and fractures (see Chapter 9.9). Here we will restrict ourselves to its analgesic applications. Rehabilitation has developed and discarded a great many approaches to stimulating benign, sensory afferents for physiological effect. Those that have withstood the test of time, though not necessarily the scrutiny of randomized controlled trials, as well as newer approaches whose use seems more predicated on novelty than empirical support are discussed in this section.

Transcutaneous electrical nerve stimulation

Transcutaneous electronic nerve stimulation (TENS) is one of the most thoroughly studied and widespread of the modalities used to modulate nociceptive drive. Its introduction provided a non-invasive means to provide the afferent sensory stimuli posited by the 'gate theory' as necessary to block nociceptive signals (Melzack and Wall, 1954). A few successful trials ensured its acceptance. Acceptance and use has not, however, completely clarified its best application or the complete characterizing of how it, or close relatives such as interferential current, achieve their effects

TENS units are typically small, programmable within limits, and consist of a power source, a set of electrodes, and one or more signal generators. The devices can produce a variety of stimuli with currents of less than 100 mA, pulse rates ranging from a few to 200 Hz, and pulse widths from 10 to a few hundred microseconds. Varying waveform modulations and stimulation parameters are chosen to increase effectiveness, improve comfort and lessen tachyphylaxis.

Electrodes are often placed over the painful area but positioning on the vicinity of afferent nerves, acupuncture points, and other sites is often assessed. Stimulation settings are similarly idiosyncratic. Two options, however, are the most common. The first ('low-intensity' or 'conventional' TENS) stimulation occurs at frequencies of about 40–80 Hz and is set at a level that is barely perceptible. The second is in many ways the reverse: frequencies are relatively slow (1–8 Hz) and intensities are set at a mildly uncomfortable level.

Response is not guaranteed and difficult to predict, and TENS studies range in quality from well-designed, prospective, randomized, controlled trials to, particularly in the earlier days, small and poorly blinded trials. Even today, trials with TENS compared with active controls are far rarer than ideal.

A number of studies in the 1970s and 1980s focused on postoperative incisional and early labour pain and found that TENS usage resulted in benefits were comparable to limited amounts of analgesics including narcotics (Chen et al., 1998; Hamza et al., 1999; Philadelphia Panel, 2001a).

Research over the subsequent years has had mixed results with more recent evidence-based clinical guidelines and systematic reviews finding that no or insufficient evidence that TENS can lessen neck or back pain (Philadelphia Panel, 2001b; Pengel et al., 2002; Khadilkar et al., 2005; Vernon et al., 2005). The situation may be somewhat more positive for knee osteoarthritis.

Cancer-related pain has, thus far, received only limited attention. As a result, while there are suggestions that TENS is capable of improving movement/weight bearing-associated cancer pain, a recent Cochrane review, despite casting a wide net for admissible studies, found that only three met its criteria for inclusion. Issues with design heterogeneity and quality were noted and while treatment was well tolerated by the subjects, the authors were unable to conclude that the evidence was strong enough to support the use of TENS (Pengel et al., 2012).

TENS relies on repetitive stimuli. As a result, a number of units have tried to avoid this issue by producing waveforms of varying shapes and frequencies. This concept has now been carried to the extreme by the introduction sof a device that is similar to conventional TENS in that its analgesic effects are mediated through transcutaneous electrical input but it differs in that its wave form randomly varies and its electrode placement can be more complex (Marineo et al., 2012). Anecdotal experience suggests benefits in mixed neuropathic and nociceptive syndromes.

TENS has few safety issues other than skin irritation and mild discomfort during use. Cardiac pacemakers appear relatively resistant to TENS signals but reasonable concerns about real or apparent introduction of dysrhythmias/malfunction restricts TENS use in this setting. It also seems prudent to avoid treatment near the carotid sinus, epiglottis, and abdomen/low back of pregnant women.

Why have TENS units continued to be used despite equivocal evidence of effectiveness? The reasons may help clinicians in deciding whether to consider TENS for their patients. First, TENS studies are heterogeneous in terms of the conditions assessed, parameter settings, and outcome measures. Thus, while systematic reviews have found limited evidence of effectiveness, they have been unable to state that the approach is ineffective. Second, side effects are minimal. Third, efficacy in both nociceptive and neuropathic pain syndromes—most patients with cancer experience a mixture of both (Zech et al., 1995; Caraceni and Portenoy, 1999)—is anecdotally and weakly empirically supported in reducing patients' numerical rating scale ratings. Fourthly, a TENS trial can be incorporated into a course of physical therapy (PT) without significantly interfering with other potentially beneficial activities, such as therapeutic exercise. Lastly, the prolonged use of TENS by a subgroup of patients suggests that it may benefit certain individuals. In all, reasonable candidates are patients whose localized pain is inadequately controlled by conventional treatments, who experience untenable medication side effects, or who prefer to trial non-pharmacological approaches. Depending on the pain syndrome, a PT-based TENS trial can be combined with counter-stimulation, myofascial release techniques, and therapeutic exercises during a single treatment session.

Counterstimulation and desensitization techniques

Other rehabilitation techniques increase benign afferent sensory drive in order to attenuate pain intensity. Some, such as desensitization, have this as their sole objective. Others, such as massage or compression garments, increase afferent sensory drive in conjunction with other treatment goals such as the control of oedema or muscle tone. Desensitization techniques warrant particular mention since they are a first-line rehabilitation medicine treatment for complex regional and neuropathic pain. Tolerance for increasingly intense and unpleasant stimuli is systematically cultivated by gently applying stimuli in an incremental fashion to steadily shift a patient's threshold for experiencing a stimulus as noxious. Desensitization techniques can be coupled with other modalities during a treatment session.

Stabilization and unloading strategies

Cancer is often associated with a decreased ability of the body to bear weight, move, or tolerate the forces placed on it by even routine activities of daily living. As a consequence, the limbs, spine, and muscles frequently become pain generators, particularly with movement. The most prevalent example is bone pain in the face of metastatic cancer. For example, a cervical vertebra with metastatic involvement may produce pain since the neck not only supports the weight of the head but also its positioning in space. Even intact musculoskeletal elements can become inflamed, hypertonic, or frankly compromised as a consequence of the biomechanical changes induced by cancer and cancer treatment (Cheville and Tchou, 2007). Suffice to mention that virtually any distorting force, such as contracted soft tissue from radiation fibrosis, pectoralis muscle tension from breast implants, or compromised core muscle strength from extensive abdominal surgery, has the potential to alter normal biomechanical relationships in a manner that stresses other musculoskeletal elements to the point that they become independent pain generators.

Stabilizing and unloading strategies are designed to reduce the forces placed upon painful bony or connective tissues. Four approaches are utilized:

1. displacing loads onto external supports

2. improving the load bearing capacity of intact anatomic elements

3. immobilizing painful joints, or

4. reducing the work required by a painful activity.

The information in the following sections is organized by therapeutic approach similar to the manner in which a therapy prescription would be structured. As will become clear, more than a single modality can be applied to each of the four listed approaches.

Assistive devices for mobility and ADL performance

A wide range of devices to assist patients with safe and autonomous mobility are available. Fig. 9.10.1 includes a single point cane, quad cane, platform walker, and rolling walker. Each has its fitting requirements as well as its strengths and weaknesses. The need for the guidance of a physical therapist and the importance of professionally supervised trials and fitting cannot be overstated if patients are to effectively utilize and incorporate these devices into their lives. Mechanized or electrical assistive devices may be required to substitute for entire activities if pain renders their performance intolerable. For example, a Hoyer lift, scooter or wheelchair may free the patient from pain during transfers and locomotion.

A mind-boggling array of assistive devices can be used to protect inflamed or otherwise vulnerable structures from ADL-related forces. Fig. 9.10.2 shows a variety of possibilities. In contrast to assistive devices for mobility, these for ADL performance generally reduce the amount of reaching, bending, or twisting required to complete a painful activity. Occupational therapists (OTs) can trial a range of ADL assistive devices during an initial evaluation on an out- or inpatient basis.

The efficacy of assistive devices for ADLs has not been well assessed in clinical trials since a strong experiential base (e.g. the use of elastic shoe laces and a long-handled shoe horn permitting a patient to don his/her shoes when they had previously been unable to do so) supports their use. Several excellent reports have quantified the off-loading achieved by various mobility assistive devices, particularly canes, and found this to exceed 30% (Blount, 1956).

Compensatory strategies

The pain-relieving benefits of compensatory strategies stem from the same theoretical basis as assistive devices: relief of forces applied to painful structures. In fact, compensatory strategies so often rely on assistive devices that it becomes almost contrived to separate them. Nonetheless, there are important distinctions that, if appreciated, may help clinicians to produce more effective and comprehensive PT and OT prescriptions.

Our daily activities consist of an orchestrated combination of coordinated and isolated movements. Often, not all the movements required to execute an activity produce pain. By deconstructing painful activities to their constituent movements, PTs and OTs can isolate those that are painful and devise alternative, 'compensatory', strategies to achieve the patient's goal. Simply helping a patient to recognize the movements that trigger pain frequently enable them to develop their own strategies. Activities that can be deconstructed in this manner vary widely from transferring into or out of a vehicle to toileting and other hygiene-related activities. Engaging caregivers, using architectural supports and durable medical equipment, as well as altering the home environment can be combined to optimize patients' non-painful functioning.

Therapeutic exercise

Muscles are dynamic and often provide the most effective means of stabilization and immobilization. There are obvious limitations to this approach (e.g. the unstable spine) but the approach, often

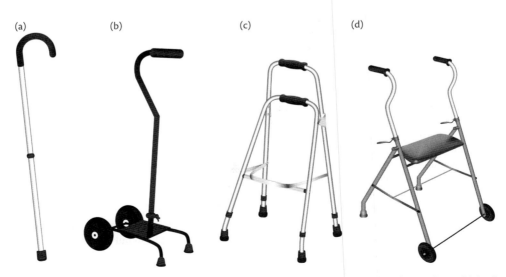

Fig. 9.10.1 Devices to assist patients with safe and autonomous mobility. (A) Single point cane; (B) quad cane; (C) platform walker and (D) rolling walker.

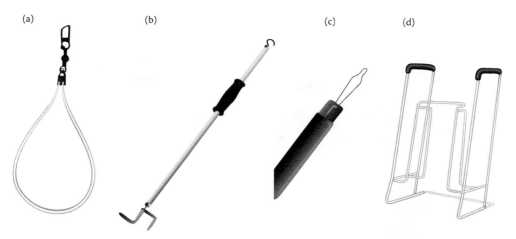

Fig. 9.10.2 Assistive devices used to protect inflamed or vulnerable structured from ADL-related forces.

termed dynamic stabilization, has been a mainstay in the treatment of low back and knee pain for years. As a result, therapeutic exercises aimed at enhancing the strength and stamina of muscles capable of splinting a painful body part can be a remarkably effective adjunct to conventional analgesia. Further consideration of the translation of the techniques of sports and musculoskeletal medicine into the realm of cancer rehabilitation seems warranted given the benefits of unloading painful areas and mobilizing the patient with metastatic disease.

Though conceptually simple, therapeutic exercises should be chosen and implemented by a PT with the skills and time to identify the painful structures or movements and to design a strengthening programme that can effectively splint or constrain the movement of a pain-generating structure. For the most part, muscles should be strengthened in a fixed position through isometric contractions that avoid pain-producing changes in muscle length or in the angle of the joint on which the muscle is acting. Common examples of isometric exercises used to stabilize pain-generating bony structures include strengthening of the abdominal and hip abductor muscles to deweight painful vertebrae and hip joints, respectively.

Orthotics

Orthotics, often referred to as braces, can be used to stabilize, deweight, and protect compromised musculoskeletal structures. Stabilization is the most common application among patients with cancer and the orthotics that perform this function typically either (a) immobilize the entire affected body part or (b) apply pressure at selected points to restrict motion. Orthotics come in myriad forms. Many are commercially available while others may require custom construction. Those used with the goal of avoiding pain in cancer care are, in large part, directed at stabilizing the neck, trunk, and low back. However, orthotics for the extremities such as moulded ankle foot orthoses '(AFOs') and spica or resting wrist splints may benefit patients with distal limb pain.

Spinal braces warrant specific mention. Often their prescription is initiated and coordinated by an orthopaedic surgeon when a patient's spine is deemed unstable. Moulded body jackets, also referred to as clam shell braces, which require custom fabrication are most frequently prescribed because of their superior immobilizing properties. While body jackets unquestionably limit motion better than other spinal orthoses, they are costly, hot,

uncomfortable, and poorly tolerated. In these cases it may be necessary to consider a less ideal alternative such as the semi-rigid braces that are often commercially available and are also capable of restricting spinal motion (Utter et al., 2010).

Less expensive, and more tolerable, alternatives include prefabricated orthoses that encompass different segments of the spine. Thoracolumbosacral orthoses such as the CASH and Jewett braces (Fig. 9.10.3) are widely available and generally well tolerated. These 'three-point braces' apply pressure at two anterior points on the upper and lower trunk and at a third point on the mid-back in between the two anterior points. A nice attribute of such off-the-shelf orthoses is that they can be trialled to assess patients' tolerance and pain control without making an expensive investment in either purchase or custom fabrication. It should be noted that while these braces do limit spinal flexion, they do little or nothing to constrain truncal extension. Fortunately, the anterior vertebral column is the most common site of metastatic involvement and pain generation. As a result, in the absence of spinal instability, the limitation of spinal flexion is the goal. If the spine is unstable, however, surgical stabilization or a body jacket should be considered.

Lumbosacral orthoses (LSOs), while most effective at the mid-lumbar level, control spinal motion from roughly the epigastrium to the lower gluteal area. LSOs are, for the most part, variations on the abdominal corset with rigid struts and other support. The off-the-shelf Bell Horn Brace, for example, is a lightweight LSO. Like abdominal binders, the Bell Horn and other LSOs are believed to alleviate pain by deweighting the spine through compression of the abdominal contents to generate a load-bearing fluid column. This sounds potentially uncomfortable, but LSOs are generally well tolerated. An advantage of most LSOs is that as they can be easily trialled without financial outlay by the patient. A number of LSOs have adrawstring or one-handed cinching mechanism which facilitates easy donning, doffing, and adjustment.

Cervical orthoses also offer a continuum from the fixed immobilization of the halo brace to the essentially tactile feedback and limited support of the soft cervical collar (Sandler et al., 1996). Between the two extremes are a range of pre-fabricated orthoses including the Miami J, Philadelphia, and sterno-occipital mandibular immobilizer brace. All are variably uncomfortable and are used principally to restrict cervical motion. If pain control,

(a) (b)

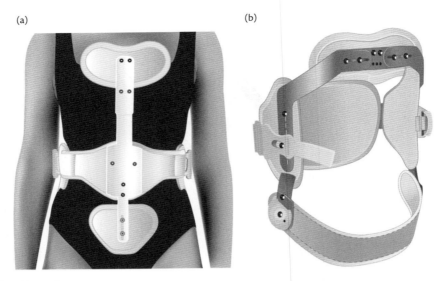

Fig. 9.10.3 Examples of CASH and Jewett braces.

rather than stabilization, is the impetus for considering a cervical orthotic, a trial of the differing options as well as a soft collar, is warranted since patients' preferences and degree of benefit can vary in unexpected ways.

Coordinating an orthotic trial is generally straightforward and within the practice scope of most OTs and PTs. Patients can also be sent directly to an orthotist, but this may require prior determination of which brace should be dispensed. Many medical centres have established alliances with orthotic suppliers. Orthotists may be available to evaluate and fit patients while hospitalized or during their outpatient oncology visits. Payers may restrict the providers from which patients may obtain their orthotics and coverage should be explored prior to initiating a trial.

Positioning

The strategic use of pillows, bolsters, the built environment, hospital beds, and adaptive equipment to support patients and constrain them to a pain-free range of motion is so common sense that it almost does not warrant mention. However, these effective approaches receive little attention in the formal guidance given to both professional and lay caregivers. For patients with severe motor deficits and weakness, stabilizing their painful areas at rest by positioning can not only reduce pain, but also protect vulnerable skin over bony prominences. Like orthotics, pillows and bolsters can be used to reduce the forces placed on compromised muscles and tissue. For example, use of pillows, arm rests, or padded bed rails to support the arms of people with treated head and neck cancers with weakened cervical and shoulder stability following neck dissections can radically reduce painful hypertonicity and myofascial pain in the residual musculature.

Modalities with physiological effects that influence nociception

Light and laser therapy

Laser therapy had been widely taken up to treat to a wide variety of soft tissue injuries and conditions. With time, the evolution of their use has grown to include a large number of non-laser monochromatic light sources and a tendency for treatments to take place with 30–150+ mW devices and with a limited number of joules/cm^2. As such, tissue temperatures are not elevated more than a few tenths of a degree Celsius and the theoretical support for their effectiveness lies in research findings that irradiation at these intensities and energies can produce a variety of effects that range from the modulation of metabolic processes and DNA synthesis to improving the healing and function of damaged nerves. These devices have been approved for use by the US Food and Drug Administration, typically as an adjunct to the treatment of pain, for the last 10 years or so.

As is true for many modalities, evaluation of clinical benefits has been difficult. A large number of clinical trials have evaluated the efficacy of laser therapy over the years with those done more recently typically having better designs and power than their earlier counterparts. While many are quite encouraging, the variety of conditions and parameter settings (e.g. wavelength and intensity) has limited systematic, evidenced-based analysis. Thus, recent evidence-based reviews on non-specific low back pain and venous stasis ulcers have been unable to support benefits (Flemming and Cullum, 2000; Yousefi-Nooraie et al., 2008). The situation is somewhat better for patients with cancer receiving treatment for oral mucositis and rheumatoid arthritis where systematic reviews have found 'limited benefits' (Brosseau et al., 2000; Clarkson et al., 2010). Even, here, however, concern is voiced for the need for additional trials to ensure an adequate evaluation.

In summary, evidence for the benefits of low-level light sources remains mixed but with some level of support above the individual study. Treatment is associated with minimal side effects.

Manual lymphatic drainage

Manual lymphatic drainage (MLD), 'lymphatic massage', or 'Vodder-type massage' is a highly specialized technique designed to enhance the sequestration and transport of lymph (see Chapter 11.3). Specific stroke duration, orientation, pressure, and sequence characterize MLD. MLD stimulates the smooth muscles in the lymph vessel walls to enhance their contractility, leading to increased removal of potentially inflammatory and pro-nociceptive macromolecules from the interstitium (Casley-Smith, 1988). Through gentle and rhythmic skin distention, congested lymph is directed to intact lymph vessels and nodal beds. Thereby, MLD permits removal of congested lymph and reduction of its adverse local effects. The massage is very light and superficial, limited to finger or hand pressures of around 30–45 mmHg. MLD treatments are initiated proximal to lymphostatic regions. Lymph is constantly directed towards functional lymphatics with strategic hand movement. Treatments gradually progress distally to terminate in the regions farthest removed from intact lymphatics, and presumably most congested.

MLD's analgesic properties have been recognized through its extensive use in the management of lymphoedema. Consequently, MLD is increasingly applied to pain syndromes in which congested lymph is thought to play a role (Ekici et al., 2009; Ebert et al., 2013). Because it is remarkably low pressure, MLD tends to be well tolerated, even among patients with moderate to severe allodynia. MLD is a cultivated skill and its clinical benefit highly practitioner dependent.

Rehabilitation approaches to managing musculoskeletal pain

The overwhelming majority of analgesic modalities utilized in rehabilitation medicine are directed towards pain arising from the soft tissues of the musculoskeletal system. These structures may contribute importantly to cancer pain syndromes through four principal mechanisms: (1) direct tumour invasion, (2) maladaptive changes induced by cancer treatment or local tumour effects, (3) exacerbation of pre-existing musculoskeletal pain and (4) secondary hypertonicity and spasm related to (2), and (3). The third, exacerbation of pre-existing pain, may be the most common across all cancer populations, though this, to the best of our knowledge, has never been subjected to epidemiological scrutiny. However, common sources of musculoskeletal pain, such as knee osteoarthritis or rotator cuff tendonitis, affect over 70% of the population. Common approaches to the treatment of musculoskeletal pain are outlined below. Often, multiple approaches are integrated in a unified treatment plan. Pain arising from tumour invasion is far more likely to definitively respond to treatment with antineoplastic therapies; however rehabilitation medicine approaches may be trailed once tumour control has been optimized.

Principals of rest, ice compression and elevation (PRICE)

PRICE, though simple, continues to be widely used because of its effectiveness and safety in controlling acute inflammation. Musculoskeletal pain of abrupt onset or with a clear precipitant, such as overuse or trauma, warrants a trial of PRICE with or without NSAIDs. Twice daily, 20-minute immersion of the affected body part, when feasible and tolerated, in a slurry of crushed ice and water will be more effective than ice packs.

Injections

Injections all share a common goal of delivering an analgesic or anti-inflammatory agent at high concentration to a pain generator in order to maximize therapeutic effects while minimizing systemic toxicity. An impressive array of pharmaceuticals is injected, but steroids and local anaesthetics remain the most common. Ultrasound guidance is increasingly used to optimize localization; however, the benefits of this approach, particularly with lipophilic injectates, have not been clearly established. Inflamed tendons, bursae, and synovium are the most common targets

When the long-term benefits of steroid injections have been subjected to high-quality and rigorous scrutiny, they appear to be less effective than PT alone, although benefits are slower to accrue with PT. To date, some of the best work has been done in lateral epicondylitis or tennis elbow (Coombes et al., 2013). There seems to be a rebound effect following the near-term anti-inflammatory benefits of the injection (Bisset et al., 2006). This is relevant to patients with cancer since their prognoses and involvement with cancer treatments vary radically. For a disease-free survivor with a good prognosis, PT in conjunction with or independent of an injection may offer greater collective benefit than an injection alone. In contrast, patients with far advanced cancer need near-term relief and may not survive to experience the more delayed and sustained benefits offered by PT.

Injections are relatively safe and toxicity free. Patients should not receive more than three per year to a single joint. Most physiatrists, orthopaedists, rheumatologists, as well as many primary care practitioners perform these procedures. However, for more specialized injections, such as those involving the smaller structures of the hand, the involvement of specialists who frequently target these joints is recommended.

Myofascial release techniques and trigger points

Myofascial pain is a painful syndrome that is most commonly located in upper back musculature and affects millions of people (Gerwin, 2001; Alvarez and Rockwell, 2002). Its most salient findings include tenderness on palpation and the presence of 'taut bands' of increased muscle tone and tenderness in association with trigger point (small areas of increased tenderness that when pressed, generate repeatable patterns of referred pain). While the nature and cause of the syndrome remains controversial, its effects on patients can be large. Massage, exercise, and trigger point/botulinum injections are the mainstays of myofascial pain treatment.

Massage, often accompanied with heat, which builds in intensity according to the patient's tolerance along with muscle tension release techniques and relaxation exercises are frequently employed. 'Spray and stretch,' a massage variant in which a cooling spay (often pentafluoropropane or tetrafluoroethane in place of the environmentally outlawed fluoromethane) is applied briefly to the trigger point and then along a line that follows the pattern of its pain radiation. Several sweeps with the spray are typically applied, followed by a gentle, sustained stretch for 30–60 seconds. The cycle of spray and stretch is repeated several times. Like most approaches to myofascial pain, multiple treatment sessions are required for sustained benefit.

Trigger point injections and dry needling mechanically stimulate the discreet taut bands that are the hallmark of myofascial pain. Controversy persists as to the benefits of introducing an injectate, such as local anaesthetic, botulinum toxin, or steroid, versus simply penetrating taut bands with a needle. No direct comparisons offer an empirical basis to choose one over the other. However, since positive benefits have been reported for approaches utilizing very narrow gauge (> 30), needles that inflict less trauma and discomfort, these may be preferred for initial trials of invasive myofascial techniques.

Therapeutic exercise plays a critical role in normalizing the biomechanical derangements that predispose patients to develop myofascial pain. Chronic muscle overuse is the most common source of myofascial pain among patients with cancer and occurs when muscles, whether through surgical alterations, radiation-induced contractures, or focal neurological/myogenic weakness, must work harder or differently than they were designed to. It may not be possible to reverse the injuries produced by the inciting trauma through stretching and strengthening activities. However, the forces on the affected muscles, as well as the intensity and chronicity of their associated pain, can generally be improved through therapeutic exercise approaches. Evaluation by a physician or therapist familiar with cancer treatment-related changes, as well as comprehensive myofascial pain management, offers the best chance of developing an appropriate and individualized exercise programme targeting all implicated muscle groups.

Therapeutic exercise

In addition to its role in the optimal control of myofascial pain and enhancing splinting capacity, therapeutic exercise is a cornerstone of all rehabilitative approaches to pain arising from muscles, tendons, and ligaments. The structured application of specific demands to muscle and connective tissues reliably elicits desirable physiological changes. Such demands may be resistive, aerobic, or tensile depending on the desired alterations in muscle anatomy and physiology. In the palliative setting, therapeutic exercise is used most commonly to strengthen painful muscle, as tolerated, to improve their resistance to over use.

Conclusion

Rehabilitation medicine offers a range of pain management approaches that may serve as beneficial adjuncts to conventional systemic and interventional analgesia. These approaches may be particularly beneficial to patients with movement-associated pain and those who are ambivalent about pharmacoanalgesia.

Online materials

Additional online materials and complete references for this chapter are available online at <http://www.oxfordmedicine.com>.

References

Alvarez, D.J. and Rockwell, P.G. (2002). Trigger points: diagnosis and management. *American Family Physician*, 65(4), 653–660.

Bisset, L., Beller, E., Jull, G., Brooks, P., Darnell, R., and Vicenzino, B. (2006). Mobilisation with movement and exercise, corticosteroid injection, or wait and see for tennis elbow: randomised trial. *BMJ*, 333(7575), 939.

Blount, W.P. (1956). Don't throw away the cane. *Journal of Bone and Joint Surgery*, 38-A(3), 695–708.

Brosseau, L., Robinson, V., Pelland, L., et al. (2002). Efficacy of thermotherapy for rheumatoid arthritis: a meta-analysis. *Physical Therapy Reviews*, 7(1), 5–15.

Brosseau, L., Welch, V., Wells, G., et al. (2000). Low level laser therapy (classes I, II and III) in the treatment of rheumatoid arthritis. *Cochrane Database of Systematic Reviews*, 2, CD002049.

Caraceni, A. and Portenoy, R.K. (1999). An international survey of cancer pain characteristics and syndromes. IASP Task Force on Cancer Pain. International Association for the Study of Pain. *Pain*, 82(3), 263–274.

Casley-Smith, J.R. (1988). The pathophysiology of lymphedema and the action of benzo-pyrones in reducing it. *Lymphology*, 21(3), 190–194.

Chen, L., Tang, J., White, P.F., et al. (1998). The effect of location of transcutaneous electrical nerve stimulation on postoperative opioid analgesic requirement: acupoint versus nonacupoint stimulation. *Anesthesia & Analgesia*, 87(5), 1129–1134.

Cheville, A.L. and Tchou, J. (2007). Barriers to rehabilitation following surgery for primary breast cancer. *Journal of Surgical Oncology*, 95(5), 409–418.

Chou, R. and Huffman, L.H. (2007). Nonpharmacologic therapies for acute and chronic low back pain: a review of the evidence for an American Pain Society/American College of Physicians clinical practice guideline. *Annals of Internal Medicine*, 147(7), 492–504.

Clarkson, J.E., Worthington, H.V., Furness, S., McCabe, M., Khalid, T., and Meyer, S. (2010). Interventions for treating oral mucositis for patients with cancer receiving treatment. *Cochrane Database of Systematic Reviews*, 8, CD001973.

Coombes, B.K., Bisset, L., Brooks, P., Khan, A., and Vicenzino, B. (2013). Effect of corticosteroid injection, physiotherapy, or both on clinical outcomes in patients with unilateral lateral epicondylalgia: a randomized controlled trial. *Journal of the American Medical Association*, 309(5), 461–469.

Denys, E.H. (1991). AAEM minimonograph #14: the influence of temperature in clinical neurophysiology. *Muscle & Nerve*, 14, 795–811.

Doering, T.J., Aaslid, R., Steuernagel, B., et al. (1999). Cerebral autoregulation during whole-body hypothermia and hyperthermia. *American Journal of Physical Medicine & Rehabilitation*, 78(1), 33–38.

Ebert, J.R., Joss, B., Jardine, B., and Wood, D.J. (2013). Randomized trial investigating the efficacy of manual lymphatic drainage to improve early outcome after total knee arthroplasty. *Archives of Physical Medicine and Rehabilitation*, 94(11), 2103–2111.

Ekici, G., Bakar, Y., Akbayrak, T., and Yuksel, I. (2009). Comparison of manual lymph drainage therapy and connective tissue massage in women with fibromyalgia: a randomized controlled trial. *Journal of Manipulative and Physiological Therapeutics*, 32(2), 127–133.

Flemming, K. and Cullum, N. (2000). Laser therapy for venous leg ulcers. *Cochrane Database of Systematic Reviews*, 2, CD001182.

French, S.D., Cameron, M., Walker, B.F., Reggars, J.W., and Esterman, A.J. (2006). Superficial heat or cold for low back pain. *Cochrane Database of Systematic Reviews*, 1, CD004750.

Gerwin, R.D. (2001). Classification, epidemiology, and natural history of myofascial pain syndrome. *Current Pain and Headache Reports*, 5(5), 412–420.

Guyton, A.C. (1986). *Textbook of Medical Physiology* (7th ed.). Philadelphia, PA: WB Saunders.

Hamza, M.A., White, P.F., Ahmed, H.E., and Ghoname, E. (1999). Effect of the frequency of transcutaneous electrical nerve stimulation on the postoperative opioid analgesic requirement and recovery profile. *Anesthesiology*, 91(5), 1232–1238.

Hurlow, A., Bennett, M.I., Robb, K.A., Johnson, M.I., Simpson, K.H., and Oxberry, S.G. (2012). Transcutaneous electric nerve stimulation (TENS) for cancer pain in adults. *Cochrane Database of Systematic Reviews*, 3, CD006276.

Khadilkar, A., Milne, S., Brosseau, L., et al. (2001). Transcutaneous electrical nerve stimulation for the treatment of chronic low back pain: a systematic review. *Spine*, 30(23), 2657–2666.

Knight, K.L. (1985). *Cryotherapy: Theory, Technique and Physiology*. Chattanooga: Chattanooga Corporation.

Lehmann, J.F., Silverman, D.R., Baum, B.R., Kirk, N.L., and Johnston, V.C. (1966). Temperature distributions in the human thigh, produced by infrared, hot pack and microwave applications. *Archives of Physical Medicine and Rehabilitation*, 47, 291–299.

Lin, Y.H. (2003). Effects of thermal therapy in improving the passive range of knee motion: comparison of cold and superficial heat applications. *Clinical Rehabilitation*, 17(6), 618–623.

Marineo, G., Iorno, V., Gandini, C., Moschini, V., and Smith, T.J. (2012). Scrambler therapy may relieve chronic neuropathic pain more effectively than guideline-based drug management: results of a pilot, randomized, controlled trial. *Journal of Pain and Symptom Management*, 43(1), 87–95.

Melzack, R. and Wall, P.D. (1965). Pain mechanisms: a new theory. *Science*, 150(3699), 971–979.

Oosterveld, F.G. and Rasker, J.J. (1994). Effects of local heat and cold treatment of surface and articular temperature of arthritic knees. *Arthritis & Rheumatology*, 31(11), 1578–1582.

Pengel, H.M., Maher, C.G., Refshauge, K.M., Pengel, H.M., Maher, C.G., and Refshauge, K.M. (2002). Systematic review of conservative interventions for subacute low back pain. *Clinical Rehabilitation*, 16(8), 811–820.

Philadelphia Panel (2001a). Philadelphia panel evidence-based clinical practice guidelines on selected rehabilitation interventions for knee pain. *Physical Therapy*, 81(10), 1675–1699.

Philadelphia Panel (2001b). Philadelphia panel evidence-based clinical practice guidelines on selected rehabilitation interventions for low back pain. *Physical Therapy*, 81(10), 1641–1674.

Sandler, A.J., Dvorak, J., Humke, T., Grob, D., and Daniels, W. (1996). The effectiveness of various cervical orthoses. An in vivo comparison of the mechanical stability provided by several widely used models. *Spine*, 21(14), 1624–1629.

Stubblefield, M.D. (2011). Radiation fibrosis syndrome: neuromuscular and musculoskeletal complications in cancer survivors. *PM&R*, 3(11), 1041–1054.

Utter, A., Anderson, M.L., Cunniff, J.G., et al. (2010). Video fluoroscopic analysis of the effects of three commonly-prescribed off-the-shelf orthoses on vertebral motion. *Spine*, 35(12), E525–529.

Vernon, H.T., Humphreys, B.K., and Hagino, C.A. (2005). A systematic review of conservative treatments for acute neck pain not due to whiplash. *Journal of Manipulative & Physiological Therapeutics*, 28(6), 443–448.

Yousefi-Nooraie, R., Schonstein, E., Heidari, K., et al. (2008). Low level laser therapy for nonspecific low-back pain. *Cochrane Database of Systematic Reviews*, 2, CD005107.

Zech, D.F., Grond, S., Lynch, J., Hertel, D., and Lehmann, K.A. (1995). Validation of World Health Organization Guidelines for cancer pain relief: a 10-year prospective study. *Pain*, 63(1), 65–76.

Psychological and psychiatric interventions in pain control

Julie R. Price, Alric D. Hawkins, Michael L. Adams, William S. Breitbart, and Steven D. Passik

Introduction to psychological and psychiatric interventions in pain control

Pain is a common problem in populations with advanced illness and has been best characterized in those with cancer or AIDS. The causes, presentation, and impact of pain may be highly complex in some patients, and effective management may require the expertise of multiple specialties, including neurology, neurosurgery, anaesthesiology, and rehabilitation medicine (Foley, 1975, 1985; Breitbart, 1990b). Psychiatric and psychological interventions are integral to the comprehensive treatment of pain and distress in these populations (Breitbart, 1989, 1990b; Massie and Holland, 1987).

The scope of the problem

Approximately 70% of cancer patients experience severe pain at some time in the course of their illness (Foley, 1985) and nearly 75% of those with advanced cancer have chronic pain (Fitzgibbon, 2001). Overall, approximately 50% of terminally ill patients are in moderate to severe pain (Weiss et al., 2001) and 25% of cancer patients may die in severe pain (Twycross and Lack, 1983). Pain prevalence varies among different types of cancer, ranging from a low of approximately 5% in leukaemia to 50–75% in cancers of the lung, gastrointestinal tract, and genitourinary system, and to 85% in cancers of the bone or cervix (Foley, 1975).

Pain is frequently under-diagnosed and inadequately treated (Twycross et al., 1973). This phenomenon presumably has multiple causes, one of which is the complex presentation of pain in populations with advanced illness. In those with cancer, this complexity is partly determined by the common experience of symptoms other than pain, one or more of which may contribute to symptom distress. In one survey, cancer patients had an average of three additional troubling physical symptoms (Grond et al., 1994) and another study observed that patients with advanced disease reported a median of 11 symptoms (Walsh et al., 2000). A global evaluation of the symptom burden allows for a more complete understanding of the impact of pain (Achte and Vanhkonen, 1971).

Pain also is a significant and often neglected problem in patients with AIDS. Although its epidemiology has likely changed in the era of antiretroviral therapy, it also is likely that earlier prevalence data continue to apply to those with poorly controlled or advanced disease. Estimates of the prevalence of pain in AIDS generally range from 30% to 90%, with prevalence increasing as the disease progresses (Breitbart et al., 1996; Norval, 2004). The incidence of pain may be as high as 88%, and 69% of patients may experience moderate to severe pain-related impairment in activities of daily living (Frich and Borgbjerg, 2000). A retrospective chart review of hospitalized patients with AIDS revealed that pain heralded the onset of the illness in 30% and was second only to fever (Lebovits et al., 1989). More than 50% required treatment for pain, including chest pain in 22%, headache in 13%, oral cavity pain in 11%, abdominal pain in 9%, and peripheral neuropathy in 6%. Another retrospective study reported that abdominal pain, peripheral neuropathy, and Kaposi's sarcoma were the three most frequent pain problems, together affecting 15% of patients (Newshan, et al., 1989). Other studies report that between 5% and 30% of AIDS patients have painful peripheral neuropathy (Snider et al., 1983; Levy et al., 1985; Cornblath and McArthur, 1988; Schofferman and Brody, 1990); this disorder has many determinants and it is likely that the prevalence is changing as the use of neurotoxic treatments declines. In a hospice setting, pain was observed in 53% of patients and the main diagnoses were peripheral neuropathy, abdominal pain, headache, and skin pain due to Kaposi's sarcoma (Schofferman and Brody, 1990). Prior to the advent of effective therapies, pain was highly prevalent even in the ambulatory AIDS population, with 43% of patients reporting pain of at least 2 weeks' duration (Rosenfeld et al., 1996); painful neuropathy accounted for 50% of pain diagnoses and lower extremity pain related to Kaposi's sarcoma was found in 45%.

The aetiologies of pain in populations with cancer, AIDS or other advanced illnesses are heterogeneous. For example, a study of ambulatory patients with AIDS before the widespread availability of antiretroviral therapy observed that 33% of pain syndromes were somatic, 35% were visceral, and 33% were neuropathic (Hewitt et al., 1997). Patients often experience different types of pain concurrently.

Multidimensional concept of pain in terminal illness

In populations with serious illness, pain often involves a complex interplay between physical causes and other aspects of human functioning, including personality, affect, cognition, behaviour, and social relations (Breitbart et al., 1993). An enlightened description of pain in terminal illness—known as 'total pain'—was proposed by Cecily Saunders (Saunders, 1967). This label describes the all-encompassing nature of pain, helps explain the inadequate effects of analgesic drugs in some patients (Hanks, 1991), and underscores the importance of psychological factors as determinants of both pain intensity and distress (Syrjala and Chapko, 1995).

The interaction of cognitive, emotional and socio-environmental factors with nociceptive aspects of pain (Fig. 9.11.1) illustrates the multidimensional nature of pain and suggests a model for multimodal intervention (Breitbart, 1990). The challenge of untangling and addressing both the physical and psychological issues involved in pain is essential to developing rational and effective management strategies. Psychosocial therapies directed primarily at psychological variables may have an impact on pain intensity or distress, while somatic therapies directed at nociception may reduce the adverse psychological aspects of pain. To manage complex chronic pain problems, both somatic and psychosocial therapies should be used in a multimodality approach (Breitbart, 1989).

Psychological factors in pain experience

Pain-related distress is complex and may be influenced by stressors faced by patients with advanced disease, such as loss of independence, disability, and fear of painful death. Distress may be influenced by medical factors, cognitions, coping capacity, personality, and social support. Daut and Cleeland (1982) showed that cancer patients who attributed a new pain to a benign cause reported less interference with their activity and pleasure than cancer patients who believed that their pain represented progression of disease. Spiegel and Bloom (1983) found that women with metastatic breast cancer experienced more intense pain if they were depressed and believed that their pain represented spreading of their cancer. The presence of a mood disturbance and beliefs about the meaning of pain are better predictors of pain levels than is the site of metastasis.

The variables that affect pain-related quality-of-life may be categorized in three domains: (1) physical well-being, (2) psychological well-being (consisting of affective factors, cognitive

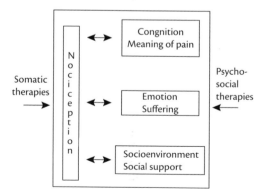

factors, spiritual factors, communication, coping, and meaning of pain or cancer), and (3) interpersonal well-being (focusing on social support or role functioning) (Padilla et al., 1990). The heterogeneity and prominence of these variables have been revealed in studies linking higher levels of pain or pain-related distress to impairment in activities of daily living, the experience of unpredictable painful episodes, negative thoughts about personal or social competence, cognitions about the cause of pain, greater anxiety or depressed mood, and more existential concerns such as fears about the future (Bond and Pearson, 1969; McKegney et al., 1981; Payne et al., 1994; Payne, 1995; Strang, 1997; Smith et al., 1998; Portenoy et al., 1999). A prospective study of cancer patients found that maladaptive coping strategies, lower levels of self-efficacy, and distress specific to the treatment or disease progression were modest but significant predictors of reported pain intensity (Syrjala and Chapko, 1995).

These data highlight the broad variation in the response to pain. A classification that was developed in populations with chronic pain and focuses on adaptation (described as 'dysfunctional', 'interpersonally distressed', or 'adaptive coping') also describes the population with cancer pain, further suggesting the importance of psychosocial factors in the pain experience (Turk et al., 1998). Psychological distress is strongly associated with the number of concerns reported by patients and concerns about pain and treatment have been particularly associated with depression (Heaven and Maguire, 1998).

Most of the aforementioned studies have been performed in the cancer population. Similar findings have been found in patients with AIDS. The perception of control over pain, emotional associations and memories of pain, fear of death, depression, anxiety, and hopelessness—all contribute to the experience of pain and increase suffering in this population (Breitbart et al., 1994). In ambulatory populations with AIDS, pain was associated with depression, functional impairment, and disability (Rosenfeld et al., 1996), and negative pain-related thoughts were associated with greater pain intensity, psychological distress, and disability (Payne et al., 1994). Patients with pain were twice as likely to have suicidal ideation (40%) than those without pain (20%), and those who felt that pain represented a threat to their health reported more intense pain than those who did not see pain as a threat (Rosenfeld et al., 1996). Singer and colleagues (Singer et al., 1993) also reported an association among the frequency of multiple pains, increased disability, and higher levels of depression.

Although these data underscore the importance of psychological variables in explaining continued pain or lack of response to therapy, it must be emphasized that the diagnosis of the physical factors responsible for pain is essential to treatment. It also is important to emphasize that the nature of psychological distress cannot be accurately determined when pain is severe. The psychologist or psychiatrist consulted on a patient with pain must review the medical evaluation of the pain and the adequacy of the analgesic management provided. If medical options for therapy are available, they always should be considered. Pain control should be considered a prerequisite to both the assessment and management of other sources of distress. Indeed, personality factors may be quite distorted by the presence of pain, and relief of pain often results in the disappearance of a perceived psychiatric disorder (Marks and Sachar, 1973, Cleeland and Tearman, 1986).

Fig. 9.11.1 The multidimensional nature of pain in terminal illness.
Reproduced from Breitbart W, and Holland JC, Psychiatric aspects of cancer pain, pp. 73–87, in K. Foley (ed.), *Advances in Pain Research*, and Therapy, (make italic) Volume 16, Raven Press, New York, USA, Copyright © 1990, with permission from Lippincott Williams & Wilkins..

Psychiatric disorders and pain in the terminally ill

In cancer populations, the prevalence of psychiatric disorders is associated with chronic pain (Ahles et al., 1983; Derogatis, 1983; Woodforde, 1989). For example, the Psychosocial Collaborative Oncology Group Study (Derogatis, 1983) found that 39% of the patients who received a psychiatric diagnosis (Table 9.11.1) reported significant pain, compared to 19% without a psychiatric diagnosis. The psychiatric disorders in those with pain were largely adjustment disorders with depressed or anxious mood (69%) and major depression (15%).

The prevalence and patterns of psychiatric disorders may vary systematically in subgroups of patients. For example, a study of patients receiving high-dose dexamethasone for epidural spinal cord compression (as much as 96 mg a day for up to a week, followed by a tapering course for up to 3 or 4 weeks) noted that the incidents of depression (22%) and delirium (24%) were much higher than a comparison group (4% and 10%, respectively) (Breitbart et al., 1993). Although there is limited information about patterns of disorders in other subpopulations, it is apparent that advanced disease itself, at least among patients with cancer, is associated with a relatively high prevalence of depression and delirium (Bukberg et al., 1984). The prevalence of severe depressive symptoms increases from approximately 25% among all cancer patients to 77% in those with advanced illness, and the prevalence of organic mental disorders (delirium) requiring psychiatric consultation increases from the range of 25% to 40% to as high as 85% during the terminal stages of illness (Massie et al., 1983). The latter finding is presumably multifactorial and partly related to the use of opioids and other drugs that can cause confusional states, particularly in the elderly and terminally ill (Bruera, 1989).

Rosenfeld, Breitbart, and colleagues (Rosenfeld et al., 1996) described the psychological impact of pain in an ambulatory AIDS population. AIDS patients with pain reported significantly greater depression and functional impairment than those without pain. Psychiatric disorders, in particular the organic mental disorders such as AIDS dementia complex, can occasionally interfere with adequate pain management. The use of an opioid in this setting may worsen dementia or cause treatment-limiting sedation, confusion, or hallucinations. This observation has suggested the judicious use of psychostimulants to diminish sedation and neuroleptics to clear confusional states. Other psychiatric disorders that have an impact on pain management in the AIDS population include substance abuse and personality disorders.

Pain and suicide

Uncontrolled pain is a major factor in suicide and suicidal ideation in the medically ill (Breitbart, 1987, 1990a; Sison et al., 1991), confirming a US public opinion survey in which 69% agreed that cancer pain could cause a person to consider suicide (Levin et al., 1985). Although relatively few cancer patients commit suicide, they are at increased risk overall (Farberow et al., 1963; Levin et al., 1985) and the majority of suicides involve patients who have severe, inadequately controlled or poorly tolerated pain (Bolund, 1985). Patients with advanced illness, who are most likely to have pain, depression or delirium, are at highest risk. A review of the psychiatric consultation data at Memorial Sloan Kettering Cancer Center showed that one-third of hospitalized cancer patients who were seen for evaluation of suicide risk received a diagnosis of major depression, approximately 20% met criteria for delirium, and more than 50% were diagnosed with an adjustment disorder (Breitbart, 1987).

Thoughts of suicide probably occur quite frequently, particularly in the setting of advanced illness (Massie et al., 1994). For many patients, these thoughts actually may be reassuring, acting as a 'steam valve' for feelings: 'If it gets too bad, I always have a way out'. Patients who have a trusting and safe relationship with a health professional commonly admit to occasional thoughts of suicide as a means of escaping the threat of being overwhelmed by pain. Persistent suicidal ideation is relatively infrequent, however, and is limited to those who are significantly depressed. Silberfarb et al. (1980) found that only three of 146 breast cancer patients had suicidal thoughts, whereas none of the 100 cancer patients interviewed in a Finnish study expressed suicidal thoughts (Achte, 1971). A study conducted at St Boniface Hospice in Winnipeg, Canada, demonstrated that only ten of 44 terminally ill cancer patients were suicidal or desired an early death, and all ten were suffering from clinical depression (Brown et al.,

Table 9.11.1 Rates of DSM-III psychiatric disorders and prevalence of pain observed in 215 cancer patients from three cancer centers

Diagnostic category	Number in diagnostic class	Percentage of psychiatric diagnoses	Number with significant pain[a]
Adjustment disorders	69	32	68
Major affective disorders	13	6	13
Organic mental disorders	8	4	8
Personality disorders	7	3	7
Anxiety disorders	4	2	4
Total with psychiatric diagnosis	101	47	39 (39%)
Total with no psychiatric diagnosis	114	53	21 (19%)
Total patient population	215	100	60 (28%)

[a] Score greater than 50 mm on a 100 mm VAS pain severity.

Source: data from Derogatis, L.R. et al., The prevalence of psychiatric disorders among cancer patients, *Journal of the American Medical Association*, Volume 249, Number 6, pp.751–7, Copyright © 1983 American Medical Association. All Rights Reserved.

1986). At Memorial Sloan Kettering Cancer Center, suicide risk evaluation accounted for 8.6% of psychiatric consultations, usually requested by staff in response to patients verbalizing suicidal wishes (Breitbart, 1987); all 71 patients who had suicidal ideation with serious intent had a psychiatric disorder (mood disturbance or organic mental disorder) and 30% had significant pain (Breitbart, 1987).

In the cancer population, pain has been associated with the desire for hastened death. In multivariate analyses, depression and hopelessness provided independent and unique contributions to the prediction of the desire for hastened death, while social support and physical functioning added significant but smaller contributions (Breitbart et al., 2000). In a study at Memorial Sloan Kettering Cancer Center, 17% of 185 patients with pain expressed suicidal ideation, with the majority reporting suicidal ideation without intent to act (Saltzburg, 1989). Interestingly, in this population of cancer patients who had significant pain, suicidal ideation was not directly related to pain intensity, but was strongly related to the degree of depression and mood disturbance. Pain was related to suicidal ideation indirectly in that patients' perception of poor pain relief was associated with suicidal ideation. Perceptions of pain relief may have more to do with aspects of hopelessness than pain itself.

Although pain may play an important role in vulnerability to suicide in populations with advanced cancer, these data suggest that factors other than pain, such as mood disturbance, delirium, loss of control and hopelessness, contribute to cancer suicide risk (Bolund, 1985). Frequency of suicidal ideation in one study was associated with poor well-being, depression, anxiety, and shortness of breath, but not with other somatic symptoms such as pain, nausea, and loss of appetite (Suarez-Almazor et al., 2002).

Although work in other populations has been limited, studies of patients with advanced AIDS also have found complex and variable relationships among pain, depression, hopelessness, and suicidal ideation, and suggest that the findings in cancer studies may be more universal. A study of men with AIDS in New York City (Marzuk et al., 1988) demonstrated a relative risk of suicide 36 times greater than that of males in the general population. Many of these patients had advanced AIDS, with Kaposi's sarcoma and other potentially painful conditions. However, the role of pain in contributing to increased risk of suicide was not specifically examined. In a study at Memorial Sloan Kettering Cancer Center (Rabkin et al., 1993), suicidal ideation in ambulatory AIDS patients was found to be highly correlated with the presence of pain, depressed mood (as measured by the Beck Depression Inventory), and low T4 lymphocyte counts. While 20% of ambulatory AIDS patients without pain reported suicidal thoughts, more than 40% of those with pain reported suicidal ideation. Only two of the 110 patients in this study reported suicidal intent. One of these two men was in the pain group; both scored highly on measures of depression. No correlations were observed between suicidal ideation and pain intensity or pain relief. The mean visual analogue scale measure of pain intensity for the group overall was 49 mm (range 5–100 mm), thus falling predominantly in the moderate range. Similar to cancer patients, suicidal ideation in AIDS patients with pain is more likely to be related to a concomitant mood disturbance than to pain intensity. Although AIDS patients are frequently found to have suicidal ideation, these thoughts are more often context-specific, occurring almost exclusively during exacerbations of the illness, when pain is severe, or at times of bereavement (Rabkin et al., 1993).

Inadequate pain management

The adequacy of pain management can be best judged when there is consensus about best practice and data that illuminate the likelihood of satisfactory pain control when treatment is optimal. From this perspective, studies in the cancer population and AIDS population may illuminate the prevalence and causes of undertreatment and suggest the seriousness of the problem in other medically ill groups. Studies suggest that pain in cancer is undertreated (Cleeland et al., 1994) and pain in AIDS is dramatically undertreated (Lebovits et al., 1989; McCormack et al., 1993; Breitbart et al., 1996). In one study of a cohort of AIDS patients treated in New York City (Breitbart et al., 1996), only 6% of patients reporting pain in the severe range (8–10 on a numerical rating scale) received a strong opioid, such as morphine. This degree of undermedication far exceeds published reports of undermedication of pain in cancer populations (Cleeland et al., 1994). Similar to the cancer population, undertreatment of AIDS-related pain may be more likely in women, those with limited education or a substance abuse history, and those who express a variety of patient-related barriers to opioid treatment (Breitbart et al., 1996, 1998). It is also clear that adjuvant agents such as the antidepressants are also dramatically underused (Lebovits et al., 1989; McCormack et al., 1993; Breitbart et al., 1996). Only 6% of patients in a sample of AIDS patients reporting pain received an adjuvant analgesic drug (i.e. an antidepressant).

Inadequate management of pain often is due to the inability to properly assess pain in all its dimensions (Foley, 1985; Breitbart 1989; Twycross and Lack, 1983). Psychological variables may be ignored, or contrariwise, may be proposed to explain pain when in fact medical factors have not been adequately appreciated. Other causes of inadequate pain management include lack of knowledge about pharmacological interventions, focus on prolonging life rather than alleviating suffering, lack of communication between doctor and patient, limited expectations of patients to achieve pain relief, patients' limited capacity to communicate, unavailability of opioid drugs, doctors' fear of opioid toxicity, and doctors' fear of amplifying addiction and substance abuse. In advanced cancer, several related factors have been noted to predict the undertreatment of pain, including a discrepancy between physician and patient in judging the severity of pain; the presence of pain that physicians did not attribute to cancer, better performance status, age of 70 or over, and female sex (Cleeland et al., 1994).

The pharmacological risks associated with opioid drugs, including respiratory depression, are too often overestimated and also can limit appropriate use of opioid analgesics. Non-specialists may not appreciate the safety of opioid therapy when careful dose selection and titration are employed. The widely accepted use of morphine to treat dyspnoea in populations with serious cardiopulmonary disease, without causing a significant deterioration in respiratory function, may be useful to cite when educating colleagues about these drugs (Bruera et al., 1990).

The adequacy of cancer pain management also can be adversely influenced by other misapprehensions. Persistent cancer pain is often ascribed to a psychological cause when it does not respond to treatment attempts. Clinical observation suggests that the complaint of 'severe' pain is relatively more likely to be viewed as having a psychological contribution. Indeed, staff members' ability to empathize with a patient's pain complaint may be limited by the report of high intensity. Grossman et al. (1991) found that while there is a high degree of concordance between patient and staff ratings of patient pain intensity at the low and moderate levels, this concordance broke down at high pain levels; specifically, the clinicians' ability to assess a patient's level of pain became unreliable when pain intensity was greater than 7 on a 0–10 scale. Physicians must be educated about the limitations of their ability to objectively assess the severity of a subjective pain experience. Additionally, patient education may be useful given the observation that patients are more likely to be believed and adequately treated if they are taught to request pain relief without behaviours that would be interpreted as emotional over-reaction.

A history of drug abuse has been repeatedly associated with the undertreatment of pain. Clinicians may overestimate the prevalence of drug abuse in populations with serious medical illness. At Memorial Sloan Kettering Cancer Center, for example, only eight (1.7%) of 468 inpatients referred for cancer pain had a history of intravenous drug abuse, and none had been actively abusing drugs during the previous year. All eight of these patients were intentionally undermedicated because of concern by staff that drug abuse was active or would recur, and adequate pain control was ultimately achieved in these patients by using appropriate analgesic dosages and intensive staff education. Although populations in other settings may have far higher prevalence of substance use disorders—for example, the base rate of substance use disorders is clearly higher in the younger HIV population (Breitbart, 2003)—clinicians should be able to reassure colleagues and others through knowledge of the true prevalence rates. Derogatis et al. (1983) assessed 215 ambulatory cancer patients for psychiatric diagnoses and found that fewer than 5% met the criteria for a substance use disorder.

Limited knowledge about the presentation, assessment, and management of tolerance, physical dependence, drug abuse and addiction may contribute to an overestimation of risk, which may, in turn, discourage the appropriate use of opioids to treat pain (Charap, 1978; Kanner and Foley, 1981; Twycross and Lack, 1983; Macaluso et al., 1988; Breitbart, 1990). For example, a patient's request for a higher dose to treat worsening pain may be perceived as a strong indicator of, tolerance, abuse, or addiction. In populations with advanced illness, however, most patients stabilize on a dose for a prolonged period, and when dose escalation is needed, it usually is linked to observable progression of disease. If pain increases as a result of disease progression, the loss of drug effect cannot be ascribed to the development of tolerance; in the absence of other findings, it should not be attributed to abuse or addiction. Like physical dependence, which is defined as the potential for abstinence if the dose is abruptly reduced or an antagonist is administered, tolerance usually is not perceived to be a clinical problem unless there is repeated loss of analgesic efficacy in the absence of disease progression.

Addiction is a neurobiological disease with a strong genetic basis, which is defined by the occurrence of craving, loss of control over drug use, compulsive use, and continuing use despite harm. Understanding the assessment strategies needed to identify these characteristics, and acknowledging the key differences between addiction and both tolerance and physical dependence,

are essential to accurately judge the true risks of opioid therapy in an individual patient.

Patients who require pain treatment with opioids or other potentially abusable drugs and either have a history of significant alcohol or drug abuse or meet criteria for a substance use disorder do pose a challenge for clinicians. This is exemplified by the management of pain in the growing segment of the AIDS population that is actively abusing intravenous drugs (Breitbart, 2003). Active drug use, particularly intravenous opioid abuse, may compromise pain therapy through (a) high tolerance to opioid analgesics needed for disease-related pain, (b) drug-seeking and manipulative behaviour, (c) lack of adherence or reliability of patient history, and (d) the risk of spreading HIV. Because subjective report may be the only indication of the presence and intensity of pain, or the degree of pain relief achieved by an intervention, patients who are assumed to lie as an element of addictive disease are at high risk to generate concern among clinicians, whose reluctance to believe the patient may lead to anger and limited pain therapy. Undertreatment is clearly a risk in this context.

Most clinicians experienced in working with medically ill patients with substance abuse history recommend clear and direct limit setting. To the extent possible, clinicians should attempt to eliminate the issue of drug abuse as an obstacle to pain management by dealing directly with the problems of opioid withdrawal and drug abuse treatment. Often, specialized substance abuse consultation services are available to help manage such patients and initiate structured drug administration, or other elements of drug treatment, at the same time that pain management is occurring. If analgesic drugs are the focus of a battle for control between the patient and physician, therapy will be compromised, especially in terminal stages of illness. In this setting, it is appropriate for clinicians to err on the side of believing a patient when they complain of pain, and present a bias toward treatment, as long as there is no clear evidence of self-destructive behaviours or drug diversion to the illicit market (see Chapter 9.5).

Psychiatric and psychological management of pain in advanced disease

Optimal treatment of pain associated with advanced illness often requires a multimodality strategy, including pharmacological, psychological, rehabilitative, and interventional approaches. The numerous psychological approaches include psychotherapeutic, cognitive behavioural, and psychopharmacologic interventions, usually in combination.

Psychotherapy and pain

When patients experience pain in the context of serious medical illness, the goals of psychotherapy are to provide support, knowledge, and skills (Table 9.11.2). Short-term supportive psychotherapy focused on the crisis created by the medical illness is a common strategy, through which the therapist provides emotional support, continuity and information, and assists in adaptation. The therapist has a role in emphasizing past strengths, supporting previously successful coping strategies, and teaching new coping skills. These new skills may include relaxation training, cognitive behavioural approaches to improve coping, self-monitoring skills, and assertiveness and communication skills. Patients can be taught about documentation, such as the effective use of a pain diary, and

Table 9.11.2 Goals and forms of psychotherapy for pain in patients with advanced disease

Goals	Form
Support—provide continuity	Individuals—supportive/crisis intervention
Knowledge—provide information	Family—patient and family are the unit of concern
Skills—relaxation, cognitive coping, communication, use of analgesics	Group—share experiences, identify successful coping strategies

about the safe and effective use of analgesics. In some cases, existential issues arise and require exploration. Communication skills are of paramount importance for both patient and family, particularly around pain and analgesic issues. The patient and family is the unit of concern, and there is a need to support a more general, long-term supportive relationship within the health-care system, in addition to providing specific psychological approaches.

Psychotherapy with the patient who has advanced illness and pain consists of active listening with supportive verbal interventions and the occasional interpretation (Cassem, 1987). Despite the seriousness of the patient's plight, it is not necessary for the psychologist or psychiatrist to appear overly solemn or emotionally restrained. Often, the relationship is strengthened by the ability of the psychotherapist to converse lightheartedly and allow the patient to talk about his life and experiences, rather than focus solely on impending death. The patient who wishes to talk or ask questions about death and pain and suffering should be allowed to do so freely, with the psychotherapist maintaining an interested, interactive stance. This work may ensue in parallel with discussions between the patient or family and other members of the treatment team, including the chaplain.

As the illness progresses, psychotherapy with the individual patient may become limited by cognitive or speech deficits. It is at this point that the focus of supportive psychotherapeutic interventions shifts primarily to the family. A common issue for the family at this point is the level of alertness of the patient. Attempts to control pain are often accompanied by sedation that can limit communication between patient and family. This can sometimes become a source of conflict, with family members disagreeing among themselves or with the patient about what constitutes an appropriate balance between comfort and alertness. It can be helpful for the physician to clarify the patient's preferences as they relate to these issues early so that conflict can be avoided and work related to bereavement can begin.

Group interventions with individual patients (even in advanced stages of disease), spouses, couples, or families are a powerful means of sharing experiences and identifying successful coping strategies. The limitations of using group interventions for patients with advanced disease are primarily pragmatic. The patient must be physically comfortable enough to participate and have the cognitive capacity to be aware of group discussion. It is often helpful for family members to attend support groups during the terminal phases of the patient's illness.

Family caregivers often assist in pain management and interventions may be targeted to enhance these efforts. In an novel intervention, Keefe (2005) tested the efficacy of a partner-guided cancer pain management protocol consisting of a three-session intervention conducted in patients' homes that integrated educational information about cancer pain with systematic training of patients and partners in cognitive and behavioural pain coping skills (see 'Cognitive behavioural techniques'); this approach produced significant increases in the partners' ratings of their self-efficacy for helping the patient control pain and self-efficacy for controlling other symptoms.

Psychotherapeutic interventions that have multiple targets may be the most useful. Based upon a prospective study of cancer pain, cognitive behavioural and psychoeducational techniques based upon increasing support and self-efficacy, as well as providing education, may help patients deal with increased pain (Syrajala et al., 1992). Distress related to the illness, self-efficacy, and coping may be associated with pain and be specifically addressed by these interventions.

Psychotherapy to diminish symptoms of anxiety and depression, factors that can intensify pain, also may be an important strategy. In a randomized controlled study, Spiegel and Bloom (1983) demonstrated that both supportive group therapy and training in hypnotic pain control exercises benefited patients with pain related to metastatic breast cancer. The supportive group focused not on interpersonal processes or self-exploration, but rather on a series of themes related to the practical and existential problems of living with cancer.

While psychotherapy in populations with advanced illness is primarily non-analytical and focuses on current issues, exploration of reactions to illness often involve insights into earlier, more pervasive life issues. Some patients choose to continue a more exploratory psychotherapy during extended periods of stable disease, or during survivorship.

Cognitive behavioural techniques

Cognitive behavioural techniques can be useful as adjuncts to the management of pain in the setting of serious medical illness (Box 9.11.1). The goal of these techniques is to guide the patient towards a sense of control over pain. Some of the specific interventions are primarily cognitive in nature, focusing on perceptual and thought processes, and others are directed at modifying patterns of behaviour that may help patients cope with pain. Specific strategies include passive relaxation with mental imagery, cognitive distraction or focusing, progressive muscle relaxation, biofeedback, hypnosis, and music therapy (Cleeland, 1987; Fishman and Loscalzo, 1987; Loscalzo and Jacobsen, 1990; Singer et al., 1993). Behavioural techniques may seek to modify physiologic pain reactions, respondent pain behaviours, or operant pain behaviours (see Table 9.11.3 for definitions).

The cognitive interventions that are used to reduce pain intensity or associated distress may attempt to modify the thoughts about the pain, introduce more adaptive coping strategies, or provide instruction through various types of relaxation techniques. Cognitive modification (cognitive restructuring) is an approach derived from cognitive therapy for depression or anxiety and is based on how one interprets events and bodily sensation. It is assumed that patients have dysfunctional automatic thoughts that reflect underlying assumptions and beliefs. In both cancer and AIDS populations, negative thoughts about pain have been shown to be significantly related to pain intensity, degree of psychological distress, and level of interference in functional

Box 9.11.1 Cognitive behavioural techniques used by pain patients with advanced disease

- Psychoeducation:
  - preparatory information
  - self-monitoring
- Relaxation:
  - passive breathing
  - progressive muscle relaxation
- Distraction:
  - focusing
  - controlled by mental imagery
  - cognitive distraction
  - behavioural distraction
- Combined techniques (relaxation and distraction):
  - passive/progressive relaxation with mental imagery
  - systematic desensitization
  - meditation
  - hypnosis
  - biofeedback
  - music therapy
- Cognitive therapies:
  - cognitive distortion
  - cognitive restructuring.

Behavioural therapies:

Modelling

Graded task management

Contingency management

Behavioural rehearsal

Table 9.11.3 Cognitive behavioural techniques: definitions and descriptions

Behavioural therapy	The clinical use of techniques derived from the experimental analysis of behaviour, i.e. learning and conditioning for the evaluation, prevention, and treatment of physical disease or physiological dysfunction
Cognitive therapy	A focused intervention targeted at changing maladaptive beliefs and dysfunctional attitudes. The therapist engages the patient in a process of collaborative empiricism, where these underlying beliefs are challenged and corrected
Operant pain	Pain behaviours resulting from operant learning or conditioning. Pain behaviour is reinforced and continues because of secondary gain, i.e. increased attention and caring
Respondent pain	Pain behaviours resulting from respondent learning or conditioning. Stimuli associated with prior painful experiences can elicit increased pain and avoidance behaviour
Cognitive restructuring	Redefinition of some or all aspects of the patient's interpretation of the noxious or threatening experience, resulting in decreased distress, anxiety, and hopelessness
Self-monitoring (pain diary)	Written or audiotaped chronicle that the patient maintains to describe specific agreed-upon characteristics associated with pain
Contingency management	Focusing the patient and family member responses that either reinforce or inhibit specific behaviours exhibited by the patient. Method involves reinforcing desired 'well' behaviours
Grade task assignments	A hierarchy of tasks, i.e. physical, cognitive, and behavioural, are compartmentalized and performed sequentially in manageable steps ultimately achieving an identified goal
Systematic desensitization	Relaxation and distraction exercises paired with a hierarchy of anxiety-arousing stimuli presented through mental imagery, or presented *in vivo*, resulting in control of fear

activities (Payne et al., 1994; Payne, 1995). By identifying and challenging dysfunctional automatic thoughts and underlying beliefs by restructuring or modifying thought processes, a more rational response to pain can occur (Fishman and Loscalzo, 1987). Examples of such automatic thoughts that have been shown to worsen pain experience are: 'The intensity of my pain will never diminish' or 'Because my pain limits my activities, I am completely helpless.' Patients can be taught to recognize and interrupt such thoughts and proceed to develop a view of the pain experience as time-limited and themselves as functional despite periods in which they are limited.

The use of cognitive restructuring may shift as the goals change in the palliative care context. In the setting of advanced illness, the goal may not be to change the patient's maladaptive thoughts, but rather, to utilize techniques designed to diminish the patient's anxiety, frustration, and anger. Helping patients to employ more adaptive coping strategies, allowing for decreased catastrophization and increase problem-solving skills, may be helpful at this stage (Fishman, 1990; Turk and Fernandez, 1990; Jensen et al., 1991).

Aside from modifying dysfunctional thoughts and attitudes, the most fundamental behavioural technique is self-monitoring. The development of the ability to monitor one's behaviours allows a person to notice their dysfunctional reactions to the pain experience and learn to control them.

Another approach, systematic desensitization (see Table 9.11.3), may be useful in extinguishing the anticipatory anxiety that can lead to avoidant behaviours, and in remobilizing inactive patients. Graded task assignment may be viewed as a type of systematic desensitization, by which function is improved by teaching patients to take small steps gradually and thereby initially avoiding the anxiety associated with the specific task until more effective coping mechanism and self-efficacy is achieved. Finally, contingency management is a method of reinforcing 'well' behaviours only; this may modify dysfunctional operant pain behaviours associated with secondary gain (Cleeland, 1987; Loscalzo and Jacobsen, 1990).

The range of cognitive behavioural interventions that may be useful in the setting of advanced illness is very broad (Breitbart and Holland, 1988) and there is some evidence that all methods are not equally effective. Cognitive strategies, including relaxation, suggestion, and distracting imagery, appear to hold the greatest promise, although research on the usage of these techniques to control pain is scant (Sellick and Zaza, 1998; Montgomery et al., 2002). The mechanisms by which these techniques relieve pain are not known and it widely accepted that a favourable response to a psychological technique should not be viewed as evidence that pain is psychogenic. All these techniques share the elements of relaxation and distraction, and this common pathway may help reduce awareness of pain, muscle tension and sympathetic arousal (Cleeland, 1987). Although studies of these interventions in populations with advanced illness are limited, the recommendation to consider a combined non-pharmacological and pharmacological pain management strategy is common, and is especially promoted with paediatric populations (Kazak et al., 1998). These interventions may be a particularly attractive part of a multimodality approach because they produce no side effects.

Patient selection for cognitive behavioural interventions for pain

The selection of patients with advanced illness and pain for trials of cognitive behavioural strategies should take into account the intensity of pain and the mental clarity of the patient. Ideal candidates have mild to moderate pain, either at baseline or as a result of analgesic drug therapy. Confusional states interfere dramatically with a patient's ability to focus attention and thus limit the usefulness of these techniques (Loscalzo and Jacobsen, 1990). Occasionally, however, these techniques can be modified so as to include mildly impaired patients. This may involve the therapist taking a more active role by orienting the patient, creating a safe and secure environment, and evoking a conditioned response to the therapist's voice or presence.

Barriers to engaging patients in cognitive behavioural therapies can be divided into physician/nurse-based barriers and patient-based barriers. Many health professionals are uncomfortable with the use of behavioural therapies. Pharmacotherapy is highly effective in the management of pain and seems simpler and easier to use than labour-intensive and time-consuming non-pharmacological interventions. Physicians and nurses have typical concerns about the practice of behavioural interventions such as: 'What if the patient laughs, doesn't buy it?' or 'It seems too theatrical, unscientific, non-medical; too New Age!' Overcoming such obstacles may yield gratifying results. Physicians working with patients with advanced illness should become aware of the effective non-pharmacological interventions and be able to make appropriate referrals to practitioners who can provide them.

Patients may be uncertain about the utility of these therapies. Some may ask, 'How can breathing take away my pain?' They may be frightened by the word 'hypnosis' and its connotations. Although hypnosis is often associated with powerful and magical properties, some patients become frightened at the prospect of losing control or being under the influence of someone else. It generally is best to introduce cognitive behavioural interventions after some rapport has been established with a patient. Although some patients may benefit from a discussion of the theoretical basis of these interventions, it is important to stress that an understanding of the mechanism is not needed for effectiveness and the outcome is most important. Apprehensions must be addressed, and patients must feel in control of the process at all times and be reassured that they can stop at any time.

Practical considerations in the use of cognitive-behavioural approaches

A general approach to using cognitive behavioural interventions with patients with advanced illness and pain involves the following: (1) assessment of the symptom, (2) choosing a cognitive behavioural strategy, and (3) preparing the patient and the setting.

The main purpose of conducting a cognitive behavioural assessment of pain is to determine what, if any, interventions are indicated (Kanner and Foley, 1981). One must initially engage the patient and establish a therapeutic alliance. A history of the pain symptom must be taken. One should review previous efforts to treat the patient's pain, and collect data regarding the nature of the pain and its impact on the patient and their family. Choosing the appropriate behavioural strategy should consider the patient's medical condition, physical and cognitive limitations, time constraints, and practical matters. For instance, patients with cognitive impairment or delirium will probably be unable to keep a pain diary or employ techniques that involve cognitive manipulation.

Muscular tension, autonomic arousal, and mental distress exacerbate pain (Cleeland, 1987; Loscalzo and Jacobsen, 1990), and a variety of techniques can be used to achieve a state of relaxation. These include passive relaxation through the focusing of attention on sensations of warmth and decreased tension in various parts of the body, progressive muscle relaxation involving active tensing and relaxing of muscles, and meditation. Other techniques that employ relaxation, as well as other cognitive therapies, include hypnosis, biofeedback, and music therapy (discussed later). Although studies of relaxation do not confirm a positive effect on chronic pain, but indicate that relaxation training can reduce some pain scores and more clearly has a positive effect on anxiety (Wallace, 1997; Carroll and Seers, 1998; Luebbert et al., 2001).

Passive relaxation, focused breathing, and passive muscle relaxation exercises involve the focusing of attention systematically on one's breathing, on sensations of warmth and relaxation, or on release of muscular tension in various body parts. Verbal suggestions and imagery are used to help promote relaxation. Muscle relaxation is an important component of the relaxation response and can augment the benefits of simple focused breathing exercises, leading to a deeper experience of relaxation and self-control.

Progressive or active muscle relaxation involves the active tensing and relaxing of various muscle groups in the body, focusing attention on the sensations of tension and relaxation. Clinically, in the hospital setting, relaxation is most commonly achieved through the use of a combination of focused breathing and progressive muscle relaxation exercises. Once patients are in a relaxed state, imagery techniques can then be used to induce deeper relaxation and facilitate distraction from or manipulation of a variety of cancer-related symptoms.

Script for passive relaxation (focused breathing)

The following script is a generic relaxation exercise, utilizing passive relaxation or focused breathing, that is based on and integrates the work of Erickson (1959), Benson (1995), and others (Loscalzo and Jacobsen, 1990).

'Why don't you begin by finding a comfortable position. Slowly allow your body to unwind and just let it go. That's it . . . I wonder if you can allow your body to become as calm as possible . . . just let it go, just let your body sink into that bed (or chair) . . . feel free to move or shift around in any way that your body needs to, to find that comfortable position. You need not try very hard, simply and easily allow yourself to follow the sound of my voice as you allow your body to find itself a safe, comfortable position to relax in.

If you like, you can gently allow your eyes to close, just let the lids cover your eyes . . . allow your eyes to sink back deeply into their sockets . . . that's it, just let them go, falling back gently and deeply into their sockets as your lids begin to feel heavier and heavier. As you allow your head to fall back deeply into the pillow, feeling the weight of your head sinking into the pillow as you breath out, just breath out, one big breath. Slowly, if you can begin to turn your attention to your breathing. Notice your breath for a few moments, how much air you take in, how much air you let out, and just breath evenly and naturally, and with the sound of my voice I wonder if you can begin to take in more air, breathing in and out, in and out, that's it, gradually breathing in and out . . . in and out . . . breathing in calmness and quietness, breathing out tiredness and frustration, that's it . . . let it go, it's not important to you now . . . breathing in quietness and control, breathing out fear and tension . . . breathing in and out . . . in and out . . . you can enjoy breathing in this relaxed way for as long as you need to. You are peaceful now as you continue to observe your even and steady breathing that is allowing you to feel gentle and calm, breathing that is allowing you to feel a gentle calm, that's it, breathing relaxation in and tension out . . . in and out . . . breathing in quietness and control, breathing out tiredness and tension . . . that's it (patient's name here) as you continue to notice the quietness and stillness of your body, why don't you take a few quiet moments to experience this process more fully.'

It may be helpful for the clinician to mark the end of an exercise by increasing the pace, raising the volume of voice, and shifting position. Additionally, it is helpful for the clinician to both pace and model for the patient. This includes positioning yourself as similarly to the patient as possible (e.g. closing eyes, assuming a position of relaxation, and breathing at the same rate). If the patient exhibits any visible anxiety or agitation, this can be briefly explored verbally, and then, if appropriate, the exercise can be continued.

Script for active or progressive muscle relaxation
This exercise involves the patient actively tensing and then relaxing specific body parts. Once again, it may be helpful if the clinician paces and models for the patient.

'Now, I wonder if you can tense up every muscle in your body . . . that's it, squeeze in the muscles . . . hold it, and then just let it go . . . once more, tense up your muscles . . . make them very tight and tense, hold it, hold it . . . and then breath out, and let your muscles relax, just let them go . . . Now, as your body begins to feel more and more relaxed, clench your jaw, squeeze it tight, clench it and then let it go . . . now open your mouth wide, as wide as it will go, stick out your tongue, stick it way out, hold it and then let it go. Feel your head becoming more and more relaxed, as it sinks down into the pillow, allowing all the tension and tightness to drift out of it . . . Now, I wonder if you can lift up your shoulders, lift them up, up to your ears, hold them there, squeezing them tightly, squeeze, and then let them drop down, just let them go . . . and then once more lift them up . . . hold it . . . then let them go . . . as you feel all

the tightness and tension in your shoulders begin to drain away . . . Now, I wonder if you can clench your hands into a fist, make a tight fist as your whole arm tightens, tense your arms as you squeeze in your fingers tighter and tighter . . . and now just let them go, once more now make a fist, a tight fist, hold it, and then let it go.'

As with passive muscle relaxation, the clinician guides the patient through the exercise, requesting the patient to tense and release specific muscles in a progressive order.

Imagery/distraction techniques
Clinically, relaxation techniques are most helpful in managing pain when combined with distraction or pleasant imagery. The use of distraction or focusing involves control over the focus of attention and can be used to make the patient less aware of the noxious stimuli (Broome et al., 1992). Keeping oneself busy is a form of behavioural distraction. Mental distraction can be used and is similar to the practice of counting sheep to aid sleep. Imagery—using one's imagination while in a relaxed state—can be used to transform pain into a warm or cold sensation. One can employ imaginative inattention by picturing oneself on a beach. One can also imaginatively transform the context of pain; for example, one could imagine oneself in battle on the football field instead of the hospital bed. Dissociated somatization, which can be employed by some patients, involves imagining that a painful body part is no longer part of their body (Fishman and Loscalzo, 1987; Breitbart, 1989, 1990; Loscalzo and Jacobsen, 1990). It is important to note that not every patient finds these techniques acceptable, and the therapist must try out a number of approaches to determine which are consistent with the patient's style.

Imagery (often referred to as guided imagery) is most effective when the specific image is obtained from the patient. The clinician may ask the patient to close his or her eyes and think of a place, an activity, or an experience where the patient felt most safe and secure. The clinician may provide suggestions for the patient such as a favourite beach scene, or a room in a house, or riding a bicycle in a state park. Once the patient identifies the scene, the clinician may ask the patient to elaborate upon the scene, asking for specific details such as the temperature, season, time of day, type of ocean (calm, or with big waves), etc. The clinician then utilizes this information and describes an image for the patient in detail. The clinician should be as flexible and as creative as possible, and elaborate upon the scene, utilizing all aspects of the senses and bodily sensations such as 'feel the suns rays touch your skin, allow your skin to feel warm and tingly all over . . .' or, 'breath in the fresh, clear air, allow it to fill your lungs with its freshness . . .' or, 'feel the fresh dew of the grass under your feet'. The clinician can focus on 'aromas in the garden' or the 'sounds of birds singing', always reminding the patient to breath evenly and steadily as he or she feels more and more relaxed and more and more in control. If possible, the clinician should avoid volunteering an image or scene for the patient because the clinician is unaware of the association or meaning the image may have for the patient. For example, a patient may have a fear of the water, and therefore a beach scene may invoke feelings of fear and loss of control.

Script for pleasant distracting imagery
The following is a generic script for a imagery exercise:

'Once you are in a comfortable position, I wonder if you can continue lying there with your eyes closed, continuing to breath in out . . . in and out to the sound of my voice. Let your mind wander . . . just let it go . . . and if any unwanted thoughts come into your mind, you can allow then to pass out as easily as they came in . . . You don't need them now . . . they are not important to you now. You have the ability to control your thoughts. You have the ability to be in control.

Slowly, I wonder if you can allow your mind to travel . . . to travel far away to your favourite beach. The beach that you have many fond memories of. I wonder if you can imagine that it's almost the end of the day and the beach is deserted . . . and the sun, while setting, is still warm, as it beats down . . . and makes your skin feel tingly and warm all over. As you begin to walk on the sand, you can feel the granules underneath your feet. Step evenly and steadily along the sand. As you look around, you can see the different colours in the sky. You can see for miles off into the distance and you feel exhilarated and free because no one is around you. You are alone and in control. As you walk closer to the edge of the ocean the sand is becoming a little damp and you can feel the dampness underneath your feet—it feels refreshing. As you continue walking, you may notice a few odds and ends on the sand maybe something that the ocean brought in . . . some shells perhaps. They may be broken from being knocked against the rocks . . . or there may be a few bits of seaweed or some jellyfish. You stop to notice them as you walk past . . . marvelling at the wonders of nature. As you get to the edge of the ocean, you can feel the tiny little ripples of water washing over your feet . . . bouncing over your feet making you feel light and fresh. The water is warm—it soothes your feet. Washing back and forth . . . back and forth. As you keep walking you see your rubber raft. This is your old dependable rubber raft. You get to the raft and you secure it in your hands and lie down on it letting your whole body sink into the raft—just let it go . . . that's it. Slowly you kick off as the raft begins to take you away. The ocean is very calm and very gentle. Your whole body begins to unwind and sink deeper and deeper into the raft as you feel more and more relaxed. This raft allows you to drift off . . . and underneath you can feel the ripples of the ocean . . . rocking back and forth . . . back and forth as you continue to float away evenly and gently. You can become aware of the sun beating down on your skin. You are aware of the sounds around you—you can hear the ocean washing against the rocks as the waves rock back and forth . . . back and forth. You can hear the gulls crying in the distance. There is a very tiny protected bay that you are floating away in. It is a very calm and peaceful day, and you are feeling more and more relaxed. You are in control now . . . and as you continue to sail away, all your troubles and problems wash right out of you. They're not important to you now. You don't need them now. What's important is that your whole body, from the tip of your toes all the way up to the top of your head, is relaxed and calm in this very safe and private place that is your own. You can continue to lie here as you rock back and forth . . . back and forth for as long as you need to.

When you are ready, you can slowly readjust yourself to the sound of my voice and I am going to count slowly backwards from ten and with each count backwards, you can become more and more familiar with where you are. Perhaps when I get to number five you may want to open your eyes or you can keep then closed for as long as you need to. Ten, nine . . . —become aware of the sounds around you . . . eight, seven . . . become aware of the temperature of the room—how does it feel?, how does your body

feel? . . . six, five . . . —you can open your eyes now if you want to or you can keep them closed . . . four, three, two, one. You can stay in this relaxed position for as long as you need to. When you feel ready you may slowly prepare to sit up.'

Hypnosis

The American Society of Clinical Hypnosis defines hypnosis as 'a state of inner absorption, concentration, and focused attention' (American Society of Clinical Hypnosis., 2013). Hypnosis can foster a way of processing information in which analytic cognition and peripheral awareness is suspended. This can lead to involuntary changes in the perception of mood and memory, which in turn can lead to biological and behavioural changes (Wickramaskera, 2003).

The hypnotic trance is essentially a state of heightened and focused concentration, and thus it can be used to manipulate the perception of pain. The depth of hypnotizability may determine the effectiveness of this approach, as well as the strategies employed during hypnosis. One-third of patients are not hypnotizable, and it is recommended that other techniques be employed for them. Of the two-thirds of patients who are identified as being less, moderately, and highly hypnotizable, three principles underlie the use of hypnosis in controlling pain (Broome et al., 1992): (1) use self-hypnosis, (2) relax, do not fight the pain, and (3) use a mental filter to ease the hurt in pain. Patients who are moderately and highly hypnotizable can often alter sensations in a painful area by changing temperature sensation or experiencing tingling. Less hypnotizable patients can often utilize an alternative focus by concentrating on a sensation in a non-affected body part or on a mental image of a pleasant scene.

Hypnosis can be a useful adjunct in the management of pain (Spiegel and Bloom,1983; Spiegel,1985; Levitan,1992; Syrajala et al.,1992; Tan, 1997; Douglas, 1999; Liossi and Hatira, 1999; Montgomery et al., 2000; Rajasekaran et al., 2005) including acute pain from mucositis, procedures, or surgery (Syrajala et al., 1992; Liossi and Hatira, 1999; Montgomery et al., 2000, 2002; Floryn et al., 2007; Wobst, 2007) and pain related to wounds, burns, and various chronic conditions (Jensen and Patterson, 2006; Hammond, 2007; Neron and Stephenson, 2007; Gevirtz, 2009; Abrahamsen et al., 2011). In 1996, the National Institutes of Health in the United States assembled a Technology Assessment Panel that reviewed the evidence to date and concluded that relaxation and hypnosis are effective in reducing chronic pain (NIH Technology Assessment Panel, 1996). The main disadvantage of hypnosis for cancer patients is that the technique frequently requires more attentional capacity than these patients generally have.

Biofeedback

Biofeedback is a behavioural therapy that teaches patients how to gain awareness and control over physiological functions for the purpose of improving health and performance. Instruments are used to measure physiological activity, such as heart function, breathing, skin temperature, muscle activity, carbon dioxide partial pressure (PCO_2), or brainwave pattern. This information is then presented, rapidly and accurately, back to the patient. Patents use this information to change their thinking, emotions, and behaviours, which in turn support the desired physiological changes. Over time, these changes can be continued without the use of the biofeedback instruments.

Myrvik et al. studied single-session biofeedback-assisted relaxation training in patients with sickle cell disease. Ten participants completed a 1-hour session and showed changes in body temperature after the training session and at 6-week follow-up. Reductions in pain frequency, even though very small, were also reported (Myrvik et al., 2012). Shapiro and Shanani showed that six of nine participants who underwent biofeedback treatment for 1–4 years showed significant improvements in functional chest pain compared with those who were not treated (Shapiro and Shanani, 2012). In a meta-analysis, reductions in frequency, duration, and intensity of tension type and migraine headaches was accomplished in children with biofeedback techniques (Trautmann et al., 2006). Fotopoulos et al. (1979) noted significant pain relief in a group of cancer patients who were taught electromyographic (EMG) and electroencephalographic (EEG) biofeedback-assisted relaxation. However, only two of 17 were able to maintain analgesia after the treatment ended. The latter finding suggests that this biofeedback technique may lack generalization to other settings, and this is viewed as a problem with biofeedback techniques. Although physical condition may make a prolonged training period impossible, especially for the terminally ill, most cancer patients could utilize EMG and temperature biofeedback techniques for learning relaxation-assisted pain control (Kazak et al., 1998).

Music, aroma, and art therapies

Music is often used to enhance well-being, reduce stress, and distract patients from unpleasant symptoms. Munro and Mount (1978) have written extensively on the use of music therapy with cancer patients, documenting clinical examples and suggesting mechanisms of action. Although there are wide variations in individual preferences, music appears to exert direct physiologic effects through the autonomic nervous system and can be particularly helpful in managing the discomfort associated with procedures (Chlan et al., 2000). Music can often capture the focus of attention like no other stimulus, offers patients a new form of expression, and helps patients distract themselves from their perception of pain, while expressing themselves in meaningful ways (Schroeder-Sheker, 1993; Magill, 2001). Some studies suggest that music may decrease the overall intensity of the patient's pain when used with analgesics, and although studies have shown mixed results, music can result in a decreased need for pain medicine in some patients (Cepeda et al., 2006).

As a general relaxation technique, aromatherapy may have an application for pain management, but studies are limited and the technique warrants further investigation.

Utilizing the scent, heliotropin, Manne et al. (1991) reported that two-thirds of the patients found the scent especially pleasant and reported much less anxiety than those who were not exposed to the scent during magnetic resonance imaging. Wilkinson et al., (2007) found short-term but not persistent benefits from aromatherapy in a group of cancer patients with depression, and Anderson and Johnson found that aromatherapy did not significantly change perineal discomfort after childbirth (Anderson and Johnson, 2005)

Art therapy can be used to reduce fear, anxiety, stress and pain, and help enhance overall sense of well-being (Nainis et al., 2006). Palliative care clinicians may use art therapy to explore issues relating to loss of control, helplessness, and hopelessness (Trauger-Querry, 2001). In addition, art therapy allows the less verbally skilled adult or children to express the fears and concerns that they have in a more comfortable fashion. The creative experience can be used as both an important means of providing support and also as an avenue for providing patients with psychological insights into their experience (Connell, 1992).

Psychotropic adjuvant analgesics for pain in the patient with advanced illness

Although randomized controlled trials of psychotropic medications have largely been done in subjects who are generally healthy, there appears to be increasing evidence that they may offer some benefit for patients requiring palliative care in the advanced stages of illness.

Antidepressants

Antidepressants may improve depression in patients with advanced cancer (Holland et al., 1998). Some of these drugs are established analgesics. Although positive effects on mood, should they occur, may be beneficial for pain, the analgesic effects produced by the latter drugs may be independent of their mood-enhancing potential (Dharmshaktu et al., 2012).

Serotonin selective reuptake inhibitors (SSRIs)

SSRIs inhibit serotonin reuptake into the presynaptic neuron, which ultimately increases synaptic concentrations of serotonin. This group includes a number of commonly used agents, such as fluoxetine, citalopram, and paroxetine. They are generally considered first-line treatments for depression, anxiety, and eating disorders. This is largely related to tolerability when compared to other agents, although they are capable of causing significant gastrointestinal side effects (which tend to be a time limited side effect), as well as increased anxiety and sexual side effects. A recent meta-analysis demonstrated the efficacy of these agents in the management of mood symptoms in palliative care patients but found limited evidence to support the superiority of any one agent when compared to others within the class (Rayner et al., 2011). There are few data supporting their efficacy as analgesics (Otto et al., 2008; Dharmshaktu et al., 2012). The SSRIs are not preferred when the primary goal of treatment is to mitigate pain.

Serotonin norepinephrine reuptake inhibitors (SNRIs)

SNRIs inhibit the neuronal reuptake of both serotonin and norepinephrine (noradrenaline), similar to the tricyclic antidepressants. Among others, they include venlafaxine and duloxetine, which are widely used as first-line agents in the treatment of depression and anxiety disorders. These drugs are generally well tolerated and have a side effect profile comparable to the SSRIs. Venlafaxine may worsen hypertension, however, and is more likely to produce withdrawal symptoms when discontinued than other drugs. In contrast to the SSRIs, this antidepressant class has substantial evidence of analgesic efficacy (Sindrup et al., 2003; Eisenberg, 2007; Attal et al., 2010; Bachman et al., 2011; Kaur, 2011); both duloxetine and another agent in this group, milnacipran, are approved in the United States as analgesics for specific disorders. Although large studies are lacking in the use of these agents in patients with pain related to cancer, there are some smaller studies that demonstrate efficacy of these agents in the treatment of neuropathic syndromes following chemotherapeutic and surgical interventions for patients being treated for cancer (Tasmuth et al., 2002; Amr and Yousef, 2010; Henry et al., 2011; Durand, 2012; Yang et al., 2012).

Tricyclic antidepressants (TCAs)

TCAs also inhibit the reuptake of serotonin and norepinephrine. The various agents in this group differ in their potency at each of these sites, as well by their affinity at the receptor sites for other neurotransmitters. There are two broad categories: the tertiary amine drugs, such as amitriptyline and imipramine, tend to cause more side effects (particularly anticholinergic effects) than the secondary amine drugs, such as nortriptyline and desipramine. All the TCAs now tend to be used as second-line agents due to the relatively better side effect profiles of the SSRIs and SNRIs. Nevertheless, there is substantial evidence that these drugs have primary analgesic effects for diverse painful conditions (Raja et al., 2002; Sindrup et al., 2003; Rahimi et al., 2009; Attal et al., 2010; Bachman et al., 2011; Kaur, 2011; Brian et al., 2012; Dharmshaktu et al., 2012). Specific evidence in populations with cancer or other serious illnesses is limited, however (Kautio et al., 2009; Arai et al., 2010; Mishra et al., 2012).

Some TCAs have been employed in non-oral formulations. An oral doxepin rinse is available that appears to offer some benefit for pain related to mucositis, although studies have been small (Epstein JP et al. 2001; Epstein JB et al. 2008). Topical doxepin is used for itch.

Monoamine oxidase inhibitors (MAOIs)

MAOIs inhibit the enzyme monoamine oxidase and include such drugs as phenelzine and selegiline, which has a transdermal preparation. These agents have largely been relegated to the treatment of refractory depression due to their potential complications, including orthostatic hypotension, interactions with other serotonergic agents leading to serotonin syndrome, and the potential for hypertensive crisis if exposed to certain medications and tyramine-containing foods. There is no support for their use as analgesics.

Other antidepressants

Mirtazapine is an antagonist at presynaptic alpha-2 receptors on noradrenergic neurons and has gained some popularity in medically ill populations due to its propensity to enhance appetite and promote sedation at lower doses (effects that tend to decrease as the dose increases), and its potential for reducing nausea. There is little evidence to support its use as an adjuvant treatment for pain.

Bupropion enhances the effects of norepinephrine and dopamine. It has current indications for the treatment of depression, smoking cessation, and attention deficit/hyperactivity disorder. It is usually activating and is well tolerated as compared to other antidepressants; it has fewer sexual side effects than the SSRIs and SNRIs. However, there is evidence of dose dependent increases in seizures, especially in patients with eating disorders. There is little evidence of analgesic efficacy, but it is sometimes tried when its profile of effects would be beneficial.

Trazodone's primary mechanism of action involves antagonism of the serotonin receptor. It has indications for the treatment of depression and anxiety, but has been relegated to the treatment of primarily insomnia due to its tendency to cause sedation. There is limited evidence supporting its use as an adjuvant for pain management.

Stimulants

Stimulant drugs such as methylphenidate and dextroamphetamine/amphetamine, are typically used in the treatment of conditions such as attention deficit/hyperactivity disorder. However, in the medically ill, they do have a role in the treatment of depression (Kaufmann et al., 1982; Bruera et al., 1987; Fernandez et al., 1987) and they be beneficial for fatigue (Bruera et al., 1987, 1989). They are not used for pain.

Mood stabilizers

Mood stabilizers describe a group of medications typically intended to treat bipolar spectrum disorders. Broadly, this group consists of lithium, antiepileptic drugs, and medications generally utilized in the treatment of psychotic disorders. The mechanisms by which these medications are effective are not entirely known. Lithium is a first-line treatment for mania and bipolar disorder, notwithstanding a narrow therapeutic window and the need for close follow-up to avoid potentially fatal toxicities, particularly in the elderly and those with chronic medical illness. It also has limiting side effects including tremor, gastrointestinal disturbance, and nephrotoxicity, amongst other issues. It is not used for the purpose of pain management.

Some antiepileptics are approved for bipolar disorder and may have utility in the treatment of neuropathic pain. These include the gabapentinoids, gabapentin (Arai et al., 2010) and pregabalin (Bril et al., 2011), and topiramate (Attal et al., 2010; Howard et al., 2011; Callaghan et al., 2012). The gabapentinoids are considered first-line agents for neuropathic pain. Other antiepileptic medications used for psychiatric indications also are occasionally considered for pain. Valproic acid and its derivatives, such as divalproex sodium, are older drugs with well-established indications for a range of neurological and psychiatric conditions. Although they are generally considered to be a first-line treatment for mania, their broader use is limited by a side effect profile that includes gastrointestinal disturbances and the potential for hepatotoxicity and hyperammonaemia. There is evidence of efficacy in neuropathic pain syndromes (Howard et al., 2011; Callaghan et al., 2012). Carbamazepine also has efficacy in the treatment of mania, but generally is not considered first line because of the potential for bone marrow suppression and hepatotoxicity, and concern about drug–drug interactions. It, too, may have efficacy in neuropathic pain, and is indicated for the treatment of trigeminal neuralgia (Eisenberg, 2007; Howard et al., 2011). Oxcarbazepine is similar to carbamazepine, but has less risk of toxicity; evidence in bipolar disorder is limited, as is evidence in pain syndromes such as trigeminal neuralgia (Eisenberg, 2007). Lamotrigine has demonstrated efficacy primarily in the management of depressive symptoms in bipolar disorder, but its use is hindered by the risk of cutaneous hypersensitivity syndromes, which necessitate a slow increase in the dose when starting therapy and avoidance of the drug in children. There is limited evidence for efficacy in neuropathic pain (Howard et al., 2011; Shaikh et al., 2011; Smith and Argoff, 2011).

Anxiolytics

Medications used for anxiety include antidepressants (as mentioned previously) and drugs that modulate the function of gamma-aminobutyric acid type A (GABA$_A$) receptors, most importantly the benzodiazepines. The latter drugs include alprazolam, clonazepam, lorazepam, diazepam, and others. Buspirone is a non-benzodiazepine serotonin agonist also indicated for anxiety. The only anxiolytic used commonly for pain in some countries is clonazepam. Evidence of efficacy is very limited, and it is reasonable to consider this agent primary for those circumstances in which anxiety complicates significant neuropathic pain.

Antipsychotics

Antipsychotic drugs are used to manage psychotic disorders, such as schizophrenia; problems such as agitation and aggression that may be complicating other psychiatric disorders; and manifestations of organic brain disorders, including frank delirium. Broadly, the group can be divided into low-potency typical, high-potency typical, and atypical. The low-potency typical drugs are typified by chlorpromazine. These drugs have low affinity for the D_2 receptor, which is seen as their primary site of action. As a result, they have a decreased likelihood of causing extrapyramidal side effects, but are more likely to cause anticholinergic side effects, which limit their utility in many chronically ill patients. The high-potency typical drugs are typified by haloperidol. They have a high affinity for the D_2 receptor and as a result tend to cause more difficulties with extrapyramidal side effects. However, they tend to cause fewer anticholinergic side effects than the low-potency agents, and fewer metabolic side effects than the atypical antipsychotics. The atypical drugs, including olanzapine and risperidone, have a variety of mechanisms and generally cause fewer extrapyramidal side effects than the typical agents. However, as a group, they tend to cause more metabolic side effects, such as glucose intolerance.

The antipsychotic drugs have a variety of indications that are beneficial in medically ill populations, including nausea (Patt et al., 1994) and delirium (Patt et al., 1994; Grover et al., 2011a, 2011b) although additional studies are needed to better support the latter (Lonergan et al., 2007; Flaherty, 2011). Their benefit in the management of pain, including cancer-related pain, is not well supported by available data (Lonergan et al., 2007; Lussier et al., 2004; Seidel et al., 2008, 2010). The exception is methotrimeprazine, which has been used as adjuvant therapy for pain with some demonstrated benefit (Patt et al., 1994).

Online materials

Complete references for this chapter are available online at <http://www.oxfordmedicine.com>.

References

Abrahamsen, R., Baad-Hansen, L., and Zachariae, R. (2011). Effect of hypnosis on pain and blink reflexes in patients with painful temporomandibular disorders. *Clinical Journal of Pain*, 27, 344–351.

Amr, Y.M. and Yousef, A.A. (2010). Evaluation of efficacy of the perioperative administration of venlafaxine or gabapentin on acute and chronic postmastectomy pain. *Clinical Journal of Pain*, 26 (5), 381–385.

Attal, N., Cruccu, G., Baron, R., *et al.* (2010). EFNS guidelines on the pharmacologic treatment of neuropathic pain 2010 revision. *European Journal of Neurology*, 17, 1113–1123.

Bachman, D.R., Barton, D.L., Watson, J.C., and Loprinzi, C.L. (2011). Chemotherapy-induced polyneuropathy: prevention and treatment. *Clinical Pharmacology and Therapeutics*, 90(3), 377–387.

Bond, M.R. and Pearson, I.B. (1969). Psychological aspects of pain in women with advanced cancer of the cervix. *Journal of Psychosomatic Research*, 13, 13–19.

Breitbart, W. (1990a). Cancer pain and suicide. In K.M. Foley, J.J. Bonica, and V. Ventafridda (eds.) *Advances in Pain Research and Therapy*, pp. 399–412. New York: Raven Press.

Breitbart, W. (1990b). Psychiatric aspects of pain and HIV disease. *Focus: A Guide to AIDS Research and Counseling*, 5, 1–2.

Breitbart, W. and Holland, J.C. (1990). Psychiatric aspects of cancer pain. In K.M. Foley, J.J. Bonica, and V. Ventafridda (eds.) *Advances in Pain Research*, pp. 73–87. New York: Raven Press.

Callaghan, B.C., Cheng, H.T., Stables, C.L., Smith, A.L., and Feldman, E.L. (2012). Diabetic neuropathy: clinical manifestations and current treatments. *The Lancet*, 11(6), 521–534.

Charap, A.D. (1978). The knowledge, attitudes, and experience of medical personnel treating pain in the terminally ill. *Mount Sinai Journal of Medicine*, 45, 561–580.

Dharmshaktu, P., Tayal, V., and Kalra, B.S. (2012). Efficacy of antidepressants as a analgesics: a review. *The Journal of Clinical Psychopharmacology*, 52(1), 6–17.

Douglas, D.B. (1999). Hypnosis: useful, neglected, available. *American Journal of Hospice and Palliative Care*, 16(5), 665–670.

Durand, J.P. (2012). Efficacy of venlafaxine for the prevention and relief of oxaliplatin-induced acute neurotoxicity: results of EFFOX, a randomized, double-blind, placebo-controlled phase III trial. *Annals of Oncology*, 23(1), 200–205.

Eisenberg, E. (2007). Antiepileptic drugs in the treatment of neuropathic pain. *Drugs*, 67(9), 1265–1289.

Floryn, N., Salazar, G.M., and Lang, E.V. (2007). Hypnosis for acute distress management during medical procedures. *International Journal of Clinical and Experimental Hypnosis*, 55, 303–317.

Gevirtz, C. (2009). Pain management of the burn patient. *Topics in Pain Management*, 24(7), 7–9.

Hammond, D.C. (2007). Review of the efficacy of clinical hypnosis with headaches and migraines. *International Journal of Clinical and Experimental Hypnosis*, 55, 207–219.

Henry, N.L., Banerjee, M., Wicha, M., *et al.* (2011). Pilot study of duloxetine for treatment of aromatase inhibitor-associated musculoskeletal symptoms. *Cancer*, 117(24), 5469–7545.

Jensen, M. and Patterson, D.R. (2006). Hypnotic treatment of chronic pain. *Journal of Behavioral Medicine*, 29, 95–124.

Kanner, R.M. and Foley, K.M. (1981). Patterns of narcotic use in a cancer pain clinic. *Annals of the New York Academy of Science*, 362, 161–172.

Kaur, H. (2011). A comparative evaluation of amitriptyline and duloxetine in painful diabetic neuropathy. *Diabetes Care*, 34(4), 818–822.

Levitan, A. (1992). The use of hypnosis with cancer patients. *Psychiatry and Medicine*, 10, 119–131.

Liossi, C. and Hatira, P. (1999). Clinical hypnosis versus cognitive behavioral training for pain management with pediatric cancer patients undergoing bone marrow aspirations. *International Journal of Clinical and Experimental Hypnosis*, 47(2), 104–116.

Macaluso, C., Weinberg, D., and Foley, K.M. (1988). *Opioid Abuse and Misuse in a Cancer Pain Population* (Abstract). In Second International Congress on Cancer Pain, Rye, NY.

McKegney, F.P., Bailey, C.R., and Yates, J.W. (1981). Prediction and management of pain in patients with advanced cancer. *General Hospital Psychiatry*, 3, 95–101.

Montgomery, G.H., DuHamel, K.N., and Redd WH. (2000). A meta-analysis of hypnotically induced analgesia: how effective is hypnosis? *International Journal of Clinical and Experimental Hypnosis*, 48(2), 138–153.

Montgomery, G.H., Weltz, C.R., Seltz, M., and Bovbjerg, D.H. (2002). Brief presurgery hypnosis reduces distress and pain in excisional breast biopsy patients. *International Journal of Clinical and Experimental Hypnosis*, 50(1), 17–32.

Neron, S. and Stephenson, R. (2007). Effectiveness of hypnotherapy with cancer patients' trajectory: emesis, acute pain, and analgesia and anxiolysis in procedures. *International Journal of Clinical and Experimental Hypnosis*, 55, 336–354.

Payne, D. (1995). *Cognition in Cancer Pain*. (Unpublished dissertation).

Payne, D., Jacobsen, P., Breitbart, W., Passik, S., Rosenfeld, B., and McDonald, M. (1994). *Negative thoughts related to pain are associated with greater pain, distress, and disability in AIDS pain*. Presentation at the American Pain Society meeting, Miami, FL.

Portenoy, R.K., Payne, D., and Jacobsen, P. (1999). Breakthrough pain: characteristics and impact in patients with cancer pain. *Pain*, 81(1–2), 129–134.

Rahimi, R., Nikfar, S., Rezaie, A., and Abdollahi, M. (2009). Efficacy of tricyclic antidepressants in irritable bowel syndrome: a meta-analysis. *World Journal of Gastroenterology*, 15(13), 1548–1553.

Raja, S.N., Haythornthwaite, J.A., Pappagallo, M., *et al.* (2002). Opioids vs. antidepressants in postherpatic neuralgia: a randomized, placebo-controlled trial. *Neurology*, 59 (7), 1015–1021.

Rajasekaran, M., Edmonds, P.M., Higginson, I.L. (2005). Systematic review of hypnotherapy for treating symptoms in terminally ill adult cancer patients. *Palliative Medicine*, 19(5), 418–426.

Sindrup, S.H., Bach, F.W., Madsen, C., *et al.* (2003). Venlafaxine vs. imipramine in painful neuropathy. *Neurology*, 60(8), 1284–1289.

Smith, W.B., Gracely, R.H., and Safer, M.A. (1998). The meaning of pain: cancer patients' rating and recall of pain intensity and affect. *Pain*, 78(2), 123–129.

Spiegel, D. (1985). The use of hypnosis in controlling cancer pain. *CA: A Cancer Journal for Clinicians*, 4, 221–231.

Spiegel, D. and Bloom, J.R. (1983). Pain in metastatic breast cancer. *Cancer*, 52, 341–345.

Strang, P. (1997). Existential consequences of unrelieved cancer pain. *Palliative Medicine*, 11(4), 299–305.

Syrajala, K., Cummings, C., and Donaldson, G. (1992). Hypnosis or cognitive behavioral training for the reduction of pain and nausea during cancer treatment: a controlled trial. *Pain*, 48, 137–146.

Tan, S.Y. and Leucht, C.A. (1997). Cognitive-behavioral therapy for clinical pain control: a 15-year update and its relationship to hypnosis. *International Journal of Clinical and Experimental Hypnosis*, 45(4), 396–416.

Tasmuth, T., Härtel, B., and Kalso, E. (2002). Venlafaxine in neuropathic pain following treatment of breast cancer. *European Journal of Pain*, 6(1), 17–24.

Twycross, R.G. and Lack, S.A. (1983). *Symptom Control in Far Advanced Cancer: Pain Relief*. London: Pitman Brooks.

Wobst, A.H. (2007). Hypnosis and surgery: past, present, and future. *Anesthesia & Analgesia*, 104, 1199–1208.

Yang, Y.H., Lin, J.K., Chen, W.S., *et al.* (2012). Duloxetine improves oxaliplatin-induced neuropathy in patients with colorectal cancer: an open label pilot study. *Supportive Care in Cancer*, 20(7), 1491–1497.

Complementary therapies in pain management

Gary Deng and Barrie R. Cassileth

Introduction to complementary therapies in pain management

Pain is one of the most important symptoms that compromise patients' quality of life (QOL). Appropriate and adequate pain management remains challenging because pharmacologic treatment, the mainstay of pain management, does not always meet patients' needs and may produce difficult side effects. Interventional approaches, such as neuraxial analgesia and neuroablative techniques, and disease-modifying therapies, such as radiotherapy, are sometimes useful, but often are unavailable or contrary to the goals of care (Cherny, 2004).

The medical treatment of pain requires continuing effort to balance analgesic effects while minimizing adverse effects (Cherny, 2000; Paice and Ferrell, 2011).Opioid side effects are very common, particularly gastrointestinal effects (e.g. constipation, nausea, and emesis) and somnolence or cognitive impairment. Despite the many strategies that may be used to improve the balance between analgesia and side effects, such balance may not always be achievable (Cherny and Portenoy, 1994; McNicol et al., 2003).

Complementary therapies offer additional treatment options that are not traditionally part of Western medical care but can be incorporated into a multimodality care plan. Some of these therapies have demonstrated a favourable benefit:risk ratio in recent research and are increasingly used as adjunct therapies integrated into mainstream care. Clinicians who manage pain in populations with serious or life-threatening illness should understand the current state of evidence for complementary modalities, such as mind–body therapies, acupuncture, and massage therapy, and should be able to make recommendations for clinical practice.

Types of pain and analgesic mechanisms of complementary therapies

In general, complementary therapies reduce pain by interfering with the processing of pain signals. Mind–body therapies reduce the perception of pain by affecting psychological factors, such as anxiety or depressed mood, that can increase pain intensity or worsen the impact of pain on QOL. Neurophysiology and neuroimaging studies since the 1970s provide evidence that the analgesic effect of acupuncture is likely mediated via modulation of endogenous opioid and other neurotransmitter pathways, activities in the limbic system of the brain, and the processing of pain signals in the central nervous system (Napadow et al., 2008; Han, 2011). The array of symptoms relieved by massage therapies points to both positive local effects on soft tissue, as well as subconscious mechanisms that control the experience of pain and emotions (Sagar et al., 2007).

Mind–body therapies

Mind–body therapies are defined as practices that focus on the interactions among the brain, mind, body, and behaviour, with the intent to use the mind to affect physical functioning and promote health (National Center for Complementary and Alternative Medicine, 2012). The most common symptoms that people turn to these therapies for are pain, dyspnoea, and fatigue (Wells et al., 2007). Mind–body therapies encompass a wide variety of specific therapies, such as hypnosis, meditation, yoga/qigong (which also has physical movement components), and music therapy.

Hypnosis is a practice by which a therapist induces, or instructs the patient on how to self-induce, a mental state of focused attention or altered consciousness between wakefulness and sleep. In this state, distractions are blocked, allowing the patient to concentrate intently on a particular subject, memory, sensation, or problem. Patients may receive suggestions, or self-suggest, changes in perceptions toward sensations, thoughts, and behaviours. In a systematic review of 21 studies (11 randomized controlled trials (RCTs), two non-RCTs, and eight case series), self-hypnosis provided pain relief in cancer patients and dying patients (Pan et al., 2000). However, a subsequent systematic review of 27 reports (one RCT, 24 case studies, and two other types of studies) concluded that the poor quality of studies evaluated, and the heterogeneity of study populations, limited further evaluation (Rajasekaran et al., 2005). More recently, a meta-analysis of 37 studies ($N = 4199$) on psychosocial interventions, including hypnosis, concluded that these modalities have a significant medium-size effect on both pain severity and pain interference with functioning, and that quality-controlled psychosocial interventions should be considered in multimodal approaches to pain management for cancer patients (Sheinfeld Gorin et al., 2012).

Importantly, there appears to be a widespread acceptance among the general public to consider the use of hypnosis to control side effects associated with cancer treatment (Sohl et al., 2010). This willingness to participate may in fact have an added impact. In a RCT evaluating a hypnotherapy intervention in a sample of patients with metastatic breast cancer (*N* = 124), the intervention group had significantly less increase in the intensity of pain and suffering over time, and highly hypnotizable participants reported greater benefits from hypnosis, employed self-hypnosis more often outside of group therapy, and used it to manage other symptoms in addition to pain (Butler et al., 2009).

Meditation involves practices that invite heightened awareness and attention to one's own sensations, surroundings, and/or inner mental processes. A particular type of meditation, mindfulness-based stress reduction (MBSR), provides the practitioner with the opportunity to develop an objective 'observer role' for emotions, feelings, and perceptions, and to create a non-judgemental 'mindful state' of conscious awareness. A meta-analysis of four RCTs and six observational studies totalling 583 participants showed that MBSR is beneficial for mood, anxiety, depression, and QOL in general, although not so much for pain specifically (Ledesma and Kumano, 2009). Several systematic reviews show similar findings (Smith et al., 2005; Matchim and Armer, 2007; Shennan et al., 2011).

Yoga and qigong are practices that combine physical movement, breath control, and meditative components. Yoga has been found to significantly improve anxiety, depression, distress, and stress in a meta-analysis of ten RCTs (Lin et al., 2011). RCTs evaluating pain as the primary end point in a palliative care setting are lacking. Similarly, qigong was found promising for stress reduction and improving QOL, but no strong data support its efficacy in treating pain specifically (Chan et al., 2012).

Music therapy takes advantage of the profound effect of music on a patient's emotional and spiritual state. Patients may listen to or participate in the performance of music and singing. There are a large number of qualitative studies demonstrating the benefit of music therapy in reducing pain and anxiety (Hilliard, 2005). A recent RCT that tested music therapist-guided autogenic relaxation and live music in 200 palliative care patients showed a significant decrease in pain scores (Gutgsell et al., 2013).

In general, mind–body therapies have the most benefit in reducing psychological complications from pain, or anxiety and distress that exacerbate the impact of pain on patients, rather than the pain itself. The side effect risk is low and most of these practices can be taught to patients for self-practice. Mind–body therapies should be considered for palliative care patients who are experiencing anxiety, distress, or sleep and mood disturbance in addition to pain.

Acupuncture

Acupuncture, a modality originating from Traditional Chinese Medicine, involves the insertion of needles into certain points on the body followed by stimulation of the needles using manual manipulation, electrical pulses, or heat. Its effects on pain are supported by numerous RCTs.

The strongest data for the analgesic effects of acupuncture comes from studies targeting pain in the absence of a serious illness. Systematic reviews and meta-analyses support its benefit in the management of joint pain (Collins et al., 2012), labour pain (Smith et al., 2011a), migraine (Linde et al., 2009a), tension headache (Linde et al., 2009b), dysmenorrhoeal (Smith et al., 2011b), and chronic pain in general (Vickers et al., 2012). For the treatment of cancer pain, a systematic review of 15 RCTs showed that

acupuncture did not generate a better effect than drug therapy (risk ratio (RR), 1.12; 95% confidence interval (CI) 0.98– 1.28; p = 0.09); acupuncture plus drug therapy demonstrated a significant improvement when compared with drug therapy alone (RR, 1.36; 95% CI 1.13– 1.64; p = 0.003) (Choi et al., 2012).

One study of particular interest is an RCT in which auricular acupuncture demonstrated superiority over sham treatment in the control of cancer pain (Alimi et al., 2003). Many of the patients in that study had persistent neuropathic pain that had not responded to other treatments. In the management of chemotherapy-induced peripheral neuropathy, both a controlled pilot study and a case series using acupuncture showed some benefit, but with very small sample sizes (Wong and Sagar, 2006; Schroeder et al., 2012). Acupuncture's effect on post-thoracotomy pain syndrome is mixed, with one study using embedded tiny needles showing no benefit (Deng et al., 2008) and another using electro-acupuncture demonstrating a reduction in opioid requirement (Wong et al., 2006).

The strongest support from clinical trials supports the efficacy of acupuncture for nausea and vomiting. A high-quality Cochrane systematic review of 11 trials (*N* = 1247) concluded that electro acupuncture has demonstrated benefit for chemotherapy-induced acute vomiting (Ezzo et al., 2006). In non-chemotherapy settings, another systematic review of more than 40 RCTs supports the effect of acupuncture in preventing or attenuating nausea and vomiting (Streitberger et al., 2006). Because the use of opioid analgesics may be associated with nausea and vomiting, acupuncture may be considered among approaches to address a common opioid toxicity.

In summary, the analgesic effect of acupuncture is supported by preclinical and clinical studies. Although its analgesic effects are better established in musculoskeletal pain and headache, and less well established for chronic pain due to cancer or other medical illnesses, the relative safety of acupuncture suggests that it should be considered in populations receiving palliative care—for both pain and nausea. Acupuncture is not associated with common opioid side effects, such as sedation, constipation, and nausea, and combining the use of both modalities appears warranted in order to manage pain in patients who do not respond favourably to opioids alone.

Massage therapy

Massage therapy involves applying pressure to muscle and connective tissue with the intent to reduce tension and pain, improve circulation, and encourage relaxation. Massage techniques most commonly used in oncology include Swedish massage, aromatherapy massage, reflexology, and acupressure. All involve manual manipulation of soft tissues of the body by a trained therapist. However, the methods of applying touch, degree of educational preparation, regulatory requirements, and underlying theoretical frameworks vary widely among these modalities.

Clinical studies show that massage therapy can reduce anxiety, depression, and pain in cancer patients. A 2009 systematic review of massage therapy for cancer palliation and supportive care examined 14 RCTs, which studied anxiety (seven RCTs; *N* = 514), depression (three RCTs; *N* = 107), or pain (six RCTs; *N* = 718) (Ernst, 2009). It concluded that massage can alleviate a wide range of symptoms: pain, nausea, anxiety, depression, anger, stress, and fatigue. However, poor methodology among the studies makes the benefits encouraging but not compelling.

An earlier systematic review focusing on cancer patients included 12 RCTs, which also used anxiety (five RCTs; $N = 236$), depression (two RCTs; $N = 63$), and pain (three RCTs; $N = 144$) as end points (Wilkinson et al., 2008). The trials used standard care, attention, or low-intensity bodywork as control interventions. The reviewers concluded the data support massage therapy as an effective adjunct in cancer supportive care to reduce anxiety, depression, and pain, with stronger evidence for its effect on anxiety than depression or pain. However, the methodological quality of most included trials was poor.

Among non-randomized trials, results from an observational study ($N = 1290$) showed that massage improved pain scores for both inpatients and outpatients by 40%, and reduced other cancer-related symptoms by approximately 50% (Cassileth and Vickers, 2004). More recently, a pilot study comparing reflexology and Swedish massage therapy for cancer survivors aged 75 or older in nursing homes found that both interventions resulted in significant declines in salivary cortisol and pain, as well as improvements in mood. Further, both interventions were well tolerated in an elderly population of cancer survivors typically excluded from trials (Hodgson and Lafferty, 2012). Another randomized pilot study found that a combination of massage and other physiotherapy can reduce pain and improve mood in patients with terminal cancer (Lopez-Sendin et al., 2012).

In palliative care, precautions must be paid to the safety of massage therapy, as some patients may have a large tumour burden or bone metastases, and could be at risk for an exacerbation of pain, fracture, bruising, or bleeding. Strong pressure should not to be applied over areas of disease involvement. In these cases, gentle light touch massage or reflexology (hand or foot massage) can still be used.

Application in clinical practice

In summary, evidence supporting the use of complementary therapies in pain management is encouraging but not definitive. In considering various treatment options for clinical practice, the strength of the evidence in favour of efficacy must be weighed against the risks and burdens to patients, and the potential alternatives or the lack thereof. From this perspective, the mind–body therapies, acupuncture, and massage therapy have a favourable record. They may improve symptoms, and the medical risk and burden they pose usually is negligible. They also encourage patient self-care and empowerment, making patients active participants in their care.

The use of complementary approaches may present financial concerns, as most of the time they are not covered by health insurance, but coverage for these therapies is expanding and reflects consumer demand along with managed care efforts to control costs. Financial barriers also may be partially overcome. Patients can be taught to practice mind–body interventions themselves, and yoga/qigong or meditation classes can be given to groups. Acupuncture also can be given in a group setting to lower unit costs, or patients can be taught to do acupressure (application of pressure, usually with a finger, on acupuncture points). Family members or caregivers can be taught to safely give massages.

The origin of pain, and the factors complicating it, should be considered when selecting from among the complementary modalities for pain. If the pain is augmented by anxiety, fear, depression, or sleep disturbance, or if the pain exacerbates psychological distress, mind–body therapies and massage therapy should be considered. If opioid therapy creates undesirable effects, such as sedation, constipation, fatigue, nausea, and emesis, the addition of acupuncture has the potential of lowering the required dose of pain medications.

Each patient's belief system and cultural background should be taken into consideration. Patients who have a strong spiritual need, who wish a more naturalistic approach to health, and patients who have experienced benefit from these therapies previously, are more open to complementary therapies and appreciate their availability as an integrated component of mainstream care. Only by considering what is truly important to a patient as an individual can we provide optimal patient-centred palliative care, improve the quality of pain management, and comfort the patient to the best of our ability.

Online materials

Complete references for this chapter are available online at <http://www.oxfordmedicine.com>.

References

Alimi, D., Rubino, C., Pichard-Leandri, E., Fermand-Brule, S., Dubreuil-Lemaire, M.L., and Hill, C. (2003). Analgesic effect of auricular acupuncture for cancer pain: a randomized, blinded, controlled trial. *Journal of Clinical Oncology*, 21, 4120–4126.

Cherny, N.I. and Portenoy, R.K. (1994). The management of cancer pain. *CA: A Cancer Journal for Clinicians*, 44, 263–303.

Choi, T.Y., Lee, M.S., Kim, T.H., Zaslawski, C., and Ernst, E. (2012). Acupuncture for the treatment of cancer pain: a systematic review of randomised clinical trials. *Supportive Care in Cancer*, 20, 1147–1158.

Ernst, E. (2009). Massage therapy for cancer palliation and supportive care: a systematic review of randomised clinical trials. *Supportive Care in Cancer*, 17, 333–337.

Ezzo, J.M., Richardson, M.A., Vickers, A., et al. (2006). Acupuncture-point stimulation for chemotherapy-induced nausea or vomiting. *Cochrane Database of Systematic Reviews*, 2, CD002285.

Gutgsell, K.J., Schluchter, M., Margevicius, S., et al. (2013). Music therapy reduces pain in palliative care patients: a randomized controlled trial. *Journal of Pain and Symptom Management*, 45(5), 822–831.

Han, J.S. (2011). Acupuncture analgesia: areas of consensus and controversy. *Pain*, 152, S41–48.

Hilliard, R.E. (2005). Music therapy in hospice and palliative care: a review of the empirical data. *Evidence-Based Complementary and Alternative Medicine*, 2, 173–178.

Ledesma, D. and Kumano, H. (2009). Mindfulness-based stress reduction and cancer: a meta-analysis. *Psycho-Oncology*, 18, 571–579.

Matchim, Y. and Armer, J.M. (2007). Measuring the psychological impact of mindfulness meditation on health among patients with cancer: a literature review. *Oncology Nursing Forum*, 34, 1059–1066.

Napadow, V., Ahn, A., Longhurst, J., et al. (2008). The status and future of acupuncture mechanism research. *Journal of Alternative and Complementary Medicine*, 14, 861–869.

Pan, C.X., Morrison, R.S., Ness, J., Fugh-Berman, A., and Leipzig, R.M. (2000). Complementary and alternative medicine in the management of pain, dyspnea, and nausea and vomiting near the end of life. A systematic review. *Journal of Pain and Symptom Management*, 20, 374–387.

Rajasekaran, M., Edmonds, P.M., and Higginson, I.L. (2005). Systematic review of hypnotherapy for treating symptoms in terminally ill adult cancer patients. *Palliative Medicine*, 19, 418–426.

Sheinfeld Gorin, S., Krebs, P., Badr, H., *et al.* (2012). Meta-analysis of psychosocial interventions to reduce pain in patients with cancer. *Journal of Clinical Oncology*, 30, 539–547.

Smith, J.E., Richardson, J., Hoffman, C., and Pilkington, K. (2005). Mindfulness-based stress reduction as supportive therapy in cancer care: systematic review. *Journal of Advanced Nursing*, 52, 315–327.

Vickers, A.J., Cronin, A.M., Maschino, A.C., *et al.* (2012). Acupuncture for chronic pain: individual patient data meta-analysis. *Archives of Internal Medicine*, 1–10.

Wilkinson, S., Barnes, K., and Storey, L. (2008). Massage for symptom relief in patients with cancer: systematic review. *Journal of Advanced Nursing*, 63, 430–439.

9.13

Paediatric pain control

Renée McCulloch and John J. Collins

Introduction to paediatric pain control

Pain is common in children requiring palliative care. It is one of the most prevalent and also the most feared symptoms (Wolfe et al., 2000; Jalmsell et al., 2006; Hechler, 2008; Feudtner et al., 2011). A child in pain can be a very distressing experience for the child, the family, and the clinician. As health-care professionals, we have a responsibility to respond, either through direct support or by seeking appropriate help.

Children treated by palliative care teams usually have pain that is a result of multiple aetiologies rather than a single cause. Pain is multidimensional, involving the emotional and sensory experience of the child within their developmental and social framework. Professionals working in the field need to be competent in the management of acute pain, chronic pain, recurring pain, procedure-related pain, and pain at the end of life. Pain is often a combination of nociceptive (visceral and/or somatic) and neuropathic pain. The expectation must be for exemplary pain control through meticulous assessment and treatment, using the skills of the multidisciplinary team. Essential to success are the development of effective communication and a trusting relationship between professionals, parent/carer, and child. An open and honest approach will allow dialogue about anxieties and misconceptions, which, if not addressed, may compromise successful treatment.

The study of pain in children started with recognition that pain is undertreated in this population (Schechter, 1989; Schechter et al., 1993). The last quarter of a century has seen unprecedented advances in the understanding and management of pain in children.

We know:

- infants can experience pain and failure to alleviate pain causes adverse physiological consequences and needless suffering

- children can experience many different types of acute, recurrent, and persistent pain

- children can describe their pain

- children's pain must be regularly monitored, evaluated, and assessed

- children may suffer prolonged pain due to disease, trauma, and psychological factors

- children in severe pain require strong analgesics for relief

- administration of opioids in children does not lead to addiction (McGrath, 1998).

Much research focus has been upon the assessment and management of acute pain and the neurophysiological basis of pain in the newborn and infants. These important strides are at the beginning of a long road to understanding and implementing evidence-based, effective pain management across the spectrum of paediatrics. Lack of resources and the significant challenge of undertaking research in children, hamper progress (McGrath and Ruskin, 2007; Berde et al., 2012). This lack of evidence extends to include children's pain during the palliative phase of illness.

Although pain is an area receiving significant attention in the literature, clinical practice is currently influenced by extrapolation of evidence from studies in acute pain in children and adult palliative care. Clinicians must be cautious about extrapolating data from different populations. Paediatric patients represent a variable and diverse subset of individuals from the premature neonate to the fully-grown, sexually mature young adult. Anatomy, physiology, cognitive responses, disease types, along with social, psychological, and environmental factors all differ. However, in spite of these concerns and the lack of 'robust evidence', a sensible and empirical approach with thorough assessment and good understanding of the disease process will enable a safe and effective therapeutic approach.

This chapter sets out some of the background and principles of pain management in children's palliative care. For the purposes of this chapter the term 'child' will include all children and adolescents up to the age of 16 years.

World Health Organization 2012 guidelines for a global strategy to improve pain management in children

Persisting pain in children is a global phenomenon recently highlighted by the World Health Organization (WHO) as 'duration of pain lasting beyond what one would expect from an acute injury'. This definition intends to cover longer-term pain related to medical illness and has no defined time frame. The latest initiative *WHO Guidelines on the Pharmacological Treatment of Persisting Pain in Children with Medical Illness* has taken the best available evidence and developed a new guideline to improve the management of persisting pain in children (WHO, 2012). As such it replaces the previous guideline *Cancer Pain and Palliative Care in Children* (WHO, 1998). The new guidelines are based upon the principle that, irrespective of whether an underlying cause can be identified, pharmacological and non-pharmacological techniques should be used to treat pain in children.

Importantly, the WHO recognizes that universal application and implementation of clinical recommendations will only occur through health system change; the significant barriers to delivering effective pain management in children are due to poor education and rigid health-care systems.

The child, pain, and palliative care

Why are children different?

Although there is no doubt that the core principles of pain management in palliative care can be shared between the adult and paediatric specialties, there are many differences that determine quite distinct practice.

Firstly, there is considerable variation in disease type and trajectory compared to adult palliative care. Approximately 60% of the paediatric palliative care team's patients have non-malignant conditions (Fraser et al., 2012; Hain et al., 2012). In developed countries, there is a range of diagnostic categories: congenital, genetic, neuromuscular, respiratory, cancer, and gastrointestinal conditions with a high prevalence of cognitive impairment (Feudtner et al., 2011). In sub-Saharan Africa overwhelming numbers of HIV-related illnesses in children are treated by paediatric palliative care teams (Amery, 2012). Long and unpredictable disease trajectories have necessitated combining efforts for proactive disease modification with palliation of symptoms.

One of the main differences between children and adults is communication. Communication is the cornerstone of effective pain management and can be a major challenge in children. Understanding and interpreting pain in verbal and non-verbal children with a range of developmental and cognitive abilities needs a different psychotherapeutic approach. Additionally, continuing cognitive and physical development throughout illness requires an informed and responsive team.

The variation and complexity of ethical dilemmas in children may offer the palliative care team significant challenge not seen in adult medicine (Nolan, 1993; McGrath, 2005). For example, although children cannot legally consent, their compliance and 'assent' are important requirements for treatment. Children should be involved in the decision-making process as much as possible (Bioethics Committee, Canadian Paediatric Society, 2004). Overprotective attitudes of health-care professionals and parents/carers can underestimate the ability of children to make informed decisions (American Academy of Pediatrics, 1995; Rylance, 1996).

Many of the medications used routinely in adult palliative medicine are not licensed for use in the paediatric population and are frequently prescribed outside the terms of the product licence. Although there are some weight-related profiles for dosing analgesic medications, many have not been studied for longer-term dosing (Hain et al., 2005). Factors that may influence prescribing include pharmacokinetics and pharmacodynamics, particularly drug clearance, changing size and surface area, mode of delivery of medication, and compliance.

When considering pain in infants and children, it is important to acknowledge how situational and social factors impact upon achieving optimal pain control. Infants and children are vulnerable as they depend upon the response of an adult to alleviate their pain. Dependence on proxy reporting and interpretation of symptoms is influenced strongly by the child's family and social structure, their culture, and beliefs. When unwell, this dependence extends to the health-care professional who also has their own social basis for understanding and interpreting the child's pain.

Finally, the role of the parents and family when a child is getting progressively worse is quite different to that of the family of the dying adult, necessitating a distinctive skill set and approach from the paediatric palliative care team. Parents often carry a particularly heavy burden due to the long-term nature of many conditions. This can result in increased incidence of depression and other psychosocial issues such as divorce and unemployment with extra burden placed upon siblings. Supporting the extended family of grandparents, parents, and siblings is an important part of the holistic care offered by the palliative care team (Davies et al., 2007).

Myths and misconceptions

It is important to address the myths and misconceptions surrounding pain in children. Unfortunately the entrenchment of these attitudes and beliefs has not only been in the general population but is frequently found within the clinical fraternity (Table 9.13.1).

Misconceptions regarding pain in the child with advanced disease abound. One of the most prevalent findings in clinical practice is the child or family or another professional questioning the use of opioid analgesia. Any combination of the misconceptions listed in Table 9.13.1 may be involved in forming this barrier and care must be taken to explore and counter these barriers.

Impact of persisting pain on the child

A child's individual experience of, and response to, pain is unique and depends upon the interplay of multiple factors. Pain behaviour is a reflection of age, gender, developmental level, previous pain experiences, family learning, and cultural background. These characteristics shape the child's interpretation and experience of pain.

There is little evidence that pain perception is modified by cultural or ethnic factors but the expression of pain by children and its subsequent interpretation by a caregiver may be affected by the sociocultural context of the patient or the caregiver (Finley et al., 2009). Therefore the meaning attributed to the pain might be governed by culture (Koffman et al., 2008).

Some of these characteristics are relatively fixed: age, developmental level, and family and cultural background. Others, such as emotional, behavioural, and cognitive factors can change dynamically, reflecting the particular circumstances when the child experiences pain (Fig. 9.13.1). These 'situational' factors represent an individual and specific interaction between the context in which the pain is experienced and the child's individual response (McGrath, 1990).

What children think, what they do, and what they might sense or feel, influences their pain experience deeply. The combination of situational factors (worsening physical function associated with disease progression, sleep deprivation, upset parents, and feeling worried and scared) that influence the meaning and context of the pain experience for the child, impacts upon the physiological response of the body (Palermo et al., 2006). The ability of the central nervous system (CNS) to respond in such a flexible and varied way, influenced by internal and external factors, both conscious and subconscious, is due to plasticity. Change in situational factors may indicate why the same pain insult, or tissue damage, can result in a varied response in different children and within the same child. It would also explain why analgesic efficacy can vary both in the same child and across groups of children with the same injury.

Pain can be caused, exacerbated, maintained, or reduced as a consequence of behavioural factors. Behaviours such as crying,

Table 9.13.1 Common myths and the scientific evidence

Myth	Scientific evidence
1. Newborns do not have a mature nervous system to experience pain	By 26 weeks, a fetus *in utero* is capable of experiencing pain. Pain pathways and the cortical and subcortical pain centres are well developed. At birth, a newborn is highly sensitive to pain (Anand, 1999)
	Response to pain in young infants has been well documented in behavioural and physiological studies and the newborn is well able to feel pain (Fitzgerald et al., 1988; Fitzgerald and McIntosh, 1989; Fitzgerald, 1991)
2. Children do not feel as much pain as adults	Children feel as much pain as adults, and perhaps even more (McGrath, 2005)
3. Children will get used to pain. If a young child experiences pain, they have no memory and it will have no lasting effect	Continuing pain has deleterious effects and causes long-term changes in the nervous system (Schmelzle-Lubiecki et al., 2007)
	Data suggest that early pain experience may produce permanent reorganization of developing neural pathways, which in turn may impact negatively on future pain experience (Anand and the International Evidence-Based Group for Neonatal Pain, 2001; Fitzgerald and Walker, 2009)
4. Children cannot explain their pain reliably	If asked, children are capable at a very young age (even at 20 months) of saying where it hurts, how much it hurts, and what makes the hurt feel better
	Children can report pain intensity at the age of 3 years
	Children as young as 4 years old can indicate pain on a body chart without being able to name their body parts (Craig and Korol, 2008)
5. If a child can be distracted, the child is not in pain	Children use distraction and play as a coping mechanism for pain (Kuttner, 1996)
6. If a child says that he/she is in pain but does not appear in pain, the child does not need relief	The child is the authority on whether or not he or she is in pain
	Adults and medical professionals:
	◆ consistently and significantly under-rate children's pain
	◆ often have concern that children exaggerate pain which causes them to discount pain
	◆ diminish the seriousness of the pain and suffering as the pain may be difficult to treat (Craig et al., 1996; Pillai Riddell et al., 2008)
7. A sleeping child is a comfortable child	Sleep may be due to exhaustion from pain. Disturbed sleep patterns are common, this does not mean the child never sleeps (Long et al., 2008)
8. Opioid analgesics are dangerous for children and may result in addiction	Opioid analgesics are powerful pain-relieving medications that are invaluable for children in pain
	Children are no more at risk of addiction than adults
	Addiction is not experienced in patients with true pain on therapeutic doses (Schechter et al., 1993)

Adapted with permission from Kuttner, L., *A Child in Pain, How to Help, What to Do*, Hartley and Marks Publishers, Vancouver, Canada, Copyright © Leora Kuttner 2004.

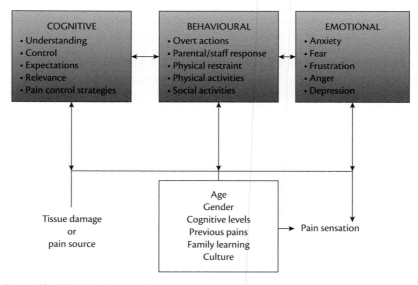

Fig. 9.13.1 The situation factors that modify children's pain perception.

Reproduced from PA McGrath and LM Hillier, Modifying the Psychological Factors that Intensify Children's Pain and Prolong Disability, in NL Schechter et al., (Eds.), *Pain in Infants, Children and Adolescents*, Second Edition, Lippincott, Williams and Wilkins, Copyright © 2002, by permission of Lippincott, Williams and Wilkins.

withdrawal, or becoming very distressed can impact negatively upon the pain experience. Emotional factors are known to have a direct impact upon the pain complaint, the persistence of pain, and the further development of pain. The emotional response of the child to pain depends upon the nature of the pain and the impact that it has on their everyday life. Feeling worried, fearful, cross, sad, and irritated will affect behaviours and therefore the ability of the child to cope with pain. Usually, increased emotional distress leads to a more intense pain experience.

It is important to try and understand the child's perception of their illness, what meaning they have attached to the pain, what their expectations are regarding the quality and severity of the pain, and what coping strategies have been tried in the past. Being able to provide accurate, age-appropriate information increases a child's sense of control and has a direct impact on their experience of pain. Offering children reasonable options and choices (e.g. 'Would you like tablets or liquid?' 'Would you like a heat pack or a massage?') with explanations about how treatments work and what to expect (e.g. 'This medicine might make you feel a bit sleepy, but this feeling should get better in a couple of days' and so on) also supports this process. Knowing how a child 'makes sense' of their pain, in terms of being linked to an internal or external causes, enables the team to understand how the child is projecting their pain and respond appropriately with pain reducing strategies.

Emotional and cognitive factors tend to feature most prominently in children receiving palliative care.

Case history

Ahmed, an 11-year-old boy with a brain tumour became more withdrawn and had aggressive mood swings. Ahmed's parents report that he often refused to take prescribed oral analgesic medications but are not sure whether he has any headaches, as he never complains of pain. Ahmed ultimately discloses that he has continuous pain from headaches with several severe episodes per day and that he often wakes from sleep with pain. He thinks that the tumour and therefore the pain, is a punishment from God that he has to bear in order to be forgiven for past wrong doings. Ahmed's pain management plan includes regular meetings with the family's spiritual advisor who clarifies the religious and existential meaning of Ahmed's illness. Ahmed is then able to comply with his analgesic regimen.

Impact of a child's pain on parents

Parents are the experts on their children. They act as an essential source of information for the health-care professional in the observation, assessment, and reporting of pain. Not only this, they are often the main carer and the most important resource for managing pain. They may guide and direct the health-care professional towards strategies that 'work' for their child.

Attitudes towards pain and behaviour patterns are often absorbed and learnt through parental role-modelling. Part of a child's response to pain stems from an inherited belief system and a familial approach to pain. Increased awareness of this can enable the health-care professional to influence the role of the parent in developing new and improving existing coping strategies.

Parents who encourage their children to engage in normal, everyday activities and support behaviours that encourage as much

'familiarity and routine' as possible, enable their child to maintain 'normality'. Children who lose their normal environment and adopt a passive role, tend to become more isolated and inevitably pain is heightened. Inadvertently, as children get sicker, the family becomes more insular and isolated from friends and relatives. As play and social interaction can help to lesson anxiety and offer some distraction from the situation, isolation can contribute to the experience of pain.

Parental education of pain mechanisms and management is important in ensuring that parents are not only able to comprehend and comply with a pain management plan, but are also equipped with the correct information to pass on to their child. Educating parents regarding rationale for treatments, how disease processes and situational factors impact upon pain, what to expect from medication in terms of benefits and side effects, and non-pharmacological pain control techniques, is absolutely vital. Parents have described the need to be 'enabled in their caring' for their child at the end of life and that this is central to coping with the stress and uncertainty of living through the death of a child (Price et al., 2011).

How parents respond to their child in pain is critically important to how both parent and child attempt to cope with pain (Palermo and Chambers, 2005). Response from carers that offer a calm and consistent approach, or encouragement to use an effective pain coping strategy will influence the experience of pain (Mitchell et al., 2007). Studies have shown that parental characteristics, such as gender and likelihood for catastrophic thoughts, as well as the threatening context of pain, play an important part in regulating parental response (Schneider et al., 2011; Caes et al., 2012).

Evaluating pain in children

Evaluation of pain is the cornerstone of good pain management in children. This process includes a detailed pain history, examination, diagnosis of the causes, and subsequent measurement of pain. The consequence of pain upon the child's activity and daily routine needs to be established. In children, understanding the impact of pain upon behaviour, relationships, development level, emotional state, sleep, and physical function is essential (Palermo, 2009).

Box 9.13.1 shows a summary of questions that are pertinent in the evaluation of childhood pain (WHO, 2012).

Level of cognitive development and expression of pain by children

How pain is perceived and expressed is modulated by various factors including the age and cognitive development of the child. Over the course of child development, change can be observed in the way pain is expressed and communicated (von Baeyer and Spagrud, 2003).

Infants

The infant is totally helpless and dependent upon the carer/parent to recognize pain behaviours. As infants have no language, facial expression and pitch of cry are the characteristics used to assess pain in infants (Grunau and Craig, 1987). Moreover, there is no single behaviour that indicates pain; more a deviation from the norms of behaviours that indicate the baby is experiencing pain. Most babies cry when they experience pain or may attempt to pull away from a painful experience or 'guard' or protect the painful limb or area (Hadjistavropoulos et al., 1994). By 6 months of age,

---

Box 9.13.1 Summary of questions by the health-care provider during clinical evaluation

- What words do the child and family use for pain?

- What verbal and behavioural cues does the child use to express pain?

- What do parents/and or caregivers do when the child has pain?

- What works best in relieving the pain?

- Where is the pain and what are the characteristics (site, severity, character of pain as described by the child/parent, e.g. sharp, burning, aching, stabbing, shooting, throbbing)?

- How did the present pain start (was it sudden/gradual)?

- Where is the pain (single/multiple sites)?

- Is the pain disturbing the child's sleep/emotional state?

- Is the pain restricting the child's ability to perform normal physical activities (sit, stand, walk, run)?

- Is the pain restricting the child's ability/willingness to interact with others, and ability to play?

Reproduced with permission from World Health Organization, *WHO guidelines on the pharmacological treatment of persisting pain in children with medical illnesses*, p.29, Copyright © World Health Organization 2012, available from <http://whqlibdoc.who.int/publications/2012/9789241548120_Guidelines.pdf>.

---

a baby will be fearful of anticipated painful situations if they have previously experienced pain in the same context (Lilley et al., 1997). Gibbons et al. have found that extremely premature babies have a similar pain response compared to babies born at older gestational ages but their responses are damped down (Gibbins et al., 2008).

Toddlers

As a baby grows and develops it starts to learn how to communicate discomfort through speech and body language. Frank reports that children rapidly develop an extensive pain language between the age of 12 and 30 months. Difference in verbal expressions make a cognitive distinction between the origins and sensory aspects of pain (Franck et al., 2010). If the child has the right descriptive language and uses terms to describe their pain ('sore', 'ouch') then they can often indicate a part of their body that is in pain. Children in this age group display fear of painful situations and often demonstrate anger, upset, and sadness if they experience pain.

Preschool children

Children aged 2–5 years can understand vocabulary for both positive and negative emotional experience (Azize et al., 2011). They think in concrete terms and as they grow, start to distinguish between the cause and the consequence of pain, particularly if they have some memory of previous painful experiences. Although they may find pain distressing, they are usually able to express themselves and may use their own specific words and terminology that can describe pain (Craig et al., 2006). With prompting they are able to understand and learn words that help describe their pain.

Children in this age group experience 'magical thinking' with blurring of boundaries between fantasy and reality. They create explanations for pain and may regard the pain as a punishment or a consequence of an unrelated event or behaviour. Creative play can be a helpful way to discover a child's understanding and interpretation of pain.

The preschool child with chronic pain may stop thinking of their pain as an abnormal perception, stop reporting the pain and become 'withdrawn'. Gauvain-Piquard has described this as the child being 'too well behaved' and becoming overwhelmed by their pain (Gauvain-Piquard, 1997). The clinician must be watchful for this observation.

School-aged children

Children between the ages of 6 and 12 years are more adept at abstract conceptualization. At 6 years old a child can define pain intensity and children from 7 to 10 years can explain why it hurts (McGrath and Craig, 1989). They are able to link cause and effect more easily and understand concepts of time. Children in this group are able to learn more detail about their pain and explanation of facts can assist understanding and allay fears and misconceptions. Younger children in this age group may perceive their pain as a punishment. Negative emotions and feelings of persecution may arise with chronic pain and internalization resulting in withdrawal and a label of 'depression' can be a feature.

Adolescents

Teenagers are able to think in an abstract way about pain. They understand the psychological element of the pain experience as well as the physical aspect. They have insight and are able to reflect upon their pain experiences in a more systematic and flexible way, drawing upon their individual coping strategies to support this process. Most adolescents shift from strategies focused upon emotion to strategies focused upon the causative problem around the age of 15 years.

Adolescence is a time of personal growth and independence. Pain, as a consequence of a persisting or progressive disease, can undermine this natural evolution. Pain can therefore become an injustice and an aggressor. Some teenagers may show signs of regression in their ability to cope with pain, particularly when there has been longer-term disease treatment and previous pain-related learned behaviours might emerge. It is important to address adolescents on an individual basis. If questioned in front of parents or peers there is often a tendency to 'play down' or deny pain in these situations. Teenagers can be very receptive to being taught coping strategies for pain management.

Response to pain in adolescents is based upon understanding (of disease, prognosis, and treatments), emotional (fear, anxiety, sorrow, and frustration) and cognitive factors (personality, beliefs, and culture). Trembly and Sullivan have shown that attachment style and cognitive-affective factors might increase vulnerability for problematic pain outcomes in adolescents. In a group of 382 high school students preoccupied and fearful attachment styles were associated with heightened pain severity, depression, pain catastrophizing, and anxiety (Tremblay and Sullivan, 2010). Worry is prevalent in youth and develops early in adolescents. Catastrophizing about pain usually can be thought of as extreme worry involving repeated thought about threat as uncontrollable and likely to have 'awful' consequences (Eccleston et al., 2012).

The child with severe cognitive impairment

There has been a growing awareness of the pain experiences of children with cognitive impairment and how pain perception may be affected in this cohort (Hunt and Burne 1995; Oberlander, 1999; Breau et al., 2003; Malviya et al., 2005). Understanding pain in a child with profound cognitive impairment is recognized as challenging, as the usual verbal and behavioural cues may not be reliable (Hunt et al., 2003). This group of children has an increased incidence of pain in their everyday lives but is reliant on parents and caregivers to recognize a problem (Breau, and Burkitt, 2009; Herr et al., 2011). Parents and carers develop a refined skill set that recognizes their child's individual emotional and behavioural cues that are suggestive of pain (Carter et al., 2002; Hunt et al., 2003). Pain is seen as an inextricable part of everyday life (Oberlander, 2001). Parents often report that pain is something that children with severe cognitive impairment learn to live with and tolerate (Fanurik et al., 1999).

The malnourished child

Attention must be paid to children with severe malnutrition as they are often developmentally delayed, perhaps through under stimulation or as a complication of an associated chronic condition. This group expresses pain in a markedly different way with lack of facial expression and verbalization and limited physical response. Under- development and indifference may instead result in whimpers or faint moans (Albertyn, 2007).

Pain severity measures

Several pain assessment measures have been developed and validated specific to the paediatric population. There is no single tool that is appropriate across all ages or all types of pain. The choice of a scale is dependent on developmental age, cognitive ability, and the necessity for carer report. Most pain scales have been developed and validated for acute pain. A significant amount of work has been published on scales for those children who cannot communicate verbally. There is no scale specifically for children receiving palliative care.

Pain measures must have well-established reliability and validity and have been used to measure pain outcome (in clinical trials) and improve clinical practice (efficacy) (Franck and Bruce, 2009). The best available evidence informing current practice is from systematic reviews by the Society of Pediatric Psychology Pain Assessment Task Force and the Paediatric Initiative on Methods Measurement and Pain Assessment in Clinical Trials (Stinson et al., 2006; von Baeyer and Spagrud, 2007; Cohen et al., 2008a, 2008b; McGrath et al., 2008; Huguet et al., 2010).

There are three approaches for measuring pain in children: self-report, observational or behavioural, and physiological. Physiological changes such as heart rate and respiratory rate are only loosely correlated to painful events and do not distinguish between pain and anxiety (Hain, 1997). The most commonly used tools rely on the quantification of pain intensity by self-report and are based upon counting or 'grading' pain severity in acute pain. Scales recommended for the quantification of acute pain and persisting pain in children over 3 years are the Faces Pain Scale –Revised, Poker Chip Tool, the Visual Analogue Scale, and the Oucher Photographic and the Numeric Rating Scale (WHO, 2012).

Table 9.13.2 Behavioural responses to pain

Behavioural indicators of acute pain	Behavioural indicators of chronic pain
Facial expression	Abnormal posture
Body movement and posture	Fear of being moved
Inability to be consoled	Lack of facial expression
Crying	Lack of interest in surroundings
Groaning	Undue quietness
	Increased irritability
	Low mood
	Sleep disruption
	Anger
	Changes in appetite
	Poor school performance

Adapted with permission from World Health Organization, *WHO guidelines on the pharmacological treatment of persisting pain in children with medical illnesses*, p.30, Copyright © World Health Organization 2012, available from <http://whqlibdoc.who.int/publications/2012/9789241548120_Guidelines.pdf>.

Observation of behavioural cues is a valid approach to acute pain severity assessment in children under 3 years old and those with impaired cognitive and verbal ability. Methods for observational measurement of acute pain are much more established than methods for longer lasting or chronic pain.

The absence of visible signs in a child with persisting pain is common. However, these observational signs may be present during an exacerbation of pain, such as on moving or on perceiving a social cue, for example, someone asking about the pain (von Baeyer and Spagrud, 2003).

There are no validated scales in children for chronic or persisting pain. Only the Douleur Enfant Gustave Roussy (DEGR) (Gauvain-Piquard et al., 1999) attempts to distinguish between acute and chronic cancer pain in children. However the DEGR takes some time to perform and further validation is required (von Baeyer and Spagrud, 2007).

Overt signs of pain tend to dissipate if pain is present longer term. There is also great variability as to the expression of persisting chronic pain in different individuals (von Baeyer and Spagrud, 2007). More complex changes in behaviour are likely to be manifest in chronic pain states, for example, low mood, increased irritability, sleep disturbance, being aggressive, and changes in appetite, all of which require knowledge of the child's baseline temperament (Palermo, 2000). Generally, sleep is of poor quality (Long et al., 2008; Palermo et al., 2008). Children with chronic pain may have negative thinking or may catastrophize about pain and experience increased pain severity and physical symptoms. Catastrophic thinking also contributes to psychological distress and functional disability (Vervoort et al., 2006).

Children who have persisting pain may display a variety of behaviours including being withdrawn, silent, and passive, and are often labelled as 'depressed' or even 'very well behaved' (Gauvain-Piquard, 1997). This psychomotor inertia has been well described and is a sign of untreated or undertreated, chronic pain. Other children may be seen as 'difficult' patients with aggressive behaviour and mood swings. Again this must be considered as pain-related behaviour if it is not the norm for the child.

Recognition of these signs and prescription of appropriate analgesia is the most appropriate approach to these issues.

Children may decide not to disclose information or under report pain if they associate the outcome as having a negative impact; for example, requiring a hospital visit or inpatient stay, necessitating an unpleasant intervention such as an injection, or causing upset or worry to their parents. Absence of signs and absence of reporting does not equate to absence of pain.

The literature is currently replete with studies regarding acute pain assessment in children. However, there has been concern in more recent publications regarding what is advocated by pain experts and researchers and what is actually delivered in clinical practice (Taylor et al., 2003; Franck and Bruce, 2009; Wadensten et al., 2011; Voepel-Lewis et al., 2012). Over the past decade, questions have been raised as to the efficacy of current interpretation of pain measurement in paediatric clinical practice (Hodgins, 2002; Mularski et al., 2006; Voepel-Lewis et al., 2011; von Baeyer et al., 2011). Franck (2009) states that 'poor compliance with pain assessment in children may not be the result of a "theory to practice gap" but may indicate unspoken resistance to methods that are overly simplistic, burdensome to patients, often inaccurate and perhaps even disrespectful of clinical expertise and experience'. Many experts acknowledge the complex influence of multiple intervening factors that influence children's pain expression and expose the challenges in interpreting individual pain scores in clinical practice (Schiavenato and Craig, 2010).

Hajistavropoulos and Craig (2002) have described the social communication model of pain for understanding pain in children. This conceptual model integrates biological, psychological, and social perspectives at the level of interaction between the child in pain and the person present (parent, carer, or professional). It presents a framework for the numerous and complicated interactions among psychological and social determinants of pain through the process of pain communication (Hadjistavropoulos et al., 2011).

This model describes four domains: the child's *experience* and *expression* of pain, together with the adult's *assessment* and *action* taken. Identification of these domains, and importantly the intra- and interpersonal factors that influence each step, enables appreciation of the complexity of assessment and organization of thought around the process. Acknowledging the social context of pain in infants and children enables identification of barriers that may prohibit adequate pain management (see Fig. 9.13.2).

Despite these areas of concern that simply highlight the complexity of the issue, the available tools for pain assessment can be used effectively in palliative care, particularly during exacerbation of pain symptoms. Rating pain before and after analgesic or non-pharmacological intervention, in addition to assessment of situational factors, can be used to assess efficacy of management.

As persisting pain in serious illness affects physical and social functioning and consequently quality of life, measures that incorporate a broader assessment may be more suitable in palliative care patients rather than single-pain intensity measures.

Pain management

Optimal pain relief in children's palliative care is achieved through the holistic assessment of the child. An integrated pharmacological and non-pharmacological approach for controlling a child's pain is shown in Fig. 9.13.3.

The pharmacological management of pain in children: the 2012 WHO approach

The 2012 guidelines have been developed by an expert working group using the best available evidence and aim to cover 'persistent' pain in children with medical illness (WHO, 2012). It is important to highlight that the WHO guidelines act as a framework and pharmacological point of reference for those working with children. The guidelines do not attempt to address the non-pharmacological approach to pain. This is relevant to palliative care teams as management of pain in children is always inclusive of the psychological, emotional and existential domains of 'total' pain.

The guidelines reiterate the key principles of pain management in children:

1. Ensure that detailed assessment has occurred.
2. Dose analgesia at regular intervals when pain is constant ('by the clock').
3. Make sure medication is available for 'break through' pain episodes.
4. Use the simplest route of administration ('by the appropriate route').
5. Tailor treatment to the individual ('by the child').

Using a two-step strategy

Modifications of the original WHO guidelines have included moving from the 'three-step analgesic ladder' (mild vs moderate vs severe pain) to a 'two-step analgesic approach' (mild pain vs moderate to severe pain).

A strong recommendation by the expert group but with very low-quality evidence, this decision-making was centred on a more effective strategy for analgesic management in children and various concerns regarding the 'weak' opioids Tramadol and codeine have been excluded from the guidelines based upon the safety and efficacy of these medications in children. There is no available evidence for the effectiveness and safety of tramadol in children. Codeine has varied metabolism across the population and in neonates and children it has a very low analgesic effect but a significant side effect profile (Williams et al., 2002; Tremlett et al., 2010). Concern regarding the use of strong opioids in children is offset by poor efficacy and unknown response to the weak opioids. In effect the 'weak' opioids are not recommended for use in paediatrics and have been replaced with a low dose of a 'Step 3' or strong opioid. The 'level' of approach is determined by severity of pain.

Step one: mild pain

Paracetamol and ibuprofen are the medicines of choice in children over the age of 3 months with mild pain.

Paracetamol

Paracetamol (acetaminophen) provides effective relief from mild pain and is widely available and well tolerated. It is also one of the few analgesics that can be used safely in neonates and children under the age of 3 months. Available in syrup, tablets, and parenteral formulations, it has a low adverse effect profile when used in appropriate doses. Doses of intravenous paracetamol for children and neonates should be based upon body weight rather than age (Van Den Anker et al., 2011; Mohammed et al., 2012).

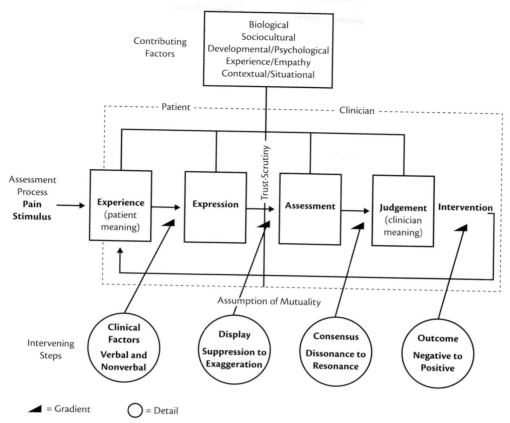

PAIN ASSESSEMNT AS A TRANSACTION

Fig. 9.13.2 Pain as a social transaction.

Hepatotoxicity is rare but can occur in vulnerable children at therapeutic doses (Haun et al., 2002). Risk factors that increase toxicity are those that can frequently be present in the paediatric palliative care population: hepatic or renal disease, malnutrition, and enzyme induction with various drugs (including carbamaz-epine; rifampicin and phenobarbitone amongst others). There are no data on the safety of long-term paracetamol administration in children.

Ibuprofen

Prescribing of ibuprofen is common in paediatric practice. Ibuprofen is safe to use in children and the risk of renal, gastrointestinal, and cardiovascular side effects is low, although care must be taken in children who are dehydrated (Southey et al., 2009). Ibuprofen must also be used cautiously in children with cancer due the increased risk of platelet dysfunction and subsequent bleeding.

Step two: moderate to severe pain

Children assessed with moderate to severe pain should have an opioid analgesic administered. The second step recommends the use of low-dose opioids for moderate pain. Risks regarding the use of strong opioids in children can be offset by effective risk management systems and importantly pain management education. The WHO guidelines reiterate that fear and lack of knowledge

regarding the use of opioids in children should not be a barrier for effective analgesia (WHO, 2012).

Opioid analgesics

It has been estimated that 60–80% of children who die require opioids for the management of pain (Zernikow et al., 2009). The palliative care physician should have confidence and familiarity with the range of opioids availability, their scientific basis for action, and side effect profile. There are occasions when children who could benefit from opioid therapy are, or their family is, unwilling to take opioids. This is usually based on misconceptions about their use and the perception that opioids mark 'the beginning of the end'. These fears need to be explored and correct information provided. Many parents need support in understanding the difference between physical dependence, tolerance, and addiction. There is no empirical evidence that children receiving opioid analgesics are at risk for addiction. Significant time and educational investment is often needed, usually on repeated consults, to allay fears and misconceptions and ensure adequate understanding for adherence to pain management plans.

There is a great variety of opioids available to the paediatric palliative care physician in some countries; however, there are no proven benefits of using alternatives to morphine in children. Morphine is well established as a first-line opioid in children as it is inexpensive and has a wide range of formulations; however,

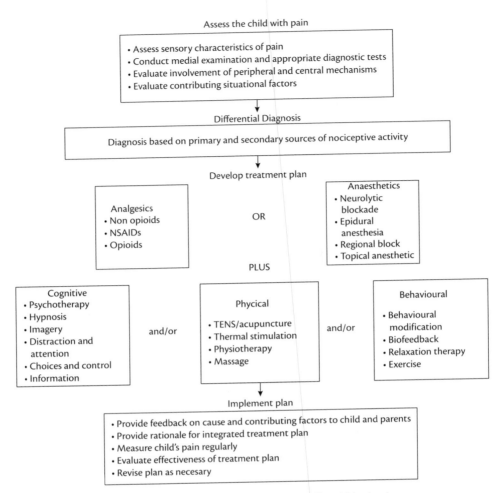

Fig. 9.13.3 A model of integrated pharmacological and non-pharmacological approach for controlling children's pain.
Adapted with from PA McGrath, Pain Control in Children, pp. 32–43, in RS Weiner (Ed.), *Innovations in Pain Management: A Practical Guide for Clinicians*, Paul M. Deutsch Press, Copyright © 1992, with permission of DC Press.

alternative strong opioids can be considered based upon scientific evidence, pain pathophysiology, safety, and availability.

Effective analgesia is achieved through gradual increase in opioid until pain relief is achieved. High-dose opioids may be needed at times (Collins et al., 1995).

Dosing at regular intervals: by the clock

When pain is severe and constant, opioid analgesia must be prescribed on a regular basis rather than 'as needed'. Theoretically the dosage interval of morphine is shorter than that of adults as the half-life of morphine in children is reduced compared to adults (Zernikow et al., 2009) Nonetheless there is wide inter-individual variability. In practice, a 4-hourly dosing schedule for immediate-release opioid works well. Some children may benefit from an 8-hourly dose of long-acting opioid preparations rather than the standard 12-hourly regimen (Hunt et al., 1999).

The exception to this 'rule' is when the half-life of the opioid is increased. This occurs in neonates and infants up to the age of 12 months who, amongst other pharmacokinetic differences, have reduced renal clearance of morphine. Neonates and infants (under 12 months) are, therefore, prescribed a lower starting dose of opioid at longer intervals, for example, 6- or 8-hourly.

Impaired renal function is another indication to approach opioid dosing cautiously. It is sensible to use immediate release opioids at a dosing schedule of 8- or 12-hourly or even as needed initially until titration of dose interval to requirements in the individual patient is established. Effectively the immediate release opioid has a longer acting duration as excretion is delayed.

Using the appropriate route of administration: by the mouth

The least invasive route, the oral route, is usually preferable in children. As such, palatability, availability of oral solutions, size of tablets, and frequency of dosing become factors to consider to ensure compliance and, consequently, good symptom management. Unless these factors are reviewed regularly, administering medication in children can become a major issue and may be a source of conflict between child and parent/carer. Endless drug regimens with poor planning and lack of individual consideration can create 'battles and barriers', affect relationships and impact on quality of life.

Some manufacturers have developed concentrated oral solutions to facilitate administration of medication for children who are unable (or unwilling) to take tablets. It is also common in paediatric practice to open capsules, to crush tablets, or to dissolve medication into solution and then to mix the powder or solution with more palatable food and drink. Consequently there may be issues regarding accuracy of dosing.

Many children with complex neurological disease, or those receiving cancer treatment, may have a gastrostomy *in situ*. Although these devices can be incredibly helpful, negating palatability and dose frequency issues, other problems may arise as several commonly used medications cannot be given via gastrostomy due to interaction between the medication and the device.

There are several situations when the enteral route might not be suitable and an alternative route must be sought, for example:

♦ poor absorption: vomiting, disordered gastrointestinal motility

♦ inability to comply: unconscious; severe nausea, poor swallow; risk of aspiration, medication refusal

♦ pain crisis requiring rapid titration of opioids.

The choice of alternative routes of administration when the oral route is not possible should be based on clinical judgement, availability, feasibility, and patient preference.

Other routes of medication administration in children

Alternative routes of administration of analgesics in children include the subcutaneous, intravenous, or transdermal routes. The intramuscular route is practically obsolete in children as the injection itself is a cause of pain and may result in under-reporting of pain.

The availability of short-gauge, indwelling, non-metallic needle systems has been very useful and made the subcutaneous route popular in paediatric practice. Ease of insertion, the possibility of numerous sites for access, and avoidance of recurrent intravenous cannulation offer obvious benefit. Drugs, and if necessary, fluid can be delivered effectively via this route.

Indwelling percutaneous intravenous catheters or central venous access devices are used frequently for children requiring long-term therapy, recurrent blood product transfusion, and/or parenteral nutrition. They can be useful in the palliative setting towards the end of life for delivery of analgesia and other medications, particularly if higher-volume infusions are needed. The risk of sepsis and the impact of the catheter on the child's activities of daily living and quality of life must be measured against the benefits and ease of intravenous access. The successful use of patient (or proxy) controlled analgesia has been reported in children at the end of life (Schiessl et al., 2008; Anghelescu et al., 2012).

The development of 'transdermal' medication patches has been particularly advantageous to children with chronic, stable opioid requirements (Hunt et al., 2001). Although the minimum quantity of opioid required for use might provide a barrier in smaller children, the more recent manufacture of lower-dose, matrix-based patches has enabled more children to gain from the clear advantages offered by this route.

Medication delivered by the rectal route may be advantageous in some instances but many children dislike this way of giving medications. It can be a very useful route in the infant and younger child to avoid parenteral routes in the short term. Additionally some immediate and sustained release opioid preparations can be readily absorbed from the rectal mucosa. Anticonvulsants have

also been reported to be given via this route in special circumstances (Anderson and Saneto, 2012).

The transmucosal route has become an increasingly popular means to deliver medication in children. Drugs absorbed through the transmucosal membrane of the nose or buccal cavity avoid the first-pass metabolism of the gastrointestinal tract and are absorbed rapidly. This mode of delivery is particularly effective for drugs such as midazolam, which is now available for this use in a concentrated buccal form. Diamorphine has also been used very effectively via this route for breakthrough pain although intranasal fentanyl has received more attention in the literature (Crellin et al., 2010; Mudd et al., 2011; Harlos et al., 2013). Although alternative opioids are available for sublingual, transmucosal, and nasal use, there are often issues regarding the practicalities of appropriate dosing, particularly in younger children when lower doses of opioid preparations for nasal, sublingual, or buccal use may be very helpful for rapid relief of symptoms. End-of-life symptoms including pain, dyspnoea, agitation, and seizures have been controlled successfully via the transmucosal routes but unfortunately literature supporting this is scarce.

Adapting treatment to the individual: by the child

This principle promotes individualized treatment according to the assessed need of the child. Finding the right dose of opioid for a child involves three phases:

Initiation: the initial starting dose of medication in an opioid naïve child is usually calculated per kilogram of body weight (up to a maximum dose of 50 kg). The WHO guidelines have added a specified age range to allow for changes in pharmacokinetics in the growing child. In a child already receiving opioids the current dose of opioid should be used as a basis for calculation.

Titration: the dose of analgesia is titrated on an individual basis. Opioid analgesics must be increased in steps until the correct dose, based on the child's response to medication. The correct dose of opioid is determined in partnership with the child and carers until the best possible pain relief is achieved, with the fewest side effects. Generally the maximum dose increase is approximately 50% of the previous total opioid dose in non-naïve opioid patients, however in an inpatient setting, with careful monitoring and repeated assessment, experienced practitioners may increase doses more rapidly (WHO, 2012).

Maintenance: is established once a dose that provides adequate relief of pain is achieved. A long-acting opioid is commenced at this point, if available. For many children, long-acting morphine preparations (granules) are convenient and offer flexible dosing. A minimum total daily dose of oral morphine 30–40 mg is required prior to commencing the lowest available dose of a fentanyl 12-microgram patch, which can prohibit use in many small children.

Internationally the availability of child appropriate dosage formulations is often very limited and prohibits optimal analgesia. Efforts to ensure availability are supported through the *WHO Model List of Essential Medicines for Children* (WHO, 2013).

Opioid switching

Opioid switching should be considered in children who have opioid dose limiting side effects. A reduction in the equianalgesic dose of the new opioid by approximately 25–30% is recommended to reduce toxicity and counter the possibility of incomplete cross-tolerance.

Opioid side effects

Children may not report adverse effects voluntarily, for example, constipation, nausea, and itching, so careful attention must be paid to these problems when assessing opioid efficacy.

Sedation is usually one of the first side effects that occur when opioids are commenced in the opioid naïve patient or when the dose is increased significantly. Drowsiness may last for a few days but then usually subsides. Warning parents and carers avoids any unnecessary worry about sedation.

If opioids are titrated appropriately, respiratory depression is a very rare occurrence. In palliative care patients, opioid toxicity is more likely to occur when there is sudden removal of a pain stimulus, such as following radiation therapy to a bone metastasis or the insertion of an intrathecal pump for metastatic spinal disease. In these situations it is helpful to revert to short-acting opioids, or an opioid infusion, to enable close monitoring of opioid requirements. The onset of renal failure and an inability to excrete opioid metabolites is another potential reason for respiratory compromise, as is the inadvertent administration of higher doses of opioid than those prescribed, such as ingestion of sustained-release medication in the place of short-acting opioids.

If sedation persists, and renal or hepatic and CNS disease are excluded, an opioid switch should be considered. Sedation may be caused by an accumulation of morphine's centrally acting metabolite, morphine-6-glucaronide, hence a different opioid such as fentanyl may have a more favourable ratio of analgesia to side effects. Rarely, paradoxical agitation can be seen in children taking opioids. Treatment is reduction in dose or switching of opioid.

If respiratory depression occurs then small, frequent doses of naloxone (an opioid antagonist) may be necessary at a starting dose, in opioid-tolerant patients, of 1 microgram per kilogram, titrated over time (e.g. every 3 minutes) until the child is breathing spontaneously. A low-dose infusion of naloxone may be required until the adverse effect of the opioid resolves. Administration of naloxone must be done with caution as reversal of analgesia will precipitate extreme pain and opioid withdrawal syndrome. Assisted ventilation for respiratory depression may be indicated in palliative care patients in this situation.

Psychostimulants such as methylphenidate have been used in adults to reverse opioid-induced sedation, despite a recent review stating that robust data are lacking (Stone and Minton, 2011). A small study in adolescents in cancer and various case reports describe use in younger populations, however concomitant adverse effects such as delirium, psychosis, and hallucinations might deter use (Yee and Berde, 1994).

The incidence of nausea seems relatively rare in paediatric palliative care and, in contrast to adult medicine, most physicians do not prescribe antiemetics automatically in conjunction with an opioid. However, its incidence may well be overlooked in children (Mashayekhi et al., 2009), as it is not a symptom children find easy to describe.

Constipation is very common in children prescribed opioids. Regular stimulant and softening laxatives should accompany all opioid therapy. There is good evidence in adults that the opioid antagonists naloxone and methylnaltrexone are effective in opioid-induced constipation without causing opioid withdrawal (Sykes, 1996; Portenoy et al., 2008; Chamberlain et al., 2009; Candy et al., 2011). There is no such evidence in children, although

there are now published paediatric cases which report successful management with these drugs (Lee and Mooney, 2012). Fentanyl has been reported as causing less constipation than other opioids (Finkel et al., 2005; Zernikow et al., 2007).

Pruritus as a side effect of opioids is not uncommon in infants and children and occurs frequently around the nose and face. Standard management for pruritus can be trialled, however if it persists an opioid switch may be required (Drake et al., 2004; Mashayekhi et al., 2009).

Myoclonus is an involuntary muscle contraction that occurs as a consequence of either opioid toxicity or long-term use of opioids. It is not infrequent in children and usually prompts opioid switching or treatment with a benzodiazepine or muscle relaxant, depending upon the circumstances.

Urinary retention is seen in children particularly after rapid dose escalation and spinal or epidural opioids. Anecdotally, children seem to experience urinary symptoms (usually hesitancy) not infrequently; however, a small case series indicated that one in seven children (14%) had overt symptoms of retention (Mashayekhi et al., 2009). External bladder massage/pressure, heat packs, voiding in a warm bath, and, if necessary, intermittent catheterization or cholinergic agent may be required. Opioid rotation is also an option.

Non-malignant pain and use of opioids

Data on the use of opioids in children with severe pain due to non-malignant conditions are limited. One retrospective review studied opioid prescription for chronic, severe non-malignant pain in a multidisciplinary paediatric pain clinic. During a 12-month period, 104 patients were seen in the clinic, of whom 49 received an opioid as part of their pain management; 11 received an opioid for more than 3 months, and five of these were still receiving an opioid at the end of the study period. Overall, there appeared to be better pain control and improved function in patients receiving opioid therapy in the context of prescription in a multidisciplinary pain clinic with close review and a multisystem approach to pain management. More data are needed to know if such therapy is safe and beneficial on a longer-term basis (Slater et al., 2010).

Adjuvant analgesics

An adjuvant analgesic is a medication that has a primary indication other than pain, but is analgesic in some painful conditions. The WHO recently reviewed the evidence for the use of adjuvant analgesic medicines in pain management for children (WHO, 2012). The use of corticosteroids as adjuvant medicines is not recommended for the treatment of persisting pain in children with medical illnesses, nor is the use of bisphosphonates for the treatment of bone pain in children, due to the low quality of evidence. Although used frequently for the management of neuropathic pain in children, it was not possible to make evidence-based recommendations for or against the use of tricyclic antidepressants (TCAs), selective serotonin reuptake inhibitors (SSRIs), or anticonvulsants as adjuvant medicines. In addition, recommendations regarding the risks or benefits of ketamine or systemic local anaesthetics as adjuvants to opioids for the treatment of neuropathic pain in children, or for the use of benzodiazepines and/or baclofen as adjuvants in the management of pain associated with muscle spasm and spasticity, could not be made based on the current literature. The quality of current evidence, and risks and benefits of different treatments are summarized in the WHO document. The need for further analgesic research in children is urgent and essential to establish the role of these medicines in paediatric pain treatment.

In reality, however, when faced with the symptoms of very sick and dying children, many of these adjuvant medications are trialled with anecdotal benefit to patients reported. Small case reports and series have been published but robust data are unavailable due to the scientific, ethical, and practical challenges in paediatric palliative medicine practice (Collins et al., 1995; Behm and Kearns, 2001; Tsui et al., 2004; Finkel et al., 2007; Dayioğlu et al., 2008). A recent expert working group has proposed more feasible analgesic study designs for children, including cross over trials and N of 1 trials in the chronic pain and palliative groups (Berde et al., 2012).

Challenging pain syndromes in paediatric palliative care

Pain aetiology in children requiring palliative care is frequently varied and dependent on underlying diagnosis and ongoing complications. A recent multisite prospective study found that the two most common principal diagnoses in 550 children referred to palliative care teams in a 3-month period were congenital disorders (49.7%) and neuromuscular disorders (39.2%) (Feudtner et al., 2011). Other large Western paediatric palliative care centres report that approximately two-thirds of their caseload has non-malignant conditions (McCulloch and Collins, 2006). However, this will depend on geography as AIDs-related illness, cancer, and infection predominate in Africa (Amery et al., 2009; Campbell, 2011; Amery, 2012).

Muscle spasm

Sporadic, episodic pain seen related to muscle spasm is common. A significant source of discomfort in children with neuromuscular conditions and severe neurological impairment, management is often multimodal and requires use of antispasmodic agents, such as dantrolene and baclofen, and non-pharmacological strategies (Tilton et al., 2010). Triggers for muscle spasm might include constipation, seizures, gastro-oesophageal reflux, and discomfort from orthotic supports (Hauer, 2010). Targeted therapies such as botulinum toxin, surgical intervention, and intrathecal drug delivery are becoming more common and may alleviate the child from the systemic side effects of medication (Hoving et al., 2007; Bonouvrié et al., 2008; Esquenazi et al., 2010).

Opioids may be considered for some children with severe chronic pain secondary to muscle spasm. However, regard must be given to the potential for children with non-malignant, life-limiting conditions to survive for many years and there should be regular review of the effectiveness of any opioid prescribed. Although anecdotal practice supports the use of opioid prescribing in children with non-malignant disorders, trial withdrawal of long-term opioids should be considered on a regular basis as the cause of the spasm may dissipate with time.

Bone pain

Bone pain is a common problem in children receiving palliative care. Its association with malignant conditions is well known, but what is often overlooked is that it is also an important problem for many children with non-malignant conditions.

In children with chronic neurological conditions such as cerebral palsy or neuromuscular conditions, bone pain associated with secondary distortion of the normal skeletal structures may occur, especially during periods of growth. It is also documented that non-ambulatory children with chronic neurological conditions have low bone density and an increased propensity to non-traumatic fracture, or fracture with minimal trauma, such as that caused by moving and handling (Khoury and Szalay, 2007). Contributing factors in children with chronic neurological features include immobility, feeding difficulties, use of anticonvulsants, and lack of exposure to sunlight (Henderson et al., 2004).

Bone pain may also be a prominent feature of inherited metabolic disorders of childhood with pathological involvement of bone from systemic disease, mucopolysaccharidosis (Rossi et al., 2011), or primary defects of structural bone proteins, osteogenesis imperfecta. Osteopenia from secondary distortion of the normal skeletal structures may occur as an effect of systemic treatments such as prolonged steroid use in cancer (Anghelescu et al., 2012).

Bone pain in a child with HIV/AIDS can be due to multiple causes including osteopenia as a result of bone loss and altered bone metabolism, cancer, and infections such as osteomyelitis or septic arthritis. Decreased bone mineral density is seen in children with HIV/AIDS (Fortuny et al., 2008), the pathogenesis of which is likely to be multifactorial, including malnutrition and mineral and vitamin deficiency.

Cancer-induced bone pain (CIBP) has been reported to be the most frequent single symptom of malignant disease (Fanurik et al., 1999). It is associated with primary bone tumours, metastatic tumour, and infiltrative bone marrow disease in haematological malignancy. In children with acute lymphoblastic leukaemia, bone pain has been reported in almost 50% of patients (Anand and the International Evidence-Based Group for Neonatal Pain, 2001).

The effective management of bone pain relies upon an individualized treatment to the identified cause and the clinical condition. This may include an appropriate orthopaedic intervention and the effective use of medication according to the two-step WHO strategy as already discussed. Although there is little evidence for the use of bisphosphonates as an adjuvant, there is increasing experience with use in children with congenital and acquired forms of osteopenia, in terms of analgesic efficacy and safety with long-term use (Stevens et al., 2006; Breau and Camfield, 2011).

Treatment of CIBP may require a multidisciplinary approach such as palliative radiotherapy alongside systemic disease-modifying treatment (chemotherapy) and supportive care (analgesic and integrative therapies). Novel approaches, such as the use of radiopharmaceuticals and interventional techniques (radioablation, magnetic resonance-guided ultrasound), have shown promising results in relieving pain in focal metastatic disease in adults and if accessible, should be considered if other treatments fail (Treede et al., 2008; Bailey et al., 2010; Wilkinson et al., 2012; Hexem et al., 2013).

Neuropathic pain

Neuropathic pain arises as a consequence of a lesion or disease affecting the somatosensory system (Treede et al., 2008). Neuropathic pain can be exceptionally severe and disabling. It is a particularly challenging diagnosis in children due to the heterogeneity of conditions, diagnostic uncertainty, and unknown trajectories (Walco et al., 2010).

If available, the child's own description provides the best indication that the pain may be of neuropathic origin. The child may describe sensory anomalies such as numbness, itching, tingling, or burning sensations. Unusual expressions such as 'shivering', 'fizzing', 'tickling', or 'pricking' should alert the clinician. Although assessment and diagnosis in adult practice is becoming more rigorous, paediatric practice is some way behind. Early work on quantitative sensory testing in children (which examines sensory perception after application of different mechanical and thermal stimuli) is establishing a paediatric reference base that may be helpful in the future to identify responders to certain treatments in accordance to the underlying pain mechanism (Voepel-Lewis et al., 2008).

The newly proposed grading system to diagnose this condition requires a history suggestive of a relevant lesion, the presence of pain with a distinct sensory distribution in a corresponding body part, indication of negative or positive sensory signs within the area, and confirmation of the lesion by a diagnostic test (Treede et al., 2008). Unfortunately, many children and infants with a possible diagnosis are not able to communicate, making it very difficult to elicit sensory changes. However, if sensory disturbances like allodynia or dysaesthesia are present consistently then these are a strong indicator that neuropathic pain is present.

Any damage to the somatosensory system presents a potential risk of the development of neuropathic pain. Damage can range from single nerve involvement to complex genetic disorders that compromise axonal transport. The clinician may need to think laterally when considering a neuropathic pain diagnosis in children, for example, the child with unstable kyphoscoliosis and vertebral instability compromising the spinal cord and nerve roots, or the population of infants and children with neurometabolic conditions and white matter anomalies that may cause lesions or disordered processes within the nervous system. Neuropathic pain has been reported following orthopaedic surgery in children with cerebral palsy (Lauder and White, 2005) and is a well-known complication of cancer and its treatment.

Peripheral neuropathy is reported to occur in about 13–34% of children with HIV/AIDS (Araújo et al., 2000). Approximately 34% of children in early or later stages of HIV advancement report symptoms and signs of peripheral neuropathy in the absence of potential neurotoxic antiretroviral drugs (Van Dyke et al., 2008). However, there is a higher prevalence of peripheral neuropathy in children with encephalopathy and symptomatic AIDS (Mherekumombe and Collins, 2014).

Cerebral irritability

Cerebral irritability is a term used to describe the clinical presentation of persistent, unremitting agitation and distress. In the paediatric palliative care setting it is most often associated with the non-verbal child with severe neurological impairment but is also seen in infants presenting with an acute illness, children with progressive, often neurodegenerative disorders (adrenoleucodystrophy, AIDS encephalopathy) and, occasionally, towards the end of life in children with malignancy. Cerebral irritability may also be confused with an agitated delirium at the end of life, although clinical management at this stage is very similar.

At present there is very little published information on this phenomenon. It describes a constellation of features, which are the end point of a variety of different processes manifesting as similar clinical symptoms and signs. These processes may be pathological or, as in many children with severe neurological conditions, of unknown aetiology, although there are various hypotheses as to potential causes in this particular group of patients, such as central neuropathic pain and visceral hypersensitivity referred to later in this chapter.

Presentation involves a variety of manifestations depending on the clinical situation; however, agitation and distress are key. Classical symptoms in an infant or non-verbal child with severe neurological impairment include an unrelenting high pitched scream and other pain related behaviours, such as an increase in tone (spasticity) and/or seizures, sleep–wake cycle disruption, autonomic dysfunction (sweating, paradoxical bradycardia), increase in secretions, vomiting, retching, and 'feed intolerance'. If these symptoms present as an acute change in behaviour, a hospital review may be required with appropriate investigations to identify the aetiology and exclude a reversible cause. However, in the neurologically impaired child, this behaviour often evolves over time with the condition and becomes a chronic pattern with a significant burden on often exhausted, parents and carers (Fig. 9.13.4).

It is a commonly held belief that cerebral irritability in a neurologically impaired child in the absence of pathology is due to an abnormal brain, and abnormal neurological processing (Klick and Hauer, 2010). In this situation it is difficult to know whether the child with severe neurological impairment and cerebral irritability is also experiencing pain. Morally and ethically the assumption has to be that pain is a feature of this condition until proven otherwise. This is endorsed by the fact that most of these children will be known to have alternative baseline behaviours when they are not distressed, or cerebral irritability mimics previous pain behaviours that have had a bona fide cause (Breau et al., 2001; Stallard et al., 2002).

Several papers have acknowledged that pain of unknown cause is often the most severe pain in children with impaired cognition (Breau et al., 2003; Hauer et al., 2007; Hauer, 2010).

Children with cerebral irritability present with their own individual narrative, symptomatology, and signs. The most important step in the management of this condition is recording a detailed history and evaluation of the child. In the case of chronic cerebral irritability, it may be necessary to request a symptom diary to establish temporal factors and understand the impact upon the child and family. Exclusion of all other causes of pain and irritability, with relevant investigations, must be undertaken. If the aetiology of acute cerebral irritation is known and reversible, then treatment will obviously be directed towards the cause.

Central pain

Central pain arises from damage to any part of the central somatosensory system, that is, those parts of the CNS that are specialized for pain perception. Conditions known to cause central neuropathic pain in adults, for example, multiple sclerosis and stroke, are rare in children. However, many other life-limiting conditions in childhood could potentially be the cause of central pain (Hain and Douglas, 2010). Neurodegenerative conditions and the consequences of hypoxic or traumatic brain injury cause a range of different types of damage to the CNS, including

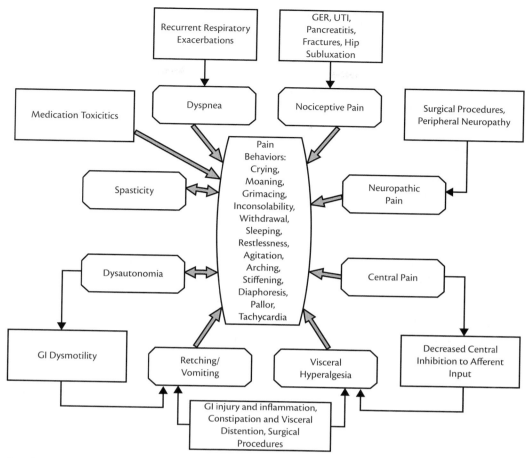

Fig. 9.13.4 Sources of pain behaviours in children with severe neurological injury.

Reproduced from *Current Problems in Pediatric and Adolescent Health Care*, Volume 40, Issue 6, Klick, J.C. and J. Hauer, Pediatric palliative care, pp.120–151, Copyright © 2010 Mosby, Inc., with permission from Elsevier, http://www.sciencedirect.com/science/journal/15385442.

disordered structure, abnormal neuronal migration and myelination, and/or abnormalities of normal neurological systems at the molecular level. A familiar clinical picture in paediatric palliative care is one of persistent screaming and distress, and alongside cerebral irritability (discussed earlier) and visceral hyperalgesia (see following sections), central pain is an important differential diagnosis when considering causes of idiopathic distress in the non-verbal child (Klick and Hauer, 2010).

Visceral hyperalgesia

Visceral hypersensitivity has been hypothesized to be a possible cause of cerebral irritability in children with severe neurological impairment (Hauer, 2010; Klick and Hauer, 2010). Gastrointestinal pain is reported commonly in children with severe cognitive impairment (Houlihan et al., 2004; Hauer, 2010). Chronic cerebral irritability in children with neurological impairment is often related temporally to gastrointestinal symptoms and signs including pain, feed intolerance, flatus, retching, and vomiting. Pain seems to be localized to bowels, gastrointestinal tract, and digestion, despite adequate treatment of constipation and gastro-oesophageal reflux.

Visceral hypersensitivity or hyperalgesia is an altered response to visceral stimulation resulting in activation of pain sensation

(Delgado-Aros and Camilleri, 2005). In contrast to other chronic pain states, visceral pain is often associated with gut motor abnormality and exaggerated intraluminal pressures and pain sensation. The presence of nociceptors in the gut wall that can be activated by a variety of modulators at lower, normally ineffective intraluminal pressures seems to be an important factor in generating pain (Buéno et al., 2000). Visceral hypersensitivity caused by abnormal gastrointestinal sensory input may also explain some of these issues in this population of children.

Zangen and colleagues have hypothesized that sensory and motor abnormalities, despite adequate management of motility and gastro-oesophageal reflux, suggest visceral hypersensitivity in the gut (Zangen et al., 2003). They studied 14 children with a lifelong history of retching and vomiting persisting after fundoplication and gastrostomy insertion, 12 of whom were impaired neurologically. Sensory anomaly and/or motility disorders were found in all 14 patients. Twelve patients had a low gastric-volume threshold for retching and seven patients had both reduced gastric volume and a motility disorder. Interventions included pain management with the intention of reducing afferent signals and/or central sensitization including amitriptyline, gabapentin, and imipramine.

Another recent report of a feeding programme for medically ill, non-verbal toddlers described the successful use of an outpatient programme based on a multidisciplinary pain rehabilitation model. The report hypothesized that pain from gastric distension and retching against a fundoplication maintained or further sensitized the peripheral nociceptive system. Pain management involved either amitriptyline or gabapentin, amongst other interventions such as jejunal feeding to reduce gastric distension. By the end of a 14-week programme all nine patients showed significant improvement in oral feeding and irritability symptoms (Davis et al., 2009).

Hauer et al. have also suggested that visceral hyperalgesia may manifest as feeding intolerance presenting with symptoms of neuro irritability (Hauer et al., 2007). The authors identified retrospectively nine children with severe global developmental impairment who experienced 'recurrent irritability that was disruptive to daily life'. All children had daily crying episodes that lasted at least an hour. Signs reported by parents included arching, crying, feed intolerance, and disrupted sleep and descriptors included irritability, pain, and agitation. Treatment with gabapentin resulted in marked improvement in all individuals. Final doses ranged from 15 to 35 mg/kg per day (Hauer et al., 2007).

Based on information from animal models which reveal gastrointestinal tract inflammation resulting in hyperexcitability of nociceptive neurons, colonic distension producing chronic visceral hypersensitivity and allodynia and hyperalgesia in newborn rats, and altered gastric motility and visceral hyperalgesia in rats with localized gastric ulceration, there are suggestions in the literature that visceral hyperalgesia in this group of patients is likely to be the result of repeated painful gastrointestinal experiences in infancy. These painful gastrointestinal experiences result in recruitment of previously silent nociceptors and sensitization of peripheral visceral afferent fibres causing pain (Zangen et al., 2003). These 'experiences' might include a history of prolonged neonatal care, gastro-oesophageal reflux, constipation, gastrostomy feeding, and fundoplication. This interesting hypothesis, that visceral hyperalgesia is a result of sensitization not of the underlying neurological impairment itself, is a plausible explanation.

Zenger has also proposed that visceral sensory processing occurs as a perinatal event or during infancy as there is evidence to suggest that newborns have neural pathways for detection, transmission and reaction to noxious stimuli but a mature descending inhibitory pathway is lacking (Fitzgerald and McIntosh, 1989; Fitzgerald, 1991; Zangen et al., 2003). One must also consider the potential effects of CNS plasticity in the abnormal but developing brain that may have aberrant neuromodulation and hence contribute significantly to the development of pathological pain pathway. There remain many unknowns within this field and it is an important area for continued investigation. Visceral hypersensitivity may, therefore, be considered as a differential diagnosis for cerebral irritability.

Pharmacological management directed at central neuropathic pain and visceral hypersensitivity has been studied poorly and, in adults, central neuropathic pain classically has been difficult to treat (Klit et al., 2009). Approaches with medication would involve usually a trial of adjuvant agents including TCAs, anticonvulsants, and N-methyl-D-aspartate receptor (NMDA) receptor antagonists (Zangen et al., 2003; Hauer et al., 2007; Davis et al., 2009).

The paucity of paediatric data on this topic is striking considering the regular prescribing of anticonvulsants in paediatric practice. A single case report of a 3-month-old infant with neurological impairment and cerebral irritability detailed improvement in tone and disposition after the infant was treated with 5 mg/kg gabapentin at night, following the failure of regular lorazepam and intermittent morphine to provide relief. Gabapentin was tolerated well and dose increases lead to further improvement (Behm and Kearns, 2001).

Benzodiazepines are used commonly for the treatment of irritability and agitation in children both at the end of life and in the context of chronic cerebral irritability. Midazolam is used often in the treatment of cerebral irritability as it is short acting and can be given easily through the buccal route. This short-term efficacy can facilitate 'breaking the cycle' of distress in cerebral agitation, particularly in children with severe neurological conditions. If multiple dosing of midazolam is required on a daily basis, then consideration should be given to a longer-acting benzodiazepine, such as clonazepam. Clonazepam has the added benefit of more anticonvulsant activity relatively, which may be helpful if seizures are a feature of increasing cerebral irritability. Due to the emergence of tolerance with prolonged use of any benzodiazepine, they are best used for a short duration of up to 4 weeks if required regularly or as a 'rescue' treatment when symptoms are particularly difficult on an intermittent basis only. Abrupt withdrawal of benzodiazepines following prolonged use will precipitate an unpleasant withdrawal syndrome and treatment should be tapered slowly as a rule.

Opioids are not a first-line medication in this situation although they have been shown to improve pain in some central neuropathic pain conditions (Dworkin et al., 2007; Attal et al., 2010). They may be appropriate as a short-term control measure for acute neuropathic pain until other agents have been introduced and titrated to effect (Rowbotham et al., 2003; O'Connor et al., 2009; Barrera-Chacon et al., 2011). However, as the use of any analgesic medication for children with cerebral irritability may be necessary for a prolonged period of time, the potential for long-term effects of using the medication must be given due consideration. In the case of a long-term opioid administration, the development of tolerance or opioid-induced hyperalgesia is a concern. Despite these measures, some children will have intractable symptoms and may require additional medications such as benzodiazepines, phenobarbitone, or agents such as levomepromazine and haloperidol.

Neural stimulation therapies including motor cortex stimulation (Fontaine et al., 2009), deep brain stimulation (Owen et al., 2006), and transcranial magnetic stimulation (Leung et al., 2009) have been reported to be successful in adults with treatment-resistant central pain; however, there are no reports of any of these methods being used in children.

Cancer pain

Progressive cancer usually results in increasing illness burden and a myriad of complex and challenging symptoms with the evidence showing pain to be a distressing and prevalent symptom towards the end of life in children with this disease (Heath et al., 2010; Pritchard et al., 2010). In a recent study of 141 parents of children who died of cancer, more than 10% considered hastening their child's death; this was more likely if their child was in pain (Dussel et al., 2010). Anticipation and continuous planning of analgesic need is crucial to effective management, particularly with the drive in many countries to provide as much care as possible outside of the hospital environment.

As disease progresses, the goals of care alter to maximize quality of life and minimize invasive treatments and procedures. Diagnoses regarding pain aetiology are based upon knowledge of disease pathology and clinical signs, with minimal imaging and, frequently, the anticipation of pain or the assumption that pain must be present, particularly in the non-verbal child.

Not infrequently, palliative chemotherapy may be offered in the hope of slowing disease progression and improving symptoms (Farah et al., 2011; Pui et al., 2011) but there is little evidence to show that it improves analgesia. There are data, however, that palliative radiotherapy with locally advanced disease can reduce analgesic requirements, particularly when it is offered in combination with other treatment modalities (Robinson, 2011; Simeoni, 2012).

There is increasing experience with anaesthetic or neurosurgical analgesic options, for example, epidural/intrathecal infusions or neurolytic blocks, when systemic analgesia has failed (Whyte and Lauder, 2012). Epidural and peripheral nerve catheters can be used successfully despite typical contraindications (thrombocytopenia, fever, spinal metastasis, vertebral fracture) and does not preclude patients from being cared for in their preferred setting (Anghelescu et al., 2010).

Polypharmacy and continual addition or increment of medication, without consideration for withdrawal or efficacy of drugs, should be avoided. Of particular concern can be the phenomenon of opioid-induced hypersensitivity (OIH). This may well go unrecognized and is significantly under-reported in children in the literature (Heger et al., 2009; Hallett and Chalkiadis, 2012).

OIH is most broadly defined as a state of nociceptive sensitization caused by exposure to opioids (Mitra, 2008). The state is characterized by a paradoxical response whereby a person receiving opioids for the treatment of pain may become more sensitive to pain and this is thought to be due to neuroplastic changes in the central and peripheral nervous system (Chu et al., 2008). It is important to note that OIH and analgesic tolerance are two distinct pharmacological phenomena that can result in similar net effects on opioid requirements. However, increasing the dose of opioid in OIH will paradoxically aggravate the problem and worsen the patient's pain. Considerable diagnostic confidence is required to reduce the opioid consumption in a child with end-stage cancer. It is therefore advisable to rotate the opioid, potentially in combination with an NMDA receptor antagonist, and methadone has been reported to have efficacy in reducing high-dose OIH (Sjøgren et al., 1994; Laulin et al., 2002; Mercadante and Arcuri, 2005).

Intractable pain

Palliative sedation in end-of-life care is an accepted but controversial means of providing relief from otherwise refractory and intolerable symptoms and distress (Chater et al., 1998; Manzini, 2011). The European Association for Palliative Care defines palliative sedation as the monitored use of medications intended to induce a state of decreased or absent awareness in order to relieve the burden of otherwise intractable suffering in an ethically acceptable manner (Cherny et al., 2009). The use of sedation in the setting of refractory pain assumes that all possible analgesic therapies have been employed and that there is no acceptable means of providing analgesia without compromising consciousness (Collins, 2010).

There is little information regarding palliative sedation in paediatrics, there are no international guidelines for children and little is known about the clinical effectiveness of sedation practice. A recent review of the paediatric literature offers some insight into practice by stating that sedation in children remains controversial and is influenced by educational, cultural, legal, moral, and health policy issues. Importantly, it highlighted that physical symptoms are described as an indication for practice but existential suffering must also be considered in the evaluation of refractoriness of symptoms (Kiman et al., 2011). Existential suffering of parents must also be acknowledged, as their distress behaviour may impact upon patient management, as explored in the study by Dussel et al. (2010)

Reports of pain and suffering at the end of life are described mainly for children with end-stage cancer, but also recognized in HIV/AIDS (Collins, 2005; Bennett and Givens, 2011). Recent studies have shown that incidence may be higher than perhaps expected in some regions. A retrospective case series of children with end-stage cancer showed that 25 of 37 patients received 'palliative sedation' for unrelieved suffering, with pain being the most common symptom cited (Postovsky et al., 2007). Also, a survey of Belgian physicians signing death certificates of all children between the ages of 1 and 17 years found that continuous, deep, and persistent sedation was used in 21.8% of all deaths; 46.8% of all none-sudden deaths (Pousset et al., 2011). Physicians had the explicit or concurrent intention of hastening death in one-quarter of cases. The incidence of continuous sedation in this study was higher than the 14.5% found in a comparable study of adults (Chambaere et al., 2010).

For the specific cohort which requires sedation for intractable pain, recommended therapeutic modalities include opioids, benzodiazepines, neuroleptic, and anaesthetic agents such as propofol (Anghelescu et al., 2012).

Conclusion

In the twenty-first century, dying children should not suffer undue pain. Although managing pain is only one of the aspects of providing palliative care for children, in reality it is a core task, as pain is the one of the most common symptoms experienced and necessitates effective action. Children's pain in palliative care has to be recognized within the wider context of progressive illness, emotional distress, and family influences. Therapy must mitigate both causative and contributing factors, use a multidisciplinary approach to address pharmacological and non-pharmacological treatments, and continually be appraised and evaluated.

Online materials

Complete references for this chapter are available online at <http://www.oxfordmedicine.com>.

References

Anand, K.J.S. (1999). Physiology of pain in infants and children. *Annales Nestle*, 57(1), 1–12.

Berde, C.B., Walco, G.A., Krane, E.J., *et al.* (2012). Pediatric analgesic clinical trial designs, measures, and extrapolation: report of an FDA Scientific Workshop. *Pediatrics*, 129(2), 354–364.

Breau, L.M., Camfield, C.S., McGrath, P.J., and Finley, G.A. (2003). The incidence of pain in children with severe cognitive impairments. *Archives of Pediatrics and Adolescent Medicine*, 157(12), 1219–1226.

Chu, L.F., Angst, M.S., and Clark, D. (2008). Opioid-induced hyperalgesia in humans: molecular mechanisms and clinical considerations. *Clinical Journal of Pain*, 24(6), 479–496.

Craig, K.D. and Korol, C.T. (2008). Developmental issues in understanding, assessing, and managing pediatric pain. In G. Walco and K. Goldschnieder (eds.) *Pediatric Pain Management in Primary Care: A Practical Guide*, pp. 9–20. Totowa, NJ: Humana Pres

Feudtner, C., Kang, T.I., Hexem, K.R., *et al.* (2011). Pediatric palliative care patients: a prospective multicenter cohort study. *Pediatrics*, 127(6), 1094–1101.

Fitzgerald, M. and Walker, S.M. (2009). Infant pain management: a developmental neurobiological approach. *Nature Clinical Practice Neurology*, 5(1), 35–50.

Hauer, J. (2010). Identifying and managing sources of pain and distress in children with neurological impairment. *Pediatric Annals*, 39(4), 198–205.

McGrath, P. (1998). Pain control. In G. Hanks, D. Doyle, N.I. Cherny, and K. Calman (eds.) *Oxford Textbook of Palliative Medicine* (2nd ed.), pp. 775–789. Oxford: Oxford University Press.

McGrath, P.A. (2005). Children—not simply 'little adults'. In H. Merskey, J. D. Loeser, and R. Dubner (eds.), *The Paths of Pain 1975–2005*, pp. 433–446. Seattle, WA: IASP Press.

McGrath, P.J., Walco, G.A., Turk, D.C., *et al.* (2008). Core outcome domains and measures for pediatric acute and chronic/recurrent pain clinical trials: PedIMMPACT recommendations. *Journal of Pain*, 9(9), 771–783.

Pui, C.H., Gajjar, A.J., Kane, J.R., Qaddoumi, I.A., and Pappo, A.S. (2011). Challenging issues in pediatric oncology. *Nature Reviews Clinical Oncology*, 8(9), 540–549.

Voepel-Lewis, T., Piscotty, R.J. Jr, Annis, A., and Kalisch, B. (2012). Empirical review supporting the application of the 'pain assessment as a social transaction' model in pediatrics. *Journal of Pain and Symptom Management*, 44(3), 446–457.

Von Baeyer, C.L. and Spagrud, L.J. (2003). Social development and pain in children. In P.J. McGrath and G.A. Finley (eds.) *The Context of Pediatric Pain: Biology, Family, Culture. Progress in Pain Research and Management* (Vol. 26), pp. 81–97. Seattle, WA: IASP Press.

Walco, G.A., Dworkin, R.H., Krane, E.J., LeBel, A.A., and Treede, R.D. (2010). Neuropathic pain in children: special considerations. *Mayo Clinic Proceedings*, 85(3 Suppl.), S33–41.

World Health Organization (2012). *WHO Guidelines on the Pharmacological Treatment of Persisting Pain in Children with Medical Illness*. Geneva: WHO. Available at: <http://whqlibdoc.who.int/publications/2012/9789241548120_Guidelines.pdf>.

Zernikow, B., Michel, E., Craig, F., and Anderson, B.J. (2009). Pediatric palliative care: use of opioids for the management of pain. *Pediatric Drugs*, 11(2), 129–151.

Common symptoms and disorders: gastrointestinal symptoms

SECTION 10

Common symptoms and
disorders: gastrointestinal
symptoms

Dysphagia, dyspepsia, and hiccup

Katherine Clark

Dysphagia

Definition of dysphagia

Dysphagia is defined as difficult swallowing which is different to odynophagia which is painful swallowing. There are two main types of dysphagia: oropharyngeal which reflects difficulty initiating swallow and oesophageal where the food bolus fails to easily traverse the oesophagus.

Dysphagia may occur as a complication of many diseases both malignant and non-malignant. It is highly likely that some people will already be dysphagic at the time of presentation to palliative care. However, there is a second cohort of people who will become dysphagic after referral to palliative care either as a complication of their life-limiting illness or because of increasing frailty. It is a reasonably prevalent condition in this population (Langmore et al., 2009).

Pathophysiology of dysphagia

Normal swallowing is a complex process. The initial phase, known as the *oral phase*, is under voluntary control. The next stage is the *transfer phase* where the solid or fluid bolus is pushed back into the pharynx by the tongue. The involuntary swallow response is evoked when the bolus enters the hypopharnyx. As a result, the larynx is elevated and pushed anteriorly, opening the upper oesophageal sphincter and allowing the tongue to push the bolus into the oesophagus, which in turn relaxes the lower oesophageal sphincter. The bolus entering the oesophagus provokes a primary peristaltic contraction which serves to both clear any residual bolus in the pharynx and propels the bolus through the oesophagus and into the stomach. The movement of the bolus along the oesophagus is assisted by secondary peristaltic actions which occur as a result of oesophageal distension. The oesophagus is divided into two sections: cervical and thoracic. The cervical oesophagus, like the oropharynx, is composed of striated muscle, unlike the thoracic oesophagus which is composed of smooth muscle.

Oropharyngeal dysphagia occurs as a result of difficulty transferring either food or fluid from either the mouth to the pharynx or from the pharynx to the oesophagus (Box 10.1.1). Problems with the oral or pharyngeal phase can result in regurgitation, coughing, or a sense of choking. Oropharyngeal dysphagia carries a high risk of aspiration and respiratory complications, malnourishment, dehydration and, as a result, poorer survival than people without dysphagia.

Aspiration refers to the complication of the passage of either food or fluids through the vocal cords leading to pneumonia. The severity of the complications depends upon the amount and type of aspirate and the capacity of the individual to subsequently clear the pulmonary tree. Aspiration of solids may lead to fatal airway obstruction. Depending upon the material aspirated, a chemical pneumonia may result if the aspirate is very acidic. The normal flora of the mouth and pharynx may result in bacterial pneumonia.

Oesophageal dysphagia occurs due to narrowing of the lumen of the oesophagus, impaired motor function, or altered oesophageal sensation. This may result in the retention of the food or fluid bolus in the oesophagus (Cook, 2009).

Causes of dysphagia

There are numerous causes of dysphagia which may be subcategorized into either oropharyngeal or oesophageal as summarized in Box 10.1.1.

Prevalence of dysphagia

Oropharyngeal dysphagia is a common problem in older populations and is expected to affect between 40% and 50% of people living in residential care. Although it is prevalent, it should not be considered part of healthy ageing and people presenting with new-onset dysphagia require careful evaluation. High-risk groups include people who have suffered a cardiovascular accident (CVA), where 25–40% of people suffering an acute unilateral stoke will have dysphagia. Up to 60% of CVA patients with dysphagia are likely to die due to nutritional and respiratory complications of their impaired swallow. Other groups at high risk of dysphagia include those with Alzheimer's disease where up to 80% of people are likely to have dysphagia and Parkinson's disease where between 50% and 80% of people are likely to be affected (Kumar, 2010).

Oesophageal dysphagia may be due to oesophageal cancer, the incidence of which is rising. Sadly, more than 50% of people who are diagnosed with oesophageal cancer will have advanced and incurable disease. At the time of diagnosis, more than 70% of these patients are likely to experience oesophageal dysphagia. More than 100 different medications have been linked to oesophageal dysphagia. This suggests such problems may well complicate the lives of people at the end of life (Pace et al., 2009).

The overall prevalence of either type of dysphagia in people at the time of referral to palliative care is not well documented. Whilst under care of the palliative care service, up to 12% of people have been identified as suffering dysphagia, some of which reflects increasing frailty. This rate may be an underestimate.

Box 10.1.1 Causes of dysphagia

Oropharyngeal

◆ Structural: malignancy, enlarged thyroid, Zencker's diverticulum

◆ Neurological: CVA, amyotrophic lateral sclerosis, brainstem tumours, bulbar poliomyelitis, multiple sclerosis, Parkinsonism, neuropathy (diabetes, alcohol, cachexia), dementias

◆ Myopathic: dermatophytosis, muscular dystrophy, polymyositis, myasthenia gravis, thyroid disease

◆ Iatrogenic: medications that must result in a myopathy (botulin toxin, procainamide, amiodarone, statins, vincristine), medications that inhibit saliva (opioids, tricyclic antidepressants, phenothiazines, atropine, hyoscine), radiotherapy to the head and neck, surgical procedures of the head and neck

◆ Poor dentition

◆ Anxiety.

Oesophageal

◆ Neuromuscular: achalasia, oesophageal spasm, scleroderma, systemic lupus erythematosus, rheumatoid arthritis, inflammatory bowel diseases

◆ Vascular: ischaemic oesophagus

◆ Structural: stricture secondary to reflux, diverticula, malignancy (oesophageal, gastric), benign tumours, external vascular compression, mediastinal masses, foreign body, mucosal injury secondary to infections (candidiasis, cytomegalovirus, HIV), mucosal injury secondary to medications (non-steroidal anti-inflammatories, alendronate, ascorbic acid, ferrous sulphate, antibiotics, theophylline), allergic disorders (eosinophilic oesophagitis), mucosal injury secondary to skin disorders (pemphigus vulgaris, pemphigoid, epidermolysis bullosa dystrophica).

Source: Data from Cook, I. J., Oropharyngeal dysphagia, *Gastroenterology Clinics of North America*, Volume 38, Issue 3, pp. 411–31, Copyright © 2009 Elsevier Inc. All rights reserved.

Presenting problems of dysphagia

Clinical problems that people with oropharyngeal dysphagia may describe include difficulty initiating swallow and then having to swallow repeatedly to effect pharyngeal clearance. People may experience a hoarse voice, nasopharyngeal regurgitation, or coughing on swallowing. Typically, these people tend to have greater problems when attempting to swallow thin fluids rather than solids. Cough on swallowing is typically due to aspiration. People may describe a sense of food being 'stuck' in both oesophageal and oropharyngeal dysphagia. When such problems occur acutely, the most likely cause is cerebrovascular. Where the onset is more gradual, the presenting problems may include weight loss, malnutrition, recurrent respiratory tract infections, and pneumonia.

In contrast, people with oesophageal dysphagia are more likely to have symptoms localized to the chest and are more likely to experience problems with solids compared to liquids. Chest pain

may accompany swallowing particularity when the underlying problem relates to reflux, narrowing of the lumen due to a structural abnormality, or a disorder of peristalsis.

Bedside examination for dysphagia

The bedside examination includes an assessment of the person's current nutritional and hydration, the possible aetiologies of the dysphagia, and the site of the pathology of the dysphagia. A comprehensive medical history can help discern whether this is an acute swallowing problem or associated with more gradual onset. Physical examination requires an examination of the neuromuscular structures that facilitate swallowing.

Bedside examination should include an assessment of whether or not the person is drowsy or confused as such changes in mentation may impair concentration necessary to safely swallow. Ask the person to identify themselves, paying attention to voice quality as dysphonia and dysarthria are signs of motor dysfunction of the structures involved in oral and pharyngeal phases of swallowing.

The oral cavity should be inspected for local problems and the state of the teeth recorded. Poor dentition increases the likelihood of aspiration pneumonia. Cranial nerves V and VII to XII should be systematically assessed. The face should be inspected for symmetry and the strength and sensation of the lips should be assessed (trigeminal and facial cranial nerves). The motor, sensory, and autonomic functions of the glossopharyngeal, vagus, and hypoglossal cranial nerves should be assessed. This includes an inspection of the uvula to ensure it is midline. The motor and sensory aspects of the gag reflex require testing. This reflex is elicited by stroking the pharyngeal mucosa with a tongue depressor. It must be noted that the absence of a gag reflex does not necessarily indicate that a patient is unable to swallow safely. Unilateral retraction of the palate during testing of the gag reflex indicates weakness of the muscles of the contralateral palate and suggests unilateral bulbar pathology. The tongue is inspected particularly in the floor of the mouth for wasting or fasciculations at rest. The person should be asked to move the tongue which should be inspected to ensure that this does not deviate to one side. The person should be asked to cough.

The bedside physical examination should include an observed swallowing test if this is deemed safe. This includes observing how well the person is able to open their mouth, how well they are able to close their mouth when taking fluid or solids, and whether or not they are able to clear the oropharynx or if food residue remains. People need to be observed to see whether or not the swallow changes with fatigue. Drooling, delayed swallow initiation, coughing, or a wet or hoarse voice quality may indicate a problem. After the swallow, observe the patient for 1 minute or more to see if a delayed cough response is present (Bours et al., 2009).

The physical examination must include a respiratory examination to identify if there are any changes to suggest respiratory complications. The physical examination when oesophageal dysphagia is the likely diagnosis is often unremarkable. In this situation, the examination should be directed to an assessment of the person's nutritional and hydration status. The oral cavity should be inspected particularly to consider infections such as candidiasis which may extend to involve the oesophagus and more distally to the stomach.

Investigations of dysphagia

If untreated, the initial investigations include biochemical and haematological parameters of hydration and nutrition (albumin, lymphocyte count, haemoglobin, and haematocrit). A cerebral computed tomography scan or magnetic resonance image may be warranted if the onset was sudden. A plain radiograph of the chest may also be indicated to exclude pneumonia. When indicated, the most useful investigations to explore oropharyngeal dysphagia include video-fluoroscopy, endoscopy, and manometry.

Barium video-fluoroscopy is a commonly used method to localize the site of pathology underlying swallowing difficulties, allowing clinicians to review oral, pharyngeal, and oesophageal structure and function. This investigation is usually organized as a collaboration between a speech pathologist and radiographer and requires the person to be able to sit upright for the duration of the study. Not surprisingly, the main complication is aspiration. However, even with this risk, this investigation has the advantage of visualizing all phases of swallowing. Together with providing important diagnostic information, the results of the study can be utilized as the basis to recommend the most tolerable diet for the patient. In people with adequate life expectancy, this investigation may help clinicians decide which people may even require parenteral feeding.

Flexible endoscopic evaluation of swallowing allows the pharynx and larynx to be directly visualized by the operator. This investigation is not considered to provide as comprehensive information as the barium swallow outlined above but does have the advantage of not exposing the patient to radiation and is not associated with the risk of aspiration. Furthermore, this can be conducted at the bedside, avoiding exposure to radiographs. One of the main disadvantages is that the oral phase of swallowing cannot be assessed.

Intraluminal manometry is used to quantify pharyngeal swallowing strength and to explore whether the upper oesophageal sphincter relaxes appropriately. Manometry is most useful when combined with the investigations listed earlier.

Oesophageal dysphagia

Gastro-oesophageal endoscopy allows visualization of the oesophageal mucosa and allows biopsies to be taken and, if needed, oesophageal dilatation and insertion of a stent. This is usually a well-tolerated investigation that can be performed under sedation. There is the potential risk of oesophageal perforation as a complication of biopsies or stent insertion.

Oesophageal pH monitoring is considered the optimal diagnostic tool to diagnose reflux disease. This is undertaken by inserting a naso-oesophageal probe which allows recording of pH levels.

Management of oesophageal dysphagia

Palliative management of dysphagia aims to maximize swallowing function, maintain adequate nutrition within the context of the stage of life, and allow people to participate in the social activities of eating and drinking. Management strategies differ depending upon whether the problem is localized to the oropharynx or the oesophagus, the chronicity of the underlying disease, and the overall prognosis.

For those with longer prognoses, the aim of management is to maximize the safe intake of an adequate diet to maintain nutrition and hydration, as malnutrition is associated with increased morbidity and mortality.

When considering the management of oropharyngeal dysphagia, for those able to participate in structured programmes, swallowing may be improved through modification of a number of factors. For example, with diet, a pureed diet is most appropriate for people who are experiencing difficulties with the oral phase of swallowing, who pocket food in the buccal recesses, or who have significant pharyngeal retention of chewed solid foods. Other recommendations include increasing the number of times food is chewed and the numbers of swallows per bolus. As well as pureeing food, increasing the thickness of fluids is recommended.

An important component of feeding is to consider how diet may best contribute to maintaining nutrition and hydration. People at risk of aspiration are much more likely to develop complications of aspiration when they are malnourished. This is because resistance to infections is compromised and defence mechanisms such as cough are impaired. Malnutrition may result in deteriorating performance status, anaemia, increased risk of pressure sores, impaired wound healing, and accelerated osteoporosis. Inadequate hydration also places people at risk of metabolic complications and aspiration, increasing the risk of pneumonia. This is because the salivary flow may be reduced therefore altering the normal flora of the oropharynx.

Ensuring good oral hygiene is important to help avoid complications of aspiration. People with impaired clearance of the oropharynx are at risk of altered colonization due to retained secretions and poor nutrition and hydration. Simple measures such as regular mouth washes and artificial salvia may be useful. When possible, medications without anticholinergic adverse effects should be prescribed.

The support of speech pathologists should be sought to consider whether a routine of exercises might be useful. Two distinct types of exercises can be considered. There are exercises aimed at improving the strength of muscles that facilitate swallowing and techniques that improve the safety of swallowing when a person is actually eating.

When trying to improve the strength of muscles involved in swallowing, the exercises are targeted to the site of the pathology. For example, lip exercises may improve a person's ability to prevent drooling when attempting to swallow. Tongue exercises may improve a person's capacity to push a food bolus towards the upper oesophageal sphincter, jaw exercises may improve mastication, and vocal cord adduction exercises can promote strengthening of weak vocal cords thereby limiting aspiration. In some situations, these exercises may be supplemented by low-current electrical stimulation that is administered by electrodes placed on the skin of the neck.

Techniques aimed at improving the safety of swallowing include advice on how to position the person during eating with the intent of improving oropharyngeal clearance and reducing the risk of aspiration. People who have delayed supraglottal closure can be taught how to voluntarily close the glottis before and during swallow thereby preventing aspiration. Other techniques include advising people to tilt their head away from the side of unilateral weakness of the tongue to force the bolus of food to the strong side.

In some situations, surgery for dysphagia may be considered. This is only in chronic situations where life expectancy is longer. Such procedures might include laryngeal closure or laryngotracheal separation-diversion. Laryngeal closure involves permanent closure of the glottis thereby avoiding aspiration. Separating the larynx from the trachea may be performed acutely by creating a tracheostomy.

For some people, such interventions are either not adequate or appropriate, resulting in a situation where the person is not able to maintain nutrition or hydration safely. Enteral or parenteral feeding might then be considered. However, initiation of parental or enteral feeding must be considered in the context of the individual with factors such as the potential reversibility of the swallowing problem, the degree to which the underlying physical disease can be modified, the wishes of the person with the swallowing problem, and the potential risks involved.

Most feeding tubes are inserted for progressive debilitating conditions such as dementia, motor neurone disease, and cancers. However, despite the fact that feeding is initiated with the aim of maintaining nutrition and avoiding malnutrition, significant complications may accompany enteral feeding.

There are different types of feeding tubes available and when considering insertion of such tubes it is important to understand the risks and benefits of each type. The simplest approach to tube enteral feeding is by inserting a nasogastric tube. This is the least invasive as people do not require sedation or surgery. It is recommended in situations when the need for enteral feeding is short or as a temporary measure until a more definitive approach can be organized. At the time of insertion, problems can include bleeding, trauma, and misplacement of the tube and oesophageal perforation. When used for longer periods, problems include discomfort, nasal ulceration, chronic sinusitis, gastro-oesophageal reflux, and aspiration pneumonia. A variation on the nasogastric tube is the oro-oesophageal tube. This refers to the temporary placement of a narrow-bore tube that remains *in situ* only for the duration of the feed. This may be a useful approach when people do not have a gag reflex and decline other approaches to feeding. However, this requires the person to be compliant and requires a significant time commitment.

More commonly in the longer term is the placement of a percutaneous gastrostomy tube. There are two different ways that such tubes may be inserted. The first is a surgical gastrostomy which requires a general anaesthetic and the second is a percutaneous endoscopic gastrostomy. This latter approach has the benefit that it may be performed under sedation. Both approaches require the insertion of a tube through the anterior abdominal wall. Insertion complications include bleeding, infections, peritonitis, or perforation of other abdominal organs. Observational studies identify that 10% of people are still likely to suffer an aspiration with other complications including infections, tube leakage, tube removal, displacement or migration, bleeding, gastric mucosal overgrowth or ulceration, metabolic and biochemical complications such as re-feeding syndrome, gastrointestinal side effects, and microbial contamination of the feeds. Approximately 50–60% of people are unlikely to survive 12 months after enteral feeding is commenced. Given these problems, an absolute contraindication to commencing supplemental feeding should be a short life expectancy. In

these situations, sensitive and knowledgeable communication with the person and their formal and informal carers is required.

More than with oropharyngeal dysphagia, approaches to the management of oesophageal dysphagia are tailored according to the process that underlies the dysphagia. Particular local interventions that require discussion include management of benign and malignant structures, with or without insertions of oesophageal stents and medical management tailored to the underlying problem.

Oesophageal strictures narrow the lumen from processes that affect the structures, function, or problems external to the oesophagus. The most common cause of oesophageal strictures is reflux disease. Whilst treatment of the cause of the stricture is recommended, local interventions including dilatation and stent placement provide palliation for both benign and malignant strictures.

The best results from dilatation alone for benign strictures are achieved when the stricture is simple (i.e. < 2 cm long), straight and an endoscope can easily be passed through it. In this scenario, most people do not require multiple dilatations. Complex strictures are typically longer, tortuous and it is difficult to pass the endoscope. It is not uncommon for people to require a minimum of three dilatations. If more than seven attempts have been made, that stricture is considered 'resistant'. Although usually well tolerated, there are complications associated with dilatation which include perforation, bleeding, and bacteraemia though such complications are expected in less than 1% of people. The more tortuous the stricture or strictures that have occurred as the result of a caustic injury are considered to place people at higher risk of complications.

Complex benign strictures are sometimes managed with oesophageal stenting. Recent observations suggest that biodegradable stents or the short-term use of stents may be useful palliation in the management of benign strictures though the evidence is less robust than the evidence for stents in malignant disease. The main complications include stent migration, difficulty in removing stents, pain, and tissue overgrowth. Although the numbers of observations available to report the benefit or otherwise of stenting in this situation are few, the risk of perforation in this group seems to be less than that experienced by people with malignant strictures (Siersema, 2008; Vlavianos and Zabron, 2012).

Malignant strictures are palliated with a combination of dilatation, stent placement, and adjuvant radiotherapy or brachytherapy. The choice depends upon the person's prognosis. Dilatation without stenting may be used when life expectancy is very short. Stenting alone is typically offered when prognosis is less than 3 months. People expected to live longer than 3 months with inoperable disease are typically offered ether brachytherapy or stenting plus radiotherapy. When a stricture is located in the mid to distal portion of the oesophagus, the main complications with stent insertion include stent migration, stent obstruction (secondary to benign or malignant overgrowth or food), and reflux that may be complicated by aspiration pneumonia. Up to 40% of people are likely to develop problems within the first 2 months of the stent insertion. However, re-stenting is likely to be successful in 90% of these people. Proximal strictures are considered more challenging to stent with a greater risk of food obstruction, fistula formation, and aspiration. It is not considered possible to stent a stricture that crosses the upper oesophageal sphincter. However, more distal to the sphincter, stenting is considered possible. A more flexible stent which exerts less force on the oesophageal wall has improved outcomes

Single-dose brachytherapy is delivered by passing an applicator into the oesophagus. The main complications are fistula formation, stricture formation, and esophagitis. Comparing patient outcomes from stenting versus brachytherapy have identified that immediate palliation is better with stents but longer-term outcomes are better with brachytherapy, including quality of life assessments (Schembre, 2010; de Wijkerslooth et al., 2011).

Problems such as infections or inflammatory conditions causing oesophageal dysphagia require targeted treatments to manage the specific problem. For example, eosinophilic esophagitis which occurs as the result of inhaled allergens requires identification of the allergen, a trial of inhaled corticosteroids, or systemic corticosteroids depending upon the severity of the presentation (Moawad et al., 2009). Other problems such as oesophageal spasm may also be managed medically. Agents that have been trialled for this include smooth muscle relaxants and calcium channel blockers. More recently sildenafil, a phosphodiesterase-5 inhibitor, has been trialled with success. However, its use is limited by the adverse effects of headache and vertigo. Botulinum toxin injections have been used to manage oesophageal spasm (Roman and Kahrilas, 2012).

Acid reflux is the main contributing factor to oesophageal dysphagia and it is likely that reflux will overlap with other causes of dysphagia. The medications most likely to be of benefit are the proton pump inhibitors (PPIs) with lesser benefit expected from histamine type 2 receptor antagonists (H_2 blockers) (van Pinxteren et al., 2005; Rosemurgy et al., 2011). Despite the use of PPIs, some people continue to suffer distressing symptoms. Although the evidence to support additional agents is less than robust, clinical guidelines recommend supplementing PPIs with a number of other agents. These include suggestions such as avoiding foods that are likely to impair gastric emptying, the use of antacids for intermittent exacerbations, and intermittent prokinetic therapy to promote gastric emptying with either metoclopramide or domperidone, barrier therapy with sucralfate or inhibiting reflux with baclofen (Armstrong and Sifrim, 2010) (see Boxes 10.1.2 and 10.1.3).

Dyspepsia

Definition of dyspepsia

Dyspepsia is a specific term that requires people to have one or more of the four specific symptoms of epigastric pain, epigastric burning, postprandial fullness, or early satiety. Dyspepsia is separate from heartburn which is defined as a sensation of retrosternal burning distinct from epigastric burning. Heartburn may accompany dyspepsia but it is considered a separate entity. Heartburn is considered pivotal for the diagnosis of reflux disease (Oustamanolakis and Tack, 2012).

Dyspepsia may be either a functional disorder where no cause for the problem may be identified or may occur as a secondary problem. The diagnosis of functional dyspepsia is typically made when other causes have been excluded: gastro-oesophageal reflux disease, peptic ulcer disease (PUD), gastric inflammatory conditions, and upper gastrointestinal tract cancers. Although clinically difficult to differentiate, people may also develop dyspeptic symptoms secondary to gastroparesis. Dyspepsia has been identified as

---

Box 10.1.2 A summary of management strategies to palliate oropharyngeal dysphagia

Managing oropharyngeal dysphagia when life is measured in months to years

- Diet changes:
- avoid thin fluids, avoid very hard or chewy foods
- pureed diet
- thickened fluids
- Nutritional support
- Adequate fluid intake to maintain hydration
- Modification of swallowing behaviours: sitting upright, swallowing three times, taking fluids from a spoon, turning the head to one side to swallow, ensuring residual food is removed from the oral cavity
- Oral hygiene
- Avoid medications likely to contribute to a dry mouth
- Targeted exercises
- Electrical stimulation
- Compensatory techniques
- Surgery
- Parenteral or enteral feeding.

Managing oropharyngeal dysphagia when life is measured in weeks

- Diet
- Positioning
- Avoidance of medications likely to contribute to sedation
- Oral care to improve dry mouth this may contribute to difficulty swallowing
- Meticulous oral hygiene after meals to reduce the risk of aspiration.

Managing oropharyngeal dysphagia in the final stages of life

- Oral hygiene
- Diet as tolerated.

---

a problem that may have a significant detrimental effect on quality of life (Aro et al., 2011).

Pathophysiology of dyspepsia

The major function of the stomach is to facilitate breakdown of solid food, and to empty this as chime into the small bowel along with indigestible foods. The proximal stomach relaxes as a vagally mediated reflex secondary to swallowing. The proximal stomach increasingly relaxes to accommodate increasing volumes whilst

> **Box 10.1.3** A summary of management strategies to palliate oesophageal dysphagia
>
> **Managing oesophageal dysphagia when life is measured in months to years**
>
> - Diet
> - Surgery
> - Stenting
> - Brachytherapy
> - Radiotherapy
> - Medication: PPIs, H$_2$ antagonists, baclofen, metoclopramide, domperidone, sucralfate
> - Botulin toxin
> - Enteral feeding.
>
> **Managing oesophageal dysphagia when life is measured in weeks**
>
> - Diet
> - Medication
> - Dilatation
> - Stenting.
>
> **Managing oesophageal dysphagia in the very final stages of life**
>
> - Diet
> - Medication: parenteral PPI, or H$_2$ antagonists, parenteral metoclopramide.
>
> Source: Data from Armstrong, D. and Sifrim, D., New pharmacologic approaches in gastroesophageal reflux disease, *Gastroenterology Clinics of North America*, Volume 39, Issue 3 pp. 393–418, Copyright © 2010 Elsevier Inc. All rights reserved.

concurrently contracting more distally to allow the food to be broken down into smaller and smaller particles. Emptying of liquid into the duodenum requires coordinated contraction of the whole stomach, though the speed at which this occurs is mediated by the pylorus.

Dyspepsia is considered a disorder of gastric motility. Dysmotility may have no identified reason with the changes in gastric emptying that accompany dyspepsia being varied. It is estimated that 25–50% of people with dyspepsia will have delayed gastric emptying but it is not clear how this affects symptoms. The underlying theory is that larger gastric volumes lead to more marked distension and therefore early satiety.

Other changes have been noted in people with functional dyspepsia including impaired accommodation of the proximal stomach in 40% of people, but the mechanism whereby this may lead to symptoms is not well categorized. Likewise, hypomotility of the gastric antrum is commonly observed but again it is unclear how this may lead to symptoms (Aro et al., 2011; Tack et al., 2011; Miwa et al., 2011). As well as functional and secondary causes of dyspepsia, there are a number of problems that can

result in dyspepsia-like symptoms as the result of disordered gastric emptying.

Causes of dyspepsia

There are numerous causes of dyspepsia which include functional and secondary. Functional dyspepsia is defined as a problem that occurs when people present with complex symptoms of pain, burning, early satiety, and postprandial fullness but no clearly identifiable cause. In contrast, secondary dyspepsia may be as the result of numerous causes as summarized in Box 10.1.4.

> **Box 10.1.4** Causes of dyspepsia
>
> **Functional**
>
> *Secondary*
>
> - Gastro-oesophageal reflux
> - Oesophagitis secondary to medications:
>   - Iron supplements, opioid analgesia, theophylline, digoxin, antibiotics, calcium channel blockers, nitrates, bisphosphonates, non-steroidal anti-inflammatory agents, corticosteroids
> - Peptic ulcer disease (PUD):
>   - *H. pylori*, NSAIDS
> - Malignancy:
>   - oesophageal cancer, gastric cancer
>   - Coeliac disease
>
> **Dyspepsia-like symptoms**
>
> - Infections:
>   - *Giardia lamblia*, *Strongyloides stercoralis*, tuberculosis
> - Inflammatory:
>   - Coeliac sprue, Crohn's disease, sarcoidosis, lymphocytic gastritis, eosinophilic gastroenteritis
> - Infiltrative:
>   - lymphoma, amyloid, Ménétrier disease
>   - recurrent gastric volvulus
>   - chronic mesenteric or gastric ischaemia
>   - ideopathic gastroparesis
> - Drug-induced gastroparesis:
>   - Opioids, medications with anticholinergic effects
> - Secondary gastroparesis:
>   - Metabolic (diabetes, hypercalcaemia, renal failure, hypothyroidism)
>   - Neurological (autonomic neuropathy
>   - Infiltrative (malignant, systemic sclerosis)
> - Other (idiopathic, post-surgical, paraneoplastic).

Prevalence of dyspepsia

Within the whole population, dyspeptic symptoms are estimated to affect between 10% and 45% of the population. There are suggestions that this higher figure may overestimate the problem of dyspepsia by the inclusion of heartburn symptoms which are not considered part of the syndrome. The prevalence of dyspepsia is not clear in palliative care patients.

Presenting problems of dyspepsia

The four cardinal symptoms diagnostic to dyspepsia are post-prandial fullness, early satiation, epigastric pain, and epigastric burning. Other symptoms may accompany these four symptoms including bloating, fullness, belching, nausea, and vomiting.

Other questions may be useful to try and understand the aetiology of the dyspepsia. Functional dyspepsia is not uncommonly accompanied by irritable bowel disease. This may present with recurrent abdominal pain or discomfort often improved by a bowel action. However, in palliative care patients, constipation is a frequently occurring co-morbidity and it is not clear how the regular use of laxatives may contribute to symptoms that mimic irritable bowel syndrome. Other questions to consider include whether or not pain is improved by eating (e.g. PUD), if there post-prandial heartburn (e.g. reflux oesophagitis), what medications the person is currently taking that might contribute to symptoms, how much weight the person has lost, and if there are other changes to appetite. Alternatively, when the dyspeptic symptoms are secondary to gastroparesis, people may also describe vomiting, often of undigested food following meals (Hasler, 2011).

Investigations of dyspepsia

The aim of investigations is help discern whether the underlying problem is functional, organic, or secondary to gastroparesis. The main reason to understand the difference is to allow the most appropriate management to be implemented. The initial steps when people present with dyspeptic symptoms include a comprehensive and focused clinical history and physical examination. Excluding functional dyspepsia requires, at a minimum, people to have an upper gastrointestinal endoscopy, 24-hour oesophageal pH monitoring, and *Helicobacter pylori* assessment.

Management of dyspepsia

Most people with functional dyspepsia do not require medications. Rather, this group are most likely to benefit from reassurance, education about the condition, and recommendations regarding dietary and lifestyle changes. Patients are generally advised to eat smaller and more frequent meals, and to avoid food with high fat content and food that aggravates their symptoms. When symptoms are severe, a trial of a PPI is warranted. Those people who are bothered by postprandial fullness and early satiety may benefit from a prokinetic agent such as domperidone or metoclopramide. More recently, acotiamide, a muscarinic receptor antagonist and cholinesterase inhibitor has been identified as an efficacious agent in the management of functional dyspepsia. In patients with bothersome symptoms that persist despite these initial therapies, a trial of a low-dose tricyclic antidepressant may be considered (Tack and Janssen, 2011).

Box 10.1.5 A summary of approaches to palliate dyspepsia

Palliation of dyspepsia when life is managed in months to years

- Identify and treat underlying cause
- Oral PPIs or H_2 antagonists for pain or burning
- Dietary advice
- Positioning
- Prokinetics when early satiety is a feature
- Antidepressants or supportive counselling.

Management of dyspepsia when life is managed in weeks

- Oral PPI or H_2 antagonists for pain or burning
- Dietary advice
- Positioning
- Prokinetics.

Management of dyspepsia in final stages of life

- Parenteral PPI, H_2 antagonists
- Parenteral metoclopramide.

Source: Data from Loyd, R. A. and McClellan, D. A., Update on the evaluation and management of functional dyspepsia, *American Family Physician*, Volume 83, Number 5, pp. 547–52, Copyright © 2011 American Academy of Family Physicians.

For people with a longer prognosis who present with dyspepsia for which an organic cause is identified, the management strategies require firstly, eradication of the underlying cause and secondly, palliation of symptoms. When people have epigastric pain or burning, the first medications of choice are any of the PPIs or alternatively, H_2 receptor blockers (Loyd and McClellan, 2011) (Box 10.1.5).

Hiccup

Definition of hiccups

Hiccup, or more correctly singultus, refers to the situation where people experience a sharp and involuntary contraction of the muscles of inspiration which causes a sudden sharp inspiration and closure of the glottis. This results in the characteristic sound which occurs when the column of air inhaled due to involuntary muscle contraction strikes the closed glottis. Even now, there is no identified physiological purpose for this phenomenon.

Prevalence of hiccups

The prevalence of hiccups has not been well articulated in palliative care. However, clinical experience suggests that this patient population is at greater risk of protracted hiccups compared to the general population. This observation is based on the fact that at any point, palliative care patients are likely to simultaneously have more than one risk factor. Hiccups are more likely to affect men compared to women with usually only one hemi-diaphragm affected.

Pathophysiology of hiccups

Despite no identified purpose, the hiccup reflex arc is a complex series of connections between an afferent limb, efferent limb, and central component. The afferent limb travels between the phrenic nerve, vagus nerve, and the sympathetic chain. The vagus nerve may be irritated anywhere along its path suggesting that hiccups may occur as the abnormalities in the head and neck structures, or thoracic or intra-abdominal structures. In addition, the afferent limb may also be stimulated by chin thrust. This is believed to be as the result of stimulation of the trigeminal nerve to the reticular formation.

The central component of hiccups remains poorly localized but probably involves connections to the fourth cerebral ventricle, the respiratory centre in the brain stem, medial reticular formation, the hypothalamus, and the phrenic nerve nuclei. Whilst there are likely to be numerous neurotransmitters, the most implicated remain dopamine and gamma-aminobutyric acid (GABA).

The efferent limb is mediated through the phrenic nerve to the diaphragm. Additionally, the external intercostal and scalenus anticus nerves cause contraction of the intercostal and scalene muscles. Lastly, the recurrent laryngeal nerve causes the glottis to close. As noted earlier, it is the column of air evoked by diaphragmatic contraction hitting the closed glottis which results in the noise form which the term hiccup is derived.

Causes of hiccups

There are multiple causes of hiccups reported in the literature with data extrapolated from case reports or case series (Woelk, 2011) (Box 10.1.6).

Presenting problems of hiccups

Hiccups have a frequency of four to 60 hiccups per minute and for each individual, there is a relatively constant rate. Higher arterial carbon dioxide levels tend to slow the frequency of hiccups.

Hiccups persisting for less than a few minutes are termed a 'bout' with hiccups persisting more than 48 hours labelled 'protracted'. Hiccups persisting for more than 1 month are considered 'intractable'. Whilst short bouts of hiccups are considered no more than a nuisance with interventions not indicated, more prolonged bouts can lead to serious complications. This is particularly so in people with serious illness already complicated by problems such as fatigue, anorexia, and weight loss. Protracted hiccups may cause sleep disturbances (Kvale and Shuster, 2006). Protracted hiccups may result in daytime drowsiness, mood disturbances such as anxiety and depression, and cognitive dysfunction. Protracted hiccups may also worsen fatigue, through a number of different mechanisms. Protracted hiccups may lead to skeletal muscle fatigue whilst concurrently interfering with people's capacity to eat and drink. In the worst case, hiccups may result in vomiting. Lastly, hiccups have been associated with aspiration and pneumonia. Protracted hiccups in a patient with a tracheostomy may lead to the life-threatening complication of respiratory alkalosis secondary to hyperventilation.

Aside from the physical implications, anecdotal reports suggest that hiccups may cause significant distress and anxiety to the person who has hiccups and to family and informal caregivers.

Investigations of hiccups

The diagnosis of hiccup is a clinical diagnosis only. Short bouts of hiccups are, by definition, self-limiting and therefore do not require investigation.

Box 10.1.6 Causes of hiccup

Central

- Vascular: cerebral aneurysm, ischaemic stroke, haemorrhagic stoke
- Space-occupying lesion: cerebral tumours, cerebral abscess
- Head trauma
- Encephalitis
- Neurodegenerative: multiple sclerosis, Parkinson's disease.

Peripheral

- Oesophageal: oesophageal dilatation, achalasia, food impaction, tumours
- Gastrointestinal: gastric distension, gastritis, reflux, peritoneal traction, small bowel obstruction, ascites
- Hepatic: liver metastases, primary liver cancers, hepatic abscess, cholecystitis
- Iatrogenic: benzodiazepines, opioids, corticosteroids, chemotherapy (e.g. cisplatinum)
- Respiratory: diaphragmatic irritation (pneumonia, pleural effusion, malignancy), subphrenic abscess
- Toxic/metabolic: renal failure, alcohol intoxication, electrolyte disturbances, hypoadrenalism
- Infectious: herpes zoster, gastrointestinal candidiasis
- Cardiovascular: myocardial ischaemia
- Perioperative: intubation, general anaesthesia, mechanical ventilation
- Psychological: anxiety, distress.

Source: Data from Woelk, C. J., Managing hiccups, *Canadian Family Physician*, Volume 57, Number 6, pp. 672–5, Copyright © 2011 the College of Family Physicians of Canada.

More protracted episodes of hiccups may require investigations.

Prior to initiation of investigations, regardless of the stage, a comprehensive history of the factors precipitating hiccups and physical examination is indicated. The physical examination should be directed to ensuring that structures of hiccup arc are considered. Basic investigations should include screening for renal failure, uraemia, and electrolytes disturbances particularly hyponatremia, hypokalaemia, and hypocalcaemia. Imaging studies should be tailored to the results of history and examination.

Management of hiccups

The main problem complicating the management of hiccups is the lack of robust studies. As a result, there are numerous medications and interventions suggested as effective for hiccups with most recommendations based on case reports.

Interventions may be pharmacological and non-pharmacological if reversible causes cannot be found (Jatoi et al., 2009) (Tables 10.1.1 and Table 10.1.2).

Table 10.1.1 A summary of non-pharmacological approaches to palliating hiccups

Intervention	Rationale for intervention
Vagal nerve stimulation using nerve stimulator	Vagus nerve stimulation
Acupuncture	Acupuncture points for hiccups are located near dermatomes related to afferent/efferent pathways, secondary synapses, or nuclei involved in the hiccup reflex arc suggesting that acupuncture may modulate the hiccup reflex
Stimulation of the palate or pharynx with a cotton applicator or catheter	Glottic stimulation
Traction on the tongue	Vagus nerve stimulation
Lifting the uvula with a spoon	Vagus nerve stimulation
Performing a Valsalva manoeuvre	Vagal nerve stimulation
Gargling or drinking ice water	Vagal nerve stimulation
Sudden fright	Sympathetic response
Breath holding	Increase $PaCO_2$
Breathing into a paper bag	Increase $PaCO_2$
Digital rectal massage	Vagus nerve stimulation

Source: Data from Jatoi, A., Palliating hiccups in cancer patients: moving beyond recommendations from Leonard the lion, *The Journal of Supportive Oncology*, Volume 7, Number 4, pp. 129–30, Copyright © 2009; Tegeler, M. L. and Baumrucker, S. J., Gabapentin for intractable hiccups in palliative care, *American Journal of Hospice and Palliative Medicine*, Volume 25, Number 1, pp. 52–4, Copyright © 2003 by SAGE Publications; Twycross, R., Baclofen for hiccups, *American Journal of Hospice and Palliative Medicine*, Volume 20, Number 4, p.262, Copyright © 2003 by SAGE Publications; and Marinella, M., Diagnosis and management of hiccups in patients with advanced cancer, *Journal of Supportive Oncology*, Volume 7, Number 4, pp. 122–28, Copyright © 2009.

Table 10.1.2 Suggested interventions to palliate hiccups

Intervention	Rationale
Dopamine antagonists: Chlorpromazine, Haloperidol, Metoclopramide	Dopamine antagonist
Anticonvulsants: Gabapentin	The proposed mechanism whereby gabapentin is believed to modify hiccups is by inhibiting the $[alpha]_2[delta]$ subunit of voltage-dependent calcium channel and increasing GABA release, which modulates diaphragmatic excitability
Phenytoin, Sodium valproate, Carbamazepine	Blockade of sodium channels
Antispasmodics: Baclofen	Smooth muscle relaxant
Anti-arrhythmia: Nifedipine	Calcium channel blockade
Intravenous lignocaine	Sodium channel blockade
Benzodiazepines: Midazolam	Muscle relaxant, anxiolytic
Nebulized lignocaine	Blockade of sensory afferents
Corticosteroid: Dexamethasone	Anti-inflammatory
Neurostimulant: Methylphenidate	Inhibition of dopamine and noradrenaline (norepinephrine) uptake

Source: Data from Jatoi, A., Palliating hiccups in cancer patients: moving beyond recommendations from Leonard the lion, *The Journal of Supportive Oncology*, Volume 7, Number 4, pp. 129–30, Copyright © 2009; Tegeler, M. L. and Baumrucker, S. J., Gabapentin for intractable hiccups in palliative care, *American Journal of Hospice and Palliative Medicine*, Volume 25, Number 1, pp. 52–4, Copyright © 2003 by SAGE Publications; Twycross, R., Baclofen for hiccups, *American Journal of Hospice and Palliative Medicine*, Volume 20, Number 4, p.262, Copyright © 2003 by SAGE Publications; and Marinella, M., Diagnosis and management of hiccups in patients with advanced cancer, *Journal of Supportive Oncology*, Volume 7, Number 4, pp. 122–28, Copyright © 2009.

Online materials

Complete references for this chapter are available online at <http://www.oxfordmedicine.com>.

References

Cook, I.J. (2009). Oropharyngeal dysphagia. *Gastroenterology Clinics of North America*, 38, 411–431.

Hasler, W.L. (2011). Gastroparesis: pathogenesis, diagnosis and management. *Nature Reviews Gastroenterology & Hepatology*, 8, 438–453.

Langmore, S.E., Grillone, G., Elackattu, A., and Walsh, M. (2009). Disorders of swallowing: palliative care. *Otolaryngologic Clinics of North America*, 42, 87–105, ix.

Loyd, R.A. and McClellan, D. A. (2011). Update on the evaluation and management of functional dyspepsia. *American Family Physician*, 83, 547–552.

Marinella, M. (2009). Diagnosis and management of hiccups in patients with advanced cancer. *Journal of Supportive Oncology*, 7, 122–128.

Miwa, H., Watari, J., Fukui, H., *et al.* (2011). Current understanding of pathogenesis of functional dyspepsia. *Journal of Gastroenterology & Hepatology*, 26(Suppl. 3), 53–60.

Oustamanolakis, P. and Tack, J. (2012). Dyspepsia: organic versus functional. *Journal of Clinical Gastroenterology*, 46, 175–190

Tack, J., Masaoka, T., and Janssen, P. (2011). Functional dyspepsia. *Current Opinion in Gastroenterology*, 27, 549–557.

Tegeler, M.L. & Baumrucker, S.J. (2008). Gabapentin for intractable hiccups in palliative care. *American Journal of Hospice & Palliative Medicine*, 25, 52–54.

Twycross, R. (2003). Baclofen for hiccups. *American Journal of Hospice & Palliative Medicine*, 20, 262; author reply 262.

Van Pinxteren, B., Sigterman, K.E., Bonis, P., Lau, J., and Numans, M.E. (2005). Short-term treatment with proton pump inhibitors, H2-receptor antagonists and prokinetics for gastro-oesophageal reflux disease-like symptoms and endoscopy negative reflux disease. *Cochrane Database of Systematic Reviews*, 11, CD002095.

Palliation of nausea and vomiting

Janet R. Hardy, Paul Glare, Patsy Yates, and
Kathryn A. Mannix

Introduction to palliation of nausea and vomiting

Nausea and vomiting (NV) are unpleasant symptoms that are reported as highly distressing by sufferers (Bliss et al., 1992; Bruera et al., 2000; Meuser et al., 2001). The symptoms are separate, but related, and arise in many life-limiting conditions such as cancer, AIDS, and hepatic or renal failure. A systematic review of symptom prevalence in various advanced diseases identified nausea prevalence rates ranging from 6–68% for people with advanced cancer, 43–49% for people with AIDS, 17–48% for people with heart disease, and 30–43% for people with renal disease (Solano et al., 2006). Less is known about the prevalence of vomiting, although when it occurs it is often in association with nausea. One study of patients with advanced cancer reported 62% had NV, 34% had isolated nausea and 4% had isolated vomiting (Stephenson and Davies, 2006). Importantly, when these symptoms are present they may significantly impact on well-being. A curvilinear relationship between nausea in cancer patients and Karnofsky performance status (PS) has been reported, with nausea at its worst when PS is rated as 40 (on a scale of 0–100) and decreasing as PS declines (Mercadante et al., 2000). A similar decrease in the prevalence and intensity of nausea at the end of life has also been documented in ambulatory cancer patients. The distress caused by the experience of nausea and, to a lesser extent, vomiting, is now better understood (Seow et al., 2011). NV has a significant impact on activities of daily living. In one study of patients with NV, over 40% rated the impact of NV on general activity and emotional well-being as higher than 5 on a 0–10-point scale (Yates et al., 2005).

Despite major advances in antiemetic drug development in the last two decades in the supportive care of patients receiving anti-cancer therapies, the incidence and severity of NV in patients with life-limiting disease remains a significant management problem. The neurophysiology of the vomiting reflex is well established in experimental animals, and is becoming better understood in man (Carpenter, 1990; Yates et al., 1998; Shelke et al., 2004; Sanger and Andrews, 2006). Several multifactorial clinical syndromes can contribute to NV in patients with advanced illness, including conditions associated with gastric stasis, biochemical disturbances, raised intracranial pressure, vestibular disturbances, and bowel dysmotility (Glare et al., 2008). Interventions aimed at reducing NV must therefore take into account the cause of the symptoms and the central emetogenic pathways involved. Treatment requires knowledge of these pathways, careful assessment of the patient, and prescribing tailored to the patient's individual needs. The physiological processes can be partly extrapolated from animal models but the management of a person experiencing nausea also demands empathy, supportive care, and attention to the patient's concerns, in addition to any pharmacological intervention deemed appropriate.

Pathways involved in emesis

Definitions

Nausea is an unpleasant subjective sensation that signals imminent vomiting, that may or may not result in vomiting. Vomiting is an objective patient experience involving the forceful elimination of the contents of the stomach by the sustained action of abdominal muscles and the opening of the gastric cardia (Shelke et al., 2004). It is important to differentiate NV from regurgitation (the passive retrograde flow of oesophageal contents into the mouth), rumination (an eating disorder), and dyspepsia (Glare et al., 2011).

Central pathways involved in emesis

Emesis is mediated centrally by two separate 'centres': the vomiting centre (VC) and chemoreceptor trigger zone (CTZ). Whilst these are anatomically distinct in experimental animals, in man the pathways are more diffuse (see Fig. 10.2.1).

The CTZ is located in the area postrema, in the floor of the fourth ventricle, where there is effectively no blood–brain barrier. Chemosensitive nerve cell projections are bathed by cerebrospinal fluid, which is in chemical equilibrium with blood in the fenestrated local capillaries (Miller and Leslie, 1994). The nature of the chemoreceptors in the CTZ remains obscure. Neural pathways project from the CTZ to the nucleus of the tractus solitarius and the reticular formation in the medulla oblongata, the location of the VC (Carpenter, 1990; Kovac, 2000; Shelke et al., 2004).

There may be a central antiemetic tone sustained by medullary neurons, inhibition of which potentiates the CTZ (Lang, 1999). An encephalinergic pathway has been hypothesized. Displacement of encephalins from their receptors by naloxone (Costello and Borison, 1977) or opioids (Yates et al., 1998) may reduce antiemetic tone, as may inhibition of encephalin synthesis by chemotherapy (Harris, 1982). This interesting hypothesis would help to explain the different emetogenic potentials of chemotherapeutic agents according to the point at which they interrupt cellular protein synthesis. The presence of medullary antiemetic tone and its influence on the CTZ remains speculative.

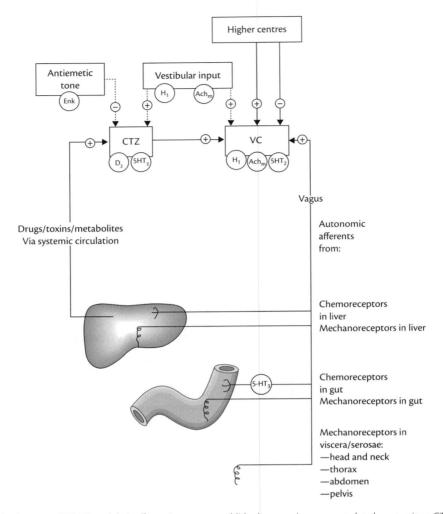

Fig. 10.2.1 The interrelationship between CTZ, VC, and their afferent inputs. —, established connections; ---, postulated connections; CTZ, chemoreceptor trigger zone; VC, vomiting centre; Enk, enkephalinergic pathways. *Receptors*: D_2, dopamine type 2; 5-HT$_{2,3}$, serotonin types 2,3; Ach$_m$, muscarinic cholinergic; H$_1$, histamine type 1.

The VC is a diffuse, interconnecting neural network that integrates emetogenic stimuli with parasympathetic and motor efferent activity to produce the vomiting reflex. It is now thought that the VC is not a distinct anatomical structure, but represents a convergence of a number of different afferent pathways in the lateral reticular formation of the medulla oblongata of the mid brainstem in close proximity to the nucleus of the tractus solitaries and area postrema at the level of the dorsal motor nucleus of the vagus nerve (Carpenter, 1990; Kovac, 2000). The integration of multiple activities mediated by several different centres is necessary for the vomiting reflex (Carpenter, 1990). This is a complex reflex, with respiratory, salivary, vasomotor, and somatic motor components. The VC acts as a central pattern generator. Sequential activation of various components of the VC, with amplification at each step, may be required to trigger vomiting. Nausea in the absence of vomiting may arise from stimuli that excite the VC without sufficient amplification to trigger the vomiting cascade. Thus, nausea usually accompanies the prodromal autonomic effects that precede vomiting. However, the degree of nausea cannot be predicted by the accompanying autonomic changes; the relative reduction in gastric contraction may not be proportional. Also, nausea is not always relieved by vomiting. This usually indicates continuing excitation of the central emetogenic pathway.

The VC receives afferents from the cerebral cortex and higher brainstem, thalamus, and hypothalamus, the vestibular system, and via the vagus and splanchnic nerves, the pharynx, gastrointestinal (GI) tract, and serosae. There is also input from the CTZ, which can only initiate vomiting via the VC (Fig. 10.2.1) (Willems and Lefebvre, 1986). The close proximity to the VC of areas in the central nervous system associated with balance, vasomotor activity, salivation, and respiration explains why vomiting is often associated with increased salivation, swallowing, sweating, pallor, tachypnoea, tachycardia, and dizziness (Kovac, 2000).

Many potential neurotransmitters and receptors have been identified in the CTZ and nucleus of the tractus solitarius. These include dopamine, serotonin, histamine, opioid, cannabinoid, and neurokinin receptors. The principal receptors at the CTZ are dopamine type 2 (D_2). At the VC the principal receptors are muscarinic cholinergic (Ach_m) and histamine type 1 (H_1) (Sanger and Andrews, 2006). Both sites exhibit serotonin type 3 (5-HT_3) receptors, and serotonin type 2 (5-HT_2) receptors appear to be important in the VC (Lang, 1999). Neurokinin type 1 (NK_1) receptors are widely distributed in the central nervous system, and particularly in those areas of the brainstem involved in emesis. These emetic neuroreceptor areas serve as sensors and are stimulated by drugs and electrolytes. This initiates a relay of neurotransmitters to the VC and the vomiting reflex (Kovac, 2000; Shelke et al., 2004). The blockade of these receptor sites is the mechanism of action of many antiemetics (Sanger and Andrews, 2006).

Nausea is reported as a highly distressing symptom. The link between nausea and mood may be related to involvement of the inferior frontal gyrus of the human cerebral cortex (Miller et al., 1996). NK_1 receptors, distributed widely in the brain are associated with regulation of mood and are also implicated in emesis. Blockade of NK_1 receptors is associated with both antidepressant (Kramer et al., 1998) and antiemetic (Navari, 2004; Gobbi and Blier, 2005) activity. Thus, the link between nausea and dysphoria may be biochemical or structural.

Afferent pathways involved in emesis

The interrelationship between the CTZ, VC, and their various afferent inputs is summarized in Fig. 10.2.1. The major afferent neural pathway from the body to the central structures is the vagus, with additional input via the splanchnic nerves, sympathetic ganglia, and the glossopharyngeal nerve. The vagus itself is stimulated via mechanoreceptors and chemoreceptors in the GI tract, serosae, and viscera (Willems and Lefebvre, 1986; Andrews et al., 1990; Lichter, 1993; Lang, 1999).

The VC receives descending fibres from higher centres that may stimulate or inhibit activation of the emetic cascade. Most vagal afferents terminate at the VC, but there is some vagal input to the CTZ (Koga and Fukuda, 1992). Projections from the vestibular nuclei, that mediate emesis, are incompletely understood, but are presumed to be similar to those that generate NV after the ingestion of toxins. This would involve the CTZ, but D_2 antagonists are not particularly effective in motion sickness. H_1 and Ach_m antagonists are more effective; they are thought to act on first-order vestibular neurons (Yates et al., 1998).

Choosing an antiemetic

The paucity of evidence to support decisions about antiemetic therapy for patients with advanced disease is well recognized (Glare et al., 2004; Ang et al., 2010). Before prescribing drugs, care should be taken to reduce the stimulus to nausea from the patient's environment. This includes avoidance of cooking smells, attention to unpleasant odours (e.g. from an infected, necrotic tumours), and presentation of small, attractive meals. Cool, fizzy drinks are often more palatable than still or hot drinks. Many patients experience a taste change so that previously innocuous foods taste nauseating.

Nausea can be relieved if it is possible to treat the underlying cause. Nausea associated with hypercalcaemia will improve following treatment with bisphosphonates, drug-related nausea with discontinuation of the drug, raised intracranial pressure with steroids or cranial irradiation, and constipation with laxatives (Ang et al., 2010). Treating the underlying cause is much more likely to relieve the symptom than antiemetics.

Two strategies have been proposed for the management of NV; mechanistic and empirical approaches. The mechanistic approach is detailed in Box 10.2.1 and is currently recommended as the ideal approach to management (Lichter, 1993; Glare et al., 2004). It involves identifying the most likely cause of the nausea and hence the pathways and receptors involved, preferably within the context of a clinical guideline (Peroutka and Snyder, 1982; Ison and Peroutka, 1986; Glare et al., 2004). Drugs known to inhibit those particular receptors are then chosen. Several uncontrolled studies have reported very high response rates when this strategy is utilized (Lichter, 1993; Bentley and Boyd, 2001; Stephenson and Davies, 2006). The difficulty with this approach is that the cause of nausea in advanced disease is often multifactorial, unclear, or of unknown origin (Kennett et al., 2005; Hardy et al., 2010). Moreover, there is no evidence to date that this approach is any more effective than using various antiemetics that cover a range of postulated pathways and receptors or in fact any well-tolerated single agent of proven efficacy irrespective of the underlying cause. This is termed the empirical approach and is equally supported by a number studies (Bruera et al., 1994, 1996, 2000; Mystakidou et al., 1998a).

Antiemetic drugs available

A wide variety of agents have antiemetic efficacy. Many are primarily used for other indications. The availability of specific drugs varies from country to country. Those that have potent, receptor-specific action are summarized in Table 10.2.1. The antiemetic efficacy

---

Box 10.2.1 The mechanistic approach to the management of nausea and vomiting

1. Identify the likely cause(s) of nausea and/or vomiting.

2. Identify the pathway by which each cause triggers the vomiting reflex.

3. Identify the neurotransmitter receptor involved in the identified pathway.

4. Choose the most potent antagonist to the receptor identified—the binding affinity of a particular antagonist predicts its antiemetic efficacy.

5. Choose a route of administration that ensures that the drug reaches its site of action—this often excludes the oral route.

6. Titrate the dose carefully, review the patient frequently.

7. *Give the antiemetic regularly.*

8. If symptoms persist, review the likely cause(s): additional treatment may be required for an overlooked cause, or alternative treatment may be suggested by a different cause becoming apparent.

9. If combining antiemetics, potential drug interactions need to be considered. For example, an antihistamine may counteract the effects of a prokinetic agent.

Table 10.2.1 Receptor-specific antiemetics of use in palliative care

Drug	Receptor and site (see text)	Indications	Dosage and routes	Side effects	Notes
Butyrophenones Haloperidol	D_2 -CTZ	Opioid induced N; chemical/metabolic N	1.5–5.0 mg/day; PO, SC	EPS, QTc; somnolence	Side effects unusual at low doses, caution in severe liver impairment
Prokinetic agents Metoclopramide	D_2 -CTZ D_2 -GIT 5-HT$_4$ -GIT (potentiation)	Gastric stasis; ileus	10–20 mg 4-hrly PO, SC, IV	EPS, restlessness, drowsiness Colic in GI obstruction	Prolonged half-life in renal failure
	5-HT$_3$ -CTZ (at high doses) -GIT	Chemotherapy	N/A		Superseded by 5-HT$_3$ antagonists
Domperidone	D_2 -CTZ D_2 -GIT	Gastric stasis, ileus	10–20 mg PO 4–8-hrly 30–90 mg PR 4–8-hrly	Colic if GIT obstructed; oesophageal pain, QTc	Does not cross BBB, extrapyramidal side effects are rare, cannot be given parenterally (cardiac toxicity)
Cisapride	5-HT$_4$ -GIT (potentiation) Ach -GIT	Gastric stasis ileus	10 mg PO 6–8-hrly 30 mg PR 6–8-hrly	Abdominal cramps; diarrhoea; cardiac arrhythmias particularly with systemic azole antifungals, QTc	Prokinetic throughout GIT, withdrawn in many countries because of cardiac toxicity
Phenothiazines (including prochlorperazine chlorpromazine, thiethylperazine)	D_2 -CTZ D_2 -GIT H_1 -VC Ach -CNS $α_1$ Ad -GIT		Prochlorperazine: 5–10 mg PO, 12.5–25 mg IM, 25 mg PR 6–8-hrly Chlorpromazine: 25–50 mg IM 4–6-hrly	Vary according to spectrum of receptor blockade, QTc	
Levomepromazine	5-HT$_2$ -CVS H_1 -VC D_2 -VC $α_1$ Ad -CTZ	Intestinal obstruction: peritoneal irritation; nausea of unknown aetiology; vestibular causes; raised ICP	5–12.5 mg/24-hrly PO, SC	Drowsiness at higher doses, orthostatic hypotension	Long half-life: once daily dosing may suffice
Antihistamines Cyclizine Cinnarizine Diphenylhydramine Promethazine	H_1 -GIT -CVS -CNS -VC -vestibular afferents -brain substance		Cyclizine: 25–50 mg 8-hrly PO/SC/PR Promethazine: 12–25 mg 8-hrly PO	Dry mouth, blurred vision, sedation, EPS Skin irritation at SC injection sites QTc	Cyclizine is least sedative but anticholinergic Avoid in the elderly
Diphenylhydramine	Ach$_m$ -VC				

Anticholinergics					
Hyoscine (scopolamine) Hydrobromide Butylbromide	-VC -GIT -GIT	Intestinal obstruction; peritoneal irritation; raised ICP; excess secretions	200–400 mcg 4–8-hrly subling/SC 500–1500 mcg/72-hour transdermal patches 20 mg PO/SC 6-hrly	Dry mouth, sedation, ileus, urinary retention, blurred vision, occasionally agitation	Useful if NV coexist with colic, illogical to give with prokinetics Does not cross BBB, antisecretory; non-sedative Poorly absorbed from the GI tract
5-HT3 antagonists					
Granisetron Ondansetron Tropisetron Polanesetron Dolasetron	-GIT -CTZ -(VC)	Chemotherapy; abdominal radiotherapy; postoperative NV	Granisetron: 3 mg slowly IV up to 8-hrly; Ondansetron: 8 mg PO or slowly IV 8-hourly; Tropisetron: 5 mg PO or slowly IV daily Palonosetron 250 mcg IV daily	Headache in 30%; constipation; diarrhoea, dizziness, QTc	Effectiveness increased by combination with dexamethasone Indicated for NV related to chemo-, radiotherapy or surgery
NK1 antagonist					
Aprepitant	NK1	Late-onset chemotherapy-related NV	125 mg 1 hour prior to chemotherapy; then 80 mg OD for the next 2 days	Hiccups; asthenia; fatigue; somnolence; anxiety; anorexia; GI upset	Only available PO

CTZ, chemoreceptor trigger zone; VC, vomiting centre; GIT, gastrointestinal tract; ICP, intracranial pressure; mcg, micrograms; NV, nausea and vomiting; PO, by mouth; PR, by rectum; SC, by subcutaneous injection; IV, by intravenous injection; IM, by intramuscular injection; occ, occasionally; OD, once daily, EPS, extrapyramidal symptoms, QTc, prolonged QT interval, EPS, extrapyramidal symptoms.

and side effects of a drug can be predicted by its binding affinity for particular receptors (Peroutka and Snyder, 1982; Ison and Peroutka, 1986).

Drugs with receptor-specification

Dopamine (D₂) antagonists

The butyrophenones (haloperidol, droperidol), phenothiazines (promethazine, prochlorperazine) and benzamides (metoclopramide, domperidone) are all D_2 antagonists. Of these, haloperidol is said to be the most potent at the CTZ (Peroutka and Snyder, 1982). Although widely used in palliative care, systematic reviews have failed to identify any randomized controlled trials that prove the efficacy of dopamine antagonists (Wallenborn et al., 2006) or droperidol in any setting (Dorman and Perkins, 2010). A prospective uncontrolled clinical trial has suggested that haloperidol provides at least partial relief in around 50% of patients with NV not related to chemotherapy or radiotherapy (Hardy et al., 2010). Metoclopramide and domperidone, whilst having some CTZ anti-dopaminergic activity, act in the gut to antagonize D_2 and stimulate 5-HT_4 receptors. Metoclopramide is a weak antagonist of peripheral 5-HT_3 receptors explaining why high doses are necessary to control chemotherapy induced NV. Local acetylcholine release, mediated by the 5-HT_4 receptor, appears to play an important role in reversing gastroparesis and bringing about normal peristalsis in the upper GI tract. At high doses, metoclopramide blocks 5-HT_3 receptors in the CTZ and gut. Extrapyramidal symptoms (akathisia, acute dystonia, pseudoparkinsonism, and tardive dyskinesia) are a concern, especially in frail older patients. Prolonged use of metoclopramide (beyond 3 months) is not recommended by the US Food and Drug Administration. A recent study has shown that single doses, even at high doses (50 mg given postoperatively) were associated with surprisingly few side effects (Wallenborn et al., 2006). The development of specific 5-HT_3 antagonists has replaced the use of this drug for acute cancer chemotherapy-induced emesis (Basch et al., 2011). Metoclopramide is one of only a few antiemetics with high-grade evidence to support its use in advanced cancer (Glare et al., 2004; Ang et al., 2010).

Any agent that is prokinetic may induce colic in an obstructed intestine. Alternatively, it is postulated that drugs of this class may help to alleviate a partial obstruction by increasing gut motility. The action of prokinetic agents in the lower oesophagus may provoke oesophageal spasm; typically, this is retrosternal and may mimic angina pectoris. Extrapyramidal reactions occur with all of the D_2 antagonists, although the incidence with domperidone is extremely low (Ison and Peroutka, 1986). Many of these agents prolong the QT interval. This may be clinically relevant in patients on other drugs with the same effect (e.g. high-dose methadone)

Olanzapine has high affinity for multiple dopaminergic and other receptors (Glare et al., 2008). It is associated with less extrapyramidal side effects at the expense of somnolence and weight gain. There are uncontrolled studies suggesting benefit in NV (Passik et al., 2002; Jackson and Tavernier, 2003; Srivastava et al., 2003).

Phenothiazines

The phenothiazines are less potent D_2 antagonists with moderate antihistaminergic and anticholinergic actions. They have varying antagonist activity at other receptors that predicts their side effect profile (e.g. chlorpromazine, an α_1 adrenergic receptor may cause hypotension and sedation whereas diphenhydramine, a phenothiazine antihistamine Ach_m receptor, may cause sedation and dry mouth). Chlorpromazine can lower seizure thresholds in patients with chronic seizures or epilepsy.

Levomepromazine blocks a wide spectrum of receptors. At higher doses, it is highly sedative and causes hypotension, but at lower doses (5–12.5 mg per 24 hours by mouth or subcutaneous infusion) it is a useful antiemetic with efficacy in uncontrolled trials similar to that of haloperidol (Eisenchlas et al., 2005; Kennett et al., 2005). Circumstantial evidence suggests that 5-HT_2 blockade may mediate levomepromazine antiemetic activity (Twycross et al., 1997). At the VC, its lower affinity for D_2 receptors may contribute to its broad-spectrum antiemetic activity. Comparative clinical trials are awaited.

Historically, prochlorperazine has been considered the drug of choice for motion sickness. In many countries, it is not licensed for parenteral use. Chlorpromazine is not effective for the prevention of motion sickness (Yates et al., 1998; Kovac, 2000) and is dose limited by sedation and hypotension (Mystakidou et al., 1998a, 1998b). Phenothiazines, along with most antiemetics are likely to worsen Parkinsonian symptoms.

Antihistamines and anticholinergics

The antihistamines act on H_1 receptors in the VC and on vestibular afferents. H_1 antagonists alleviate NV induced by vestibular disorders and motion sickness but not that related to chemotherapy (Shelke et al., 2004). Cyclizine is less sedating than the anticholinergic hyoscine (hyoscyamine, scopolamine) hydrobromide, which blocks Ach_m receptors in the VC and peripherally (Ison and Peroutka, 1986). Although very widely used, the evidence to support the efficacy of this drug is very weak (Glare et al., 2004). Hyoscine hydrobromide can be given sublingually, subcutaneously, and transdermally. Its side effects are those of parasympathetic blockade, which may be beneficial (drying of secretions, reduction of colic) or troublesome (dry mouth, ileus, urinary retention, blurred vision). Hyoscine butylbromide (Buscopan®) does not have central antiemetic action as it does not cross the blood–brain barrier. In the gut, its anticholinergic properties reduce peristalsis and inhibit exocrine secretions, thus contributing to the palliation of colic and nausea in intestinal obstruction (De Conno et al., 1991). Promethazine has little anticholinergic activity. It is sedating and can cause skin irritation when delivered subcutaneously. According to Beers criteria (The American Geriatrics Society Beers Criteria Update Expert, 2012), the drug should be avoided in the elderly as clearance is reduced, resulting in increased risk of confusion, dry mouth, and other anticholinergic side effects.

5-HT₃ receptor antagonists

The discovery of selective 5-HT_3 receptor antagonists has been one of the most significant developments in supportive care in recent times and has revolutionized antiemetic prescribing for chemotherapy-induced nausea and vomiting (CINV). The initial early promise of this class of drugs in the 1980s has proved successful for acute-onset emesis in chemotherapy, although later-onset nausea remained a problem (Lichter, 1993; Gardner et al., 1995; Navari et al., 1999) until the development of the NK_1 receptor blockers (see 'NK_1 receptor antagonists'). Evidence of benefit for the 5-HT$_3$ inhibitors has subsequently been shown for both radiotherapy (Feyer et al., 2011) and postoperative emesis (Carlisle and Stevenson, 2006) and these drugs are licensed specifically for these indications in many countries. Although extremely effective for the indications as specified above, no definitive place has been demonstrated for 5-HT$_3$ antagonists in the management of NV from other causes. An increasing body of evidence suggests that they may be as effective as many of the other agents in common use (Mystakidou et al., 1998a; Porcel et al., 1998; Hardy et al., 2002; Weschules et al., 2006).

5-HT$_3$ receptors have been demonstrated in the CTZ and VC centrally, and on terminals of vagal afferents in the gut peripherally. The emetogenic action of serotonin derived from enterochromaffin cells appears to be by direct stimulation of local vagal 5-HT$_3$ receptors. High abdominal vagotomy abolishes emesis induced by abdominal irradiation, and blood serotonin levels are rarely raised during emesis, although raised urinary levels of the serotonin metabolite 5-hydroxindole acetic acid reflect the timing and severity of emesis after chemotherapy (Cubeddu et al., 1995). Antagonists of 5-HT$_3$ block vagal afferent activity. A reflex increase in vagal efferent activity may be caused, and this has been shown to give rise to temporary (and inconsequential) bradyarrhythmias in patients receiving repeated doses of these drugs, although not in healthy volunteers (Upward et al., 1990; Watanabe et al., 1995). Several 5-HT$_3$ antagonists are currently available (see Table 10.2.1). Oral formulations are as effective and safe as intravenous. All are equivalent with respect to antiemetic activity and safety (Basch et al., 2011) and share similar adverse events (headache, constipation, and transient elevations of serum aminotransferases). Palonosetron was developed because of its longer serum half-life and higher binding affinity to the 5-HT$_3$ serotonin receptor. It is preferred in some centres as it can be given as a single dose. Dolasetron and its major metabolite, and granisetron are the most specific 5-HT$_3$ receptor antagonists. Ondansetron and tropisetron show some affinity for other receptors including α-adrenergic, other 5-HT and opioid μ receptors.

In contrast to ondansetron, the metabolism of granisetron is not subject to induction by cytochrome P450 inducers (Upward et al., 1990). All are licensed for use in children, and adverse effects are few. Evidence-based antiemetic guidelines issued by the American Society of Clinical Oncology make no distinction between the different agents available, suggesting that cost should dictate local practice. They also recommend the use of cheaper oral preparations rather than intravenous treatment as first line.

NK$_1$ receptor antagonists

These drugs have proven efficacy in control of late emesis from chemotherapy (Hesketh et al., 2003a; Basch et al., 2011) and are now included in international CINV antiemetic guidelines (Roila et al., 2010; Basch et al., 2011). While it is generally accepted that acute CINV is mainly due to release of serotonin within the GI tract, delayed CINV is thought to be occur following release of substance P in the brainstem (Darmani et al., 2009). An analysis of the timing of the effect demonstrates differential stimulation of 5-HT$_3$ receptors during the first 8 hours following emetogenic chemotherapy, followed by onset of stimulation of NK$_1$ receptors and loss of response to 5-HT$_3$ antagonists (Hesketh et al., 2003b). Aprepitant, the first commercial

NK$_1$ receptor antagonist antiemetic made available, is an oral preparation. Fosaprepitant dimeglumine is now available in a water soluble injectable formulation (Huang and Korlipara, 2010). The role of NK$_1$ receptor antagonists in palliative care settings is yet to be explored.

Other antiemetic drugs

Corticosteroids

Corticosteroids are known to possess intrinsic antiemetic properties and to enhance the effect of other antiemetics (Basch et al., 2011). Their mechanism of action is unclear and may be multiple. Corticosteroids may enhance antiemetic tone in the medulla by: reducing the permeability of the blood–brain barrier to chemicals that antagonize medullary antiemetic tone (such as chemotherapy agents), depleting the inhibitory amine γ-aminobutyric acid (GABA) in medullary antiemetic neurons, and/or reducing leu-encephalin release in the brainstem. Alternatively, the mode of action may relate to their established effects of reducing inflammation and oedema through eicosanoid metabolism (Sanger and Andrews, 2006). They do not ameliorate acute apomorphine or ipecacuanha-induced emesis (Sanger and Andrews, 2006).

The anti-inflammatory effects of corticosteroids in reducing tumour-associated oedema is thought to reduce the stimulus to emesis from peripheral autonomic stretch receptors or from intracranial tumours. Steroids may hasten the resolution of bowel obstruction and therefore the vomiting associated with this condition (Feuer and Broadley, 2000). Dexamethasone has efficacy against postoperative NV equivalent to ondansetron and droperidol (Apfel et al., 2004).

Cannabinoids

Anecdotal reports of a lower incidence of chemotherapy-induced emesis amongst marijuana smokers led to clinical trials of cannabinoids. Subsequently, the antiemetic activity of cannabinoids in both animals and humans has been well documented (Gonzalez-Rosales and Walsh, 1997; Parker et al., 2011). Two oral formulations, dronabinol and nabilone, are approved by the US Food and Drug Administration for use in CINV refractory to conventional antiemetic therapy. These drugs have shown superiority to dopamine antagonists in preventing CINV (Slatkin, 2007). This activity may occur at doses lower than those that lead to psychotropic side effects.

The mechanism of action of the cannabinoids has recently been explored with the discovery of the endocannabinoid system (Parker et al., 2011). Cannabinoid agonists act mainly on peripheral CB$_1$ receptors to decrease intestinal motility but may act centrally to attenuate emesis. Cannabinoid receptors have been detected within the dorsal vagal complex (Devane et al., 1992; Van Sickle et al., 2003). Some antiemetic effects of synthetic cannabinoids are reversed by naloxone, raising the possibility that some of their mechanism of action is on opioid μ receptors.

The use of the currently licensed cannabinoids is limited by psychomimetic side effects, particularly dysphoria in the elderly. This effect is said be reduced by low-dose phenothiazines but the resulting drowsiness may undermine any therapeutic advantage of the cannabinoids (Cunningham et al., 1985). Euphoria is more common than dysphoria in younger patients, and there are reports of the successful use of nabilone for intractable nausea in AIDS patients, who tend to be younger than adults with cancer, and in children receiving chemotherapy (Dalzell et al., 1986; Green et al., 1989; Flynn and Hanif, 1992).

Benzodiazepines

Benzodiazepines have been used in chemotherapy antiemetic combinations, generally for the treatment and prevention of anticipatory nausea. However, there are no prospective trials to establish their effectiveness in this setting (Basch et al., 2011). Although they have little antiemetic activity per se, in drug combinations they reduce anxiety and the likelihood of anticipatory nausea. They decrease the anxiety and restlessness associated with anaesthesia and surgery thereby may decrease postoperative NV (Diflorio, 1992). These drugs are sedative and sometimes amnesic when used in effective doses, which limits their usefulness for patients with chronic nausea (Potanovich et al., 1993).

Octreotide

Octreotide is a somatostatin analogue that exerts wide-ranging potent inhibition of endocrine and exocrine secretions, promoting reabsorption of electrolytes in the gut (Lamberts et al., 1996) with both inhibition and restoration of normal GI transit (Soudah et al., 1991; Fallon, 1994). It is thus commonly used in an attempt to reduce the vomiting associated with bowel obstruction. Inhibition of exocrine secretion in the gut reduces distension, thus potentially contributing to diminished nausea (Mystakidou et al., 2002; Ripamonti et al., 2000; Laval et al., 2012).

Propofol

Propofol, an intravenous anaesthetic agent, has been noted to protect against postoperative emesis (Barst, 1990; Raftery and Sherry, 1992). Furthermore, subhypnotic doses of propofol have antiemetic action in postanaesthetic and chemotherapy-induced emesis (Scher et al., 1992; Borgeat et al., 1994). The duration of antiemetic action of an intravenous low-dose bolus outlasts the very short duration of hypnosis that would be introduced by a far larger dose, suggesting that hypnosis or anxiolysis are not the mechanisms of antiemetic action. Propofol has a widespread central nervous system depressant effect and it is possible that its antiemetic action is at a subcortical level, in either the CTZ or within the VC complex. The observation that propofol is less successful as an antiemetic following vagal-stimulating abdominal surgery suggests that its site of action may be the CTZ.

Opioids

As opioid receptors are abundant in the CTZ, it is thought that opioids or encephalins may possess antiemetic properties (Shelke et al., 2004). Patients will often complain of nausea when first commenced on opioids, probably through stimulation of receptors in the area postrema. The resolution of NV after a few days may be attributed to the antiemetic activity of opioids once they have crossed the blood–brain barrier (Yates et al., 1998). Opioids can induce or block emesis in experimental models and both actions can be antagonized by naloxone (Costello and Borison, 1977). Experimentally, intravenous fentanyl in subanaesthetic doses abolishes emesis due to morphine, cisplatin, and copper sulphate,

an effect that is reversed by naloxone (Barnes et al., 1991). The release of endogenous opioids during emesis could be part of the physiological mechanism by which the vomiting reflex is terminated (Yates et al., 1998). In clinical practice, the persistent nauseating properties of the opioids are well known and it remains doubtful whether these agents may have any role as antiemetics.

Mirtazapine

Mirtazapine is an antidepressant with some 5-HT$_3$ receptor antagonist activity. There are anecdotal reports of its benefit in the management of NV (Pae, 2006).

Non-drug measures of palliation of nausea and vomiting

Psychological techniques and massage

Most of the authoritative research on psychological techniques for palliation of emesis has been conducted amongst chemotherapy patients, which is not necessarily analogous to the situation of nauseated patients with disease not related to the treatment of cancer. However, these studies have shown that patients can learn techniques such as progressive muscle relaxation and guided mental imagery, and use these during the stress of chemotherapy with good effect (Cotanch, 1991; Burish and Tope, 1992; Fallowfield, 1992). Cognitive therapy has been used to help relieve the psychological morbidity arising from physical symptoms in advanced cancer (Moorey and Greer, 2002). Behavioural therapy with systematic desensitization is recommended for the management of anticipatory nausea (Basch et al., 2011).

One review of mind–body interventions for management of symptoms at the end of life identified 11 studies of massage interventions of which three reported improved outcomes for patients experiencing nausea. The review also identified 16 studies of meditation-based interventions for symptom management, of which six reported benefits for patients experiencing nausea. However, the methods and results were often inconsistent across studies, with many studies including mixed samples of patients who did not have advanced illness (Lafferty et al., 2006). Nevertheless, the possibility of adapting such techniques for the needs of nauseated patients with advanced diseases warrants further exploration (see Chapter 9.11).

Transcutaneous electrical nerve stimulation

Transcutaneous electrical nerve stimulation (TENS) has been shown to enhance the effect of antiemetic drugs. The TENS effect is blocked by naloxone, suggesting that it is mediated by endogenous opioid peptides (Saller et al., 1986). In a more recent study, TENS reduced the incidence of nausea and emesis after laparoscopic cholecystectomy when compared to placebo (Silva et al., 2012) (see Chapter 9.9).

Acupuncture and acupressure

There is some evidence for the benefit of acupuncture and acupressure when used in conjunction with standard antiemetics during chemotherapy (Ezzo et al., 2006; Bao, 2009) and to reduce postoperative NV (Lee and Fan, 2009). The benefit of acupuncture is lost if administered under general anaesthetic (Vickers, 1996). Acupressure prolongs the effect of acupuncture, and the use of TENS in place of traditional acupuncture needles at the P6 acupuncture point is a practical technique for self-use by patients, being only slightly less effective than the use of traditional needles (Dundee et al., 1991). The P6 (Neiguan) acupuncture point is located in the midline of the palmar aspect of each wrist, approximately 3 cm from the palmar crease (see Chapter 9.12).

Dietary modification, ginger, fish oil, and aromatherapy

There is limited published evidence about dietary modifications to minimize NV for people with advanced illness. However, avoiding sights, sounds, and smells that can trigger NV, and respecting an individual's preferences and food choices are major considerations in advanced illness (Yates, 2012). Ginger has been used to treat nausea in a range of settings. No additional benefit was found over and above modern-day antiemetics (5-HT$_3$ antagonists and aprepitant) in a randomized controlled trial of CINV (Zick et al., 2009). Aromatherapy is less effective than standard antiemetics in postoperative NV (Hines et al., 2012). Fish oil supplements provided no benefit with respect to nausea in patients with advanced cancer (Bruera et al., 1987, 2003).

Clinical syndromes associated with nausea and vomiting

Table 10.2.2 summarizes some common or important causes of NV in patients receiving palliative care. They are grouped according to the pathway that mediates emesis, and are similarly grouped in the following discussion. In advanced cancer, there are a number of factors that are predictors of NV. These include: female gender (Walsh et al., 2000); GI symptoms such as local pathology or intestinal obstruction (Mercadante et al., 2000); age under 65 years (Walsh et al., 2000); specific tumour types such as gynaecological, stomach, oesophageal, and breast cancers (Vainio and Auvinen, 1996); the presence of metastases in the lung, pleura, peritoneum (Morita et al., 1999); and opioid medication (Meuser et al., 2001).

It must be emphasized, however, that in advanced disease, NV may have more than one cause, stimulating symptoms by more than one pathway (Hardy et al., 2010; Kennett et al., 2005). Sometimes, apparently appropriate treatment fails to relieve symptoms, necessitating a search for additional and less obvious causes. Sometimes, a cause cannot be identified. Into this category are likely to fall those with cancer-associated autonomic failure. Growth factors and other tumour products may be emetogenic; their actions are still only partly understood, but it is likely that such factors would act via the CTZ. Tumours arising outside the areas described in Table 10.2.2 may generate emesis via the same pathways, for example, head and neck tumours cause pressure effects which trigger autonomic relays to the VC. The key to good management of NV is a high index of suspicion, an understanding of the pathways involved, regular antiemetics, and the setting of realistic goals.

Chemical causes of emesis

Drug-induced nausea may arise by chemical action at the CTZ, by serotonin release in the gut, through GI irritation or gastric stasis, or a combination of these (Table 10.2.3).

Transient nausea mediated by the CTZ accompanies the introduction or increase of morphine in about one-third of patients (Campora et al., 1991) and can lead to chronic nausea in some patients on opioids. A number of clinical characteristics and specific genetic polymorphisms have been shown to be associated with the variability in NV amongst cancer patients receiving opioids (Laugsand et al., 2011). Most patients on opioids experience a degree of opioid-induced gastric stasis and associated constipation.

Multiple neurotransmitters are thought to be involved in the aetiology of CINV. Acute CINV is primarily related to the release of 5-HT within the GI tract while the delayed phase is related to the release of substance P in the brainstem (Darmani et al., 2009). Cytotoxic-induced nausea is mediated by the CTZ and by 5-HT$_3$ receptors on vagal gut afferents. Selective blockade of 5-HT$_3$ receptors in the gut is highly effective for immediate-onset emesis (Gregory and Ettinger, 1998). These drugs may also act at the CTZ. The addition of drugs that target other sites (e.g. corticosteroids and NK$_1$ receptor antagonists) enhances the effectiveness of treatment, particularly for delayed-onset emesis.

Metabolic causes of nausea include organ failure and hypercalcaemia, that may progress insidiously. Nausea in this scenario may be controlled using a central D$_2$ blocker.

Gastrointestinal causes of emesis

Pharyngeal irritation may cause retching, nausea, or cough-induced vomiting. The oropharynx is richly innervated by the glossopharyngeal nerve and vagus, and is highly sensitive to touch. Tenacious sputum or candida overlying the pharyngeal mucosa can stimulate the VC via these afferents. People with AIDS may also have mucosal lesions of cytomegalovirus or herpes simplex. Appropriate antimicrobial therapy is indicated for infections of mouth, pharynx, oesophagus, or respiratory tract. Sticky sputum may be loosened by inhalations, and irritating nocturnal cough causing retching and disturbed sleep may be palliated by the application of local anaesthetic spray to the pharynx (with appropriate caution about eating and drinking for the next few hours).

Delayed gastric emptying may arise from physiological abnormalities or mechanical resistance to emptying. Mechanical resistance includes ascites, hepatomegaly, pre-pyloric inflammation, duodenal ulceration or tumour, and pancreatic cancer. Resistance may be partial or there may be complete obstruction. Physiological abnormalities include anticholinergic effects of drugs (Table 10.2.3), and autonomic failure. The symptoms are listed in Table 10.2.2, they may not all occur and the diagnosis can easily be missed.

Complete gastric outlet obstruction is managed as high intestinal obstruction (see Chapter 14.3). Other causes of delayed emptying are managed by attention to optimizing gastric emptying and reducing stimulus to gastric stretch. The prokinetic agents metoclopramide and domperidone normalize the rate of gastric and upper intestinal peristalsis, increase lower oesophageal tone (thus reducing reflux), and relax the pylorus. Gastric and upper intestinal transit time is thus shortened. The prokinetic agent cisapride increases the rate of peristalsis throughout the GI tract. This drug has been withdrawn in several countries because of concerns about cardiotoxicity. Reduction in volume of meals and drinks and inhibition of gastric secretion using

H_2 blockers, proton pump inhibitors, or octreotide will reduce gastric stretch, thus reducing both the diaphragmatic irritation that gives rise to hiccup and the vagal stimulation that gives rise to nausea and pain.

Stretch and distortion of the GI tract activates mechanoreceptors in the bowel wall. Similar receptors are present in visceral capsules and in parietal serosal surfaces. Their afferent input is to the VC via the vagus and splanchnic nerves. Mechanoreceptors may be triggered by tumour distorting an organ, stretching or directly invading serosa or mesentery, or by increased transmural pressure in a hollow viscus proximal to a site of obstruction, such as the ureter or colon. This is, therefore, a common complication of advanced intra-abdominal, retroperitoneal, or pelvic malignancy. Local inflammation may potentiate afferent nerve receptors in the GI tract, mediating emesis in bowel infections such as cryptosporidiosis in AIDS patients.

If reversal of the cause of emesis is not possible, nausea may be palliated by using antiemetics active at the VC. Control of vomiting may be more difficult to achieve with obstruction in the GI tract. This is discussed in more detail in Chapter 14.3.

Constipation, with resultant colonic stretch, is assumed to be a cause of nausea and anorexia in advanced disease, although there are no studies to prove this. Management is of the constipation, although antiemetics acting at the VC may help to reduce the nausea. Concomitant anticholinergic agents should be avoided or reduced as they will exacerbate the constipation.

Cranial causes of emesis

Raised intracranial pressure may present with NV before headache is apparent. Meningeal irritation can also trigger emesis. Clinical associations are with intracerebral tumours (primary and secondary), bone metastases to skull (base of skull metastases may give rise to cranial nerve symptoms and signs), intracranial bleeding, and cerebral oedema. High-dose corticosteroids are the treatment of choice. An antiemetic acting at the VC may be necessary in addition. Palliative radiotherapy, chemotherapy, or surgery should be considered.

Other causes of emesis

Motion sickness can occur when sensory inputs regarding body position in space are contradictory, or are different from those predicted from experience and is dependent on signals from the vestibular system (Yates et al., 1998). Movement-associated emesis may be triggered by distorted or distended viscera exerting increased traction upon their mesentery during movement. Movement-associated nausea may also occur as a side effect of opioids, related to increased vestibular sensitivity. Centrally mediated emesis must be distinguished from passive regurgitation of gastric contents during movement in a terminally ill patient, which is usually related to gastroparesis. Placement of a nasogastric tube to aspirate the stomach dry of fluid and gas may be necessary to relieve this symptom.

Anxiety-induced emesis is a common experience in healthy people. The patient with advanced disease may be able to identify anxiety as the trigger to nausea, or carers may notice an association between symptoms and stressful situations or conversations. Other causes of emesis must be excluded as far as possible before attributing NV to anxiety. Treatment is by identifying anxiety as a trigger and then working collaboratively with the patient to increase

relaxation, identify and manage anxiety-provoking thoughts, and establishing workable coping strategies (Fallowfield, 1992; Moorey and Greer, 2002). A number of behavioural techniques have been found to be effective including progressive relaxation, systematic desensitization, hypnosis, and cognitive and internal distraction (Shelke et al., 2004). Benzodiazepines may be useful as short-term adjuvants. Some patients benefit from tricyclic antidepressants with secondary anxiolytic properties, such as amitriptyline.

Anticipatory emesis is a conditioned response in some patients who have suffered nausea and/or vomiting provoked by a previous experience. Several studies have confirmed that the development of anticipatory NV involves elements of classical conditioning (Shelke et al., 2004). Any reminder of their previous experience may trigger emesis, such as television pictures of hospitals, hospital smells, or visits by hospital personnel. In the case of chemotherapy-induced NV, correlates and determinants of anticipatory nausea include female sex, young age, high levels of anxiety, distress, limited ability to cope, a history of alcoholism, or the experience of strange tastes during chemotherapy (Morrow and Rosenthal, 1996). It can be refractory to treatment and is best managed by ensuring good control of emesis from the first cycle of chemotherapy. Management is as for anxiety-induced emesis.

Intractable nausea

As with pain, the pathways of emesis are incompletely documented. Identification and reversal of the cause and administration of appropriate antiemetics given regularly and prophylactically (rather than only when the patient is reporting nausea) leads to control in most patients. In a minority, NV continues unabated. There are few published data about these patients. In those with cachexia and chronic nausea, one group has identified a subgroup of people with a degree of autonomic failure (Bruera et al., 1987).

Appropriate goal setting is important. It is unwise to expect or to promise total relief of NV, especially in cases of mechanical obstruction (e.g. bowel obstruction). Most patients will be content with some relief of nausea, even if intermittent vomiting continues, provided they have been informed that this is a possible outcome.

When all apparently appropriate measures have failed to relieve symptoms, and combinations of antiemetics directed at different receptors have proved ineffective, empirical use of drugs acting at a range of different receptors such as levomepromazine may offer relief to some patients. Good clinical trials of therapy for patients with refractory nausea are indicated.

Future developments

Progress has been made in the recognition of nausea as an important symptom that must be evaluated separately from vomiting. This has improved the quality of the data emerging from chemotherapy-related emesis and postoperative NV studies.

Patients' perceptions are different from those of nurses observing them, and there is a need for an agreed tool for measurement of NV (Olver et al., 1994). The development of tools for self-evaluation of symptoms by patients, and the identification of biological markers for emesis, would enhance the evaluation of antiemetic strategies. A comprehensive review of available tools for rating NV in palliative care concluded that an ideal measurement tool for the assessment of NV and retching has not yet been developed (Saxby et al.,

Table 10.2.2 Common syndromes involving nausea and vomiting in patients requiring palliative care

Syndrome	Causes	Key features	Pathway and receptors	Treatment possibilities
Chemically induced nausea	◆ Drugs: opioids, digoxin, anticonvulsants, antibiotics, cytotoxics ◆ Toxins: food poisoning, ischaemic bowel, e.g. gut obstruction, ? tumour products ◆ Metabolic: organ failure, hypercalcaemia, ketoacidosis	Of drug toxicity or of underlying disease, plus constant nausea, variable vomiting	Chemical action stimulates D_2 ($\pm 5\text{-HT}_3$) in CTZ Chemotherapy → serotonin release in GI tract → 5-HT_3 receptors on vagus Chemotherapy → NK_1 receptor activation in brain	◆ Stop or reduce the offending drug ◆ Treat the underlying cause ◆ Haloperidol ◆ 5-HT_3 antagonists for chemotherapy or irradiation induced NV ◆ NK_1 antagonist for delayed emesis with chemotherapy

Gastric stasis	◆ Anticholinergic drugs, opioids
	◆ Ascites
	◆ Hepatomegaly
	◆ Peptic ulcer
	◆ Gastritis
	  • Stress
	  • Drugs
	  • Radiotherapy
	◆ Autonomic failure
		Epigastric pain, fullness, nausea, early satiety, flatulence, acid reflux, hiccup, large volume vomits (possibly projectile) gastric regurgitation, other features of autonomic failure	Gastric mecho-receptors
			↓
			Vagal afferents
			↓
			VC
			
			H₁; Achm
				◆ Treat the underlying causes
				◆ Prokinetic agents
				◆ Reduce gastric secretions:
				  • H_2 blocker
				  • proton pump inhibitor
				  • Octreotide
				◆ Aid eructation: dimeticone

Stretch/distortion of GI tract	◆ Constipation ◆ Intestinal obstruction ◆ Mesenteric metastases	Altered bowel habit, nausea, vomiting, may be faeculent, colic	Gut/serosal Mechanoreceptors ↓ Vagal afferents ↓ VC	◆ Treat underlying cause ◆ Active bowel management ◆ Corticosteroids may reduce swelling associated with a tumour mass
Serosal stretch/ irritation	e.g.: ◆ Liver metastases ◆ Ureteric obstruction ◆ Retroperitoneal cancer	Of underlying condition, nausea, occasional vomiting	H_1; Achm	◆ Cyclizine ◆ Hyoscine butylbromide if bowel paralysis is acceptable
Irritation of GI tract	◆ e.g. cryptospordiosis	Profuse diarrhoea, nausea, occasional vomiting.		
Raised intracranial pressure/meningism	◆ Cerebral oedema ◆ Intracranial tumour ◆ Intracranial bleeding ◆ Meningeal infiltration by tumour ◆ Skull metastases ◆ Cerebral infections (AIDS)	Headache (diurnal); papilloedema, photophobia may be absent. Nausea may be diurnal; neurological signs may be absent	May be direct stimulation of cerebral H_1 meningeal mechanoreceptors ↓ VC H_1; Achm	◆ Treat underlying cause ◆ High-dose corticosteroids may reduce cerebral oedema ◆ Cyclizine ◆ Levomepromazine

(continued)

Table 10.2.2 Continued

Syndrome	Causes	Key features	Pathway and receptors	Treatment possibilities
Movement-associated emesis	◆ Opioids (more common in ambulant patients) ◆ Gut distortion ◆ Gastroparesis → passive regurgitation	Nausea and/or sudden vomits on movement/turning in bed	Opioid-induced sensitivity of vestibular afferents H_1; Ach_m Gut mechanoreceptors ↓ vagal afferents ↓ VC H_1;Ach_m	◆ Treat the underlying cause ◆ Nasogastric aspiration in terminal gastroparesis ◆ Cyclizine ◆ Cinnarizine ◆ Hyoscine hydrobromide ◆ Prochlorperazine
Anxiety-induced emesis	◆ Anxiety: • about self • about others • about disease • about symptoms ◆ Anticipatory emesis with cytotoxics	'Waves' of nausea, ± vomiting, reminders trigger nausea; may be relieved by distraction	Cortex ↓ VC H_1; Ach_m	◆ Address the anxiety ◆ Psychological techniques ◆ Relaxation ◆ Benzodiazepines may be useful

D_2, dopamine type 2 receptor; 5-HT_3, serotonin type 3 receptor; H_1, histamine type 1 receptor; Achm—muscarinic cholinergic receptor; CTZ, chemoreceptor trigger zone; VC, vomiting centre; GI, gastrointestinal.

Table 10.2.3 Causes of drug-induced nausea

Mechanism	Drugs	
Activation of chemo-receptor trigger zone	Opioids	Cytotoxics
	Digoxin	Imidazoles
	Anticoagulants	Antibiotics
Gastrointestinal irritation	Non-steroidal anti-inflammatory drugs	Antibiotics
		Cytotoxics
	Iron supplements	
Gastric stasis	Tricyclics	Opioids
	Phenothiazines	Anticholinergics

2007) although numerical rating scales have been used to measure other subjective symptoms and are likely to be just as relevant for nausea (Hjermstad et al., 2011).

Much of the research to date has attempted to identify key neurotransmitter receptors and find ways of interfering with their action. The underlying assumption of this approach is that a particular transmitter or receptor is pivotal and that a stimulus to emesis operates via one predominant pathway (Sanger and Andrews, 2006). This seems unlikely in a palliative care population. Improved outcomes in the management of CINV have followed the use of several drugs in combination (i.e. a 5-HT$_3$ antagonist plus an NK$_1$ inhibitor and dexamethasone) to suppress more than one pathway. Whether this approach may be of benefit for the control of NV not related to chemotherapy and whether a combination of antiemetics is any better than a broad-spectrum single agent remains unknown.

Recent work around symptom clusters (Skerman et al., 2012) has highlighted the need to maximize treatment of those symptoms commonly associated with NV (e.g. anorexia, dyspepsia, and fatigue). It would be of interest to explore whether a more holistic approach to NV would lead to improved outcomes.

Online materials

Complete references for this chapter are available online at <http://www.oxfordmedicine.com>.

References

Bao, T. (2009). Use of acupuncture in the control of chemotherapy-induced nausea and vomiting. *Journal of the National Comprehensive Cancer Network*, 7, 606–612.

Basch, E., Prestrud, A.A., Hesketh, P.J., et al. (2011). Antiemetics: American Society of Clinical Oncology clinical practice guideline update. *Journal of Clinical Oncology*, 29, 4189–4198.

Bliss, J.M., Robertson, B., Selby, P.J., et al. (1992). The impact of nausea and vomiting upon quality of life measures. *British Journal of Cancer*, 66, S14–S29.

Bruera, E., Belzile, M., Neumann, C., Harsanyi, Z., Babul, N., and Darke, A. (2000). A double-blind, crossover study of controlled-release metoclopramide and placebo for the chronic nausea and dyspepsia of advanced cancer. *Journal of Pain and Symptom Management*, 19, 427–435.

Burish, T.G. and Tope, D.M. (1992). Psychological techniques for controlling the adverse side effects of cancer chemotherapy: findings from a decade of research. *Journal of Pain and Symptom Management*, 7, 287–301.

Carpenter, D.O. (1990). Neural mechanisms of emesis. *Canadian Journal of Physiology and Pharmacology*, 68, 230–236.

Cotanch, P.H. (1991). Use of nonpharmacological techniques to prevent chemotherapy-related nausea and vomiting. *Recent Results in Cancer Research*, 121, 101–107.

Dorman, S. and Perkins, P. (2010). Droperidol for treatment of nausea and vomiting in palliative care patients. *Cochrane Database of Systematic Reviews*, 10, CD006938.

Ezzo, J.M., Richardson, M.A., Vickers, A., et al. (2006). Acupuncture-point stimulation for chemotherapy-induced nausea or vomiting. *Cochrane Database of Systematic Reviews*, 2, CD002285.

Feuer, D.J. and Broadley, K.E. (2000). Corticosteroids for the resolution of malignant bowel obstruction in advanced gynaecological and gastrointestinal cancer. *Cochrane Database of Systematic Reviews*, 2, CD001219.

Feyer, P.C., Maranzano, E., Molassiotis, A., et al (2011). Radiotherapy-induced nausea and vomiting (RINV): MASCC/ESMO guideline for antiemetics in radiotherapy: update 2009. *Support Care Cancer*, Supp 1; S5–14

Glare, P., Pereira, G., Kristjanson, L.J., Stockler, M., and Tattersall, M. (2004). Systematic review of the efficacy of antiemetics in the treatment of nausea in patients with far-advanced cancer. *Supportive Care in Cancer*, 12, 432–440.

Glare, P.A., Dunwoodie, D., Clark, K., et al. (2008). Treatment of nausea and vomiting in terminally ill cancer patients. *Drugs*, 68, 2575–2590.

Hardy, J., Daly, S., McQuade, B., et al. (2002). A double-blind, randomised, parallel group, multinational, multicentre study comparing a single dose of ondansetron 24 mg p.o. with placebo and metoclopramide 10 mg t.d.s. p.o. in the treatment of opioid-induced nausea and emesis in cancer patients. *Supportive Care in Cancer*, 10, 231–236.

Hesketh, P.J., Grunberg, S.M., Gralla, R.J., et al. (2003a). The oral neurokinin-1 antagonist aprepitant for the prevention of chemotherapy-induced nausea and vomiting: A multinational, randomised, double-blind, placebo-controlled trial in patients receiving high-dose cisplatin—The Aprepitant Protocol 052 Study Group. *Journal of Clinical Oncology*, 21, 4112–4119.

Hines, S., Steels, E., Chang, A., and Gibbons, K. (2012). Aromatherapy for treatment of postoperative nausea and vomiting. *Cochrane Database of Systematic Reviews*, 4, CD007598.

Hjermstad, M.J., Fayers, P.M., Haugen, D.F., et al. (2011). Studies comparing numerical rating scales, verbal rating scales, and visual analogue scales for assessment of pain intensity in adults: a systematic literature review. *Journal of Pain and Symptom Management*, 41, 1073–1093.

Kennett, A., Hardy, J., Shah, S., and A'Hern, R. (2005). An open study of methotrimeprazine in the management of nausea and vomiting in patients with advanced cancer. *Supportive Care in Cancer*, 13, 715–721.

Mercadante, S., Casuccio, A., and Fulfaro, F. (2000). The course of symptom frequency and intensity in advanced cancer patients followed at home. *Journal of Pain and Symptom Management*, 20, 104–112.

Morrow, G.R. and Rosenthal, S.N. (1996). Models, mechanisms and management of anticipatory nausea and emesis. *Oncology*, 53(Suppl. 1), 4–7.

Mystakidou, K., Befon, S., Liossi, C., and Vlachos, L. (1998a). Comparison of the efficacy and safety of tropisetron, metoclopramide, and chlorpromazine in the treatment of emesis associated with far advanced cancer. *Cancer*, 83, 1214–1223.

Peroutka, S.J. and Snyder, S.H. (1982). Antiemetics: neurotransmitter receptor binding predicts therapeutic actions. *The Lancet*, 1, 658–659.

Roila, F., Herrstedt, J., Aapro, M., et al. (2010). Guideline update for MASCC and ESMO in the prevention of chemotherapy- and radiotherapy-induced nausea and vomiting: results of the Perugia consensus conference. *Annals of Oncology*, 21(Suppl. 5), v232–243.

Sanger, G.J. and Andrews, P.L. (2006). Treatment of nausea and vomiting: gaps in our knowledge. *Autonomic Neuroscience*, 129, 3–16.

Shelke, A.R., Mustian, K.M., and Morrow, G.R. (2004). The pathophysiology of treatment-related nausea and vomiting in cancer patients: current models. Indian *Journal of Physiology and Pharmacology*, 48, 256–268.

Solano, J.P., Gomes, B., and Higginson, I.J. (2006). A comparison of symptom prevalence in far advanced cancer, AIDS, heart disease, chronic obstructive pulmonary disease and renal disease. *Journal of Pain and Symptom Management*, 31, 58–69.

Stephenson, J. and Davies, A. (2006). An assessment of aetiology-based guidelines for the management of nausea and vomiting in patients with advanced cancer. *Supportive Care in Cancer*, 14, 348–353.

Vainio, A. and Auvinen, A. (1996). Prevalence of symptoms among patients with advanced cancer: an international collaborative study. Symptom Prevalence Group. *Journal of Pain and Symptom Management*, 12, 3–10.

Walsh, D., Donnelly, S., and Rybicki, L. (2000). The symptoms of advanced cancer: relationship to age, gender, and performance status in 1,000 patients. *Supportive Care in Cancer*, 8, 175–179.

Yates, P., Clavarino, A., Mitchell, G., *et al.* (2005). Understanding factors contributing to nausea in advanced cancer: clinical and patient perspectives. *EJC Supplements*, 3, 446–446.

Constipation and diarrhoea

Nigel P. Sykes

Definition of constipation and diarrhoea

A working definition of constipation is 'the passage of small, hard faeces infrequently and with difficulty' (Larkin et al., 2008). The often-referred-to Rome Criteria (Longstreth et al., 2006), designed for gastroenterological research into idiopathic constipation, require that a constipated patient should have had for at least 3 months two or more of the following: straining during at least 25% of defecations, a sensation of anorectal obstruction during at least 25% of defecations, lumpy or hard stools at least 25% of the time, and fewer than three bowel movements per week.

Patients, however, differ in the weights they give to different aspects of this symptom cluster and the length of time over which they have to persist before they consider themselves constipated. Therefore they may consider themselves constipated when a doctor using the Rome Criteria would not (Probert et al., 1994). The importance of constipation in the context of cancer is as a symptom—or a syndrome—rather than as a disease, and it is therefore appropriate that we should be hearing the patient's complaint of constipation and understanding what they mean by it rather than trying to validate their opinion by comparison with external norms.

Prevalence of constipation and diarrhoea

In the general population, around 10% will report themselves to have constipation (Connell et al., 1965; Everhart et al., 1989), with the highest prevalences tending to be associated with older age and female gender. Physical illness is a risk factor for constipation: 63% of elderly people in hospital have been found to be constipated, compared with 22% of the same age group living at home (Wigzell, 1969). Constipation is more common in people terminally ill with cancer than in those dying of other causes (Cartwright et al., 1973), and about 50% of patients admitted to British hospices complain of it. There is evidence that constipation is inadequately treated in both cancer units (Laugsand et al., 2011) and palliative care (Goodman et al., 2005). As a result, constipation rivals pain in prevalence (Potter et al., 2003) and as a source of distress (Dunlop, 1989) in this patient group.

Normal intestinal physiology

Bowel function is the result not only of the state of intestinal motility but also of its fluid handling.

Intestinal motility

Gut contents spend 2–4 hours in the small bowel, whereas transit time through the colon is usually 24–48 hours and may be considerably longer: nearly half of a hospice population had transit times of between 4 and 12 days (Sykes, 1990).

Small and large intestines each have their own characteristic motility patterns, but throughout the gut most muscle movements mix the contents rather than propel them. This facilitates enzymatic and bacterial breakdown of food and absorption of the resulting nutrients and of water.

The colon shows episodes of forward peristalsis, resulting in mass movements of gut contents, about six times per day grouped into two peaks, a larger one associated with wakening and breakfast and a smaller one associated with the midday meal (Bassotti and Gaburri, 1988). The frequency is reduced by inactivity.

Gut muscle layers form a syncytium through which depolarization spreads from pacemaker areas. The myenteric nerve plexus coordinates motility, which is also under external neuronal influence, particularly via the parasympathetic system. High spinal cord transection mainly abolishes the motility response to food, but low cord or pelvic outflow lesions produce colonic dilation and slowing of transit in the descending and distal transverse colon.

Autonomic neuropathy can occur as a non-metastatic manifestation of malignancy, particularly in association with small cell carcinoma of the lung and carcinoid tumours. The resulting neural damage most commonly causes gastroparesis, but can also be associated with severe constipation (Walsh and Nelson, 2002).

The two principal neurotransmitters involved in the control of peristalsis appear to be acetylcholine (ACh) and vasoactive intestinal peptide (VIP). Peristalsis movements have two components, ascending contraction and descending relaxation; ACh mediates the first of these and VIP the second. Both ACh and VIP neurons are modulated by other agents of which endogenous opioids are one group. Both exogenous opioids and drugs with anticholinergic effects will therefore have the capacity to disrupt peristalsis and precipitate constipation.

Intestinal fluid handling

About 7 L of fluid are secreted into the gut each day, to which are added at least 1.5 L of dietary fluid. Most of this is reabsorbed by the small bowel, especially the jejunum, but over 1 L is left to enter the colon. As daily stool water content is around 200 mL and the difference between constipation and diarrhoea in terms of fluid excretion is only about 100 mL per day, the fine tuning of fluid absorption by the colon is very important in maintaining a convenient bowel habit.

Fluid handling reflects a dynamic state of absorption and secretion in the gut wall. Most secretion occurs from the mucosal crypt cells and absorption takes place in the villous cells. Through the enteric nervous system mechanical stimulation of mucosal sensory neurons activates secretion as well as stimulating blood flow and smooth muscle contraction. 5-hydroxytryptamine (5-HT), substance P, and neurokinins 1 and 2 are involved in the sensory side of the reflex and VIP is the secretomotor neurotransmitter (Cooke et al., 1997). The presumed physiological importance of this linkage is the enhancement of digestion through greater mixing and dilution of luminal contents and the increased absorption that has been shown to accompany an increase in motility.

Causes of constipation

Constipation in patients with progressive disease is usually multifactorial. Thus, an ill person with poor food intake, impaired mobility, and a requirement for opioid analgesia has three reasons to be constipated. A list of the constipating factors most relevant to palliative medicine is given in Box 10.3.1. Of these, other than in patients undergoing cancer chemotherapy where some regimens commonly have constipation as an adverse effect, the most important are the secondary effects of disease and the use of opioids.

In advanced cancer, the use of morphine and the other opioid analgesia is probably the greatest single constipating factor which can be isolated, but there is a background of widespread constipation arising from debility. In one study, 63% of advanced cancer patients not taking morphine required laxatives, a figure similar to that found in the ill elderly, but 87% of those receiving morphine needed them and used a higher average dose (Sykes, 1998).

The functional effect of opioids is to reduce peristaltic propulsion, but to enhance non-propulsive contractions. Opioids also cause constipation through changes in intestinal fluid handling. In part these changes result simply from the additional time available for water absorption because luminal contents are slowed down but, in addition, opioids cause inhibition of secretomotor neurons so that less fluid enters the gut. The result is drier, harder, and smaller stools that are more difficult to pass (Bannister et al., 1987). Opioids also reduce sensations of gut distension, including rectal distension. This may help to precipitate faecal impaction, especially in older patients in whom rectal sensitivity may already be impaired as a result of ageing.

Most opioids are probably similar in their constipating potency. However, there is evidence that transdermal fentanyl is somewhat less constipating than morphine (Radbruch et al., 2000) or oxycodone (Ackerman et al., 2004), the same probably being also true of other lipophilic opioids such as buprenorphine and alfentanil that require only relatively small doses to be given in order to achieve central nervous system penetration. Methadone analgesia has been associated with lower laxative requirements than the use of either morphine (Daeninck and Bruera, 1999) or hydromorphone (Mancini et al., 2000). This has been attributed to the effects of methadone being only partly mediated through opioid receptors as a result of its N-methyl-D-aspartate receptor activity. Tramadol and tapentadol, also opioids whose actions are partly mediated via other receptor types, may also be less constipating than morphine but are also less potent analgesics.

A group of drugs frequently used in palliative care that exacerbate constipation are those with anticholinergic effects, such as tricyclics, antihistamines, and neuroleptics. This effect is unsurprising, given the role of ACh as the chief stimulant neurotransmitter for peristalsis.

Box 10.3.1 Causes of constipation in palliative medicine

Malignancy

Directly due to tumour:

- Intestinal obstruction due to (i) tumour in the bowel wall or(ii) external compression by abdominal or pelvic tumour
- Damage to lumbosacral spinal cord, cauda equina or pelvic plexus
- Hypercalcaemia.

  Due to secondary effects of disease:

- Inadequate food intake
- Low-fibre diet
- Dehydration
- Weakness
- Inactivity
- Confusion
- Depression
- Unfamiliar toilet arrangements.

Drugs

- Opioids
- Drugs with anticholinergic effects:
  - Hyoscine
  - Phenothiazines
  - Tricyclic antidepressants
  - Antiparkinsonian agents
- Antacids (calcium and aluminium compounds)
- Diuretics
- Anticonvulsants
- Iron
- Antihypertensive agents
- Vincristine.

Concurrent disease

- Diabetes
- Hypothyroidism
- Hypokalaemia
- Hernia
- Diverticular disease
- Rectocele
- Anal fissure or stenosis
- Anterior mucosal prolapse
- Haemorrhoids
- Colitis.

Diagnosis

Assessment

It is the frequency and difficulty of defecation that are the basis for the diagnosis of constipation and, given the normal variability of bowel habit, should be compared with the pre-illness pattern. Abdominal examination and, unless there has been a recent full evacuation, rectal examination, will help to avoid the major pitfalls in the diagnosis of constipation in palliative medicine. These are:

Impaction, presenting as diarrhoea, often with incontinence

This occurs characteristically in elderly patients in whom confusion or rectal insensitivity leads to the formation of a large faecal mass that is impossible to pass spontaneously. Semi-liquid faecal material from higher in the colon seeps past the mass, appearing as diarrhoea and, if the closing pressure of the anal sphincters has been exceeded by the mass, faecal leakage or incontinence. Most faecal impactions are low enough to be apparent on rectal examination.

Intestinal obstruction by tumour or adhesions

Known intra-abdominal malignant deposits, previous intestinal surgery, alternating constipation and diarrhoea, gut colic, and nausea and vomiting combine to suggest the presence of intestinal obstruction. A similar picture can, however, occur in severe constipation. The distinction is important, as attempts to clear 'constipation' which is actually obstruction, by use of stimulant laxatives can cause severe pain. A plain abdominal radiograph may help clarify the diagnosis.

Nausea

Some patients rapidly experience nausea, with or without vomiting, in the presence of intestinal hold-up (Twycross and Lack, 1986a). Unexplained nausea or vomiting should prompt enquiry and examination for constipation.

Abdominal pain

The effort of colonic muscle to propel hard faeces commonly causes abdominal pain, frequently colicky in nature. Such pain may be particularly marked—and difficult to diagnose—where abdominal or pelvic tumour exists, presumably as a result either of pressure on the tumour from distended gut or because of partial intestinal obstruction. Abdominal palpation may reveal faecal masses in the line of the descending colon and even that of the more proximal colon and caecum. The distinction between tumour and faecal masses can be hard to make. Faeces will usually indent, if the patient will tolerate sufficiently firm pressure, and may give a crepitus-like sensation because of entrained gas. They also move, given time. Occasionally an abdominal radiograph is needed to distinguish tumour from stool.

The complete absence of stool on rectal examination implies colonic inertia. Rectal examination may also uncover rectal tumour, a rectocele, solitary rectal ulcer, or anal stenosis. A lax anal sphincter may indicate spinal cord damage associated with colonic hypotonia. If a rectocele or compression from pelvic tumour masses is suspected, vaginal examination may be justifiable.

Examination of the stool itself can be useful. Small, hard pellets suggest slow colonic transit, ribbon-like stools suggest stenosis or haemorrhoids, and blood or mucus suggests tumour, haemorrhoids, or coexisting colitis.

Urinary incontinence

Faecal impaction is a well-recognized precipitant of urinary incontinence in the elderly, and the recent onset of incontinence should indicate abdominal and rectal examination as the first investigative steps.

Investigations

Investigations are rarely needed in the assessment of constipation in palliative medicine. Abdominal radiography may distinguish between constipation and obstruction if there is persisting doubt, but is rarely necessary and should certainly not be a standard procedure.

Blood tests are even more rarely needed but, but if the clinical picture is suggestive, corrected calcium levels and thyroid function tests should be performed.

Measurement tools

Patients' perception of their constipation can be formally assessed by use of visual analogue (VAS) or verbal rating scales, or questionnaires. A discrete response modification of the VAS and a verbal rating scale have each been found to have validity and to be easy to use in a palliative care setting (Sykes, 2001). Since the most common cause of diarrhoea in palliative care is the treatment of constipation (Twycross and Lack, 1986b) it is appropriate that any subjective measure of bowel function includes the ability to assess not only constipation but also diarrhoea as well. This is easily applied with VAS and adjectival scales, but is lacking in the questionnaires that have been validated only for the assessment of constipation, such as the well-established Constipation Assessment Scale (McMillan and Williams, 1989), the PAC-SYM (Patient Assessment of Constipation Symptoms) (Frank et al., 1999), or the newer Constipation Severity Instrument (Varma et al., 2008). In contrast, the Victoria Bowel Performance Scale was designed for use in palliative care and assesses both constipation and diarrhoea equally (Downing et al., 2007). It has proved acceptable to staff in this setting and capable of influencing improvement in constipation management (Hawley et al., 2011).

The aspects of bowel function that are objectively measurable by direct assessment are stool frequency and form. Simply counting the number of occasions when some stool has been passed may be misleading in making a diagnosis of the presence or absence of constipation: a frequent loose stool may indicate not diarrhoea but faecal impaction with overflow. What is more helpful is to count only episodes of formed stool leading to a sense of reasonably complete rectal evacuation. The basis of comparison is the individual's previous normal pattern, as the range of normal bowel movement frequency is very wide, ranging from three to 21 stools per week (Connell et al., 1965).

The shape of the stools is a guide to their consistency and has also been shown to be correlated with bowel transit time in both idiopathic constipation and palliative care cancer populations (O'Donnell et al., 1990; Sykes, 1990). With the aid of illustrated charts, of which the Bristol Stool Form Scale (Fig. 10.3.1) is best known, patients can estimate stool form reliably for themselves as an adjunct to recording stool frequency.

Scoring systems for radiological assessment of constipation exist, including in palliative care (Bruera et al., 1994), but have been heavily criticized for their unreliability (Jackson et al., 2009).

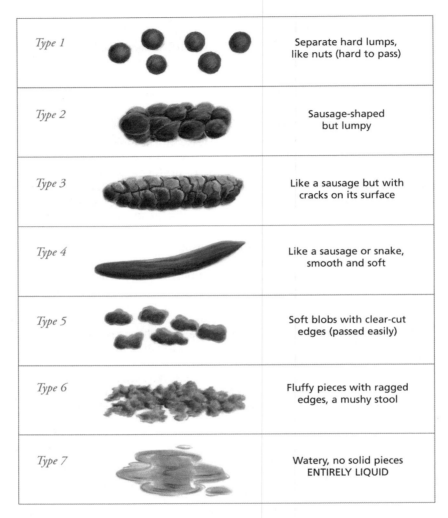

THE BRISTOL STOOL FORM SCALE

Type 1		Separate hard lumps, like nuts (hard to pass)
Type 2		Sausage-shaped but lumpy
Type 3		Like a sausage but with cracks on its surface
Type 4		Like a sausage or snake, smooth and soft
Type 5		Soft blobs with clear-cut edges (passed easily)
Type 6		Fluffy pieces with ragged edges, a mushy stool
Type 7		Watery, no solid pieces ENTIRELY LIQUID

Fig. 10.3.1 The Bristol Stool Form Scale.
Reproduced by kind permission of Dr K.W. Heaton, formerly Reader in Medicine at the University of Bristol. © 2000–2014 Norgine group of companies.

Treatment

Good overall symptom management sets the best context for relief of constipation. Thus, tackling pain and breathlessness with the aid of both drugs and physiotherapy will maximize mobility; control of nausea and provision of a tailored diet containing as much fibre as tolerable will maximize dietary intake; and encouragement of fluids will minimize dehydration. The sum effect of all these interventions will be to normalize as far as possible the gut's working environment.

Despite these measures most patients with advanced disease will need additional assistance in order to avoid constipation. Some will wish to use non-pharmaceutical methods initially or on an ongoing basis. Herbal remedies may contain the same types of chemical as proprietary laxatives and so will have a similar effectiveness, albeit less predictable because less standardized. However, there is little or no evidence for other complementary approaches to constipation, whose principal contribution is likely to be to the overall sense of well-being of the patient rather than the specific relief of their constipation. The best support is for abdominal massage, which can equal the effect of a regular laxative regimen but at a significantly greater cost in terms of staff time (Emly et al., 1998).

The predominant action of laxative agents can be characterized as either softening the stool or stimulating peristalsis. Clinical experience has suggested that, although initially a softening laxative alone may be adequate, more severe constipation tends to respond best to a combination of the two types (Larkin et al., 2008). There is some experimental support for this view from a study conducted on healthy volunteers using a model of opioid-induced constipation. Here the combination of a stimulant and a softening laxative resulted in fewer adverse effects, such as colic, and a lower medication burden than the use of either type of laxative on its own (Sykes, 1997). However, a study in cancer patients failed to show a clear advantage to the addition of a softener (docusate) to a stimulant (senna) (Hawley and Byeon, 2008) and the stimulant sodium picosulfate has been found to be effective and well tolerated when used as a single agent in a palliative care population ((Twycross et al., 2006).

A systematic review of laxative use in the elderly found that any laxative would increase bowel frequency by about 1.4 stools per week compared with placebo (Petticrew et al., 1997). Given the lack of evidence for true differences in efficacy and their generally mediocre palatability (Morrison and Pirrello, 2011), the choice of laxative should be strongly influenced by patient preference and by cost.

Stimulant laxatives

Examples include senna, bisacodyl, dantron, and sodium picosulfate. These drugs differ in the extent to which they require activation by colonic bacteria and are subject to hepatic recirculation. They all act on the myenteric plexus to stimulate intestinal contraction. Concerns about carcinogenicity with continued use appear to be unsupported in practice (Nusko et al., 2000). However, dantron is subject to a limited licence in some countries for this reason and also has the potential to cause perianal skin rashes in incontinent patients.

$5\text{-}HT_4$ agonists, of which tegaserod is currently licensed in some countries, may also be considered stimulant laxatives in that they reinforce normal enteric neuronal stimulation of peristalsis (Kamm et al., 2005). Whether they are effective in situations where the enteric nervous system is damaged, as in some cases of cancer-related constipation, has not been demonstrated.

Softening laxatives

All these preparations primarily soften the stool, making it easier to pass, but do so by different mechanisms.

Osmotic agents retain water within the gut lumen. Sugars, such as lactulose, act in their native form in the small bowel before being broken down by colonic flora to organic acids whose pH-lowering effect is speculated to enhance motility and secretion in the proximal colon (Jouet et al., 2008). In practice, lactulose is a relatively weak laxative and gives rise to flatulence in about 20% of patients. Conversely, inorganic osmotic substances such as magnesium hydroxide or sulphate are not absorbed and so maintain their osmotic potency throughout the intestine. They also appear capable of stimulating peristalsis and at higher doses give a pronounced purgative effect.

Surfactants such as docusate or poloxamer increase water penetration of the stools. Docusate also promotes water, sodium, and chloride secretion in the jejunum and colon, but its efficacy has been questioned (Hurdon et al., 2000).

Macrogols, such as polyethylene glycol, render water unabsorbable by the gut. Their effect therefore depends on the volume of water in which they are dissolved. Secondarily this also contributes to stimulation of gut contraction as a reflex response to distension. Macrogols are now one of the best-evidenced groups of laxatives (American College of Gastroenterology, 2005) and have been shown to be an effective oral treatment for faecal impaction (Culbert et al., 1998), but this may require the daily consumption of a litre of the solution, which not all patients can tolerate.

Chloride channel activator: lubiprostone is to date the only example of this mode of action. Acting on type 2 chloride channels on the apical surface of the luminal epithelium, it increases secretions without electrolyte disturbance. A secondary effect on motility is claimed and both small and large bowel transit is accelerated (Camilleri et al., 2006).

Bulk-forming agents such as psyllium and methyl cellulose increase the size of stools partly by providing material that resists bacterial breakdown and hence remains in the gut, and partly by providing a substrate for bacterial growth and gas production. Effective in mild constipation, they are less helpful in cancer patients for three main reasons. First, they need to be taken with at least 200–300 mL of water; this and their consistency are unacceptable to many people who feel unwell. Second, if taken with inadequate water, a viscous mass may result, which can complete an incipient malignant obstruction. Third, their effectiveness in severe constipation is doubtful.

The key to using general laxatives such as those mentioned above is to titrate the dose against response. This implies that there is in place some disciplined follow-up of patients' perception of their bowel function, preferably assisted by recording of the frequency and type of bowel actions passed. Common practice has been to initiate laxative therapy with a softening agent. However, there is growing evidence that a stimulant laxative which, although principally having a motor effect will also to some extent soften stool through both reducing the time available for water absorption and a direct secretory action, may be a more effective single-agent choice. Addition of a softener is indicated if colic occurs.

If oral laxatives are inadequate, recourse can be had to rectal interventions: suppositories, enemas, or, at the last resort and with appropriate analgesia and sedation, manual evacuation of the rectum. Anything introduced into the rectum may induce defecation via the ano-colic reflex, but suppositories may additionally have an osmotic softening action (glycerine or sodium phosphate) or may locally stimulate peristalsis (bisacodyl). Enemas may lubricate (olive or arachis oils) or soften via osmotic (sorbitol, sodium phosphate, or sodium citrate) or surfactant (sodium docusate, sodium lauryl, or alkyl sulphoacetate) actions. Attention to laxative dosing can halve the use of enemas and suppositories (Sykes, 1991). This is important not only because of the staff time involved but also because rectal laxatives are widely disliked, with only 17% preferring suppositories or enemas to oral laxatives. Nevertheless, it has been reported that among late-stage cancer patients 72% have received suppositories and 65% an enema, with no less than 40% continuing to receive them on an ongoing basis (Droney et al., 2008).

Newer developments

The limitations of existing general laxatives have led to interest in finding specific agents for opioid-induced constipation. As the constipating action of opioids is predominantly peripheral in man, mediated via opioid receptors in the gut itself, an opioid antagonist could prevent or relieve this provided it did not reach the opioid receptors in the central nervous system responsible for analgesia. Two opioid antagonists are currently licensed for this indication.

Methylnaltrexone is a quaternary derivative of the mu-opioid antagonist naltrexone whose polarity prevents it from crossing the blood–brain barrier. It is administered by subcutaneous injection and in a series of 134 patients who were taking regular opioids and had advanced disease was significantly (p < 0.0001) more likely than placebo to induce a bowel action. Median time to response was 0.5 hours (Thomas et al., 2008). For patients who had not responded to the first dose the chance of a bowel movement response to a second dose was 35% and to those who had not responded to either of the first two doses there was a 26% response rate to a third dose (Chamberlain et al., 2009). If no response has been obtained after three methylnaltrexone doses it is appropriate to seek other remedies. The overall response rate in this sample was about 50%, probably indicating the important role of other constipating factors even where opioids are involved. The observed adverse effects did not suggest any methylnaltrexone antagonism of central effects of opioids.

Methylnaltrexone appears appropriate to use when constipation is associated with opioid use, has not been satisfactorily controlled with general laxatives by mouth and either an enema or suppositories are being considered (Fig. 10.3.2). For a few people, methylnaltrexone may become their routine therapy for constipation but the excess cost over existing laxatives is considerable, and it seems likely that for most patients the role of methylnaltrexone will be to remove an accumulation of stool and allow a fresh start to be made on laxative therapy in order to establish an effective regimen.

Early work with naloxone administered orally for opioid-induced constipation found an unacceptable occurrence of opioid withdrawal or return of pain, despite the drug having only a 1–3% bioavailability by this route (Sykes, 2005). However, an oral sustained-release combination of oxycodone and naloxone in a fixed 1:2 dose ratio has been licensed as an analgesic with the claimed advantage of reducing the risk of opioid-induced constipation. There is evidence that it reduces the perceived severity of constipation and also increases bowel movement frequency (Vondrackova et al., 2008). The ability to improve constipation while preserving analgesia compared with use of oxycodone alone was confirmed in a group of cancer patients (Ahmedzai et al., 2011). These studies did not show an excess of opioid withdrawal effects, perhaps as a result of the lower peak of naloxone absorption achieved through use of the sustained-release mechanism rather than the immediate-release formulation employed in previous studies. It might be noted that the low oral bioavailability of naloxone depends on rapid metabolism by the liver: in hepatic impairment blood levels can be very much greater. Patients with impaired liver function were excluded from trials of the oxycodone/naloxone combination.

A suggested guide to the management of constipation in palliative care is given in Fig. 10.3.2.

Diarrhoea

Diarrhoea is the passage of frequent loose stools with urgency. Objectively, it has been defined as the passage of more than three unformed stools (Bristol stool forms 5–7 (see Figure 10.3.1)) within a 24-hour period. Patients, however, may describe as 'diarrhoea' a single loose stool, frequent small stools of normal or even hard consistency, or faecal incontinence. As with constipation, a complaint of diarrhoea requires careful clarification.

Prevalence of diarrhoea

Diarrhoea is a complaint of 7–10% of cancer patients on admission to a hospice and 6% of similar patients in hospital. It is, therefore, a far less common problem in palliative medicine than constipation when cancer patients are being considered, but 27% of symptomatic HIV-infected patients have been reported to suffer diarrhoea (Rolston et al., 1989) (for management of HIV-related diarrhoea, see Chapter 15.1.).

Clinical manifestations and diagnostic considerations

Diarrhoea persisting for over 3 weeks is said to be chronic and is often linked to serious organic disease. Most diarrhoea is acute, lasting only a few days, and is generally the result of gastrointestinal infection (Box 10.3.2), possibly including overgrowth by *Candida*.

However, the commonest cause of diarrhoea in palliative medicine is an imbalance of laxative therapy (Twycross and Lack, 1986b). This particularly occurs when laxative doses have been increased to clear a backlog of constipated stool. The diarrhoea normally settles within 24–48 hours if laxatives are temporarily stopped, after which they should be reinstated at a lower dose. Meanwhile the diarrhoea may be distressing, especially if it leads to faecal incontinence.

A variety of other common drugs can also precipitate diarrhoea, either commonly, as in the case of antacids and antibiotics, or idiosyncratically, as in the case of non-steroidal anti-inflammatory agents or iron preparations. Sorbitol, used as a sweetener in some 'sugar-free' elixirs, is easily overlooked as a cause of diarrhoea in sensitive patients. Those receiving enteral feeding appear particularly prone, sorbitol being more than twice as likely to be the cause of diarrhoea as the feed itself (Edes et al., 1990).

Malignant intestinal obstruction and faecal impaction are the next most common causes of diarrhoea in this patient group. Complete intestinal obstruction produces intractable constipation, but partial obstruction may present with either diarrhoea or alternating diarrhoea and constipation. This clinical picture can also result from severe constipation caused by opioid analgesia, where it has been dubbed the 'narcotic bowel syndrome' (Sandgren et al., 1984). Faecal impaction results in fluid stool leaking past the mass, often with anal leakage or incontinence. In elderly patients hospitalized for non-malignant disease, faecal impaction can account for 55% of instances of diarrhoea (Kinnunen et al., 1989), emphasizing the need for careful attention to regular laxative therapy in any ill, relatively immobile population.

Many disease-modifying medication used in the palliative management of advanced cancer can cause diarrhoea. Certain cytotoxic chemotherapy agents most commonly 5-fluorouracil, capecitabine, and irinotecan (CPT-11) can cause severe diarrhoea through epithelial necrosis and inflammation leading to a loss of absorptive surface and an imbalance between absorptive and secretory cells (Kornblau et al., 2000). Interleukin-2 therapy can also cause severe watery diarrhoea. Additionally, almost all of the recently developed small-molecule-targeted therapies cause

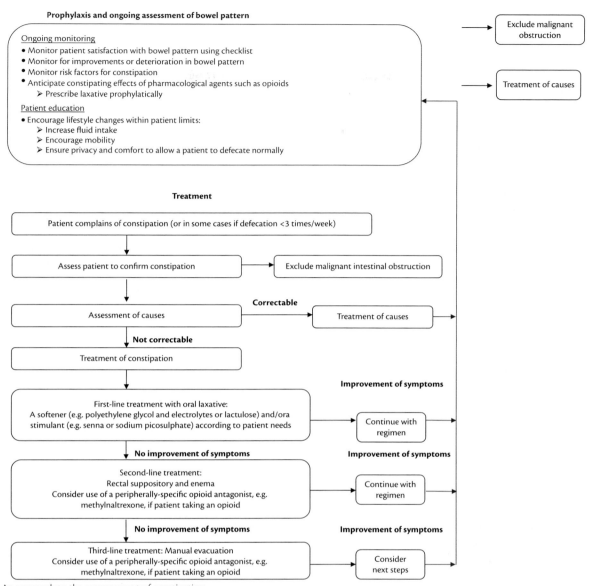

Fig. 10.3.2 An approach to the management of constipation.

Adapted with permission from Larkin P, et al., The management of constipation in palliative care: clinical practice recommendations, *Palliative Medicine*, Volume 22, Issue 7, pp. 796–807, Copyright © 2008 SAGE Publications Ltd.

diarrhoea as a side effect. Diarrhoea, which can be severe, has been reported in 30–50% of patients receiving bortezomib, erlotinib, gefitinib, sorafenib, sunitinib, and imatinib, and the m-Tor inhibitors temsirolimus and everolimus. The monoclonal therapies targeting the epidermal growth factor receptor, cetuximab and panitumumab, both cause diarrhoea in 10–20% of patients which may be severe in a small subset of patients.

High volume diarrhoea can be a feature of graft-versus-host disease (GVHD) resulting from an allogeneic stem cell or bone marrow transplant into an immuno-compromised recipient, and may be life-threatening. The diarrhoea can persist into chronic GVHD, where rather than the intense mucosal inflammation seen in acute GVHD the cause may be infection, motility disturbance, or malabsorption secondary to pancreatic insufficiency (Lee et al., 2003).

Radiotherapy involving the abdomen or pelvis is liable to cause diarrhoea, with a peak incidence in the second or third week of therapy and continuing for some time after cessation of the course. Damage to intestinal mucosa by radiation results in the release of prostaglandins and the malabsorption of bile salts, both of which increase peristaltic activity. Chronic radiation enteritis rarely presents as diarrhoea.

Uncommonly, another iatrogenic cause of diarrhoea relevant to palliative care is coeliac plexus blockade, which can be associated with the onset of profuse, long-lasting watery diarrhoea. This possibly results from anatomical variations in the innervation of the gut so that in certain individuals interruption of the coeliac plexus has an excessive influence on bowel activity (Dean and Reed, 1991).

Box 10.3.2 Causes of diarrhoea in palliative medicine

- Drugs:
  - Laxatives
  - Antacids
  - Antibiotics
  - Chemotherapy
  - NSAID, especially mefenamic acid, diclofenac, indomethacin
  - Mitomycin
  - Iron preparations
  - Disaccharide-containing elixirs
- Radiation
- Graft-versus-host disease
- Obstruction:
  - Malignant
  - Faecal impaction
  - Narcotic bowel syndrome
- Malabsorption:
  - Pancreatic carcinoma
  - Gastrectomy
  - Ileal resection
  - Colectomy
- Tumour:
  - Colonic or rectal carcinoma
  - Pancreatic islet cell tumours
  - Carcinoid tumours
- Concurrent disease:
  - Diabetes mellitus
  - Hyperthyroidism
  - Inflammatory bowel disease
  - Irritable bowel syndrome
  - Gastrointestinal infection
- Diet:
  - Bran
  - Fruit
  - Hot spices
  - Alcohol.

Malabsorption sufficient to cause diarrhoea may occur in carcinoma of the head of the pancreas or after gastrectomy or ileal resection. Failure of pancreatic secretion leads to reduced fat absorption and consequent steatorrhoea. Gastrectomy can also produce steatorrhoea, presumably as a result of poor mixing of food with pancreatic and biliary secretions. However, the accompanying vagotomy causes increased faecal secretion of bile acids

in some patients, resulting in increased water and electrolyte secretion in the colon and hence a chologenic diarrhoea, compounding the problem.

A different type of malabsorption that can be seen in palliative care patients treated with antibiotics, or as a complication of gut infection such as *Clostridium difficile*, is lactose intolerance secondary to changes in the intestinal flora. This will gradually correct itself but meanwhile a lactose-free diet produces prompt resolution of the diarrhoea (Noble at al., 2002).

Ileal resection reduces the gut's ability to reabsorb bile acids, of which up to 97% are normally recirculated, again producing chologenic diarrhoea, which is characteristically watery and explosive. If less than 100 cm of terminal ileum is removed, fat malabsorption generally does not occur, as the liver can compensate for the increased biliary loss. A resection of over about 100 cm results in relative bile acid deficiency and hence fat malabsorption, exacerbating the diarrhoea. Ileal resection also produces a disaccharidase deficiency proportional to the length of removed and thus an osmotic diarrhoea due to carbohydrate malabsorption.

Partial colectomy produces little, if any, persistent diarrhoea. However, total or almost total colectomy results in a high volume of liquid effluent that rapidly diminishes over 7–10 days but still remains at 400–800 mL/day owing to the small intestine's inability to compensate fully for the loss of the colon's water absorbing capacity. For this reason an ileostomy is normally fashioned. Such patients require an average of an extra litre of water per day and about 7 g of extra salt to compensate, with special care needed in hot weather. Iron and vitamin supplementation is also indicated. Similar symptoms can also result from an enterocolic fistula, caused either by cancer or as a result of operation (Mercadante, 1992). Alteration of gut anatomy by surgery may also promote diarrhoea through bacterial overgrowth.

A colonic or rectal tumour can precipitate diarrhoea through causing partial intestinal obstruction, or loosen stools through increased mucus secretion. Rarely, endocrine tumours cause a secretory diarrhoea. The WDHA syndrome (watery diarrhoea hypokalaemia achlorhydria) is associated with tumours of the pancreatic islet cells and of the sympathetic nervous system, including the adrenal glands, and can occur with bronchogenic carcinomas. VIP is thought to be the causative hormone both here and in the diarrhoea of the Verner–Morrison syndrome encountered in childhood ganglioneuroblastoma. Diarrhoea occurs also in the Zollinger– Ellison syndrome, seen with pancreatic islet cell tumours secreting gastrin, and in carcinoid tumours, where serotonin, prostaglandins, bradykinin, and VIP secretions have all been implicated.

Apart from concurrent gastrointestinal disease, the ability of dietary factors to cause diarrhoea should be remembered. Excessive dietary fibre may produce diarrhoea and fruits may do so both by this means and by their content of specific laxative factors.

Assessment

A complaint of diarrhoea demands a careful history, detailing first of all the frequency of defecation, the nature of the stools, and the time course of the problem. Together, these often indicate the diagnosis. Defecation described as 'diarrhoea', which occurs only once or twice a day, suggests anal incontinence. Profuse watery stools are characteristic of colonic diarrhoea, whereas the pale, fatty, offensive stools of steatorrhoea indicate malabsorption due to a pancreatic or small intestinal cause. The sudden advent of diarrhoea following a period of constipation, perhaps with little warning of impending defecation, should raise the suspicion of faecal impaction.

Both current and recent medication should be sought. If laxatives are to blame, the error may be of insufficiently regular therapy, resulting in alternating constipation and diarrhoea, or an excessive dose. Too much of a predominantly peristalsis-stimulating laxative tends to produce colic and urgency, and too much of a predominantly stool-softening agent may cause faecal leakage, although at high doses lactulose and docusate have the ability to produce colic and watery diarrhoea in some patients.

The occurrence of pyrexia, blood in the stools, or dehydration as features of diarrhoea should be watched out for, as they signal the presence of potentially life-threatening complications and the need for more intensive support and intervention. In a palliative care context this situation is principally likely to arise as a result of recent cytotoxic chemotherapy. Diarrhoea in the presence of neutropenia should suggest the presence of neutropenic enterocolitis in which mucosal ulceration occurs, allowing bacterial and fungal invasion and consequent septicaemia as well as the possibility of intestinal perforation. Incidence has been reported to be 5% or more in adults receiving chemotherapy for solid malignancies and the condition carries a mortality of 30–50% (Ullery et al., 2009).

Examination and investigations

Examination should exclude the possibilities of faecal impaction and intestinal obstruction, and should therefore include rectal examination and abdominal palpation for faecal masses. If there is doubt, an abdominal radiograph will make the distinction, but this is rarely necessary.

Steatorrhoea is generally clearly suggested in the history and readily confirmed on examination of the stool. Persistent watery diarrhoea, without systemic upset, which would suggest an infective cause, may be more difficult to diagnose. If in doubt, the stool osmolality and sodium and potassium concentrations should be measured. The anion gap, the difference between the stool osmolality and double the sum of the cation concentrations, is over 50 mmol/L in osmotic diarrhoea, because of the presence of an additional non-absorbed solute, for example, a disaccharide from a medicinal elixir. An anion gap of below 50 mmol/L shows secretory diarrhoea, resulting from active secretion of fluid and electrolytes, as in the WDHA syndrome. Ileal resection gives rise to a mixed picture, which will become purely secretory if the patient can be fasted.

In any persistent diarrhoea, haematology and blood chemistry should be checked.

Diarrhoea occurring within 3 days of inpatient admission may be due to community-acquired bacterial enteric pathogens such as *Salmonella*, *Shigella*, or *Campylobacter*, or to viral infection. After this point the infection is likely to have originated in the inpatient unit and stool culture is usually unrewarding; repeating the culture does not improve the diagnostic yield (Chitkara et al., 1996). *Clostridium difficile* is the most commonly detected cause of nosocomial diarrhoea and is associated with antibiotic treatment, particularly quinolones or cephalosporins. It affects predominantly the over 65 age group, in whom its incidence in the United States more than doubled between 2000 and 2005 (Lessa et al., 2012). This rise has been accompanied by an increase in multidrug resistance. Although there is evidence that stricter antibiotic and hospital hygiene policies are slowing the rate of rise in incidence, *Clostridium difficile* diarrhoea is still common and may be life-threatening unless diagnosed and treated with appropriate antimicrobials as directed by stool sample analysis.

Management approaches

Supportive treatment

Other than in HIV infection or as a result of chemotherapy, diarrhoea in palliative medicine is rarely severe or prolonged enough to cause significant risk through dehydration. If rehydration *is* needed, the oral route is superior to the intravenous. Proprietary rehydration solutions, containing appropriate electrolyte concentrations and a source of glucose to facilitate active electrolyte transport across the gut wall, are adequate for all but the most severe diarrhoea. Any diarrhoea will benefit from a diet of clear liquids, such as flat lemonade or ginger ale, and simple carbohydrates, as in toast or crackers. Some infective causes of diarrhoea cause transient lactase deficiency and so milk should be avoided in these circumstances (Noble et al., 2002). Protein and, later, fats are reintroduced gradually to the diet as the diarrhoea resolves.

NCI grade 3 or 4 diarrhoea, characterized by pyrexia, neutropenia, dehydration or bloody stools, requires inpatient management with intravenous fluid support, octreotide with or without opioid antidiarrhoeals (see 'General treatment'), assessment of stool for the presence of infection (*Clostridium difficile*, *Salmonella*, *Escherischia coli*, and *Campylobacter*) and antibiotic treatment as indicated (Benson et al., 2004). Neutropenic colitis may also involve fungal infection, principally by *Candida* spp., and there is some indication of reduced mortality if antifungal therapy is provided (Cardona Zorrilla et al., 2006). Management may also entail administration of granulocyte colony-stimulating factor or resection of the affected bowel (Ullery et al., 2009) and hence should be carried out in a setting where such options are available.

Specific treatment

Specific treatments exist for several causes of diarrhoea. Pancreatin is a combination of amylase, lipase, and protease, which is available in several forms for pancreatic enzyme replacement. The effective dose varies widely between individuals and it may be more effective if gastric acidity is reduced with an H_2-receptor antagonist, in which case enteric-coated preparations should not be used.

Cholestyramine is a bile acid-binding resin that is effective in controlling chologenic diarrhoea provided ileal resection has not been too extensive. It is often found unpalatable. Sulfasalazine appears in clinical practice guidelines for prophylaxis of radiation-induced diarrhoea (Rubenstein et al., 2004), while both cholestyramine (Condon et al., 1996) and aspirin (Mennie et al., 1975) have been claimed to be effective for its treatment. However, 5-aminosalicylic acid (Baughan et al., 1993) and mesalazine (Resbuet et al., 1997) have been found ineffective for this type of diarrhoea.

Carcinoid syndrome diarrhoea often responds to general antidiarrhoeals, but peripheral serotonin antagonists, such as methysergide or the less toxic cyproheptadine, have been used against more severe diarrhoea and, sometimes, the accompanying malabsorption. $5-HT_3$ antagonists may also have a role in this type of diarrhoea (Saslow et al., 1998).

Metronidazole remains the first-line antibiotic for *Clostridium difficile* diarrhoea, and can reasonably be tried also in situations where diarrhoea is suspected to be due to bacterial overgrowth, where it may produce a prompt resolution.

General treatment

Non-specific antidiarrhoeal agents are numerous, but are either absorbent, adsorbent, mucosal prostaglandin inhibitors, opioids, or somatostatin derivatives. These agents may make illness due to *Shigella* and *Clostridium difficile* worse and so should be used with caution if these organisms are known to be present, or if there is blood in the stool, or fever.

Absorbent agents absorb water to form a gelatinous or colloidal mass that gives a thicker consistency to loose stools. Examples are pectin and bulk-forming agents such as methyl cellulose. Bulk-forming agents may have a delay of up to 48 hours in onset of antidiarrhoeal action and are poorly tolerated in ill patients. They have proved useful in the management of colostomies but exacerbate electrolyte loss from ileostomies. The use of pectin is time-honoured and there is some evidence of effectiveness in children (de la Motte et al., 1997).

Adsorbent agents non-specifically take up dissolved or suspended substances, such as bacteria, toxins, and water, on to their surfaces. All are naturally occurring minerals, for example, kaolin and attapulgite. Attapulgite has been shown to be better than placebo in acute diarrhoea although significantly less effective than loperamide (DuPont et al., 1990). Kaolin is often combined with morphine as an antidiarrhoeal mixture and there is no evidence for efficacy separate from that of the opioid.

Mucosal prostaglandin inhibitors inhibit intestinal water and electrolyte secretion. Bismuth subsalicylate has a direct antimicrobial effect on enterotoxigenic *Escherichia coli*, but no more than that of wine (Weisse et al., 1995), and is used for treatment of non-specific acute diarrhoea. Aspirin is used as a specific antidiarrhoeal treatment for radiation-induced diarrhoea, and mesalazine for ulcerative colitis.

Opioid agents act via specific gut opioid receptors to reduce peristalsis, and possibly water and electrolyte secretion, in the colon. The opioids are the mainstay of general antidiarrhoeal treatment in palliative medicine and a requirement for morphine analgesia may obviate the need for any additional antidiarrhoeal medication. Loperamide is the opioid antidiarrhoeal of choice, as it does not reach or cross the blood–brain barrier significantly and so causes few adverse effects, at least in adults (Ruppin, 1987). It is significantly more effective than diphenoxylate or codeine, both of which are prone to cause systemic opioid effects. Diphenoxylate is available only in combination with atropine in order to limit its abuse potential. Codeine is cheap.

In man, approximate equivalent antidiarrhoeal doses are 200 mg/day of codeine, 10 mg/day of diphenoxylate, and 4 mg/day of loperamide (Twycross and Lack, 1986b). Despite the research evidence, clinical experience suggests that the individual response to opioids for diarrhoea can be as idiosyncratic as that for pain, and in some patients codeine has superior antidiarrhoeal properties to the other opioids without causing excessive nausea or drowsiness. Opioids increase anal sphincter pressure, and loperamide and codeine have been shown to improve continence in patients with diarrhoea suffering from faecal incontinence (Palmer et al., 1980).

Somatostatin analogues mimic the activity of the natural gut hormone on intestinal epithelial receptors to inhibit secretion and peristalsis. Octreotide has been shown to be effective in cryptosporidial diarrhoea and diarrhoea due to the carcinoid, Zollinger–Ellison, and Verner–Morrison syndromes as well as to ileostomy (Riley and Fallon, 1994) or enterocolic fistula (Mercadante, 1992). Subcutaneous injection of octreotide may be painful, but continuous subcutaneous infusion is generally well tolerated and the drug can be combined with morphine, diamorphine, haloperidol, midazolam, or hyoscine without apparent loss of efficacy (Riley and Fallon, 1994). Mixing with cyclizine may cause precipitation.

Octreotide is established as an effective therapy for severe secretory diarrhoea, particularly that related to HIV infection, where doses up to 1500 micrograms/24 hours have been found necessary (Romeu et al., 1991). Expert consensus has recommended octreotide dose titration as high as 1500 micrograms/24 hours for chemotherapy-induced diarrhoea (Benson et al., 2004). Lanreotide has a far more prolonged duration of action and so requires neither frequent injections nor an infusion device, but is also less flexible for use in the continually changing clinical situations of palliative care.

New developments

Calcium carbonate 3.6 g/day reduced stool frequency by a mean of 49% and faecal wet weight by 50% over 12 weeks in 15 post-gut-resection patients. No change in plasma calcium concentrations was found (Steinbach et al., 1996). Results in healthy subjects have been variable and it was ineffective in nelfinavir-associated diarrhoea in HIV-positive patients (Jensen-Fangel et al., 2003).

There is increasing interest in the use of probiotics, or beneficial microorganisms, for the management of diarrhoea. *Lactobacillus* spp. are the most commonly used. There is some evidence that probiotics can be effective in infective diarrhoea in adults (Hickson, 2011) and in the management of acquired lactose intolerance (Noble et al., 2002).

The pathogenesis of diarrhoea frequently involves neurohumoral mechanisms controlling water secretion. Antagonists to 5-HT and substance P may prove clinically useful in the future, as may peptide YY and neuropeptide Y, both of which reduce intestinal fluid secretion and inhibit gut transit (Tough et al., 2011).

Online materials

Additional online materials and complete references for this chapter are available online at <http://www.oxfordmedicine.com>.

References

Connell, A.M., Hilton, C., Irvine, G., Lennard-Jones, J.E., and Misiewicz, J.J. (1965). Variation in bowel habit in two population samples. *British Medical Journal*, ii, 1095–1099.

Droney, J., Ross, J., Gretton, S., Welsh, K., Sato, H., and Riley, J. (2008). Constipation in cancer patients on morphine. *Supportive Care in Cancer*, 16, 453–459.

Goodman, M., Low, J., and Wilkinson, S. (2005). Constipation management in palliative care: a survey of practices in the UK. *Journal of Pain and Symptom Management*, 29, 238–244.

Hawley, P., Barwich, D., and Kirk, L. (2011). Implementation of the Victoria Bowel Performance Scale. *Journal of Pain and Symptom Management*, 42, 946–953.

Hawley, P.H. and Byeon, J.J. (2008). A comparison of sennosides-based protocols with and without docusate in hospitalised patients with cancer. *Journal of Palliative Medicine*, 11, 575–581.

Hurdon, V., Viola, R., and Schroder, C. (2000). How useful is docusate for patients at risk of constipation? A systematic review of the evidence in the chronically ill. *Journal of Pain and Symptom Management*, 19, 130–136.

Jackson, C.R., Lee, R.E., Wylie, A.B., Adams, C., and Jaffray, B. (2009). Diagnostic accuracy of the Barr and Blethyn radiological scoring systems for childhood constipation assessed using colonic transit time as the gold standard. *Pediatric Radiology*, 39, 664–667.

Kornblau, S., Benson, A.B., Catalano, R., *et al.* (2000). Management of cancer treatment-related diarrhea: issues and therapeutic strategies. *Journal of Pain and Symptom Management*, 19, 118–129.

Larkin, P., Sykes, N., Centeno, C., *et al.* (2008). The management of constipation in palliative care: clinical practice recommendations. *Palliative Medicine*, 22, 796–807.

Longstreth, G.F., Thompson, W.G., Chey, W.D., Houghton, L.A., Mearin, F., and Spiller, R.C (2006). Functional bowel disorders. *Gastroenterology*, 130, 1480–1491.

Mancini, I.L., Hanson, J., Neumann, C.M., and Bruera, E.D. (2000). Opioid type and other predictors of laxative dose in advanced cancer patienTS : a retrospective study. *Journal of Palliative Medicine*, 3, 49–56.

Nusko, G., Schneider, B., Schneider, I., Wittekind, C., and Hahn, E.G. (2000). Anthranoid laxative use is not a risk factor for colorectal neoplasia: results of a prospective case control study. *Gut*, 46, 651–655.

O'Donnell, L.J.D., Virjee, J., and Heaton, K.W. (1990). Detection of pseudodiarrhoea by simple clinical assessment of intestinal transit rate. *BMJ*, 300, 439–440.

Radbruch, L., Sabatowski, R., Loick, G., *et al.* (2000). Constipation and the use of laxatives: a comparison between transdermal fentanyl and oral morphine. *Palliative Medicine*, 14, 111–119.

Sykes, N.P. (1997). A volunteer model for the comparison of laxatives in opioid-induced constipation. *Journal of Pain and Symptom Management*, 11, 363–369.

Sykes, N.P. (1998). The relationship between opioid use and laxative use in terminally ill cancer patients. *Palliative Medicine*, 12, 375–382.

Sykes N.P. (2005). Using oral naloxone in the management of opioid bowel dysfunction. In C. S. Yuan (ed.) *Handbook of Opioid Bowel Syndrome*, pp. 175–195. New York: Haworth.

Thomas, J., Karver, S., Cooney, G.A., *et al.* (2008). A randomised, placebo-controlled trial of subcutaneous methylnaltrexone for the treatment of opioid-induced constipation in patients with advanced illness. *The New England Journal of Medicine*, 358, 2332–2334.

Walsh, D. and Nelson, K.A. (2002). Autonomic nervous system dysfunction in advanced cancer. *Supportive Care in Cancer*, 10, 523–528.

10.4

Jaundice, ascites, and encephalopathy

Jeremy Keen

Introduction to jaundice, ascites, and encephalopathy

For many people, jaundice will occur as part of an episode of acute, self-limiting, viral hepatitis but in the context of chronic hepatic disease or malignancy, the development of jaundice or ascites is usually an ominous indicator of advanced disease.

In two reported studies of individuals admitted to hospital with jaundice, 24% and 42% of patients with malignancy and 23% with cirrhosis died during their first admission (Whitehead et al., 2001; Bjornsson et al., 2003). The necessity of a willingness to adopt a 'palliative approach' to the care of such individuals is obvious.

This chapter will discuss three features of liver impairment that may be encountered in those for whom palliative care is appropriate but the review of ascites will concentrate on causes other than cirrhosis and portal hypertension.

Jaundice

The approach to the investigation and management of jaundice developing during palliative care should follow a logical progression which aids the difficult ethical decision-making which often arises. An indication of the frequency of disorders causing jaundice and a commonly used classification system are shown in Tables 10.4.1 and 10.4.2.

Pre-hepatic jaundice

Pre-hepatic causes of jaundice include Gilbert's syndrome, an inherited disorder characterized by mild chronic unconjugated hyperbilirubinaemia in the absence of liver disease or overt haemolysis. Between 3% and 10% of the general population may be affected by this syndrome and may demonstrate elevated bilirubin levels in response to stresses including fasting and comorbidity (Bosma et al., 1995). Therapeutic interventions for malignancy in individuals with Gilbert's may lead to hyperbilirubinaemia and mild jaundice (Wasserman et al., 1997; Engin et al., 2003; Ruiz-Arguelles et al., 2005) and there has been debate as to whether individuals with Gilbert's are more prone to toxic side effects with certain cytotoxic agents (Mandala et al., 2004). Prolonged parenteral nutrition has also been associated with hyperbilirubinaemia in individuals with Gilbert's syndrome (Au et al., 2004).

Hepatic jaundice

Hepatic causes of jaundice include any process which interferes with the excretion of conjugated bilirubin into the biliary system.

Table 10.4.1 Causes of jaundice in a series of 121 patients in Wales (Whitehead et al., 2001) and 171 patients in Sweden (Bjornsson et al., 2003)

Cause of jaundice	Wales (%)	Sweden (%)
Malignancy	35	33
Septicaemia	22	2.5
Cirrhosis	21	11
Gall stones	13	16
Drugs	6	1
Autoimmune hepatitis	1.5	2.5
Viral hepatitis	1.5	3.5

Source: Data from Whitehead MW et al., The causes of obvious jaundice in South West Wales: perceptions versus reality, *Gut*, Volume 48, Issue 3, pp.409-413, Copyright © 2001 and Bjornsson E et al., Severe jaundice in Sweden in the new millennium: causes, investigations, treatment and prognosis, *Scandinavian Journal of Gastroenterology*, Volume 38, Issue 1, pp.86–94, Copyright © 2003.

Such processes have either resulted in widespread necrosis of hepatocytes (hepatocellular jaundice) or impairment of bile excretory mechanisms (cholestatic jaundice). Worldwide, chronic viral and alcohol-related hepatitis are the major causes of hepatic jaundice. According to the most recent data, over 200 000 individuals

Table 10.4.2 A classification system for jaundice, with examples

Pre-hepatic	Hepatic	Post-hepatic
Gilbert's syndrome	Tumour infiltration	*Malignant:*
Haemolysis	Viral hepatitis	Pancreas
Haematoma	Drug toxicity	Ampulla
	(including alcohol)	Cholangiocarcinoma
	Cholestasis:	Lymphadenopathy
	Drugs	*Benign:*
	Septicaemia	Gall stones
	Parenteral nutrition	Chronic pancreatitis
	Graft-versus-host disease	Biliary stricture
	Venous outflow block:	
	Severe heart failure	
	Budd–Chiari syndrome	

in the United Kingdom are living with chronic hepatitis C infection. The number of hospital admissions and deaths with hepatitis C-related end-stage liver disease and hepatocellular carcinoma more than tripled between 1998 and 2010 (Health Protection Agency, 2012) and it is now one of the most common indications for liver transplant.

It is important to be aware of the existence and characteristics of chronic hepatitic viral infection in any individual for whom immunosuppressive therapy is being considered. Fulminant liver failure is a well-recognized complication of chemotherapy and other immunosuppressive therapy (allowing viral reactivation and proliferation) or, more frequently, its discontinuation (allowing a rebound immune and inflammatory response) (Xunrong et al., 2001; Esteve et al., 2004). Importantly, given their widespread use in palliative care, reactivation of hepatitis B infection has been related to the use of corticosteroids for comorbid conditions (Koga et al., 1992; Hammond et al., 1999) and the inclusion of steroids in cytotoxic regimens (Cheng et al., 2003; Yeo et al., 2004).

Hepatic failure after chronic infection with hepatitis B and/or C viruses is now a major cause of death for individuals infected with HIV (Williams, 2006). The Data Collection on Adverse Events of Anti-HIV Drugs study, which followed over 23 000 HIV-infected persons from three continents reported that 14.5% of deaths were from liver-related causes (Echejoh et al., 2006). Two post-mortem series from Nigeria and India noted the presence of tuberculous granulomata within the liver of individuals with AIDS as the most frequent abnormal histological finding (Amarapurkar and Sangle, 2005; Echejoh et al., 2006) and cholestatic, non-obstructive, jaundice has been described as a consequence of hepatic involvement in tuberculosis (Ghoda, 2005).

Drug-induced liver disease

Of hospital admissions for non-obstructive jaundice 2–7% have been reported to be drug induced (Ryder and Beckingham, 2001). Although most drug effects simply lead to an increase in serum liver enzymes, there is a significant mortality associated with the development of jaundice. Drug-induced liver disease accounts for over 50% of cases of acute liver failure in the United States of which approximately 70% relate to paracetamol overdose and the remainder a result of idiosyncratic reaction to one of over 600 medicinal compounds that have been reported to cause hepatotoxicity of one form or another (Bissell et al., 2001). A recent Swedish audit reported that 77 of 1164 new referrals to a hepatology clinic were deemed to have drug-induced liver disease with 29 having clinical jaundice (De Valle et al., 2006). Flucloxacillin, diclofenac, and ciprofloxacin were the most frequently associated drugs with mean lengths of exposure of 10, 23, and 6 days respectively.

Jaundice in drug-induced liver disease can be both hepatocellular and cholestatic such that histological findings include acute hepatocyte necrosis, chronic hepatitis, vascular injury, and bile ductular injury. Raised serum hepatic enzyme levels will usually rapidly return to normal after withdrawal of the offending drug (a reduction of 50% after 2 weeks and to baseline by 4 weeks is a general rule), but induced immune-mediated cholestatic reactions do have the potential for chronicity despite drug withdrawal (Table 10.4.3).

Complementary medications may be responsible for up to 5% of drug-induced liver disease and include preparations such as

Table 10.4.3 Drugs associated with immune-mediated liver disease

Hepatocellular reactions	Cholestatic/mixed reactions
Allopurinol	Amoxicillin/clavulanic acid
Germander (& other herbal medications)	Chlorpromazine/levomepromazine
	Erythromycin
Halothane	Tricyclic antidepressants
Minocycline	Fluoxetine
Phenytoin	Acetylcholinesterase inhibitors

germander and mistletoe (Harvey and Colin-Jones, 1981; Laliberte and Villeneuve, 1996).

There appears to be little evidence that there is an increased risk of drug-related hepatotoxicity in individuals with pre-existing liver disease although they are at increased risk of systemic drug toxicity secondary to slowed metabolism. For example, individuals with cirrhosis tolerate therapeutic doses of paracetamol without deterioration in liver function (Dart et al., 2000; Ford-Dunn, 2005). Exceptions include an increased rate of hepatotoxicity with the anti-androgens flutamide and cyproterone in those with chronic hepatitis B or C infection (Pu et al., 1999).

Sepsis

Cholestatic, non-obstructive jaundice is a feature of chronic liver disorders such as primary biliary cirrhosis and sclerosing cholangitis but can also occur as a result of sepsis and/or shock (21% of cases of jaundice in one study in the United Kingdom (Moseley et al., 2001)). Cholestasis may result from hypotension and low hepatic blood flow but also from direct inhibition of bile secretion by endotoxin and inflammatory cytokines (interleukin-1, interleukin-6, and tumour necrosis factor alpha (TNF-α)) (Moseley, 2004).

Cardiac failure and the liver

Eight patients out of 661 presenting with jaundice in a recent series were found to have cardiac failure as their main diagnosis (van Lingen et al., 2005). Although jaundice is clearly a rare presentation of heart failure, altered liver function is common in severe heart failure. It is thought to be mainly a result of sinusoidal congestion although significant hypotension (usually secondary to infarction or valvular disease) can lead to an ischaemic hepatitis signalled by a massive rise in aminotransferases and prolonged prothrombin time. Hepatic congestion produces a cholestatic derangement of liver enzymes thought to represent secondary damage to the bile canaliculae as a result of sinusoidal disruption (Cogger et al., 2003). Sinusoidal congestion is most marked in tricuspid valve regurgitation and a clear correlation between severity of regurgitation and serum levels of alkaline phosphatase (ALP) and gamma-glutamyl transferase (GGT) has been demonstrated (Lau et al., 2002).

Venous occlusion

A rapid onset of jaundice can occur in the venous occlusion of the Budd–Chiari syndrome although a chronic form of the syndrome resulting in the usual symptoms of chronic liver disease is more usual (Zimmerman et al., 2006). Venous obstruction can occur at any point from the hepatic venules to the right atrium and is particularly associated with disorders which produce a hypercoagulable state such as the myeloproliferative disorders, polycythaemia rubra vera and essential thrombocytosis. Malignancy is clearly associated with Budd–Chiari syndrome both through increased thrombogenicity and local obstruction of the venous system by solid tumours. Untreated acute Budd–Chiari syndrome requires an urgent and aggressive approach to management, if appropriate in the context of the individual's disease status. Inferior vena caval stenting and transjugular intrahepatic portosystemic shunt formation are relatively uninvasive procedures that can be of significant benefit in selected individuals. In those unsuitable for interventional procedures, a decision regarding anticoagulant therapy is required but the outlook with medical therapy alone is bleak with a mortality of over 80% in one series (McCarthy et al., 1985).

Obstructive jaundice

Obstruction of the biliary tract can occur at any point from within the liver to the ampulla of Vater. To give rise to jaundice this usually occurs at the confluence of the major ducts at the porta hepatis or more distally.

In two population studies of the causes of obstructive jaundice, gall stones were found to be responsible in 13% and 16% of individuals but carcinoma of the head of the pancreas, cholangiocarcinoma, and metastatic disease were most commonly identified (Luman et al., 2001; Bjornsson et al., 2003). Hepatocellular carcinoma is being

increasingly diagnosed as a cause of jaundice given the prevalence of chronic viral hepatitis and cirrhosis.

Symptoms related to jaundice

Studies involving patients who have undergone procedures to relieve biliary obstruction give some indication of the symptoms related to hyperbilirubinaemia. In addition to the expected clearing of jaundice and relief of pruritus, significant improvements were noted in anorexia, indigestion, sleep pattern, and global health scores (Ballinger et al., 1994; Luman et al., 1997). A Canadian study demonstrated a significant association between the degree of reduction in bilirubin levels after stenting and an improvement in social function and mental health as assessed by the SF-36 Health Survey Questionnaire (Abraham et al., 2002).

Malignant obstructive jaundice is classically thought to be 'painless' and therefore distinguished from benign causes such as gallstones. However, a study of elderly patients with biliary duct obstruction reported that 32% of those with a malignant cause alone presented with abdominal pain (Ashton et al., 1998).

Investigation of jaundice

It has been estimated that a thorough history, physical examination, and biochemical liver function tests are sufficient for making an accurate diagnosis of the type of liver disease in at least 80% of patients Table 10.4.4, (Kamath, 1996). During palliative care, the history should elucidate the primary disease process and set the onset of

Table 10.4.4 Clinical characteristics of jaundice of differing aetiologies

Clinical factors	Haemolytic	Hepatocellular	Intrahepatic Cholestatic	Post-hepatic Cholestatic ('obstructive')
Symptoms	Asymptomatic or backache, arthralgia	Nausea, vomiting, anorexia, pyrexia	Deep jaundice, Dark urine, light stools Pruritus	Deep jaundice, Dark urine, light stools Pruritus, cholangitis Biliary colic
Physical	Splenomegaly	Tender hepatomegaly	Tender hepatomegaly	Hepatomegaly Palpable gallbladder
Liver function tests				
Bilirubin	< 100μmol/L	Variable	Variable may be >500 μmol/L	<500 μmol/L
ALT	Normal	> 5-fold increase	2-to 5-fold increase	< 2-to 3-fold increase but 3- to 5-fold increase with cholangitis
ALP	Normal	<2- to 3-fold increase	>3- to 5-fold increase	>3- to 5-fold increase
Prothrombin time	Normal	Prolonged	Prolonged	Prolonged
Corrected by Vitamin K?	—	No	Variable	Yes
Dilated bile ducts on ultrasound?	No	No	No	Yes

ALT, alanine aminotransferase; ALP, alkaline phosphatase.

Adapted with permission from Mayo Clinic Proceedings, Volume 71, Issue 11, Kamath PS, Clinical approach to the patient with abnormal liver test results, pp.1089–1094, Copyright © 1996 Mayo Foundation for Medical Education and Research, with permission from Elsevier, http://www.sciencedirect.com/science/journal/00256196.

jaundice in the context of other markers of disease status. A drug history from the patient including non-prescription items is clearly vital.

Physical examination may confirm signs of chronic liver disease, portal hypertension, and/or intra-abdominal malignancy and may give clues as to current liver function. It is important to assess cognitive function for signs of associated encephalopathy. In all cases, signs of infection must be looked for within the biliary tree or peritoneum (if ascites is present) particularly if the patient is immunosuppressed by chronic infection, including HIV, or drugs (including corticosteroids). Infective cholangitis is associated with a significant mortality rate.

Blood tests

A clinical diagnosis of jaundice is confirmed by elevated serum levels of bilirubin. Should there be no derangement of liver enzymes to suggest cholestasis or hepatocellular injury then relative levels of unconjugated and conjugated bilirubin can be measured to distinguish between pre-hepatic and hepatic causes of jaundice. A review of over 1000 patients presenting with obstructive jaundice found serum bilirubin levels of higher than 100 µmol/l had sensitivity and specificity for a malignant aetiology of 71.9% and 86.9% respectively (Garcea et al., 2011). The performance of serum bilirubin levels in terms of distinguishing benign from malignant causes of obstructive jaundice in comparison with a variety of imaging techniques is shown in Table 10.4.5. Elevated levels of ALP and GGT with relatively normal, or only moderately increased, levels of aspartate transaminase and alanine transaminase would be a typical finding in cholestatic jaundice (Table 10.4.4). Isolated elevation of ALP is unusual in cholestasis and if present may reflect bone disease. Isolated raised GGT may indicate a drug effect. Serum albumin levels and prothrombin time reflect, in part, the synthetic functioning of the liver and evidence of coagulopathy is vital information prior to performing invasive investigations and therapeutic procedures.

Table 10.4.5 Distinguishing a benign from malignant cause of obstructive jaundice: serum bilirubin levels compared with other assessment modalities

Modality	Patients, N	Sensitivity, %	Specificity, %
Bilirubin, µmol/L	1026		
> 100		71.9	88.0
> 250		31.9	98.0
CA19-9	776	68.4	72.5
MRCP[a]	4711	95.0	97.0
ERCP	220	74.0	94.0
EUS	3532	78.0	84.0
PET-CT	46	89.0	74.0

[a] Includes patients with jaundice secondary to stone disease.

CT, computed tomography; ERCP, endoscopic retrograde cholangiopancreatography; EUS, endoscopic ultrasonography; MRCP, magnetic resonance cholangiopancreatography; PET-CT, positron emission tomography

Reproduced from Garcea G, et al., Bilirubin levels predict malignancy in patients with obstructive jaundice, *HPB*, Volume 13, Issue 6, pp. 426–430, Copyright © 2011 International Hepato-Pancreato-Biliary Association, with permission from John Wiley & Sons, Inc.

Imaging

Imaging the individual with jaundice aims to visualize the liver and biliary tree as an aid to confirming or identifying the underlying diagnosis as well as determining the location and extent of disease and the potential for treatment.

Ultrasound

Ultrasound scanning remains the first imaging investigation of choice in the patient with jaundice. It can be used at the bedside, does not involve radiation, and is relatively cheap. In a patient with obstructive jaundice, ultrasound will detect bile duct dilatation with a sensitivity and specificity of between 95% and 99% (Stott et al., 1991; Stroszczynski and Hunerbein, 2005). However, ultrasound is highly operator dependent and is problematic in obese patients and in situations where bowel gas overlies the region studied. Indeed, a review of reports of the use of standard transcutaneous ultrasound imaging to determine the level and the aetiology of biliary obstruction reported a range of respective accuracies of 27–95% and 23–88% (Blackbourne et al., 1994). The diagnosis of carcinoma of the ampulla is particularly difficult with transabdominal ultrasound with sensitivities of as low as 5% reported. However, endoscopic ultrasonography is proving more sensitive for detecting pancreatic cancers than computed tomography (CT), magnetic resonance imaging, or endoscopic retrograde cholangiopancreatography (ERCP).

Computed tomography

Given the advantages of ultrasound, the principal role of CT in the investigation of obstructive jaundice is to determine the extent and stage of disease to inform treatment options. However, CT with intravenous contrast allows better imaging of the liver parenchyma in hepatocellular causes of jaundice. The introduction of spiral CT and, more recently, multidetector CT, has resulted in improved resolution for the detection and characterization of small obstructing lesions to levels approaching magnetic resonance and direct cholangiography.

Magnetic resonance cholangiopancreatography

Magnetic resonance cholangiopancreatography (MRCP) is non-invasive, does not involve exposure to radiation, and does not require intravenous injection of contrast medium (Fig. 10.4.1). A large systematic review of the diagnostic ability of MRCP in biliary obstruction reported a pooled sensitivity of 95% for the demonstration of the level of obstruction and an 88% sensitivity in distinguishing between benign and malignant lesions (Romagnuolo et al., 2003). MRCP can, therefore, demonstrate the level of obstruction as accurately as direct cholangiography but avoids the risks associated with cannulation of the biliary tract. MRCP also allows simultaneous imaging of the abdomen to determine the extent of disease and has therefore been proposed as the complete diagnostic study (Pavone et al., 1999).

Many centres will use MRCP, if available, after initial ultrasound assessment leaving ERCP or percutaneous transhepatic cholangiography (PTC) to be used only when therapeutic interventions are required. Developments in CT techniques will continue to challenge magnetic resonance and relative cost-effectiveness will need regular review.

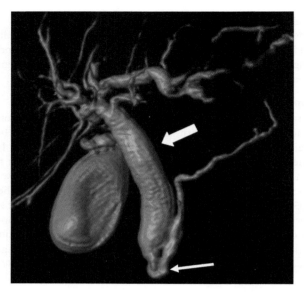

Fig. 10.4.1 A volume-rendered image from MRCP in a 49-year-old man with jaundice showing dilatation of the pancreatic duct (thin arrow) and common bile duct (thick arrow). The features are suggestive of a periampullary mass. Reproduced with permission from Patel HT et al., Cholangiopancreatography at 3.0T, *Radiographics*, Volume 29, Issue 1, pp.1689–1706, Copyright © 2009 Radiological Society of North America.

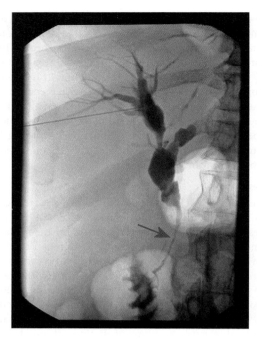

Fig. 10.4.2 Percutaneous transhepatic cholangiogram showing a long stricture of the common bile duct (arrow) caused by a cholangiocarcinoma. Endoscopic cholangiography and bile duct stenting had proved impossible but a stent was successfully deployed via the percutaneous route.

Cholangiography

Both ERCP and PTC allow imaging, cytological sampling, and palliative drainage of the biliary system via dilatation and stent insertion. Access to the biliary tree via the percutaneous route is usually only attempted when the level of biliary obstruction is proximal to the common hepatic duct or when distorted anatomy, often due to previous surgery or the presence of local tumour, precludes ERCP (Fig. 10.4.2).

Both procedures are associated with potentially fatal complications including bacterial cholangitis, bleeding, and bile leakage with acute pancreatitis being a particular complication of ERCP. However, the incidence of adverse events in both approaches is low, being reported in 0.5–5% of patients and is, to an extent, operator dependent (Bilbao et al., 1976; Harbin et al., 1980).

Management of jaundice

Antitumour therapy for sensitive malignancies may allow at least temporary relief of jaundice in those thought fit enough to receive a likely net benefit. Treatment can be considered even in the presence of incipient hepatic failure resulting from widespread tumour infiltration. Careful drug selection and dose titration is required but significant improvements in symptoms and survival can be achieved (Gurevich and Akerley, 2001; Schull et al., 2003).

Uncontrolled studies of biliary drainage procedures for obstructive jaundice suggest the potential for significant and rapid improvement in symptoms, particularly pruritus, pain, nausea, anorexia, and in overall quality of life (Larssen et al., 2002; Larssen et al., 2011; Barkay et al., 2013). However, a recent case report illustrates the need for careful individual assessment in advanced disease (Dy et al., 2012). In certain individuals, if biliary drainage is combined with post-procedural antitumour therapy, rapid predictable improvement in symptom control can be combined with potential prolonged survival and stent patency (Qian et al., 2006).

Jaundice resulting from superinfection or malignancy in individuals with AIDS may well respond to specific treatment if adequate doses of antibacterial, antiviral, antifungal, or cytotoxic chemotherapy can be tolerated.

Biliary drainage procedures

Obstructive jaundice is present at the time of presentation in 70–80% of individuals with pancreatic carcinoma and 85% are deemed unsuitable for curative resection (Andtbacka et al., 2004). In one review of over 8000 patients with unresectable carcinoma of the pancreas, those who underwent a surgical bypass procedure allowing biliary drainage had a significant improvement in quality and length of survival (Sarr and Cameron, 1982). Patients deemed unfit for surgery should be considered for biliary stenting via endoscopic or percutaneous routes. One study of quality of life related to endoscopic biliary drainage demonstrated increased quality of life post drainage but only in those individuals with pre-procedure serum bilirubin levels below 222 µmol/L (Ballinger et al., 1994). The authors proposed, therefore, that careful assessment is carried out prior to stent insertion in those with very high serum bilirubin levels.

Individuals with high bile duct obstruction or distorted duodenal anatomy may require a percutaneous approach either for stent placement or to allow external drainage of bile for symptomatic relief and to widen the choice, if appropriate, of systemic cytotoxic agents that maybe administered (Covey and Brown, 2006a). Chronic loss of bile through the drain can lead to nutritional deficiencies and if stents cannot be deployed then an attempt to pass an internal-external catheter via guidewire manipulation may be made. This catheter has side holes positioned proximal to the obstruction and the tip lies within the bowel to allow drainage of bile either externally or internally (Covey and Brown, 2006b).

Nutrition

Chronic cholestasis can lead to malabsorption of fat-soluble vitamins. Vitamin K deficiency contributes to the prolonged clotting time that may be associated with jaundice (O'Brien et al., 1994). The international normalized ratio should be regularly checked in jaundiced patients and vitamin K given either parenterally or orally (both routes, interestingly, seem as effective (Green et al., 2000)). Even in patients with end stage disease this intervention may reduce the likelihood of distressing haemorrhage.

Pruritus

Pruritus is one of the most distressing symptoms experienced by individuals with jaundice. Successful management is rare and the symptom so impacting on quality of life that severe pruritus is an indication for liver transplant in chronic liver disease.

The self-rated severity of itching or observed scratching behaviour does not correlate with serum bilirubin levels or the stage of chronic liver disease. Itch may be mild or severe, localized or generalized, but a pattern in which itch typically starts on the palms of the hands and soles of the feet before becoming more generalized has been described (Twycross et al., 2003). Itching in cholestasis appears to follow a circadian rhythm being at its worst between 1200 and 1800 hours (Bergasa et al., 1995) and one small pilot study suggested a benefit of bright-light therapy directed towards the eyes to disrupt this rhythm (Bergasa et al., 2001).

The pathogenesis of pruritus in jaundice is thought to involve either the stimulation of peripheral itch receptors within the skin, by an increased level of circulating bile acids and other pruritogens, or via central neural mechanisms resulting from alterations in neurotransmitters such as endogenous opioids, serotonin, and gamma-aminobutyric acid (GABA).

Opioid systems

Pruritus, although a rare side effect of systemically administered opioids, has been reported to occur in between 30% and 100% of individuals after epidural or intrathecal infusion (Szarvas et al., 2003). Increased plasma levels of opioid peptides have been recorded in individuals with primary biliary cirrhosis (Thornton and Losowsky, 1988) and animal models suggest increased hepatic synthesis of encephalins in cholestatic states. Furthermore, animals display naloxone-reversible scratching behaviour when given plasma extracts from humans with cholestasis and pruritus (but not from those without pruritus) (Jones and Zylicz, 1993).

Published reports describe a significant improvement in cholestatic pruritus, by both subjective and objective assessment, after the intravenous infusion of naloxone (Bergasa et al., 1992, 1995) and with the oral opioid antagonists naltrexone and nalmefene (Carson et al., 1996; Wolfhagen et al., 1997; Bergasa et al., 1998; Terg et al., 2002). Various protocols have been suggested to lessen the withdrawal-like reactions that can occur with antagonist therapy even in individuals not receiving exogenous opioids (Jones and Zylicz, 2001; Jones et al., 2002). Many individuals receiving palliative care will, however, require exogenous opioids for pain control. Trials in postoperative anaesthesia have demonstrated a reduction in opioid-induced side effects, including pruritus, without loss of pain control or increased opioid requirements, by the addition of low-dose naloxone to morphine for intravenous infusion (Cepeda et al., 2004; Maxwell et al., 2005). Interestingly, one small trial reports a significant decrease in pruritus associated with perioperative intrathecal analgesia with morphine if low-dose, intravenous buprenorphine was co-administered (Beltrutti et al., 2002). A small case series found significant relief from cholestatic pruritus in two out of five patients treated with buprenorphine but intolerable side effects in three patients (Juby et al., 1994).

Recent attention has switched to the potential role of central and peripheral kappa opioid receptors in the regulation of pruritus. It is thought, in very general terms, that activation of kappa receptors inhibits mu receptor activity. The serum and hypothalamic levels of the endogenous kappa agonist, dynorphin A, have been shown to be reduced after bile duct ligation in animal models (Inan and Cowan, 2005) and cessation of scratching behaviour has been demonstrated in animals given the kappa agonist, nalfurafane (Inan and Cowan, 2006). Nalfurafane has been clinically trialled for the relief of uraemic pruritus and there are case reports of the use of butorphanol, a partial kappa agonist, in cholestatic and paraneoplastic itch (Phan et al., 2012).

Serotoninergic systems

There are close links between the central opioidergic and serotonergic transmission systems. Although early reports suggested substantial beneficial effects of serotonin type 3 (5-HT$_3$) receptor antagonists, such as ondansetron, in cholestatic pruritus (Raderer et al., 1994; Schworer et al., 1995) more recent controlled trials have suggested only modest or no benefit (Muller et al., 1998; O'Donohue et al., 2005). Case series have attested to the potential benefit of the serotonin re-uptake inhibitor sertraline in cholestatic pruritus (Browning et al., 2003). Sertraline at doses of 75–100 mg per day is now recommended by the guidelines of the American Association for the Study of Liver Diseases as fourth-line treatment (after cholestyramine, rifampicin and naltrexone) of cholestatic pruritus associated with primary biliary cirrhosis (Lindor et al., 2009).

GABAergic systems

Opioids antagonize the central inhibitory effects of GABA and several groups have shown recent interest in the use of propofol, a GABA agonist to reduce spinal opioid-induced pruritus. An early, small randomized trial showed benefit of subhypnotic doses of propofol in cholestatic pruritus (Borgeat et al., 1993). Phenobarbitone has been shown in two case series to improve itch in cholestasis associated with pregnancy and chronic liver disease (Bloomer and Boyer, 1975; Heikkinen et al., 1982). This effect may be related to enzyme induction effects on the liver but phenobarbitone is also a central GABA agonist. Another GABA enhancer, midazolam, gave prolonged relief of cholestatic pruritus when given by continuous infusion, without undue sedation, in one case report (Prieto, 2004).

Lysophosphatidic acid and autotaxin

Perhaps the most significant recent contribution to the advancement of an understanding of the pathogenesis of cholestatic pruritus has come from the identification of high levels of lysophosphatidic acid (LPA) in the serum of individuals with cholestatic itch (Kremer et al., 2010) A correlation has been shown between the serum levels of LPA and the severity of itch and intradermal injection of the compound induces scratching behaviour in animal models. The same group have also identified markedly elevated activity of autotaxin, a lysophospholipase enzyme that converts lysophosphatidylcholine to active LPA, in the serum of pruritic individuals when compared to serum from those without pruritus (Kremer et al., 2012). Furthermore, the group demonstrated that a response to conventional approaches to pruritic management (bile acid chelators, rifampicin, biliary drainage) correlated directly with a lowering of serum autotaxin activity. Interestingly, rifampicin has been shown to reduce levels of autotaxin *in vivo* by down-regulating gene transcription via agonism of the pregnane X receptor (Jones, 2012). However, other disease states demonstrate high levels of autotaxin activity but without associated pruritus. Therefore, there is likely to be a co-factor, possibly either bile acids or endogenous opioids, working with LPA at the level of the pruritogenic peripheral neurons.

Drawing on these observations, Jones has proposed a model to describe the possible pathogenesis of cholestatic pruritus and to highlight points at which therapeutic agents may be targeted (Fig. 10.4.3).

TGR5

The close relationship between pain and itch sensory transmission in the peripheral and central nervous systems has been very recently described by a large international research group (Alemi et al., 2013). In animal models they report that bile acids can induce both itch and analgesia through the activation of G-protein-coupled plasma membrane bile acid receptors (TGR5) expressed on peripheral sensory neurons and in the spinal cord. Scratching behaviour did not occur in *Tgr5*-knockout mice given

intradermal injections of bile acids and an exaggerated response was noted in mice that over-expressed the gene.

The research group acknowledged both the evidence of a role for autotaxin and LPA in cholestatic pruritus and the lack of evidence of a direct correlation between levels of circulating bile acids and the severity of pruritus. It is likely, therefore, that pruritogens in addition to bile acids, such as LPA, are involved in the generation of pruritus in a pathway still to be fully elucidated.

Removal of pruritogens

Early studies of the management of cholestatic pruritus focussed on lowering plasma levels of bile acids by reducing intestinal reabsorption with chelating agents such as cholestyramine (Datta and Sherlock, 1963; Di Padova, 1984). Such agents are unlikely to be helpful in complete biliary duct obstruction. Cholestyramine is not very palatable, can lead to bloating and constipation and can bind and interfere with the absorption of numerous drugs. A relatively new chelating agent, colesevelam, seemed to be well tolerated and to relieve cholestatic pruritus in one small study (Berg, 2001) but a recent larger randomized control trial found no benefit over placebo (Kuiper et al., 2010).

Cholestyramine and other similar agents may bind other pruritogens that are more influential in the generation of pruritus than bile acids. A study of extracorporeal plasma separation and anion adsorption demonstrated a significant reduction in cholestatic pruritus but which did not correlate to reduction in plasma levels of bile acids (Pusl et al., 2006). Other extracorporeal techniques

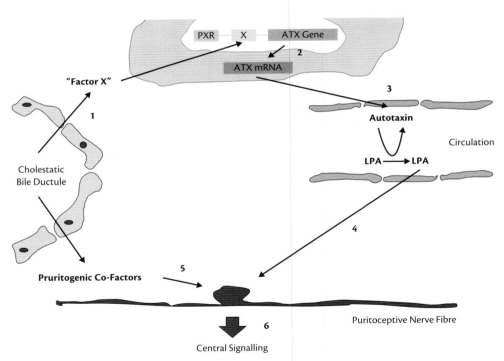

Fig. 10.4.3 A possible model for the pathogenesis of pruritus in cholestasis. A putative Factor X, found in increased levels in cholestasis (1) can, in turn, increase circulating levels of autotaxin (ATX) by either upregulating transcription or by decreasing breakdown (2) The resulting increased cleavage of lysophosphatidylcholine (LPC), generates increased levels of lysophosphatidic acid (LPA) (3). LPA has a direct action on puritoceptive nerve fibres (4). However, high levels of ATX are present in conditions other than cholestasis without associated pruritus. Jones therefore suggests the need for a co-factor, 'Factor Y' (5, possibly endogenous opioids) to act with LPA to stimulate pruritic signalling.

for removing pruritogens have been suggested including haemodialysis (Hoek et al., 1982), charcoal haemoperfusion (Lauterburg et al., 1980), plasmapheresis (Warren et al., 2005) and albumin dialysis (Parés et al., 2010).

Enzyme induction

Hepatic enzyme inducers such as flumecinol, rifampicin and phenobarbitone have been advocated in the management of cholestatic pruritus although their mechanism of action is unknown (Bloomer and Boyer, 1975; Ghent and Carruthers, 1988). Rifampicin is the only member of this group that is used regularly in the management of cholestatic itch. However, it has potential activity at multiple points on the pruritic pathway including the alteration of bowel flora, inhibition of bile acid uptake by hepatocytes (Bachs et al., 1989), central opioid antagonism (Bergasa et al., 2004), and most recently described, the reduction in circulating levels of autotaxin (Jones, 2012).

Antihistamines

Histological evidence of mast cell activity within the skin of jaundiced individuals is limited and conflicting. However, clinical observation suggests that antihistamines are generally ineffective in relieving the itch associated with jaundice, with any benefit reported most likely to reflect an improvement in sleep through their sedative action.

Non-pharmacological measures

In pruritus of cholestasis the value of topical emollients and environmental measures to cool and lessen sweating is unclear. Most benefit may be obtained from keeping finger nails cut short and wearing cotton gloves at night to lessen damage to the skin through scratching.

Ascites

The development of ascites as a complication of either chronic liver disease or malignancy not only heralds a poor prognosis in terms of survival but also can be associated with multiple distressing symptoms resulting from increased intra-abdominal pressure.

Cirrhosis is the precursor to ascites in approximately 75% of individuals, malignancy is the main cause in 10%, and cardiac failure and tuberculosis in 3% and 2% of individuals respectively (Rosenberg, 2006). There are several excellent published reviews of the pathogenesis of ascites and its management in individuals with cirrhosis to which the reader is directed (Gines et al., 2004; Moore and Aithal, 2006). The literature concerning malignant ascites is not as extensive or consensual and this form of ascites will become the focus for the ensuing section of the chapter.

Malignant ascites

A survey of Canadian physicians and their management of malignant ascites produced comments such as 'generally impossible to manage', 'it is a frustrating clinical situation', and 'a practical and effective solution is needed' (Lee et al., 1998).

The main frustrations in the management of ascites relate to questions such as the role of diuretic therapy, imaging and the method of paracentesis, each of which remain poorly tested in formal trials. However, recent interest in the pathophysiology of ascites formation may lead to more individualized and novel methods of management.

Incidence/prevalence

Problems related to the presence of malignant ascites are present in 3.6–6% of patients admitted to palliative care units (Preston, 1995; Keen and Fallon, 2002). Malignant ascites is most frequently associated with a primary diagnosis of ovarian carcinoma and less frequently with endometrial, breast, colonic, gastric, pancreatic, or unknown primary carcinoma (Ringenberg et al., 1989; Malik et al., 1991; Parsons et al., 1996). The presence of ascites is usually an indicator of advanced disease and, unfortunately, is detectable at the time of initial diagnosis in over half of the patients in whom it develops (Garrison et al., 1986). Patients with ovarian cancer, however, do have a longer mean survival from the time of development of ascites when compared to those with other malignancies (Parsons et al., 1996). This may relate to ascites being a complication of relatively early stage ovarian cancer and its relative sensitivity to cytotoxic chemotherapy.

Control of ascites often requires repeated inpatient episodes that, in one series of patients with ovarian cancer, showed a rapid increase in frequency over the last year of life to a median of seven admissions in the last 3 months (von Gruenigen et al., 2003).

Symptoms related to ascites

Symptoms requiring palliation relate to increased intra-abdominal pressure; discomfort of the abdominal wall, dyspnoea, anorexia, early satiety, nausea and vomiting, oesophageal reflux, poor mobility, insomnia related to general discomfort, pain in the groins and subcostal regions, and lower limb oedema. Abdominal compartment syndrome with resultant multisystem failure has also been reported (Etzion et al., 2004). Easily overlooked can be the significant negative effect of abdominal distension on body image.

Pathophysiology of ascites

Ascites formation in cirrhosis occurs predominantly as a result of a cascade of events including portal hypertension and consequent splanchnic vasodilatation that results in both sodium and fluid retention and an increase in intestinal capillary pressure and permeability (Gines et al., 2004). In contrast, it is tumour invasion of the visceral or parietal peritoneum that is the major cause of ascites in individuals with malignancy (Rosenberg, 2006).

Ascites accumulates as a result of an imbalance in the normal state of influx and efflux of fluid from the peritoneal cavity. A decreased rate of fluid efflux may occur as a result of blockage of open ended diaphragmatic lymphatics by tumour and this has been shown histologically in association with malignant ascites in animal models (Feldman et al., 1972).

It is unlikely that a reduced rate of fluid efflux alone is sufficient to cause the accumulation of massive amounts of ascitic fluid. Indeed, the rate of efflux has been shown to increase to rates approaching 80 mL/hour as ascites accumulates and intra-abdominal pressure increases (Hirabayashi and Graham, 1970).

The rate of fluid influx into the peritoneal space may be increased in malignancy as a result of two distinct mechanisms. Each mechanism will result in ascitic fluid of different biochemical properties and may respond to different modes of treatment.

1. Increased hepatic venous pressure, as an anatomical consequence of multiple hepatic metastases, or single large (sometimes benign) tumours causing a Budd–Chiari syndrome (Sebastian et al., 2004). An increase in venous pressure results in both fluid leakage into the peritoneum from the sinusoids and, via an

increase in plasma renin concentration, to the retention of salt and water by the kidneys. The ascitic fluid resulting from this mechanism is similar to that seen as a result of cirrhosis and has the properties of a *transudate*.

2. An *exudate*, of relatively high protein concentration, may be produced as a result of increased vascular permeability. Peritoneal tumour neovasculature is thought to be intrinsically leaky allowing extravasation of fluid. Additionally, neovascularization of the otherwise normal parietal peritoneum has been observed in patients with malignant ascites and ovarian carcinoma (Beecham et al., 1983).

The permeability of normal microvessels, such as those which line the peritoneal cavity, can be increased by a variety of tumour or inflammatory cell derived cytokines including transforming growth factors alpha and beta, epidermal growth factor, and vascular endothelial growth factor (VEGF) (De Simone, 1999). VEGF also stimulates angiogenesis, facilitating tumour growth and, potentially, the observed neovascularization of normal peritoneum. Animal experiments have demonstrated a significant relationship between the degree of tumour cell expression of VEGF and observed levels of angiogenesis and ascites production (Yoneda et al., 1998; Huang et al., 2000). VEGF has been detected in high concentrations in malignant as opposed to non-malignant ascites and associated with metastases from a variety of primary sites (Verheul et al., 1999; Zebrowski et al., 1999; Verheul et al., 2000).

In an individual patient, the relative contribution of these two principal mechanisms of ascitic fluid production can be estimated from the calculation of the serum–ascites albumin gradient. The serum–ascites gradient is calculated by subtracting the albumin concentration of the ascitic fluid from that within a serum specimen obtained on the same day. The gradient correlates with the portal venous pressure with a value of 11g/L or higher being indicative of a transudate and the presence of portal hypertension (Runyon, 1994). This may be of importance in assessing the likelihood of response to diuretic therapy with an aldosterone antagonist.

The formation of chylous ascites is a complication of retroperitoneal tumour spread or its treatment and arises either from damage to lymphatic vessels or through obstruction of lymphatic flow through lymph nodes or the pancreas.

Diagnosis of ascites

The diagnosis of the presence of ascites relies on a relevant clinical history and examination (Williams and Simel, 1992). Where there is doubt, usually with typical symptoms present in a patient with an obese abdomen or with potential bowel obstruction, ultrasound scanning can detect as little as 100 mL of free fluid in the peritoneum (Regnard and Mannix et al., 1970). The presence of ascites in a patient with known malignancy cannot always be assumed to be secondary to the presence of intra-abdominal tumour and other causes, such as cirrhosis, congestive heart failure, nephrotic syndrome, tuberculosis and pancreatitis must be excluded

Management of ascites

Guidelines and treatment algorithms for management of problems such as ascites have been developed and are helpful (Regnard and Mannix, 1989; Stephenson and Gilbert, 2002) but the temptation is to manipulate every patient into particular protocols and lose sight

of individual risk:benefit analyses. Furthermore, the evidence underpinning common approaches is weak at best. A recent systematic review of the management of malignant ascites detected 32 studies, of which none were randomized trials and 26 were non-analytical studies such as case series (Becker et al., 2006).

Antitumour therapy

Specific antitumour therapy should always be considered, particularly for individuals developing ascites with known ovarian or breast carcinoma. Malik et al. (1991) demonstrated complete clearance or significant reduction of ascites in 46% of patients with ovarian cancer treated with systemic cytotoxic chemotherapy. Significant response in ovarian cancer can be observed with second- and even third-line chemotherapy, so should always be considered.

Cytotoxic agents have been given intraperitoneally from as early as the 1950s (Weisberger et al., 1955). A resurgence of interest has accompanied the development of hyperthermic intraperitoneal chemotherapy (HIPEC) that appears to allow greater tissue penetration and lowers levels of drug resistance (Witkamp et al., 2001). A multi-institutional analysis of the outcome of 52 individuals treated with laparoscopic HIPEC demonstrated complete resolution of ascites in 94% with a mean hospital stay of 2.3 days and complicated by only two minor wound infections and a deep venous thrombosis (Valle et al., 2009).

Chylous ascites, when associated with retroperitoneal lymphoma and a consequent disruption of normal lymphatic drainage pathways, may be expected to show some response to chemotherapy if it be first- or second-line treatment.

The success of the intracavitary instillation of a variety of agents in the control of malignant pleural effusions has encouraged a similar approach to the treatment of malignant ascites. There have been numerous small trials and case series reporting the use of radioisotopes, cytotoxics, and more recently, biological agents and response modifiers to reduce ascitic fluid formation (Box 10.4.1). One phase II study found that intraperitoneal instillation of the corticosteroid, triamcinolone hexacetonide, resulted in a significant slowing of ascites accumulation (Mackey et al., 2000). The effect was noted particularly in patients with an albumin serum–ascites gradient of less than 11 g/L. The authors postulated the effect to have been mediated through a steroid-induced reduction of the secretion of VEGF.

Other approaches

Initial pre-clinical trials with anti-VEGF antibodies, anti-VEGF receptor antibodies, and an inhibitor of VEGF receptor tyrosine kinase activity (Xu et al., 2000) have been reported to show a reduction in ascites formation in animal models. Transfection of a mutated gene controlling production of VEGF has decreased ascites production in mice (Huang et al., 2000). Clinical trials of the humanized VEGF antibody, bevacizumab, given both systemically and intra-peritoneally have been promising (Numnum et al., 2006; Kobold et al., 2009). More recently, aflibercept, a decoy VEGF receptor that binds and neutralizes VEGF, has shown good inhibitory effects on ascites production but parenteral therapy in phase II trials was associated with a relatively high level of side effects, principally intestinal perforation (Colombo et al., 2012; Gotlieb et al., 2012).

TNF has been found to block re-accumulation of ascites in an animal model by inhibiting the expression of VEGF mRNA

Box 10.4.1 Agents reported to have been employed for intraperitoneal instillation in the management of peritoneal malignancy and ascites	
◆ Thiotepa	◆ ^{198}Au
◆ Fluorouracil	◆ ^{32}CrPO$_4$
◆ Mustine	◆ Interferon alpha
◆ Bleomycin	◆ Interferon beta
◆ Cisplatinum	◆ Tumour necrosis factor
◆ Catumaxomab	◆ Interleukin-2
◆ Carboplatin	◆ Radiolabelled monoclonal antibodies
◆ Etoposide	◆ Metalloproteinase inhibitors
◆ Mitomycin C	◆ Corticosteroids
◆ Adriamycin	◆ *Corynebacterium parvum*
◆ Docetaxel	◆ OK-432 (extract from Streptococcus pyogenes).
◆ Mitoxantrone	

(Gotlieb et al., 2000) and an early clinical study suggested benefit from the administration of recombinant TNF-α (Rath et al., 1991). VEGF expression and associated angiogenesis has also been shown to be reduced by ketoprofen (Sakayama et al., 2004), green tea (Kojima-Yuasa et al., 2003) and angiotensin-converting enzyme inhibitors (Yoshiji et al., 2004).

The use of octreotide, the somatostatin analogue, to reduce the volume of ascites has been proposed but the results of small case series have been variable (Cairns and Malone, 1999; Cairns and Malone et al., 2012). The physiological mechanism remains unclear although there is some evidence that octreotide may be an inhibitor of VEGF (Cascinu et al., 2009). A small case series did report the successful control of chylous ascites with the combination of octreotide and a fat-free diet (Mincher et al., 2005).

Diuretic therapy

Diuretic therapy remains the mainstay of control of ascites of non-malignant origin where 90% of patients would be expected to respond to treatment (Runyon, 1994). The role of diuretics in the management of malignant ascites remains controversial. A very small study of the use of diuretics in patients with ascites and either massive hepatic metastases, 'peritoneal carcinomatosis', or chylous ascites only demonstrated a reduction in estimated ascitic volume in the group with hepatic metastases (Pockros et al., 1992). Each patient with hepatic metastases had raised plasma renin levels, a high serum–ascites albumin gradient, and responded to the aldosterone antagonist, spironolactone.

It seems appropriate to consider a trial of diuretics in individuals with malignant ascites and a high serum–ascites albumin gradient. Amiloride has a faster onset of action than spironolactone and although not a classical mineralocorticoid receptor antagonist appears to interfere with aldosterone activity and to have a similar effect to spironolactone on endothelial cells (Oberleithner et al., 2004). If spironolactone is used, the initial addition of a loop diuretic may speed the clinical response during the accumulation period (Amiel et al., 1984).

In addition to the usual potential side effects of diuretic therapy in a frail population, hepatic encephalopathy may be triggered in patients with limited residual hepatic function.

Paracentesis

Abdominal paracentesis affords quick symptomatic relief in a population that often has a relatively short prognosis and for whom diuretic therapy, if effective, may include a lag period and be associated with significant side effects.

The reported techniques and equipment used for the procedure are numerous and allows palliative care physicians full expression of their creativity. A Cochrane Review published in 2010 could find no evidence to support particular methods of paracentesis with no answers to questions relating to the length of time that a drain should remain in place, the use of intravenous replacement of fluid, the clamping of drains, and the recording of vital observations during drainage (Keen et al., 2010).

Stephenson and Gilbert reported the successful introduction of guidelines for paracentesis into an oncology unit that resulted in reductions in the use of ultrasound to mark sites for drainage, the mean duration of drainage, and the length of inpatient stay (Stephenson and Gilbert, 2002). Catheters were left in for no more than 6 hours with up to 5 L being drained and intravenous fluids only considered if patients were hypotensive, dehydrated, or known to have severe renal impairment.

The debate over the use of replacement parenteral fluid stems from the large experience of the potential problems associated with paracentesis in patients with hepatic cirrhosis. In the absence of a serum–ascites gradient of 11g/L or greater, complications of paracentesis are rare in patients with malignant ascites and fluid maybe drained off relatively rapidly with no need to routinely administer intravenous colloid or albumin. Indeed, the use of vacuum bottles allowing several litres to be removed in a matter of minutes, with apparently few complications, has been reported to be particularly useful in the outpatient clinic or even the patient's home (Moorsom, 2001). Patients without peripheral oedema or with a high serum–ascitic albumin gradient who do not respond to diuretics may be particularly prone to hypovolaemia. Intravascular volume can be replenished by intravenous infusion of either colloid or plasma protein solution should hypotension develop.

A study of 35 patients with ascites and ovarian cancer demonstrated a direct correlation between the measured value of intraperitoneal pressure and the severity of symptoms reported (Gotleib et al., 1998). The most significant drop in intra-abdominal pressure occurs with the removal of the first few litres of fluid. One study confirmed that in a group of patients from whom a mean of 5.3 L were drained over 24 hours no further improvement in symptom scores occurred after the first 2 hours of drainage (McNamara, 2000). It would have been of interest if perception of body image had been factored into these studies.

Since symptoms can often be relieved by the removal of relatively small volumes of ascites over a short time period this is to be recommended, particularly in the very frail with a limited prognosis. One to 2 L of fluid can be removed simply over 30 minutes via a plastic intravenous cannula. The insertion of the cannula into the peritoneal cavity is simple and if used in conjunction with infiltration of local anaesthetic is a relatively comfortable procedure. The removal of such a modest volume is unlikely to cause symptomatic hypovolaemia and the use of a small cannula for a short time is highly unlikely to cause local complications.

Clearly without antitumour therapy ascites is likely to re-accumulate and should the prognosis be more than a few days then regular moderate volume paracenteses through a temporary catheter will be required to allow the individual a reasonable time period between admissions with acceptable symptom control.

There has been increasing evidence of the effectiveness, safety, tolerability, and potential financial savings afforded by the use of implanted 'permanent' peritoneal catheters allowing regular ascitic drainage at home (Fig. 10.4.4). Indeed in England and Wales, the National Institute for Health and Care Excellence (NICE) issued a report in 2012 recommending the use of this system in the NHS for individuals with malignant ascites likely to require repeated large volume paracenteses for palliation of symptoms (NICE, 2012). The system results in financial savings if regular large volume paracenteses involve an overnight stay in hospital but not if usually performed on a day-case or outpatient basis.

The most likely complications of the drainage of malignant ascites include bowel perforation, peritonitis, and localized cellulitis surrounding the drain site. One study reported two deaths from peritonitis in a series of 127 paracenteses in 100 patients (Parsons et al., 1996). Infection was a particular problem in an early case series of patients with permanent implanted drains (Belfort et al., 1990). However, a more recent series of ten patients treated with tunnelled PleurX® (Denver Biomedical, Denver, Colorado) catheters recorded no catheter-related infections with a mean catheter survival of 70 days (Richard et al., 2001). Two case reports of the prolonged use implanted catheters for 17 and 18 months, with twice weekly and daily drainage respectively, each described only one episode of infection treated with antibiotics and not necessitating catheter removal (Bui et al., 1999; Brooks and Herzog, 2006).

Anecdotal experience would suggest that many patients feel extremely tired for several days following paracentesis and both hyponatraemia and a progressive fall in plasma albumin concentration with repeated paracenteses have been recorded in some series, although not all.

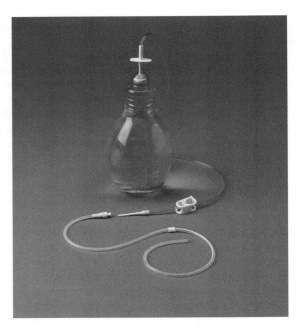

Fig. 10.4.4 PleurX® catheter and vacuum flask for repeated, rapid, drainage of ascites. Once the catheter has been inserted individuals with ascites, or their carers, can continue to perform intermittent drainage at home.

Patients with severely compromised hepatic function are at particular risk of hepatic failure and encephalopathy over the first 24 hours after ascitic drainage.

Peritoneovenous shunting

Potential problems of repeated paracentesis such as intravascular hypovolaemia, hypoalbuminaemia, infection, and visceral damage, and the expense, discomfort, and inconvenience of repeated hospital admissions have prompted the development of alternative drainage procedures. Peritoneovenous shunting was established in the mid 1970s (Le Veen et al., 1974) and remains the most common procedure performed.

Two forms of shunt have been commonly used, the original Le Veen (production now discontinued) and the Denver shunt. The shunts are designed to allow drainage of ascites into the central venous system, usually via the internal jugular or femoral veins. They may be placed surgically, laparoscopically, or percutaneously with one study reporting no difference in performance or complication rate on direct comparison of these methods (Clara et al., 2004).

A review of published case series that described the placement of a total of 353 Denver shunts reported that they provided 'effective palliation' in approximately 75% of cases (White et al., 2011). Complications occurred in 38% of patients including shunt occlusion (24%) and disseminated intravascular coagulation (9%). Shunt patency averaged 87 ± 57 days and 74% of patients died with functioning shunts. Shunt lumen occlusion appears to occur more frequently during drainage of malignant ascites than cirrhotic ascites and usually occurs as a result of thrombosis of the venous terminal or from debris in the peritoneal end of the shunt.

Other complications include postoperative fluid overload with pulmonary oedema, thromboembolism, vena caval thrombosis, hepatic encephalopathy, peritonitis, and tumour seeding to the subcutaneous tissues of the anterior abdominal wall.

The potential effects of the introduction of tumour cells from the peritoneal cavity into the circulation via the shunt have been examined in a small series of post-mortem examinations (Markey et al., 1984). The study reported a variety of observations but concluded that metastases, although occurring in some patients as a direct result of shunt placement, are not clinically significant and do not alter prognosis.

Peritoneovenous shunts are clearly unsuitable for patients with loculated ascites and are not advised if the ascites is haemorrhagic or chylous, or the patient has poor cardiac or renal function, or a tendency to hepatic encephalopathy. Portal hypertension, massive pleural effusion, and coagulation disorders are relative contraindications (Markey et al., 1979; Qazi and Savlov, 1982).

A reported series of patients with ascites and non-gynaecological primary tumours showed the best outcomes of peritoneovenous shunts to occur in patients with normal renal function and tumours of non-gastrointestinal primary origin (Bieligk et al., 2001). One study measured 'quality of life' by a single question and visual analogue scale and found a non-significant trend to an improvement with either paracenteses or shunts but no difference between the two methods of drainage, despite a progressive reduction in serum albumin in the group treated by serial paracenteses (Gough and Balderson, 1993).

The relatively long survival of patients with ascites and gynaecological malignancies and the potential savings in terms of repeated hospitalizations for paracenteses should make perito-neovenous shunting an option to be considered in all cases.

Summary

Despite numerous small studies of the intraperitoneal adminis-tration of various cytotoxic agents, radioisotopes, and immune/biological response modifiers, management of malignant ascites continues to rely upon the use of diuretics, abdominal paracente-sis, and peritoneovenous shunts. There is increasing interest in the use of 'long-term' indwelling drainage catheters to alleviate the need for repeated hospital attendance.

However, it is from recent studies into the pathophysiology of ascites production in intra-abdominal malignancy that new and specific ways to slow or halt ascitic fluid production are likely to emerge. In particular, the present interest in the role of vascular endothelial growth factor in tumour angiogenesis, peritoneal neo-vascularization, and resultant ascites production has highlighted a possible new target for therapy.

Hepatic encephalopathy

Hepatic encephalopathy manifests as a complex neuropsychi-atric disturbance often developing as a consequence of progres-sive liver disease with cirrhosis. It may occur as a complication of acute liver failure associated with acute cerebral oedema or may also result from portosystemic bypass with no intrinsic hepatocellular disease. Abnormal cognitive and motor function and psychiatric disorders are characteristic with severity varying from mild abnormalities, detected only by formal psychometric testing, to deep coma. Signs of neuromotor impairment include hyper-reflexia, rigidity, myoclonus, and asterixis.

An international working party has proposed a nomenclature that defines hepatic encephalopathy with respect to both the underlying hepatic abnormality and the associated duration and characteristics of neurological signs and symptoms (Mullen, 2007).

Whilst encephalopathy is most often associated with chronic liver disease it can complicate a diagnosis of malignancy. Rarely, hepatic failure and encephalopathy can result from massive infil-tration by primary or metastatic tumour but the prognosis in such cases is usually measured in days (Alexopoulou et al., 2006). Individuals with hepatocellular carcinoma, as reported by a study from Hong Kong, had a median survival of 1 month following the first presentation with encephalopathy (Cheung et al., 2006).

Encephalopathy is a sign of decompensation in cirrhosis and is related to the development of significant portosystemic venous shunting. The first episode of encephalopathy is associated with a subsequent estimated 1-year survival of 42% and a 3-year survival of 23% (Bustamante et al., 1999). Individuals with raised serum bilirubin, ALP, potassium, and urea along with reduced albumin and prothrombin activity have a significantly worse prognosis. The survival of all individuals with chronic liver disease after their first episode of acute encephalopathy is less than that associated with liver transplantation which should therefore always be con-sidered at this stage in the disease process.

Pathogenesis of hepatic encephalopathy

A raised blood ammonia level can be found in over 90% of indi-viduals with clinical signs of hepatic encephalopathy. Although two studies have demonstrated a correlation between blood levels of ammonia and severity of encephalopathy (Ong et al., 2003; Odeh et al., 2005), other studies have failed to demonstrate such a relationship and it is likely that there are other variable factors involved, in addition to hyperammonaemia, in the patho-genesis of encephalopathy.

Ammonia is generated in the small intestine by the action of glutaminase on glutamine and in the colon by the activity of bacte-rial urease. Individuals with normal liver function will metabolize over 90% of the ammonia entering the portal system (Mas, 2006). Raised levels of ammonia in the systemic circulation come prin-cipally from either portosystemic shunting or from a reduction in the processing capacity of the liver. In individuals with hepatic failure an intestinal protein load either from the diet or from, for example, oesophageal variceal haemorrhage, will significantly increase ammonia levels and can produce overt encephalopathy.

The mechanism by which increased circulating blood ammo-nia leads to encephalopathy remains unclear. Recent evidence suggests that the observed oedema of glial cells that accompanies hyperammonaemia, and which can be exacerbated by other fac-tors known to predispose to hepatic encephalopathy, is likely to be important (Haussinger and Schliess, 2008). Ammonia read-ily passes through the blood–brain barrier and can be detoxi-fied, in astrocytes, by scavenging processes producing glutamine from glutamate. Increased cerebral metabolism of ammonia has been demonstrated by positron emission tomography in individuals with hepatic encephalopathy (Lockwood, 2002). Increased intracellular levels of osmotically active glutamine cause intra-astrocytic oedema. This oedematous change has been found to occur primarily within the frontal and occipital white matter, the globus pallidus, the putamen, and the anterior limb of the internal capsule (Haussinger and Schliess, 2008). It is thought that astrocytic oedema may cause alterations in cell function and gene expression in part through oxidative stress-dependent modi-fications of proteins and RNA. Alteration of GABAergic and glu-tamatergic neurotransmission systems may be examples of such effects on cell function. Enhanced GABA$_A$ receptor activity that is only partially reversed by a benzodiazepine antagonist such as flumazenil, is one of several possible pathways involved in the gen-eration of hepatic encephalopathy.

In addition to ammonia, intestinal bacteria produce other potential central neurotoxins such as benzodiazepine-like com-pounds, mercaptans, phenols, and short- and medium-chain fatty acids, all of which have been found in relatively high levels in indi-viduals with chronic liver disease (Williams, 2007).

Elevated serum levels of manganese have also been detected in individuals with cirrhosis and encephalopathy and autopsy specimens have demonstrated increased deposition of manga-nese within the basal ganglia (Rose et al., 1999). It has been pos-tulated that the deposition of manganese, a known neurotoxin, may cause, either directly or via effects on dopamine receptors, the extrapyramidal signs and symptoms noted in some individu-als with encephalopathy. Manganese may also act synergistically with ammonia to increase the activity of GABAergic neurotrans-mission (Jones and Basile, 1998).

Episodes of acute hepatic encephalopathy in chronic liver dis-ease can be precipitated by a variety of factors, most frequently infection, alcohol, or other sedative drugs, gastrointestinal haem-orrhage, electrolyte disturbance, dehydration, and constipation (Box 10.4.2). Infection can precipitate delirium in any individual

Box 10.4.2 Common precipitating factors of hepatic encephalopathy

- Infection
- Drugs (benzodiazepines, opioids, alcohol and other sedatives)
- Gastrointestinal bleeding
- Excessive dietary protein
- Constipation
- Dehydration
- Uraemia
- Hypokalaemia
- Hypoglycaemia
- Anaemia
- Hypoxia.

ut those with chronic liver disease seem particularly susceptible. It has been postulated that inflammatory cytokines produced in response to infection may affect the central nervous system at several different levels and, in synergism with hyperammonaemia, precipitate frank encephalopathy. Interleukins 1 and 6 and TNF-α have been particularly implicated (Blei, 2004). Another theory suggests that the reduced cerebral blood flow associated with bacteraemia may augment the existing reduced cerebral flow associated with chronic liver disease (Blei, 2004).

Diagnosis of hepatic encephalopathy

The diagnosis of hepatic encephalopathy could be thought of as one of exclusion given the many possible causes of delirium associated with abnormal neurological signs. Other metabolic disorders, infection, cerebrovascular events, and intracranial space-occupying lesions may all present in a similar fashion. However, in individuals with known liver disease, the existence of a precipitating factor and/or a prior history of hepatic encephalopathy the diagnosis can usually be safely made. The presence of asterixis ('liver flap'), fetor hepaticus, and extrapyramidal signs help strengthen the diagnosis but are not always present. Elevated blood ammonia levels may confirm the degree of underlying liver disease and susceptibility to encephalopathy.

Other objective diagnostic methods have been described including the measurement of visual and auditory evoked potentials (Sandford and Saul, 1988), electroencephalography, and, more recently, actigraphy (Hourmand-Ollivier et al., 2006).

An International Working Party has recommended the use of the West Haven criteria (Table 10.4.6) and Glasgow Coma scales for grading and monitoring established encephalopathy (Mullen, 2007).

Covert encephalopathy

An estimated 50–80% of individuals with cirrhosis will have subclinical encephalopathy, without classic clinical signs and demonstrated only by altered formal psychometric testing. These individuals are not only at increased risk of acute episodes of frank encephalopathy (Mullen, 2007) but also have associated impaired daily functioning,

disturbed sleep patterns, and a predisposition to other dangers such as road traffic accidents (Kappus and Bajaj, 2011). The potential to reverse such 'covert encephalopathy', or to at least delay progression to overt encephalopathy, means recognition of the condition is important (Cordoba et al., 1998; Groeneweg et al., 1998).

Psychometric testing has been recommended by an International Working Party as a reliable method of detecting and monitoring covert encephalopathy. The group recommended the use of at least two instruments including either the number connection tests-A and/or B, the block design test or the digit symbol test (Quero et al., 1996).

Management of encephalopathy

The care of individuals with encephalopathy will be similar to that given to those with delirium. The environment and approach taken by care staff is particularly important for individuals likely to be disorientated and at risk of falls. The family and other lay carers are likely to need particular support and should be included in care procedures wherever possible.

Precipitating factors of encephalopathy in chronic liver disease have been well described (Table 10.4.6) and investigation and treatment should firstly be directed at such factors. A careful history is required with particular note taken of symptoms suggestive of an infection or upper gastrointestinal haemorrhage and a review made of recent psychotropic drug use, prescribed and otherwise.

Table 10.4.6 West Haven criteria of altered mental state in hepatic encephalopathy

Stage 0	Lack of detectable changes in personality or behaviour
	Impairment noted only on formal psychomotor testing
	Asterixis absent
Stage 1	Mild lack of awareness
	Shortened attention span
	Altered sleep pattern
	Mild asterixis or tremor
Stage 2	Lethargy
	Disorientation
	Inappropriate behaviour
	Slurred speech
	Obvious asterixis
Stage 3	Somnolent but rousable
	Gross disorientation
	Bizarre behaviour
	Asterixis generally absent
	Increased muscle tone and hyper-reflexia
Stage 4	Coma
	Decerebrate posturing

Reproduced from Ferenci P et al., Hepatic encephalopathy—definition, nomenclature, diagnosis, and quantification: final report of the working party at the 11th World Congresses of Gastroenterology, Vienna, 1998, *Hepatology*, Volume 37, Issue 3, pp. 716-21, Copyright © 2002 American Association for the Study of Liver Diseases, with permission from John Wiley & Sons, Inc.

It is generally agreed that the production of ammonia and possibly other, as yet undefined, neurotoxins by intestinal bacteria is key to the pathogenesis of hepatic encephalopathy. Most proposed therapeutic options are therefore directed towards a reduction in ammonia production or increased clearance through dietary manipulation, non-absorbable disaccharides, and broad-spectrum antibiotics.

Diet

A high-protein diet can increase ammonia production and precipitate encephalopathy and in the acute stages restriction of dietary protein intake is usually suggested. However, in the longer term, protein restriction can aggravate encephalopathy, and in the setting of the increased catabolic rate that is often present in chronic liver disease, can lead to a reduced skeletal muscle mass with a consequent reduced ability to detoxify ammonia (Blei and Cordoba, 2001). A recent International Working Group has suggested an optimal diet comprises 1.2–1.5 g/kg/day of mainly vegetable protein along with a late-night snack of complex carbohydrates to minimize protein metabolism (Amodio et al., 2013).

Disaccharides

The cornerstone of the medical management of encephalopathy has for many years been the use of non-absorbable disaccharides, such as lactulose. Lactulose is not broken down by intestinal enzymes so reaches the colon where it is metabolized by bacteria to acetic and lactic acid. Intestinal bacteria will preferentially take up carbohydrate over protein so that lactulose or any other carbohydrate in the diet will potentially reduce bacterial ammonia production. Additionally, as result of bacterial metabolism, acidification of the intestinal contents converts ammonia to non-diffusible ammonium, helps catharsis and excretion of potential toxins and may aid a change in microbial population from urease producing bacteria to acidophilic non-urease producing organisms (Bass, 2007). The use of additional probiotic and synbiotic preparations to further aid the change in intestinal flora has also been proposed, but whilst trials suggest benefit they have been of generally poor quality (McGee et al., 2011; Shukla et al., 2011). Protocols for the use of lactulose usually suggest titration of dosing to produce two or three soft stools per day. Lactulose can produce nausea, bloating, abdominal cramps, and, in cases of excessive diarrhoea, dehydration and hypernatraemia which can exacerbate encephalopathy. Despite the regular use of disaccharides such as lactulose in the management of hepatic encephalopathy for many years, a recent Cochrane systematic review found only modest benefit overall and no significant benefit when only high quality trials were included in the analysis (Als-Nielsen et al., 2004c). The authors concluded there was insufficient evidence to support or refute the use of disaccharides in encephalopathy and, additionally, in head-to-head trials antibiotics were superior to disaccharides in terms of improved symptoms and lowered ammonia levels.

Antibiotics

Antibiotics to reduce the numbers of urease-producing bacteria in the intestine have been employed in the management of encephalopathy for many years. The use of neomycin, metronidazole, ampicillin and, more recently, rifaximin have been described (Festi et al., 2006). The evidence for the use of neomycin and metronidazole is modest and there is concern over the prolonged use of these agents because of the risk of toxicity. Rifaximin is a broad-spectrum, poorly-absorbed, antibiotic with a tolerability comparable to placebo (Huang and DuPont, 2005). Several trials have demonstrated its efficacy in relieving symptoms of encephalopathy, reducing blood ammonia levels and improving electroencephalographic abnormalities (Festi et al., 2006). One recent study demonstrated lower serum levels of ammonia, benzodiazepine-like substances, and endotoxin in individuals treated with rifaximin (Lighthouse et al., 2004). Interestingly this same study demonstrated that clinical improvement could be maintained by sequential administration of rifaximin followed by a probiotic mixture of lactobacilli and bifidobacter.

Neurotransmitters

Although endogenous or bacterial-derived benzodiazepine-like substances are thought to be involved in the pathogenesis of encephalopathy, studies of the use of the antagonist, flumazenil, have shown a short-lived effect at best (Als-Nielsen et al., 2004a). The use of this approach is probably limited to managing encephalopathy precipitated by the intake of benzodiazepine medications.

The presence of extrapyramidal signs in some individuals with hepatic encephalopathy has generated a small number of studies into the use of the dopaminergic agonists such as L-dopa and bromocriptine. A recent Cochrane systematic review concluded that there was insufficient evidence to recommend their use (Als-Nielsen et al., 2004b).

Miscellaneous

The maintenance of circulating blood volume by correction of dehydration (often caused by overuse of diuretics) is important to maintain adequate renal excretion of ammonia (Shawcross and Jalan, 2005).

Skeletal muscle reduces circulating ammonia through the synthesis of glutamine and L-ornithine L-aspartate can provide intermediates that increase glutamate availability. Several studies suggest that administration of L-ornithine L-aspartate can improve the symptoms of encephalopathy (Shawcross and Jalan, 2005).

The administration of phenylbutyrate provides an alternate pathway of nitrogen excretion whereby glutamine is conjugated and excreted by the kidney with no production of ammonia. Early studies have been promising (Rockey et al., 2014).

The role of external detoxification devices akin to dialysis in renal failure has been proposed for individuals with hepatic encephalopathy. Artificial support systems such as MARS (molecular adsorbents recirculating system) and bioartificial systems have been shown in a systematic review of a small number of trials to significantly improve symptoms of encephalopathy and are under continued investigation (Liu et al., 2004). Interestingly one trial showed significant improvement in encephalopathy with MARS without changes in blood levels of ammonia (Sen et al., 2004).

Liver transplantation should always be considered when hepatic encephalopathy develops in chronic liver disease. Unfortunately signs and symptoms do not always resolve indicating that permanent organic cerebral changes can occur (Mas, 206).

There is a recent awakening of interest in the management of hepatic encephalopathy prompted by advances in molecular biology and imaging techniques. The role of anti-inflammatory agents, *N*-methyl-D-aspartate receptor antagonists, L-carnitine, sodium benzoate and phenylacetate, manganese chelators, and zinc supplementation are all under investigation.

Summary

At present, given the relative lack of evidence for any of the medical interventions described, it is imperative that any individual presenting with hepatic encephalopathy is, if appropriate given the context of the associated disease process, intensively investigated for precipitating factors. Close attention paid to treating infections, dehydration, acid–base and electrolyte disturbances, and constipation is likely to have the most significant impact on the clinical situation. If no precipitating factors are identified or symptoms are persistent, then antibiotics such as neomycin or particularly rifaximin, if available, should receive a trial of therapy. The care of individuals with covert hepatic encephalopathy continues to be a worthy subject of debate.

Online materials

Complete references for this chapter are available online at <http://www.oxfordmedicine.com>.

References

Abraham, N.S., Barkun, J.S., and Barkun, A.N. (2002). Palliation of malignant biliary obstruction: a prospective trial examining impact on quality of life. *Gastrointestinal Endoscopy*, 56, 835–841.

Alemi, F., Kwon, E., Poole, D.P.J., *et al.* (2013) The TGR5 receptor mediates bile acid-induced itch and analgesia. *Journal of Clinical Investigation*, 123, 1513–1530.

Als-Nielsen, B., Gluud, L.L., and Gluud, C. (2004c). Nonabsorbable disaccharides for hepatic encephalopathy. *Cochrane Database of Systematic Reviews*, 2, CD003044.

Amodio, P., Bemeur, C., Butterworth, R., *et al.* (2013) The nutritional management of hepatic encephalopathy in patients with cirrhosis: International Society for Hepatic Encephalopathy and Nitrogen Metabolism Consensus. *Hepatology*, 58, 325–36.

Ballinger, A.B., McHugh, M., Catnach, S.M., Alstead, E.M., and Clark, M.L. (1994). Symptom relief and quality of life after stenting for malignant bile duct obstruction. *Gut*, 35, 467–470.

Barkay, O., Mosler, P., Schmitt, C.M., *et al.* (2013). Effect of endoscopic stenting of malignant bile duct obstruction on quality of life. *Journal of Clinical Gastroenterology*, 47, 526–531.

Becker, G., Galandi, D., and Blum, H.E. (2006). Malignant ascites: systematic review and guideline for treatment. *European Journal of Medicine*, 42, 589–597.

Beecham, J.B., Kucera, P., Helmkamp, B.F., and Bonfiglio, T.A. (1983). Peritoneal angiogenesis in patients with ascites. *Gynecologic Oncology*, 15, 142.

Bergasa, N.V. (2004). An approach to the management of the pruritus of cholestasis. *Clinics in Liver Disease*, 8, 55–66.

Bergasa, N.V., Alling, D.W., Talbot, T.L., *et al.* (1995). Effects of naloxone infusions in patients with the pruritus of cholestasis. A double-blind, randomized, controlled trial. *Annals of Internal Medicine*, 123, 161–167.

De Simone, G.G. (1999). Treatment of malignant ascites. *Progress in Palliative Care*, 7, 10–16.

Di Padova, C., Tritapepe, R., Rovagnati, P., *et al.* (1984) Double-blind placebo-controlled clinical trial of microporous cholestyramine in the treatment of intra and extra-hepatic cholestasis: relationship between itching and serum bile acids. *Methods and Findings in Experimental and Clinical Pharmacology*, 6, 773–776.

Dy, S.M., Harman, S.M., Braun, U.K., *et al.* (2012). To stent or not to stent: an evidence-based approach to palliative procedures at the end of life. *Journal of Pain and Symptom Management*, 43, 795–801.

Festi, D., Vestito, A., Mazzella, G., Roda, E., and Colecchia, A. (2006). Management of hepatic encephalopathy: focus on antibiotic therapy. *Digestion*, 73(Suppl. 1), 94–101.

Ford-Dunn, S. (2005). Managing patients with cancer and advanced liver disease. *Palliative Medicine*, 19, 563–565.

Garcea, G., Ngu, W., Neal, C.P., *et al.* (2011). Bilirubin levels predict malignancy in patients with obstructive jaundice. *HPB*, 13, 426–430.

Garrison, R.N., Kaelin, L.D., Galloway, R.H., and Heuser, L.S. (1986). Malignant ascites. Clinical and experimental observations. *Annals or Surgery*, 203, 644–651.

Gines, P., Cardenas, A., Arroyo, V., and Rodes, J. (2004). Management of cirrhosis and ascites. *The New England Journal of Medicine*, 350, 1646–1654.

Haussinger, D. and Schliess, F. (2008) Pathogenetic mechanisms of hepatic encephalopathy. *Gut*, 57, 1156–1165.

Health Protection Agency (2012). *Hepatitis C in the UK. 2012 Report.* [Online] Available at: <http://www.hpa.org.uk/webc/HPAwebFile/HPAweb_C/1317135237219>.

Jones, D.E. (2012). Pathogenesis of cholestatic itch: old questions, new answers, and future opportunities. *Hepatology*, 56, 1194–1196.

Jones, E.A. and Zylicz, Z. (2005). Treatment of pruritus caused by cholestasis with opioid antagonists. *Journal of Palliative Medicine*, 8, 1290–1294.

Jones, E.A., Neuberger, J., and Bergasa, N.V. (2002). Opiate antagonist therapy for the pruritus of cholestasis: the avoidance of opioid withdrawal-like reactions. *Quarterly Journal of Medicine*, 95, 547–552.

Kamath, P.S. (1996). Clinical approach to the patient with abnormal liver test results. *Mayo Clinic Proceedings*, 71, 1089–1094.

Kappus, M.R. and Bajaj, J.S. (2011). Covert hepatic encephalopathy: not as minimal as you might think. *Clinical Gastroenterology and Hepatology*, 10, 1208–1219.

Keen, A., Fitzgerald, D., Bryant, A., and Dickinson, H.O. (2010) Management of drainage for malignant ascites in gynaecological cancer. *Cochrane Database of Systematic Reviews*, 1, CD007794.

Kremer, A.E., van Dijk, R., Leckie, P., *et al.* (2012) Serum autotaxin is increased in pruritus of cholestasis, but not of other origin, and responds to therapeutic interventions. *Hepatology*, 56, 1391–400.

Larssen, L., Medhus, A.W., Hjermstad, M.J., *et al.* (2011). Patient-reported outcomes in palliative gastrointestinal stenting: a Norwegian multi-center study. *Surgical Endoscopy*, 25, 3162–3169.

Lee, C.W., Bociek, G., and Faught, W. (1998). A survey of practice in management of malignant ascites. *Journal of Pain and Symptom Management*, 16, 96–101.

Lindor, K.D., Gershwin, M.E., Poupon, R., *et al.* (2009) Primary biliary cirrhosis. *Hepatology*, 50, 291–308.

Luman, W., Cull, A., and Palmer, K.R. (1997). Quality of life in patients stented for malignant biliary obstructions. *European Journal of Gastroenterology & Hepatology*, 9, 481–484.

Malik, I., Abubakar, S., Rizwana, I., Alam, F., Rizvi, J., and Khan, A. (1991). Clinical features and management of malignant ascites. *Journal of the Pakistan Medical Association*, 41, 38–40.

Moorsom, D. (2001). Paracentesis in a home care setting. *Palliative Medicine*, 15, 169–170.

Mullen, K.D. (2007). Review of the final report of the 1998 Working Party on definition, nomenclature and diagnosis of hepatic encephalopathy. *Alimentary Pharmacology & Therapeutics*, 25(Suppl. 1), 11–16.

National Institute for Health and Clinical Excellence (2012). *The PleurX Peritoneal Catheter Drainage System for Vacuum-Assisted Drainage of Treatment-Resistant, Recurrent Malignant Ascites*. NICE medical technology guidance MTG9. London: NICE.

Phan, N.Q., Lotts, T., Antal, A., *et al.* (2012) Systemic kappa opioid receptor agonists in the treatment of chronic pruritus: a literature review. *Acta Dermato-Venereologica*, 92, 555–560.

Pockros, P.J., Esrason, K.T., Nguyen, C., Duque, J., and Woods, S. (1992). Mobilization of malignant ascites with diuretics is dependent on ascitic fluid characteristics. *Gastroenterology*, 103, 1302–1306.

Prieto, L.N. (2004). The use of midazolam to treat itching in a terminally ill patient with biliary obstruction. *Journal of Pain and Symptom Management*, 28, 531–532.

Quero, J.C., Hartmann, I.J., Meulstee, J., Hop, W.C., and Schalm, S.W. (1996). The diagnosis of subclinical hepatic encephalopathy in patients with cirrhosis using neuropsychological tests and automated electroencephalogram analysis. *Hepatology*, 24, 556–560.

Rosenberg, S.M. (2006). Palliation of malignant ascites. *Gastroenterology Clinics of North America*, 35, 189–199.

Runyon, B.A. (1994). Care of patients with ascites. *The New England Journal of Medicine*, 330, 337–342.

Shawcross, D. and Jalan, R. (2005). Dispelling myths in the treatment of hepatic encephalopathy. *The Lancet*, 365, 431–433.

Stephenson, J. and Gilbert, J. (2002). The development of clinical guidelines on paracentesis for ascites related to malignancy. *Palliative Medicine*, 16, 213–218.

Szarvas, S., Harmon, D., and Murphy, D. (2003). Neuraxial opioid-induced pruritus: a review. *Journal of Clinical Anesthesia*, 15, 234–239.

Twycross, R., Greaves, M.W., Handwerker, H., *et al.* (2003). Itch: scratching more than the surface. *Quarterly Journal of Medicine*, 96, 7–26.

White, M.A., Agle, S.C., Padia, R.K., and Zervos, E.E. (2011). Denver peritoneovenous shunts for the management of malignant ascites: a review of the literature in the post LeVeen Era. *American Surgeon*, 77, 1070–1075

Williams, J.W., Jr and Simel, D.L. (1992). The rational clinical examination. Does this patient have ascites? How to divine fluid in the abdomen. *Journal of the American Medical Association*, 267, 2645–2648.

Williams, R. (2006). Global challenges in liver disease. *Hepatology*, 44, 521–526.

Williams, R. (2007). Review article: bacterial flora and pathogenesis in hepatic encephalopathy. *Alimentary Pharmacology & Therapeutics*, 25(Suppl. 1), 17–22.

Aetiology, classification, assessment, and treatment of the anorexia-cachexia syndrome

Vickie E. Baracos, Sharon M. Watanabe, and Kenneth C. H. Fearon

Introduction to aetiology, classification, assessment and treatment of the anorexia-cachexia syndrome

The anorexia-cachexia syndrome is a complex multidimensional problem and, until recently (Evans et al., 2008; Fearon et al., 2011), there has been no generally agreed classification system or treatment algorithm. This had led clinicians to feel that perhaps it was not worth trying to grapple with the difficult problem of assessment and treatment of patients with cachexia. Recent progress in our understanding of the underlying biology and the development of new biological therapeutic targets has led to a new era of hopeful optimism. The aim of this chapter is to resolve some of these issues and provide (a) the reader with some background principles to classification, (b) a simple approach to patient assessment and a robust algorithm for basic multimodal treatment, and (c) an overview of the evidence base for different pharmacological interventions.

Cachexia affects a wide spectrum of patients with a variety of chronic diseases including cancer, chronic heart failure, end-stage renal failure, rheumatoid arthritis, and HIV. The common feature of cachexia is that it is not possible to completely reverse the syndrome with conventional nutritional support. Whilst undoubtedly there are common mechanisms of wasting in each of these conditions, there are many unique aspects which are too complex to explore in a single chapter. The present chapter focuses primarily on the patient with cancer. It is hoped that the principles outlined will provide a platform on which to build an approach for other groups of patients. To this end, comment is added in 'Pharmacological treatment' section on specific pharmacological interventions where the latter have been tested in large groups of cachectic patients with chronic diseases other than cancer.

Before approaching classification and therapeutics, it is useful to have some understanding of the pathophysiology of cachexia as these principles should underpin the logic behind the clinical management of patients. Cachexia is characterized by a negative energy and protein balance driven by a variable combination of reduced food intake and abnormal metabolism. Thus it is important to assess and manage actively both food intake and abnormal metabolism in all patients. Cancer cachexia may be considered initially an adaptive response to access body stores of energy and protein. Mobilization of skeletal muscle and adipose tissue is a highly organized response. Inflammation is widely agreed to be a unifying mechanism for the entire cluster of sickness behaviours (asthenia, increased slow wave sleep, mood alteration, lethargy, depression, anorexia, fever, anhedonia, cognitive impairment, hyperalgesia, and decreased social interaction), including loss of fat and muscle. Inflammation is generated in the brain, by the tumour, by tissues in the locale of the tumour and by a diversity of host cells including skeletal muscle, adipose tissue, and cells of the immune system and liver. The specific identity of the inflammatory and neuro-endocrine mediators participating in cancer cachexia is emerging (Fearon et al., 2012).

It is also important to recognize that cachexia in general, and muscle wasting in particular, does not occur in isolation. Other factors that can exacerbate muscle wasting include co-morbid conditions (e.g. cardiac failure, chronic obstructive pulmonary disease (COPD), and chronic renal failure), old age (age-related sarcopenia), physical deconditioning, hypogonadism, insulin resistance, nutritional deficiency, drugs, and medical interventions (including all major cancer therapies: surgery, radiotherapy and chemotherapy). Given such clinical complexity, there has been a drive to establish specific clinics to deal with cachexia and this is something that may develop further in the future.

Classification

A conceptual framework for classification

Cachexia is a syndrome of involuntary weight loss, which may progress through various phases (pre-cachexia, cachexia syndrome, refractory cachexia (Fearon, K., Strasser, F., Anker, S., et al. (2011). Definition and classification of cancer cachexia: an international consensus. The Lancet Oncology, 12, 489–495)) and culminate in a grossly emaciated state (severe cachexia). The depletion pertains to body weight and its major elements which constitute the physiological stores of energy and protein in the body (i.e. adipose tissue and skeletal muscle). Varying degrees of depletion are associated with quantifiable risks. The health risks that have been considered range from functional loss (e.g. physical function, immune function), morbidity (e.g. injuries from falls, infections), increased

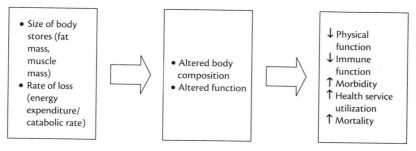

Fig. 10.5.1 The timing and magnitude of the clinical risks associated with cachexia are determined, in part, by the size of the initial body stores and the rate at which they are lost.

health service utilization and associated costs (e.g. hospital stay, emergency room visit) to mortality (Fig. 10.5.1). The timing of the emergence of and the magnitude of the clinical risks associated with body weight loss are affected by the patients' initial body weight (constituting the stores that may be mobilized) and the dynamic rate of loss of these constituents.

Weight and weight loss classification

The designation of clinically underweight is consistent with the notion of depletion of body reserves below a functionally important threshold. The simplest and most widely understood classification scheme is the World Health Organization (WHO) (WHO, 2000) categories of body mass adjusted for stature (body mass index (BMI): weight (kg)/height (m^2)) are widely used to classify clinically important deviations of body weight (Table 10.5.1). In addition to the risks from a variety of morbidities and mortality from secondary causes, depletion to a BMI in the vicinity of 10–11 kg/m^2 is, of itself, fatal (Rigaud et al., 2000). It should be noted that in patients over 65 years of age, a somewhat higher limit for underweight (20 kg/m^2) is generally accepted. During weight loss, individuals may pass through a zone conventionally referred to as 'normal', 'healthy', or 'ideal' body weight. However, depending on the intensity of weight loss, severe depletion will occur sooner or later; this situation is neither healthy nor ideal.

Healthy adults are highly resistant to weight reduction and the appearance of involuntary weight loss is both a fundamental abnormality of physiological regulation and a cardinal diagnostic criterion of cancer cachexia. Various classification schemes for weight loss have been developed with different intent. The National Cancer Institute's Common Toxicity Criteria (Cancer Therapy Evaluation Program, 2006) are used widely to define cancer- and cancer therapy-associated toxicity and these define the total degree of loss relative to stable body weight as follows: grade 0, up to 4.9% loss; grade 1, 5–9.9%; grade 2, 10–19.9%; and grade 3, 20% or higher. Grade 4 (life-threatening) weight loss is not defined. The scored Patient-Generated Subjective Global Assessment (PG-SGA) (Ottery 1996), a tool designed to screen for malnutrition, includes a grading system incorporating four weight loss grades that can be based on a 1-month or 6-month weight history, whichever is available (Table 10.5.2). These different grading systems provide one possible explanation for the considerable confusion amongst oncologists as to what constitutes a clinically significant degree of weight loss (Spiro et al., 2006). A recent analysis of an international sample of over 11,000 patients with advanced stages of cancer (Martin et al., in press) provides a

Table 10.5.1 WHO classification of body mass adjusted for stature: body mass index (BMI)

	BMI (kg/m^2)
Severely underweight	<16
Moderately underweight	16–17
Mildly underweight	17–18.5[a]
Normal	18.5–25
Overweight	25–30
Class I obesity	30–35
Class II obesity	35–40
Morbid obesity	>40

[a] Range extended 17–20 in elderly.

Reproduced with permission from World Health Organization (WHO) Technical Report Series, Obesity: preventing and managing the global epidemic, Issue 894, pp.1–253, Copyright © 2000, available from http://whqlibdoc.who.int/trs/WHO_TRS_894_(part1).pdf.

Table 10.5.2 Weight loss score from the Patient-Generated Subjective Global Assessment

Grade	1-month loss	6-month loss
0	0–1.9%	0–1.9%
1	2.0–2.9%	2.0–5.9%
2	3.0–4.9%	6.0–9.9%
3	5.0–9.9%	10.0–19.9%
4	≥ 10%	≥ 20%

Reproduced from Nutrition Volume 12, Issue 1, Supplement, Ottery, F.D., Definition of standardized nutritional assessment and interventional pathways in oncology, pp.S15–19, Copyright © 1996, with permission from Elsevier, http://www.sciencedirect.com/science/journal/08999007.

grading system based on BMI and percentage weight loss, allowing both the degree of depletion of BMI and the rate of their loss to be simultaneously incorporated. BMI and weight loss were entered into a multivariate analysis controlling for age, sex, cancer site, stage, and performance status and their relationships to overall survival were examined to develop a grading system based on their prognostic weight. Five categories of BMI (< 20.0, 20.0–21.9,

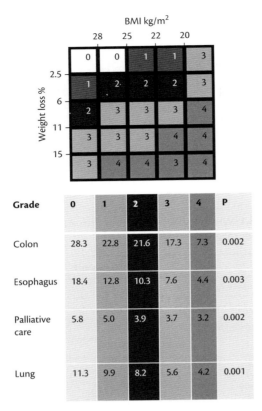

Fig. 10.5.2 (BMI-adjusted) Weight loss grade. Grading scheme is based on groupings showing distinct median survival. Different colours denote distinct survival (P < 0.001; adjusted for age, sex, disease site, stage and performance status).

22.0–24.9, 25.0–27.9, ≥ 28.0 kg/m²) differed in overall survival (P < 0.001). Five categories of weight behavior also differed in survival (P < 0.001): (weight stable (+2.4 to −2.4%) and weight loss −2.5 to −5.9%, −6.0 to −10.9%, −11.0 to −14.9%, ≥ −15.0%). Grade (0–4) was assigned according to the combined prognostic weight of BMI and weight loss (Fig. 10.5.2).

Measurement of tissue wasting

It is clear that the main constituents of body weight, adipose and lean tissues, merit separate consideration. This adds new orders of complexity to our understanding of wasting syndromes. Both muscle protein and adipose tissues can be considered as independent physiologic stores. The presence of a large adipose tissue reserve, at least up to a certain point, is a favourable prognostic factor in patients embarking on different types of wasting syndromes. By itself, depletion of muscle mass is associated with health risks, including frailty, functional problems in gait and balance, risk of falls, inability to complete tasks of daily living, extended hospital stay and infectious and non-infectious complications in hospital, as well as overall mortality (Baumgartner et al., 1998; Morley et al., 2001; Roubenoff, 2003; Kyle et al., 2005; Cosqueric et al., 2006). These health risks are seen to be independent of adiposity and are present in normal body weight ranges, as well as in obese persons. Skeletal muscle wasting may be under-recognized in the context of epidemic obesity. Overweight and obese patients may already have substantial ongoing muscle depletion (sarcopenic obesity) at the time of presentation.

The independent significance of muscle wasting requires some clinical capacity to determine muscle mass. Individuals within a population present with different degrees of muscularity, and this feature is variously expressed in the literature depending on the methods used for its determination. Whole-body muscle mass may be evaluated using image-based approaches, and is often expressed in the same units as BMI (kg skeletal muscle/m²). Methods such as whole-body computed tomography (CT) or magnetic resonance image analysis are required to determine this value. Dual energy X-ray absorptiometry may be used to quantify muscle in the arms and legs only, expressed as total appendicular skeletal muscle (kg/m²). Anthropometrics constitute a simple tool to estimate skeletal muscle stores, as mid-arm muscle circumference. It should be noted that there are important methodological considerations. Ease of determination is often counterbalanced by low precision. Upper arm measurements are prone to inter-observer variation. Scoring fatness and muscularity on physical examination has utility in the hands of a highly trained observer, but is otherwise difficult to standardize. Mid-arm muscle circumference is based on the assumption that the upper arm is perfectly cylindrical, which it is evidently not. The image-based methods enjoying high precision and the ability to discriminate muscle and adipose tissues require instrumentation, money, and time. Cut-off points have been proposed for clinically important depletion of skeletal muscle (sarcopenia) (i.e. below the 5th percentile for healthy adults). Sex-specific cut points for severe muscle depletion have been suggested, according to the available methods of assessment: mid upper-arm muscle area by anthropometry (men < 32 cm², women < 18 cm²); appendicular skeletal muscle index determined by dual-energy X-ray absorptiometry (men < 7.26 kg/m²; women < 5.45 kg/m²); lumbar skeletal muscle index determined from oncology CT imaging (men < 55 cm²/m²; women < 39 cm²/m²); whole-body fat-free mass index without bone determined by bioelectrical impedance (men < 14.6 kg/m²; women < 11.4 kg/m²). This series of options includes methods with clinical utility as well as options for specialized or research-related investigations.

Multiple-factor classification systems

The definition of cachexia is a multifactorial syndrome characterized by an ongoing loss of skeletal muscle mass (with or without loss of fat mass) that cannot be fully reversed by conventional nutritional support and which leads to progressive functional impairment (Fearon et al., 2011). Reduced food intake is caused by primary anorexia (i.e. central nervous system level) and may be compounded by secondary impairments to oral intake. Concurrent hypermetabolism, hypercatabolism and hypoanabolism aggravate the associated weight loss and are provoked by systemic inflammation and catabolic factors that may act peripherally and via the central nervous system. Cachexia is thus a multidimensional problem and therefore it may not be possible to reflect the physiological change and clinical risks the patient sustains by a single measurement (e.g. loss of weight or skeletal muscle mass). On the basis that risk derives from several key elements in the cachexia syndrome, a classification system based on weight loss (> 10%), reduced food intake (< 1500 kcal/day) and systemic inflammation (serum C-reactive protein concentration > 10 mg/L) has been proposed (Fearon et al., 2006). Patients with all three features have increased physiological impairment and reduced survival. Of key clinical importance is that patients with early stage of disease who demonstrate these features are at high risk of early demise and are therefore a key group to target for early and effective intervention. The current international consensus classification system (Fearon et al., 2011) includes these three essential features but has extended the assessment domains to include anorexia/intake, reserves (including muscle mass), catabolic drivers (e.g. systemic inflammation) and functional and psychosocial impairment.

Clinical assessment and treatment strategy

When medical or nursing professionals who have not received specific training are confronted with a patient who requires nutritional assessment the prospect can seem daunting. Moreover, the purpose of such assessment is often muddled since no clear link between assessment and treatment has been provided. The purpose of this section is to provide a clear, logical framework for patient assessment and to link this with a simple treatment algorithm.

Patients lose weight as a result of reduced food intake, abnormal metabolic activity, or, most commonly, a combination of the two. Weight loss reflects that the patient has a negative energy balance (resulting in loss of fat mass: the main energy reserve) and a negative protein balance (resulting in loss of skeletal muscle: the main protein reserve). The purpose of nutritional assessment (Fig. 10.5.3) is to determine to what extent *stores* have been depleted, what contribution to this loss has been due to reduced food *intake*, what impact such changes are having on the patient's *performance*, and what *potential* there is for reversal of the situation. In turn, the potential for reversal is partly dependent on the nature of catabolic drivers including such factors as systemic inflammation and tumour progression. Each of these domains can be considered in relation to the patient's clinical journey (i.e. past, present, and future). The Scored PG-SGA (Ottery 1996) is a validated screening tool designed specifically for patients with cancer

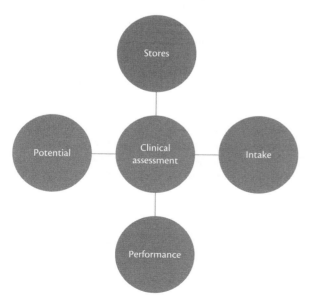

Fig. 10.5.3 Patients should be assessed briefly, if found to be at risk more detailed assessment is warranted and overall management should be guided by performance status

and is recommended by the Oncology Nutrition Dietetic Practice Group of the American Dietetic Association, and Oncology Nursing Society. Several elements of this instrument have practical utility for patient assessment, including the weight loss history (Table 10.5.2), the dietary intake component, checklist of 13 'nutrition impact' symptoms, and functional capacity component.

Stores (including muscle mass): the primary variables that are assessed readily are weight and weight loss history. Key questions include: height and current weight (kg), previous stable weight, duration of weight loss, and calculation of percentage weight loss. Weight loss grade 3 or 4 (Table 10.5.2) and/or a BMI less than 18.5 kg/m^2 are indicators of depletion of energy and/or protein reserves. As indicated previously, in the relatively near future it may be possible in routine practice to derive a direct measure of muscle wasting from diagnostic cross sectional imaging.

Intake: routine clinical assessment with the PG-SGA includes basic questions concerning type and amount of intake, loss of appetite, presence of early satiety, and other symptoms impeding dietary intake. This level of assessment is intended for non-specialists, and is useful for deciding when to refer patients to a nutrition health-care professional (dietitian or specialist in clinical nutrition). A detailed diet history or diet diary is a specialized assessment which usually undertaken by a dietician. The information from such assessments can be used to estimate total energy and macronutrient intakes.

Performance/psychosocial impact: every clinical, medical, or surgical oncologist is used to assessing the performance status of patients. The functional capacity component of the PG-SGA, is a version of the Eastern Cooperative Oncology Group (ECOG) performance status score; alternatively either the WHO or Karnofsky scales may be used. Knowledge whether the patient is active and mobile is vital in determining not only how depletion of stores/intake is affecting quality of life but also what the nature of therapy should be. Bed-bound patients suffer from anabolic resistance and in these circumstances it is very difficult to improve muscle mass/function. *It is also important to consider the psychosocial impact of cachexia both on the patient and their family* (Oberholzer et al., 2013). Physical activity may be impaired by the loss of muscle tissue, concentration, and alertness diminished by fatigue, and mood dominated by lethargy and increasing indifference. Patients may become isolated due to shrinking physical, mental, and emotional activity. Some families exhaust themselves by trying to fight the patient's visible loss of weight and power; urging him or her to eat despite the absence of appetite and finally experiencing frustration, helplessness, and fear.

Catabolic drivers (potential for reversal): knowledge of the patient's tumour type, stage of disease, and purpose of current cancer therapy can give a ready impression of prognosis and the purpose of nutritional intervention. The presence or absence of systemic inflammation (serum C-reactive protein > 10mg/L) may also identify the patient who requires early nutritional/metabolic support (Fearon et al., 2006). For the patient with relatively stable disease and with more than 2 months to live it is reasonable to plan nutritional intervention. For the patient whose disease is progressing rapidly and has less than 2–3 months to live, symptomatic management (e.g. steroids) is perhaps more appropriate (refractory cachexia). It is also important to consider carefully the patients' expectations concerning the future benefits of any intervention. The burden of intervention (e.g. daily intake of oral nutritional supplements) has to match what the patient is willing to consider in the light of possible gains.

Intervention strategy

A simple treatment algorithm is outlined in Fig. 10.5.4. For those not at nutritional risk (e.g. weight stable, adequate macronutrient stores, normal appetite/intake, good performance status, and stable disease) it would be reasonable simply to review or ask the patients to seek further advice if they lose weight. For patients at nutritional risk (grade 3 or 4 weight loss, BMI <18.5, evidence of depletion of lean body mass, reduced appetite/intake), it is vital to undertake a screen for reversible causes of anorexia/reduced food intake and to ensure that their underlying primary disease and co-morbidities are being managed optimally. Key variables to consider in relation to secondary causes of reduced intake include oral ulceration, intestinal obstruction, constipation, diarrhoea, nausea, vomiting, uncontrolled pain, and side effects of drugs. Metabolism-related variables include the development of diabetes or malabsorption (e.g. both common associations with advanced pancreatic cancer) and which if not managed with insulin/pancreatic enzyme supplements will result in continuing weight loss independent of any nutritional intervention.

The next stage in assessment involves consideration of the patient's performance status, prognosis, and expectations. For patients reaching an end-of-life phase and whose main complaint is anorexia, it would be reasonable to consider the prescription of oral steroids or megestrol acetate. For patients with a better prognosis (including those undergoing palliative chemotherapy/radiotherapy) and who are not bed-bound consideration should be given to the following four specific domains:

Oral intake

Cancer patients are often anxious about whether their diet has contributed to the development of cancer or whether it may modify the course of established illness. In general it is important to emphasize the need for a broad balanced diet and to explain the importance of maintaining a normal food intake in order to undergo cancer therapy or to optimize quality of life. It is vital to explore what patients consider to be a normal diet and to identify the principal daily source of protein in the diet. Two key basics in dietary advice are (a) that the average daily calorie deficit in a weight-losing cancer patient is of the order of 250–400 kcal/day and (b) that it is vital to maintain protein intake at a high level in order to either stabilize or replete diminished skeletal muscle mass. Protein intake should generally be maintained between 1–1.5g/kg/day (Wolfe, 2006). In order to achieve this intake, patients will generally need to consume red or white meat or fish on a daily basis and supplement this with dairy products (e.g. milk or cheese). An alternative approach is to take an energy- and protein-dense oral nutritional supplement. A 250 mL carton with 1.5 kcal/mL should contain sufficient calories and protein to make up the average daily deficit. However, significant repletion of a patient with depleted stores will probably require consumption of two such supplements per day. Patients will often benefit from specialist dietary assessment and advice from a

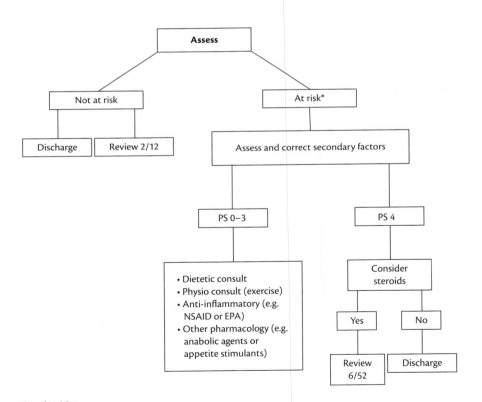

Fig. 10.5.4 Cachexia intervention algorithm.

* At risk defined by the presence of persistent weight loss, reduced dietary intake,

dietician especially if they continue to lose weight after initial management.

Exercise

The average physical activity levels of advanced cancer patients still attending the outpatient clinic is reduced by about 40–50% (Dahele et al., 2007). Many patients with advanced cancer are elderly and may have significant co-morbidity. Thus, the idea of resistance exercise training to optimize muscle mass is beyond their capacity. However, it is vital to explain to patients the value of daily exercise to counteract muscle wasting. Simply maintaining mobility and going out for a regular daily walk are reasonable goals to set. Motivated patients may benefit from the advice of a physiotherapist.

Anti-inflammatory

There is growing evidence concerning the role of systemic inflammation in most forms of cachexia. Inflammatory mediators contribute to both reduced food intake and metabolic change. There is no ideal anti-inflammatory strategy that has been proven to be of benefit in cachexia. However, two common approaches are either non-steroidal anti-inflammatory drugs (NSAIDs) (Preston et al., 1995) or fish oil (eicosapentaenoic acid (EPA), docosahexaenoic acid). NSAIDs with a low incidence of gastrointestinal side effects such as ibuprofen (400 mg three times daily) can be taken long term with or without gastric mucosal protection. Fish oil represents a 'natural' alternative and may appeal more to some patients. A total dose of 1.5–2.0 g/day EPA is recommended and can be taken either as fish oil capsules (Wigmore et al., 1996) or as a fish oil enriched oral nutritional supplement (Fearon et al., 2003; Moses et al., 2004).

Other specific pharmacological agents

See following section on 'Pharmacological treatment'.

Pharmacological treatment

Pharmacological approaches to wasting syndromes have a number of specific treatment targets and have been evaluated in a variety of diseases, including cancer, AIDS, and COPD. Such pharmacological treatments have been assessed in randomized clinical trials, and there are a number of high-quality systematic reviews (i.e. Cochrane Database) available summarizing the evidence. The reader is referred to these reviews for full details. The results of the systematic reviews are summarized in the following paragraphs, with information from subsequently published trials added. The section on cancer is the most extensive and an attempt to group the agents according to evidence/benefit has been made. With the introduction of effective antiretroviral therapy for HIV, the clinical problem of progressive wasting in this condition has mostly resolved in Western society. An abbreviated summary of the evidence for the management of HIV-related anorexia-cachexia is therefore presented.

Cancer

In 2005, Yavuzsen and colleagues published a systematic review of pharmacological therapies for cancer-associated anorexia and weight loss in adult patients with non-haematological malignancies. Fifty-five randomized controlled trials were included. Only two classes of drugs (progestins and corticosteroids) were found to have sufficient evidence to support their use in cancer patients. Studies with other agents had mixed outcomes, positive results in only a single trial, or were not adequately controlled. Note was made of heterogeneity amongst trials with respect to outcome measures, assessment tools, treatment duration, and timing of assessment (Yavuzsen et al., 2005).

Approaches well supported by evidence
Progestins

In the Yavuzsen review, the largest number of studies involved progestins (29 trials conducted in a total of 4139 patients). Twenty-three trials in 3436 patients involved megestrol acetate (MA) at doses of 160–1600 mg per day for 2 weeks to 2 years. Results for appetite and weight gain favoured MA over placebo. Five trials comparing different doses suggested that the optimal dose is between 480 and 800 mg per day. The influence of MA on quality of life was minimal.

Five trials compared MA with other drugs. MA was equivalent to corticosteroids and significantly better than dronabinol and fluoxymesterone for appetite stimulation. Compared with cisapride, MA was associated with significantly less weight loss and better appetite. Ibuprofen plus MA was significantly better than MA plus placebo at maintaining weight. A study comparing MA with EPA will be discussed later.

Six trials in 703 patients involved medroxyprogesterone acetate (MPA) at doses of 300 mg to 1200 mg per day for 6–12 weeks. Significant advantages were demonstrated for MPA versus placebo in terms of appetite improvement, increased caloric intake, and weight gain or attenuation of weight loss. Effects on quality of life were inconsistent (Yavuzsen et al., 2005).

In 2005, Berenstein and Ortiz published a systematic review of MA for the treatment of anorexia-cachexia syndrome in patients with cancer, AIDS or other underlying pathologies. Thirty-four randomized controlled trials involving 4826 patients were identified. Twenty-six were performed in cancer patients, while the remainder were in patients with AIDS, chronic obstructive lung disease, and cystic fibrosis, as well as in the elderly. Compared with placebo, relative risks for appetite improvement and weight gain in cancer patients were 3.03 (95% confidence interval (CI) 1.83–5.01) and 2.14 (95% CI 1.41–3.24), respectively. Oedema of the lower limbs was the only side effect that occurred at a significantly greater frequency with MA compared with placebo (relative risk 1.74, 95% CI 1.29–2.35) (Berenstein and Ortiz, 2005).

Corticosteroids

Corticosteroids were the subject of six studies conducted in a total of 637 patients, in the Yavuzsen review. Three trials in 402 patients used methylprednisolone orally or intravenously at doses of 32–125 mg per day for 1–8 weeks. Versus placebo, significant improvements were seen in appetite and quality of life, but not weight.

One trial in 61 patients involved prednisolone 10 mg per day for 6 weeks. Compared with placebo, appetite and well-being were significantly improved. Two trials in 184 patients used dexamethasone 3–8 mg per day for 4 days or until time of death. A transient improvement in appetite compared to placebo was seen.

Due to their well-known adverse effects, particularly with longer duration of use, corticosteroids may be more suitable for patients with a short life expectancy, especially if they have other symptoms that may be alleviated by this drug such as pain or nausea.

New approaches with limited supportive evidence
Androgenic steroids

Two trials examining the effects of androgenic steroids in a total of 512 patients were included in the review by Yavuzsen. The first compared chemotherapy plus nandrolone 200 mg intramuscularly weekly for 4 weeks versus chemotherapy alone. The nandrolone-treated patients demonstrated a trend towards less weight loss. The second trial, mentioned previously, compared fluoxymesterone with megestrol acetate or dexamethasone. Fluoxymesterone was inferior in terms of appetite and weight gain.

Eicosapentaenoic acid

In 2007, Dewey and colleagues published a systematic review that included five trials in a total of 587 patients, examining the effects of EPA given at doses of 1–6 g per day for 1 week to 3 months. Three studies compared EPA to placebo. Improvements were not shown for weight, lean body mass, quality of life, appetite, or total energy intake in patients treated with EPA. Two studies compared EPA to active treatment controls. One compared an EPA-containing nutritional supplement to a nutritional supplement without EPA; differences were not seen between arms for lean body mass and nutritional intake. The other compared EPA plus placebo, MA plus placebo, and EPA plus MA; appetite was not improved with EPA. Combined data from these two studies showed no benefit of EPA for weight gain or quality of life. The review concluded that there were insufficient data to establish whether oral EPA is better than placebo (Dewey et al., 2007).

Subsequently, a trial was published in which 518 patients were randomized to receive EPA 2 g per day, EPA 4 g per day, or placebo for 8 weeks; trends to improvement in weight and lean body mass were seen in patients treated with EPA 2 g per day (Fearon et al., 2006). In a double-blind randomized trial ($N = 40$), administration of EPA during chemotherapy for lung cancer was associated with better quality of life, performance status, and physical activity (van der Meij et al., 2012).

Ghrelin

A single-centre randomized double-blind placebo-controlled double-crossover trial was performed in 20 patients. They received ghrelin 2 micrograms per kg or 8 micrograms per kg intravenously prior to lunch on days 1 and 8, placebo on days 4 and 11, or vice versa. Patient preference scores tended to favour ghrelin. No differences between treatments were seen for nutritional intake, symptoms, adverse effects, or tolerability (Strasser et al., 2008).

In another study, 31 patients with metastatic gastrointestinal cancer were randomized in a double-blind manner to ghrelin 10 micrograms per kg or 0.5 micrograms per kg subcutaneously daily for 8 weeks. In the high-dose group, versus the low-dose group, appetite scores were significantly better, and there was a trend to less fat-free mass loss and improved energy balance. There were no differences in food intake, quality of life or physical activity (Lundholm et al., 2010).

Anamorelin

A pilot study was published, examining the short-term effects of anamorelin, a novel oral mimetic of ghrelin. Sixteen patients with incurable cancer and involuntary weight loss participated in this multicentre, randomized, double-blind, placebo-controlled, crossover trial. Treatment consisted of anamorelin 50 mg or placebo daily for 3 days, followed by a washout period of 3–7 days, then the alternative treatment for 3 days. Compared to placebo

treatment, anamorelin treatment was associated with significant advantages in terms of weight gain, and improvement in appetite and total symptom and quality of life scores. The drug was well-tolerated (Garcia et al., 2013). Results of a series of phase III trials are awaited.

Insulin

A single-centre, randomized, open-label trial was conducted to evaluate the effect of adding long-acting insulin to 'best available support', which consisted of indomethacin if erythrocyte sedimentation rate and C-reactive protein were elevated, erythropoietin if haemoglobin was below normal, and oral or parenteral nutritional supplementation if oral intake was reduced. One hundred and thirty-eight patients with advanced gastrointestinal malignancies were entered and followed until death or withdrawal from the study. Insulin treatment was associated with significantly higher carbohydrate but not overall caloric intake. Body weight and lean tissue mass did not differ, but trunk and leg fat was significantly higher with insulin treatment. Metabolic efficiency during exercise was significantly better with insulin treatment, but not maximum exercise capacity, maximum work load or physical activity. Quality of life was not different between groups. Survival was significantly longer in insulin-treated patients, suggesting that tumour growth was not stimulated (Lundholm et al., 2007).

Adenosine 5'-triphosphate

In a single-centre trial, 58 stage IIIB or IV non-small cell lung cancer patients were randomized in an unblinded manner to receive adenosine 5'-triphophate (ATP) and supportive care, or supportive care alone. ATP was administered by 30-hour intravenous infusion every 2 weeks for seven doses, and then every 4 weeks for three doses. Treatment was given on an inpatient basis. Compared with placebo, ATP was associated with significantly less weight loss, improved upper and lower extremity strength, better quality of life, increased energy intake and greater appetite (Agteresch et al., 2000, 2002).

Combined therapy

A single-centre, randomized, open-label phase III clinical trial of five different arms of treatment was conducted in 332 patients, who received one of (1) MPA 500 mg or MA 320 mg per day, (2) EPA 2.2 g per day in a nutritional supplement, (3) L-carnitine 4 g per day, (4) thalidomide 200 mg per day, or (5) the combination of the four treatments. All patients also received polyphenols, lipoic acid, carbocysteine, vitamin E, vitamin A, and vitamin C. The MPA/MA and EPA arms were stopped early at interim analysis due to inferiority. The combination arm was found to be significantly superior for increase in lean body, decrease in resting energy expenditure, decrease in fatigue, and increase in appetite. Toxicity was negligible and comparable (Mantovani et al., 2010).

The same group published a single-centre, randomized, open-label phase III clinical trial of combined treatment for cachexia in patients with gynaecological cancers. One hundred and forty-four gynaecological cancer patients with progressive or recurrent disease after one of more lines of chemotherapy and weight loss received either a combined treatment of the antioxidant agents alpha lipoic acid 600 mg and carbocysteine 2.7 g per day, L-carnitine 4 g per day, and MA 320 mg per day, or MA 320 mg per day alone. Significant differences were seen in favour of combined treatment for increase in lean body mass, decrease in resting energy expenditure, decrease in fatigue, and improvement in quality of life. Toxicity was negligible and comparable (Maccio et al., 2012).

The same group also published a single-centre, randomized, open-label phase III non-inferiority study, the aim of which was to simplify combined treatment. Sixty patients with advanced cancer, weight loss, and abnormal proinflammatory cytokine and/or C-reactive protein levels received L-carnitine 4 g per day plus celecoxib, or L-carnitine plus celecoxib plus MA 320 mg per day for 4 months. All patients also received polyphenols, lipoic acid, carbocysteine, vitamin E, vitamin A, and vitamin C. Both groups demonstrated a significant gain in lean body mass, without a difference between arms. Neither arm showed a change in total daily physical activity. Significant improvement in the 6-minute walk test was seen in both arms, without a difference between arms. Grip strength did not change in either arm. Resting energy expenditure, fatigue, performance status, and Glasgow Prognostic Score decreased in both arms. Body weight tended to increase in the arm with MA. Appetite improved in both arms. Adverse effects were negligible and comparable (Madeddu et al., 2012).

Enobosarm

Enobosarm is a selective androgen modulator, which is a new class of non-steroidal, tissue-specific, anabolic agents. In a multicentre, randomized, double-blind phase 2 trial, 159 weight-losing patients with stages II–IV cancer of various types received enobosarm 1 mg, enobosarm 3 mg, or placebo for up to 113 days. One hundred patients were evaluable for efficacy. Patients in both enobosarm groups demonstrated significant improvements in total lean body mass and physical function (i.e. stair climb time and stair climb power) compared to baseline, whereas patients in the placebo group did not. The drug appeared to be well tolerated (Dobs et al., 2013).

Approaches shown to have little or no benefit
Melatonin

The review by Yavuzsen included two trials examining the effects of melatonin in a total of 186 patients, using doses of 20 mg per day for 1 to 16 weeks. Patients on melatonin lost significantly less weight than control patients. No improvement was seen in nutritional intake and appetite (Yavuzsen et al., 2005).

In a subsequent single-centre study, patients with advanced lung or gastrointestinal cancer were randomized in a double-blind manner to melatonin 20 mg daily or placebo for 28 days. The study was closed after an interim analysis of 48 patients revealed no significant differences between groups for appetite, weight, lean body mass, symptoms, or quality of life (Del Fabbro et al., 2013).

Tumour necrosis factor alpha inhibitors

In a multicentre proof-of-concept study, 63 patients were randomized in a double-blind manner to etanercept 25 mg or placebo subcutaneously twice weekly for up to 24 weeks. The study was terminated early when none of the patients in either arm achieved the primary endpoint of weight gain of 10% or more of baseline. No differences were seen in weight gain, appetite, quality of life, or overall survival (Jatoi et al., 2007).

In a multicentre phase II study, 89 patients with locally advanced or metastatic adenocarcinoma of the pancreas were randomized in a double-blind fashion to infliximab plus gemcitabine. There were no differences in the primary endpoint of change in lean body mass

at 8 weeks, nor in overall survival, progression-free survival, performance status, or 6-minute walk test (Wiedenmann et al., 2008).

Another multicentre, randomized, double-blind, placebo-controlled trial was conducted in elderly or poor performance status patients with metastatic non-small cell lung cancer. All patients received docetaxel and were randomized to infliximab. The trial was stopped after 61 patients had been entered due to slow accrual; in addition, no patient in either arm achieved the primary endpoint of 10% or higher weight gain. Moreover, infliximab-treated patients had worse fatigue, and functional and physical well-being. There were no differences in tumour response, survival, or toxicity (Jatoi et al., 2010).

Thalidomide

In 2012, Reid and colleagues published a systematic review that identified three randomized controlled trials of thalidomide for cancer cachexia, conducted in a total of 406 patients. Due to the small number of studies and high heterogeneity among them, meta-analysis was not possible. Overall, the review concluded that there is insufficient evidence to refute or support the use of thalidomide for the management of cachexia in advanced cancer patients (Reid et al., 2012).

Subsequently, a single-centre study was published in which 31 patients were randomized in a double-blind manner to thalidomide 100 mg or placebo for 14 days. The trial was hampered by poor accrual and high attrition. No differences between groups were seen in symptoms, body composition, resting metabolic rate or cytokines (Yennurajalingam et al., 2012).

Amino acids

A multicentre study was published in which 49 patients were randomized in a double-blind manner to beta-hydroxy-beta-methylbutyrate 3 g, L-arginine 14 g, and L-glutamine 14 g, or a nitrogen content-matched non-essential amino acid mixture orally daily for 24 weeks. At 4 weeks, the active treatment group demonstrated an increase in fat-free mass that was significantly different from control patients; there was also a trend to greater weight gain. Only nine patients completed 24 weeks; a trend to greater weight and fat-free mass gain in the active treatment group was apparent. No differences were seen in quality of life (May et al., 2002).

In another multicentre, randomized, double-blind trial, 472 patients received β-hydroxyl β-methyl butyrate, glutamine, and arginine mixture or placebo orally twice a day for 8 weeks. The non-compliance rate was high, resulting in only 197 analysable patients. No differences were seen in percentage change in lean body mass, fatigue, or quality of life. In the area under the curve analysis, patients on the active arm demonstrated a strong trend towards higher lean body mass throughout the study (Berk et al., 2008).

Cannabinoids

The review by Yavuzsen included one trial in 469 patients comparing dronabinol 5 mg per day versus MA 800 mg per day versus the combination. Improvement in appetite was significantly greater with MA than with dronabinol alone. There was no additional benefit to combining the drugs.

In a subsequent multicentre trial, 243 patients were randomized in a double-blind manner to receive cannabis extract, dronabinol 2.5 mg, or placebo twice a day for 6 weeks. The study was terminated after the first interim analysis because of insufficient differences in the primary endpoint of appetite change between active treatment and placebo arms (Strasser et al., 2006).

In a two-centre proof-of-principle trial, 46 advanced cancer patients with chemosensory alteration and decreased food intake were randomized in a double-blind manner to dronabinol or placebo for 18 days. The drug could be titrated to a maximum of 20 mg per day. Compared to the placebo group, dronabinol-treated patients demonstrated significant improvements in chemosensory enhancement, appetite, and protein intake (Brisbois et al., 2011).

HIV

Anabolic steroids

In 2005, Johns and colleagues published a systematic review of randomized controlled trials of anabolic steroids for the treatment of weight loss in HIV-infected individuals. Thirteen randomized controlled trials were included. Drugs studied were testosterone, nandrolone, oxandrolone, and oxymetholone. The trials involved different routes of delivery, doses, duration of therapy, and methodology of reporting adverse events. Meta-analysis of change from baseline in lean body mass in 532 analysable patients revealed a weighted mean difference of 1.3 kg (95% CI 0.6–2.0) in favour of anabolic steroid therapy. Meta-analysis of change from baseline in body weight in 629 analysable patients showed a weighted mean difference of 1.1 kg (95% CI 0.3–2.0) in favour of anabolic steroid therapy. Adverse events were usually reported as mild and reversible (Johns et al., 2005).

Subsequent to the systematic review, additional trials have been published. In a multicentre trial, 262 men were randomized in a double-blind manner to oxandrolone 20, 40, or 80 mg or placebo orally daily for 12 weeks. All patients then received oxandrolone 20 mg daily in an open-label fashion. At 12 weeks or the last measurement, weight gain was greater in the oxandrolone 40 mg per day group than the placebo group. Increase in body cell mass was greater in the oxandrolone 40 mg and 80 mg per day groups than the placebo group. There were no differences in quality of life and total work output. By 24 weeks, weight gain was not different between groups. Oxandrolone treatment was accompanied by significant increases in transaminases and low-density lipoprotein and decreases in high-density lipoprotein (Grunfeld et al., 2006).

Two randomized, double-blind trials have compared nandrolone 150 mg, testosterone 250 mg, or placebo intramuscularly every 2 weeks for 12 weeks. A multicentre trial conducted in 303 men revealed that lean body mass increased significantly more with nandrolone versus placebo. Also, weight gain and patient perception of benefit were significantly better with nandrolone versus testosterone and placebo (Gold et al., 2006). A single-centre trial conducted in 104 men showed that weight gain was significantly greater with nandrolone and testosterone versus placebo. There was no difference between arms in adverse events (Sardar et al., 2010).

Recombinant human growth hormone (rhGH)

In a review article, it was noted that gains in weight and lean body mass with rhGH in randomized controlled trials were in the order of 3 kg, and the most common adverse events were blood glucose elevation, arthralgia, myalgia, and peripheral oedema (Gelato et al., 2007).

Dronabinol

In a multicentre trial, 139 patients were randomized in a double-blind manner to dronabinol 2.5 mg or placebo twice daily for 6 weeks. Appetite and nausea improved significantly with dronabinol compared to placebo, with a trend to weight gain and improvement in mood and performance status. However, there was a significantly higher frequency of central nervous system adverse events with dronabinol compared to placebo (Beal et al., 1995).

Megestrol acetate

In a multicentre trial, 271 patients were randomized in a double-blind manner to MA 100, 400, or 800 mg, or placebo daily for 12 weeks. Maximum weight change, percentage of patients gaining at least 5 lb and mean change in lean body mass were significantly greater in the group that received MA 800 mg daily, compared with the group that received placebo. Also, perception of well-being, change in caloric intake and improvement in appetite were significantly greater in this group (Von Roenn et al., 1994).

In another multicentre trial, 100 patients were randomized in a double-blind manner to MA 800 mg or placebo daily for 12 weeks. Changes in caloric intake, protein intake, weight, fat mass, and well-being scores significantly favoured MA. There were no differences between groups in lean body mass, performance status and survival (Oster et al., 1994).

Thalidomide

In a multicentre randomized double-blind study, 104 men received either thalidomide 100 mg, thalidomide 200 mg, or placebo daily for 8 weeks. Weight gain in the thalidomide 100 mg group but not the 200 mg group was significantly different from the placebo group. More patients had dropped out of the 200 mg group due to adverse events, the most common of which was rash. No differences were seen in body composition, caloric intake or tumour necrosis factor alpha levels (Kaplan et al., 2000).

Amino acids

A single-centre trial was undertaken to determine whether glutamine supplementation and select antioxidants could satisfy an increased glutamine requirement and thus reverse body cell mass loss in patients with AIDS. Twenty-six patients were randomized in a double-blind manner to glutamine 40 mg with selected antioxidant nutrients or placebo orally daily for 12 weeks. Glutamine-treated patients had a significantly greater increase in body cell mass and body weight compared to control patients (Shabert et al., 1999).

In another single-centre trial, 58 patients were randomized in a double-blind fashion to arginine 14 g, glutamine 14 g and hydroxyl beta-methylbutyrate 3 g or placebo daily for 8 weeks. The amino acid-treated group gained significantly more weight and lean body mass compared to the placebo group (Clark et al., 2000).

Multiple agents

In a multicentre, open-label trial, 52 patients were randomized to dronabinol 2.5 mg twice daily, MA 750 mg daily, the two agents together, or the dronabinol plus MA at a lower dose of 250 mg daily for 12 weeks. Patients who received MA at the higher dose gained significantly more weight than those who didn't. There were no differences between arms with respect to performance status, quality of life, mood, hunger, or adverse events (Timpone et al., 1997).

Forty patients were randomized in a multicentre study to MA 800 mg daily or oxandrolone 10 mg twice daily for 2 months in an unblinded manner. Weight, BMI, fat, and lean body mass increased significantly in both groups, with no differences between groups (Mwamburi et al., 2004).

A multicentre, randomized, double-blind trial was undertaken in 79 men who received MA 800 mg daily plus testosterone 200 mg or placebo every two weeks for 12 weeks. Both groups experienced increased weight, lean body mass, and fat mass, but there were no differences between groups in magnitude or composition of weight gain (Mulligan et al., 2007).

Chronic obstructive pulmonary disease
Anabolic steroids

In a single-centre trial, 230 patients with moderate to severe COPD who were admitted to an inpatient pulmonary rehabilitation programme were randomized to placebo intramuscularly every 2 weeks for four doses, placebo injections plus nutritional supplementation, or nandrolone (50 mg for men and 25 mg for women) intramuscularly every 2 weeks for four doses plus nutritional supplementation. The injections were given in a double-blind manner. Patients in both groups that received nutritional supplementation experienced significant weight gain compared to those in the placebo group. However, patients who did not receive nandrolone gained fat mass, whereas those who also received nandrolone gained fat-free mass. Maximal inspiratory pressure improved significantly in both treatment groups at 4 weeks, but was sustained only in combination group at 8 weeks (Schols et al., 1995).

In a single-centre, randomized, double-blind trial, 23 male patients with stable COPD received testosterone 250 mg intramuscularly plus stanozolol 12 mg or placebo orally daily for 27 weeks. Both groups received daily inspiratory muscle training from weeks 9 to 18, and exercise training on a cycle ergometer from weeks 18 to 27. Lean body mass increased from baseline in the anabolic steroid group, but was not significantly different from the placebo group. Both groups demonstrated increased maximal inspiratory pressure, which was greater in the anabolic steroid group but not significantly different from the placebo group. There were no significant changes in 6-minute walking distance or maximal oxygen consumption in either group. No adverse effects were apparent (Ferreira et al., 1998).

In a single-centre, randomized, double-blind trial, 63 male patients with stable COPD received nandrolone 50 mg or placebo on days 1, 15, 29, and 43. All patients participated in an 8-week inpatient pulmonary rehabilitation programme. Patients who were depleted in fat-free mass received oral nutritional supplements. Treatment with nandrolone resulted in a significantly greater increase in fat-free compared to placebo. Physical functioning improved in both groups, without differences between groups. Health status as measured by the St George's Respiratory Questionnaire improved in the nandrolone group but not in the placebo group, although the difference between groups was not significant. In a post hoc analysis, patients on oral glucocorticoids who received nandrolone had a significantly greater improvement in maximal inspiratory pressure compared to the placebo group. Also, peak workload improved to a significantly greater extent compared to the placebo group (Creutzberg et al., 2003).

Fifty-three men with stable COPD and serum testosterone at the lower range of normal were randomized to the following groups: (1) placebo without resistance training, (2) testosterone 100 mg weekly without resistance training, (3) placebo with resistance training focused on muscles of ambulation, and (4) testosterone with resistance training. The interventions lasted for 10 weeks, and the drug component was double-blind and placebo-controlled. Patients receiving testosterone demonstrated a significantly greater increase and decrease in lean body mass and fat mass, respectively. The increase in lean body mass tended to be greater in testosterone-treated patients who received resistance training versus those who didn't, but the difference was not significant. Measures of leg strength and fatigability improved significantly in all three active intervention groups compared to the non-intervention group, with the greatest improvement seen in the group that received both testosterone and resistance training. There was no increase in respiratory muscle strength or whole-body exercise endurance in any group (Casaburi et al., 2004).

A single-centre randomized double-blind trial was undertaken in 29 male ambulatory patients with stable moderate to severe COPD who were not participating in a pulmonary rehabilitation programme. Patients received testosterone 250 mg or placebo intramuscularly every four weeks for 26 weeks. No changes were seen in pulmonary function, respiratory symptoms, mood, disability scores or body weight. Fat-free mass increased and sexual function improved in the testosterone group, with a significant difference from the placebo group. No adverse effects were noted (Svartberg et al., 2004).

In a single-centre randomized double-blind trial, ambulatory patients with stable severe COPD who were not participating in a pulmonary rehabilitation programme received nandrolone (50 mg in men and 25 mg in women) or placebo every 2 weeks for 16 weeks. The study was terminated after interim analysis of results of first 16 patients showed no differences in any nutritional, functional or quality of life outcomes (Sharma et al., 2008).

Megestrol acetate

In a multicentre trial, 145 patients were randomized to MA 800 mg or placebo daily for 8 weeks in a double-blind manner. The MA group gained significantly more weight compared to the placebo group. The weight gain was determined to be fat mass. $PaCO_2$ decreased and PaO_2 increased significantly in the MA group compared to the placebo group, consistent with stimulation of ventilation. There were no differences between groups in respiratory muscle strength. Distance walked in 6 minutes and dyspnoea score were significantly worse with MA compared to placebo, but body image and appetite scores were significantly better (Weisberg et al., 2002).

Growth hormone

A single-centre randomized double-blind trail was conducted in stable COPD patients attending an inpatient pulmonary rehabilitation programme. Sixteen patients received either rhGH 0.15 IU per kg or placebo subcutaneously daily for 3 weeks. The rhGH group demonstrated significant advantages in lean body mass and resting energy expenditure compared to the placebo group. No differences were seen in body weight, caloric intake, respiratory or peripheral muscle strength, maximal power during incremental exercise, dyspnoea, or mood.

Six-minute walking distance was significantly worse in rhGH-treated patients (Burdet et al., 1997).

Polyunsaturated fatty acids (PUFAs)

A single-centre, randomized, double-blind trial was undertaken in 102 stable COPD patients admitted to an inpatient pulmonary rehabilitation centre. They received a PUFA blend 9 g or placebo daily for 8 weeks. All patients who were nutritionally depleted also received liquid nutritional supplementation. PUFA-treated patients showed significantly greater increase in peak workload and duration of submaximal bicycle ergometry test, compared to placebo-treated patients. No differences were apparent in body composition, muscle strength or lung function (Broekhuizen et al., 2005).

Agents under investigation

Current trials in progress and investigational new agents can be found at <http://www.clinicaltrials.gov>. Current investigations appearing under the search term *anorexia* encompassed continuing interest in progestational agents at various doses/combinations with other therapies, as well as new agents including atypical neuroleptics (olanzapine, mirtazapine), creatine, as well as various herbal preparations. Trials appearing under the search term *cachexia* encompassed further elaborations within current drug classes (e.g. ghrelin, synthetic ghrelin, small molecule ghrelin receptor agonists), multimodal therapeutic strategies as well as new agents especially muscle-specific agents (selective androgen receptor modulators, antagonists to myostatin) and monoclonal antibodies to interleukin 1α and interleukin 6.

Conclusion and future perspectives

At the present time there is a basis to adopt a proactive approach to screening, assessment and early intervention for involuntary weight loss in cancer cachexia. There are clinically useful evaluations and the efficacy of a number of treatments has been established in randomized clinical trials. A future goal will be to further improve surveillance, especially the development of more clinically practical ways of assessing body composition so that losses of lean body mass and skeletal muscle may be detected early. A number of investigational new drugs are appearing in phase I–III clinical trials and these are targeted at stimulation of appetite in the hypothalamus as well as skeletal muscle anabolism. These agents provide further promise of slowing down or reversing weight loss and functional loss. Investigations of nutrient requirements are required to define the unique needs of patients with cachexia syndromes and underpin the development of nutritional recommendations or nutritional support products.

Online materials

Complete references for this chapter are available online at <http://www.oxfordmedicine.com>.

References

Beal, J.E., Olson, R., Laubenstein, L., *et al.* (1995). Dronabinol as a treatment for anorexia associated with weight loss in patients with AIDS. *Journal of Pain and Symptom Management*, 10, 89–97.

Berenstein, E.G. and Ortiz, Z. (2005). Megestrol acetate for the treatment of anorexia-cachexia syndrome. *Cochrane Database of Systematic Reviews*, 2, CD004310.

Del Fabbro, E., Dev, R., Hui, D., Palmer, L., and Bruera, E. (2013). Effects of melatonin on appetite and other symptoms in patients with advanced cancer and cachexia: a double-blind placebo-controlled trial. *Journal of Clinical Oncology*, 31, 1271–1276.

Dewey, A., Baughan, C., Dean, T., Higgins, B., and Johnson, I. (2007). Eicosapentaenoic acid (EPA, an omega-3 fatty acid from fish oils) for the treatment of cancer cachexia. *Cochrane Database of Systematic Reviews*, 1, CD004597.

Dobs, A.S., Boccia, R.V., Croot, C.C., *et al.* (2013). Effects of enobosarm on muscle wasting and physical function in patients with cancer: a double-blind, randomized controlled phase 2 trial. *Lancet Oncology*, 14, 335–345.

Fearon, K.C.H., Barber, M.D., Moses, A.G., *et al.* (2006). Double-blind, placebo-controlled, randomized study of eicosapentaenoic acid diester in patients with cancer cachexia. *Journal of Clinical Oncology*, 24, 3401–3407.

Johns, K.K.J., Beddall, M.J., and Corrin, R.C. (2005). Anabolic steroids for the treatment of weight loss in HIV-infected individuals. *Cochrane Database of Systematic Reviews*, 4, CD005483.

Martin, L., Senesse, P., Gioulbasanis, I., *et al.* (2014). Diagnostic criteria for the classification of cancer-associated weight loss. *Journal of Clinical Oncology*, ii: JCO.2014.56.1894. [Epub ahead of print] PMID: 25422490.

Oster, M.H., Enders, S.R., Samuels, S.J., *et al.* (1994). Megestrol acetate in patients with AIDS and cachexia. *Annals of Internal Medicine*, 121, 400–408.

Reid, J., Mills, M., Cantwell, M., Cardwell, C.R., Murray, L.J., and Donnelly, M. (2012). Thalidomide for managing cancer cachexia. *Cochrane Database of Systematic Reviews*, 4. CD008664.

Strasser, F., Luftner, D., Possinger, K., *et al.* (2006). Comparison of orally administered cannabis extract and delta-9-tetrahydrocannabinol in treating patients with cancer-related anorexia-cachexia syndrome: a multicenter, Phase III, randomized, double-blind, placebo-controlled clinical trial from the Cannabis-In-Cachexia-Study-Group. *Journal of Clinical Oncology*, 24, 3394–400.

Yavuzsen, T., Davis, M.P., Walsh, D., LeGrand, S., and Lagman, R. (2005). Systematic review of the treatment of cancer-associated anorexia and weight loss. *Journal of Clinical Oncology*, 23, 8500–8511.

Von Roenn, J.H., Armstrong, D., Kotler, D.P., *et al.* (1994). Megestrol acetate in patients with AIDS-related cachexia. *Annals of Internal Medicine*, 121, 393–399.

SECTION 11

Common symptoms and disorders: skin problems

Skin problems in palliative care

Patricia Grocott, Georgina Gethin, and Sebastian Probst

Introduction to skin problems in palliative care

Skin problems are prevalent in patients with advanced disease who are receiving palliative care. Nursing aspects include the management of skin breakdown and wounds together with related symptoms, and promoting patient comfort and dignity, thereby enhancing the quality of life of patients and families. Palliative wound care encompasses the nursing care of patients, of all ages, with a weakened skin barrier together with the management of wounds caused by advanced and intractable diseases and conditions.

Framework for palliative wound care practice

Palliative wound care acknowledges the psychosocial impact of wounds on the individual concerned, their family and friends, and also their clinicians. It is driven by patient and family goals, which are integrated with three wound management components to reduce the impact of wounds on all concerned:

◆ management of palliation of the underlying cause of the wound

◆ management of wound-related symptoms

◆ management of the wound and peri-wound skin.

These components will be illustrated in this chapter in relation to good skin care, pressure ulcers, and fungating malignant wounds.

Palliative wound care patients

As with other aspects of palliative care, there is a concern that patients should not be labelled 'palliative' unless their situation warrants this. That said, the components of palliative wound care we propose are essentially components of appropriate patient care, which could complement curative wound care protocols. The difference between curative and palliative wound care, in our view, has more to do with goal setting and outcome measures than radically different clinical interventions. For example, palliative wound care goals include the management of odour, exudate, bleeding, pain, and the maintenance of an intact dressing system, which are interim goals towards wound healing by secondary intention (Dealey, 2012). Wound healing may also be achievable, demonstrated by Maida et al. (2012) in their survey of patients in a regional palliative care programme in Canada. The potential for complete healing of pressure ulcers of grade II and above, skin tears, and diabetic and venous ulcers increased the longer the

patients lived. Deep pressure ulcers, arterial wounds, and malignant wounds, however, did not heal (Maida et al., 2012).

The following are examples of skin damage and wounds in palliative care:

◆ pressure ulcers

◆ moisture lesions

◆ skin tears

◆ dry irritated skin

◆ malignant fungating wounds

◆ fistulae

◆ blistering skin conditions, for example, epidermolysis bullosa, bullous pemphigoid.

Patients' experiences of living with wounds

A cluster of qualitative research studies demonstrate the profound impact that wounds have on patients, carers, and professionals. Nurses have described caring for patients with this condition as an intense and unforgettable experience (Alexander, 2010). Patients reported an overwhelming sense of vulnerability of living within a body that cannot be trusted or one that was continually changing (Piggin and Jones, 2007). Patients also described delaying seeking medical help as they were feeling a sense of shame and blame (Lund-Nielsen et al., 2011) until their situations became unmanageable. Their problems included unpleasant wound odour, wound pain, bleeding and/or itching, as well as other fears related to being diagnosed with advanced cancer.

Uncontrolled wounds are distressing and burdensome for patients and families (Probst et al., 2012) and are linked to a poorer quality of life (Lo et al., 2012). Uncontrolled wound exudate and odour lead to a loss of self-confidence and progressive social isolation. For some this extends to keeping the wound a secret from family members (Probst et al., 2013). The concept of the unbounded body, depicting the erosion of physical boundaries and progressive spiritual loss, is used by researchers to explain patients' experiences of living with uncontrolled wounds (Lawton 2000; Probst et al., 2013).

Lawton (2000) observed that body boundaries could be reinstated, and individuals could regain a sense of control and well-being, with local wound management and continence interventions. Lund-Nielsen (2005) has demonstrated the positive impact of systematic approaches to dressing and managing fungating wounds, as has Grocott (2000). However, the systems evaluated by Grocott (2000) were experimental and have not been commercialized. Probst et al.'s (2012, 2013) study, which included family members who were also carers, indicates that there is an ongoing struggle to contain advanced malignant wounds with currently available products, together with a lack of coherent professional advice and guidance on wound care interventions.

With regard to another condition giving rise to palliative care needs—epidermolysis bullosa (EB)—Grocott et al. (2013) have demonstrated the burden of skin and wound care on the individuals with this condition and their carers. A shared problem between people with EB and those with fungating wounds is the mismatch between the size and shape of EB and fungating wounds, and current dressings, which are designed to cover individual discrete wounds. Pre-sized and shaped dressings need to be patch-worked across extensive wounds, and are inherently unstable.

With regard to the management of symptoms such as malodour, which will be discussed further in the section of this chapter on symptom management, evidence from a recent international survey indicates that a myriad of interventions to control this very distressing symptom are not found effective (Gethin et al., 2014). A linked explanation of these findings may be that there is a similar mismatch between the size and scale of the wounds, the malodour problem, and the presentation of commercially available preparations for managing the source of the malodour. The fact that clinicians resort to unlicensed use of licensed materials (e.g. crushing metronidazole tablets into a hydrogel to line a large necrotic cavity) and the use of shaving foam and cat litter to absorb and mask odour, are evidence of desperate measures.

To overcome the limitations of current dressings in providing adequate and stable coverings for extensive wounds, Grocott et al. (2012, 2013) have worked in partnership with adults with EB, their carers, a designer, and a manufacturer to find solutions for whole-body wounds, based on the EB experiences. This research has resulted in dressing retention garments, which have been commercialized through international health services supply chains (Grocott et al., 2013a). A next stage of this research is to develop body-wrap disposable dressings for use with the dressing retention garment in a two-layer system.

Clinical assessment, decision-making, and evaluation

Clinical assessment, routine documentation, and evaluation are particularly important in palliative wound care where the evidence base is not established. Regarding the assessment of palliative wounds, five assessment scales have been identified: the Toronto Symptom Assessment System for Wounds, the Schulz Malignant Fungating Wound Assessment Tool, the Wound Symptoms Self-Assessment Chart (WOSSAC), the TELER System, and the Hopkins Wound Assessment Tool (Haisfield-Wolfe, 1999; Naylor, 2002; Maida et al., 2009; Grocott et al., 2011). Five 'core' symptoms are assessed by all the scales, these include odour, pain, exudate, itching, and bleeding. WOSSAC and TELER also include psychosocial aspects and impact on daily life. The structures of the five scales vary in the number of items used, their measurement, as well as in their mode of application. These scales can help clinicians to assess wounds and derive interventions in a systematic way, thereby improving professional practice and patient outcomes.

Patients with a weakened skin barrier: good skin care

General skin problems in advanced disease are largely attributable to skin that is weakened by the effects of chronic disease and ageing, performance status, multiple co-morbidities, and the iatrogenic effects of treatments, such as systemic glucocorticoid use (Maida et al., 2012). If the many factors that predispose palliative care patients to skin problems are taken into account it may be possible to mitigate their effects. Nursing care is clearly not able to prevent and resolve all the problems of advanced disease, for example, immobility and anorexia. However, dedicated interventions to prevent morbidity resulting from these problems, for example, pressure ulcers, skin tears, and dry skin conditions, may be possible.

Good skin care aims to maintain and replenish the skin by cleansing, hydrating and moisturizing, and protecting. If the patient's skin is to remain intact and free of distressing symptoms, knowledge and skill is required in the selection and use of skin cleansers, creams, and barrier products, together with dedicated and consistent care (Voegeli, 2012).

Skin cleansing

It is well recognized that the use of soap and water to clean the skin, with paper and cloth towels to dry the skin, can strip the skin of natural oils. The high alkaline content of soaps can alter the pH and the protective acid mantle of the skin. This disturbs the balance of normal skin flora, thereby reducing its protective function against colonization by pathogenic bacteria, which enter the body through breaks in the weakened skin (Voegeli, 2012).

A number of skin cleansers are available that are formulated to minimize alteration of skin pH and maximize the protective function of the skin. These products come in the form of emulsions, foams, and sprays. Some of the preparations also include a barrier product.

Moisturizing and hydrating

Moisturizing products such as emollients are designed to maintain or increase the hydration of the skin by trapping moisture under the barrier provided by the emollient itself. The choice of a lotion or an ointment depends on patients' preferences. Ointments take time to be absorbed into the skin and can leave a greasy feel, whereas lotions are rapidly absorbed. Ointments can also interfere with the action of disposable pads for the management of incontinence, as discussed later.

Protecting

Barrier products, such as barrier creams, have some effect on hydrating and moisturizing the skin, but their main function is to form a thin layer on the skin surface to protect the skin from excoriating body fluids. They need to be replenished whenever the skin is cleaned.

Pressure ulcers and moisture lesions

There is an extensive literature on the prevention and management of pressure ulcers, including clinical guidelines, which can be drawn on to guide pressure-relieving strategies and local wound management. There is also increasing recognition that excessive moisture, maceration, and excoriation cause skin breakdown in patients who are not mobile and also suffer from continence problems (European Pressure Ulcer Advisory Group and National Pressure Ulcer Advisory Panel (EPUAP and NPUAP), 2009, 2010). Pressure ulcers and moisture lesions can coexist if each predisposing risk factor is not managed optimally.

The focus in this section is to put general principles of pressure relief, prevention, and management of moisture and excoriating skin damage, and ulcer management into the context of palliative wound care.

Prevention of pressure ulcers is inextricably linked with treatment. When pressure damage occurs, interventions that relieve pressure need to be put in place, together with additional measures to manage broken skin and wounds, including:

♦ pressure relief and management of any friction or shear forces

♦ good skin care

♦ wound management

♦ continence and fistula management.

Pressure damage prevention

Assessment of patients at risk of pressure damage is an important aspect of prevention. The use of risk assessment tools needs to be combined with clinical judgement and patients' preferences. The Hunters Hill Marie Curie Centre risk assessment tool has been developed specifically for palliative care patients who are, in the main, at considerable risk of developing pressure ulcers (Chaplin, 2010). Patients require regular repositioning on pressure redistribution devices (mattresses, seating), regardless of the quality of the device. Repositioning is also essential to maintain movement in joints, to help prevent contractures and pain from immobility, and for psychological reasons. The frequency of position change will be based on assessment of risk, the general condition of the patient, and the equipment being used.

Skin condition is the best indicator of how often position changes need to occur. This is assessed by lightly pressing an area of skin on which the patient was lying prior to turning. The skin should go white (blanche) and then return to its normal colour. The time taken to return to normal should be no longer than twice the length of time for which the finger pressure was applied. A fixed red mark that does not fade within 20 minutes after pressure has been relieved is indicative of pressure damage, loss of tissue viability, and varying degrees of skin breakdown and ulceration (EPUAP and NPUAP, 2009).

Patients with no evidence of pressure damage simply require good skin care and ongoing monitoring. However, pressure ulcers can still occur in spite of rigorous assessment and monitoring, and the use of first-class pressure-relieving devices for beds and chairs.

The development of a pressure ulcer is understandably distressing for patients, families and clinicians. Once an ulcer is established, care and management revolve around pressure relief, local wound management, including the management of moisture, and symptom management.

The nature and stage of the damage dictates treatment interventions together with curative or palliative goals. Pressure ulcers comprise devitalized tissue following interruption of the blood supply. The management plan will be guided by whether the aim is to heal the wound or to palliate. Strategies for healing and palliation are discussed in the section on local wound management and symptom control, using the conceptual framework of wound bed preparation (WBP). See Table 11.1.1.

Prevention of skin damage from moisture

Moisture lesions can be confused with sacral pressure ulcers, because of their location. However, the skin damage is associated with body fluids (urine, faeces, sweat) as opposed to pressure and shear (Bianchi, 2012). If the patient also has a pressure ulcer, the exudate from the ulcer will contribute further to the moisture damage unless it is managed effectively with local wound management strategies. In conjunction with good skin care, interventions to prevent and manage moisture lesions include the management of urinary and faecal incontinence with the following medical devices (EPUAP and NPUAP, 2009).

Disposable pads and close-fitting underwear or self-seal nappies

The pads are based on baby nappy technology and comprise a fluid handling system (super absorbent and gelling material with hydrophobic skin contact layer) designed to wick the urine away from the skin and contain it within the pad. Faecal matter will remain on the skin side of the pad. It is essential to change soiled pads as soon as possible to maintain patient dignity and also skin integrity.

Urinary catheters

Catheters may be used on an intermittent basis, by self-catheterization, or an indwelling catheter may be used on longer-term basis whereby the urine is collected into a drainage bag. Patients may find catheterization preferable to the use of pads; the choice needs to rest with the patient.

Anal or stoma bags

A variety of bags are available to collect faeces and fistula fluid. The practicality of using these is very dependent on the position of the anus, stoma, or fistula, the amount and consistency of the effluent, and the ability to get a good seal around the anus, stoma, or fistula, otherwise there will be leakage. This will not only embarrass the patient but also cause skin damage. Further discussion on the management of fistulae is provided in the section on fungating wounds and in Chapter 8.4.

Faecal management systems

These systems are based on the principles of a closed catheter system, whereby a flexible tube is inserted into the anus and the faeces are drained into a collection bag. Again their use will be based on an individual decision with the patient and carefully supervised by practitioners experienced in the use of these devices. Consideration needs to be given to the positioning of the patient to avoid blocking the drainage tube. Faecal management systems have been found to be helpful in situations where there is high faecal output and also a risk of cross infection, with *Norovirus* and *Clostridium difficile*, for example (see Chapters 4.12 and 10.3).

Fungating malignant wounds

Fungating malignant wounds are caused by tumour infiltration of the skin and its supporting blood and lymph vessels. The tumours may be locally advanced, metastatic, or recurrent. Unless they can be treated by single or combination anti-cancer treatments, there

Table 11.1.1 TIME, wound bed preparation, a range of potential nursing interventions, methods, and generic products for palliative wound care

TIME	Wound bed preparation: palliative nursing interventions	Methods and generic products for palliative wound care
TISSUE **Necrotic**	Debride the necrotic tissue	Autolytic debridement: hydrogel dressings Biological debridement: larval therapy Mechanical debridement: ultrasound and water irrigation devices Surgical and sharp debridement: scalpel, scissors, forceps by trained tissue viability nurse or surgeon Chemical debridement: active dressings: medical grade honey Enzymatic debridement: collagenase agents (European Wound Management Association (2013ab))

	Consider promoting and maintaining dry scab in the following circumstances:
	   Life expectancy is short
	   Multiple wounds over the body
	   Head and neck wounds
		Apply astringent antiseptics: potassium permanganate (see Box 11.1.1)

Granulating	Promote and protect fragile granulating tissue	Apply semi-occlusive, non-gauze-based dressings: foam dressings with a low adherent wound contact layer
Epithelializing	Protect epithelializing tissue	Apply low-adherent moisture conserving primary dressings: soft silicone-based atraumatic dressings
INFECTION and/or **INFLAMMATION**	Debride the dead tissue which harbours bacteria, *unless scab formation is indicated* Apply antimicrobial dressings and solutions to remove bacteria	Select an option from the TISSUE debridement section above Select from the range of antimicrobial dressings: medical grade honey; polyhexamethylene biguanide (PHMB) impregnated dressings (European Wound Management Association, 2013a)
Moisture	Use dressing products to remove exudate from the wounds, without allowing the wound to dry out and stick to the dressings If wound has very high fluid output and dressing changes are a burden to the patient, consider topical negative pressure devices. These need to be used by trained personnel and with caution to prevent the potential for bleeding, particularly if applied to fungating malignant wounds (Ford-Dunn 2006)	Two-layer dressing system: low adherent primary dressing and secondary absorbent or super-absorbent pad Alginate or methylcellulose dressings with secondary absorbent or super absorbent pad Low-adherent foam dressings Topical negative pressure device
EDGE	**E**dge of wound epithelializing to cover granulation tissue **E**dge of wound free of non-viable tissue and debris in non-healing wounds	Monitor outcomes from the above to achieve optimal condition of wound edge in healing and non-healing wounds

Source: Data from Leaper DJ et al., Extending the TIME concept: what have we learned in the past 10 years?, *International Wound Journal*, Volume 9, Supplement 2, pp.1–19, Copyright © 2012; Ford-Dunn, S, Use of vacuum assisted closure therapy in the palliation of a malignant wound, *Palliative Medicine*, Volume 20, Issue 4, pp.477–78, Copyright © 2006 and F. Gottrup et al., (Ed.) *Antimicrobials and Non-healing Wounds: Evidence, controversies and suggestions*, EWMA Document, MA Healthcare Ltd, London, UK, Copyright © 2013, http://ewma.org/english/publications.html

is the potential for massive skin damage. This occurs through a combination of tumour growth, loss of local blood supply, consequent loss of tissue viability, and local infections. The dead tissue is colonized by anaerobic and aerobic bacteria, which are associated with malodour, exudate, and potential for further tissue damage.

Fungating tumours present with proliferative tissue growth, progressing to ulceration as and when the blood supply to the area is interrupted. The wounds can be full thickness, also extending into adjacent structures, most notably muscle.

Diagnosis is based on histological assessment and the treatment aim is to control tumour growth, control bleeding, and promote wound closure whenever possible. Fungating tumours that are sensitive to conventional anti-cancer treatments can be resolved. Unfortunately tumour recurrence with fungation is not uncommon. Without treatment, fungation can extend catastrophically and is associated with significant co-morbidity (Grocott et al., 2013b).

Commonly available treatment options include surgery, radiotherapy, photodynamic therapy, immunotherapy, and systemic treatment of the primary cancer with chemotherapy (see Chapter 12.3). Whilst these treatments may to an extent be successful, their burden to the patient can be considerable and the likelihood of the resultant of fungating lesion healing is relatively low.

Advances in palliative treatments, however, offer the potential to manage cutaneous and subcutaneous metastases, for example, electrochemotherapy (ECT). This physical drug delivery system, using electroporation to deliver low doses of non-permeant or poorly permeant chemotherapeutic agents (bleomycin and cisplatin) directly into the tumour cells, is demonstrating positive palliative outcomes, regardless of tumour aetiology. Standard operating procedures for administering ECT have been validated (Marty et al., 2006). There is growing evidence of favourable patient outcomes in terms of complete and objective responses with minimal and transient side effects, such as mild erythema localized to the treatment site, acceptability to patients, and the ability to re-treat if the problem recurs. Symptom management with ECT (bleeding, exudate, odour) is also reported (Matthiessen et al., 2012; Teissié et al., 2012).

Without curative or palliative treatment, fungating wounds advance relentlessly. The nursing management of these wounds is complex, requiring a range of specialist skills such as stoma care, continence care, lymphoedema management, nutrition and parenteral feeding, symptom control, and local wound management (see Chapters 4.12, 11.1, 11.3).

Local wound management

Wound dressings and devices in conjunction with symptom management can significantly relieve the physical and psychosocial problems, and the overall impact of a wound. However, as already discussed, there are limitations in the performance of dressing systems currently available for the extensive wounds that fall within the remit of palliative care.

Local wound management is determined by the location, size, and shape of the wounds together with presenting problems. Current practice in wound care, including the manufacturing focus for wound dressings, is substantially based on the theory of moist wound healing (Winter, 1962). This theory explains the profound influence on epithelialization of restricting the evaporation of water from the wound surface. It does not explain the management of advanced, exudating wounds (Grocott, 2000).

Tissue hypoxia in pressure ulcers and fungating wounds is a significant factor in local wound management because of the consequential dead tissue, exudate, and odour. The activity of anaerobic bacteria, which proliferate in these hypoxic conditions, combined with facultative aerobic species is attributed to the characteristic symptoms of malodour and another distressing symptom, profuse exudate. Exudate production is also attributed to bacterial enzymes (proteases) and their role in the autolytic processes of tissue breakdown and liquefaction together with local oedema and lymphoedema (Ford-Dunn, 2006).

WBP is a framework to guide and structure a local wound management strategy that is increasingly adopted in clinical care together with the acronym, TIME (Leaper et al., 2012). TIME summarizes the four components of WBP and requires assessment and monitoring of the following:

♦ **T**issue management

♦ **I**nfection and inflammation management

♦ **M**oisture balance

♦ **E**dge of wound in terms of how this advances inwards to cover the broken area.

Table 11.1.1 illustrates the components of WBP and TIME applied to palliative wound care, together with a diverse range of possible local wound management strategies, for example, wound debridement or preservation/promotion of a dry scab. The application of such strategies should be based on individualized assessment of needs.

Essentially, WBP is a framework for managing the local wound environment including clinical signs of bacterial overload, infection, the state of wound tissue, exudate, and the peri-wound skin. The rationale underpinning WBP is that if healing is the goal, the wound bed needs to be free of bacteria and harmful enzymes that may delay healing. If palliation is the goal, clearance of dead tissue and management of bacterial overload can reduce odour, exudate, and damage to the peri-wound skin.

Correction of cellular dysfunction and cellular imbalance refers to a number of factors including cell senescence and the overexpression of proteolytic enzymes. Enzyme imbalance can apparently be corrected with advanced wound products such as topical proteinase modulating agents. However, dysfunction at the cellular level is challenging to address in practical and measurable ways, and the evidence base for the effectiveness of these agents, which are costly, remains weak.

WBP emphasizes the removal of dead tissue (unless preservation of natural scab is indicated) and the control of symptoms such as exudate and odour.

Debridement of dead tissue

Dead tissue is unsightly and a focus for bacteria. Bacteria metabolize dead tissue and the by-products of this metabolism are malodorous. This is a natural autolytic process of dead tissue removal. A number of methods have been advanced to speed the removal of dead tissue. These include surgical, larval, enzymatic, and mechanical methods (European Wound Management Association, 2013b).

Debridement in long-term wounds will need to be repeated. Therefore careful attention needs to be paid to the choice of method, so that it minimizes side effects and is acceptable to the patient. In addition, the clinical gains to the individual patient need to be assessed critically. For example, patients with extensive wounds covered with scabs may not benefit from debridement if life expectancy is short and the consequent exudate profuse. In these circumstances, the aim will be to maintain a dry wound environment.

The use of medical-grade honey dressings to debride and deodorize a range of extensive, complex wounds, including fungating lesions, has been reported (Molan, 2005). For some patients, the introduction of honey into a wound can be painful, attributed to the osmotic pull exerted by the honey on fluid and tissues within the wound. The pain may be transient as the honey liquefies. However, for some patients this symptom is intolerable and alternative debriding agents such as hydrogels or iodine preparations will be indicated. Because honey promotes autolysis, the devitalized tissue is liquefied and separated from the wound bed. This exudate has to be contained with wound dressings otherwise the patient experiences a further unpleasant problem or the aggravation of an existing problem. The management of exudate is discussed further in the following section, as is the use of honey in the section on malodour.

Exudate

Without control of exudate the physical and psychosocial impact of a wound is compounded by leakage, soiling, frequent dressing changes or re-padding, peri-wound maceration, and odour. Effective control of exudate substantially reduces the wound management problems, and patients can regain a degree of independence and control over their daily lives.

As previously mentioned, there are circumstances when maintaining a dry scab over the wound is the kindest option for the patient. If a complete scab cannot be achieved or maintained, and if the wound surface can be dried to slow the rate of volume of

Box 11.1.1 Case example: patient with a large, exuding, fungating wound of the face

The patient had an aggressive facial cancer, which resulted in a large crater in the centre of her face. The crater was lined with dry dead tissue. The dead tissue started to liquefy causing exudate to dribble down her face, and into her mouth. The wound management goal was to dry the wound to a scab, and to minimize the intrusion of dressing changes. Potassium permanganate-soaked[a] gauze dressings were applied, and left for 20 minutes. They were removed and a permeable silicone foam dressing was applied to line the cavity, to prevent dressing adherence, and to allow free passage of air to the wound to maintain the scab. Until scab formation was achieved, the potassium permanganate-soaked dressings were applied twice a day. Thereafter they were applied as needed. This dressing protocol was simple and quick to apply, and achieved the goal of scab formation to minimize the distress caused by uncontrolled exudate.

[a] Potassium permanganate solution is an astringent antiseptic that can dry broken skin that is oozing fluid. The solution can stain the skin and nails and therefore needs to be used with care (Palliativedrugs.com (2014).

exudate produced, the wound may be manageable, and the patient may not be subject to the distress and embarrassment that a wet wound can generate (McManus, 2007) (see Box 11.1.1).

Fistula management

The management of fluid from fistulae is particularly challenging with immense variation in presentations between patients. A fistula is an abnormal track that communicates between two hollow organs. An enterocutaneous fistula is a connection between a hollow organ and the skin. There are multiple causes of fistulae. For example, they may develop as a complication of surgery, infection, radiotherapy, and progressive malignant disease.

The nursing care of patients with fistulae follows substantially the principles of stoma care. These principles are:

◆ Prevention of skin excoriation with barrier products.

◆ Collection of effluent in closed stoma devices or wound manager devices.

◆ Management of odour in a closed device; the use of odour-neutralizing sprays when bags are emptied and changed.

◆ Nutrition and fluids to maintain a balance between intake and loss, which may require enteral or parenteral feeding.

◆ Supportive care to protect the patient's sense of self, autonomy, and ability to socialize (see also Chapter 4.12).

The location and advancement of the fistula can preclude the application of a stoma device. Clinicians are challenged in these circumstances to find novel approaches to manage the lesions. Custom-built solutions need to be found using stomahesive pastes and hydrocolloid dressings to which a drainage bag(s) can be attached. Alternatively it may be possible to fit silicone mesh dressings over a fistula. The dressing, which can be left *in situ* for 3–4 days unless clogged with debris, can assist in directing the flow of fluid into a super absorbent pad with a waterproof backing, which also assists with preserving the integrity of the skin,. The pads will need to be fixed with an adhesive, waterproof tape, or film to avoid leakage. Given that the pads will need to be changed several times a day, when heavily soiled, the skin under the adhesive needs to be protected with repeat applications of a barrier product.

Management of wound-related symptoms

Symptom management measures are both systemic and local. The measures focused on in this chapter are predominantly linked to local wound management. The key issue here is that the management of advanced wounds is complex and requires an interdisciplinary approach. The patients need to be referred to palliative care teams who have specialist knowledge and expertise in the art and science of symptom control.

Symptoms specifically related to the wound include pain, soreness and irritation from excoriated skin conditions, pruritus, odour, spontaneous bleeding, and haemorrhage. Frequently more than one problem needs to be managed at a given time. For example, it is well known that wounds can bleed, be malodorous, and painful. If the wounds become infected, problems of pain, odour, and bleeding are exacerbated, the wound extends, and the frequency of dressing changes increases, including the amount of product required. Accurate diagnosis and treatment can reduce the severity of the problems to all concerned.

Pain

The causes of pain may be multiple, and include emotional factors. Pain associated with pressure ulcers and fungating wounds is generally of a mixed aetiology. Patients can experience stinging, burning, aching, and sharp pain, depending on the size, position, and nature of the wound. Some will have no pain at all, others just at dressing changes, whilst some will have constant pain.

Pain management requires careful assessment, administration of combinations of drugs, monitoring of pain levels, and emotional support (see Section 9).

Analgesia can be given systemically and/or locally. For pain at dressing changes, a short-acting analgesic can be administered and repeated if the dressing change is lengthy.

The local application of analgesia for pain from damaged and ulcerated skin, such as topical opioids, is not supported by high-quality studies. Opioids were considered to act systemically until receptors were identified in inflamed peripheral tissues. A systematic review of the evidence to support the use of topical opioids concluded that the evidence does not provide clear, detailed recommendations for clinical practice. For example, the evidence is lacking in terms of the wounds that are most suitable, the choice of opioid, the carrier, the starting dose, titration, or interval of administration (LeBon et al., 2009). Concerns about the systemic uptake of opioids may be allayed by a small experimental study by Ribeiro et al. (2004) who found that when applied topically to ulcers, morphine was not absorbed unless the ulcer had a large surface area. They concluded that the analgesic effects are likely to be mediated locally, not systemically (Ribeiro et al., 2004).

Current published literature on the prescribing and use of topical opioids is based on individual case reports and small randomized controlled trials involving patients with a variety of painful wounds. In the face of this lack of research, a concentration of morphine: hydrogel 1:1000 (0.1%) has been adopted as normal practice, as suggested in the literature (Graham et al., 2013). We have observed that the wetness of the wound environment can result in the gel sliding off the wound. Frequency of dressing changes and replacement gel must therefore increase commensurately.

Soreness and irritation from macerated and excoriated skin conditions

As indicated earlier in the section on good skin care, exudate and body fluids cause predictable and inevitable damage to the skin in the form of inflammation, pruritus, and progressive damage to the tissues. The interventions indicated earlier are applicable to the prevention and treatment of maceration and excoriation from exudate in relation to pressure ulcers and fungating wounds. To maintain skin integrity, interventions need to cover the area of skin that is vulnerable, repeating the process at dressing and pad changes.

Cutaneous pruritic irritation

This form of irritation is quite distinct from the irritation caused by maceration. It is a creeping, intense itching sensation attributed to a number of diseases and disorders, such as cholestatic liver disease and tumours. Inflammatory breast disease with cutaneous infiltration is a particular example. Pruritus can be extremely disabling and difficult to treat. It is generally not responsive to antihistamines. It is worth considering non-pharmacological interventions. For example, the intensity of pruritus can be diminished with the use of transcutaneous electrical nerve stimulation (TENS). The application of TENS is worked out according to receptor sites in the skin and involves a degree of trial and error. It is therefore important to involve experts in the administration of this treatment, being careful not to raise patients' expectations (see Chapter 9.9). In addition, drawing on research into the management of pruritic dermatological conditions, personal clothing, and bed linen that wicks away heat and moisture can help to dampen this very debilitating symptom (Senti et al., 2006).

Malodour

The impact of malodorous wounds on patients, carers, and health-care professionals is quite profound (Gethin, 2011). Indeed, strong environmental odours have been shown to be related to increased levels of stress and negative mood (Avery Hoton et al., 2009). Wound odour has been described as 'repulsive', 'that stinking thing', 'rotten', and, in the absence of treatment strategies, some patients resort to a range of measures including decreasing fluid intake in an attempt to manage this problem (Lo et al., 2008; Probst et al., 2012, 2013).

The causative agents in malodour include a mixture of volatile agents produced by aerobic and anaerobic bacteria together with a mixture of amines and diamines such as cadaverine and putrescine that are produced by the metabolic processes of other proteolytic bacteria (Thomas et al., 1998). More recently, dimethyl trisulphide (DMTS) (a compound also emitted from vegetables and some microorganisms) has been identified as a source of odour in fungating wounds (Shirasu et al., 2009). In addition, dead tissue also provides a source of malodour. While agents such as metronidazole, charcoal, aloe vera, and honey have been reported to decrease malodour there is no consensus or guidelines to manage this distressing symptom.

A survey aimed to determine, from an international perspective, those measures that clinicians currently use to manage and assess malodorous wounds, revealed the significance of the problem and also the lack of effective strategies to combat the odour (Gethin et al., 2014). In all, 1444 clinicians from a range of disciplines and specialties across 36 countries participated. Results reveal a lack of strategies to assess and manage malodour as only 12% currently assess odour, yet 83% report this as being a major problem for both the patient and caregiver. A total of 3671 words were suggested to describe odour and seemed to represent repulsion to malodour with words such as 'offensive', 'pungent', 'foul', 'putrid', and 'rotten' being among the most commonly cited.

The following systemic and topical approaches are the most commonly used to attempt to deal with malodour.

Systemic antibiotics

These are used to reduce bacterial colonization and thereby to control the offensive odour from volatile metabolic end-products. One of the limitations of systemic antibiotics is the increasing incidence of antibiotic resistance. A further limitation is their side effects which may be debilitating.

Topical antimicrobials

Topical agents, such as metronidazole gels and the silver impregnated dressings, are alternatives to the systemic route, though they tend to be more expensive than systemic antibiotics (European Wound Management Association, 2013a). There are practical issues around the application of topical agents and dressings to extensive wounds to achieve sufficient inhibitory concentration of the active ingredients of the agents to deodorize. The issues include the size of the wounds and a lack of tissue penetration to bacteria located below the surface. In addition, the site of the wound may limit the efficacy of topical gels, which are absorbed into dressings and pads. Perineal wounds are an example of wounds that are particularly difficult to manage. Although metronidazole is widely used (Gethin et al., 2014) there is a lack of guidelines or consistency in the method and strength of application. A recent systematic review of topical agents, which included metronidazole, to control odour of malignant fungating wounds identified ten studies of which only two were controlled studies (da Costa Santos et al., 2010). Of these, the sample size was small ($N = 11$) and the method of topical application differed across all studies. The review highlighted the need for further research to determine the optimal method and strength of application to achieve odour control in malignant fungating wounds.

Debridement of dead tissue

The rationale for removal of dead tissue is covered in the section on local wound management and Table 11.1.1.

Adsorption of volatile malodorous chemicals by charcoal cloth

Activated charcoal dressings act as filters to absorb the volatile malodorous chemicals from the wound, before they pass into the air. They must therefore be fitted as a sealed unit or the volatile malodorous chemicals simply escape into the air. Air-tight charcoal garments may overcome this limitation when the wounds are extensive or sited in body curves which are difficult to dress. In addition, charcoal is inactivated if it becomes wet, therefore the dressings need to be applied as the outer dressing, and changed if wet (Hampton, 2008). Charcoal dressings are the second most frequently cited dressing for management of malodour but it is recognized that more methodologically refined studies are required to raise the level of evidence and grade of recommendation for use (da Costa Santos et al., 2010).

The case report by Ford-Dunn (2006) illustrates the benefits of a topical negative pressure system to combat malodour and manage exudate in a malignant wound

Infection

As with other interventions in palliative wound care, the aim is to provide maximum comfort and minimum distress to the patient. If a wound is showing no signs of improvement, and the patient's condition is sufficiently good to allow for wound healing, heavy bacterial colonization and infection may be root causes. Signs of local infection, such as advancing redness of the skin with heat, are sufficient to consider the wound infected, and to initiate topical antimicrobial dressing products.

It may not be necessary or indicated to take a wound swab if the patient's prognosis is short, particularly if they are unable to take oral antibiotics. Systemic medication of proven sensitivity to the culture from the wound swab is otherwise indicated for the management of infection as bacteria have invaded local tissues. Topical agents can additionally help to reduce the microbial load on the wound, and assist the management of exudate and odour.

The role of wound dressings in infected wounds is threefold:

◆ to contain the infection and prevent contamination to and from the wound

◆ to keep anti-microbial agents in contact with the wound

◆ to contain exudate and odour.

Some of the advanced dressings such as silver-impregnated products can be left *in situ* for several days as they are designed to release the active antimicrobial agent over a specified time period. The manufacturers' guidance assists decisions around frequency of changes when using these products. Exudate levels will, however, dictate the frequency of changes required on an individual basis (European Wound Management Association, 2013a).

Bleeding

On rare occasions tumours will erode a major vessel, causing a fatal bleed. These situations are extremely distressing to witness and manage. Death will normally occur within a few minutes and the patient will lose consciousness some time before that.

Attention to the following can reduce the incidence of more minor bleeding at the dressing changes:

◆ dressing application and removal techniques

◆ maintenance of humidity at the wound/dressing interface

◆ cleaning techniques.

Particularly for fungating wounds, when capillaries are visible on the surface, mechanical damage and bleeding can occur with fibrous materials such as alginates. Alternative non-fibrous systems include silicone wound contact dressings with dressing pads, or gel sheets. In addition, radiotherapy may be used palliatively to control spontaneous bleeding from eroding blood vessels. Additionally, through observation, Gehl and Geertsen (2006) have identified an antivascular or blood-stemming effect of ECT on bleeding tumours, with almost immediate effect and no regression (Gehl and Geertsen, 2006). It is therefore important to have

contacts with oncology centres for rapid patient referrals for effective control of bleeding.

Topical measures such as adrenaline 1:1000 are also applied. Surgical haemostatic sponges are alternative, practical emergency measures for controlling fast capillary bleeding though they appear expensive on a unit cost basis. Sucralfate suspension is also advocated by palliative care specialists as an off-licence, cost-effective alternative.

Conclusion

Palliative wound care can be complex and is best addressed using an interdisciplinary approach, drawing on colleagues who can contribute specific knowledge, skills, and experience to problem-solve for the patients. The mainstays of palliative wound management comprise treatment of underlying causes wherever possible, local wound management, and symptom control. These are crucial to the physical and psychological well-being of the patients and families. There remain significant limitations in the evidence to underpin palliative wound care interventions. In addition, the design and presentation of medical devices for palliative wound care need to take into account the extensive nature of the skin damage and wounds that occur as a result of advanced disease.

Online materials

Complete references for this chapter are available online at <http://www.oxfordmedicine.com>.

References

Alexander, S.J. (2010). An intense and unforgettable experience: the lived experience of malignant wounds from the perspectives of patients, caregivers and nurses. *International Wound Journal*, 7, 456–465.

Da Costa Santos, C.M., de Mattos Pimenta, C.A., and Nobre, M.R.C. (2010). A systematic review of topical treatments to control the odor of malignant fungating wounds. *Journal of Pain and Symptom Management*, 39, 1065–1076.

European Pressure Ulcer Advisory Group and National Pressure Ulcer Advisory Panel (2009). *Treatment of Pressure Ulcers: Quick Reference Guide*. [Online] Available at: <http://www.epuap.org/guidelines/>.

European Pressure Ulcer Advisory Group and National Pressure Ulcer Advisory Panel (2010). *Pressure Ulcer Prevention: Quick Reference Guide*. [Online]. Available at: <http://www.epuap.org/guidelines/>.

European Wound Management Association (2013a). *Antimicrobials and Non-healing Wounds Evidence, Controversies and Suggestions*. [Online] Available at: <http://ewma.org/english/publications/ewma-documents/ewma-antimicrobial-document.html>.

European Wound Management Association (2013b). *Debridement: An updated overview and clarification of the principle role of debridement*. [Online] Available at: <http://ewma.org/english/publications.html>.

Gehl, J. and Geertsen, P.F. (2006). Palliation of haemorrhaging and ulcerated cutaneous tumours using electrochemotherapy. *European Journal of Cancer Supplements*, 4, 35–37.

Gethin, G. (2011). Management of malodour in palliative wound care. *British Journal of Community Nursing*, 16, S28–36.

Gethin, G., Grocott, P., Probst, S., and Clarke, E. (2014). Current practice in the management of wound odour: an international survey. *International Journal of Nursing Studies*, 51(6), 865–874.

Graham, T., Grocott, P., Probst, S., Wanklyn, S., Dawson, J., and Gethin, G. (2013). How are topical opioids used to manage painful cutaneous lesions in palliative care? A critical review. *Pain*, 154, 1920–1928.

Grocott, P., Blackwell, R., Currie, C., Pillay, E., and Robert, G. (2013a). Co-producing novel wound care products for epidermolysis bullosa; an empirical case study of the use of surrogates in the design and prototype development process. *International Wound Journal*, 10, 265–273.

Grocott, P., Blackwell, R., Currie, C., *et al.* (2013b). Woundcare research for epidermolysis bullosa: designing products with the users. *Dermatological Nursing*, 12, 30–35.

Grocott, P., Blackwell, R., Weir, H., and Pillay, E. (2013b). Living in dressings and bandages: findings from workshops with people with epidermolysis bullosa. *International Wound Journal*, 10, 274–284.

Grocott, P., Gethin, G., and Probst, S. (2013a). Malignant wound management in advanced illness: new insights. *Current Opinion in Supportive and Palliative Care*, 7, 101–105.

Lawton, J. (2000). *The Dying Process: Patients' experiences of palliative care*. Routledge. London.

LeBon, B., Zeppetella, G., and Higginson, I.J. (2009). Effectiveness of topical administration of opioids in palliative care: a systematic review. *Journal of Pain and Symptom Management*, 37, 913–917.

Leaper, D.J., Schultz, G., Carville, K., Fletcher, J., Swanson, T., and Drake, R. (2012). Extending the TIME concept: what have we learned in the past 10 years? *International Wound Journal*, 9(Suppl. 2), 1–19.

Lo, S.F., Hayter, M., Hu, W., Tai, C.Y., Hsu, M.Y., and Li, Y.F. (2012). Symptom burden and quality of life in patients with malignant fungating wounds. *Journal of Advanced Nursing*, 68(6), 1312–1321.

Lund-Nielsen, B., Midtgaard, J., Rorth, M., Gottrup, F., and Adamsen, L. (2011). An avalanche of ignoring—a qualitative study of health care avoidance in women with malignant breast cancer wounds. *Cancer Nursing*, 34, 277–285.

Marty, M., Sersa, G., Garbay, J.R., *et al.* (2006). Electrochemotherapy—an easy, highly effective and safe treatment of cutaneous and subcutaneous metastases: results of ESOPE (European Standard Operating Procedures of Electrochemotherapy) study. *European Journal of Cancer Supplements*, 4, 3–13.

Matthiessen, L.W., Johannesen, H.H., Hendel, H.W., Moss, T., Kamby, C., and Gehl, J. (2012). Electrochemotherapy for large cutaneous recurrence of breast cancer: a phase II clinical trial. *Acta Oncologica*, 51, 713–721.

Palliativedrugs.com (2014). *Palliative Care Formulary*. [Online] Available at: <http://www.palliativedrugs.com/palliative-care-formulary.html>.

Probst, S., Arber, A., and Faithful, S. (2013). Malignant fungating wounds—the meaning of living in an unbounded body. *European Journal of Oncology Nursing*, 17(1), 38–45.

Probst, S., Arber, A., Trojan, A., and Faithful, S. (2012). Caring for a loved one with a malignant fungating wound. *Supportive Care in Cancer*, 20(12), 3065–3070.

Ribeiro, M.D.C., Joel, S.P., and Zeppetella, G. (2004). The bioavailability of morphine applied topically to cutaneous ulcers. *Journal of Pain and Symptom Management*, 27, 434–439.

Teissié, J., Escoffre, J.M., Paganin, A., *et al.* (2012). Drug delivery by electropulsation: recent developments in oncology. *International Journal of Pharmaceutics*, 423, 3–6.

Winter, G. (1962). Formation of the scab and the rate of epithelialisation of superficial wounds in the skin of the young domestic pig. *Nature*, 193, 294.

Pruritus and sweating in palliative medicine

Mark R. Pittelkow, Charles L. Loprinzi, and Thomas P. Pittelkow

Introduction to pruritus and sweating in palliative medicine

Itching (pruritus) and sweating (perspiration, diaphoresis) are physiological functions of the skin that normally serve human existence well. Itching is the sensory input arising from the skin and mucous membranes that alerts man to potentially harmful insults from physical, chemical, and biological sources. The reflex of scratching is closely linked to the perception of itch, and in most situations functions effectively as an aversive motor response to relieve the sensation and protect the skin. Similarly, sweating is a well-developed and finely coordinated sudomotor response designed to regulate body temperature and prevent hyperthermia.

However, both pruritus and sweating have the potential to function aberrantly and develop into pathological conditions that create significant suffering and morbidity. Since these skin responses encompass both normal and abnormal functions, effective treatments to alleviate or eliminate the pathological component are challenging. In this chapter we provide a practical overview of the normal function and pathophysiology of pruritus and sweating, and offer a variety of therapeutic options and general comforting measures for patients experiencing these maladies.

Pruritus

Terminology

Itch and pruritus are terms used to describe both physiological and pathological sensory perception. Itch is a distinctive and common cutaneous sensation that arises from the superficial layers of the skin and mucous membranes. It is often fleeting, and the sensation may pass relatively unnoticed since the reflex action of scratching is largely involuntary and typically relieves the temporary discomfort.

Itch (itching, itchy, or itchiness) and pruritus (from the Latin *prurire*, to itch) are generally considered to have equivalent meanings. Itch and related descriptions such as 'terrible itching' are terms commonly used by the patient to convey this distinctive symptom. However, subtle differences in the terminology of itch and pruritus have evolved in the medical literature. In this respect, the terms itch and pruritus have been used to characterize the spectrum of unique cutaneous sensations ranging from the physiological response to severe pathological symptoms (Winkelmann, 1961; Winkelmann and Muller, 1964; Gilchrest, 1982; Denman, 1986; Bernhard, 1994). Physiological itch is the short-lived cutaneous response to the usual events of living, while pruritus is more closely associated with pathological itch (Winkelmann and Muller, 1964; Bernhard, 1994). Use of the term pruritus represents the symptomatic level or quality of itch that is defined as an intense cutaneous discomfort occurring with pathological change in the skin or body and eliciting vigorous scratching.

The definition of pruritus or itch is subjective and not entirely precise. Although the general sensation is well known and implicitly understood, many patients with more severe symptoms assimilate itch with various other discomforting or unpleasant sensation. The term itch frequently encompasses a range of descriptive or qualifying terms such as tickle, prickle, pins and needles, burning, stinging, chafed, raw, aching, and even 'painful' sensations (Bernhard, 1994).

To avoid confusion and to focus on the palliative medicine perspective, the terms itch and pruritus are used interchangeably to describe this pathological symptom. Patients experiencing pruritus may develop this symptom only mildly and transiently, or itching may be so severe and unrelenting that it preoccupies and completely disrupts their daily existence. It must be recognized that itch or pruritus is variable in its perceived quality and intensity. As with pain, the perception and tolerance of pruritus and the response to this sensation depends significantly on the individual's physical and emotional states, the functional level of activity, adaptive coping mechanisms, and the overall outlook. Attempts to develop questionnaires that assess severity of pruritus have been developed based on modified pain questionnaires (Yosipovitch et al., 2001). These quantitative measuring tools will be useful to better standardize symptoms and treatment responses.

Anatomy and physiology

Pruritus is a discrete sensation and a primary sensory modality arising from the activation and integration of cutaneous sensory neural receptors, afferent pathways, and central nervous system processing centres (Paus et al., 2006) (Fig. 11.2.1). In the past, itch

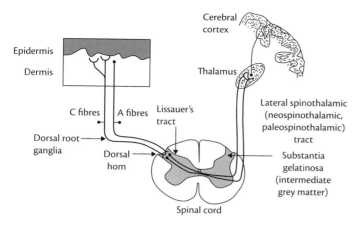

Fig. 11.2.1 Pathway for transmission of itch sensation. The C fibres terminate in substantia gelatinosa. Spinothalamic relay axons cross and ascend contralaterally at the spinal level of entering sensory neurons. Larger-diameter A fibres and other interneuronal and central pathways may modulate signalling information.

was considered to be a low-threshold form or submodality of pain based on various clinical and experimental observations. Both pain and itch are induced by noxious stimuli and therefore are designated 'nociceptive'.

A prevailing theory was that itch and pain were related sensations that differed only in the strength of the stimulus, with itch being a response to a weak stimulus and pain being elicited by a stronger stimulus. Further investigation of pain and pruritus not only revealed similarities but also clearly demonstrated the distinctive differences between these two sensations. Recent research has conclusively demonstrated that itch and pain are represented by distinct nerve fibres. Itch neurons are specific type C fibres in skin, each having a wide innervation territory, thin axon, and very low conduction velocity (Schmelz et al. 1997). The central neural pathway for itch has also been recently localized to spinothalamic lamina I neurons that are selectively sensitive to histamine (Andrew and Craig, 2001).

Many definitions of pruritus specifically include the reflex action of scratching. Scratching illustrates the distinctive sensation of pruritus, and the scratching reflex is routinely elicited and intimately coupled to itch. Scratching is regarded as a protective reflex, much as withdrawal (flexion) and guarding are comparable reflexes in response to painful stimuli.

Pruritogenic stimuli

Pruritus is induced in skin by various stimuli. Both exogenous and endogenous factors have the capacity to elicit itch (Hägermark, 1992; Wallengren, 1993). Most experimental and spontaneous triggering factors are mediated via the exogenous or external route. Cutaneous sensory nerves which convey the pruritic signal become activated through the application of either physical or chemical stimuli to the skin (Fig. 11.2.2). Many physical stimuli induce pruritus, including pressure, thermal stimulation, low-intensity electrical stimulation, formation of suction blisters, and epicutaneous application of caustic substances.

Chemical stimuli include histamine, proteases, prostaglandins, and neuropeptides (Pauset al., 2006). Delivery of histamine to the upper layers of skin by injection or iontophoresis has been a quantitative and reproducible method of examining pruritus experimentally. Histamine is also secreted in skin by mast cells. It acts directly on free nerve endings in skin.

Proteases such as trypsin, chymotrypsin, papain, and kallikrein have the ability to induce pruritus when injected into skin. For example, the spicules of the plant cowage (*Mucuna pruriens*) contain an endopeptidase. These fine spicules are an active ingredient of itching powder and induce an itching sensation when they penetrate into the epidermal layers or dermoepidermal junction of skin. Other natural proteases produced in cells and tissues of the body or by microorganisms such as bacterial or fungal microflora of the skin also have the potential to induce pruritus.

Mediators of pruritus

The nerve fibres that conduct signals representing itch are located predominantly at the epidermal–dermal junction and have free endings extending into the epidermis (Wallengren, 1993). The afferent sensory neurons that mediate these separate stimuli are distinct subsets of pruritogenic fibres (Dhand and Aminoff, 2014). Many of these nerve fibres contain neuropeptides such as substance P, neurokinin A, and calcitonin gene-related peptide (Fig. 11.2.2). Other neuropeptides contained in nerves deeper in the dermis and located around blood vessels include vasoactive intestinal peptide and neuropeptide Y. Substance P, which is the best-characterized pruritogenic neuropeptide, is a sensory transmitter of nociception. It is localized to sensory nerve endings in the skin and is abundant in the prevertebral ganglia, the dorsal roots of the spinal cord, and the brain. Administration of substance P intrathecally causes intense scratching that can be blocked by an antagonist. Nerve fibres containing substance P appear to transmit direct synaptic sensory impulses for the itch sensation.

Capsaicin, an alkaloid derived from the common pepper plant, is a well-known stimulant of erythema and pain when applied to mucous membrane or skin. It depletes substance P from the sensory nerves and excites the type C polymodal nerve fibres conveying pain. However, after initial stimulation, capsaicin blocks C fibre conduction and mediates neuronal toxicity which eventually decreases fibre density. These activities of capsaicin have stimulated the use of this agent for the treatment of pruritus (Bernstein, 1992).

Neuromediators directly influence vascular permeability and erythema (Fig. 11.2.2). They also activate release of other mediators such as interleukins, prostaglandins, bradykinin, serotonin, and histamine from infiltrating leucocytes and tissue-localized mast cells. Together, these neural and cellular mediators induce the sensation of itch, augment local activation of inflammatory responses that often accompany itch, and create areas of hyper-responsiveness around the primary stimulus zone for itch. For example, the phenomenon of 'itchy skin' (alloknesis) may be due to regional hyper-responsiveness as well as a lowering of the threshold to itch stimuli at the level of the spinal cord. Additionally, neuromediator release is probably augmented through antidromic nerve stimulation.

Cutaneous neural input

Human skin is supplied principally by nerve fibre networks composed of A and D myelinated fibres and thin type C

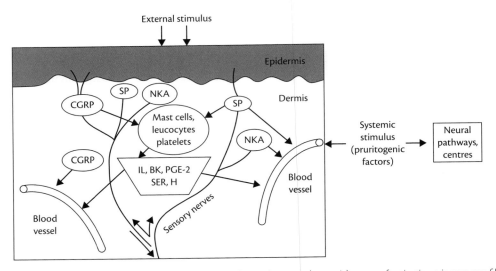

Fig. 11.2.2 Stimuli of itch in skin or at peripheral and central neural sites. External or endogenous (systemic) routes of activation trigger nerve fibre stimulation in the skin and the release of neuropeptides including substance P (SP), neurokinin A (NKA), and calcitonin gene-related peptide (CGRP). These mediators trigger inflammatory cells in the skin to release histamine (H), bradykinins (BK), serotonin (S), interleukins (IL), and prostaglandin E_2 (PGE-2). Vascular permeability, inflammatory cell infiltration, and nerve stimulation are evoked by stimuli.

unmyelinated fibres. Afferent type C fibres include C mechano-receptors, cold thermoreceptors, C polymodal, and C itch nociceptors. Itch is primarily conveyed by the C itch fibres which represent approximately 15–20% of unmyelinated nerve fibres in skin. The remaining polymodal C fibres constitute about 80% of all afferent C fibres (Fig. 11.2.1). The exact location and unique identity of the itch receptor is unknown, but it is likely resides in free nerve endings.

Itch, therefore, is separate from the slow, aching, dull, or burning pain that is conducted by type C polymodal fibres (Winkelmann, 1988; Handwerker et al., 1991). Myelinated A delta nociceptors conveying sharp pain also have been identified. Physiological and pharmacological studies have shown that separate independent sensory channels conduct itch and pain stimuli. The latency between stimulation and onset of the sensation of pain coincides with the relatively low rates of conduction (2 m/s) by the neurons that serve these sensory functions. Itch fibres have very slow velocities of 0.5–0.7 m/s (Schmelz et al., 1997; Andrew and Craig, 2001). Some investigators have suggested separating 'itch' into the 'pricking' sensation carried by myelinated fibres and the 'burning' sensation conveyed by unmyelinated fibres. This classification of sensations correlates with the two different systems of sensation described by Head (Head, 1905) in 1905 as the epicritic or specific well-defined sensation that mediates spontaneous itch and the protopathic or diffuse poorly localized sensation that conveys the perception of itchy skin. On the basis of current scientific knowledge pain and itch are largely separable cutaneous sensations. However, there is evidence of secondary neuron interactions with 'itch-specific' fibres being suppressed by coactivation of pain nociceptors using agents such as capsaicin.

In addition to the external or exogenous pathway for initiation of the itch sensation, there is considerable clinical evidence for the endogenous activation of pruritus (Winkelmann, 1961; Winkelmann and Muller, 1964; Gilchrest, 1982; Denman, 1986; Bernhard, 1994) (Fig. 11.2.2). The endogenous route for stimulation of pruritus represents a major and clinically relevant pathway; however, it is poorly understood. The potential sites of stimulation (the peripheral nervous system, the spinal cord, and/or the central nervous system), the inciting agents and mediators, and the relative overlap of exogenous versus endogenous activation pathways remain to be clearly delineated and applied effectively in the clinical setting. The systemic or endogenous stimuli for itch have been only partially characterized, and the biochemical causes for pruritus associated with a spectrum of systemic illnesses, including metabolic disease, organ failure, and various malignancies, continue to be ill-defined and vexing problems. One recently identified and novel endogenous mediator is lysophosphatidic acid which is markedly elevated in cholestatic pruritus and is an intense pruritogen when injected into the skin (Oude Elferink et al., 2011).

Several substances have been shown to mediate different or opposing effects on itch when tested experimentally. Their activities depend on the route of administration and their specific responses at the peripheral, spinal cord, and/or central nervous system levels. These observations support the concept of itch as a neural message that is interpreted in the context of signal reception, transmission, and modulation at each level of the nervous system.

Opioid and serotonergic mediators

Opioids are one example of substances that exert separate and potentially disparate responses in modulating the transmission and perception of itch and pain at different levels of the nervous system (Lowitt and Bernhard, 1992; Bernhard, 1994). Uncovering the existence of central opioid receptors led to the discovery of encephalins, endogenous pentapeptides that bind to these receptors. Opioids are powerful analgesics that mimic the effects of enkephalins. However, opioids mediate both excitatory and modulatory effects on pruritus at several levels. At the spinal level, enkephalins released from short spinal interneurons and opioids stimulate an inhibitory presynaptic signal transmitted to primary afferents that modulates secondary transmission of itch. However, within some regions of the central nervous system, opioids directly trigger itch. Clinically, intrathecal or epidural morphine has been known to induce localized or generalized itching. At the peripheral level within skin, opioids stimulate mast cell degranulation and release of histamine which produces itch. Furthermore, based on the recent identification and characterization of itch-specific primary nerve fibres, opioids may induce itching by blocking the painful stimuli that suppress activity of central itch neurons.

Central activation of itch by opioids appears to play a dominant role in some diseases, since opioid antagonists have been shown to exert significant antipruritic effects (Lowitt and Bernhard, 1992; Bergasa et al., 1995). The parenterally administered opioid antagonist naloxone inhibits induction of itch following histamine injection of skin. Pruritus of cholestatic liver disease (primary or secondary biliary cirrhosis) can be dramatically reduced with naloxone or the oral antagonist nalmephene (Khandelwal and Malet, 1994; Paus et al., 2006).

Serotonergic compounds are another group of agents that modulate effects on pruritus primarily at the peripheral level, although receptors for serotonin are present in the peripheral and central nervous systems. Cutaneous injection but not intravenous infusion of a serotonergic agonist increases the scratching reflex in animals. Peripheral serotonin receptors in humans are presumed to play a role in the mediation of pruritus. Temperature-dependent pruritus experienced by patients with polycythaemia vera may be stimulated by serotonin. Serotonin reuptake inhibitors, specifically paroxetine, have recently been reported to be useful for treatment of polycythemia vera-related pruritus (Diehn and Tefferi, 2001). Of potential clinical significance, generalized pruritus of hepatic cholestatic disease and chronic renal insufficiency have been relieved dramatically with intravenous administration of the type 3 serotonin ($5\text{-}HT_3$) receptor antagonist ondansetron (Schworer and Ramadori, 1993; Radereret al., 1994). However, other recent placebo-controlled studies have refuted this finding in uraemic pruritus (Ashmore et al., 2000). Nonetheless, opioid and serotonin receptor antagonists have revealed the complex mechanisms involved in transmitting signals for pruritus at the peripheral and central nervous system levels.

Pathogenic correlates in management of pruritus

The similarity of the symptoms of exogenous and endogenous forms of pruritus has prompted empirical use of similar treatment measures for both types of conditions. Frequently, however, effective therapy for pruritus caused by one condition is not particularly beneficial for pruritus of another cause. Also, treatments that ameliorate or relieve pruritus induced by exogenous agents have limited or minimal effects on alleviating pruritus of endogenous cause. This is probably related to the site and mode of activity of these treatments and their limitations in targeting the receptors, mediators, or central neural pathways that control expression of endogenous versus exogenous pruritus.

The nuclei of the afferent C itch and polymodal nerves reside in the dorsal root ganglia and axon extensions that synapse in the dorsal horn of the substantia gelatinosa (Fig. 11.2.1). Secondary neurons cross the spinal cord to the contralateral spinothalamic tract of the venterolateral quadrant before ascending to the thalamus. Lamina I of the spinothalamic tract contains type C itch fibres (Andrew and Craig, 2001). There is also evidence in animals that pathways in addition to the anterolateral system can transmit pruritogenic stimuli. Both the ventral posterior inferior nucleus and the ventral periphery of the ventral posterior lateral nucleus of the thalamus contain itch fibres projecting from lamina I (Andrew and Craig, 2001). The synaptic neurons within the thalamus project to the somatosensory cortex of the postcentral gyrus. Scratching is the spinal reflex in response to itching but also has input from higher neural centres.

Perception of itch has the potential to be modulated at the level of the spinal cord and, probably at other levels, by additional neural input as described for pain by Melzack and Wall (1965). The description of 'a gate control system that modulates sensory input from the skin before it evokes pain perception' can also be applied to the perception of itch.

A fibre impulse conduction is self-regulated by a negative feedback pathway that tends to dampen continued firing. It also interrupts summation of sensations of itch and pain conveyed by the C itch and polymodal fibres. The 'gate' has the ability to control neural transmission. Gate closure is envisaged to produce inhibition at the spinal cord level such that stimulation of A fibres by scratching would induce or enhance inhibition of conduction. Although the gate-control theory has been intensively evaluated and revised over the past three decades and its operational functionality has been challenged, practical application based on this theory appears to have been made in the control of pain and itch using transcutaneous electrical nerve stimulation (Carlsson et al., 1975; Monk, 1993).

Clinical evaluation and treatment of pruritus

The clinical approach to pruritus can present a considerable diagnostic as well as therapeutic challenge. To formulate a simple clinical strategy for diagnosis and treatment of pruritus, pathological itch can be classified as primary or secondary (Table 11.2.1). Secondary pruritus is caused by either dermatological or systemic disease (Winkelmann, 1961; Winkelmann and Muller, 1964; Gilchrest, 1982; Bernhard, 1994). Pruritus can be further separated into localized and generalized forms based on the location and extent of body surface involvement. In most cases, localized pruritus is due to cutaneous infections or other regionalized expressions of dermatological disease. As a comprehensive classification to better understand the wide ranging causes and interventions for pruritus, The International Forum for the Study of Itch (<http://www.itchforum.net>) has adopted these broad categories: dermatologic, systemic, neurogenic, and psychogenic (Yosipovitch and Bernhard, 2013).

Generalized or diffuse pruritus typically presents more troublesome symptoms for the patient and a greater challenge for the physician. Diffuse pruritus is usually related to a dermatological or systemic disorder affecting the entire skin surface. However, even pruritus which is generalized or diffuse exhibits symptoms that may be accentuated and localized to certain regions of the body, and these symptoms may fluctuate, migrate, or extend over time.

Table 11.2.1 Pruritus: causes, distribution, and classification

Aetiology	Distribution	Classification
Primary	Localized	Dermatologic
Idiopathic	Generalized, diffuse	Systemic
Essential		Neurogenic
Secondary		Psychogenic
Dermatological		
Systemic		

Primary pruritus

Primary or idiopathic pruritus is identified in the majority (> 70%) of patients where dermatological disease (secondary pruritus) has been excluded as a cause for itching (Paul et al., 1987). Idiopathic pruritus may be fairly limited in extent and intensity. Symptoms can be reasonably controlled by conscientious skin care and topical soothing measures. However, other cases of primary pruritus prove to be quite extensive, severe, and chronic. The diagnosis of primary pruritus is established following a thorough medical and dermatological evaluation to exclude secondary causes of itching.

Evaluation and management of idiopathic pruritus is frequently a frustrating experience for the patient and physician as possible causes and beneficial treatments are sought. When no clear aetiology is delineated, both the patient and physician may experience disappointment. With severe idiopathic pruritus, there is also lingering uncertainty whether an occult disease, particularly malignancy, may eventually be uncovered. However, several clinical studies have shown that only a small percentage of patients referred to dermatologists for generalized pruritus will develop a malignancy during follow-up evaluation (Kantor and Lookingbill, 1983; Paul et al., 1987). The majority manifest haematological malignancies, particularly lymphomas, and therefore periodic clinical surveillance is warranted. However, the duration and severity of chronic primary pruritus may be sufficiently debilitating for palliative intervention and the identification of effective therapies to become the principal goals.

Secondary pruritus—dermatological

Secondary pruritus is associated with a variety of disorders including both dermatological and systemic diseases (Boxes 11.2.1 and 11.2.2). For example, contact dermatitis is a common characteristic skin disease that has itching and scratching as its hallmarks. Box 11.2.1 lists the major dermatological entities that are accompanied by pruritus. Some disorders, such as scabies, insect bites, folliculitis, and allergic contact dermatitis, are caused by exogenous agents that elicit pruritus. Other conditions, including atopic dermatitis, bullous pemphigoid, lichen planus, psoriasis, and urticaria, are endogenously mediated inflammatory skin conditions that exhibit variably intense symptoms of pruritus.

The mechanisms that induce itching have been partially characterized for some of these disorders. Specific inflammatory cell types, such as mast cells, lymphocytes, and eosinophils, play important roles in the pathogenesis of specific diseases and the

---

Box 11.2.1 Skin diseases associated with pruritus

Aquagenic pruritus
Atopic dermatitis (eczema)
Bullous pemphigoid
Contact dermatitis (allergic and irritant)
Cutaneous T-cell lymphoma (mycosis fungoides, Sézary's syndrome)
Dermatitis herpetiformis
Drugs (dermatitis medicamentosa)
Folliculitis
Grover's disease (focal acantholytic dermatosis)
Insect bites
Lichen planus
Lichen simplex chronicus
Mastocytosis
Miliaria
Pediculosis
Pityriasis rosea
Prurigo
Prurigo nodularis
Pruritus ani and vulvae
Psoriasis
Scabies
Sunburn
Systemic parasitic infection (onchocerciasis, trichinosis, echinococcosis)
Urticaria, dermographism
Xerosis (asteatosis).

---

development of pruritus. Neuropeptides, cytokines, and proteases, among other mediators, are the main cellular products initiating pruritus (Fig. 11.2.3). These mediators probably act in addition to specific neurotransmitters which directly convey a pruritogenic signal to the itch receptor. Treatment of the specific skin condition and elimination of any offending exogenous agent(s) typically alleviate the symptoms of pruritus. When dealing with pruritus which may be skin related, it is crucial to identify and classify any primary skin lesions and obtain appropriate skin sample specimens or skin biopsies. This information is often very helpful in establishing a diagnosis. The correct diagnosis and appropriate therapy for dermatological disorders should be sought through specialist consultation and is well described in standard dermatology textbooks.

Cutaneous diseases which cause pruritus should not be overlooked. For example, unrelenting pruritus caused by scabies infestation, sometimes lasting for months to years, has been mistakenly attributed to concurrent malignancy. Other cutaneous infections, irritant or allergic contact dermatitis, or autoimmune blistering diseases such as bullous pemphigoid have been repeatedly observed to develop during the course of malignancies or other systemic illnesses. By recognizing that pruritus is due to a supervening dermatological condition, prompt and appropriate treatment can be instituted and the skin disease and pruritus both resolve. Therefore the periodic evaluation and re-evaluation of the causes of idiopathic or poorly controlled pruritus may uncover new information that will significantly benefit total patient care and improve overall comfort.

Box 11.2.2 Systemic disorders associated with pruritus

Biliary and hepatic disease:

Biliary atresia

Primary biliary cirrhosis

Sclerosing cholangitis

Extrahepatic biliary obstruction

Cholestasis of pregnancy

Drug-induced cholestasis

Chronic renal failure—uraemia

Drugs:

Opioids

Amphetamines

Cocaine

Acetylsalicylic acid

Quinidine

Niacinamide

Etretinate, Acitretin

Other medications

Subclinical drug sensitivity

Endocrine diseases:

Diabetes insipidus

Diabetes mellitus

Parathyroid disease

Thyroid disease (hypothyroidism, thyrotoxicosis)

Haematopoietic diseases:

Hodgkin's and non-Hodgkin's lymphoma

Cutaneous T-cell lymphoma (mycosis fungoides, Sézary's syndrome)

Systemic mastocytosis

Multiple myeloma

Polycythaemia vera

Iron-deficiency anaemia

Infectious diseases:

Syphilis

Parasitic

HIV

Fungal

Malignancy:

Breast, stomach, lung, etc.

Carcinoid syndrome

Neurological disorders:

Distal small-fibre neuropathy

Stroke

Multiple sclerosis

Tabes dorsalis

Brain abscess/tumours

Psychosis, psychogenic causes

Delusions of infestation (parasitosis).

Some dermatological conditions provide instructive lessons on the aetiology and limitations of managing pruritus. For example, prurigo nodularis is a distinctive pruritic dermatosis that can be chronic and is often recalcitrant to therapy (Doyle et al., 1979). The symptom of pruritus appears to play a more central role in the pathogenesis and propagation of this disease and there is increasing evidence that the primary form has a neurogenic aetiology. The pruritus of prurigo nodularis largely localizes to the nodular lesions that appear to develop and become more prominent as a result of scratching. Cutaneous nerve elements are accentuated and aberrantly located within the epidermis and dermis within the lesions and are often difficult to block effectively or eliminate. These factors probably account for the refractory nature of the condition to various treatments. Clinical and therapeutic observations on prurigo nodularis potentially have aetiological and practical relevance to non-dermatological disorders that are associated with pruritus since some of these conditions may also be quite refractory to many therapeutic measures directed at alleviating the itch.

Secondary pruritus—systemic

Pruritus is a feature of a broad range of systemic diseases (Box 11.2.2). For some diseases, specific medical or surgical treatment provides cure of the illness and pruritus. However, with many of the chronic systemic diseases, patients may survive for long periods with adequate control of the illness. Unfortunately, pruritus often continues to be a major symptom and may cause considerable morbidity. Several excellent reviews have recently been published that examine the criteria and evidence to recommend various skin directed or parenteral agents for treatment of pruritus due to various systemic (systemic or neurogenic) causes (Weisshaar et al., 2012; Xander et al., 2013).

Topical antipruritic agents

A variety of topical medications have been developed through the years to provide symptomatic relief of itching (Arndt et al., 1995; Devers and Galer, 2000). Many of the active ingredients have long been known to ease the symptoms of itch. A list of the common therapeutic antipruritic lotions, creams, and gels, together with their active ingredients, is given in Table 11.2.2. Topical medications are not convenient to apply to the entire body surface on a routine basis, but even patients with more generalized pruritus often have localized areas of accentuated itching that are more troublesome to control. Therefore topical agents have a role in treating both regionalized accentuation of generalized pruritus and localized itching.

Phenol in dilute solution (0.5–2%) alleviates pruritus by anaesthetizing cutaneous nerve endings. Phenol is potentially neurotoxic and hepatotoxic, and should be avoided in pregnancy and in

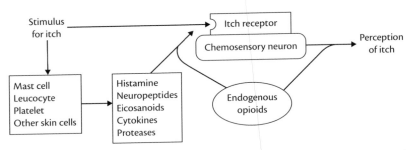

Fig. 11.2.3 Factors mediating itch: direct or indirect activation of itch receptor by specific pruritogens. The itch signal is transmitted to a chemosensory neuron which is activated and conveys perception centrally in the nervous system. Endogenous opioids, among other factors, modulate pruritogenic signals.
Adapted from Bernhard, J.D, *Itch: Mechanisms and Management of Pruritus*, McGraw-Hill, New York, USA, Copyright © 1994, with permission of the author.

Table 11.2.2 Topical antipruritic agents

Preparation	Active ingredient
Dodd's lotion	Phenol, glycerine, zinc oxide
Lerner's lotion	Ethyl alcohol, glycerine, zinc oxide
Salol	Phenol, acetylsalicylic acid
Sarna®	Menthol, camphor, phenol
Schamberg's lotion	Menthol, phenol, zinc oxide
Topic gel	Benzyl alcohol, ethyl alcohol, menthol, phenol
Wibi lotion	Menthol
Crude coal tar 3–10% solution	Crude coal tar
Caladryl®	Diphenhydramine, calamine, camphor
Pramosone®, Prax®	Pramoxine
Quotane®	Dimethisoquin
EMLA™	Lignocaine, prilocaine
Lignocaine patch	Lignocaine
Zonalon®	Doxepin
Zostrix®	Capsaicin

Source: data from Fransway, A.F. and Winkelmann, R.K., Treatment of pruritus, *Seminars in Dermatology*, Volume 7, Number 4, pp. 310–25, Copyright © 1988.

infants under 1 year of age. Menthol and camphor relieve itching by counter-irritant and anaesthetic properties. Menthol (typically 0.25–2%, but can be as high as 16%) produces a cool sensation, and camphor (typically 1–3%, but can be as high as 9%) exerts similar effects. Zinc oxide, coal tars, calamine, glycerine, and salicylates also have been used in many preparations with reported benefit, although their specific modes of action have not been elucidated.

Pramoxine hydrochloride is a topical anaesthetic similar to dyclonine that has been used as the sole ingredient or has been compounded with hydrocortisone or menthol and is available as an aerosol, foam, cream, gel, or lotion. Newer anaesthetic prescription medications include EMLA™ cream, a combination of the caine drugs lignocaine (lidocaine) and prilocaine which are absorbed transcutaneously and produce anaesthesia as well as abolish itch. Lignocaine patches (Lidoderm®) are also available that can be applied to problematic pruritic areas (Devers and Galer, 2000). Combinations of amitriptyline (1–2%) and ketamine (0.5–5%) compounded for

topical application in solutions, gels, and creams have been shown to possess significant antipruritic and dysaesthesia-relieving activities when applied topically (two to five times daily) to limited (< 10%) body surface areas (Poterucha et al., 2013a, 2013b). Doxepin has been demonstrated to be effective in relieving the itch of skin disease and may be useful for pruritus of various aetiologies. Capsaicin has been reported to be effective in localized neurogenic pruritus of various causes and has demonstrated benefit in other conditions accompanied by itch. Initial applications of the medication produce burning sensations and other discomfort. The patient must be alerted to these sensations and coaxed to continue if sustained use is planned and benefit is to be obtained.

Systemic therapies and other treatments

A plethora of systemic medications and various other modalities have been used in the treatment of pruritus (Winkelmann and Muller, 1964; Gilchrest, 1982; Winkelmann, 1982; Denman, 1986; Fransway and Winkelmann, 1988; Lorette and Vaillant, 1990). These agents are organized and listed in Box 11.2.3 according to their standard pharmacological activities. On examining this list, it becomes apparent that no drug has ever been successfully developed, tested, and produced exclusively or even primarily for pruritus. This fact alone reveals the potential difficulties that are encountered in the pharmacological treatment of chronic and severe cases of pruritus. All too frequently, patients requiring palliative relief from intractable itching are subjected to trials of various medicines in an attempt to discover which one 'works best' for them. With persistence and luck, a particular drug or modality can be identified that offers benefit and has tolerable side effects. Combinations of systemic and topical agents often seem to provide the best relief. Clinical experience has also shown that certain medications or treatment modalities seem to provide more consistent benefit for specific types of secondary pruritus, as is the case for ultraviolet B (UVB) phototherapy and the pruritus of chronic renal failure. Unfortunately, few controlled clinical studies have ever been conducted on the palliative management of pruritus, and a well-developed and simple clinical management strategy does not exist. Therefore, as outlined above, the practical aspects of establishing the probable cause(s), selecting a treatment, and assessing its benefit, side effects, and potential risks must all be addressed routinely as part of the process of providing palliative care for the patient with pruritus. In addition, several simple measures can be adopted to give patients and their skin some relief from the anguish of itching and the injury of scratching.

Box 11.2.3 Pruritus therapies

Anti-inflammatory agents
  Corticosteroids
  H_1, H_2, H_3 blocking agents
  Salicylates
  Cromolyn
  Thalidomide
Vasoactive drugs
  α-blockers
  β-blockers (e.g. propranolol)
Central and peripheral nervous system agents
Anaesthetic agents:
  Lignocaine etc.
  Propofol
  Ketamine
Antidepressant agents (tricyclic, SSRI(34)):
  Neuroleptic agents
  Tranquillizing agents
  Sedatives
  Opioid antagonists (naloxone, naltrexone, nalmephene)
  Serotonin antagonists (ondansetron)
Analgesic (non-conventional, voltage-gated calcium channel)
Neurokinin receptor antagonist agents:
  Aprepitant
GABA agonists-voltage-gated calcium channel modulators:
  Gabapentin
  Pregabalin
Sequestrants:
  Cholestyramine
  Charcoal
  Heparin (IV)
Miscellaneous
Disease-specific drugs and therapies:
  Cholestatic disease (Jones and Bergasa, 2000): rifampicin, methyltestosterone ursodeoxycholic acid, partial external biliary diversion (Fransway and Winkelmann, 1988; Ghent and Carruthers, 1988; Whitington and Whitington, 1988; Gregorio et al., 1993)
  Uraemia: erythropoietin, parathyroidectomy, ultraviolet B phototherapy (Gilchrist et al., 1977; Hampers et al., 1986; Marchi et al., 1992)
  Polycythaemia vera: α-interferon (Finelli et al., 1993), paroxetine (Diehn and Tefferi, 2001)
  Neurofibromatosis (neurofibroma): ketotifen (Riccardi, 1993)
Phototherapy: ultraviolet A, ultraviolet B, photochemotherapy (PUVA) (Gilchrist et al., 1977; Fransway and Winkelmann, 1988)
Transcutaneous nerve stimulation (Carlsson et al., 1975; Monk, 1993)
Plasma exchange, apheresis (Fransway and Winkelmann, 1988)
Acupuncture (Fransway and Winkelmann, 1988)
Psychotherapy, biofeedback, relaxation techniques (Fransway and Winkelmann, 1988).

Pruritus of malignancy

Itching associated with malignancy presents special challenges and dilemmas. It can be among the most severe and recalcitrant forms of secondary pruritus. Patients with malignancy-associated pruritus represent a significant percentage of those requiring palliation, and many may manifest this symptom at some time during their illness. However, the frequency, chronicity, and severity of pruritus associated with malignancy and its response to treatment are difficult parameters to determine, and they have not been examined systematically and reported in the literature. For example, the percentage of patients for whom the symptoms of itching have been relieved by primary treatment of the malignancy versus those who have benefited from symptomatic therapies has not been defined in this population of patients. As a result, a single, specific, and effective treatment plan for pruritus of malignancy is not available.

Symptomatic skin care

Patients with itching of malignancy may manifest different types of pruritic skin lesions that warrant individualized therapies. Many patients will demonstrate excoriations due to scratching and injury of the skin from fingernails or other implements (brushes etc.). Other patients show discrete papular, crusted, or excoriated lesions more characteristic of prurigo. As a routine, close trimming and filing of sharp edges of fingernails as well as wearing cotton gloves, if necessary, are initial steps to minimize further skin injury. Tepid (not too warm or too hot) baths are usually soothing and temporarily relieve the itch. Patients often relate that a hot bath or shower feels more relaxing and offers symptom relief, but the itch is worse afterwards due in part to vasodilation and the accentuated neural response of cutaneous heating. Immediately following the bath and a light towelling, the patient or caregiver should lubricate the skin with a fragrance-free, cream-base emollient containing phenol or menthol if this is found to be beneficial. Applying a cream results in better maintenance of skin hydration and lessens the chance of further aggravation of pruritus from xerosis. Wearing clothing that is loose fitting, less irritating (e.g. avoid wools), and minimizes heat retention and sweating (e.g. avoid synthetics) can also be helpful in lessening the frequency and intensity of itch. Cotton fabric clothing usually meets these requirements.

For patients with numerous excoriations and crusting due to scratching, application of tap water wet dressings (or cotton long underwear soaked in water) to the affected areas several times daily for 1–2 h provides temporary relief and hastens healing of injured skin. A low- to medium-potency corticosteroid cream containing 1–2.5% hydrocortisone can be applied to the skin prior to the wet dressings for topical anti-inflammatory action. A more potent corticosteroid such as triamcinolone 0.05–0.1% in a cream base can be used for 7–10 days as needed on an intermittent basis, but prolonged use should be avoided to prevent atrophy and bruising of the skin, secondary skin infections, or hypothalamic–pituitary–adrenal suppression.

Oral corticosteroids

Various systemic anti-inflammatory agents are useful in the management of pruritus. Oral corticosteroids often improve the symptoms of itching for patients with primary or secondary pruritus. In many patients, the specific activity is unknown. The corticosteroid may inhibit release of pruritogens, inflammatory factors, or neuromediators, or it may block pruritogen activity or alter its metabolism. As with topical steroids, prolonged use has significant adverse side effects. However, in cases where the duration of treatment is limited, an oral corticosteroid can provide much sought relief of itching.

Antihistamines

Antihistamines are another class of agent that offers benefit in treatment of itching. More than 30 different antihistaminic compounds of at least six different classes are available over the counter or by prescription. Although antihistamines provide minimal benefit for some patients with problematic itching such as that associated with Hodgkin's disease, obstructive jaundice, or uraemic pruritus, they have a good safety profile and should be used at full dose to attempt amelioration of pruritus. For example, pruritus is an early manifestation of HIV infection, and antihistamines, sometimes at high dosages, are used to control symptoms. Studies have shown superior efficacy of sedating over low-sedating antihistamines for relieving itch. Low-sedating antihistamines (e.g. fexofenadine, cetirizine, and loratadine) should be reserved for the histamine-mediated whealing disorders that are accompanied by pruritus. Longer-acting antihistamines with central nervous system sedation are preferred for control of itch. These include chlorpheniramine, diphenhydramine, clemastine, hydroxyzine, and cyproheptadine. Agents of different classes should be tried if an antihistamine of one class is not effective. Sometimes, combination of agents from different classes is efficacious when a single agent is ineffective.

Other drug therapies

Cromones and thalidomide are anti-inflammatory agents that have been reported to be useful in pruritus associated with several different types of chronic or malignant disease. Disodium chromoglycate improves the flushing and pruritus of systemic mast cell disease (Soter et al., 1979). It also has been reported to improve the pruritus of Hodgkin's disease when other therapies have failed (Leven et al., 1979). Thalidomide has been found to relieve the intractable pruritus and development of skin lesions in prurigo nodularis (Winkelmann et al., 1984). More recently, thalidomide (100 mg/day) was found to produce significant relief of uraemic pruritus (Silva et al., 1994). This drug is used primarily in the treatment of leprosy reactions and graft-versus-host disease. Because of its neuropathic and teratogenic side effects, thalidomide is not routinely available for prescription. However, selected patients who require only a limited course of therapy and can be monitored regularly may be candidates for thalidomide when an alternative medication is sought.

Many drugs have effects on the peripheral or central nervous system, and some of these agents have been found to be very useful in the treatment of itching from many causes. Anaesthetic agents administered by the intradermal, intravenous, or intra-arterial routes have effects similar to topical anaesthetics in blocking sensory input and transmission, including the sensation of pruritus. Parenteral lignocaine (200 mg in 100 mL saline by an intra-arterial line) alleviates refractory pruritus in hepatic cholestasis and chronic renal failure (Tapia et al., 1977; Levy and Catalano, 1985). Hypotension, cardiovascular effects, seizures, and psychosis are possible side effects. Recently, the anaesthetic sedative propofol, used at subhypnotic doses (15 mg) daily when itch was most severe or by continuous infusion at 1–1.5 mg/kg/hour, produced significant reduction in pruritus due to cholestatic disease of pancreatic neoplasia, hepatic and bile duct metastasis, cholangitis, and primary biliary cirrhosis (Borgeat et al., 1993,

1994). A rapid onset of action within 5–10 minutes was observed. Propofol also relieves pruritus from spinal morphine administration, and it is postulated that propofol blocks effects of opioid-like pruritogens at the spinal level (Borgeat et al., 1992). Parenterally administered agents such as lignocaine, propofol, and naloxone are of relatively limited use in chronic pruritus. However, if acute severe episodes of pruritus become incapacitating, these agents can often provide much sought relief and re-establish some measure of symptom control.

Antidepressant drugs, including doxepin, amitriptyline, nortriptyline, and imipramine, have antihistaminic effects as well as psychoactive and analgesic properties that make them useful in the management of various pain and itch states. Serotonin reuptake inhibitors such as paroxetine have demonstrated significant activity in controlling recalcitrant types of pruritus, especially secondary to polycythemia vera (Diehn and Tefferi, 2001), as well as various other advanced cancers (Zylicz et al., 1998). Neuropathic pain with protopathic features of diffuse burning itch as well as the sensation of pain is improved by chronic antidepressant treatment (Willner and Low, 1993). These medications may also benefit patients with pruritus where depression appears to be playing a role in the prominence or severity of symptoms Fried, 1994). Neuroleptic medications, including pimozide and haloperidol as well as risperidone, drugs useful in the management of delusions of infestation (parasitosis), may play a therapeutic role in some clinical situations. Although not indicated for the primary treatment of organic pruritus, these agents may be useful when patients exhibit delusional ideation in conjunction with their disease process. Treatment improves the symptoms of psychosis and diminishes the mental fixation on pruritus (Fried, 1994).

Sedative medications such as diazepam have been shown to be ineffective in reducing experimental itch, although mechanically induced pruritus was eliminated with this agent (Hagermark, 1975; Lorette and Vaillant, 1990). Sedatives in conjunction with other antipruritic agents appear to offer greater relief if the patient is experiencing anxiety as part of the chronic pruritic reaction. In addition to the sedative effects of antihistamines such as hydroxyzine, doxepin, and diphenhydramine, specific anxiolytic agents, including buspirone, clomipramine, and benzodiazepines such as alprazolam, can be used when anxiety appears to be playing a role in magnifying the symptoms of pruritus. Long-term treatment with benzodiazepines should be avoided as there is a risk of habituation (Fried, 1994).

The opioid and serotonin antagonists, as reviewed earlier, have been found to be very effective in selected types of chronic pruritus. The opioid antagonists have been evaluated most extensively in the clinical setting of pruritus of cholestasis where they show significant benefit in symptom relief (Jones and Bergasa, 1990; Bergasa et al., 1995). Naloxone must be administered parenterally. Naltrexone and nalmephene are orally active agents which may be useful as longer-term therapeutic agents for chronic pruritus. Some studies have clearly demonstrated benefit for cholestatic pruritus (Jones and Bergasa, 2000), though randomized, blinded, and placebo-controlled studies in uraemic pruritus seem to indicate no significant improvement in symptoms (Pauli-Magnus et al., 2000). Serotonin (5-HT) antagonists are few in number and less well evaluated in pruritus. However, the 5-HT$_3$ receptor antagonist ondansetron shows promise as the first in a new class of agents to alleviate the symptoms of generalized pruritus in patients with cholestasis and chronic renal failure (Schworer and Ramadori, 1993; Raderer et al., 1994), although recent studies have refuted its efficacy in uraemic pruritus (Ashmore et al., 2000).

Gabapentin and the newer analogue, pregabalin are anticonvulsant drugs with analgesic activity but with no appreciable anti-inflammatory activities. These novel agents have recently been shown to bind to the alpha 2-delta-1 subunit of the voltage-dependent calcium channel and mediate analgesic properties in the brain and spinal cord levels. Both agents have activity in neuropathic pain, and recent clinical evidence indicates effectiveness in pruritus due to uraemic states as well as other types of primary and secondary pruritus, including pruritus following burn injury.

Sequestrants such as cholestyramine or charcoal administered orally or heparin administered by intravenous infusion have been reported to be helpful in the treatment of obstructive biliary pruritus (Fransway and Winkelmann, 1988). Cholestyramine was also observed to improve itching in polycythaemia vera and uraemia. These treatments may be useful as adjuvant or alternative therapies during the management of chronic pruritus due to these diseases.

A variety of miscellaneous therapies are listed in Box 11.2.3, which also includes additional disease-specific medications reported to benefit chronic pruritus and other treatment modalities such as phototherapy, transcutaneous nerve stimulation, plasma exchange, and acupuncture. Pertinent references reporting the benefit of specific therapies are cited for each modality. For example, several medications and physical modalities have been found to relieve the pruritus of chronic renal failure. Despite our lack of knowledge regarding specific pruritogenic factors and their expression and activity in chronic renal failure, UVB phototherapy often provides symptomatic relief. UVB phototherapy is well tolerated, has few side effects, and can be administered at many dermatological practices or regional clinical phototherapy centres. A combination of narrow-band UVB and crotamiton has been reported to alleviate pruritus of metastatic breast carcinoma to the skin (Holme and Mills, 2001). Erythropoietin and thalidomide have been reported to improve uraemic pruritus. Interferon-α and rifampicin have been found to be effective for polycythemia vera and malignant cholestatic pruritus, respectively (Price et al., 1998; Lengfelder et al., 2000). Parenteral lignocaine is typically reserved for severe recalcitrant episodes of pruritus in uraemic patients unresponsive to other measures.

The multitude and variety of medications and sundry other therapeutic modalities reviewed in this chapter attest to the magnitude, severity, and chronicity of pruritus. All these drugs and therapies have been successful, to some extent, in ameliorating or abolishing this troublesome symptom. In managing the symptom of pruritus as well as the disease, it behoves the physician to make the best possible assessment of the specific physical and emotional factors that may be contributing to the intensity and character of a patient's problem of itch. With reassurance, flexibility, creativity, persistence, and a demonstrated concern by the physician, most patients will find relief and comfort.

Sweating

Anatomy and physiology

Sweating is a physiological sudomotor response of skin that has pathological counterparts. Abnormalities of sweating can be classified in terms of quantitative or qualitative dysfunction. From the perspective of palliative care, the most troublesome sudomotor symptoms relate to inappropriate or excessive sweating which occurs as part of malignant disease or its treatment. To understand the aetiological factors contributing to abnormal sweating and its palliative management, the anatomy and physiology of the peripheral and central thermoregulatory systems of the human are presented and reviewed.

Sweating or perspiration is a unique function of the skin of humans and apes that allows evaporative heat loss and regulation of body temperature in a hot environment or during physical exertion. Other mammals must pant, seek a cooler location, rest, or splash the skin with water to lower body temperature thermally. The crucial function and efficiency of sweat production is witnessed in individuals with the inherited disorder anhidrotic ectodermal hypoplasia who are unable to rely on evaporative heat loss through sweating. Physical inactivity, a cool ambient environment, or wetting the clothing or skin with water substitutes for sweating in order to achieve thermoregulation. Another group of persons particularly susceptible to the adverse consequences of thermal stress are young infants and the sedentary elderly who fail to sweat sufficiently and are also more likely to develop and succumb to hyperthermia.

Temperature regulation

Sweating is an important component of the elaborate thermoregulatory system of humans that is shown diagrammatically in Fig. 11.2.4 (Ogawa and Low, 1992). The hypothalamus integrates inputs from central and peripheral thermoreceptors with the efferent response mechanisms, particularly sweating. The two types of thermosensitive neurons, warm-sensitive and cold-sensitive, are located in the preoptic and anterior hypothalamus (POAH). Warm-sensitive neurons respond to a rise in peripheral body temperature and are more abundant than cold-sensitive neurons which are activated by a decrease in peripheral temperature.

Body temperature is sensed at several crucial sites within the body, including specific thermoreceptors in the skin, spinal cord, and brainstem as well as thermal responses from the abdominal viscera. The POAH integrates thermal information from these sites and others in the body. Body temperature appears to be regulated to match a set-point. An abnormal upward shift of the set-point is believed to be the mechanism for production of fever. Additional control of the central thermoregulatory centre is mediated at several other sites in the brain with projections to the POAH, including the midbrain reticular formation, the raphe nucleus, the amygdala, the hippocampal formation, the sulcal prefrontal cortex, and the medial forebrain bundle. Thermoregulatory control of the hypothalamus can be modified by higher brain activity such as sleep, mental stress, and emotional excitement.

Hypercapnia, plasma osmolality, intravascular volume changes, and dehydration also alter the body temperature and set-point. Chemical mediators, including neurotransmitters such as catecholamines and acetylcholine and the eicosanoid prostaglandin E, play central roles in the control of normal thermoregulation as well as in the expression of fever. Hypothalamic peptides, including thyrotropin-releasing hormone, bombesin, neurotensin, adrenocorticotropic hormone, and vasopressin, are also important in the modulation of central thermoregulation.

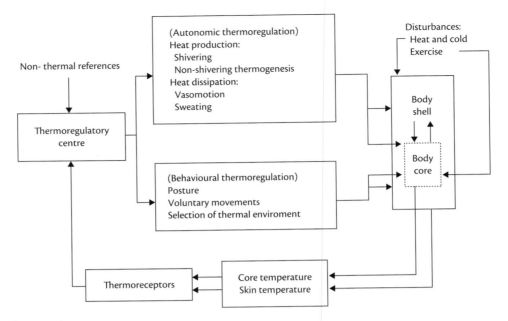

Fig. 11.2.4 The human thermoregulatory system.
Reproduced from Ogawa, T. and Low, P. A., Autonomic regulation of temperature and sweating, pp. 79–91, in Low, P. A. (Ed), *Clinical Autonomic Disorders: Evaluation and Management*, Little Brown, Boston, USA, Copyright © 1992, with permission from Lippincott Williams & Wilkins.

Autonomic control

The afferent input and efferent responses of thermoregulation are complex but are intimately coupled and controlled by both peripheral and central mechanisms (Fig. 11.2.5). The main thermoregulatory response affecting vasomotion and sweating is mediated through the autonomic system. The cutaneous vasculature is innervated mainly by adrenergic vasoconstrictor nerve fibres. Vasodilation and constriction are coordinated with sweating responses and interact to control blood flow and dissipate or preserve body heat. Sympathetic efferent pathways descend from the hypothalamus through the brainstem to the spinal cord and the preganglionic neurons. From here the fibres exit the cord and enter the sympathetic chain. Postganglionic sympathetic axons innervate sweat glands, blood vessels, and pilomotor muscles in skin. Eccrine glands are innervated by cholinergic fibres. Sweating is produced by both thermal and mental stimulation of eccrine glands, but the distribution and inciting factors causing the sudomotor response are different. Thermal sweating results from excess temperature that is perceived by the body. A local thermal stimulus will generate a uniform sweat response over the body surface while sparing the palms and soles.

The palms and soles show a baseline sweat pattern in the waking state, and mental excitement and stress will increase the rate. This response is called mental sweating. Mental sweating is controlled by the cerebral neocortex limbic system as well as by the hypothalamus. Thermal and mental sweating have some overlap in their central control but are also coordinated independently. General body surface sweating can be affected by various mental stresses. Mental sweating may augment or depress the thermal response of sweating over the body surface, but always increases sweating of the palms and soles. Axillary and, in some individuals, forehead sweating have a lower threshold to stimulation and are often active when there is no thermal sweating elsewhere.

Thermal sweating normally occurs uniformly over the body. Various factors, including body position, exercise, dehydration, sweat gland blood flow, ambient humidity, gender, and age, have also been shown to exert significant effects on the distribution, rate of production, activation thresholds, and other functional aspects of sweating. These factors must be taken into consideration in determining whether sweating responses are physiological or pathological.

Hyperhidrosis

In considering the palliative aspects of sweat dysfunction, most patients are typically bothered by hyperhidrosis (excessive sweating) or the distinctive symptom of nocturnal diaphoresis (night sweats) (Lea and Aber, 1985). A variety of underlying disorders contribute to localized or generalized hyperhidrosis (Table 11.2.3). Hyperhidrosis can be further classified as primary or secondary. It also should be appreciated that it may be a compensatory response to anhidrosis at other body sites. Therefore the cause of hyperhidrosis should be determined if possible, and attempts should be made to alleviate underlying abnormalities that may induce pathological states of excessive or insufficient sweat production.

Clinical evaluation

Determination of sweating abnormalities can be based on the clinical history and examination, or on more comprehensive evaluations such as thermoregulatory sweat testing or specific measurements such as quantitative sudomotor axon reflex tests (QSART) (Fealey, 1992). QSART measures the pattern of sweat response and discriminates whether abnormalities in sweat production are pre- or postganglionic. Postganglionic abnormalities demonstrate alterations in the QSART while disturbances at the preganglionic level typically spare QSART function.

Thermoregulatory sweat testing assesses the integrity of the peripheral and central sympathetic sudomotor pathways

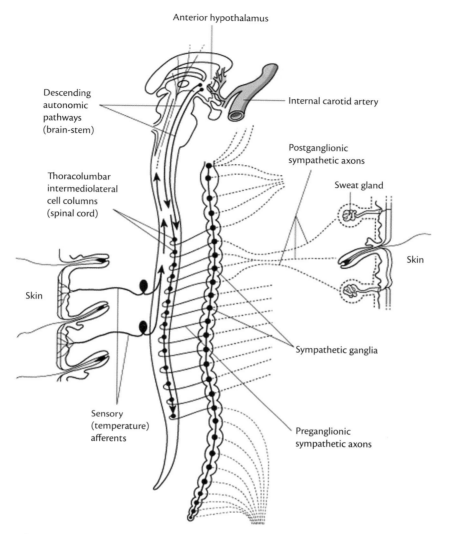

Fig. 11.2.5 Autonomic thermoregulatory sweat pathways: afferent and efferent limbs integrating temperature sensation and sudomotor response.
Reprinted from *Mayo Clinic Proceedings*, Volume 64, Issue 6, Robert D. Fealey et al., Thermoregulatory Sweating Abnormalities in Diabetes Mellitus, pp.617–628, Copyright © 1989 Mayo Foundation for Medical Education and Research, with permission from Elsevier, http://www.sciencedirect.com/science/journal/00256196.

(Fealey, 1992). Thermal stimulation is achieved by raising the skin temperature and the central or core body temperature. An environmentally controlled cabinet that warms the ambient air temperature to 45–50°C and also heats the skin with infrared lamps is used to raise central (oral or tympanic membrane) temperature and skin temperature to levels that stimulate sweating. Sweating on the skin surface is visualized with a special indicator powder containing iodinated corn starch, iodine solution, or alizarin-red-containing corn starch and sodium carbonate. Reduced or absent sweating can be delineated clearly (Fig. 11.2.5), and the distribution and extent of sweat loss is useful in further characterizing potential pathological abnormalities of the pre- or postganglionic pathways (Fig. 11.2.6) or the end organ, that is, the sweat glands (Fig. 11.2.7).

Disruption of the sympathetic chain or white rami produces localized loss of sweating as can be seen with a Pancoast tumour involving the apical lung (Fig. 11.2.6). In contrast, irritation of the sympathetic chain by encroachment of a neoplasm such as bronchial carcinoma, mesothelioma, or osteoma may also produce ipsilateral hyperhidrosis (Walsh et al., 1976).

Stroke rarely causes contralateral hyperhidrosis if large infarcts affect both the superficial and deep cerebral structures. Basilar artery strokes have been known to produce focal symmetrical sweating.

Generalized or regionalized hyperhidrosis

Generalized hyperhidrosis occurs with various systemic diseases, including endocrine disorders, menopause, infections, lymphomas and other cancers, carcinoid syndrome, and drug withdrawal (Fealey, 1992). Endocrine disturbances observed to cause excessive sweating include acromegaly, diabetes mellitus, diabetes insipidus, hypopituitarism, hypoglycaemia thyrotoxicosis, and phaeochromocytoma. Drugs reported to cause hyperhidrosis include opioid analgesics such as morphine, diamorphine, methadone, butorphanol, and pentazocine, antidepressants such as fluoxetine, aciclovir, and naproxen. If patients experience significant symptoms of sweat excess as a result of a particular medication, switching to an alternative drug may provide significant relief. Although the mechanism producing hyperhidrosis is not clearly understood and may be different for each of these causes,

Table 11.2.3 Hyperhidrosis

Localized hyperhidrosis	Generalized hyperhidrosis
Essential (primary)	*Systemic illness*
Neurogenic:	Phaeochromocytoma
Spinal cord disease	Thyrotoxicosis
Peripheral neuropathy	Hypopituitarism
Cerebrovascular disease (stroke)	Diabetes insipidus
Intrathoracic neoplasms or masses	Diabetes mellitus
Unilateral circumscribed	Acromegaly
Cold-induced	Hypoglycaemia
Associated with cutaneous lesions	Carcinoid syndrome
Gustatory	Menopause
	Tuberculosis
	Lymphoma
	Endocarditis
	Angina
	Malignancy
	Nocturnal
	Episodic
	Medication-induced

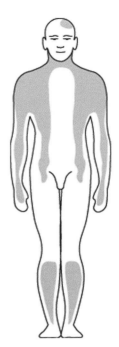

Fig. 11.2.7 Loss of sweating in the distribution of the truncal radiation port. Anhidrosis is caused by damage to the dermis and loss of sweat gland function.
Reproduced from Fealey, R.D., The thermoregulatory sweat test, pp. 217–29, in Low, P. A. (Ed), *Clinical Autonomic Disorders: Evaluation and Management*, Little Brown, Boston, USA, Copyright © 1992, with permission from Lippincott Williams & Wilkins.

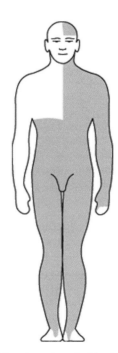

Fig. 11.2.6 Anhidrosis (light-coloured areas) of the right head, upper trunk, and upper extremity due to a right-sided Pancoast tumour. Distal sweat loss is due to peripheral neuropathy.
Reproduced from Fealey, R.D., The thermoregulatory sweat test, pp. 217–29, in Low, P. A. (Ed), *Clinical Autonomic Disorders: Evaluation and Management*, Little Brown, Boston, USA, Copyright © 1992, with permission from Lippincott Williams & Wilkins.

a downward shift of the set-point of the POAH could stimulate inappropriate sweating.

The patient may confuse excessive regionalized sweating with generalized hyperhidrosis. Compensatory hyperhidrosis may occur within normal sweat-producing areas of the skin in response to anhidrosis that involves other areas of the skin. The patient may not notice the loss of sweating, but, rather, experiences discomfort from the exaggerated sweating response. In this case, detection of the underlying cause of the loss of sweating would guide further treatment and appropriate management for symptomatic hyperhidrosis.

Treatment of sweating

The management of hyperhidrosis is based on identifying the primary cause underlying the abnormal sweat response as well as eliminating any potential aggravating factors that may further augment sweating. Primary hyperhidrosis will not be considered in the discussion of the palliative management of sweating. A variety of therapies offer benefit in treatment of primary hyperhidrosis but are not usually applicable to management of secondary hyperhidrosis (White, 1986). For primary localized hyperhidrosis, endoscopic thoracic sympathectomy or botulinum toxin injections into the affected skin regions are the most popular therapies (Heckmann et al., 2001; Vallieres, 2001).

Hot flushes

Hot flushes are a prominent cause of excessive sweating in patients with cancer. A detailed discussion of the proposed pathophysiological mechanisms for this problem is outside the scope of this chapter, but can be found elsewhere (Casper and

Yen, 1985; Charig and Rundle, 1989; Quella et al., 1994). Hot flushes classically occur in menopausal women and are associated with oestrogen depletion. Breast cancer survivors are not exempt from this clinical problem; in fact, they are more at risk for several reasons. First, adjuvant chemotherapy given to premenopausal women can frequently result in premature ovarian failure with all the sequelae of oestrogen-depletion problems; second the commonly used anti-oestrogen, tamoxifen, causes hot flushes as its most common toxicity; third, commonly used aromatase inhibitors also cause hot flushes; and fourth, general clinical practice has been to deny hormone replacement therapy to these women because of theoretical concerns that oestrogen replacement might harm them.

Given that breast cancer is a commonly diagnosed cancer whose incidence is rising, particularly among younger women, and that hot flushes are a very common clinical problem, what therapeutic options are available? Potential options can be grouped into two classes: hormonal and non-hormonal. Non-hormonal options will be considered first.

Non-hormonal treatment options for women

Twenty-five years ago, the most common non-hormonal treatment option for treating hot flushes was Bellergal®. This is a mixture of phenobarbital and belladonna alkaloids. Review of studies, however, show minimal suggestions of efficacy for hot flushes (Bergmans et al., 1987).

Clonidine is the next non-hormonal agent that was studied and utilized for hot flushes. Well-conducted, placebo-controlled trials demonstrated that it reduces hot flushes more than does a placebo (Goldberg et al., 1994; Pandya et al., 2000). However, it only reduces hot flushes by about one hot flash per person per day, on average. It is also associated with toxicities, such as dry mouth, constipation, and sleeping troubles. Thus, it is not very useful for most women.

In the 1990s, data became available looking at the newer antidepressants as agents to decrease hot flushes. A placebo-controlled clinical trial looked at venlafaxine in a dose-finding study (Loprinzi et al., 2000). This demonstrated that venlafaxine, at a target dose of 75 mg per day (with an initiation dose of 37.5 mg per day), decreased hot flushes by about 60% from baseline, compared to a 27% reduction with a placebo arm. This agent does cause some toxicities, with nausea and vomiting being the biggest problem. In 5–10% of patients this is severe enough to prevent continuation of this medication. In the rest of them, however, the nausea generally abates with continuation of the drug for longer than one week.

Multiple additional antidepressants have been studied, illustrating that paroxetine (Stearns et al., 2000, 2003, 2005), desvenlafaxine (Deecher et al., 2006, 2007; Speroff et al., 2008; Archer et al., 2009), citalopram (Barton et al., 2003, 2010), and escitalopram (Defronzo Dobkin et al., 2009; Freedman et al., 2011; Freeman et al., 2011; Carpenter et al., 2012) can decrease hot flushes to a similar degree as does venlafaxine. Fluoxetine and sertraline appear to also reduce hot flushes, but to a less substantial degree than is seen with venlafaxine and paroxetine (Loprinzi et al., 2002; Suvanto-Luukkonen et al., 2005; Kimmick et al., 2006). An individual patient pooled analysis confirmed that the available randomized trials demonstrated that antidepressants does decrease hot flushes (Loprinzi et al., 2009b).

There is concern that some of these antidepressants should not be used with tamoxifen as it interferes with an enzyme (CYP 2D6) which is utilized to convert tamoxifen to its active metabolite, endoxifen (Stearns et al., 2003). This concern was first noted with paroxetine. Fluoxetine also appears to be a strong inhibitor of CYP 2D6. Venlafaxine and citalopram have not been considered to be strong inhibitors of this enzyme, but are the topic of current investigation.

Subsequent to information regarding antidepressant use, data became available demonstrating that gabapentin also reduces hot flushes. At a target dose of 900 mg per day, it reduces hot flushes by about 50–60% (Guttuso et al., 2003; Pandya et al., 2005). An individual patient pooled analysis confirmed that the available randomized trials demonstrated that gabapentin does decrease hot flushes (Loprinzi et al., 2009b). An additional placebo-controlled trial demonstrated that a related agent, pregabalin, also decreases hot flushes to a similar degree (Loprinzi et al., 2010).

A recent trial compared the use of venlafaxine versus gabapentin in breast cancer survivors, in a randomized cross-over trial. This study revealed that the women preferred venlafaxine over gabapentin at a 2:1 ratio (p = 0.01) (Bordeleau et al., 2010).

There are other non-hormonal agents that have been studied, such as black cohosh and vitamin E, that do not appear to be very efficacious (Barton et al., 1998; Pockaj et al., 2006).

Hormonal agents

Soy products have been examined in multiple placebo-controlled clinical trials. The bulk of the information available suggests that soy is not very helpful for reducing hot flushes (Quella et al., 2000). There have been some studies which have reported positive results and, eventually, further investigation might define some soy product that does help hot flushes. Nonetheless, until this has been done, soy phytoestrogens should not be recommended as therapy for hot flushes.

Progestational agents, however, do clearly decrease hot flushes. A placebo-controlled trial examined 40 mg/day of megestrol acetate versus a placebo (Loprinzi et al., 1994b). This demonstrated an approximately 85% reduction of hot flushes, with low doses of megestrol acetate, results similar to what would be expected with oestrogen therapy. These results were replicated by an independent study group, which also supported that 20 mg/day was an effective dose (Goodwin et al., 2008). A subsequent clinical trial compared oral megestrol acetate to intramuscular medroxyprogesterone acetate (MPA) (Bertelli et al., 2002). Both of these agents appeared similarly advantageous, with a suggestion that the MPA was slightly better. Another trial compared a single intramuscular dose of MPA to continuous oral venlafaxine. MPA reduced hot flushes more substantially then did venlafaxine (Loprinzi et al., 2006).

There are hypothetical concerns with regards to the use of low doses of progestational agents in women with breast cancer (Loprinzi et al., 2006). There are some data to suggest that it might promote breast cancer growth, while there are other data suggesting that it might actually have antitumor activity. Many oncologists have been concerned about giving this therapy to women with a history of breast cancer, especially hormonal receptor positive breast cancer.

Oestrogen also decreases hot flushes by approximately 80–90% (North American Menopause Society, 2004) but increased concerns were raised with combined hormonal therapy (oestrogen plus progesterone) with the publication of the Women's Health Initiative (Rossouw et al., 2002). This therapy increased the risk of breast cancer and increased the risk of cardiovascular trouble, including thromboembolic problems. This raised concern for the use of this therapy, both in women with breast cancer and women without a history of breast cancer. A subsequent Women's Health Initiative trial reported on the use of oestrogen therapy alone (without a progestational agent) in women who had had a hysterectomy (Anderson et al., 2004). In this situation there was no increased risk of breast cancer, with a suggestion that there was actually a decreased incidence of breast cancer in women receiving Premarin*, when compared to the placebo group. There are mixed reports with regards to the safety of oestrogen use in women with a history of breast cancer (Vassilopoulou-Sellin et al., 1997, 1999, 2002; Dew et al., 1998; Col et al., 2001). All in all, oestrogen is frequently not utilized in patients with a history of breast cancer because of the concerns noted above.

Another group of cancer patients who suffer from hot flushes are men who have had androgen ablation therapy for prostate cancer. Hot flushes affect approximately 75% of such men and can be a very substantial problem (Charig and Rundle, 1989; Quella et al., 1994). Noting that there have not been near as many hot flash trials performed in men, as there have been in women, it has been proposed, as a general principle, that hot flash treatment in women can relatively well provide direction for what works in men (Loprinzi and Wolf, 2010).

Nonetheless, some hot flash studies have been done in men. A placebo-controlled trial demonstrated that clonidine does not appear to decrease hot flushes in men (Loprinzi et al., 1994a, 1994b). A randomized, placebo-controlled, dose-finding, double-blinded clinical trial evaluated gabapentin for treating hot flushes in men, reporting results similar to what has been observed in women (Loprinzi et al., 2009a; Moraska et al., 2010). Additionally, pilot trials support that venlafaxine and paroxetine appear to help hot flushes in men as well as it does in women (Roth and Scher, 1998; Quella et al., 1999; Loprinzi et al., 2004). Lastly, low-dose megestrol acetate alleviates hot flushes in men as well as it does in women, with about an 85% reduction in hot flushes. It should be noted that megestrol acetate has occasionally been associated with rising prostate-specific antigen concentrations, however (Burch and Loprinzi, 1999; Sartor and Eastham, 1999). Therefore, it is reasonable to try one or more of the non-hormonal agents first, saving progestational agents for patients who do not get relief from non-hormonal agents.

Treatment of other causes of sweating

Another cause of sweating is related to fever. Sweating is a physiological response to fever, and documented fevers that elicit diaphoresis either during or following the episodes need to be investigated and treated appropriately. Sweating can be a prominent clinical problem in patients with advanced cancer who have tumour fever. Antipyretic agents such as aspirin and paracetamol (acetaminophen) appear to reduce fever by resetting the POAH set-point, and these agents improve symptoms, including sweating, that are associated with fever. At times, however, patients with tumour fever are relatively asymptomatic while they are febrile, but they may perspire and chill during defervescence. A simple solution to this problem is to discontinue antipyretic medications. Asymptomatic fever may continue but symptomatic periods of defervescence decrease. Another method of treating tumour fever is to use non-aspirin-containing non-steroidal anti-inflammatory drugs (NSAIDs) such as naproxen. These drugs can be remarkably successful in alleviating tumour fevers and associated sweating (Chang and Gross, 1984; Tsavaris et al., 1990; Chang and Hawley, 1995). While the efficacy may cease after a period of weeks or months, switching to another NSAID may again induce defervescence (Tsavaris et al., 1990).

Sweating may be a chronic and prominent concern for many patients who do not have any malignancy or infectious aetiology. Even in patients with malignancy, where antipyretic therapies have either been instituted or discontinued to attempt symptom relief, diaphoresis may continue to be a major symptom. Various medications, including H_2-antagonists, have been tried empirically in attempts to provide relief. Although a specific mechanism of action is not well defined and documented clinical trials are lacking, clinical experience has indicated marked benefit from cimetidine (400–800 mg twice daily) in both idiopathic and malignancy-associated sweating. Whether other newer H_2-blockers exhibit a better or worse clinical response is not known.

Thalidomide is another medication that may exert significant benefit in reducing sweating as well as improving other symptoms and syndromes of advanced cancer, such as cachexia, nausea, and insomnia (Peuckmann et al., 2000). Both low-dose (100 mg orally every night) and high-dose (300 mg twice daily) thalidomide have been reported to improve sweating in the majority of affected patients (Deaner et al., 2000; Eisen, 2000). Thalidomide has been shown to reduce tumour necrosis factor-α production as well as modulate other interleukins and cytokines. Besides peripheral neuropathy, severe constipation, headache, cutaneous eruptions-skin sloughing, and oedema have been reported. However, the relative safety of the drug in advanced cancer favours judicious use. Other medications to be considered for management of excessive sweating in general as well as night sweats include thioridazine, nabilone, mirtazapine, desloratidine, and benztropine (Mold et al., 2012). It is hoped that improved therapies will follow as the peripheral and central neural controls of sweating become better understood.

Online materials

Additional online materials and complete references for this chapter are available online at <http://www.oxfordmedicine.com>.

References

Bernhard, J.D. (1994). *Itch: Mechanisms and Management of Pruritus*. New York: McGraw-Hill.

Fealey, R.D. (1992). The thermoregulatory sweat test. In P.A. Low (ed.) *Clinical Autonomic Disorders: Evaluation and Management*, pp. 217–229. Boston MA: Little Brown.

Fransway, A.F. and Winkelmann, R.K. (1988). Treatment of pruritus. *Seminars in Dermatology*, 7, 310–325.

Gilchrest, B.A. (1982). Pruritus: pathogenesis, therapy, and significance in systemic disease states. *Archives of Internal Medicine*, 142, 101–105.

Heckmann, M., Ceballos-Baumann, A.O., and Plewig, G. (2001). Botulinum toxin A for axillary hyperhidrosis (excessive sweating). *The New England Journal of Medicine*, 344, 488–493.

Ogawa, T. and Low, P. (1992). Autonomic regulation of temperature and sweating. In P.A. Low (ed.) *Clinical Autonomic Disorders: Evaluation and Management*, pp. 79–91. Boston MA: Little Brown.

Paus, R., Schmelz, M., Bíró, T., and Steinhoff, M. (2006). Frontiers in pruritus research: scratching the brain for more effective itch therapy. *Journal of Clinical Investigation*, 116, 1174–1186.

Vallieres, E. (2001). Endoscopic upper thoracic sympathectomy. *Neurosurgery Clinics of North America*, 12, 321–327.

Wallengren, J. (1993). The pathophysiology of itch. *European Journal of Dermatology*, 3, 643–647.

White, J.W. (1986). Treatment of primary hyperhidrosis. *Mayo Clinic Proceedings*, 61, 951–956.

Yosipovitch, G. and Bernhard, J.D. (2013). Chronic pruritus. *New England Journal of Medicine*, 368, 1625–1634.

Lymphoedema

Vaughan Keeley

Introduction to lymphoedema

Lymphoedema is a chronic oedema developing as a result of failure of the lymphatic system to drain fluid and other substances, such as proteins, from the tissues. It typically affects the limbs but can involve any part of the body.

The management of all types of lymphoedema is largely palliative in nature in that there are no surgical or other treatments which offer a cure for the problem in the vast majority of cases.

This chapter will focus on oedema associated with advanced cancer and other diseases, encountered towards the end of life with some reference to cancer treatment-related lymphoedema, as this may also be present in people with advanced disease. Further details on cancer treatment-related lymphoedema are available in the online appendix of this chapter.

Although the literature on this topic remains sparse (Beck et al., 2012), there is a growing recognition of the problem (Towers et al., 2010). The International Lymphoedema Framework (ILF) (a charity established to aim to improve the management of lymphoedema and related disorders worldwide) recently published a 'position document' on 'The Management of Lymphoedema in Advanced Cancer and Oedema at the End of Life' (ILF, 2010).

Physiology of chronic oedema

Tissue fluid formation

The amount of fluid in the tissues depends upon the balance between fluid entering by capillary filtration and that leaving by lymphatic drainage. Under normal circumstances the two are balanced and there is no oedema. If capillary filtration exceeds lymphatic drainage, then oedema develops (Levick and McHale, 2003).

Capillary filtration and lymphatic drainage

The amount of capillary filtration depends upon the so-called Starling forces across the capillary wall:

- the hydrostatic pressure gradient across the capillary wall which tends to push fluid out of the capillary
- the colloid osmotic (oncotic) pressure due to plasma proteins which tends to draw fluid into the capillary.

The net effect of these opposing forces, together with the permeability of the capillary wall, will determine the rate of flow out of the capillary. Fluid within the tissue (interstitial) space then drains away via the lymphatics. The flow into the lymphatics will depend upon similar forces.

The previous understanding of capillary filtration and re-absorption as described by Starling, whereby fluid is filtered out of the arteriolar end of the capillary and a large proportion reabsorbed in the venous end of capillary, is no longer felt to be true in the steady state for most capillary beds (Levick and Michel, 2010). In the new model, in most capillary beds, once fluid has entered the interstitial space, it is drained away via the lymphatics only and not via re-absorption into the veins. This emphasizes the central role of lymphatics in maintaining tissue fluid homeostasis and in oedema formation. The old model is still found in most medical text books but the new concepts are being increasingly recognized.

The flow along the lymphatics is dependent upon a number of factors:

- an intrinsic 'pumping' effect of smooth muscle within the walls of larger lymph vessels, the direction of flow being determined by valves
- extrinsic compression of the lymphatics by skeletal muscle activity, similar to that which enhances venous flow
- fluid is re-absorbed from the lymphatics into the veins in lymph nodes, such that the flow in efferent lymph vessels is less than in the afferent vessels which carry lymph to the lymph nodes.

Oedema formation

Oedema occurs when capillary filtration exceeds lymphatic drainage. This can occur in a number of circumstances:

1. Failure of lymphatic drainage (lymphoedema)—this can result from:
   - mal-development of the lymphatics (primary lymphoedema)
   - damage to the lymphatics from surgery, radiotherapy, infection, trauma, and cancer (secondary lymphoedema)
   - malfunction of the lymphatics due to reduced extrinsic compression by skeletal muscles in conditions resulting in immobility, for example, paraparesis (this causes a mixed aetiology oedema as there will also be reduced venous drainage, which leads to increased capillary filtration).

2. Increased venous pressure (causing increased capillary hydrostatic pressure and capillary filtration rate) in:
   - deep vein thrombosis (DVT) and post-thrombotic syndrome
   - chronic venous hypertension secondary to varicose veins
   - heart failure,
   - chronic immobility (see above).

3. Hypoalbuminaemia (resulting in increased capillary filtration as the plasma colloid osmotic pressure is reduced), for example, in:

 ◆ advanced cancer

 ◆ advanced liver disease

 ◆ nephrotic syndrome.

Oedema in advanced cancer

In the oedema of advanced cancer, the swelling can have a particularly complex aetiology which may include:

◆ lymphatic damage due to treatment or malignant lymphadenopathy

◆ venous obstruction due to extrinsic venous compression by tumour or by intrinsic obstruction by thrombosis or tumour, including that of large veins such as the superior vena cava or inferior vena cava

◆ hypoalbuminaemia

◆ lymphovenous malfunction due to immobility (dependency oedema)

◆ general fluid retention due to drugs, for example, corticosteroids.

Clinical features

General features of chronic oedema

In lymphoedema, the oedema which is soft and pitting initially becomes firmer and pits less easily. This is due to the accumulation of adipose tissue and fibrosis, which arises from a chronic inflammatory process (Brorson and Svensson, 1998; Daroczy et al., 2003).

By contrast, in chronic venous oedema, chronic lipodermatosclerosis is a common finding along with ulceration. There is a loss of subcutaneous tissue with fibrosis which typically distorts the shape of the leg causing the 'inverted champagne bottle' appearance (Mortimer and Burnand, 2004).

In conditions with mixed aetiology, the skin and subcutaneous changes can also be mixed.

Skin changes of lymphoedema

Although these changes are characteristic of lymphoedema, they are more typical of longstanding chronic lymphoedema and are usually not seen in oedema which develops in association with advanced cancer due to the time course of development (see later). They may, however, be present in patients who have previously developed cancer treatment-related lymphoedema or those with other long-term conditions leading to immobility.

At first the skin appears normal or a little stretched but again with time various changes occur.

Typical skin changes in lymphoedema include the following:

◆ Skin thickening.

◆ Hyperkeratosis: build-up of the horny layer of the skin.

◆ Lymphangiectasia: dilated lymph vessels which appear on the skin surface like small blisters, which if damaged can leak lymph (lymphorrhoea).

◆ Papillomata: these skin lesions are similar to lymphangiectasia but also contain fibrous tissue, giving them a firmer consistency; they often occur in groups producing a cobblestone-like appearance to the skin.

◆ Increased skin creases: these can become very deep in severe particularly around the joints swelling causing deformity of the limb.

◆ Chronic inflammation: this leads to erythema of the skin and can be similar to the chronic lipodermatosclerosis seen in venous disease.

◆ Stemmer's sign (usually positive): this is the inability to pick up a fold of skin over the proximal phalanx second toe in lymphoedema of the leg and reflects the skin and subcutaneous tissue changes described above. In normal toes Stemmer's sign is negative, that is, one can pick up a fold of skin at the toe base.

These skin changes are usually more obvious in leg lymphoedema than in the arm but can occur anywhere.

Pain

The limb often feels heavy and the skin stretched or tight. Patients may experience pain which is often described as an ache, tightness, or heaviness rather than a severe sharp pain (Badger et al., 1998). Typically, the pain is worse when the swelling is worse such as towards the evening in active patients with leg lymphoedema. In addition, the weight of the limb can cause pain at its root typified by shoulder pain in patients with arm oedema.

Impaired mobility/use of limb

Lymphoedema can impair the use of a limb by the weight of the swelling making it more difficult to move or by causing stiffness due to firm swelling around the joints. This is particularly problematic in the leg with stiffness of the ankle joint resulting in restricted contraction of the calf muscles and thus impairment of the muscle pump which would normally aid venous and lymphatic flow. This in turn exacerbates the swelling.

Psychological aspects

Many patients experience significant distress as a result of their lymphoedema (Woods, 2000). This may include alteration of body image, loss of independence, loss/change of employment, and difficulty in finding suitable clothes and shoes to wear.

Frid et al. (2006) found that for those in the late stages of cancer, the impact of oedema was worsened due to feelings of hopelessness, disgust, and social isolation.

Specific situations

Advanced breast cancer

Oedema in advanced breast cancer can be particularly distressing. It can occur as a result of recurrent disease in the axilla, when it may be associated with a brachial plexopathy which, by causing paralysis of the arm, can exacerbate the swelling.

In addition, metastatic cancer can develop in the skin of the chest wall (cancer en cuirasse) and upper arm. This tends to obstruct the skin lymphatics and may cause gross oedema of the arm with the skin becoming tense, stretched, and fragile. In these circumstances the limb can become useless, heavy, and painful. The fingers and hand can become deformed and may look like a 'boxing glove'. The skin can break, leading to profuse lymphorrhoea and predisposing to infection and ulceration (Fig. 11.3.1).

The extreme nature of the oedema in this situation is probably explained by the combination of damage to the deeper lymphatics by surgery, radiotherapy, and possibly tumour and damage to the superficial skin lymphatics by tumour. It is believed that the

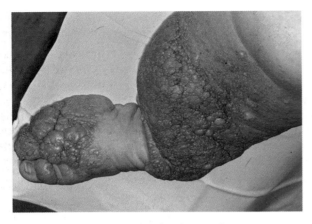

Fig. 11.3.1 Severe skin changes in a lymphoedematous leg.

superficial lymphatics act as a collateral system of drainage when the deeper system is damaged, a process exploited by the compression and massage techniques used in the treatment of lymphoedema. When these are blocked by tumour, the collateral routes are no longer available so severe oedema develops. There may be additional factors such as extrinsic compression of the axillary vein which can contribute to the swelling.

Advanced pelvic and abdominal cancer

Gross oedema of the legs, genitalia, and abdomen can occur in patients with advanced pelvic and abdominal cancers.

The clinical features may include:

- soft, pitting or firm oedema of the leg(s)
- stretched, shiny, fragile skin
- lymphorrhoea
- ulceration
- genital oedema—scrotal and penile or vulval
- pitting oedema of the abdominal wall
- ascites
- dilated veins on the abdominal wall in inferior vena caval obstruction
- Stemmer's sign may be negative.

There may be no skin changes typical of chronic lymphoedema, unless there has been a preceding treatment-related oedema.

Gross oedema can severely restrict mobility. Patients may be unable to walk, climb stairs, get up from a chair, or lift their own legs on to their bed. This may exacerbate existing problems resulting from the muscle weakness of advanced cancer.

Patients may find the appearance of their limbs and genitalia difficult to cope with. Furthermore, in men, penile oedema may lead to problems with micturition and sexual function. It may be difficult to insert a catheter per urethram, if needed, so sometimes a suprapubic catheter is necessary.

The oedema can be part of a 'pelvic syndrome' which includes other symptoms such as neuropathic pain, bladder spasms, fistulae, haemorrhage, and malodorous discharge (Sanz and del Valle, 2007).

Facial oedema in advanced head and neck cancer

Previous treatment of head and neck cancer with radiotherapy and neck dissections can cause lymphoedema, commonly in the submental region. However, with recurrent disease, extensive soft oedema may develop. This can include the whole face and eyelids. This can result in the inability to open the eyes particularly first thing in the morning when the oedema is at its worst due to gravitational effects if the individual has been lying down in bed during the night. Speech and swallowing can also be affected.

End-stage heart failure

Peripheral oedema is a usual feature of chronic heart failure but may be extensive and include ascites in severe cases. Immobility contributes to the oedema. Sometimes as the heart failure worsens and hypotension develops, there can be a slight improvement (as capillary filtration is reduced). Hypoalbuminaemia can also contribute to worsening oedema.

End-stage renal disease

'Fluid overload' is a feature of end-stage renal disease even with dialysis. Hypoalbuminaemia secondary to proteinuria can contribute to the oedema, as can immobility.

End-stage respiratory disease

In this situation, right heart failure (cor pulmonale), immobility, and hypoalbuminaemia from anorexia/cachexia may contribute to oedema formation. Patients who sleep in a chair at night due to dyspnoea are particularly prone to dependency oedema of the legs.

End-stage liver disease

Venous hypertension due to fluid retention caused by hyperaldosteronism and portal hypertension with ascites, hypoalbuminaemia, and immobility cause oedema in advanced liver disease.

End-stage neurological disease

Immobility is the main contributing factor in this situation. Typically as the neurological condition progresses, oedema increases as a result of deteriorating mobility.

Investigations

In the palliative care setting the diagnosis is usually clear, but factors which can contribute to the clinical picture of oedema, such as coexisting heart failure, need to be considered. In patients with advanced cancer, investigations may aid the consideration of palliative treatments such as chemotherapy/radiotherapy (see below) or help to determine the prognosis and thereby, guide management.

Investigations which may be helpful in the assessment of oedema in palliative care can be seen in Table 11.3.1.

The choice of any investigations will depend upon the initial clinical assessment.

Other tests may be necessary to confirm that it is safe to carry out planned compression treatments by assessing the ankle brachial pressure index (ABPI), Doppler wave form examination, or arterial ultrasound studies to investigate possible peripheral vascular disease.

Treatment

General principles

The current management of lymphoedema and other chronic oedema is largely based upon a combination of physical techniques:

- compression
- massage

Table 11.3.1 Assessment of oedema in palliative care

Investigation	To assess
Blood tests	
Full blood count	Anaemia
Urea and electrolytes	Renal function
Liver function tests	Hepatic disease
Plasma proteins	Hypoalbuminaemia
Brain natriuretic peptide	Heart failure
Ultrasound examinations	
Venous system	Venous disease, incompetence, thrombosis
Abdomen	Intra-abdominal disease
Axilla/breast	Axilla/breast cancer recurrence
Computed tomography/ magnetic resonance scans	Extent of malignancy

- exercise
- skin care.

This approach is known by various terms including decongestive lymphoedema therapy (DLT) and combined decongestive therapy (CDT).

Although there is evidence that the combination of these techniques is effective in reducing the volume of limb oedema and the incidence of cellulitis in chronic lymphoedema (Ko et al., 1998), there are few reports on the effectiveness of each component (Badger et al., 2004). As a consequence, an international consensus approach has been taken to produce a guidance document, *Best Practice for the Management of Lymphoedema* (Lymphoedema Framework, 2006).

Compression

Compression is a key component of management. It is provided in a number of ways: bandaging, elastic compression garments, and intermittent pneumatic compression pumps.

Multilayer lymphoedema bandaging

This technique comprises a series of layers of bandage applied to a swollen limb, which creates a graduated compression with the pressure reducing from the distal to proximal part of the limb.

Compression bandages need to be applied by skilled trained practitioners as, if incorrectly used, they may cause damage to the skin and subcutaneous tissues.

They are particularly useful for the initial management of lymphoedema to reduce swelling and improve limb shape before applying an elastic compression garment. They are also used if there is broken, ulcerated, or fragile skin and for the control of lymphorrhoea.

In patients with oedema of advanced cancer and lymphorrhoea, a modified lower-pressure 'palliative bandage' can help control symptoms of heaviness and leakage (Crooks et al., 2007).

Elastic compression garments

Graduated elastic compression garments are used in the long-term management of lymphoedema and other chronic oedemas. They are available 'off the shelf' or 'made to measure' and in a number of different strengths of compression and materials. They may, however, not be suitable for people with extensive oedema in advanced disease, particularly those with fragile skin.

Intermittent pneumatic compression pumps

Although the use of intermittent compression pumps had largely 'gone out of fashion' in the management of lymphoedema in the United Kingdom, interest is being regained with the development of more sophisticated devices. These multichamber devices inflate in a sequential fashion and provide a massage effect from the distal part of the limb to the proximal, said to mimic manual lymphatic drainage (MLD) (see following section).

Massage techniques

Manual lymphatic drainage

This is a technique of light superficial massage which improves lymphatic drainage. It is carried out by trained professionals as part of a programme of management, usually combined with other modes of treatment, particularly compression.

It seems to be particularly useful in the management of midline oedemas such as breast, trunk, genital, and head and neck oedema and where there is swelling at the root of an oedematous limb. These are all areas where it is difficult to create effective compression garments.

MLD is said to be contraindicated in acute cellulitis, severe heart failure, renal failure, hypertension, ascites, superior vena caval obstruction, around primary tumours, and metastases (Badger et al., 2004). In the latter, it is considered theoretically possible that MLD facilitates metastatic spread (Godetter et al., 2006). However, in the oedema of advanced cancer, MLD may be helpful in providing symptomatic relief (Pinell et al., 2008). In this situation, it seems reasonable to use MLD if the benefit is likely to outweigh the risks and the patient gives informed consent.

Simple lymphatic drainage

This is a technique based upon MLD but which patients and carers can be taught to apply themselves. Again there is little research evidence for its effectiveness but many patients find it helpful. It is usually carried out daily and the patient or carer needs to be motivated to do it regularly.

Skin care

The aim of skin care is to maintain the integrity of the skin and minimize the risk of infection. The routine use of moisturizers is recommended for all patients, with oilier preparations being used if the skin is particularly dry or doesn't respond to simple preparations (e.g. aqueous cream).

Other conditions such as eczema and tinea should be treated appropriately.

Exercise

Muscular activity is known to improve lymphatic and venous drainage. However, for patients with advanced disease, opportunities for exercise are likely to be limited.

Outcome measures

The conventional outcome measure of the treatment of lymphoedema of the limbs is an improvement in limb volume. Limb volumes may be measured by a tape measure method or an opto-electronic device such as the Perometer˚. In the former, a series of circumferences is measured along the limb and these are converted into a calculated volume.

In patients with oedema in advanced cancer, the aims of treatment are not usually focused on volume reduction and therefore other measures of symptom improvement such as the relief of pain and improvement in mobility and quality of life may be more relevant.

Other treatments

Drug treatments also have little place in management. Diuretics such as frusemide (furosemide) seem to be ineffective in lymphoedema although they may have a place where there is also fluid retention where heart failure is a component.

Skin taping (e.g. kinesio tape) is increasingly used in the management of lymphoedema, particularly mid-line oedema. This tape is believed to stimulate lymph flow as the skin moves against it. There is little research evidence for its use.

Management of oedema in advanced cancer

The general principles of symptom management in palliative care can be applied to oedema in advanced cancer:

◆ determining the underlying cause(s)

◆ considering potentially reversible factors including psychosocial issues

◆ deriving treatment options, taking into account likely prognosis

◆ ensuring the burdens of treatment do not outweigh the benefits

◆ enabling patients and their carers to make an informed decision.

Potentially reversible factors and their treatment are summarized in Table 11.3.2.

Details of a number of these approaches can be found elsewhere in this book or in a textbook of general medicine. Some factors, for example, hypoalbuminaemia are difficult to reverse.

Corticosteroids can sometimes be helpful in relieving lymphatic and extrinsic venous obstruction. It is usual to give a trial of high-dose steroids, for example, dexamethasone 6 mg twice daily for 1 week to assess effectiveness. After this the drug can either be discontinued if ineffective or 'down-titrated' to the minimum effective dose, balancing benefit against unwanted effects.

Table 11.3.2 Potentially reversible factors in oedema of advanced cancer and their management

Factor	Possible management
Anaemia	Blood transfusion
Ascites	Paracentesis
Fluid-retaining drugs	Discontinue if possible, consider diuretics
Superior vena caval obstruction	Metal stent, corticosteroids and radiotherapy, chemotherapy
Inferior vena caval obstruction	Corticosteroids, stent insertion
Heart failure	Diuretics, digoxin, angiotensin-converting enzyme inhibitors, beta blockers
Lymphadenopathy	Corticosteroids, consider anticancer treatment

If there are no reversible factors or the unwanted effects of treatment outweigh the benefits, then a purely symptomatic approach may be necessary. This may include:

◆ analgesia

◆ skin care

◆ modified, supportive bandaging for comfort or controlling lymphorrhoea

◆ shaped tubular bandage, for example, tubigrip if unable to tolerate an elastic compression garment

◆ support and positioning, for example, the use of a Lancaster sling to support a paralysed swollen arm with a brachial plexopathy

◆ passive movements to help reduce stiffness

◆ gentle massage techniques (MLD, SLD)

◆ aids to mobility and function.

The skin is often very fragile in patients with advanced disease and the oedema can be very extensive so the physical management techniques described previously need to be modified accordingly. (For details see ILF (2010) and Crooks et al. (2007).) The aim of treatment is comfort rather than limb volume reduction.

Compression techniques should be used with care in those with extensive oedema in advanced cancer, particularly those with hypoalbuminaemia. In this situation, in our clinical experience, oedema can be displaced to other areas, for example, from the legs to the trunk/genitalia.

Some patients, for example, those with advanced breast cancer, may have associated fungating lesions. If a compression bandage is applied to an oedematous arm with an ipsilateral fungating breast lesion, there may be an increase in any discharge from the lesion. This can be distressing for patients and it is important to warn them about this possibility.

Further details on the management of fungating and other wounds in oedema of advanced disease can be found in the ILF position document (ILF, 2010).

Needle drainage of oedema

There has been renewed interest in the physical drainage of oedema fluid in patients with advanced cancer. A good symptomatic response has been reported in eight patients with severe oedema using subcutaneous needles draining into a closed bag system (Clein and Pugachev, 2004). No patients developed an infection but the median survival was only 2 weeks. There would normally be concerns about introducing needles into a lymphoedematous limb because of the risk of infection and worsened swelling. However, this technique may have a place in selected patients with advanced cancer, a short prognosis and severe symptomatic oedema which has been unresponsive to other conventional approaches.

Oedema in non-cancer advanced disease/end-of-life care

There is little in the literature which describes the specific management of oedema in advanced cardiac, renal, respiratory, hepatic, and neurological disease. The general approaches described above are appropriate but specific techniques such as the use of diuretics in heart failure need to be considered (see Chapter 15.3).

Evidence base for treatments in palliative care

A recent systematic review of the evidence for various treatment modalities in the palliative care of cancer-related lymphoedema

(Beck et al., 2012) confirmed the paucity of large well-designed studies. There were no randomized controlled trials found, with most reports relating to case studies of needle drainage, MLD, DLT, compression and kinesio taping. All were rated as 'effectiveness not established' by the reviewers.

Complications of lymphoedema and their treatment

Cellulitis

Clinical features

Patients with lymphoedema are more prone to developing cellulitis in the affected limb (Mortimer and O'Donnell, 2003).

The typical clinical presentation is the onset of flu-like symptoms which may include malaise, fever, myalgia, nausea, vomiting, and headaches. This usually precedes symptoms in the affected limb which can include pain, redness, and increased swelling. On examination, the patient may have a red, warm, tender swollen limb or part of the limb. There may be lymphangitis, lymphadenitis, and in severe cases the skin may blister and desquamate in places. In very severe cases, this may progress to necrotizing fasciitis.

This classical presentation is, however, not seen in a number of patients who may have a variety of different rashes in the affected limb and variable systemic symptoms.

There may be evidence of a likely portal of entry of infection, for example, a scratch or cut, insect bite, skin cracking due to tinea pedis (athlete's foot), an ingrowing toenail, dermatitis, etc. However, in many cases there is no obvious source. It has been postulated that in some cases the infection arises at a distant site, for example, tonsillitis.

The cause of most of these infections is believed to be beta haemolytic streptococci but it is not easy to prove this with swabs or blood cultures. Indeed, the degree of uncertainty as to the aetiology of these episodes has led to them also being known as 'acute inflammatory episodes'. Some episodes may be inflammatory rather than infective but because of the often rapid progression of symptoms which can result in hospital admission for intravenous (IV) antibiotics, it is usual practice at present to treat them as infective.

The differential diagnosis includes acute DVT, acute inflammatory skin conditions such as eczema, and acute lipodermatosclerosis arising from acutely increased venous pressure.

The propensity to develop these infections is believed to be related to a local immune paresis in lymphoedematous limbs, as normally functioning lymphatics are an essential part of the local immune response to infection (Mallon et al., 1997).

Management

Antibiotic treatment is aimed at the beta-haemolytic *Streptococcus*. Many patients who present early can be managed with oral antibiotics and rest at home but some with severe cellulitis may need to be admitted to hospital for IV antibiotics, either at presentation or if their condition progresses despite appropriate oral antibiotics.

There is no research evidence at present as to the best antibiotic regimen but a group of clinicians in the United Kingdom has produced a 'consensus' guideline (British Lymphology Society and the Lymphoma Support Network 2013).

The recommended antibiotics are

- For management at home:
  - Amoxicillin 500 mg 8-hourly (or erythromycin 500 mg 6-hourly if allergic to penicillin).
  - Clindamycin 300 mg 6-hourly—if not responding satisfactorily to amoxicillin after 48 hours
  - Flucloxacillin 500 mg 6-hourly may be added if there is a suspicion of a staphylococcal infection, for example, folliculitis, crusted dermatitis.
  - Antibiotics should be continued for at least 14 days or until signs of inflammation have resolved.

- For management in hospital:
  - Flucloxacillin 2 g 6-hourly IV.
  - Clindamycin 600 mg 6-hourly IV—if penicillin allergic or if poor response to flucloxacillin after 48 hours.

Antibiotics can be changed to the oral route when temperature is normal for 48 hours and the inflammation is much resolved. NB Local hospital antibiotic guidelines determine the choice of regimen.

It is worth taking swabs from any area of broken skin but the results may be unhelpful. Blood tests (white cell count, erythrocyte sedimentation rate, and C-reactive protein) may be helpful in monitoring progress as is marking and dating the edge of the rash/erythema.

Bed rest seems to improve the rate of recovery. Compression garments used to treat the lymphoedema may need to be removed temporarily because of discomfort but, ideally, this should be for as short a time as possible. Massage should be avoided in the acute episode.

In end-of-life care, the appropriateness of the use of oral or IV antibiotics in symptom relief should be considered.

Lymphorrhoea

Lymphorrhoea is the leakage of lymph from an oedematous limb through defects in the skin. It can result from direct trauma, for example, cuts and abrasions, or from rupture of cutaneous lymphangiectasia or papillomata.

The leakage can be quite profuse and distressing for patients. Any damage to the skin is also likely to increase the risk of infection and therefore lymphorrhoea should be treated promptly.

Lymphorrhoea is best treated by the application of a compression bandage with absorbent padding but the compression applied may need to be modified in patients with fragile skin, for example, in advanced cancer (Anderson, 2003). The bandage may need to be changed several times per day to begin with because of 'strike through' but often the leakage can be sealed within a few days. However, in some situations, particularly with severe oedema and skin breakdown, the leakage may be persistent and require prolonged bandaging.

Conclusions

Although in some countries, for example, the United Kingdom, a number of palliative care services treat people with all types of chronic oedema, the most commonly encountered forms in the palliative care setting are those related to cancer treatments and those associated with advanced disease, especially cancer, towards the end of life.

Currently, the standard treatment usually involves a combination of physical treatments (DLT or CDT). However, this usually needs to be adapted in advanced disease, ensuring that realistic outcome goals are set and that the burden of treatment does not outweigh the benefit. The conventional holistic palliative care approach is important in this as in the management of other symptoms.

Online materials

Additional online materials and complete references for this chapter are available online at <http://www.oxfordmedicine.com>.

References

Anderson, I. (2003). The management of fluid leakage in grossly oedematous legs. *Nursing Times*, 99, 54–56.

Badger, C.M., Mortimer, P.S., Regnard, C.F.B., *et al.* (1998). Pain in the chronically swollen limb. *Progress in Lymphology*, 11, 243–246.

Badger, C., Preston, N., Seers, K., and Mortimer, P. (2004). Physical therapies for reducing and controlling lymphoedema of the limbs. *Cochrane Database of Systematic Reviews*, 4, CD003141.

Beck, M., Wanchai, A., Stewart, B.R., Cormier, J.N., and Armer, J.M. (2012). Palliative care for cancer-related lymphoedema: a systematic review. *Journal of Palliative Medicine*, 15(7), 821–827.

British Lymphology Society and the Lymphoma Support Network (2013). *Guidelines on the Management of Cellulitis in Lymphoedema*. [Online] Available at: <http://www.thebls.com/consensus.php>.

Brorson, H. and Svensson, H. (1998). Liposuction combined with controlled compression therapy reduces arm lymphoedema more effectively than controlled compression therapy alone. *Plastic and Reconstructive Surgery*, 102, 1058–1067.

Clein, L.J. and Pugachev, E. (2004). Reduction of edema of lower extremities by subcutaneous controlled drainage: eight cases. *American Journal of Hospice and Palliative Medicine*, 21 (3), 228–232.

Crooks, S., Locke, J., Walker, J., and Keeley, V. (2007). Palliative bandaging in breast cancer-related arm oedema. *Journal of Lymphoedema*, 2(1), 50–54.

Daroczy, J., Wolfe, J., and Mentzel, T. (2003). Pathology. In N. Browse, K. Burnand, and P. Mortimer (eds.) *Diseases of the Lymphatics*. pp. 65–101. London: Arnold.

Frid, M., Strang, P., Friedrichsen, M.J., and Johansson, K. (2006). Lower limb lymphodema: experiences and perceptions of cancer patients in the late palliative stage. *Journal of Pallliative Care*, 22, 5–11.

Godetter, K., Mondry, T., and Johnstone, P. (2006). Can manual treatment of lymphoedema promote metastasis? *Journal of the Society for Integrative Oncology*, 4, 8–12.

International Lymphoedema Framework (2010). *The Management of Lymphoedema in Advanced Cancer and Oedema at the End of Life.* [Online] Available at: <http://www.lympho.org>.

Ko, D.S.C., Lerner, R., Klose, G., and Cosimi, A.B. (1998). Effective treatment of lymphoedema of the extremities. *Archives of Surgery*, 133, 452–458.

Levick, J. and McHale, N. (2003). The physiology of lymph production and propulsion. In N. Browse, K. Burnand, and P. Mortimer (eds.) *Diseases of the Lymphatics*, pp. 44–64. London: Arnold.

Levick, J.R. and Michel, C.C. (2010). Microvascular fluid exchange and the revised Starling principle. *Cardiovascular Research*, 87, 198–210.

Lymphoedema Framework (2006). *Best Practice for the Management of Lymphoedema. International Consensus.* London: MEP Ltd.

Mallon, E., Powell, S., Mortimer, P., and Ryan, T.S. (1997). Evidence for altered cell-mediated immunity in postmastectomy lymphoedema. *British Journal of Dermatology*, 137, 928–933.

Mortimer, P.S. and Burnand, K.S. (2004). Diseases of the veins and arteries: leg ulcers. In T. Burns, N. Cox, C. Griffith, and S. Breathnach (eds.) *Rook's Textbook of Dermatology* (7th ed.), pp. 25–26. Oxford: Blackwell Publishing.

Mortimer, P. and O'Donnell, T. (2003). Principles of medical and physical treatment. In N. Browse, K. Burnand, and P. Mortimer (eds.) *Diseases of the Lymphatics*, pp. 167–178. London: Arnold.

Pinell, X.A., Kirkpatrick, S.A., Hawkins, K., Mondry, T.E., and Johnstone, P.A. (2008). Manipulative therapy of secondary lymphoedema in the presence of locoregional tumours. *Cancer*, 112, 950–954.

Sanz, A. and del Valle, M.L. (2007). The pelvic syndrome: tumours involving the pelvis. *European Journal of Palliative Care*, 14(6), 226–229.

Towers, A., Hodgson, P., Shay, C., and Keeley, V. (2010). Care of palliative patients with cancer-related lymphoedema. *Journal of Lymphoedema*, 5(1), 72–80.

Woods, M. (2000). Psychosocial aspects of lymphoedema. In R. Twycross, K. Jenns, and J. Todd (eds.) *Lymphoedema*, pp. 89–96. Oxford: Radcliffe Medical Press.

SECTION 12

Issues in populations with cancer

Issues in populations with cancer

The oncologist's role in delivering palliative care

Nathan I. Cherny and Stein Kaasa

Introduction to the oncologist's role in delivering palliative care

The division of cancer care into initial primary anti-tumour therapies followed by hospice or palliative care for patients who have progressive disease is anachronistic (World Health Organization, 1990). Since the goals of medical oncology extend beyond the reduction of tumour burden and the deferral of death and incorporate a quality of life dimension, there is need for a continuum in patient care in which both primary therapies and palliative interventions are integrated according to the clinical circumstances of the patient. For most patients, it is the oncologist who assumes the role of the physician primarily responsible for the provision and coordination of cancer care. This role is enormously challenging (Box 12.1.1) and it demands a wide range of cognitive, clinical, and interpersonal skills and a readiness to work collaboratively with professionals from other disciplines including palliative care.

Traditionally, the study and practice of medical oncology has focused on the development and implementation of anti-cancer therapies. By virtue of these endeavours, along with measures to provide for early diagnosis, substantial improvements in long- and short-term survival have been achieved for a number of cancers such as the germ cell tumours, lymphomas, early-stage breast and colorectal cancer, and the leukaemias. More sobering, however, are the observations that the cure rate for cancer remains less than 60% and that cancer continues to account for over 25% of all adult deaths (Siegel et al., 2012). Many patients are not cured, and for them the issues regarding the quality of their remaining time are critical, irrespective of the clinical course of their illness or the duration of survival.

Palliative and supportive care in medical oncology

Recommendations on the integration of palliative medicine and medical oncology

An expert committee of the World Health Organization on cancer pain and palliative care has emphasized the need for the integration of efforts directed at maintaining the patient's quality of life in all stages of cancer treatment (World Health Organization, 1990). This report emphasized that factors causing patient distress exist from the time of diagnosis and that supportive and palliative interventions are needed concurrently with efforts to control the underlying cancer. This holds true for patients undergoing curative, life-prolonging, and palliative anti-cancer treatments. This approach has been widely endorsed by numerous national and professional bodies (Foley and Gelband, 2001; National Institute for Clinical Excellence, 2004; Smith et al., 2012; Greer et al., 2013).

The National Comprehensive Cancer Network (NCCN) Clinical Practice Guidelines in Oncology (NCCN Guidelines®) emphasize the importance of palliative care as part of comprehensive cancer care:

Palliative care is a special kind of patient- and family-centered health care that focuses on the effective management of pain and other distressing symptoms, while incorporating psychosocial and spiritual care according to the patient/family needs, values, beliefs, and cultures. The goal of palliative care is to anticipate, prevent, and reduce suffering and to support the best possible a quality of life for patients and their families, regardless of the state of the disease or the need for other therapies. Palliative care begins at diagnoses and should be delivered concurrently with disease-directed, life-prolonging therapies and should facilitate patient autonomy, access to information, and choice. Palliative care becomes the main focus of care when disease-directed, life-prolonging therapies are no longer effective, appropriate, or desired. Palliative care should be initiated by the primary oncology team and then augmented by collaboration with an interdisciplinary team of palliative care experts. (National Comprehensive Cancer Network, 2014)

In recent years the importance of this integration has been emphasized by several randomized studies involving patients with advanced cancer that demonstrated that integrating specialty palliative care with standard oncology care leads to significant improvements in quality of life and care and possibly survival (Jordhoy et al., 2001; Brumley et al., 2007; Gade et al., 2008; Bakitas et al., 2009; Temel et al., 2010; Zimmermann et al., 2012).

Supportive or palliative care: defining terms

There has been much confusion regarding the definitions of supportive care and palliative care. The most widely accepted formal definition of palliative care, which was drafted by two oncologists (Neil MacDonald and Eduardo Bruera), is that of the World Health Organization (World Health Organization, 2002, 2007). It states:

Palliative care is an approach that improves the quality of life of patients and their families facing the problem associated with life-threatening illness, through the prevention and relief of suffering by means of early identification and impeccable assessment and

---

Box 12.1.1 The clinical roles of the medical oncologist

Preventative oncology

- Counselling:
  - diet
  - cigarette smoking
  - alcohol
  - environmental
- Screening.

Diagnostic evaluation

- Primary evaluation of the patient with suggestive clinical findings
- Cancer staging
- Physiological staging
- Goals of care appropriate to tumour type and stage and patient physiological staging.

Communication

- Disclosure full and partial
- Treatment counselling
- Prognostic counselling
- Eliciting advanced directives
- Patient and family support
- Psychological support
- Advanced directives.

Anti-tumour therapies

- Indications
- Selection of optimal therapeutic modality
- Safe administration
- Prevention and management of adverse effects.

Symptom control

- Physical symptoms
- Psychological symptoms
- Complications of cancer
- Complications of treatment.

Social

- Optimization of social supports.

Care of the dying patient

- Physical symptoms
- Psychological symptoms.

---

treatment of pain and other problems, physical, psychosocial and spiritual. Palliative care:

- provides relief from pain and other distressing symptoms;
- affirms life and regards dying as a normal process;

- intends neither to hasten nor postpone death;
- integrates the psychological and spiritual aspects of patient care;
- offers a support system to help patients live as actively as possible until death;
- offers a support system to help the family cope during the patient's illness and in their own bereavement;
- uses a team approach to address the needs of patients and their families, including bereavement counseling, if indicated;
- will enhance quality of life, and may also positively influence the course of illness;
- is applicable early in the course of illness, in conjunction with other therapies that are intended to prolong life, such as chemotherapy or radiation therapy, and includes those investigations needed to better understand and manage distressing clinical complications.'

The European Society of Medical Oncology (ESMO) has adopted pragmatic definitions that distinguish supportive and palliative care and emphasizes the discrete sub-entity of end-of life care. According to these definitions, supportive care aims to optimize the comfort, function, and social support of the patient and their family at all stages of the illness. Palliative care is care that aims to optimize the comfort, function, and social support of the patient and their family when cure is not possible. Although the clinical scenarios suggested by these definitions obviously overlap, it is the context of incurability, with all of its implications for the patent and family, that grounds palliative care as a special entity. Supportive care is needed by every patient continuously; palliative care focuses on the special needs of patients who are either incurable or who have a very low likelihood of cure.

From this perspective, 'end-of-life care' or 'terminal care' is defined as palliative care when death is imminent (Fig. 12.1.1). End-of-life care acknowledges that the intensity of physical, psychological, existential, spiritual, and family issues may be magnified by the patient's approaching death.

Ultimately, however, the distinction between supportive care and palliative care is largely semantic, and it should be emphasized that the terms are used differently by various specialists across countries (Cherny, 2009). Regardless of the definition, the fundamental reality is that patients with cancer, and their families, may express unmet physical, psychosocial, or spiritual needs at any point during the course of the illness. These needs require specific interventions that aim to reduce distress, enhance coping, or otherwise improve the individual's quality of life (Cherny, 2009).

The oncologist's role in palliative care

Both the American Society of Clinical Oncology (ASCO) (Smith and Schnipper, 1998; Ferris et al., 2009; Smith et al., 2012) and ESMO (Cherny et al., 2003) have policy statements outlining the responsibilities of medical oncologists in the care of patients with incurable cancer and the integration of oncology and palliative care. ASCO states that it is the oncologist's responsibility to care for their patient along a continuum that starts at the moment of diagnosis and extends throughout the course of the illness. In addition to appropriate anti-cancer treatment, this includes symptom control and psychosocial support during all phases of care, including the last phase of life (Smith and Schnipper,

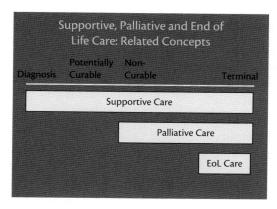

Supportive, Palliative and End of Life Care: Related Concepts

| Diagnosis | Potentially Curable | Non-Curable | | Terminal |

Supportive Care

Palliative Care

EoL Care

Fig. 12.1.1 Trajectories of illness.

1998; Ferris et al., 2009). The ESMO policy statement reiterates these points and defines the role of the oncologist in palliative care (Box 12.1.2).

The oncological management of advanced cancer

The judicious use of disease modifying treatments can potentially prolong survival and improve comfort and function. As treatment options become more varied, complex and expensive, the balancing of benefits and burdens in considering these primary treatment options is becoming increasingly challenging (Markman, 2003; Harrington and Smith, 2008). Decision-making must take into account a range of relevant issues, including goals of care, likelihood of benefit, likelihood of harm, and the desires, beliefs, and understanding of the patient and family (Hairon, 2008). Addressing the relative roles of disease-modifying approaches requires familiarity with key concepts of patient benefit, quality of life, and risk/benefit analysis (Detmar et al., 2002). When the therapeutic index of anti-tumour therapies is diminished and the likelihood of benefit is outweighed by either the risk or the burden of the treatments, it is the oncologist who must help steer the patients and the family to a care programme that focuses on symptom management and other efforts to reduce suffering, help coping, maintain quality of life, and prepare for the end of life (see below) (Harrington and Smith, 2008; Cheng et al., 2013; Schenker et al., 2014).

Communication with patients and family members

Given the complexity of the goals of care, patient and family expectations, and the range of therapeutic options, communication with patients and their families is a critical element of the oncologist's role in caring for patients with incurable cancer. Communication is challenging and requires patience and refined interpersonal and counselling skills to facilitate effective, informed decision-making.

A variety of communication tasks usually are undertaken by the oncologist. The diagnosis, prognosis, and treatment options must be explained and this may involve discussions about the potential risks and benefits of treatment options, the role of palliative care, and the necessity for discontinuing anti-tumour therapies when appropriate. In performing these tasks, oncologists need the skills to deal with intense emotions, highly distressed patients, and family members with fears, anger, and anticipatory grief.

Box 12.1.2 ESMO policy regarding the role of the oncologist in the provision of supportive and palliative care

1. The Medical Oncologist must be skilled in the supportive and palliative care of patients with cancer and in end-of-life care.

2. The oncologist must address the need for an appropriate medical nursing and para-medical infrastructure to address the special needs of these patients and their families.

3. It is the responsibility of the medical oncologist to assess and evaluate physical and psychological symptoms of patients under their care and to ensure that these problems are adequately addressed.

4. The delivery of high-quality supportive and palliative care requires cooperation and coordination with physicians of other disciplines (including radiotherapy, surgery, rehabilitation, psych-oncology, pain medicine and anaesthesiology, palliative medicine, etc.) as well as with paramedical clinicians (including nursing, social work, psychology, physical and occupational therapy, chaplains, and others).

5. In the care of dying patients the medical oncologist must:

   ◆ Respect the dignity of both patient and caregivers

   ◆ Be sensitive to and respectful of the patient's and family's wishes

   ◆ Use the most appropriate measures that are consistent with patient choices

   ◆ Make alleviation of pain and other physical symptoms a high priority

   ◆ Recognize that good care for the dying person requires quality medical care, but also entails services that are family- and community-based to address, for example, psychological, social, and spiritual/religious problems.

   ◆ Offer continuity (the patient should be able to continue to be cared for, if so desired, by his/her primary care and medical oncology providers)

   ◆ Advocate access to therapies which are reasonably expected to improve the patient's quality of life and ensure that patients who choose alternative and non-traditional treatments not be abandoned

   ◆ Provide access to palliative care and hospice care

   ◆ Respect the patient's right to refuse treatment, as expressed by the patient or an authorized surrogate

   ◆ Respect the physician's professional responsibility to discontinue some treatments when appropriate, with consideration for both patient and family preferences

   ◆ Promote clinical and evidence-based research on providing care at the end of life.

The management of the complications of cancer

Oncologists must be expert in the evaluation and management of the complications of cancer and anti-cancer therapies. Some common complications are listed in Box 12.1.3.

Evaluation and management of physical, psychosocial, and spiritual disturbances

Patients with advanced cancer commonly have multiple symptoms and other sources of suffering. To address their needs, oncologists must be expert in the evaluation and management of the common physical symptoms, including pain, dyspnoea and cough, fatigue, nausea and vomiting, constipation, diarrhoea, insomnia and itch. In addition, psychological and existential distress is common and oncologists must be prepared to assess and help manage the varied sources of these concerns.

There is extensive evidence suggesting that cancer patients' informational and emotional needs are commonly underestimated and that depression, in particular, is often undetected or undertreated (Breitbart et al., 2000; Pereira and Bruera, 2001; Hotopf et al., 2002; Rhondali et al., 2012). Many patients who develop psychological distress do not spontaneously disclose these problems (Maguire, 2002). There is a notion that 'good patients' don't complain. Furthermore, cancer patients may believe their emotional response to be an inevitable reaction to having a cancer diagnosis. Paradoxically, the most distressed patients may be least likely to acknowledge or discuss their emotional concerns (Greenley et al., 1982).

Oncologists ought to be familiar with the assessment of common psychological problems, such as anxiety, depression, delirium, suicidality and desire for death, death anxiety, and anticipatory grief (Passik et al., 1998; Holland, 2003; Rhondali et al., 2012). Where possible, they should be familiar with anxiolytic and antidepressant pharmacotherapy and they should work closely with mental health clinicians to help address these issues.

Ensuring a care continuum

Abandonment and discontinuity of care are a cause of great distress to cancer patients (Back et al., 2009). As the physician typically responsible for the primary care of the major medical problems faced by the patient, the oncologist should ensure that the patient has an ongoing and adequate care plan, particularly as the role for anti-tumour therapies diminishes and the patient approaches the end of life.

Interdisciplinary cancer care

The needs of patients with advanced cancer are too complex to be cared for by any one person. In the setting of advanced cancer, the oncologist must work with an interdisciplinary team to build a care plan around the individual needs of the patient and family (Borneman et al., 2008; Viola et al., 2009). In addition to other oncological and medical subspecialists, interdisciplinary cancer care often will involve collaboration with social workers, mental health professionals, chaplains, physical therapists, occupational therapists, speech therapists, palliative care clinicians, and others.

Palliative care research

Quality of life research has had important impact on the evaluation of oncological interventions and the quality of life is a now widely accepted clinical outcome worthy of evaluation (Minasian

---

Box 12.1.3 Complications of cancer

Neurological
- Tumour infiltration:
  - peripheral nerve
  - cranial nerve
  - nerve plexus
  - spinal cord
  - leptomeninges
  - brain
- Paraneoplastic.

Pulmonary
- Airway obstruction
- Pleural effusion
- Superior vena cava compression
- Diffuse pulmonary metastases
- Haemoptysis.

Musculoskeletal
- Bone pain
- Pathological fractures.

Gastrointestinal
- Obstruction:
  - oropharyngeal
  - oesophageal
  - gastric outlet
  - small bowel
  - large bowel
  - pancreatic duct
- Bleeding
- Ascites.

Hepatobiliary
- Obstruction
- Infiltration

Genitourinary
- Obstruction:
  - ureteric
  - bladder outlet
- Bleeding.

Metabolic
- Hypercalcaemia
- Hyponatraemia
- Cachexia
- Anasarca.

Vascular
- Obstruction:
  - venous
  - lymphatic
- Thrombosis
- Ischaemia
- Haemorrhage.

> **Box 12.1.4** Common ethical issues in the care of patients with advanced cancer
>
> ◆ Ethical issues related to disclosure of diagnosis and prognosis
> ◆ Ethical issues in decision-making: paternalism, autonomy, informed consent
> ◆ Ethical issues relating conflicts of interest
> ◆ Ethical issues when patients refuse or demand treatment
> ◆ The right to adequate relief of physical and psychological symptoms and its implications
> ◆ Consent: informed, uninformed
> ◆ Ethical issues at the end of life:
>   • sedation for refractory symptoms
>   • hydration and nutrition at the end of life
>   • Do not resuscitate orders
>   • use of invasive palliative approaches, that is, nephrostomy or dialysis.
>   • foregoing treatment
>   • euthanasia, assisted suicide.

et al., 2007). Oncologists should be familiar with some of the methodologies involved in the measurement of pain (Caraceni et al., 2002) and other physical and psychological symptoms, such as dyspnoea (Bausewein et al., 2007), fatigue (Stein et al., 2004; Wu et al., 2006), nausea and vomiting (Aaronson et al., 1993), depression and anxiety (Moorey et al., 1991; Maher et al., 1996; Fossa and Dahl, 2002), and desire for death (Chochinov et al., 1995). Though most oncologists will not conduct palliative care research, appreciation for the strategies used to study quality of life and its component domains is important, even if only to assist in judging the level of evidence for the interventions that may be applied to address sources of distress.

Ensuring sound ethical practice

Patients with advanced and incurable illness are in a vulnerable position and there are multiple ethical issues that arise in their care. Medical oncologists must be familiar with common ethical problems that arise (Box 12.1.4) and the ethical principles that assist in their resolution.

Transitioning oncology patients to palliative care

In the setting of far advanced and increasingly refractory cancer, one of the most challenging aspects of the oncologists role is to help patients and their families deal with the transitioning to care that is increasingly focused on palliation rather than disease modification (Schofield et al., 2006). Talking to patients and families about dying and palliative care is not easy, especially when patients and/or families want to continue aggressive therapy (Neff et al., 2003; Matsuyama et al., 2006; Otani et al., 2011). This transition to increasingly palliative care is a stressful experience; for many patients it implies impending death and it often triggers fears of

helplessness and abandonment by the medical profession. One can diminish the trauma of this process by gradually introducing palliative care as a legitimate and important focus of care at an earlier stage of the disease trajectory alongside efforts to modify the natural history of the disease This approach recognizes that with disease progression, treatment goals will evolve from seeking a cure, to control of disease and complications, maintaining physical functioning and quality of life, and ultimately to symptom control.

When to raise the issue

In general, it is preferable to introduce the concept of palliative care as care focused on optimizing the quality of life and introducing access to a multidisciplinary team early after the diagnosis of advanced cancer (Morita et al., 2004). This approach is widely supported by data derived from patients and their family members (Hagerty et al., 2004, 2005). Discussion of this kind need to include a review of the information needs and desires of the patient.

The setting

Sensitive discussions of this kind should be carried out in a supportive private environment and patients should be encouraged to invite their significant others to be present. Where possible the place should be a quiet, comfortable, and private location, and adequate uninterrupted time should be available for questions and discussion, and the patients should be encouraged to invite their significant others to be present (Butow et al., 1996; Ptacek and Eberhardt, 1996).

Assess patients' information needs

As a starting point it is important to evaluate the patient's understanding of his/her illness and their understanding of the goals of the treatments that they have undergone until this point. Open-ended questions can be used to evaluate how the patient is coping physically and emotionally and regarding major concerns. Patients' information needs vary greatly and one wants to find the balance between delivering information necessary for understanding and decision-making and an 'assault of truth' whereby patients are given more information than they want or desire (Clayton et al., 2005c).

Several studies have shown that a small proportion of people do not want a lot of information (Sapir et al., 2000; Hagerty et al., 2004; Clayton et al., 2005c). A survey of 126 metastatic cancer patients (Hagerty et al., 2004) found that 33% wanted to discuss 'dying and palliative care services' when first told cancer had spread; 19% said in the next few consultations; 33% said later, upon (their) request; 11% said never; and 10% were unsure. Almost half wanted the oncologist to initiate the discussion, 20% wanted the oncologist to check first if the patient wanted to know, and 24% wanted the oncologist to address the issue only if the patient asked. For some patients, there will be a 'necessary collusion' in which these issues will not be addressed forthrightly, but rather with the passage of time and evolution of the disease (Groopman, 2005; Helft, 2005).

Talking about prognosis

In these dialogues it is common for patients to ask questions about prognosis. The motivation underlying queries about prognosis are not always clear. Whereas many patients want information about their anticipated future so they can plan accordingly, others are seeking reassurance that things are not so serious or hopeless. It is important to try to understand the patient's motive in seeking this information.

In discussing prognosis, clinicians often describe median survival data or 5-year survival data. Median survival information can be particularly misleading as it is a point descriptor that does not describe interindividual variability, which may be great. Similarly, 5-year survival data may not give adequate information about true anticipated likelihood of survival. If, indeed, prognostic information is required, the following principles are useful (The Michigan Physician Guide to End-of-Life Care, 2001; Clayton et al., 2005a):

1. *Be honest.* If you don't know, say so. It may be useful to describe a worst case and a best case scenario.

2. *Use averages.* 'One third of people will still be doing well a year from now and half will live about 6 months. However, you are unique and I don't know exactly what course this disease will take.'

3. *Emphasize the limits of predictions.* 'No one can really be sure what this will mean for you as an individual. We can't predict surprises and it is prudent to make plans both for the best, but also to cover options if things don't go well.'

4. *Commit to non-abandonment.* Reassure the patient you will continue to care for him or her, whatever happens.

5. *Caution patients and their families that unexpected events can happen.* Suggest that it is worth while to get their affairs in order so they won't be totally unprepared if something unexpected does happen. 'Let's hope and work for the best but, at the same time, prepare for things in case the situation does not go as well as what we hope for.'

6. *Avoid nihilism.* Never tell a patient 'There's nothing more that can be done' or ' Do you want everything done?' There is ALWAYS something to be done. Though chemotherapy may have a higher likelihood of harm than help, there is still much that must be done to help the life yet to be lived. Discuss what can be done to make it better (and what might make it worse).

7. *Initiate end of life planning.* Sensitively bring up the important subject of advance care planning

Adapted with permission of The Michigan Physician Guide to End-of-Life Care, *Michigan, USA, Copyright © 2001, available from <http://www.michigan.gov/documents/mdch/EOL__ COMPLETE_317766_7.pdf>*

Discussing anti-tumour therapies when cure is not possible

It is intrinsically difficult to tell a patient and their family that there is no treatment that offers the possibility of cure (Otani et al., 2011). Despite progress in non-curative anti-tumour therapies in some conditions, in many diseases the potential benefit of therapy is small and when benefit is derived, it is often of short duration. Many patients in this setting undertake sometimes burdensome treatments based on exaggerated expectations of potential treatment benefits (Weeks et al., 1998). In counselling such patients it is important to outline treatment options including those that do not involve potentially burdensome anti-tumour treatments. As well as presenting potential benefits

of anti-tumour therapies, it is appropriate to discuss the likelihood of help and of harm.

Situations in which cure is not possible are heterogeneous. In some instances, such as metastatic breast, colorectal cancer, ovarian or small cell lung cancer, there may be a moderate to high likelihood of prolonging survival. In other situations, such as gastric or pancreatic cancer and most of the soft tissue sarcomas, substantial survival prolongation is less likely. In the latter situations informed consent requires that patients understand the limited likelihood of benefit and patients should almost always be offered the options of palliation without chemotherapy or the option of participating in an experimental therapy (if one is available).

These recommendations are supported by the findings of a study of the recordings of the initial oncological consultations of 118 cancer patients with incurable disease. Analysis of these consultations found that whereas 84.7% of patients were informed about the aim of anti-cancer treatment, that their disease was incurable (85%) and about life expectancy (58%), only a minority of consultations included discussion of an alternative to anti-cancer treatments (44%), discussion on the impact of anti-cancer treatment on quality of life (36%), or an offer of management choice (30%) (Gattellari et al., 2002). In only 10% of consultations did the oncologist check the patient's understanding.

Introducing palliative care options

After indicating that further curative treatment has a low chance of being effective and that the aims of the treatment are disease control and optimizing quality of life, the clinician should introduce the option of effective palliative treatment options to help improve the quality of life. For patients wishing to continue disease-modifying treatments, it needs to be explained that this is not an 'either/or' choice, but rather a situation in which the best care will incorporate a balanced approach between the two parallel strategies.

Maintaining hope

Being told that a cancer cannot be cured is devastating for most people and in this setting patients believe it is crucial that doctors help them find some way of maintaining hope as well as giving them honest information about their disease (Clayton et al., 2005b). Indeed, many patients and their families are avoidant of discussions about prognosis or curability for fear that the discussion may undermine or destroy hope.

Hope has been defined as an expectation that there will be a positive outcome in the future (Nunn, 1996). Commonly, however, it is associated with unrealistic expectations. Magical thinking and hope for miracles are a transcultural phenomenon and, in the context of a poor prognosis, it is not necessarily inappropriate for a patient to hope for a cure even if it is highly unlikely, but messages of hope from health professionals should focus on more realistic events, such as long periods of remission, response to treatments and excellent symptom control. Strategies that successfully promote appropriate hope may make a critical contribution to discussing the transition from curative to palliative care.

Deliberately fostering false hope of a cure, when a cure is not possible, may hinder patients and their family from making appropriate treatment and lifestyle decisions in order to make the best use of their remaining time together. Hence, it is critical that the messages of hope provided to patients are appropriate.

In a survey of 156 patients with advanced and incurable illness (Hagerty et al., 2005), doctor behaviours that augmented hope included offering the most up-to-date treatment (90%), appearing to know all there is to know about the patient's cancer (87%), and saying that pain will be controlled (87%). The majority of patients indicated that the doctor appearing to be nervous or uncomfortable (91%), giving the prognosis to the family first (87%), or using euphemisms (82%) would not facilitate hope.

Qualitative data derived from interviews with patients and their caregivers (Clayton et al., 2005b) revealed several hope enhancing themes: (1) emphasize what can be done (particularly control of physical symptoms, emotional support, care and dignity, and practical support), (2) explore realistic goals, and (3) discuss issues related to day-to-day living. Dr Joanne Lynne suggests making seven commitments to patients (Lynn, 2000):

1. You will have the best of medical treatment, aiming to prevent exacerbation, improve function and survival, and ensure comfort.

2. You will never have to endure overwhelming pain, shortness of breath, or other symptoms. Symptoms will be anticipated and prevented when possible, evaluated and addressed promptly, and controlled effectively. Severe symptoms—such as shortness of breath—will be treated as emergencies. Sedation will be used when necessary to relieve intractable symptoms near the end of life.

3. Your care will be continuous, comprehensive, and coordinated. You and your family can count on having certain professionals to rely upon at all times and on an appropriate and timely response to your needs. The transitions between services, settings, and personnel will be minimized in number and made to work smoothly.

4. You and your family will be prepared for everything that is likely to happen in the course of your illness. If necessary you will receive supplies and training needed to handle predictable events.

5. Your wishes will be sought and respected, and followed whenever possible. You will be given information about the available choices and you will be encouraged to be an active participant in decision making. You will have the right to refuse treatments.

6. We will help you and your family consider your personal and financial resources, and we will respect your choices about the use of your resources.

7. We will do all we can to see that you and your family will have the opportunity to make the best of every day. We are committed to treat you as a person, not a disease. What is important to you is important to us as part of the care team. We will endeavor to respond to your physical, psychological, social, and spiritual needs as well as those of your family. Indeed we will be there to support your family throughout this period and after your death.

Adapted with permission from The National Coalition on Health Care and The Institute for Healthcare Improvement, Promises to keep: Changing the way we provide care at the end of life, Accelerating Change Today (A.C.T.), Cambridge, Massachusetts: Institute for Healthcare Improvement, Copyright © 2000, available at <http://www.IHI.org>.

Logistical considerations in provision of oncological palliative care

Oncology, hospice, and palliative medicine—the division of labour

The integration of oncological care and palliative care requires familiarity with a range of therapeutic options, appropriate patient evaluation, and a collaborative therapeutic relationship with the patient and other members of an interdisciplinary care team. Care planning and goal setting may be facilitated by considering the natural history of cancer in five phases (Box 12.1.5). The changing status of the patient along this continuum influences the coordination and implementation of palliative interventions.

The medical oncologist is almost always the coordinating health-care provider during the first three phases: the diagnostic work-up, attempts at curative therapy, and the phase of ambulatory palliative care, during which the patient continues to attend the cancer clinic. During the latter phase, community-based nursing and medical providers are often introduced to provide additional services outside of the health-care institution and in anticipation of diminished mobility. A large majority of cancer patients live at home during most of the course of the illness. Programmes to extend palliative care services into the home are widely available. Oncologists should familiarize themselves about the existing programmes, refer patients appropriately, and provide continuity of care. In the United States, home-based end-of-life care often is provided by a certified hospice programme. In the US version of hospice, the oncologist can choose to remain the physician of record throughout the period of end-of-life care, or can become a consultant (Schonwetter, 1996).

During the fourth phase, when the patient has advanced illness and may not be ambulatory, and during the fifth, end-of-life care, new decisions often are required about the site of care and level of help required by the patient and family. Patients may be treated at home, in a nursing home, in an inpatient palliative care facility such as a hospice residence, or if indicated, an acute care hospital. Decisions regarding the site of care are influenced by the nature and severity of the prevailing clinical problems, the extent of home-based medical and nursing resources, the availability of community facilities, the goals of care, and patient preference (Hinton, 1994a, 1994b).

The role of the oncologist during these latter phases is determined by similar considerations. In some instances, the oncologist will remain the primary provider of palliative care until the patient dies. In other instances, there should be a smooth transition of care as other services play a progressively greater role and the oncologist becomes a supportive figure. By maintaining

Box 12.1.5 Five phase in the natural history of cancer
1. Diagnostic: ambulatory or inpatient
2. Curative primary therapy
3. Ambulatory palliative therapy
4. Sedentary palliative therapy- interactional
5. Sedentary palliative therapy- non-interactional.

continuity in care, the oncologist can ensure that cancer-related issues are adequately addressed and also can limit concerns about abandonment that can magnify patient and family distress (Quill and Cassel, 1995).

Models of care

There is no one best way for oncologists and specialist palliative care services to work together. Rather a number of different models have been developed (Greer et al., 2013):

Sequential care model

In this model the patients is cared for by the oncology service as long as there is potential benefit in disease-modifying treatment. When it is clear that there is no further benefit to be derived from this treatment, the responsibility for the patient's ongoing care is transferred to the palliative care service. Of course, the palliative care service may be consulted earlier, when the patient is under primary oncological management, and similarly, should anti-tumour interventions be required (such as palliative radiotherapy) when the patient is being followed primarily by the palliative care services, expert oncological consultation is available. In this model of care, end-of-life care is coordinated by the palliative care service.

The advantages of this model of care are that it is characterized by clear delineation of responsibility. It enables the oncologist to focus on the dominant aspects of his professional tasks and allows him to fulfil his obligations to provide palliative care and continuity of care by a process of benevolent transfer of primary responsibility to a palliative care team. Successful implementation if this model requires close cooperation between the oncology and palliative care services, good communication to minimize patient feelings of abandonment, and timely referral of patients.

Oncologist-based palliative care

In this model, the oncologist assumes the role of coordinating care and providing both anti-cancer and palliative care services, thus seeing the patient through from diagnosis until death (Cherny, 2003). This approach emphasizes the importance of the oncologist/patient relationship and the notions of continuity of care and non-abandonment. Oncologists undertaking this approach need to be highly skilled in palliative care and in interdisciplinary care, including interaction with a palliative care support team. Even oncologists who are highly skilled in palliative care may sometimes benefit from expert input and this should be sought when difficult problems arise.

The major advantage of this approach is its emphasis on continuity of care. The success of this model is dependent on the level of palliative care skills and sophistication of the oncologist, and his/her ability to balance competing intellectual and practical interests. This approach is augmented by having a strong relationship with a care team, including a palliative medicine expert for backup in difficult cases.

Concurrent model

In this model, patients with advanced cancer are jointly cared for by both oncology and palliative medicine specialists in a similar way that medical, surgical, and radiation oncologists traditionally work together (Meyers et al., 2004). The relative role of the oncology or palliative medicine physician is determined by the

prevailing problems and, indeed, case management responsibilities may be handled by either and are usually determined by the circumstances of the patient.

This model emphasizes the duality of advanced cancer care and the need for continuity of care, both with regard to disease modification and palliative care. Successful implementation of this approach requires close cooperation and open communication between oncology and palliative medicine clinicians. This approach is strongly supported by data demonstrating improved patient outcomes (Jordhoy et al., 2001; Brumley et al., 2007; Gade et al., 2008; Bakitas et al., 2009; Temel et al., 2010; Zimmermann et al., 2012).

Palliative care delivery in major cancer centres

A survey of 142 cancer centres in the United States found that the overwhelming proportion of centres had palliative care services, but in many cases these services were very limited in their scope (Hui et al., 2010). Although this penetration is also seen in Canada, the United Kingdom, and Australia, integration of palliative care and oncology is the exception rather than the rule in many other parts of the world.

Beyond minimal requirements (Box 12.1.6), ESMO has developed an incentive programme to recognize centres that demonstrate a high level of integration between medical oncology and palliative care (Cherny et al., 2010). To be eligible for accreditation as a 'designated centre' 13 criteria must be met (Box 12.1.7). These criteria set a gold standard for integration. As of 2014, 174 centres across Europe, North America, Asia, and the Middle East have been accredited with achieving this level of care. Processes for the development of integrated services in major cancer centres have been described (Bruera and Sweeney, 2001; Walsh, 2001; Hydeman, 2013; Marchetti et al., 2013).

Box 12.1.6 Proposed minimal requirements for palliative care in cancer centres

1. Cancer patients receiving active therapy in cancer centres, especially those with advanced cancer, should be routinely assessed regarding the presence and severity of physical and psychological symptoms and the adequacy of social supports.

2. When inadequately controlled symptoms are identified they must be evaluated and treated with the appropriate urgency (depending on the nature and severity of the problem).

3. Cancer centres must provide skilled emergency care of inadequately relieved physical and psychological symptoms.

4. Cancer centres must ensure an ongoing programme of palliative and supportive care for patients with advanced cancer who are no longer benefited by anti-tumour interventions.

5. Cancer centres should incorporate social work and psychological care as part of routine care.

6. When patients require inpatient end of life care, the cancer centre staff either provide the needed inpatient care or arrange adequate care in an appropriate hospice or palliative care service.

Box 12.1.7 Criteria for optimal supportive and palliative care in a cancer centre

1. The centre provides closely integrated oncology and palliative care clinical services.
2. The centre is committed to a philosophy of continuity of care and non-abandonment.
3. The centre provides high-level home care with expert back-up and coordination of home care with primary cancer clinicians.
4. The centre incorporates programmatic support of family members.
5. The centre provides routine patient assessment of physical and psychological symptoms and social supports and has an infrastructure that responds with appropriate interventions in a timely manner.
6. The centre incorporates expert medical and nursing care in the evaluation and relief of pain and other physical symptoms.
7. The centre incorporates expert care in the evaluation and relief of psychological and existential distress.
8. The centre provides emergency care of inadequately relieved physical and psychological symptoms.
9. The centre provides facilities and expert care for inpatient symptom stabilization.
10. The centre provides respite care for ambulatory patients for patients unable to cope at home or in cases of family fatigue.
11. The centre provides facilities and expert care for inpatient end-of-life care and is committed to providing adequate relief of suffering for dying patients.
12. The centre participates in basic or clinical research related to the quality of life of cancer patients.
13. The centre is involved in clinician education to improve the integration of oncology and palliative care.

The development of palliative care services requires appropriate resource allocation for staffing, physical space, and necessary supports. Thought should be given to the development of processes such as joint meetings to facilitate good integration between oncology and palliative care services. Tumour boards for patients with advanced cancer, radiology conferences, and interdisciplinary psychosocial conferences to discuss challenging cases, afford excellent opportunities to forge collaborative working relationships and balanced discussion.

Where oncological palliative care is delivered in the cancer centre

Since most patients with advanced cancer receive a trial of therapy in an ambulatory office-based setting or radiotherapy centre, the incorporation of onsite palliative care assessment and intervention programmes provides an excellent opportunity to assess the need for palliative interventions, and to address physical or psychosocial needs.

With the changing patterns of oncological care delivery, oncology inpatient wards increasingly are occupied by patients needing symptom control or terminal care (Salminen et al., 2008) and the administration of palliative care has become a major part of inpatient oncology care (Ferris et al., 2009).

In some inpatient and outpatient settings, palliative care consultation services can help deliver specialist palliative care in a manner similar to other consultation services. When a patient is admitted to the hospital, this service can assist oncologists by providing expert back-up in the management of difficult cases. Back-up of this type may take the form of advice, direct participation in management, or sometimes in the transfer of case management. Palliative care consultations can have major impact on physician education and practice among oncologists (Hanson et al., 2008; Weissman et al., 2008; Zhukovsky et al., 2009).

Dedicated acute inpatient palliative care units, if available, can provide a high level of expertise in palliative interventions, such as symptom control, and comprehensive end-of-life care (Mercadante et al., 2008; Albanese et al., 2013; Eti et al., 2014). Oncologists can admit patients to acute palliative care units in hospitals for symptom evaluation and management, respite, management of treatment complications, or terminal care.

Barriers to coordination between oncology and palliative care

Different cultures of care

It has been pointed out that palliative care and oncology have substantially different histories and cultures of care (McKenzie, 1998). These differences may account for some of the difficulties sometimes encountered in integration of these approaches. Whereas palliative care grew out of the hospice movement, which tends to the physical and emotional needs of patients and their families rather than focusing on the diseases themselves, modern oncology has developed out of the specialist biomedical model with a strong emphasis on addressing the disease processes with view to cure patients or to prolong their lives. Whereas interdisciplinary care is inherent to palliative care, in oncology despite the growing prevalence of multidiscipline clinics and tumour boards, the concept of the 'patient care team' has not yet been universally adopted. Indeed, the ESMO survey of oncologist practice in the management of incurable cancer patients indicates that it is relatively underdeveloped and uncommon (Cherny and Catane, 2003).

Delays in referral for palliative care consultations

Very often the timing of referrals to specialized palliative care services, including palliative care units, inpatient hospices, and home-based palliative care programmes, is very delayed until patients have a very severe symptom burden or, often, until patients are close to death (Cheng et al., 2005; Ferrell, 2005; Morita et al., 2005). In a survey of bereaved family members of cancer patients (Morita et al., 2005), half of the respondents regarded the timing of referrals as late or very late, and indeed the median admission period was less than 1 month (22 days), and approximately 20% of the patients died within 1 week. The reasons for this are complex: persistent beliefs that palliative care has an alternative philosophy of care incompatible with cancer therapy, beliefs that providing palliative care is the oncologist's role, lack of knowledge about locally available services, oncologist and patient reluctance to address issues implying incurability, optimism that third- or fourth-line salvage treatments will prolong survival or improve quality of life, fears that a palliative care referral will undermine hope or shortens the patient's life, and insufficient in-advance discussion about preferred end-of-life care with physicians (Morita et al., 2005; Schenker et al., 2014). Oncologists sometimes express reluctance about palliative care referrals for fear that anti-tumour treatment strategies will be challenged (often by palliative care clinicians with limited familiarity with oncological care strategies) or that the patient will be 'stolen' (Cherny and Catane, 2003; Ferrell, 2005; Schenker et al., 2014; Von Roenn et al., 2013).

Another reason for delayed referral is the oncologist's failure to recognize the deterioration in the patient's clinical course. There are data to suggest that oncologists are commonly overoptimistic and overestimate survival substantially (Christakis and Lamont, 2000). Indeed, a meta-analysis of the 13 available studies showed that cancer physicians tended to overestimate prognosis by at least 30% (Glare et al., 2003). To add to this, when patients request information about prognosis, many physicians consciously overstate the prognosis even beyond their own (inflated) estimate (Lamont and Christakis, 2001).

Abandonment

Unfortunately, when a patient's disease reaches an advanced stage, a point at which symptom management becomes more necessary, some oncologists relinquish their role in the care of the patient because radiotherapy and chemotherapy have nothing more to contribute (Dias et al., 2003). Sadly, it is not uncommon to hear patients relate that the oncologist said that 'there is nothing further can be done'. In many cases, not only is there no continuity of care, but in many cases, palliative care options are not presented. For some patients, situations of this ilk undermine hope and the desire to live (Kissane et al., 1998).

Territoriality

There is anecdotal evidence that professionals in various disciplines looking after patients with cancer may never meet one another, and oncologists, family physicians, and palliative care specialists often do not appreciate the challenges other physicians face (McKenzie, 1995, 1998). The survey of European oncologists revealed that many oncologists believe that palliative care colleagues do not understand cancer care at a level sufficient to render informed advice, and a small proportion of oncologists feel that palliative care physicians will 'steal' patients (Cherny and Catane, 2003).

Palliative care education for oncologists

Current shortcomings in oncologist education

In 1998, the ASCO performed a large-scale survey of US oncologists about their experiences in providing palliative care (Emanuel et al., 2000; Hilden et al., 2001). The survey questionnaire consisted of 118 questions. A total of 3227 oncologists responded. There were no significant differences between the percentages of medical, radiation, surgical, or paediatric oncologists who responded as a proportion of their representation in ASCO. In this survey, the most frequent sources of palliative care education were trial and error during clinical practice (90%), from colleagues during clinical practice (73%), from a role model during oncology fellowship

training (71%), and from a traumatic experience with a patient. The ASCO survey found that the oncologists did not obtain adequate information from their colleagues and role models, despite reporting these people as the most frequent educational resource: 81% said they had inadequate mentoring or coaching in how to discuss poor prognosis, 65% said they received inadequate information about controlling symptoms, and less than 10% thought all of their formal training during medical school, internships, residency, and fellowship combined was 'very helpful'.

In a 2004 survey, ASCO trainees rated end-of-life education less highly than their general fellowship training. They viewed their attendings as more expert in non-end-of-life care than in terminal care. Of those who had performed bone marrow biopsy, feedback on this technique was more likely to have occurred than feedback on an end-of-life discussion (73% vs 56%; p = 0.0006). Regarding pain management, 94% of fellows felt prepared to manage pain in the dying, 75% assessed pain in their patient who died most recently, 41% were explicitly taught when to rotate opioids, and only 30% performed an opioid conversion correctly (Buss et al., 2007).

In a survey of ESMO members regarding their involvement in palliative care, 42% of respondents reported that they had not received adequate training in palliative care during their residency. This finding is consistent with previously published data regarding the training of medical oncologists in the management of cancer pain (Larue et al., 1995; Gerrard et al., 1999; Sapir et al., 1999), communication skills (Baile et al., 1997; Fallowfield and Jenkins, 1999), and palliative care (Gerrard et al., 1999; Gilewski, 2001). In response to the statement 'most medical oncologists I know *are* expert in the management of the physical and psychological symptoms of advanced cancer', more respondents disagreed (41.8%) than agreed (37.5%). This finding suggests that most oncologists have a low assessment of their colleagues' readiness to manage the physical and psychological symptoms of advanced cancer, a perception that is consonant with the findings regarding training.

Curricular requirements of ASCO and ESMO

There is universal recognition for the need to provide training in palliative care for all oncologists. This has been incorporated into the 'Global Core Curriculum in Medical Oncology' that was developed and endorsed by ASCO and ESMO (Hansen et al., 2004) and in the ESMO document describing the core elements of oncology training in palliative and supportive care (Cherny et al., 2003).

In 2010, the ESMO palliative care working group and the ASCO task force on palliative care made a joint submission for the revision of the palliative care content of the Global Core Curriculum in Medical Oncology. These recommendations are presented in Box 12.1.8. These recommendations distinguish between three levels of desired proficiency:

1. *Expert*: refers to a high level of academic and practical knowledge. At the completion of training, oncology graduates should be expert in the oncological management of advanced cancer, the management of complications of cancer and the evaluation and management of physical symptoms of cancer and cancer treatment.

2. *Skilled*: refers to effective clinical competence. This level of proficiency is required for communication with patients and family members.

Box 12.1.8 Proposal for the core curriculum submitted jointly from Professor Nathan I. Cherny on behalf of the ESMO PCWG and Professor Jamie Von Roenn, Chair of the ASCO Task Force on Pain and Symptom Management

The palliative care role of the oncologist

It is the oncologist's responsibility to care for their patient along a continuum that starts at the moment of diagnosis and extends throughout the course of the illness. In addition to appropriate anti-cancer treatment, this includes symptom control, psychosocial support and the coordination of services to provide continuity of care and family support during all phases of care, including the last phase of life.

Interdisciplinary care

Trainees should be aware that the management of patients with advanced cancer will usually require close cooperation with clinicians of other disciplines including nurses, social workers, anaesthesiologists, palliative care clinicians, psychologists, psychiatrists, chaplains, rehabilitation, physical therapy, occupational therapy, speech therapy and dietitians.

Trainees should be skilled at interdisciplinary care planning and coordination. They must be familiar with the roles of clinicians from other disciplines and indications for referral of requests for assistance.

The oncological management of advanced care

Medical oncologists must be expert in the appropriate selection and use of anti-tumour therapies as palliative techniques when cure is no longer possible. They should be familiar with key concepts of patient benefit, quality of life and risk/benefit analysis.

Pain

Trainees must be expert in the assessment and management of cancer pain.

1. Pain assessment: trainees should be skilled in the comprehensive assessment of pain from cancer and its treatment. They should have an understanding of the use of pain scales. They should understand the mechanisms and pathophysiology of cancer pain syndromes, understand the concept of 'total pain,' and be familiar with the clinical features of the full range of cancer pain syndromes and the diagnostic approaches to identify them.

2. Pharmacotherapy: trainees should have an understanding of the pharmacology and toxicity of non-opioid and opioid medications commonly used in the management of cancer pain. They should be experienced in the initiation of analgesic therapy, monitoring patients for adequacy of pain relief and titration of analgesics. They must be skilled in the evaluation and management of opioid adverse effects such as constipation, nausea and vomiting, drowsiness, confusion and myoclonus. Trainees should be familiar with the use of adjuvant analgesics for the management of neuropathic, visceral and bone pain. They must be familiar with approaches to the management of breakthrough pain

3. Primary therapies: trainees must be familiar with the role of primary anti-cancer treatments for the relief of pain, including the roles of radiotherapy and surgery. Specific examples include the role of radiotherapy and/or surgery in the setting of spinal cord compression and impending fractures.

4. Difficult pain syndromes: Trainees must be familiar with the range of options available to patients with difficult or refractory pain syndromes including the indications for experts consultations with a pain or palliative medicine specialist, invasive or neuroablative procedures and sedation as an option of last resort for dying patients with refractory pain.

Symptom evaluation and management

Trainees should be familiar with the use of scales to evaluate common physical symptoms in patients with cancer. The trainees should be expert in the evaluation and management of common symptoms including dyspnea, nausea and vomiting, constipation, diarrhea and cancer related fatigue.

1. Dyspnea: trainees should be familiar with the differential diagnosis of dyspnea in the patient with advanced cancer. Trainees should be able to identify potentially remediable causes and be familiar with specific treatment modalities. Trainees should be familiar with the use of opioids for the management of symptomatic dyspnea.

2. Nausea and vomiting: trainees should be familiar with the differential diagnosis of nausea and vomiting in the setting of advanced cancer and be able to identify potentially remediable causes. Trainees should have an understanding of the mechanism of action of antiemetics and their appropriate use for symptom control.

3. Constipation: trainees should be familiar with the factors that contribute to constipation in patients with advanced cancer. Trainees should be able to distinguish constipation from bowel obstruction. Trainees should be familiar with approaches to prevent constipation, provide supportive counseling and prescribe rational pharmacotherapy for the treatment of constipation.

4. Cancer-related fatigue: trainees should be familiar with the factors that contribute to fatigue in patients with advanced cancer and the expected occurrence and duration of treatment-related fatigue. Trainees should be able to identify potentially remediable causes and recommend appropriate pharmacologic and supportive approaches for fatigue.

Box 12.1.8 Continued

5. Diarrhea: trainees should be familiar with the differential diagnosis of diarrhea in patients with advanced cancer. Trainees should be able to identify potentially remediable causes and identify patients at high risk for obstruction. Trainees should be familiar with treatment strategies for the various causes of diarrhea in patients with advanced cancer. In particular, trainees should be familiar with treatment strategies for chemotherapy- and radiation therapy-induced diarrhea and neutropenic enterocolitis.

6. Delirium: trainees should be familiar with the differential diagnosis of delirium in patients with advanced cancer. Trainees should be able to identify its medical causes. Trainees should be familiar with treatment strategies for the various causes of delirium in patients with advanced cancer and with the symptomatic management of delirium with antipsychotic medications.

7. Anorexia/cachexia and starvation: trainees should be able to differentiate between starvation and cancer cachexia. They should be familiar with the pathophysiology of cancer cachexia with the phases or early cachexia, cancer cachexia and refractory late cachexia. They should be able to formulate rational therapeutic plans for patients with starvation syndromes and cancer cachexia, recognizing the potential benefits, limitations of benefit and risks of the various treatment options.

Management of the complications of cancer

Trainees must be expert in the evaluation and management of the complications of cancer including:

1. Bone metastases: indications for radiotherapy and surgery, the role of biological treatments, radiopharmaceuticals and the use of bisphosphonates.

2. *CNS metastases, brain and leptomeningeal metastases: indications for steroids, surgery, radiotherapy, and shunts. Use and limitations of intrathecal or systemic chemotherapy.*

3. Neurological dysfunction: primary, metastatic, paraneoplastic and iatrogenic.

4. Liver metastases and biliary obstruction: management of obstruction including percutaneous and endoscopic stenting.

5. Malignant effusions pleural, peritoneal and pericardial. Trainees should be skilled at paracentesis and thoracocentesis. They should be familiar with the role of surgical approaches including percardiocentesis, pericardial window, shunts, and pleuradhesis.

6. Obstruction of hollow viscera: esophagus, airways, gastric outlet, small and large bowel, ureters. They should be familiar with medical management of bowel obstructions and the indications for surgical, radiotherapeutic and gastroenterological approaches to esophageal, bowel and ureteric obstruction.

7. Metabolic consequences of cancer: hypercalcemia, hyponatremia, renal failure.

8. Anorexia and cachexia: dietary counseling, the use of appetite stimulants, the role of enteral and parenteral feeding.

9. Hematologic consequences: anemia, neutropenia, thrombocytopenia, clotting diathesis.

10. Sexual dysfunction.

Communication

Trainees must be skilled in effective and compassionate communication with cancer patients and their families. Specific skills include:

1. Explaining diagnosis and treatment options.

2. Disclosure of diagnosis.

3. Defining goals of care.

4. Explaining issues relating to prognosis.

5. Explaining the potential risk and benefits of treatment options.

6. Counselling skills to facilitate effective, informed decision-making.

7. Explaining the role of palliative care and it relevance in all phases of the illness trajectory.

8. The care of distressed family members: fear, anticipatory grief, bereavement care.

9. Convening and leading of family meetings.

10. Discussing transitions in care; e.g., initiation of hospice, discontinuation of chemotherapy.

Palliative rehabilitation

Trainees must be aware that palliative cancer care aims to improve function as well as comfort and that rehabilitation may have an important part in optimal care, even for patients with incurable disease. Trainees should be familiar with the role of rehabilitation in patients with deficits in speech, swallowing, breathing, cognition and all forms of motor function.

Box 12.1.8 Continued

Cultural competence

Trainees should be familiar with the impact of culture on the management of patients with cancer. Trainees should be able to discuss specific cultural-based preferences with patients and their families. Trainees should appreciate the need for cultural sensitivity. Trainees should be familiar with the need for individual assessment of patient's desire for disclosure and full participation in decision-making processes.

Evaluation and management of psychological and existential symptoms of cancer

Trainees should understand the psychosocial influence of cancer. Trainees should be aware of available resources and recognize when intervention is indicated at all stages of disease. Trainees should appreciate the spiritual conflicts associated with the diagnosis and treatment of cancer. Trainees should learn to recognize adaptive and maladaptive behavior in coping with disease. Trainees should recognize acceptable coping mechanisms by patients and families within the context of the cancer diagnosis.

Trainees should be familiar with the indication and uses of psychotropic drugs.

Trainees should have knowledge of the bereavement process.

Trainees should have an appreciation of the physician's personal coping.

Trainees must be familiar with the evaluation and management of the common psychological and existential symptoms of cancer including:

1. Distress

2. Anxiety

3. Depression

4. Demoralization

5. Loss of dignity

6. Delirium

7. Suicidality, desire for death and requests for euthanasia or assisted suicide

8. Death anxiety

9. Anticipatory grief

10. Uncertainty

Self-care

1. Trainees should recognize the factors that contribute to burnout and compassion fatigue.

2. Trainees should be able to differentiate depression from burnout.

3. Trainees should develop a plan for self-care that includes recognizing and monitoring for symptoms of burnout, addressing symptoms if they occur, maintaining work-life balance and seek consultation if the symptoms are progressive or severe.

End-of-life care

1. Advanced care planning: Trainees should be equipped to discuss advanced care planning with patients with advanced and incurable illnesses and their family members.

2. Communication: Trainees should be skilled in the effective and empathic communication of impending death with patients and their family members. Trainees should be able to discuss discontinuation of antineoplastic therapies, transitions in care, the anticipated clinical course, signs and symptoms of imminent death and the strategy to ensure optimal patient comfort as well as family support

3. End-of-life care planning: Trainees should be aware that it is the responsibility to ensure that care planning is undertaken interpersonally, or by another member of the interdisciplinary team. They should be aware of options for end-of-life care including home-based care, inpatient care and hospice care and should be able to help negotiate care preferences with the patient and their family.

4. Non-abandonment: Trainees should be aware that many patients and families are concerned that their oncologist will abandon them at the end of life and should be aware of the need to maintain availability and support.

5. Symptom management: Trainees must be familiar and skilled in the management of common symptoms at the end of life including pain, dyspnea, delirium, death rattle, and anguish. Trainees must be familiar with the identification of refractory symptoms and indications for, and use of sedation in the management of refractory symptoms at the end of life.

Box 12.1.8 Continued

Ethical issues in the management of patients with cancer

Trainees must be familiar with common ethical problems that arise in the management of advanced cancer and ethical principles that assist in their resolution. They should be familiar with:

1. Ethical issues related to disclosure of diagnosis and prognosis.

2. Ethical issues in relation to decision-making: autonomy, relational autonomy, indications for paternalism, assessment for decision-making capacity, surrogate decision-making, principles of shared decision-making

3. The right to adequate relief of physical and psychological symptoms and its implications.

4. Consent: informed, uninformed.

5. Ethical issues at the end of life: sedation for refractory symptoms, hydration and nutrition at the end of life, DNR, use of invasive palliative approaches; i.e., nephrostomy or dialysis.

6. Ethical issues related to foregoing treatment.

7. Ethical issues relating to requests for euthanasia or assisted suicide.

Palliative care research

Medical oncologist must be familiar with palliative care research methodologies that are applicable to patients with advanced cancer including:

1. Quality of life research.

2. Pain measurement and research.

3. Measurement of other physical and psychological symptoms: dyspnea, fatigue, cachexia, nausea and vomiting, depression and anxiety, and desire for death.

4. Needs evaluation.

5. Decision-making research.

6. Psychosocial research.

7. Care delivery research; particularly with reference to integrating oncology in palliative care

8. Palliative care audit.

Reproduced from *Proposal for the core curriculum*, submitted jointly from Prof. Nathan I. Cherny on behalf of the ESMO PCWG and Prof. Jamie Von Roenn, Chair of the ASCO Task Force on Pain and Symptom Management, with permission from the authors.

---

3. *Familiar*: is the lowest level of required competence. It refers to familiarity with core concepts to the level of being able to adequately evaluate the patient, initiate basic therapy, and communicate with clinical experts. At the completion of training, oncology graduates should be familiar with evaluation and management of psychological and existential symptoms of cancer, interdisciplinary care of patients with advanced cancer, palliative care research principles, ethical issues in the management of patients with cancer, and strategies to identify and prevent burnout.

Educational materials for oncologists

Remarkably, despite the frequent role as primary care provider to cancer patients with advanced illness, oncologists are not a regular target audience for educational materials on palliative care. Nonetheless, special educational materials have been developed and should be widely promoted. Among these materials are the following:

ESMO Handbook of Advanced Cancer Care: this is a small practical handbook developed and distributed by ESMO, written by oncologists and clinicians working with cancer patients, outlining major issues in palliative care as they apply to the cancer patient. It addresses a wide range of issues in decision-making, physical, and psychological management issues.

Evidence-based clinical guidelines: in the United States, both the NCCN (<http://www.nccn.org>) and the National Cancer Institute (NCI; <http://www.cancer.gov/cancertopics/pdq/supportivecare>) have developed online resources to deliver up-to-date, evidence-based guidelines for elements of palliative care. The NCI's supportive care subsection of the PDQ includes monographs covering common physical and psychological symptoms in patients with advanced cancer. The NCCN Guidelines* offer a thoughtful evidence-based approach to several aspects of supportive and palliative care for cancer patients. The guidelines on 'Palliative Care and Distress Management' are particularly commended (<http://www.nccn.org/professionals/physician_gls/f_guidelines.asp#supportive>).

EPEC-O: ASCO, in collaboration with the National Cancer Institute and EPEC (Education for Physicians in End-of-Life Care), has developed a curriculum in end-of-life care specific to oncologists. This well-developed programme aims to equip oncologists with the attitudes, knowledge, and skills to provide the best possible palliative care for their patients. The educational materials, which are available on DVD includes three plenary sessions and 32 PowerPoint presentations with background information for the instructors. The multimedia materials make excellent use of trigger films to stimulate discussion and to highlight important points.

Optimizing Cancer Care—The Importance of Symptom Management Vols I and II: these are curricular materials that have been published and marketed by ASCO. This is a well-developed (but expensive) educational resource that covers 29 supportive care topics, including effective communication, and physical and psychological symptom assessment and management. It uses an array of teaching tools—treatment scenarios, annotated slides, algorithms, and a table of medications.

Initiatives to improve oncologist understanding and involvement in palliative care

Oncology conferences: there is an encouraging trend to greater incorporation of palliative care content in major oncology meetings. Additionally, many of the international and national oncology organizations now organize conferences and workshops on palliative and supportive care issues.

Incorporation of palliative care issues in major oncological journals: journal content of the major oncological journals reflects, to some degree, professional priorities. Although all of the major oncological journals cover palliative care issues to some degree, they remain marginalized issues in most of the journals. Of the major oncology journals, the outstanding exception is the *Journal of Clinical Oncology*. In addition to publishing more than 600 reports of clinical trials in the area of palliative care and quality of life, it created a new section in 2000, which is entitled 'The Art of Oncology: When the Tumor Is Not the Target' and focuses on issues of patient–physician communication, ethical decision-making, and symptom control in the management of advanced cancer.

Working towards the future

The advancement of medical oncologist awareness, knowledge, practice, and research in palliative medicine will require an elevation of the relative priority of palliation as a goal of cancer care. This, in turn, will need to be reflected in resources allocation, programme development, and clinical practice.

Palliative medicine as an oncological subspecialty: there is a need for more oncologists with advanced training in palliative medicine. The prevalence of patients in need of this sort of specialty service suggests that each department would benefit from at least one oncologist with palliative medicine expertise. For the medical oncologist, an enhanced familiarity with palliative medicine can extend the clinician's therapeutic repertoire, diminish the stress of caring for patients who have incurable cancer, improve patient outcomes, and provide new avenues for clinical research and reward (Epstein and Morrison, 2012).

Elevating the priority of palliation: this process requires a paradigm shift at all levels of the cancer medicine infrastructure. Given the current infrastructure for career development and resource allocation for clinical and research programmes in medical oncology, initiatives such as those undertaken by ASCO and ESMO are needed to raise the priority of palliative medicine.

Development of clinical programmes: individual institutions must be encouraged to develop expert services to provide a clinical service and role models, and to conduct clinical and basic research in the palliative care of cancer patients. Services should incorporate clinical resources to address problems related to physical and psychological symptoms.

Research: palliative medicine opens a vast array of potential research questions. Symptom palliation, ethics, communication, coping needs, emotional and spiritual care, and the palliative effects of primary antineoplastic therapy are all valid research directions for oncologists. The clinical trials expertise that currently exists in the oncology community should be used to address specific symptom control problems (such as dyspnoea, nausea, and delirium) or complications of cancer (such as neoplastic plexopathies, or bowel obstruction).

The individual clinician: every oncologist can focus their attention on the palliative needs of their own patients. Practice guidelines, journals, consultants, and other resources are available to help address these issues. Physicians can remind themselves, their colleagues, and students to think about physical and psychological symptom control and patient supports at all stages of the illness and not just in the terminal phase. Oncologists can develop relationships with local hospice organizations to ensure close cooperation and smooth transition with continuity of care for patients referred for hospice care. Those involved with teaching can emphasize the evaluation and management of physical and psychological symptoms, communication skills, attitudes, and the care of dying patients.

Conclusion

The integration of palliative medicine and medical oncology, in practice and in education, can provide a better standard of patient care, reduce the risk of oncologist burnout, and increase the likelihood of patient family and physician satisfaction. There need be no gulf between these disciplines and only together do they represent truly comprehensive cancer care. The realization of this fusion will require the participation of individual clinicians, programme directors, and the policymakers for cancer centres, professional organizations, and the health-care regulatory authorities. It is a logical next step in the evolution of medical oncology.

Acknowledgments

Online materials

Complete references for this chapter are available online at <http://www.oxfordmedicine.com>.

References

Back, A.L., Young, J.P., McCown, E., *et al.* (2009). Abandonment at the end of life from patient, caregiver, nurse, and physician perspectives: loss of continuity and lack of closure. *Archives of Internal Medicine*, 169, 474–479.

Bakitas, M., Lyons, K.D., Hegel, M.T., *et al.* (2009). Effects of a palliative care intervention on clinical outcomes in patients with advanced cancer: the Project ENABLE II randomized controlled trial. *Journal of the American Medical Association*, 302, 741–749.

Buss, M.K., Lessen, D.S., Sullivan, A.M., Von Roenn, J.H., Arnold, R.M., and Block, S.D. (2007). A study of oncology fellows' trainign in end-of-life care. *Journal of Supportive Oncology*, 5, 237–242.

Cheng, M.J., King, L.M., Alesi, E.R., and Smith, T.J. (2013). Doing palliative care in the oncology office. *Journal of Oncology Practice*, 9, 84–88.

Cherny, N.I. and Catane, R. (2003). Attitudes of medical oncologists toward palliative care for patients with advanced and incurable cancer: report on a survery by the European Society of Medical Oncology Taskforce on Palliative and Supportive Care. *Cancer*, 98, 2502–2510.

Cherny, N.I., Catane, R., and Kosmidis, P. (2003). ESMO takes a stand on supportive and palliative care. *Annals of Oncology*, 14, 1335–1337.

Cherny, N., Catane, R., Schrijvers, D., Kloke, M., and Strasser, F. (2010). European Society for Medical Oncology (ESMO) Program for the integration of oncology and Palliative Care: a 5-year review of the Designated Centers' incentive program. *Annals of Oncology*, 21, 362–369.

Clayton, J.M., Butow, P.N., and Tattersall, M.H. (2005c). When and how to initiate discussion about prognosis and end-of-life issues with terminally ill patients. *Journal of Pain and Symptom Management*, 30, 132–144.

Epstein, A.S. and Morrison, R.S. (2012). Palliative oncology: identity, progress, and the path ahead. *Annals of Oncology*, 23(Suppl. 3), 43–48.

Foley, K. and Gelband, H. (2001). *Improving Palliative Care for Cancer: Summary and Recommendations*. Washington, DC: National Academies Press.

Gade, G., Venohr, I., Conner, D., *et al.* (2008). Impact of an inpatient palliative care team: a randomized control trial. *Journal of Palliative Medicine*, 11, 180–190.

Greer, J.A., Jackson, V.A., Meier, D.E., and Temel, J.S. (2013). Early integration of palliative care services with standard oncology care for patients with advanced cancer. *CA: A Cancer Journl for Clinicians*, 63, 349–363.

Harrington, S.E. and Smith, T.J. (2008). The role of chemotherapy at the end of life: 'when is enough, enough?' *Journal of the American Medical Association*, 299, 2667–2678.

Hui, D., Elsayem, A., De La Cruz, M., *et al.* (2010). Availability and integration of palliative care at US cancer centers. *Journal of the American Medical Association*, 303, 1054–1061.

Hydeman, J. (2013). Improving the integration of palliative care in a comprehensive oncology center: increasing primary care referrals to palliative care. *Omega*, 67, 127–134.

Lynn, J. (2000). Sick to death and not going to take it any more. In P.Q. Schoeni (ed.) *Promises to Keep: Changing the Way We Provide Care at the End of Life*, pp. 1–4. Boston, MA: The National Coalition for Health Care, The Institute for Health Care Improvement.

Marchetti, P., Voltz, R., Rubio, C., Mayeur, D., and Kopf, A. (2013). Provision of palliative care and pain management services for oncology patients. *Journal of the National Comprehensive Cancer Network*, 11(Suppl. 1), S17–27.

Matsuyama, R., Reddy, S., and Smith, T.J. (2006). Why do patients choose chemotherapy near the end of life? A review of the perspective of those facing death from cancer. *Journal of Clinical Oncology*, 24, 3490–3496.

McKenzie, M.R. (1998). Oncology and palliative care: bringing together the two solitudes. *Canadian Medical Association Journal*, 158, 1702–1704.

Mercadante, S., Intravaia, G., Villari, P., *et al.* (2008). Clinical and financial analysis of an acute palliative care unit in an oncological department. *Palliative Medicine*, 22, 760–767.

National Comprehensive Cancer Network (2014). *Palliative Care*. [Online] Available at: <http://www.nccn.org/professionals/physician_gls/pdf/palliative.pdf> Referenced with permission from the NCCN Clinical Practice Guidelines in Oncology (NCCN Guidelines®) for Palliative Care V.1.2014. © National Comprehensive Cancer Network, Inc 2014. All rights reserved. Accessed 16 December, 2014. To view the most recent and complete version of the guideline, go online to NCCN.org. NATIONAL COMPREHENSIVE CANCER NETWORK®, NCCN®, NCCN GUIDELINES®, and all other NCCN Content are trademarks owned by the National Comprehensive Cancer Network, Inc.

National Institute For Clinical Excellence (2004). *Improving Supportive and Palliative Care for Adults with Cancer: The Manual*. London: National Health Service.

Quill, T.E. and Cassel, C.K. (1995). Nonabandonment: a central obligation for physicians. *Annals of Internal Medicine*, 122, 368–374.

Salminen, E., Clemens, K.E., Syrjanen, K., and Salmenoja, H. (2008). Needs of developing the skills of palliative care at the oncology ward: an audit of symptoms among 203 consecutive cancer patients in Finland. *Supportive Care in Cancer*, 16, 3–8.

Smith, T.J. and Schnipper, L J. (1998). The American Society of Clinical Oncology Program to improve end-of-life care. *Journal of Palliative Medicine*, 1, 221–230.

Smith, T.J., Temin, S., Alesi, E.R., *et al.* (2012). American Society of Clinical Oncology provisional clinical opinion: the integration of palliative care into standard oncology care. *Journal of Clinical Oncology*, 30, 880–887.

Temel, J.S., Greer, J.A., Muzikansky, A., *et al.* (2010). Early palliative care for patients with metastatic non-small-cell lung cancer. *The New England Journal of Medicine*, 363, 733–742.

Viola, D., Leven, D.C., and Lepere, J.C. (2009). End-of-life care: an interdisciplinary perspective. *American Journal of Hospice and Palliative Medicine*, 26, 75–78.

Von Roenn, J.H., Voltz, R., and Serrie, A. (2013). Barriers and approaches to the successful integration of palliative care and oncology practice. *Journal of the National Comprehensive Cancer Network*, 11(Suppl 1), S11–16.

Weeks, J.C., Cook, E.F., O'Day, S., *et al.* (1998). Relationship between cancer patients' predictions of prognosis and their treatment preferences. *Journal of the American Medical Association*, 279, 1709–1714.

Weissman, D.E., Meier, D.E., and Spragens, L.H. (2008). Center to Advance Palliative Care palliative care consultation service metrics: consensus recommendations. *Journal of Palliative Medicine*, 11, 1294–1298.

World Health Organization (1990). *Cancer Pain Relief and Palliative Care*. Geneva: World Health Organization.

Zhukovsky, D.S., Herzog, C.E., Kaur, G., Palmer, J.L., and Bruera, E. (2009). The impact of palliative care consultation on symptom assessment, communication needs, and palliative interventions in pediatric patients with cancer. *Journal of Palliative Medicine*, 12, 343–349.

Zimmermann, C., Swami, N., Rodin, G., and Al., E. (2012). Cluster-randomized trial of early palliative care for patients with metastatic cancer. *Journal of Clinical Oncology*, 30(Suppl.), Abstract 9003.

Disease-modifying therapies in advanced cancer

Dirk Schrijvers

Introduction to disease-modifying therapies in advanced cancer

Diagnosis of cancer can be in an early or advanced stage. The stage at diagnosis depends on several factors such as the region where the patient is living (more advanced disease in developing countries); the health-care system and the implementation of screening programmes; patient factors such as cancer awareness, beliefs, and financial resources; and cancer-related factors such as visibility (ulcerations) and early physical complaints (e.g. bleeding and pain).

If a patient is diagnosed with advanced-stage disease, the possibilities of treatment and the outcome of treatment depends on several factors such as the health-care resources, knowledge and attitudes of both the professional health-care giver, the patient, and the non-professional caregiver, the availability of different treatment modalities (e.g. surgery, radiotherapy, and medication) and the type of cancer.

In regions with sufficient health-care resources, disease-modifying therapies can be proposed to the patient in combination with palliative care.

Aims of therapy

When an advanced-stage cancer is diagnosed and health-care resources are available, a disease-modifying therapy might be considered. Before discussing such a treatment, it is important that the patient is informed about his or her condition to participate in the decision process.

Different aims of therapy can be postulated in patients with advanced disease, depending on their condition and wishes and the disease itself.

If the condition of the patient is very weak (e.g. Eastern Cooperative Oncology Group Performance status ≥ 3) the likelihood of benefit from anticancer treatment is limited and in many instances treatment should be withheld because it may compromise well-being without contributing to improved quality or duration of survival. Several instruments have been developed to determine the frailty of a patient (Luciano et al., 2010) and expected toxicity (Extermann et al., 2012) in relation to treatment and the patient should be evaluated before any diagnostic and treatment procedure to avoid unnecessary examinations and harm to the patient.

If the condition of the patient permits, an anticancer treatment may be proposed. The aim of the treatment may be curative or palliative. Even in patients with advanced disease, treatment may be given with the aim of curing (= curative intent) the patient with certain cancer types (Box 12.2.1) while for other conditions, cure is not an option and anticancer treatment can be given to improve or stabilize the quality of life and sometimes prolong life (= palliative treatment).

The aim of the treatment should be clearly explained to the patient and the caregiver(s) with information regarding acute and late side effects to ensure that the patient can make an informed decision and consent to the proposed treatment plan.

Disease-modifying therapies in advanced cancer

Surgery

While in the past, surgery was mainly used in patients with localized disease or with palliative intent (e.g. derivations), it now has a place in the treatment of patients with advanced disease to achieve cure or better disease control. It has an important impact on treatment outcome in combination with other treatment modalities and the treatment proposal should be discussed beforehand in a multidisciplinary team.

Local disease

Even in patients with advanced disease, the removal of the primary tumour can be used to influence the course of the disease.

In a treatment with *curative intent*, surgery on the primary tumour is standard practice in patients with metastatic testicular cancer (e.g. orchiectomy), ovarian cancer (e.g. removal of both ovaries together with all peritoneal disease), and metastatic thyroid cancer (total thyroidectomy) and improves treatment outcome.

The beneficial effect of removing the primary tumour in *palliative setting* has also been shown in certain tumour types:

- In patients with metastatic renal cell carcinoma, nephrectomy can result in the disappearance of lung metastases and in patients treated with interferon, prior nephrectomy improves overall survival. This improved survival might be the result of deprivation of angiogenic factors secreted by the primary tumour (Karam and Wood, 2011).

- In patients with breast cancer (Pérez-Fidalgo et al., 2011; Hartmann et al. 2014) and colorectal cancer (Verhoef et al., 2011) there is limited data to suggest that removal of the local tumour may have a beneficial effect on survival.

Box 12.2.1 Advanced stage cancer that can be treated with curative intent

Chemotherapy:

- acute lymphoblastic leukaemias (children)
- acute myeloid leukaemia
- choriocarcinoma
- high-grade non-Hodgkin's lymphoma
- Hodgkin's disease.

Combination of chemotherapy and surgery:

- breast cancer
- germ cell tumours of testis and ovary
- colorectal cancer
- epithelial ovarian cancer
- Ewing's sarcoma
- osteosarcoma
- rhabdomyosarcoma
- Wilms' tumour.

Combination of chemotherapy and radiotherapy:

- anal cancer
- cervical cancer
- head and neck cancer
- lymphoma
- non-small cell lung cancer
- small-cell lung cancer.

Regional disease

Lymph node invasion has a prognostic role in most tumours and determines subsequent adjuvant treatment in many tumour types. In some tumour types (e.g. intermediate and high-risk endometrial cancer (Neubauer and Lurain, 2011), malignant melanoma (Rager et al., 2005), non-small cell lung cancer (Bakir et al., 2011), and bladder cancer (Brunocilla et al., 2011)), lymph node dissection and removal of all involved lymph nodes contributes to a better overall survival.

Distant metastatic/recurrent disease

Surgery is also used more frequently in patients with synchronous and/or metachronous metastatic disease and selected patients with solid tumours can be cured by complete resection of metastases if the primary tumour is controlled.

- In some patients with *lung* metastasis, metastasectomy can be considered if the primary tumour is controlled, no extra-thoracic lesions are present with the exception of hepatic lesions that can be resected completely, metastases are technically resectable, and the general and functional risks are acceptable (Hornbech et al., 2011). Long-term survival has been reported after metastasectomy of lung metastases in patients with testicular cancers, osteosarcoma, soft tissue sarcoma, renal cell carcinoma, and colorectal cancer (Hornbech et al., 2011).

- While curative resections of *liver* metastasis have been reported in patients with colorectal cancer, its value in other tumour types (e.g. breast cancer and melanoma) has not been clearly demonstrated (Zani and Clary, 2011).

- Resection of solitary *brain* metastasis in combination with whole-brain irradiation of different tumour types has also been reported to be beneficial in patients with a good performance status (Scoccianti and Ricardi, 2012) resulting in improved function and duration of survival.

- Metastasectomy of painful lesions in the adrenal gland and bone may improve comfort but there is no evidence of improved survival.

Radiotherapy

External beam radiotherapy is another local treatment modality that has a place in the treatment of patients with advanced cancer (see Chapter 12.4). It is indicated in the palliative treatment of metastatic lesions causing symptoms such as pain due to bone metastasis or compressive complications by metastatic disease (e.g. pathological enlarged lymph nodes, brain metastasis). In addition to its palliative effects, radiotherapy has also an impact on disease outcome and overall survival in selected (loco-regional) advanced cancers.

- In patients with extensive disease *small cell lung cancer*, combination of loco-regional radiotherapy with chemotherapy improves local control and survival compared to chemotherapy alone (Jeremic et al., 2010). In patients with extensive disease small cell lung cancer and a response to chemotherapy, prophylactic whole-brain irradiation leads to a significant reduction in symptomatic brain metastases and improved survival (Slotman et al., 2007).

- Radiotherapy has also a role in the multimodality treatment of patients with *solitary brain metastasis* and the combination of surgery and whole-brain radiation improves tumour control at the original metastatic site and in the brain overall when compared to surgical resection alone (Scoccianti and Ricardi, 2012).

- In patients with loco-regional recurrent *head and neck cancer*, re-irradiation of the head and neck region with or without chemotherapy can induce long-time disease control although toxicity can be excessive.

While radioactive isotopes have been used in the control of painful diffuse bone metastases in palliative care setting, some isotopes are able to modify the course of metastatic disease. In patients with *thyroid cancer*, radioactive iodine has been used to control metastatic disease; Yttrium (^{90}Y)-edotreotide (Reiners et al., 2011) improves symptoms and survival in patients with metastatic *carcinoid tumours* (Bushnell et al., 2010), and radium 223 is able to improve survival in castration-resistant *prostate cancer* patients and bone metastasis only (Parker et al., 2011). Microspheres labelled with ^{90}Y are being tested in the local treatment of primary and metastatic *liver malignancies* (Uthappa et al., 2011).

Medication use

Several drugs are used in the treatment of cancer and are classified as (anti)hormones, cytotoxic or chemotherapeutic agents, targeted agents, and immunomodulatory drugs.

(Anti)Hormones

Some cancers are hormone sensitive and their biological behaviour can be modified by hormonal manipulations.

Breast cancer

In 70% of breast cancers, oestrogen and/or progesterone receptors are present and these tumours can be treated with hormonal manipulations in adjuvant and metastatic setting to modify the course of the disease. In oestrogen receptor (ER)-positive postmenopausal women with loco-regional disease, treatment with aromatase inhibitors and/or anti-oestrogens (e.g. tamoxifen) improves disease-free and overall survival. Postmenopausal women with ER-positive metastatic disease without prior endocrine therapy or with a previous treatment with tamoxifen should be offered an aromatase inhibitor. In pre- or perimenopausal women with ER-positive tumours not previously treated with hormonal therapy, tamoxifen and ovarian suppression should be offered as first-line treatment while ovarian suppression should be added to women previously treated with tamoxifen at disease progression (National Institute for Health and Clinical Excellence, 2009). When starting (anti)hormonal treatment, side effects (e.g. hot flushes, arthralgia, second tumours, and osteoporosis) should be taken into account for selection of the hormonal therapy.

Endometrial cancer

Endometrial cancer is considered to be a hormone-driven cancer. A trial of hormonal therapy may be helpful to palliate symptoms (Kokka et al., 2010).

Prostate cancer

Prostate cancer is usually a hormone-sensitive tumour that can be influenced by hormonal manipulations. In patients with advanced prostate cancer, androgen deprivation therapy (ADT) by orchiectomy, luteinizing hormone-releasing hormone agonists or antagonists, and diethyl-stilbestrol has a high likelihood of inducing a remission, thus delaying progression, relieving and preventing complications, and palliating symptoms effectively.

The timing of starting ADT should be individualized. Although immediate ADT at diagnosis significantly reduces disease progression and the complication rate compared with deferred ADT at the time of symptomatic progression, it does not induce a clear survival benefit. Side effects of ADT are sexual dysfunction, hot flushes, osteoporosis with fractures, metabolic syndrome, and cardiovascular morbidity and mortality (Heidenreich et al., 2012). Hormonal manipulations are also effective in patients who have developed castration-resistant prostate cancer and an overall survival benefit has been shown with abiraterone acetate, a cytochrome 17-complex inhibitor that completely inhibits testosterone production in all tissues as well as some newer anti-androgens.

Thyroid cancer

Patients with advanced differentiated thyroid cancer may benefit from L-thyroxine treatment at doses that suppress serum thyroid stimulating hormone (TSH) levels. TSH is thought to increase tumour growth but the optimal reduction of TSH concentration to reduce tumour recurrences and improve survival is unknown. Aggressive TSH suppression is indicated in patients with high-risk disease or recurrent tumours, whereas less aggressive TSH suppression is reasonable in low-risk patients (Biondi and Cooper, 2010). Side effects of high-dose L-thyroxine include

cardiovascular (e.g. arrhythmia, heart failure, hypertension, myocardial infarction, palpitation, and tachycardia), central nervous system (e.g. anxiety, emotional lability, fatigue, fever, headache, hyperactivity, insomnia, irritability, and nervousness), gastrointestinal (e.g. abdominal cramps, appetite increased, diarrhoea, vomiting, and weight loss), neuromuscular (e.g. muscle weakness and tremor), and skeletal (e.g. decreased bone mineral density,) complications.

Neuroendocrine tumours

Low-grade neuroendocrine tumours may be treated with somatostatin analogues (e.g. octreotide or lanreotide) to improve symptoms such as flushing and diarrhoea and influence disease evolution (Grozinsky et al., 2008) and in patients with metastatic enteropancreatic neuroendocrine tumours progression-free survival (Caplin et al., 2014).

Cytotoxic agents

Cytotoxic agents interfere with cell cycle processes and have been used since the 1940s in the treatment of early and advanced cancer. Patient selection is of utmost importance since the therapeutic index between activity and toxicity is very narrow. Most of these treatments induce severe acute and sometimes late side effect that have to be taken into account when deciding on the use of chemotherapy.

In the curative setting, cytotoxic agents are mostly used in combination schedules and/or with other treatment modalities (e.g. surgery, radiotherapy). In high-risk patients with local or loco-regional disease their aim is to improve cure rates. Adjuvant chemotherapy with curative intent is given in patients with breast, colorectal, non-small cell lung, or testicular cancer while chemoradiation is used in locally advanced cervical, anal, and head and neck cancer. In patients with advanced metastatic cancer such as testicular cancer, germ cell tumours, non-Hodgkin and Hodgkin lymphoma, and certain haematological malignancies, chemotherapy can be given with curative intent (Box 12.2.1).

In most patients with advanced disease, the aim of chemotherapy is not cure but disease control to improve quality of life or sometimes overall survival. In several tumour types, chemotherapy is able to improve overall survival and quality in life when given as first-line treatment. In a number of tumour types, second- and even third-line chemotherapy is able to influence cancer evolution positively compared to best supportive care or standard treatment (Table 12.2.1).

Targeted agents

Due to a better insight into processes involved in carcinogenesis, a group of drugs targeting specific pathways has been developed and is used in the treatment of cancers. These drugs are able to induce tumour responses in previously treatment-unresponsive disease and have a disease-modifying potential in patients with specific dysregulations of a pathway. Although they are considered to be specific, they induce toxicities that, although different from those due to chemotherapy, are a burden for the patient or can be life-threatening.

One of the first agents in this group was imatinib and this drug changed the disease evolution of patients with gastrointestinal stromal tumours (GIST) and chronic myeloid leukaemia. There were few treatment options for these patients to induce long-term remission and the use of imatinib acting as a blocker of the

Table 12.2.1 Improved quality of life and/or survival with an anti-cancer therapy compared with best supportive care/placebo/standard treatment in randomized trials in patients with advanced solid cancers

Tumour type	First-line therapy	Second- and third-line therapy
Adrenal cortex	Mitotane[a]	
Bladder	Platinum-based + gemcitabine	Vinflunine[b]
Breast	(Hormones, sequential chemotherapy) Doxorubicin + docetaxel; taxane + trastuzumab[c]; aromatase inhibitor + trastuzumab; liposomal doxorubicin	Docetaxel[b], capecitabine + docetaxel; trastuzumab[c], T-DM1**, exemestane + everolimus
Carcinoid	Somatostatine analogue + interferon α	
Colorectal	Fluoropyrimidine-based[b], irinotecan-based + cetuximab, oxaliplatin-based + cetuximab, fluoropyrimidine-based + bevacizumab; oxaliplatin-based + panitumumab***, capecitabine	Irinotecan-based[b], cetuximab***; irinotecan-based + panitumumab***; panitumumab***[b], capecitabine-based, regorafenib
Gastric	5-fluorouracil-based; platinum-based + docetaxel; fluoropyrimidine-platinum + trastuzumab[c], capecitabine-based	
Gastro-intestinal stromal tumour	Imatinib'	Sunitinib[b], regorafenib°
Head and neck	Platinum-based + Cetuximab Platinum-based + docetaxel	
Kaposi sarcoma	Liposomal doxorubicin	Liposomal doxorubicin
Liver	Sorafinib[b]	
Melanoma	Interferon α, interferon α + bevacizumab, vemurafinib, dabrafenib + trametinib	Ipilumumab[b]
Mesothelioma	Platinum + pemetrexed	
Non-small cell lung	Platinum-based[b]; platinum-based + docetaxel; platinum-based + bevacizumab; platinum-based + pemetrexed gefitinib[d]; erlotinib[d]	Docetaxel[b]; pemetrexed, erlotinib[b]/gefitinib[b], crizotinib[g]
Ovary	Platinum-paclitaxel-based, platinum-paclitaxel-based + bevacizumab	Topotecan; liposomal doxorubicin
Pancreas	Gemcitabine[b]; gemcitabine + erlotinib	
Pancreatic neuroendocrine tumours	Somatostatin analogues + sunitinib[b]; everolimus[b]	
Prostate*	Docetaxel + prednisone*, abiraterone acetate	Abiraterone acetate[b], cabazitaxel, enzalutamide, radium-223
Renal cell	Interferon α, interleukin, sunitinib, pazopanib[b]; temsirolimus	Sorafinib[b], everolimus[b]; pazopanib[b]
Small cell lung	Platinum-based	Topotecan[b]
Thyroid—medullary	Vandetanib[b]	

[a] phase II study; [b] placebo-controlled or best supportive care only; [c] HER-2 overexpressing tumours; [d] activating epidermal growth factor receptor tyrosine kinase mutations; [e] Ras wild type; [f] castration-resistant prostate cancer.; [g] alk mutation.

mutated protein BCR-ABL was able to turn these difficult-to-treat and fatal diseases into chronic conditions.

Bosutinib is also a drug that interferes with this system.

Other agents targeting *independency of growth signals* have been used to treat several tumour types. The epidermal growth factor receptor (EGFR) can be influenced by monoclonal antibodies (e.g. cetuximab and panitumumab) or tyrosine kinase inhibitors (e.g. gefitinib, erlotinib, and afatinib) in patients with advanced disease. They are currently used in the treatment of metastatic cancers such as non-small cell lung cancer, head and neck cancer, and colorectal cancer. Some of these medications are used in combination with cytotoxic agents and patient selection should not only be based on specific mutations but also according to the patient's frailty. Common side effects are skin toxicity and diarrhoea.

Another target influencing tumour growth is HER-2. Trastuzumab, a monoclonal antibody against HER-2 is used in combination with chemotherapy to treat advanced breast and gastric cancer while the dual tyrosine kinase inhibitor lapatinib is used as single agent in metastatic breast cancer. Cardiotoxicity is of major concern and combination with cardiotoxic chemotherapy is contraindicated.

In malignant melanoma, 50% of patients have an activating mutation in the serine/threonine-protein kinase *B-raf* gene (BRAF) and inhibition of mutated B-raf protein by vemurafenib or dabrafenib leads to an overall survival benefit in this group of patients. Trametinib is a MEK protein kinase inhibitor that is registered for the treatment of patients with unresectable or metastatic melanoma with a BRAF V600 mutation.

Angiogenesis is another important target. Several medications against parts of the process of angiogenesis are used. They comprise interference with hypoxia-inducible factor, a transcription factor, by influencing the mTOR pathway (e.g. everolimus, temsirolimus); the vascular endothelial growth factor (VEGF) that induces angiogenesis (e.g. bevacizumab and aflibercept); and the VEGF receptor (e.g. sorafinib, sunitinib, pazopanib, and axitinib). This group of drugs is active against renal cell carcinoma, (neuro)endocrine tumours, colorectal, breast, and ovarian cancer with improvement of progression-free and overall survival. The main side effects are hypertension, thrombotic events, proteinuria, and bleeding.

Other pathways have been discovered (e.g. evading growth suppressors, resisting cell death or apoptosis, enabling replicative immortality, activating invasion, and metastasis) and many drugs are being explored to influence these pathways and improve patient outcome.

Immune system modulatory drugs

The immune system is an important factor in the control of cancer and medication interfering with this system has shown activity in patients with advanced cancer.

High-dose interleukin-2 is used in selected patients with malignant melanoma and renal cell carcinoma. The activity is difficult to predict but some patients reach a durable response. However, toxicity is impressive (e.g. 71% grade 3–4 hypotension; 52% chills, 34% confusion, 42% rash, 67% diarrhoea, and 43% dyspnoea with 24% pulmonary congestion).

Interferon is used in patients with advanced hairy cell leukaemia, lymphoma (follicular), malignant melanoma, and AIDS-related Kaposi's sarcoma. Again, systemic toxicities can be serious.

In patients with malignant melanoma, immune modulation by ipilimumab, a monoclonal antibody against the immune modulatory antigen CTLC-4, can induce durable responses with manageable skin and liver toxicity. Several drugs interfering with the programmed death receptor system on immune modulatory T cells are being tested and expected to be active in patients with solid tumours.

Oncological literacy

Palliative care clinicians do not need to be cancer experts. However, high-level integration between oncological care and palliative care requires familiarity with contemporary approaches to disease modification that can improve patient well-being. Palliative care clinicians ought to be familiar with web-based resources to access contemporary updates of standard oncological treatments for the diseases that they are encountering, especially when involved with upstream or early intervention palliative care programmes. Excellent web-based guidelines are available from the National

Comprehensive Cancer Network (NCCN; <http://www.nccn.com>), the US National Cancer Institute (NCI; <http://www.cancer.gov/cancertopics/pdq>), the European Society for Medical Oncology (ESMO Guidelines) (<http://www.esmo.org/Guidelines-Practice/Clinical-Practice-Guidelines>) and eviQ Cancer Treatments Online (<http://www.eviq.org.au>).

Conclusion

In oncology, many new treatments have been introduced that have changed the dismal and short prognosis in patients with advanced disease. While some patients with advanced disease can be cured, the use of these treatments in patients with advanced non-curable disease is often beneficial. However, patient selection is of utmost importance and treatment decisions should be taken in a multidisciplinary team. It is important that these patients are evaluated by an oncologist to give them the best information on their disease and the possible interventions, so that patient and caregivers can make an informed decision about further treatment and care.

References

Bakir, M., Fraser, S., Routledge, T., and Scarci, M. (2011). Is surgery indicated in patients with stage IIIa lung cancer and mediastinal nodal involvement? *Interactive CardioVascular and Thoracic Surgery*, 13(3), 303–310.

Biondi, B. and Cooper, D.S. (2010). Benefits of thyrotropin suppression versus the risks of adverse effects in differentiated thyroid cancer. *Thyroid*, 20(2), 135–146.

Brunocilla, E., Pernetti, R., and Martorana, G. (2011). The role of pelvic lymph node dissection during radical cystectomy for bladder cancer. *Anticancer Research*, 31(1), 271–275.

Bushnell, D.L., Jr, O'Dorisio, T.M., O'Dorisio, M.S., *et al.* (2010). 90Y-edotreotide for metastatic carcinoid refractory to octreotide. *Journal of Clinical Oncology*, 28(10), 1652–1659.

Caplin, M.E, Pavel, M., Ćwikła, J.B., *et al.* (2014). Lanreotide in metastatic enteropancreatic neuroendocrine tumors. *The New England Journal of Medicine*, 371(3), 224–233.

Extermann, M., Boler, I., Reich, R.R., *et al.* (2012). Predicting the risk of chemotherapy toxicity in older patients: the Chemotherapy Risk Assessment Scale for High-Age Patients (CRASH) score. *Cancer*, 118(13), 3377–3386.

Grozinsky-Glasberg, S., Shimon, I., Korbonits, M., and Grossman, A.B. (2008). Somatostatin analogues in the control of neuroendocrine tumours: efficacy and mechanisms. *Endocrine-Related Cancer*, 15(3), 701–720.

Hartmann, S., Reimer, T., Gerber, B., and Stachs, A. (2014). Primary metastatic breast cancer: the impact of locoregional therapy. *Breast Care (Basel)*, 9(1), 23–28.

Heidenreich, A., Bastian, P.J., Bellmunt, J., *et al.* (2012). *Guidelines on Prostate Cancer.* European Association of Urology. [Online] Available at: <http://www.uroweb.org/guidelines/online-guidelines/>.

Hornbech, K., Ravn, J., and Steinbrüchel, D.A. (2011). Current status of pulmonary metastasectomy. *European Journal Cardio-Thoracic Surgery*, 39(6), 955–962.

Jeremic, B., Casas, F., Wang, L., and Perin, B. (2010). Radiochemotherapy in extensive disease small cell lung cancer ED-SCLC. *Frontiers of Radiation Therapy and Oncology*, 42, 180–186.

Karam, J.A. and Wood, C.G. (2011). The role of surgery in advanced renal cell carcinoma: cytoreductive nephrectomy and metastasectomy. *Hematology/Oncology Clinics of North America*, 25(4), 753–764.

Kokka, F., Brockbank, E., Oram, D., Gallagher, C., and Bryant, A. (2010). Hormonal therapy in advanced or recurrent endometrial cancer. *Cochrane Database of Systematic Reviews*, 12, CD007926.

Luciani, A., Ascione, G., Bertuzzi, C., *et al.* (2010). Detecting disabilities in older patients with cancer: comparison between comprehensive geriatric assessment and vulnerable elders survey-13. *Journal of Clinical Oncology*, 28(12), 2046–2050.

National Institute for Health and Clinical Excellence (2009). *Advanced Breast Cancer: Diagnosis and Treatment*. Cardiff: National Collaborating Centre for Cancer.

Neubauer, N.L. and Lurain, J.R. (2011). The role of lymphadenectomy in surgical staging of endometrial cancer. *International Journal of Surgical Oncology*, 2011, 814649.

Parker, C., Heinrich, D., O'Sullivan, J.M., *et al.* (2011). Overall survival benefit of radium-223 chloride (Alpharadin) in the treatment of patients with symptomatic bone metastases in castration-resistant prostate cancer: a phase III randomized rial (ALSYMPCA). *European Journal of Cancer*, 47(Suppl. 2), Abstract 1LBA.

Pérez-Fidalgo, J.A., Pimentel, P., Caballero, A., *et al.* (2011). Removal of primary tumor improves survival in metastatic breast cancer. Does timing of surgery influence outcomes? *Breast*, 20(6), 548–554.

Rager, E.L., Bridgeford, E.P., and Ollila, D.W. (2005). Cutaneous melanoma: update on prevention, screening, diagnosis, and treatment. *American Family Physician*, 72(2), 269–276.

Reiners, C., Hänscheid, H., Luster, M., Lassmann, M., and Verburg, F.A. (2011). Radioiodine for remnant ablation and therapy of metastatic disease. *Nature Reviews Endocrinology*, 7(10), 589–595.

Scoccianti, S. and Ricardi, U. (2012). Treatment of brain metastases: review of phase III randomized controlled trials. *Radiotherapy and Oncology*, 102(2), 168–179.

Slotman, B.J., Faivre-Finn, C., Kramer, G.W., *et al.* (2007). Prophylactic cranial irradiation in small cell lung cancer. *The New England Journal of Medicine*, 357, 664–672.

Uthappa, M.C., Ravikumar, R., and Gupta, A. (2011). Selective internal radiation therapy: 90Y (yttrium) labeled microspheres for liver malignancies (primary and metastatic). *Indian Journal of Cancer*, 48(1), 18–23.

Verhoef, C., de Wilt, J.H., Burger, J.W., Verheul, H.M., and Koopman, M. (2011). Surgery of the primary in stage IV colorectal cancer with unresectable metastases. *European Journal of Cancer*, 47(Suppl. 3), S61–66.

Zani, S. and Clary, B.M. (2011). A role for hepatic metastasectomy in stage IV melanoma and breast cancer: reestablishing the surgical modality. *Oncology*, 25(12), 1158–1164.

Radiotherapy in symptom management

Peter J. Hoskin

Introduction to radiotherapy in symptom management

The majority of cancer patients, particularly those with common tumours such as lung, breast, and prostate, require radiation therapy one or more times during the course of their disease. More than 40% of radiation treatments are given with palliative intent for control of local symptoms (Willams and Drinkwater, 2009).

General principles of radiotherapy

Radiobiology

Radiotherapy uses ionizing radiation to damage DNA. The most frequently used forms of ionizing radiation are X-rays produced from an X-ray machine or linear accelerator and gamma rays produced from a radioactive source. Biologically, these have identical effects. Particle radiation also is sometimes used, particularly electrons for superficial treatments and beta particles from systemic radioisotopes. Proton therapy is not indicated in palliative treatments.

Radiation causes both direct and indirect damage to DNA. Direct damage includes base deletions and breaks in the DNA chain, and indirect damage results from toxic free radicals produced from the interaction between radiation and water molecules in the cell. Indirect damage is the more important cause of cell death, which may occur from either reproductive failure or apoptosis following derangement of cell regulatory mechanisms. When very high single doses (> 10 Gy) of radiation are delivered, damage to endothelial cells occurs and the resulting interruption in blood flow may be another mechanism for cellular injury.

In clinical practice, radiation is delivered to maximize tumour cell kill whilst minimizing normal tissue damage by exploiting differences between normal and malignant cells. Cancer cells are less able than normal cells to repair 'sublethal' radiation damage, and differences in repair capacity account, in part, for variation in radiosensitivity. Factors that influence response other than repair capacity include oxygenation (hypoxic cells are relatively radioresistant), the number of cells actively dividing (cells in certain phases of the cell cycle are more sensitive than others; non-cycling cells are relatively radioresistant), and the rate of repopulation within the tumour. These parameters of repair, re-oxygenation, repopulation, and redistribution within the cell cycle, are the fundamental influences on the cellular response to radiation.

Palliative versus radical radiotherapy

The aim of radical radiotherapy is complete eradication of tumour cells within the treated volume, which must encompass the entire extent of the tumour. This must be done in a manner that also minimizes long-term normal tissue damage. In contrast, the aim of palliative radiotherapy is the control of symptoms with minimum associated acute radiation reaction.

These two very different aims result in different philosophies in the delivery of radiation. To minimize normal tissue damage during radical radiotherapy, the radiation dose is built up by delivering treatment on a daily basis over several weeks. In this way, high doses of radiation close to, or beyond, those tolerated by surrounding normal tissues can be given. Conventional treatment schedules deliver a single dose of radiation, often called a fraction, on a daily basis, Monday to Friday. This treatment may be accelerated, that is, given two or three times a day over a relatively shorter period, to produce greater tumour damage by reducing the opportunity for tumour repopulation. Treatment acceleration is limited by the increase in the acute reaction of normal tissue. *Hyperfractionation*, which delivers the total dose in an increased number of fractions over the same period dividing the usual daily dose into two or three smaller doses, may be employed to deliver higher doses with greater sparing of normal tissues.

Although fractionated and hyperfractionated radiotherapy requires 6–8 weeks and is arduous for the patient, it is justified when cure is the aim. For patients with limited life expectancy, however, more pragmatic schedules are appropriate. Sixty to 80% of tumour cells are killed by the first one or two radiation doses, and when the intent of treatment is palliative, this initial effect may be more than adequate for long-term symptom control. Indeed, in some scenarios, for example, metastatic bone pain, symptom response is independent of tumour shrinkage. Most palliative radiotherapy can be delivered in one or two treatments and rarely is it necessary to extend a course of treatment beyond 1–2 weeks. The delivery of short, relatively low-dose schedules results in less acute reaction and a minimal risk of late damage to normal tissues within the expected life span of the patient.

Radiotherapy in clinical practice

The most common type of radiotherapy is external beam irradiation (Table 12.3.1). In a modern radiotherapy department, most treatments are performed by a linear accelerator (Fig. 12.3.1) and comprise high-energy X-rays or an electron beam for superficial

Table 12.3.1 Types of external beam radiotherapy

	Energy	Source	Depth of penetration	Clinical use
Superficial X-rays	50–150 kV	X-ray tube	5–10 mm	Surface skin tumours
Orthovoltage X-rays	250–500 kV	X-ray tube	15–30 mm	Surface tumours
				Superficial bones, e.g. ribs, sacrum
Electrons	4–20 MeV	linear accelerator	15–70 mm	Surface tumours
				Superficial bones, e.g. ribs, sacrum
				Lymph nodes
Megavoltage X-rays	4–25 MV	linear accelerator	3–20 cm	Main source of radiation beams for sites other than above
Gamma rays	2.5 MV	cobalt source	5–10 cm	All sites except superficial skin

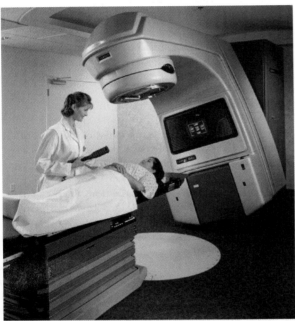

Clinac® Accelerators: Clinac 23EX with MLC-120 and PortalVision™

Fig. 12.3.1 Treatment with a modern linear accelerator.
Image courtesy of Varian Medical, United Kingdom.

Table 12.3.2 Isotope use in brachytherapy

Intracavitary	Iridium	Intrauterine
	Cobalt	Intravaginal
		Endo-oesophageal
		Endobronchial
		Endorectal
Interstitial	Iridium	Tongue, floor of mouth
	Cobalt	Buccal mucosa
		Breast
		Anal canal
		Vulva/vagina
Surface (Mould)	Iridium	Skin
	Cobalt	Penis

lesions. Alternative means to deliver radiation—brachytherapy and systemic radioisotopes—are used in specific circumstances. In brachytherapy, the radioactive source is placed directly onto or within the area to be treated (Table 12.3.2). Systemic radioisotopes target a specific tissue or pathophysiology, for example, radioiodine for thyroid cancer and strontium for bone metastases.

To direct radiation as accurately as possible to the tumour whilst minimizing exposure to normal tissue requires a systematic process that defines the treatment volume and optimal technique. This is called 'planning' and includes the following steps:

- Immobilization: it is necessary to immobilize the patient when small movements could result in the irradiation of critical structures, for example, the eye. Although a simple technique, such as sandbags, may suffice, more complex treatments may require a plastic shell with an individualized face mask.

- Treatment volume localization: superficial lesions can be easily defined on examination but deep-seated tumours require radiographic localization. Although computed tomography (CT) scanning, which enables accurate three-dimensional reproduction of the anatomical region of interest, is now used for most planning situations, plain radiography with a treatment simulator is sufficient in many common palliative scenarios, such as bone metastases or a primary lung tumour. The simulator is an X-ray machine identical to the therapy machine in its geometric specifications and movement, which emits a diagnostic X-ray beam and produces an image of the proposed therapeutic beam.

- Dosimetric planning: once the volume has been defined, the means of treatment delivery is determined. For simple treatments, such as those for bone metastases, a single beam or two opposing beams to treat a block of tissue will be all that is required. For internal volumes, more complex, three- or four-field arrangements may be optimal. Even more complex planning, which may employ intensity-modulated radiotherapy (IMRT) or stereotactic techniques, is required in some situations, such as treatment close to the spinal cord, retreatments close to critical organs, and treatment of oligometastases (fewer than three metastases) when higher doses may be considered.

◆ Verification: the defined beam arrangement must be checked on the patient before treatment delivery. Beam position may be checked by imaging on the treatment machine using the megavoltage treatment beam, or on modern linear accelerators, using integrated kilovoltage CT imaging. With simple superficial fields, clinical measurement and observation are adequate. Accurate documentation of the beam position with indelible marking of defined skin entry points on the patient will facilitate this and ensure accurate day-to-day reproducibility when more than one fraction is to be given

A linear accelerator produces high-energy radiation at a rate of around 1 Gy per minute. This means that most treatments, even those using large single fractions in the palliative setting, last for only a few minutes. There are no accompanying symptoms provided the patient is comfortable at the outset. Many patients require help in achieving the required position and lying still during treatment. Unfortunately, many patients experience discomfort related to immobilization, the use of hard wooden flat couch, and the need for staff to leave the patient isolated whilst radiation delivery is taking place. The judicious administration of an analgesic or anxiolytic drug prior to treatment always should be considered.

Side effects of radiotherapy

The side effects of radiotherapy are categorized into two groups based on their timing relative to the radiation exposure. Acute effects occur during treatment and may persist for several weeks. Late effects are rarely seen before 9 months after treatment and the risk of a late complication continues indefinitely. The common clinical manifestations of acute and late radiation toxicity are shown in Table 12.3.3.

Acute toxicity is due to loss of epithelial cells. This results in skin erythema or desquamation, and depending on the site of treatment, oropharyngeal mucositis, oesophagitis, cystitis, or gastrointestinal irritation. Repair of the denuded surface with new epithelial cells occurs once treatment is completed, provided that the underlying stem cell population has not been damaged irreparably. Recovery usually occurs within a period of a few days or weeks. On rare occasions, however, there may be persistent damage, which is termed 'consequential damage'. This most often occurs in vulnerable sites, such as the back or the lower leg, where skin healing appears less efficient. Poor healing after radiotherapy may also be seen where there is secondary infection or trauma, and it is these events that predispose to the rare occurrence of radionecrosis.

Late effects cause of treatment-related loss of function and even mortality in patients receiving radical radiotherapy. For every tissue a 'tolerance dose' is defined, up to which late damage is not expected in the 'normal' population. One of the reasons for the complex planning systems which have evolved for radiation delivery is the strenuous effort required to avoid exceeding these doses whilst delivering effective doses to nearby tumour. Unfortunately there are genetically predisposed individuals to radiation damage where even a conventional tolerance dose may result in late damage.

Late radiation injury is due to vascular damage, specifically progressive endarteritis obliterans. This results in closure of small blood vessels and potential tissue ischaemia. Although the clinical

Table 12.3.3 Acute and late effects of radiation

Site	Acute effect	Late effect[a]
Skin	Erythema	Atrophy, fibrosis
	Desquamation	Telangiectasia
		Necrosis
Gastrointestinal tract	Nausea, anorexia	Stricture
	Vomiting	Telangiectasia, bleeding
	Diarrhoea	Perforation
		Malabsorption
		Chronic enteritis, colitis, proctitis
Bladder	Sterile cystitis	Reduced volume
		Telangiectasia, bleeding
		Urethral or ureteric stricture
		Fistula
Oral cavity	Mucositis	Mucosal atrophy
Pharynx	Dry mouth	Telangiectasia, bleeding
	Taste loss	Dental caries
		mandibular necrosis
Lung	Pneumonitis	Fibrosis
Central nervous system	Transient demyelination (Lhermitte's sign)	Myelitis
		Necrosis
		Local oedema
Eye	Keratitis	Cataract
		Entropion or ectropion
		Dry eye

[a] In most patients only minor late effects are seen. These are minimized by reducing the dose of radiation delivered to sensitive structures with the treated region to known safe 'tolerance' doses. Late effects are not expected after palliative radiotherapy.

manifestations may be relatively minor, such as the commonly observed appearance of skin or mucosal atrophy or telangiectasia, more serious consequences may occur. In the pelvis, the bowel or bladder may be damaged, resulting in fibrosis and bowel perforation or fistula formation between the bladder, bowel, or vagina. In the central nervous system, there is very limited ability to repair damage and catastrophic necrosis may occur if dose limits are exceeded.

Management of radiation side effects

Acute side effects are common and management is focused on relief of symptoms whilst allowing the affected area to heal. Mild skin reactions require no active treatment. Local applications are generally best avoided. Desquamation will rarely if ever be seen after palliative doses. The use of topical preparations such as gentian violet is to be discouraged, and talcum powder and proprietary creams containing metallic salts should be avoided at all costs during treatment as these can enhance the reaction. Starch powder, as found in proprietary baby powders, may be helpful in keeping the surrounding skin dry and comfortable.

Nausea during irradiation to the abdomen or pelvis usually responds to antiemetic therapy such as metoclopramide 10 mg 6–8-hourly, ondansetron 8 mg twice daily, or granisetron 2 mg daily. If antiemetics are ineffective, a small dose of a corticosteroid such as prednisolone 10–30 mg daily may be valuable. Prophylactic therapy may be helpful. For example, single radiation doses given to the lumbar spine or pelvis produce an exit dose of radiation to the abdomen, and a prophylactic regimen of dexamethasone 8 mg and ondansetron 8 mg or granisetron 2 mg given 30 minutes before treatment is effective in avoiding severe symptoms.

Radiation-induced acute diarrhoea may respond to a low residue diet, avoiding fruit and other fibre-containing foods. When required, loperamide or codeine phosphate on a regular basis three to four times daily is helpful.

Radiation cystitis is more difficult to ameliorate. The use of an alpha blocker such as tamsulosin may be helpful when there is severe bladder spasm. Potassium citrate or cranberry juice are both time-honoured remedies, which may be of supportive value but have no evidence for efficacy. When there is significant dysuria or strangury, systemic analgesics are also of value. Secondary infection should always be excluded.

Oropharyngeal mucositis occurs when treating the head and neck region. It is important to maintain a high level of oral hygiene, using regular chlorhexidine mouthwashes and prophylactic anti-candidal preparations with nystatin suspension or clotrimazole gel. Local relief of pain may be achieved using soluble aspirin or benzydamine mouthwashes. If symptoms are severe and nutritional intake is compromised, enteral feeding via a nasogastric fine bore tube or more commonly a percutaneous gastrostomy, may be required. Radical high-dose treatment to the oral cavity, particularly if the salivary glands are included in the treatment volume, can result in troublesome mouth dryness and loss of taste, and predispose to dental caries and osteoradionecrosis of the jaw. Pre-treatment dental assessment and meticulous hygiene using fluoride dental gel during and after treatment is important in these patients. These measures are not required for simple low-dose palliative treatments, such as radiation to a metastasis in the mandible. Oropharyngeal effects are worse in those patients who smoke or imbibe alcohol, and if possible, these should be avoided during treatment.

Pneumonitis may occur, even after palliative treatment to the lungs. Patients develop dry cough and dyspnoea up to four months after treatment and have a radiograph showing patchy shadowing conforming to the geometry of the radiation field (Fig. 12.3.2). A 2–3-week course of systemic steroids and antibiotics for secondary infection is recommended. Symptoms may continue and late radiation fibrosis may occur.

It is always important to anticipate likely acute side effects, explain them to the patient, and encourage the prophylactic use of antiemetics, antidiarrhoeal drugs, and mouthwashes. The patient should also be reassured that these are temporary events which will resolve following completion of radiotherapy.

Combined modality treatment

Combined modality treatment refers to the administration of chemotherapy during a course of radical radiotherapy to enhance the effects. Substantial Level I evidence supports this practice for cancers of the oesophagus (Herskovic et al., 1992), anal canal

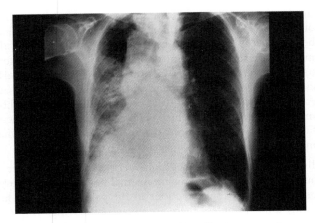

Fig. 12.3.2 Interstitial pneumonitis in the right and lower zones on chest radiograph after palliative radiotherapy for carcinoma of the bronchus.

(Ryan et al., 2000), uterine cervix (Thomas, 1999), lung (Komakil et al., 2000) and head and neck (Munro, 1995). Other treatment strategies involve the administration of chemotherapy before (neo-adjuvant) or more commonly after (adjuvant) radiotherapy to control micro-metastases whilst the radiotherapy obtains local control of the more bulky primary site. These approaches are used in the management of breast cancer, bladder cancer, small cell lung cancer, colorectal cancer, and lymphoma.

Radiotherapy and symptom control

Radiotherapy is effective for many cancer-related symptoms, particularly those due to pressure or infiltration by a tumour (Table 12.3.4).

Bone pain

Radiotherapy may be indicated for bone metastases because of bone pain, pathological fracture, or pressure on nerves. It is a highly effective treatment for local pain and achieves durable pain control for the majority of patients. Those with advanced illness can benefit from simple, short treatment schedules, and if pain recurs in those who survive longer, retreatment can be used.

There is extensive evidence supporting the efficacy of radiation for bone pain. Although a fractionated course of treatment delivering 20–30 Gy over 1–2 weeks is preferred by some centres, especially where there is concern over possible fracture or nerve compression, meta-analyses that include more than 3000 patients conclude that single-fraction treatments delivering 8 Gy generally yield comparable results (Fig. 12.3.3) (McQuay et al., 1997; Sze et al., 2003; Wu et al., 2003; Chow et al, 2012). One large randomized trial revealed a response rate of around 80% and pain control maintained out to 12 months (Bone Pain Trial Working Party, 1999) (Fig. 12.3.4). Pain improves progressively for weeks after treatment; about half of patients achieve pain relief within the first 2–4 weeks and others experience adequate relief after 6–8 weeks (Fig. 12.3.4).

Meta-analyses indicate that a higher proportion of patients require retreatment after single-dose treatments than after fractionated treatments. In most trials, about 25% of patients who receive single doses undergo retreatment. This is not a justification for more prolonged treatments, however. The Dutch bone pain trial (van der Linden et al., 2004) confirmed that single-dose

Table 12.3.4 Indications for radiotherapy in symptom palliation

Symptom	Cause
Pain	
Bone pain	Bone metastases
Visceral pain	Soft tissue metastases
Neuropathic pain	Bone metastases
	Soft tissue primary or metastases
	Intrinsic tumour in nerve tissue
Local pressure	
Spinal canal compression	Extradural metastases
	Bone metastases
Cranial nerve palsies	Skull base bone metastases
	Meningeal metastases
	Intrinsic brain tumour
Obstruction	
Bronchus	Intrinsic bronchial tumour
	Extrinsic lymphadenopathy
Oesophagus	Intrinsic bronchial tumour
	Extrinsic lymphadenopathy
Superior vena cava	Primary mediastinal tumour
	Primary lung or oesophageal tumour
	Metastatic mediastinal lymphadenopathy
Hydrocephalus	Malignant meningitis
	Primary or metastatic brain tumour
Limb swelling	Metastatic lymphadenopathy
Bleeding	
Haemoptysis	Primary bronchial tumour
	Metastatic bronchial or lung tumour
Haematuria	Primary tumour in kidney,
	Ureter, bladder, prostate
Vaginal bleeding	Primary tumours of vagina, cervix or uterus
	Metastases in vagina
Rectal bleeding	Primary anal or colorectal tumours

radiotherapy is equivalent to multifraction treatment for localized bone pain, even with the requirement for retreatment. The probability of response after re-treatment is around 80%, similar to that after primary treatment, and the effect is not always predicted by the initial response (Huisman et al., 2012). For this reason, re-irradiation should be considered when pain returns after a previous good response and when the initial response is unsatisfactory. The best dose for retreatment is uncertain and is the subject of a recently completed randomized trial comparing single-dose retreatment with multifraction retreatment (Chow et al., 2006).

The treatment techniques for bone metastasis are usually simple. Superficial bones such as the clavicle, ribs, and sacrum may be treated with a direct field using orthovoltage X-rays or electrons and other sites are treated using a linear accelerator or cobalt beam. Under optimal conditions, the site is localized using a treatment simulator based on clinical examination and radiographic or bone scan evidence of metastatic disease. Increasingly, CT simulation is used to more accurately define the field (Haddad et al., 2004). It is particularly important to document carefully the field margin, since most patients will have multiple sites of metastasis and overlap of fields should be avoided at the time of later treatment. This is especially important in the treatment of spinal metastases. If sequential treatments are required, overlapping fields increase the risk of overdosage to the spinal cord, which may culminate in radiation myelitis and irreversible neurological deterioration developing within 6–9 months from treatment. This is not a concern if patients have a short prognosis, in which case a decision to accept an overlap may be made, with the full knowledge of the patient, if it is perceived that benefit from treatment in the short term outweighs any theoretical hazard of later myelitis.

Patients with multiple sites of disease and pain that is diffuse or multifocal may be considered for wide field radiotherapy or radioisotope therapy. Wide field radiotherapy delivers treatment to an area that may include up to half the body, using doses of 6 Gy to the upper half-body, where the lungs limit higher doses, or 8 Gy to the lower half-body. The response rate is around 80% and pain relief is maintained until death in the majority of patients (Salazar et al., 1986, 2001). There is no advantage to higher doses, although one randomized trial recommended 8 Gy in 2 fractions as the optimum dose (Salazar et al., 2001).

Inevitably, wide field treatment is associated with greater toxicity than local field irradiation. About two-thirds of patients have nausea, vomiting, or diarrhoea, and the majority of patients have a period of bone marrow suppression, which may require blood transfusions but rarely causes clinically relevant neutropenia or thrombocytopenia. Spontaneous recovery is expected, and indeed, sequential treatment of upper and lower half-bodies is possible given a 4–6-week gap for marrow recovery. The most serious consequence of upper hemibody irradiation is the development of radiation pneumonitis, which may be avoided by limiting the dose to 6 Gy through the lungs.

Radioactive isotopes that selectively concentrate at sites of bone metastasis also may be used for diffuse or multifocal bone pain. The ideal isotope delivers radiation by releasing beta particles with a short range of only a few millimetres, thereby concentrating the dose within the immediate area of uptake (Table 12.3.5). Low-energy gamma release is also desirable as this enables imaging of the isotope distribution with a gamma camera. Single injections of strontium (Hoskin, 1994) or samarium (Sartor et al., 2004) are used most often, and samarium, which has no gamma release, requires no restrictions on the patient other than careful disposal of urine. Both these compounds are highly effective, with response rates similar to wide field external beam irradiation and fewer side effects (Hoskin, 1994). Their efficacy has been demonstrated predominantly in prostate cancer, but bone metastases from other primary sites, in particular breast and lung, are also effectively treated. Even metastases from osteosarcoma, which retains an osteblastic response, may concentrate these isotopes and be effectively treated. The treatments are costly, however, and they are relatively underused, particularly in less wealthy health

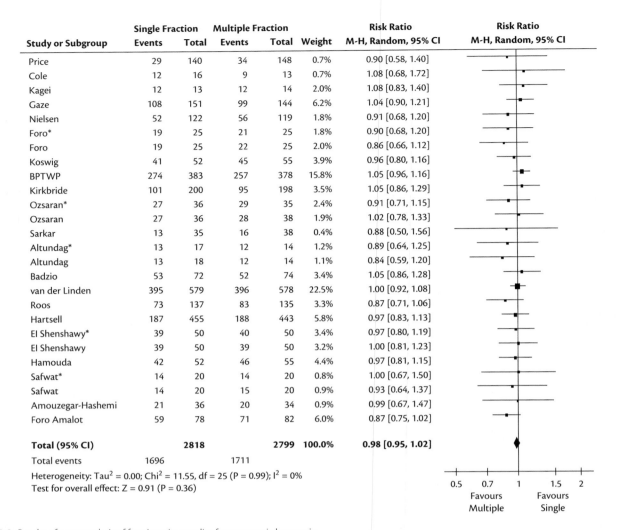

| Study or Subgroup | Single Fraction | | Multiple Fraction | | Weight | Risk Ratio M-H, Random, 95% CI | Risk Ratio M-H, Random, 95% CI |
	Events	Total	Events	Total			
Price	29	140	34	148	0.7%	0.90 [0.58, 1.40]	
Cole	12	16	9	13	0.7%	1.08 [0.68, 1.72]	
Kagei	12	13	12	14	2.0%	1.08 [0.83, 1.40]	
Gaze	108	151	99	144	6.2%	1.04 [0.90, 1.21]	
Nielsen	52	122	56	119	1.8%	0.91 [0.68, 1.20]	
Foro*	19	25	21	25	1.8%	0.90 [0.68, 1.20]	
Foro	19	25	22	25	2.0%	0.86 [0.66, 1.12]	
Koswig	41	52	45	55	3.9%	0.96 [0.80, 1.16]	
BPTWP	274	383	257	378	15.8%	1.05 [0.96, 1.16]	
Kirkbride	101	200	95	198	3.5%	1.05 [0.86, 1.29]	
Ozsaran*	27	36	29	35	2.4%	0.91 [0.71, 1.15]	
Ozsaran	27	36	28	38	1.9%	1.02 [0.78, 1.33]	
Sarkar	13	35	16	38	0.4%	0.88 [0.50, 1.56]	
Altundag*	13	17	12	14	1.2%	0.89 [0.64, 1.25]	
Altundag	13	18	12	14	1.1%	0.84 [0.59, 1.20]	
Badzio	53	72	52	74	3.4%	1.05 [0.86, 1.28]	
van der Linden	395	579	396	578	22.5%	1.00 [0.92, 1.08]	
Roos	73	137	83	135	3.3%	0.87 [0.71, 1.06]	
Hartsell	187	455	188	443	5.8%	0.97 [0.83, 1.13]	
El Shenshawy*	39	50	40	50	3.4%	0.97 [0.80, 1.19]	
El Shenshawy	39	50	39	50	3.2%	1.00 [0.81, 1.23]	
Hamouda	42	52	46	55	4.4%	0.97 [0.81, 1.15]	
Safwat*	14	20	14	20	0.8%	1.00 [0.67, 1.50]	
Safwat	14	20	15	20	0.9%	0.93 [0.64, 1.37]	
Amouzegar-Hashemi	21	36	20	34	0.9%	0.99 [0.67, 1.47]	
Foro Amalot	59	78	71	82	6.0%	0.87 [0.75, 1.02]	
Total (95% CI)		**2818**		**2799**	**100.0%**	**0.98 [0.95, 1.02]**	
Total events	1696		1711				

Heterogeneity: Tau^2 = 0.00; Chi^2 = 11.55, df = 25 (P = 0.99); I^2 = 0%
Test for overall effect: Z = 0.91 (P = 0.36)

Fig. 12.3.3 Results of meta-analysis of fractionation studies for metastatic bone pain.
Reproduced from *Clinical Oncology*, Volume 24, Issue 2, Chow E. et al., Update on the Systematic Review of Palliative Radiotherapy Trials for Bone, pp.112–124, Copyright © 2011 The Royal College of Radiologists, with permission from Elsevier, http://www.sciencedirect.com/science/journal/09366555.

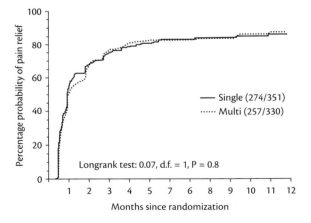

Fig. 12.3.4 Probability of pain relief seen after local radiotherapy for metastatic bone pain
Reproduced from *Radiotherapy and Oncology*, Volume 52, Issue 2, Bone Pain Trial Working Party, 8 Gy single fraction radiotherapy for the treatment of metastatic skeletal pain: randomised comparison with a multifraction schedule over 12 months of patient follow-up, pp.111–121, Copyright © 1999 Elsevier Science Ireland Ltd., with permission from Elsevier, http://www.sciencedirect.com/science/journal/01678140.

ecomonies, despite their established efficacy, convenience, and favourable toxicity profile.

Radioisotope treatment can cause transient bone marrow depression, but this is rarely of clinical significance provided patients have a normal blood count at the start of therapy. These compounds are cleared by renal excretion and patients must be continent of urine to prevent contamination, or be prepared to have an indwelling catheter for the duration of radioactive excretion. Renal impairment is a relative contraindication because reduced clearance can prolong radiation exposure and potentially exacerbate bone marrow toxicity.

In contrast to patients with multiple metastases, those with only one or two (oligometastases) are potential candidates for local therapy using a high enough dose to achieve both pain relief and local tumour control. This may be accomplished using stereotactic body radiotherapy, which enables localization of very high-dose radiation in a small area. An example of such a treatment to a solitary metastasis in the pubis is shown in Fig. 12.3.5. The evidence base for such treatments is evolving; good pain relief with local control rates of 60–70% at 1 year have been reported (Lo et al., 2010).

Table 12.3.5 Radioisotopes available for treatment of metastatic bone pain

Tumour specific	Bone specific	Bisphosphonate conjugates
131I	89Sr	153Sm
	223Ra	186Re
		188Re

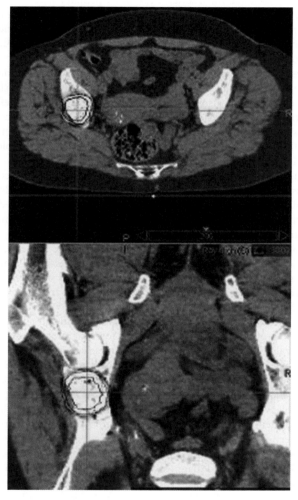

Fig. 12.3.5 Stereotactic radiotherapy plan to treat a solitary pelvic metastasis; note how the isodose lines conform tightly to the region of the metastasis enabling high-dose delivery with minimal dose to surrounding tissues.

The mechanism by which radiation achieves pain control is not clear. Tumour shrinkage may not be necessary. Although a considerable proportion of malignant cells within a tumour mass are undoubtedly killed after small single doses of radiation, rapid tumour shrinkage is not routinely observed. Pain relief may be seen within 24 hours, particularly after hemibody irradiation and there is no relationship between pain relief and histological types of tumour correlating with variations in radiosensitivity. There also has been no clear dose response effect above 8 Gy. Osteoclast activation may be another important factor, as suggested by the efficacy of bisphosphonate drugs. Following radiotherapy, changes

in biochemical markers of osteoclast activity occur and these may predict response (Hoskin et al., 2000).

The increased understanding of the pathophysiology of metastatic bone pain has led to further developments in treatment. Current research is seeking to evaluate the role of pregabalin with radiotherapy and new agents such as denosumab directed at RANKL (ligand for the receptor activator of nuclear factor kappa B), a pivotal molecule in osteoclast activation are also under evaluation.

Although there is some evidence that radiotherapy can prevent the later development of pain metastases or pain, there is no routine role for prophylactic treatment. Inadvertent treatment of the thoracic spine when a breast is irradiated has been shown to reduce the instance of subsequent bone metastases. Hemibody irradiation and strontium therapy both modestly reduce subsequent episodes of bone pain (Poulter et al., 1992; Porter et al., 1993). There is stronger evidence in favour of bisphosphonate treatment, which is now routinely given for myeloma and high-risk patients with breast cancer (Diel et al., 1998; McCloskey et al., 1998).

The relative roles of radiotherapy and bisphosphonates, and the interaction between them, in the overall management of bone metastases have yet to be adequately defined and are currently an active area of research (Hoskin, 2003). Early results from a recent randomized trial suggest that radiotherapy and ibandronate are equivalent in achieving pain control with some suggestion of a synergistic effect (Hoskin et al., 2011)

Pathological fracture

When surgery is not possible or indicated for pathological fracture, local irradiation remains a valuable tool to achieve local pain relief and enable bone healing. Although there are no data to define the optimal dose, single dose of 8 Gy is adequate when the object of treatment is pain relief alone; about two-thirds of patients achieve pain relief. In practice most patients will receive courses delivering 20–30 Gy in 5–10 fractions over 1–2 weeks. Remineralization is reported in one-third of patients after doses of 40–50 Gy delivered in 4–5 weeks, but anecdotally, also occurs after lower doses of only 20 Gy in 2 weeks.

Radiotherapy may also be indicated postoperatively following internal fixation to prevent further progression of the remaining metastatic tumour and enable healing of the bone around the prosthesis. Although there are few data to support this common practice, a non-randomized study suggests better functional recovery when radiotherapy is given (Townsend et al., 1995). Conventionally, fields covering the entire length of the prosthesis or intramedullary nail are used because of the perceived risk of tumour dissemination through the marrow cavity by the operative procedure. Patients with widespread metastatic disease, limited survival, and adequate pain control gain little benefit from postoperative radiotherapy.

Neurological symptoms and disorders

Spinal cord and cauda equina compression

Spinal cord or cauda equina compression may cause catastrophic loss of limb function and sphincter control (see Chapters 14.1 and 12.5). As tumour compresses neurological tissue in the spinal canal, there is early venous engorgement and oedema followed by mechanical compression that ultimately leads to irreversible damage. About one-quarter of cases occur due to direct encroachment of the spinal canal by tumour in a vertebral body and the rest are attributable to blood borne extradural or intradural metastases (Fig. 12.3.6) (Pigott et al., 1994). Approximately 70% of cases involve thoracic cord, 20% the lumbosacral region, and 10% the cervical cord.

Early diagnosis and treatment is the major determinant of outcome. Spinal cord or cauda equina compression should be suspected in any patient with sensory or motor findings in the limbs or urinary symptoms, in particular where there is backache or known vertebral metastasis. Prompt visualization of the spinal

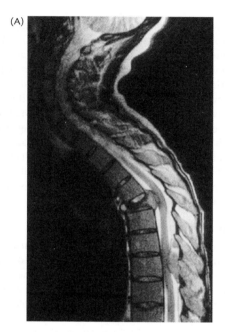

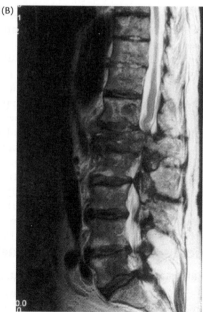

Fig. 12.3.6 Magnetic resonance imaging of spinal cord compression demonstrating (A) both extradural and vertebral collapse with adjacent compression and (B) direct infiltration of the canal from bone metastases in the spine.

canal using magnetic resonance imaging is the optimal management, even if recent investigations have shown no evidence of metastatic disease. If magnetic resonance imaging (MRI) is unavailable or contraindicated because of metal implants or a pacemaker, CT imaging should be used. If MRI is negative and the clinical findings are suggestive, a lumbar puncture is needed to exclude meningeal carcinomatosis.

The commonest causes of spinal cord compression are tumours of the breast, lung, or prostate, each of which accounts for about 20% of patients in most series. Most other primary sites have also been associated with spinal canal involvement, with the next two commonest being kidney and lymphoma. If a patient with metastatic disease presents with spinal cord compression, it is usually reasonable to assume that this will be the same disease process unless there are atypical features to suggest a second primary. Patients with spinal cord or cauda equina compression and no history of metastatic disease require a histological diagnosis before treatment. In one series, 48% of patients with spinal cord compression had no previous history of malignant disease (Shaw et al., 1980). In most cases, a CT-guided fine-needle aspirate cytology specimen or needle biopsy will be sufficient (Findlay, 1988).

The initial management of spinal cord or cauda equina compression includes administration of a corticosteroid and local irradiation to the spinal site. The corticosteroid doses used in practice vary greatly but are generally relatively high, for example, dexamethasone 4 mg every 6 hours or higher.

Both radiotherapy and decompressive surgery are effective in the initial management of spinal cord compression. Primary treatment of some tumours, such as lymphoma and small cell lung cancer, includes chemotherapy. One randomized trial that compared radiotherapy with decompressive surgery via an anterior approach followed by radiotherapy showed significant advantage for the group receiving surgery, both for functional status and survival. The population in this trial was selected for those with good performance status, absent metastases elsewhere and a single level of spinal cord compression; patients with these characteristics should be referred for surgery followed by radiotherapy, if possible. Whilst no randomized comparison of the two modalities of treatment with sufficient numbers to provide a true comparison has been undertaken, no advantage of surgery over radiotherapy has been demonstrated in published series where patients have a previously confirmed diagnosis of malignant disease and no evidence of vertebral collapse. The role of postoperative radiotherapy has not been tested but a non-randomized comparison has suggested that better pain relief is seen after radiotherapy or where radiotherapy is given postoperatively (Findlay, 1984).

In patients who have extensive vertebral collapse with intrusion to the spinal canal, radiotherapy is of little value in re-establishing neurological function, and surgery using an anterior approach and spinal stabilization also must be considered. This procedure is far more invasive than radiotherapy and has significant operative morbidity and even mortality, but results in selected patients are superior to either laminectomy or radiotherapy alone, with 62–83% of patients being able to walk and 71% achieving pain relief (Siegal and Siegal, 1985; Moore and Uttley, 1989). Many of these patients, however, are in poor general condition, as shown by a 30% mortality in one series of 26 consecutive patients operated on for pain or neurological deficits. Careful selection of patients for surgical referral is required (Patchell et al., 2005).

When primary radiotherapy is the treatment of choice, the technique in most cases is simple, using a single posterior field to encompass the vertebral level and a suitable margin. With accurate localization using MRI, one vertebral body or 3 cm above and below the area of cord compression is adequate. Problems may arise where there are multiple sites of compression, particularly if anatomically distant. In some patients, more than one radiation field may be required to cover the sites. When there is a large paravertebral mass, more complex planning may be necessary to ensure complete coverage. Two or three angled fields to cover the tumour volume, taking care to avoid sensitive paravertebral structures such as the kidneys, may be needed.

Most patients with good performance status will receive fractionated courses of treatment, delivering 20–30 Gy in 5–10 fractions. Most patients who have lost ambulation for more than 24 hours will not regain it, and in these cases, a single dose of 8–10 Gy often is given for pain relief, without any expectation of neurological recovery. In other selected cases, particularly those with a localized, potentially curable tumour, such as a solitary plasmacytoma, higher doses of up to 40 or 50 Gy over 3–5 weeks may be delivered.

The outcome of radiotherapy depends primarily upon the speed of diagnosis and neurological status at initiation of treatment. When patients begin treatment while ambulatory, more than three-quarters retain the ability to walk; of those who are paraparetic, only 42% become ambulant and 20–25% deteriorate during treatment. More than three-quarters have pain relief, compared with only one-third following laminectomy. Histology may influence outcome, patients with myeloma and lymphoma having a better outcome than those with breast cancer, who in turn respond better than those with lung or kidney tumours. There is some evidence that these patients may benefit from higher-dose radiotherapy (Rades et al., 2011).

Since the outcome of treatment is best when diagnosis is made very early there would be considerable advantages in predicting those patients at risk of spinal cord compression and treating them prophylactically. MRI can detect vertebral metastasis at very early stages when minor encroachment into the spinal canal is clinically asymptomatic and not detectable on plain radiographs. Other predictors for spinal canal compression reported in small cell lung cancer are local back pain associated with positive bone scan in the spine or cerebral metastasis with a positive bone scan; these situations are associated with cord compression in 36% and 25%, respectively (Goldman et al., 1989). Early use of radiotherapy would be likely to have a positive effect on outcomes, and in some centres, there is an aggressive policy of prophylactic irradiation for spinal metastasis on this basis. There is some evidence from the use of bisphosphonates that prophylactic treatment of subclinical bone metastasis can reduce spinal complications and similar observations have been made using early antiandrogen treatment in prostate cancer.

Brain metastasis

Up to 10% of all cancers metastasize to the brain, the most common primary sites being the lung and breast; approximately one-third of these will be solitary deposits (see Chapter 14.1). Disability from brain metastasis is disproportionate to the bulk of the tumour. A very small deposit on the motor cortex can be catastrophic for the patient, whilst a deposit of similar size would have little effect in the lung or liver. Because the spread of malignant cells to the brain is via blood, isolated brain metastases are relatively unusual; the typical patient has widespread metastatic disease. Careful patient assessment and selection of those who may benefit from active treatment is therefore essential, recognizing that for a proportion this will herald the terminal phase of an advanced malignancy for which local treatment will have little benefit.

After confirmation of the diagnosis by CT or MRI, steroids are used to help control raised intracranial pressure and reduce symptoms due to oedema rather than tumour infiltration. There is evidence that high-dose steroids in this setting contribute significantly to morbidity and total doses of 4–8mg dexamethasone daily may be adequate. If the patient does not have known metastatic disease, a histological diagnosis is needed; whilst it is preferable to biopsy a site other than the brain, an intracranial needle biopsy will be needed if a solitary brain lesion is the first manifestation of malignancy.

Further management depends upon the general condition of the patient, underlying primary site, and the distribution of the brain metastases (Fig. 12.3.7). Solitary metastases usually reflect a more favourable prognosis, and in selected patients with no detectable systemic disease, surgical removal gives good local and long-term control. Postoperative radiotherapy is usually recommended on the basis of two randomized trials, which showed a significant reduction in brain recurrence (but no impact on survival because of a high incidence of death from progressive systemic disease); a third larger trial has failed to confirm this advantage for postoperative radiotherapy (Tsao et al., 2012).

Localized high-dose radiotherapy using radiosurgery is an alternative to surgical excision. There has been no formal comparison between the two, but where surgery is limited by the site of metastasis and proximity to critical structures, it may be considered an alternative. Radiosurgery uses either a dedicated multisource cobalt unit (gamma knife) or a stereotactic high-energy X-ray unit to deliver single doses of 15–20 Gy. The role of whole-brain radiotherapy after radiosurgery, analogous to the use of postoperative radiotherapy, remains uncertain, but is recommended in some centres. Recent studies suggest that post-radiosurgery treatment may reduce the likelihood of relapse outside the initial site of treatment, it imparts no survival benefit and may result in impaired neurocognitive functioning (Linskey et al., 2010). Unfortunately, the 1-year survival of patients with solitary brain metastases is 30–50%, despite effective local control with surgery or radiosurgery. Most patients succumb to the effects of distant metastasis and careful selection and screening is required before embarking upon aggressive local therapy of this type.

Whole-brain radiotherapy is well established as an effective palliative treatment for multiple cerebral metastases, yielding benefit for headache, motor and sensory loss, and confusion in about 80% of patients; a complete response occurs in 35–55% (Linskey et al., 2010). Median survival after irradiation is less than 6 months, reflecting the fact that brain metastasis often heralds widespread advanced metastatic disease. Twenty per cent of patients who embark upon a course of radiotherapy for brain metastases fail to complete the course, which highlights the need for careful selection in determining which patients may benefit from radiotherapy. Those with multiple metastases outside the central nervous system and those with poor performance status and rapidly progressive disease are most likely to succumb within the period of treatment (Table 12.3.6).

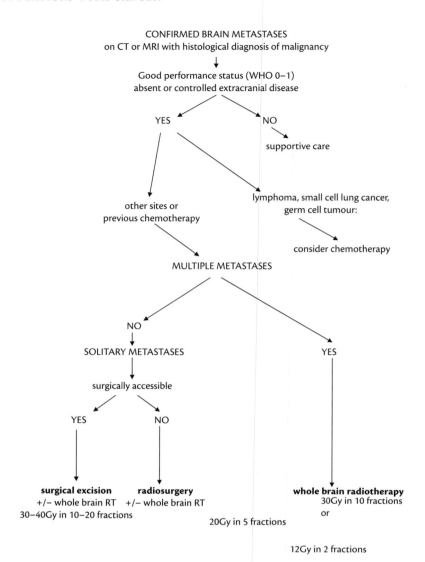

Fig. 12.3.7 Algorithm for the management of brain metastases.

Table 12.3.6 Prognostic factors influencing survival after irradiation of brain metastases

Increased survival	Decreased survival
Brain first site of relapse	Multiple lobes involved
Brain sole site of relapse	> 3 metastases
Long disease-free interval prior to brain relapse	Meningeal disease
Primary site in brain	
Performance status 0/1	
Age < 60 years	

Treatment techniques for multiple brain metastases are simple, using lateral fields from each side (parallel opposed fields) covering the entire intracranial contents. A series of randomized trials have shown no benefit for doses greater than 20–30 Gy in 1–2 weeks (Borgelt et al., 1982) and there is one trial which has shown similar effects after12 Gy in 2 fractions compared to 30 Gy in 10 fractions (Priestman et al., 1996). For patients with advanced disease and only moderate performance status, a simple two fraction schedule can be recommended.

There is usually little acute toxicity from a short palliative course of whole-brain radiotherapy for multiple brain metastases, but an unfortunate and unavoidable effect is complete alopecia. Although hair returns within 2–3 months, some patients are highly distressed by the change, and for some, alopecia is an unacceptable cost of treatment. Mild scalp erythema may also occur, particularly around the external pinnae. Most patients continue steroids through treatment in an effort to prevent transient rises in intracranial pressure. Following completion of cranial irradiation, steroid treatment should be tapered, and if possible, discontinued to minimize long-term side effects. Over the longer term, some patients who receive cranial irradiation experience deterioration in neurocognitive function; this is an important consideration in patients likely to survive for a prolonged period.

About a quarter patients experience persistent or recurrent cerebral metastasis. Re-treatment with radiotherapy following a dose of 20–30 Gy carries a risk of radiation damage to the brain and there is often reluctance to consider re-irradiation for recurrent disease. Without treatment, however, progressive morbidity and ultimately death from brain metastasis will occur. Neurological sequelae from radiation damage may take many months if not years to manifest and the risks of low dose re-treatment (a further 20–30 Gy in 2–3 weeks) may be worth taking for selected patients who have a good initial response to treatment. Similarly, recurrence at a solitary site can be an indication for stereotactic re-irradiation.

Primary brain tumours

Primary brain tumours usually are treated by surgery, radiotherapy, or both with curative intent. Grade III or IV astrocytomas are extremely malignant and have a prognosis of only a few months if untreated. Palliative radiotherapy for the latter patients may be of value and the best results occur in those aged younger than 60 who have no neurological deficits and present with seizures. In patients with good performance status, high-dose treatment delivering 60 Gy in 30 fractions with adjuvant and concomitant temozolamide, improves median survival from 12.1 months to 14.6 months and 2 year survival from 10.4% to 26.5% compared to radiotherapy alone (Stupp et al., 2005). In those with poor performance status, significant neurological deficits and older age, significant benefit from a high dose treatment schedule is rarely seen and short schedules delivering doses of 20–30 Gy over 1–3 weeks should be considered (Thomas et al., 1994).

Diffuse meningeal carcinomatosis is generally a pre-terminal event, with a median survival of only a few weeks if untreated. It may present with symptoms and signs of multifocal radiculopathy or cranial neuropathy, or with headache or backache. There may be raised intracranial pressure. Common primary sites breast and lung, and central nervous system relapse of leukaemia also typically presents with malignant meningitis. The diagnosis is suspected on MRI and confirmed by cerebrospinal fluid sampling.

Intensive treatment may be indicated where there is a treatable underlying malignancy. In the case of acute leukaemia and lymphoma, sustained remissions may be achieved by the use of intrathecal chemotherapy using methotrexate and cytosine arabinoside, sometimes combined with craniospinal irradiation (radiotherapy to the entire brain and spinal cord) or cranial irradiation alone. Such treatment is no small undertaking and may be associated with significant morbidity due to bone marrow depression, nausea and vomiting, and alopecia. In children, there are also the associated issues of impaired spinal growth and intellectual development after radiotherapy to the spine and brain respectively. Furthermore it is unfortunately the case that despite initial remission, central nervous system relapse of lymphoma or leukaemia is generally associated with a poor overall prognosis,

The outlook for meningeal carcinomatosis from solid tumours is even worse and even intensive therapy with intrathecal chemotherapy and craniospinal irradiation will extend prognosis from a few weeks to a few months, much of which may be taken up with treatment (Wasserstrom et al., 1982). On this basis judicious local irradiation to specific sites causing symptoms, such as the skull base when cranial nerves are involved or the segments of the spinal cord related to nerve root symptoms, delivering a dose of 20 Gy in 5 fractions, offers a more pragmatic approach, potentially palliating symptoms whilst minimizing the morbidity and duration of treatment in a universally fatal condition.

Cranial nerve palsies

Cranial neuropathy may arise from intrinsic metastasis in the brainstem, infiltration of the leptomeninges, compression by extradural deposits, or bone involvement in the skull base. The management of intrinsic metastasis and leptomeningeal metastasis has been discussed above; results of whole-brain irradiation show an overall response rate of 78% and a complete response rate of 42% (Vikram and Chu, 1979). Local irradiation of the skull base when diffuse bone involvement has resulted in cranial nerve compression, yields improvement in 50–78% of patients, which is maintained until death in around 80%. In general, patients with skull base metastasis have a better prognosis (median survival of 10–20 months) than those with intrinsic central nervous system metastases, their (Vikram and Chu, 1979; Hall et al., 1983).

Peripheral nerve symptoms

Tumour compression of nerve roots, nerve plexus, or peripheral nerves can result in motor or sensory loss, or neuropathic pain, in the distribution of the nerve. A large randomized trial that evaluated the efficacy of local radiotherapy in neuropathic pain observed an overall response rate of 57%, with 26% achieving a complete response at three months after treatment (Roos et al., 2005). In keeping with the experience of uncomplicated bone metastases, single doses of 8 Gy were not inferior to more prolonged fractionated doses. Lumbosacral neuropathic pain responded to palliative doses of radiotherapy with complete pain relief within one month in 85–100% of patients (Russi et al., 1993). Pelvic irradiation for pain relief for recurrent colorectal cancer is successful in up to 80% of patients, with no difference detected between a 3-week course of treatment delivering 45 Gy and a single dose of 10 Gy (James et al., 1983). Treatment to apical lung tumours or axillary recurrence of breast cancer causing upper limb pain due to brachial plexus neuropathy is successful in up to 77% of patients using typical doses of 20–30 Gy in 1–2 weeks (Ampil et al., 1985).

Choroidal and orbital metastasis

Metastases to the eye are unusual but may cause distressing proptosis, pain and visual disturbance. Unless treated, there is progressive deterioration and ultimately loss of vision. The most common intraocular site is the choroid and the most common tumour types are breast (> 50%) and lung (30%); about 25% are bilateral. After diagnosis by fundoscopy or slit lamp examination, radiotherapy delivering doses of 30–40 Gy in 2–4 weeks can improve vision in up to 86% of patients (Rudoler et al., 1997; Wiegel et al., 2002). Asymptomatic lesions should also be treated to preserve vision. Local tumour control is reported in 98% of treated patients.

Metastasis at other intra-orbital sites are less common and may arise haematogenously or through direct invasion from other head and neck sites, in particular the nasopharynx, nasal cavity, and sinuses. Palliative irradiation may prevent or relieve local symptoms from pressure and infiltration.

Radiotherapy to the eye and orbit requires meticulous attention to technique, avoiding as far as possible direct irradiation of the cornea, which can result in painful keratitis. Whenever possible, the lens also should be shielded to prevent cataracts, which may be induced after only 5–10 Gy. Radiation cataracts may take many years to evolve and should not be considered a reason for avoiding radiation to the orbit in the context of palliative treatment.

Cerebral lymphoma

The incidence of primary lymphoma of the central nervous system, a rare extranodal non-Hodgkin lymphoma, has increased in recent years due to its association with advanced HIV infection. It may cause headache, fits, cranial nerve palsies, or other focal neurological signs. Initial treatment with a steroid may achieve good symptom palliation and some tumour regression, but the mainstay of modern treatment is chemotherapy, typically using high-dose methotrexate, which results in a median survival of 10–18 months (Laperriere et al., 1997). The role of whole-brain radiotherapy in addition to chemotherapy in radical treatment has been questioned, particularly in the light of late effects on cognitive function in survivors. It is currently under investigation. Whole-brain radiotherapy has a role in primary treatment for older patients unable to tolerate intensive chemotherapy. Doses of 40–50 Gy may be given (Schultz and Bovi, 2010), but late changes in neurocognitive function are common. In advanced cases, those with relapse after chemotherapy, with poor performance status or with a significant co-morbidity, a short treatment delivering a dose of 30 Gy in 10 fractions over 2 weeks will be of value.

Obstructive symptoms

Mediastinal compression and superior vena cava obstruction

The syndrome of superior vena cava obstruction (SVCO) may arise due to occlusion by extrinsic compression, intraluminal thrombosis, or direct invasion of the vessel wall. The majority of cases are due to malignant tumour within the mediastinum but other rare causes which should be excluded include aortic aneurysm, chronic mediastinitis, trauma, or thrombosis following central venous catheterization. Approximately 3% of patients with carcinoma of the bronchus and 8% of those with lymphoma develop SVCO; of those with SVCO, 75% have primary bronchial carcinomas (40% small cell lung cancer) and 15% have lymphoma.

The extent to increased venous pressure above the site of obstruction produces symptoms depends on the efficiency of collateral vessels, particularly the internal mammary vessels, pulmonary veins, and the thoracic and vertebral venous plexuses. Obstruction above the azygos vein produces a lesser effect than obstruction below this level. Impeded venous drainage from the head can cause headaches, somnolence, and dizziness; more rarely convulsions result from cerebral hypertension. Oedema and pressure within the mediastinum may cause dysphagia, dyspnoea, cough, or hoarseness. Examination may reveal fixed engorgement of arm and neck veins with visible dilatation of superficial skin veins, cyanosis, and facial oedema.

Whilst potentially a hazardous condition, emergency treatment rarely is needed, and it is important to have a full and accurate assessment of the underlying disease, together with a histological diagnosis, in order to ensure that correct therapy is instigated. Presentation with SVCO is not a contraindication to radical curative treatment when this is appropriate, for example, mediastinal Hodgkin lymphoma, and it is important not to compromise management by inappropriate emergency treatment. A policy of delayed treatment until definitive tissue diagnosis can be achieved has been evaluated in a large review of 1986 patients presenting with SVCO which found that only one death could be directly attributed to venous obstruction (caused by aspiration of blood after epistaxis) (Ahman, 1984). Although biopsy within a region of raised venous pressure raises concerns about the risk of haemorrhage, in practice bronchoscopy, mediastinoscopy or lymph node biopsy are performed without major complications and should be undertaken unless there is life-threatening large airways obstruction.

Management of SVCO should address both symptoms and the cause of the obstruction. Steroids are usually administered, such as dexamethasone 12–16 mg daily, although there is no good objective data to support this practice. In some cases, prompt symptom relief may be possible with bronchoscopy and stenting, or the insertion of a superior vena cava stent (Lanciego et al., 2001). Chemotherapy is appropriate for some tumour types, in particular small cell lung cancer, Hodgkin's disease, non-Hodgkin's lymphoma, and germ cell tumours. For other tumours, radiotherapy to the mediastinum covering the tumour mass and adjacent lymph nodes areas where appropriate is indicated. If a stent is placed, this is followed by radiotherapy. In the palliative setting, it is usual to deliver doses of 20–30 Gy in 1–2 weeks, but where the primary tumour is localized and radical treatment would otherwise be indicated, a radical course of radiotherapy or chemoradiation should not be denied the patient.

Symptomatic relief following irradiation for SVCO is reported in 50–95% of patients within the first 2 weeks of treatment. Treatment may have little effect upon the obstruction to blood flow in the superior vena cava, which persists in three-quarters of patients. This suggests that the development of collaterals, rather than the physical release of compression from the superior vena cava, is most important in achieving the observed clinical improvement (Ahman, 1984). Long-term survival is determined by the underlying disease, rather than the syndrome itself, with the exception of the relatively rare instance of large airway obstruction or cerebral oedema when urgent treatment is required.

Lung collapse secondary to bronchial obstruction

The most common cause of complete bronchial occlusion leading to collapse of lung is intrinsic carcinoma of the bronchus. Less often, occlusion results from extrinsic compression by mediastinal nodal invasion by carcinoma or lymphoma. When obstruction occurs rapidly, dyspnoea and cough occur, and treatment is aimed at restoring the patency of the bronchus. For intrinsic tumours, this may be best achieved by local treatment, such as cryotherapy or laser therapy via a bronchoscope. For extrinsic tumours appropriate radiotherapy or chemotherapy is indicated. As with SVCO, presentation with bronchial obstruction does not preclude radical treatment in those patients where that would be appropriate. Lymphoma and small cell lung cancer are best treated with primary chemotherapy and localized non-small cell lung cancer may benefit from radical doses of radiotherapy given either as an accelerated schedule such as CHART (continuous hyperfractionated accelerated radiotherapy) or within a chemoradiation programme (Fairchild et al., 2009). For poor performance status patients and those with distant metastasis palliative radiotherapy or chemotherapy is indicated. In large randomized trials, a single dose of 10 Gy is equivalent to a more prolonged schedule in terms of both symptom control and survival, with a reduced risk of acute morbidity (MRC Lung Cancer Working Part, 1991, 1992). There is an intermediate group of good performance status patients with advanced tumours who may have a small but significant survival advantage from higher-dose radiotherapy. Randomized trials comparing 17 Gy in 2 fractions with either 39 Gy in 13 fractions or 20 Gy in 5 fractions showed a significant survival advantage of around 2 months for the higher dose schedules (Bezjak et al., 2002; Goldstraw et al., 2011). In this setting, radiotherapy may be given before or after palliative chemotherapy, which also may have an important role in symptom control and improving quality of life (Goldstraw et al., 2011).

An alternative method of delivering radiotherapy in the bronchial lumen is endobronchial irradiation. This may be particularly appropriate for patients relapsing after previous external beam irradiation. In this brachytherapy technique, a fine plastic catheter is placed alongside the tumour-bearing region of bronchus (Fig. 12.3.8) and a high dose rate afterloading machine passes a radioactive source, iridium 192, along the catheter to dwell within the area bearing tumour where treatment is required. This technique can be combined with either laser therapy or cryotherapy to restore the lumen where there is complete bronchial obstruction. In a randomized controlled trial comparing endobronchial brachytherapy with external beam radiotherapy (Stout et al., 2000), there was no difference in survival or symptom control scores for cough, haemoptysis, shortness of breath, or hoarseness, but external beam radiotherapy was found to be superior for symptoms of chest pain, anorexia, tiredness and nausea, and brachytherapy was better for dysphagia. The standard dose is 15 Gy at 1 cm and the major advantage of brachytherapy is that it can be given as a single procedure often possible as an outpatient day case.

Dysphagia

Pain and difficulty in swallowing is a common symptom in patients with advanced cancer within the mediastinum. This may be due to intrinsic tumour arising from the wall of the oesophagus, hypopharynx (piriform fossa, post-cricoid region, and posterior pharyngeal wall), and stomach. Alternatively there may be extrinsic compression from mediastinal lymph nodes or tumours in the thymus, thyroid gland, or adjacent bronchus. Postmortem data shows that around 80% of patients presenting with dysphagia have intrinsic tumour within the oesophagus. One study showed multiple levels of obstruction in almost a quarter of these patients (Sykes et al., 1998). Symptoms may be ameliorated with analgesics and anticholinergic drugs to reduce secretions, and nutrition can be maintained by a percutaneous gastrostomy. Where there is widespread metastatic disease in poor performance patients more active treatment may be inappropriate and unsuccessful, but in selected patients with good performance status and limited disease, surgical intervention or if not appropriate laser resection or stenting should be considered.

Given the risk of procedure-related morbidity and mortality, external beam irradiation also may be considered as a means of relieving dysphagia. A typical radiation field is shown in Fig. 12.3.9, and the usual dose is 20–30 Gy in 1–2 weeks. Swallowing is re-established in more than 80% of patients and maintained for a mean duration of 6 months (Wara et al., 1976). The disadvantage of radiotherapy in this setting is the time required to attain relief, which can be several weeks, and the initial period of enhanced dysphagia because of acute oesophagitis. Higher doses of radiotherapy delivering 50 Gy in 5 weeks or more may give a higher and more durable response and should be considered for patients who

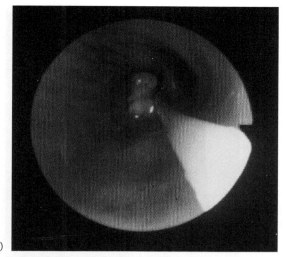

(A)

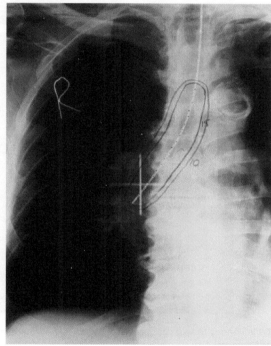

(B)

Fig. 12.3.8 View of (A) an endobronchial catheter being passed through a fibreoptic bronchoscope for endobronchial brachytherapy and (B) a subsequent X-ray showing catheter position.

have good performance status and limited disease (Leslie et al., 1992). If radical treatment is performed, chemoradiation with cisplatin and 5-fluorouracil during the course of radiotherapy has been shown to be superior to radiotherapy alone (Herskovic et al., 2012).

An alternative technique is endo-oesophageal radiotherapy, which is similar to that of endobronchial brachytherapy (Fig. 12.3.8). A high-dose afterloading source can be passed through a fine catheter that fits inside a nasogastric tube, which is passed through the area of oesophageal constriction. The outpatient procedure typically takes only a few minutes. Used alone, sustained improvement in swallowing is reported in 54% of patients (Brewster et al., 1995). This technique has also been

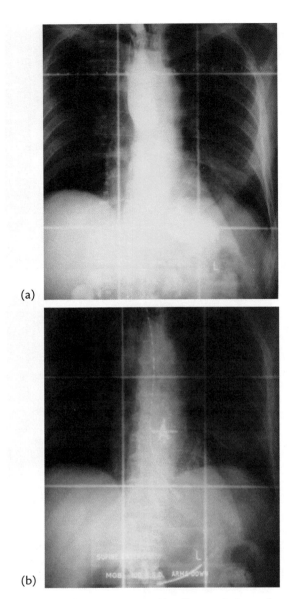

(a)

(b)

Fig. 12.3.9 Planning films to treat inoperable palliative radiotherapy for dysphagia from carcinoma of oesophagus using (A) external beam fields and (B) endobronchial brachytherapy showing the treatment catheter *in situ*.

used in an attempt to achieve high local doses in combination with external beam radiotherapy for radical treatment. One randomized trial suggests there may be a survival advantage to this approach over the use of stents, with equivalent control of dysphagia (Shenfine et al., 2005). In addition to acute toxicity there may be later side effects, of which oesophageal stricture is the most troublesome; this occurs in less than 5% patients (Shenfine et al., 2005). Late deterioration in swallowing usually is caused by tumour recurrence.

Urinary tract obstruction

Urinary tract obstruction may arise because of obstruction of the renal pelvis, ureter, bladder, or urethra at any point (see Chapter 8.4). The most satisfactory means of re-establishing renal drainage is a procedure to bypass the obstruction using a nephrostomy,

ureteric stents, or transurethral resection of an intrinsic urethral tumour. The role of radiotherapy is restricted to cancer patients for whom a procedure is technically not possible or otherwise inappropriate, and to those who have had a procedure and require treatment of the underlying cause. Common neoplasms include cervix, bladder, or prostate, and recurrent colorectal tumour. It is important to ascertain the primary site, and in the setting of para-aortic lymphadenopathy, obtain histological confirmation given the need to determine chemosensitivity of the lesion. In some instances, for example, lymphoma and germ cell tumour, primary chemotherapy with curative intent will be appropriate.

Primary tumours of the cervix, prostate, or bladder without lymph node or distant metastasis are treated with high radiation doses to achieve tumour shrinkage and re-establish urinary flow with the expectation that a proportion of patients will have long-term disease control or even cure. Cervical cancer may be treated by radical chemoradiation and intrauterine brachytherapy, bladder cancer requires doses 55 Gy in 20 daily fractions or 60–65 Gy in 6–6½ weeks, and prostate cancer may be treated radically with doses of 74–78 Gy in 32–34 fractions. Shorter and lower dose schedules may be chosen in advanced disease. In one series of patients with carcinoma of the prostate presenting with urinary retention, radiotherapy alone was sufficient to restore normal urinary drainage in 84%, with a mean time to catheter removal from completion of radiotherapy of 10 weeks (Wells et al., 1996). In practice, most patients with advanced prostate cancer also are treated with androgen deprivation therapy and similar regression may be achieved with this approach in the short term.

In some instances intraluminal or interstitial radiotherapy may have a role in urinary obstruction. A specific example is suburethral metastasis from endometrial carcinoma. This is a recognized pattern of spread from submucosal vaginal lymphatic invasion to the urethra meatus. Techniques are also available to deliver intraluminal brachytherapy to the urethra for recurrent prostate cancer or bladder base tumours.

Limb oedema

Limb oedema in a patient with advanced cancer may result from venous obstruction, lymphatic obstruction, or both (see Chapter 11.3). This may be compounded by general debility, immobility, and poor nutrition with accompanying hypo-albuminaemia. In a proportion of patients, post-radiation changes may cause lymphatic obstruction; upper limb oedema occurs in more than 30% of patients undergoing both axillary surgery and radiotherapy for breast cancer.

Local radiotherapy may be of value in the treatment of limb oedema when enlarged malignant axillary, inguinal, or pelvic nodes are the cause of obstruction. The best results are obtained with early treatment, when the circulatory obstruction can be reversed. Relatively low doses of 20–30 Gy in 1–2 weeks are used, taking care to preserve wherever possible a channel of unirradiated skin and soft tissue through which lymph drainage can be maintained despite post-radiation changes.

Hydrocephalus

Obstructive hydrocephalus is an uncommon manifestation of cancer within the central nervous system and may result from primary or secondary tumours that obstruct the cerebrospinal fluid at any point in the ventricular system. Typically, it occurs when tumours of either the midbrain or the posterior fossa obstruct the aqueduct or fourth ventricle; it may also be secondary to malignant meningitis. Patients present with features of raised intracranial pressure together with focal neurological symptoms, depending upon the site of the tumour. Rapid relief of hydrocephalus may be gained by inserting an intraventricular shunt and patients with advanced disease may need no further treatment to achieve temporary symptom control. Where surgery is not feasible or where there are multiple intracerebral lesions, palliative radiotherapy should be given in the same way as discussed for the management of brain metastases in the previous section. Advanced primary central nervous system tumours of the mid brain and posterior fossa are also treated by radiotherapy usually delivering doses of 50–55 Gy given over 6–7 weeks.

Haemorrhage

Haemoptysis

Haemoptysis is a common symptom of bronchial carcinoma, occurring in about 50% of patients at presentation, and may also accompany pulmonary metastasis (see Chapter 8.7). It is distressing for the patient, although rarely of haemodynamic significance unless a major vein or bronchial artery is eroded. Haemoptysis is an indication for local radiotherapy and control rates of up to 80% are reported with palliative doses, using either external beam treatment or endobronchial brachytherapy as discussed above. Randomized trials show that a single dose of 10 Gy external beam is as effective as other more prolonged schedules, with less acute morbidity (MRC Lung Cancer Working Party, 1992).

Haemoptysis is not a contraindication to radical treatment in patients with localized bronchial carcinoma. Screening for this possibility should always occur prior to embarking upon palliative irradiation. Patients with stage I or II non-small cell lung cancer (no involvement of mediastinal lymph nodes) should be considered for high-dose radiotherapy using either accelerated schedules such as CHART or chemoradiation (Fairchild et al., 2009). Some patients with good performance status and stage III disease, (mediastinal node involvement) may also benefit from high-dose chemoradiation. Patients with small cell lung cancer may receive combined chemotherapy, mediastinal radiotherapy, and prophylactic cranial irradiation.

The management of haemoptysis due to pulmonary metastasis is more difficult. Local irradiation is only of value where a specific site of haemorrhage can be identified or where there is only a solitary metastasis. Bronchoscopic confirmation of the origin of bleeding is therefore needed when there are multiple metastases; arbitrary irradiation of the particular area of metastatic disease is not to be recommended, although low-dose whole-lung irradiation delivering a dose of 25 Gy in 20 fractions over 4 weeks has been used in the past for widespread metastasis from radiosensitive tumours such as Ewing's sarcoma or Wilms' tumour. In general, however, chemotherapy or hormone therapy is the preferred treatment in this setting and only when this has failed should palliative irradiation be explored.

There is no proven advantage in terms of survival for treating the asymptomatic patient with inoperable lung cancer. Nonetheless, there is evidence that tumours greater than 10 cm in diameter, whether primary or metastatic, carry a significant risk of haemorrhage and it has been suggested that such lesions should receive prophylactic treatment.

Haematuria

Haematuria may be related to bleeding from primary or metastatic disease at any site along the urinary tract (see Chapter 8.4). Careful localization of the site of bleeding through intravenous urography, CT scanning, or cystoscopy is necessary for treatment planning. In patients with advanced cancer, bleeding is usually caused by a lesion in the bladder, which may be primary or secondary to local infiltration of an advanced rectal or uterine carcinoma, advanced renal cell carcinoma or urethral infiltration by carcinoma of the prostate. Other causes that may be relevant to the cancer patient are infective cystitis, chemical cystitis associated with certain chemotherapy agents such as cyclophosphamide or ifosfamide, bladder telangiectasia as a late change following high-dose radiotherapy to the bladder (or adjacent pelvic organs), and rarely, thrombocytopenia or a blood coagulation defect.

The main role of radiotherapy in this setting is to achieve haemostasis in patients with inoperable or recurrent tumours. When conservative measures, such as bladder irrigation, administration of antifibrinolytic drugs such as tranexamic acid, or cystoscopic diathermy, are unsuccessful, modest doses of irradiation delivered to a small volume encompassing the site of haemorrhage may be successful. A large randomized trial comparing 35 Gy in 10 fractions with 21 Gy given in 3 fractions on alternate days over one week has shown equivalent symptomatic improvement of bladder-related symptoms in patients with advanced bladder cancer invading muscle, with no excess toxicity from the shorter 21 Gy schedule (Duchesne et al., 2000). Haematuria was improved in 50% of patients at completion of treatment and 63% at 3 months after treatment. The same doses and techniques can be used for prostatic cancer causing urethral or bladder base infiltration and haemorrhage. In poor performance status patients, single doses of 8–10 Gy may be equally effective and 17 Gy in 2 fractions has also been reported as a useful schedule in this setting, with a 59% response rate for haematuria (Srinivasan et al., 1994).

As with other sites haematuria may be the presentation of a potentially curable primary bladder or prostatic carcinoma, and full assessment of the patient both in terms of their tumour and general status is important before deciding upon palliative treatment. For advanced tumours of the bladder, radical radiotherapy delivers doses of 55 Gy in 4 weeks or 60–65 Gy in 6–6½ weeks. Radical radiotherapy to the prostate gland delivers doses in excess of 70 Gy in 7 weeks. In selected cases, brachytherapy can be used.

Haematuria due to locally advanced inoperable renal carcinoma may also benefit from local irradiation. The tolerance of the normal kidney to radiation is low and even with modest palliative doses, the kidney will have loss of function. It is therefore important to ensure that renal function from the contralateral kidney is normal before treatment. Doses of 10 Gy as a single dose, 21 Gy in 3 fractions over 1 week, or 20–30 Gy over 1–2 weeks have all been used in this setting; there are few published data on the expected response rate.

Treatment of the bladder or prostate may result in diarrhoea because of the inevitable inclusion of some of the rectum in the treatment volume. In the Medical Research Council randomized trial of palliative radiotherapy in bladder cancer there was a 5% incidence of mild diarrhoea not requiring medication and a 2% incidence of moderate diarrhoea requiring medication for control (Duchesne et al., 2000). Treatment of the kidney may include stomach or small bowel, resulting in nausea, vomiting and diarrhoea. Careful explanation and reassurance about these side effects, together with ready availability of anti-diarrhoeal agents and antiemetics, is an important part of management.

Uterine and vaginal bleeding

Tumours of the uterus, including endometrial and cervical cancer, and uterine sarcomas, frequently present with abnormal vaginal bleeding. This is rarely excessive but occasionally major haemorrhage is the presenting feature. Haemorrhage may be due to recurrent or locally advanced tumours of the cervix or uterus, local infiltration from advanced cancers of the bladder or rectum, or metastatic mucosal deposits along the vaginal wall typical of the pattern of spread from endometrial cancer. Haemorrhagic mucosal deposits are also a particular feature of vulval or vaginal melanoma.

Radiotherapy is of value in obtaining control of bleeding, using either external beam irradiation or intracavitary brachytherapy as appropriate. When bleeding is the primary presentation of advanced cervical cancer, then radical chemoradiation is often appropriate, delivering external beam treatment to a dose of around 50 Gy in 5 weeks with cisplatin followed by intracavitary brachytherapy to the cervix and para-cervical tissues. Similarly, when locally advanced bladder, rectal or uterine tumours are the cause and previous radiotherapy has not been given, palliative pelvic doses are effective, using a schedule of 21 Gy in 3 fractions or 20–30 Gy over 1–2 weeks. If previous radiotherapy had been given, low doses, for example, single doses of 8 Gy or short courses of up to 20 Gy in 5 fractions, may be considered, although there may be risks of additional late bowel damage associated with this. These decisions must be balanced between the severity of symptoms and the anticipated life expectancy of the patient.

Where bleeding is from small volume disease, such as nodules at the vaginal vault or along the vaginal mucosa, intracavitary brachytherapy may be optimal. Vaginal sources in the form of either ovoids or a vaginal tube can be introduced directly into the vagina and used to carry a radiation source, usually iridium (Fig. 12.3.10) (Hoskin and Coyle, 2011). The use of intracavitary brachytherapy in this way enables a high surface dose to be given to the mucosa but with a rapid fall off in dose away from the source so that critical structures such as bladder and rectum are relatively spared from the radiation dose. It is able to treat only to a depth of 5–10 mm, and for larger tumours, an interstitial implant may be necessary. This requires general anaesthesia and the placement of afterloading radioactive tubes. It enables high dose treatment to be delivered locally within the tumour, even where previous radiotherapy has been given to the pelvis, and may provide highly effective palliation in the difficult situation of progressive tumour in the vulvo-vaginal tissues.

Gastrointestinal haemorrhage

Symptomatic gastrointestinal haemorrhage from the upper or lower gastrointestinal tract may arise from a primary neoplasm of the stomach, large bowel or rectum, or from direct invasion by locally advanced tumour in adjacent structures such as the uterus, bladder, or prostate. Blood borne metastasis to the bowel are rare, but metastatic malignant melanoma is a recognized cause of haemorrhagic deposits within the small bowel wall and Kaposi's sarcoma, seen with HIV infection, may cause a similar problem.

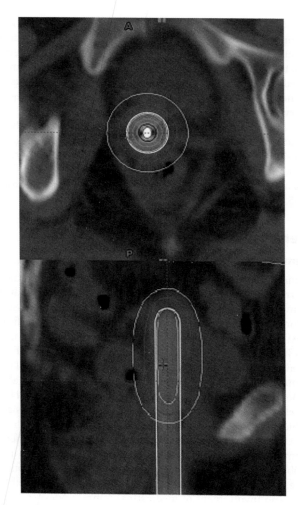

Fig. 12.3.10 X-ray and CT planning films of intravaginal applicator used to treat symptomatic recurrent vaginal tumour showing (A) transaxial and (B) sagittal views. Red line denotes prescription isodose; note low surrounding dose to bowel, bladder, and rectum.

Modest doses of radiotherapy to a site of haemorrhage within the bowel will often achieve effective and durable control of bleeding. In the lower bowel, tumours in the rectum and colon are usually readily identified and localized within a treatment volume. Treatment of the stomach may be more difficult both because it can be a relatively mobile structure and also because the sensitivity of surrounding tissues, in particular liver, small bowel, and kidneys, limits tolerance and the dose that can be delivered safely. Localization of tumours within the small bowel also can be difficult because of its mobility. Radiation to the stomach or small bowel can have considerable associated morbidity with nausea, vomiting, and diarrhoea.

External beam radiotherapy for bleeding from recurrent colorectal cancer has been reported to achieve an overall response rate of 85%, with complete control of bleeding in 63% of patients following a dose of 30–35 Gy in 10 fractions over 2 weeks (Taylor et al., 1987). An alternative approach is again to use intraluminal brachytherapy, similar to the technique used for vaginal bleeding. A tube can be passed into the rectum through which a radioactive source can be placed to deliver a high surface dose to the rectal mucosa and associated tumour area. This approach has the advantage of being delivered as a single outpatient procedure when high dose rate afterloading brachytherapy is used, the actual technique being little different to a sigmoidoscopic examination. Control of bleeding is achieved in 64% (Corner et al., 2010). It is however limited to accessible tumours in the lower sigmoid colon, rectum, and anal canal.

Chest wall and other skin lesions

Locoregional recurrence remains a significant problem in patients with breast cancer, occurring in 7–10% of those with early disease and up to 40% of those presenting with advanced local disease. Although post-operative irradiation at the time of primary treatment significantly reduces the likelihood of locoregional relapse, some patients develop progressive locoregional tumour on the chest wall which will fungate and bleed. If total mastectomy is possible, this may be the best procedure to surgically clear recurrent tumour on the chest wall. In many cases, however, the tumour will be fixed and inoperable, and associated with multiple satellite nodules across the chest, often involving the contralateral breast or extending laterally across the mid-axillary line on to the back. Chemotherapy may be used, but if no previous radiotherapy had been given and there is no evidence of distant metastasis, high dose local irradiation may be appropriate, delivering doses of up to 60 Gy in 6 weeks. In patients with distant metastasis and a poor prognosis, shorter schedules of 10 Gy in 1 fraction or longer courses of 20–30 Gy in 1–2 weeks may be used. Often it is not possible to encompass the entire extent of clinically detectable disease and in these circumstances those causing greatest symptoms may be targeted.

Recurrence at the site of previous irradiation may still present the option of further radiotherapy to a limited area of symptomatic tumour since the risks of skin necrosis are negligible compared with the effects of progressive fungating tumour within the skin. Superficial X-ray treatment or low energy electrons to fungating or bleeding chest wall nodules is often highly effective and a single dose of 8–10 Gy or a longer course delivering 20–30 Gy over 1–2 weeks is commonly used. More complex techniques using a surface mould in which radioactive sources are placed over the involved area, or interstitial brachytherapy in which large tumour masses are implanted with radioactive needles or afterloading applicator tubes, can also be considered.

Skin nodules may also be a manifestation of primary tumours in other sites. These reflect blood borne metastasis and therefore radical treatment is usually inappropriate but local treatment to symptomatic nodules is of value. Techniques and doses similar to those discussed above for recurrent breast cancer are employed.

Primary skin tumours may also present with locally advanced inoperable disease. Bleeding and fungation are likely to become major problems in the management of these patients and local radiotherapy is of value in their control. In the absence of metastasis, and in the case of basal cell carcinomas which do not metastasize, high radical doses may be considered using appropriate techniques with either electrons of appropriate energy to treat to the depth of the tumour or tangential X-ray beams to cover the tumour volume. Doses of 60 Gy in 6 weeks or equivalent are given to large tumours where this is appropriate in the light of the patient's general performance status. For patients with poor performance status or metastatic disease shorter courses delivering doses of 20–30 Gy in 1–2 weeks may be considered and will

be effective in achieving growth delay and stopping haemorrhage. Melanoma characteristically presents with haemorrhagic tumours and may in more advanced cases result in multiple skin nodules. Local radiotherapy delivering higher doses of 30 Gy in 5–6 fractions treating twice weekly is often used with good effect (Overgaard, 1986).

Other local tumour effects

Fungation

Fungation of a superficial tumour mass is a distressing feature of locally advanced cancer (see Chapters 11.1 and 14.4). As noted, it is seen most commonly in chest wall recurrence after breast carcinoma and with metastatic lymph nodes in the neck or groin. Local irradiation is most valuable in the prevention of fungation at a time when the overlying skin is intact. A palliative course of treatment delivering 20–30 Gy in 1–2 weeks will usually delay growth within a tumour mass sufficient to prevent fungation. Higher dose may be appropriate if the local tumour is the sole manifestation of malignancy. The most common scenario of this type is the presence of a cervical lymph node containing squamous carcinoma from the head and neck region or inguinal lymph nodes with squamous carcinoma from the perineal region. Occasionally, large lymph nodes may present without an obvious underlying primary tumour. Radical radiotherapy to malignant nodes from an unknown primary in the neck can achieve long term control in this setting with overall 5-year survival figures of 20–30% in selected series (Fletcher, 1990).

Once fungation has occurred successful treatment is more difficult. Combined with nursing care and administration of analgesics and antibiotics, local irradiation may still be of value in reducing the underlying tumour bulk, arresting surface haemorrhage and drying the surface as the process of healing is allowed to commence. This will make nursing care simpler and relieve the patient from the distress of local haemorrhage.

Kaposi's sarcoma

Kaposi's sarcoma is now most commonly seen as a feature of HIV infection and is the most common AIDS-related malignancy. It may also be seen in sporadic cases when it typically presents in the skin of the lower limbs in European men. Multiple skin lesions are usual but extracutaneous disease is also common affecting the oral cavity and gastrointestinal tract. The characteristic purplish raised plaques may bleed and ulcerate. In contrast to other soft tissue sarcomas, Kaposi's is markedly radiosensitive and small doses of irradiation will result in complete regression of lesions in up to 70% of patients (Munro and Stewart, 1989). There is good evidence that single doses are as effective as more prolonged schedules and superficial irradiation delivering 8 Gy to symptomatic sites is recommended.

Liver metastases

In most instances, the presence of liver metastasis heralds the terminal phases of advanced cancer. Clinical symptoms include anorexia, malaise, and weight loss alongside local pain and discomfort from hepatic enlargement and stretching of the liver capsule. Pain may be acute where there is rapid expansion of the liver or haemorrhage into a metastasis.

A subgroup of patients who have liver oligometastases with only one to three lesions in the setting of a controlled or absent primary and no other metastatic sites may benefit from radical treatment. Surgical resection is indicated where technically feasible. In inoperable oligometastases, then stereotactic radiotherapy may be used to deliver an ablative dose of radiation. A range of dose fractionation schedules have been reported from single doses of 14–26 Gy to fractionated schedules delivering 30–55 Gy in 3–5 fractions. There is no consensus on the optimal dose schedule but high local control rates from 56% to 100% are reported in cohort studies with little acute or late toxicity (Lo et al., 2010). High-frequency ultrasound has recently introduced a further treatment option for superficial metastases

Local radiotherapy may also be of value in the setting of multiple metastases particularly in those patients with good performance status and normal bilirubin and where the primary site is other than stomach or pancreas (Leibel et al., 1981). If the primary tumour is chemosensitive, this is usually the first line of approach, but for other patients palliative low-dose radiotherapy may provide valuable relief of symptoms. Two prospective randomized trials have demonstrated relief of hepatic pain in 80% of patients, with complete relief in 55% and improvements in nausea, vomiting, fever, and night sweats in 45% (Borgelt et al., 1981; Leibel et al., 1981).

The liver has limited tolerance to radiation. Non-stereotactic hepatic radiotherapy may be associated with side effects, and when doses greater than 30 Gy are given, there is a risk of inducing radiation hepatitis. Toxicity is related not only to dose but also the volume of liver included in the treatment volume. Unless there is diffuse infiltration of the entire organ, uninvolved liver should be excluded from the radiation volume. With doses of 30 Gy delivered in 2–3 weeks, relatively mild self-limiting toxicity is reported with lethargy and nausea being the predominant symptoms.

Splenomegaly

Symptomatic splenomegaly from malignant diseases is usually associated with haematological malignancies, in particular chronic granulocytic leukaemia and certain types of non-Hodgkin's lymphoma. It is also a feature of myelodysplasia. Surgical removal of the spleen is the preferred management, but in advanced disease or in patients with poor performance status this may not be appropriate and local irradiation is an effective means of palliation. Symptoms due to local bulk (causing pain and discomfort) and hypersplenism (causing consumption of red cells and platelets) benefit from treatment. Pain relief is reported in over 90% of patients and durable size reduction in 60% (Paulino and Reddy, 1996). When treatment is for hypersplenism, then caution is required as high doses may precipitate pancytopenia. Single doses of 1 Gy or less delivered at weekly intervals are recommended to a total dose of between 3 and 10 Gy with weekly assessment before each treatment to evaluate the effect on the peripheral blood count and the degree of splenic shrinkage. The spleen containing lymphoma or leukaemia is often extremely sensitive to radiation and whilst standard doses of 20–30 Gy in 10–15 fractions will be needed precautions should be taken against the effects of rapid tumour lysis ensuring the patient is well hydrated and giving allopurinol to prevent hyperuricaemia.

Hypercalcaemia

Hypercalcaemia complicates the clinical course of around 10% of all patients with malignant disease particularly those with common epithelial tumours such as breast, prostate and lung cancer.

Whilst it frequently occurs in patients with widespread metastatic disease, no clear correlation with the extent of bone metastasis is usually demonstrated and most cases arise due to the production of chemical agents promoting osteoclastic reabsorption of bone, in particular parathyroid hormone-related protein. The initial management of a patient with hypercalcaemia secondary to advanced cancer includes rehydration, diuresis, and the introduction of bisphosphonates. However, whilst an initial reduction of serum calcium is usually achieved, rebound hypercalcaemia frequently follows requiring further intensive treatment and often a refractory phase is entered after several episodes. Where a potential source of the chemical agent can be identified such as locally advanced endobronchial carcinoma, local irradiation to reduce its production and enable stabilization of blood calcium levels may be of value. Standard palliative doses are usually delivered as described above and whilst anecdotally a valuable treatment in this setting no published data is available for accurate estimates of response.

Paraneoplastic phenomena

The most common paraneoplastic syndromes occur association is with primary carcinoma of the bronchus. These arise in around 2% of patients and include neuropathies, myopathies, myasthenia (the Eaton–Lambert syndrome) and cutaneous manifestations such as acanthosis nigricans, erythema gyratum, or hairy man syndrome. These symptoms reflect secretion of a humeral agent, possibly an auto-antibody. The para-endocrine syndromes are associated with ectopic production of adrenocorticotropic hormone, antidiuretic hormone, human chorionic gonadotrophin, 5-hydroxytryptamine, or thyroid stimulating hormone, as well as those mentioned above in the context of hypercalcaemia. If there is an identifiable local tumour and surgical excision is not possible or appropriate, local irradiation may result in improvement and resolution of the paraneoplastic symptoms as the tumour regresses. In advanced disease, only palliative doses may be appropriate, but in localized disease the presence of a paraneoplastic syndrome should not exclude consideration of radical treatment. As with hypercalcaemia, there is no good data on precise response rates to treatment in this setting.

Conclusion

Local irradiation is a valuable treatment for palliation of local symptoms, with consistently high response rates in the relief and control of bone pain, neurological symptoms, obstructive symptoms, and haemorrhage. Short treatments and simple techniques can minimize disruption and acute morbidity for the patient with advanced cancer whilst enabling control of symptoms.

Online materials

Complete references for this chapter are available online at <http://www.oxfordmedicine.com>.

References

Ahman, F.R. (1984). A reassessment of the clinical implications of the superior vena caval syndrome. *Journal of Clinical Oncology*, 2, 961–968.

Bone Pain Trial Working Party (1999). 8 Gy single fraction radiotherapy for the treatment of metastatic skeletal pain: randomised comparison with a multifraction schedule over 12 months of patient follow-up. *Radiotherapy and* Oncology, 52: 111–121.

Chow, E., Zeng, L., Salvo, N., Dennis, K., Tsao, M., and Lutz, S. (2012). Update on the systematic review of palliative radiotherapy trials for bone. *Clinical Oncology* 24, 112–124.

Duchesne, G.M., Bolger, J.J., Griffiths, G.O., *et al.* (2000). A randomized trial of hypofractionated schedules of palliative radiotherapy in the management of bladder carcinoma: results of Medical Research Council Trial BA09. *International Journal of Radiation Oncology, Biology, Physics*, 47, 379–388.

Fairchild, A., Harris, K., Barnes, E., et al. (2009). Palliative thoracic radiotherapy for lung cancer: a systematic review. *Journal of Clinical Oncology*, 26, 4001–4011.

Goldstraw, P., Ball, D., Jett, J.R., *et al.* (2011). Non small cell lung cancer. *The Lancet*, 378, 1727–1740.

Herskovic, A., Russell, M., Liptay, M., Fidler, M.J., and Al-Sarratt, M. (2012). Esophageal cancer advances in treatment results for locally advanced disease. Annals of Oncology, 2012; 23: 1095–1103.

Huisman, M., van den Bosch, M.A.A.J., Wijlemans, J.W., *et al.* (2012). Effectiveness of reirradiation for painful bone metastases: a systematic review and meta-analysis. *International Journal of Radiation Oncology, Biology, Physics*, 84, 8–14.

Lo, S.S., Achilles, F.J., Chang, E.L., *et al.* (2010). Stereotactic body radiotherapy: a novel treatment modality. *Nature Reviews Clinical Oncology*, 7, 44–54.

Patchell, R., Tibbs, P.A., Regine, W.F., *et al.* (2005). Direct decompressive surgical resection in the treatment of spinal cord compression caused by metastatic cancer: a randomised trial. *The Lancet*, 366, 643–648.

Roos, D., Turner, S.L., O'Brien, P.C. *et al.* (2005). Randomized trial of 8 Gy in 1 versus 20 Gy in 5 fractions of radiotherapy for neuropathic pain due to bone metastases(Trans-Tasman Radiation Oncology Group, TROG 96.05). *Radiotherapy and Oncology* 2005; 75, 54–63.

Ryan, D.P., Compton, C.C., and Mayer, R.J. (2000). Carcinoma of the anal canal. *The New England Journal of Medicine*, 342, 792–800.

Salazar, O.M., Sandhu, T., Da Motta, N.W., *et al.* (2001). Fractionated half-body irradiation (HBI) for the rapid palliation of widespread, symptomatic, metastatic bone disease: a randomized phase III trial of the International Atomic Energy Agency (IAEA). *International Journal of Radiation Oncology, Biology, Physics*, 50, 765–775.

Stupp, R., Mason, W.P., van den Bent, M.J., *et al.* (2005). Radiotherapy plus concomitant and adjuvant temozolamide for glioblastoma. *The New England Journal of Medicine*, 352, 987–996.

Tsao, M.N., Lloyd, N., Wong, R.K., *et al.* (2012). Whole brain radiotherapy for the treatment of newly diagnosed multiple brain metastases. *Cochrane Database of Systematic Reviews*, 4, CD003869.

Willams, M. and Drinkwater, K. (2009). Geographical variation in radiotherapy services across the UK in 2007 and the effect of deprivation. *Clinical Oncology*, 21, 431–440.

The role of general surgery in the palliative care of patients with cancer

Brian Badgwell and Robert S. Krouse

Role of the surgeon in palliative care of the cancer patient

Palliation is increasingly becoming recognized as an important component of care of the cancer patient for general surgeons. In fact, studies from tertiary cancer centres have shown that 12.5% of cases were done with a palliative intent while 40% of inpatient surgical consultations met the criteria for palliative evaluation (Krouse et al., 2001; Badgwell et al., 2009). Additionally, in a survey of cancer surgeons, it was estimated that 21% of all surgical procedures for cancer patients are for palliation (McCahill et al., 2002). The diverse surgical indications to improve the quality of life (QOL) in advanced cancer patients include hormonal imbalance, malignant fluid re-accumulation, obstructions, tumour bleeding or other local complications, and pain (Markman, 1995). These may be due to the many various primary or metastatic cancers.

Goals of surgery

Definition of success

The benefits and risks of surgical procedures are always of paramount importance, and are crystallized in the patient with advanced cancer. The benefits of palliative surgery should always focus on QOL, symptom control, and symptom prevention (Markman, 1995). One must also consider that there will frequently be a secondary benefit: survival. This is clearly an important goal of patients and families, even in the setting of incurable disease. Unfortunately, the literature frequently focuses exclusively on survival as an endpoint, leaving surgeons with little information on an intervention's impact on QOL.

A major dilemma for the surgeon caring for a patient with a terminal cancer is measures of success. The surgical literature has been a poor guide for decision-making for this population of patients. Outcome measures related to QOL and symptom distress are not clearly defined and documented. Historically, what little focus there is on palliation in the surgical literature has been remiss in examining appropriate QOL outcomes. In fact, from 1990 to 1996, QOL measurements have been included in only 17% of reports of palliative procedures in the surgical literature and only 12% examined pain (Miner et al., 1999). This is in contrast to the more common outcome measures of physiologic response

(69%), survival (64%), and morbidity and mortality (61%). While it is imperative to understand these outcomes, they should not be the primary focus of palliative procedures, as they may not equate with an improvement in QOL. It is possible that palliative surgery would have no effect on general QOL surveys such as the Short Form-36 (SF-36) or Functional Assessment of Cancer Therapy-General (FACT-G) (Ware and Sherbourne 1992; Cella et al., 1993). Future studies will hopefully include targeted measures based upon the indication for surgical intervention and the symptoms that the patients are seeking to improve.

For patients contemplating palliative surgery, the primary decision-making factor has been shown to be the physical impact of uncontrolled symptoms. Secondary factors included the social impact of symptoms and maintenance of hope (Ferrell et al., 2003). Similarly, a study of patients with malignant gastric outlet obstruction requested patients to list and rank factors influencing their choice of palliative intervention (Schmidt et al., 2009). Patients listed physician's recommendation and the desire to eat and drink normally as the most important factors influencing their decision. Such studies may ultimately identify the optimal outcome in palliative surgical assessment (Badgwell et al., 2012).

Pre-emptive surgical palliation

Palliative surgery is most often considered in the setting of an active symptom. Prevention of symptoms in the palliative setting may also be a goal of palliative surgery (Markman, 1995). Many symptoms related to tumours are known to occur, but it is less understood if or when the symptom will actually occur. Therefore, it is not always clear when or if a procedure would be helpful. Appropriate pre-emptive palliative surgery must consider prognostication related to a particular symptom, as well as the lifespan of a patient. For example, in the setting of biliary obstruction where a surgical bypass is attempted, one must also consider a gastric bypass to alleviate the risk of a patient having a gastric outlet obstruction prior to death. Another example may be with nodal dissections in the setting of positive sentinel node mappings, especially if distant disease is noted. A nodal dissection will have little effect on long-term survival, but this procedure may alleviate the risk of nodal recurrence and the suffering this may cause. Therefore, while there is frequently no clear direction for surgeons in these settings, pre-emptive palliative procedures should be considered in settings where tumour-related morbidity can be anticipated. Although this remains an area of active controversy in research endeavours, invasive procedures to prevent symptoms to improve QOL for patients with incurable illness has been included in the American College of Surgeons Surgical Palliative Care Task Force definition of palliative surgery (Cady et al., 2005). As always, the inherent risks of an operation must be considered, but these are more difficult to assess when the benefits are ultimately unknown.

Surgical risks

With every goal of success must be an understanding of risk. While all treatments contain risk, this is magnified related to a surgical procedure. It is further highlighted with patients who are facing the end of life. There are multiple preoperative considerations to ensure a successful palliative procedure with limited morbidity and mortality. This includes nutritional status. Albumin level is frequently an excellent tool to decide when not to operate. It is mandatory to assess the overall status of patients, including other medical problems and amount and location of primary or metastatic disease. This issue will clearly affect overall risk.

Complications will occur even with the most fastidious care, especially if the patient is debilitated related to the cancer or underlying conditions. Surgical morbidity may include complications unrelated to the surgical site, such as pneumonia, deep venous thrombosis, ileus, and heart failure. With meticulous care, these can often be avoided. Related to the procedure itself, pain is a major issue that occurs in the perioperative setting, and may persist throughout the patient's course. Epidural, patient-controlled analgesia, and local anaesthetic pumps may improve pain control and ultimate outcomes. Related to the surgical site, wound complications must always be considered. For example, it has been noted that lymph node dissections may have high rates of wound problems (47% for axillary node and 71% after inguinal node dissections) (Serpell et al., 2003). Issues such as seromas and infections may be long-term problems that take weeks to months to heal. Lymphatic leaks may necessitate frequent drainage or catheter placement. Patients with advanced cancers may not ever heal their wounds. Postoperative infections and non-healing wounds can also delay or prevent other treatment options. These issues must be discussed in detail prior to an operation. As new innovations are utilized, outcomes will continue to improve for surgical patients.

Acceptance of major disfigurement and lifestyle changes are most pronounced in the immediate postoperative setting. For example, the shock of a permanent stoma may be overwhelming for many patients. While QOL problems related to ostomies may diminish with time (Persson et al., 2005), this may not be possible for the patient facing the end of life.

A poor surgical outcome may be that symptoms worsen after a procedure. In addition, hospital stays may be longer if complications occur. Importantly, an invasive procedure may hasten someone's death, which is the ultimate poor outcome.

Surgical palliative care problems for cancer patients: indications, options, and outcomes

Malignant bowel obstruction (MBO)

Indications of MBO

MBO is the most common indication for palliative surgical consultation (Badgwell et al., 2009) (see also Chapter 14.3). It occurs most frequently with ovarian and colorectal cancers, but occurs with other abdominal and occasionally with non-abdominal malignancies. MBO may be related to tumour, its treatment (e.g. radiation enteritis), or benign aetiologies (e.g. adhesions or internal hernia). One problem in evaluating MBO outcomes in the literature is the myriad of definitions that are utilized. An accepted definition that allows for comparison across studies and hopefully can provide the framework for a clinical trial is the following: (a) clinical evidence of a bowel obstruction via history, physical exam, or radiographic examination, (b) bowel obstruction beyond the ligament of Treitz, (c) intra-abdominal primary cancer with incurable disease, or (d) non-intra-abdominal primary cancer with clear intraperitoneal disease (Anthony et al., 2007). The goals of treatment include relieving nausea and vomiting, allowing oral intake, alleviating pain, and permitting the patient to return to their chosen care setting. Persistent obstructions in the face of conservative therapy (usually nasogastric decompression, hydration, and bowel rest) or evidence of complete obstructions are indications that a surgical procedure should be considered. Surgery should be contemplated for all patients with MBO except those who are actively dying.

Options for MBO

There are a myriad of situations one might encounter in the operating room; typically the approach is unknown until exploring the abdomen. The optimal procedure is that which is the quickest, safest, and most efficacious in alleviating the obstruction. If due to adhesions, adhesiolysis might be the optimal surgical procedure. Bowel resection may lead to the best outcome (Aranha et al., 1981; Legendre et al., 2001), although bypass may be a better option when resection is not possible due to tumour burden or deemed unsafe due to operative risks. In the setting of carcinomatosis, the placement of a gastrostomy tube for intermittent venting might be optimal. An intestinal stoma may be necessary after resection or to adequately bypass the blockage. Laparoscopic procedures may be attempted, although this approach may be difficult due to adhesions, carcinomatosis, or bowel dilatation. Cytoreductive procedures (resection of intraperitoneal tumour) frequently carry a high morbidity and usually are only considered with very low-grade tumours, such as pseudomyxoma peritonei. Many patients are deemed inoperable (6.2–50%) (Feuer et al., 1999). This may be due to poor operative risk or contraindications to surgery. Poor operative risk must be assessed based on co-morbidities (e.g. cardiac and pulmonary function), amount and location of metastatic disease (e.g. overwhelming metastasis to the liver), and current functional status (e.g. Karnofsky < 50%). Potential contraindications for surgery in patients with incurable cancer and MBO include ascites (> 3 L) and particularly ascites that rapidly recurs after drainage, carcinomatosis, multiple obstructions, or a palpable intra-abdominal mass (Ripamonti, 1994).

Endoscopic approaches for MBO

Endoscopic procedures are suited for patients who are poor operative candidates or who decline an open operative intervention. They also may obviate the need for an intestinal stoma. The major approaches include stenting and percutaneous endoscopic gastrostomy (PEG) tube placement. Stenting may include procedures to initially canalize the lumen (e.g. laser or balloon dilatation). PEG tubes are generally well tolerated 'venting' procedures that can alleviate symptoms of intractable vomiting and nausea for upper GI obstructions (Campagnutta and Cannizzaro, 2000). A study from MD Anderson Cancer Center, Texas, United

States, found that percutaneous gastrostomy tubes were utilized for palliation in 23% of small bowel obstructions in patients with advanced malignancy (Badgwell et al., 2011). In combination with other medical techniques, both open and percutaneous gastrostomy offers the possibility of intermittent oral intake.

Outcomes of MBO

Although it is recognized that improvement in QOL after surgery is variable (42–85%) (Feuer et al., 1999; Miner et al., 2002), there is no consistent parameter used to determine this clinical outcome; operations may offer an advantage of an increased survival. Surgical risks must be carefully considered prior to an operation, as morbidity (42%) (Makela et al., 1991) and mortality (5–32%) (Makela et al., 1991; Feuer et al., 1999; Legendre et al., 2001) are common, and the re-obstruction rate is high (10–50%) (Feuer et al., 1999; Miner et al., 2003). Poor prognostic indicators for surgical intervention include ascites, carcinomatosis, palpable intra-abdominal masses, multiple bowel obstructions, prior obstructions, and very advanced disease with poor performance status.

Endoluminal wall stents have a high success rate for relief of symptoms (64–100%) in complete and incomplete colorectal obstructions (Harris et al., 2001), and in over 70% of upper intestinal malignant obstructions including gastric outlet, duodenal, and jejunal obstructions (Soetikno and Carr-Locke 1999). While risks include perforation (0–15%), stent migration (0–40%), or re-occlusion (0–33%), stents can frequently lead to adequate palliation for long periods of time (Harris et al., 2001). Stent occlusion by tumour in-growth is usually amenable to another endoscopic intervention. Complications related to PEGs are rare, even when puncturing other organs (Campagnutta and Cannizzaro, 2000). The presence of significant ascites is a relative contraindication.

Gastric outlet obstruction

Indications of gastric outlet obstruction

There is some controversy as to when to do a surgical procedure for gastric outlet obstruction. Typically, these procedures are considered in the setting of persistent nausea, vomiting, eructation, and early satiety. They also may be considered when there is evidence of duodenal compression on radiographic or endoscopic evaluations. Stents for gastric outlet obstruction are noted to be quite successful (approximately 90%) with rare complications (Kim et al., 2001; Kaw et al., 2003), making an operative approach less common. If the stent fails due to tumour in-growth or migration (around 10%), another stent can often be placed (Kim et al., 2001; Kaw et al., 2003). Unfortunately, few centres have clinicians with the technical ability to accomplish this procedure successfully.

In the setting where a biliary bypass is planned, there is some controversy as to whether to do a pre-emptive gastric bypass (gastrojejunostomy) in the asymptomatic patient. Late gastric obstruction occurs from 9% to 23% (Holbrook et al., 1990; Huguier et al., 1993; Coene et al., 1994), and this must be considered at the time of biliary bypass. If the patient is of good performance status with limited disease (no or minimal metastasis), then a pre-emptive procedure may be indicated.

Options for gastric outlet obstruction

The surgical options for gastric outlet obstruction are a bypass procedure (gastrojejunostomy) or a resection (antrectomy or pancreaticoduodenectomy). There are several technical variations of a gastrojejunostomy, but the results are similar. This can be achieved via open or laparoscopic techniques (Choi, 2002). A distal gastric tumour may also be resected with a palliative intent. Percutaneous gastrostomy is also an option, with some centres reporting use in almost a quarter of their patients with gastric outlet obstruction and advanced malignancy (Miner et al., 2002).

Outcomes of gastric outlet obstruction

If endoscopic expertise is available, stenting is often preferable for gastric obstruction. If endoscopic stenting fails for the gastric outlet blockage or is unavailable, open or laparoscopic bypass is warranted. For those undergoing laparoscopic exploration for resection and found to be unresectable, it is reasonable to discontinue the procedure and then attempt an endoscopic procedure. If the expertise is unavailable, an operative bypass is warranted. If exploration via an open procedure reveals that the patient is unresectable, it is reasonable to bypass the patient.

It has been shown that symptomatic patients (vomiting prior to operation) typically have a poor outcome (approximately 90% did not have relief of symptoms) to gastric bypass. In comparison, if patients were not symptomatic but had evidence of impending obstruction, only about 40% had a poor outcome (Weaver et al., 1987). One consideration as to the reason for this is that symptomatic patients are potentially sicker with a greater tumour burden.

Gastric outlet obstruction has been safely treated with a laparoscopic gastrojejunostomy. In fact, for unresectable gastric cancer this technique has been shown to have less suppression of immune function, less pain, shorter hospital stays, lower postoperative morbidity, and earlier recovery of bowel movements than an open procedure (Choi, 2002).

Antrectomy along with gastrojejunostomy in the setting of unresectable pancreatic cancer has been shown to have excellent results until death in one small series (Lucas et al., 1991). There is limited evidence in the literature to support this procedure in the setting of gastric outlet obstruction, and a simpler bypass may be more reasonable.

Wounds/fistulae

Indications of wounds/fistulae

There are multiple different kinds of wounds related to advanced cancer that require the involvement of a general surgeon and wound problems represent approximately 10% of all palliative surgical consultations (Badgwell et al., 2009). These are often directly related to tumours, but may be due to treatments such as surgical procedures or radiation therapy. Tumour-related wounds can be seen with primary, recurrent, or nodal manifestations of tumours. Primary cancers that frequently lead to wound problems include breast cancer, skin cancers, soft tissue sarcomas, or soft tissue manifestations of other cancers (e.g. lung cancer). Special consideration must be taken related to the primary tumour type. As treatment approaches are frequently multidisciplinary, it is important for the surgeon to include other specialists, including medical and radiation oncologists, in the decision-making. Procedure-related wounds may be due to node dissections, local resections, or simple incisions. Radiation may lead to non-healing ulcers at resection sites. Finally, due to debilitation, patients may have pressure sores which complicate their overall course and lead to suffering. In the debilitated patient, pressure sores are more likely to occur. It is unlikely that there would be an indication for a major procedure for this complication, although minor procedures may be helpful.

Fistulae, like wound problems, may occur in patients who are facing the end of life for various reasons. Fistulae are a heterogeneous group of problems. A fistula is simply a communication of one structure to another, including bowel to bowel, bowel to skin, or pancreas to skin. Fistulae may be a complication of procedures, such as pancreatic fistulae after a resection, or due to other treatments, such as a radiation therapy leading to enterocutaneous fistulae. These problems may be extremely difficult to cure, especially in the setting near death. Indications for surgical options are rare.

Options for wounds/fistulae

Prevention of wounds is of primary importance. For example, resection of a nodal or soft tissue metastasis can simply be excised to avoid the potential wound problems that will ensue if ignored. Another preventative consideration is related to pressure wounds. This entails ensuring patients are not stationary for long periods of time. Once a pressure sore has started, it can be difficult or impossible to heal.

Many wounds, especially related to radiation injury or in the severely malnourished, may not heal. Therefore, this should not be a goal of treatment, but focus should be on control of pain, odour, and mess. Wound care is of primary importance. This may include local debridement as indicated to keep the wound as clean as possible. While surgical options for wounds are limited, operative intervention has been reported in 38% and primarily involves incision and drainage or debridement (Badgwell et al., 2009). Only a minority of patients are able to undergo wide excision and closure of tumours causing wound problems.

One example of a chronic wound problem is chest wall complications of breast tumours. There are many articles in the nursing literature regarding local wound care. Chemotherapy, especially if the patient is chemo-naive, is an option. Radiation therapy, although unlikely to have a great effect with a very large tumour, is possible. Of course, surgical resection is an alternative. The term 'toilet' mastectomy is used in the setting of a fungating incurable breast cancer to remove the tumour with the intent of wound control. It is always important to know the previous treatments to better understand possible success. This will also help to identify the optimal reconstruction alternatives as well as the extent of resection that is possible. The surgical literature is not very helpful in directing the extent of resection, and this must be based on surgeon judgement.

Reconstruction options include primary closure, skin grafts, and an omental flap with skin graft, musculocutaneous flaps or free flaps. The major surgical complications that must be considered include infection, open wounds, and flap loss.

Additional morbid options are possible based on the site of the tumour and medical status of the patient. These may include amputations, limb perfusions, and major head and neck resections. While these options may seem quite radical in the setting of palliation, they may be reasonable solutions based on symptoms and if the patient can withstand a large procedure.

While treatment options for fistulae in the patient with advanced cancer may not significantly differ from those not facing the end of life, there are many issues in this population that necessitate special consideration. As with the non-advanced cancer patient, controlling fistulae is the most important treatment. For cutaneous fistulae, this may be through the utilization of stoma bags, drains, or active wound care. For internal fistulae, such as bowel communicating to bowel or bladder, the specific anatomy of the communication is paramount to decide if a surgical option is reasonable.

Outcomes of wounds/fistulae

There have been many reports concerning local wound care for tumour-related wounds. Most of these are in nursing journals. This component of care is extremely important, and has been shown to have great impact on QOL. For example, controlling odour and seepage has been shown to lead to less isolation, greater comfort, and increased psychosocial well-being (Lund-Nielsen et al., 2004). This straightforward approach to some wounds will lead to the best outcomes for many patients facing the end of life.

Multiple reports have focused on chest wall resections for breast cancer. These were either related to recurrent disease or an initial presentation of a fungating breast tumour. Many different reconstruction techniques have been shown to be efficacious, including myocutaneous or omental flaps. The recurrence rates in this setting may be high. In one small series it was noted to be 73% (Cheung et al., 1997), and 20% to 52% in some of the larger series (Flook et al., 1989; Sweetland et al., 1995; Downey et al., 2000; Henderson et al., 2001). The majority of these recurrences were quite small though, and could be locally excised or observed in patients who already had other major metastatic disease. Local wound morbidity is variable, and most are quite minor, such as local skin necrosis in a skin graft which will not have great impact on the patient's life. Importantly, if there is major local wound morbidity, this could have a profound effect on the patient for the remainder of their life.

Related to amputation, there are multiple small reports that do indicate good to excellent palliation (Paz, 2004). Complications may be over 50%, including flap necrosis, infection, and death. Complication rates will depend on the extent of amputation. In addition to amputation, limb perfusion most commonly utilizing melphalan with or without tumour necrosis factor-alpha (TNF-α) has been advocated in some centres for melanoma or sarcoma recurrences. Complete response rates are 45–72%, usually greater if TNF-α was used (Noorda et al., 2006). Importantly, it has been shown that QOL can be excellent, with reasonable long-term function.

Related to fistulae, there is little evidence specific to the end-of-life patient. Therefore, non-surgical techniques are usually optimal. One can look to the non-palliative literature for guidance, but in patients with limited survival, this is unlikely to be a sufficient guide.

Biliary obstruction

Indications of biliary obstruction

Tumours causing obstruction of the extrahepatic bile duct may also occur all along the biliary tree, most likely at the ampulla of Vater (see also Chapter 10.4). Blockages must be treated expediently as this will lead to hyperbilirubinaemia which may become symptomatic, leading to pruritus, bleeding diathesis, and liver failure. Surgical involvement today is often in the instances of a failed endoscopic retrograde cholangiography procedure (ERCP) stenting or inoperability at the time of surgical exploration for a presumed resection with a curative intent. There are multiple studies comparing methods, especially stenting versus surgery (Bornman et al., 1986; Shepherd et al., 1988; Andersen et al., 1989; Dowsett et al., 1989;

Smith et al., 1994; Moss et al., 2006; Moss et al., 2007). Endoscopic stenting has been shown to have similar success rates as surgery with less morbidity. However, the risk of recurrent biliary obstruction prior to death is higher in patients undergoing endoscopic stent placement. One approach is to perform endoscopic stent placement in patients considered to have short life spans with limited potential for recurrent obstruction and perform surgical bypass for patients with less aggressive tumours, longer expected life expectancy, and limited access to endoscopic expertise for treatment of recurrent obstruction. Metal stents are reported to have improved patency compared to plastic stents yet there is currently insufficient evidence to make a statement comparing metal stents to surgery. If the bile duct is entered via the ERCP but a stent could not be placed, it may necessitate a relatively urgent surgical procedure due to the potential cholangitis risk. If urgent surgery is not realistic due to patient co-morbidities, overall status, or operating room availability, a transhepatic drain placed by an interventional radiologist is indicated. If a laparoscopic exploration is first undertaken for a potentially resectable mass and metastatic disease is noted, it is reasonable to abort the procedure with the hope that a less morbid endoscopic stenting can be accomplished. Also, if endoscopic stenting fails or is unavailable, open or laparoscopic bypass is warranted. If at open exploration the patient is found to be unresectable, it is reasonable to proceed with a surgical intervention.

Options for biliary obstruction

There are multiple surgical options to bypass the biliary system. They include cholecystojejunostomy, choledochojejunostomy, or choledochoduodenostomy. In addition, the bypass may be performed higher along the duct to the hepatic duct (above the cystic duct). While these procedures may be undertaken with a laparoscope, few surgeons have the technical skills for this procedure (Krouse, 2004). Importantly, in the appropriate operative candidate, a pancreaticoduodenectomy (Whipple procedure) is an option. While the surgeon should not proceed with a Whipple procedure if there are clear signs of metastasis to the liver or other organs or invasion of major vascular structures, many surgeons will complete the procedure if there is limited local nodal disease.

Outcomes of biliary obstruction

The overall morbidity of surgical bypass is almost 20%, and the recurrence rate is 0–15% (Bornman et al., 1986; Shepherd et al., 1988; Andersen et al., 1989; Dowsett et al., 1989; Smith et al., 1994). It has been shown that choledochoduodenostomy has the fewest complications at only 3% (Potts et al., 1990). Of course, the ability to mobilize the duodenum may not be possible in all patients. There have been several reports of laparoscopic biliary bypass of malignant biliary obstructions, mainly via cholecystojejunostomy, although hepaticojejunostomy also might be performed (Gentileschi et al., 2002), though it requires expertise available in only a few centres. Palliative pancreaticoduodenectomies are infrequently performed and likely represent a prohibitive risk for surgery, although there is little data upon which to base such decisions.

Bleeding

Indications of bleeding

Tumour-related bleeding is frequently difficult to treat, especially with patients who may have a coagulopathy related to illness or treatments. Bleeding may be related to superficial tumours such as recurrent breast, head and neck, or sarcomas. Symptoms related

to deeper tumours include haemoptysis (e.g. primary or metastatic lung tumours), haematemesis (e.g. gastric cancer), melena or haematochezia (e.g. colorectal tumours), vaginal bleeding (e.g. cervical or endometrial carcinomas), or haematuria (e.g. renal or bladder tumours). Surgical intervention for gastrointestinal bleeding is infrequently required in palliative surgical evaluation (14%) and most often involves bowel resection (Miner et al., 2002). Indications for surgical involvement will be related to location of the tumour and whether another approach is less morbid and has a reasonable chance at success. Non-surgical options include radiation therapy, arterial embolization, endoscopic procedures and bronchoscopic techniques.

Options for bleeding

Obviously, there are multiple reasons for bleeding leading to a very heterogeneous group of patients, and the optimal surgical option will depend mainly on the location and reason for bleeding. For example, if there is superficial tumour bleeding, direct suturing may be possible. It must be considered though, that the bleeding may be diffuse and simple suturing may not be efficacious. Therefore, resection may be indicated. For deeper tumours, such as colon tumours, a resection may more clearly be the best option. Rectal tumours, which necessitate larger, more complex procedures and probably an intestinal stoma, may be better served first with non-surgical attempts (e.g. radiation therapy or interventional radiology embolization). The success of alternative approaches will be based on the availability and expertise at each institution.

Outcomes of bleeding

The outcomes to the treatment of bleeding depend specifically on the treatment approach and the aetiology of the bleeding. Resecting a bleeding tumour will universally stop the bleeding, but there may be added surgical morbidity and mortality than if the operation was performed in the non-emergent setting. Other options to temporize the situation or attempt to alleviate the need for an operation, such as an embolization procedure, may carry a greater risk of recurrence of bleeding but will often be less morbid than a major operation. Of course, this may be quite variable and depends on the tumour location.

Malignant ascites

Indications of malignant ascites

Ascites may be due to overwhelming liver metastasis, cirrhotic liver disease, or carcinomatosis (see also Chapter 10.4). It can be a difficult management problem, and treatment may be determined by the extent of ascites, condition of patient, or aetiology. If ascites is minimal, no therapy is indicated. Treatments will be necessary with larger volumes of ascites, which can lead to discomfort, fullness, or respiratory problems. Surgical options should be considered if diuretics no longer are helping or percutaneous aspirations are becoming painful and frequent. In addition to improving patient comfort, a reasonable indication for surgical interventions is to ease the burden of care. If the patient has very advanced disease, simpler approaches should be initiated. If the patient has a longer lifespan, more invasive techniques may be considered.

Options for malignant ascites

Probably the simplest surgical techniques are the insertion of permanent intraperitoneal drainage catheters. This will allow serial drainage of fluid by the patient or their caretaker. Catheters can be placed surgically or by the interventional radiology team via computed tomography (Mercadante et al., 1998) or ultrasound guidance (O'Neill et al., 2001). Multiple types of catheters have been used, including a pigtail catheter, peritoneal dialysis catheters (e.g. Tenkoff catheter), pleural cavity catheters (e.g. Pleurx® catheter), fenestrated port-a-catheters, and even a Foley catheter (Richard et al., 2001; Rosenblum et al., 2001; Barnett and Rubins 2002; Iyengar and Herzog 2002; Kuruvillea et al., 2002). The patient and/or caregiver can be trained to drain excess peritoneal fluid when the patient is symptomatic.

Another option for malignant ascites is a peritoneovenous shunt. The two most common are the LeVeen or Denver® shunt. Ascitic fluid travels from the peritoneal cavity into the venous circulation due to higher peritoneal pressures. Surgeons are often apprehensive to perform this procedure due to the historical catastrophic complications, including sepsis, disseminated intravascular coagulation (DIC), heart failure, and pulmonary embolism leading to a rapid death. In addition, patients often die within 1 month of their procedure due to their poor general condition (Smith et al., 1989).

Hyperthermic intraperitoneal chemotherapy (HIPEC), without cytoreduction, is an accepted approach for palliation of malignant ascites with good early data. In addition, this procedure can be performed laparoscopically in an attempt to minimize complications (Valle et al., 2009). A much more invasive surgical technique includes a major debulking of carcinomatosis followed by intraperitoneal hyperthermic chemotherapy. This procedure is only available at specialized institutions but will likely be infrequently performed for palliation in the future based on the results emerging from HIPEC without cytoreduction and laparoscopic HIPEC (Facchiano et al., 2012).

Outcomes of malignant ascites

The success rates for permanent intraperitoneal catheters functioning until death is quite high (90%) (O'Neill et al., 2001; Barnett and Rubins, 2002). There is low procedural morbidity. The major complications are obstruction and infection, and are around 17% (O'Neill et al., 2001; Barnett and Rubins, 2002), although catheter sepsis has been reported to be 35% (Lee et al., 2000). To avoid infection there must be meticulous insertion technique, close patient follow-up, and liberal use of antibiotics (O'Neill et al., 2001). In fact many catheter-related infections can be treated with antibiotics (Kirk et al., 1993). Sometimes the catheters may need to be removed due to infection, occlusion or leakage around the catheter. Leakage has been reported to be alleviated by continuous drainage (Barnett and Rubins, 2002) or a suture around the drain (Lee et al., 2000).

While the incidence of major complications may be less common than previously reported for peritoneovenous shunts, the overall complication rate can be quite high (14–51%) (Smith et al., 1989; Bieligk et al., 2001; Zanon et al., 2002). DIC is the major complication that most frequently will lead to patient death. It has been reported from 5% to 10% of these procedures. Congestive heart failure is another major complication. The more common complication is shunt occlusion. The advantage of the Denver® shunt over the LeVeen shunt is that the Denver® shunt has a pump to help the shunt remain patent (26% Denver® vs 50% LeVeen shunt occlusion rates) (Bieligk et al., 2001). Denver® shunts have been shown to have quite high function of these shunts until death

(96%) (Zanon et al., 2002). The risk of infection is variable (0–18%) (Zanon et al., 2002), and this may lead to shunt removal if not relieved with antibiotics. Importantly, relief of symptoms can be as high as 87.5% (Zanon et al., 2002). Therefore, a peritoneovenous shunt may be an excellent option in properly selected patients.

In the carcinomatosis patient, cytoreduction and intraperitoneal chemotherapy can have dramatic effects on ascites. In one report, 79% of patients did not have recurrence for the remainder of their life (median survival 7.6 months) (Loggie et al., 2000). Surprisingly, their group has also shown that this procedure can lead to an acceptable QOL and return of function status for many patients (McQuellon et al., 2007). Palliative treatment of malignant ascites with cytoreduction and HIPEC may be of historical interest only as the contribution from cytoreduction may be minimal based on reports of laparoscopic HIPEC. Laparoscopic HIPEC without cytoreduction is a less technically demanding procedure with a shorter length of stay and decreased risk of surgical complications. A recent systematic review of 76 patients undergoing palliative laparoscopic HIPEC reported the procedure was considered successful in 72 patients (95%), defined as complete regression of ascites, with no deaths and a morbidity rate of 12% (Bieligk et al., 2001). Laparoscopic HIPEC appears to be safe and highly effective for the treatment of malignant ascites. The morbidity, although low, suggests this procedure is best utilized in settings of ascites refractory to less aggressive treatments (Cavazzoni et al., 2013). The improvement in ascites and lack of a need for catheters or follow-up procedures is encouraging but it should be noted that none of the studies of palliative laparoscopic HIPEC have included symptom assessment or QOL outcomes measures.

Splenomegaly

Indications of splenomegaly

Splenectomy due to splenomegaly may be on an urgent/emergent basis due to injury, or in an elective setting related to symptomatic splenic hypertrophy. Splenomegaly may have profound symptoms due to a mass effect, most commonly on the stomach leading to early satiety. Large spleens may also compress other structures, such as the kidney. In addition, splenomegaly may lead to an increased chance of injury, with consideration of a prophylactic splenectomy to avoid such a complication. Related to splenic trauma, in the non-palliative setting it is common to try to preserve the spleen and avoid an operation. In the context of a patient facing the end of life, splenic preservation is less of a priority and may be more dangerous. Therefore, urgent splenectomy is usually indicated in this setting, provided the patient is an operative candidate. For symptomatic splenomegaly, the choice of treatment is usually related to the anticipated survival of the patient and the estimated operative risks. If the patient is felt to have a survival of at least 3–6 months, an operation is usually the best alternative as the recurrence rate related to radiation for haematological disorders is quite high (Weinmann et al., 2001). If survival is predicted to be low, it is reasonable to attempt radiation therapy.

Options for splenomegaly

Splenectomy can frequently be accomplished via laparoscopy. Laparoscopically, splenic tissue is removed via morcellation. This is acceptable as margin of resection is not of significance in this setting. Some feel that laparoscopic splenectomy is the procedure of choice for elective spleen removal (Rosen et al., 2002). Massive splenomegaly may make a laparoscopic procedure difficult or impossible. Open splenectomy may carry a higher morbidity and mortality, especially in this sick population. In the setting of splenic trauma, a laparoscopic approach may not be reasonable.

Outcomes of splenomegaly

Laparoscopic splenectomy has been reported to carry a complication rate of 13%, and a mortality of 1%, with decreased hospitalization and pain (Brodsky et al., 2002). These rates are likely to be higher in the setting of advanced cancer. Use of a hand port (the introduction of a surgeon's hand into the peritoneal cavity to assist the procedure) may greatly facilitate the operation, and is advocated by some surgeons especially for significantly enlarged spleens (Hellman et al., 2000; Targarona et al., 2001; Ailawadi et al., 2002; Rosen et al. 2002). While port-site splenosis has been documented (Kumar and Borzi, 2001), this is unlikely to be an issue for patients facing the end of life. Only a surgeon skilled in the procedure should undertake laparoscopic splenectomy in a patient with massive splenomegaly (Terrosu et al., 2002; Targarona et al., 2000). No matter how a spleen is removed, obstructive symptoms such as early satiety should ultimately be resolved. There is little data on palliative splenectomy in advanced cancer patients upon which to base treatment decisions. The majority of reports focus on splenectomy in patients with myelofibrosis with myeloid metaplasia. In a study from the Mayo Clinic, Minnesota, United States, 76% of patients experienced a palliative benefit, although morbidity was 28% with a 7% mortality rate (Mesa et al., 2006). Until better evidence-based guidelines are available, surgeons will continue to rely on their best estimation of operative risks, which are considerable, in relation to the anticipated symptom improvement in the background of life expectancy.

Hormonal control of hepatic metastases of neuroendocrine tumours

Indications of hormonally active tumours

The surgical goals of treating hormonally active tumours (i.e. metastatic gastrointestinal carcinoid, insulinoma, gastrinoma, VIPoma) are to limit or minimize the endocrine symptoms or to lessen the medications patients are currently taking. Nonfunctional endocrine tumours may lead to fatigue or pain, and it may be reasonable to attempt an intervention to relieve these symptoms. When surgery is not an option or felt to be too high risk in a patient that is not achieving acceptable palliation with biotherapy, transarterial embolization (alone or with chemotherapy) is a good palliative treatment modality.

Options for hormonally active tumours

Invasive options for symptomatic endocrine tumours are based on location of the tumour, type of tumour, and alternative treatment options. For pancreatic neuroendocrine tumours, aggressive surgical treatment of the primary tumour is usually indicated (Schurr et al., 2007). For metastatic gastrinoma, total gastrectomy may also be indicated, although newer medications may alleviate the necessity for such a drastic procedure. While somatostatin analogues frequently modulate symptoms in the setting of liver metastases, it may be short-lived and necessitate increasing doses. The major invasive options for liver metastasis include surgical debulking or ablative techniques. Surgical debulking may necessitate a major hepatectomy or segmental ('wedge') resections. The major ablative technique currently utilized is radiofrequency

ablation (RFA), which is associated with low morbidity and mortality (Erce and Parks, 2003). RFA also allows options to perform open, laparoscopic or radiologist-guided procedures. Finally, it has even been suggested that liver or multivisceral transplantation is a therapeutic option for metastatic neuroendocrine tumours (Olausson et al., 2007).

Outcomes of hormonally active tumours

In addition to minimizing treatment-related complications and shortening hospital stays, ablative techniques can also offer improved QOL in the treatment of pain and tumour hormone output. Anecdotal accounts and small series have shown RFA to be useful in treating metastatic endocrine tumours, but the long-term outcomes are not yet known. Laparoscopic RFA has been shown to achieve symptomatic improvement in patients with secreting neuroendocrine tumours (Siperstein et al., 1997; Berber et al., 2002). This technique does not require an advanced skill set, but does have a learning curve to efficiently complete procedures. The laparoscopic approach should be considered for patients with symptomatic neuroendocrine liver metastases, although the procedure may be difficult to accomplish in the setting of extensive adhesions.

While ablation of metastatic neuroendocrine tumours is an option for some patients with bulky disease, radical resection with or without ablation must still be an alternative for these patients. As there is a more defined long-term history with radical resection of metastatic hepatic tumours, it should remain the first choice of care in the appropriately selected patient. The surgery must accomplish a significant reduction of tumour bulk to have a symptomatic response, although this number is difficult to quantify (Gronbech et al., 1992). Nevertheless, cytoreductive surgery for selected patients with carcinoid tumours does seem to accomplish a symptomatic advantage related to relief/prevention of obstructions or relief of the carcinoid syndrome (Chamberlain et al., 2000; Gulec et al., 2002). Resection and ablative techniques, when followed by a somatostatin analogue, can lead to extremely high rates of long-term symptom-free survival (Chung et al., 2001).

There are limited reports of liver or multivisceral transplantation in the setting of metastatic neuroendocrine tumours. A recent report has shown a 5-year survival of 90% ($N = 15$) (Olausson et al., 2007). The QOL benefit is unclear. While this may be a consideration, the experience is quite small and therefore should be attempted with trepidation.

Future directions

Technology

As technology improves for the surgical treatment of tumours for cure, this will also have impact on palliative care. For example, the use of RFA techniques, chemoembolization, and radioactive TheraSphere® for primary hepatomas and metastatic colorectal cancers also has a role for the less common endocrine metastases. Many other technologies, including minimally invasive techniques can effectively treat complications related to tumours or their care with less morbidity.

Education

While education of the surgeon has been lacking, its importance is being increasingly recognized, which will lead to improved patient care. The reasons for a lack of focus on end-of-life care in surgical residency programmes are multifaceted, and are based in the culture of surgeons and the clinical dilemmas they face. First, many surgeons may not feel comfortable or competent with end-of-life issues. This is in part due to the 'cut to cure' mentality that has been passed on through the generations. Medical students over the years have been drawn to surgery because they want to 'fix' the problem. In the setting of the cancer patient with advanced disease, where cure is not an option, then QOL must be the focus as the problem to be 'fixed'.

While all medical specialties have been remiss in the teaching of palliative care, general surgery has been especially deficient. Surgical textbooks are inferior to all others in ensuring that end-of-life topics are addressed. One investigation revealed that 71.8% of all end-of-life topics were not included in the leading surgery textbooks (Rabow et al., 2000). Furthermore, in a survey by the Society of Surgical Oncology, 48% of respondents said they had had no palliative care training while in medical school (McCahill et al., 2002), and 30% of the respondents had had no training in these issues during their residency or fellowship training. Almost 80% reported 10 hours or less of such instruction during all of their training. This confirms a previous report that surgical training is deficient in adequately educating residents in end-of-life care (Rappaport et al., 1991). Of greatest concern, however, is the lack of postgraduate CME in end-of-life care, as 23.6% of surgeons with a special interest or focus in cancer said that they have had no continuing education in palliative care.

The American College of Surgeons has recognized the need for increased palliative surgical education and has created an education tool to assist residents and surgeons in improving palliative care for surgical patients and their families (American College of Surgeons 2009). In addition, the American College of Surgeons created the Surgical Palliative Care Task Force, now the Committee on Surgical Palliative Care, as part of their Division of Education to meet the Promoting Excellence in End-of-Life Care National Program Office priorities by gathering data and developing tools to help surgeons become more effective in palliative care.

Research

There is currently a paucity of prospective palliative studies in the surgical literature (Miner et al., 1999). This is for many reasons, including ethical considerations in surgical palliative care studies (Krouse et al., 2003). Issues such as vulnerability of patients or the clinician as the researcher are not exclusive to palliative research, but they certainly are highlighted in the advanced cancer setting. There are matters unique to palliative research itself, such as the lack of clarity of the risk-benefit relationship. Another concern is with randomization, which can be quite difficult, especially if there is a placebo arm. A placebo arm is likely impossible in a palliative surgery trial. Finally, there are issues unique to surgical palliative research in that surgery is obviously quite invasive. In addition, once a procedure is completed it is difficult or impossible to reverse, unlike a chemotherapy trial where the medication can be stopped.

In addition to ethics, there are other barriers to surgical research on those with advanced cancer. These include surgeon and procedure variability, patient and family agreement to participate in a trial, the consent process (especially if there are mental status changes or no family member available), inaccessibility of patients

based on referring practitioner bias or patients being in hospice care, and the high attrition rate associated with palliative surgical interventions. This has proved difficult in outcomes assessment for prospective observational studies comparing operative to non-operative management. In a recent prospective observational study of patients undergoing palliative surgical consultation, 40% of the patients died prior to completion of the study at 3 months (Badgwell et al., 2013).

Research in the advanced cancer patient is important to pursue to improve patient care related to treatment alternatives, but also to improve the care by the surgical team. In assessing QOL in extremity sarcoma trials, it was observed that the very act of trying to determine what QOL means to people seemed to have had a humanizing effect on the investigative team (Sugarbaker et al., 1982). Therefore, additional importance placed on palliative care through research could lead to greater importance of QOL issues for surgeons.

Importantly, as standard methods of research may not be applicable or possible in the palliative surgery setting, researchers must consider alternative methodologies to examine optimal care questions. This likely will mean utilizing comparative effectiveness techniques to include alternative outcome measures (rather than survival, mortality, and morbidity), as well as novel statistical manoeuvres to assess surgical treatment benefit. In addition, surgical questions beyond the outcomes of an actual operation should be examined, such as costs, communication issues, and symptom prevention.

Conclusions

Palliative procedures are an important component of the practice for general surgeons who care for cancer patients. It is imperative to understand the surgical and non-surgical options afforded each patient. If a surgical procedure is considered, the patient, family, and treating teams must have a firm understanding of realistic goals of success which focus on QOL. In addition, the chances of attaining those goals must be understood. Finally, the risks of the procedure, including worsening of symptoms and death must be clearly described. As long as these criteria are met, surgical procedures may be undertaken in the setting of terminal cancer. In addition, surgeons should maintain follow-up with the patient whether they operate or not. If an alternative approach is attempted, there may be evolution of disease and surgical intervention may be subsequently indicated. Importantly, the surgeon should continue to follow their patient if at all possible, even if no surgical procedure is undertaken, especially if a relationship has been established. Care of patients by a surgeon includes much more than the operations they perform.

Online materials

Complete references for this chapter are available online at <http://www.oxfordmedicine.com>.

References

American College of Surgeons (2009). *Surgical Palliative Care: A Resident's Guide*. [Online] Available at: <http://www.facs.org/palliativecare/surgicalpalliativecareresidents.pdf>.

Badgwell, B.D., Smith, K., Liu, P., Bruera, E., Curley, S.A., and Cormier, J.N. (2009). Indicators of surgery and survival in oncology inpatients requiring surgical evaluation for palliation. *Supportive Care in Cancer,* 17, 727–734.

Ferrell, B.R., Chu, D.Z., Wagman, L., *et al.* (2003). Online exclusive: patient and surgeon decision making regarding surgery for advanced cancer. *Oncology Nursing Forum,* 30, E106–114.

Feuer, D.J., Broadley, K.B., Shepherd, J.H., and Barton, D.P. (1999). Systematic review of surgery in malignant bowel obstruction in advanced gynecological and gastrointestinal cancer. *Gynecologic Oncology,* 75, 313–322.

Krouse, R.S., Nelson, R.A., Ferrell, B.R., *et al.* (2001). Surgical palliation at a cancer center. *Archives of Surgery,* 136, 773–778.

Legendre, H., Vahhuyse, F., Caroli-Bose, F.X., and Pector, J.C. (2001). Survival and quality of life after palliative surgery for neoplastic gastrointestinal obstruction. *European Journal of Surgery,* 27, 364–367.

McCahill, L.E., Krouse, R., Chu, D., *et al.* (2002). Indications and use of palliative surgery: results of Society of Surgical Oncology survey. *Annals of Surgical Oncology,* 2, 104–112.

Miner, T.J., Jaques, D.P., Tavaf-Motamen, H., and Shriver, C.D. (1999). Decision making on surgical palliation based on patient outcome data. *American Journal of Surgery,* 177, 150–154.

Ripamonti, C. (1994). Management of bowel obstruction in advanced cancer. *Current Opinions in Oncology,* 6, 351–357.

Valle, M., van der Speeten, K., and Garofalo, A. (2009). Laparoscopic hyperthermic intraperitoneal preoperative chemotherapy (HIPEC) in the management of refractory malignant ascites: a multi-institutional retrospective analysis in 52 patients. *Journal of Surgical Oncology,* 100, 331–334.

Orthopaedic surgery in the palliation of cancer

John H. Healey and David McKeown

Introduction to orthopaedic surgery in the palliation of cancer

Orthopaedic surgery is a powerful tool in the palliation of pain and disability in cancer patients who develop metastasis to bone, with the capacity to maintain quality of life and, occasionally, extend life. Even in late-stage disease, orthopaedic surgery plays an important role in cancer care and may be the definitive method to relieve pain and maintain patient independence, as well as assist in terminal care. In order to guide the complex decision-making in the care of these patients, the clinician must employ a broad understanding of metastatic bone disease and a specific understanding of appropriate surgical techniques. This chapter provides the context in which to evaluate patients with metastatic bone disease and offers management guidelines for common disease patterns.

Bone metastases are a significant source of morbidity and mortality among cancer patients. Annually, approximately half of patients who die from cancer have metastatic disease (American Cancer Society, 2006). Progression of primary carcinoma to bone is most commonly associated with breast, prostate, lung, kidney, and thyroid cancers (Coleman, 2001). Metastasis to bone occurs during the course of disease in 75–85% of patients with advanced prostate or breast cancer, in as many as 40% of patients with lung cancer, and in about 25% of those with renal cancer (Coleman, 1997). Improvements in treatment during the past few decades have prolonged the survival of patients with advanced disease. The long-term survival of patients with metastatic bone disease varies according to the type of primary lesion, with a median survival of 40 months for prostate cancer, 24 months for breast cancer, 48 months for thyroid cancer, and less than 6 months for lung cancer (Rubens and Coleman, 1995). In certain situations, surgical intervention can provide better or more prompt pain relief than available medical interventions; thus, providing pain relief to patients with metastatic disease is a common role of the orthopaedic surgeon in palliative cancer care.

Patient presentation

In addition to pathological fractures and bone pain, metastatic bone disease can lead to hypercalcaemia, spinal instability, and spinal cord compression. Knowledge of these potentially life-threatening complications is essential for all clinicians caring for patients with metastatic bone disease. Although a patient can present with any of these processes, the most common presenting sign or symptom of metastatic bone disease is pain.

Bone pain from cancer invasion can result from the mechanical instability that occurs at sites of osteoclastic bone destruction, triggered by the release of cytokines and growth factors by tumour cells. Bone pain can also result from tumour cell stimulation of primary sensory afferent nerve fibres (Goblirsch et al., 2005). Sensory afferent fibres are abundant within the periosteum and the medullary canal of bones, in close proximity to blood vessels within the haversian canals. Neurochemical studies of protein production within the spinal cord and afferent nerve fibres have shown that cancer-induced bone pain differs from neuropathic and inflammatory type pain (Honore et al., 2000). Mechanical and structural stability also play a substantial role in bone pain. The same microenvironment that contributes to nerve sensitization has a major impact on structural stability. The pH of the tumour microenvironment is known to be acidic, and osteoclasts resorb bone in a locally acidic environment (Healey, 2007). Thus, the acidity of the tumour microenvironment ultimately promotes significant bone resorption, though the degree varies in different primary cancers. Pain will occur when the structure has been affected to such a degree that microfractures propagate or the nerve supply within the periosteum is activated (Weilbaecher et al., 2011; Yoneda et al., 2011).

Bone metastases most frequently arise within the axial skeleton. Metastases to the appendicular skeleton occur most commonly in the femur and humerus (Harrington, 1997), with less frequent incidence of metastases in more distal regions. Pain in the axial skeleton may be diffuse and poorly localized, while in the appendicular skeleton, it is often more discrete. In both situations, abnormal stimulation of afferent nerve fibres can cause night pain or pain at rest, for which anti-inflammatory agents provide insufficient relief. If bone pain worsens with functional activities or weight bearing, there may be a mechanical component, as functional pain frequently indicates a bone at risk for fracture.

The clinician must identify and distinguish between localized pain within the axial or appendicular skeleton and radicular pain that radiates most commonly from the spine. Patients with radicular pain arising from metastases near the spinal nerve root will often complain of shooting pain into their legs or arms and may report symptoms of spinal stenosis or spinal canal compromise, characterized by improvement in pain with bending forward. On examination, reproduction of the patient's symptoms will occur with a straight leg raise test for the lower extremities or a positive

Spurling's test for symptoms in the upper extremities. Deep tendon reflexes and pathological reflexes must be carefully examined to rule out myelopathic symptoms as well.

Evaluation of a patient with a bone lesion

For symptomatic bone lesions from metastatic disease, patients will typically present with (a) known widely disseminated metastatic disease, (b) a known primary and a new bone lesion, or (c) an unknown primary and a bone lesion. Each scenario must be addressed differently.

In patients known to have widely disseminated metastatic disease, biopsy of a bone lesion is unnecessary. It is more important to identify the location of the pain, the type of pain, and the severity of bone involvement. In a patient with a known primary who was otherwise disease free but who now presents with a new bone lesion, imaging studies to identify other possible bone and/or visceral metastases must be undertaken and should include the initial primary site; the chest, abdomen, and pelvis; and the rest of the skeleton. In this situation, a biopsy of the most easily accessible metastatic site should be performed to confirm disease recurrence.

In patients who present with an unknown primary and a bone lesion, the other sites of involvement must be identified. Computed tomography (CT) of the chest, abdomen, and pelvis should be used to evaluate the visceral system for a primary site of involvement and/or additional metastases. A bone scan should also be performed to identify any other skeletal metastases.

Imaging of patients with metastatic bone disease

Plain radiographs

Initial evaluation of a patient with bone pain should be performed via plain radiography, with at least two views of the area of interest. Plain X-rays are especially useful in evaluating the overall structural integrity of the bone, identifying patients who can benefit from surgery, and for planning surgical interventions or areas of radiation treatment. However, plain radiography is an insensitive method for metastasis detection, as a minimum lesion diameter of 1 cm and bone mineral loss of at least 50% are required (Salvo et al., 2009). In home care and hospice environments, however, plain X-rays are a practical, cost-effective method for the initial evaluation of new pain or functional loss.

The patterns of bone destruction visible on plain radiographs may help guide treatment, and are often characterized as moth-eaten, permeative, or geographic. A moth-eaten appearance often occurs with multiple myeloma and indicates a slightly more aggressive process. A permeative pattern is seen with the most aggressive bone destruction, while a geographic pattern may indicate a slow-growing tumour process.

Bone scintigraphy

Bone scintigraphy can be extremely useful in detecting other bone lesions throughout the skeleton. It utilizes a technetium-labelled diphosphonate, which is incorporated into the hydroxyapatite mineral matrix of bone. Hence, bone scintigraphy will detect the disease progression only when new bone formation is occurring. For instance, lesions from multiple myeloma will often be cold on bone scan, despite bone destruction, due to the lack of new bone deposition. Similarly, highly aggressive lesions that do not involve new bone deposition, such as lung carcinoma or melanoma metastases, will not be detected by bone scintigraphy. Although scintigraphy detects bone disease with a sensitivity of approximately 72–75% (Eustace et al., 1997; Hahn et al., 2011), it lacks specificity and does not provide information about structural integrity.

Computed tomography

CT is very useful for evaluating the structural integrity of bone and is helpful in preoperative planning, particularly for pelvis and spine lesions. It can also detect occult fractures in the setting of a metastatic lesion, which can be difficult to see on magnetic resonance imaging (MRI) because of marrow oedema caused by the tumour itself. It is more useful than plain radiographs because it better delineates bone involvement of a lesion and can reveal soft tissue extension.

Magnetic resonance imaging

MRI, which provides excellent contrast between normal bone marrow and tumour-involved marrow space, is a valuable tool for studying the anatomic characteristics of a metastatic lesion to bone. However, it lacks the ability to provide detailed information about the structural integrity of the bone. Therefore, it is best used in conjunction with plain films and/or CT scan. MRI of the entire spine with sagittal images is now the most efficient way to conduct an overall evaluation of the patient. It helps to avoid missing a critical remote lesion that is producing neurogenic or referred pain.

Positron emission tomography

Positron emission tomography (PET) scan is a nuclear study that utilizes ^{18}F radioactive-labelled fluorodeoxyglucose, a glucose analogue, as a tracer element. Cells with high metabolic activity, such as tumour cells, demonstrate higher tracer uptake and visually are easily distinguished from cells with normal or low metabolic activity.

PET imaging likely has diagnostic potential in the setting of metastatic bone disease, but investigations of its utility are ongoing. Like MRI and bone scintigraphy, PET does not provide information on the structural integrity of the bone and must be used in conjunction with plain radiography or CT imaging.

Therapeutic considerations in patients with metastatic bone disease

When treating metastatic bone disease, the goal is to increase the quality of the patient's remaining life, through increasing mobility, improving function, and decreasing tumour burden and pain. Often, throughout this process, multiple treatment modalities, such as systemic bisphosphonate treatment, local and global radiation therapy, hormonal therapy, and chemotherapy, must be appropriately coordinated.

Bone pain can result from local environment changes, caused by the tumour itself, that cause abnormal stimulation of afferent nerve fibres, or it can be associated with the mechanical weakening of bone. Therefore, surgical interventions can reduce pain either by mechanical stabilization of a metastatic site or by decreasing the tumour burden at a given site. The ultimate goal of almost all orthopaedic interventions in patients with metastatic disease is immediate weight bearing as tolerated, which facilitates the quickest return to normal function.

The vast majority of surgical interventions in patients with metastatic bone lesions are for the treatment of impending or existing pathological fractures. In rare instances, patients with impending or existing pathological fractures are too sick to undergo surgery or their life expectancies are too short to benefit from surgical intervention. In these patients, casting or splinting the areas of involvement may provide mechanical pain relief but will usually not provide improved function. The cast or splint should be well padded and free of any areas of increased pressure to prevent skin breakdown and ulceration. Casts should be avoided for limbs with lymphoedema, as they can cause tissue damage or compartment syndrome.

In almost all other instances, impending and existing pathological fractures should be surgically stabilized, ideally prior to actual fracture. Surgical intervention is more easily performed in this setting and the patient will experience less pain. Because pathological fractures have a poor healing rate, surgical fixation is essential for providing long-term stability to the area (Fig. 12.5.1).

It is important to note that not all fractures sustained by patients with advanced cancer are pathological tumour-related fractures. Elderly cancer patients and patients who have received androgen deprivation therapy for prostate cancer can develop osteoporotic fractures. In one population-based study, patients with prostate cancer who were treated with luteinizing hormone-releasing hormone agonists had a 19% incidence of non-pathological fractures and only a 6% incidence of pathological fracture (Krupski et al., 2004).

Classification and characterization of impending pathological fractures

Much research in orthopaedics has been devoted to identifying factors that accurately predict the likelihood of a pathological fracture developing from a metastatic lesion. Metastatic lesions that are at low risk for pathological fracture are often best treated with non-surgical systemic interventions and radiation therapy.

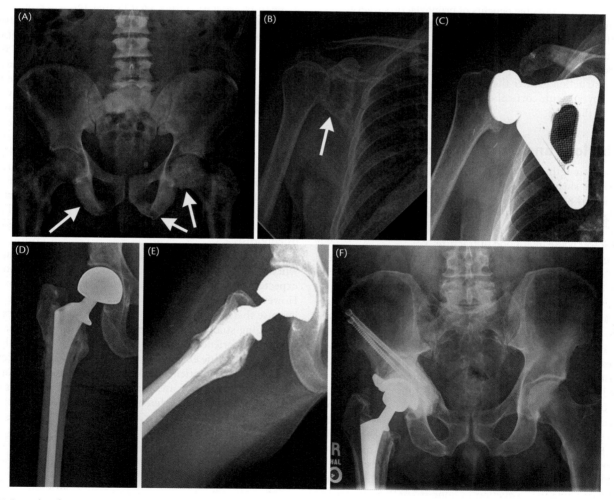

Fig. 12.5.1 Examples of metastatic bone lesions and surgical fixation techniques. (A) A patient with metastatic prostate cancer who developed multiple osteoblastic lesions of the pelvis and proximal femur. (B) Metastatic renal carcinoma of the right scapula, with involvement of the glenoid and entire scapula; (C) a titanium scapular replacement was used to reconstruct the area after resection of the native scapula. (D–E) A hemiarthroplasty was performed on this 40-year-old female with metastatic breast cancer to the proximal femur. A cemented long-stem component was used; note that only one side of the joint was replaced with a large head that articulates with the native acetabulum. (F) A patient with metastatic breast cancer involving the proximal femur and acetabulum was treated with a total hip arthroplasty, including a Harrington reconstruction of the acetabulum. The large pins and surrounding cement provide support for the cup component of the arthroplasty.

Patients with lesions not at risk for fractures treated in this manner have less morbidity and equal or better pain control. It is essential in the treatment of patients with metastases to distinguish these two groups of patients.

In 1989, Mirels published the first scoring system for predicting the likelihood of pathological fracture in patients with metastatic lesions (Mirels, 1989). He then analysed 78 metastatic lesions in 38 patients with various malignancies. All lesions were evaluated prior to irradiation. All patients were followed for 6 months. Patients with a score of 7 had a fracture probability of only 4%. Those with a score of 6 or less experienced no fractures during his study period. A score of 8 was associated with a fracture probability of 15%, with a false positive rate of 6%, and patients with a score of 9 had a 33% probability of fracture and a 0% false positive rate. He concluded that all patients with scores of 9 or higher should undergo prophylactic stabilization of the involved bone, while all patients with scores of 7 or less can be treated with irradiation and subsequent monitoring. For those with a score of 8, he advised further imaging studies to better characterize the lesion's extent in order to determine possible benefits of prophylactic surgery.

Unfortunately, Mirels' rating system does not include several factors that are considered important for assessing pathological fracture risk. At Memorial Sloan Kettering Cancer Center, New York City, surgery is performed in any patient with endosteal cortical destruction greater than 50%, with functional pain after radiotherapy, or with cortical defects larger than 2.5 cm or the diameter of the bone.

Bone biology and biomechanics

The overall strength and structural properties of bone are determined by the shape and distribution of cortical and cancellous bone. Cortical bone has a greater density than cancellous bone and a higher resistance to deformation and failure under given stresses. Therefore, the greater the amount of cortical bone present, the lower is the likelihood of fracture.

Bone is comprised of an organic matrix (40% total content of bone) and an inorganic matrix (60%). The organic matrix is made of collagen (90%), matrix proteins (10%), and proteoglycans (< 1%). The inorganic matrix is composed largely of calcium hydroxyapatite. Collagen in bone provides most of the tensile strength, while the calcium hydroxyapatite provides most of the compressive strength. Tumour-induced osteolysis occurs when cytokines from tumour cells stimulate osteoclast activity. The osteoclasts reabsorb the organic and inorganic components of bone and release free calcium from the calcium hydroxyapatite into the circulation. Lytic lesions trigger greater removal of both the mineral and organic components of bone, leading to greater losses in strength and stiffness. Blastic lesions, however, do not disturb the mineral content of bone and only act to disrupt the normal trabecular framework of the cancellous bone, resulting in a lower likelihood of fracture. Chemotherapy and radiation therapy also contribute to a reduction in bone strength by impairing both osteoblast and osteoclast function and compromising bone repair mechanisms (Hopewell, 2003).

Bone fracture from metastatic disease can occur through one of two processes. First, smaller osteolytic defects in the cortex can lead to stress risers, which are areas of bone where stresses are concentrated around a small hole. A 62% reduction in a bone's bending strength has been associated with a lesion diameter to bone diameter ratio of only 0.2 (McBroom et al., 1988). With smaller lesions, torsional strength is reduced more than compressive or bending strength. Torsional loads to bone occur most frequently during normal daily activities that involve turning or pivoting from a standing position. Activity such as getting up from a chair to transfer can also lead to high torsional loads. The other mechanism of bone fracture results from an open section defect that forms when a larger metastatic lesion creates a hole in the bone larger than the bone's diameter.

The location of a skeletal metastatic lesion greatly influences the likelihood of fracture. The upper extremities are generally subjected to lower stress loads than the lower extremities; therefore, lower-extremity lesions are much more likely to fracture. The proximal femur is also a majority metaphyseal area where cortical bone is thin and cancellous bone comprises the bulk of the structural integrity of the bone. Hence, the proximal femur is the most common site of pathological fracture in the appendicular skeleton.

Metastatic lesions affect not only the strength of bone, but also its healing capacity. Other factors that influence bone healing in patients with metastatic disease are radiation exposure to the area, use of systemic chemotherapy, type of surgical fixation, and histology of the lesion. In a classic study by Gainor and Buchert, bone healing in the setting of pathological fractures was examined in 129 pathological fractures. The overall fracture healing rate was 35% for all cancer types and correlated positively with longer patient survival. Multiple myeloma had the highest healing rate (67%), followed by renal cancer (44%) and breast cancer (37%) (Gainor and Buchert, 1983). Lung cancer patients with pathological fractures had the poorest healing rate; all patients died before healing had occurred. The treatment of internal fixation combined with radiotherapy resulted in the highest union rate in this study (Gainor and Buchert, 1983). Other factors that can influence bone healing in the setting of pathological fracture are nutritional status, use of hormone therapy, and pre-existing osteoporosis.

The surgical procedure chosen should provide stabilization that will last the patient's lifetime; therefore, proper assessment of life expectancy is necessary to make the best decision (Box 12.5.1). However, prediction of survival is fraught with uncertainty, because there are no reliable objective standards. Factors including staging studies, laboratory factors, patient performance status, and experienced clinical judgement account for only half of the variance of life expectancy (Honore et al., 2000). Recent work suggests that the patient's self-assessment may contribute to the accuracy of prediction, and that Bayesian analysis shows the best predictive value across different cultures (Forsberg, 2012).

Box 12.5.1 Factors predicting life expectancy

- Multiple bone involvement
- Parenchymal organ involvement
- Low absolute neutrophil count
- Hypoalbuminaemia
- Anaemia
- Hypercalcaemia.

Types of orthopaedic surgical interventions

Tumour excision

Reducing the tumour burden is an important part of orthopaedic treatment of metastatic lesions and can be accomplished through either intralesional or extralesional excision. Intralesional excision, which is the more common treatment choice, provides significant pain reduction and is associated with fewer fixation failures and a lower risk of tumour progression at the involved site.

Marginal or wide excision has been advocated for certain tumours. Marginal excision removes the bulk of the tumour by excising it just at the border where normal and abnormal tissue meet. Microscopic disease often remains, but the tumour burden is greatly reduced. Marginal excision is often performed in conjunction with arthroplasty.

Wide excision of a metastatic lesion may occasionally be indicated, particularly for patients with a long projected period of survival, such as those with renal, thyroid, or breast cancer. Complete resection of an isolated tumour can reduce the risk of local recurrence to the area and, consequently, the need for further surgery. Such a treatment strategy can improve long-term pain control in these patients (Althausen et al., 1997).

Prosthetic joint replacement (arthroplasty)

Joint arthroplasty, which is performed most frequently in the knee, hip, shoulder, and elbows, involves resection of either one side (hemiarthroplasty) or both sides (total arthroplasty) of the joint surface with prosthetic replacement of the resected joint components. In fractures that involve the epiphyseal surface of joints, healing is exceedingly poor. In such cases, the best treatment is resection of the lesion and prosthetic replacement of the joint; this strategy provides the best long-term outcome. If both sides of the joint are involved, then total joint replacement should be considered. After resection and curettage of the lesion, the prosthetic components are cemented into the remaining bone. The stem of the prosthetic component should always bypass any distal lesions by at least twice the diameter of the involved bone to prevent later periprosthetic fracture. Cement is almost always used in the setting of malignancy because the bone ingrowth required for achieving stability with a non-cemented component will typically not occur.

Plate fixation

Plate fixation provides load-bearing stability to a fracture site by supporting the weight transmitted through the bone until union of the fracture occurs. The disadvantage of this type of stabilization is that the repeated weight-bearing stresses affecting the plate can lead to screw and plate breakage. If tumour progression occurs at the site of the plate, then the screws used to stabilize the plate may also dislodge from the bone in a loss of fixation. Plates are useful devices in places where bone healing is expected to occur in a relatively short period of time; however, this rarely occurs in pathological fractures. Plates are best used in bones that cannot accommodate intramedullary devices, as in severely sclerotic medullary cavities, or to augment another type of fixation.

Intramedullary fixation

In intramedullary fixation, a rod or nail is placed down the centre of the medullary cavity of the bone. Intramedullary devices are load-sharing devices, partially bearing the weight transmitted through the bone. Because the device is in the centre of the bone, where most forces are directed, the device is subjected to less bending force than plate fixation, making fracture much less likely in the setting of slower bone healing and allowing for more immediate weight bearing. Intramedullary devices are particularly useful in diaphyseal fractures, as they are fixed proximally and distally with interlocking screws to help create torsional control at the fracture site. The implanted device can also be augmented with cement to provide additional torsional stability and prevent failure in the setting of disease progression. Any metastatic lesion should be curetted prior to insertion of the intramedullary device to help prevent seeding the rest of the bone with tumour cells.

Bone cement

Bone cement is a very useful adjuvant stabilizer of a fracture site. In a well-delineated lesion, the cement can fill the defect that remains after excision and curettage of the lesion. Bone cement has very strong compressive force resistance and can be used in conjunction with any of the above-mentioned devices to improve the torsional and compressive strength of the fixation. The barium contrast used in the cement also facilitates plain-radiograph monitoring of disease progression or recurrence at the site of cement placement. An additional benefit is the emission of large quantities of heat as the cement solidifies in the bone, destroying tumour cells and further reducing tumour burden.

In 1976, Harrington and colleagues reported on 323 patients treated with cement augmentation of conventional intramedullary fracture fixation techniques (Harrington et al., 1976). They reported 94% return to function and 85% satisfactory pain relief in their patient population.

Amputation

Amputation has a very limited role in the treatment of patients with metastatic disease. The current indications include a limb that cannot be reconstructed due to extensive disease involvement or in situations where complications of the disease leave no other options. These complications include fungating masses, recurrent infections that cannot be controlled with antibiotics, and intractable pain in a limb that has failed treatment by other conventional methods. The most common malignancies to metastasize to the hands and feet are lung, renal, and oesophageal (Healey et al., 1986). An amputation can often provide lasting pain relief for the patient with good functional outcomes.

Anatomic considerations

The type of fixation used to stabilize a fracture site or site of metastasis is dependent on the site of bone involvement. These anatomic considerations are important in choosing the correct type of stabilization in a patient.

Epiphyseal fractures

Epiphyseal fractures, which occur at the ends of long bones near or involving the articular surface, have a very poor healing rate and are not easily stabilized in the setting of malignancy. They are best treated with cemented arthroplasty, which provides a stable, pain-free joint and allows the patient to tolerate immediate weight bearing.

Metaphyseal fractures

Metaphyseal fractures create quite a dilemma in orthopaedic oncology. They frequently occur at sites where intramedullary fixation is difficult, due to insufficient bone on the joint side of the fracture to provide adequate torsional or translational stability. Therefore, the options that remain are usually plate fixation or arthroplasty. As mentioned previously, plate fixation has a high failure rate (22%) when used alone (Wedin et al., 2012). Plates are better suited for patients with radiosensitive tumours that will heal after surgery with radiation treatment, by providing support to the limb during fracture healing. Plates are also suitable for patients with longer life expectancies who can tolerate partial or non-weight bearing for a period of time, while the fracture heals. Rarely can full weight bearing be allowed on a bone that is stabilized with only a plate and screws. Cement augmentation can improve stability when plate fixation is the chosen form of treatment.

Diaphyseal fractures

Diaphyseal lesions are usually well treated with intramedullary nails. In most situations the site of malignant involvement should be opened for complete curettage of the tumour, which will reduce tumour burden and prevent its further dissemination. Once curetted, the site can be filled with bone cement after nail insertion to provide further compressive strength to the area.

In bones that have both diaphyseal and epiphyseal or metaphyseal involvement, arthroplasty for the periarticular involvement should be performed and a cemented long-stem device should be used. The cemented long-stem component of the joint prosthetic device will provide stability to a diaphyseal lesion similar to the intramedullary nail.

Upper extremity

Upper-extremity metastases comprise approximately 20% of all bone metastases. Although the upper extremities are typically subjected to less weight bearing, in many instances, the patient must use the upper extremities for weight bearing during transfers and for using walkers or other mobility aids if necessary. Treatment goals for pathological lesions of the upper extremity are (a) to enable use of the limb in carrying out these basic activities of daily living and (b) to relieve pain.

Pathological fractures of the humerus occur more frequently in torsion than as a result of compressive loads. Obtaining torsional stability is an essential goal in treating humeral fractures. Fractures that involve the periarticular surfaces of the humerus can usually be treated with cemented arthroplasty. In the proximal humerus, if there is tumour in the greater and/or lesser tuberosities of the proximal humerus, then maintenance of rotator cuff attachments and function may be impossible. If the greater and lesser tuberosities cannot be spared, attempts to reattach the rotator cuff using synthetic material like mesh or polyethylene terephthalate (Dacron®) can be performed with variable success. Patients without rotator cuff function will still have a relatively pain-free arm and will retain enough use of the elbow and hand to carry out most activities of daily living, but they will likely be unable to perform activities requiring over-the-head arm movements.

Elbow replacement for distal humeral metastases can provide pain relief and adequate function. For diaphyseal lesions of the humerus, cemented intramedullary devices have the greatest success. In one series of 59 patients treated for pathological fractures of the humerus with either cemented intramedullary nailing or prosthetic replacement, all patients had good pain relief, but patients treated with intramedullary fixation augmented with cement had the best functional outcomes (Bickels et al., 2005).

Most lesions of the scapula and clavicle can be treated with radiation therapy, although irradiation of the lung and other vital organs may be a concern with higher doses. For lesions that are unresponsive to radiation therapy, resection and/or reconstruction may be required. The clavicle is an expendable bone and frequently can be resected without serious functional sequelae. Metal scapula replacements can be used when resection of the entire scapula, including the glenoid, is necessary for tumour control. Smaller portions of the scapula can be resected without prosthetic reconstruction.

Lower extremity

The femur is the third most common site of skeletal metastases. Fractures of the femur account for two-thirds of all pathological long-bone fractures. The proximal femur accounts for 90% of all pathological femur fractures (Sim, 1992). Forces within the proximal femur can be as high as 8 N with certain activities, which may explain why fractures to this region are so frequent (Jacofsky and Haidukewych, 2004). Any reconstruction to this area also must be able to support significant loads.

Metastatic lesions of the proximal femur involving the femoral neck should be treated with arthroplasty. The advantages of hemiarthroplasty over total joint arthroplasty are a shorter operative time, less blood loss, and less risk of postoperative dislocation. However, total hip replacement should be considered when there is evidence of disease within the acetabulum. Peritrochanteric lesions can be treated with arthroplasty as well. Treatment of pathological peritrochanteric fractures with intramedullary nails that include cephalomedullary screws can sometimes provide further stability proximally in the neck region, but the long-term results of these constructs in this setting are still unknown; hence, the standard of care remains joint replacement (Steensma, 2012).

Lesions below the lesser trochanter should be treated like femoral shaft fractures with intramedullary nail stabilization. Lesions very distal in the femur near the knee joint should be treated with cemented total knee arthroplasty or, if well contained and not involving the epiphyseal region, can be treated with curettage, cement, and plate fixation.

Tibial lesions comprise about 4.5% of skeletal metastases (Kelly et al., 2003). In a retrospective study of 25 patients with impending and pathological fractures in the tibia, 23 were proximal or diaphyseal and two were distal lesions. Well-contained metaphyseal lesions not involving the epiphysis were treated with curettage, cement, and plate fixation, while diaphyseal lesions were treated with intramedullary nailing and cement augmentation. Two patients with aggressive metaphyseal lesions extending into the epiphysis underwent endoprosthetic replacement. All patients experienced good pain relief and there was only a 4% failure rate in this series of patients (Kelly et al., 2003).

Pelvis and acetabulum

Metastatic disease to the pelvis and acetabulum are frequent causes of pain and mechanical instability in patients with cancer.

Conventional total hip arthroplasty can fail when there is inadequate bone stock on the acetabular side to support the metal and polyethylene cup component of the implant. The bone stock must be evaluated via CT scan of the pelvis and acetabulum to determine the appropriate treatment option. Only in situations where there is limited disease and intact superior, medial, and anterior and posterior cortices can a conventional total hip arthroplasty, with cementing of the cup component, be performed. When bone is deficient, acetabular reconstruction usually requires protection with a protrusio ring and transferring force transfer past the deficient bone with pins and cement constructs (Marco, 2000).

The most difficult scenarios involve patients with complete destruction of the acetabulum with significant disease involvement of the medial wall, superior dome, and anterior and posterior columns. For such patients, the acetabulum either needs to be completely resected and replaced or supplemental fixation around the acetabulum must be provided. The saddle prosthesis, which was originally created for large acetabular defects following failed conventional total hip arthroplasty, has been used in the setting of pelvic reconstructions for metastatic disease as well as after resection of primary bone tumours of the pelvis. Successful implantation requires a portion of retained ilium as the weight-bearing component of the reconstruction. Although there has been some success in patients with metastatic disease, its use has been fraught with complications. Any concern about disease progression into the ilium precludes use of this device, since a minimum of 2 cm of adequate bone within the ilium located close to the sacroiliac joint is required for stability of this construct. Even with adequate bone remaining, limb shortening, device dislocation, infection, and periprosthetic fracture are frequent complications (Aljassir et al., 2005). This type of reconstruction should be reserved for select patients with intermediate life expectancies.

When solid iliac bone remains, pins or screws can be secured into it and the defect filled with cement and a large anti-protrusio cup to relieve mechanical pain and prevent acetabular cup migration.

Minimally invasive and adjuvant treatment options

Kyphoplasty and vertebroplasty

Vertebroplasty and kyphoplasty are both techniques used to treat painful compression fractures in the spine due to osteoporosis or malignancy. Both vertebroplasty and kyphoplasty are minimally invasive techniques performed through percutaneous instrumentation. Both techniques involve the injection of bone cement posteriorly through the spinal pedicles into the vertebral body. The cement stabilizes the fractured vertebral body, preventing further collapse and reducing mechanical pain created at the site of fracture.

In kyphoplasty, a balloon is first inserted through the pedicle into the vertebral body and then inflated. This re-expands the collapsed vertebra and creates an open space for the injection of cement into the vertebral body. One advantage of kyphoplasty is that some of the height of the vertebral body is restored, improving spinal biomechanics and preventing collapse of other weakened adjacent vertebra. Another advantage is a lowered risk of cement extrusion into the spinal canal, because the space created by the balloon allows for lower-pressure cement injection (Masala et al., 2003). Both techniques provide significant pain relief in patients

with metastatic spinal disease and pain non-responsive to other treatments (Masala et al., 2003).

These techniques should only be considered in patients who have no evidence of cord compromise from tumour involvement and who, aside from pain, have an otherwise normal neurological exam. These techniques are minimally invasive, but are not without risks, including cement migration into the spinal canal, fat embolization, and abnormal cardiovascular response to the cement monomer.

Cryotherapy

In cryosurgery, liquid nitrogen is used to achieve a fast freeze followed by slow thaw, resulting in intracellular protein denaturation, water crystallization, cell membrane destabilization, and, ultimately, cell death. Cryotherapy can be used as the primary treatment for a lesion or as an adjuvant to other surgical techniques.

Newer percutaneous techniques now exist in which a probe is used to introduce liquid nitrogen or an argon beam into the area of involvement (Simon and Dupuy 2005), and have been used in areas of soft-tissue metastases with good success. The technique is less useful in bone metastases, due to the difficulty of probe insertion into bone, and it cannot be used to treat larger lesions, because the probes can only cover a small area of involvement. With percutaneous techniques, bone cement cannot be used to stabilize the area, making them even less desirable in areas where fracture is a concern.

Radiofrequency ablation

Radiofrequency (RF) ablation makes use of alternating electrical current with the same frequency range as radio waves (460–480 kHz) (Simon and Dupuy, 2005). A small electrode, placed near or directly into the target tissue, emits a current that produces ion vibration within the tissue, leading to increased local temperatures and thermal necrosis of the tissue.

The size of the lesion influences the efficacy of RF ablation. Tumours larger than 5 cm can be adequately treated with this technique (Simon and Dupuy, 2005) and it is a good alternative to surgical stabilization for isolated small painful lesions in the extremity. Similarly, lesions within the flat bones of the pelvis and remaining axial skeleton may respond well to this treatment and not require further surgical intervention.

The most common complications associated with RF ablation include skin necrosis, unplanned tissue damage, and fracture at the site of involvement (Simon and Dupuy, 2005). In areas where impending pathological fracture is a concern, surgical intervention is required and RF ablation is not appropriate.

Embolization

Embolization is used to reduce blood flow to vascular tumours. The technique is usually performed by the interventional radiologist and involves the injection of small particles or stainless steel coils into vascular pedicles feeding into tumours, ultimately resulting in diminished blood flow to the lesion and local tissue necrosis. Hypervascular tumours are most responsive to this technique. Renal and thyroid carcinomas are the two most common hypervascular tumours that metastasize to bone, and both haemorrhage significantly when surgically disrupted. Embolization can be used as primary treatment of lesions in areas at low risk of fracture or can be performed 24–72 hours prior to further surgical stabilization and tumour excision. Several studies have shown a significant reduction in intraoperative blood loss and transfusion requirement with use of preoperative embolization (Roscoe et al., 1989; Chatziioannou et al., 2000; Pazionis et al., 2014).

Conclusion

Orthopaedic surgical intervention can be quite successful in reducing pain and improving function in patients with metastatic bone disease, particularly when combined with other treatment modalities. All patients who undergo surgery for treatment of bone metastases should be considered for postoperative radiation therapy as well as systemic treatment with bisphosphonates, hormone therapy, and/or chemotherapy whenever appropriate (Hillner et al., 2000; Saad et al., 2006). This requires the integration of all modalities of oncologic care and coordination of all teams caring for the patient.

The physician's goal when treating patients with metastatic bone disease is to cure some, help most, and provide comfort for all. Proper fracture care is a fundamental element in achieving this goal.

Online materials

Complete references for this chapter are available online at <http://www.oxfordmedicine.com>.

References

Coleman, R.E. (2001). Metastatic bone disease: clinical features, pathophysiology and treatment strategies. *Cancer Treatment Reviews*, 27(3), 165–176.

Forsberg, J.A., Wedin, R., Bauer, H.C., *et al.* (2012). External validation of the Bayesian Estimated Tools for Survival (BETS) models in patients with surgically treated skeletal metastases. *BMC Cancer*, 12(1), 493.

Goblirsch, M.J., Zwolak, P., and Clohisy, D.R. (2005). Advances in understanding bone cancer pain. *Journal of Cellular Biochemistry*, 96(4), 682–688.

Hahn, S., Heusner, T., Kummel, S., *et al.* (2011). Comparison of FDG-PET/CT and bone scintigraphy for detection of bone metastases in breast cancer. *Acta Radiologica*, 52(9), 1009–1014.

Harrington, K.D. (1997). Orthopedic surgical management of skeletal complications of malignancy. *Cancer*, 80(8 Suppl.), 1614–1627.

Healey, J.H. (2007). Cancer pain management in orthopedic surgery. In R.F. Schmidt and W.D. Willis (eds.). *Encyclopedia of Pain*, pp. 255–257. Berlin: Springer.

Hillner, B.E., Ingle, J.N., Berenson, J.R., *et al.* (2000). American Society of Clinical Oncology guideline on the role of bisphosphonates in breast cancer. American Society of Clinical Oncology Bisphosphonates Expert Panel. *Journal of Clinical Oncology*, 18(6), 1378–1391.

Honore, P., Luger, N.M., Sabino, M.A., *et al.* (2000). Osteoprotegerin blocks bone cancer-induced skeletal destruction, skeletal pain and pain-related neurochemical reorganization of the spinal cord. *Nature Medicine*, 6(5), 521–528.

Masala, S., Fiori, R., Massari, F., and Simonetti, G. (2003). Vertebroplasty and kyphoplasty: new equipment for malignant vertebral fractures treatment. *Journal of Experimental & Clinical Cancer Research*, 22(4 Suppl.), 75–79.

Mirels, H. (1989). Metastatic disease in long bones: a proposed scoring system for diagnosing impending pathologic fractures. *Clinical Orthopaedics and Related Research*, 249, 256–264.

Marco, R.A.W., Sheth, D.S., Boland, P.J., Wunder, J.S., Siegel, J.A., and Healey, J.H. (2000). Functional and oncological outcome of acetabular reconstruction for the treatment of metastatic disease. *Journal of Bone and Joint Surgery*, 82A(5), 642–651.

Pazionis, T.J., Papanastassiou, I.D., Maybody, M., and Healey, J.H. (2014). Embolization of hypervascular bone metastases reduces intraoperative blood loss: a case-control study. *Clinical Orthopaedics and Related Research*, 472(10), 3179–3187.

Simon, C.J. and Dupuy, D.E. (2005). Image-guided ablative techniques in pelvic malignancies: radiofrequency ablation, cryoablation, microwave ablation. *Surgical Oncology Clinics of North America*, 14(2), 419–431.

Steensma, M., Boland, P.J., Morris, C.D., Athanasian, E., and Healey, J.H. (2012). Endoprosthetic treatment is more durable for pathologic proximal femur fractures. *Clinical Orthopaedics and Related Research*, 470(3), 920–926.

Wedin, R., Hansen, B.H., Laitinen, M., *et al.* (2012). Complications and survival after surgical treatment of 214 metastatic lesions of the humerus. *Journal of Shoulder and Elbow Surgery*, 21(8), 1049–1055.

Weilbaecher, K.N., Guise, T.A., and McCauley, L.K. (2011). Cancer to bone: a fatal attraction. *Nature Reviews Cancer*, 11(6), 411–425.

Interventional radiology in the palliation of cancer

Tarun Sabharwal, Nicos I. Fotiadis, and Andy Adam

Introduction to interventional radiology in the palliation of cancer

Over the past four decades, a variety of invasive diagnostic and therapeutic procedures have been developed by radiologists. The term 'interventional radiology' most appropriately refers to therapeutic procedures performed under imaging guidance (Adam, 1998). The emergence of this specialty has been made possible by enormous technological advances in relation to catheter and instrument design and manufacture, imaging systems, and radiological expertise. Interventional radiological procedures have virtually replaced several more invasive and hazardous surgical alternatives. Other interventional techniques offer completely new therapeutic options. Some diagnostic radiological procedures are frequently followed by therapeutic manoeuvres. For example, percutaneous antegrade pyelography, performed to delineate the site and nature of renal obstruction, is usually followed immediately by the placement of a nephrostomy drainage catheter. Purely diagnostic procedures, such as percutaneous biopsy, will not be discussed in any detail, as they are largely inappropriate for the patient with a known neoplastic process receiving palliative care.

All interventional procedures carry some risk, which is related to the underlying condition, the nature of the procedure, and the experience of the radiologist. Therefore, it is important in patients with advanced malignant disease receiving palliative care to contemplate only those procedures that will alleviate symptoms, and in which the potential benefits outweigh the risks (Bogda, 2003).

Interventional radiology can make a significant contribution to the palliation of patients with irresectable malignant tumours, as many of the procedures can relieve symptoms without the need for general anaesthesia, a prolonged stay in hospital, or the discomfort associated with recovery from a surgical operation. The vast majority of procedures are performed using local anaesthesia and mild sedation. The emphasis in this chapter is on the indications, contraindications, and likely outcomes, rather than on detailed technical descriptions.

Therapeutic interventional radiological procedures

A summary of procedures that may be useful in patients undergoing palliative care is shown in Table 12.6.1.

Percutaneous puncture and drainage procedures

Utilizing fluoroscopy, ultrasound, computed tomography (CT), or magnetic resonance imaging (MRI) guidance it is possible to image and drain obstructed renal and biliary systems, cysts, abscesses, and effusions.

Renal tract

Antegrade pyelography and percutaneous nephrostomy are used in the management of a variety of situations, including malignant obstruction of the urinary tract, haemorrhagic cystitis secondary to chemotherapy (where it is desirable to divert the urine to 'rest' the bladder), and in patients with recto-vaginal or recto-vesical fistula caused by pelvic malignancy. Diversion of urinary flow may assist in healing of the fistulas, ease nursing problems, and allow patients to become 'dry'.

The pelvicalyceal system is initially punctured under ultrasound guidance with a fine-gauge needle through which radiographic contrast medium is instilled to demonstrate the anatomy and determine the level of obstruction. Urine can be aspirated for microbiological and cytological examinations. Percutaneous nephrostomy entails the insertion into the collecting system of a pigtail configuration catheter with multiple, large side-holes. If drainage is to be of short duration, an external bag may be satisfactory; however, if long-term drainage is required and if it is possible to cross the area of obstruction, an internal stent is preferred (Pingound, 1980), as it allows the patient to be free of 'bags'. It is noteworthy that, in most cases, it is possible to manipulate a catheter across an area of apparently complete obstruction. Although a contrast study may indicate total obstruction, a hydrophilic guidewire can usually be advanced through the 'obstruction', as it finds the (very narrow) lumen and follows it. The balloon catheter can then be advanced over the guidewire to dilate the stricture and restore patency before a stent is inserted.

In patients with pelvic malignancy and fistulas to the perineum it may prove necessary to combine nephrostomy with ureteric embolization using steel coils or segments of gelatine sponge to prevent any urine reaching the skin of the perineum. A catheter can be manipulated into the ureter and embolic materials, such as steel coils and sterile sponge, can be injected to occlude the ureter (Gaylord and Johnsrude, 1989).

Table 12.6.1 Interventional radiological procedures

Procedure	Examples of indications
Drainage	Malignant obstruction of renal and biliary tract, pleural effusions, and ascites
Stenting	Malignant gastrointestinal, biliary, ureteric and airway obstruction, superior or inferior vena caval obstruction, etc.
Feeding	Venous access—Hickman lines peripherally-inserted central catheter (PICC) lines
	Percutaneous gastrostomy
Extraction	Retrieval or re-siting of venous lines
Infusion	Regional, selective infusion of chemotherapeutic agents
Embolization	Hormone-producing metastases, primary hepatocellular carcinoma, skeletal metastases, etc.
Neurolysis	Coeliac axis block in pancreatic cancer
Vertebroplasty	Vertebral metastasis, multiple myeloma, and osteoporosis
Tumour ablation	Liver, renal, lung, bony, and soft tissue tumours

Biliary tract

Patients with obstructive jaundice due to irresectable malignant biliary strictures can be palliated by the insertion of an endoprosthesis (stent) (Fig. 12.6.1). Stents may be inserted endoscopically for lesions affecting the low common bile duct or percutaneously in patients with lesions at the hilum of the liver or when endoscopic retrograde cholangiopancreatography (ERCP) fails to relieve the obstruction. In most cases unilateral drainage is usually sufficient for relieving jaundice and pruritus. The procedure is usually carried out under fluoroscopic and ultrasound guidance. Self-expandable metallic stents are now widely available and generally preferable to the conventional plastic endoprosthesis. Such stents can be inserted using a small introducing catheter (5–7 French diameter) and yet they achieve a large internal diameter (10 mm) when released across the obstructing lesion.

The large calibre of these devices ensures that the rate of occlusion is lower than that of a plastic endoprosthesis. The overall failure rate of plastic stents is in the region of 30–40%, whereas that of metallic stents is 10–15%. The frequency of cholangitis is approximately 30% in patients with plastic stents and approximately 10% in patients with metallic endoprostheses (Morgan and Adam, 2001). Occluded plastic stents can be replaced using a variety of endoscopic or percutaneous techniques. Occluded metallic endoprostheses cannot be removed but their patency can be restored by the introduction of a second device inserted coaxially within the first. Unless life expectancy is very short, it is well worth considering restoring the patency of an occluded stent, as this can greatly improve the patient's quality of life (Davids et al., 1992).

Malignant pleural effusions

Malignant pleural effusions (MPEs) can produce significant respiratory symptoms and diminished quality of life in patients with terminal malignancies. A patient who presents with a MPE should first have a diagnostic and therapeutic thoracocentesis. This can be done under ultrasound guidance. It is important to assess for symptom improvement and the ability of the lung to re-expand. The fluid will re-accumulate in almost all patients, at which time local treatment is needed. This typically consists of tube thoracostomy, usually followed by instillation of a sclerosing agent (doxycycline, bleomycin, or talc) to chemically induce pleurodesis (Patz et al., 1996). A tunnelled pleural catheter, the Denver Pleurx® catheter (Denver Biomaterials, Inc., Golden, CO) is also available for those patients who are ineligible or fail sclerotherapy. This is a 66-cm long 15.5 French soft silicone catheter with a polyester cuff to promote fibrosis to the subcutaneous tissue and multiple side-holes to enhance drainage. A valve in its hub is opened only when a dilator is passed through it. This prevents inadvertent entry of air or leakage of fluid. The drainage system consists of a vacuum bottle with a pre-connected tube that has a dilator at its

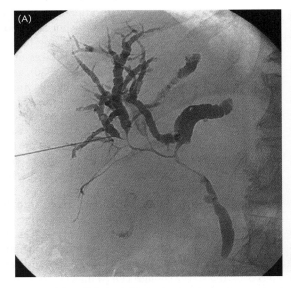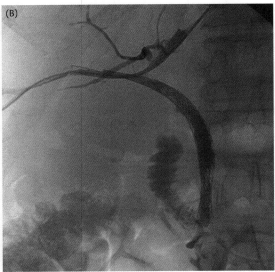

Fig. 12.6.1 Percutaneous biliary drainage. (A) Percutaneous cholangiogram showing stricture of the central bile ducts and proximal common bile duct due to cholangiocarcinoma (Klatskin tumour), and dilated intrahepatic ducts. (B) Biliary drainage with two metallic endoprosthesis.

end to pass into the hub of the catheter. Drainage will typically take no longer than 15 minutes and should be performed at least every other day. In the outpatient setting, this can be done by a visiting nurse, family members, or the patient (Pollak et al., 2001).

Malignant ascites

The accumulation of large volume ascites is a common occurrence for patients with intraperitoneal spread of tumour. These patients have a very poor prognosis, with anticipated mean survival ranging from 1 to 4 months. Patients often experience symptoms of abdominal pressure, shortness of breath, nausea, early satiety, and limited mobility because of the mass effect of the fluid. Management of symptoms is palliative and methods used include percutaneous drainage, diuretics, shunt placement, and intraperitoneal drug therapy. Paracentesis is not only the most common treatment method used by physicians, but also the most effective at relieving symptoms (Becker et al., 2006). Unfortunately, management of recurrent ascites with paracentesis requires frequent trips to the hospital and has greater risk of complications associated with multiple needle passes into the abdomen. There is an increasing number of published reports which show that a 15.5 French tunnelled draining catheter, the Pleurx® Catheter, provides effective palliation with a complication rate similar to that for large volume paracentesis, while obviating the need for frequent trips to the hospital for repeated percutaneous drainage (Tapping et al., 2012).

Dilatation/stenting techniques

These techniques are employed for the treatment of a variety of malignant strictures and occlusions in many systems, including the gastrointestinal tract, the respiratory system, and the renal and biliary tract.

Gastrointestinal tract

Oesophagus

The aim of palliation in patients with inoperable oesophageal cancer is to relieve dysphagia with minimal morbidity and mortality,

and thus improve quality of life. The use of a self-expanding metal stent (SEMS) is a well-established modality for palliation of dysphagia in such patients (Sabharwal et al., 2004). Placement of the stent can be achieved under fluoroscopic (Fig. 12.6.2) or endoscopic guidance, or both. The procedure is relatively straightforward with negligible mortality and low morbidity. Advantages of radiological placement of oesophageal stents include (Sabharwal, 2005):

◆ accurate positioning under X-ray guidance

◆ ability to traverse even tight stenoses or occlusions

◆ ability to use small-calibre catheters and wires which minimizes the risk of perforation and bleeding.

New advances in oesophageal stent technology include smaller introductory devices, more flexible stents, retrievable stents which can be used as a bridge to surgery, biodegradable stents, and devices with an anti-reflux valve which are used for stenting across the gastro-oesophageal junction (Katsanos et al., 2010).

Covered metallic stents are also very useful in the management of malignant oesophageal fistulas. Unlike fistulas associated with benign diseases, which may heal with conservative therapy, fistulas associated with malignant lesions do not heal spontaneously. Without definitive treatment, most patients succumb to malnutrition and thoracic sepsis within weeks. Radiological insertion of a covered metallic stent can result in immediate sealing of the fistula and the patient can drink fluids a few hours after the procedure, resuming a normal diet on the following day (Morgan et al., 1997).

Gastroduodenal and colorectal

SEMSs are playing an increasingly important role in the treatment of gastroduodenal obstruction and acute colonic obstruction (Katsanos et al., 2011). Patients with these conditions are often elderly and frail with dehydration and electrolyte imbalance. Self-expanding stents offer a non-surgical therapeutic alternative that rapidly relieves the obstruction and improves their clinical condition, with a high success rate and low morbidity (Fig. 12.6.3). This may be a temporizing measure allowing stabilization of the patient prior to definitive surgery, or alternatively, patients who

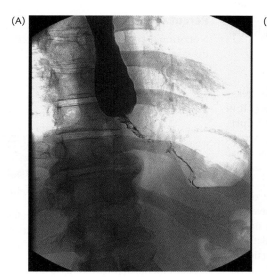

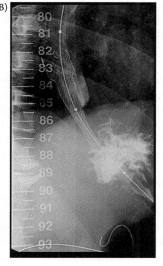

Fig. 12.6.2 Oesophageal stenting.

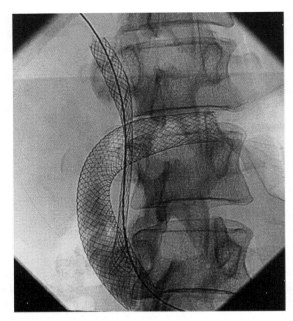

Fig. 12.6.3 Concurrent percutaneous biliary (Wallstent®) and gastroduodenal (enteral) stent in patient with inoperable pancreatic cancer.

are not surgical candidates, the stent may provide adequate palliation (Sebastian et al., 2004).

Tracheobronchial

Malignant airways obstruction can cause considerable distress to patients. When surgical resection is not possible, SEMSs can provide good palliation. This procedure is best carried out under general anaesthesia, as a combined effort between an interventional radiologist and a bronchoscopist. Bronchoscopic visualization is used to determine the position of the stricture, the limits of which are marked with a radio-opaque marker. The stricture is then dilated under fluoroscopic guidance. Following dilatation, a SEMS is released across the stricture, again under fluoroscopic guidance. This can result in significant symptomatic improvement and prevent collapse and/or infection and abscess formation beyond an obstructing lesion (Tan et al., 1996). Placement of plastic-covered metallic stents in the trachea is an effective method of managing tracheo-oesophageal fistulae unsuitable for treatment with covered oesophageal stents (Morgan et al., 1997).

Venous obstruction

The superior vena cava syndrome often presents as a very distressing pre-terminal event in patients with thoracic malignancy. It is most commonly related to mediastinal neoplasia, particularly primary and secondary lung tumours and lymphoma. The obstruction, which can be partial or complete, can be caused by caval compression and/or invasion by tumour and is frequently complicated by venous thrombosis.

Superior venocavography delineates the site and extent of the obstruction. If extensive thrombosis is present, selective intravenous thrombolysis with a catheter placed within the thrombus is undertaken under local anaesthesia. Percutaneous transfemoral dilatation of the narrowed superior vena cava is followed by the insertion of a self-expandable metallic endoprosthesis. Flow is restored immediately, providing excellent and immediate palliation of symptoms

(Lanciego et al., 2009). This procedure can be performed prior to, in conjunction with, or after therapy, including radiotherapy or chemotherapy. It can also be performed in conjunction with airway stenting (Fig. 12.6.4). Malignant involvement of the inferior vena cava can be managed in a similar fashion. All patients with malignant superior or inferior vena caval obstruction should be considered for this relatively straightforward and usually successful procedure, which can readily improve their quality of life.

Percutaneous insertion of an *inferior vena cava filter* is indicated in patients with recurrent pulmonary embolism refractory to or unsuitable for treatment with anticoagulation therapy and in those patients with free-floating thrombus in the inferior vena cava (Hammond et al., 2009).

Feeding techniques

Venous access

Central venous access may be essential in some patients with terminal disease for feeding and the delivery of medication, palliative chemotherapy or analgesia. A variety of long-term venous access systems (e.g. tunnelled central venous catheters, peripherally inserted central catheters (PICCs), and venous ports), have been developed for insertion under fluoroscopic and ultrasound guidance. The procedure is now usually performed in the radiology department under local anaesthesia and strict asepsis (Adam, 1995). The main advantage over the surgical venous cut-down technique is that performing the procedure under fluoroscopic guidance ensures that the tip of the catheter is always in the correct position and virtually eliminates the need for repositioning the catheter at a later date. The procedure is rapid, well tolerated by the patient, and associated with high success and low complication rates. In our experience, it is virtually always possible to gain venous access using interventional radiological methods. The rate of occurrence of pneumothorax when using a subclavian approach is approximately 1%. This complication is very rare when access is gained via the internal jugular vein. The long-term complications of occlusion and infection of the catheter are not significantly different from those observed when a surgical method of venous access is used (Adam, 1995).

Percutaneous gastrostomy

Nutritional support may be required in patients with end-stage disease. This sometimes raises difficult questions, particularly in relation to parenteral nutrition. Enteric feeding is generally a simpler option and can be accomplished by the insertion of gastrostomy tubes. The insertion of a feeding gastrostomy tube either under fluoroscopic (Fig. 12.6.5) or endoscopic guidance and local anaesthesia can significantly improve the patient's well-being and ease of management, often avoiding the need for uncomfortable psychologically distressing nasogastric tubes and intravenous lines. A gastrostomy tube can be readily managed in the home environment by the patient's family and carers as well as by nursing staff (Lowe et al., 2012).

Gastro-jejunostomy tubes are preferable when there is gastric outlet obstruction or in cases of gastro-oesophageal reflux.

Extraction techniques

Developments in intravenous feeding therapy and monitoring techniques have led to a vast increase in the number of indwelling venous

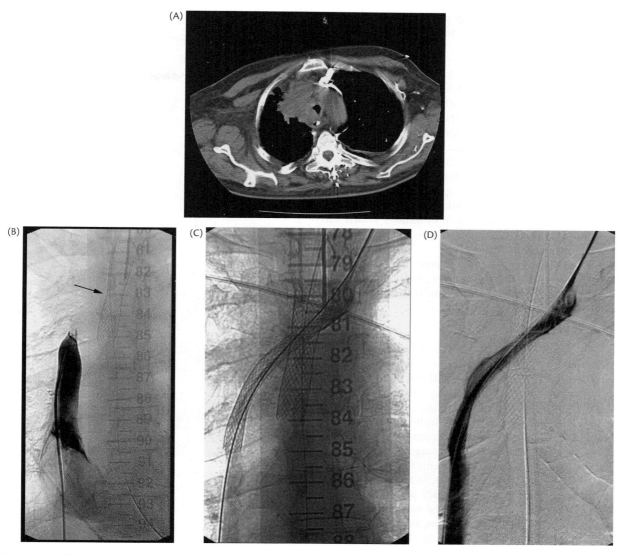

Fig. 12.6.4 Tracheal and superior vena cava (SVC) stenting. (A) Computed tomography shows a Pancoast tumour occluding the SVC and compromising the trachea. (B) A tracheal stent was inserted initially (arrow) and a venogram reveals the obstructed SVC. (C) A metallic Wallstent® has been placed across the obstructed SVC. (D) Completion venogram shows patency of the SVC stent and also the widely opened tracheal stent.

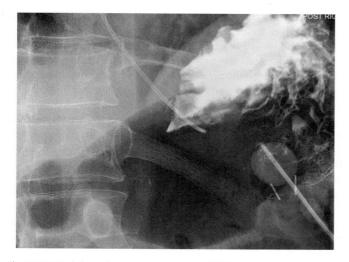

Fig. 12.6.5 Radiologically inserted gastrostomy (RIG).

cannulas and catheters. Unfortunately, these occasionally break or become disconnected and a part or all of the catheter is 'lost' within the venous system. It is important to retrieve these intravascular foreign bodies as they not only perforate vascular structures and cause dysrhythmias but also act as a seat of infection, particularly in immunosuppressed patients. Surgical retrieval of catheter fragments is hazardous (and sometimes impractical), necessitating a thoracotomy. It is almost invariably possible to retrieve these catheter fragments, which usually lodge within the right side of the heart or the pulmonary arteries, percutaneously under fluoroscopic guidance. Detailed descriptions of all the retrieval techniques available are beyond the scope of this chapter but any interventional radiologist offering a comprehensive vascular service is well advised to become acquainted with the various methods and have the necessary equipment available (Wolf et al., 2008).

The ability to snare or 'catch' the end of a catheter can also be of value when the tip of an indwelling central venous catheter has become displaced into the jugular vein. It is usually possible to 'pull' such a catheter back into a correct position using a percutaneous vascular approach under local anaesthesia.

Infusion techniques

The ability of the radiologist accurately to site a catheter into virtually any blood vessel within the body has brought into play the concepts of regional infusion of chemotherapeutic agents, monoclonal antibodies and isotopes. The principle underlying these techniques is that a high dose of the therapeutic agent is delivered to the tumour(s) with minimal side effects. Recent advances include the addition of embolic materials (see embolization section, below) and the microencapsulation of cytotoxic agents to achieve gradual and sustained release. Lipiodol® has been used for many years in combination with cytotoxic drugs for the treatment of certain hepatic tumours; it is retained in tumour vessels and also acts as a contrast agent, thus allowing monitoring of tumour response to treatment using CT imaging.

These techniques have been used with varying degrees of success to treat primary and metastatic liver tumours, bone neoplasms, cerebral neoplasms, sarcomas, melanomas, and pelvic neoplasms (Lewandowski et al., 2011).

Vascular embolization

The deliberate occlusion of arteries and/or veins by the injection of embolic agents through selectively placed catheters, is one of the major therapeutic applications of interventional radiology in the patient with neoplastic disease. This technique has been employed in the management of severe and disabling symptoms from a very wide variety of tumours throughout the body. Embolization, which usually involves a percutaneous technique with local anaesthesia, offers an attractive alternative to surgery under general anaesthesia and, in some situations, is the only therapeutic option available. A wide variety of embolic agents are available. The broad categories of substances used include particulate emboli (sterile sponge, polyvinyl alcohol, and the newer clear acrylic microspheres), mechanical emboli (balloons, steel coils), and liquids (n-butyl cyanoacrylate (glue), absolute alcohol, Lipiodol®). The appropriate agent or combination of agents depends on the lesion to be treated and its site (with particular reference to adjacent vulnerable vascular structures).

Embolization can be used definitively to stop internal bleeding and pre-operatively to assist effective, safe surgery, but in many cases it is used palliatively to alleviate distressing symptoms (Fig. 12.6.6).

Palliative embolization

Embolization can be used to control pain, haemorrhage, and hormone production as well as to reduce tumour bulk. The technique may be used as the primary mode of treatment in inoperable malignancy and embolization of metastatic deposits has, in some situations, been shown to extend survival times in advanced disease (Lovet and Bruix, 2003). Tumours in all sites have been treated in this fashion (liver, kidney, bone, lung, soft tissues, nervous system, and gastrointestinal tract). Hormone secreting neoplasms such as metastatic neuroendocrine tumours show the greatest therapeutic response to arterial embolization. Appropriate pharmacological blockade is necessary during the embolization to avoid the effects of a dramatic outpouring of hormone as the tumour is deprived of its blood supply. The beneficial effects of embolization may become apparent within a matter of hours. In embolization procedures it

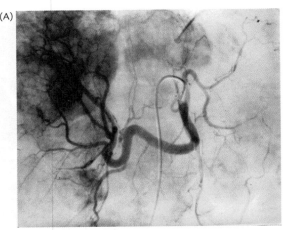

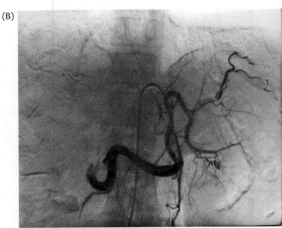

Fig. 12.6.6 Hepatic embolization for metastatic carcinoid tumour. (A) The arterial parenchymal phase shows hepatic enlargement and reveals multiple tumour deposits. (B) Post-embolization arteriogram shows that the arterial supply has been obliterated. The patient's symptoms (flushing and diarrhoea) were dramatically alleviated by this procedure.

is important that adequate premedication is given prior to the procedure, including broad-spectrum antibiotics. In many situations, for example, liver and bone, it is necessary to continue antibiotics for 10 days after the procedure to prevent sepsis developing in the devascularized tissue.

A major advance in tumour embolization has been the development of transcatheter arterial chemoembolization (TACE). In this technique embolic materials are mixed with chemotherapeutic drugs; the emboli cause ischaemia of the tumour cells and by increasing the transit time through the tumour vascular bed, the contact time between the cytotoxic agent and the neoplastic cells is prolonged, resulting in a greater therapeutic effect.). At present TACE is considered to be the mainstay of treatment for unresectable hepatocellular carcinoma (HCC). It provides significantly prolonged survival in selected patients with preserved liver function and adequate performance status (Lover and Bruix, 2003). Prolonged survival can be achieved in selected patients with a combination of local ablative techniques (percutaneous ethanol injection (PEI), radiofrequency ablation (RFA)) and TACE (Marelli et al., 2006). TACE also has been used as a bridge for orthotopic liver transplantation.

Drug-eluting beads, polyvinyl alcohol-based microspheres that can be loaded with various types of chemotherapeutic agents, have more recently been developed in effort to improve the pharmacokinetic profile of the chemotherapeutic agents administered during TACE (Varela et al., 2007). Such a system loaded with doxorubicin has shown promising results in patients with unresectable HCC with an advantageous pharmacokinetic profile, reduced adverse effects, and improved tumour response as shown by imaging when compared with conventional TACE (Lammer et al., 2010).

After embolization of large tumour masses, patients may experience some discomfort and pain and they may have a fever for a few days accompanied by a feeling of malaise and an elevated white cell count. This combination of signs and symptoms has been called the *post-embolization syndrome*, and is an indicator of the presence of necrotic tissue. Sustained pyrexia should alert the clinician to the possibility of abscess formation and blood cultures plus regional ultrasound should or CT be performed.

Neurolysis

Alcohol injection is useful in the palliation of intractable pain which occasionally accompanies retroperitoneal malignancy. Pain associated with pancreatic and gastric cancer can be severely debilitating with significant impairment in quality of life. Frequently, this chronic abdominal pain does not respond adequately to conventional analgesics including opioids. Coeliac plexus neurolysis and coeliac plexus block are aimed at either selectively destroying the coeliac plexus or temporarily blocking visceral afferent nociceptors to alleviate chronic pain. Both techniques require injection of the chosen agent at the coeliac axis. Agents most commonly used include alcohol for neurolysis and bupivacaine and triamcinolone for temporary block. The procedure is performed percutaneously either under CT or fluoroscopic guidance. Between 70% and 85% of patients experience pain relief lasting from 1 month up to 1 year post procedure (Kambadakone et al., 2011). Complications include transient diarrhoea, orthostasis, and transient increase in pain but the incidence of these is low. Major complications occur in less than 1% of patients and include retroperitoneal bleeding, abscess formation, and transient or permanent paraplegia (Kambadakone et al., 2011).

Bone strengthening techniques

Percutaneous vertebroplasty, kyphoplasty and osteoplasty

Percutaneous vertebroplasty is a therapeutic, image-guided procedure that involves injection of polymethylmethacrylate (bone cement) into a partially collapsed vertebral body, in an effort to relieve pain and provide stability (Gangi et al., 1994). This procedure is being used for patients with intractable debilitating pain due to vertebral compression fractures that is refractory to conventional therapies such as analgesic use, bed rest, and bracing. Neoplastic causes of vertebral compression fractures include bone metastases, multiple myeloma, lymphoma and aggressive haemangiomas. Up to 80% of patients with pain unresponsive to conventional medical treatment experience a significant degree of pain relief (Gangi et al., 2006).

Percutaneous vertebroplasty is performed under conscious sedation or general anaesthesia, and may be carried out as an outpatient procedure or may require a short hospital stay. CT and/or fluoroscopic guidance is used. The patient lies in the prone position, and then a large-bore (10–15 gauge) needle is placed into the vertebral body, through a transpedicular route for the lumbar spine or a intercostovertebral route for the thoracic spine. Access to cervical lesions is via an anterolateral approach. Once positioned in the vertebral body acrylic bone cement, usually methyl methacrylate, mixed with contrast medium, is then injected into the affected vertebra. This material is viscous to minimize leakage into adjacent structures or blood vessels. The whole procedure usually takes 1–2 hours. Non-steroidal anti-inflammatory drugs can be used for 2–4 days after vertebroplasty to minimize the inflammatory reaction to the acrylic compound. Pain relief is expected within 24 hours of the procedure. Complication rates are lower than 2% for osteoporotic indications and lower than 10% for malignant indications and include temporary or permanent neurologic deficit, infection, bleeding from puncture site, and allergic reaction (Gangi et al., 2006).

Kyphoplasty is a refinement of the vertebroplasty procedure. In addition to the reduction of fracture-related pain, some or all of the height is restored to the compressed vertebral body. Normalizing the height of the fractured vertebra reduces the focally exaggerated curvature of the spine (i.e. kyphosis). This effect, in turn, results in an aesthetic improvement, improved posture, and a reduced risk of fracture of the adjacent vertebra as a result of abnormal load bearing. The restoration of a more normal appearing configuration of the vertebral body and improvement in the load-bearing physics is accomplished with the intravertebral inflation of one or two high-pressure balloon tamps prior to the infusion of methylmethacrylate (Sabharwal et al., 2006).

Osteoplasty involves the injection of bone cement into a painful lytic pelvic lesion in patients who are unable to tolerate surgery and conventional treatments (radiotherapy, opioids) fail (Fig. 12.6.7). It achieves immediate bone strengthening, reduces the risk of pathological fracture, and improves mobility and pain control (Sabharwal, 2006). Contraindications include local infection and uncorrected coagulopathy. The major complication encountered when treating acetabular lesions is intra-articular injection. The risk is minimized by continuous monitoring the bone-filling procedure with fluoroscopic guidance.

Percutaneous tumour ablation

Ablation refers to local (rather than systemic) methods that destroy the tumour without removing it. These techniques are usually reserved for patients with recurrent malignancy in areas of previous radiation therapy, localized metastatic disease, and primary neoplasms in patients who are poor surgical candidates. They are not always considered curative but can produce survival rates equal to surgery in people with small tumours. Percutaneous techniques of local tumour ablation may be categorized into three major groups: injection (ethanol, acetic acid, hot saline), heating (RFA, electrocautery, interstitial laser therapy, microwave coagulation therapy, high-intensity focused ultrasound), and freezing (cryotherapy). Advantages of the ablative therapies compared to surgical resection include reduced morbidity and mortality, low cost, and the ability to perform procedures on an outpatient basis (Ahmed et al., 2011). All these techniques induce cell death by coagulative necrosis.

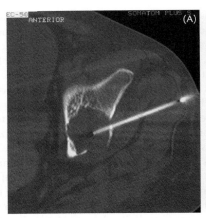
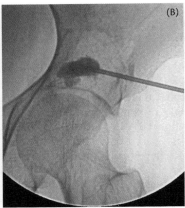
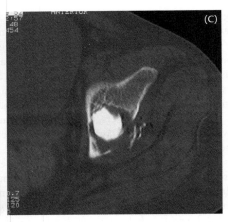

Fig. 12.6.7 Symptomatic metastatic left acetabular deposit that was injected with cement for consolidation and pain relief. (A) Insertion of the needle under CT guidance into the lesion. (B) Injection of cement under fluoroscopic guidance. (C) CT confirming good fill with no leaks.

Percutaneous liver tumour ablation

The liver is the organ with the greatest number of patients eligible for treatment with percutaneous tumour ablation given the large number of patients with primary or secondary hepatic malignancies and the low number eligible for surgical resection. Multiple minimally invasive techniques have been developed including PEI, interstitial laser photocoagulation (ILP), microwave, cryotherapy, focused ultrasound, and RFA. Thermal ablation is the most widely used techniques both for HCC and hepatic metastasis (Gillams, 2008).

Thermal ablation

Lesional heating techniques such as RFA and ILP affect tumour necrosis by hyperthermia. RF electrodes or laser fibres are inserted into the tumour under ultrasound, CT, or MRI guidance.

ILP produces thermal coagulation by conversion of absorbed light energy into heat (Nikfarjam and Christophi, 2003). In RFA, alternating current induces ionic agitation, which results in frictional heat production within the tissues. The size and shape of the necrotic lesion produced by RF has been shown to be a function of the probe gauge, length of the exposed tip, temperature along the exposed electrode, and duration of therapy. Strategies aiming at increasing the volume of tissue coagulation include the use of multi-probe electrodes and saline enhancement (Ahmed et al., 2011). Cooling the electrode with saline during the ablation prevents charring of the liver and reduces the impedance of the tissues adjacent to the electrode. In turn, this permits dissemination of heat further out into the tumour and increases the area of coagulation. The procedure is tolerated well and causes either no or only slight and transient abnormalities of liver function tests. Serious complications are rare and consist mainly of intraperitoneal haemorrhage and liver abscess formation.

The follow-up of patients after all forms of percutaneous tumour ablation includes a combination of imaging, tumour marker assay, and selected use of fine-needle aspiration biopsy. It is useful to follow serial levels of alpha-fetoprotein or carcino-embryonic antigen, in the case of HCC or metastatic disease, respectively, only when the serum levels of these markers are elevated prior to the initiation of therapy. The immediate goal of imaging is to assess whether complete necrosis has been achieved. Ultrasound does not usually provide useful information, as the echogenicity of fibrosis and neoplastic tissue overlap. Contrast enhanced-MRI and contrast enhanced-CT are capable of demonstrating remaining viable tumour requiring treatment. However, in difficult cases, positron emission tomography/CT scanning may provide additional information (Thulkar et al., 2012).

Several clinical series using different methods of RFA have been reported. The results appear to be promising, showing a 35% 5-year survival rate and 70% complete ablation rate for selected patients with colorectal metastasis (Gillams and Lees, 2009) and a 43%, 5-year survival rate for patients with HCC (Yan et al., 2008). RF thermal ablation is a quick, relatively safe, and highly effective technique for bulky primary and secondary malignant hepatic tumours. Also, it holds great promise as a technique for local tumour eradication. However, it is difficult to create an adequate tumour-free margin around larger (> 5 cm) tumours and failure to do so results in incomplete ablations and tumour recurrence.

RF thermal ablation has many potential advantages over existing therapies. It is far more effective for debulking tumours than is radiation therapy or systemic chemotherapy. Unlike surgical resection, it is minimally invasive and can be repeated as necessary to treat new tumours. It has far fewer complications than chemoembolization and could be used in conjunction with other systemic and local treatments.

Radiofrequency ablation of renal and adrenal masses

In patients with renal or adrenal tumours, recurrent malignancy in areas of prior radiation treatment, localized metastatic disease and primary neoplasms in patients who are poor surgical candidates RFA may be a suitable treatment option. Renal cell carcinomas are often incidental findings in older patients in which the standard of care has been total or partial nephrectomy. The growth pattern in many renal cell carcinomas can be slow and the risk of metastasis variable. VHL and hereditary RCC may also be successfully treated with RFA, which preserves kidney function (Gervais et al., 2005).

Patient selection should include those with known contraindications to partial or complete nephrectomy due to co-morbid conditions or advanced age, and small tumour burden. Centrally located masses may be harder to treat and the complication rate may be higher. This is likely related to the higher blood flow in

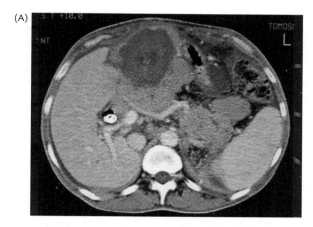

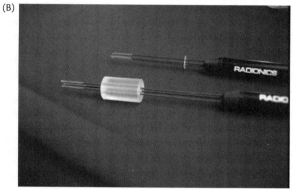

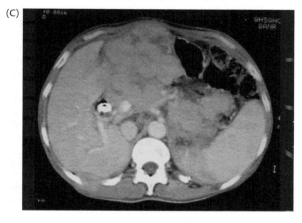

Fig. 12.6.8 RFA of a pancreatic secondary tumour. Patient had inoperable disease with metastatic melanoma and suffered with symptoms of severe abdominal pain and bowel obstruction. (A) CT scan of abdomen demonstrating large tumour in the head of the pancreas thought to be responsible for current symptoms. (B) Triple-cooled RF probe that was used for percutaneous RFA therapy. (C) Follow-up CT scan (1 week later) showed a low attenuation area within the tumour mass that represents necrosis; the pancreatic tumour lesion is smaller and there was now less mass effect. Patient's symptoms were significantly alleviated.

the renal hilum that prevents complete thermocoagulation due to a heat sink effect. Complications in the kidney include haemorrhage, urinoma, abscess, paraesthesias, transient haematuria, and pain. Ureteral stricture may occur with a tumour touching the ureter. RFA has also been found to be effective for the control of persistent haematuria in patients with kidney tumours (Neeman et al., 2005).

Treatment options for primary and metastatic adrenal tumours are limited. For adrenocortical carcinoma, chemotherapy and radiation therapy play a limited role. However, repeat surgical resection may prolong survival. Extrapolation from these data suggests that local adrenal tumour destruction with RFA may improve survival in selected patients. Phaeochromocytoma, aldosteronoma, and metastases to the adrenal may also be treated with RFA, with the appropriate endocrine evaluation and blockade for phaeochromocytoma (Wood et al., 2003).

Radiofrequency ablation of lung tumours

First reported in 2000 (Dupuy et al., 2000), RFA for primary and metastatic lung tumours is now gaining momentum. Results are encouraging particularly when palliation for pain or mass lesion is needed. Pneumothorax rates appear to be in the range of 10–20%, with other complications less common, such as bleeding, fistula, haemoptysis, subcutaneous emphysema, effusions, fever, infection, and pain (Kashima et al., 2011).

The surrounding air in adjacent normal lung parenchyma may provide insulation for the thermal lesion, making cooking easier or faster than in the well-vascularized liver.

Radiofrequency ablation of painful metastases

Early reports show promise for RFA of painful soft tissue tumours that are resistant to conventional radiation and pharmacological therapies. RFA has been found to be effective for short-term local control of painful soft tissue tumours and of bone metastases in multiple locations, decreasing or obviating the need for opioids (Dupuy et al., 2010). Other examples of the role of RFA in palliative care include the relief of distressing symptoms of bowel obstruction, abdominal distension, and pain from a large pancreatic mass (Fig. 12.6.8).

Better methods of imaging guidance and more sophisticated equipment are likely to increase the importance of percutaneous tumour ablation in the future.

Conclusions

This chapter was not intended to be an exhaustive list of every procedure that can be performed but to give an overall impression of the vast range of interventional techniques available. The patient undergoing palliative care should not be subjected to any unnecessary procedures or instrumentation. However, there are many readily performed, well-tolerated, and safe interventional procedures which can significantly alleviate distressing symptoms, improve the quality of remaining life, and ease the nursing burden. Further detailed information can be obtained from the many reviews, journals, and books on the subject, some of which are included in the reference list.

References
Adam, A. (1995). Insertion of long term central venous catheters: time for a new look. *British Medical Journal*, 311, 341–342.
Adam, A. (1998). The definition of interventional radiology (or, 'When is a barium enema an interventional procedure?'). *European Radiology*, 8, 1014–1015.
Ahmed, M., Brace, C.L., Lee, F.T., Jr, and Goldberg, S.N. (2011). Principles of and advances in percutaneous ablation. *Radiology*, 258(2), 351–369.
Becker, G., Galandi, D., and Blum, H.E. (2006). Malignant ascites: systematic review and guideline for treatment. *European Journal of Cancer*, 42(5), 589–597.

Bogda, K. (2003). Radiological interventions: special considerations in cancer patients. In C.E. Ray, M.E. Hicks, and N.H. Patel (eds.) *SIR Syllabus: Interventions in Oncology*, pp. 1–7. North Fairfax, VA: Society of Interventional Radiology.

Davids, P.H.P., Groen, A.K., Rauws, E.A., Tygtat, G.N., and Huibregtse, K. (1992). Randomized trial of self-expanding metal stents versus polyethylene stents for distal malignant biliary obstruction. *The Lancet*, 340, 1488–1492.

Dupuy, D.E., Liu, D., Hartfeil, D., *et al.* (2010). Percutaneous radiofrequency ablation of painful osseous metastases: a multicenter American College of Radiology imaging network trial. *Cancer* 116(4), 989–997.

Dupuy, D.E., Zagoria, R.J., Akerley, W., *et al* (2000). Percutaneous radiofrequency ablation of malignancies in the lung. *American Journal of Roentgenology*, 175, 1263–1266.

Gangi, A., Kastler, B.A., and Dietemann, J.L. (1994). Percutaneous vertebroplasty guided by a combination of CT and fluoroscopy. *American Journal of Neuroradiology*, 15(1), 83–86.

Gangi, A., Sabharwal, T., Irani, F.G, Buy, X., Morales, J.P, and Adam, A. (2006). Quality assurance guidelines for percutaneous vertebroplasty. *CardioVascular and Interventional Radiology*, 29, 173–178.

Gaylord, G. and Johhsrude, I.S. (1989). Transrenal ureteral occlusion with Gianturco coils and gelatin sponge. *Radiology*, 172, 1047–1048.

Gervais, D.A., McGovern, F.J., Arellano, R.S., McDougal, W.S., and Mueller, P.R. (2005). Radiofrequency ablation of renal cell carcinoma: part 1, indications, results, and role in patient management over a 6-year period and ablation of 100 tumours. *American Journal of Roentgenology*, 185, 64–71.

Gillams, A.R. and Lees, W.R. (2009). Five-year survival in 309 patients with colorectal liver metastasis treated with radiofrequency ablation. *European Radiology* 19(5), 1206–1213.

Hammond, C.J., Bakshi, D.R., Currie, R.J., *et al.* (2009). Audit of the use of IVC filters in the UK: experience from three centres over 12 years. *Clinical Radiology*, 64(5), 502–510.

Kambadakone, A., Thabet, A., Gervais, D.A., Mueller, P.R., Arellano, R.S. (2011). CT-guided celiac plexus neurolysis: a review of anatomy, indications, technique, and tips for successful treatment. *Radiographics*, 31(6), 1599–1621.

Kashima, M., Yamakado, K., Takaki, H., *et al.* (2011). Complications after 1000 lung radiofrequency ablation sessions in 420 patients: a single center's experiences. *American Journal of Roentgenology*, 197(4), W576–580.

Katsanos, K., Sabharwal, T., and Adam, A. (2010). Stenting of the upper gastrointestinal tract: current status. *CardioVascular and Interventional Radiology*, 33(4), 462–473.

Katsanos, K., Sabharwal, T., and Adam, A. (2011). Stenting of the lower gastrointestinal tract: current status. *CardioVascular and Interventional Radiology* 34(3), 462–473.

Lammer, J., Malagari, K., Vogl, T., *et al.* (2010). Prospective randomized study of doxorubicin eluting-bead embolization in the treatment of hepatocellular carcinoma: results of the PRECISION V study. *CardioVascular and Interventional Radiology*, 33(1), 41–52.

Lanciego, C., Panqua, C., Chacon, J.I., *et al.* (2009). Endovascular stenting as the first step in the overall management of malignant superior vena cava syndrome. *American Journal of Roentgenology*, 193(2), 549–558.

Lewandowski, R.J., Geschwind, J.F., Liapi. E., and Salem, R. (2011). Transcatheter intra-arterial therapies: rationale and overview. *Radiology*, 259(3), 641–657.

Llovet, J.M. and Bruix, J. (2003). Systematic review of randomized trials for unresectable hepatocellular carcinoma: chemoembolization improves survival. *Hepatology*, 37, 429–442.

Lowe, A.S., Lassch, H.U., Stephenson, S., *et al.* (2012). Multicentre survey of radiologically inserted gastrostomy feeding tube (RIG) in the UK. *Clinical Radiology*, 67(9), 843–854.

Marelli, L., Stigliano, R., Triantos, C., *et al.* (2006). Treatment outcomes for hepatocellular carcinoma using chemoembolization in combination with other therapies. *Cancer Treatment Reviews*, 32, 594–606.

Morgan, R.A. and Adam, A. (2001). Malignant biliary disease: percutaneous interventions. *Techniques in Vascular and Interventional Radiology*, 4(3), 147–152.

Morgan, R.A., Ellul, J.P., Denton, E.R., Glynos, M., Mason, R.C., and Adam A. (1997). Malignant esophageal fistulas and perforations: management with plastic-covered metallic endoprostheses. *Radiology*, 204(2), 527–532.

Neeman, Z., Sarin, S., Coleman, J., Fojo, T., Wood, B.J. (2005). Radiofrequency ablation for tumor-related massive hematuria. *Journal of Vascular and Interventional Radiology*, 16(3), 417–421.

Nikfarjam, M. and Christophi, C. (2003). Interstitial laser thermotherapy for liver tumours. *British Journal of Surgery*, 90(9), 1033–1047.

Patz, E.F., McAdams, H.P., Goodman, P.C., Blackwell, S., and Crawford, J. (1996). Ambulatory sclerotherapy for malignant pleural effusions. *Radiology*, 199(1), 133–135.

Pingoud, E.G., Bagley, D.H., Zeman, R.K., Glancy, K.E., and Pais, O.S. (1980). Percutaneous antegrade bilateral ureteral dilation and stent placement for internal drainage. *Radiology*, 134, 780.

Pollak, J.S., Burdge, C.M., Rosenblatt, M., *et al.* (2001). Treatment of malignant pleural effusions with tunneled long-term drainage catheters. *Journal of Vascular and Interventional Radiology*, 12, 201–208.

Sabharwal, T., Morales, J.P., Irani, F., and Adam, A. (2005). Quality assurance guidelines for placement of oesophageal stents. *CardioVascular and Interventional Radiology*, 28, 284–288.

Sabharwal, T., Morales, J.P., Salter, R., and Adam, A. (2004). Esophageal cancer: self-expanding metallic stents. *Abdominal Imaging*, 29, 1–9.

Sabharwal, T., Salter, R., Adam, A., and Gangi, A. (2006). Image-guided therapies in orthopedic oncology. *Orthopedic Clinics of North America*, 37, 105–112.

Sebastian, S., Johnston, S., Geoghegan, T., Torreggiani, W., and Buckley, M. (2004). Pooled analysis of the efficacy and safety of self expanding metal stenting in malignant colorectal obstruction. *American Journal of Gastroenterology*, 99, 2051–2057.

Tan, B.S., Watkinson, A.F., Dussek, J.E., and Adam, A. (1996). Metallic endoprosthesis for malignant tracheo-bronchial obstruction: initial experience. *CardioVascular and Interventional Radiology*, 19, 91–96.

Tapping, C.R., Ling, L., and Razack A. (2012). Pleurx drain use in the management of malignant ascites: safety, complications, long-term patency and factors predictive of success. *British Journal of Radiology*, 85, 623–628.

Thulkar, S., Chawla, M., Sharma, P., Malhotra, A., and Kumar R. (2012). 18F-FDG PET/CT in evaluation of radiofrequency ablation of liver metastasis. *Clinical Nuclear Medicine*, 37(5), 498–501.

Varela, M., Real, M.I., Burrel, M., *et al.* (2007). Chemoembolization of hepatocellular carcinoma with drug eluting beads: efficacy and doxorubicin pharmacokinetics. *Journal of Hepatology*, 46, 474–481.

Wolf, F., Schernthaner, R.E., Dirisamer, A., *et al.* (2008). Endovascular management of lost or misplaced intravascular objects: experience of 12 years. *CardioVascular and Interventional Radiology*, 31(3), 563–568.

Yan, K., Chen, M.H., Yang, W., *et al.* (2008). Radiofrequency ablation of hepatocellular carcinoma: long term outcome and prognostic factors. *European Journal of Radiology*, 67(2), 336–347.

Wood, B.J., Abraham, J., Hvizda, J.L., Alexander, H.R., and Fojo, T. (2003). Radiofrequency ablation of adrenal tumours and adrenocortical carcinoma metastases. *Cancer*, 97, 554–560.

SECTION 13

Cancer pain syndromes

Cancer pain syndromes: overview

Nathan I. Cherny

Acute pain syndromes

Cancer-related acute pain syndromes are most commonly due to diagnostic or therapeutic interventions (Stull et al., 1996; Jain and Chatterjee, 2010) and they generally pose little diagnostic difficulty. Although some tumour-related pains have an acute onset (such as pain from a pathological fracture), most of these will persist unless effective treatment for the underlying lesion is provided.

Acute pain associated with diagnostic and therapeutic interventions

Many investigations and treatments are associated with predictable, transient pain. For those patients with a pre-existing pain syndrome, otherwise innocuous manipulations can also precipitate incident pain.

Acute pain associated with diagnostic interventions
Lumbar puncture headache

Lumbar puncture (LP) headache is the best characterized acute pain syndrome associated with a diagnostic intervention. This syndrome is characterized by the delayed development of a positional headache, which is precipitated or markedly exacerbated by upright posture. Less commonly dural puncture may also cause back pain, arm pain, thoracic pain, and bowel and bladder dysfunction (Schabel et al., 2000; Ho et al., 2005). The pain is believed to be related to reduction in cerebrospinal fluid volume, due to ongoing leakage through the defect in the dural sheath, and compensatory expansion of the pain-sensitive intracerebral veins (Levine and Rapalino, 2001). The incidence of headache is related to the calibre of the LP needle (0–2% with 27–29-gauge, 0.5–7% with 25–26-gauge, 5–8% with 22-gauge, 10–15% with 20-gauge, and 20–30% with 18-gauge needles) (Bonica, 1953; McConaha et al., 1996; Lambert et al., 1997).

The risk of LP headache can be reduced by several strategies: when using a regular bevelled needle, longitudinal insertion of the needle bevel, which induces less trauma to the longitudinal elastic fibres in the dura, may reduce the incidence of headache (Kempen and Mocek, 1997).

Non-traumatic, conical tipped needles with a lateral opening are associated with a substantially lesser risk of post-LP headaches than regular cannulae (Prager et al., 1996; Corbey et al., 1997; Lambert et al., 1997; Vallejo et al., 2000; Toyka et al., 2002). The evidence that recumbency after LP reduces the incidence

of this syndrome is controversial (Gonzalez, 2000; Ebinger et al., 2004).

LP headache, which usually develops hours to several days after the procedure, is typically described as a dull occipital discomfort that may radiate to the frontal region or to the shoulders. Pain is commonly associated with nausea and dizziness. The duration of the headache is usually 1–7 days (Lybecker et al., 1995; Vilming and Kloster, 1998), and routine management relies on rest, hydration, and analgesics (Evans, 1998). Persistent headache may necessitate application of an epidural blood patch (Evans, 1998). Although a controlled study suggested that prophylactic administration of a blood patch may reduce this complication (Martin et al., 1994), the incidence and severity of the syndrome do not warrant this routinely. Severe headache has also been reported to respond to treatment with intravenous or oral caffeine (Morewood, 1993).

Transthoracic needle biopsy

Transthoracic fine-needle aspiration of intrathoracic mass is generally a non-noxious procedure. Severe pain has, however been associated with this procedure when the underlying diagnosis was a neurogenic tumour (Jones et al., 1993).

Transrectal prostatic biopsy

Transrectal ultrasound-guided prostate biopsy is an essential procedure in the diagnosis and management of prostate cancer. In a prospective study, 16% of the patients reported pain of moderate or greater severity and 19% would not agree to undergo the procedure again without anaesthesia (Irani et al., 1997). Subsequent studies have demonstrated low rate of severe pain (Sheikh et al., 2005). When present, pain may persist up to 4 weeks after the biopsy (Naughton et al., 2000). Periprostatic lidocaine infiltration (Jones et al., 2003; Stravodimos et al., 2007; Gurbuz et al., 2010), intrarectal introduction of lidocaine cream 2% (Kandirali et al., 2009; Skriapas et al., 2009; Issa et al., 2000), and unilateral pudendal nerve block (Adsan et al., 2004; Bhomi et al., 2007) may reduce the pain associated with this procedure.

Mammography pain

Breast compression associated with mammography can cause moderate, and rarely severe, pain (Leaney and Martin, 1992; Aro et al., 1996). The duration of the pain is generally short (Sapir et al., 2003). Unless patients are adequately counselled and treated, occasional patients will refuse repeat mammograms because of pain (Leaney and Martin, 1992). Pain may be reduced by using a lesser level of compression (Chida et al., 2009). In a systematic review the only intervention to significantly reduce the pain was of patient-controlled compression (Miller et al., 2002).

Acute pain associated with therapeutic interventions
Postoperative pain

Acute postoperative pain is universal unless adequately treated. Unfortunately, undertreatment is endemic despite the availability of adequate analgesic and anaesthetic techniques (Anonymous, 2008b; Sommer et al., 2008; Wu and Raja, 2011). Guidelines for management have been reviewed (NHS Quality Improvement Scotland, 2004; Savoia et al., 2010; Wu and Raja, 2011). Postoperative pain that exceeds the normal duration or severity should prompt a careful evaluation for the possibility of infection or other complications.

Radiofrequency tumour ablation

Radiofrequency tumour ablation is commonly used in the management of liver metastases. It is also increasingly used in other settings including adrenal metastases and renal tumours as well as in lung, bone, breast, and bone tumours. Percutaneous ablation of liver tumours may be associated with severe right upper quadrant abdominal pain or pain radiating to the right shoulder (Zagoria et al., 2002; Buscarini and Buscarini, 2004) in 5–10% of patients. Pain has also been reported after radiofrequency ablation of renal lesions (Baker et al., 2007) and it is presumably possible with the use of this approach in other sites.

Cryosurgery

Cryotherapy is commonly applied in the management of skin, cervical, and prostatic tumours. Topical cryotherapy typically causes a local painful reaction that decreases in severity over 2–7 days (Wang et al., 2001; Thai et al., 2004). Cryosurgery of the cervix in the treatment of intraepithelial neoplasm commonly produces an acute cramping pain syndrome. The severity of the pain is related to the duration of the freeze period and it is not diminished by the administration of prophylactic non-steroidal anti-inflammatory drugs (NSAIDs) (Harper, 1994). Cryotherapy for prostate cancer may uncommonly result in persistent pain (Ismail et al., 2007) which may sometimes be related to abscess formation (Wu and Jones, 2010).

Other interventions

Invasive interventions other than surgery are commonly used in cancer therapy and may also result in predictable acute pain syndromes. Examples include the pains associated with tumour embolization techniques (Yu et al., 2008; Aliberti et al., 2011) radioembolization of liver tumours (Sato et al., 2008), and chemical pleurodesis (Antunes et al., 2003; Shaw and Agarwal, 2004).

Acute pain associated with analgesic techniques
Local anaesthetic infiltration pain

Intradermal and subcutaneous infiltration of lidocaine produces a transient burning sensation before the onset of analgesia. This can be modified with the use of buffered solutions (Hanna et al., 2009) or by warming of the solution (Hogan et al., 2011). Slowing rate of injection does not diminish injection pain (Scarfone et al., 1998).

Opioid injection pain

Intramuscular (IM) and subcutaneous (SC) injections are painful. When repetitive dosing is required, the IM route of administration is not recommended (NHS Quality Improvement Scotland, 2004; Savoia et al., 2010; Wu and Raja, 2011). The pain associated with SC injection is influenced by the volume injected and the chemical characteristics of the injectant.

Opioid headache

Rarely, patients develop a reproducible generalized headache after opioid administration. Although its cause is not known, speculation suggests that it may be caused by opioid-induced histamine release.

Spinal opioid hyperalgesia syndrome

Intrathecal and epidural injection of high opioid doses is occasionally complicated by pain (typically perineal, buttock, or leg), hyperalgesia, and associated manifestations including segmental myoclonus, piloerection, and priapism. This is an uncommon phenomenon that remits after discontinuation of the infusion (De Conno et al., 1991; Cartwright et al., 1993).

Spinal injection pain

Back, pelvic, or leg pain may be precipitated by epidural injection or infusion. The incidence of this problem has been estimated at approximately 20% (Naumann et al., 1999; Willis and Doleys, 1999). It is speculated that it may be caused by the compression of an adjacent nerve root by the injected fluid (De Castro et al., 1991; Buchser and Chedel, 1992). Similar problems have been described with intrathecal injections associated with pericatheter fibrosis (Gaertner et al., 2003)

Acute pain associated with anticancer therapies
Acute pain associated with chemotherapy infusion techniques
Intravenous infusion pain

Pain at the site of cytotoxic infusion is a common problem. Four pain syndromes related to intravenous infusion of chemotherapeutic agents are recognized: venous spasm, chemical phlebitis, vesicant extravasation, and anthracycline-associated flare. Venous spasm causes pain that is not associated with inflammation or phlebitis, and which may be modified by application of a warm compress or reduction of the rate of infusion. Chemical phlebitis can be caused by cytotoxic medications including amsacrine, dacarbazine, carmustine (Hundrieser, 1988; Mrozek-Orlowski et al., 1991), vinorelbine (Rittenberg et al., 1995; de Lemos, 2005; Porzio et al., 2008), as well as the infusion of potassium chloride and hyperosmolar solutions (Pucino et al., 1988). The pain and linear erythema associated with chemical phlebitis must be distinguished from the more serious complication of a vesicant cytotoxic extravasation (Bertelli, 1995; Boyle and Engelking, 1995; Langer, 2010). Vesicant extravasation may produce intense pain followed by desquamation and ulceration (Sauerland et al., 2006; Wickham et al., 2006). Finally, a brief venous flare reaction is often associated with intravenous administration of the anthracycline, doxorubicin. The flare is typically associated with local urticaria and occasional patients report pain or stinging (Vogelzang, 1979; Curran et al., 1990).

Hepatic artery infusion pain

Cytotoxic infusions into the hepatic artery (for patients with hepatic metastases) are often associated with the development of a diffuse abdominal pain (Kemeny, 1991; Barnett and Malafa, 2001). Continuous infusions can lead to persistent pain. In some patients, the pain is due to the development of gastric ulceration or erosions (Shike et al., 1986), or cholangitis (Batts, 1998). If the latter complications do not occur, the pain usually resolves with discontinuation of the infusion. A dose relationship is suggested by the observation that some patients will comfortably tolerate reinitiating of the infusion at a lower dose (Kemeny, 1992).

Intraperitoneal chemotherapy pain

A transient mild abdominal pain, associated with sensations of fullness or bloating is reported by approximately 25% of patients after intraperitoneal chemotherapy (Almadrones and Yerys, 1990; Jaaback and Johnson, 2006; American College of Obstetricians and Gynecologists, 2008a). A further 25% of patients reports moderate or severe pain necessitating opioid analgesia or discontinuation of therapy (Almadrones and Yerys, 1990). Moderate or severe pain is usually caused by chemical serositis or infection (Jaaback and Johnson, 2006). Chemical serositis is a common complication of intraperitoneal of the anthracycline agents mitoxantrone and doxorubicin and with taxol, but it is relatively infrequent with 5-flurouracil (5-FU) or cis-platinum. Pain may indicate suboptimal drug distribution within the abdominal cavity. Some patients experience discomfort related to sensing abdominal distention, or from intercostal nerve irritation (Topuz et al., 2000). Abdominal pain associated with fever and leucocytosis in blood and peritoneal fluid is suggestive of infectious peritonitis.

Intravesical chemo- or immunotherapy

Intravesical bacillus Calmette–Guérin (BCG) therapy for transitional cell carcinoma of the urinary bladder usually causes a transient bladder irritability syndrome characterized by frequency and/or micturition pain (Palou et al., 2001; Shelley et al., 2003, 2004). Similarly, intravesical doxorubicin (Matsumura et al., 1992), mitomycin C (Shelley et al., 2004), and thiotepa (Choe et al., 1995) can also cause a painful chemical cystitis. Rarely, intravesical BCG treatment may trigger a painful polyarthritis sometimes associated will a full blown Reiter's syndrome (Pardalidis et al., 2002; Okamoto et al., 2010) or localized regional or systemic infections with abscess formation (Alvarez-Mugica et al., 2009; Harving et al., 2009).

Acute pain associated with chemotherapy toxicity
Mucositis

Severe mucositis is an almost invariable consequence of the myeloablative chemotherapy and radiotherapy that precedes bone marrow transplantation, but it is less common with standard intensity therapy (Peterson and Lalla, 2010). The cytotoxic agents most commonly associated with mucositis are cytarabine, doxorubicin, etoposide, 5-FU, and methotrexate. Pretreatment oral pathology and poor dental hygiene increase the risk of chemotherapy-induced mucositis. Younger patients have a relatively greater risk of chemotherapy-induced stomatitis, perhaps related to a higher epithelial mitotic rate. Damaged mucosal surfaces may become superinfected with microorganisms, such as *Candida albicans* and herpes simplex (Peterson and Lalla, 2010). The latter complication is most likely in neutropenic patients, who are also predisposed to systemic sepsis arising from local invasion by aerobic and anaerobic oral flora.

Corticosteroid-induced perineal discomfort

A transient burning sensation in the perineum is described by some patients following rapid infusion of large doses (20–100 mg) of dexamethasone (Perron et al., 2003). Clinical severity is variable and may be severe (Neff et al., 2002). Experience suggests that this syndrome is prevented by slow infusion.

Steroid withdrawal pseudorheumatism

The withdrawal of corticosteroids may produce a pain syndrome which manifests as diffuse myalgias, arthralgias, and tenderness of muscles and joints. These symptoms occur with rapid or slow withdrawal and may occur in patients taking these drugs for long or short periods of time. Treatment consists of reinstituting the steroids at a higher dose and withdrawing them more slowly (Rotstein and Good, 1957, Weissman et al., 1991).

Painful peripheral neuropathy

Chemotherapy-induced painful peripheral neuropathy, which is usually associated with vinca alkaloids, cis-platinum, oxaliplatin, and paclitaxel can have an acute course. The vinca alkaloids (particularly vincristine) are also associated with other, presumably neuropathic, acute pain syndromes, including pain in the jaw, legs, arms, or abdomen that may last from hours to days (Sandler et al., 1969; Rosenthal and Kaufman, 1974; Legha, 1986; McCarthy and Skillings, 1992). Vincristine-induced orofacial pain in the distribution of the trigeminal and glossopharyngeal nerves occurs in approximately 50% of patients at the onset of vincristine treatment (Rose, 1967; McCarthy and Skillings, 1992). The pain, which is severe in about half of those affected, generally begins 2–3 days after vincristine administration and lasts for 1–3 days. It is usually self-limiting and if recurrence occurs, it is usually mild (McCarthy and Skillings, 1992). Vinorelbine is associated with mild paraesthesias in about 20% of patients and severe neuropathy is rare (Scalone et al., 2004). The neuropathy associated with paclitaxel neuropathy is dose related and is generally subacute in onset with resolution after the completion of therapy (Loprinzi et al., 2011); however, in a proportion of cases it can be severe and persistent (Argyriou et al., 2006a). Most patients treated with oxaliplatin experience symptoms of acute neurotoxicity including paraesthesias and dysaesthesias of the hands, feet, and perioral region and muscle cramps (Argyriou et al., 2013).

Headache

Intrathecal methotrexate in the treatment of leukaemia or leptomeningeal metastases produces an acute meningitic syndrome in 5–50% of patients (Weiss et al., 1974). Headache is the prominent symptom and may be associated with vomiting, nuchal rigidity, fever, irritability, and lethargy. Rarely, it may present as a polyradiculopathy (Pascual et al., 2008). Symptoms usually begin hours after intrathecal treatment and persist for several days. Patients at increased risk for the development of this syndrome include those who have received multiple intrathecal injections and those patients undergoing treatment for proven leptomeningeal metastases (Weiss et al., 1974). The syndrome tends not to recur with subsequent injections.

Systemic administration of L-asparaginase for the treatment of acute lymphoblastic leukaemia may cause a thrombosis of cerebral veins or dural sinuses in 1–2% of patients (Eloraby, 2009; Wani et al., 2010). Headache is the most common initial symptom, and seizures, hemiparesis, delirium, vomiting, or cranial nerve palsies may also occur. The diagnosis is established by magnetic resonance imaging (MRI) scan (Kieslich et al., 2003).

Trans-retinoic acid therapy, which may be used in the treatment of acute promyelocytic leukaemia (APML), can cause a transient severe headache (Visani et al., 1996; Avvisati and Tallman, 2003). The mechanism may be related to pseudotumour cerebri induced by hypervitaminosis A.

Diffuse bone pain

Trans-retinoic acid therapy in patients with APML often produces a syndrome of diffuse bone pain (Avvisati and Tallman, 2003; Pilatrino et al., 2005). The pain is generalized, of variable intensity, and closely associated with a transient neutrophilia. The latter observation suggests that the pain may be due to marrow expansion.

Taxol-induced arthralgia and myalgia

Administration of paclitaxel generates a syndrome of diffuse arthralgias and myalgia in 10–20% of patients (Garrison et al., 2003; Loprinzi et al., 2007, 2011). They are related to individual doses; associations with the cumulative dose and infusion duration are less clear. Diffuse pain in joints and muscle generally appear 1–2 days after the infusion and lasted for a median of 4–5 days. Pain is commonly located in the back, hips, shoulders, thighs, legs, and feet. The pain is often exacerbated by weight bearing, walking, or tactile contact. Steroids may reduce tendency to myalgia and arthralgias (Markman et al., 1999).

5-flurouracil-induced anginal chest pain

Patients receiving 5-FU may develop ischaemic chest pain (Tsibiribi et al., 2006; Saif et al., 2009). Although the overall risk is generally considered low (1–2%), this is debated and there is some evidence suggesting risk as high as 20% (Saif et al., 2009). Overall the risk is higher with patients receiving continuous infusion than those receiving bolus therapy and patients with pre-existing ischaemic heart disease (Labianca et al., 1982). It is widely speculated that coronary vasospasm may be the underlying mechanism (Wacker et al., 2003; Shoemaker et al., 2004; Saif et al., 2009). Similar ischaemic cardiotoxicity has been reported in patients receiving the 5-FU prodrug capecitabine (Cardinale et al., 2006; Sestito et al., 2006; Monsuez et al., 2010).

Palmar–plantar erythrodysaesthesia syndrome

(Also called acral erythema, hand–foot syndrome, toxic erythema of the palms and soles, and Burgdof's syndrome.) This is a painful rash seen in association with continuously infused 5-FU, capecitabine (Gressett et al., 2006), and liposomal doxorubicin (Alberts and Garcia, 1997). It has also been reported with paclitaxel (Vukelja et al., 1993), the tyrosine kinase inhibitors sorafenib and sunitinib (Lipworth et al., 2009), and the mTOR inhibitor everolimus (Balagula et al., 2010). It is characterized by the development of a tingling or burning sensation in the palms and soles followed by the development of an erythematous rash. The pathogenesis is unknown. Management often requires the discontinuation of therapy and symptoms may be more manageable at lower doses of therapy. Symptomatic measures are often required (Bellmunt et al., 1988) and treatment with pyridoxine has been reported to induce resolution of the lesions (Fabian et al., 1990).

Post-chemotherapy gynaecomastia

Painful gynaecomastia can occur as a delayed complication of chemotherapy. Testis cancer is the most common underlying disorder (Aki et al., 1996; Uygur and Ozen, 2003), but it has been reported after therapy for other cancers as well (Glass and Berenberg, 1979; Trump et al., 1982). Gynaecomastia typically develops after a latency of 2–9 months and resolves spontaneously within a few months. Persistent gynaecomastia is occasionally observed (Trump et al., 1982).

Chemotherapy-induced acute digital ischaemia

Raynaud's phenomenon or transient ischaemia of the toes is a common complication of bleomycin, vinblastine, and cisplatin (PVB) treatment for testicular cancer (Aass et al., 1990). Rarely, irreversible digital ischaemia leading to gangrene has been reported after bleomycin (Elomaa et al., 1984). Capecitabine and vincristine have been implicated in case reports (Gottschling et al., 2004; Coward et al., 2005).

Chemotherapy-induced tumour pain

Pain at the site of tumour is reported to occur in some patients (7%) after treatment with vinorelbine. Typically, pain begins within a few minutes of the vinorelbine infusion, is moderate to severe in intensity and requires analgesic therapy. Premedication with ketorolac may prevent recurrence in some cases (Colleoni et al., 1995; Kornek et al., 1996; De Marco et al., 1999).

Acute pain associated with hormonal therapy
Luteinizing hormone-releasing factor tumour flare in prostate cancer

Initiation of luteinizing hormone-releasing factor (LHRF) hormonal therapy for prostate cancer produces a transient symptom flare in 5–25% of patients (Chrisp and Goa, 1991; Chrisp and Sorkin, 1991). The flare is presumably caused by an initial stimulation of luteinizing hormone release before suppression is achieved. The syndrome typically presents as an exacerbation of bone pain or urinary retention; spinal cord compression and sudden death have been reported (Thompson et al., 1990). Symptom flare is usually observed within the first week of therapy, and lasts 1–3 weeks in the absence of androgen antagonist therapy. Co-administration of an androgen antagonist during the initiation of LHRF agonist therapy can prevent this phenomenon (Labrie et al., 1987).

Hormone-induced pain flare in breast cancer

Any hormonal therapy for metastatic breast cancer can be complicated by a sudden onset of diffuse musculoskeletal pain commencing within hours to weeks of the initiation of therapy (Plotkin et al., 1978). Other manifestations of this syndrome include erythema around cutaneous metastases, changes in liver function studies, and hypercalcaemia. This may be associated with increased metabolic activity at tumour sites that can be detected on positron emission tomography (PET) scan (Mortimer et al., 2001). The underlying mechanism is not understood and the flare reaction is often predictive of later tumour response to the hormonal therapy.

Aromatase inhibitor-induced arthralgias

Aromatase inhibitor medications used in the hormonal therapy of breast cancer may cause a multifocal arthralgia syndrome in 10–20% of patients (Chlebowski, 2009). This most commonly manifests as early morning stiffness and hand/wrist pain. Pain intensity is variable and in some patients it interferes in daily activities. Occasionally it justifies discontinuation of treatment due to severe symptoms (Chlebowski, 2009). The possible mechanisms are unclear but an association with the development of osteoporosis has been noted (Muslimani et al., 2009). Treatment options for arthralgia (primarily NSAIDs) are often inadequate, and areas of active research include high-dose vitamin D and new targeted therapies to inhibit bone loss.

Acute pain associated with immunotherapy

Interferon-induced acute pain

Virtually all patients treated with interferon experience an acute syndrome consisting of fever, chills, myalgias, arthralgias, and headache (Quesada et al., 1986). The syndrome usually begins shortly after initial dosing and frequently improves with continued administration of the drug (Quesada et al., 1986). Doses of 1–9 million units of alpha-interferon are usually tolerated, but doses greater than or equal to 18 million units usually produce moderate to severe toxicity (Quesada et al., 1986). Acetaminophen pre-treatment is often useful in ameliorating these symptoms.

Acute pain associated with bisphosphonates

Bisphosphonate-induced bone pain

Bisphosphonates are widely used in the care of patients with bony metastases. Infusion of bisphosphonates is commonly associated with the development of multifocal bone pain and/or myalgia. Typically, pain occurs within 24 hours of infusion and may last up to 3 days. Pain intensity is variable and may be severe. The condition is self-limiting but may require analgesic therapy (Coukell and Markham, 1998; Lipton, 2007).

Acute pain associated with growth factors

Granulocyte-macrophage colony-stimulating factor (GM-CSF) and granulocyte colony-stimulating factor (G-CSF) commonly produce mild to moderate bone pain and constitutional symptoms such as fever, headache, and myalgias during the period of administration (Vial and Descotes, 1995; Veldhuis et al., 1995). In studies of G-CSF in dose-dense chemotherapy the prevalence of pain is 20–30% (Paciucci et al., 2002; Venturini et al., 2005) and similar prevalence is seen with pegylated G-CSF (Hill et al., 2006). Pain intensity is variable and may be severe. Co administration of dexamethasone may reduce the prevalence and severity of bone pain (Heuft et al., 2004).

Subcutaneous administration of recombinant human erythropoietin (r-HuEPO) alpha is associated with pain at the injection site in about 40% of cases (Frenken et al., 1991). Subcutaneous injection of r-HuEPO alpha is more painful than r-HuEPO beta (Morris et al., 1994). Alpha erythropoietin injection pain can be reduced by dilution of the vehicle with benzyl alcohol saline, reduction of the volume of the vehicle to 1.0–0.1 mL (Frenken et al., 1994) or addition of lidocaine (Alon et al., 1994).

Acute pain associated with radiotherapy

Incident pains can be precipitated by transport and positioning of the patient for radiotherapy. Other pains can be caused by acute radiation toxicity, which is most commonly associated with inflammation and ulceration of skin or mucous membranes within the radiation port. The syndrome produced is dependent upon the involved field: head and neck irradiation can cause a stomatitis or pharyngitis (Rider, 1990), treatment of the chest and oesophagus can cause an esophagitis (Vanagunas et al., 1990), and pelvic therapy can cause a proctitis, cystitis-urethritis, vaginal ulceration, or radiation dermatitis.

Oropharyngeal mucositis

Radiotherapy-induced mucositis is invariable with doses above 1000 cGy, and ulceration is common at doses above 4000 cGy. Although the severity of the associated pain is variable, it is often severe enough to interfere with oral alimentation. Painful mucositis can persist for several weeks after the completion of the treatment (Scully et al., 2003, 2004).

Acute radiation enteritis and proctocolitis

Acute radiation enteritis occurs in as many as 50% of patients receiving abdominal or pelvic radiotherapy. Involvement of the small intestine can present with cramping abdominal pain associated with nausea and diarrhoea (Andreyev et al., 2005). Pelvic radiotherapy can cause a painful proctocolitis, with tenesmoid pain associated with diarrhoea, mucous discharge, and bleeding (Babb, 1996; Andreyev et al., 2005). These complications typically resolve shortly after completion of therapy, but may have a slow resolution over 2–6 months (Nussbaum et al., 1993; Babb, 1996; Andreyev et al., 2005). Acute enteritis predicts for an increased risk of late-onset radiation enteritis (see following paragraphs).

Early-onset brachial plexopathy

A transient brachial plexopathy has been described in breast cancer patients immediately following radiotherapy to the chest wall and adjacent nodal areas (Salner et al., 1981; Pierce et al., 1992) and after mantle radiotherapy for Hodgkin's disease (Churn et al., 2000). In retrospective studies, the incidence of this phenomenon has been variably estimated as 1.4–20% (Salner et al., 1981; Pierce et al., 1992); clinical experience suggests that lower estimates are more accurate. The median latency to the development of symptoms was 4.5 months (3–14 months) in one survey (Salner et al., 1981). Paraesthesias are the most common presenting symptom, and pain and weakness occur less frequently. The syndrome is self-limiting and is not predictive of the subsequent development of delayed onset, progressive plexopathy.

Subacute radiation myelopathy

Subacute radiation myelopathy is an uncommon phenomenon that may occur following radiotherapy of extraspinal tumours (Ang and Stephens, 1994; Schultheiss, 1994). It is most frequently observed involving the cervical cord after radiation treatment of head and neck cancers and Hodgkin's disease. In the latter case, patients develop painful, shock-like pains in the neck that are precipitated by neck flexion (Lhermitte's sign); these pains may radiate down the spine and into one or more extremities. The syndrome usually begins weeks to months after the completion of radiotherapy, and typically resolves over a period of 3–6 months (Ang and Stephens, 1994)

Radiotherapy-induced pain flare

Palliative radiotherapy of bone metastases causes a temporary increase in bone pain in 30–40% of patients immediately after radiotherapy (Loblaw et al., 2007; Hird et al., 2009a). This is better treated with prophylactic medication rather than management with breakthrough pain medications. A single 8 mg dose of dexamethasone before radiotherapy has been effective in reducing the severity and prevalence of pain (Hird et al., 2009c).

The radiopharmaceuticals strontium-89, rhenium-186 hydroxyethylidene diphosphonate, and samarium-153 are systemically administered beta-emitting calcium analogues that are taken up by bone in areas of osteoblastic activity and which may help relieve pain caused by blastic bony metastases (McEwan, 1997). A 'flare' response, characterized by transient worsening of pain 1–2 days after administration, occurs in 15–20% of patients (Robinson et al., 1995). This flare usually resolves after 3–5 days and most effected patients subsequently develop a good analgesic response (Robinson et al., 1995).

Acute pain associated with infection

Acute herpetic neuralgia

A significantly increased incidence of acute herpetic neuralgia occurs among cancer patients, especially those with haematological or lymphoproliferative malignancies and those receiving immunosuppressive therapies (Portenoy et al., 1986; Rusthoven et al., 1988; Insinga et al., 2005). The pain, which may be continuous or lancinating, usually resolves within 2 months (Galer and Portenoy, 1991). Pain persisting beyond this interval is referred to as post-herpetic neuralgia (PHN) (see 'Post-herpetic neuralgia' section). Patients with active tumour are more likely to have a disseminated infection (Rusthoven et al., 1988). In those predisposed by chemotherapy, the infection usually develops less than 1 month after the completion of treatment. The dermatomal location of the infection is often associated with the site of the malignancy (Rusthoven et al., 1988). The infection also occurs twice as frequently in previously irradiated dermatomes as non-radiated areas (Dunst et al., 2000).

Acute pain associated with vascular events

Acute thrombosis pain

Thrombosis is the most frequent complication and the second cause of death in patients with overt malignant disease (Ashrani and Heit, 2009; Rana and Levine, 2009). Thrombotic episodes may precede the diagnosis of cancer by months or years and represent a potential marker for occult malignancy (Prandoni and Piccioli, 2006). Postoperative deep vein thrombosis is more frequent in patients operated for malignant diseases than for other disorders, and both chemotherapy and hormone therapy are associated with an increased thrombotic risk (Ashrani and Heit, 2009; Rana and Levine, 2009).

Possible prothrombic factors in cancer include the capacity of tumour cells and their products to interact with platelets, clotting and fibrinolytic systems, endothelial cells, and tumour-associated macrophages. Cytokine release, acute phase reaction, and neovascularization may contribute to *in vivo* clotting activation (Sood, 2009). Data from a very large cohort of 66 329 cancer patients demonstrated that bone, ovary, brain, and pancreas cancers are associated with the highest incidence thrombosis and that distant metastases, chemotherapy and hormonal therapy all led to a 1.5–2.5 times increased risk (Blom et al., 2006).

Lower-extremity deep venous thrombosis

Pain and swelling are the commonest presenting features of lower extremity deep vein thrombosis (Criado and Burnham, 1997; Qaseem et al., 2007). The pain is variable in severity and it is often mild. It is commonly described as a dull cramp, or diffuse heaviness. The pain most commonly affects the calf but may involve the sole of the foot, the heel, the thigh, the groin, or pelvis. Pain usually increases on standing and walking. On examination, suggestive features include swelling, warmth, dilatation of superficial veins, tenderness along venous tracts, and pain induced by stretching (Criado and Burnham, 1997).

Rarely, patients may develop tissue ischaemia or frank gangrene, even without arterial or capillary occlusion; this syndrome is called phlegmasia cerulea dolens. It is most commonly seen in patients with underlying neoplasm (Hirschmann, 1987; Lorimer et al., 1994) and it is also seen proximal to inferior vena cava filters (Cookson and Caldwell, 2012; Kiefer and Colletti, 2013). Clinically it is characterized by severe pain, extensive oedema, and cyanosis of the legs. Gangrene can occur unless the venous obstruction is relieved. Intravenous thrombolytic therapy (Tardy et al., 2006) may be more effective than traditional treatments with anticoagulation and thrombectomy (Perkins et al., 1996). Until recently, the mortality rate for ischaemic venous thrombosis was about 30–40%, the cause of death usually being the underlying disease or pulmonary emboli (Vysetti et al., 2009)

Upper-extremity deep venous thrombosis

The three major clinical features of upper-extremity venous thrombosis are oedema, dilated collateral circulation, and pain (Flinterman et al., 2008). Approximately two-thirds of patients have arm pain. Among patients with cancer the most common causes are central venous catheterization and extrinsic compression by tumour (Flinterman et al., 2008). Although much less common, phlegmasia of the upper limb has been reported (Bedri et al., 2009; Petritsch et al., 2012). Although thrombosis secondary to intrinsic damage usually responds well to anticoagulation alone and rarely causes persistent symptoms, when extrinsic obstruction is the cause, persistent arm swelling and pain are commonplace (Flinterman et al., 2008).

Superior vena cava obstruction

Superior vena cava (SVC) obstruction is most commonly caused by extrinsic compression by enlarged mediastinal lymph nodes (Rice et al., 2006; Wilson et al., 2007; Wan and Bezjak, 2009). In contemporary series, lung cancer and lymphomas are the most commonly associated conditions. Increasingly, thrombosis of the SVC is caused by intravascular devices (Morales et al., 1997; Rice et al., 2006) particularly with left-sided ports and when the catheter tip lies in the upper part of the vena (Puel et al., 1993). Patient usually present with facial swelling and dilated neck and chest wall veins. Chest pain, headache, and mastalgia are less common presentations.

Acute mesenteric vein thrombosis

Acute mesenteric vein thrombosis is most commonly associated with hypercoagulability states. Rarely, it has been associated with extrinsic venous compression by malignant lymphadenopathy (Traill and Nolan, 1997), extension of venous thrombosis (Vigo et al., 1980), as a result of iatrogenic hypercoagulable state (Sahdev et al., 1985) or as an adverse effect of pancreatic resection (Zyromski and Howard, 2008).

Superficial thrombophlebitis

Superficial thrombophlebitis is more common among patients with cancer and may be a presenting symptom of cancer (Mouton et al., 2009; van Doormaal et al., 2010). It presents with the development of a palpable tender cord in the course of a superficial vein; often associated with erythema of the overlying skin. Duplex ultrasound should be considered to rule out occult deep venous thrombosis, particularly when the greater or lesser saphenous veins are involved (Blumenberg et al., 1998).

Trousseau's syndrome or migratory thrombophlebitis is a rare condition characterized by a recurrent and migratory pattern and involvement of superficial veins, frequently in unusual sites such as the arm or chest (Varki, 2007).

Chronic pain syndromes

Most chronic cancer-related pains are caused directly by the tumour. Data from the largest prospective survey of cancer pain syndromes revealed that almost one-quarter of the patients experienced two or more pains. Over 90% of the patients had one or more tumour related pains and 21% had one or more pains caused by cancer therapies. Somatic pains (71%) were more common than neuropathic (39%) or visceral pains (34%) (Caraceni and Portenoy, 1999). Bone pain and compression of neural structures are the two most common causes.

Bone pain

Bone metastases are the most common cause of chronic pain in cancer patients. Cancers of the lung, breast, and prostate most often metastasize to bone, but any tumour type may be complicated by painful bony lesions. Although bone pain is usually associated with direct tumour invasion of bony structures, more than 25% of patients with bony metastases are pain free (Wagner, 1984), and patients with multiple bony metastases typically report pain in only a few sites.

Differential diagnosis

Bone pain due to metastatic tumour needs to be differentiated from less common causes. Non-neoplastic causes in this population include osteoporotic fractures (including those associated with multiple myeloma), focal osteonecrosis, which may be idiopathic or related to chemotherapy, corticosteroids, or radiotherapy (see following paragraphs) and osteomalacia (Gray et al., 1992; Shane et al., 1997). Rarely, a paraneoplastic osteomalacia, which is associated with elevated levels of fibroblast growth factor 23, can mimic multiple metastases (Woznowski et al., 2008; Zadik and Nitzan, 2012).

Multifocal or generalized bone pain

Bone pain may be focal, multifocal, or generalized. Multifocal bone pains are most commonly experienced by patients with multiple bony metastases. A generalized pain syndrome is occasionally produced by replacement of bone marrow (Jonsson et al., 1990; Wong et al., 1993; Hesselmann et al., 2002; Lin et al., 2002; Hussain and Chui, 2006). This bone marrow replacement syndrome has been observed in haematogenous malignancies and, less commonly, in solid tumours (Cohen et al., 1982; Wong et al., 1993; Hussain and Chui, 2006) and brain tumours (Didelot et al., 2006; Cordiano et al., 2011). This syndrome can occur in the absence of abnormalities on bone scintigraphy or radiography, increasing the difficulty of diagnosis. It is best demonstrated on MRI scanning (Ollivier et al., 2006) or using PET scanning techniques (Evangelista et al., 2012).

Vertebral syndromes

The vertebrae are the most common sites of bony metastases. More than two-thirds of vertebral metastases are located in the thoracic spine; lumbosacral and cervical metastases account for approximately 20% and 10%, respectively. Multiple level involvement is common, occurring in greater than 85% of patients (Constans et al., 1983).

The early recognition of pain syndromes due to tumour invasion of vertebral bodies is essential, since pain usually precedes compression of adjacent neural structures and prompt treatment of the lesion may prevent the subsequent development of neurologic deficits. Several factors often confound accurate diagnosis; referral of pain is common, and the associated symptoms and signs can mimic a variety of other disorders, both malignant (e.g. paraspinal masses) and non-malignant.

Atlantoaxial destruction and odontoid fracture

Nuchal or occipital pain is the typical presentation of destruction of the atlas or fracture of the odontoid process. Pain often radiates over the posterior aspect of the skull to the vertex and is exacerbated by movement of the neck, particularly flexion (Bilsky et al., 2002; Lakemeier et al., 2009). Pathological fracture may result in secondary subluxation with compression of the spinal cord at the cervicomedullary junction. This complication is usually insidious and may begin with symptoms or signs in one or more extremity. Typically, there is early involvement of the upper extremities and the occasional appearance of so-called 'pseudo-levels' suggestive of more caudal spinal lesions; these deficits can slowly progress to involve sensory, motor, and autonomic function (Sundaresan et al., 1981).

C7–T1 syndrome

Invasion of the C7 or T1 vertebra can result in pain referred to the interscapular region. These lesions may be missed if radiographic evaluation is mistakenly targeted to the painful area caudal to the site of damage. Additionally, visualization of the appropriate region on routine radiographs may be inadequate due to obscuration by overlying bone and mediastinal shadows. Patients with interscapular pain should therefore undergo radiography of both the cervical and the thoracic spine.

T12–L1 (thoracolumbar junction) syndrome

A T12 or L1 vertebral lesion can refer pain to the ipsilateral iliac crest or the sacroiliac joint. Imaging procedures directed at pelvic bones can miss the source of the pain.

Sacral syndrome

Severe focal pain radiating to buttocks, perineum, or posterior thighs may accompany destruction of the sacrum (Nader et al., 2004). The pain is often exacerbated by sitting or lying and is relieved by standing or walking (Payer, 2003). Tumour can spread laterally to involve muscles that rotate the hip (e.g. the pyriformis muscle). This may produce severe incident pain induced by motion of the hip, or a malignant 'pyriformis syndrome', characterized by buttock or posterior leg pain that is exacerbated by internal rotation of the hip. Local extension of the tumour mass may also involve the sacral plexus (see following paragraphs).

Back pain and epidural compression

Epidural compression of the spinal cord or cauda equina is a common neurologic complication of cancer. In a large retrospective series, 0.23% of cancer patients had epidural compression at the presentation of their disease and 2.5% of patients dying of cancer had at least one admission for cord compression in the 5 years preceding death (Loblaw et al., 2012). Breast, lung, and prostate cancers each account for 20–25% of events (Loblaw et al., 2012). Most epidural compression is caused by posterior extension of vertebral body metastasis to the epidural space. Occasionally, epidural compression is caused by tumour extension from the posterior arch of the vertebra or infiltration of a paravertebral tumour through the intervertebral foramen.

Untreated, epidural compression leads inevitably to neurological damage. Effective treatment can potentially prevent these complications. The most important determinate of the efficacy of treatment is the degree of neurological impairment at the time therapy is initiated. Seventy-five per cent of patients who begin treatment while ambulatory remain so; the efficacy of treatment declines to 30–50% for those who begin treatment while markedly paretic, and is 10–20% for those who are plegic (Prasad and Schiff, 2005). Despite this, delays in diagnosis are commonplace (Loblaw et al., 2005; Abrahm et al., 2008).

Back pain is the initial symptom in almost all patients with epidural compression (Posner, 1987; Dugas et al., 2011), and in 10% it is the only symptom at the time of diagnosis (Greenberg et al., 1980). Since pain usually precedes neurologic signs by a prolonged period, it should be viewed as a potential indicator of epidural compression, which can lead to treatment at a time that a favourable response is most likely. Back pain, however, is a non-specific symptom that can result from bony or paraspinal metastases without epidural encroachment, from retroperitoneal or leptomeningeal tumour, epidural lipomatosis due to steroid administration (Stranjalis et al., 1992) or from a large variety of other benign conditions. Since it is not feasible to pursue an extensive evaluation in every cancer patient who develops back pain, the complaint should impel an evaluation that determines the likelihood of epidural compression and thereby selects patients appropriate for definitive imaging of the epidural space. The selection process is based on symptoms and signs and the results of simple imaging techniques.

Suggestive clinical features

Some pain characteristics are particularly suggestive of epidural extension (Helweg-Larsen and Sorensen, 1994). Rapid progression of back pain in a crescendo pattern is an ominous occurrence (Rosenthal et al., 1992). Radicular pain, which can be constant or lancinating has similar implications (Helweg-Larsen and Sorensen, 1994). It is usually unilateral in the cervical and lumbosacral regions and bilateral in the thorax, where it is often experienced as a tight, belt-like band across the chest or abdomen (Helweg-Larsen and Sorensen, 1994). The likelihood of epidural compression is also greater when back or radicular pain is exacerbated by recumbency, cough, sneeze, or strain (Ruff and Lanska, 1989). Other types of referred pain are also suggestive, including Lhermitte's sign (Ventafridda et al., 1991) and central pain from spinal cord compression, which usually is perceived some distance below the site of the compression and is typically a poorly localized, non-dermatomal dysaesthesia (Posner, 1987).

Weakness, sensory loss, autonomic dysfunction, and reflex abnormalities usually occur after a period of progressive pain (Helweg-Larsen and Sorensen, 1994). Weakness may begin segmentally if related to nerve root damage or in a multisegmental or pyramidal distribution if the cauda equina or spinal cord, respectively, is injured. The rate of progression of weakness is variable; in the absence of treatment, following the onset of weakness one-third of patients will develop paralysis within 7 days (Barron et al., 1959). Without effective treatment, sensory abnormalities, which may also begin segmentally, may ultimately evolve to a sensory level, with complete loss of all sensory modalities below the site of injury. The upper level of sensory findings may correspond to the location of the epidural tumour or be below it by many

segments (Helweg-Larsen and Sorensen, 1994). Ataxia without pain is the initial presentation of epidural compression in 1% of patients; this finding is presumably due to early involvement of the spinocerebellar tracts (Gilbert et al., 1978).

Bladder and bowel dysfunction generally occur late, except in patients with a conus medullaris lesion who may present with acute urinary retention and constipation without preceding motor or sensory symptoms (Helweg-Larsen and Sorensen, 1994).

Other features that may be evident on examination of patients with epidural compression include scoliosis, asymmetrical wasting of paravertebral musculature, and a gibbus (palpable step in the spinous processes). Spinal tenderness to percussion, which may be severe, often accompanies the pain.

Imaging modalities

Definitive imaging of the epidural space confirms the existence of epidural compression (and thereby indicates the necessity and urgency of treatment), defines the appropriate radiation portals, and determines the extent of epidural encroachment (which influences prognosis and may alter the therapeutic approach). The options for definitive imaging include MRI, myelography, and computed tomography (CT) myelography or spiral CT without myelographic contrast.

MRI is non-invasive and offers accurate imaging of the vertebrae, intraspinal, and paravertebral structures. When available it is generally the preferred mode of evaluation (Loblaw et al., 2005). Whenever possible, total spine imaging should be performed since multiple level involvement is common and other sites may be clinically occult. In a study of 65 patients with cord compression, 32 (49%) showed multiple level involvement and of these, 28 (66%) were clinically occult (Heldmann et al., 1997). MRI has multiple advantages: metastases can be distinguished from other pathological processes involving the axial skeleton, epidural and intradural space, and spinal cord. This is particularly true for bacterial abscesses, leptomeningeal carcinomatosis, intradural extramedullary or, rarely, intramedullary metastases or primary tumours and infectious or inflammatory myelitis.

MRI is relatively contraindicated in patients with severe claustrophobia and certain metallic implants, and is absolutely contraindicated for patients with cardiac pacemakers or aneurysm clips. Several other groups who may not be suitable for MRI include very obese patients and those with severe kyphosis or scoliosis.

CT: similar to MRI, CT scanning is non-invasive, and it provides excellent visualization of the vertebrae, vertebral structural integrity, paravertebral soft tissues, and of the vertebral foraminae. The improved resolution observed with contemporary spiral techniques facilitate very clear imaging of the spinal canal contents. CT scanning of regions identified by either plain radiography or bone scan usually provides excellent visualization of cortical integrity, the intervertebral foraminae, and canal contents and correlation studies with MRI findings demonstrated very high sensitivity and specificity (Crocker et al., 2011). Bone and soft tissue windows are used in a complementary manner; bone windows allow evaluation of bony integrity and, in particular, of cortical breach, and soft-tissue windows are used to evaluate the contents of the spinal canal. Using this approach one can reserve more expensive and less readily available MRI imaging for equivocal cases, when leptomeningeal metastases are suspected, or when total spinal imaging is required.

With the improved resolution of standard CT techniques, post-myelographic CT is a technique that is now rarely used. Besides immediate patient discomfort, myelography is often complicated by post-procedure side effects that include back pain, headache, vomiting, seizures, and adverse neurobehavioral reactions. The risk of adverse effects is related to the gauge and type of needle used (Wilkinson and Sellar, 1991), the contrast medium (Killebrew et al., 1983), and the anatomy of the epidural compression.

Pain syndromes of the bony pelvis and hip

The pelvis and hip are common sites of metastatic involvement. Lesions may involve any of the three anatomic regions of the pelvis (ischiopubic, iliosacral, or periacetabular), the hip joint itself, or the proximal femur (Papagelopoulos et al., 2007). The weight-bearing function of these structures, essential for normal ambulation, contributes to the propensity of disease at these sites to cause incident pain with walking and weight bearing.

Hip joint syndrome

Tumour involvement of the acetabulum or head of femur typically produces localized hip pain that is aggravated by weight bearing and movement of the hip (Singh et al., 2006). The pain may radiate to the knee or medial thigh, and occasionally, pain is limited to these structures (Sim, 1992). Medial extension of an acetabular tumour can involve the lumbosacral plexus as it traverses the pelvic sidewall. Evaluation of this region is best accomplished with CT or MRI, both of which can demonstrate the extent of bony destruction and adjacent soft tissue involvement more sensitively than other imaging techniques (Vijayanathan et al., 2009), PET/CT approaches assist by identifying disease activity (Vijayanathan et al., 2009). Important differential diagnoses include avascular necrosis, radicular pain (usually L1) or, occasionally, occult infections.

Acrometastases

Acrometastases, metastases in the hands and feet are rare and often misdiagnosed or overlooked. In the feet, the larger bones containing the higher amounts of red marrow, such as the os calcis, or talus are usually involved (Kouvaris et al., 2005; Bahk et al., 2006). Symptoms may be vague and can mimic other conditions, such as osteomyelitis, gouty rheumatoid arthritis, Reiter's syndrome, Paget's disease, osteochondral lesions, and ligamentous sprains.

Arthritides

Hypertrophic pulmonary osteoarthropathy

Hypertrophic pulmonary osteoarthropathy (HPOA) is a paraneoplastic syndrome that incorporates clubbing of the fingers, periostitis of long bones, and occasionally a rheumatoid-like polyarthritis (Martinez-Lavin, 1997). Periostitis and arthritis can produce pain, tenderness, and swelling in the knees, wrists, and ankles. The onset of symptoms is usually subacute, and it may precede the discovery of the underlying neoplasm by several months. It is most commonly associated with non-small cell lung cancer; however, even in that setting it is uncommon (Ito et al., 2010). Rarely, it may be associated with benign mesothelioma, pulmonary metastases from other sites, smooth muscle tumours of the oesophagus, breast cancer, and metastatic nasopharyngeal cancer.

HPOA is diagnosed on the basis of physical findings, radiological appearance, and radionuclide bone scan (Greenfield et al., 1967; Sharma, 1995; Martinez-Lavin, 1997). Effective anti-tumour therapy is sometimes associated with symptom regression (Hung et al., 2000; Kishi et al., 2002; Ito et al., 2010), bisphosphonate therapy may help relieve symptoms (Suzuma et al., 2001; Amital et al., 2004), and there are case reports of resolution after vagotomy (Treasure, 2006; Ooi et al., 2007)

Other polyarthritides

Rarely, rheumatoid arthritis, systemic lupus erythematosus, and an asymmetrical polyarthritis may occur as paraneoplastic phenomena that resolve with effective treatment of the underlying disease (Racanelli et al., 2008). A syndrome of palmar plantar fasciitis and polyarthritis characterized by palmar and digital with polyarticular painful capsular contractions, has been associated with ovarian (Shiel et al., 1985; Giannakopoulos et al., 2005), breast (Saxman and Seitz, 1997), and gastric (Enomoto et al., 2000) cancers.

Muscle pain

Muscle cramps

Persistent muscle cramps in cancer patients are usually caused by an identifiable neural, muscular, or biochemical abnormality (Siegal, 1991). In one series of 50 patients, 22 had peripheral neuropathy, 17 had root or plexus pathology (including six with leptomeningeal metastases), two had polymyositis and one had hypomagnesaemia. In this series, muscle cramps were the presenting symptom of recognizable and previously unsuspected neurologic dysfunction in 27 of 42 (64%) of the identified causes (Steiner and Siegal, 1989). Cramps have been reported as an adverse effect of imatinib (Breccia et al., 2005), goserelin (Ernst et al., 2004), and vincristine (Haim et al., 1994).

Skeletal muscle tumours

Soft tissue sarcomas arising from fat, fibrous tissue, or skeletal muscle are the most common tumours involving the skeletal muscles. Skeletal muscle is one of the most unusual sites of metastasis from any malignancy. They occur disproportionally at sites of prior muscle trauma (Magee and Rosenthal, 2002). Lesions are usually painless but they may present with persistent ache.

Headache and facial pain

Headache in the cancer patient results from traction, inflammation, or infiltration of pain-sensitive structures in the head or neck. Early evaluation with appropriate imaging techniques may identify the lesion and allow prompt treatment, which may reduce pain and prevent the development of neurological deficits (Vecht et al., 1992).

Intracerebral tumour

The prevalence of headache in patients with brain metastases or primary brain tumours is 60–90% (Chidel et al., 2000; El Kamar and Posner, 2004; Kirby and Purdy, 2007) and headache is often the first presenting symptom of patients with brain tumours or metastases (Argyriou et al., 2006b; Wilne et al., 2006; Kirby and Purdy, 2007) and is often associated with dizziness (Hird et al., 2009b). Among 183 patients with new-onset chronic headache, as an isolated symptom, investigation revealed underlying tumour in 15 cases (Vazquez-Barquero et al., 1994). The headache is presumably produced by traction on pain-sensitive vascular and dural tissues. Patients with multiple metastases and those with posterior fossa metastases are more likely to report this symptom (Kirby and Purdy, 2007). The pain may be focal, overlying the site of the lesion, or generalized. Headache has lateralizing value, especially in patients with supratentorial lesions (Suwanwela et al., 1994; Argyriou et al., 2006b; Kirby and Purdy, 2007). Posterior fossa lesions often cause a bi-frontal headache. The quality of the headache is usually throbbing or steady, and the intensity is usually mild to moderate (Suwanwela et al., 1994; Argyriou et al., 2006b).

Among children, headache is the most common presenting symptom of brain tumours (Wilne et al., 2006) The clinical features predictive of underlying tumour include sleep-related headache, headache in the absence of a family history of migraine, vomiting, absence of visual symptoms, headache of less than 6 months' duration, confusion, and abnormal neurologic examination findings (Medina et al., 1997; Wilne et al., 2006). The headache is often worse in the morning and is exacerbated by stooping, sudden head movement, or Valsalva manoeuvres (cough, sneeze or strain) (Suwanwela et al., 1994).

Leptomeningeal metastases

Leptomeningeal metastases, which are characterized by diffuse or multifocal involvement of the subarachnoid space by metastatic tumour occur in 1–8% in patients with systemic cancer (Grossman and Krabak, 1999; Taillibert et al., 2005). Non-Hodgkin's lymphoma and acute lymphocytic leukaemia both demonstrate predilection for meningeal metastases (Nolan and Abrey, 2005); the incidence is lower for solid tumours alone (Bruno and Raizer, 2005). Of solid tumours, adenocarcinomas of the breast and small cell lung cancer predominate (Bruno and Raizer, 2005).

Leptomeningeal metastases present with focal or multifocal neurological symptoms or signs that may involve any level of the neuraxis (Wasserstrom et al., 1982; Grossman and Krabak, 1999; van Oostenbrugge and Twijnstra, 1999; Yamanaka et al., 2011). The most common presenting symptoms are headache, cranial nerve palsies (Yamanaka et al., 2011), and radicular pain in the low back and buttocks (van Oostenbrugge and Twijnstra, 1999). More than one-third of patients presents with evidence of cranial nerve damage, including double vision, hearing loss, facial numbness, and decreased vision (Wasserstrom et al., 1982; van Oostenbrugge and Twijnstra, 1999; Yamanaka et al., 2011). Less common features include seizures, papilloedema, hemiparesis, ataxic gait, and confusion (Balm and Hammack, 1996).

The headache is variable and may be associated with changes in mental status (e.g. lethargy, confusion, or loss of memory), nausea, vomiting, tinnitus, or nuchal rigidity. Pains that resemble cluster headache (DeAngelis and Payne, 1987) or glossopharyngeal neuralgia with syncope (Sozzi et al., 1987) have also been reported.

Increasingly, gadolinium-enhanced MRI imaging of the neuroaxis is the investigation of choice when leptomeningeal metastases are suspected. Compared to CSF cytology examination, MRI probably is more sensitive but it is less specific as false positive cytologies are rare (Straathof et al., 1999). When headache is the presenting feature, gadolinium-enhanced MRI examination of the brain, is the initial imaging investigation, especially if signs of cranial nerve involvement are present (Collie et al., 1999; Straathof et al., 1999). If this is non-diagnostic and if the pain

distribution indicates spinal involvement, sensitivity is enhanced by performing an examination of the whole spine. There is evidence that gadolinium-enhanced spinal MRI may be positive in almost 50% of patients without clinical findings related to the spinal region and in 60% of patients with negative cerebrospinal fluid (CSF) cytology (Gomori et al., 1998). Additionally, findings of contrast enhancement of the basilar cisterns, parenchymal metastases, hydrocephalus without a mass lesion, or spinal subarachnoid masses or enhancement may all have therapeutic implications (Grossman and Krabak, 1999).

The diagnosis of leptomeningeal metastases may be confirmed through analysis of the CSF. The CSF may reveal elevated pressure, elevated protein, depressed glucose, and/or lymphocytic pleocytosis. Ninety per cent of patients ultimately show positive cytology, but multiple evaluations may be required. After a single LP, the false-negative rate may be as high as 55%; this falls to only 10% after three LPs (Olson et al., 1974; Wasserstrom et al., 1982; Kaplan et al., 1990). Despite these measures, CSF cytology is persistently negative in as many as 20% of patients with clinically or radiographically unequivocal leptomeningeal involvement presumably because the malignant cells adhere to the leptomeninges rather than float in the CSF. The sensitivity and specificity of CSF cytology may be enhanced by the use of fluorescence *in situ* hybridization (FISH) (van Oostenbrugge et al., 1998, 2000) or immunocytochemical techniques (Thomas et al., 2000). Tumour markers, such as lactic dehydrogenase (LDH) isoenzymes (Wasserstrom et al., 1982), carcinoembryonic antigen (Liu et al., 2009), beta-2-microglobulin (Twijnstra et al., 1987), and tissue polypeptide antigen (Soletormos and Bach, 2001) may help to delineate the diagnosis. Flow cytometry for detection of abnormal DNA content may be a useful adjunct to cytological examination (Schinstine et al., 2006).

Untreated leptomeningeal metastases cause progressive neurologic dysfunction at multiple sites, followed by death in 4–6 weeks. Current treatment strategies, which includes radiation therapy to the area of symptomatic involvement, corticosteroids, and intraventricular or intrathecal chemotherapy or systemic chemotherapy, are of limited efficacy and in general patient outlook remains poor (Clarke et al., 2010).

Base of skull metastases

Base of skull metastases are associated with well-described clinical syndromes (Greenberg et al., 1981; Laigle-Donadey et al., 2005), which are named according to the site of metastatic involvement: orbital, parasellar, middle fossa, jugular foramen, occipital condyle, clivus, and sphenoid sinus (Fig. 13.1.1). Cancers of the breast, lung, and prostate are most commonly associated with this complication (Greenberg et al., 1981; Hawley et al., 1999; Laigle-Donadey et al., 2005), but any tumour type that metastasizes to bone may be responsible. When base of skull metastases are suspected, axial imaging with CT (including bone window settings) is the usual initial procedure (Greenberg et al., 1981; Laigle-Donadey et al., 2005). MRI is more sensitive for assessing soft tissue extension, and CSF analysis may be needed to exclude leptomeningeal metastases.

Orbital syndrome

Orbital metastases usually present with progressive pain in the retro-orbital and supraorbital area of the affected eye (Ben Simon et al., 2006; Ahmad and Esmaeli, 2007). Blurred vision and

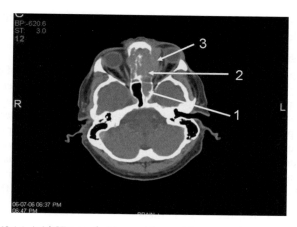

Fig. 13.1.1 Axial CT scan of a 54-year-old man with tumour arising in paranasal sinuses (arrow 1) with extension to the orbit (arrow 2) and nasopharynx (arrow 3).

diplopia may be associated complaints. Signs may include proptosis, chemosis of the involved eye, external ophthalmoparesis, ipsilateral papilloedema, and decreased sensation in the ophthalmic division of the trigeminal nerve.

Parasellar syndrome

The parasellar syndrome typically presents as unilateral supraorbital and frontal headache, which may be associated with diplopia (Yi et al., 2000). There may be ophthalmoparesis (Besada et al., 2007) or papilloedema, and formal visual field testing may demonstrate hemianopsia or quadrantinopsia.

Middle cranial fossa syndrome

The middle cranial fossa syndrome presents with facial numbness, paraesthesias, or pain, which is usually referred to the cheek or jaw (in the distribution of second or third divisions of the trigeminal nerve) (Lossos and Siegal, 1992). The pain is typically described as a dull continual ache, but may also be paroxysmal or lancinating. On examination, patients may have hypaesthesia in the trigeminal nerve distribution and signs of weakness in the ipsilateral muscles of mastication. Occasional patients have other neurological signs, such as abducens palsy (Greenberg et al., 1981; Bullitt et al., 1986).

Jugular foramen syndrome

The jugular foramen syndrome usually presents with hoarseness or dysphagia. Pain is usually referred to the ipsilateral ear or mastoid region and may occasionally present as glossopharyngeal neuralgia, with or without syncope (Greenberg et al., 1981; Laigle-Donadey et al., 2005). Pain may also be referred to the ipsilateral neck or shoulder. Neurologic signs include ipsilateral Horner's syndrome, and paresis of the palate, vocal cord, sternocleidomastoid, or trapezius. Ipsilateral paresis of the tongue may also occur if the tumour extends to the region of the hypoglossal canal.

Occipital condyle syndrome

The occipital condyle syndrome presents with unilateral occipital pain that is worsened with neck flexion (Loevner and Yousem, 1997; Moris et al., 1998; Martinez Salamanca et al., 2006). The patient may complain of neck stiffness. Pain intensity is variable, but can be severe. Examination may reveal a head tilt, limited movement of the neck, and tenderness to palpation over the occipitonuchal junction. Neurological findings may include ipsilateral

hypoglossal nerve paralysis and sternocleidomastoid weakness (Capobianco et al., 2002).

Clivus syndrome

The clivus syndrome is characterized by vertex headache, which is often exacerbated by neck flexion. Lower cranial nerve (VI–XII) dysfunction may develop (Ulubas et al., 2005; Malloy, 2007) and may become bilateral (Fink et al., 1987).

Sphenoid sinus syndrome

A sphenoid sinus metastasis often presents with bi-frontal and or retro-orbital pain, which may radiate to the temporal regions (Lawson and Reino, 1997). There may be associated features of nasal congestion and diplopia (Mickel and Zimmerman, 1990). Physical examination is often unremarkable, although unilateral or bilateral sixth nerve paresis can be present.

Painful cranial neuralgias

As noted, specific cranial neuralgias can occur from metastases in the base of skull or leptomeninges. They are most commonly observed in patients with prostate and lung cancer (Gupta et al., 1990; McDermott et al., 2004). Invasion of the soft tissues of the head or neck, or involvement of sinuses can also eventuate in such lesions. Each of these syndromes has a characteristic presentation. Early diagnosis may allow effective treatment of the underlying lesion before progressive neurologic injury occurs.

Glossopharyngeal neuralgia

Glossopharyngeal neuralgia has been reported in patients with leptomeningeal metastases (Sozzi et al., 1987), the jugular foramen syndrome (Greenberg et al., 1981), or head and neck malignancies (Metheetrairut and Brown, 1993; Pfendler, 1997; Ribeiro et al., 2007). This syndrome presents as severe pain in the throat or neck, which may radiate to the ear or mastoid region. Pain may be induced by swallowing. In some patients, pain is associated with sudden orthostasis and syncope (Weinstein et al., 1986; Metheetrairut and Brown, 1993; Ribeiro et al., 2007).

Trigeminal neuralgia

Trigeminal pains may be continual, paroxysmal, or lancinating. Pain that mimics classical trigeminal neuralgia can be induced by tumours in the middle or posterior fossa (Bullitt et al., 1986; Cheng et al., 1993; Barker et al., 1996; Hirota et al., 1998; Benoliel et al., 2007) or leptomeningeal metastases (DeAngelis and Payne, 1987). Sometimes, pain may be caused by perineural spread without evidence of a discrete mass (Boerman et al., 1999). Continual pain in a trigeminal distribution may be an early sign of acoustic neuroma (Payten, 1972). All cancer patients who develop trigeminal neuralgia should be evaluated for the existence of an underlying neoplasm.

Orthostatic headache with cervical spine metastases

Headache triggered by upright posture has been described in patients with metastases of the upper cervical spine with compression of the C2 or C3 nerve roots (Kim et al., 2008).

Ear and eye pain syndromes
Otalgia

Otalgia is the sensation of pain in the ear, while referred otalgia is pain felt in the ear but originating from a non-otologic source (Siddiq and Samra, 2008). The rich sensory innervation of the ear derives from four cranial nerves and two cervical nerves which also supply other areas in the head, neck, thorax, and abdomen. Pain referred to the ear may originate in areas far removed from the ear itself. Otalgia may be caused by acoustic neuroma (Morrison and Sterkers, 1996) and metastases to the temporal bone or infratemporal fossa (Hill and Kohut, 1976; Shapshay et al., 1976; Leonetti et al., 1998). Referred otalgia is reported among patients with tumours involving the oropharynx or hypopharynx (Scarbrough et al., 2003).

Eye pain

Blurring of vision and eye pain are the two most common symptoms of choroidal metastases (De Potter, 1998). More commonly, chronic eye pain is related to metastases to the bony orbit (Shih et al., 2007), intraorbital structures such as the rectus muscles (Weiss et al., 1984; Friedman et al., 1990), the optic nerve (Laitt et al., 1996), or the cavernus sinus (Rodriguez et al., 2007). Physical examination should include evaluation of visual fields, oculomotor function, fundi, and a careful evaluation for evidence of exophthalmos.

Oral cancer pain

Studies in patents with newly diagnosed oral cancer commonly reported significant levels of spontaneous pain and functional restriction with either talking or eating restriction associated with the pain (Lam and Schmidt, 2011).

Uncommon causes of headache and facial pain

Headache and facial pain in cancer patients may have many other causes. Unilateral facial pain can be the initial symptom of an ipsilateral lung tumour (Sarlani et al., 2003; Evans, 2007; Navarro et al., 2010). Presumably, this referred pain is mediated by vagal afferents. Facial squamous cell carcinoma of the skin may present with facial pain due to extensive perineural invasion (Schroeder et al., 1998). Patients with Hodgkin's disease may have transient episodes of neurological dysfunction that has been likened to migraine (Dulli et al., 1987). In some cases this may be a reversible posterior leucoencephalopathy syndrome (RPLS) which is characterized by headache, conscious disturbance, seizure, and cortical visual loss with neuroimaging finding of oedema in the posterior regions of the brain (Miyazaki et al., 2004).

Headache may occur with cerebral infarction or haemorrhage, which may be due to non-bacterial thrombotic endocarditis or disseminated intravascular coagulation. Headache is also the usual presentation of sagittal sinus occlusion, which may be due to tumour infiltration, hypercoagulable state or treatment with L-asparaginase therapy (Sigsbee et al., 1979). Headache due to pseudotumour cerebri has also been reported to be the presentation of SVC obstruction in a patient with lung cancer (Portenoy et al., 1983). Tumours of the sinonasal tract may present with deep facial or nasal pain (Marshall and Mahanna, 1997).

Neuropathic pains involving the peripheral nervous system

Neuropathic pains involving the peripheral nervous system are common. The syndromes include painful radiculopathy, plexopathy, mononeuropathy, or peripheral neuropathy.

Painful radiculopathy

Radiculopathy or polyradiculopathy may be caused by any process that compresses, distorts or inflames nerve roots. Painful radiculopathy is an important presentation of epidural tumour and leptomeningeal metastases (see earlier paragraphs).

Post-herpetic neuralgia

The precise clinical definition of PHN has been a matter of dispute. There is agreement that acute herpetic neuralgia refers to pain preceding or accompanying the eruption of rash that persists up to 30 days from its onset. Some authorities refer to all persistent pain as PHN, others describe a subacute herpetic neuralgia that persists beyond healing of the rash but which resolves within 4 months of onset, reserving the term PHN to pain persisting beyond 4 months from the initial onset of the rash (Dworkin and Portenoy, 1996). One study suggests that PHN is two to three times more frequent in the cancer population than the general population (Rusthoven et al., 1988).

Cervical plexopathy

Among cancer patients cervical plexus injury is frequently due to tumour infiltration or treatment (including surgery or radiotherapy) to neoplasms in this region (Jaeckle, 1991). Tumour invasion or compression of the cervical plexus can be caused by direct extension of a primary head and neck malignancy or neoplastic (metastatic or lymphomatous) involvement of the cervical lymph nodes (Jaeckle, 1991). Pain may be experienced in the preauricular (greater auricular nerve) or postauricular (lesser and greater occipital nerves) regions, or the anterior neck (transverse cutaneous and supraclavicular nerves). Pain may refer to the lateral aspect of the face or head, or to the ipsilateral shoulder. The overlap in the pain referral patterns from the face and neck may relate to the close anatomic relationship between the central connections of cervical afferents and the afferents carried in cranial nerves V, VII, IX and X in the upper cervical spinal cord.

Associated features can include ipsilateral Horner's syndrome or hemidiaphragmatic paralysis. The diagnosis must be distinguished from epidural compression of the cervical spinal cord and leptomeningeal metastases. MRI or CT imaging of the neck and cervical spine is usually required to evaluate the aetiology of the pain.

Brachial plexopathy

The two most common causes of brachial plexopathy in cancer patients are tumour infiltration and radiation injury. Less common causes of painful brachial plexopathy include trauma during surgery or anaesthesia, radiation-induced second neoplasms, acute brachial plexus ischaemia, and paraneoplastic brachial neuritis.

Malignant brachial plexopathy

Plexus infiltration by tumour is the most prevalent cause of brachial plexopathy. Malignant brachial plexopathy is most common in patients with lymphoma, lung cancer, or breast cancer. The invading tumour usually arises from adjacent axillary, cervical, and supraclavicular lymph nodes (lymphoma and breast cancer), or from the lung (superior sulcus tumours or so-called Pancoast tumours) (Kori et al., 1981; Kori, 1995; Jaeckle, 2004). Pain is nearly universal, occurring in 85% of patients, and often precedes neurologic signs or symptoms by months (Kori, 1995). Lower plexus involvement (C7, C8, T1 distribution) is typical, and is reflected in the pain distribution, which usually involves the elbow, medial forearm and fourth and fifth fingers. Pain may sometimes localize

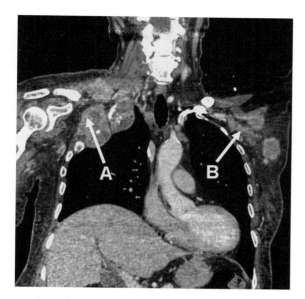

Fig. 13.1.2 Coronal CT reconstruction of a patient with bilateral brachial plexopathy. Arrow A: bulky metastases arising from ribs compressing inferior right plexus. Arrow B: tumour infiltrates deposited on left plexus.

to the posterior arm or elbow. Severe aching is usually reported, but patients may also experience constant or lancinating dysaesthesias along the ulnar aspect of the forearm or hand.

Tumour infiltration of the upper plexus (C5–C6 distribution) is less common. This lesion is characterized by pain in the shoulder girdle, lateral arm, and hand. Seventy-five per cent of patients presenting with upper plexopathy subsequently develop a panplexopathy, and 25% of patients present with panplexopathy (Kori et al., 1981).

Cross-sectional imaging is essential in all patients with symptoms or signs compatible with plexopathy (Fig. 13.1.2). Although comparative data on the sensitivity and specificity of MRI to CT in evaluating lesions of the brachial plexus is not available, MRI is widely thought to be the best choice for evaluating the anatomy and pathology of the brachial plexus (van Es et al., 2010). Limited experience has been reported for PET-CT imaging (Luthra et al., 2006).

Electrodiagnostic studies may be helpful in patients with suspected plexopathy, particularly when neurological examination and imaging studies are normal (Ferrante and Wilbourn, 2002). Although not specific for tumour, abnormalities on electromyography (EMG) or somatosensory-evoked potentials may establish the diagnosis of plexopathy, and thereby confirm the need for additional evaluation.

Patients with malignant brachial plexopathy are at high risk for epidural extension of the tumour (Portenoy et al., 1989; Jaeckle, 1991). Epidural encroachment can occur as the neoplasm grows medially and invades vertebrae or tracks along nerve roots through the intervertebral foramina. In the latter case, there may be no evidence of bony erosion on imaging studies. The development of Horner's syndrome, evidence of panplexopathy, or finding of paraspinal tumour or vertebral damage on CT or MRI are highly associated with epidural extension and should lead to definitive imaging of the epidural tumour (Portenoy et al., 1989; Jaeckle, 1991).

Radiation-induced brachial plexopathy

Two distinct syndromes of radiation-induced brachial plexopathy have been described: (1) early-onset transient plexopathy (see earlier paragraphs) and (2) delayed-onset progressive plexopathy. Delayed-onset progressive plexopathy can occur 6 months to 20 years after a course of radiotherapy that included the plexus in the radiation portal. In contrast to tumour infiltration, pain is a relatively uncommon presenting symptom (18%), and when present, is usually less severe (Kori et al., 1981). After supraclavicular node radiotherapy there is a progressively increasing incidence over time which rises to 56% after 20 years (Bajrovic et al., 2004). Weakness and sensory changes predominate in the distribution of the upper plexus (C5, C6 distribution) (Mondrup et al., 1990; Olsen et al., 1990; Vecht, 1990; Schierle and Winograd, 2004; Jaeckle, 2010). Radiation changes in the skin and lymphoedema are commonly associated.

The typical appearance of radiation fibrosis of the plexus on CT studies is a diffuse infiltration and loss of tissue planes without a mass lesion (Cascino et al., 1983). There is often associated lymphoedema in the arm, evident on CT, and occasionally, radiation necrosis of the clavicle or rib or humeral head occurs at the adjacent level (Schulte et al., 1989). Tumour infiltration of the plexus cannot be differentiated from radiation fibrosis by CT studies when diffuse infiltration is noted. On MRI the most common findings observed with radiation fibrosis are thickening and diffuse enhancement of the brachial plexus without a focal mass and/or soft-tissue changes with low signal intensity on both T1- and T2-weighted images (Wittenberg and Adkins, 2000).

Electrodiagnostic studies in patients with radiation fibrosis typically include widespread infraclavicular demyelinating conduction blocks on motor nerve conduction studies, and myokymic discharges and fasciculation potentials on needle electrode examination (Ferrante, 2004, 2012). Widespread myokymia is strongly suggestive of radiation-induced plexopathy (Flaggman and Kelly, 1980; Albers et al., 1981; Lederman and Wilbourn, 1984; Harper et al., 1989; Roth et al., 1988). Although a careful history, combined with neurologic findings and the results of tomographic and electrodiagnostic studies can strongly suggest the diagnosis of radiation-induced injury, repeated assessments over time may be needed to confirm the diagnosis. Rare patients require surgical exploration of the plexus to exclude neoplasm and establish the aetiology.

The natural history of brachial plexus fibrosis is variable. Motor dysfunction may be incomplete, or may progress to a severe paresis (Killer and Hess, 1990; Olsen et al., 1990; Olsen et al., 1993). In a long-term follow-up study of 71 patients radiated to 57 Gy, 11 of the 12 surviving patients had severe arm paralysis (Johansson et al., 2000). Even with advanced radiation fibrosis, severe pain is relatively uncommon and its presence should prompt evaluation of the patient for recurrent tumour (Kori et al., 1981).

Uncommon causes of brachial plexopathy

Malignant peripheral nerve tumour or a second primary tumour in a previously irradiated site can account for pain recurring late in the patient's course (Binder et al., 2004). Pain has been reported to occur as a result of brachial plexus entrapment in a lymphoedematous shoulder (Vecht, 1990), and as a consequence of acute ischaemia many years after axillary radiotherapy (Gerard et al., 1989). An idiopathic brachial plexopathy has also been described in patients with Hodgkin's disease (Lachance et al., 1991). Paraneoplastic brachial plexopathy associated with anti-amphiphysin antibodies has been described (Coppens et al., 2006).

Lumbosacral plexopathy

In the cancer population, lumbosacral plexopathy is usually caused by neoplastic infiltration or compression. Radiation-induced plexopathy also occurs, and occasional patients develop the lesion as a result of surgical trauma, infarction, cytotoxic damage, infection in the pelvis or psoas muscle, abdominal aneurysm, or idiopathic lumbosacral neuritis. Polyradiculopathy from leptomeningeal metastases or epidural metastases can mimic lumbosacral plexopathy.

Malignant lumbosacral plexopathy

The primary tumours most frequently associated with malignant lumbosacral plexopathy include colorectal, cervical, breast, sarcoma, and lymphoma (Jaeckle et al., 1985). Most tumours involve the plexus by direct extension from intrapelvic neoplasm; metastases account for only one-quarter of cases. Rarely, plexopathy can arise by perineural spread from a prostate cancer along prostatic nerves into the lumbosacral plexus (Ladha et al., 2006).

Pain is, typically, the first symptom and it is experienced by almost all patients at some point, and it is the only symptom in almost 20% of patients. The quality is aching, pressure-like, or stabbing; dysaesthesias are relatively uncommon. Most patients develop numbness, paraesthesias, or weakness weeks to months after the pain begins. Common signs include leg weakness that involves multiple myotomes, sensory loss that crosses dermatomes, reflex asymmetry, focal tenderness, leg oedema, and positive direct or reverse straight-leg raising signs.

A lower plexopathy is most common accounts for just over 50% of patients with malignant lumbosacral plexopathy (Jaeckle et al., 1985). It is usually caused by direct extension from a pelvic tumour, most frequently rectal cancer, gynaecological tumours, or pelvic sarcoma. Pain may be localized in the buttocks and perineum, or referred to the posterolateral thigh and leg. Associated symptoms and signs conform to an L4–S1 distribution. Examination may reveal weakness or sensory changes in the L5 and S1 dermatomes and a depressed ankle jerk. Other findings include leg oedema, bladder or bowel dysfunction, sacral or sciatic notch tenderness, and a positive straight-leg raising test. A pelvic mass may be palpable.

An upper plexopathy occurs in almost one-third of patients with lumbosacral plexopathy (Jaeckle et al., 1985). Pain may be experienced in the back, lower abdomen, flank or iliac crest, or the anterolateral thigh. Examination may reveal sensory, motor, and reflex changes in a L1–4 distribution.

A subgroup of these patients present with a syndrome characterized by pain and paraesthesias limited to the lower abdomen or inguinal region, variable sensory loss, and no motor findings. CT scan may show tumour adjacent to the L1 vertebra (the L1 syndrome) (Jaeckle et al., 1985) or along the pelvic sidewall, where it presumably damages the ilioinguinal, iliohypogastric, or genitofemoral nerves.

Another subgroup has neoplastic involvement of the psoas muscle and presents with a syndrome characterized by upper lumbosacral plexopathy, painful flexion of the ipsilateral hip, and positive psoas muscle stretch test; this has been termed the malignant psoas syndrome (Stevens and Gonet, 1990; Agar et al., 2004). Similarly,

pain in the distribution of the femoral nerve has been observed in the setting of recurrent retroperitoneal sarcoma (Zografos and Karakousis, 1994) and tumour in the iliac crest can compress the lateral cutaneous nerve of the thigh producing a pain that mimics meralgia paraesthetica (Tharion and Bhattacharji, 1997).

Sacral plexopathy may occur from direct extension of a sacral lesion or a presacral mass (Payer, 2003). This may present with predominant involvement of the lumbosacral trunk, characterized by numbness over the dorsal medial foot and sole and weakness of knee flexion, ankle dorsiflexion, and inversion. Other patients demonstrate particular involvement of the coccygeal plexus, with prominent sphincter dysfunction and perineal sensory loss. The latter syndrome occurs with low pelvic tumours, such as those arising from the rectum or prostate.

A panplexopathy with involvement in a L1–S3 distribution occurs in almost one-fifth of patients with lumbosacral plexopathy (Jaeckle et al., 1985). Local pain may occur in the lower abdomen, back, buttocks, or perineum. Referred pain can be experienced anywhere in distribution of the plexus. Leg oedema is extremely common. Neurological deficits may be confluent or patchy within the L1–S3 distribution and a positive straight leg raising test is usually present.

Cross-sectional imaging, with either CT or MRI, is the preferred diagnostic procedure to evaluate lumbosacral plexopathy (Fig. 13.1.3). Scanning should be done from the level of the L1 vertebral body, through the sciatic notch. Limited data suggests superior sensitivity MRI over CT imaging. Definitive imaging of the epidural space adjacent to the plexus should be considered in the patient who has features indicative of a relatively high risk of epidural extension including bilateral symptoms or signs, unexplained incontinence, or a prominent paraspinal mass.

Radiation-induced lumbosacral plexopathy

Radiation fibrosis of the lumbosacral plexus is a rare complication that may occur from 1 to over 30 years following radiation treatment. The use of intracavitary radium implants for carcinoma of the cervix may be an additional risk factor (Stryker et al., 1990; Gonzalez-Caballero et al., 2000). Radiation-induced plexopathy typically presents with progressive weakness and leg swelling; pain is not usually a prominent feature (Thomas et al., 1985; Stryker et al., 1990). Weakness typically begins distally in the L5–S1 segments and is slowly progressive. The symptoms and signs may be bilateral (Thomas et al., 1985). If CT scanning demonstrates a lesion, it is usually a non-specific diffuse infiltration of the tissues. Electromyography may show myokymic discharges (Thomas et al., 1985).

Uncommon causes of lumbosacral plexopathy

Lumbosacral plexopathy may occur following intra-arterial cis-platinum infusion (see following paragraphs) and embolization techniques. This syndrome been observed following attempted embolization of a bleeding rectal lesion. Raised intrapelvic pressure due to a collection (Lin et al., 2009) or even a massively distended bladder or rectum may sometimes cause a plexus compression syndrome with radicular pain. Benign conditions that may produce similar findings include haemorrhage or abscess in the iliopsoas muscle (Chad and Bradley, 1987), abdominal aortic aneurysms, diabetic radiculoplexopathy, vasculitis, and an idiopathic lumbosacral plexitis analogous to acute brachial neuritis (Chad and Bradley, 1987).

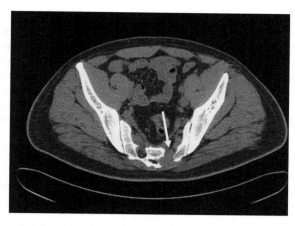

Fig. 13.1.3 Axial CT scan image of a 29-year-old male with known renal cell cancer and pain radiating into his left buttock. CT demonstrated a soft tissue lesion in the foramen of S2 (arrowed).

Painful mononeuropathy

Tumour-related mononeuropathy

Tumour-related mononeuropathy usually results from compression or infiltration of a nerve from tumour arising in an adjacent bony structure. The most common example of this phenomenon is intercostal nerve injury in a patient with rib metastases. Other examples include the cranial neuralgias previously described, sciatica associated with tumour invasion of the sciatic notch, and common peroneal nerve palsy associated with primary bone tumours of the proximal fibula and lateral cutaneous nerve of the thigh neuralgia associated with iliac crest tumours.

Other causes of mononeuropathy

Cancer patients also develop mononeuropathies from many other causes. Post-surgical syndromes are well described (see following paragraphs) and radiation injury of a peripheral nerve occurs occasionally. Rarely, cancer patients develop nerve entrapment syndromes (such as carpal tunnel syndrome) related to oedema or direct compression by tumour (Desta et al., 1994).

Painful peripheral neuropathies

Painful peripheral neuropathies have multiple causes, including nutritional deficiencies, other metabolic derangements (e.g. diabetes and renal dysfunction), neurotoxic effects of chemotherapy, and, rarely, paraneoplastic syndromes.

Paraneoplastic painful peripheral neuropathy

Paraneoplastic painful peripheral neuropathy can be related to injury to the dorsal root ganglion (also known as subacute sensory neuronopathy or ganglionopathy) or injury to peripheral nerves (Grisold and Drlicek, 1999; Oki et al., 2007). These syndromes may be the initial manifestation of an underlying malignancy. Except for the neuropathy associated with myeloma (Kissel and Mendell, 1996; Rotta and Bradley, 1997), their course is usually independent of the primary tumour (Dalmau and Posner, 1997; Grisold and Drlicek, 1999).

Subacute sensory neuronopathy is characterized by pain (usually dysaesthetic), paraesthesias, sensory loss in the extremities, and severe sensory ataxia (Brady, 1996). Although it is usually associated with small cell carcinoma of the lung (van Oosterhout et al., 1996), other tumour types, including breast cancer (Peterson

et al., 1994), Hodgkin's disease (Plante-Bordeneuve et al., 1994), and other solid tumours are rarely associated. The pain usually develops before the tumour is evident and its course is typically independent.

Coexisting autonomic, cerebellar, or cerebral abnormalities are common (Brady, 1996). An antineuronal IgG antibody ('anti-Hu'), which recognizes a low-molecular-weight protein present in most small cell lung carcinomas, has been associated with the condition (Dalmau and Posner, 1997). A number of other paraneoplastic antibodies have been identified these include anti-CV2 (Antoine et al., 2001) and anti-Ri (Fasolino et al., 2004).

A sensorimotor peripheral neuropathy, which may be painful, has been observed in association with diverse neoplasms, particularly Hodgkin's disease and paraproteinaemias (Kelly and Karcher, 2005). Clinically evident peripheral neuropathy occurs in approximately 15% of patients with multiple myeloma, and electrophysiological evidence of this lesion can be found in 40% (Kissel and Mendell, 1996). The pathophysiology of the neuropathy is unknown.

Pain syndromes of the viscera and miscellaneous tumour-related syndromes

Pain may be caused by pathology involving the luminal organs of the gastrointestinal or genitourinary tracts, the parenchymal organs, the peritoneum, or the retroperitoneal soft tissues. Obstruction of hollow viscus, including intestine, biliary tract, and ureter, produces visceral nociceptive syndromes that are well described in the surgical literature (Silen, 1983). Pain arising from retroperitoneal and pelvic lesions may involve mixed nociceptive and neuropathic mechanisms if both somatic structures and nerves are involved.

Hepatic distention syndrome

Pain sensitive structures in the region of the liver include the liver capsule, blood vessels, and biliary tract. Nociceptive afferents that innervate these structures travel via the coeliac plexus, the phrenic nerve, and the lower right intercostal nerves. Extensive intrahepatic metastases, or gross hepatomegaly associated with cholestasis, may produce discomfort in the right subcostal region, and less commonly in the right mid-back or flank (Harris et al., 2003) (Fig. 13.1. 4). Referred pain may be experienced in the right neck or shoulder, or in the region of the right scapula (Mulholland et al., 1990).

Occasional patients who experience chronic pain due to hepatic distension develop an acute intercurrent subcostal pain that may be exacerbated by respiration. Physical examination may demonstrate a palpable or audible rub. These findings suggest the development of an overlying peritonitis, which can develop in response to some acute event, such as a haemorrhage into a metastasis (La Fianza et al., 1999).

Midline retroperitoneal syndrome

Retroperitoneal pathology involving the upper abdomen may produce pain by injury to deep somatic structures of the posterior abdominal wall, distortion of pain sensitive connective tissue, vascular and ductal structures, local inflammation, and direct infiltration of the coeliac plexus. The most common causes are pancreatic cancer (Kelsen et al., 1995; Grahm and Andren-Sandberg, 1997; Kelsen et al., 1997) and retroperitoneal lymphadenopathy

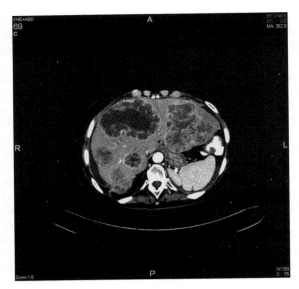

Fig. 13.1.4 CT scan of a 53-year-old woman with right upper quadrant abdominal pain caused by multiple liver metastases.

(Krane and Perrone, 1981; Neer et al., 1981; Sponseller, 1996), particularly coeliac lymphadenopathy (Schonenberg et al., 1991).

In some instances of pancreatic cancer, obstruction of the main pancreatic duct with subsequent ductal hypertension generates pain which can be relieved by stenting of the pancreatic duct (Tham et al., 2000).

The pain is experienced in the epigastrium, in the low thoracic region of the back, or in both locations. It is often diffuse and poorly localized. It is usually dull and boring in character, exacerbated with recumbency, and improved by sitting. The lesion can usually be demonstrated by CT, MRI, or ultrasound scanning of the upper abdomen (Fig. 13.1.5).

Intestinal obstruction

(Also see Chapter 14.3.)

Abdominal pain is an almost invariable manifestation of intestinal obstruction, which may occur in patients with abdominal or pelvic cancers (Ripamonti et al., 2008; Dolan, 2011). The factors

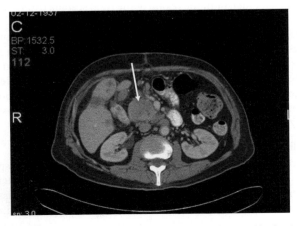

Fig. 13.1.5 Axial CT scan of a 72-year-old man with epigastric and back pain caused by cancer in the head of the pancreas (arrowed).

that contribute to this pain include smooth muscle contractions, mesenteric tension, and mural ischaemia. Obstructive symptoms may be due primarily to the tumour, or more likely, to a combination of mechanical obstruction and other processes, such as autonomic neuropathy and ileus from metabolic derangements or drugs. Both continuous and colicky pains occur which may be referred to the dermatomes represented by the spinal segments supplying the affected viscera. Vomiting, anorexia, and constipation are important associated symptoms.

Peritoneal carcinomatosis

Peritoneal carcinomatosis occurs most often by transcoelomic spread of abdominal or pelvic tumour; excepting breast cancer, haematogenous spread of an extra-abdominal neoplasm in this pattern is rare. Carcinomatosis can cause peritoneal inflammation, mesenteric tethering, malignant adhesions, and ascites, all of which can cause pain. Pain and abdominal distension are the most common presenting symptoms. Adhesions can also cause obstruction of hollow viscus, with intermittent colicky pain (Averbach and Sugarbaker, 1995). CT scanning may demonstrate evidence of ascites, omental infiltration, and peritoneal nodules.

Malignant perineal pain

Tumours of the colon or rectum, female reproductive tract, and distal genitourinary system are most commonly responsible for perineal pain (Stillman, 1990; Boas et al., 1993; Hagen, 1993; Miaskowski, 1996; Rigor, 2000). Severe perineal pain following resection of pelvic tumours often precede evidence of detectable disease and should be viewed as a potential harbinger of progressive or recurrent cancer (Stillman, 1990; Boas et al., 1993; Rigor, 2000). There is evidence to suggest that this phenomenon is caused by microscopic perineural invasion by recurrent disease (Seefeld and Bargen, 1943). The pain, which is typically described as constant and aching, is often aggravated by sitting or standing, and may be associated with tenesmus or bladder spasms (Stillman, 1990).

Tumour invasion of the musculature of the deep pelvis can also result in a syndrome that appears similar to the so-called tension myalgia of the pelvic floor (Sinaki et al., 1977). The pain is typically described as a constant ache or heaviness that exacerbates with upright posture. When due to tumour, the pain may be concurrent with other types of perineal pain. Digital examination of the pelvic floor may reveal local tenderness or palpable tumour.

Adrenal pain syndrome

Large adrenal metastases, common in lung cancer, may produce unilateral flank pain, and less commonly, abdominal pain. Pain is of variable severity, and it can be severe (Berger M.S. et al., 1995). Adrenal metastases can be complicated by haemorrhage which may cause severe abdominal pain (Karanikiotis et al., 2004) (Fig. 13.1.6).

Ureteric obstruction

Ureteric obstruction is most frequently caused by tumour compression or infiltration within the true pelvis (Harrington et al., 1995; Russo, 2000). Less commonly, obstruction can be more proximal, associated with retroperitoneal lymphadenopathy, an isolated retroperitoneal metastasis, mural metastases, or intraluminal metastases. Cancers of the cervix, ovary, prostate, and rectum are most commonly associated with this complication. Pain

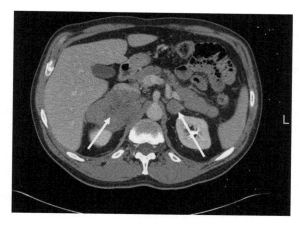

Fig. 13.1.6 Axial CT scan image of a 62-year-old male with small cell lung cancer and pain radiating into his right loin. CT demonstrated bilateral adrenal metastases. The right lesion is much larger than that on the left.

may or may not accompany ureteric obstruction. When present, it is typically a dull chronic discomfort in the flank, with radiation into the inguinal region or genitalia (Little et al., 2003). If pain does not occur, ureteric obstruction may be discovered when hydronephrosis is discerned on abdominal imaging procedures or renal failure develops. Ureteric obstruction can be complicated by pyelonephritis or pyonephrosis, which often present with features of sepsis, loin pain, and dysuria. Diagnosis of ureteric obstruction can usually be confirmed by the demonstration of hydronephrosis on renal sonography. The level of obstruction can be identified by pyelography, and CT scanning techniques will usually demonstrate the cause (Russo, 2000).

Ovarian cancer pain

Moderate to severe chronic abdominopelvic pain is the most common symptom of ovarian cancer; it is reported by almost two-thirds of patients in the 2 weeks prior to the onset or recurrence of the disease (Portenoy et al., 1994). Pain is experienced in the low back or abdomen (Goff et al., 2004; Webb et al., 2004). In patients who have been previously treated it is an important symptom of potential recurrence (Portenoy et al., 1994).

Lung cancer pain

Even in the absence of involvement of the chest wall or parietal pleura, lung tumours can produce a visceral pain syndrome. In a large case series of lung cancer patients, pain was unilateral in 80% of the cases and bilateral in 20%. Among patients with hilar tumours the pain was reported to the sternum or the scapula. Upper and lower lobe tumours referred to the shoulder and to the lower chest respectively (Marino et al., 1986; Marangoni et al., 1993). As previously mentioned, early lung cancers can generate ipsilateral facial pain (Sarlani et al., 2003). It is postulated that this pain syndrome is generated via vagal afferent neurons.

Other uncommon visceral pain syndromes

Sudden onset severe abdominal or loin pain may be caused by non-traumatic rupture of a visceral tumour. This has been most frequently reported with hepatocellular cancer (Miyamoto et al., 1991) but also with other liver metastases (Marini et al., 2002). Kidney rupture due to a renal metastasis from an adenocarcinoma

of the colon (Wolff et al., 1994), splenic rupture in acute leukaemia (Rajagopal et al., 2002), rupture of adrenocortical cancers (Stamoulis et al., 2004) and metastasis-induced perforated appendicitis (Ende et al., 1995) have been reported. Torsion of pedunculated visceral tumours can produce a cramping abdominal pain.

Paraneoplastic nociceptive pain syndromes

Tumour-related gynaecomastia

Tumours that secrete chorionic gonadotrophin (HCG), including malignant and benign tumours of the testis (Daniels and Layer, 2003; Duparc et al., 2003; Foppiani et al., 2005) and rarely cancers from other sites (Wurzel et al., 1987; Nishiyama et al., 1992; Forst et al., 1995; Liu et al., 1999), may be associated with chronic breast tenderness or gynaecomastia. Approximately 10% of patients with testis cancer have gynaecomastia or breast tenderness at presentation and the likelihood of gynaecomastia is greater with increasing HCG level (Tseng et al., 1985). Breast pain can be the first presentation of an occult tumour (Haas et al., 1989; Mellor and McCutchan, 1989; Cantwell et al., 1991).

Paraneoplastic pemphigus

Paraneoplastic pemphigus is a rare mucocutaneous disorder associated with non-Hodgkin's lymphoma and chronic lymphocytic leukaemia. The condition is characterized by widespread shallow ulcers with haemorrhagic crusting of the lips, conjunctival bullae and, uncommonly, pulmonary lesions. Characteristically, histopathology reveals intraepithelial and subepithelial clefting and immunoprecipitation studies reveal autoantibodies directed against desmoplakins and desmogleins (Camisa et al., 1992; Allen and Camisa, 2000).

Paraneoplastic Reynaud's syndrome

Paraneoplastic is a rare manifestation of solid tumours. It has been reported with lung cancer, ovarian cancer, testicular cancer, and melanoma (Wilmalaratna and Sachdev, 1987; Borenstein et al., 1990; DeCross and Sahasrabudhe, 1992).

Chronic pain syndromes associated with cancer therapy

Most treatment-related pains are caused by tissue-damaging procedures. These pains are acute, predictable and self-limited. Chronic treatment-related pain syndromes are associated with either a persistent nociceptive complication of an invasive treatment (such as a postsurgical abscess), or more commonly, neural injury. In some cases, these syndromes occur long after the therapy is completed, resulting in a difficult differential diagnosis between recurrent disease and a complication of therapy.

Post-chemotherapy pain syndromes
Toxic peripheral neuropathy

Chemotherapy-induced peripheral neuropathy is a common problem, which is typically manifested by painful paraesthesias in the hands and/or feet, and signs consistent with an axonopathy, including 'stocking-glove' sensory loss, weakness, hyporeflexia, and autonomic dysfunction (Ocean and Vahdat, 2004). The pain is usually characterized by continuous burning or lancinating pains, either of which may be increased by contact (Windebank and Grisold, 2008; Kautio et al., 2011). The drugs most commonly associated with a peripheral neuropathy are the vinca alkaloids (especially vincristine), cis-platinum, oxaliplatin, and paclitaxel. Procarbazine, carboplatin, ixabepilone, misonidazole and hexamethylmelamine are less common causes. Data from several studies indicates that the risk of neuropathy associated with cis-platinum and oxaliplatin can be diminished by amifostine (Spencer and Goa, 1995; Penz et al., 2001), glutathione (Cascinu et al., 1995, 2002), and calcium and magnesium infusion at the time of treatment (Gamelin et al., 2004). Conflicting data exists regarding the potential efficacy of prophylactic vitamin E in reducing paclitaxel neuriopathy (Argyriou et al., 2006a; Kottschade et al., 2011).

Avascular (aseptic) necrosis of femoral or humeral head

Avascular necrosis (AVN) of the femoral or humeral head may occur either spontaneously or as a complication of intermittent or continuous corticosteroid therapy (Cook et al., 2001; Virik et al., 2001) or high-dose chemotherapy with bone marrow transplantation (Fink et al., 1998). Osteonecrosis may be unilateral or bilateral. Involvement of the femoral head is most common and typically causes pain in the hip, thigh, or knee. Involvement of the humeral head usually presents as pain in the shoulder, upper arm, or elbow. Pain is exacerbated by movement and relieved by rest. There may be local tenderness over the joint, but this is not universal. Pain usually precedes radiological changes by weeks to months; bone scintigraphy and MRI are sensitive and complementary diagnostic procedures For the detection of radiographically occult AVN, radionuclide bone scanning and MRI are both sensitive methods but, MRI is preferred because it has greater sensitivity and a greater specificity than bone scanning (DeSmet et al., 2000). Early treatment consists of analgesics, decrease or discontinuation of steroids, and sometimes surgery. With progressive bone destruction, joint replacement may be necessary.

Plexopathy

Lumbosacral or brachial plexopathy may follow cis-platinum infusion into the iliac artery (Castellanos et al., 1987) or axillary artery (Kahn et al., 1989), respectively. Affected patients develop pain, weakness, and paraesthesias within 48 hours of the infusion. The mechanism for this syndrome is thought to be due to small-vessel damage and infarction of the plexus or nerve. The prognosis for neurologic recovery is not known.

Raynaud's phenomenon

Among patients with germ cell tumours treated with cisplatin, vinblastine, and bleomycin, persistent Raynaud's phenomenon is observed in 20–30% (Berger C.C. et al., 1995). This effect has also been observed in patients with carcinoma of the head and neck treated with a combination of cisplatin, vincristine, and bleomycin (Kukla et al., 1982). Pathophysiological studies have demonstrated that a hyper-reactivity in the central sympathetic nervous system results in a reduced function of the smooth muscle cells in the terminal arterioles (Hansen et al., 1990).

Chronic pain associated with hormonal therapy
Gynaecomastia with hormonal therapy for prostate cancer

Chronic gynaecomastia and breast tenderness are common complications of antiandrogen therapies for prostate cancer (McLeod and Iversen, 2000). The incidence of this syndrome varies among drugs; it is frequently associated with diethylstilbestrol and bicalutamide, is less common with flutamide and cyproterone and is uncommon among patients receiving luteinizing hormone-releasing hormone agonist therapy. Gynaecomastia in

the elderly must be distinguished from primary breast cancer or a secondary cancer in the breast (Olsson et al., 1984; Ramamurthy and Cooper, 1991).

Aromatase inhibitor pain syndromes

Aromatase inhibitor therapy in the treatment of hormones responsive breast cancer is often by musculoskeletal pain and stiffness. Common manifestations include hand osteoarthritis, tendonitis, trigger finger, and carpal tunnel syndrome. In one series of 51 patients, arthralgia and/or bone pain was reported in 61% of patients. Pain was severe in 30%, continuous in 41%, central in 50%, peripheral in 79%, and resulted in discontinuation of the drug in 20% of patients (Presant et al., 2007). The mechanism is not known (Moxley, 2010). Additionally other pain syndromes including Raynaud's syndrome (Bertolini et al., 2011) and carpal tunnel syndrome have also been observed (Nishihori et al., 2008).

Chronic pain associated with bisphosphonate therapy
Osteonecrosis of the jaw

Osteonecrosis of the jaw is described as an intraoral complication after administration of intravenous nitrogen-containing bisphosphonates. It is an uncommon complication whose incidence rate has climbed in recent years (Migliorati et al., 2010). It is defined as an unexpected development of necrotic bone in the oral cavity, and is commonly associated with administration of the bisphosphonates pamidronate and zoledronate. Clinical features include local pain, soft-tissue swelling, and/or loose teeth. Symptoms can mimic routine dental problems such as decay or periodontal disease (Migliorati et al., 2010; Yamashita et al., 2010). Osteonecrosis of the jaw is also often correlated with previous dental procedures, such as tooth extractions, during bisphosphonate therapy. Symptoms can mimic routine dental problems such as decay or periodontal disease (Migliorati et al., 2010). To reduce this risk clinical dental examination and a panoramic jaw radiograph should be performed before patients begin bisphosphonate therapy; dental treatment and other oral procedures should be completed before initiating bisphosphonate therapy and patients should be informed and instructed on the importance of maintaining good oral hygiene and having regular dental assessment (Migliorati et al., 2010).

Chronic diffuse pain

In June 2008, the US Food and Drug Administration issued a special warning regarding the possibility of severe and sometimes incapacitating bone, joint, and/or muscle (musculoskeletal) pain in patients taking bisphosphonates. The severe musculoskeletal pain may occur within days, months, or years after starting a bisphosphonate. Some patients have reported complete relief of symptoms after discontinuing the bisphosphonate, whereas others have reported slow or incomplete resolution. The risk factors for and incidence of severe musculoskeletal pain associated with bisphosphonates are unknown (Lenzer, 2008).

Chronic post-surgical pain syndromes

Surgical incision at virtually any location may result in chronic pain. Although persistent pain is occasionally encountered after nephrectomy, sternotomy, craniotomy, inguinal dissection, and other procedures, these pain syndromes are not well described in the cancer population. In contrast, several syndromes are now clearly recognized as sequelae of specific surgical procedures. The predominant underlying pain mechanism in these syndromes is neuropathic, resulting from injury to peripheral nerves or plexus.

Breast surgery pain syndromes

Chronic neuropathic pain of variable severity is a common sequela of surgery for breast cancer. Although chronic pain has been reported to occur after almost any surgical procedure on the breast from lumpectomy to radical mastectomy, it is most common after procedures involving axillary dissection (Vecht et al., 1989; Vecht, 1990; Hladiuk et al., 1992; Maunsell et al., 1993), occurring in 25–70% of patients (Keramopoulos et al., 1993; Maunsell et al., 1993; Tasmuth et al., 1995, 1996; Carpenter et al., 1998; Warmuth et al., 1998; Kakuda et al., 1999; Smith et al., 1999; Kuehn et al., 2000; Taylor, 2004; Vilholm et al., 2008).

The risk for, and severity of, pain is correlated positively with the number of lymph nodes removed (Hack et al., 1999; Johansson et al., 2000; Hack et al., 2010), presence of tumour in the upper outer quadrant of the breast (Vilholm et al., 2008) and is inversely correlated with age (Warmuth et al., 1998; Hack et al., 1999; Smith et al., 1999, Vilholm et al., 2008; Hack et al., 2010). There is conflicting data as to whether preservation of the intercostobrachial nerve during axillary lymph node dissection can reduce the incidence of this phenomenon (Temple and Ketcham, 1985; Salmon et al., 1998; Freeman et al., 2003; Torresan et al., 2003; Taylor, 2004; Ivanovic et al., 2007).

The incidence is reduced, but not avoided, when axillary dissection is avoided either by sentinel node excision without full dissection (Schulze et al., 2006; Baron et al., 2007; Langer et al., 2007; Lucci et al., 2007; Hack et al., 2010) or when nodes are irradiated without dissection (Albrecht et al., 2002).

The pain is usually characterized as a constricting and burning discomfort localized to the medial arm, axilla, and anterior chest wall (Wood, 1978; Granek et al., 1983; Vecht et al., 1989; Paredes et al., 1990; van Dam et al., 1993). Pain may begin immediately or as late as many months following surgery. The natural history of this condition appears to be variable, and both subacute and chronic courses are possible (International Association for the Study of Pain: Subcommittee on taxonomy, 1986, Ernst et al., 2002). The onset of pain later than 18 months following surgery is unusual, warranting careful evaluation to exclude recurrent disease. On examination, there is often an area of numbness within the region of the pain (van Dam et al., 1993; Schell, 2006; Baron et al., 2007; Ivanovic et al., 2007). Chronicity of pain is related to the intensity of the immediate postoperative pain (Stevens et al., 1995; Tasmuth et al., 1996), postoperative complications, and subsequent treatment with chemotherapy and radiotherapy (Tasmuth et al., 1995).

It is most commonly associated with neuropraxia of the intercostobrachial nerve during the process of axillary lymph node dissection (Vecht et al., 1989; Bratschi and Haller, 1990; van Dam et al., 1993). There is marked anatomic variation in the size and distribution of the intercostobrachial nerve, and this may account for some of the variability in the distribution of pain observed in patients with this condition (Assa, 1974).

This syndrome must be differentiated from post-mastectomy phantom breast pain (Rothemund et al., 2004), neuroma pain (Jung et al., 2003), post-mastectomy frozen shoulder (Johansen et al., 2000; Deutsch and Flickinger, 2001), axillary web syndrome (Moskovitz et al., 2001), and breast cellulitis (Hughes et al., 1997). In some cases of pain after breast surgery, a trigger point can be palpated in the axilla or chest wall.

Post-radical neck dissection pain

Chronic neck and shoulder pain after radical neck dissection is common (Dijkstra et al., 2001; Whale et al., 2001; Laverick et al., 2004; Donatelli-Lassig et al., 2008). Shoulder pain is most often caused by damage to the spinal accessory nerve (CN XI) (van Wilgen et al., 2003; Laverick et al., 2004). In other cases it can result from musculoskeletal imbalance in the shoulder girdle following surgical removal of neck muscles (Talmi et al., 2000). Similar to the droopy shoulder syndrome (Swift and Nichols, 1984), this syndrome can be complicated by development of a thoracic outlet syndrome or suprascapular nerve entrapment, with selective weakness and wasting of the supraspinatus and infraspinatus muscles (Brown et al., 1988).

Escalating pain in patients who have undergone radical neck dissection may signify recurrent tumour or soft tissue infection. These lesions may be difficult to diagnose in tissues damaged by radiation and surgery. Repeated CT or MRI scanning may be needed to exclude tumour recurrence. Empiric treatment with antibiotics should be considered (Bruera and MacDonald, 1986; Coyle and Portenoy, 1991; Reinbolt et al., 2005).

Post-thoracotomy pain

There are several patterns of post-thoracotomy pain:

Prolonged post-thoracotomy pain: this is the most common pattern. Pain has been reported most profound around the scar, and 82–90% of pain patients relate their pain directly to the surgical site (Wildgaard et al., 2009). The pain is primarily described as aching, tender, with numbness and to a lesser degree burning (Wildgaard et al., 2009). It is usually caused by trauma and compression to the intercoastal nerves, fractured and compressed ribs, inflammation of the chest muscles, atrophy of chest muscles, or scar tissue rubbing (Hopkins and Rosenzweig, 2012). Neuropathic component to the pain, related to intercostal nerve damage is very common (Guastella et al., 2011). Although it usually resolves after within 2 months after surgery, it may persist for up to 10 years (Grosen et al., 2013).

Increasing pain: a second group (16%) experienced pain that persisted following the thoracotomy, then increased in intensity during the follow-up period. Local recurrence of disease and infection were the most common causes of the increasing pain.

Recurrent pain: chest wall pain that recurs following resolution of the postoperative pain is often due to recurrent neoplasm. In one series, the development of recurrent or increasing post-thoracotomy pain was due to recurrent or persistent tumour in greater than 95% of patients (Kanner, 1982) . This finding was corroborated in a study which evaluated the records of 238 consecutive patients who underwent thoracotomy which identified recurrent pain 20 patients, all were found to have tumour regrowth (Keller et al., 1994).

Patients with recurrent or increasing post-thoracotomy pain should be carefully evaluated, preferably with a chest CT scan or MRI. Chest radiographs are insufficient to evaluate recurrent chest disease. In some patients, post-thoracotomy pain appears to be caused by a taut muscular band within the scapular region. In such cases, pain may be amenable to trigger point injection of local anaesthetic (Hamada et al., 2000).

Postoperative frozen shoulder

Patients with post-thoracotomy or post-mastectomy pain are at risk for the development of a frozen shoulder (Maunsell et al.,

1993). This lesion may become an independent focus of pain, particularly if complicated by reflex sympathetic dystrophy. Adequate postoperative analgesia and active mobilization of the joint soon after surgery are necessary to prevent these problems.

Phantom pain syndromes

Phantom limb pain is perceived to arise from an amputated limb, as if the limb were still contiguous with the body. Phantom pain is experienced by 60–80% of patients following limb amputation but is only severe or persistent in 5–10% of cases (Ehde et al., 2000; Nikolajsen and Jensen, 2000; Flor, 2002; Burgoyne et al., 2012). The incidence of phantom pain is significantly higher in patients with a long duration of pre-amputation pain and those with pain on the day before amputation (Weinstein, 1994; Nikolajsen et al., 1997b; Burgoyne et al., 2012). Patients who had pain prior to the amputation may experience phantom pain that replicates the earlier one (Katz and Melzack, 1990).

Phantom pain is more prevalent after tumour related than traumatic amputations, and postoperative chemotherapy is an additional risk factor (Smith and Thompson, 1995; Flor, 2002). The pain may be continuous or paroxysmal and is often associated with bothersome paraesthesias. The phantom limb may assume painful and unusual postures and may gradually telescope and approach the stump. Phantom pain may initially magnify and then slowly fade over time. There is growing evidence that preoperative or postoperative neural blockade reduces the incidence of phantom limb pain during the first year after amputation (Pavy and Doyle, 1996; Enneking and Morey, 1997; Katz, 1997; Nikolajsen et al., 1997a; Karanikolas et al., 2011).

Some patients have spontaneous partial remission of the pain. The recurrence of pain after such a remission, or the late onset of pain in a previously painless phantom limb, suggests the appearance of a more proximal lesion, including recurrent neoplasm (Chang et al., 1997).

Phantom pain syndromes have also been described after other surgical procedures. Phantom breast pain after mastectomy, which occurs in 15–30% of patients (Kroner et al., 1989; Kwekkeboom, 1996; Tasmuth et al., 1996; Rothemund et al., 2004, Bjorkman et al., 2008; Steegers et al., 2008), also appears to be related to the presence of preoperative pain (Kroner et al., 1989). The pain tends to start in the region of the nipple and then spread to the entire breast. The character of the pain is variable and may be lancinating, continuous or intermittent (Kroner et al., 1989; Rothemund et al., 2004). A phantom rectum pain syndrome occurs in approximately 15% of patients who undergo abdominoperineal resection of the rectum (Ovesen et al., 1991; Boas et al., 1993). Phantom rectal pain may develop either in the early postoperative period or after a latency of months to years. Late-onset pain is almost always associated with tumour recurrence (Boas et al., 1993, Ovesen et al., 1991). Rare cases of phantom bladder pain after cystectomy and phantom eye pain after enucleation have also been reported.

Stump pain

Stump pain occurs at the site of the surgical scar several months to years following amputation (Davis, 1993). It is usually the result of neuroma development at a site of nerve transection. This pain is characterized by burning or lancinating dysaesthesias, which are often exacerbated by movement or pressure and blocked by an injection of a local anaesthetic. Pain that is associated by signs of local inflammation may indicate abscess formation.

Postsurgical pelvic floor myalgia

Surgical trauma to the pelvic floor can cause a residual pelvic floor myalgia, which like the neoplastic syndrome described previously, mimics so-called tension myalgia (Sinaki et al., 1977). The risk of disease recurrence associated with this condition is not known, and its natural history has not been defined. In patients who have undergone anorectal resection, this condition must be differentiated from the phantom anus syndrome (see 'Burning perineum syndrome').

Chronic post-radiation pain syndromes

Chronic pain complicating radiation therapy tends to occur late in the course of a patient's illness. These syndromes must always be differentiated from recurrent tumour.

Radiation-induced brachial and lumbosacral plexopathies

Radiation-induced brachial and lumbosacral plexopathies were described previously in this chapter.

Chronic radiation myelopathy

Chronic radiation myelopathy is an uncommon late complication of spinal cord irradiation (Macbeth et al., 1996). The latency is highly variable but is most commonly 12–14 months. The most common presentation is a partial transverse myelopathy at the cervicothoracic level, sometimes in a Brown-Séquard pattern (Schultheiss and Stephens, 1992). Sensory symptoms, including pain, typically precede the development of progressive motor and autonomic dysfunction (Schultheiss and Stephens, 1992). The pain is characterized as a burning dysaesthesia localized to the area of spinal cord damage or below. Imaging studies, particularly MRI, are important to exclude an epidural metastases and demonstrate the nature and extent of intrinsic cord pathology, which may include atrophy, swelling, or syrinx. On MRI the signs of radiation myelitis include high-intensity signals on T2-weighted images or gadolinium enhancement of T1-weighted images (Alfonso et al., 1997). The course of chronic radiation myelopathy is characterized by steady progression over months, followed by a subsequent phase of slow progression or stabilization.

Chronic radiation enteritis and proctitis

Chronic enteritis and proctocolitis occur as a delayed complication in 2–10% of patients who undergo abdominal or pelvic radiation therapy (Yeoh and Horowitz, 1987; Nussbaum et al., 1993). The rectum and rectosigmoid are more commonly involved than the small bowel, a pattern that may relate to the retroperitoneal fixation of the former structures. The latency is variable (3 months–30 years) (Yeoh and Horowitz, 1987; Nussbaum et al., 1993; Tagkalidis and Tjandra, 2001). Chronic radiation injury to the rectum can present as proctitis (with bloody diarrhoea, tenesmus, and cramping pain), obstruction due to stricture formation, or fistulae to the bladder or vagina. Small bowel radiation damage typically causes colicky abdominal pain, which can be associated with chronic nausea or malabsorption. Barium studies may demonstrate a narrow tubular bowel segment resembling Crohn's disease or ischaemic colitis. Endoscopy and biopsy may be necessary to distinguish suspicious lesions from recurrent cancer (Chi et al., 2005).

Radiation cystitis

Radiation therapy used in the treatment of tumours of the pelvic organs (prostate, bladder, colon/rectum, uterus, ovary, and vagina/

vulva) may produce a chronic radiation cystitis (Pavlidakey and MacLennan, 2009). The late sequelae of radiation injury to the bladder can range from minor temporary irritative voiding symptoms and asymptomatic haematuria to more severe complications such as gross haematuria, contracted non-functional bladder, persistent incontinence, and fistula formation. The clinical presentation can include frequency, urgency, dysuria, haematuria, incontinence, hydronephrosis, pneumaturia, and faecaluria.

Lymphoedema pain

One-third of patients with lymphoedema as a complication of breast cancer or its treatment, experience pain and tightness in the arm (Newman et al., 1996; Hamner and Fleming, 2007) and pain is a major part of the morbidity among affected patients (McWayne and Heiney, 2005). In some patients, pain is caused by a secondary rotator cuff tendonitis caused by internal derangement of tendon fibres caused by impingement, functional overload, and intrinsic tendinopathy. Conservative treatment with NSAIDs and physiotherapy is a safe and effective treatment (Herrera and Stubblefield, 2004). Some patients develop nerve entrapment syndromes of the carpal tunnel syndrome or brachial plexus (Ganel et al., 1979; Vecht, 1990). Severe or increasing pain in a lymphoedematous arm is strongly suggestive of tumour invasion of the brachial plexus (Kori et al., 1981; Kori, 1995).

Burning perineum syndrome

Persistent perineal discomfort is an uncommon delayed complication of pelvic radiotherapy. After a latency of 6–18 months, burning pain can develop in the perianal region; the pain may extend anteriorly to involve the vagina or scrotum (Minsky and Cohen, 1988; Mannaerts et al., 2002). In patients who have had abdominoperineal resection, phantom anus pain and recurrent tumour are major differential diagnoses.

Post-prostate brachytherapy pelvic pain

Brachytherapy patients with prostate cancer may produce a chronic radiation-related pelvic pain syndrome that is exacerbated by urination or perineal pressure. Data suggests that it may be partly related to higher central prostatic radiation doses (Wallner et al., 2004).

Osteoradionecrosis

Osteoradionecrosis is another late complication of radiotherapy. Bone necrosis, which occurs as a result of endarteritis obliterans, may produce focal pain. Overlying tissue breakdown can occur spontaneously or as a result of trauma, such as dental extraction or denture trauma (Epstein et al., 1987, 1997). Delayed development of a painful ulcer must be differentiated from tumour recurrence.

Conclusion

Adequate assessment is a necessary precondition for effective pain management. In the cancer population, assessment must recognize the dynamic relationship between the symptom, the illness, and larger concerns related to quality of life. Syndrome identification and inferences about pain pathophysiology are useful elements that may simplify this complex undertaking.

References

Abrahm, J.L., Banffy, M.B., and Harris, M.B. (2008). Spinal cord compression in patients with advanced metastatic cancer: 'all I care about is walking and living my life'. *Journal of the American Medical Association*, 299, 937–946.

Amital, H., Applbaum, Y.H., Vasiliev, L., and Rubinow, A. (2004). Hypertrophic pulmonary osteoarthropathy: control of pain and symptoms with pamidronate. *Clinical Rheumatology*, 23, 330–332.

Anonymous (2008b). Postoperative pain undertreated in the United States. *Journal of Pain and Palliative Care Pharmacotherapy*, 22, 92–93.

Argyriou, A.A., Chroni, E., Polychronopoulos, P., et al. (2006b). Headache characteristics and brain metastases prediction in cancer patients. *European Journal of Cancer Care (England)*, 15, 90–95.

Benoliel, R., Epstein, J., Eliav, E., Jurevic, R., and Elad, S. (2007). Orofacial pain in cancer: part I—mechanisms. *Journal of Dental Research*, 86, 491–505.

Bilsky, M.H., Shannon, F.J., Sheppard, S., Prabhu, V., and Boland, P.J. (2002). Diagnosis and management of a metastatic tumor in the atlantoaxial spine. *Spine*, 27, 1062–1069.

Bruno, M.K. and Raizer, J. (2005). Leptomeningeal metastases from solid tumors (meningeal carcinomatosis). *Cancer Treatment Research*, 125, 31–52.

Caraceni, A. and Portenoy, R.K. (1999). An international survey of cancer pain characteristics and syndromes. IASP Task Force on Cancer Pain. International Association for the Study of Pain. *Pain*, 82, 263–274.

Chidel, M.A., Suh, J.H., and Barnett, G.H. (2000). Brain metastases: presentation, evaluation, and management. *Cleveland Clinic Journal of Medicine*, 67, 120–127.

Clarke, J.L., Perez, H.R., Jacks, L.M., Panageas, K.S., and Deangelis, L.M. (2010). Leptomeningeal metastases in the MRI era. *Neurology*, 74, 1449–1454.

Crocker, M., Anthantharanjit, R., Jones, T.L., et al. (2011). An extended role for CT in the emergency diagnosis of malignant spinal cord compression. *Clinical Radiology*, 66, 922–927.

Dijkstra, P.U., Van Wilgen, P.C., Buijs, R.P., et al. (2001). Incidence of shoulder pain after neck dissection: a clinical explorative study for risk factors. *Head & Neck*, 23, 947–953.

Dolan, E.A. (2011). Malignant bowel obstruction: a review of current treatment strategies. *American Journal of Hospice and Palliative Care*, 28(8), 576–582.

Dugas, A.F., Lucas, J.M., and Edlow, J.A. (2011). Diagnosis of spinal cord compression in nontrauma patients in the emergency department. *Academic Emergency Medicine*, 18, 719–725.

Ehde, D.M., Czerniecki, J.M., Smith, D.G., et al. (2000). Chronic phantom sensations, phantom pain, residual limb pain, and other regional pain after lower limb amputation. *Archives of Physical Medicine and Rehabilitation*, 81, 1039–1044.

Ernst, M.F., Voogd, A.C., Balder, W., Klinkenbijl, J.H., and Roukema, J.A. (2002). Early and late morbidity associated with axillary levels I-III dissection in breast cancer. *Journal of Surgical Oncology*, 79, 151–155.

Evangelista, L., Panunzio, A., Polverosi, R., et al. (2012). Early bone marrow metastasis detection: the additional value of FDG-PET/CT vs. CT imaging. *Biomedicine & Pharmacotherapy*, 66, 448–453.

Ferrante, M.A. (2004). Brachial plexopathies: classification, causes, and consequences. *Muscle & Nerve*, 30, 547–568.

Garrison, J.A., Mccune, J.S., Livingston, R.B., et al. (2003). Myalgias and arthralgias associated with paclitaxel. *Oncology (Williston Park)*, 17, 271–277.

Hird, A., Chow, E., Zhang, L., et al. (2009a). Determining the incidence of pain flare following palliative radiotherapy for symptomatic bone metastases: results from three Canadian cancer centers. *International Journal of Radiation Oncology, Biology, Physics*, 75, 193–197.

Jaeckle, K.A. (2010). Neurologic manifestations of neoplastic and radiation-induced plexopathies. *Seminars in Neurology*, 30, 254–262.

Kautio, A.L., Haanpaa, M., Kautiainen, H., Kalso, E., and Saarto, T. (2011). Burden of chemotherapy-induced neuropathy-a cross-sectional study. *Supportive Care in Cancer*, 19(12), 1991–1996.

Langer, S.W. (2010). Extravasation of chemotherapy. *Current Oncology Reports*, 12, 242–246.

Loblaw, D.A., Mitera, G., Ford, M., and Laperriere, N.J. (2012). A 2011 updated systematic review and clinical practice guideline for the management of malignant extradural spinal cord compression. *International Journal of Radiation Oncology, Biology, Physics*, 84, 312–317.

Loblaw, D.A., Wu, J.S., Kirkbride, P., *et al.* (2007). Pain flare in patients with bone metastases after palliative radiotherapy—a nested randomized control trial. *Supportive Care in Cancer*, 15, 451–455.

Migliorati, C.A., Woo, S.B., Hewson, I., *et al.* (2010). A systematic review of bisphosphonate osteonecrosis (BON) in cancer. *Supportive Care in Cancer*, 18, 1099–1106.

Moxley, G. (2010). Rheumatic disorders and functional disability with aromatase inhibitor therapy. *Clinical Breast Cancer*, 10, 144–147.

Peterson, D.E. and Lalla, R.V. (2010). Oral mucositis: the new paradigms. *Current Opinion in Oncology*, 22, 318–322.

Wu, C.L. and Raja, S.N. (2011). Treatment of acute postoperative pain. *The Lancet*, 377, 2215–2225.

Yamashita, J., Mccauley, L.K., and Van Poznak, C. (2010). Updates on osteonecrosis of the jaw. *Current Opinion in Supportive and Palliative Care*, 4, 200–206.

13.2

Cancer-induced bone pain

Lesley A. Colvin and Marie T. Fallon

Introduction to cancer-induced bone pain

Bone is the third most common site of metastatic disease, after liver and lung, with approximately 75% of these patients suffering from related pain (Ibrahim et al., 2013). Cancer-induced bone pain (CIBP) is a major clinical problem, with limited options for predictable, rapid, and effective treatment for some of the elements without unacceptable adverse effects. When treating the different components of CIBP, background pain may respond reasonably well to opioids, whereas both spontaneous and movement-evoked pain may be much more problematic. Our understanding of how current therapy acts is based mainly on studies in non-cancer pain syndromes, which are likely to be quite different, not only in clinical presentation, but also in terms of pathophysiology. It can be difficult to study the specific neurobiological changes associated with CIBP, although development of laboratory models of isolated bone metastases has allowed more specific study of pain mechanisms in this syndrome. Most of the previous models involved systemic disease, making it difficult to determine the specific changes associated with CIBP. In order to evaluate our current therapies properly and direct the development of new therapies logically, it is important to understand the underlying mechanisms of CIBP (Portenoy, 2011).

Animal models

The laboratory models of CIBP, developed within the past 10–15 years, involve focal inoculation of tumour cells into the intramedullary cavity of a single bone in rodents. This results in the growth of an isolated bone metastasis, without any of the systemic effects associated with widespread tumour, as was seen in previous models. These models allow measurement of behavioural signs of pain behaviour as well as study of pathophysiological changes and appear to correlate well with the clinical syndrome.

A range of sites such as humerus, femur, and calcaneus have been used, with tumour cell lines varying from osteosarcoma to breast, prostate, and melanoma (Schwei et al., 1999; Medhurst et al., 2002; Wacnik et al., 2003; Seong et al., 2004; Zhang et al., 2005). The underlying changes in nociceptive pathways are unique and quite distinct from those seen in other pain states, such as neuropathic or inflammatory pain (Honore et al., 2000). There is also some evidence that tumour type may have subtle changes on nociceptive processing in CIBP, with evidence that cortical destruction is not necessary for CIBP to develop (Sabino et al., 2003; Luger et al., 2005). It is clear that there are complex interactions between tumour, the tumour environment, nociceptive processing, and other factors (e.g. genetic) that will define precisely the nature of CIBP and response to treatment in any one individual (Mantyh et al., 2002).

Pain processing

In order to understand the pathophysiology of CIBP, it is useful to consider the neurobiology of nociception prior to the occurrence of tissue injury. Much of our understanding of this is based on basic science research, although brain imaging techniques are providing exciting evidence of alterations in many areas of the brain. This confirms earlier laboratory work with direct clinical evidence of how pain perception is processed at a cortical level. The International Association for the Study of Pain (IASP) definition of pain as 'an unpleasant sensory and emotional experience associated with actual or potential tissue damage or described in terms of such damage' is useful in reminding us that pain is more than nociception and involves a balance between sensory, cognitive, and affective components (Merskey, 1986). The traditional concept of sensory input being processed in the brain, with little interaction between spinal and cortical response is incomplete, as increasing evidence from brain imaging studies indicates significant potential for bi-directional modulation between sensory input and cortical activity (Ploghaus et al., 1999; Longe et al., 2001; Tracey et al., 2002).

It was not until the 1960s that nociceptors were first identified and the gate control theory of pain was introduced by Melzack and Wall (1965). This theory emphasized the importance of spinal modulation, with continuous interaction between small- and large-diameter afferents, local spinal neurons, and descending systems from the brain.

A basic outline of the nociceptive system is shown in Fig. 13.2.1, showing the neuraxis (the peripheral and central nervous system) involved in sensory processing and giving a framework for understanding the changes occurring in CIBP. Importantly, this is a dynamic system, with the potential for significant alterations at all levels within the system dependent on sensory input, tumour effects, and treatment.

Peripheral processing

Painful stimuli, whether mechanical, thermal, or chemical, may activate nociceptors (non-specialized free nerve endings) on particular sensory neurons (or primary afferent fibres). Sensory neurons vary in function, size, and conduction velocity, as outlined in Table 13.2.1, with generation of action potentials in C and A-delta fibres in response to noxious stimuli (Besson and Chaouch, 1987).

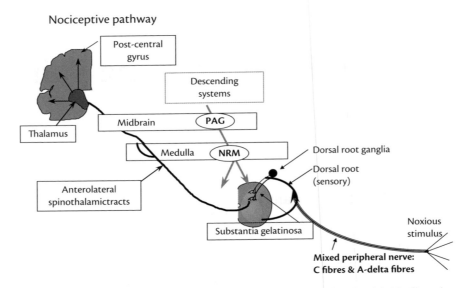

Fig. 13.2.1 Nociceptive pathway: peripheral noxious stimuli activate nociceptors, generate action potentials in C and A delta fibres, that may result in neuronal activity within the brain and pain perception. Descending systems from the brain modulate this process, as do local interneurons within the spinal cord. NRM, nucleus raphe magnus; PAG, periaqueductal grey matter.

Table 13.2.1 Classification of sensory neurons

Fibre type	Diameter (μm)	Conduction velocity (m/s)	Sensory modality
A-beta: large, myelinated	6–15	30–100	Light touch, proprioception
A-delta: small, myelinated	2–6	12–30	Noxious and innocuous sensory
C: unmyelinated	0.5–2	0.5–2.0	Pain, temperature; also post-ganglionic autonomic

The sensory fibres ascend towards the spinal cord in mixed nerves. Close to the spinal cord, the sensory fibres split into the dorsal root and enter the spinal cord. The cell bodies of all sensory fibres are situated close to the spinal cord, in the dorsal root ganglia. This is where the cell nucleus lies and where neurotransmitters essential for synaptic transmission are synthesized, before peripheral and central transport to axon terminals (Willis and Coggeshall, 1991).

Peripheral receptors and ion channels

A range of receptors has been identified on the peripheral terminations of sensory neurons. These are important in transduction of noxious mechanical, thermal, and chemical stimuli, with the potential for modulating pain processing providing potential sites of action for analgesics. These include mechanically gated ion channels, which have a role in mechanical transduction, and the transient receptor potential (TRP) family of ion channels, involved in noxious heat and cold processing. For example, the vanilloid receptor (TRPV1) is activated by noxious heat stimuli. Some receptors may also detect alterations in pH (acid-sensing ion channels) and may be more active when there has been tissue injury (Burnstock and Wood, 1996; Price et al., 2001; Welsh et al., 2002; Bandell et al., 2004; Wang and Woolf, 2005; Wemmie et al., 2006; Cortright et al., 2007; Fleetwood-Walker et al., 2007; Sluka et al., 2007). Sodium channels are essential in transmission of neuronal action potentials, with a number of subtypes that may

alter in CIBP (Liu et al., 2011; Dib-Hajj et al., 2013). In addition, there are several types of receptor detecting noxious chemical stimuli such as prostaglandins, endothelins (ETs), nerve growth factor (NGF), and bradykinin, as may be found in response to tissue injury (Kidd and Urban, 2001; Marceau and Regoli, 2004; Urch, 2004; Voilley, 2004). Peripheral opioid receptors are also found and may have a role in certain pain states, including CIBP (Janson and Stein, 2003; Menendez et al., 2003).

Central processing

Spinal cord

After entering the dorsal horn, the majority of C fibres and A-delta fibres synapse, in a somatotopic manner, in laminae I and II of the superficial dorsal horn (the substantia gelatinosa), with some A-delta fibres terminating in lamina V (Handwerker et al., 1975; Cervero and Iggo, 1980; Swetl and Woolf, 1985; Woold and Fitzgerald, 1986). The sensory fibres synapse with second-order projection neurons that ascend to the brain in specific tracts. These second-order neurons vary in their response, with, for example, nociceptive specific (NS) neurons, responding only to noxious stimuli, and wide dynamic range (WDR) neurons, responding to innocuous and noxious stimuli. Complex modulation of second-order activity occurs both via intrinsic spinal mechanisms and descending systems (Willis and Coggeshall, 1991; Coghill et al., 1993; Biella and Sotgui, 1995; Stamford, 1995). At a local level within the spinal cord, there are a range of inhibitory mechanisms at a spinal level which may be augmented by descending inhibitory pathways from the brain (Fig. 13.2.1), acting to reduce nociceptive transmission (Besson and Chaouch, 1987; Antal et al., 1996; Dickenson, 2002).

Within the spinal cord, the main neurotransmitter involved in fast synaptic transmission in the spinal cord is glutamate, acting at a range of ionotropic (ion channels) and metabotropic (G-protein coupled) receptors. Normally, the alpha-amino-3-hydroxyl-5-methyl-4-isoxazole propionic acid (AMPA) receptor is involved in nociceptive transmission. The main inhibitory neurotransmitters, predominantly found in local interneurons and descending projection neurons, are glycine and gamma-aminobutyric acid (GABA) (Antal et al., 1996; Todd, 1996; Wiensenfeld-Hallin et al., 1997; Baba et al., 2003). Neuropeptides, such as substance P, are also released in response to noxious stimulation, with some endogenous opioid peptides acting to reduce onward transmission of noxious input (Allen et al., 1997; Duggan et al., 1998; Costigan and Woolf, 2002).

Spinal connections and supraspinal pathways

Ascending spinal tracts

After synapsing in the dorsal horn, second-order spinal neurons mainly cross to the opposite side of the spinal cord and ascend in the spinothalamic tracts to thalamic nuclei, conveying predominantly noxious information (Giesler et al., 1994; Todd, 2002). There are also spinomesencephalic tracts, originating from cells in laminae I, V, and VI to the mesencephalic tegmentum region, which includes the periaqueductal grey area (PAG) (Menetrey et al., 1982).

Descending systems

The concept of descending inhibitory pathways, or 'descending noxious inhibitory control' first originated from Melzack and Wall's gate control theory of pain (Wall, 1967; Morgan, 1994). There are several areas within the brainstem that the descending pathways originate from, including the medullary nucleus raphe magnus (NRM) and rostral ventromedial medulla (RVM). The NRM contains endogenous opioids and has been shown to have an anti-nociceptive effect, with a major descending serotonergic input to the dorsal horn (Basbaum and Fields, 1984; McGaraughty and Heinricher, 2002; Polgar et al., 2002). In the midbrain, the PAG is also involved in opioid-mediated analgesia and the locus coeruleus (LC) in modulating nociceptive transmission, via its actions on the parafascicular neurons (PF) of the thalamus (Gray and Dostrovsky, 1983; Mokha et al., 1985; Men et al., 1996; Zhang et al., 1997; Sonohata et al., 2004).

There is accumulating evidence for the existence of both anti- and pro-nociceptive pathways from the RVM, via a mechanism that may involve the N-methyl-D-aspartate (NMDA) receptor (Suzuki et al., 2004).

If there is persistent noxious input, such as may occur in CIBP, this may increase activity of this system contributing to increased spinal excitability. There is also some evidence of an indirect connection of the RVM with the anterior cingulate cortex, normally associated with the affective–motivational aspects of pain perception. Thus alterations in the balance of inhibition and facilitation from the brainstem, which may itself be modulated by higher centres, can alter inherent excitability at the level of the spinal cord (for review, see Porreca et al., 2002).

Cortical processing

Multiple areas of the brain are activated in response to pain, reflecting the complex nature of pain perception. In the clinical setting, the use of brain imaging techniques, such as functional magnetic resonance imaging (fMRI), is expanding and providing insights into our understanding of pain perception. Cortical responses to nociceptive stimuli can be demonstrated (the most consistently activated areas include the insular and the anterior cingulate regions) as well as the considerable top-down regulation of the context on peripheral nociceptive stimuli (Berman et al., 1998; Davis, 2000; Peyron et al., 2000; Bingel et al., 2011; Lee and Tracey, 2013). It is clear that there are many complex bidirectional interactions between the brain and the spinal cord in pain processing (Tracey et al., 2002; Eccleston and Crombez, 2005).

Mechanisms of cancer-induced bone pain
Peripheral factors

Evidence from the animal models of CIBP demonstrates wide-ranging alterations in the peripheral environment around the site of the bony metastasis and subsequent sensory processing. The relationship between the site of bone metastasis, the sensory nerves, and the surrounding microenvironment plays a key role in CIBP.

The complex interaction between the tumour itself and the development of CIBP may be modulated by tumour type, site, and degree of bony destruction (Dore-Savard et al., 2013). CIBP may occur prior to evidence of bony destruction, with clear signs of pain behaviours found in animal models (Luger et al., 2005). Other factors, both local and central, must play a role in the generation of pain in CIBP. The type of tumour clearly influences the likelihood of bony metastases occurring, although the relationship to CIBP has not been described (Halvorson et al., 2006; Alarmo et al., 2008).

Local changes in sensory neurons

Direct pressure and compression of surrounding structures, including the sensory nerves innervating the bone and periosteum, will occur with tumour growth. Both myelinated and unmyelinated primary afferent neurons innervating the marrow and mineralized bone may be injured and sensitized in CIBP (Peters et al., 2005). Although not examined in CIBP, a rodent bone fracture model found that the periosteum is densely innervated by a meshwork of calcitonin gene-related peptide (CGRP) containing fibres. This subgroup of C fibres is thought to be involved in nociceptive transmission and could thus contribute to the marked movement-related pain that is such a challenging component of CIBP (Martin et al., 2007). It has also been shown that purinergic receptors (P2X3) on these fibres are upregulated in CIBP and may contribute to peripheral sensitization, although the role of purines in CIBP may be less important than in some other chronic pain states, such as inflammation (Gilchrist et al., 2005; Hansen et al., 2012).

The capsaicin receptor, TRPV1, is increased on sensory neurons close to the tumour site and also within the dorsal root ganglia, preferentially in CGRP-containing neurons. TRPV1 antagonists reduce pain behaviour in CIBP models (Men et al., 1996; Ghilardi et al., 2005; Niiyama et al., 2007; Gui et al., 2013).

Ion channel changes in sensory neurons occur in CIBP: There is a decrease in some types of K⁺ channels (KCNQ2 and -3) in small-diameter neurons, associated with the development of CIBP and neuronal excitability (Zheng et al., 2013). Sodium channel subtypes also change and may be associated with generation of spontaneous ectopic discharges in CIBP, similar to that seen in neuropathic pain (where they are thought to be linked with the generation of spontaneous pain) (Schafers et al., 2008; Ke et al., 2012; Qiu et al., 2012).

Inflammation

In the area of bony metastases, a range of pro-hyperalgesic mediators, commonly associated with inflammation, is released from the tumour and associated immune system cells, including macrophages, neutrophils, and T cells. This includes prostaglandins, ETs, bradykinin, tumour necrosis factor (TNF) alpha and a number of growth factors, such as transforming growth factor beta (TGF-β) all of which are likely to contribute to CIBP (Wagner and Myers, 1996; Woolf et al., 1996; DeLeo et al., 1997; Cain et al., 2001; Sabino et al., 2002). These will not only sensitize peripheral nociceptors to subsequent stimuli, but also have a direct action on specific receptors on the primary sensory neurons in the area. For example, TGF-β may promote proliferation of prostate cancer cells, activate osteoclasts, and has been implicated in the development of bone metastases (Buijs et al., 2007; Sato et al., 2008). Interleukin 1(IL-1) beta has been shown to be upregulated in a rodent model: electroacupuncture decreased this increase in IL-1 beta as well as reducing pain behaviours (Zhang et al., 2007). Bradykinin antagonist may have a therapeutic role and non-steroidal anti-inflammatory drugs (NSAIDs) may also modulate CIBP. Of the growth factors, there is some evidence that nerve growth factor (NGF) has a particular role in CIBP, with a potential therapeutic option in the form of an anti-NGF antibody (Halvorson et al., 2005; Sevcik et al., 2005; Jimenez-Andrade et al., 2007). Pre-treatment with anti-NGF was found to reduce pain behaviours and reduce sensory sprouting and neuroma formation (Jimenez-Andrade et al., 2011).

Factors secreted by the tumour may include not only cytokines and other pro-inflammatory mediators, but also substances such as formaldehyde, with resultant increases in pain (Coluzzi et al., 2011; Liu et al., 2013).

CIBP, at least peripherally, seems to display a combination of neuropathic pain, either due to direct tumour compression or ischaemia, plus peripheral sensitization as is found in inflammatory pain, with release of cytokines and other mediators.

Bone microenvironment

Other factors specific to the bone, its response to tumour implantation, and the effect of the microenvironment must also be considered (Marguiles et al., 2006). Within the tumour there may be low oxygen levels, an acidic pH, and high extracellular calcium concentrations (Kingsley et al., 2007). When tumour cells spread to bone, the balance of bone turnover is disrupted, with an increase in bone resorption, formation of abnormal bone matrix and disruption of the precise balance between osteoclast and osteoblast activity, such that normal regulatory mechanisms are lost (Boyle et al., 2008; Peyruchaud et al., 2013).

An increase in osteoclasts and their activity results in increased degradation of bone matrix, by secretion of acid and lytic enzymes. Bone resorption is increased correspondingly. The RANK (receptor

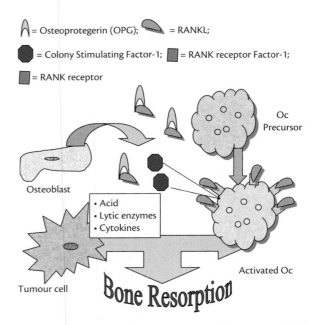

Fig. 13.2.2 Schematic diagram of bone and tumour cell interaction. The balance between OPG and RANKL is disrupted with a relative reduction in OPG and thus an increase in osteoclast activation and hypertrophy resulting in increased bone resorption. Oc, osteoclast.

for activator of nuclear factor kappa B) signalling pathway plays a key role in this process. The TNF-related cytokine, RANK ligand (RANKL), expressed on osteoblasts, and colony stimulating factor (CSF)-1 combine to stimulate production of activated osteoclasts. This process is normally controlled via a negative feedback loop, involving osteoprotegerin (OPG), a secreted soluble receptor that is also a member of the TNF family. OPG acts by sequestering RANKL, preventing osteoclast activation and reducing bone resorption (Boyle et al., 2008). This feedback loop is disrupted in CIBP, with a marked osteoblastic inflammatory response, increased secretion of a range of cytokines increasing osteoclast activity, and an increased ratio of RANKL to OPG (Nagae et al., 2007; Kinder et al., 2008) (Fig. 13.2.2).

Agents that interfere with osteolysis may therefore improve therapy of CIBP. This includes not only currently available agents such as bisphosphonates, but also novel agents that would alter the balance of bone metabolism to reduce CIBP. These include OPG-type drugs, anti-NGF, and other agents that interfere with intracellular pathways in osteoclasts (Medhurst et al., 2001; Walker et al., 2002; Clohisy and Mantyh, 2004; Roudier et al., 2006; Jimenez-Andrade et al., 2007; Tsubaki et al., 2007).

Central factors

While it is clear that peripheral changes, due to tumour effects on the bone, drive or at least initiate central responses, it is not understood at all how much the central changes contribute to the degree of severity of the pain syndrome. It is known from other chronic pain states that changes in spinal pain processing, with central sensitization, and wind up, play a major role in the development of chronic pain (Woolf, 2007).

What has been found in animal models of CIBP is that the central changes are quite different from either inflammatory or neuropathic pain (Honore and Mantyh, 2000).

Glial cells

A particular feature that has been noted is an increase in glial cells, with a marked astrocytosis in the spinal cord on the side of the lesion. Interventions to reduce glial activation have been shown to correlate with reductions in pain behaviour and reduced spinal cord cytokines (Wang et al., 2011). Increases in extracellular signal regulated kinase occurs in both astrocytes and microglia and is associated with allodynia, while the microglial inhibitor, minocycline, reduces brain-derived neurotrophic factor levels and CIBP behaviour (Zhang et al., 2005; Wang et al., 2012a, 2012b).

The central neuroinflammation that seems to occur in CIBP may be mediated via the Toll-like receptor-4, which has also been implicated in central neuroinflammatory effects of opioids (Watkins et al., 2005; Mao-Ying et al., 2012). An increase in T-cell death-associated gene 8 (TDAG8) protein expression was found in CIBP, with knockdown of TDAG8 reducing spinal protein kinase A activity and reducing CIBP (Hang et al., 2012).

Current standard clinical treatment for bone pain, local radiotherapy, will reduce glial activity in the spinal cord, as well as reversing some of the abnormal neurochemistry (Vet et al., 2006). There is increasing interest in the interaction between the immune system and sensory neurons in the generation of chronic pain syndromes and it seems likely that this may be particularly relevant to CIBP (Scholz and Woolf, 2007).

Glutamate and neuronal responsiveness

Metabotropic glutamate receptors are found on glial cells within the spinal cord and may contribute to pain behaviour, in addition to more well-defined glutamate receptors, such as the NMDA receptor (Saito et al., 2006).

The likely involvement of glutamate, one of the main excitatory neurotransmitters in the spinal cord, has been confirmed by the efficacy of gabapentin in CIBP models, with a presynaptic effect on glutamate release (Donovan-Rodriguez et al., 2005).

Gabapentin has also been found to reduce activity of a particular type of dorsal horn neuron—the WDR neuron. WDR neurons appear to alter in CIBP, with increased responsiveness to mechanical and thermal stimuli in addition to ongoing spontaneous activity (Urch et al., 2003; Donovan-Rodriguez et al., 2005; Khasabov et al., 2007). An alteration in descending pathways from the brainstem to the spinal cord has also been found, with an increase in activity of pro-nociceptive pathways, as can occur in other chronic pain states (Porreca et al., 2002; Donovan-Rodriguez et al., 2006).

Opioids

Clinically, opioids may control some elements of CIBP well, but have significant limitations in controlling aspects of breakthrough pain, which is common in CIBP. There may be a neurobiological basis for this, with alterations in the endogenous opioid systems found in animal models of CIBP.

Mu opioid receptors (MOR) have been found to decrease in specific subpopulations of primary afferent neurons in the dorsal root ganglia. These neurons were predominantly CGRP or TRPV1-containing neurons, known to be involved in CIBP. This reduction in MOR expression seemed to correlate to a reduced analgesic response to intrathecal morphine and was not seen in an inflammatory model (Yamamoto et al., 2008). The dose–response curve for morphine is shifted to the right, with greater doses needed to reduce pain behaviour compared to inflammatory pain, suggesting fundamental differences in the underlying mechanisms (Luger et al., 2002). Prolonged morphine treatment may increase pain behaviour, associated with an increase in CGRP neurons in the dorsal root ganglia and increased osteoclast activity (King et al., 2007). Conversely, another group found that chronic systemic morphine had greater efficacy than acutely administered morphine (Urch et al., 2005). There is also evidence that binding to MORs may be attenuated in CIBP, with a variable effect between opioids resulting in differential analgesic effects, where oxycodone binding was minimally attenuated and its analgesic effect was more than morphine (Nakamura et al., 2013).

Other opioid receptors may also be important, with evidence for an analgesic effect of kappa agonists (Kim et al., 2011). The pro-nociceptive opioid peptide, dynorphin, increases markedly in the dorsal horn of the spinal cord (Honore et al., 2000). This may contribute to an increase in the activity of descending facilitatory systems from the brain (Vanderah et al., 2001; Porreca et al., 2002).

Summary of pre-clinical aspects of CIBP

The advent of locally restricted bone metastases models has allowed us to begin defining the underlying mechanisms related to CIBP, separate from the systemic effects of widespread tumour. There are complex interactions between local factors at the site of tumour metastasis to bone, with inflammatory and neuropathic processes, contributing to the response that is elicited within the central nervous system. The spinal cord changes occurring in CIBP appear to be unique and distinct from other chronic pain states. Improved understanding of all these processes should aid development of novel targeted therapies that may improve our clinical armamentarium for managing this challenging clinical problem.

Clinical features

Introduction to clinical features

Pain as a result of metastatic spread to bone is a significant clinical problem for patients, their carers, and health-care professionals (Fallon and McConnell, 2007). Bone pain can have a significant impact on physical, psychological, and social functioning (and so overall quality of life) (Rusteon et al., 2005). CIBP can be difficult to manage and treatment may require the use of multiple types of interventions (Clare et al., 2005). The optimum use of the World Health Organization (WHO) analgesic ladder is critical for successful management of CIBP. This, of course, means using the ladder as outlined in Chapter 9.4 but remembering that the ladder was never intended for use in isolation of other methods of cancer pain relief. CIPB provides a classical paradigm for the WHO analgesic ladder, sitting within a wider context of other pain-relieving techniques (Fig. 13.2.3).

Epidemiology

Bone is the most common source of pain in patients with malignant disease with studies suggesting that approximately 28% of hospice inpatients, 34% of patients in a cancer pain clinic, and 45% of advanced cancer patients followed up at home, are affected by pain from bone metastases (Twycross and Fairfield, 1982; Banning et al., 1991a; Portenoy and Lesage, 1999; Loeser, 2000). Studies also suggest that lesions in bone account for 30–35% of

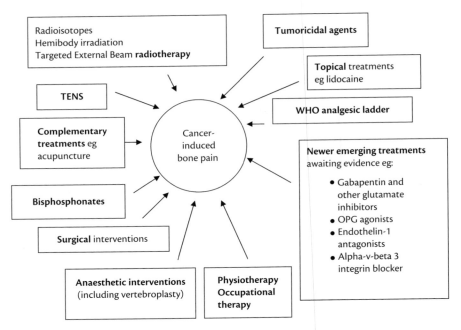

Fig. 13.2.3 CIBP requires a multimodality approach individualized for each patient.

all cancer pains in patients with advanced disease (Twycross and Fairfield, 1982; Grond et al., 1996). Some patients will experience multiple sites of pain due to bone metastases.

However, not everyone will have pain as a result of bone metastases. For example, one-third of patients with metastatic breast disease affecting the skeleton, do not complain of pain (Front et al., 1979). The mechanisms which mediate the onset of pain in some metastases but not others in the same patient are poorly understood, however the local tumour and its immediate environment must play an important role.

Clinical characteristics

Descriptors of cancer-related bone pain are varied, but it is generally accepted that there is a triad of background pain, spontaneous pain at rest, and movement-related pain. Movement-related pain is a form of incident pain and along with spontaneous pain at rest are types of breakthrough pain (Mercadante and Arcuri, 1998; Urch, 2004).

Breakthrough pain is referred to as 'transitory exacerbation of pain experienced by the patient who has relatively stable and adequately controlled baseline pain' (Portenoy et al., 2004). Spontaneous pain refers to episodes of breakthrough pain that occur unexpectedly at rest. In contrast, movement-related pain (also known as incident pain or 'precipitated pain') refers to episodes of breakthrough pain that are related to specific events

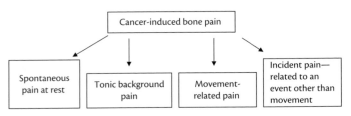

Fig. 13.2.4 Clinical characteristics of CIBP.

(Davies, 2006). Movement-related pain is the more common form of incident pain in patients with CIBP, however other types of incident pain, such as pain on coughing or breathing, associated with rib or sternal metastases, are common (Fig. 13.2.4).

Background pain

Temporal pattern of pain

Background pain can be intermittent initially, but rapidly progresses to become constant in nature. Once established it is usually unrelenting.

Site of pain

In a study where 41% of participants had pain due to neoplastic damage to bones and joints, 13% had vertebral (including sacral) pain, 7.1% had pelvic pain, 6.8% had pain in the chest wall from rib lesion(s), 3.9% had pain in the long bones, and 10.2% had generalized bone pain from multiple bone metastases (Caraceni and Portenoy, 1999). The skeleton was affected in slightly different patterns depending on the primary site of the tumour (Table 13.2.2).

Radiation of pain

Usually the pain is localized to a specific area (and frequently there is point tenderness over the affected area of bone). In other cases, pain may be referred (Mercadante, 1997). For example, a metastatic deposit in the hip may result in pain in the knee area; a lesion in the T12/L1 site may cause pain felt in the iliac crest or sacro-iliac joint (either unilaterally or bilaterally); a cervical spine metastasis may have pain referred to the occipital region or the skull vertex (Loeser, 2000).

Another feature which is recognized in CIBP is the phenomenon of a 'migratory pattern of pain', where pain might appear in one area of the body at a given time, then move to a completely different part of the body with total resolution of the pain at the original site (Pollen and Schmidt, 1979).

Table 13.2.2 Prevalence of different pain syndromes in patients with different tumours

Cancer diagnosis	Pain syndrome					
	Skull	Vertebral	Pelvis and long bones	Generalized bone pain	Chest wall	Pathological fracture
All tumours	5.2	13.0	10.5	11.4	6.8	5.0
Breast	2.1	20.9	12.5	25.3	9.7	8.3
Lower GI tract	1.9	10.6	17.4	0	0.9	1.9
Upper GI tract	1.9	4.8	0.9	0.9	0	0
Head & neck	21.6	4.5	6.3	5.4	0.9	0.9
Leukaemia/lymphoma	0	4.7	11.9	14.2	0	0
Lung	4.6	18.0	8.8	10.4	20.7	7.7
Prostate	1.5	21.5	26.1	40.0	4.6	3.0
Uterus	0	4.2	4.2	0	2.8	0

Reproduced from Caraceni A and Portenoy RK, *PAIN®*, Volume 82, Issue 3, pp.263–274, Copyright © 1999. This table has been reproduced with permission of the International Association for the Study of Pain® (IASP). The table may not be reproduced for any other purpose without permission.

Quality (character) of pain

Background pain is often described as a dull ache (Colleau, 2002). However, the descriptions of the pain were variable in a study of patients with bone pain from metastatic prostate cancer (Pollen and Schmidt, 1979). Recent work has suggested that it may be more commonly associated with terms like 'sharp', 'throbbing', and 'tingling' (Laird et al., 2011).

Intensity (severity) of pain

The intensity of bone pain is independent of tumour type, location, number and size of metastases, gender, and age of patient (Oster et al., 1978).

In a study of patients with bone pain from metastatic prostate cancer, 60% had 'severe' pain, 30% had 'moderate' pain, and the rest described their pain as being 'mild (Pollen and Schmidt, 1979). Bone pain usually increases in intensity over time (Mercadante, 1997).

A study of hospitalized patients with advanced cancer demonstrated that, while 49% of patients with bone metastases reported severe pain, only 31% of patients without bone involvement reported a similar level of pain (Brescia et al., 1999). This concurs with the clinical impression that CIBP often presents a therapeutic challenge.

Exacerbating factors of pain

As discussed above, exacerbation of pain is often related to specific events ('incident pain'). Incident pain can be further divided into (a) volitional pain—precipitated by a voluntary act (e.g. walking) and (b) non-volitional—precipitated by an involuntary act (e.g. coughing) (Davies, 2006). However, for practical purposes, it is the individual patient's history which is key as there clearly exists an overlap between these categories. We suggest always using explicit terms to describe the different categories of CIBP outlined in Fig. 13.2.4.

Relieving factors of pain

A variety of different non-pharmacological, pharmacological, oncological, and other types of interventions have been used to treat bone pain. These interventions are discussed below and outlined in Fig. 13.2.3.

Other features of pain

As bone pain due to cancer becomes more established, mechanical allodynia can develop, resulting in pain from a stimulus or activity which was normally not painful, for example, moving in bed (Clohisy and Mantyh, 2003). Recent studies also suggest that cancer-related bone pain can result in paraesthesia (altered sensation), dynamic allodynia (perception of pain in response to light brushing of the skin), static allodynia (perception of pain in response to pressure), or thermal hyperalgesia (pain at normal, low, and high temperature thresholds) (Medhurst et al., 2002; Menendez et al., 2003a). Interestingly, normalization of thermal hyperalgesia and hypoalgesia have been shown to be associated with successful pain relief from palliative radiotherapy and improved function (Scott et al., 2012; Sande et al., 2013).

Breakthrough pain: epidemiology

An IASP survey found that breakthrough pain was present according to clinicians in 65% of patients with cancer-related pain (Caraceni and Portenoy, 1999; Caraceni et al., 2004). However, breakthrough pain was more likely to be reported in English-speaking countries, which may reflect factors more to do with the definition, than the recognition, of the phenomenon.

Bone pain is a major source of breakthrough pain and has been reported as the predominant source of incident pain (Caraceni et al., 2004). In the aforementioned survey, breakthrough pain was significantly associated with certain pain syndromes, including those due to vertebral lesions and lesions in the pelvis, long bones, or joints. Thus, of the patients with vertebral pain syndrome, 85% had breakthrough pain. Similarly, of the patients with pelvis and long bone lesions, 78% had breakthrough pain.

The clinical features of breakthrough pain vary from individual to individual (Portenoy et al., 2004). Nevertheless, breakthrough pain is often reported to be frequent in occurrence, acute in onset, short in duration, and moderate to severe in intensity (Portenoy and Hagen, 1990; Portenoy et al., 1999; Zeppetella et al., 2000). Zeppetella et al. reported a mean number of four episodes per day (range 0–14 episodes per day) among hospice inpatients with pain (Zeppetella, 2000). Portenoy et al. found the median interval between onset and peak of pain to be 3 minutes, with a range of 1 second to 30 minutes (Portenoy et al., 1999). In addition, Portenoy and Hagen reported a median duration of 30 minutes (range 1–240 minutes) amongst hospital inpatients with pain (Portenoy and Hagen, 1990). The clinical features of breakthrough pain often mirror the clinical features of the background pain; however, they may differ.

The clinical features of breakthrough pain may also vary within an individual. For example, patients may experience both spontaneous pain and incident pain. In the study by Portenoy et al. almost two-thirds of patients could identify a precipitant for their pain, such as weight-bearing and/or movement (Portenoy et al., 1999). However, nearly half of patients also stated that their pain could be unpredictable at times.

Patients with breakthrough pain have more intense background pain that those without breakthrough pain (Portenoy et al., 1999; Caraceni et al., 2004). Moreover, the study by Portenoy et al. confirms that patients with breakthrough pain have greater functional impairment (as measured on the interference scale of the Brief Pain Inventory) when compared to patients without such pain (Portenoy et al., 1999). In addition, patients with breakthrough pain have significantly increased levels of depression and anxiety (as measured by the Beck Depression Inventory and the Beck Anxiety Inventory) when compared with patients without such pain.

While the tonic background pain is usually controlled with opioid analgesia, the other two components, spontaneous or movement related (including incident pain which is not movement related), are problematic because:

1. There is a mismatch between temporal onset of pain in relation to temporal onset of analgesia from opioids.

2. Resolution of pain in relation to duration of opioid analgesia again has a mismatch. While immediate (normal) release morphine may have analgesic effects for up to 4 hours, spontaneous and movement-related pain can resolve in less than 30 minutes in 50% of patients, rendering the patient more susceptible to opioid side effects

3. There is evidence of poor opioid responsiveness of some aspects of the underlying neurophysiology of the spontaneous and movement-related pain components (Martin et al., 2007; Yamamoto et al., 2008; Laird et al., 2011). This may mean that some patients may fail to achieve adequate analgesia with even the 'ideal' formulation of opioid.

The combination of the above factors indicates that opioid side effects, especially sedation, are more likely to dominate over analgesia. In any pain syndrome where there are sudden, short-lived, peaks of pain, over and above a stable background pain, the opioid side effects are more likely to be problematic. In particular, such patients may become opioid toxic.

Opioid toxicity

Opioid toxicity is a spectrum which at one extreme may involve sleepiness, poor concentration, and vivid dreams while at the other end of the spectrum may involve hallucinations, confusion, agitation, and even a paradoxical increase in pain known also as hyperalgesia. A survey of inpatients in a regional cancer centre showed 50% of patients to have some symptoms of opioid toxicity,

most of which were not identified by staff (Isherwood et al., 2012). Significant opioid toxicity is associated with a 50% mortality and it is known clinically, that in those patients who recover, the distress experienced was profound. It is therefore very important to avoid opioid toxicity and to develop treatments which minimize this risk.

Current management of CIBP

Currently, NSAIDs and palliative radiotherapy form the key strategies which complement simple or opioid analgesia in CIBP relief. The evidence base for these strategies, along with emerging newer strategies is discussed below; however, a major problem with the evidence base is the lack of information on which components of CIBP are helped by which treatments. Many studies of bone pain treatment have used single-item scales such as a visual analogue scale to assess pain, which may give an inadequate assessment of the true clinical significance of treatments, with some interest in developing more comprehensive standardized assessments for clinical trials (Caissie et al., 2012; Matza et al., 2012; Zeng et al., 2012a, 2012b).

The standard approach to the management of CIBP is a combination of analgesia and radiotherapy. While it is accepted that radiotherapy is the gold standard treatment for pain relief in CIBP, there are a significant number of patients who fail to receive adequate analgesia. A systematic review showed external beam radiotherapy, whether single or multiple fractions, produced 50% pain relief in 41% of patients and complete pain relief at 1 month in 24% of patients (McQuay et al., 2000). However, many patients are too frail to attend for palliative radiotherapy or it is too late to reasonably expect pain relief before death.

We know that current therapeutic regimens leave up to 45% of patients with inadequate and under-managed pain control (de Wit et al., 2001; Meuser et al., 2001).

For such reasons, an improved understanding of the pathophysiological mechanisms underlying, in particular, spontaneous pain at rest and movement-related pain, are important. The development of effective pharmacological interventions to act as adjuvants or synergists to palliative radiotherapy to improve the degree of pain relief, in addition to providing analgesia to those too unwell to benefit from palliative radiotherapy, is an important area of research.

Opioid-based therapy does remain the basis for most analgesia in CIBP and in theory there are two aspects to the optimization of opioid analgesia. Firstly, to establish the best opioid for an individual, based on the pharmacogenomic principle of interindividual variation in balance between analgesia and side effects and secondly, to assess the optimal pharmacokinetic:pharmacodynamic profile from the opioids available (Quigley, 2004). There is more weight given to the first aspect in relation to chronic background pain, however more weight is given to the second in relation to spontaneous pain at rest and movement-related pain. For example, a patient may use a long-acting opioid preparation, such as morphine, for background pain and a fast-acting fentanyl preparation for breakthrough pain.

A subgroup of patients experience uncontrolled CIBP only after considerable and predictable movement, such as a long walk. This group is often satisfied to use a standard opioid such as immediate (normal)-release morphine, 30 minutes in advance of such activity.

Conversely, in those patients whose pain, or the exacerbating factor, is unpredictable and of fast onset, unacceptable side effects are likely to occur with standard opioids. In such cases a faster, short-acting opioid is more appropriate. Most of the evidence for opioids with faster onset of analgesia and faster peak plasma analgesic levels is limited to fentanyl (Zeppetella and Ribeiro, 2006).

Non-steroidal anti-inflammatory drugs

The use of NSAIDs in CIBP has been questioned due to the lack of robust, clinical evidence (Fucella et al., 1975; Stambaugh et al., 1988; Sunshine and Olson, 1988; Staquet, 1989; Estape et al., 1990; Minotti et al., 1998). The COX2 (an inducible isoform of cyclooxygenase (COX) enzyme involved in prostaglandin synthesis) specific inhibitors may in theory be of greater therapeutic potential due to their anti-tumour/antiangiogenesis properties (Shengetal, 1997; Sumitani et al., 2001). In an animal model of CIBP acute treatment with a highly selective COX2 inhibitor attenuated both background and movement-related pain, whilst chronic treatment additionally reduced tumour burden and osteoclast destruction (Sabino et al., 2002). Clearly the use and availability of COX2 inhibitors has fluctuated since they were first available because of concerns with some drugs within this class. A systematic review of randomized controlled clinical trials of NSAIDs for cancer pain was published in 2004 (McNicol et al., 2004; Zeppetella, 2007). It included 42 trials involving 3084 patients. The review concluded that NSAIDs were effective for the short-term treatment of cancer pain and that there was no clear evidence to support a superior efficacy or safety of one NSAID over another. It included 14 trials involving patients with bone metastases, although the authors were unable to conclude from the data presented whether NSAIDs have a specific role in CIBP.

The results of this systematic review were in keeping with the results of an earlier systematic review of the literature on NSAIDs for cancer pain and a concurrent evidence-based review of the literature on the generic treatment of cancer pain (Eisenberg et al., 1994; Carr et al., 2004). It should be noted that many of the trials included in these reviews are single-dose studies and few of the trials evaluate the efficacy or safety of NSAIDs beyond a few days of treatment.

In summary, therefore, despite good pre-clinical evidence, there is a lack of clinical evidence for a specific role for NSAIDs in the management of CIBP. Despite this, some clinicians continue to regard NSAIDs as an important part of CIBP management unless contraindications exist.

Breakthrough pain

Here we are referring to all types of breakthrough pain, other than that caused by inadequate around-the-clock analgesia to control background pain or 'end-of-dose' failure. It is a heterogeneous phenomenon, although it is typically of fast onset and short duration as previously discussed.

Despite implementation of guidelines, patients continue to have inadequate pain control and often express a variety of problems secondary to this. Breakthrough pain associated with CIBP can be particularly difficult to control (Banning et al., 1991b).

Three principles have been proposed for the management of general breakthrough pain, not specifically related to bone metastases (Portenoy, 1997):

1. Implementation of primary therapies for the underlying aetiology of the pain

2. Optimizing around-the-clock analgesia

3. Specific pharmacological or non-pharmacological interventions for the breakthrough pain.

It is generally agreed that one of the main problems with breakthrough pain due to bone metastases is that multiple breakthrough doses of opioid to control pain on movement and/or spontaneous pain at rest, usually leave the patient with frank, unacceptable opioid side effects, especially sedation, or with frank opioid toxicity. However, it has been suggested that increasing around-the-clock medication may prevent or limit breakthrough pain associated with CIBP (Mercadante et al., 2004a). Twenty-five patients admitted to a palliative care unit with movement-related breakthrough pain were titrated with intravenous morphine to background pain relief. The morphine dose was then increased further until patients began to experience unacceptable side effects at which point the increase was either stopped, or the morphine dose reduced. Patients remained as inpatients for an average of 5 days, and the breakthrough pain intensity on a 0–10 scale fell from an average of 9.2 before titration to 4.6 at the time of discharge. Most patients tolerated the higher dose of morphine. Translation of these findings to other settings may be limited by the fact that inpatients are often less mobile and there may be particular characteristics in this group which are not representative of CIBP patients in general.

The commonest method of managing breakthrough pain continues to be the use of so-called rescue medication ('breakthrough medication'). Ideally, rescue medication should have an onset/duration of action appropriate for the pain, should have a potency of effect appropriate for the pain and be easily administered. Rescue medication should be offered soon after the pain has started in cases of unpredictable pain, and before the pain has started in cases of predictable pain.

Opioids are commonly used as rescue medication. Morphine, hydromorphone, and oxycodone are the most common oral opioids used, and a fixed proportion of the daily dose is usually advised (e.g. the 4-hourly dose equivalent or 10–20% of the total daily dose) (Hanks et al., 2001). One study formally addressed the use of a fixed dose of rescue medication (Mercadante et al., 2004b): 48 patients using oral morphine for background cancer pain, and admitted to a palliative care unit, were treated with intravenous morphine, equivalent to one-fifth of the around-the-clock dose, for management of their breakthrough pain. A total of 172 episodes of pain were assessed and most patients had a 33% reduction in their pain within 18 minutes. Although most patients had somatic cancer pain, there was no specific reference to CIBP.

Non-opioids such as NSAIDs could have a role in the management of breakthrough pain as their mode of action suggests that they could be efficacious. However, with an onset of action of approximately 30 minutes, a relatively long duration of action, and dose-limiting adverse effects, they are not ideally suited to the management of breakthrough pain. There are no studies to suggest that they are effective in this clinical scenario.

A systematic review on the use of opioids for breakthrough pain identified four studies, each concerned with the application of oral transmucosal fentanyl citrate (OTFC) (Zeppetella and Ribeiro, 2006). These studies confirmed the efficacy of this delivery system for the management of breakthrough pain (Farrar et al., 1988; Christie et al., 1998; Portenoy et al., 1999; Coluzzi et al.,

2001). However, all of the studies failed to demonstrate a relationship between the effective dose of OTFC and the effective dose of around-the-clock medication and, as a result, the optimum dose of OTFC is determined by titration. This differs from usual practice of prescribing one-sixth of the 24-hour opioid dose as a breakthrough dose. It is, however, hardly surprising that when an opioid dose is carefully titrated for breakthrough pain in the context of a clinical trial, that the individual effective doses vary between patients and rarely work out as one-sixth of the 24-hour opioid dose. Although one of these OTFC studies did describe the number of patients with CIBP (Christie et al., 1998), none of the studies distinguished between CIBP and non-CIBP in their analyses which perhaps leaves a question over the favourable efficacy of OTFC or other fentanyl equivalents over standard opioids for breakthrough pain in CIBP.

Bisphosphonates for bone pain

Over the years, a number of different bisphosphonates have been developed, with the newer agents exhibiting increased potency as compared to the original agents (Wong, 2007). There are an increasing number of studies on bisphosphonates in the management/prevention of CIBP and other skeletal-related events (SRE), including pathological fracture, spinal cord compression, and hypercalcaemia (Krempien et al., 2005; Stewart, 2005).

Structure of bisphosphonates

With side-chain modifications from a simple methyl group (CH_3) to progressively longer alkyl chains, successive generations of bisphosphonates have been developed, each with increasing potency to inhibit osteoclast-mediated bone resorption.

Bisphosphonates have a number of actions, which account for their anti-resorptive properties (Santini et al., 2003; Green, 2004). They inhibit dissolution of hydroxyapatite crystals, have an effect on osteoclasts and osteoblasts, and also can have an effect on the underlying tumour. Different bisphosphonates have a different range of activities.

Bisphosphonates can inhibit the differentiation of stem cells to osteoclasts, affect the structure and function of osteoclasts, and cause apoptosis of osteoclasts (Santini et al., 2003). The latter actions rely on the bisphosphonate being taken up into the osteoclast by a process of endocytosis. Bisphosphonates also affect the interaction between osteoclasts and osteoblasts via the OPG RANK and RANKL axis. The normal RANK–RANKL balance is described in the basic science section of this chapter.

In addition, bisphosphonates can inhibit the growth of tumour cells, stimulate the immune system (against the tumour), and cause apoptosis of tumour cells (Santini et al., 2003). The inhibition of growth is achieved by a reduction in the adhesion of tumour cells to bone, a reduction in the secretion of tumour growth factors into the bone (secondary to a reduction in bone resorption), and an inhibition of tumour angiogenesis.

Bisphosphonates delay the development of skeletal events, particularly in patients with breast cancer, multiple myeloma, and prostate cancer (Bloomfield, 1998; Michaelson and Smith, 2005). A positive effect of delaying skeletal events is clearly a reduction in pain (e.g. pathological fracture).

However, bisphosphonates can also improve pain secondary to established bone lesions: many patients only respond after months of treatment, whilst other patients respond soon after treatment is initiated. The mechanism by which bisphosphonates cause long-term pain relief is likely to be due to their effect on bone resorption (and healing of the bone lesions) (Sevcik et al., 2004). The mechanism by which bisphosphonates cause short-term pain relief is unclear, but is likely to be related to their effect on tumour growth factors and other nociceptive agents.

A Cochrane systematic review addressing the (acute) analgesic effect of bisphosphonates was first published by Wong and Wiffen (2002). The data were subsequently updated to create a Health Technology Report for the Canadian Coordinating Center of Health Technology Assessment (Wong et al., 2004). The data were further updated by Wong.

Fifty-six trials fulfilled the selection criteria for the most recent analysis. The data support the fact that bisphosphonates provide moderate relief of pain within 12 weeks of therapy. The odds ratio (OR) for the best response within 12 weeks was 1.87 (95% confidence interval (CI) 1.23–2.86). The time-course of the effect was not immediate. While there was a trend towards pain relief at weeks 4 and 8, this only became statistically significant at week 12.

A more recent systematic review and meta-analysis found a reduction in SREs and improved pain control when bisphosphonates were added to another oncological treatment such as chemotherapy or radiotherapy (RR 1.18; 95% CI 1.0–1.4) (Lopez-Olivo et al., 2012)

It is not possible to say from the studies available if there is a different analgesic effect with different primary tumour sites.

Results for different bisphosphonates

Five randomized trials provided direct comparisons between different bisphosphonates. All of them compared pamidronate against a different bisphosphonate: three compared it with clodronate (Zhang et al., 1997; Diel et al., 1999; Jagdev et al., 2001) and two against zoledronate (Berensen et al., 2001; Rosen et al., 2001). Based on the limited data available, pamidronate appears to be a better choice than clodronate with a greater response rate and a greater magnitude of pain relief. Further studies are necessary to elucidate the relative merits of pamidronate and the more potent bisphosphonates, such as ibandronate and zoledronate (Cameron et al., 2006).

Clinical data tolerability

Bisphosphonate side effects commonly described include flu-like syndromes and injection site reactions. Randomized trials with standard doses did not identify excessive gastrointestinal toxicities, although concern has been raised about this (Lanza, 2002).

Renal toxicity is another important area. Rapid infusions may result in renal toxicity, especially in patients with renal compromise. Pamidronate infusions (90 mg) are typically delivered over a period of 2 hours, while zoledronate infusions (2 mg) are typically delivered over 15 minutes. Ibandronate does not appear to possess the same renal toxicity concerns and can be used in patients with varying degrees of renal impairment (Jackson, 2005; von Moos, 2005). Adverse ocular events including uveitis, scleritis, and conjunctivitis have been reported with amino-bisphosphonate use, particularly pamidronate use (Leung et al., 2005).

Bisphosphonate-associated osteonecrosis of the mandibular and maxillary bone has been described (Migliorati et al., 2005). The pathophysiology of this condition is unknown, but the risk factors include dental extraction, local trauma, local infection, and systemic chemotherapy. The condition has been reported with pamidronate and zoledronate and usually appears after many months of treatment. Appropriate prophylactic dental assessment and management, along with antibiotic therapy if indicated, are keystone to minimizing occurrence of this complication.

Summary of clinical use of bisphosphonates in CIBP

Bisphosphonates delay the development of skeletal events, particularly in patients with breast cancer, multiple myeloma, and prostate cancer. A positive effect of delaying these skeletal events is an overall reduction in pain secondary to bone resorption and its complications (e.g. pathological fracture). In addition, bisphosphonates also provide relief of bone pain, although the magnitude of the effect is modest in the short term and can take up to 12 weeks to work. Currently there are numerous small studies which suggest a potential role for bisphosphonates in acute CIBP relief; however, the studies are very heterogeneous and all use different outcome measurements. Further work is underway to evaluate the utility of the potent bisphosphonates such as ibandronate in achieving acute pain relief (Ibrahim et al., 2013). A double-blind, randomized controlled trial of single-dose ibandronate versus palliative radiotherapy for management of CIBP has been completed by Peter Hoskin and his team and is soon to report.

Radiotherapy

External beam radiotherapy is by far the most commonly used radiation modality in the management of bone pain: the most common type of treatment is local field radiotherapy (van As and Huddart, 2007) (see Chapter 12.3). Wide field radiotherapy and radioisotopes are used in treating disseminated bone metastases.

In 2000, the Cochrane group published on the use of radiotherapy for painful bone metastases. The review included data from 20 randomized controlled trials; 15 other studies were excluded for various methodological reasons. The trials were not sufficiently alike to allow pooling of data and therefore no meta-analysis was performed. Nevertheless, the authors concluded that radiotherapy provides effective analgesia for bone metastases. Over 40% of patients could expect at least 50% pain relief at 1 month and 20% could expect complete relief (McQuay et al., 2000). There was no discernible difference between fractionation schedules, or between different doses using the same schedule.

The Bone Pain Trial Working Group led a study to compare treatment with an 8 Gy single fraction and a multiple fraction regimen of either 20 Gy in five fractions or 30 Gy in 10 fractions (98% of patients in the multiple fraction arm received 20 Gy in five fractions and only 2% of patients received 30 Gy in 10 fractions) (Anonymous, 1999).

There was no difference between the arms in the time to first improvement in pain, time to complete pain relief, or time to increase in pain at any time over the 12-month follow-up period. There was also no difference in the acute toxicity of a single fraction of 8 Gy and the multiple-fraction regimens. Although retreatment was more common in the single-fraction arm, this was felt possibly to be due to clinicians being more likely to re-treat after a single-fraction than after a multiple-fraction regimen (Anonymous, 1999). In general, the equal efficacy, patient convenience, and lower cost should make a single 8 Gy fraction the standard treatment for palliation of pain from bone metastases. A review of studies of the efficacy of reirradiation for CIBP found variable study quality, but around 58% of patients did derive some additional analgesic benefit (Huisman et al., 2012).

Wide field radiotherapy

Wide field radiotherapy can be done in several ways, including radiation to the entire upper half of the body, radiation to the entire lower half of the body, radiation to the mid-section (from the lower chest to the upper thighs), and sequential hemi-body radiation in which half the body is irradiated in one session and the other half of the body is irradiated in a later session (4–6 weeks later). The latter procedure allows enough time for the bone marrow from the un-irradiated half of the body to re-populate the marrow cavity in the irradiated half of the body (van As and Huddart, 2007).

A number of radioisotopes have been used in the treatment of bone metastases (e.g. phosphorus-32, strontium-89, samarium-153, rhenium-186). In a systematic review and meta-analysis of radiopharmaceuticals in the treatment of CIBP (mainly from prostate or breast) approximately 70% of patients had some analgesic benefit with toxicity occurring in up to 15% of those treated (D'angelo et al., 2012). There is continued interest in this form of therapy with newer agents being developed (Yuan et al., 2013). Despite evidence, they are not widely used currently and while there are a number of potential reasons for low use of radioisotopes, cost may be an issue in many countries.

Chemotherapy

Chemotherapy can also be of considerable value in the management of metastatic bone pain where a tumour is chemosensitive. Examples would include myeloma, both small cell and non-small cell lung cancer, and breast cancer, where the natural history of these tumours is for widespread dissemination including bone as a common site of metastasis (Table 13.2.3).

Hormone therapy

Hormone therapy is also of value in hormone-sensitive tumours and both breast cancer and prostate cancer commonly spread to bone; in the latter this is the most common site and pattern of metastasis. Quite dramatic responses can be achieved within a few days of starting anti-androgen therapy in prostate cancer.

Response in metastatic breast cancer is generally slower and additional measures for pain relief are usually required in the first few weeks of starting hormone therapy. Hormone therapy, as with any other treatment which may induce acute new activity in bone, may be associated with a transient flare-up of pain which needs to be managed with appropriate manipulation of analgesia (Fig. 13.2.5).

Physiotherapy and occupational therapy

Many of the techniques in maximizing pain control through a multidisciplinary team approach discussed in Chapter 4.15 are integral to the adequate care of patients with CIBP. Life can be made infinitely easier for the patient who has difficulty mobilizing and problems in such areas as toileting and bathing, by the introduction of specific mobilizing techniques along with appropriate individualized aides.

Interventional analgesia

Vertebral cementoplasty

Instability of vertebrae due to metastatic disease can cause significant pain. Vertebral collapse causes pain per se, but structural change may also risk nerve root compression (Farquhar-Smith,

Table 13.2.3 Chemosensitivity of primary tumours commonly metastasizing to bone

Primary site	Sensitivity[a]
Myeloma	High
Bronchus	High
Breast	High
Rectum	Mid
Oesophagus	Mid/low
Prostate	Low
Thyroid	Low
Kidney	Low

[a] High = > 50% response rate; mid = 25–50% response rate; low = < 25% response rate.

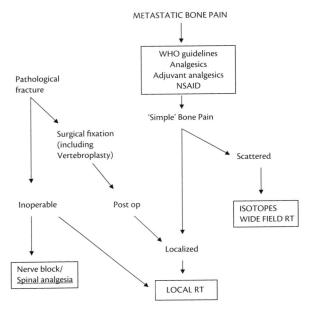

Fig. 13.2.5 Management of metastatic bone pain.

2007). Percutaneous vertebral cementoplasty (also known as percutaneous vertebroplasty) under radiological control has been used to reduce pain and treat vertebral body collapse (Gangi et al., 1996). Access to this technique depends on local expertise.

The analgesic mechanism of this technique is not explained solely by treating collapse, since as little as 2 mL of methylmethacrylate cement can achieve good pain relief (Gangi et al., 2003). Stabilization of microfractures, and subsequent reduction in mechanical forces through the bone, have been postulated as analgesic mechanisms (Legroux-Gerot et al., 2004). Analgesia could also be secondary to cytotoxic and thermal destruction of tumour cells, and interference with tumour blood supply.

A study of patients with intractable pain from vertebral myeloma found that 97% of patients had at least a 'moderate' reduction in pain following percutaneous vertebral cementoplasty (Cortet et al., 1997). The improvement in pain of 36/37 patients in this study was unrelated to the proportion of vertebral filling, reiterating the importance of tumour destruction rather than anatomical correction (Cotton et al., 1996).

Complications

Cement leak is a potential problem, which can encroach upon the epidural space, risking root or cord compression, and also chemothermal damage (Gangi et al., 2003). Cement embolism may also occur if there is evidence of a venous leak. In a case series of 868 percutaneous cementoplasty procedures for malignant and non-malignant vertebral body collapse, epidural leak was only observed in 15 cases (three had neuropathic pain) and asymptomatic pulmonary embolism in two cases (Gangi et al., 2003).

It is interesting that injection of methylmethacrylate is not restricted to the vertebrae and has been reported to be successful in the management of bone pain involving the pelvic bones (Cotton et al., 1995, 1996).

Lesioning of isolated metastases

There is some interest in targeted lesioning of isolated painful bony metastases using either radiofrequency (RF), or cryoablation. A small multicentre study of computed tomography-guided RF ablation did find some evidence of efficacy and this may have potential for single lesions (Guenette et al., 2013). Another multicentre study, again with relatively small numbers (I = 69) of cryoablation with follow-up to 6 months found sustained pain relief, although there was one episode of osteomyelitis (Callstrom et al., 2013).

Spinal analgesia

Generally, where patients suffer uncontrolled CIBP despite optimal pharmacological and non-pharmacological management, then either epidural or intrathecal analgesia should be considered. This is discussed in more detail in Chapter 9.4; however, it involves infusion of small amounts of opioid combined with local anaesthetic, sometimes in combination with clonidine.

Local anaesthetic is particularly useful for movement and other incident-related pains.

It is important that patients who have a pathological fracture but who are too unwell and close to death to consider internal fixation, are assessed urgently for an epidural or intrathecal line. Such patients often suffer extreme pain on even slight movement and their end-of-life care can be improved by interventional analgesia.

Orthopaedic interventions

Surgery for pathological fracture

The aim of fixing pathological fractures is different from that of traumatic (non-pathological) fractures (Al-Hakim et al., 2007) (see Chapter 12.5). Bone healing in these situations is impaired and often the fragments do not unite together. It is, therefore, a priority that the operation involves a method of fracture fixation that can allow immediate return to normal function.

Surgery for impending fracture

Some malignant bone lesions cause symptoms in the absence of a fracture; such lesions are at risk of fracturing at some point in the future (although many do not fracture and the symptoms settle with conservative measures). In general, metastases in long bones progress to fractures in 25% of cases (although this rises to approximately 60% in the proximal femur).

The criteria for operating on impending fractures vary. A widely used method is Mirels' scoring system (Table 13.2.4). This uses

Table 13.2.4 Mirels' scoring system for impending pathological fracture (Mirels, 1989)

Variable	Score		
	1	**2**	**3**
Site	Upper limb	Lower limb	Peritrochanteric
Pain	Mild	Moderate	Functional
Lesion	Blastic	Mixed	Lytic
Size[a]	< 1/3	1/3 to 2/3	> 2/3

[a] Maximum destruction of cortex in any view as seen on plain X-ray.

Reproduced with permission from Mirels H., Metastatic Disease in Long Bones A Proposed Scoring System for Diagnosing Impending Pathologic Fractures, *Current Orthopaedic Practice*, Volume 249, pp.256–264, Copyright © 1989 Lippincott-Raven Publishers.

four factors related to the likelihood of a malignant bone lesion fracturing. These include:

* the site of the lesion
* the amount of pain caused by the lesion
* whether the lesion is blastic, lytic, or a combination
* the size and involvement of the lesion (defined as the maximum amount of cortex destroyed).

A score of 1–3 is given for each variable, so that the lowest total score is 4 and the highest total score is twelve. A score of 7 or lower indicates that surgery is not needed, whereas a score of 9 or more indicates that surgery is warranted; a score of 8 means that the decision has to be taken in the context of the patient and his/her disease.

However, patients with severe pain every time they weight-bear, in spite of appropriate analgesics, radiotherapy, and other appropriate measures, may benefit from surgery, no matter what their calculated score.

There is mixed evidence to support the case that the outcome for surgical management of impending pathological fractures is better than that for actual fractures. Ward et al. reported a significant difference in favour of patients with impending fractures in terms of perioperative blood loss, shorter hospital stay, greater likelihood of discharge home instead of temporary step-down facilities, and higher rates of unassisted ambulation (Ward et al., 2003). In contrast, Dijkstra et al. reported no significant difference in outcomes such as pain relief, physical function, complications, and survival (Dijkstra et al., 1994). The decision about surgical intervention has to be highly individualized while taking into account the accepted, but limited, evidence base.

New approaches under evaluation

Glutamate inhibitors and NMDA antagonists

On the basis that CIBP has neuropathic and inflammatory components and clinical and laboratory evidence of central wind-up, it is not surprising that inhibitors of glutamate release have been considered and investigated. It is known that in animal studies, gabapentin reverses dorsal horn changes associated with CIBP resulting in relief of spontaneous and movement-related pain

(Donovan-Rodriguez et al., 2005). The specific role of pregabalin as adjuvant drug therapy in CIBP is under evaluation in a double-blind randomized, placebo-controlled study on a background of standardized best supportive care (Delaney et al., 2008). This is a good example of translational research in palliative medicine and follows on from Dickenson's group's preclinical work (Donovan-Rodriguez et al., 2005).

Inhibitors of the NMDA glutamate receptor complex may also be of interest, especially if NMDA subtype inhibitors are developed. At present the non-specific NMDA antagonist, ketamine, is used in some difficult to manage cases.

Osteoprotegerin

OPG is a promising target, which may act through reduction of osteoclast function to diminish tumour-induced bone destruction. Indeed early clinical work with OPG is interesting and may hold future promise (Gramoun et al., 2007). A single subcutaneous dose of AMGN-0007 (a recombinant construct of OPG) suppressed bone resorption as indicated by a rapid, sustained and profound decrease of urinary N-terminal telopeptide of collagen (NTX)/creatinine in multiple myeloma and breast carcinoma patients. Changes were comparable to those with pamidronate.

Denosumab

Denosumab is a human monoclonal antibody that binds to and inhibits RANKL (see Fig. 13.2.2), thus reducing osteoclastic activity. There have been a number of clinical trials of denosumab in osteoporosis and also in malignant disease. In a phase III study comparing denosumab to zoledronate in patients with advanced cancer, there was a reduced need for radiotherapy, in addition to less worsening of pain and a lower opioid requirement (Vadhan-Raj et al., 2012; Cleeland et al., 2013).

Endothelin-1 antagonists

Androgen refractory prostate cancer continues to evade effective treatment. The potent vasoconstrictor ET-1 is produced by prostate cancer and appears to have a role in prostate cancer progression and morbidity. Based on preclinical and clinical trial data, the ET axis is emerging as potentially important in this response (Body et al., 2003). Drugs targeting the endothelin axis, such as the potent ET_A receptor antagonists atrasentan, have been studied in large clinical trials and appear to have an impact on disease progression and morbidity. The role of the ET axis in prostate cancer deserves further investigation in the laboratory and clinic. Laboratory studies of ET_A in CIBP have demonstrated analgesic effects on both background and movement-evoked pain (Peters et al., 2005).

Monoclonal antibodies for nerve growth factor

NGF is a neurotrophin that regulates the structure and function of neurons. A humanized monoclonal antibody against NGF has been developed by two different pharmaceutical companies.

Tanezumab has been used in hip osteoarthritis studies with superior pain relief and improvement in physical function compared to placebo (Brown et al., 2013). Phase II studies have been completed in CIBP and the results are awaited. This may be a completely novel and opioid-sparing way of managing CIBP, however trial results are awaited.

Future concepts

Alphavbeta3 ($\alpha v\beta 3$) integrin blocker

The integrin $\alpha v\beta 3$ mediates cell-matrix interactions (Nelson 2003). Vitaxin®, a humanized monoclonal antibody that blocks human and rabbit $\alpha v\beta 3$ integrins, is in clinical trials for metastatic melanoma and prostate cancer. Vitaxin® decreases bone resorption by impairing osteoclast attachment, without affecting osteoclast multinucleation. Data also show that the inhibitory effects of Vitaxin® on osteoclasts can be modulated by factors known to alter the conformation of $\alpha v\beta 3$. The effects of Vitaxin® on reducing osteoclast activity may have future clinical utility in the management of CIBP.

Summary

CIBP remains a clinical challenge if we aim to achieve pain relief without unacceptable opioid side effects. An accurate assessment followed by an individualized management plan is key. A multimodality approach is required. Standard analgesic approaches using the WHO guidelines along with palliative radiotherapy as appropriate form the basis of management; however, every patient should be assessed with all modalities in mind. Clearly the patient's general physical condition, primary tumour diagnosis, extent of bone disease, previous treatments, and treatment response, along with specific features such as the likelihood of pathological fracture, are among the factors which will influence management decisions.

It is encouraging that we are emerging into an era where, largely due to an improved pre-clinical understanding of CIBP along with new drug development, we are likely to see the emergence of an improved evidence-based armamentarium for this challenging and frequent clinical problem.

References

Al-Hakim, W., Jagiello, J., and Briggs, T. (2007). Orthopaedic interventions. In A. Davies (ed.) *Cancer-related Bone Pain*, pp. 99–114. Oxford: Oxford University Press.

Alarmo, E.L., Korhonen, T., Kuukasjarvi, T., *et al.* (2008). Bone morphogenetic protein 7 expression associates with bone metastasis in breast carcinomas. *Annals of Oncology*, 19, 308–314.

Allen, B.J., Rogers, S.D., Ghilardi, J.R., *et al.* (1997). Noxious cutaneous thermal stimuli induce a graded release of endogenous substance P in the spinal cord: imaging peptide action in vivo. *Journal of Neuroscience*, 17, 5921–5927.

Anonymous (1999). 8 Gy single fraction radiotherapy for the treatment of metastatic skeletal pain: randomized comparison with a multifraction schedule over 12 months of patient follow-up. Bone Pain Trial Workshop Party. *Radiotherapy and Oncology*, 52, 111–121.

Antal, M., Petko, M., Polgar, E., Heizmann, C.W., and Stormmathisen, J. (1996). Direct evidence of an extensive gabaergic innervation of the spinal dorsal horn by fibers descending from the rostral ventromedial medulla. *Neuroscience*, 73, 509–518.

Baba, H., Ji, R.R., Kohno, T., *et al.* (2003). Removal of GABAergic inhibition facilitates polysynaptic A fiber-mediated excitatory transmission to the superficial spinal dorsal horn. *Molecular & Cellular Neurosciences*, 24, 818–830.

Bandell, M., Story, G.M., Hwang, S.W., *et al.* (2004). Noxious cold ion channel TRPA1 is activated by pungent compounds and bradykinin. *Neuron*, 41, 849–857.

Banning, A., Sjogren, P., and Henriksen, H. (1991a). Pain causes in 200 patients referred to a multidisciplinary cancer pain clinic. *Pain*, 45, 45–48.

Banning, A., Sjogren, P., and Henriksen, H. (1991b). Treatment outcome in a multidisciplinary cancer pain clinic. *Pain*, 47, 129–134.

Basbaum, A.I. and Fields, H.L. (1984). Endogenous pain control systems—brainstem spinal pathways and endorphin circuitry. *Annual Review of Neuroscience*, 7, 309–338.

Berensen, J.R., Rosen, L.S., Howell, A., *et al.* (2001). Zoledronic acid reduced skeletal-related events in patients with osteolytic metastases. *Cancer*, 91, 1191–1120.

Berman, H.H., Kim, K.H.S., Talati, A., and Hirsch, J. (1998). Representation of nociceptive stimuli in primary sensory cortex. *Neuroreport*, 9, 4179–4187.

Besson, J.-M. and Chaouch, A. (1987). Peripheral and spinal mechanisms of nociception. *Physiological Review*, 67, 67–186.

Biella, G. and Sotgui, M.L. (1995). Evidence that inhibitory mechanisms mask inappropriate somatotopic connections in the spinal cord of normal rat. *Journal of Neurophysiology*, 74(2), 495–505.

Bingel, U., Wanigasekera, V., Wiech, K., *et al.* (2011). The effect of treatment expectation on drug efficacy: imaging the analgesic benefit of the opioid remifentanil. *Science Translational Medicine*, 3, 70ra14.

Bloomfield, D.J. (1998). Should bisphosphonates be part of the standard therapy of patients with multiple myeloma or bone metastases from other cancers? An evidence-based review. *Journal of Clinical Oncology*, 16, 1218–1225.

Body, J.J., Greipp, P., Coleman, R.E., *et al.* (2003). A phase 1 study of AMGN-0007, a recombinant osteoprotegerin construct, in patients with multiple myeloma or breast carcinoma related bone metastases. *Cancer*, 97 (3 Suppl.), 887–892.

Boyle, W.J., Simonet, W.S., and Lacey, D.L. (2008). Osteoclast differentiation and activation. *Nature*, 423, 337–342.

Brescia, F.J., Adler, D., Gray, G., Ryan, M.A., Cimino, J., and Mamtani, R. (1999). Hospitalized advanced cancer paints: a profile. *Journal of Pain and Symptom Management*, 5, 221–227.

Brown, M.T., Murphy, F.T., Radin, D.M., *et al.* (2013). Tanezumab reduces osteoarthritic hip pain. *Arthritis and Rheumatism*, 65(7), 1795–1803.

Buijs, J.T., Henriquez, N.V., van Overveld, P.G., *et al.* (2007). TGF-beta and BMP7 interactions in tumour progression and bone metastasis. *Clinical & Experimental Metastasis*, 24, 609–617.

Burnstock, G. and Wood, J.N. (1996). Purinergic receptors: their role in nociception and primary afferent neurotransmission. *Current Opinion in Neurobiology*, 6, 526–532.

Cain, D.M., Wacnik, P.W., Turner, M., *et al.* (2001). Functional interactions between tumor and peripheral nerve: changes in excitability and morphology of primary afferent fibers in a murine model of cancer pain. *Journal of Neuroscience*, 21, 9367–9376.

Caissie, A., Zeng, L., Nguyen, J., *et al.* (2012). Assessment of health-related quality of life with the European Organization for Research and Treatment of Cancer QLQ-C15-PAL after palliative radiotherapy of bone metastases. *Clinical Oncology (Royal College of Radiologists)*, 24, 125–133.

Callstrom, M.R., Dupuy, D.E., Solomon, S.B., *et al.* (2013). Percutaneous image-guided cryoablation of painful metastases involving bone: multicenter trial. *Cancer*, 119, 1033–1041.

Cameron, D., Fallon, M., and Diel, I. (2006). Ibandronate: its role in metastatic breast cancer. *The Oncologist*, 11(Suppl. 1), 27–33.

Caraceni, A., Martini, C., Zecca, E., *et al.* (2004). Breakthrough pain characteristics and syndromes in patients with cancer pain. An international survey. *Palliative Medicine*, 18, 177–183.

Caraceni, A. and Portenoy, R.K. (1999). An international survey of cancer pain characteristics and syndromes. *Pain*, 82, 263–274.

Carr, D.B., Goudas, L.C., Balk, E.M., Bloch, R., Ioannidis, J.P., and Lau, J. (2004). Evidence report on the treatment of pain in cancer patients. *Journal of the National Cancer Institute, Monographs*, 32, 23–31.

Cervero, F. and Iggo, A. (1980). The substantia gelatinosa of the spinal cord: a critical review. *Brain*, 103, 717–772.

Christie, J.M., Simmonds, M., Patt, R., *et al.* (1998). Dose-titration, multicenter study of oral transmucosal fentanyl citrate for the treatment of breakthrough pain in cancer patients using transdermal fentanyl for persistent pain. *Journal of Clinical Oncology*, 16, 3238–3245.

Clare, C., Royle, D., Saharia, K., *et al.* (2005). Painful bone metastases: a prospective observational cohort study. *Palliative Medicine*, 19, 521–525.

Cleeland, C.S., Body, J.J., Stopeck, A., *et al.* (2013). Pain outcomes in patients with advanced breast cancer and bone metastases: results from a randomized, double-blind study of denosumab and zoledronic acid. *Cancer*, 119, 832–838.

Clohisy, D.R. and Mantyh, P.W. (2003). Bone cancer pain. *Clinical Orthopaedics and Related Research*, (415 Suppl.), S279–288.

Clohisy, D.R. and Mantyh, P.W. (2004). Bone cancer pain and the role of RANKL/OPG. *Journal of Musculoskeletal Neuronal Interactions*, 4(3), 293–300.

Coghill, R.C., Mayer, D.J., and Price, D.D. (1993). The roles of spatial recruitment and discharge frequency in spinal coding of pain: a combined electrophysiological and imaging investigation. *Pain*, 53, 295–309.

Colleau, S.M. (2002). Palliation of bone pain in cancer; facts and controversies. *Cancer Pain Release*, 15, 1.

Coluzzi, F., Mandatori, I., and Mattia, C. (2011). Emerging therapies in metastatic bone pain. *Expert Opinion on Emerging Drugs*, 16, 441–458.

Coluzzi, P.H., Schwartzberg, L., Conroy, J.D., Jr, *et al.* (2001). Breakthrough cancer pain: a randomized trial comparing oral transmucosal fentanyl citrate (OTFC) and morphine sulphate immediate release (MSIR). *Pain*, 91, 123–130.

Cortet, B., Cotton, A., Boutry, N., *et al.* (1997). Percutaneous vertebroplasty in patients with osteolytic metastases or multiple myeloma. *Revue du Rhumatisme (English Edn)*, 64, 117–183.

Cortright, D.N., Krause, J.E., and Broom, D.C. (2007). TRP channels and pain. *Biochimica et Biophysica Acta*, 1772, 978–988.

Costigan, M. and Woolf, C.J. (2002). No DREAM, No pain. Closing the spinal gate. *Cell*, 108, 297–300.

Cotton, A., Deprez, X., Migaud, H., Chabanne, B., Duquesnoy, B., and Chastenet, P. (1995). Malignant acetabular osteolyses: percutaneous injection of acrylic bone cement. *Radiology*, 197, 307–310.

Cotton, A., Dewatre, F., Cortet, B., *et al.* (1996). Percutaneous vertebroplasty for osteolytic metastases and myeloma: effects of the percentage of lesion filling and the leakage of methyl methacrylate at clinical follow-up. *Radiology*, 200, 525–530.

D'angelo, G., Sciuto, R., Salvatori, M., *et al.* (2012). Targeted 'bone-seeking' radiopharmaceuticals for palliative treatment of bone metastases: a systematic review and meta-analysis. *The Quarterly Journal of Nuclear Medicine & Molecular Imaging*, 56, 538–543.

Davies, A. (2006). Introduction. In A. Davies (ed.) *Cancer-related Breakthrough Pain*, pp. 1–11. Oxford: Oxford University Press.

Davis, K.D. (2000). The neural circuitry of pain as explored with functional MRI. *Neurological Research*, 22, 313–317.

De Wit, R., van Dam, F., Loonstra, S., *et al.* (2001). The Amsterdam Pain Management Index compared to eight frequently used outcome measures to evaluate the adequacy of pain treatment in cancer patients with chronic pain. *Pain*, 91, 339–349.

Delaney, A., Fleetwood-Walker, S.M., Colvin, L.A., and Fallon, M. (2008). Translational medicine: cancer pain mechanisms and management. *British Journal of Anaesthesia*, 101(1), 87–94.

DeLeo, J.A., Colburn, R.W., and Rickman, A.J. (1997). Cytokine and growth factor immunohistochemical spinal profiles in two animal models of mononeuropathy. *Brain Research*, 759, 50–57.

Dib-Hajj, S.D., Yang, Y., Black, J.A., and Waxman, S.G. (2013). The Na(V)1.7 sodium channel: from molecule to man. *Nature Reviews Neuroscience*, 14, 49–62.

Dickenson, A.H. (2002). Gate control theory of pain stands the test of time. *British Journal of Anaesthesia*, 88, 755–757.

Diel, I.J., Marschner, N., Kindler, M., *et al.* (1999). Continual oral versus intravenous interval therapy with bisphosphonates in patients with breast cancer and bone metastases. *Proceedings of the Annual Meeting of the American Society of Clinical Oncology*, Abstract 488.

Dijkstra, S., Wiggers, R., Van Geel, B.N., and Boxma, H (1994). Impending and actual pathological fractures in patients with bone metastases of the long bones. A retrospective study of 233 surgically treated fractures. *European Journal of Surgery*, 160, 535–542.

Donovan-Rodriguez, T., Dickenson, A.H., and Urch, C.E. (2005). Gabapentin normalizes spinal neuronal responses that correlate with behavior in a rat model of cancer-induced bone pain. *Anesthesiology*, 102, 132–140.

Donovan-Rodriguez, T., Urch, C.E., and Dickenson, A.H. (2006). Evidence of a role for descending serotonergic facilitation in a rat model of cancer-induced bone pain. *Neuroscience Letters*, 393, 237–242.

Dore-Savard, L., Beaudet, L.N., Tremblay, L., Xiao, Y., Lepage, M., and Sarret, P. (2013). A micro-imaging study linking bone cancer pain with tumor growth and bone resorption in a rat model. *Clinical & Experimental Metastasis*, 30(2), 225–236.

Duggan, A.W., Hendry, I.A., Morton, C.R., Hutchison, W.D., and Zhao, Z.Q. (1988). Cutaneous stimuli releasing immunoreactive substance P in the dorsal horn of the cat. *Brain Research*, 451, 261–273.

Eccleston, C. and Crombez, G. (2005). Attention and pain: merging behavioural and neuroscience investigations. *Pain*, 113, 7–8.

Eisenberg, E., Berkey, C.S., Carr, D.B., Mosteller, F., and Chalmers, T.C. (1994). Efficacy and safety of non-steroidal anti-inflammatory drugs for cancer pain: a meta-analysis. *Journal of Clinical Oncology*, 12, 2756–2765.

Estape, J., Vinolas, N., Gonzalez, B., *et al.* (1990). Ketorolac, a new non-opioid analgesic: a double-blind trial versus pentazocine in cancer pain. *Journal of International Medical Research*, 18, 298–304.

Fallon, M.T. and McConnell, S. (2007). Clinical features. In A. Davies (ed.) *Cancer-related Bone Pain*, pp. 17–26. Oxford: Oxford University Press.

Farquhar-Smith, P. (2007). Anaesthetic and interventional techniques. In A. Davies (ed.) *Cancer-related Bone Pain*, pp. 85–97. Oxford: Oxford University Press.

Farrar, J.T., Cleary, J., Rauck, R., Busch, M. and Nordbrock, E. (1998). Oral transmucosal fentanyl citrate: randomized, double-blinded, placebo-controlled trial for treatment of breakthrough pain in cancer patients. *Journal of the National Cancer Institute*, 90, 611–616.

Fleetwood-Walker, S.M., Proudfoot, C.J., Garry, E.M., Allchorne, A., Vinuela-Fernandez, I., and Mitchell, R. (2007). Cold comfort pharm. *Trends in Pharmacological Sciences*, 28(12), 621–628.

Front, D., Schneck, S.O., Frankel, A., and Robinson, E. (1979). Bone metastases and bone pain in breast cancer. *Journal of the American Medical Association*, 242, 1747–1478.

Fuccella, L.M., Conti, F., Corvi, G., *et al.* (1975). Double-blind study of the analgesic effect of indoprofen (K 4277). *Clinical Pharmacology & Therapeutics*, 17, 277–283.

Gangi, A., Dietemann, J.L., Schultz, A., Mortazavi, R., Jeung, M.Y., and Roy, C. (1996). Interventional radiologic procedures with CT guidance in cancer pain management. *Radiographics*, 16, 1289–1304.

Gangi, A., Guth, S., Imbert, J.P., Marin, H., and Dietemann, J.L. (2003). Percutaneous vertebroplasty: indications, technique and results. *Radiographics*, 23, e10.

Ghilardi, J.R., Rohrich, H., Lindsay, T.H., *et al.* (2005). Selective blockade of the capsaicin receptor TRPV1 attenuates bone cancer pain. *Journal of Neuroscience*, 25, 3126–3131.

Giesler, G.J., Jr, Katter, J.T., and Dado, R.J. (1994). Direct spinal pathways to the limbic system for nociceptive information. *Trends in Neurological Sciences*, 17, 244–250.

Gilchrist, L.S., Cain, D.M., Harding-Rose, C., *et al.* (2005). Re-organization of P2X3 receptor localization on epidermal nerve fibers in a murine model of cancer pain. *Brain Research*, 1044, 197–205.

Gramoun, A., Shorey, S., Bashutski, J.D., *et al.* (2007). Effects of Vitaxin, a novel therapeutic in trial for metastatic bone tumors, on osteoclast functions in vitro. *Journal of Cellular Biochemistry*, 102, 341–52.

Gray, B.G. and Dostrovsky, J.O. (1983). Descending inhibitory influences from periaqueductal gray, nucleus raphe magnus, and adjacent reticular-formation.1. effects on lumbar spinal-cord nociceptive and nonnociceptive neurons. *Journal of Neurophysiology*, 49, 932–947.

Green, J.R. (2004). Bisphosphonates: preclinical review. *The Oncologist*, 9(Suppl. 4), 3–13.

Grond, S., Zech, D., Diefenbach, C., Radbruch, L., and Lehmann, K.A. (1996). Assessment of cancer pain: a prospective evaluation in 2266 cancer patients referred to a pain service. *Pain*, 64, 107–114.

Guenette, J.P., Lopez, M.J., Kim, E., and Dupuy, D.E. (2013). Solitary painful osseous metastases: correlation of imaging features with pain palliation after radiofrequency ablation—a multicenter American college of radiology imaging network study. *Radiology*, 268, 907–915.

Gui, Q., Xu, C., Zhuang, L., *et al.* (2013). A new rat model of bone cancer pain produced by rat breast cancer cells implantation of the shaft of femur at the third trochanter level. *Cancer Biology & Therapy*, 14, 193–199.

Halvorson, K.G., Kubota, K., Sevcik, M.A., *et al.* (2005). A blocking antibody to nerve growth factor attenuates skeletal pain induced by prostate tumor cells growing in bone. *Cancer Research*, 65(20), 9426–35.

Halvorson, K.G., Sevcik, M.A., Ghilardi, J.R., Rosol, T.J., and Mantyh, P.W. (2006). Similarities and differences in tumor growth, skeletal remodeling and pain in an osteolytic and osteoblastic model of bone cancer. *Clinical Journal of Pain*, 22, 587–600.

Handwerker, H.O., Iggo, A., and Zimmermann, M. (1975). Segmental and supraspinal actions on dorsal horn neurons responding to noxious and non-noxious skin stimuli. *Pain*, 1, 147–165.

Hang, L.H., Yang, J.P., Yin, W., *et al.* (2012). Activation of spinal TDAG8 and its downstream PKA signaling pathway contribute to bone cancer pain in rats. *European Journal of Neuroscience*, 36, 2107–2117.

Hanks, G.W., De Conno, F., Cherny, N., *et al.* (2001). Morphine and alternative opioids in cancer pain: the EAPC recommendations. *British Journal of Cancer*, 84, 587–593.

Hansen, R., Nasser, A., Falk, S., *et al.* (2012). Chronic administration of the selective P2X3, P2X2/3 receptor antagonist, A-317491, transiently attenuates cancer-induced bone pain in mice. *European Journal of Pharmacology*, 688, 27–34.

Honore, P. and Mantyh, P.W. (2000). Bone cancer pain: from mechanism to model to therapy. *Pain Medicine*, 1, 303–309.

Honore, P., Rogers, S.D., Schwei, M.J., *et al.* (2000). Murine models of inflammatory, neuropathic and cancer pain each generates a unique set of neurochemical changes in the spinal cord and sensory neurons. *Neuroscience*, 98, 585–598.

Honore, P., Schwei, J., Rogers, S.D., *et al.* (2000). Cellular and neurochemical remodeling of the spinal cord in bone cancer pain. *Progress in Brain Research*, 129, 389–397.

Huisman, M., van den Bosch, M.A., Wijlemans, J.W., *et al.* (2012). Effectiveness of reirradiation for painful bone metastases: a systematic review and meta-analysis. *International Journal of Radiation Oncology, Biology, Physics*, 84, 8–14.

Ibrahim, T., Farolfi, A., Mercatali, L., Ricci, M., and Amadori, D. (2013). Metastatic bone disease in the era of bone-targeted therapy: clinical impact. *Tumori*, 99, 1–9.

Kim, W.M., Jeong, C.W., Lee, S., Kim, Y.O., Cui, J.H., and Yoon, M.H. (2011). The intrathecally administered kappa-2 opioid agonist GR89696 and interleukin-10 attenuate bone cancer-induced pain through synergistic interaction. *Anesthesia & Analgesia*, 113, 934–940.

Jackson, G.H. (2005). Renal safety of ibandronate. *The Oncologist*, 10(Suppl. 1), 14–18.

Jagdev, S.P., Purohit, P., Heatley, S., Herling, C., and Coleman, R.E. (2001). Comparison of the effects of intravenous pamidraonte and oral clodronate on symptoms and bone resorption in patients with metastatic bone disease. *Annals of Oncology*, 12, 1433–1438.

Janson, W. and Stein, C. (2003). Peripheral opioid analgesia. *Current Pharmaceutical Biotechnology*, 4, 270–274.

Jimenez-Andrade, J.M., Ghilardi, J.R., Castaneda-Corral, G., Kuskowski, M.A., and Mantyh, P.W. (2011). Preventive or late administration of anti-NGF therapy attenuates tumor-induced nerve sprouting, neuroma formation, and cancer pain. *Pain*, 152, 2564–2574.

Jimenez-Andrade, J.M., Martin, C.D., Koewler, N.J., *et al.* (2007). Nerve growth factor sequestering therapy attenuates non-malignant skeletal pain following fracture. *Pain*, 133, 183–196.

Ke, C.B., He, W.S., Li, C.J., Shi, D., Gao, F., and Tian, Y.K. (2012). Enhanced SCN7A/Nax expression contributes to bone cancer pain by increasing excitability of neurons in dorsal root ganglion. *Neuroscience*, 227, 80–89.

Khasabov, S.G., Hamamoto, D.T., Harding-Rose, C., and Simone, D.A. (2007). Tumor-evoked hyperalgesia and sensitization of nociceptive dorsal horn neurons in a murine model of cancer pain. *Brain Research*, 1180, 7–19.

Kidd, B.L. and Urban, L.A. (2001). Mechanisms of inflammatory pain. *British Journal of Anaesthesia*, 87, 3–11.

Kinder, M., Chislock, E., Bussard, K.M., Shuman, L., and Mastro, A.M. (2008). Metastatic breast cancer induces an osteoblast inflammatory response. *Experimental Cell Research*, 314, 173–183.

Kingsley, L.A., Fournier, P.G., Chirgwin, J.M., and Guise, T.A, (2007). Molecular biology of bone metastasis. *Molecular Cancer Therapeutics*, 6, 2609–2617.

King, T., Vardanyan, A., Majuta, L., *et al.* (2007). Morphine treatment accelerates sarcoma-induced bone pain, bone loss, and spontaneous fracture in a murine model of bone cancer. *Pain*, 132, 154–168.

Krempien, R., Niethammer, A., Harms, W., and Debus, J. (2005). Bisphosphonates and bone metastases: current status and future directions. *Expert Review of Anticancer Therapy*, 5, 295–305.

Laird, B.J., Walley, J., Murray, G.D., Clausen, E., Colvin, L.A., and Fallon, M.T. (2011). Characterization of cancer-induced bone pain: an exploratory study. *Supportive Care in Cancer*, 19, 1393–1401.

Lanza, F.L. (2002). Gastrointestinal adverse effects of bisphosphonates: etiology, incidence and prevention. *Treatments in Endocrinology*, 1, 37–43.

Lee, M.C. and Tracey, I. (2013). Imaging pain: a potent means for investigating pain mechanisms in patients. *British Journal of Anaesthesia*, 111, 64–72.

Legroux-Gerot, I., Lormeau, C., Boutry, N., Cotton, A., Duquesnoy, B., and Cortet, B. (2004). Long-term follow-up of vertebral osteoporotic fractures treated by percutaneous vertebroplasty. *Clinical Rheumatology*, 23, 310–317.

Leung, S., Ashar, B.H., and Miller, R.G. (2005). Bisphonate-associated scleritis: a case report and review. *Southern Medical Journal*, 98, 733–735.

Liu, J., Liu, F.Y., Tong, Z.Q., *et al.* (2013). Lysine-specific demethylase 1 in breast cancer cells contributes to the production of endogenous formaldehyde in the metastatic bone cancer pain model of rats. *PLoS ONE*, 8, e58957.

Liu, M., Oh, U., AND Wood, J.N. (2011). From transduction to pain sensation: defining genes, cells, and circuits. *Pain*, 152, S16–S19.

Loeser, J.D. (2000). Cancer pain: assessment and diagnosis. In J.J. Bonica and J.D. Loeser (eds.) *Bonica's Management of Pain*, pp. 634–641. Philadelphia, PA: Lippincott Williams & Wilkins.

Longe, S.E., Wise, R., Bantick, S., *et al.* (2001). Counter-stimulatory effects on pain perception and processing are significantly altered by attention: an fMRI study. *Neuroreport*, 12, 2021–2025.

Lopez-Olivo, M.A., Shah, N.A., Pratt, G., Risser, J.M., Symanski, E., and Suarez-Almazor, M.E. (2012). Bisphosphonates in the treatment of patients with lung cancer and metastatic bone disease: a systematic review and meta-analysis. *Supportive Care in Cancer*, 20, 2985–2998.

Luger, N.M., Mach, D.B., Sevcik, M.A., and Mantyh, P.W. (2005). Bone cancer pain: from model to mechanism to therapy. *Journal of Pain and Symptom Management*, 29, S32–S46.

Luger, N.M., Sabino, M.A., Schwei, M.J., *et al.* (2002). Efficacy of systemic morphine suggests a fundamental difference in the mechanisms that generate bone cancer vs inflammatory pain. *Pain*, 99, 397–406.

Mantyh, P.W., Clohisy, D.R., Koltzenburg, M., and Hunt, S.P. (2002). Molecular mechanisms of cancer pain. *Nature Reviews Cancer*, 2, 201–209.

Mao-Ying, Q.L., Wang, X.W., Yang, C.J., *et al.* (2012). Robust spinal neuroinflammation mediates mechanical allodynia in Walker 256 induced bone cancer rats. *Molecular Brain*, 5, 16.

Marceau, F. and Regoli, D. (2004). Bradykinin receptor ligands: therapeutic perspectives. *Nature Reviews Drug Discovery*, 3, 845–852.

Marguiles, A., Klimberg, V., Bhattacharrya, S., Gaddy, D., and Suva, L.J. (2006). Genomics and proteomics of bone cancer. *Clinical Cancer Research*, 12, 6217s–6221s.

Martin, C.D., Jimenez-Andrade, J.M., Ghilardi, J.R., and Mantyh, P.W. (2007). Organization of a unique net-like meshwork of CGRP+ sensory fibers in the mouse periosteum: implications for the generation and maintenance of bone fracture pain. *Neuroscience Letters*, 427, 148–152.

Matza, L.S., Fallowfield, L.J., Chung, K.C., Currie, B.M., Van, B.K., and Patrick, D.L. (2012). Patient-reported outcome instruments used to assess pain and functioning in studies of bisphosphonate treatment for bone metastases. *Supportive Care in Cancer*, 20, 657–677.

McGaraughty, S. and Heinricher, M.M. (2002). Microinjection of morphine into various amygdaloid nuclei differentially affects nociceptive responsiveness and RVM neuronal activity. *Pain*, 96, 153–162.

McNicol, E., Strassels, S., Goudas, L., Lau, J., and Carr, D. (2004). Non-steroidal anti-inflammatory drugs, alone or combined with opioids for cancer pain: a systematic review. *Journal of Clinical Oncology*, 22, 1975–1992.

McQuay, H.J., Collins, S.L., Carroll, D., *et al.* (2000). Radiotherapy for the palliation of painful bone metastases. *Cochrane Database of Systematic Reviews*, 2, CD001793.

Medhurst, S., Bowes, M., Kidd, B.L., *et al.* (2001). Antinociceptive effects of the bisphosphonate, zoledronic acid, in a novel rat model of bone cancer pain. *British Journal of Pharmacology*, 134, 156P.

Medhurst, S.J., Walker, K., Bowes, M., *et al.* (2002). A rat model of bone cancer pain. *Pain*, 96, 129–140.

Melzack, R. and Wall, P.D. (1965). Pain mechanisms: a new theory. *Science*, 150, 971–979.

Men, D.S., Matsui, A., and Matsui, Y. (1996). Somatosensory afferent inputs release 5-HT and NA from the spinal cord. *Neurochemical Research*, 21, 1515–1519.

Menendez, L., Lastra, A., Fresno, M.F., *et al.* (2003a). Initial thermal heat hypoalgesia and delayed hyperalgesia in a murine model of bone cancer pain. *Brain Research*, 969, 102–109.

Menendez, L., Lastra, A., Hidalgo, A., Meana, A., Garcia, E., and Baamonde, A. (2003b). Peripheral opioids act as analgesics in bone cancer pain in mice. *Neuroreport*, 14, 867–869.

Menetrey, D., Chaouch, A., Binder, D., and Besson, J.M. (1982). The origin of the spinomesencephalic tract in the rat—an anatomical study using the retrograde transport of horseradish-peroxidase. *Journal of Comparative Neurology*, 206, 193–207.

Mercadante, S. (1997). Malignant bone pain: pathophysiology and treatment. *Pain*, 69, 1–18.

Mercadante, S. and Arcuri, E. (1998). Breakthrough pain in cancer patients: pathophysiology and treatment. *Cancer Treatment Reviews*, 24, 425–432.

Mercadante, S., Villari, P., Ferrera, P., Bianchi, M., and and Casuccio, A. (2004b). Safety and effectiveness of intravenous morphine for episodic (breakthrough) pain using a fixed ratio with the oral daily morphine dose. *Journal of Pain and Symptom Management*, 27, 352–359.

Mercadante, S., Villari, P., Ferrera, P., and Casuccio, A. (2004a). Optimization of opioid therapy for preventing incident pain associated with bone metastases. *Journal of Pain and Symptom Management*, 28, 505–510.

Merskey, H. (1986). IASP Subcommittee on Taxonomy: classification of chronic pain. *Pain*, 3, S216–S222.

Meuser, T., Pietruvk, C., Radbruch, L., *et al.* (2001). Symptoms during cancer pain treatment following WHO-guidelines: a longitudinal follow-up study of symptom prevalence, severity and etiology. *Pain*, 91, 247–257.

Michaelson, M.D. and Smith, M.R. (2005). Bisphosphonates for treatment and prevention of bone metastases. *Journal of Clinical Oncology*, 23, 8219–8224.

Migliorati, C.A., Schubert, M.M., Peterson, D.E., and Seneda, L.M. (2005). Bisphosphonate-associated osteonecrosis of mandibular and maxillary bone: an emerging oral complication of supportive cancer therapy. *Cancer*, 104, 83–93.

Minotti, V., de Angelis, V., Righetti, E., *et al.* (1998). Double-blind evaluation of short-term analgesic efficacy of orally administered diclofenac, diclofenac plus codeine, and diclofenac plus imipramine in chronic cancer pain. *Pain*, 74, 133–137.

Minotti, V., Patoia, L., Roila, F., *et al.* (1989). Double-blind evaluation of analgesic efficacy of orally administered diclofenac, nefopam, and acetylsalicylic acid (ASA) plus codeine in chronic cancer pain. *Pain*, 36, 177–183.

Mirels, H. (1989). Metastatic disease in long bones. A proposed scoring system for diagnosing impending pathological fractures. *Clinical Orthopaedics and Related Research*, 249, 256–264.

Mokha, S.S., McMillan, J.A., and Iggo, A. (1985). Descending control of spinal nociceptive transmission. Actions produced on spinal multireceptive neurones from the nuclei locus coeruleus (LC) and raphe magnus (NRM). *Experimental Brain Research*, 58, 213–226.

Morgan, N.M., Gogas, K.R., and Basbaum, A.I. (1994). Diffuse noxious inhibitory controls reduce the expression of noxious stimulus-evoked fos-like immunoreactivity in the superficial and deep laminae of the rat spinal cord. *Pain*, 56, 347–352.

Nagae, M., Hiraga, T., and Yoneda, T. (2007). Acidic microenvironment created by osteoclasts causes bone pain associated with tumor colonization. *Journal of Bone & Mineral Metabolism*, 25, 99–104.

Nakamura, A., Hasegawa, M., Minami, K., *et al.* (2013). Differential activation of the u-opioid receptor by oxycodone and morphine in pain-related brain regions in a bone cancer pain model. *British Journal of Pharmacology*, 168, 375–388.

Nelson, J.B. (2003). Endothelin inhibition: novel therapy for prostate cancer. *Journal of Urology*, 170, S65–S67.

Niiyama, Y., Kawamata, T., Yamamoto, J., Omote, K., and Namiki, A. (2007). Bone cancer increases transient receptor potential vanilloid subfamily 1 expression within distinct subpopulations of dorsal root ganglion neurons. *Neuroscience*, 148, 560–572.

Oster, M.W., Visel, M., and Turgeon, L.R. (1978). Pain in terminal cancer patients. *Archives of Internal Medicine*, 138, 1801–1802.

Peters, C.M., Ghilardi, J.R., Keyser, C.P., *et al.* (2005). Tumor-induced injury of primary afferent sensory nerve fibers in bone cancer pain. *Experimental Neurology*, 193, 85–100.

Peyron, R., Laurent, B., and Garcia-Larrea, L. (2000). Functional imaging of brain responses to pain. A review and meta-analysis. *Neurophysiologie Clinique-Clinical Neurophysiology*, 30, 263–288.

Peyruchaud, O., Leblanc, R., and David, M. (2013). Pleiotropic activity of lysophosphatidic acid in bone metastasis. *Biochimica et Biophysica Acta*, 1831, 99–104.

Ploghaus, A., Tracey, I., Gati, J.S., *et al.* (1999). Dissociating pain from its anticipation in the human brain. *Science*, 284, 1979–1981.

Polgar, E., Puskar, Z., Watt, C., Matesz, C., and Todd, A.J. (2002). Selective innervation of lamina I projection neurones that possess the neurokinin 1 receptor by serotonin-containing axons in the rat spinal cord. *Neuroscience*, 109, 799–809.

Pollen, J.J. and Schmidt, J.D. (1979). Bone pain in metastatic cancer of prostate. *Urology*, 13, 129–134.

Porreca, F., Ossipov, M.H., and Gebhart, G.F. (2002). Chronic pain and medullary descending facilitation. *Trends in Neurosciences*, 25, 319–325.

Portenoy, R. (2011). Clinical perspectives on preclinical models of bone pain: questions and promises. *Pain*, 152, 2455–2456.

Portenoy, R.K. (1997). Treatment of temporal variations in chronic cancer pain. *Seminars in Oncology*, 5, S16, 7–12.

Portenoy, R.K., Forbes, K., Lussier, D., and Hanks. G. (2004). Difficult pain problems: an integrated approach. In D. Doyle, G. Hanks, N. Cherny, and K. Calman (eds.) *Oxford Textbook of Palliative Medicine* (3rd ed.), pp. 438–458. Oxford: Oxford University Press.

Portenoy, R.K. and Hagen, N.A (1990). Breakthrough pain: definition, prevalence and characteristics. *Pain*, 41, 273–281.

Portenoy, R.K. and Lesage, P. (1999). Management of cancer pain. *The Lancet*, 353, 1695–1700.

Portenoy, R.K., Payne, R., Coluzzi, P., *et al.* (1999). Oral transmucosal fentanyl citrate (OTFC) for the treatment of breakthrough pain in cancer patients; a controlled dose titration study. *Pain*, 79, 303–312.

Portenoy, R.K., Payne, D., and Jacobsen, P. (1999). Breakthrough pain: characteristics and impact in patients with cancer pain. *Pain*, 81, 129–134.

Price, M.P., McIlwrath, S.L., Xie, J., *et al.* (2001). The DRASIC cation channel contributes to the detection of cutaneous touch and acid stimuli in mice. *Neuron*, 32, 1071–1083.

Qiu, F., Jiang, Y., Zhang, H., Liu, Y., and Mi, W. (2012). Increased expression of tetrodotoxin-resistant sodium channels Nav1.8 and Nav1.9 within dorsal root ganglia in a rat model of bone cancer pain. *Neuroscience Letters*, 512, 61–66.

Quigley, C. (2004). Opioid switching to improve pain relief and drug tolerability. *Cochrane Database of Systematic Reviews*, 3, CD004847.

Rosen, L.S., Gordon, D., Kaminski, M., *et al.* (2001). Zolendronic acid versus pamidronate in the treatment of skeletal metastases in patients with breast cancer or osteolytic lesions of multiple myeloma: a phase III double-blind, comparative trial. *Cancer Journal*, 7, 377–387.

Roudier, M.P., Bain, S.D., and Dougall, W.C. (2006). Effects of the RANKL inhibitor, osteoprotegerin, on the pain and histopathology of bone cancer in rats. *Clinical & Experimental Metastasis*, 23, 167–175.

Rusteon, T., Moum, T., Padilla, G., Paul, S., and Miaskowski, C. (2005). Predictors of quality of life in oncology outpatients with pain from bone metastasis. *Journal of Pain and Symptom Management*, 20, 234–242.

Sabino, M.A., Ghilardi, J.R., Jongen, J.L., *et al.* (2002). Simultaneous reduction in cancer pain, bone destruction, and tumor growth by selective inhibition of cyclooxygenase-2. *Cancer Research*, 62, 7343–7349.

Sabino, M.C., Ghilardi, J.R., Feia, K.J., *et al.* (2002). The involvement of prostaglandins in tumorigenesis, tumor-induced osteolysis and bone cancer pain. *Journal of Musculoskeletal Neuronal Interactions*, 2, 561–562.

Sabino, M.A., Luger, N.M., Mach, D.B., Rogers, S.D., Schwei, M.J., and Mantyh, P.W. (2003). Different tumors in bone each give rise to a distinct pattern of skeletal destruction, bone cancer-related pain behaviors and neurochemical changes in the central nervous system. *International Journal of Cancer*, 104, 550–558.

Saito, O., Aoe, T., Kozikowski, A., Sarva, J., Neale, J.H., and Yamamoto, T. (2006). Ketamine and N-acetylaspartylglutamate peptidase inhibitor exert analgesia in bone cancer pain. *Canadian Journal of Anaesthesia*, 53, 891–898.

Sande, T.A., Scott, A.C., Laird, B.J., *et al.* (2014). The characteristics of physical activity and gait in patients receiving radiotherapy in cancer induced bone pain. *Radiotherapy & Oncology*, 111(1), 18–24.

Santini, D., Vaspasiani Gentilucci, U., Vicenzi, B., *et al.* (2003). The anti-neoplastic role of bisphosphonates: from basic research to clinical evidence. *Annals of Oncology*, 14, 1468–1476.

Sato, S., Futakuchi, M., Ogawa, K., *et al.* (2008). Transforming growth factor beta derived from bone matrix promotes cell proliferation of prostate cancer and osteoclast activation-associated osteolysis in the bone microenvironment. *Cancer Science*, 99, 316–323.

Schafers, M., Sommer, C., Geis, C., Hagenacker, T., Vandenabeele, P., and Sorkin, L.S. (2008). Selective stimulation of either tumor necrosis factor receptor differentially induces pain behavior in vivo and ectopic activity in sensory neurons in vitro. *Neuroscience*, 157, 414–423.

Scholz, J. and Woolf, C.J. (2007). The neuropathic pain triad: neurons, immune cells and glia. *Nature Neuroscience*, 10(11), 1361–1368.

Schwei, M.J., Honore, P., Rogers, S.D., *et al.* (1999). Neurochemical and cellular reorganization of the spinal cord in a murine model of bone cancer pain. *Journal of Neuroscience*, 19, 10886–10897.

Scott, A.C., McConnell, S., Laird, B., Colvin, L., and Fallon, M. (2012). Quantitative Sensory Testing to assess the sensory characteristics of cancer-induced bone pain after radiotherapy and potential clinical biomarkers of response. *European Journal of Pain*, 16, 123–133.

Seong, J., Park, H.C., Kim, J., Kim, U.J., and Lee, B.W. (2004). Radiation-induced alteration of pain-related signals in an animal model with bone invasion from cancer. *Annals of the New York Academy of Sciences*, 1030, 179–186.

Sevcik, M.A., Luger, N.M., Mach, D.B., *et al.* (2004). Bone cancer pain: the effects of the bisphosphonate alendronate on pain, skeletal remodeling, tumor growth and tumor necrosis. *Pain*, 111, 169–180.

Sevcik, M.A., Ghilardi, J.R., Peters, C.M., *et al.* (2005). Anti-NGF therapy profoundly reduces bone cancer pain and the accompanying increase in markers of peripheral and central sensitization. *Pain*, 115(1–2), 128–141.

Sheng, H., Shao, J., Kirkland, S.C., *et al.* (1997). Inhibition of human colon cancer cell growth by selective inhibition of cyclooxygenase-2. *Journal of Clinical Investigation*, 99, 2254–2259.

Isherwood, R.J., Haraldsottir, E., Allan, G., Colvin, L., and Fallon, M. (2012). Opioid toxicity: the patient experience. EAPC, Trondheim. *Palliative Medicine*, 26(4), 572.

Sluka, K.A., Radhakrishnan, R., Benson, C.J., *et al.* (2007). ASIC3 in muscle mediates mechanical, but not heat, hyperalgesia associated with muscle inflammation. *Pain*, 129, 102–112.

Sonohata, M., Katafuchi, T., Yasaka, T., Doi, A., Kumamoto, E., and Yoshimura, M. (2004). Actions of noradrenaline on substantia gelatinosa neurones in the rat spinal cord revealed by in vivo patch recording. *Journal of Physiology*, 555, 515–526.

Stambaugh, J, Drew J, Stambaugh J, *et al.* (1988). A double-blind parallel evaluation of the efficacy and safety of a single dose of ketoprofen in cancer pain. *Journal of Clinical Pharmacology*, 28, S34–S39.

Stamford, J.A. (1995). Descending control of pain. *British Journal of Anaesthesia*, 75, 217–227.

Staquet, M.J. (1989). A double-blind study with placebo control of intramuscular ketorolac tromethamine in the treatment of cancer pain. *Journal of Clinical Pharmacology*, 29, 1031–1036.

Stewart, A.F. (2005). Clinical practice. Hypercalcaemia associated with cancer. *The New England Journal of Medicine*, 352, 373–379.

Swett, J.E. and Woolf, C.J. (1985). The somatotopic organization of primary afferent terminals in the superficial laminae of the dorsal horn of the rat spinal-cord. *Journal of Comparative Neurology*, 231, 66–77.

Sumitani, K., Kamijo, R., Toyoshima, T., *et al.* (2001). Specific inhibition of cyclooxygenase-2 results in inhibition of proliferation of oral cancer cell lines via suppression of prostaglandin E2 production. *Journal of Oral Pathology & Medicine*, 30, 41–47.

Sunshine, A. and Olson, N.Z. (1988). Analgesic efficacy of ketoprofen in postpartum, general surgery, and chronic cancer pain. *Journal of Clinical Pharmacology*, 28, S47–S54.

Suzuki, R., Rahman, W., Hunt, S.P., and Dickenson, A.H. (2004). Descending facilitatory control of mechanically evoked responses is enhanced in deep dorsal horn neurones following peripheral nerve injury. *Brain Research*, 1019, 68–76.

Todd, A.J. (1996). GABA and glycine in synaptic glomeruli of the rat spinal dorsal horn. *European Journal of Neuroscience*, 8, 2492–2498.

Todd, A.J. (2002). Anatomy of primary afferents and projection neurones in the rat spinal dorsal horn with particular emphasis on substance P and the neurokinin 1 receptor. *Experimental Physiology*, 87, 245–249.

Tracey, I., Ploghaus, A., Gati, J.S., *et al.* (2002). Imaging attentional modulation of pain in the periaqueductal gray in humans. *Journal of Neuroscience*, 22, 2748–2752.

Tsubaki, M., Kato, C., Manno, M., *et al.* (2007). Macrophage inflammatory protein-1alpha (MIP-1alpha) enhances a receptor activator of nuclear factor kappaB ligand (RANKL) expression in mouse bone marrow stromal cells and osteoblasts through MAPK and PI3K/Akt pathways. *Molecular & Cellular Biochemistry*, 304, 53–60.

Twycross, R.G. and Fairfield, S. (1982). Pain in far advanced cancer. *Pain*, 14, 303–310.

Urch, C. (2004). The pathophysiology of cancer-induced bone pain: current understanding. *Palliative Medicine*, 18, 267–274.

Urch, C.E., Donovan-Rodriguez, T., and Dickenson, A.H. (2003). Alterations in dorsal horn neurones in a rat model of cancer-induced bone pain. *Pain*, 106, 347–356.

Urch, C.E., Donovan-Rodriguez, T., Gordon-Williams, R., Bee, L.A., and Dickenson, A.H. (2005). Efficacy of chronic morphine in a rat model of cancer-induced bone pain: behavior and in dorsal horn patho-physiology. *Journal of Pain*, 6, 837–845.

Vadhan-Raj, S., von MR, Fallowfield LJ, *et al.* (2012). Clinical benefit in patients with metastatic bone disease: results of a phase 3 study of denosumab versus zoledronic acid. *Annals of Oncology*, 23, 3045–3051.

Van As, N. and Huddart, R. (2007). Radiotherapy. In A. Davies (ed.) *Cancer-related Bone Pain*, pp. 75–84. Oxford: Oxford University Press.

Vanderah, T.W., Ossipov, M.H., Lai, J., Malan, T.P., and Porreca, F. (2001). Mechanisms of opioid-induced pain and antinociceptive toler-ance: descending facilitation and spinal dynorphin. *Pain*, 92, 5–9.

Vit, J.P., Ohara, P.T., Tien, D.A., *et al.* (2006). The analgesic effect of low dose focal irradiation in a mouse model of bone cancer is associated with spinal changes in neuro-mediators of nociception. *Pain*, 120, 188–201.

Voilley, N. (2004). Acid-sensing ion channels (ASICs): new targets for the analgesic effects of non-steroid anti-inflammatory drugs (NSAIDs). *Current Drug Targets – Inflammation & Allergy*, 3, 71–79.

Von Moos, R. (2005). Bisphosphonate treatment recommendations for oncologists. *Oncologist*, 10(Suppl. 1), 19–24.

Wacnik, P.W., Kehl, L.J., Trempe, T.M., Ramnaraine, M.L., Beitz, A.J., and Wilcox, G.L. (2003). Tumor implantation in mouse humerus evokes movement-related hyperalgesia exceeding that evoked by intramus-cular carrageenan. *Pain*, 101, 175–186.

Wagner, R. and Myers, R.R. (1996). Schwann cells produce tumor necrosis factor alpha: expression in injured and non-injured nerves. *Neuroscience*, 73, 625–662.

Walker, K., Medhurst, S.J., Kidd, B.L., *et al.* (2002). Disease modifying and anti-nociceptive effects of the bisphosphonate, zoledronic acid in a model of bone cancer pain. *Pain*, 100, 219–229.

Wall, P.D. (1967). The laminar organization of dorsal horn and effects of descending impulses. *Journal of Physiology*, 188, 403–423.

Wang, H. and Woolf, C.J. (2005). Pain TRPs. *Neuron*, 46, 9–1.

Wang, L.N., Yang, J.P., Zhan, Y., *et al.* (2012a). Minocycline-induced reduction in brain-derived neurotrophic factor expression in rela-tion to cancer-induced bone pain in rats. *Journal of Neuroscience Research*, 90, 672–681.

Wang, L.N., Yao, M., Yang, J.P., *et al.* (2011). Cancer-induced bone pain sequentially activates the ERK/MAPK pathway in different cell types in the rat spinal cord. *Molecular Pain*, 7, 48.

Wang, X.W., Li, T.T., Zhao, J., *et al.* (2012b). Extracellular signal-regulated kinase activation in spinal astrocytes and microglia contributes to cancer-induced bone pain in rats. *Neuroscience*, 217, 172–181.

Ward, W.G., Holsenbeck, S., Dorey, F.J., Spang, J., and Howe, D. (2003). Metastatic disease of the femur: surgical treatment. *Clinical Orthopaedics and Related Research*, 415(Suppl.), S230–244.

Watkins, L.R., Hutchinson, M.R., Johnston, I.N., and Maier, S.F. (2005). Glia: novel counter-regulators of opioid analgesia. *Trends in Neurosciences*, 28, 661–669.

Welsh, M.J., Price, M.P., and Xie, J. (2002). Biochemical basis of touch perception: mechanosensory function of degenerin/epithelial Na+ channels. *Journal of Biological Chemistry*, 277, 2369–2372.

Wemmie, J.A., Price, M.P., and Welsh, M.J. (2006). Acid-sensing ion chan-nels: advances, questions and therapeutic opportunities. *Trends in Neurosciences*, 29, 578–586.

Wiesenfeld-Hallin, Z., Aldskogius, H., Grant, G., Hao, J.X., Hokfelt, T., and Xu, X.J. (1997). Central inhibitory dysfunctions: mechanisms and clinical implications. *Behavioral and Brain Sciences*, 20, 420–425.

Willis, W.D. and Coggeshall, R.E. (1991). *Sensory Mechanisms of the Spinal Cord*. New York: Plenum Press.

Woolf, C.J. (2007). Central sensitization: uncovering the relation between pain and plasticity. *Anesthesiology*, 106, 864–867.

Woolf, C.J. and Fitzgerald, M. (1986). Somatotopic organization of cutane-ous afferent terminals and dorsal horn neuronal receptive fields in the superficial and deep laminae of the rat lumbar spinal cord. *Journal of Complementary Neurology*, 251, 517–531.

Woolf, C.J., Ma, Q.-P., Allchorne, A., and Poole, S. (1996). Peripheral cell types contributing to the hyperalgesic action of nerve growth factor in inflammation. *The Journal of Neuroscience*, 16(9), 2716–2723.

Wong, R. (2007). Bisphosphonates for bone pain. In A. Davies (ed.) *Cancer-related Bone Pain*, pp. 61–74. Oxford: Oxford University Press.

Wong, R., Shukla, V., Mensinkai, S., and Wiffen, P (2004). *Bisphosphonate Agents for the Management of Pain Secondary to Bone Metastases: A Systematic Review of Effectiveness and Safety.* Technology Report Number 45. Ottawa: Canadian Coordinating Office for Health Technology Assessment.

Wong, R. and Wiffen, P.J. (2002). Bisphosphonates for the relief of pain secondary to bone metastases. *Cochrane Database of Systematic Reviews*, 2, CD002068.

Yamamoto, J., Kawamata, T., Niiyama, Y., Omote, K., and Namiki, A. (2008). Down-regulation of mu opioid receptor expression within distinct subpopulations of dorsal root ganglion neurons in a murine model of bone cancer pain. *Neuroscience*, 151, 843–853.

Yuan, J., Liu, C., Liu, X., *et al.* (2013). Efficacy and safety of 177Lu-EDTMP in bone metastatic pain palliation in breast cancer and hormone refractory prostate cancer: a phase II study. *Clinical Nuclear Medicine*, 38, 88–92.

Zeng, L., Chow, E., Bedard, G., *et al.* (2012a). Quality of life after palliative radiation therapy for patients with painful bone metastases: results of an international study validating the EORTC QLQ-BM22. *International Journal of Radiation Oncology, Biology, Physics*, 84, e337–e342.

Zeng, L., Chow, E., Zhang, L., *et al.* (2012b). An international prospec-tive study establishing minimal clinically important differences in the EORTC QLQ-BM22 and QLQ-C30 in cancer patients with bone metastases. *Supportive Care in Cancer*, 20, 3307–3313.

Zeppetella, J. (2007). Conventional analgesics for bone pain. In A. Davies (ed.) *Cancer-related Bone Pain*, pp. 53–58. Oxford: Oxford University Press.

Zeppetella, G., O'Doherty, C.A., and Collins, S. (2000). Prevalence and characteristics of breakthrough pain in cancer patients admit-ted to a hospice. *Journal of Pain and Symptom Management*, 20, 87–92.

Zeppetella, G. and Ribeiro, M.D. (2006). Opioids for the management of breakthrough (episodic) pain in cancer patients. *Cochrane Database of Systematic Reviews*, 1, CD004311.

Zhang, C., Yang, S.W., Guo, Y.G., Qiao, J.T., and Dafny, N. (1997). Locus coeruleus stimulation modulates the nociceptive response in parafas-cicular neurons: an analysis of descending and ascending pathways. *Brain Research Bulletin*, 42, 273–278.

Zhang, L., Guan, Z., and He, Y. (1997). Randomized comparative clinic trial of treatment of bone metastatic diseases by infusion of pamidro-nate and clodronate. *Chinese Journal of Cancer*, 16, 340–432.

Zhang, R.X., Li, A., Liu, B., *et al.* (2007). Electroacupuncture attenuates bone cancer pain and inhibits spinal interleukin-1 beta expression in a rat model. *Anesthesia & Analgesia*, 105, 1482–1488.

Zhang, R.X., Liu, B., Wang, L., *et al.* (2005). Spinal glial activation in a new rat model of bone cancer pain produced by prostate cancer cell inoculation of the tibia. *Pain*, 118, 125–136.

Zheng, Q., Fang, D., Liu, M., *et al.* (2013). Suppression of KCNQ/M (Kv7) potassium channels in dorsal root ganglion neurons contributes to the development of bone cancer pain in a rat model. *Pain*, 154, 434–448.

13.3

Management issues in neuropathic pain

Nanna Brix Finnerup and Troels Staehelin Jensen

Introduction to management issues in neuropathic pain

Neuropathic pain is a heterogeneous group of chronic pain conditions arising from a lesion or disease of the peripheral or central somatosensory nervous system (Jensen et al., 2011). The responsible lesion may be of any type and occur at any location along the sensory transmission pathways. Neuropathic pain is commonly divided into peripheral and central neuropathic pain, and further classified according to anatomical site and disease (Table 13.3.1).

Neuropathic pain may be challenging therapeutically and have a substantial impact on quality of life, sleep, and mood. Treatment often is difficult and may involve interventions distinct from those typically used for nociceptive pains. Given these challenges, awareness of the various neuropathic pain syndromes and an

Table 13.3.1 Classification of neuropathic pain

Peripheral	Central
Mono- and polyneuropathy	
diabetes	Multiple sclerosis
alcohol	
HIV	
chemotherapy	
other	
Plexopathy	Neoplasms
Radiculopathy	Spinal cord injury
Nerve injury:	
postsurgical	Syringomyelia
post-traumatic	
Amputation:	
phantom limb pain	Myelopathy
stump pain	
Root avulsion	Stroke
Post-herpetic neuralgia	
Trigeminal neuralgia	
Neoplasms	

understanding of issues related to assessment and treatment may lead to better recognition and improved outcomes.

Clinical characteristics

Neuropathic pain may develop immediately after a nerve injury or disease or occur as a late effect, often after several months. The pain is likely to be chronic and is characterized by spontaneous and evoked types of pain perceived in areas of sensory abnormality, either hyposensitivity and/or hypersensitivity. In certain cases, neuropathic pain may develop as an acute pain, for example, cold-evoked pain after treatment with the chemotherapeutic drug, oxaliplatin.

Spontaneous pain may be ongoing, with a constant or fluctuating pain intensity, or dominated by pain paroxysms of short duration with pain-free intervals or a less intense background pain. Other sensations, such as paraesthesia (abnormal sensation that is not painful or unpleasant) and dysaesthesia (unpleasant abnormal sensation) may be present spontaneously or occur only when evoked by a stimulus (Merskey and Bogduk, 1994). Allodynia is a type of evoked pain that is elicited by a non-noxious stimulation. Dynamic mechanical allodynia or touch-evoked allodynia is the most common form, but allodynia to cold or warm may also be present. Hyperalgesia, which describes an increased response to a stimulus that is normally painful, also is often present but usually not described as a symptom by the patient.

Definition and diagnosis of neuropathic pain

Neuropathic pain is defined as pain caused by a lesion or disease of the somatosensory system (Jensen et al., 2011). To diagnose neuropathic pain, an effort must be made to demonstrate a nervous system lesion, a relevant onset of pain related to this, and a location of pain in areas of sensory disturbance that are neuroanatomically compatible with the lesion (Treede et al., 2008). The diagnosis cannot rely on single pain descriptors and is not always easy to confirm in the absence of clear diagnostic criteria. The diagnosis may be particularly challenging when sensory loss is masked by areas of hypersensitivity, and when neuropathic and nociceptive components to the pain occur together. The latter is often the case in cancer patients, where nociceptive muscle, bone, visceral pain, etc. is often mixed with neuropathic pain, making the clinical picture difficult to elucidate (Vadalouca et al., 2012).

A medical history, including a detailed pain history and a careful medical and neurological examination, is essential (Haanpaa et al., 2011). The neurological examination is essential for the diagnosis of neuropathic pain and should include a careful sensory examination evaluating decreased or increased responses to touch, vibration, pinprick, and thermal stimuli, as well as a mapping of the distribution of the sensory dysfunction. At times, additional diagnostic testing, such as scanning with computed tomography or magnetic resonance imaging, electromyography and nerve conduction velocity testing, or nerve biopsy may be indicated. Electromyography and nerve conduction velocity testing only assess large-fibre function and may be supplemented with quantitative sensory testing using thermal testing to identify a small fibre neuropathy.

Tools have been developed for identifying patients with neuropathic pain based on clusters of symptoms and signs: the Leeds Assessment of Neuropathic Symptoms and Signs (LANNS scale) (Bennett 2001), the ten-item questionnaire DN4 (Bouhassira et al., 2005), the Neuropathic Pain Questionnaire (NPQ) (Krause and Backonja 2003), painDETECT (Freynhagen et al., 2006), and the ID-Pain (Portenoy 2006). While these questionnaires, which include descriptors like burning pain, painful cold, electric shocks, pins and needles, tingling, numbness, and itching, are useful for epidemiological research, the diagnosis of neuropathic pain cannot be confirmed on the basis of these tools alone, but should always be accompanied by a clinical examination (Haanpaa et al., 2011).

Neuropathic pain syndromes

Neuropathic pain may occur in many advanced progressive diseases. Any disease affecting the nervous system, including cancer, HIV/AIDS, stroke, herpes zoster, diabetic polyneuropathy, chemotherapy-induced neuropathy, and multiple sclerosis may cause neuropathic pain. Description of all neuropathic pain syndromes is beyond the scope of this chapter and only some with special reference to palliative care will be mentioned here.

Neuropathic pain syndromes have become an increasing problem in cancer patients, affecting up to 40% of patients (Caraceni and Portenoy, 1999; Forman, 2004). In a recent systematic review including 22 studies and 13 683 patients with active cancer and pain, 19% (95% confidence interval (CI) 9.4–28.4%) had neuropathic pain, and a liberal estimate of 39.1% (95% CI 28.9–49.5%) was calculated when patients with mixed pain were included (Bennett et al., 2012). This study also suggested that a greater proportion of neuropathic pain in cancer patients is caused by cancer treatment or comorbid disease compared with all cancer pain. Neuropathic pain conditions may persist independently of the cancer and affect the quality of life in disease-free cancer survivors. In those with active disease, painful mononeuropathy or plexopathy often is caused by direct infiltration of peripheral nerves by the cancer. Neuropathic pain is also a frequent complication of treatment of cancer including cancer surgery (Kehlet et al., 2006; Nikolajsen and Jensen, 2006; Gartner et al., 2009; Hoimyr et al., 2011; Wildgaard et al., 2011) and radio therapy. Polyneuropathy may occur in association with malnutrition or paraneoplastic syndromes, which may affect as many as 5% of patients (Forman, 2004). Probably of more importance is painful peripheral polyneuropathy as a complication of treatment with specific types of chemotherapy (Forman, 2004). Chemotherapy-induced neuropathy usually is a dose-dependent, cumulative side effect with the 'glove-and-stocking' distribution. Symptoms include sensory loss, paraesthesia, dysaesthesia, and pain sometimes accompanied with muscle weakness. Oxaliplatin-induced neuropathy is characteristic as it has an acute phase characterized with cold allodynia and pricking dysaesthesia affecting hands and feet but also characteristic pharyngolaryngeal dysaesthesia with sensations of shortness of breath or swallowing difficulties induced by cold drinks (Leonard et al., 2005; Binder et al., 2007; Attal et al., 2009).

Distal sensory, predominantly axonal, polyneuropathy is the most common form of neuropathy associated with HIV and occurs in about one-third of patients (Evans et al., 2011). Immunological dysfunction secondary to the HIV infection itself and toxicity caused by nucleoside antiretroviral agents are thought to be the two most important mechanisms (Evans et al., 2011).

Central pain develops in about 8% of stroke patients, 25% of patients with multiple sclerosis, and 40–50% of patients with spinal cord injury; brain and spinal cord tumours, and other diseases affecting the central nervous system, are other, less common, causes of central pain (Klit et al., 2009; Wasner 2010).

Herpes zoster is due to reactivation of varicella zoster infection and occurs most often in later life and in immunocompromised patients, such as those with HIV infection. The most common and disabling complication is post-herpetic neuralgia, which is characterized by steady burning and paroxysmal, lancinating pain in the affected dermatome, often associated with allodynia.

Pharmacological treatment of neuropathic pain

Treating neuropathic pain remains a great challenge. The drugs that are used commonly for these disorders have limited response rates, and typically responders experience only partial reduction in pain at tolerable doses. Neuropathic pain treatment is often symptomatic, but in some cases, for example, in the use of corticosteroids for the treatment of compression of spinal cord or peripheral nerve, the underlying cause of neuropathic pain can be treated. Today, more than 170 randomized controlled trials (RCTs) support decision-making and provide a basis for evidence-based treatment algorithms (Finnerup et al., 2010). Few comparative drug trials exist, however, and the most rational approach to comparing treatments involves calculation of the number needed to treat (NNT) and the number needed to harm (NNH) from clinical trials data. NNT is calculated as the number of patients needed to treat with a certain drug to obtain one patient with a defined degree of pain reduction (usually 50%) and is calculated as the reciprocal of the absolute risk reduction. NNH is likewise calculated as the reciprocal of the absolute difference in risk, with risk defined as side effects or dropouts. In the following, only double-blind RCTs will be considered.

Anticonvulsants

Anticonvulsant drugs are used primarily for the treatment of epilepsy. They have several pharmacological actions that can interfere with processes involved in neuronal hyperexcitability, either by decreasing excitatory or increasing inhibitory transmission, thereby exerting a net neuronal depressant effect. These effects may underlie the analgesic effects that some of these drugs exert in neuropathic pain states.

Gabapentin and pregabalin

Gabapentin and pregabalin are structurally related compounds. Their analgesic effect in neuropathic pain is thought to be mediated through antagonism of the $\alpha_2\delta$ subunit of voltage-dependent calcium channels at presynaptic sites (Sills 2006).

The effects of gabapentin and pregabalin are well established in post-herpetic neuralgia, painful diabetic neuropathy, and spinal cord injury pain (Finnerup et al., 2010), and also in neuropathic cancer pain (Mishra et al., 2012). Both drugs seem equally effective, with NNTs ranging from 4.2 to 6.4. The pain relief is rapid, within the first or second week, and often accompanied by improvements in sleep and quality of life measures. The effects of gabapentin in HIV neuropathy and peripheral nerve injury are inconclusive (Phillips et al., 2010).

Both gabapentin and pregabalin are generally well tolerated. Neither drug has any known drug–drug interactions. Somnolence and dizziness are the most common side effects and peripheral oedema, weight gain, nausea, vertigo, asthenia, dry mouth, and ataxia may occur. Side effects may resolve over time or improve with dose reduction. Gabapentin is usually administered three times daily. Dosing is initiated slowly, for example, starting with 300 mg the first day and increased by 300 mg every 1–7 days. The final daily dose is between 1800 and 3600 mg, but side effects may limit dose escalation. Pregabalin may be initiated with 75 or 150 mg daily and increased every 3–7 days by 150 mg, up to 600 mg in two divided doses. Both gabapentin and pregabalin undergo renal excretion and renal impairment requires dosage adjustment. Pregabalin has anxiolytic effects in patients with generalized anxiety disorders (Frampton and Foster, 2006) and may therefore be the first drug choice in patients with anxiety. It is still unknown whether patients failing to respond to one of these drugs will benefit from the other.

Other anticonvulsants

The main action of carbamazepine, and its analogue oxcarbazepine, is blocking of sodium channels. Carbamazepine and oxcarbazepine are first-line drugs for trigeminal neuralgia (Zakrzewska and McMillan, 2011). Newer trials comparing oxcarbazepine to carbamazepine have reported comparable analgesic effects, but fewer side effects during oxcarbazepine treatment. Additional studies have not confirmed clinically significant effects on other neuropathic pain conditions (Finnerup et al., 2010).

Carbamazepine treatment is associated with cognitive side effects, drowsiness, dizziness, ataxia, diplopia, and, in elderly patients, confusion (Rogvi-Hansen and Gram, 1995). Other side effects include rash, nausea, weight gain, and hyponatraemia. Slow titration is needed to minimize side effects. In rare cases, severe blood dyscrasia may be seen and a full blood count should be obtained prior to treatment and continuously throughout treatment. Carbamazepine has several drug interactions and is contraindicated in patients with atrioventricular block and hepatic insufficiency. Oxcarbazepine is generally better tolerated but side effects include drowsiness, ataxia, diplopia, dizziness, headache, hyponatraemia, rash, and nausea. Carbamazepine is usually initiated with 300 mg/day and increased by 100 mg every other day to a maximum dosage of 1500–2000 mg/day. The starting dose of oxcarbazepine may be 600 mg/day, increased by 150–300 mg every other day to 1500–3000 mg/day.

Lamotrigine and valproate have limited roles in the treatment of neuropathic pain as results from RCTs are conflicting (Finnerup et al., 2010).

Antidepressants

Antidepressants have a well-established beneficial effect on various neuropathic pain states. Antidepressants used in neuropathic pain treatment include tricyclic antidepressants (TCAs) (e.g. amitriptyline and imipramine) and the selective serotonin noradrenaline reuptake inhibitors (SNRIs) (duloxetine and venlafaxine). The analgesic effects of the selective serotonin reuptake inhibitors (SSRIs) are less certain (Sindrup et al., 2005). Antidepressants relieve pain in non-depressed patients, and it is well established that their pain-relieving effects are independent of their antidepressant effects. However, because of this dual effect, antidepressants may be the first drug of choice in patients with a coexisting depression.

Tricyclic antidepressants

Several randomized controlled trials have documented the effect of TCAs in different neuropathic pain conditions with NNT values ranging from 2.1 to 2.8 (Finnerup et al., 2010) and are also suggested effective in neuropathic cancer pain (Mishra et al., 2012). As the majority of TCA trials are small cross-over trials with results that are not based on the intention-to-treat population and with low placebo responses, the NNT values cannot be directly compared with those from gabapentin, pregabalin, and duloxetine trials. In HIV-related neuropathy, amitriptyline failed to relieve neuropathic pain in two randomized trials (Phillips et al., 2010). Nortriptyline up to 100 mg/day was evaluated in the treatment of cis-diamminedichloroplatinum (CDDP)-induced dysaesthesia in a randomized trial (Hammack et al., 2002). Nortriptyline only provided modest relief of dysaesthesia and pain.

Anticholinergic side effects are common during TCA therapy and include dry mouth, constipation, urinary retention, sweating, and blurred vision. The risk of somnolence and confusion may be present when initiating treatment, and the risk is increased in elderly patients and others predisposed to such side effects, including patients treated with concomitant centrally acting drugs. Orthostatic hypotension and gait disturbances are concerns, especially in the elderly. Combination with class IC antiarrhythmics or SSRIs that are metabolized by cytochrome P450 2D6 may cause toxic serum levels of TCAs. TCAs are contraindicated in patients with epilepsy.

The most serious side effect of TCAs is cardiotoxicity. TCAs are contraindicated in patients with heart failure and cardiac conduction blocks, and an electrocardiogram is needed before initiating treatment. A recent large retrospective cohort study found that TCAs in doses of 100 mg or more daily were associated with increased relative risk of sudden cardiac death, which suggests that such doses should be used cautiously, particularly in patients with an elevated baseline risk of sudden death (Ray et al., 2004). The secondary amines (desipramine and nortriptyline) may be better tolerated than tertiary amines (imipramine, amitriptyline, and clomipramine), with imipramine causing fewer sedating side effects than amitriptyline (McQuay et al., 1996).

Initiation of TCA treatment is best done slowly, starting with 25 mg daily (10 mg in the elderly) and slowly increasing (25 mg every 3–7 days) up to 50–150 mg daily. There is a large pharmacokinetic variability in the metabolic pathways of TCAs due to a genetic polymorphism of the enzymes that metabolize these drugs. Some patients may therefore attain high plasma drug concentrations at normal doses, while others may have subtherapeutic concentrations at such doses, and monitoring of serum drug concentrations may be helpful in guiding treatment.

Selective serotonin noradrenaline reuptake inhibitors

Recent randomized trials have documented the effect of venlafaxine and duloxetine in painful diabetic polyneuropathy and chemotherapy-induced painful peripheral neuropathy (Finnerup et al., 2010; Smith et al., 2013). The combined NNT from these five trials of SNRIs in painful polyneuropathy was 5.0 (3.9–6.8). The effect of duloxetine was present from week 1, and the most effective dose, associated with fewest side effects, was 60 mg once daily. Only one randomized trial has studied bupropion in neuropathic pain (Semenchuk and Davis 2000). Results were positive. This drug is less sedating than other antidepressants and therefore tolerated better in patients with fatigue or sedation.

The SNRIs are generally well tolerated, and side effects tend to decrease with continued treatment (Stahl et al., 2005). The most common side effect is nausea. Other side effects include somnolence, dizziness, constipation, anorexia, and hyperhidrosis. Sexual dysfunction with decreased libido, ejaculation failure, and erectile dysfunction related to serotonergic actions has been reported for the SNRIs, as well as for the SSRIs (Stahl et al., 2005). Regular monitoring of blood pressure is recommended during venlafaxine treatment due to risk of elevated blood pressure. Duloxetine should not be used in patients with hepatic dysfunction, and venlafaxine dose should be decreased in patients with renal or hepatic insufficiency. Duloxetine can be started at 30 mg once daily and increased to 60 mg once daily after one week, and venlafaxine should be initiated with 37.5 mg and increased by 75 mg weekly up to 150–225 mg daily.

Topical lidocaine

Randomized trials have shown positive effects of a lidocaine patch 5% in post-herpetic neuralgia and mixed peripheral focal neuropathy with allodynia (Meier et al., 2003; Rowbotham et al., 1996).

Side effects from the lidocaine patch are mild, usually skin irritation. Lack of systemic side effects is favourable, particularly in the treatment of the elderly and in patients prone to side effects. It also may be useful as add-on therapy due to the lack of interference with systemic treatment. Although there is minimal absorption, it should not be used in patients taking oral class I antiarrhythmic drugs. A maximum of three to four patches should be applied for 12 hours per day.

Opioids in neuropathic pain

Neuropathic pain responds to opioids with an effect size similar to antidepressants and gabapentin/pregabalin with no proven difference between various opioids (oxycodone, morphine, methadone, levorphanol, and tramadol) (Raja et al., 2002; Arbaiza and Vidal 2007; Finnerup et al., 2010). The combined NNT in peripheral neuropathic pain range from 2.6 to 5.1. In a recent evidence-based guideline for the use of opioid analgesics in the treatment of cancer pain, there was a weak recommendation that patients receiving step II opioids who do not achieve adequate analgesia and have side effects that are severe or unmanageable, might benefit from switching to an alternative opioid, although there are no RCTs to support this (Quigley 2004; Caraceni et al., 2012). In chronic non-cancer pain, opioids are not first-line analgesics and long-term therapy is generally considered only after other reasonable therapies have failed to provide adequate pain relief (Kalso et al., 2003).

Other pharmacological agents

N-methyl-D-aspartate receptor (NMDA) antagonists

NMDA antagonists given as intravenous infusions have been shown to relieve varied types of neuropathic pain, but the effects of oral NMDA antagonists, such as dextromethorphan, riluzole and memantine, have been less convincing because of low response rates and unfavourable therapeutic indices (Finnerup et al., 2010). In cancer patients on morphine therapy, IV ketamine improved analgesia, but the study also pointed out the need to take central adverse effects into account (Mercadante et al., 2000). A recent RCT could not, however, confirm the efficacy of ketamine for opioid refractory cancer pain, although it did suggest that some patients could be 'good responders' (Salas et al., 2012).

Cannabinoids

Cannabinoids have recently been studied in a few RCTs with positive outcomes (Lynch and Campbell, 2011). Cannabinoids were generally well tolerated with gradually increasing doses. Side effects include dizziness, drowsiness, impaired psychomotor function, and dry mouth, especially during the run-in period, and other psychoactive effects like dysphoria (Rice, 2008). Cannabinoid use is associated with concerns about abuse and addiction as well as legal and regulatory issues. Cannabinoids have antiemetic effects and improve appetite, and may therefore be considered for treating neuropathic pain in patients with AIDS-related wasting disease or in the palliative care of patients with nausea and decreased appetite (Hall et al., 2005).

Capsaicin

Capsaicin is thought to act by depleting substance P from primary afferent nociceptors. Recently, studies have found at least a 12-week modest pain reduction following application of a single high-concentration capsaicin patch on painful polyneuropathy and post-herpetic neuralgia (Finnerup et al., 2010; Wallace and Pappagallo 2011). The effect size is rather small and the application of capsaicin is painful and requires prior application of a local anaesthetic, but the treatment has long-term effect and no or only limited systemic exposure and systemic side effects, suggesting that it may be a safe treatment option. A cutaneous patch of capsaicin 8%, has been given marketing authorization in Europe with the indication: 'treatment of peripheral neuropathic pain in non-diabetic adults' and US Food and Drug Administration approval for post-herpetic neuralgia (Wallace and Pappagallo, 2011).

Botulinum toxin type A

Botulinum toxin has been found to have antihyperalgesic effects and thus may be of potential value in treating chronic pain conditions. Botulinum toxin type A injected intradermally in the painful area has been shown to relieve painful neuropathy (Ranoux et al., 2008; Yuan et al., 2009). Besides pain upon application, the treatment had no further local or systemic side effects. Future studies are needed to determine if the long-term effect is consistent.

Combination therapy

If treatment with a single drug is only partly effective, other drugs may be added. In patients with painful diabetic neuropathy or post-herpetic neuralgia, high quality studies have documented greater pain relief and less pain interference with the combination of gabapentinoids and TCAs or opioids, than the single drugs alone (Gilron et al., 2005, 2009; Achar et al., 2010). Also in patients with cancer related neuropathic pain, gabapentin (400 mg) in combination with imipramine (20 mg) as add-on therapy caused a greater pain reduction than in patients in the monotherapy groups (Arai et al., 2010).

In the late stages of cancer, three-quarters of patients have pain, and will usually be treated with opioids when decisions regarding adding other analgesics are made (Lussier et al., 2004), but if patients do not have nociceptive pain, initiation with an antidepressant or gabapentinoid is advised. In cancer patients treated with opioids for nociceptive cancer pain, adding an additional analgesic for neuropathic pain may also allow for reduction of opioid dose. In mixed cancer patients with neuropathic pain partially controlled with opioids, amitriptyline had no pain-relieving effect and was associated with adverse effects (Mercadante et al., 2002). The treatment period was, however, short (1 week) and the dose was relatively low (up to 50 mg daily). In another RCT in cancer patients with neuropathic pain already treated with opioids, gabapentin improved analgesia (Caraceni et al., 2004). In a systematic review including also open-label studies, the addition of an antiepileptic or antidepressant to existing opioid analgesia was shown to result in modest improvement in pain, but also to cause significantly more adverse events (Bennett, 2011). It was suggested that better outcomes might be achieved if opioid doses are reduced initially when first-line drugs for neuropathic pain is commenced and both drugs are then titrated according to response.

While some combinations reduce side effects, others may cause intolerable side effects. Sedation, dizziness, nausea, and other side effects needs to be monitored carefully and it is important to be aware of specific side effects, for example, the serotonergic syndrome that may occur when combining, for example, tramadol with serotonin reuptake inhibitors.

Because of possible additive side effects, risk of medication overuse, and noncompliance, it is generally preferable to minimize polypharmacy (Gilron and Max 2005). Therefore, when combination therapy is needed, sequential add-on therapy is recommended in patients who show a partial response to the first or both drugs given alone and a rational approach is to use drugs with complementary modes of actions. During the course of pain treatment, the level and character of the pain, and side effects should be monitored and dose adjustments should be made. Despite common clinical practice and rationale for combination therapy, we still lack important information on combination therapy including which drugs to combine, optimal dosing and dose titration methods, combinations that include non-pharmacological treatment, responder analysis, long-term effects and side effects, adherence to therapy, and cost-effectiveness.

Pre-emptive treatment

Chronic postoperative pain may be limited when minimally invasive techniques are used, presumably with less risk of damaging major nerves (Kehlet et al., 2006). Although pre-emptive or preventive analgesia may be able to accomplish the same result, studies that have evaluated the use of aggressive or multimodal analgesia in the perioperative period have yielded contradictory results regarding the effect on chronic pain (Kehlet et al., 2006).

Few studies in non-surgical neuropathic pain have evaluated the effect of early treatment in preventing or reducing pain. A study that compared low-dose amitriptyline 25 mg daily with placebo during the initial 90 days after eruption of herpes zoster, found that the active drug reduced pain prevalence at 6 months by more than 50% (Bowsher, 1997). In the prevention of chemotherapy-induced neuropathy, venlafaxine reduced the number of patients experiencing acute neurologic toxicity following oxaliplatin treatment (Durand et al., 2012). These studies were small and results need to be replicated in larger prospective trials. In another study, amitriptyline with a target dose of 100 mg daily for the duration of the chemotherapy did not prevent neuropathy (Kautio et al., 2009). However, in this study, neuropathic symptoms were mild and outcomes were not limited to pain but included also loss of sensory and motor function, which are probably less likely to be prevented by amitriptyline. Neuroprotective agents may, combined with chemotherapy regimens, protect peripheral nerves from chemotherapeutic injury with preserved control of malignancy (Forman, 2004). Such agents, for example, vitamin E or sulphur-containing thiol drugs, are under investigation as neuroprotective agents preventing chronic neuropathy caused by chemotherapy or antiviral AIDS treatment.

Non-pharmacological treatment

When chronic pain is severe or associated with a high level of disability, concurrent treatment with multiple modalities via a multidisciplinary approach may be preferred. There is increasing evidence for the effect of cognitive behavioural therapy in chronic pain (Morley et al., 1999; Turk and Flor, 2006). Cognitive behavioural therapy includes a variety of approaches, including cognitive reconstructuring and coping strategies, problem solving, relaxation training, attention–diversion techniques, assertiveness training, and modification in activity and exposure to feared activities.

Physiotherapy may be indicated in some patients with neuropathic pain to alleviate complications related to immobility or to other effects of the neurological disease. Nociceptive pain contributing to overall pain intensity and disability may be reduced by techniques that may include correcting poor posture, dystonia and contractures, passive mobilization, stretching and massage, and active exercise. The evidence for the use of different non-pharmacological management strategies, for example, massage, acupuncture, fitness and mind–body techniques, to enhance pain management of neuropathic pain associated with cancer has been summarized (Cassileth and Keefe, 2010). Other non-pharmacological treatments such as sympathetic blockade, spinal cord and motor cortex stimulation, and neurosurgery may be considered in severe refractory pain, but depend on many factors such as pain type, and life expectancy.

General treatment principles

A broad approach to the treatment of chronic neuropathic pain is essential. Patients may be elderly; may have concurrent medical problems and impairments, depression, sleep disturbances, or psychosocial problems; and may be treated with multiple drugs with unwanted side effects. The diagnosis of the neuropathic pain syndrome and the presumptive underlying mechanisms is the first important step and requires a thorough assessment. The diagnosis of neuropathic pain is not always easy, and often neuropathic pain coexists with other types of pain, particularly in palliative care. Whenever possible, the underlying disease should be treated. Whether or not the underlying mechanisms causing the pain can be treated, symptomatic treatment of pain and related disability should be offered. Realistic expectations for the outcome of a given treatment should be discussed with the patient, explaining that often only partial pain relief from neuropathic pain can be expected.

As analgesic therapies are applied, the effects are unpredictable and patients with the same disease or same symptom may respond differently to the same treatment. There is little evidence to support the use of specific drugs for specific symptoms and at the present time, treatment of neuropathic pain is a 'trial-and-error' process. Although a mechanism-based treatment approach has been suggested, future trials will tell whether pain mechanisms can be identified in an individual patient, and whether specific symptoms and signs, or clusters, will be able to predict response to certain treatments.

Treatment algorithm

Although a general treatment algorithm may be proposed, each treatment has to be individualized to each patient, taking into account all co-morbidities and drug interactions. Most randomized controlled trials are performed in patients with diabetic polyneuropathy and post-herpetic neuralgia, and to what extent a treatment, which is found effective in one neuropathic pain condition, can be expected to relieve other conditions, is unknown (Dworkin et al., 2011). Based on experience, it seems likely that efficacy demonstrated in one condition can be extrapolated to others (Hansson and Dickenson 2005). There are clearly exceptions, however, and the existing studies, albeit very limited, suggest that some disorders, such as HIV-related pain, may be more difficult to treat, although these studies may have had low assay-sensitivity because of high placebo responses.

During the course of pain treatment, the level and character of the pain, and side effects should be monitored. If there is no effect of a first-line drug, the treatment should be switched to another first-line drug, then ultimately to a second line drug. In case of partial pain relief, another drug with complementary mechanisms can be added. Treatment algorithms for neuropathic pain have recently been updated (Attal 2010; Attal et al., 2010; Dworkin et al., 2010).

First-line treatments

In patients with trigeminal neuralgia, carbamazepine and oxcarbazepine are the first drug choices. In other neuropathic pain conditions, tricyclic antidepressants, SNRIs (duloxetine or venlafaxine), or calcium channel $\alpha_2\delta$ agonists (gabapentin or pregabalin) are the first drug choices. In patients with focal peripheral neuropathy with allodynia, topical lidocaine patch is also a first-line drug. Antidepressants may be the first drug choice in patients with depression, and both TCAs and calcium channel $\alpha_2\delta$ agonists may be considered in patients with sleep disturbances. Pregabalin may be the first choice in patients with anxiety.

Second-line treatments

Opioids (including tramadol) may be considered if there is no, or insufficient, effect of first-line drug classes and may be first line in episodic pain or in patients with co-existing cancer-related non-neuropathic pain. Switching from one opioid to another may improve pain relief. Combination therapy may be considered in patients with insufficient effect from one drug.

References

Attal, N. (2010). Management of neuropathic cancer pain. *Annals of Oncology*, 21, 1134–1135.

Attal, N., Cruccu, G., Baron, R., *et al.* (2010). EFNS guidelines on the pharmacological treatment of neuropathic pain: 2010 revision. *European Journal of Neurology*, 17, 1113–e88.

Bennett, M.I. (2011). Effectiveness of antiepileptic or antidepressant drugs when added to opioids for cancer pain: systematic review. *Palliative Medicine*, 25, 553–559.

Bennett, M.I., Rayment, C., Hjermstad, M., Aass, N., Caraceni, A., Kaasa, S. (2012). Prevalence and aetiology of neuropathic pain in cancer patients: a systematic review. *Pain*, 153, 359–365.

Caraceni, A. and Portenoy, R.K. (1999). An international survey of cancer pain characteristics and syndromes. IASP Task Force on Cancer Pain. International Association for the Study of Pain. *Pain*, 82, 263–274.

Caraceni, A., Zecca, E., Bonezzi, C., *et al.* (2004). Gabapentin for neuropathic cancer pain: a randomized controlled trial from the Gabapentin Cancer Pain Study Group. *Journal of Clinical Oncology*, 22, 2909–2917.

Caraceni, A., Hanks, G., Kaasa, S., *et al.* (2012). Use of opioid analgesics in the treatment of cancer pain: evidence-based recommendations from the EAPC. *The Lancet Oncology*, 13, e58–e68.

Cassileth, B.R. and Keefe, F.J. (2010). Integrative and behavioral approaches to the treatment of cancer-related neuropathic pain. *Oncologist*, 15(Suppl. 2), 19–23.

Dworkin, R.H., O'Connor, A.B., Audette, J., *et al.* (2010). Recommendations for the pharmacological management of neuropathic pain: an overview and literature update. *Mayo Clinic Proceedings*, 85, S3–14.

Evans, S.R., Ellis, R.J., Chen, H., *et al.* (2011). Peripheral neuropathy in HIV: prevalence and risk factors. *AIDS*, 25, 919–928.

Finnerup, N.B., Sindrup, S.H., Jensen, T.S. (2010). The evidence for pharmacological treatment of neuropathic pain. *Pain*, 150, 573–581.

Forman, A.D. (2004). Peripheral neuropathy and cancer. *Current Oncology Reports*, 6, 20–25.

Gartner, R., Jensen, M.B., Nielsen, J., Ewertz, M., Kroman, N., Kehlet, H. (2009). Prevalence of and factors associated with persistent pain following breast cancer surgery. *Journal of the American Medical Association*, 302, 1985–1992.

Haanpaa, M., Attal, N., Backonja, M., *et al.* (2011). NeuPSIG guidelines on neuropathic pain assessment. *Pain*, 152, 14–27.

Hall, W., Christie, M., Currow, D. (2005). Cannabinoids and cancer: causation, remediation, and palliation. *The Lancet Oncology*, 6, 35–42.

Jensen, T.S., Baron, R., Haanpaa, M., *et al.* (2011). A new definition of neuropathic pain. *Pain*, 152, 2204–2205.

Kalso, E., Allan, L., Dellemijn, P.L., *et al.* (2003). Recommendations for using opioids in chronic non-cancer pain. *European Journal of Pain*, 7, 381–386.

Lussier, D., Huskey, A.G., Portenoy, R.K. (2004). Adjuvant analgesics in cancer pain management. *Oncologist*, 9, 571–591.

Merskey, H. and Bogduk, N. (1994). *Classification of Chronic Pain: Descriptions of Chronic Pain Syndromes and Definitions of Pain Terms*. Seattle, WA: IASP Press.

Mishra, S., Bhatnagar, S., Goyal, G.N., Rana, S.P., and Upadhya, S.P. (2012). A comparative efficacy of amitriptyline, gabapentin, and pregabalin in neuropathic cancer pain: a prospective randomized double-blind placebo-controlled study. *American Journal of Hospice and Palliative Care*, 29, 177–182.

Morley, S., Eccleston, C., Williams, A. (1999). Systematic review and meta-analysis of randomized controlled trials of cognitive behaviour therapy and behaviour therapy for chronic pain in adults, excluding headache. *Pain*, 80, 1–13.

Phillips, T.J., Cherry, C.L., Cox, S., Marshall, S.J., and Rice, A.S. (2010). Pharmacological treatment of painful HIV-associated sensory neuropathy: a systematic review and meta-analysis of randomised controlled trials. *PLoS ONE*, 5, e14433.

Quigley, C. (2004). Opioid switching to improve pain relief and drug tolerability. *Cochrane Database of Systematic Reviews*, 3, CD004847.

Rice, A.S. (2008). Should cannabinoids be used as analgesics for neuropathic pain? *Nature Clinical Practice Neurology*, 4, 654–655.

Salas, S., Frasca, M., Planchet-Barraud, B., *et al.* (2012). Ketamine analgesic effect by continuous intravenous infusion in refractory cancer pain: considerations about the clinical research in palliative care. *Journal of Palliative Medicine*, 15, 287–293.

Smith, E.M., Pang, H., Cirrincione, C., *et al.* (2013). Effect of duloxetine on pain, function, and quality of life among patients with chemotherapy-induced painful peripheral neuropathy: a randomized clinical trial. *Journal of the American Medical Association*, 309, 1359–1367.

Treede, R.D., Jensen, T.S., Campbell, J.N., *et al.* (2008). Neuropathic pain: redefinition and a grading system for clinical and research purposes. *Neurology*, 70, 1630–1635.

Vadalouca, A., Raptis, E., Moka, E., Zis, P., Sykioti, P., and Siafaka, I. (2012). Pharmacological treatment of neuropathic cancer pain: a comprehensive review of the current literature. *Pain Practice*, 12, 219–251.

13.4

Visceral pain

Victor T. Chang

Introduction to visceral pain

Visceral pain is pain that arises from in or around internal organs. This chapter provides a brief overview of visceral nociception and pain pathophysiology, visceral pain syndromes, and therapeutic approaches.

Visceral nociception

The central nervous system receives sensory information from visceral organs and their surrounding tissues through afferent nerves that run in parallel with the efferent autonomic nerves that comprise the sympathetic and parasympathetic systems. Visceral nerves are predominantly unmyelinated C fibres and some thinly myelinated A fibres. The larger nerves within which these afferents run include the vagus, the pelvic nerves, and the spinal nerves.

The vagus nerve conveys efferent parasympathetic activity and information from the visceral organs in the chest and the abdomen, up to the level of the proximal colon. Vagal nerve cell bodies are located in the nodose and jugular ganglia and terminate in the nucleus tractus solitarius in the dorsal medulla. Emerging data suggests that the vagus nerve may convey nociceptive information related to mucosal inflammation (Kollarik et al., 2010). The parasympathetic nerves in the lower bowel and pelvic organs carry afferent fibres that innervate these structures. The cell bodies are in pelvic ganglia. These nerves proceed as pelvic nerves to the sacral cord.

The sympathetic system similarly has afferent fibres running in parallel to the efferent sympathetic nerves. The cell bodies of the sensory fibres from the abdominal viscera are found in the coeliac, hypogastric, and sacral plexuses, and impulses proceed from these structures to the dorsal horn of the thoracolumbar spinal cord. The coeliac plexus is the largest prevertebral ganglion and typically is located anterior to the crura of the diaphragm and L1. There are usually two coeliac ganglia, but up to five have been noted (Ward et al., 1979); the ganglia vary in location (Yang et al., 2011). The superior and inferior hypogastric plexus are located in the retroperitoneum from L4 to S1, and carry visceral afferent impulses from the pelvic viscera and the left colon to the dorsal horn. The superior hypogastric plexus is located anterior to L5 and the Inferior hypogastric plexus at the level of the sacrococcygeal junction. For further anatomical details, readers are referred to Bonica et al. (2001) and Wesselman et al. (1997).

Afferent fibres from the periphery project primarily to second order neurons in laminae I, II, V, and X in the dorsal horn. In contrast to input from somatic structures, this visceral input has wide arborization in the spinal cord; fibres extend to other segments and the contralateral cord. Furthermore, unlike somatic pathways, the second order visceral afferents may also project to other adjacent segments and join other contralateral tracts to the brain, such as the spinothalamic, spinomesencephalic, and spinoparabrachial tracts. An ipsilateraldorsal column pathway has been described where spinal neurons in lamina X ascend by the dorsal columns to the contralateral thalamus by the gracile or cuneate pathways (Willis et al., 1999).

In the brain, visceral nociceptive fibres project to the thalamic ventral posterolateral and posteromedial nuclei, and then the somatosensory cortex, prefrontal cortex, perigeniculate areas of the anterior cingulate cortex, amygdala, and laterally to the insula. The density of visceral fibre projection to the somatosensory cortex is significantly less than for cutaneous fibres.

There are features that distinguish the anatomical organization of the visceral nociceptive system from that of the somatosensory system. Among the most important are the following: The innervation density in the periphery is much lower for visceral nerves than somatic nerves. Both visceral and somatic afferent nerves may converge on the same second order neurons in the dorsal horn of the spinal cord, but the visceral sensory afferent nerves project to a larger number of levels in the spinal cord than somatic nerves, and to the contralateral side, and one visceral sensory neuron may innervate two different visceral organs, especially in the pelvis (Christianson et al 2007).

The vast majority of visceral sensations never reach consciousness and the relationship between conscious experience and visceral nociceptor activity, like many other elements of visceral neural functioning, remain an area of investigation (Robinson and Gebhart, 2008). Functionally, visceral nociceptors are thought to be polymodal, potentially responsive to different kinds of noxious stimuli, such as distention, ischaemia, and electrical stimulation (Ness and Gebhart, 1990). From work on bowel preparations, there also may be mechanosensory, chemosensory, and temperature receptors. Three kinds of mechanosensory nociceptors have been described: those that respond to a range of distention pressures including normal pressures (tonic), those that respond to high levels of distention (high threshold), and those that are silent but become activated in the presence of inflammation. These nociceptors are located in the different layers of the walls and muscles of internal organs (Brierley, 2010). Chemoreceptors and thermoreceptors are present in the mucosa and the muscular layers.

The various components of the   sensory system transmit different types of information, and concurrent activation of these components may account for the symptoms that commonly accompany pain. For example, the afferent nerves running with the sympathetic nerves carry acute nociceptive input, whereas activation of afferents travelling in the vagal pathway may contribute to the nausea and bloating that often occurs with abdominal pain. In the mouse, differences in afferent fibre composition have been found between colonic lumbar splanchnic and pelvic nerves (Brierley et al., 2004), and bladder splanchnic and pelvic nerves (Xu and Gebhart, 2008).

The visceral nociceptive system, like the somatic pathways, has a complex neurochemistry. In the rat, for example, there are specific pelvic nerve fibres that transmit pain, are capable of sensitization, and respond specifically to kappa opioids (Gebhart, 2000). Cell bodies in the nodose ganglion stain positively for transient receptor potential voltage-gated (TRPV) channel 1 and calcitonin gene-related peptide (CGRP), and are less likely to stain for isolectin B4. Other visceral nociceptors do not stain for any of these or other peptides. In the digestive tract, the majority of afferent fibres stain for CGRP, and members of the TRPV receptor family (Christianson and Davis, 2010). Although it is possible to identify likely nociceptors on the basis of this neurochemical staining, functional response to noxious stimuli remains the most reliable way to identify a visceral nociceptor (Robinson and Gebhart, 2008).

Many types of ion and voltage-gated channels also have been identified in visceral nociceptors. Among those that appear important are sodium channels that are tetrodotoxin resistant.

In the brain, functional magnetic resonance imaging images suggest that the regions activated by somatic pain are also activated by visceral pain, but in a slightly different pattern (Strigo et al., 2003; Dunckley et al., 2005). One study suggested that pregabalin may affect brainstem processing of visceral pain (Sikandar and Dickenson, 2011). The locus coeruleus complex, the periaqueductal grey area and the rostral ventral medulla activate descending pathways, and there is evidence for some visceral pain states that the descending spinal pathways can exhibit both inhibitory and facilitatory effects on nociception. These signals are mediated by pre- and post-alpha 2 adrenergic receptors and presynaptic 5-HT$_3$ receptors (Sikandar and Dickenson, 2012). Other potential mediators include the autonomic nervous system, the hypothalamic pituitary tract (Knowles and Aziz, 2009), and hormones such as oestrogen (Sanoja and Cervero, 2010).

Pathophysiology of visceral pain

Like somatic pain, visceral pain presumably occurs as a result of many potential mechanisms. Although understanding of these mechanisms is still very limited, speculation has focused on three broad types: peripheral activation, peripheral sensitization, and central sensitization.

Peripheral activation

Physiologic stimuli include distention, inflammation, torsion, and ischaemia. In the laboratory, additional stimuli include electricity, and the application of various inflammatory and noxious substances, such as hydrochloric acid, bradykinin, and capsaicin.

In the heart, ischaemia leads to a drop in the pH and increased lactate levels. Acid sensing ion channel 3 (ASIC 3) is activated by acidaemia (Yagi et al., 2006) and sensitized by lactate (Immke and McCleskey, 2001). TRPV channels may also be activated by ischaemia (Pan and Chen, 2004).

In the gut, afferents may be activated by physical stimuli, such as high distention pressures or contractions (Sarna, 2007), or the release of compounds that serve as ligands for receptors, such as substance P, CGRP, and products from inflammatory cells.

Mechanosensory transduction may be mediated by TRPV channels (Brierley et al., 2008, 2009), while chemosensory transmission may be mediated by serotonin, TRPV receptors (Brierley et al., 2010), tetrodotoxin resistant sodium channel Na$_v$1.8 (Cervero and Laird, 2004), and ASIC channels. Another relevant mechanism is cleavage and activation of the proteinase activated receptor (PAR) by trypsin. In pancreatic cancer, an inflammatory perineural invasion by pancreatic cancer cells leads to hypertrophy and increased arborization of the sensory nerves (Bapat et al., 2011), a process which also occurs in chronic pancreatitis. While much of this knowledge pertains to animal models of visceral pain, studies in human tissue support these findings (Peiris et al., 2011).

In the bladder and other pelvic organs, distention leads to ATP release, which in turn binds to and activates purinergic receptors P2X2/3 on the afferent nerves (Wang et al., 2005).

Peripheral sensitization

Peripheral sensitization refers to changes in the functioning of a primary afferent nerve that may include a reduced threshold to peripheral activation, spontaneous activation, or an increase in the magnitude of the response after it is activated. This sensitization may accompany inflammation or exposure to specific compounds, or follow peripheral nerve trauma. Visceral afferent nerves are sensitized by inflammatory or adrenergic compounds (Bueno and Fioramonti, 2002) and this may persist long after the initial event. Experimentally, this is accomplished by applying irritants or excitatory compounds such as ATP, bradykinin, or capsaicin. Recent studies suggest that cytokines and other mediators of inflammation can lead to peripheral sensitization (Benson et al., 2012).

This phenomenon may be relevant to the concept of visceral hyperalgesia. Ongoing work is aimed at defining the roles of a wide array of inflammatory products and candidate receptors for different organs and nerves, with interest in the role of serotonin receptors, sodium channels, nitric oxide and TRPV channels (Christianson et al., 2009; Page et al., 2009; Blackshaw et al., 2010).

Central sensitization

Central sensitization is operationally defined as an amplification of neural signalling within the central nervous system. Like peripheral sensitization, it is a process that can result in the experience of spontaneous pain, the perception of pain related to non-noxious stimuli, or hypersensitivity to noxious events. Examples of visceral pain that are believed to be related to central sensitization include oesophageal non-cardiac chest pain and chronic pancreatitis (Woolf, 2011). The N-methyl-D-aspartate (NMDA) receptor is important for central sensitization to visceral pain (Willert et al., 2004).

Clinical aspects of visceral pain

In the United States, unexplained abdominal pain is the most frequent cause of medical visits by the general population (Shaheen et al., 2006). In two large surveys of cancer pain patients, 16% of patients had purely visceral pain, mixed somatic and visceral pain occurred in 12%, and mixed visceral and neuropathic pain was noted in 3% (Caraceni et al., 1996; Grond et al., 1996).

Pain that occurs in association with injury to visceral structures may have distinctive clinical features (Cervero and Laird, 1999). If it is related to obstruction or injury to hollow viscus, the pain tends to be poorly localized and described as vague, gnawing, or crampy; the pain may become intermittently severe in association with visceral contractions. In contrast, injury to solid organs or to organ capsules or related fascia tends to be better localized and described as sharp or stabbing; it. All types of visceral pain may be referred in specific patterns and also may be associated with autonomic symptoms, such as nausea and vomiting. Visceral pain may be accompanied by highly aversive emotional reactions.

In a comparison of pain caused by cutaneous heat with pain caused by oesophageal balloon distention, subjects undergoing oesophageal distention used a wider range of descriptors, more affective descriptors, and reported more anxiety (Strigo et al., 2002). Descriptors used by patients in experimental studies include nauseating, suffocating, and deep. Burning pain has been described for oesophageal and bladder pain.

Referred pain

Because visceral and somatic afferent fibres can converge on the same lamina in the spinal cord, nociceptive impulses from a visceral site may be processed by higher brain centres as emanating from the corresponding somatic site, or viscerosomatic 'referred' pain. The referral sites are specific: in balloon distention studies, oesophageal distention leads to painful sensations in the chest and back (Strigo et al., 2002), distention of the cervix leads to perceived pain in the lower abdomen and the lower back (Bajaj et al., 2002), and bladder distention is referred to the suprapubic area (Ness et al., 1998). The area of referred pain can increase over time or with evolution of the visceral injury. Hyperalgesia and allodynia on stimulation of the skin or gentle palpation may develop in the area of referred pain.

Three general patterns of visceral referral pain have been identified (Fig. 13.4.1). The first is pain in the thoracic region referred from cardiac or oesophageal injury. The second is pain in the upper abdominal wall, which may be referred from the upper abdominal organs (stomach, pancreas, and liver). The third is pain in the lower abdominal wall related to injury of pelvic organs, including colon, bladder, or uterus; the kidney also may refer pain to this location. Other referral sites are equally well known. For example, injury to the region of the porta hepatis may refer pain to the region of the ipsilateral scapula and injury to the diaphragm may refer pain to the ipsilateral shoulder.

Visceral pain also may be referred to other visceral organs. This phenomenon originally was termed viscero-visceral referral; more recently, it has been known as cross organ sensitivity (Brumovsky and Gebhart, 2010). Afferents from different visceral organs can converge at the spinal, brainstem, or thalamic levels. For example, coronary artery disease and disease of the biliary tree have a common afferent input into the T5 spinal level, and afferents from the intestine and pelvis may converge at the T10–L1 spinal level. Although the clinical significance of this phenomenon remains to be determined, it raises the possibility that pain that localized to one organ may be related, at least in part, to a disorder affecting another (Giamberardino et al., 2010).

The complex pain complaints that may occur as a result of visceral disease are mirrored by the potential for equally complex physical findings. Referral sites can become tender and demonstrate cutaneous hypersensitivity—allodynia, hyperesthesia, or hyperalgesia. Some patients experience tenderness that predominates at the referral site. For example, the finding of cutaneous allodynia along the lower abdomen can be the most prominent

finding initially in those with injury to pelvic organs (Jarrell et al., 2011). Appreciation of these phenomena will reduce the risk that an evaluation for the source of a pain will go astray.

Visceral pain syndromes

Numerous visceral pain syndromes have been identified and can be categorized by region of the body affected by the pain-producing disorder (see Chapter 13.1). The following syndromes are representative.

Pain related to thoracic disorders

Many serious illnesses affect thoracic viscera, including the heart, its blood supply, and the great vessels; the lungs, airways, and pleura; or other mediastinal structures such as lymph nodes. The pain syndromes that result are highly variable and determined by the location of injured viscera, the nature of the injury, the course of the illness, pain referral patterns, and other factors.

Persistent pain is usually ipsilateral to the affected hemithorax. Mediastinal injury also can be broadly distributed across one or both hemithoraces, or can result in pain that is experienced more focally in the region of the thoracic spine, across one or both shoulders, or substernally.

Pain syndromes related to thoracic disease often have a time course determined by the progression of the underlying illness. Some, such as refractory angina, may have a prolonged and fluctuating course. Refractory angina may complicate ischaemic heart disease and may co-occur with congestive heart failure. The prevalence of this pain syndrome is expected to increase as patients with heart disease live longer and the population ages (Kim et al., 2002; McGillon et al., 2012).

Pain related to intra-abdominal disorders

For specialists in palliative medicine, the visceral pain disorders related to intra-abdominal disease most likely to be encountered include pain related to a neoplasm in the upper mid-retroperitoneum, such as the pancreas; the diffuse pain associated with bowel obstruction; and pain related to injury of specific structures, such as capsular pain.

Pain may arise from an inflammatory perineural invasion by pancreatic cancer cells (Bapat et al., 2011) and has been reported in up to 75% of patients with advanced pancreatic cancer. Risk factors for the development of abdominal pain are tumour size, invasion of the anterior capsule, and invasion of intrapancreatic nerves (Okusaka et al., 2001). Pain severity may have prognostic significance in patients with resectable pancreatic cancer (Ceyhan et al., 2009). Patients complain of a boring, well-localized upper abdominal pain that may radiate to the back. Most patients ultimately have a component of pain shooting towards the mid-thoracic spinal level; a small minority of patients have back pain without the anterior component. Physical exam may demonstrate an abdominal mass and inability to lie flat. Computed tomography (CT) scans and endoscopic ultrasound are helpful in defining the anatomy of the lesions and the coeliac plexus.

Bowel obstruction is characterized by fluctuating abdominal pain, distention, regurgitation or nausea and vomiting, and absence of bowel movements. Chronic obstruction is seen most commonly in patients with ovarian, cervical, or gastric primary sites. Sometimes, the main site of the obstruction can be localized and mechanical

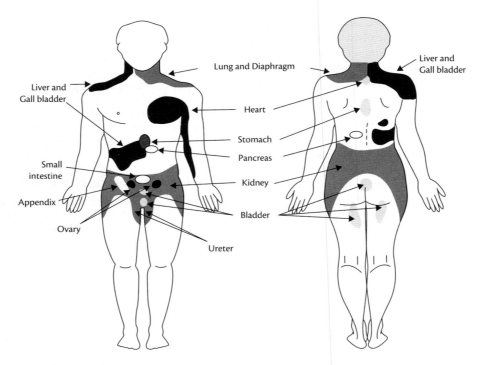

Fig. 13.4.1 Patterns of referred pain from visceral organs.

Reproduced from Mark I. Johnson, *Transcutaneous Electrical Nerve Stimulation (TENS): Research to support clinical practice*, Oxford University Press, Oxford, UK, Copyright © 2014, by permission of Oxford University Press.

strategies, such as stenting or surgical decompression, may be considered. In the context of advanced illness, the goals of care usually focus on symptom relief. The pain is usually crampy and may rise and fall during the day. The distress associated with the pain may be intense, driven by the associated symptoms, inability to eat, and concerns about progressive illness or impending death.

Some pain syndromes are causally related to capsular injury. These include the hepatic distention syndrome and pain from large adrenal masses. Marked and/or rapid enlargement of the spleen and lymph nodes can also lead to pain. In the hepatic distention syndrome, patients complain of a steady pressure sensation in the right upper quadrant. Physical examination shows an enlarged liver and imaging demonstrates hepatic lesions. Patients with massively enlarged adrenal glands from tumours will complain of flank discomfort, which may radiate to the ipsilateral inguinal region.

Enlarged retroperitoneal lymphadenopathy can cause severe back pain, which can be focal or diffuse. This pain syndrome is most prevalent among those with lymphomas or germ cell tumours. Lymphadenopathy was the most common cause of visceral pain in a study of patients with haematological malignancies (Niscola et al., 2007). Patients with lymphomas may experience a flare of pain related to enlarged lymph nodes after drinking alcohol (Atkinson et al., 1976). In patients with long standing myeloproliferative diseases and splenomegaly, splenic infarction may develop and result in left upper quadrant pain, which is often characterized as a continuous pain with exacerbations of stabbing pain. The spleen is usually prominent on examination, and its size may prevent patients from bending or sitting.

Other abdominal pain syndromes are less common. Abdominal pain from herpes zoster infections has been reported in bone marrow transplant recipients, sometimes accompanied by a complex of syndrome of inappropriate antidiuretic hormone secretion (SIADH), and rash (David et al., 1998; Koc et al., 2000). Zoster also can cause a more typical dermatomal neuropathic pain (Tribble et al., 1993). Some pain syndromes are related to antineoplastic therapies. For example, persistent abdominal pain may follow tumour embolization procedures involving lesions in the liver, kidney, spleen, or uterus; in the acute phase, pain often is associated with fever, nausea, vomiting, and leucocytosis (Brown et al., 2009). No risk factors have been identified (Patel et al., 2000), and symptoms usually resolve with supportive care after a few days. Radiation-related pain syndromes include radiation enteritis, radiation proctitis, and radiation prostatitis. Finally, pain has been associated with placement of oesophageal stents (Golder et al., 2001), and there are anecdotal observations suggesting that pain also may accompany biliary or colonic stent placement (Gianotti et al., 2013). Migration of stents can lead to pain associated with visceral perforation (Gould et al., 1988).

Pain related to pelvic disorders

Some of the pain syndromes that occur with intra-pelvic pathology, such as chronic bowel obstruction, were noted earlier. Other pain syndromes also occur from diseases in this region, particularly locally advanced neoplasms affecting gynaecological structures, prostate, or rectum. These disorders may cause persistent perineal or deep pelvic pain, and may be accompanied by tenesmus or by urinary urgency or bladder spasms. Perineal pain within 1 year of surgery for pelvic tumour should be evaluated for relapse and distinguished from patients with phantom pain (Stillman, 1990; Boas et al., 1993).

Therapeutic approaches for visceral pain

The approach to pain management in the patient with a visceral pain syndrome largely parallels the treatment of other types of chronic pain. There are several distinctions, however, as summarized below.

Opioid therapy is the mainstay approach for chronic pain that is moderate or severe. In rodent studies of bladder and colon distention, mu and kappa agonist opioids inhibited mechanoreceptor responses (Su et al., 1997a, 1997b); subsequent work points to a kappa-like receptor in visceral afferents. Morphine also affects modulation of visceral pain through its effect on the rostroventral medulla in the rat (Friedrich and Gebhart, 2003). Although some of these preclinical findings suggest that kappa agonist opioids may be preferable in visceral pain, there is no clinical evidence to substantiate this. Oxycodone interacts with both kappa and mu receptors, and in a small randomized comparison of oxycodone with morphine in patients with pancreatic cancer, no difference was seen (Mercadante et al., 2010). However, there are suggestive experimental human data. In a human experimental model with different types of pains, oxycodone did provide better pain relief than morphine in patients with visceral pain (Staahl et al., 2006). A comparison of oxycodone with KR665, a kappa opioid agonist, using a similar experimental design showed more pain relief with KR665 (Arendt-Nielsen et al., 2009). A study of another kappa specific opioid, asimadoline, in patients with irritable bowel syndrome showed improvement in the asimadoline arm (Mangel et al., 2008). More research is needed to determine whether there may be selective opioid effects related to receptor binding profile. The development of kappa receptor opioid agonists remains an area of great interest (Vanderah, 2010).

Patients with visceral pain resulting from obstruction of a hollow viscus often are considered for trials of adjuvant analgesics intended to reduce spasm of smooth muscle. Most of the data comes from studies of oesophageal spasms, biliary colic, renal colic, irritable bowel syndrome and overactive bladder, and comparatively little has been studied in populations with serious illnesses and the use of non-opioid and opioid analgesics continues to be emphasized. Indeed, non-steroidal anti-inflammatory drugs have been recommended for biliary colic (Colli et al., 2012). Based largely on anecdotal experience, anticholinergic agents, such as hyoscine (scopolamine), are used for pain related to bowel obstruction (Ripamonti et al., 2000; Tytgat, 2008); dicyclomine, which has both anticholinergic and muscle relaxant properties, has been used for irritable bowel syndrome (Ruepert et al., 2011); and oxybutynin, another anticholinergic drug, has been used for patients with bladder spasm (Kennelly, 2010; Madhuvrata et al., 2012).

With the identification of relevant neurotransmitters, interest in new classes of medications has increased (Bueno et al., 2007; Blackshaw et al., 2010; Burnstock, 2012). A trial of tetrodotoxin has been promising (Hagen et al., 2011), for example, and other agents have been considered in specific disease states. These include JAK-2 inhibitors (Hagen et al., 2010; Mesa et al., 2013) for patients with symptomatic myelofibrosis, steroids for capsule distention and for bowel obstruction (Philip et al., 1995; Feuer and Broadley, 2000), octreotide for bowel obstruction (Mercadante and Porzio, 2012) or capsule distention (Pistevou-Gombake et al., 2003), intravenous phentolamine for pancreatic cancer (Yasukawa et al., 2007), and ranolazine for angina (Yasukawa et al., 2006). Readers

are referred to Davis (2012) and Holzer and Holzer-Petesche (2009) for more details.

Some visceral pain syndromes may be best approached through specific interventions. The challenge in these cases often relates to an informed balancing of potential benefit against the burdens of the approach and the risks in the context of advanced illness. Offering a strategy of shared decision-making, which may involve both the patient and the family, appears to be the best approach.

Stents have been increasingly used as a non-surgical means of relieving oesophageal obstruction (Madhusudhan et al., 2009), bowel obstruction (Nagula et al., 2010; Larssen et al., 2011), and pain from pancreatic cancer-related duct stenosis (Costamagna et al., 1999). Surgical interventions include thoracic splanchnicectomy for upper abdominal pain (Krishna et al., 2001) and intractable angina (Khogali et al., 1999), and surgical decompression for bowel obstruction (Feuer et al., 2000; Kucukmetin et al., 2010).

So-called interventional pain procedures involve injections or infusions through catheters that re intended to block afferent input from a painful site. The coeliac plexus block is commonly employed in an effort to interrupt pain transmission from upper abdominal structures. There are numerous techniques, the most common of which include radiographically guided bilateral posterior percutaneous injections and an endoscopic ultrasound-guided transoesophageal injection. A neurolytic solution, such as phenol or alcohol, is injected, and successful cases experience pain reduction that typically lasts until death. An important but unresolved issue is timing of the block relative to titration of medications (De Oliveira et al., 2004).

Other interventional approaches are used to manage various types of visceral pain. For example, bilateral superior hypogastric block can relieve intra-abdominal and pelvic pain, but extensive retroperitoneal disease is a risk factor for poor pain control (Plancarte et al., 1997; Cariati et al., 2002). Ganglion impar block, sacral nerve root blocks, and saddle blocks may be useful in patients with visceral perineal pain (Plancarte, 1983; De Medicis et al., 2001; Slatkin and Rhiner, 2003) (see Chapter 9.8).

Rarely, neurosurgical approaches are considered for refractory visceral pain. For example, a T10 myelotomy for pelvic visceral pain can be performed by transecting the dorsal column pathway surgically (Viswanathan et al., 2010) or with CT guidance (Vilela Filho et al., 2001) (see Chapter 9.8).

Other pain therapies used very uncommonly in visceral pain involve implantation of devices. Spinal cord stimulation has been studied in small cohorts as a way to implement modulation of the dorsal columns and improve pain control in chronic pancreatitis (Kapural et al., 2011), intractable angina (Mesa and Yakovlev, 2008; Taylor et al., 2009), and testicular pain (Nouri and Brish, 2011). Neuraxial analgesia involves placement of an intrathecal or epidural catheter for long-term infusion of various analgesic compounds, including opioids, local anaesthetics, clonidine and others. There are a variety of techniques, and if the local expertise exists to evaluate them for the patient with refractory pain, there may be advantages in doing so given the flexibility of the approach and its' lack of risk relative to neurolysis (see Chapter 9.9).

Finally, radiofrequency ablation has been employed for visceral pain resulting from recurrent bladder cancer (Campbell et al., 2005) and rectal cancer (Lefevre et al., 2008). It presupposes an ability to identify the peripheral neural anatomy close to the size of the structure involved, a task that may prove difficult when the anatomy has been distorted by locally advanced disease.

For patients with cancer, antineoplastic therapy may have analgesic consequences. Radiation therapy is used commonly for pain, including visceral pain. For example, radiation has been used to palliate pain from hepatic metastases (Bydder et al., 2003), pancreatic cancer (Morganti et al., 2003), recurrent gynaecological cancers (Smith and Koh, 2001), bladder cancer (Yi et al., 2007), and from an enlarged spleen in myeloproliferative disease (McFarland et al., 2003).

Visceral pain is associated with emotional reactions and psychological approaches to pain control should be considered as important adjuncts to pharmacotherapy and interventions, as they are in other types of pain. In patients with angina pectoris, angina during daily life was associated more with the psychological distress associated with chest pain than with inducible myocardial ischaemia, whereas chest pain during exercise stress testing was related to myocardial ischaemia (Sullivan et al., 2008). In patients with gastrointestinal cancer pain, communication with caregivers and ambivalence in expressing emotion were important determinants of pain severity, mediated in part by the catastrophizing response (Keefe et al., 2003; Porter et al., 2005). Conversely, self-efficacy of the caregiver during interactions with the patient was associated with decreased pain. Interventions to assist the patient and the caregiver may be helpful in patients with visceral pain (see Chapter 9.11).

Conclusion

Distinguishing features of the visceral pain system have been delineated at many levels. Organ-specific and tissue-specific nociceptive signalling, and the pathophysiological changes that affect these processes and sustain pain in the setting of illness, are undergoing investigation and may inform specific treatment strategies for these pain syndromes in the future. For the present, there are numerous therapeutic options and the expectation should be that most patients can achieve satisfactory relief if treatment is carefully considered and implemented appropriately.

References

Arendt-Nielsen, L., Olesen, A.E., Staahl, C., et al. (2009). Analgesic efficacy of peripheral kappa-opioid receptor agonist CR665 compared to oxycodone in a multi-modal, multi-tissue experimental human pain model: selective effect on visceral pain. Anesthesiology, 111, 616–624.

Atkinson, K., Austin, D.E., McElwain, T.J., et al. (1976). Alcohol pain in Hodgkin's disease. Cancer, 37, 895–899.

Bajaj, P., Drewes, A.M., Gregersen, H., et al. (2002). Controlled dilatation of the uterine cervix—an experimental visceral pain model. Pain, 99, 433–442.

Bapat, A.A., Hostetter, G., Von Hoff, D.D., et al. (2011). Perineural invasion and associated pain in pancreatic cancer. Nature Reviews Cancer, 11, 695–707.

Benson, S., Kattoor, J., Wegner, A., et al. (2012). Acute experimental endotoxemia induces visceral hypersensitivity and altered pain evaluation in healthy humans. Pain, 153, 794–799.

Blackshaw, L.A., Brierley, S.M., and Hughes, P.A. (2010). TRP channels: new targets for visceral pain. Gut, 59, 126–135.

Boas, R.A., Schug, S.A., and Acland, R.H. (1993). Perineal pain after rectal amputation: a five year follow-up. Pain, 52, 67–70.

Bonica, J.J. and Graney, D.O. (2001). General considerations of abdominal pain. In J.D Loeser, S.H. Butler, C.R. Chapman, and C.D. Turk (eds.) Bonica's Management of Pain (3rd ed.), pp. 1243–1251. New York: Lippincott Williams & Wilkins.

Brierley, S.M. (2010). Molecular basis of mechanosensitivity. Autonomic Neuroscience, 153, 58–68.

Brierley, S.M., Hughes, P.A., Page, A.J., et al. (2009). The ion channel TRPA1 is required for normal mechanosensation and is modulated by algesic stimuli. Gastroenterology, 137, 2084–2095.

Brierley, S.M., Jones, R.C. 3rd, Gebhart, G.F., et al. (2004). Splanchnic and pelvic mechanosensory afferents signal different qualities of colonic stimuli in mice. Gastroenterology, 127, 166–178.

Brierley, S.M., Page, A.J., Hughes, P.A., et al (2008). Selective role for TRPV4 ion channels in visceral sensory pathways. Gastroenterology, 134, 2059–2069.

Brown, D.B., Geschwind, J.F., Soulen, M.C., et al. (2009). Society of Interventional Radiology position statement on chemoembolization of hepatic malignancies. Journal of Vascular and Interventional Radiology, 20(7 Suppl.), S317–323.

Brumovsky, P.R. and Gebhart, G.F. (2010). Visceral organ cross-sensitization—an integrated perspective. Autonomic Neuroscience, 153, 106–115.

Bueno, L., De Pontin, F., Fried, M., et al. (2007). Serotonergic and non-serotonergic targets in the pharmacotherapy of visceral hypersensitivity. Neurogastroenterology & Motility, 19(Suppl. 1), 89–119.

Bueno, L. and Fioramonti, J. (2002). Visceral perception: inflammatory and non-inflammatory mediators. Gut, 51(Suppl. 1), i19–i23.

Burnstock, G. (2012). Targeting the visceral purinergic system for pain control. Current Opinion in Pharmacology, 12, 80–86.

Bydder, S., Spry, N.A., Christie, D.R.H., et al. (2003). A prospective trial of short-fractionation radiotherapy for the palliation of liver metastases. Australian Radiology, 47, 284–288.

Campbell, C., Soulen, M.C., Horii, S.C., et al. (2005).Transrectal radiofrequency ablation for pelvic recurrence of bladder cancer: case report and review of complications. Journal of Vascular and Interventional Radiology, 16, 1027–1032.

Caraceni, A. and Portenoy, R.K. (1996). An international survey of cancer pain characteristics and syndromes. IASP Task Force on Cancer Pain. Pain, 82, 263–274.

Cariati, M., De Martini, G., Pretolesi, F., et al. (2002). CT-guided superior hypogastric block. Journal of Computer Assisted Tomography, 26, 428–431.

Cervero, F. and Laird, J.M. (1999). Visceral pain. The Lancet, 353(9170), 2145–2148.

Cervero, F. and Laird, J.M. (2004). Understanding the signaling and transmission of visceral nociceptive events. Journal of Neurobiology, 61, 45–54.

Ceyhan, G.O., Bergmann, F., Kadihasanoglu, M., et al. (2009). Pancreatic neuropathy and neuropathic pain—a comprehensive pathomorphological study of 546 cases. Gastroenterology, 136, 177–186.

Christianson, J.A., Bielefeldt, K., Alter C., et al. (2009). Development, plasticity and modulation of visceral afferents. Brain Research Reviews, 60, 171–186.

Christianson, J.A., Davis, B.M. (2010). The role of visceral afferents in disease. In L. Kruger and A.R. Light (eds.) Translational Pain Research: From Mouse to Man, pp. 51–76. Boca Raton, FL: CRC Press.

Christianson, J.A., Liang R., Ustinova, E.E., et al. (2007). Convergence of bladder and colon sensory innervation occurs at the primary afferent level. Pain, 128, 235–243.

Colli, A., Conte, D., Valle, S.D., et al. (2012). Meta-analysis: nonsteroidal anti-inflammatory drugs in biliary colic. Alimentary Pharmacology & Therapeutics, 35, 1370–1378.

Costamagna, G., Alevras, P., Palladino, F., et al. (1999). Endoscopic pancreatic stenting in pancreatic cancer. Canadian Journal of Gastroenterology, 13, 481–487.

David, D.S., Tegtmeier, B.R., O'Donnell, M.R., et al. (1998). Visceral varicella-zoster after bone marrow transplantation: report of a case series and review of the literature. American Journal of Gastroenterology, 93, 810–813.

Davis, M.P. (2012). Drug management of visceral pain: concepts from basic research. Pain Research and Treatment, 2012, 265605

De Medicis, E. and de Leon-Casasola, O. (2001). Ganglion impar block: critical evaluation. Techniques in Regional Anesthesia and Pain Management, 5, 120–122.

De Oliveira, R., dos Reis, M.P., and Prado, W.A. (2004). The effects of early or late neurolytic sympathetic plexus block on the management of abdominal or pelvic cancer pain. *Pain*, 110, 400–408.

Dunckley, P., Wise, R.G., Fairhurst, M., *et al.* (2005). A comparison of visceral and somatic pain processing in the human brainstem using functional magnetic resonance imaging. *Journal of Neuroscience*, 25, 7333–7341.

Feuer, D.J. and Broadley, K.E. (2000). Corticosteroids for the resolution of malignant bowel obstruction in advanced gynecological and gastrointestinal cancer. *Cochrane Database of Systematic Reviews*, 2, CD001219.

Feuer, D.J., Broadley, K.E., Shepherd, J.H., *et al.* (2000). Surgery for the resolution of symptoms in malignant bowel obstruction in advanced gynaecological and gastrointestinal cancer. *Cochrane Database of Systematic Reviews*, 4, CD002764.

Friedrich, A.E. and Gebhart, G.F. (2003). Modulation of visceral hyperalgesia by morphine and cholecystokinin from the rat rostroventral medial medulla. *Pain*, 104, 93–101.

Gebhart, G.F. (2000). J.J. Bonica Lecture—2000: Physiology, pathophysiology, and pharmacology of visceral pain. *Regional Anesthesia and Pain Medicine*, 25, 632–638.

Giamberardino, M.A., Costantini, R., Affaitati, G., *et al.* (2010). Viscero-visceral hyperalgesia: characterization in different clinical models. *Pain*, 151, 307–322.

Gianotti, L., Tamini, N., Nespoli, L., *et al.* (2013). A prospective evaluation of short-term and long-term results from colonic stenting for palliation or as abridge to elective operation versus immediate surgery for large-bowel obstruction. *Surgical Endoscopy*, 27, 832–842.

Golder, M., Tekkis, P.P., Kennedy, C., *et al.* (2001). Chest pain following oesophageal stenting for malignant dysphagia. *Clinical Radiology*, 56, 202–205.

Gould, J., Train, J.S., Dan, S.J., *et al.* (1988). Duodenal perforation as a delayed complication of placement of a biliary endoprosthesis. *Radiology*, 167, 467–469.

Grond, S., Zech, D., Diefenbach, C., *et al.* (1996). Assessment of cancer pain: a prospective evaluation in 2266 cancer patients referred to a pain service. *Pain*, 64, 107–114.

Hagen, N.A., Lapointe, B., Ong-Lam, M., *et al.* (2011).A multicentre open-label safety and efficacystudy of tetrodotoxin for cancer pain. *Current Oncology*, 18, e109–116.

Holzer, P. and Holzer-Petesche, U. (2009). Emerging pharmacological therapies. In M.A. Gimaberadino (ed.) *Visceral Pain*, pp. 51–62. New York: Oxford University Press.

Immke, D.C. and McCleskey, E.W. (2001). Lactate enhances the acid-sensing Na+ channel on ischemia-sensing neurons. *Nature Neuroscience*, 4, 869–870

Jarrell, J., Giamberardino, M.A., Robert, M., *et al.* (2011). Bedside testing for chronic pelvic pain: discriminating visceral from somatic pain. *Pain Research and Treatment*, Article ID 692102.

Kapural, L., Cywinski, J.B., and Sparks, D.A. (2011). Spinal cord stimulation for visceral pain from chronic pancreatitis. *Neuromodulation*, 14, 423–426

Keefe, F.J., Lipkus, I., Lefebvre, J.C., *et al.* (2003). The social context of gastrointestinal cancer pain: a preliminary study examining the relation of patient pain catastrophizing to patient perceptions of social support and caregiver stress and negative responses. *Pain*, 103, 151–156.

Kennelly, M.J. (2010). A comparative review of oxybutynin chloride formulations: pharmacokinetics and therapeutic efficacy in overactive bladder. *Reviews in Urology*, 12, 12–19.

Khogali, S.S., Miller, M., Rajesh, P.B., *et al.* (1999). Video-assisted thoracoscopic sympathectomy for severe intractable angina. *European Journal Cardio-Thoracic Surgery*, 16(Suppl. 1), S95–98.

Kim, M.C., Kini, A., and Sharma, S.K. (2002). Refractory angina pectoris. Mechanism and therapeutic options. *Journal of the American College of Cardiology*, 39, 923–934.

Knowles, C.H. and Aziz, Q. (2009). Basic and clinical aspects of gastrointestinal pain. *Pain*, 141, 191–209.

Koc, Y., Miller, K.B., Schenkein, D.P., *et al.* (2000). Varicella zoster virus infections following allogeneic bone marrow transplantation: frequency, risk factors, and clinical outcome. *Biology of Blood and Marrow Transplantation*, 6, 44–49.

Kollarik, M., Ru, F., and Brozmanova, M. (2010). Vagal afferent nerves with the properties of nociceptors. *Autonomic Neuroscience: Basic and Clinical*, 153, 12–20.

Krishna, S., Chang, V.T., Shoukas, J., *et al.* (2001).Video-assisted thoracoscopic sympathectomy-splanchnicectomy for pancreatic cancer pain. *Journal of Pain and Symptom Management*, 22, 610–616.

Kucukmetin, A., Naik, R., Galaal, K., *et al.* (2010). Palliative surgery versus medical management for bowel obstruction in ovarian cancer. *Cochrane Database of Systematic Reviews*, 7, CD007792.

Larssen, L., Medhus, A.W., Hjermstad, M.J., *et al.* (2011). Patient-reported outcomes in palliative gastrointestinal stenting: a Norwegian multicenter study. *Surgical Endoscopy*, 25, 162–169.

Lefevre, J.H., Parc, Y., Lewin, M., *et al.* (2008). Radiofrequency ablation for recurrent pelvic cancer. *Colorectal Disease*, 10, 781–784.

Madhusudhan, C., Saluja, S.S., Pal, S., *et al.* (2009). Palliative stenting for relief of dysphagia in patients with inoperable esophageal cancer: impact on quality of life. *Diseases of the Esophagus*, 22, 331–336.

Madhuvrata, P., Cody, J.D., Ellis, G., *et al.* (2012). Which anticholinergic drug for overactive bladder symptoms in adults. *Cochrane Database of Systematic Reviews*, 1, CD005429.

Mangel, A.W., Bornstein, J.D., Hamm, L.R., *et al.* (2008). Clinical trial: asimadoline in the treatment of patients with irritable bowel syndrome. *Alimentary Pharmacology & Therapeutics*, 28, 239–249.

McFarland, J.T., Kuzma, C., Millard, F.E., *et al.* (2003). Palliative irradiation of the spleen. *American Journal of Clinical Oncology*, 26, 178–183.

McGillon, M., Arthur, H.M., Cook, A., *et al.* (2012). Management of patients with refractory angina: Canadian Cardiovascular Society/Canadian Pain Society Joint Guidelines. *Canadian Journal of Cardiology*, 28, S20–S41.

Mercadante, S. and Porzio, G. (2012). Octreotide for malignant bowel obstruction: twenty years after. *Critical Reviews in Oncology/Hematology*, 83, 388–392.

Mercadante, S., Tirelli, W., David, F., *et al.* (2010). Morphine versus oxycodone in pancreatic cancer pain: a randomized controlled study. *Clinical Journal of Pain*, 26, 794–797.

Mesa, J.E. and Yakovlev, A.E. (2008). Treatment of intractable angina pectoris utilizing spinal cord stimulation. *Reviews in Cardiovascular Medicine*, 9, 70–74

Mesa, R.A., Gotlib, J., Gupta, V., *et al.* (2013). Effect of ruxolitinib therapy on myelofibrosis-related symptoms and other patient-reported outcomes in COMFORT-I: a randomized, double-blind, placebo-controlled trial. *Journal of Clinical Oncology*, 31, 1285–1292.

Morganti, A.G., Trodella, L., Valentini, V., *et al.* (2003). Pain relief with short term irradiation in locally advanced carcinoma of the pancreas. *Journal of Palliative Care*, 19, 258–262.

Nagula, S., Ishill, N., Nash, C., *et al.* (2010). Quality of life and symptom control after stent placement or surgical palliation of malignant colorectal obstruction. *Journal of the American College of Surgeons*, 210, 45–53.

Ness, T.J. and Gebhart, G.F. (1990). Visceral pain: a review of experimental studies. *Pain*, 41, 167–234.

Ness, T.J., Richter, H.E., Varner, R.E., *et al.* (1998). A psychophysical study of discomfort produced by repeated filling of the urinary bladder. *Pain*, 76, 61–69.

Niscola, P., Cartoni, C., Romani, C., *et al.* (2007). Epidemiology, features and outcome of pain in patients with advanced hematological malignancies followed in a home care program: an Italian survey. *Annals of Hematology*, 86, 671–676.

Nouri, K.H. and Brish, E.L. (2011). Spinal cord stimulation for testicular pain. *Pain Medicine*, 12, 1435–1438.

Okusaka, T., Okada, S., Ueno, H., *et al.* (2001). Abdominal pain in patients with resectable pancreatic cancer with reference to clinicopathologic findings. *Pancreas*, 22, 279–284.

Page, A.J., O'Donnell, T.A., Cooper, N.J., *et al.* (2009). Nitric oxide as an endogenous peripheral modulator of visceral sensory neuronal function. *Journal of Neuroscience*, 29, 7246–7255.

Pan, H.L. and Chen, S.R. (2004). Sensing tissue ischemia: another new function for capsaicin receptors? *Circulation*, 110, 1826–1831.

Patel, N.H., Hahn, D., and Rapp, S. (2000). Hepatic artery embolization: factors predisposing to postembolization pain and nausea. *Journal of Vascular and Interventional Radiology*, 11, 453–460.

Peiris, M., Bulmer, D.C., Baker, M.D., et al. (2011). Human visceral afferent recordings: preliminary report. *Gut*, 60, 204–208.

Philip, J., Lickiss, N., Grant, P.T., et al. (1999). Corticosteroids in the management of bowel obstruction on a Gynecological Oncolgy Unit. *Gynecologic Oncology*, 74, 68–73.

Pistevou-Gombake, K., Eleftheriadis, N., Plataniotis, G.A., et al. (2003). Octreotide for palliative treatment of hepatic metastases from non-neuroendocrine primary tumors: evaluation of quality of life using the EORTC QLQ-C30 questionnaire. *Palliative Medicine*, 17, 257–262.

Plancarte, R., deLeon-Casasola, O.A., El-Helaly, M., et al. (1997). Neurolytic superior hypogastric plexus block for chronic pelvic pain associated with cancer. *Regional Anesthesia*, 22, 562–568.

Porter, L.S., Keefe, F.J., Lipkus, I., et al. (2005). Ambivalence over emotional expression in patients with gastrointestinal cancer and their caregivers: associations with patient pain and quality of life. *Pain*, 117, 340–348.

Ripamonti, C., Mercadante, S., Groff, L., et al. (2000). Role of octreotide, scopolamine butylbromide, and hydration in symptom control of patients with inoperable bowel obstruction and nasogastric tubes: a prospective randomized trial. *Journal of Pain and Symptom Management*, 19, 23–34.

Robertson, D.H. (1983). Transacral neurolytic nerve block: an alternative approach to perineal pain. *British Journal of Anesthesia*, 55, 873–875.

Robinson, D.R. and Gebhart, G.F. (2008). Inside information—the unique features of visceral sensation. *Molecular Interventions*, 8, 242–253.

Ruepert, L., Quartero, A.O., de Wit, N.J., et al. (2011). Bulking agents, antispasmodics and antidepressants for the treatment of irritable bowel syndrome. *Cochrane Database of Systematic Reviews*, 8, CD003460.

Sanoja, R. and Cervero, F. (2010). Estrogen-dependent changes in visceral afferent sensitivity. *Autonomic Neuroscience: Basic and Clinical*, 153, 84–89.

Sarna, S.K. (2007). Enteric descending and afferent neural signaling stimulated by giant migrating contractions: essential contributing factors to visceral pain. *American Journal of Physiology – Gastrointestinal and Liver Physiology*, 292, G572–581.

Shaheen, N.J., Hansen, R.A., Morgan, D.R., et al. (2006). The burden of gastrointestinal and liver diseases. *American Journal of Gastroenterology*, 101, 2128–2138.

Sikandar, S. and Dickenson, A.H. (2011). Pregabalin modulation of spinal and brainstem visceral nociceptive processing. *Pain*, 152, 2312–2322.

Sikandar, S. and Dickenson, A.H. (2012). Visceral pain—the ins and outs, the ups and downs. *Current Opinion in Supportive and Palliative Care*, 6, 17–26.

Slatkin, N.E. and Rhiner, M. (2003). Phenol saddle blocks for intractable pain at end of life: report of four cases and literature review. *American Journal of Hospice & Palliative Care*, 20, 62–66.

Smith, S.C. and Koh, W.J. (2001). Palliative radiation therapy for gynaecological malignancies. *Best Practice & Research Clinical Obstetrics & Gynaecology*, 15, 265–278.

Staahl, C., Christrup, L.L., and Andersen, S.D. (2006). A comparative study of oxycodone and morphine in a multi-modal, tissue-differentiated experimental pain model. *Pain*, 123, 28–36.

Stillman, M.J. (1990). Perineal pain. Diagnosis and management, with particular attention to perineal pain of cancer. In K.M. Foley, J.J. Bonica, and V. Ventafridda (eds.) *Advances in Pain Research and Therapy* (Vol. 16), pp. 359–377. New York: Raven Press Ltd.

Stone, P.H., Gratsiansky, N.A., Blokhin, A., et al. (2006). Antianginal efficacy of ranolazine when added to treatment with amlodipine. The ERICA (Efficacy of ranolazine in chronic angina) trial. *Journal of the American College of Cardiology*, 48, 566–575.

Strigo, I., Duncan, G.H., Boivin, M., et al. (2003). Differentiation of visceral and cutaneous pain in the human brain. *Journal of Neurophysiology*, 89, 3294–3303.

Strigo, I.A., Bushnell, M.C., Boivin, M., et al. (2002). Psychophysical analysis of visceral and cutaneous pain in human subjects. *Pain*, 97, 235–246.

Su, X., Sengupta, J.N., and Gebhart, G.F. (1997a). Effects of kappa opioid receptor-selective agonists on responses of pelvic nerve afferents to noxious tension. *Journal of Neurophysiology*, 78, 1003–1012.

Su, X., Sengupta, J.N., and Gebhart, G.F. (1997b). Effects of opioids on mechanosensitive pelvic nerve afferent fibers innervating the urinary bladder of the rat. *Journal of Neurophysiology*, 77, 1566–1580.

Sullivan, M.D., Ciechanowski, P.S., Russo, J.E., et al. (2008). Angina pectoris during daily activities and exercise stress testing: the role of inducible myocardial ischemia and psychological distress. *Pain*, 139, 551–561.

Taylor, R.S., De Vries, J., Buchser, E., et al. (2009). Spinal cord stimulation in the treatment of refractory angina: systematic review and meta-analysis of randomized controlled trials. *BMC Cardiovascular Disorders*, 9, 13

Tribble D.R., Church P., and Frame J.N. (1993). Gastrointestinal visceral motor complications of dermatomal herpes zoster: report of two cases and review. *Clinical Infectious Diseases*, 17, 431–436.

Tytgat, G.N. (2008). Hyoscine butylbromide—a review on its parenteral use in acute abdominal spasm and as an aid in abdominal diagnostic and therapeutic procedures. *Current Medical Research and Opinion*, 24, 3159–3173.

Vanderah, T.W. (2010). Delta and kappa opioid receptors as suitable drug targets for pain. *Clinical Journal of Pain*, 26(Suppl. 10), S10–15.

Verstovsek, S., Kantarjian, H., Mesa, R.A., et al. (2010). Safety and efficacy of INCB018424, a JAK1 and JAK2 inhibitor, in myelofibrosis. *The New England Journal of Medicine*, 363, 1117–1127.

Vilela Filho, O., Araujo, M.R., Florencio, R.S., et al. (2001). CT-guided percutaneous punctate midline myelotomy for the treatment of intractable visceral pain: a technical note. *Stereotactic and Functional Neurosurgery*, 77,177–182.

Viswanathan, A., Burton, A.W., Rekito, A., et al. (2010). Commissural myelotomy in the treatment of intractable visceral pain: technique and outcomes. *Stereotactic and Functional Neurosurgery*, 88, 374–382.

Wang, E.C., Lee, J.M., Ruiz, W.G., et al (2005). ATP and purinergic receptor-dependent membrane traffic in bladder umbrella cells. *Journal of Clinical Investigation*, 115, 2412–2422.

Ward, E.M., Rorie, D.K., Nauss, L.A., et al. (1979). The celiac ganglia in man: normal anatomic variations. *Anesthesia & Analgesia*, 58, 461–465.

Wesselmann, U., Burnett, A.L., Heinberg, L.J. (1997). The urogenital and rectal pain syndromes. *Pain*, 73, 269–294.

Willert, R.P., Woolf, C.J., Hobson, A.R., et al. (2004). The development and maintenance of human visceral pain hypersensitivity is dependent on the N-methyl-D-aspartate receptor. *Gastroenterology*, 126, 683–692.

Willis, W.D., Al-Chaer, E.D., Quast, M.J., et al. (1999). A visceral pain pathway in the dorsal column of the spinal cord. *Proceedings of the National Academy of Sciences of the United States of America*, 96, 7675–7679.

Woolf, C.J. (2011). Central sensitization: implications for the diagnosis and treatment of pain. *Pain*, 152(3 Suppl.), S2–15.

Xu, L. and Gebhart, G.F. (2008). Characterization of mouse lumbar splanchnic and pelvic nerve urinary bladder mechanosensory afferents. *Journal of Neurophysiology*, 99, 244–253.

Yagi, J., Wenk, H.N., Naves, L.A., et al. (2006). Sustained currents through ASIC3 ion channels at the modest pH changes that occur during myocardial ischemia. *Circulation Research*, 99,501–509.

Yang, I.Y., Oraee, S., Viejo, C., et al. (2011). Computed tomography celiac trunk topography relating to celiac plexus block. *Regional Anesthesia and Pain Medicine*, 36, 21–25.

Yasukawa, M., Yasukawa, K., Kamiizumi, Y., et al. (2007). Intravenous phentolamine infusion alleviates the pain of abdominal visceral cancer, including pancreatic carcinoma. *Journal of Anesthesia*, 21, 420–423.

Yi, S.K., Yoder, M., Zaner, K., et al. (2007). Palliative radiation therapy of symptomatic recurrent bladder cancer. *Pain Physician*, 10, 285–210.

13.5

Management issues in chronic pain following cancer therapy

Martin Chasen and Gordon Giddings

Introduction to management issues in chronic pain following cancer therapy

The extended phase of cancer survivorship commences after completion of initial anti-cancer treatment and includes regular follow-up examinations with or without maintenance or intermittent anticancer therapy. The permanent survival phase follows the extended phase and continues until death (Levy et al., 2008).

The American Cancer Society have stated that their goal is to make cancer into a chronic disease state in which long-term control is possible, even in the absence of a conventional cure (Burton et al., 2007). At a global level, the incidence of 26 cancers in 2008 was estimated at 12.7 million new cancers by GLOBOCAN series of the International Agency for Research on Cancer (World Health Organization (WHO), 2008). Survival at 5 years after diagnosis is the widely used benchmark for prevalence. Accordingly, there were an estimated 24.6 million people worldwide living with cancer in 2002 (Parkin et al., 2005; WHO, 2005). As of January 2008, it is estimated that there are 11.9 million cancer survivors in the United States. This represents approximately 4% of the population, with approximately 15% of these cancer survivors being diagnosed 20 or more years earlier (Howlader and Noone, 2009).

Improved cancer surveillance, more accurate diagnoses, more efficacious treatment, as well as longer follow-up, have led to an increased life expectancy for patients and increased number of 'cancer cured' people. It is predicted that this number of cancer survivors will increase in the future. A public health effort to address cancer survivorship supports the Healthy People 2010 goal to increase the proportion of cancer survivors who are living 5 years or longer after diagnosis to 70% (US Department of Health and Human Services, 2010).

The report from the Institute of Medicine 'From Cancer Patient to Cancer Survivor: Lost in Transition' mentions that although the number of patients surviving cancer is increasing, it is unknown what this will mean to the health and well-being of these people (National Research Council, 2005).

Survivors face numerous physical, psychological, social, spiritual, and financial issues following their diagnosis and treatment and for the remaining years of their lives. The health-care challenges of survivors are being now recognized as unique. In addition to the acute effects of the surgical, radiation, and chemotherapy treatments, many permanent phase survivors are at risk for developing late or long-term side effects from their primary treatments. These long-term effects have a bearing on obtaining optimal physical, psychological, and cognitive functioning for survivors—which is the goal of rehabilitation for patients with cancer (Chasen and Dippenaar, 2008). Survivors of cancer have significantly poorer health outcomes across many burden of illness outcomes for many years after the diagnosis of cancer (Miaskowski and Dibble, 1995; Siddall and Cousins, 2004). More than 6 million survivors are older than 65 years, thus translating into a growing elderly patient population of cancer survivors who suffer from co-morbidities that affect their general well-being (Deimling et al., 2007). For many survivors, a high prevalence of physical symptoms, in addition to symptoms in other life domains will diminish their quality of life (Alfano and Rowland, 2006).

Pain is recognized as impacting on all dimensions of quality of life (Cleeland, 1984; Miaskowski and Dibble, 1995; Siddall and Cousins, 2004; Burton et al., 2007) and is one of the most distressing symptoms for patients with cancer (Patrick et al., 2003; Sun et al., 2008). Pain, may, in some cases of head and neck cancer patients predict for survival (Funk et al., 2012). Up to 40% of 5-year cancer survivors report pain (Nelson et al., 2001; Anderson et al., 2002). Experiencing pain was related to poorer general health ($p = 0.001$) and physical ($p < 0.001$), role ($p < 0.01$), and social ($p < 0.001$) functioning in a group of patients who had survived cancer (Green et al., 2011).

Patients under-recognize pain and are often unsure if optimum pain control is achievable (Green et al., 2002, 2003). They are concerned about distracting attention away from treatment and believe that pain is indicative of progressive disease (Turk, 2002; Green et al., 2003, 2009; Greenberg et al., 2003; Stewart et al., 2003; Howlader and Noone, 2009). In addition, members of the interdisciplinary team often fail to assess the patient's pain adequately or to recognize under reporting (Anderson et al., 2000; Nelson et al., 2001). Many professionals lack knowledge of the principles of pain relief, side effect management, or understanding of key concepts like addiction, tolerance, dosing, and communication (Green et al., 2009). Epidemiological data including incidence and prevalence of chronic pain in the different cancer types have not been reported consistently and pain treatment strategies such as the WHO pain ladder has not been validated for patients with cancer who have chronic pain (Burton et al., 2007).

Aetiology of pain in cancer survivors

Chronic pain in cancer survivors can arise because of damage to tissue caused by the cancer and/or the cancer therapy: surgery, chemotherapy, steroids, hormones, and radiation (Table 13.5.1). In addition, survivors may have pain from chronic conditions such as post-herpetic neuralgia, rheumatic diseases and diabetic neuropathy. At one centre, up to 40% of visits to a Cancer Survivors Pain and Palliative Care Program were due to chronic pain.

Chronic pain in cancer survivors can be divided into three pathophysiologic categories: somatic, visceral, and neuropathic (Levy et al., 2008):

1. Somatic pain occurs as a result of excitation of nociceptive receptors in the skin, serosa, and musculoskeletal system. This pain is usually confined, sharp, and aggravated by movement. Examples of somatic pains in cancer survivors include osteoporotic fractures, musculoskeletal imbalance with degenerative arthritis, and avascular necrosis of the femoral head.

2. Visceral pain is generated by nociceptive receptors in the walls of both visceral hollow and solid organs. These receptors respond to stretching and produce an ache over the organ as well as a referred pain. Examples include partial small bowel obstruction from adhesions and odynophagia from oesophageal narrowing.

3. Neuropathic pain arises from injury to the peripheral and/ or central nervous system, and can be both spontaneous and evoked by a stimulus. Neuropathic pain is the most common type of pain in cancer survivors and it poses a challenge due to the severity, persistence, and resistance to simple analgesics. The description by patients is vivid and includes: 'itching', 'pins and needles', 'electric', 'holding a snow ball', 'burning', 'hot poker iron', amongst others. Neuropathic pain is localized to specific dermatomes, nerve root distribution, or peripheral, distal extremities (Levy et al., 2008).

4. Chronic neuropathic pain, resulting from nerve injury, is a challenging clinical problem which often cannot be adequately treated by current analgesics without unacceptable side effects. It greatly reduces quality of life, even more so than other chronic pain states with a negative impact on mobility, function, mood, and general well-being (Jensen et al., 2007). The prevalence of neuropathic pain is likely to be underestimated but studies from North America, Europe and the United Kingdom have found between 8% and 17% of the population may suffer from pain of predominantly neuropathic origin (Torrance et al., 2006; Toth et al., 2009; Doth et al., 2010). Neuropathic pain associated with cancer treatment is an increasing challenge. As the incidence of cancer increases and survival improves with better oncological management, there is an increasing number of patients having to live with the long-term effects of treatment-related neuropathic pain such as chemotherapy-induced peripheral neuropathy (CIPN) or scar pain (Cavaletti et al., 2011; Naleschinski et al., 2012).

CIPN affects up to 96% of patients who receive potentially neurotoxic chemotherapy (e.g. platinums, taxanes, vinca-alkaloids, and bortezomib), resulting in dose-reduction or early cessation of potentially life-prolonging treatment for up to 50% (Vasey et al., 2004; Richardson et al., 2006; Argyriou et al., 2008; Storey et al., 2010). Symptoms are commonly in a glove and stocking distribution and include spontaneous pain, paraesthesia, allodynia (non-painful stimuli causing pain), hyperalgesia (increased sensitivity to painful stimuli), hypoaesthesia (numbness), and impaired proprioception, causing difficulty with day-to-day functioning such as fastening buttons, handling coins, walking and driving. One year following cessation of treatment approximately 50% of patients still have symptoms which both limits future treatment options for patients with relapsed/metastatic disease and leaves many with long-term pain or disability despite being cured of cancer. In our centre 57% of colorectal cancer patients still had symptoms of neuropathy 6 months after completing treatment with curative intent (WHO, 2005).

Estimates for persistent neuropathic pain after cancer surgery vary, with post-mastectomy and post-thoracotomy pain occurring in 30–60% of patients (Kehlet et al., 2006). One large study after breast cancer surgery found almost half of patients had persistent pain 2–3 years later, with this being moderate to severe in nearly a quarter of (Gartner et al., 2009). In our own centre approximately 30% of patients had persistent post-mastectomy pain, with a threefold increase in risk conferred by adjuvant chemotherapy (Sheridan et al., 2012). Recent guidelines suggest the use of objective quantifiable tests such as Quantitative Sensory Testing as clinical biomarkers to strengthen the diagnosis of neuropathic pain, which is made on history and examination (Smith et al., 2007; Cruccu et al., 2010; Haanpaa et al., 2011).

Treatment of neuropathic pain relies on early identification, understanding of the initiating and sustaining pathophysiological mechanisms and use of a range of therapeutic approaches (Attal et al., 2011). Evidence is accumulating which suggests the neurosensory characteristics of the pain may be the most important factor in predicting a treatment response, rather than the underlying aetiology (Dworkin et al., 2011; Selph et al., 2011). Current systemic therapy is mainly oral antidepressants or anticonvulsants; however, treatment often requires titration over months and is limited by variable efficacy and unacceptable side effects (Liu and Qin, 2011).

Chronic pain by disease type

Head and neck cancer

Cervical lymph node metastases in this setting have been treated commonly with radical neck dissection, which involves the removal of the ipsilateral spinal accessory nerve (cranial nerve CN) XI), internal jugular vein, and sternocleidomastoid muscle, in addition to ipsilateral cervical lymph node groups. Though performed commonly, this procedure carries with it significant morbidity.

The 'shoulder syndrome' manifests as continuous pain, shoulder tilt and drop, limitations in shoulder retraction, anterior flexion movements and active shoulder abduction, winged scapula and abnormal electromyographic findings (Ewing and Martin, 1952). Compromise or injury to the spinal accessory nerve (CN XI) can result in sensory paraesthesias and numbness. It has been observed that patients who have undergone neck dissections sparing the spinal accessory nerve, report less shoulder and neck pain than those in whom it was sacrificed. Spinal accessory nerve preservation has also been correlated with lower consumption of analgesics (Terrell et al., 2000).

Table 13.5.1 Sources of chronic pain in cancer survivors

	Chemotherapy/corticosteroids	Surgery	Radiation	Hormonal	Bisphosphonates	Cancer
Type of pain	Two major types: 1. *Acute paraesthesias* 2. *Chronic dysaesthetic pain*—often presents as 'stocking-glove' distribution	Chronic postoperative pain Characterized by type of surgery: thoracotomy breast surgery modified-radical neck dissection limb amputations nephrectomy inguinal lymph node dissection Common mechanism: central sensitization	*Several types of pain* Plexophathies Peripheral nerve entrapment Myelopathy Enteritis Proctitis Cystitis Visceral strictures Osteoradionecrosis Accelerated osteoporosis Secondary malignancies	Osteoporosis secondary to hormonal treatments of breast and prostate CA Cancer-therapy related bone loss is severe and occurs at a higher rate than typical osteoporosis	Usually well tolerated May increase risk of osteonecrosis of the jaw (ONJ) Incidence range: 1–11% 3% > 2 years 11% > 4 years	
Characteristics	*Acute paraesthesias* Typically resolves once chemotherapy is discontinued 15–50% of cases become chronic *Chronic paraesthesias* Risk of chronic pain due to cumulative toxicity Agents with prominent neurotoxic side effects Cisplatin, oxaliplatin, vincristine, vinblastine, paclitaxel, docetaxel	*Variability in pain incidence* Phantom breast pain: 13–25% Phantom limb pain: 30–80% Typically presents 2–12 months post-surgery Intensity of acute postoperative pain predicts chronic pain	Manifest months or years after treatment is completed		ONJ symptoms: localized pain, swelling, loosening of teeth, exposed bone, non-healing oral ulcers, purulent gingival discharge, numbness or heaviness of the jaw Chronic and diffuse bone pain may also occur	
Effects	*Chronic peripheral neuropathy* Risk of deconditioning and musculoskeletal pain *Myopathy* Somatic pains and weakness			Increased risk of vertebral and non-vertebral fractures; resulting in pain and disability Aseptic necrosis of the femoral heads and hip Fractures		

Source: Data from Levy et al., Management of chronic pain in cancer survivors, *Cancer Journal*, Volume 14, Issue 6, pp. 401–409, Copyright © 2008, with permission from Lippincott Williams & Wilkins, Inc.

Nonetheless, chronic pain has been demonstrated even with sparing of the spinal accessory nerve, as evidenced by electromyographic studies. This is most commonly secondary to expansive dissection, vigorous traction, intraoperative trauma, and ischaemia (Sakorafas et al., 2010). Morbidity is compounded if there is a delay in the diagnosis post surgery.

Osteonecrosis of the jaw is a known potential adverse effect of head and neck irradiation. It can be exacerbated by the use of steroids and chemotherapeutic agents, infection, periodontal disease, and poor dental hygiene. It has been associated more recently with the use of high doses of intravenous bisphosphonates in several studies, with the mandible being the most commonly affected site.

Rectal cancer

Patients who have had radiation to the pelvis for rectal cancer can be at risk of the development of 'pelvic pain syndrome'. Aetiologies for this syndrome may include chronic radiation enteritis or proctitis, chronic cystitis, pelvic insufficiency fractures, and neuropathies which may manifest as burning perineum syndrome (Levy et al., 2008).

Chronic radiation enteritis can happen in up to 15% of patients receiving abdominal or pelvic irradiation. The onset of symptoms may occur up to 18 months post radiation treatment, and commonly include crampy, colicky abdominal pain accompanied by tenesmus, bloody diarrhoea, emesis, and anorexia or weight loss.

Cystitis, the product of chronic effects of bladder irradiation, results from endothelial ischaemic damage and interstitial fibrosis, and may lead to a diminution in bladder capacity. Clinically, urgency and dysuria may be observed.

Pelvic insufficiency fractures are an uncommon side effect of chemotherapy and radiation treatment for rectal cancer, however they can lead to significant morbidity. Pain is usually intense and of acute onset, most commonly affecting the abdomen, low back, pelvis, hip, buttock or thigh. Studies indicate a 3-year average of 3.1%, and females and Caucasians appear to be at higher risk (Herman et al., 2009). Burning perineum syndrome refers to pain that has developed in the perianal region as a result of radiation that may expand to encompass the scrotum or vagina. It is a rare complication, and onset is usually 6 to 18 months following radiation (Minsky and Cohen, 1988).

Sarcoma

Depending on the disease presentation, limb-sparing surgery may be an option for soft tissue sarcomas occurring in an extremity, and thus amputation may not be necessary. Certain situations will, however, dictate limb amputation.

One of the more frequent complications post amputation is phantom limb pain (PLP), the perception of painful sensations in an amputated extremity. Though the exact mechanism is unknown, it is believed to be secondary to spinal plasticity and cerebral reorganization following an insult. Onset is typically within days to weeks of amputation, but can be delayed for months or years. It has been shown to occur acutely in over half of amputees, with higher levels of extremity amputation increasing the risk of greater pain intensity. Incidence is higher following traumatic amputation as opposed to surgical amputation (Ramachandran and Hirstein, 1998). Other risk factors include the presence of pre-amputation pain, persistent stump pain, noxious intraoperative stimuli and acute postoperative pain (Ramachandran and

Hirstein, 1997). PLP is less common in children and congenital amputees. Phantom limb pain can be varied in presentation, but may be shooting, stabbing, cramping, burning, or itchy in nature. Pain is often localized to the distal portion of the amputated extremity, and many patients report that the affected limb is in a contorted or awkward position. Some patients have also reported exacerbations with cold temperature, stress, fatigue, urination, and defecation. Psychological factors are not correlated with its occurrence, but may be exacerbating rather than causative in nature.

Genitourinary

Prostate cancer

The treatment modalities available for prostate cancer have expanded within the last several years. Standard treatment is androgen deprivation therapy, either surgical (orchidectomy) or medical (gonadotropin-releasing hormone (GnRH) agonist treatment). The intended outcome of GnRH agonist treatment is hypogonadism, which is a significant cause of acquired osteoporosis in males. GnRH agonists have been shown to decrease bone mineral density of the hip and spine by approximately 2–3% per year during initial treatment. Similarly, surgical orchidectomy for prostate cancer is often followed by severe osteoporosis and increased risk of hip fracture and vertebral fracture. Risk factors include Caucasian race, low bone mineral density, and treatment duration of at least 1 year with GnRH agonists (Smith et al., 2005; Saylor et al., 2011). This increased risk starts almost immediately and can persist for several years (Daniell, 1997).

Chronic testicular pain is a well-known potential complication of treatment for testicular cancer. This includes chronic pelvic pain syndrome (pelvic pain either continuous or recurrent for at least 6 months) and phantom testes syndrome (pain in the removed testis), with the presence of preoperative pain in the removed testes as a positive risk factor (Puhse et al., 2010). A higher incidence of genital pain during and after intercourse has also been recorded (Puhse et al., 2008).

Breast cancer

Treatments for breast cancer now commonly include surgery for axillary node dissection and primary tumour staging, radiation, hormonal (anti-oestrogen) therapy, and/or chemotherapy. Up to half of patients post mastectomy experience chronic pain, which can lead to significant encroachments on a patient's quality of life due to physical and emotional distress. Chronic neuropathic pain following mastectomy has been well documented and can be characterized by four different types of pain syndrome:

1. *Phantom breast syndrome* (PBS). PBS is a condition in which patients have the sensation of residual breast tissue which is often painful, but can also include non-painful sensations. Patients may complain of persistent pain and discomfort, numbness or tingling, pressure, burning, and throbbing among other neuropathic symptoms. Onset may be delayed up to one year post surgery, and the condition can persist for several years following surgery (Jamison et al., 1979) with an incidence ranging between 13% and 44% (Jamison et al., 1979; Kroner et al., 1989, 1992). Common risk factors for the development of PBS are severe acute postoperative pain and greater postoperative use of analgesics (Tasmuth et al., 1996). Other factors believed

to contribute include age under 40 years, psychosocial status, premenopausal state, parity, and those who have had a preoperative history of breast sensations (Staps et al., 1985; Gartner et al., 2009). In addition, it is important to remember that patients who have undergone both breast-conserving surgery or reconstructive breast surgery can also have a post-surgical pain syndrome, consisting of various neuropathic components.

2. *Neuroma pain* is pain in the area of a surgical scar on the breast, chest, or arm aggravated or intensified by touch or percussion. A neuroma is a benign growth of nerve tissue at the severed ends of sensory nerves, which may become entrapped by scar tissue. It can result in dysaesthesia to the overlying skin secondary to atypical connections of regenerating nerves. The estimated prevalence of neuroma pain is approximately 23–49%.

3. *Intercostobrachial neuralgia* (ICN) refers to post-surgical pain experienced in the distribution of the intercostobrachial nerve either with or without axillary node dissection. This most commonly results in pain, allodynia or hyperalgesia in the axilla, anterior chest wall or medial upper arm. Given the substantial inter-individual variation in distribution of the intercostobrachial nerve, the risk of damage to the nerve is relatively high, regardless of surgical procedure or method. Prevalence estimates range as high as 40% (Granek et al., 1984; Smith et al., 1999).

4. *Other nerve injury pain.* It is postulated that other nerves may be involved in the development of post-mastectomy pain syndrome. This is evidenced by the prevalence of chronic post-surgical pain in patients who have undergone mastectomy without accompanying axillary node dissection and with documented sparing of the intercostobrachial nerve (Carpenter et al., 1999).

5. *Radiation-induced pain syndromes.* It has been well documented that adjunctive radiation in breast cancer patients increases their risk of developing a chronic pain syndrome. The most common cause of pain in this setting includes radiation-induced plexopathy, especially brachial plexopathy. Brachial plexopathy is often heralded by numbness and paraesthesias of the hands and fingers, followed by weakness and increasing pain. It is thought to result from a combination of direct cell damage from ionizing radiation and progressive ischaemic changes which may lead to fibrosis surrounding the nerves of the brachial plexus, fibrous thickening of the neurilemmal sheath, demyelination, and fibrous replacement of nerve fibrils (Qayyum et al., 2000). Onset of symptoms of plexopathy may be delayed for months to years in some cases. Other less common causes include osteoradionecrosis of the chest wall, fractures, and secondary malignancies (Paice, 2011).

6. *Peripheral neuropathy.* The most common cause of peripheral neuropathy in the breast cancer population is the use of chemotherapeutic agents. Those that have been most frequently implicated include vinca alkaloids (e.g. vincristine), taxanes (paclitaxel and docetaxel), and platinum-derived compounds such as carboplatin. Peripheral neuropathy is often the dose limiting side effect of these agents (Reyes-Gibby et al., 2009). Symptoms can include numbness, tingling, pain, and other paraesthesias. The majority of breast cancer patients do experience improvement in their neuropathic symptoms over time;

however, in some patients it is irreversible. Sensory polyneuropathy is the usual presentation, but it can progress to cranial nerve palsies, motor weakness, and autonomic dysfunction (Rowinsky et al., 1993).

7. *Pain related to breast implants and surgical reconstruction.* There is some evidence to suggest that women who have undergone breast reconstruction are at a higher risk post surgery for chronic pain than those who have not. One study found the incidence of pain at 1 year following mastectomy with reconstruction to be appreciably higher (49%) than those with mastectomy alone (31%) or who had undergone breast reduction (22%). Breast reconstruction also correlated with higher pain intensity (Wallace et al., 1996) with submuscular implant placement associated with more chronic pain than subglandular implants. There has been no demonstrated relationship between the type of implant used (saline vs silicone) and the development of chronic pain (Wallace et al., 1996).

Lung cancer

Chronic post-thoracotomy pain syndrome (PTPS) is a persistent or recurrent pain in the area of a thoracotomy incision for at least 2 months following surgery (International Association for the Study of Pain, Subcommittee on Taxonomy, 1986). It is believed to be secondary to intercostal nerve damage as well as suboptimal control of acute pain in the immediate postoperative period. Aggressive rib retraction may also contribute by leading to costovertebral and costochondral dislocation. Neuroma formation and tumour recurrence have also been cited. The syndrome is characterized by significant burning pain with other associated neuropathic features postoperatively with a very slow resolution in the following months and years. Unfortunately, it does not appear to decrease appreciably with time. There is a relatively high incidence of ipsilateral arm and shoulder dysfunction. The incidence of PTPS is reported at approximately 80% at 3 months, 75% at 6 months, and 61% 1 year after surgery (Perttunen et al., 1999). One study found that approximately 30% of patients continued to report pain at 5 years post thoracotomy with no significant decrease in pain intensity (Dajczman et al., 1991). Preoperative epidural analgesia has been shown to be more effective at reducing the incidence and intensity of the resultant chronic pain than postoperative epidural analgesia (Obata et al., 1999).

Haematological/stem cell transplantation

Haematological malignancy survivors are at an increased risk of developing chronic pain syndromes due to several potential treatment related complications. These pain syndromes are of particular concern in the setting of stem cell transplantation, given the treatment intensity. Patients may experience significant bone pain as a result of prolonged steroid therapy as treatment for graft-versus-host disease. This may lead to an increased incidence of osteonecrosis and osteoporosis. Haemorrhagic cystitis is another painful condition, which can result from certain conditioning regimens, especially those containing cyclophosphamide and total body irradiation. The immune-suppressing calcineurin inhibitors used prophylactically post stem cell transplant to prevent graft rejection (i.e. cyclosporine, tacrolimus) can have neurotoxic side effects with an incidence between 5% and 30%. Profound immune suppression post transplant leaves patients susceptible to a number of opportunistic infections, such as herpes zoster, with the potential subsequent development of post herpetic neuralgia (Niscola et al., 2008).

Treatments

Despite numerous advances in the course of the last several years, the management of chronic pain in cancer survivors is often suboptimal, secondary to the complex neurophysiology of many chronic pain syndromes and a relative paucity of education and resources within many oncological settings. It requires an inter-professional approach that details a comprehensive assessment with ongoing reassessment to guide the implementation and integration of pharmacological and non-pharmacological measures. This facilitates the elucidation and revision of the pain source, alteration of the perception of pain, and inhibition of pain transmission to the central nervous system (Ferrer-Brechner et al., 1985), thereby helping to optimize patient quality of life.

Opioid therapy is one of the foundations of cancer pain treatment. Its role in the management of neuropathic as well as nociceptive pain has been confirmed in several clinical trials (Eisenberg et al., 2005). Though morphine remains the most widely used opioid, there is presently no evidence to suggest that one opioid is better than another as a first-line agent. Opioid therapy can be administered through several routes, including oral, transdermal and, most commonly, parenteral. Opioids can also be delivered via the buccal, submucosal, and intranasal routes (rapid onset opioids), and rectally for the control of episodes of breakthrough pain, in addition to regularly scheduled or long-acting preparations. Methadone may have a distinctive role in the management of chronic pain in cancer survivors due to its action as an opioid agonist and *N*-methyl-D-aspartase (NMDA) receptor antagonist, which can inhibit central sensitization and may moderate allodynia and hyperalgesia in certain neuropathic pain syndromes. In occasional situations, neuraxial (epidural or intrathecal) delivery of opioids may be appropriate for some particularly challenging pain syndromes when resources permit.

When opioids are used as a singular treatment, higher doses may be required. This may lead to adverse effects such as constipation and sedation, as well as long-term complications, which can include tolerance, opioid-induced neurotoxicity, physical dependency, and pituitary axis suppression. Clearly in susceptible individuals, psychological dependence may become an issue. Optimal management of neuropathic pain usually involves the administration of a neuropathic analgesic medication, used either alone or in combination with opioids for synergistic effect, which may reduce the risk of opioid-induced neurotoxicity. Those used most commonly in this setting include antidepressants, anticonvulsants, and non-steroidal anti-inflammatory drugs (NSAIDs).

Tricyclic antidepressants (TCAs) such as nortriptyline and desipramine are used most commonly in the setting of neuropathic pain, as they have a lower incidence of anticholinergic and cardiac side effects (QT prolongation) as compared to amitriptyline. Usually days to weeks of treatment are required before a measurable degree of analgesia is achieved. Newer classes of antidepressants including serotonin and norepinephrine (noradrenaline) reuptake inhibitors (i.e. duloxetine and venlafaxine) can also have a role in the modulation of neuropathic pain, however selective serotonin reuptake inhibitors (SSRIs) have not been proven to be as effective (Sindrup et al., 2005). (See Chapter 13.3.)

Anticonvulsant medications commonly used in the management of neuropathic pain include gabapentin, carbamazepine, and pregabalin. Carbamazepine is thought to exert its analgesic effect through the reduction of conductance in sodium channels and may have a particular role in the management of trigeminal neuralgia. Gabapentin and pregabalin are similar in their mechanism of action, which appears to be delivered via interaction with the $\alpha2-\delta$ protein subunit of voltage-gated calcium channels. Pregabalin displays linear absorption as opposed to gabapentin, giving it a more predictable dose response range and a generally faster time to therapeutic titration. The efficacy of other anticonvulsants for neuropathic pain has not been reliably established in clinical trials.

Anti-inflammatory agents (NSAIDs, steroids) have been employed in several chronic pain syndromes in cancer survivors. They are mostly used in association with opioids for musculoskeletal pain; however they are not viable options for long-term treatment due to side effects. Other potential treatments being explored include topical analgesics such as lidocaine and the NMDA receptor antagonists such as ketamine. These treatments require further research.

Non-pharmacological management of chronic pain in the cancer survivor

Non-pharmacological treatment options should be used in combination with medications where appropriate, with a view to minimizing medication side effects and optimizing function and quality of life.

The basic concept of a true multidisciplinary, interdisciplinary treatment team to manage and address the challenges and the various needs of cancer survivors, including pain, is a natural progression based on the cancer rehabilitation philosophy. The latter's objective being, through an interdisciplinary approach, to empower individuals who are experiencing loss of function, fatigue, pain, malnutrition, psychological distress, and other symptoms, as a result of cancer or its treatment to improve their own quality of life (Chasen and Dippenaar, 2008). Such teams have shown efficacy in treating chronic pain in the general population (Shealy, 2013). The results have been profound with at least one-third returning to work, their average pain intensity decreasing an average of 70% and their mood improving in 90% of patients. This same interdisciplinary treatment prototype also can be applied to cancer survivors (Robbins et al., 2003). Team members should include physicians, nurses, physical, occupational, and vocational therapists in addition to dietitians, social workers, and psychologists. The different disciplines involved in the care of these patients constitute the team. It is vital that communication within the team is open, direct, and supportive. Herein lies the strength of collaboration between team members. They will learn of the different assessment approaches, the importance that patients place on various symptoms and the effects these symptoms have on the domains of the patients' quality of life, specifically relating to pain. With the patient and the caregiver placed as the end target of all therapeutic interventions, the combined collaborative efforts of the team are synergistic in their effect. Regular roundtable discussions are a key component of this teamwork (Chasen and Jacobsen, 2013). At times, spiritual counsellors or religious personnel can be of importance. In addition, group educational sessions during which dialogue is encouraged is important to empower participants to play an active role in their own management. Attention to all symptoms including, loss of appetite, loneliness, fatigue and their relationship to pain are all key components that need to be addressed. Social isolation, existential distress, and family disharmony should all be considered an integral cause of pain. The adult 'Damocles syndrome', characterized by a state of long-term uncertainty, stress, and anxiety of having disease recurrence, experienced by the patients who have survived cancer and their families must also be considered. Cancer survivors can be physically de-conditioned after the treatments which have caused weight loss, muscle loss (sarcopenia), muscle weakness, and also be psychologically de-conditioned which expresses as a result of a change in body image, a loss of previous role within the family and work spheres, as well as having to face morbidity and mortality. All of these factors contribute to the 'total pain' of the patient. Patients with chronic pain are prone to develop 'maladaptive behaviours' (McCracken and Eccleston, 2003). These behaviours are manifested by the following cycle. Pain causes diminished activity. This leads to progressive de-conditioning, which gives rise to reduced socialization, altered sleep/awake cycle and medication and drug abuse.

Within the expertise of the various members of the interdisciplinary rehabilitation team, cancer survivors with chronic pain are instructed and trained to build stamina and endurance to counter the muscle de-conditioning, to recognize stressful situations and utilise learned, effective coping strategies. The effect of exercise training and comprehensive health improvement programmes, has been suggested to improve quality of life, particularly in chronic breast or chest-wall pain (Wong et al., 2012). By building on past, successful experiences of the patient, existential meaning can be found and utilized in order to surmount current suffering.

Other types of pain

For patients experiencing moderate to severe pain following neck dissection, acupuncture resulted in an improvement of a third of patients on a composite scale. Biogenetics as developed by Shealy, synthesizes techniques of self- regulation with emphasis on positive attitude, a belief in self, relaxation, hypnosis, massage, yoga, and transcutaneous electrical nerve stimulation (TENS), which may help to build strength and stamina (Pujol and Monti, 2007). Psychosocial interventions can include hypnosis, cognitive behavioural therapy, desensitization strategies, guided imagery, and mindfulness-based stress reduction (Keefe et al., 2005).

Conclusion

Pain can be a common experience for many cancer survivors and may develop due to a number of aetiologies. The experience and perception of pain is affected by not only physical but also psychological, cognitive, cultural, and environmental factors, which are specific to each individual. The repercussions of pain which is managed suboptimally can be extensive, and in some cases even lead to increased mortality. Substantial improvements have been made in the outcomes and survival rates of patients with many different types of cancer over the past several years, yet with this the complexity of their pain syndromes continues to increase. Though

many cancer survivors can return to relatively satisfactory levels of quality of life, chronic pain can remain a persistent issue for some, and may be underreported and therefore diagnosed and treated suboptimally. It is recognized that cancer survivors experience a greater incidence of comorbidities and psychosocial sequelae. The evidence base is increasing for a number of treatments for cancer survivors to address their pain issues and improve their quality of life. Each cancer survivor is unique and responses to pain management strategies can be diverse. Additional resources should also be focused on equipping patients with the skills to cope with chronic or persistent pain, thereby creating a more efficient transition from active treatment to survivorship. Empowerment of the cancer survivor is a key element of any successful strategy as is collaboration among team members. Respect for survivors' individuality is also paramount to any successful outcome.

Acknowledgement

The authors thank Ms Samantha Zinkie for her review and comments.

Online materials

Complete references for this chapter are available online at <http://www.oxfordmedicine.com>.

References

Alfano, C.M. and Rowland, J.H. (2006). Recovery issues in cancer survivorship: a new challenge for supportive care. *Cancer Journal*, 12, 432–443.

Argyriou, A.A., Polychronopoulos, P., Iconomou, G., Chroni, E., and Kalofonos, H.P. (2008). A review on oxaliplatin-induced peripheral nerve damage. *Cancer Treatment Reviews*, 34, 368–377.

Attal, N., Bouhassira, D., Baron, R., *et al.* (2011). Assessing symptom profiles in neuropathic pain clinical trials: can it improve outcome? *European Journal of Pain*, 15, 441–443.

Burton, A.W., Fanciullo, G., and Beasley, R. (2007). Chronic pain in the cured cancer patient. In J. Rusko and H. Cooper (eds.) *Cancer Pain Management*, pp. 155–161. New York: McGraw Hill Medical.

Burton, A.W., Fanciullo, G.J., Beasley, R.D., and Fisch, M.J. (2007). Chronic pain in the cancer survivor: a new frontier. *Pain Medicine*, 8, 189–198.

Cavaletti, G., Alberti, P., Frigeni, B., Piatti, M., and Susani, E. (2011). Chemotherapy-induced neuropathy. *Current Treatment Options in Neurology*, 13, 180–190.

Chasen, M.R. and Dippenaar, A.P. (2008) Cancer nutrition and rehabilitation-its time has come! *Current Oncology*, 15, 117–122.

Chasen, M.R. and Jacobsen, P. (2013). Rehabilitation in cancer. In I.N. Oliver (ed.) *The MASCC Textbook of Cancer Supportive Care and Survivorship*, pp. 389–398. New York: Springer.

Cruccu, G., Sommer, C., Anand, P., *et al.* (2010). EFNS guidelines on neuropathic pain assessment: revised 2009. *European Journal of Neurology*, 17, 1010–1018.

Deimling, G.T., Bowman, K.F., and Wagner, L.J. (2007). The effects of cancer-related pain and fatigue on functioning of older adult, long-term cancer survivors. *Cancer Nursing*, 30, 421–433.

Doth, A.H., Hansson, P.T., Jensen, M.P., and Taylor, R.S. (2010). The burden of neuropathic pain: a systematic review and meta-analysis of health utilities. *Pain*, 149, 338–344.

Dworkin, R.H., Turk, D.C., Katz, N.P., *et al.* (2011). Evidence-based clinical trial design for chronic pain pharmacotherapy: a blueprint for ACTION. *Pain*, 152, S107–S115.

Eisenberg, E., McNicol, E.D., and Carr, D.B. (2005). Efficacy and safety of opioid agonists in the treatment of neuropathic pain of nonmalignant origin: systematic review and meta-analysis of randomized controlled trials. *Journal of the American Medical Association*, 293, 3043–3052.

Funk, G.F., Karnell, L.H., and Christensen, A.J. (2012). Long-term health-related quality of life in survivors of head and neck cancer. *Archives of Otolaryngology – Head and Neck Surgery*, 138, 123–133.

Gartner, R., Jensen, M.B., Nielsen, J., *et al.* (2009). Prevalence of and factors associated with persistent pain following breast cancer surgery. *Journal of the American Medical Association*, 302, 1985–1992.

Green, C.R., Montague, L., and Hart-Johnson, T.A. (2009). Consistent and breakthrough pain in diverse advanced cancer patients: a longitudinal examination. *Journal of Pain and Symptom Management*, 37, 831–847.

Green, C.R., Hart-Johnson, T., and Loeffler, D.R. (2011). Cancer-related chronic pain: examining quality of life in diverse cancer survivors. *Cancer*, 117, 1994–2003.

Keefe, F.J., Abernethy, A.P., and Campbell, L. (2005). Psychological approaches to understanding and treating disease-related pain. *Annual Review of Psychology*, 56, 601–630.

Kehlet, H., Jensen, T.S., and Woolf, C.J. (2006). Persistent postsurgical pain: risk factors and prevention. *The Lancet*, 367, 1618–1625.

Kroner, K., Knudsen, U.B., Lundby, L., and Hvid, H. (1992). Long-term phantom breast syndrome after mastectomy. *Clinical Journal of Pain* 8, 346–350.

Levy, M.H., Chwistek, M., and Mehta, R.S. (2008). Management of chronic pain in cancer survivors. *Cancer Journal*, 14, 401–409.

Naleschinski, D., Baron, R., and Miaskowski, C. (2012). Identification and treatment of neuropathic pain in patients with cancer. *Pain Clinical Updates*, 20, 1–5.

National Research Council (2005). *From Cancer Patient to Cancer Survivor: Lost in Transition*. Washington, DC: The National Academies Press.

Niscola, P., Romani, C., Scaramucci, L., *et al.* (2008). Pain syndromes in the setting of haematopoietic stem cell transplantation for haematological malignancies. *Bone Marrow Transplantation*, 41, 757–764.

Pujol, L.A. and Monti, D.A. (2007). Managing cancer pain with nonpharmacologic and complementary therapies. *Journal of the American Osteopathic Association*, 107, ES15–ES21.

Reyes-Gibby, C.C., Morrow, P.K., Buzdar, A., and Shete, S. (2009). Chemotherapy-induced peripheral neuropathy as a predictor of neuropathic pain in breast cancer patients previously treated with paclitaxel. *Journal of Pain*, 10, 1146–1150.

Richardson, P.G., Briemberg, H., Jagannath, S., *et al.* (2006). Frequency, characteristics, and reversibility of peripheral neuropathy during treatment of advanced multiple myeloma with bortezomib. *Journal of Clinical Oncology*, 24, 3113–3120.

Robbins, H., Gatchel, R.J., Noe, C., *et al.* (2003). A prospective one-year outcome study of interdisciplinary chronic pain management: compromising its efficacy by managed care policies. *Anesthesia & Analgesia*, 97, 156–62.

Shealy, C.C.R. (2013). Multidisciplinary pain clinics. In R. Weiner (ed.) *Pain Management: A Practical Guide for Clinicians* (5th ed.), pp. 35–44. Boca Raton, FL: St. Lucie Press.

Sindrup, S.H., Otto, M., Finnerup, N.B., and Jensen, T.S. (2005). Antidepressants in the treatment of neuropathic pain. *Basic & Clinical Pharmacology & Toxicology*, 96, 399–409.

Smith, B.H., Macfarlane, G.J., and Torrance, N. (2007). Epidemiology of chronic pain, from the laboratory to the bus stop: time to add understanding of biological mechanisms to the study of risk factors in population-based research? *Pain*, 127, 5–10.

Sun, V., Borneman, T., Piper, B., Koczywas, M., and Ferrell, B. (2008). Barriers to pain assessment and management in cancer survivorship. *Journal of Cancer Survivorship*, 2, 65–71.

Torrance, N., Smith, B.H., Bennett, M.I., and Lee, A.J. (2006). The epidemiology of chronic pain of predominantly neuropathic origin. Results from a general population survey. *Journal of Pain*, 7, 281–289.

Toth, C., Lander, J., and Wiebe, S. (2009). The prevalence and impact of chronic pain with neuropathic pain symptoms in the general population. *Pain Medicine*, 10, 918–929.

SECTION 14

Cancer-associated disorders

Neurological problems in advanced cancer

Augusto Caraceni, Cinzia Martini, and Fabio Simonetti

Introduction to neurological problems in advanced cancer

Neurological complications are frequent in populations with advanced cancer. An adequate neurological assessment is always important in addressing pain, cognitive symptoms, and peripheral and central nervous system (CNS) complications.

Intracranial hypertension

General aspects

Intracranial pressure (ICP) is the result of the balance between the liquid (cerebrospinal fluid (CSF), blood interstitial fluid) and solid content of the cranium. It is not constant but depends on systemic blood pressure; its changes are maintained within narrow limits. The normal brain can tolerate small variations usually without clinical consequences.

An adult's cranium is a fixed vault so an increase in one of the three components—brain, blood, CSF—causes a reduction in one of the others.

Pathological processes, such as tumours, abscesses, or haematomas, increase intracranial contents that compress brain parenchyma. They also disrupt the blood–brain barrier, which may lead to increased intracranial blood volume. If this occurs slowly, there may be no increase in ICP, at least temporarily. This is due to compensatory mechanisms, such as enhanced CSF reabsorption, reduced intracranial blood volume, and increased drainage through the lymphatic and circulatory system. When these mechanisms are insufficient or if the process is acute, ICP rises rapidly and may cause death, with or without brain distortion or herniation (see below).

Clinical findings

The clinical picture of increased ICP is characterized by an altered state of consciousness, headache, nausea and vomiting, papilloedema, and, at times, focal signs. An altered state of consciousness is the most frequent sign, starting with psychomotor retardation, and slowing of verbal and motor responses. This can progress to stupor and then coma.

Headache progresses and can be severe. It usually is diffuse, more intense in the supine position, and worse in the morning immediately after awakening. It can awaken the patient from sleep, and also is worsened by head movements, cough, and the Valsalva manoeuvre. Nausea and vomiting frequently accompany the headache. Vomiting may be projectile in children with posterior fossa lesions, which can directly stimulate the trigger zone in the fourth ventricle.

Papilloedema is a specific sign of increased ICP but its sensibility is low, so it often is absent, even in severe cases. Among the focal signs that occur frequently in those with increased ICP, the most frequent is diplopia due to paralysis of the abducens nerve. This nerve, with its long intracranial course, is particularly sensitive to traction or compression. Other signs may occur in either the sensory or motor systems. Seizures also may occur in the setting of increased ICP.

In children, increased ICP often is accompanied by non-specific findings or may manifest as irritability, labile mood, negativity, or aggressive or hostile behaviours. A focal sign relatively more common in children is the 'sunset' sign; downward ocular deviation, eyelids retraction due to compression of the quadrigeminal plate.

Acute pressure symptoms

In the setting of intracranial hypertension, the physiological fluctuation in ICP can be interrupted suddenly by abnormal pressure waves, including waves of very high pressure, or plateau waves (Lundberg, 1960). These pressure waves, which usually last seconds to minutes, may be accompanied by acute pressure symptoms that are sudden acute neurological symptoms or worsening of general neurological conditions (Box 14.1.1).

Herniation

Dural reflections of the falx cerebri and tentorium cerebelli divide the cranial box into compartments, and raised ICP can result in pressure gradients between compartments. These pressure gradients can, in turn, lead to shifts of brain parenchyma or herniations: subfalcial, tentorial, upward cerebellar, and cerebellar pressure cone. These can be merely a relief for crowding or a sign of overfilled sovratentorial and posterior fossa compartments, but when they occur rapidly, or interfere with CSF circulation and cause hydrocephalus, they can be life-threatening.

Brain oedema and treatment of increased ICP

Brain oedema

In both primary and secondary brain tumours, oedema is an important cause of increased ICP. The underlying pathogenic mechanism of oedema is the loss of osmotically active substances

---

Box 14.1.1 Signs and symptoms of ICP waves

- Altered state of consciousness, agitation, delirium
- Headache, neck pain
- Focal or generalized seizures
- Cerebellar fits (opisthotonus)
- Decerebration (hypertonus, extension, and internal rotation of four limbs)
- Amaurosis, mydriasis
- II, IV, VI nerve paralysis, conjugated eye deviation
- Nystagmus, tinnitus
- Myoclonus of face and limb muscles
- Dysarthria, dysphagia
- Pyramidal signs, paraesthesiae
- Cardiovascular or respiratory disturbances, yawning
- Hyperthermia, face cyanosis, flushing, pallor, sweating
- Nausea, vomiting, hiccup, sialorrhoea, diarrhoea, incontinence.

---

such as albumin from the circulatory system into the brain interstitial tissue, which is caused by disruption of the blood–brain barrier within the tumour and in the surrounding cerebral parenchyma. According to the classic classification (Klatzo, 1967), there are four broad types of brain oedema:

- *Vasogenic oedema* is caused by an increase of the extracellular space. It results from increased capillary permeability and can be produced by any lesion that damages the blood–brain barrier.

- *Cytotoxic oedema* is caused by an increase of intracellular volume. It results from ischaemic or hypoxic cellular damage. Cellular dysfunction of the ion pump system produces intracellular accumulation of sodium followed by influx of extracellular fluid. It is now referred to as cellular swelling.

- *Interstitial oedema* is caused by an increase of the extracellular space due to blockade of CSF reabsorption at any level.

- *Osmotic oedema* is caused by an increase in the water content of the brain parenchyma due to plasma hypo-osmolarity. This may occur, for example, in water intoxication or in SIADH.

Tumour-induced brain oedema is sustained mainly, at least initially, by vasogenic mechanisms. Interstitial and osmotic oedema are rare and do not apply to the perturbations produced by a tumour.

Treatment of increased ICP

Conservative management of cerebral oedema has two main goals: maintenance of cerebral perfusion pressure (CPP) and reduction of vasogenic oedema (Rosner et al 1995). CPP is defined as mean arterial pressure minus ICP. Intracranial processes can impair CPP by increasing ICP and disrupting cerebrovascular autoregolation. The consequences of reduced CPP are cerebral ischaemia, compensatory and dilatation of cerebral vessels, with further increase of ICP. Since hypovolaemia reduces arterial pressure and therefore CPP, the patient with elevated ICP does not require fluid restriction, but should be kept euvolaemic with adequate fluid intake.

Interventions that assist in maintaining CPP and reducing vasogenic oedema are varied. Consideration of these interventions depends on the goals of care. Aggressive management strategies, such as assisted ventilation to lower the partial pressure of carbon dioxide may not be considered when the goals are purely palliative.

Positioning: a neutral head position should be adopted, with the head at least 30° above the heart to facilitate venous drainage from the head.

Infusion of hypertonic solutions: rapid reduction of ICP and cerebral oedema with hypertonic solutions has been utilized since 1925 (Howe, 1925). Nowadays, used hyperosmolar solutions are mannitol, and hypertonic saline (Ropper, 2012).

Hyperosmolar solutions are only effective if the blood–brain barrier is intact; action is by removal of water from normal brain parenchyma, as ICP is lowered in proportion to the volume of undamaged brain. There is little value on oedema around a lesion where the blood–brain barrier is damaged. In addition such solutions do not have a role in asymptomatic cerebral oedema.

Mannitol is the most commonly used agent (Ropper, 2012). Its activity is based initially on an increase in blood flow, leading to improved cerebral perfusion. Only later does it create an osmolar gradient between blood and brain and extract water from the cerebral compartment. Usually more water than sodium is eliminated, resulting in hypovolaemia and hyponatraemia. There is no interaction between mannitol and glucose metabolism. There are a number of other actions associated with the therapeutic effect of mannitol, including a diuretic effect, an increase in red cell deformability, and a rapid reduction of the diameter of arterioles and small veins of the brain surface. Mannitol is not metabolized and is excreted by the kidneys; with moderate reduction of glomerular filtration, it can accumulate in the central compartment. Although it can be administered orally, bioavailability is very poor and the usual approach is intravenous (IV) infusion, aiming to achieve concentrations higher than 5 mmol/L, which are active osmotically and persist for 4–6 hours. Mannitol 18% or 20% solutions are used and the suggested dose regimen for both adults and children is 1 g/kg delivered over 15–30 minutes immediately, then 0.25 g/kg every 6 or 8 hours. The regimen can vary according to the severity of symptoms and the presence of acute and symptomatic brain herniation. Daily doses should never be higher than 150–200 g/day. Renal disease, congestive heart failure, and intracerebral haemorrhage may contraindicate the use of mannitol. Mannitol therapy should never extend for more than 3–4 days. Salt and water balance should be monitored carefully to avoid dehydration and hypotension. Hyperosmolality should also be prevented by cessation of therapy at values of 320 mOsmol/kg.

Hypertonic saline used in the past only for craniocerebral trauma is now used for increased ICP not responsive to mannitol. It is as effective in lowering ICP as mannitol. Besides osmotic action, it has a vasoregulatory immunological action. Doses: NACL 3%: 5–10 mL/kg in 5–10'; NACL 23.4%: 30 mL/dose, repeatable. When hypertonic solution is used for a longer period than a few days, a risk for rebound effect exists. This rebound effect is, in part, a consequence of the osmotic agents entering the intracranial compartment, with inversion of the osmotic gradient between blood, extracellular fluid, and brain.

Table 14.1.1 Relative potency of different drugs

	Anti-inflammatory activity	Duration of action, hours	Equivalent dose, mg
Cortisone	0.8	8–12	25
Prednisone	4	12–36	5
6 α-Methylprednisolone	5	12–36	4
Dexamethasone	25	36–54	0.75
Betamethasone	30	36–54	0.75
Cortisol	1	8–12	20

Corticosteroids: corticosteroids initially gained a wide application in treating ICP (Galicich and French, 1961). The mechanism of action is based fundamentally on their ability to block the outflow of blood components from the capillary bed into the brain tissue at the site of blood–brain barrier damage. Dexamethasone does not reduce the water content of the swelling brain tissue (as mannitol does), and reduction of ICP does not occur before 48–72 hours. Nonetheless, it is common to observe a clinical improvement before this and within the first 24 hours.

Doses and administration schedules of corticosteroids have never been established by specific guidelines. It is, therefore, worthwhile considering the relative potency of the different drugs and their pharmacological characteristics (Schimmer and Parker, 2006) (Table 14.1.1).

Sodium retention activity is 1 for cortisol, 0.8 for hydrocortisone, 0.8 for prednisone and methylprednisolone, and 0 for betamethasone and dexamethasone.

Dexamethasone is found in higher concentrations within the CSF compared with other corticosteroids because it is less bound to plasma proteins. This should be taken into account when switching from one steroid to another, in addition to the data shown in Table 14.1.1. The dose of dexamethasone used in metastatic or primary brain tumours varies according to the clinical findings and degree of oedema, from 4 mg every 6 hours to 96 mg/day in patients with more severe symptoms or impending herniation. Once the patient is stabilized clinically, the total dose can be given in one or two daily doses, as suggested by the drug's pharmacokinetic profile. In children, the suggested initial dose of dexamethasone is 1 mg/kg followed by doses of 0.4–1 mg/kg in one or more daily doses. Clinical experience suggests that higher doses can be administered safely, if needed.

Although it is common for steroids to be continued indefinitely, continuation of steroid therapy must always be under constant review. Steroids should not be continued if there is no clear medical indication for therapy, or the clinical benefit is exceeded by side effects. Steroid side effects are significant and some may add to the disability of patients (e.g. weakness due to myopathy). Box 14.1.2 lists the side effects of corticosteroids. Although not all are relevant to short-term management of symptoms in palliative care, many can seriously impact on the quality of life of patients and require careful balancing with therapeutic effects. If a steroid is no longer indicated, it should be tapered and discontinued.

Seizures in patients with advanced illness

A seizure is a transient occurrence of signs or symptoms due to abnormal excessive or synchronous neuronal activity in the brain (Fisher et al., 2005).

Seizures are encountered not infrequently in palliative medicine. They may be caused by structural disease of the brain, non-structural causes, or both. Structural problems include metastatic cerebral lesions and infectious causes. The most common non-structural causes include metabolic derangement and drug toxicity (Delanty et al., 1998).

Seizure definition and classification

Seizures are classified according to their electroencephalographic (EEG) features as partial or focal, which applies to any seizure related to an initiating focus that can be identified in a specific brain area, and generalized, which refers to seizures that appear to begin bilaterally. Seizures that originate as truly generalized electrical discharges are defined as primary generalized seizures; those that begin locally and evolve into generalized tonic–clonic seizures are termed secondary generalized seizures.

Depending on the level of consciousness during attacks, partial or focal seizures are classified as follows:

Simple partial seizures are associated with a normal level of consciousness. Only a selective area of the cortex participates in the seizure activity, causing symptoms that depend on the function of that part of the cortex. Therefore, partial motor, sensory, autonomic, and affective seizures are possible. At times when symptoms of this kind precede the onset of a generalized seizure they are called an 'aura'.

Complex partial seizures combine focal symptoms with an altered state of consciousness. These are the most common type of seizures in adults and probably the most common encountered in palliative care. The patient seems awake but is not meaningfully engaged with the environment. If there is verbal output, questions are not answered appropriately and the patient may repeat words or sentences. Eyes can be fixed or rolling purposelessly. The patient may be immobile or engaged in repetitive behaviours (motor automatisms), such as grimacing, snapping fingers, chewing, running, or undressing. If physically restrained, behaviours can become hostile or aggressive. The seizure lasts on average 3 minutes and is followed by a post-ictal phase, which can include somnolence, delirium, and headache, and can last for several hours. After complete recovery, the patient has no recall of the event, but sometimes may remember the aura. The partial complex seizure can itself be preceded by an aura, which may be equivalent to a simple partial seizure.

Generalized seizures can be non-convulsive, which also are called absence or *petit mal*; or convulsive, which are known as tonic–clonic or *grand mal* seizures.

Generalized tonic–clonic (grand mal) seizures start with a sudden loss of consciousness, at times accompanied by shouting (due to forced air expiration by sudden contraction of the diaphragm). Diffuse muscle rigidity follows, which is accompanied by cyanosis. After a short time, myoclonus and muscle fasciculations occur and the patient can bite his or her tongue. The latter clonic phase typically lasts 2 minutes or less, but more prolonged episodes can occur. At the end, post-ictal phase presents with deep sleep and slow deep breathing. Later the patient gradually awakens, often complaining of headache.

Box 14.1.2 Acute and chronic side effects of corticosteroids

- *Infections (especially relevant if associated with chemotherapy)*: reactivation of tuberculosis, candida, pneumocystis pneumonia.

- *Metabolic disturbances*: hyperglycaemia, electrolyte imbalances, fluid retention, hyperlipidaemia.

- *Dystrophic reaction*: delay in wound healing, purpura, dermal atrophy, acne.

- *Myopathy*: weakness affects mainly the pelvic girdle muscles, but also head flexor and shoulder muscles are affected. Muscle enzymes and electromyogram are normal. On the contrary, cretinuria is elevated. Myopathy occurs as early as 2 weeks of starting dexamethasone, manifesting with difficulties in climbing stairs and standing from a sitting position. Some authors suggest that substitution with non-fluorinated steroids (methylprednisolone or prednisone) is effective in reducing myopathic effects.

- *Bone*: osteoporosis probably due to the reduced intestinal absorption of calcium and reduced tubular reuptake with increased calciuria. These mechanisms cause hypocalcaemia, which reflects on parathyroid activation and subsequent increased bone re-absorption. Phenobarbital causes osteopathy and so it is preferable to use different anticonvulsants in combined therapies.

- *Aseptic bone necrosis* (usually of the femoral head). Two hypotheses have been proposed to explain this complication. Fat embolism due to altered lipid metabolism and osteomedullary ischaemia. Bone necrosis has been seen after relatively short-term treatment with dexamethasone (cumulative doses of 220 mg) (McCluskey and Gutteridge, 1982).

- *GI side effects*: peptic ulcer disease: the use of steroids alone in patients in good general condition is not associated with damage to the GI tract. There are, however, specific risk factors that are associated with peptic ulceration and bleeding, such as, very high doses, systemic neoplasm, previous peptic ulcer, and combined use of non-steroidal anti-inflammatory drugs (NSAIDs). It is also well known that patients with intracranial lesions are at risk of GI bleeding (Cushing, 1932). Prophylaxis with proton pump inhibitors is therefore suggested in patients at increased risk.

- *Hiccup*: chronic hiccup has been observed in association with the use of dexamethasone or high-dose methylprednisolone. The physiopathology of this effect is unknown (LeWitt et al., 1982).

- *Psychiatric* (Vanelle et al., 1990): euphoria with mild insomnia. Hyperalert reaction: anxiety can be associated with confusion. Steroid psychosis: can have hypomanic, depressive, and psychotic features with high inter- and intraindividual variability. This reaction is usually seen within 2 weeks of therapy at doses above 40 mg of prednisone per day. The steroid dose should be tapered and symptoms usually subside spontaneously in about 3 weeks.

- *Anaphylaxis*: has been observed after IV methylprednisolone (Freedmann et al., 1981).

- *Ocular toxicity*: glaucoma (Garbe et al., 1997), cataract.

- *Perineal burning sensation* (Baharav et al., 1986).

- *Endocrine effects*: adrenal suppression is seen after 10 days of therapy with doses in excess of 7.5 mg prednisone per day. It is therefore useful to follow some practical suggestions to minimize this effect (Helfer and Rose, 1989). Morning administration matches the physiological zenith of adrenocorticotropic hormone (ACTH) secretion while evening administration favours the inhibition of ACTH secretion. Single administration should be preferred and when possible on alternate days. Before withholding therapy, it is important to check adrenal function (morning cortisol and response to ACTH stimulation).

- *Steroid withdrawal syndrome*: this syndrome can occur with sudden discontinuation of therapy and includes, pseudo-rheumatism, headache, lethargy, nausea, vomiting, postural hypotension, and papilloedema (Dixon and Christy, 1980).

- *Epidural lipomatosis*: this complication can cause slowly developing spinal cord compression (Jalladeau et al., 2000).

- *Pseudo-tumour cerebri*: papilloedema and headache can occur without focal neurological signs and normal CSF. It has been described in patients with Addison's disease and after steroid withdrawal and it has also been reported after chronic steroid use (Walker and Adamkiewicz, 1964).

Treatment

Prophylactic therapy of seizures in palliative medicine usually should not be undertaken if the patient has never had seizures. Although prophylactic anticonvulsant treatment in patients with primary brain tumours or metastases may be considered in selected cases, very few studies have addressed the efficacy of this approach and one randomized clinical trial confirmed that prophylactic treatment did not prevent seizures in patients with brain metastases who had never had seizures (Glantz et al., 1994).

Pharmacological therapy

The ideal anticonvulsant drug for palliative care should have no metabolic interactions, lack significant side effects, and also have parenteral formulations, so few drugs are available. General characteristics of antiepileptic drugs (AEDs) are summarized in Table 14.1.2 together with the recommended dosage. Blood levels of some anticonvulsants should be monitored because of the unpredictability of metabolic changes and drug interactions, but it must be remembered that clinical response and not blood levels should guide dosage.

Table 14.1.2 Main indications and therapeutic dosing schedules of some anticonvulsants used in palliative medicine

Drug	Indication	Therapeutic daily dose	Schedule
Phenobarbital	Broad spectrum	1–5 mg/kg in adults; 3–8 mg/kg in children	Every night at bedtime
Phenytoin	Broad spectrum and status epilepticus	200–400 mg in adults; 4–8 mg/kg children	q8–12 h
Sodium valproate	Broad spectrum and status epilepticus	1000–3000 mg in adults; 30–60 mg/kg in children	q12 h
Levetiracetam	Broad spectrum and status epilepticus	750–3000 mg in adults; 20–60 mg/kg in children	q12 h
Lacosamide	Refractory focal seizures or secondary generalized, and refractory status epilepticus	200–400 mg; 4–12 mg/kg in children	q12–24 h

Phenobarbital is available in oral and parenteral formulations. It is effective in both partial and generalized tonic–clonic seizures. It is metabolized by liver cytochrome P450 and has a very slow plasma clearance (4–5 days), which can be prolonged by liver disease. It has a wide therapeutic index but can cause drowsiness, ataxia, and severe rash (Stevens–Johnson syndrome and the more extensive toxic epidermal necrolysis, Lyell syndrome). It can interfere with the metabolism of several chemotherapy agents and in chronic use is associated with pseudo-rheumatism, which can worsen the symptoms of a concurrent steroid-induced osteoporosis.

Phenytoin is the first-line drug in simple and complex partial seizures, and in generalized tonic–clonic seizures. Dosing can vary from 4 to 8 mg/kg/day in two to three daily administrations, preferably after eating. The IV formulation of phenytoin, or fos-phenytoin, can be systemically loaded and provide rapid control of seizures. The advantages of phenytoin are the relative lack of sedative effects, and good tolerability at higher than recommended doses. Side effects due to chronic use include ataxia, gastrointestinal (GI) disturbances, gingival hypertrophy, hirsutism, osteoporosis, and megaloblastic anaemia. The use of phenytoin also may be problematic due to variation in blood levels produced by the administration of many other drugs that interfere with liver metabolism, absorption, or protein binding. Interactions have been demonstrated with ciclosporin, cis-platinum, and paclitaxel. Significant pharmacokinetic interaction is found with concurrent dexamethasone, which can reduce phenytoin plasma levels by 50%. Severe allergic reactions involving rash, hypersensitivity reactions, liver toxicity, and myelosuppression have been reported, but are rare.

Sodium valproate is active in most types of generalized seizures (tonic, myoclonic, absence, tonic–clonic), including secondary generalized partial seizures. Doses start at 250–500 mg/day and are increased by 250 mg/week up to 1000–3000 mg/day. In children, the initial dose is 10–15 mg/kg/day, increased by the same incremental

doses. Dose escalation can occur more quickly if needed, and an IV formulation is available in some countries, which can allow tolerable loading doses. Common side effects of sodium valproate are tremors, sedation, ataxia, GI symptoms, and thrombocytopenia. Liver enzymes and blood ammonia can be increased. Although severe liver toxicity can occur (usually in the first 6 months of therapy), all reported cases occurred in children under the age of 3 years who also were receiving other anticonvulsants.

Levetiracetam is used for partial and secondary generalized tonic–clonic seizures. The drug is well tolerated, and the most frequent side effects are somnolence, asthenia, and dizziness. The starting dose may be the same as the minimally effective dose of 750–1000 mg/daily, increasing to 40–40 mg/kg in children and 3000 mg in adults.

Lacosamide is approved as adjunctive treatment for focal seizures, with or without secondary generalization, that do not respond to other AEDs. Lacosamide does not affect the plasma concentration of carbamazepine, sodium valproate, clonazepam, and levetiracetam, but its tolerability may be adversely affected by a sodium-blocking AED such as carbamazepine, sodium valproate, lamotrigine, or topiramate. Lacosamide usually does not cause sedation, and cardiac side effects are comparable to those of other AEDs, but dizziness is frequent, especially at high doses. The drug is well absorbed after oral administration and it may be started at dose of 50 mg twice a day, increasing weekly by 100 mg up to a maintenance dose of 200–600 mg/day.

Status epilepticus

Mechanistically, status epilepticus represents the failure of the natural homeostatic seizure-suppressing mechanisms responsible for seizure termination (Engel, 2006). As defined for adults and children older than age 5, status epilepticus is a seizure that lasts 30 minutes or more, or two or more seizures that occur without complete recovery of consciousness in between. Although the definition requires a continuous seizure for 30 minutes, it should be recognized that the likelihood of spontaneous resolution of a seizure becomes small after 5 minutes. For this reason, the treatment used for status epilepticus should be considered whenever a seizure lasts 5 minutes or more.

Clinical characteristics of status epilepticus

Status epilepticus may be classified by the type of seizure (Engel, 2006). The broadest classification distinguishes non-convulsive status epilepticus from convulsive status epilepticus. Non-convulsive status epilepticus can manifest as an absence type and as a partial complex type. The most common convulsive status epilepticus in populations with advanced illness presents as continuous or repeated tonic–clonic seizures. *Non-convulsive status epilepticus* is characterized by EEG seizure activity without convulsive activity. It is a significant cause of impaired consciousness in patients with complex toxic–metabolic encephalopathies, occurring in 8% of comatose patients, according to recent data (Towne et al., 2000).

Partial complex non-convulsive status epilepticus may be particularly challenging to diagnose and treat. Seizure activity may fluctuate and often originates from a temporal cortical area that may not be evident on routine EEG. The syndrome may present as a confusional state with variable clinical findings. It may be continuous or frequently recurrent, or discontinuous, with recurrent

Table 14.1.3 Suggested algorithm for the management of status epilepticus in supportive care patient when cardiorespiratory problems and drug–drug interaction are a concern

Minutes	Treatment
0	Stabilize the patient: ABC, protect Airway—ensure Breathing—maintain the Circulation.
> 5 Additional drug therapy may be not required if seizure stops and the cause of status epilepticus is treated	*Lorazepam* IV, 0.1–0.15 mg/kg in children and 4–8 mg in adult (depending on body weight), at a rate of 2 mg/min; may repeat once after 20 minutes, **or** *midazolam* IV 0.2 mg/kg as bolus, continuous venous infusion of 0.1–0.6 mg/kg/h. Midazolam is well absorbed also IM and SC, and can be given at the same doses when venous access in not feasible; *midazolam* as oral or atomized nasal preparations is also an alternative, at dose of 0.5 mg/kg, 2.5 mg for children, 6–12 months old; 5 mg 1–4 years; 7.5 mg 5–9 years; 10 mg for children 10 years or older, **or** IV *diazepam* 0.15–0.25 mg/kg, at rate of 5 mg/min, until a total of 20 mg in adults; may repeat once after 5min; *rectal diazepam*, 0.5 mg/kg or 2.5 mg for children 6–12 months old; 5 mg for 1–4 years; 7.5 mg 5–9 years; 10 mg for children 10 years, or more. **then** IV *valproic acid* 20–30 mg/kg infused over 15 minutes. However, higher doses, up to 25–60 mg/kg, at 3 mg/kg/min, have been used without serious side effects. This bolus must be followed by continuous infusion of 1–2 mg/kg/h*, **or** IV *levetiracetam*: 20–30 mg/kg in 100 mL of NaCl 0.9% or 5% glucose infused in 30 minutes: then, after 12 hours, the same in two divided doses. **If status epilepticus does not respond, consider** IV *phenytoin* 15 (in the elderly)–20 mg/kg, at infusion rate of no more than 50 mg/min in adults or 1 mg/kg/min in children (monitor for hypotension and electrocardiographic QT prolongation), in *normal saline*, followed by a dose of 4–8 mg/kg/daily oral or IV. If ineffective, give supplemental IV *phenytoin* 5 mg/kg, which can be repeated up to a total dose of 30 mg/kg. * In some guidelines, phenytoin is suggested before valproic acid, but a number of papers have documented the successful use of IV valproate in status epilepticus, without serious cardiovascular side effects; fosphenytoin is better tolerated than phenytoin, but is not available in all countries. **and** *phenobarbital* IV, 20 mg/kg, infusion rate of 60 mg/min; caution with respiratory depression, mostly in patients treated before with benzodiazepines; if ineffective, supplemental IV *phenobarbital* 5–10 mg/kg
> 60: refractory status epilepticus	**First consider:** *Lacosamide: children* 2–2.5 mg/kg infused in 15 minutes then the same dose bid; *adults*: 200–400 mg in 15 minutes, then 200 mg twice a day *Otherwise refractory status epilepticus* to be treated in intensive care unit, where the patient can be treated with general anaesthesia, propofol, pentobarbital, or others drugs (Fernandez and Claassen, 2012)

Source: Data from Fernandez, A., and Claassen, J., Refractory status epilepticus, *Current Opinion in Critical Care*, Volume 18, Issue 2, pp.127–131, Copyright © 2012 Lippincott Williams & Wilkins. All rights reserved.

partial complex seizures and recovery of consciousness between episodes. The duration of a status episode is highly variable and can be as long as weeks. In 40% of cases, the episode is shorter than 24 hours; in another 40%, the episode lasts from 1 to 10 days. The clinical manifestations may take the form of a prolonged delirium, with or without psychotic behaviours and automatisms, or have a more baffling presentation. Some patients have minimal difficulty answering questions but demonstrate affective changes, such as fear, or paranoid ideation.

Convulsive status epilepticus takes the form of continuous or frequently recurrent abnormal motor movements with alteration of consciousness. The risk of cerebral damage and serious complications, including cerebral oedema with increased ICP and acute brain herniations acidosis and rhabdomyolysis, usually demands an emergent approach to management (Chen and Wasterlain, 2006). Treatment has a high rate of success if initiated early, before neuronal injury and time-dependent pharmacoresistence develop. A suggested algorithm for the management of status epilepticus is given in Table 14.1.3.

Lorazepam (Riviello et al., 2013) is considered the drug of choice for the initial emergent management of convulsive status epilepticus. The mean time to clinical effect is 3 minutes. The half-life is 10–15 hours, but effective brain levels are maintained for 8–24 hours. It has no active metabolites. It should be infused IV not faster than 2 mg/min, to reduce the risk of respiratory depression. It is well absorbed also after intramuscular (IM) administration.

Diazepam enters the brain in a few seconds but because of its high lipid solubility, redistribution to all body tissues is rapid, with a consequent fall in brain concentration. Its anticonvulsant effect is therefore very brief and a second dose may be necessary after only 20–30 minutes. Rectal formulations are available. Recommended doses are 10 mg in adults and 5 mg (0.5 mg/kg) in children. Rectal administration at these doses does not cause respiratory depression. After IM administration, absorption is very variable and unpredictable and this route should generally be avoided.

Midazolam is water soluble, has a very short half-life, and has no active metabolites. Its onset of action is 3 minutes after IV administration, and 5 minutes and 15 minutes, respectively, after IM and oral administration. The good IM absorption is an important advantage in cases of difficult venous access or in pre-hospital setting (Silbergleit et al., 2012). In refractory status epilepticus, the initial dose is 0.2 mg/kg (concomitant use of opioids or recent use of other benzodiazepines involves lower doses, i.e. 0.05 mg/kg) followed by 0.05–0.5 mg/kg/h IV infusion. Higher dose may be used in refractory status epilepticus without significant morbidity.

Sodium valproate is available as a parenteral formulation and provides an alternative to phenytoin. Studies confirm the efficacy and safety of valproate infusion, including infusion at high doses in patients with repetitive seizures. Valproate is relatively contraindicated in cirrhosis or hepatic failure, and liver function should be monitored during therapy. However, fatalities have been reported only in children under 2 years who were concurrently treated with other anticonvulsant drugs.

Levetiracetam: IV levetiracetam seems to be effective and safe in the treatment of acute repeated seizures and status epilepticus in children (McTague et al., 2012). It can be used as first choice or add-on if sodium valproate has been already in use or fails. This drug has no interactions because it has no hepatic metabolism.

Phenytoin when given intravenously, has a relatively rapid onset of action (10–20 minutes). It has no sedative effects, does not cause respiratory depression, and has a long duration of action. It may be used to abort the seizure in benzodiazepine-refractory status epilepticus. In the latter situation, it may be given IV infusion at a rate that should not exceed 50 mg/min. After diluting phenytoin in saline, the solution should be infused within 1 hour. The loading dose usually is 20 mg/kg but could be less, and is 15 mg/kg in elderly patients. A loading dose of 15–20 mg/kg can be also administered orally but poor gastric tolerability limits the use of this route in some patients. Side effects may be related to excessively fast infusion rates, as may occur in emergency situations, and include cardiac arrhythmias, hypotension, and CNS depression. The 'purple glove syndrome' is due to the high pH of the drug (–13), which manifests as blue discolouration and distal oedema near the site of infusion about 2 hours after administration. After the loading dose, the duration of the therapeutic effect is about 24 hours. Blood levels can be checked 120 minutes after the end of the infusion.

IV phenobarbital is an option if benzodiazepines, valproic acid, levetiracetam, or phenytoin fail. The peak clinical effect is delayed for 20–60 minutes after administration.

Lacosamide has been used as add-on treatment in refractory status epilepticus when standard drugs failed, and it was effective and safe (Sutter et al., 2013).

Delirium

Delirium has been defined as a transient organic brain syndrome characterized by the acute onset of disordered attention and cognition, accompanied by disturbances of cognition, psychomotor behaviour, and perception (Caraceni and Grassi, 2011) (see also Chapter 17.5). Delirium is considered to be a single taxonomic entity, and the *Diagnostic and Statistical Manual of Mental Disorders*, fourth edition (DSM-IV) proposes specific diagnostic criteria for its diagnosis and confirms that delirium is to be considered primarily a disturbance of consciousness (Box 14.1.3) (APA, 2000).

Delirium may be considered to be a stereotyped response of the brain to a spectrum of insults and as a distinctive state on

---

Box 14.1.3 Summary of DSM-IV criteria for diagnosing delirium due to a general medical condition

A. Disturbance of consciousness with reduced ability to focus, sustain, and shift attention.

B. Change in cognition (such as memory deficit, disorientation, language disturbances, or perception disturbances not better explained by a pre-existing stabilized or evolving dementia).

C. The disturbance develops over a short period of time and tends to fluctuate during the course of the day.

D. There is evidence from the history, physical examination, or laboratory findings that the disturbance is caused by the direct physiological consequences of a general medical condition.

Source: Data from American Psychiatric Association, *Diagnostic and statistical manual of mental disorders*, Fourth Edition, Text revision DSM IV-TR, American Psychiatric Press, Washington DC, USA, Copyright © 2000.

---

the continuum between normal wakefulness and stupor and coma (Engel and Romano, 1959). Other terms for this condition include 'encephalopathy' and 'acute confusional state'. The latter descriptions are used commonly by neurologists to describe acute changes in mental status.

Clinical diagnosis

The diagnosis of delirium requires that consciousness and attention are assessed together with cognitive function and performance. The Mini Mental State Examination (MMSE) is the most widely used method and can be applied to bedside patient assessment. It assesses cognitive function but is not a diagnostic tool. It screens for cognitive failure and can be abnormal in dementia as well as in delirium, or in other disorders that affect cognitive performance.

In contrast to the MMSE, the Confusion Assessment Method is a diagnostic system that can be used to apply the DSM criteria for the diagnosis of delirium. It is very sensitive and specific when applied by trained personnel (Inouye et al., 1990). More recently the Nursing Delirium Screening Scale (NUDESC) has been proposed as a useful instrument for screening delirium cases to be used by nurses; its role in palliative care still needs to be elucidated fully (Gaudreau et al., 2005).

The Delirium Rating Scale (DRS) (Trzepacz et al., 2001) and the Memorial Delirium Assessment Scale (MDAS) (Breitbart et al., 1997) are instruments specifically designed to assess delirium and its severity. These tools can be used to evaluate a range of symptoms that occur in patients with delirium.

Subtle changes frequently precede the onset of delirium. These minor symptoms and behavioural changes may go unnoticed, only to be recalled later in family or staff interviews. A patient who becomes restless, anxious, depressed, irritable, angry, or emotionally labile may be manifesting these premonitory symptoms of delirium. The differential diagnosis is complex, however, and includes adjustment disorder and any of a large number of neurological conditions, including dementia.

The first of the DSM-IV diagnostic criteria for delirium relates to disturbance of consciousness and impaired attention. This disturbance can be highly variable, characterized by increased or decreased arousal, or merely by distractibility and reduced responsiveness. Three clinical variants of delirium have been described based on the type of arousal disturbance: hypoalert–hypoactive, hyperalert–hyperactive, and mixed type (with fluctuations from hypoalert to hyperalert) (Liptzin and Levkoff, 1992; Caraceni and Grassi, 2011).

Attention is affected also by specific changes in the patient's ability to concentrate, which can be subtle. Attention disturbances may be evidenced by an inability to maintain a conversation or to attend to its flow, language abnormalities, and difficulties in writing (Wallesch and Hundsaltz, 1994).

The second DSM criterion for delirium relates to the presence of changed cognition. This may take the form of disorientation, memory deficits, or disturbances of language, reasoning, or perception. It is important to recognize that a diagnosis of delirium may be established in the presence of any one of these cognitive abnormalities.

Language abnormalities are frequent in delirium and are often compounded by the presence of incoherent reasoning. Language may lack fluency and spontaneity, and conversation may be prolonged and interrupted by long pauses or repetitions. Writing abilities are affected early and more severely than other language-related skills (Chédru and Geschwind, 1972; Macleod and Whitehead, 1997). Delirium affects reasoning and patients frequently demonstrate irrelevant or rambling thinking, abnormal conceptualization, and altered insight.

Perceptual abnormalities (hallucinations and illusions) and delusions, but also may be typical of delirium, especially in some subtypes such as delirium tremens or other types of hyperactive delirium. These disturbances in perception are systematically assessed in the DRS and the MDAS.

Delusions may be associated with hallucinations. These delusions are frequently poorly organized and characterized by paranoid features (Wolf and Curran, 1935; Lipowski, 1990).

Delirium can interfere significantly with family and staff understanding of patient's suffering. A small study of 14 patients with cancer pain and severe cognitive failure found that during episodes of agitated cognitive failure, pain intensity, as assessed by a nurse, was significantly higher than the patient's assessment had been before and after the episode (Bruera et al., 1992). Upon complete recovery, none of these patients recalled having had any discomfort during the episode.

The third and fourth criteria for diagnosis of delirium relates to the time course and organic aetiology of the disturbance. For diagnosis, there must be evidence confirming that the disturbance has developed over a short period of time and tends to fluctuate during the course of the day. Fluctuation in the clinical manifestations of delirium is usually apparent in disturbance of the sleep–wake cycle. The phenomenon known as 'sundowning' refers to the worsening of symptoms toward evening and probably has to do with sleep–wake abnormalities that are aggravated by environmental factors. The organic aetiology will be discussed below.

In addition to mental status changes, neurological examination of the patient with delirium may identify findings associated with diffuse brain dysfunction, such as multifocal myoclonus and asterixis. Some findings may be relatively specific for one or more aetiologies. For example, tremulousness is typical of alcohol withdrawal states; miosis and mydriasis suggest opioid toxicity and anticholinergic toxicity, respectively; and tachypnoea may be a manifestation of a central process, or of sepsis or hypoxaemia.

Frequency

Prevalence of delirium ranges from 20–30% of patients when admitted to palliative care services to 60–80% of those in the last days of life (Caraceni et al., 2000; Hosie et al., 2013), figures are higher than in the hospitalized elderly population (Francis et al., 1990). Altered mental state is the second most common reason for neurological consultation at a tertiary cancer centre (Clouston et al., 1992; Ljubisavljevic and Kelly, 2003).

In a study by Gagnon et al., 20% of 89 consecutively hospitalized cancer patients were delirious on admission and, among the others, 32% developed delirium subsequently (Gagnon et al., 2000). In a sample of 104 patients admitted to an acute palliative care unit, Lawlor et al. diagnosed delirium in 44 patients (42%), and of the remaining 60, delirium developed in 45% (Lawlor et al., 2000). Reversal of delirium occurred in 46 (49%) of 94 episodes in 71 patients and terminal delirium occurred in 46 (88%) of the 52 deaths (Lawlor et al., 2000). Reversibility of delirium was observed in 27% of episodes occurring during hospice admission (Leonard et al., 2008).

Aetiological factors in delirium and multifactorial risk model

Risk factors

Disease-related and sociodemographic factors that may predispose to delirium or predict its occurrence have not been well documented in cancer patients. In one study, dyspnoea, anorexia, presence of brain metastases, performance status, and physician estimated prediction of survival were associated with the diagnosis of delirium but only univariate statistics were applied (Johnson et al., 1992).

Inouye and colleagues have proposed a multifactorial model for delirium in the hospitalized elderly (Inouye et al., 1999). The model involves the interaction between 'baseline vulnerability' and 'precipitating' factors. In this model, baseline vulnerability is defined by the predisposing factors at the time of admission to hospital, and the precipitating factors are the noxious events that occurred during hospitalization. The factors that Inouye et al. specifically demonstrated to be contributory to baseline vulnerability in the elderly include visual impairment, severity of illness, cognitive impairment, and an elevated serum urea nitrogen/creatinine ratio of 18 or greater (dehydration) (Inouye et al., 1999). Other studies have implicated risk factors, including, age, dementia, depression, alcohol abuse, the preoperative use of anticholinergic drugs, poor functional status, and markedly abnormal preoperative serum sodium, potassium, or glucose levels (Schor et al., 1992; Gaudreau et al., 2005). Among medications, neuroleptics, opioids, and anticholinergic drugs (Schor et al., 1992; Caraceni et al., 2000, 2011; Gaudreau et al., 2005) have also been implicated as risk factors for delirium.

Aetiology

In cancer patients, the potential aetiologies of delirium, as distinct from 'risk factors', may be divided into direct effects related to tumour involvement and indirect effects. The latter category includes drugs, electrolyte imbalance, cranial irradiation,

Box 14.1.4 Aetiological factors implicated in the onset of delirium in patients with cancer

- ◆ Primary CNS tumour
- ◆ Secondary CNS tumour:
  - brain metastases
  - meningeal metastases
- ◆ Non-metastatic complications of cancer:
  - metabolic encephalopathy due to hepatic, renal, or pulmonary failure
  - electrolyte abnormalities
  - glucose abnormalities
  - infections
  - haematological abnormalities
  - nutritional deficiency (thiamine, folic acid, vitamin B_{12} deficiency)
  - vasculitis
  - paraneoplastic neurological syndromes
- ◆ Toxicity of antineoplastic therapies
- ◆ Chemotherapy and biological therapies: methotrexate, cisplatin, vincristine, procarbazine, asparaginase, citosina arabinoside, 5-fluorouracil, ifosfamide, tamoxifene (rare), etoposide (high doses), nitrosurea (high doses or arterial route), bevacizumab, rituximab
- ◆ Radiation to brain: acute and delayed encephalopathy
- ◆ Toxicity of other drugs
- ◆ Anticholinergics: belladonna alkaloids, scopolamine, atropine, hyoscine
  - drugs with established anticholinergic activity: tricyclic antidepressants, diphenhydramine, promethazine, triesifenidile, chlorpromazine, and other neuroleptics: hyoscine butylbromide
  - anxiolytics, hypnotics
  - steroids, opioids, digitalis, ciprofloxacin, aciclovir, ganciclovir, NSAIDs, anticonvulsants, H_2 blockers, omeprazole, interferons, interleukins, ciclosporin, levodopa, lithium
- ◆ Other diseases not related to neoplasms:
  - CNS diseases or trauma
  - cardiac disease
  - lung disease
  - endocrine pathology
  - alcohol or drug abuse or withdrawal.

organ failure, nutritional deficiencies, vascular complications, paraneoplastic syndromes, and many other factors (Box 14.1.4).

A survey of 140 confused cancer patients referred for a neurology consultation demonstrated a single cause of the altered mental status in 31% and multiple causes in 69%; the median number of probable contributing factors in each patient was three (Tuma and DeAngelis, 2000). Drugs, especially opioids, were associated with altered mental status in 64% of patients, metabolic abnormalities in 53%, infection in 46%, and recent surgery in 32%. A structural brain lesion was the sole cause of encephalopathy in 15% of patients. Two-thirds of the patients in this survey recovered cognitive function when the cause of the delirium was treated.

In the study by Lawlor and colleagues of 104 patients with advanced cancer admitted to a palliative care unit (Lawlor et al., 2000), the median number of precipitating factors was three, and 49% of patients had delirium that was reversible. Although the use of psychoactive medications, predominantly opioids, was the precipitating factor that was independently associated with reversibility of the delirium, the authors concluded that more than one factor (e.g. opioid medication and dehydration) usually requires attention if the delirium is to be reversed (Lawlor et al., 2000). In the study by Gaudreau et al. (2005) the use of opioids at doses of 90 mg of daily oral morphine or more was associated independently at multivariate analysis with the risk of delirium. Other studies have demonstrated that drug interactions with opioid metabolism and metabolic failure (especially renal impairment) can produce unexpected toxicities, especially in the patient with advanced disease (Fainsinger et al., 1993; Bortolussi et al., 1994; Caraceni and Grassi, 2011).

Cognitive compromise is probably one of the most common presenting symptoms or signs of brain (Posner, 1995) and leptomeningeal metastases (Weitzener et al., 1995). Non-convulsive epileptic status, which can occur in association with complex metabolic problems and also with ifosfamide encephalopathy, is a condition that also can result in altered consciousness manifesting with delirium (Towne et al., 2000).

In reviewing the causes of delirium, it is important to recognize that many are common and potentially reversible in the population with advance illness. These factors include, among others, dehydration, borderline renal function, infections, metabolic disturbances, drug withdrawal, and the use of psychoactive medications such as opioids (Tuma and DeAngelis, 2000; Gaudreau et al., 2005; Leonard et al., 2008; Caraceni et al., 2011).

General assessment recommendations

Clinical assessment should include careful physical and neurological examination. Specific mental status assessment can follow the above-mentioned recommendations and can be helped by the systematic use of the NuDESC MMSE, DRS, MDAS, or CAM (Inouye et al., 1990; Breitbart et al., 1997; Trzepacz et al., 2001; Gaudreau et al., 2005). Aetiological screening should involve a rational and stepwise implementation of procedures (Table 14.1.4). The completeness of the list is not incompatible with a policy of avoiding procedures which are considered inappropriate for the individual patient.

Treatment

Symptomatic management often is required both in reversible and irreversible cases, and is based on non-pharmacological and pharmacological therapies.

Environmental interventions

In a classic study by Inouye et al., systematic reorientation and a risk-modifying protocol reduced the incidence of delirium among

Table 14.1.4 Screening process for delirium aetiology in advanced cancer

Toxic factors	Bedside screen of medication profile
	Urine or blood drug screening
Sepsis	Temperature
	Blood/urine and other cultures for infection screen
	Leucocyte count
	Urinalysis
	Red cell count
Glucose-oxidative brain deficiency	Pulse oximetry
	Blood gases and acid–base balance
	Blood glucose
Electrolyte imbalances	Serum electrolytes (Na, K, Cl, Mg, Ca)
Renal failure	Urea, creatinine, creatinine clearance
Liver failure	Liver function tests
	Ammonia
CNS vascular, infectious or structural lesion	Disseminated intravascular coagulation screening and coagulation profile
	CSF examination: blood, glucose, proteins, lymphocytes, leucocytes, malignant cells, culture
	Brain CT or MRI
Paraneoplastic disease	Autoantibodies anti-Hu, Yo, Ma, etc.
Cofactor deficiency malnutrition	Vitamin B_{12} levels—administer Vitamin B_1 1 g/day[a]
Endocrine dysfunction	Thyroid hormone and thyroid-stimulating hormone
	Adrenal function

[a] Because the determination of vitamin B_1 levels is problematic, it is reasonable to supplement vitamin B_1 in every patient with poor nutritional status.

elderly hospitalized patients (Inouye et al., 1999). A calm, quiet environment, with good light, is important to allow for potential recovery and to help the patient to reorientate to time and space. The process may be further assisted by placing a clock or calendar where the patient can see them, and by permitting the patient to see or touch a well-known object from the patient's house. Presence in the room of family members can be advantageous.

Communication with patient and family

In managing the delirious patient, a close collaboration between staff and family is fundamental. Special attention needs to be focused on communication. Family members may be particularly stressed by observing the change of the patient's usual behaviour and by a new barrier to communication. The family must be informed about the characteristics of delirium, including fluctuation of cognitive function, its relationship with the disease conditions, potential for reversibility, role of therapies, and short-term prognosis.

Family members may require special care as they react to what they interpret as the patient's suffering or pain. The behaviour of families, particularly those strained by the burden of caregiving,

can swing from requests to withdraw medication to advocating sedation; caregiver distress may be compounded by personal problems in facing suffering and death (Buss et al., 2007; Morita et al., 2007; Caracenie and Grassi, 2011).

It is very important to clarify the potential aetiological role of existing therapies. For example, it is customary to blame opioid medications for mental changes that are actually caused by the complex interaction of several factors.

In communicating with the patient, the clinician should show empathy and to ask simple questions ('Do you feel confused?'). The patient may be fearful and should be reassured. As needed, logic and rational communication should be supplanted by more direct non-verbal communication. The patient should be encouraged to communicate with well-known family members, and this communication should focus more on affective aspects than on discussions that could confuse or frighten the delirious patient.

Pharmacological therapy

Agitated delirium often requires pharmacological treatment to control behaviours that could result in harm for the patient and others, and to treat hallucinations or delusions that may be contributing to patient suffering. The treatment of hypoactive deliria is more debatable and will depend on individual clinical judgement.

The usual first-choice drug for agitated delirium is haloperidol (Canadian Coalition for Seniors' Mental Health, 2006; Campbell et al., 2009), since it has relatively low sedating potency and fewer anticholinergic and cardiovascular effects than other neuroleptics. Table 14.1.5 gives guidelines for the use of haloperidol and alternative drugs.

Haloperidol has been used via IV infusion, although it is not licensed for this route of administration (Canadian Coalition for Seniors' Mental Health, 2006). Very high IV doses have been safely administered. Therapeutic effects in hyperactive delirium typically are seen at doses of 6–12 mg/day; difficult cases may require higher doses or sedation with other drugs. Careful titration of the dose at the bedside is the most important recommendation to improve outcome. ECG monitoring should be considered before and during haloperidol therapy to monitor possible prolongation of the Q–T interval that can occasionally occur with most neuroleptics; torsade de pointe has been described as a rare complication of haloperidol administration via the IV and oral routes (Jackson et al., 1997).

Alternative neuroleptics can be used if greater sedation is desired or haloperidol is contraindicated. Droperidol and chlorpromazine are relatively sedating, and recently, risperidone, clozapine, quetiapine, ziprasidone, and olanzapine have been used (Caraceni and Grassi, 2011). Benzodiazepines are first-choice agents in the treatment of delirium related to alcohol or other sedative-hypnotic withdrawal. They also can be added in cases of delirium when anxiolytic and sedative effects are considered particularly desirable or in cases unresponsive to neuroleptic medications. They should be used cautiously, however, because they can worsen delirium, especially in the elderly (Campbell et al., 2009), they should not be used in hepatic encephalopathy.

In the management of delirium in the setting of advanced illness, more than one drug may be needed. In one case series of 39 patients, only 20% could be managed by haloperidol alone (Stiefel et al., 1992). When sedation is necessary to control symptoms, the combination of an opioid with a neuroleptic and an antihistamine

Table 14.1.5 Pharmacological therapy of delirium (regimens suggested for general guidance; each case will need specific dose adjustment)

Haloperidol; oral	0.5–5 mg every 8–12 h; a dose of 2 mg/day can be efficacious in mild cases
Haloperidol; SC, IM, or IV	0.5–2 mg per dose titrating dose to clinical effect hourly IV infusion 0.2–1 mg/h with careful titration to clinical effect can be used in difficult cases. ECG monitoring is recommended
Chlorpromazine; oral, IM, or IV	12.5–50 mg every 8–12 h. More sedating, anticholinergic, and hypotensive effects; ECG monitoring is mandatory
Clozapine; oral	12.5–50 mg at night (monitoring of blood cell count is needed) very sedative, has less extrapyramidal effects than other neuroleptics
Risperidone; oral	From 0.5–1 mg/day up to 2–4 mg/day. It has extrapyramidal effects
Olanzapine; OS IM	5 mg every night at bedtime to be titrated up to clinical effect
Quetiapine; OS	25 mg every 12 h More sedating, orthostatic hypotension, to be titrated to effect, useful in mild cases with insomnia
Lorazepam; oral, SL, or IV	0.5–2 mg every 6–8 h if sedating anxiolytic effects required
Midazolam; SC or IV	20–100 mg 24 h IV or SC continuous infusion for sedation in refractory cases. 3–5 mg IV priming dose if rapid sedation is required. Start IV infusion with 1 mg/h, dose should be frequently titrated to effect
Promethazine; IM or IV	50 mg every 8–12 h; antihistamine more sedative; useful if sedation desired and for night-time sleep

Table 14.1.6 Cancer-related and treatment related neurological diagnoses in 851 patients with cancer

Diagnosis	Percentage
Brain metastasis	15.9
Metabolic or drug-related encephalopathy	10.2
Pain associated with bone metastasis	9.9
Epidural tumour	8.5
Tumour plexopathy	5.8
Leptomeningeal metastasis	5.1
Chemotherapy peripheral neuropathy	3.2
Radiculopathy	2.7
Base-of-skull metastasis	2.7
Seizures due to metastasis	2.7
Seizures not due to metastasis	1.8
Paraneoplastic syndromes	1.2
Intracranial haemorrhage related to thrombocytopenia	1.3
Radiation myelopathy	1.2
Radiation plexopathy	1.1
Intracranial haemorrhage from tumour	0.6

A total of 1042 diagnoses were given with up to three per patient. Among the non-cancer-related diagnoses, cerebrovascular disease, headache, and degenerative spine disease were the most common diagnoses.

Source: Data from Clouston, P.D. et al., The spectrum of neurological disease in patients with systemic cancer, Annals of Neurology, Volume 31, Issue 3, pp. 268–73, Copyright © 1992.

such as promethazine can be particularly effective. Alpha 2 agonists (clonidine or dexmedetomidine) can be useful to obtain controlled sedation; they can be used in combination with neuroleptics and opioids and do not have respiratory depressant effects. Their use in palliative care is still based on personal experience (Alfonso and Reis, 2012).

Other neurological complications of cancer

Neurological complications are estimated to occur in up to 20% of patients with cancer. In a large consultation survey conducted at a comprehensive cancer centre, the most frequent complaints were pain and altered mental status (Table 14.1.6) (Ljubisavljevic and Kelly, 2003).

Brain metastases
Pathology

Intracranial metastases are found at autopsy in about 25% of patients who died of cancer (Posner, 1995). Other common intracranial lesions involve the skull and meninges. There is evidence that the incidence of brain metastases and leptomeningeal metastases is increasing, because of better control of systemic disease and longer survival, which allow 'sanctuary' cells in the CNS to evolve into clinically significant lesions. Lung cancer, melanoma,

and breast cancer are the primary tumours most frequently associated with metastatic spread to the brain parenchyma. Tumours such as melanoma usually cause multiple lesions, while breast cancer more often causes single lesions (some 50% of breast cancer patients have a single lesion and 20% two lesions). Brain metastases can cause symptoms by compression, local destruction, irritation of brain tissue, brain oedema, and bleeding. The most common effect of a metastatic lesion is brain oedema and increased ICP. Focal symptoms can be due to oedema or bleeding. As discussed previously, typical presentations include cognitive failure, focal signs, seizures, and the syndrome of intracranial hypertension.

Clinical course

After clinical presentation of a brain metastasis, the median survival is about 2 months if no treatment is given, depending on tumour type (Posner, 1995). Patients who have access to brain radiotherapy and respond favourably to this modality usually die of their systemic disease. Patients who do not receive radiotherapy or do not respond often die of direct effects of the brain metastasis (Boogerd et al., 1993).

The signs and symptoms of brain metastases are highly variable. Symptoms can present progressively and deceptively, or alternatively, can be sudden, and 'stroke-like'. It should be remembered that in many patients formal neurological tests of strength and mental function will reveal signs of changes in the CNS that are not otherwise apparent (Posner, 1995).

Headache is an important symptom of brain metastasis. The headache usually is aching in quality and moderate to severe in intensity. It is caused by compression or traction of intracranial pain-sensitive structures. With supratentorial lesions, it is often bifrontal, although it can occur on one side—always that of the tumour.

Headache occurs more frequently during the night and in early morning, and is more severe with infratentorial lesions that affect CSF circulation, causing hydrocephalus and increased ICP.

Treatment

The treatment of a brain metastasis requires a careful assessment of the type of cancer and its sensitivity to radiation and chemotherapy, the neurological status of the patient, the extent of systemic disease, symptoms, and other complications and comorbidities, expectations concerning quality of life with and without treatment, and both the goals of care expressed at the time of diagnosis and the broader values of the patient. It should be understood that the provision of supportive treatment only is among the therapeutic options available.

Surgery is indicated only for single metastases with limited or no systemic disease, especially with radio-resistant tumours (Kaal et al., 2005). Whole-brain irradiation produces neurological improvement in the majority of patients but survival after treatment is only 4–6 months. Metastases from breast and lung cancers usually have a relatively good response to radiotherapy, showing both clinical and radiological improvement. Clinical improvement in the absence of radiological improvement is relatively common during treatment of metastases from melanoma, colon cancer, or renal cancer.

Newer techniques for focal radiation may be of benefit. Focal brain irradiation or 'radiosurgery' can have a role in treating single, or occasionally two, brain metastases, sometimes in combination with whole brain irradiation. The aim of this strategy is eradication of disease from the brain and radiosurgery is used as a substitute for surgery in this context (Kaal et al., 2005).

Corticosteroids

Treatment with steroids is recommended for all symptomatic patients with brain metastases or primary brain tumour. The main therapeutic effect is probably related to a reduction in peri-tumoral oedema from partial restoration of the blood–brain barrier. Steroids are also recommended for all patients undergoing brain irradiation. Treatment should start 48 hours before radiation. A regimen of dexamethasone 8–16 mg/day in one single administration, which is tapered beginning the 2nd week of radiation is recommended. Tapering should be gradual (2–4 mg every 5th day).

Higher steroid doses can be given acutely if symptoms recur (e.g. restarting 16 mg/day) or if there are signs of increased ICP or cerebral herniation (e.g. 16–100 mg IV once, followed again by tapering). If a steroid cannot be discontinued, the dose should be tapered to the minimum required for symptom control. Dexamethasone taper and discontinuation should always be attempted after completion of radiation treatment, since in most patients steroids are not necessary to preserve neurological function.

Spinal cord compression

Pathology

Most cases of epidural spinal cord compression in populations with cancer are caused by a vertebral body metastasis invading the epidural space posteriorly and compressing the spinal cord or cauda equina. Invasion of the epidural space through the intervertebral foramina by a paraspinal lesion also can occur, and is relatively more likely in lymphoma and neuroblastoma; the absence of a bony lesion on radiography in these cases can lead to misdiagnosis. Very rarely, spinal cord syndromes are due to epidural or cord metastases.

Spinal cord, including conus medullaris, and cauda equina lesions have similar aetiologies, mechanisms, and clinical implications, and are therefore usually considered together.

Clinical course

Epidural spinal cord compression is a frequent problem in patients with cancer, occurring in 25% of patients with lung cancer, 16% with prostate cancer and 11% of patients with myeloma. It is a neurological emergency, as functional outcome is dependent on the degree of neurological impairment at diagnosis, the promptitude of therapy and the initial response to therapy. Other factors important in prognosis are tumour histology and rate of progression of the neurological symptoms. The importance of early diagnosis cannot be overemphasized; symptoms are usually present for some weeks before the neurological emergency occurs. Pain precedes other neurological symptoms in almost every case, but diagnosis is often delayed until the onset of neurological symptoms and signs.

Pain of long duration, which suddenly changes its characteristics, should prompt re-evaluation and spinal imaging. Pain in a crescendo pattern is particularly worrying, as are pain aggravated by lying down, pain associated with the Valsalva manoeuvre, and radicular pain (pain occurring or radiating in a dermatomal distribution).

Other clinical features, are impaired deambulation for lower limb paralysis, ataxia or sensory loss, and altered function of bladder, and less frequently, bowel.

The occurrence of a Lhermitte's sign also should raise concern about the possibility of tumour compression of the spinal cord. A Lhermitte's sign, also described as 'barber's chair sign' in the British literature, is a shock-like sensation passing down the trunk and one or more extremities when the neck is flexed. It also may occur spontaneously or be precipitated by sudden limb movements, or by coughing or sneezing. It is due to demyelination or compression of the posterior column of the spinal cord in the cervical or upper thoracic regions. Lhermitte's sign is frequent in multiple sclerosis, but it is not uncommon in cancer-related spinal cord dysfunction. In the cancer population, the differential diagnosis ranges from relatively benign conditions such as transient radiation myelopathy and cisplatin injury, to severe complications such as cord compression and progressive radiation myelopathy (Ventafridda et al., 1991).

Diagnosis

Neurological examination discloses signs related to the location of the compressive lesion. If the spinal cord is involved (typically with lesions at or above, the T12–L1 spinal level), signs are consistent with myelopathy and usually begin with paraesthesiae, or sensory loss in the feet, which ascends as the compression worsens. Weakness of hip flexors, and then other lower extremity muscles, also occurs. The sensory signs are helpful in defining the level of the compression (Table 14.1.7) (Hellmann et al., 2013). If the lesion is at the T12–L1 level, a conus medullaris syndrome may be the presenting phenomenology, with early loss of sphincter control and 'saddle'

Table 14.1.7 Localizing signs with spinal cord lesions

Sign	Clinical level		
	Cord	Conus and epiconus medullaris	Cauda equina
Motor	Paraparesis usually flaccid	If epiconus involved L5–S3 weakness	Never pyramidal signs
	Pyramidal signs can be present	If conus S2–S3 weakness	Often asymmetrical weakness
Reflexes	Absent or hyperactive	Patellar hyperactive	Hypoactive
		Ankle hypoactive	Asymmetrical
Babinski sign	Usually present	Present only if lesion of epiconus	Never present
Sensory	Symmetrical level of dermatomal level sensory loss (locates compression within two dermatomes, or more, above the sensory level)	If conus S2–S5 'saddle' sensory loss. If epiconus L4–S5	Asymmetrical findings in the lower extremities and perineum
Sphincter control	Can be initially preserved	Early involved sometimes selectively	Can be preserved

sensory symptoms or signs. A more caudal lesion causes a cauda equine syndrome, which is usually prominently asymmetric, with weakness or sensory changes affecting one leg more than another.

Emergency imaging of the spinal cord and canal should be carried out in patients with cancer and back pain who have symptoms of myelopathy (including conus medullaris) or cauda equine syndrome.

Ideally, this should be done when the characteristic back pain is noted and before significant neurological signs ensue (Portenoy et al., 1989).

Figure 14.1.1 summarizes the clinical and radiological findings that should prompt either immediate treatment or spinal cord imaging with magnetic resonance imaging (MRI), the results of which will dictate the treatment modality (Hellmann et al., 2013). Although MRI is the best imaging procedure in these patients, myelography or computed tomography (CT) still has a place when MRI is unavailable. There may be multiple lesions and the whole spine should be evaluated.

Treatment

If the goals of care support aggressive treatment of epidural spinal cord or cauda equine compression, corticosteroids and radiation should be offered (Ingham et al., 1993; Spinazzé et al., 2005) (see also Chapter 12.3). Steroids can reduce pain, preserve neurological function, and improve functional outcome after definitive treatment (Sorensen, et al., 1994). Dexamethasone in high doses is recommended for high-degree lesions, as shown by severe or rapidly progressing neurological abnormalities, or by MRI evidence of a severe lesion). A low-dose regimen should be used for low-degree lesions, as suggested by stable or slowly progressing neurological findings, or by MRI or myelography. One high-dose regimen included an initial IV bolus of 100 mg followed by a tapering schedule of 96 mg orally for 3 days and subsequent halving of the dose every 3rd day until the end of radiation treatment (Spinazzé et al., 1994; Posner, 1995). The use of such high doses for severe epidural spinal cord compression has been questioned (Vecht et al., 1989), and lower doses between 16 and 32 mg are often clinically used. If surgery is considered, posterior laminectomy alone is now seldom if at all indicated (Findlay, 1984). A more rational surgical approach for anteriorly compressing lesions is vertebral body resection (Harrington, 1988), but the procedure requires intact vertebral elements above and below the affected level to stabilize the spine after surgery. Surgery is the first choice where the site of the primary tumour is unknown, where there is relapse after radiation treatment, and in cases of spinal instability or vertebral

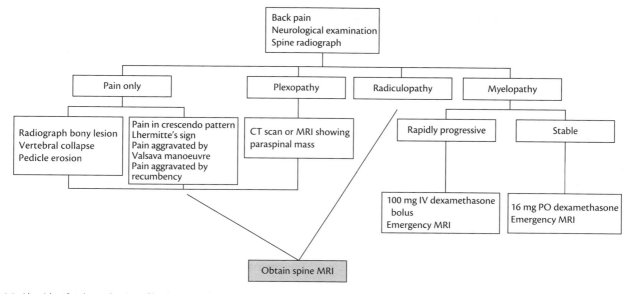

Fig. 14.1.1 Algorithm for the evaluation of back pain in the patient with cancer.

displacement. It should also be considered when neurological symptoms progress during radiotherapy, in plegia of rapid onset, and when the tumour is not likely to be radiosensitive.

Some series showed impressive results with vertebral resection. In one series, 13 of 36 paraplegic patients regained ambulation (Harrington, 1988). One controlled clinical trial suggests that surgery can be the first choice for selected patients with better prognoses (Patchell et al., 2005). Careful individual indication is key, prognosis and expected quality of life should influence the decision.

Leptomeningeal metastases

Pathology

Leptomeningeal metastases (also known as carcinomatous meningitis or meningeal carcinomatosis) are caused by the dissemination of cancerous cells throughout the subarachnoid space. These cells can reach the meninges through the general circulation or the perineural spaces along nerve roots, by direct invasion from epidural lesions, or by direct seeding from existing brain tumours (Chamberlain, 2006). Meningeal involvement can be multifocal or diffuse, and either visible on imaging as discrete masses or not visible on imaging because of microscopic infiltration.

Clinical course

Leptomeningeal metastases were once considered an unusual complication of systemic cancer (1–8% of cases at autopsy) (Posner, 1995) but these are increasingly seen nowadays, usually as a result of breast or lung cancer, lymphoma, leukaemia, or melanoma. Life expectancy is usually short, ranging from 3 to 6 months in patients who have received intensive treatment. Many patients are not offered treatment and their survival is shorter (Posner, 1995; Chamberlain, 2006).

The clinical findings associated with leptomeningeal disease may relate to CNS or peripheral nervous system dysfunction, or some combination. The clinical syndromes are highly variable. The pathophysiology includes abnormality in the flow and absorption of CSF (which can result in hydrocephalus), direct involvement of the cranial and peripheral nerve meningeal sheets, competition with brain metabolism, invasion of the brain parenchyma or nerve roots, and areas of focal ischaemia.

The most common symptoms are headache, change in mental status, and radicular-type pain (Posner, 1995; Formaglio and Caraceni, 1998; Chamberlain, 2006), but cranial nerve involvement, seizures, polyradiculopathy, and cauda equina syndrome also occur in varying combinations. Multiple symptoms, from involvement of different levels of the neuraxis, are often seen.

Diagnosis

Diagnosis is usually confirmed from examination of the CSF (Chamberlain, 2006). While malignant cells may not be apparent in the first sample of CSF, other abnormalities are usually found, such as high opening pressure, high protein content, increased white cell count, or low glucose content. In one series, only 3% of the first samples were completely normal (Chamberlain, 2006). Other markers and immunocytochemical techniques have not been found to have clinical value (Chamberlain, 2006). Repeated lumbar punctures often are

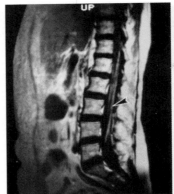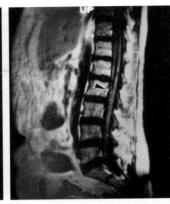

Fig. 14.1.2 MRI, gadolinium enhanced. The white enhancement of the meningeal sheath around the cauda equina (left side, arrow) and the thecal sac (right side arrow) due to meningeal infiltration.

needed to establish the diagnosis. Contrast-enhanced MRI also can be useful (Formaglio and Caraceni, 1998) (Fig. 14.1.2), as the only sign of leptomeningeal metastases may be slight enhancement of the meninges due to blood–brain barrier disruption or focal enlargement of roots.

Therapy

Traditionally, treatment modalities have been based on a combination of corticosteroids, radiotherapy, and intrathecal or intraventricular chemotherapy. Systemic chemotherapy may also be helpful in some cases with appropriate tumour histology. In one series, only 23% of treated patients could be regarded as long-term survivors. Intrathecal chemotherapy did not achieve better results than systemic chemotherapy (median survival 23 months) (Siegal et al., 1994; Chamberlain, 2006), and caused a treatment-related leucoencephalopathy in 58% of cases. The role of intrathecal chemotherapy is questionable particularly in solid tumours.

Base of the skull and cranial nerve syndromes

Lesions at the base of the skull are commonly caused by metastasis from breast, prostate, and other tumours (Greenberg et al., 1981) or from local invasion by advanced head and neck tumours (Vecht et al., 1992) (see Chapter 13.1). Symptoms secondary to bone lesions are commonly associated with alterations of cranial nerve function. Headache at the site of the lesion or referred to the vertex or to the entire affected side of the head is also frequent (Greenberg, 1981; Posner, 1995). The best imaging procedure for all these syndromes is CT scan with bone window studies. Treatment with radiation is indicated, to control pain and neurological dysfunction. Any combination of pain related to the involvement of the cranial and facial bone and of the trigeminal nerve associated with other cranial nerve dysfunction should receive careful clinical evaluation (Foley, 1979; Greenberg et al., 1981; Weinstein et al., 1986; Vecht et al., 1992).

Trigeminal nerve and the 'numb-chin syndrome'

The most common presentation is a constant dull, well-localized pain related to the underlying disease of bone and other somatic structures. This pain may be associated with paroxysmal episodes of lancinating or throbbing pain. The quality of the pain only rarely can mimic classical trigeminal neuralgia, an atypical facial pain is more common (Cheng et al., 1993). Atypical trigeminal pain and sensory abnormalities in the peripheral distribution of the V nerve, occasionally associated with incomplete lesions of the VII nerve, have been reported with different facial neoplasms (Cheng et al., 1993).

Involvement of the mental nerve does not usually produce pain but can cause the 'numb chin syndrome' of mental anaesthesia. This is a sign of disease of the jaw or, more frequently, of the base of the skull, leptomeninges carcinomatosis, and local perineural spread of lip carcinoma. The symptom can occur months before the discovery of a bony lesion (Burt et al., 1992).

Glossopharyngeal nerve

The typical patient has throat and neck pain, which radiates to the ear and is aggravated by swallowing. Pharyngeal and other carcinomas of the neck can present with odynophagia with reflex otalgia. Severe pain may be associated with syncope (Weinstein et al., 1986). Although it has been described with leptomeningeal disease, it commonly results from local nerve infiltration in the neck or base of the skull.

Radiculopathy

Radiculopathy is usually caused by the compression of nerve roots by vertebral, paraspinal lesions, or by leptomeningeal metastases. The pain of a root lesion is usually focal and radiates in the distribution of the affected root. It is sometimes difficult to distinguish a polyradiculopathy from a plexus lesion; CT and MRI are useful for imaging non-bony paraspinal lesions. MRI is necessary for imaging the epidural space.

Herpes zoster and post-herpetic neuralgia are common in patients with cancer and should always be considered in the differential diagnosis of painful radiculopathies.

Cervical plexopathy

Infiltration of the cervical plexus by tumour can be a result of compression by head and neck neoplasms or metastases to cervical nodes. Symptoms usually include local lancinating or dysaesthetic pain referred to the retro-auricular and nuchal areas, the shoulder, and the jaw. Sensory abnormalities define the affected (greater auricular and greater occipital) nerves (Vecht et al., 1992). The differential diagnosis should include post-radical neck dissection syndrome. The diagnosis in patients with head and neck cancer may be difficult because of the postoperative and post-radiation changes often found in these patients. CT or MRI scan is appropriate, and imaging of the cervical spine and paraspinal structures is very important in distinguishing between bony lesions, cervical radiculopathy, and epidural spinal cord compression.

Brachial plexopathy

Five per cent of the neurological consultations at a comprehensive cancer centre were found to be initiated by brachial plexopathy (Burt et al., 1992). It occurs most often with breast and lung carcinoma, and with lymphoma. The plexus can be compressed or infiltrated by tumour lying in contiguous structures, such as axillary or supraclavicular nodes, or the apex of the lung. Pain is the first symptom in 85% of patients (Kori

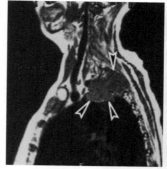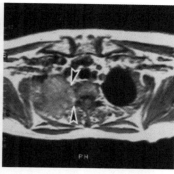

Fig. 14.1.3 MRI image. Lung tumour in the upper lobe compressing the lower trunk of the brachial plexus. Pain was reported in the inner aspect of the arm and paraesthesiae in the 5th and 4th finger. Left side: the arrows show the tumour mass invading the tissue planes in the area of the brachial plexus. Right side: the tumour is invading the left upper lobe, the arrows show the tumour invading one thoracic vertebral body.
Reproduced from *Hematology and Oncology Clinics of North America*, Volume 10, Issue 1, Caraceni, A., Clinicopathologic correlates of common cancer pain syndromes, pp.57–78, Copyright © 1996 W. B. Saunders Company, with permission from Elsevier, http://www.sciencedirect.com/science/journal/08898588

et al., 1981), preceding other neurological symptoms or signs by weeks or months.

Breast and lung malignancies typically affect the lower plexus (C7–T1) (Fig. 14.1.3) and cause pain in the shoulder, elbow, hand, and the fourth and fifth finger. Lung tumours can affect the intercostobrachial nerve, giving rise to a pain syndrome and associated sensory disturbances in the axilla (C8–T1–T2). The upper brachial plexus (C5–C6) can also be affected, especially by breast cancer, when pain is usually referred to the paraspinal region, shoulder, biceps region, elbow, and hand; burning dysaesthesia in the index finger or thumb is common. The hallmark of the syndrome is the neuropathic nature of the pain with numbness, paraesthesia, allodynia, and hyperaesthesia.

CT scan with narrow sections and contrast enhancement is effective in imaging soft tissue and bony structures in the plexus area. All patients with symptoms of brachial plexopathy should have a scan of the contiguous paravertebral region before radiation therapy, since extension of disease in this region is common (13/41 cases in one series). MRI is particularly useful in imaging the contiguous epidural space. While use of both techniques can give helpful complementary information in doubtful cases, sometimes neither is helpful even in cases of proven metastatic plexopathy (Krol, 1993). Comparative data on specificity and sensitivity of the two techniques are lacking.

Epidural invasion eventually will occur in some patients with brachial plexopathy (Fig. 14.1.4). Imaging of the epidural space is essential when patients develop Horner's syndrome, panplexopathy, vertebral body erosion, or a paraspinal mass detected on CT scan. These are often hallmark symptoms of tumour progression into the epidural space.

Radiation fibrosis is important in the differential diagnosis of brachial plexopathy in cancer (Table 14.1.8), particularly in patients who have had radiotherapy and who present with upper plexus signs. Positron emission tomography (PET) scan can be very helpful in distinguishing fibrosis from tumour. Pain is often less prominent in patients with radiation-induced plexopathy.

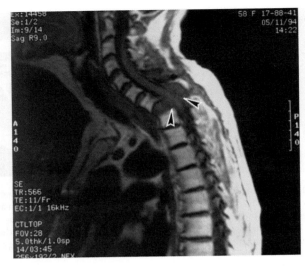

Fig. 14.1.4 MRI image in the same case as shown in Fig. 14.1.3. The tumour is invading the epidural canal and compressing the spinal cord.

Reproduced from *Hematology and Oncology Clinics of North America*, Volume 10, Issue 1, Caraceni, A., Clinicopathologic correlates of common cancer pain syndromes, pp.57–78, Copyright © 1996 W. B. Saunders Company, with permission from Elsevier, http://www.sciencedirect.com/science/journal/08898588.

exploration of the plexus is necessary to rule out fibrosis, a new primary tumour, a radiation-induced tumour, or recurrent cancer.

Lumbosacral plexopathy

Lumbosacral plexopathy is one of the most disabling complications of cancer. Although it is commonly associated with colorectal, cervical, and other pelvic malignancies (bladder, uterus, prostate, sarcoma, lymphoma), it can also be caused by breast or lung cancer, or melanoma. Retroperitoneal tumours (e.g. sarcoma, metastatic nodal tumours) may affect the lumbosacral plexus or its roots more proximally.

The presenting symptom in almost all cases (93%) (Jaeckle et al., 1985) is pain in the buttocks or the legs. Pain often precedes other symptoms by weeks or months. It is usually followed by numbness, paraesthesia, weakness, and, later, leg oedema. The pain is usually aching or pressure-like in quality, and is rarely burning or dysaesthetic. In one series (Jaeckle et al., 1985), an upper plexopathy (L1–L4) was found in about one-third of cases, a lower plexopathy (L4–S1) in one-half of cases, and panplexopathy (L1–S3) in about 20% (Table 14.1.9).

Other structures can be involved. These include nerve roots from proximal extension of the tumour, or contiguous structures,

Table 14.1.8 Differential diagnosis of brachial plexopathy

	Tumour infiltration	**Radiation fibrosis**
Incidence of pain	89%	18%
Severity of pain	Severe in 98%	Mild to moderate
Dose of radiotherapy	—	> 6000 cGy large fractions (> 1900 cGy/day)
Latency	Not indicative	> 6 months, < 5 years
Course	Progressive neurological dysfunction	Progressive weakness
	Pain progression with dysaesthetic quality	Pain stabilizing with onset of weakness
	C7–T1 distribution[a]	C5–C6 distribution
Claude Bernard–Horner syndrome	Can be present	Absent
CT scan findings[b]	Mass with tissue infiltration	Diffuse infiltration of tissue planes
MRI scan findings[b]	High signal intensity mass on T2-weighted images	Low signal intensity lesion on T_2-weighted images
Electromyography findings	Denervation no myokymia	Myokymia

[a] The distribution of the neurological findings can be helpful in some cases but it is not always indicative (see text for more details).

[b] The use of both techniques may provide complementary information. No method is totally credible in differentiating fibrosis from tumour. PET scan nowadays can be an important diagnostic tool.

Table 14.1.9 Clinical findings in lumbosacral plexopathy due to cancer

	Upper plexopathy	**Lower plexopathy**	**Panplexopathy**
Local pain	Lower abdomen	Buttock, perineum	Lumbosacral
Referred pain	Flank, iliac crest	Hip and ankle	Variable
Radicular pain	Anterolateral thigh	Posterolateral thigh, leg	Variable
Paraesthesiae	Anterior thigh	Perineum, thigh, sole	Anterior thigh, leg, foot
Motor and reflex changes	L2–L4	L5–S1	L2–S2
	Proximal leg weakness	Distal leg weakness	Weakness can affect different muscle groups and reflexes
	Patella reflex	Ankle reflex	
Sensory loss	Anterolateral thigh	Posterior thigh, sole	Anterior thigh, leg
Tenderness	Lumbar	Sciatic notch, sacrum	Lumbosacral
Positive SLRT			
Direct	50%	50%	83%
Reverse	15%	50%	83%
Leg oedema	41%	37%	83%
Rectal mass	25%	43%	15%
Anal sphincter weakness	0	50%	0

SLRT, straight leg raising test or Lasegue manoeuvre.

Adapted with permission from Jaeckle et al., The natural history of lumbosacral plexopathy in cancer, *Neurology*, Volume 35, Issue 1, pp.8–15, Copyright © 1985 American Academy of Neurology.

Although electrodiagnostic studies and imaging may distinguish radiation-induced plexopathy from malignant invasion (Harper et al., 1989), this differential diagnosis sometimes is difficult. In these cases, PET scan can be very useful but, at times, surgical such as the sympathetic chain or the psoas muscle. Selective involvement of the L1, iliohypogastric, ilioinguinal, or genitofemoral nerves can produce pain and paraesthesia in the inguinal and scrotal region.

A sacral plexopathy, often overlapping a sacral polyradiculopathy, can be produced from direct extension of a presacral mass invading the sacrum, as sometimes occurs with rectosigmoid and bladder carcinomas. The coccygeal plexus is usually affected in patients with sphincter dysfunction and perineal 'saddle' sensory loss.

Tumour is often found in the lumbar vertebrae, sacrum, or pelvis of patients with lumbosacral plexopathy (45/76 patients) and epidural extension is also common, especially with retroperitoneal tumours. Hydroureter or hydronephrosis is extremely common at diagnosis (Jaeckle et al., 1985; Thomas et al., 1985).

Lumbosacral plexopathy can occur after pelvic irradiation. Thomas et al. (1985) reported that radiation-induced lumbosacral plexopathy very rarely presents with pain and has a median latency of 5 years from radiotherapy. Motor involvement is bilateral in 80% of cases and electromyography can be a useful diagnostic tool. Other differential diagnoses include leptomeningeal carcinomatosis, and cauda equina compression.

MRI and CT scanning both image the lumbosacral plexus effectively. CT gives more information on the bony structures, while MRI is more accurate for soft tissues. The assessment should extend from L1 through the true pelvis (Jaeckle et al., 1985), and should include the spine and adjacent pelvic soft tissues.

Mononeuropathy

Mononeuropathy is less common than plexopathy or radicular lesions (Anoine and Camdessanche, 2007). It is caused by compression or infiltration of a nerve by bony lesions, or by soft tissue masses in the limbs. Intercostal nerve neuropathy from invasion of the chest wall is the most common of the mononeuropathies caused by cancer. Obturator, femoral, and sciatic neuropathies are seen when tumour involves the soft tissue along the nerve distribution in the pelvis and thigh. Peroneal mononeuropathy can occur with bony lesions of the head of the fibula and sarcoma of the popliteal fossa. Ulnar and radial neuropathies result from bony lesions in the elbow or humerus. These mononeuropathies must be distinguished from traumatic or compressive lesions, and from nutritional–metabolic lesions of nerves.

Palliative treatment of peripheral nerve compression

Management of pain is often difficult in these syndromes; opioids are indicated and adjuvants for neuropathic pain should be used for specific indications. Clinical experience suggests that dexamethasone can be particularly effective for pain due to compression and oedema of peripheral nerves.

Peripheral polyneuropathy

Polyneuropathy in cancer patients can be caused by chemotherapy, metabolic disturbance or nutritional deficiency, or paraneoplastic syndromes (Box 14.1.5) (Lipton et al., 1991; Anoine and Camdessanche, 2007).

Peripheral neuropathy is characterized by a stocking-glove distribution of negative sensory and positive sensory symptoms. Loss of sensation may predominate, or there may be painless paraesthesia or distressing burning dysaesthesia, allodynia, and hyperalgesia. Early sensory loss and later motor signs (weakness) are

---

Box 14.1.5 Polyneuropathies and peripheral neuropathies

Related to cancer

- Myeloma associated neuropathies
- Paraneoplastic sensory neuronopathy (Denny-Brown)
- Sensory-motor peripheral neuropathy
- Nutritional factors (cachexia-associated neuromyopathy[a]), vitamin B_{12} folate, deficiency, piridoossine
- Cancer-related metabolic dysfunction: hepatic, renal
- Infiltration of peripheral nerves (lymphomas, leukaemias)[b]
- Vascular (haemorrhagic or ischaemic) peripheral nerve lesion.[b]

Related to chemotherapy and radiation

- Vincristine
- Vinblastine
- Vinorelbine
- Cisplatin
- Oxaliplatin
- Paclitaxel
- Suramin
- Epothilones
- Thalidomide
- Bortezomid
- Radiation to limbs with worsening of vincristine neuropathy.

Non-cancer related

- Metabolic dysfunction: diabetes.

[a] Very frequent.
[b] Mononeuritis multiplex.

---

characteristic of some drug-induced sensorimotor neuropathies (vincristine, paclitaxel). Sensory involvement can be selective in neuropathies associated with cisplatin or paraneoplastic syndromes. Often the only early sign of polyneuropathy is reduction or loss of the ankle reflex. Muscle cramps may be associated with neuropathy and can sometimes be prominent symptoms in vincristine neuropathy. Muscle cramps are relatively frequent in cancer.

Paraneoplastic sensory neuropathy and sensory neuropathy caused by vincristine or paclitaxel is often more painful than that caused by cisplatin. Cisplatin induces a sensory neuropathy mainly affecting the cells of the dorsal root ganglia. There is predominant involvement of the large fibre functions (proprioception), which causes sensory ataxia rather than pain. Vinca alkaloids and paclitaxel produce a mostly sensory axonopathy with some motor component. New antineoplastic drugs that interfere with specific metabolic pathways, such as bortezomid, also have distinct toxic effects on the peripheral nervous system (Anoine and Camdessanche, 2007).

Clinical examination is usually sufficient for diagnosis of a polyneuropathy, although nerve conduction studies and

Table 14.1.10 Paraneoplastic neurological syndromes

Location of syndrome	Reference
Brain and cranial nerves	
Limbic encephalitis	Gultekin et al., 2000
Brainstem encephalitis	Barnett et al., 2001
Cerebellar degeneration	Peterson et al., 1992; Cao et al., 1999
Opsoclonus—myoclonus	Bataller et al., 2001
Visual syndromes	
Cancer-associated retinopathy	Goldstein et al., 1999
Optic neuritis	Lieberman et al., 1999
Chorea	Croteau et al., 2001
Parkinsonism	Golbe et a1., 1989
Spinal cord	
Necrotizing myelopathy	Rudnicki and Dalmau, 2000
Inflammatory myelitis	Babikian et al., 1985; Hedges et al., 1988
Motor neuron disease (amyotrophic lateral sclerosis)	Younger, 2000
Subacute motor neuronopathy	Schold et al., 1979
Stiff-person syndrome	Brown and Marsden, 1999; Silverman, 1999
Dorsal-root ganglia	
Sensory neuronopathy	Graus et al., 2001
Peripheral nerves	Antoine et al., 1999; Rudnicki and Dalmau, 2000
Autonomic neuropathy	Lee et al., 2001
Acute sensorimotor neuropathy	
Polyradiculoneuropathy (Guillain–Barré syndrome)	Lisak et al., 1977
Brachial neuritis	Lachance et al., 1977
Chronic sensorimotor neuropathy	Antoine et al., 1999
Vasculitic neuropathy	Blumenthal et al., 1998
Neuromyotonia	Vincent, 2000; Lahrmann et al., 2001
Neuromuscular junction	
Lambert–Eaton myasthenic syndrome	Carpentier and Delattre
Myasthenia gravis	Vernino et al., 1999
Muscle	
Polymyositis or dermatomyositis	Stockton et al., 2001
Necrotizing myopathy	Levin et al., 1998
Myotonia	Pascual et al., 1994

electromyography may provide additional information (Lipton et al., 1991). Treatment is palliative, with analgesics and adjuvants.

Paraneoplastic neurological syndromes

Paraneoplastic neurological syndromes (PNSs) are a group of neurological disorders that occur in patients with malignant tumour in which an immune-mediate mechanism and not a direct effect of the cancer is the cause. PNSs are rare, affecting less than 1/10 000 of patients with cancer, except Lambert–Eaton myasthenic syndromes (LEMSs) which affect about 3% of patients with small cell lung cancer, and myasthenia gravis, which affects about 15% of patients with tymoma. They can affect central or peripheral nervous systems, neuromuscular junction, or muscle (Darnell and Posner, 2003; Viaccoz and Honnorat, 2013) (Table 14.1.10)

Many PNSs are now recognized. For some of them with well-characterized onco-neuronal antibodies, the nature of the tumour is suggested by the antibody itself; for others the mechanism of the disease is less known, but all are severe and can affect patients' quality of life, even if the underlying tumour is healed or stable. The specific antibodies and their pathogenic role need to be evaluated carefully by highly specialized professionals (Darnell and Posner, 2003; Viacozz and Honnorat, 2013).

In general, neurological symptoms and signs develop acutely and are severe. Subtle, long-lasting symptoms are not usually caused by paraneoplastic syndromes. Only examination of CSF and immunofluorescence techniques for testing circulating autoantibodies can aid diagnosis because MRI scans are often normal and only LEMSs and myasthenia gravis have neurophysiological classic features.

The clinical course is independent of that of the original tumour, which in 50% of cases is found after the onset of neurological symptoms. The associated tumour often is small and slow growing, and may have a relatively benign course. Spontaneous remissions have been seen, but the syndrome is usually irreversible.

Online materials

Complete references for this chapter are available online at <http://www.oxfordmedicine.com>.

References

Alfonso, J. and Reis, F. (2012). Dexmedetomidine: current role in anesthesia and intensive care. *Revista Brasileira de Anestesiologia*, 62(1), 118–133.

American Psychiatric Association (2000). *Diagnostic and Statistical Manual of Mental Disorders* (4th ed., text revision). Washington, DC: American Psychiatric Press.

Anoine, J.C. and Camdessanché, J.P. (2007). Peripheral nervous system involvement in patients with cancer. *The Lancet Neurology*, 6, 75–86.

Antoine, J.C., Mosnier, J.F., Absi, L., Convers, P., Honnorat, J., and Michel, D. (1999). Carcinoma associated paraneoplastic peripheral neuropathies in patients with and without anti-onconeural antibodies. *Journal of Neurology, Neurosurgery & Psychiatry*, 67, 7–14.

Babikian, V.L., Stefansson, K., Dieperink, M.E., *et al.* (1985). Paraneoplastic myelopathy: antibodies against protein in normal spinal cord and underlying neoplasm. *The Lancet*, 2, 49–50.

Baharav, E., Harpaz, D., Mittelman, M., *et al.* (1986). Dexamethasone-induced perineal irritation. *The New England Journal of Medicine*, 314, 315–316.

Barnett, M., Prosser, J., Sutton, I., *et al.* (2001). Paraneoplastic brain stem encephalitis in a woman with anti-Ma2 antibody. *Journal of Neurology, Neurosurgery & Psychiatry*, 70, 222–225.

Bataller, L., Graus, F., Saiz, A., and Vilchez, J.J. (2001). Clinical outcome in adult onset idiopathic or paraneoplastic opsoclonus-myoclonus. *Brain*, 124, 437–443.

Batchelor, T., Taylor, L., Thaler, H., *et al.* (1997). Steroid myopathy in cancer patients. *Neurology*, 48, 1234–1238.

Blumenthal, D., Schochet, S., Jr, Gutmann, L., Ellis, B., Jaynes, M., and Dalmau, J. (1998). Small-cell carcinoma of the lung presenting with Paraneoplastic peripheral nerve microvasculitis and optic neuropathy. *Muscle & Nerve*, 21, 1358–1359.

Boogerd, W., Vos, V.W., Hart, A.A.M., *et al.* (1993). Brain metastases in breast cancer; Natural history, prognostic factors and outcome. *Journal of Neuro-Oncology*, 15, 165–174.

Bortolussi, R., Fabiani, F., Savron, V., *et al.* (1994). Acute morphine intoxication during high-dose recombinant interleukin-2 treatment for metastatic renal cell cancer. *European Journal of Cancer*, 30(12), 1905–1907.

Breitbart, W., Rosenfeld, B., Roth, A., *et al.* (1997). The memorial delirium assessment scale. *Journal of Pain and Symptom Management*, 13, 128–137.

Brown, P. and Marsden, C.D. (1999). The stiff man and stiff man plus syndromes. *Journal of Neurology*, 246, 648–652.

Bruera, E., Fainsinger, R.L., Miller, M.J., *et al.* (1992). The assessment of pain intensity in patients with cognitive failure: a preliminary report. *Journal of Pain and Symptom Management*, 7, 267–270.

Burt, R.K., Sharfam, W.H., Karp, B.I., *et al.* (1992). Mental neuropathy (numb chin syndrome). A harbinger of tumor progression or relapse. *Cancer*, 70, 877–881.

Buss, M.K., Vanderwerker, L.C., Inouye, S.K., *et al.* (2007). Associations between caregiver-perceived delirium in patients with cancer and generalized anxiety in their caregivers. *Journal of Palliative Medicine*, 10, 1083–1092.

Campbell, N., Boustani, M.A., Ayub, A., *et al.* (2009). Pharmacological management of delirium in hospitalized adults—a systematic evidence review. *Journal of General Internal Medicine*, 24(7), 848–853.

Canadian Coalition for Seniors' Mental Health (2006). *National Guidelines for Seniors' Mental Health: The Assessment and Treatment of Delirium*. [Online] Available at: <http://www.ccsmh.ca/en/guidelinesusers.cfm>.

Cao, Y., Abbas, J., Wu, X., Dooley, J., and van Amburg, A.L. (1999). Anti-Yo positive paraneoplastic cerebella degeneration associated with ovarian carcinoma: case report and review of the literature. *Gynecologic Oncology*, 75, 178–183.

Caraceni, A. and Grassi, L. (2011). *Delirium Acute Confusional States in Palliative Medicine* (2nd ed.). Oxford: Oxford University Press.

Caraceni, A., Nanni, O., Maltoni, M., *et al.* (2000). The impact of delirium on the short-term prognosis of advanced cancer patients. *Cancer*, 89, 1145–1148.

Carpentier, A.F. and Delattre, J.Y. (2001). The Lambert-Eaton myasthenic syndrome. *Clinical Reviews in Allergy & Immunology*, 20:155–158.

Chamberlain, M.C. (2006) Neoplastic meningitis. *The Neurologist*, 12, 179–187.

Chédru, F. and Geschwind, N. (1972). Disorders of higher cortical functions in acute confusional states. *Cortex*, 8, 395–411.

Chen, J.W.Y. and Wasterlain, C.G. (2006). Status epilepticus: pathophysiology and management in adults. *The Lancet Neurology*, 5, 246–256.

Cheng, T.M., Cascino, T.L., and Onofrio, B.M. (1993). Comprehensive study of diagnosis and treatment of trigeminal neuralgia secondary to tumors. *Neurology*, 43, 2298–2302.

Clouston, P.D., De Angelis, L., and Posner, J.B. (1992). The spectrum of neurological disease in patients with systemic cancer. *Annals of Neurology*, 31, 268–273.

Croteau D, Owainati A, Dalmau J, Rogers LR. (2001). Response to cancer therapy in a patient with a paraneoplastic choreiform disorder. *Neurology*, 57, 719–722.

Cushing, H. (1932). Peptic ulcers and the interbrain. *Surgery, Gynecology and Obstetrics*, 55, 1–35.

Darnell, R.B. and Posner, J. B. (2003). Paraneoplastic syndromes involving the nervous system. *The New England Journal of Medicine*, 349, 1543–1554.

Delanty, N., Vaughan, C., and French, J. (1998). Medical causes of seizures. *The Lancet*, 352, 383–390.

Dixon, R.A. and Christy, N.P. (1980). On the various forms of corticosteroid withdrawal syndrome. *American Journal of Medicine*, 68, 224–230.

Duncan, J.S., Sander, J.W., Sisodiya, S.M., *et al.* (2006). Adult epilepsy. *The Lancet*, 367, 1087–1100.

Engel, G.L. and Romano, J. (1959). Delirium: a syndrome of cerebral insufficiency. *Journal of Chronic Diseases*, 9, 260–277.

Engel, J., Jr. (2006). Report of the ILAE Classification Core Group. *Epilepsia*, 47, 1558–1568.

Fainsinger, R., Schoeller, T., Boiskin, M., *et al.* (1993). Palliative care round: cognitive failure (CF) and coma after renal failure in a patient receiving captopril and hydromorphone. *Journal of Palliative Care*, 9, 53–55.

Fernandez, A. and Claassen, J. (2012). Refractory status epilepticus. *Current Opinion in Critical Care*, 18, 127–131.

Findlay, G.F. (1984). Adverse effects of the management of malignant spinal cord compression. *Journal of Neurology, Neurosurgery, and Psychiatry*, 47, 761–768.

Fisher, R.S., van Emde Boas, W., Blume, W., *et al.* (2005). Epileptic seizures and epilepsy. Definition proposed by the International League against Epilepsy (ILAE) and the International Bureau for Epilepsy (IBE). *Epilepsia*, 46, 470–472.

Foley, K.M. (1979). Pain syndromes in patients with cancer. In J.J. Bonica and V. Ventafridda (eds.) *Advances in Pain Research and Therapy* (Vol. 2), pp. 59–75. New York: Raven Press.

Formaglio, F. and Caraceni, A. (1998). Meningeal metastases clinical aspects and diagnosis. *Italian Journal of Neurological Sciences*, 19, 133–149.

Francis, J., Martin, D., and Kapoor, W.N. (1990). A prospective study of delirium in hospitalized elderly. *Journal of the American Medical Association*, 263, 1097–1101.

Freedmann, M., Schocket, A., Chapel, N., *et al.* (1981). Anaphylaxis after intravenous methylprednisolone administration. *Journal of the American Medical Association*, 245, 607–608.

Gagnon, P., Allard, P., Masse, B., *et al.* (2000). Delirium in terminal cancer: a prospective study using daily screening, early diagnosis and continuous monitoring. *Journal of Pain and Symptom Management*, 19, 412–426.

Galicich, J.H. and French, L.A. (1961). Use of dexamethasone in the treatment of cerebral edema resulting from brain tumors and surgery. *American Practitioner and Digest of Treatment*, 12, 169–174.

Garbe, E., LeLorier, J., Boivin, J.-F., *et al.* (1997). Risk of ocular hypertension or open-angle glaucoma in elderly patients on oral glucocorticoids. *The Lancet*, 350, 979–982.

Gaudreau, J., Gagnon, P., Harel, F., Tremblay, A., and Roy, M. (2005). Fast, systematic and continuous delirium assessment in hospitalized patients: the nursing delirium screening scale. *Journal of Pain and Symptom Management*, 29(4), 368–375.

Gaudreau, J., Gagnon, P., Roy, M., and Tremblay, A. (2005). Psychoactive medications and risk of delirium in hospitalized cancer patients. *Journal of Clinical Oncology*, 23(27), 6712–6718.

Glantz, M., Cole, B.F., Friedberg, M.H., *et al.* (1994). Double blind randomized, placebo-controlled trial of anticonvulsants prophylaxis in adults with newly diagnosed brain metastases. *Proceedings of the American Society of Clinical Oncologists*, 13, 176.

Golbe, L.I., Miller, D.C., and Duvoisin, R.C. (1989). Paraneoplastic degeneration of the substantia nigra with dystonia and parkinsonism. *Movement Disorders*, 4, 147–152.

Goldstein, S.M., Syed, N.A., Milam, A.H., Maguire, A.M., Lawton, T.J., and Nichols, C.W. (1999). Cancer-associated retinopathy. *Archives of Ophthalmology*, 117, 1641–1645.

Graus, F., Keime-Guibert, F., Reñe, R., *et al.* (2001). Anti-Hu-associated paraneoplastic encephalomyelitis: analysis of 200 patients. *Brain*, 124, 1138–1148.

Greenberg, H.S., Deck, M.D., Vikram, B., *et al.* (1981). Metastasis to the base of the skull: clinical findings in 43 patients. *Neurology*, 31, 530–537.

Gultekin, S.H., Rosenfeld, M.R., Voltz, R., Eichen, J., Posner, J.B., and Dalmau, J. (2000). Paraneoplastic limbic encephalitis: neurological symptoms, immunological findings and tumour association in 50 patients. *Brain*, 123, 1481–1494.

Harper, C.M., Thomas, J.E., Cascino, T.L., *et al.* (1989). Distinction between neoplastic and radiation-induced brachial plexopathy, with emphasis on EMG. *Neurology*, 39, 502–506.

Harrington, K.D. (1988). Anterior decompression and stabilization of the spine as treatment for vertebral collapse and spinal cord compression from metastatic cancer. *Clinical Orthopaedics*, 233, 177–197.

Hedges, T.R., Schoene, W.C., and Albert, D.M. (1988). Case records of the Massachusetts General Hospital (Case 14-1988). *The New England Journal of Medicine*, 318, 903–915.

Helfer, E. and Rose, L. (1989). Corticosteroids and adrenal suppression. Characterising and avoiding the problem. *Drugs*, 38, 838–845.

Hellmann, M. A., Djaldetti, R., Luckman, J., and Dabby, R. (2013). Thoracic sensory level as a false localizing sign in cervical spinal cord and brain lesions. *Clinical Neurology and Neurosurgery*, 115, 54–56.

Hosie, A., Davidson, P.M., Agar, M., Sanderson, C.R., and Phillips, J. (2013). Delirium prevalence, incidence, and implications for screening in specialist palliative care inpatient settings: a systematic review *Palliative Medicine*, 27, 486–498.

Howe, H. (1925). Reduction of normal cerebrospinal fluid pressure by intravenous administration of hypertonic solutions. *Archives of Neurology and Psychiatry*, 14, 315–326.

Ingham, J., Beveridge, A., and Cooney, N.J. (1993). The management of spinal cord compression in patients with advanced malignancy. *Journal of Pain and Symptom Management*, 8, 1–6.

Inouye, S.K., Bogardus, S., Jnr, Charpentier, P., *et al.* (1999). A multicomponent intervention to prevent delirium in hospitalized older patients. *The New England Journal of Medicine*, 340(9), 669–676.

Inouye, S.K., van Dyck, C.H., Alessi, C.A., *et al.* (1990). Clarifying confusion: the confusion assessment method. A new method for detection of delirium. *Annals of Internal Medicine*, 113, 941–948.

Jackson, T., Ditmanson, L., and Phibbs, B. (1997). Torsade de pointes and low-dose oral haloperidol. *Archives of Internal Medicine*, 157, 2013–2015.

Jaeckle, K.A., Young, D.F., and Foley, K.M. (1985). The natural history of lumbosacral plexopathy in cancer. *Neurology*, 35, 8–15.

Jalladeau, E., Carpentier, A., Napolitano, M., *et al.* (2000). Lipomatosi epidurale cortico-induite. *Revue Neurologique*, 156, 517–519.

Johnson, J.C., Kerse, N.M., Gottlieb, G., *et al.* (1992). Prospective versus retrospective methods of identifying patients with delirium. *Journal of the American Geriatrics Society*, 40, 316–319.

Kaal, C.A., Niel, C.G.J.H., and Vecht, C.J. (2005). Therapeutic management of brain metastasis. *The Lancet Neurology*, 4, 289–298.

Klatzo, I. (1967). Neuropathological aspects of brain edema. *Journal of Neuropathology and Experimental Neurology*, 26, 1–14.

Kori, S.H., Foley, K.M., and Posner, J.B. (1981). Brachial plexus lesions in patients with cancer 100 cases. *Neurology*, 31, 45–50.

Krol, G. (1993). Evaluation of neoplastic involvement of brachial and lumbar plexus: Imaging aspects. *Journal of Back and Musculoskeletal Rehabilitation*, 3, 35–43.

Lachance, D.H., O'Neill, B.P., Harper, C.M., Jr, Banks, P.M., and Cascino, T.L. (1991). Paraneoplastic brachial plexopathy in a patient with Hodgkin's disease. *Mayo Clinic Proceedings*, 66, 97–101.

Lahrmann, H., Albrecht, G., Drlicek, M., *et al.* (2001). Acquired neuromyotonia and peripheral neuropathy in a patient with Hodgkin's disease. *Muscle & Nerve*, 24, 834–838.

Lawlor, P.G., Gagnon, B., Mancini, I., *et al.* (2000). Occurrence, causes and outcome of delirium in patients with advanced cancer. *Archives of Internal Medicine*, 160(6), 786–794.

Lee, H.R., Lennon, V.A., Camilleri, M., and Prather, C.M. (2001). Paraneoplastic gastrointestinal motor dysfunction: clinical and laboratory characteristics. *American Journal of Gastroenterology*, 96, 373–379.

Leonard, M., Raju, B., Conroy, M., *et al.* (2008). Reversibility of delirium in terminally ill patients and predictors of mortality. *Palliative Medicine*, 22, 848–854.

Levin, M.I., Mozaffar, T., Al-Lozi, M.T., and Pestronk, A. (1998). Paraneoplastic necrotizing myopathy: clinical and pathologic features. *Neurology*, 50, 764–767.

LeWitt, P., Barton, N., and Posner, J. (1982). Hiccup with dexamethasone therapy. *Annals of Neurology*, 12, 405–406.

Lieberman, F.S., Odel, J., Hirsch, J., Heinemann, M., Michaeli, J., and Posner, J. (1999). Bilateral optic neuropathy with IgGkappa multiple myeloma improved after myeloablative chemotherapy. *Neurology*, 52, 414–416.

Lipowski, Z.J. (1990). *Delirium: Acute Confusional States*. New York: Oxford University Press.

Lipton, R.B., Galer, B.S., Dutcher, J.P., *et al.* (1991). Large and small fibre type sensory dysfunction in patients with cancer. *Journal of Neurology, Neurosurgery, and Psychiatry*, 54, 706–709.

Liptzin, B. and Levkoff, S.E. (1992). An empirical study of delirium subtypes. *British Journal of Psychiatry*, 161, 843–845.

Lisak, R.P., Mitchell, M., Zweiman, B., Orrechio, E., and Asbury, A.K. (1977). Guillain–Barré syndrome and Hodgkin's disease: three cases with immunological studies. *Annals of Neurology*, 1, 72–78.

Ljubisavljevic, V. and Kelly, B. (2003). Risk factors for development of delirium among oncology patients. *General Hospital Psychiatry*, 5, 345–352.

Lundberg, N. (1960). Continuous recording and control of ventricular fluid pressure in neurosurgical practice. *Acta Psychiatrica et Neurologica Scandinavica*, 36(Suppl. 149), 1–193.

Macleod, A.D. and Whitehead, L.E. (1997). Dysgraphia in terminal delirium. *Palliative Medicine*, 11, 127–132.

McCluskey, J. and Gutteridge, D. (1982). Avascular necrosis of bone after high doses of dexamethasone during neurosurgery. *British Medical Journal*, 284, 333–334.

McTague, A., Kneen, R., Kumar, R., Spinty, S., and Appleton, R. (2012). Intravenous levetiracetam in acute repetitive seizures and status epilepticus in children: experience from a children hospital. *Seizure*, 21, 529–534.

Morita, T., Akechi, T., Ikenaga, M., *et al.* (2007) Terminal delirium: recommendations from bereaved families' experiences. *Journal of Pain and Symptom Management*, 34, 579–589.

Pascual, J., Sanchez-Pernaute, R., Berciano, J., and Calleja, J. (1994). Paraneoplastic myotonia. *Muscle & Nerve*, 17, 694–695.

Patchell, R., Tibbs, P., Regine, W., *et al.* (2005). Direct decompressive surgical resection in the treatment of spinal cord compression caused by metastatic cancer: a randomized trial. *The Lancet*, 366, 643–648.

Peterson, K., Rosenblum, M.K., Kotanides, H., and Posner, J.B. (1992). Paraneoplastic cerebellar degeneration. I. A clinical analysis of 55 anti-Yo antibody positive patients. *Neurology*, 42, 1931–1937.

Portenoy, R.K., Galer B.S., Salamon, O., *et al.* (1989). Identification of epidural neoplasm. Radiography and bone scintigraphy in the symptomatic and asymptomatic spine. *Cancer*, 64, 2207–2213.

Posner, J.B. (1995). *Neurologic Complications of Cancer*. Contemporary Neurology Series, Vol. 45. Philadelphia, PA: F.A. Davis.

Riviello, J.J., Claassen, J., La Roche, S.M., *et al.* (2013).Treatment of status epilepticus: an international survey of experts. *Neurocritical Care*, 18, 193–200.

Ropper, A.H. (2012). Hyperosmolar therapy for raised intracranial pressure. *The New England Journal of Medicine*, 367, 746–752.

Ropper, A.H. and Samuels, M.A. (2009). *Adams and Victor's Principles of Neurology* (9th ed.). New York: McGraw-Hill.

Rosner, M., Rosner, S., and Johnson, A. (1995). Cerebral perfusion pressure: management protocol and clinical results. *Journal of Neurosurgery*, 83, 949–962.

Rudnicki, S.A. and Dalmau, J. (2000). Paraneoplastic syndromes of the spinal cord, nerve, and muscle. *Muscle & Nerve*, 23, 1800–1818.

Schimmer, B. and Parker, K. (2006). Adrenocorticotropic hormone: adrenocortical steroids and their synthetic analogs; inhibitors of the synthesis and actions of adrenocortical hormones. In L.B. Brunton, J.S. Lazo, and K.L. Parker (eds.) *Goodman & Gilman's The Pharmacological Basis of Therapeutics*, pp. 1587–1612. New York: McGraw-Hill.

Schold, S.C., Cho, E.S., Somasundaram, M., and Posner, J.B. (1979). Subacute motor neuronopathy: a remote effect of lymphoma. *Annals of Neurology*, 5, 271–287.

Schor, J.D., Levkoff, S., Lipsitz, L., *et al.* (1992). Risk factors for delirium in hospitalized elderly. *Journal of the American Medical Association*, 267(6), 827–831.

Siegal, T., Lossos, A., and Pfeffer, M.R. (1994). Leptomeningeal metastases. Analysis of 31 patients with sustained off-therapy response following combined-modality therapy. *Neurology*, 44, 1463–1469.

Silbergleit, R., Durkalski, V., Lowenstein, D., *et al* (2012). Intramuscular versus intravenous therapy for prehospital status epilepticus. *The New England Journal of Medicine*, 366, 591–600.

Silverman, I.E. (1999). Paraneoplastic stiff limb syndrome. *Journal of Neurology, Neurosurgery & Psychiatry*, 67, 126–127.

Sorensen, P.S. Helweg-Larsen, S., Mouridsen, H., and Hansen, H.H. (1994). Effect of high-dose dexamethasone in carcinomatous metastatic spinal cord compression treated with radiotherapy. A randomized trial. *European Journal of Cancer*, 30A(1), 22–27.

Spinazzé, S., Caraceni, A., and Schrijvers, D. (2005). Epidural spinal cord compression. *Critical Reviews in Oncology/Hematology*, 56, 397–406.

Stiefel, F., Fainsinger, R., and Bruera, E. (1992). Acute confusional states in patients with advanced cancer. *Journal of Pain and Symptom Management*, 7, 94–98.

Stockton, D., Doherty, V.R., and Brewster, D.H. (2001). Risk of cancer in patients with dermatomyositis or polymyositis, and follow-up implications: a Scottish population-based cohort study. *British Journal of Cancer*, 85, 41–45.

Sutter, R., Marsch, S., and Rüegg, S. (2013) Safety and efficacy of intravenous lacosamide for adjunctive treatment of refractory status epilepticus: a comparative cohort study. *CNS Drugs*, 27, 321–329.

Thomas, J.E., Cascino, T.L., and Earl, J.D. (1985). Differential diagnosis between radiation and tumor plexopathy of the pelvis. *Neurology*, 35, 1–7.

Towne, A., Waterhouse, E., Boggs, J., *et al.* (2000). Prevalence of nonconvulsive status epilepticus in comatose patients. *Neurology*, 54, 340–345.

Trzepacz, P.T., Mittal, D., Torres, R., *et al.* (2001). Validation of the delirium rating scale-revised-98: comparison with the delirium rating scale and the cognitive test for delirium. *Journal of Neuropsychiatry and Clinical Neurosciences*, 13, 229–242.

Tuma, R. and DeAngelis, L.M. (2000). Altered mental status in patients with cancer. *Archives of Neurology*, 57, 1727–1731.

Vanelle, J.-M., Aubin, F., and Michel, F. (1990). Les complications psychiatriques de la corticotherapie. *La Revue du Praticien*, 40, 556–558.

Vecht, C.J., Haaxma-Reiche, H., van Putten, W.L.J., *et al.* (1989). Initial bolus of conventional versus high-dose dexamethasone in metastatic spinal cord compression. *Neurology*, 39, 1255–1257.

Vecht, C.J., Hoff, A.M., Kansen, P.J., *et al.* (1992). Types and causes of pain in cancer of the head and neck. *Cancer*, 70, 178–184.

Ventafridda, V., Caraceni, A., Martini, C., *et al.* (1991). On the significance of Lhermitte's sign in oncology. *Journal of Neuro-Oncology*, 10, 133–137.

Vernino, S., Auger, R.G., Emslie-Smith, A.M., Harper, C.M., and Lennon, V.A. (1999). Myasthenia, thymoma, presynaptic antibodies, and a continuum of neuromuscular hyperexcitability. *Neurology*, 53, 1233–1239.

Viaccoz, A., and Honnorat, J. (2013). Paraneoplastic neurological syndromes: general treatment overview. *Current Treatment Options in Neurology*, 15, 2150–2168.

Vincent, A. (2000). Understanding neuromyotonia. *Muscle & Nerve*, 23, 655–657.

Walker, A. and Adamkiewicz, J. (1964). Pseudotumor cerebri associated with prolonged corticosteroid therapy. *Journal of the American Medical Association*, 188, 779–784.

Wallesch, C.W. and Hundsaltz, A. (1994). Language function in delirium: a comparison of single word processing in acute confusional state and probable Alzheimer's disease. *Brain & Language*, 46, 592–606.

Weinstein, R.E., Herec, D., and Friedman, J.H. (1986). Hypotension due to glossopharyngeal neuralgia. *Archives of Neurology*, 40, 90–92.

Wolf, H.G. and Curran, D. (1935). Nature of delirium and allied states. The disergastic reaction. *Archives of Neurology and Psychiatry*, 33, 1175–1215.

Younger, D.S. (2000). Motor neuron disease and malignancy. *Muscle & Nerve*, 23, 658–660.

Endocrine and metabolic complications of advanced cancer

Mark Bower, Louise Robinson, and Sarah Cox

Paraneoplastic syndromes

Hypercalcaemia

Hypercalcaemia is the commonest life-threatening metabolic disorder associated with cancer. It usually occurs in patients with advanced disseminated malignancy and produces a number of distressing symptoms. The treatment of hypercalcaemia of malignancy frequently ameliorates these symptoms, and for this reason the diagnosis should always be sought.

Pathogenesis

Three related mechanisms contribute to hypercalcaemia:

1. increased osteoclastic bone resorption
2. decreased renal clearance of calcium
3. enhanced calcium absorption from the gut.

All three occur in malignancy and contribute to a greater or lesser extent. Bone resorption in malignant hypercalcaemia is universal and related to both local factors produced in response to metastases and humoral factors produced by tumours. It is mediated by osteoclasts that resorb bone at their ruffled border where cellular proton pumps secrete hydrogen and chloride ions that dissolve hydroxyapatite. In addition, osteoclasts produce lytic proteases including lysosomal proteases, metalloproteinases, and cystine proteases that dissolve bone matrix. Decreased renal calcium excretion occurs with low glomerular filtration rates and/or increased tubular reabsorption of calcium in response to parathyroid hormone or its relatives. Haematological neoplasms rarely produce 1,25-dihydroxycholecalciferol ($1,25(OH)_2D_3$, calcitriol) causing increased gastrointestinal absorption of calcium.

RANKL/RANK/OPG

The final common pathway of osteolysis at the molecular level involves a triad of osteoprotegerin (OPG), receptor activator of nuclear factor kappa B (RANK) and receptor activator of nuclear factor kappa B ligand (RANKL). Bone destruction in the presence of osteolytic skeletal metastases is not caused directly by tumour cells but by osteoclasts. The tumour cells either directly produce RANKL or stimulate bone stromal cells to produce RANKL. RANKL is an osteoclast activating factor that stimulates the RANK membrane receptor on osteoclast precursors. In conjunction with macrophage colony stimulating factor, RANKL causes the differentiation of precursors into osteoclasts and the fusion and activation of osteoclasts into functional multinucleated osteoclasts that mediate bone resorption. OPG is a soluble decoy receptor for RANKL that inhibits RANK by competing for RANKL binding. OPG production is decreased in myeloma and metastatic prostate cancer. This RANKL/RANK/OPG equilibrium is disrupted by cytokines, chemokines and prostaglandins, uncoupling the usual homeostatic balance between osteoclastic bone resorption and osteoblastic bone formation. In addition, osteotropic factors such as $1,25(OH)_2D_3$ and parathyroid hormone-related protein (PTHrP) as well as interleukins 1 and 6 enhance RANKL expression and diminish OPG expression.

Parathyroid hormone

In most cases of malignancy-associated-hypercalcaemia, cytokine-mediated osteoclastic bone resorption appears to be the dominant factor; however, in up to 20% of cases no bone metastases are present, so-called humoral hypercalcaemia of malignancy. In these patients, ectopic secretion of factors by the tumour accounts for the disturbance of calcium homeostasis. Humoral hypercalcaemia of malignancy resembles primary hyperparathyroidism biochemically, with hypercalcaemia, hypophosphataemia, renal phosphate wasting, increased tubular resorption of calcium, and enhanced osteoclastic bone resorption. Although true ectopic secretion of parathyroid hormone (PTH) has been described in non-parathyroid tumours, it is very rare indeed.

Parathyroid hormone-related protein

PTHrP is a 16 kDa peptide that resembles PTH in bioactivity but has different immunoreactivity. PTHrP (1-141) and PTH bind same PTH receptor 1 with equal affinity. Whilst PTH is only expressed in parathyroid glands, PTHrP is found in several tissues including keratinocytes, placenta, breast tissue, parathyroid glands, fetal liver and brain. PTHrP plays a central role in endochondrial bone formation, breast morphogenesis and transplacental calcium flux (Lanske et al., 1996; Vortkamp et al., 1996; Strewler et al., 2000).

PTHrP immunoperoxidase staining is strongly positive in human squamous cell carcinomas from various sites (Danks et al., 1989). Moreover, PTHrP mRNA expression was detected in all tumours from patients with humoral hypercalcaemia of malignancy but not in any tumours from normocalcaemic patients (Honda et al., 1988). Furthermore, cancer patients with hypercalcaemia have elevated serum PTHrP measured by immunoassay (> 2.5 pg/mL) (Budayr et al., 1989). Thus PTHrP assays may facilitate the diagnosis of the cause of hypercalcaemia (Hutchesson et al.,

1993). PTHrP may also have a limited role as a prognostic tumour marker, predicting the development of bone metastases in women with breast cancer (Bouizaret al., 1993).

At least 80% of patients with solid tumours and hypercalcaemia have elevated serum levels of PTHrP (Wysolmerski and Broadus, 1994) including over 60% of patients with bone metastases (Grill et al., 1991). Nevertheless, PTHrP cannot explain all the biochemical findings in humoral hypercalcaemia of malignancy. In contrast to primary hyperparathyroidism, there is impaired intestinal calcium absorption, low $1,25(OH)_2D_3$ levels and osteoclastic bone resorption is far more prominent. These features suggest that other factors (probably cytokines) have an important role in humoral hypercalcaemia of malignancy, even in the absence of bone metastases.

Vitamin D

Gut absorption of calcium and vitamin D levels generally are suppressed in patients with humoral hypercalcaemia of malignancy. However, a number of cases of Hodgkin's disease, non-Hodgkin's lymphoma, and human T-cell lymphotrophic virus type 1 (HTLV-1)-associated adult T-cell leukaemia/lymphoma (ATLL) have been reported with ectopic production of $1,25(OH)_2D_3$ resulting in hypercalcaemia (Seymour and Gagel, 1993). The mechanism is thought to involve extra-renal hydroxylation of $25(OH)D_3$ by 1 alpha-hydroxylase to $1,25(OH)_2D_3$ (Davies et al., 1994) and this has implications for therapy. Hypercalcaemia of malignancy is usually associated with low calcium absorption and hence dietary calcium restriction is unnecessary; however, with elevated $1,25(OH)_2D_3$ levels, a low-calcium diet is needed to control hypercalcaemia.

Epidemiology

One in ten cancer patients develops hypercalcaemia and malignancy accounts for about half the cases of hypercalcaemia amongst hospital inpatients. Hypercalcaemia occurs most frequently with myeloma, breast, lung, and renal cancers, and up to 20% of cases occur in the absence of bone metastases. Most patients with hypercalcaemia of malignancy have disseminated disease and 80% die within 1 year. The median survival is just 3–4 months. Thus hypercalcaemia is usually a complication of advanced disease and its treatment should be directed at symptom palliation, but occasionally patients with myeloma or metastatic breast cancer present with hypercalcaemia.

Clinical features

The clinical manifestations of hypercalcaemia are myriad and many symptoms that may have been attributed to the underlying malignancy may resolve on correction of the hypercalcaemia. Although the severity of symptoms is not correlated with degree of elevation of serum calcium, most patients initially develop malaise and lethargy followed by thirst, nausea, and constipation before neurological (drowsiness and confusion) and cardiological features appear (Table 14.2.1). A diagnosis of hypercalcaemia can only be made by biochemical investigation and all symptomatic patients with malignancy should have their serum calcium measured if treatment is likely to be appropriate.

Treatment

In parallel with the advances in the understanding of the pathogenesis of hypercalcaemia have come improvements in therapy, especially the introduction of bisphosphonates that are more effective, less toxic, and easier to administer. They represent a

Table 14.2.1 Clinical features of hypercalcaemia of malignancy

General	Gastrointestinal	Neurological	Cardiological
Dehydration	Anorexia	Fatigue	Bradycardia
Polydipsia	Weight loss	Lethargy	Atrial arrhythmias
Polyuria	Nausea	Confusion	Ventricular arrhythmias
Pruritus	Vomiting	Myopathy	Prolonged P–R interval
	Constipation	Hyporeflexia	Reduced Q–T interval
	Ileus	Seizures	Wide T waves
		Psychosis	
		Coma	

major improvement in palliative therapy for cancer patients. The treatment of hypercalcaemia should be determined on the basis of attributable symptoms and the corrected serum calcium calculated from the formula:

$$\text{Corrected calcium} = \text{measured calcium} + ([40 - \text{serum albumin (g/L)}] \times 0.02)$$

Rehydration followed by the administration of calcium lowering agents is the mainstay of therapy. Low calcium diets are unpalatable, impractical and exacerbate malnutrition. They have no place in palliative therapy. Drugs promoting hypercalcaemia (thiazide diuretics, vitamins A and D) should be withdrawn.

Intravenous fluids

Dehydration due to polyuria and vomiting is a prominent feature of hypercalcaemia and intravenous rehydration is an essential component of acute therapy for severe or symptomatic hypercalcaemia. Although large volumes of fluid will lower serum calcium, patients rarely achieve normocalcaemia and careful monitoring to avoid fluid overload is necessary. In view of this, 2–3 L per day of fluid is now the accepted practice with daily serum electrolyte measurement to prevent hypokalaemia and hyponatraemia. Loop diuretics are often prescribed as an adjunct to intravenous fluids and cause calciuresis. However there is little evidence of any benefit and they may exacerbate hypovolaemia, hypokalaemia, and hypomagnesaemia and are best avoided.

Corticosteroids

Glucocorticoids have been widely used in cancer-related hypercalcaemia and rapidly inhibit osteoclastic bone resorption *in vitro* as well as reducing calcium absorption from the gut. However, their limited clinical benefit is chiefly confined to tumours that respond to the cytostatic effects of steroids, such as myeloma, lymphoma, leukaemia, and, occasionally, breast cancer when hypercalcaemia occurs as a flare effect caused by endocrine therapy. Thus their role in severe hypercalcaemia is limited to haematological malignancies and oral prednisolone 40–100 mg/day is usually effective in these circumstances, although it may take 4–10 days to lower the serum calcium.

Bisphosphonates

Bisphosphonates are synthetic pyrophosphate analogues characterized by a phosphorus–carbon–phosphorus bond, making them resistant to enzymatic hydrolysis. They reduce bone resorption by binding hydroxyapatite crystals with a high affinity and inhibiting osteoclast function leading to disappearance of the ruffled border, decreased acid production, and altered enzyme activity (Sato et al., 1991; Zimolo et al., 1995). In hypercalcaemia of malignancy, bisphosphonates cause a gradual fall in serum calcium over a few days. Bisphosphonates do not alter PTHrP levels, renal calcium reabsorption, RANKL, or OPG levels and so they may fail to control humoral hypercalcaemia of malignancy without bone metastases (Walls et al., 1994; Zojer et al., 2005). There is a correlation between the responsiveness to pamidronate and plasma PTHrP levels; non-responders have levels above 75 pg/mL. Hence PTHrP measurement may identify patients requiring higher or more frequent doses of bisphosphonates (Zimolo, 1994).

The most commonly prescribed bisphosphonate is pamidronate, administered as a single infusion of 90 mg administered at 1 mg/minute, irrespective of the serum calcium level, and repeated every 3–4 weeks (Hillner et al., 2003). First-generation bisphosphonates (e.g. etidronate, clodronate) have been superseded by more potent third-generation preparations including ibandronate (4 mg intravenous infusion over 2 hours) (Ralston et al., 1997; Pecherstorfer et al., 2003) and zoledronate (Body et al., 1999; Major et al., 2001) that are effective in humoral hypercalcaemia of malignancy. Zoledronate corrects hypercalcaemia in more patients, faster and for longer than pamidronate, as well as only requiring a 15-minute infusion (Major et al., 2001). The differences between pamidronate and zoledronate are not marked, however, and the choice is based largely on cost and convenience. In our unit, intravenous pamidronate is used for inpatients whilst outpatients are treated with the briefer zoledronate infusions. A randomized study comparing ibandronate and pamidronate suggested similar efficacy but longer duration of normocalcaemia with ibandronate, although the study used stratified dosing based on serum calcium levels (Pecherstorfer et al., 2003).

In addition to these actions, intravenous bisphosphonates have valuable analgesic activity in patients with metastatic bone pain and reduce skeletal morbidity in patients with breast cancer and myeloma. Osteonecrosis of the jaw is a recognized complication of bisphosphonate therapy associated with prolonged use, older age, and a history of recent dental extraction. Symptoms can mimic dental problems and patient may develop severe pain. The usual management is with antibiotics and surgical debridement (Migliorati et al., 2006).

Calcitonin

Calcitonin is secreted by the parafollicular cells of the thyroid gland, although its physiological role in calcium homeostasis remains undefined. In much higher pharmacological doses, calcitonin reduces osteoclastic bone resorption and increases calciuresis, thereby reducing serum calcium. It is effective in around a third of patients and usually causes a fall in calcium within 4 hours (compared to 48 hours for bisphosphonates), but normocalcaemia is rare and the effect is short lived, usually requiring daily repeat dosing. Doses of up to 8 IU/kg salmon calcitonin may be injected subcutaneously or intramuscularly every 6–12 hours and this therapy has minimal toxicity (nausea is the most frequent side effect and occasional hypersensitivity reactions are seen).

Plicamycin

Plicamycin (formerly mithramycin), a cytotoxic antibiotic, is toxic to osteoclasts by blocking RNA synthesis and hence reduces bone resorption, producing prompt and effective lowering of serum calcium. It is administered as an intravenous bolus or 2-hour infusion at a dosage of 25 micrograms/kg. It produces normocalcaemia within 3 days in 80% of patients and is usually repeated weekly. The disadvantage of this highly effective treatment is its toxicity; cumulative nephrotoxicity and hepatotoxicity occur and thrombocytopenia is common; nausea is frequent and may be reduced when plicamycin is given as an infusion. Plicamycin is now used very rarely.

Phosphates

Oral phosphates may be effective in mild hypercalcaemia, by a combination of effects on calcium metabolism. The usual recommended dose is 0.5–3 g/day phosphate (as sodium cellulose phosphate powder) and this frequently causes nausea and diarrhoea. Intravenous phosphate is a highly effective therapy for acute life-threatening hypercalcaemia and the onset of hypocalcaemic action is more rapid than with any other agent. However, the severe toxicity of parenteral phosphate includes extensive extraskeletal calcification and hence it has been abandoned in all but exceptional cases. Recommended dosing is 1.5 g (50 mmol) elemental phosphate diluted in 1 L of saline over 6–8 hours and should preferably be given in intensive care where the patient's cardiac and renal function can be monitored closely.

Gallium nitrate

Gallium nitrate is incorporated into bone, rendering hydroxyapatite less soluble (Bockman et al., 1990). It inhibits bone resorption directly without killing osteoclasts and is not associated with the nausea or myelosuppression caused by plicamycin. Gallium is highly effective, producing normocalcaemia in 80% of patients with hypercalcaemia of malignancy. Randomized double-blind trials have demonstrated the superiority of gallium compared to calcitonin (Warrell et al., 1988), etidronate (Warrell et al., 1991), and pamidronate (Cvitkovic et al., 2006). The main drawback of gallium is that it requires continuous intravenous infusion (100–200 mg/m² per day) for 5 days and it causes nephrotoxicity. Gallium nitrate is not licensed in the United Kingdom.

Future approaches

Two promising new approaches are emerging for the management of hypercalcaemia of malignancy. Denosumab is a fully human monoclonal antibody to RANKL that is used in the management of postmenopausal women with osteoporosis (McClung et al., 2006) and reduces skeletal events in patients with bone metastases and myeloma (Fizazi et al., 2009; Henry et al., 2011). Denosumab is currently under trial for hypercalcaemia of malignancy. Circulating levels of ionized calcium ion are monitored and regulated via cell surface calcium sensing receptors (CASR). Calcium sensor mimetics or calcimimetics are small organic molecules that potentiate the effect of calcium on the CASR and suppress PTH secretion. Cinacalcet, the first drug in this class, alleviates hypercalcaemia in secondary hyperparathyroidism (Block et al., 2004) and parathyroid carcinoma.

Treatment summary

Symptomatic or severe hypercalcaemia requires intravenous rehydration with 2–3 L per day followed by a single infusion of pamidronate at 1 mg/minute according to the corrected serum calcium. This combination will control hypercalcaemia in most patients simply, promptly, and with minimal toxicity. The majority of patients will remain normocalcaemic for 2–4 weeks

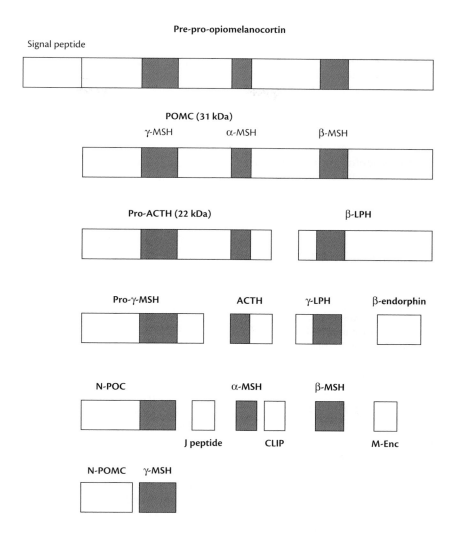

Fig. 14.2.1 Pro-opiomelanocortin (POMC)-derived peptides. CLIP, corticotropin-like intermediate lobe peptide; Enc, encephalin; MSH, melanocyte stimulating hormone; LPH, lipotropin; POC, pro-opiocortin; POMC, pro-opiomelanocortin.

with encouragement of oral hydration. In the absence of effective treatment of the malignancy, however, hypercalcaemia will recur and the serum calcium should be rechecked every 3–4 weeks. Maintenance pamidronate infusions over 2 hours or zoledronate over 5 minutes can be managed on an outpatient basis. Second-line therapy for humoral hypercalcaemia of malignancy resistant to bisphosphonates should probably be with gallium nitrate, although this is rarely available.

Cushing's syndrome

Whilst ectopic secretion of adrenocorticotrophic hormone (ACTH) by non-endocrine derived tumours is not uncommon, clinically overt paraneoplastic Cushing's syndrome is rare. ACTH and at least nine other active peptide hormones are produced from the pro-opiomelanocortin (*POMC*) gene.

Pathogenesis

The *POMC* gene can produce numerous different peptides as a consequence of using alternative gene promoters and post-translational modification and many of these products have been identified in

tumours. The main peptide products include the melanocyte stimulating hormones (α-MSH, β-MSH, and γ-MSH) and the N-terminal peptide precursor (NPP or pro-γ-MSH), the corticotrophins (ACTH and corticotropin-like intermediate peptide or CLIP), the lipotropins (β-lipotropin or β-LPH and γ-LPH) and the endorphins (β-endorphin and met-encephalin). It is remarkable that all these peptides are derived from a single gene (see Fig. 14.2.1).

Excessive ACTH production, whether as ACTH or the larger peptide pro-ACTH, leads to Cushing's syndrome. Melanocyte-stimulating hormones (MSHs) regulate skin pigmentation by affecting directly dermal melanocyte growth and melanin production. Hence ectopic secretion of any peptide containing MSH may lead to generalized hyperpigmentation but this symptom is rarely distressing. No clear clinical correlates have been described that relate to excessive production of endorphins or lipotropins.

Epidemiology

Ectopic ACTH secretion by a tumour accounts for only 5–15% of cases of Cushing's syndrome and the cancer is frequently occult at presentation (Boscaro et al., 2001; Barbosa et al., 2005). For this reason the differential diagnosis between an ACTH secreting pituitary adenoma and ectopic ACTH production is important clinically although biochemical overlap often makes distinguishing them difficult. Half the cases of ectopic ACTH syndrome are due to lung cancer, divided evenly between small cell lung cancer and bronchial carcinoids (Isidori et al., 2006). Islet cell tumour of the pancreas (16%), and thymic carcinoids (10%) make up most of the remaining cases (Beuschlein and Hammer, 2002). The levels of ACTH may decline in response to chemotherapy or radiotherapy (Abeloff et al., 1981), but any correlation between declining ACTH levels and tumour response is only anecdotal, and elevation of ACTH may persist in long-term survivors following chemotherapy (Hansen et al., 1980a).

Clinical features

The typical presentation is of a middle-aged, male smoker with features of severe hypercortisolism and hypokalaemic metabolic alkalosis. Patients have muscle weakness or atrophy, oedema, hypertension, mental changes, glucose intolerance, and weight loss. When ectopic ACTH production arises from a slower growing tumour (e.g. bronchial carcinoid or thymoma) the other classical features of Cushing's syndrome may be present including truncal obesity, moon facies and cutaneous striae, often making the clinical distinction from pituitary-dependant Cushing's disease impossible. Furthermore, biochemical tests do not always differentiate reliably a pituitary corticotroph adenoma from an ectopic tumour as the source of ACTH.

Diagnosis

In addition to the clinical features, the diagnosis of Cushing's syndrome may be confirmed by demonstrating abnormality of at least two of these first-line tests: elevated 24-hour urinary free cortisol, failure of cortisol suppression in the low-dose overnight dexamethasone (1 mg at midnight and plasma cortisol measured at 8 a.m.) test, and raised late evening salivary cortisol (Nieman et al., 2008). After establishing the diagnosis, an elevated plasma ACTH supports the diagnosis of ACTH-dependent Cushing's syndrome due to a pituitary adenoma (Cushing's disease) or ectopic ACTH secretion by a tumour. Failure of 8 am cortisol to suppress, following high-dose dexamethasone (2 mg four times daily for 2 days, or 8 mg at midnight) and very high levels of ACTH (> 200 pg/mL), suggest an ectopic source of ACTH. However, half of the cases of ectopic ACTH from carcinoid tumours suppress with high dose dexamethasone and have ACTH levels in the lower range. In difficult cases, a corticotrophin-releasing hormone (CRH) stimulation test, selective venous catheterization of inferior petrosal venous sinus with ACTH estimations, and two-site directed IRMA for pro-ACTH and ACTH measurements may be necessary to determine the source of ACTH (Orth, 1995; Boscaro et al., 2001). Recently both somatostatin analogue scintigraphy (de Herder et al., 1994) and [99]technetium methoxyisobutylisonitrile (MIBI) imaging (Jacobsson et al., 1994) have been used for localization of ectopic ACTH-producing tumours.

Further difficulties in differential diagnosis have arisen with the description of ectopic CRH secretion by tumours giving rise to Cushing's syndrome (Carey et al., 1984). In these circumstances, ectopically secreted CRH stimulates the normal pituitary to secrete excess ACTH resulting in Cushing's syndrome.

Treatment

The mainstay of palliative therapy for Cushing's syndrome due to ectopic ACTH production is inhibition of steroid synthesis, although inhibition of ACTH release and blocking glucocorticoid receptors have also been attempted. Several steroid synthesis inhibitors are available and successful use in these circumstances has been reported with ketoconazole, metyrapone, mitotane, etomidate, and octreotide. On rare occasions, laparoscopic bilateral adrenalectomy or adrenal artery embolization may be necessary to control symptoms (Boscaro et al., 2001).

The imidazole antifungal ketoconazole inhibits the first step in cortisol biosynthesis by inhibiting cytochrome P450 (CYP) 11A1 enzyme that catalyses side chain cleavage, as well as some of the other enzymes that catalyse adrenal steroidogenesis. It is the best tolerated of the steroid synthesis inhibitors, with potential side effects including nausea, headaches, pruritic rashes and liver failure. Case reports document its successful use in Cushing's syndrome due to ectopic ACTH secretion (Hoffman and Boigham, 1991; Winquist et al., 1995) and it is effective in half the patients with ectopic ACTH secretion (Tritos and Biller, 2012).

Metyrapone inhibits 11-β-hydroxylase (CYP11B1), the final step in cortisol and corticosterone synthesis and has been shown to be effective in ectopic ACTH syndrome at doses of 250–750 mg four times a day. The short half-life of metyrapone and gastrointestinal toxicity (chiefly nausea) are drawbacks and very high levels of ACTH may over-ride the effects of metyrapone. For these reasons it has been suggested that metyrapone should be used in conjunction with ketoconazole.

Mitotane is an adrenal cytotoxic which irreversibly inhibits 11-β-hydroxylase and 18-hydroxylase thus reducing glucocorticoid, mineralocorticoid and androgen production. It produces focal atrophy and necrosis of the zona fasiculata and zona reticularis. Doses of 1–12 g/day in four divided doses have been used and it is active also against primary adrenal cancers. Mitotane is a toxic drug with gastrointestinal side effects (anorexia, nausea, vomiting, diarrhoea) reported in 80% of patients and lethargy and somnolence in 40% (Wajchenberg et al., 2000). Mitotane often takes several weeks to effect cortisol levels.

Etomidate is an intravenous anaesthetic that also inhibits 11-β-hydroxylase and has been used to control hypercortisolaemia in patients unable to take oral medication (Johnson and Canada, 2007).

Octreotide, a long-acting somatostatin analogue that activates predominantly somatostatin receptor (SSTR) 2, may suppress ectopic ACTH secretion via SSTR on pituitary corticotrophs and ectopic ACTH secreting tumours (Woodhouse et al., 1993; Pivonello et al., 2005). Whilst the effects of octreotide in Cushing's disease are limited, a new somatostatin analogue, pasireotide which has broader receptor activation (including SSTR 1, 2, 3, and 5) has shown promise (Feelders et al., 2010).

Mifepristone is a progesterone partial agonist that inhibits the type 2 glucocorticoid receptor that has been used successfully in both Cushing's syndrome patients and those with ectopic ACTH secretion (Castinetti et al., 2009).

Treatment summary

The initial treatment for ectopic ACTH secretion should be ketoconazole 200 mg three times a day rising to 400 mg three times a day. If this fails to control cortisol levels, add metyrapone 250 mg two or three times a day rising to doses of up to 4.5g a day. Further options thereafter include mitotane, octreotide, mifepristone, or pasireotide. The efficacy of treatment must be monitored as hypoadrenalism may ensue and this is most easily achieved by measuring 24-hour urinary cortisol excretion. As levels return to normal in these patients, hormone replacement therapy is frequently necessary. Regimens similar to those used in Addison's disease should be used (e.g. hydrocortisone 20 mg at 8 a.m. and 10 mg at 6 p.m., fludrocortisone 0.05–0.15 mg daily).

Syndrome of inappropriate antidiuresis

Hyponatraemia, usually defined as serum Na^+ less than 135 mmol/L, is a common finding in association with advanced malignancy and many factors may contribute, including cardiac and hepatic failure, hyperglycaemia, and diuretics. However, the detection of concentrated urine in conjunction with hypo-osmolar plasma suggests abnormal renal free water excretion and the presence of the nephrogenic syndrome of inappropriate antidiuresis (SIAD) (Feldman et al., 2005). This acronym is more suitable than 'SIADH' since there is no vasopressin secretion in approximately 15% of cases (Verbalis, 1989).

Pathogenesis

The vasopressin gene encodes a peptide product that includes both the nine-amino acid arginine vasopressin (AVP) and a 90-amino acid peptide, vasopressin-specific neurophysin II (NP II). The AVP-NP II polypeptide is transported by axonal streaming from the hypothalamus to the posterior pituitary gland where it is cleaved and secreted as AVP and NP II. Three AVP receptors have been identified (V_{1A}, V_{1B}, and V_2); V_2 receptors are located on renal collecting duct cells and mediate the antidiuretic activity. Following ligand binding, V_2 receptor activation results in the insertion of aquaporin-2 (AQP2) water channels into the apical plasma membrane of collecting duct cells. Aquaporins are a group of membrane channels that allow the passage of free water but not ions across cell membranes. Thus enhanced AQP2 expression in the collecting ducts increases water reabsorption and leads to reduced free water excretion.

Epidemiology

Stimulation of hypothalamic–pituitary secretion of AVP or a direct effect on distal nephrons accounts for most cases of SIAD. However, in paraneoplastic SIAD, tumours secrete ectopic AVP or vasopressin-like peptides (Smitz et al., 1988). SIAD is most frequently associated with small cell lung cancer or carcinoid tumours but has also been described in gastrointestinal and genitourinary cancers as well as lymphomas and sarcomas (Ellison and Berl, 2007). Among 523 patients with small cell lung cancer, 9% had clinically evident SIAD, 32–44% elevated plasma AVP, and 53–68% abnormal renal handling of water loads (Comis et al., 1980; Hansen et al., 1980b). Although correction of hyponatraemia may correlate with tumour response (Cohen et al., 1978; Vanhees et al., 2000) complete restoration of normal renal water handling is rare even when complete remission is achieved (Srensen et al., 1987).

Clinical features

Significant symptoms of hyponatraemia appear at plasma sodium levels below 120 mmol/L with confusion progressing to stupor, coma, and seizures as levels fall. Nausea, vomiting, and focal neurological deficits may also occur. The clinical features depend both on the levels of plasma sodium and the rate of decline; with gradual falls in sodium the brain cells are able to compensate against cerebral oedema by secreting potassium and other intracellular solutes. Asymptomatic hyponatraemia, therefore, suggests chronic SIAD rather than acute SIAD. The division into chronic and acute SIAD is of therapeutic importance as their management differs (Hojer, 1994).

Diagnosis

The diagnosis of SIAD requires the demonstration of plasma hyponatraemia and hypo-osmolality in the presence of concentrated urine and normal extracellular fluid volume (Box 14.2.1). There are a number of causes of SIAD, including ectopic AVP production by tumours, and several may play a role in hyponatraemia in patients with advanced malignancy. Pulmonary, meningeal, and cerebral infections are common causes and drug-induced SIAD may also present in patients with cancer. Most drugs cause SIAD by stimulating hypophyseal secretion of AVP, although prostaglandin synthesis inhibitors directly inhibit renal tubular excretion of free water. The list of drugs implicated is long and includes morphine, phenothiazines, tricyclic antidepressants, and non-steroidal anti-inflammatory drugs, all frequently used in palliative care, as well as the cytotoxic drugs vincristine and cyclophosphamide, and nicotine. The possibility of drug-related SIAD should always be considered before invoking ectopic AVP secretion by tumours and in most cases the hyponatraemia resolves when the drug is stopped. When SIAD presents with no identifiable cause, a thorough search for occult malignancy (especially small cell lung cancer) should be undertaken, as SIAD may be the presenting symptom and may precede radiological evidence by up to 1 year (Cohen et al., 1984).

Treatment

The management of SIAD depends upon the rate of onset of hyponatraemia and the presence of neurological complications. Acute SIAD with an onset over 2–3 days and falls in serum

---

Box 14.2.1 Diagnosis of syndrome of inappropriate diuresis (SIAD)

Essential criteria to establish this diagnosis

1. Plasma hypo-osmolality (plasma osmolality < 275 mOsm/kg H_2O and plasma sodium < 135mmol/L)

2. Concentrated urine (plasma osmolality > 100 mOsm/kg H_2O)

3. Normal plasma/extracellular fluid volume

4. High urinary sodium (urine sodium > 20 mEq/L) on a normal salt and water intake

5. Exclude (a) hypothyroidism, (b) hypoadrenalism (c) diuretics.

Supportive criteria for this diagnosis

6. Abnormal water load test (unable to excrete > 90% of a 20 mL/kg water load in 4 hours, and/or failure to dilute urine to osmolality < 100 mOsm/kg H_2O)

7. Elevated plasma arginine vasopressin.

sodium in excess of 0.5 mmol/L per day are associated with neurological sequelae and require prompt correction by intravenous hypertonic saline. In contrast, the mainstay of therapy for chronic asymptomatic SIAD is fluid restriction, with or without demeclocycline, urea or aquaretic vaptans.

Acute hyponatraemia with neurological symptoms has a mortality of 5–8%, partly reflecting the underlying pathology. Rapid correction of hyponatraemia by intravenous hypertonic saline, causes osmotic demyelination, leading to central pontine and extrapontine myelinosis. Central pontine myelinosis usually presents 1–2 days after correcting hyponatraemia with quadriparesis and bulbar palsy and is related to the rapidity of correction of sodium. A safe balance between over-zealous correction causing irreversible myelinosis and the considerable mortality of uncorrected SIAD is required (Ellison and Berl, 2007). Hypertonic saline infusions should correct serum sodium at a rate of 0.5 mmol/L per hour although a correction rate of up to 2 mmol/L per hour is said to be safe (Ayus et al., 1982). The total rise in serum sodium should not exceed 25 mmol/L and correction should stop once the serum sodium exceeds 120 mmol/L and symptoms have resolved. To achieve a correction rate of 0.5 mmol/L per hour requires $0.3 \times$ body weight in kg (mmol Na^+/hour). Hypertonic (twice normal) saline solution of 1.8% contains 0.3 mmol/L Na^+. So the correct rate of infusion is 1 mL/kg body weight per hour of 1.8% sodium chloride (Adrogue and Madias, 2000). Although more complex formulae may prove more accurate, they tend to be more difficult to calculate (Nguyen and Kurtz, 2005).

The mainstay of treatment of chronic asymptomatic SIAD is fluid restriction: intake should be limited to 500 mL/day and urine output should not exceed 500 mL/day. This takes several days to influence hyponatraemia. In the context of palliative care, fluid restriction is frequently undesirable as it is unpleasant for patients and onerous for their carers.

The tetracycline analogue demeclocycline (desmethylchlortetracycline) causes nephrogenic diabetes insipidus and alleviates chronic SIAD. Demeclocycline administered orally in two divided doses equivalent to 900–1200 mg/day will reverse chronic SIAD over 3–4 days and should be followed by a maintenance dosage of 600–900 mg/day. The main side effects are gastrointestinal disturbances and hypersensitivity reactions, although reversible nephrotoxicity may occur with prolonged use, especially when hepatic function is impaired.

Urea is an osmotic diuretic increasing free water excretion and reducing natriuresis by raising intramedullary urea levels. It controls SIAD when given intravenously or orally but is poorly tolerated. Oral urea should be given once daily at a dose of 30 g, dissolved in orange juice to mask the taste. There is no need to fluid restrict patients treated with oral urea because of its diuretic properties (Decaux et al., 1993).

Recently non-peptide vasopressin receptor antagonists have been developed including oral selective V_2 receptor antagonists (tolvaptan, satavaptan, and lixivaptan) and intravenous V_{1A}/V_2 receptor antagonists (conivaptan). This class of drugs has been christened the vaptan aquaretics in recognition of their different mechanism of diuresis compared to the saliuretic actions of more familiar diuretics. In conjunction with modest fluid restriction vaptans have proven safe and effective in the treatment of chronic euvolaemic hyponatraemia (Decaux et al., 2008; Robertson, 2011). Oral tolvaptan and intravenous conivaptan are currently licensed for the treatment of euvolaemic hyponatraemia (Gross et al., 2011).

Non-islet cell tumour hypoglycaemia

Tumour-related hypoglycaemia is a frequent complication of pancreatic beta islet cell tumours which secrete insulin, but occurs uncommonly with non-islet cell tumours, usually due to secretion of insulin-like growth factors (Gorden et al., 1981).

Pathogenesis

The two insulin-like growth factors (IGF-1 and IGF-2) share sequence homology with insulin and influence cellular growth, differentiation and metabolism. In many cases of non-islet cell tumour hypoglycaemia, tumours secrete an abnormal precursor of IGF-2 (known as big IGF-2) (Zapf et al., 1992). Unlike insulin, IGFs are bound to at least six IGF plasma binding proteins and normally bind to two cell surface receptors (IGFR-1 and IGFR-2). At high levels of IGF-2 there is a specificity spill-over so that lower affinity binding to insulin receptors occurs, causing hypoglycaemia.

Rarely, non-islet cell tumour hypoglycaemia has been reported to be due to insulin secretion by cervical cancers (Seckl et al., 1999) and the production of antibodies to insulin (Redmon et al., 1992) and insulin receptors (Walters et al., 1987).

Epidemiology

Non-islet cell tumours associated with hypoglycaemia are usually large (average 2.4 kg), retroperitoneal or intrathoracic, often with liver invasion, and growing over several years. Histologically, half these tumours are mesenchymal (mesothelioma, neurofibroma, fibrosarcoma, leiomyosarcoma, rhabdomyosarcoma, neurofibrosarcoma, haemangiopericytoma, and spindle cell carcinoma), 20% hepatoma, 5–10% adrenal carcinoma (chiefly androgen-secreting), and 5–10% gastrointestinal tumours.

Clinical features

Hypoglycaemia may be a presenting symptom, but more commonly occurs with advanced disease. The clinical manifestations comprise cerebral hypoglycaemia and secondary secretion of catecholamines. Neurological findings include agitation, stupor, coma, and seizures which usually follow exercise or fasting and occur most often in the early morning and late afternoon. Focal neurological deficits may be present.

Tumour-related hypoglycaemia should be differentiated from other causes of hypoglycaemia including drugs (e.g. sulphonylureas), hypoadrenalism, hypopituitarism, and liver failure. In advanced malignancy the most common cause of hypoglycaemia is continued oral hypoglycaemic medication in long-standing diabetics.

Treatment

Reversing life-threatening or symptomatic hypoglycaemia requires intravenous glucose infusion. Hyperosmolar glucose solutions in excess of 10% should be administered via central lines; serum glucose levels require frequent monitoring to ensure optimal correction of hypoglycaemia. Up to 2000 g/day may be required to control tumour-related hypoglycaemia. Debulking surgery and effective chemotherapy frequently improve paraneoplastic hypoglycaemia and should therefore be considered even in a palliative context. Dietary supplementation with frequent feeding, including during the night, may control symptoms of mild paraneoplastic hypoglycaemia. Corticosteroids in high doses, parentral glucagon and human growth hormone have all been of benefit in some patients, whilst diazoxide, which inhibits insulin secretion, and somatostatin have been ineffective (Teale and Wark, 2004). Arterial embolization of tumours may also palliate paraneoplastic hypoglycaemia.

Future approaches

The discovery of the role of IGFs in the pathogenesis of non-islet cell tumour hypoglycaemia suggests that IGF antagonists may reduce the dependence on continuous glucose infusions to control hypoglycaemia (Pollak, 2012).

Enteropancreatic hormone syndromes

Enteropancreatic hormone production is relatively uncommon in malignancy; however, there is a variety of clinical syndromes associated with hormone secretion by endocrine tumours of the pancreas and less frequently tumours arising in other organs. The majority of pancreatic islet cell tumours are malignant (with the exception of most insulinomas) and frequently metastases are present at diagnosis. Surgical excision of small localized tumours is optimal treatment and unresectable malignant secretory tumours may respond to chemotherapy. However, in many patients the distressing clinical manifestations arising from excessive secretion of gastrointestinal peptides require palliation and this may be difficult to achieve. These tumours often secrete more than one polypeptide hormone and may switch hormone production during follow-up.

Treatment

The clinical manifestations listed according to the major hormone product of secretory endocrine tumours are shown in Table 14.2.2, along with palliative endocrine manoeuvres. The control of insulinoma-related hypoglycaemia is similar to the management of paraneoplastic hypoglycaemia (see above), except that diazoxide may be a valuable additional agent in insulinoma. Diazoxide inhibits insulin release from beta islet cells but may cause salt and water retention and so is usually prescribed with chlorothiazide. Palliation of acid hypersecretion in Zollinger–Ellison syndrome is achieved most effectively by proton pump inhibitors. High-dose histamine H_2 receptor antagonists may also be useful. The symptomatic control of other secretory tumours has been revolutionized by the introduction of long-acting somatostatin analogues.

Somatostatin, a widely distributed neuroendocrine peptide, acts via five receptors, has a short duration of action, and requires intravenous administration (Kulke and Mayer, 1999). These shortcomings have been overcome by the use of an eight-amino acid synthetic analogue octreotide that is given by subcutaneous injection. A depot formulation of octreotide (Sandostatin® LAR®) and a longer-acting analogue lanreotide (Somatuline LA®) are now available.

The control of clinical symptoms associated with enteropancreatic hormone hypersecretion can be achieved by 100–600 micrograms octreotide subcutaneously daily in many patients with endocrine pancreatic tumours. Once adequate symptom control has been achieved, patients may switch to the longer acting Sandostatin® LAR® or lanreotide. The response to octreotide depends upon the presence of somatostatin receptors on tumours and this has been exploited for tumour localization using *in vivo* scintigraphy with labelled octreotide (Ricke et al., 2001). Somatostatin analogues provide valuable palliation in insulinomas, glucagonomas, gastrinomas, and VIPomas but fail generally to control tumour growth. Octreotide therapy is well tolerated; although initially abdominal cramps and diarrhoea

Table 14.2.2 Clinical manifestations of secretory endocrine tumours

Tumour	Major feature	Minor feature	Common sites	Malignant	MEN associated	Palliative therapies
Insulinoma	Neuroglycopenia (confusion, fits)	Permanent neurological deficits	Pancreas (β cells) > 99%	10%	4–5%	Frequent feeding Glucose Glucagon Diazoxide and chlorothiazide Octreotide (if scan +ve)
Gastrinoma (Zollinger–Ellison syndrome)	Peptic ulceration	Diarrhoea, Weight loss Malabsorption Dumping	Pancreas (δ cells) 25% Duodenum 70%	> 50%	20–25%	Gastrectomy Proton pump inhibitors H_2 receptor antagonists Octreotide
VIPoma (WDHA or Werner–Morrison syndrome)	Watery diarrhoea Hypokalaemia Achlorhydria	Hypercalcaemia Hyperglycaemia Hypomagnesaemia	Pancreas (α–δ cells) 90% Neuroblastoma SCLC Phaeochromocytoma	> 50%	6%	Octreotide Glucocorticoids Potassium and bicarbonate during attacks
Glucagonoma	Migratory necrolyic erythema Mild diabetes mellitus Muscle wasting Anaemia	Diarrhoea Thromboembolism Stomatitis Hypoaminoacidaemia Encephalitis	Pancreas (α cells) 99%	> 70%	1–20%	Octreotide Oral hypoglycaemics Prophylactic anticoagulation

H_2, histamine type 2; MEN, multiple endocrine neoplasia; SCLC, small cell lung cancer; VIP, vasoactive intestinal polypeptide; WDHA, watery diarrhoea, hypokalaemic achlorhydria.

may occur, significant steatorrhoea and malabsorption have not been observed. Amongst the more recent advances in the management of these tumours is the use of radiolabelled somatostatin analogues (Kaltsas et al., 2005).

Carcinoid syndrome

Carcinoid tumours arise from serotonin-producing cells, principally in the gastrointestinal tract, pancreas, and lungs, but occasionally in the thymus and gonads. The incidence is 1.5 per 100 000 and carcinoid syndrome develops in 6–18% of patients with these tumours and these patients almost invariably have hepatic metastases (Feldman, 1987; Modlin and Sandor, 1997; Kulke and Mayer, 1999). The features of carcinoid tumours vary by their sites of origin (see Table 14.2.3).

The cardinal feature of carcinoid syndrome is the combination of diarrhoea and flushing and may be associated with endomyocardial fibrosis, asthma, and pellagra. One-third of patients develop late cardiac manifestations, typically involving the right side of the heart and leading to pulmonary valve stenosis and tricuspid valve regurgitation. Asthma and pellagra are less common. The pellagroid rash arises secondary to diversion of tryptophan for 5-hydroxytryptamine (5-HT) synthesis rather than nicotinamide production (Vinik et al., 1989). The clinical features are mediated by several potentially active substances secreted by carcinoid tumours including 5-HT, 5-hydroxytryptophan, kallikrein, tachykinins (substance P, neuropeptide K), prostaglandins, catecholamines, and histamine. The diagnosis is established by measuring the urinary excretion of 5-hydroxyindoloacetic acid. However, platelet 5-HT levels are a more sensitive diagnostic test and are unaffected by diet (Kema et al., 1992). Tumour localization may be achieved using somatostatin receptor scintigraphy or by positron emission tomography (PET) scanning after injecting ^{11}C-labelled 5-hydroxytryptophan (Jensen, 2000).

Pharmacological control of carcinoid syndrome is primarily achieved by inhibiting the synthesis, release and peripheral action of circulating tumour products, principally 5-HT. The choice of drugs remains empirical in view of the varied profiles of substances released by tumours. Parachlorophenylalanine and methyldopa block 5-HT synthesis, but are poorly tolerated and, therefore, rarely used. There are seven families of serotonin receptors (5-HT_{1-7}) but the relevance of the different receptors to the clinical manifestations is uncertain and is obscured by the secretion of multiple products by these tumours. Cyproheptadine (4–7 mg three times daily) blocks 5-HT_2 receptors and improves diarrhoea in 60% of patients and flushing in 47% with a mean duration of response of 8 months. In contrast, ketanserin (40–160 mg once daily) ameliorates flushing in 50% but only 20% derive relief from diarrhoea. Selective 5-HT_3 receptor inhibitors have been shown to reduce diarrhoea in carcinoid syndrome. Metoclopramide and cisapride stimulate gastric motility via the 5-HT_4 receptor and antagonists of this receptor, which are in development, may prove useful in palliating carcinoid syndrome.

Somatostatin analogues are the first line of treatment for patients with carcinoid syndrome. Octreotide in doses of 50–150 micrograms two or three times daily, subcutaneously, reduces 5-HT secretion and activity. It controls both flushing and diarrhoea in the carcinoid syndrome and produces initial relief of symptoms in 80% of patients (Kvols and Reubi, 1993). Sandostatin® LAR® and lanreotide, a related peptide, are long-acting analogues that have been found to be efficacious (di Bartolomeo et al., 1996; Rubin et al., 1999; O'Toole et al., 2000). Tumour shrinkage rarely occurs however, and the effects of treatment diminish with time.

Palliative debulking surgery may be offered to selected patients with metastatic disease, as it can delay the development of the carcinoid syndrome. Hepatic artery embolization similarly can produce good symptom palliation. Chemotherapy and alpha interferon have also been used successfully to palliate symptoms in carcinoid syndrome (Jensen, 2000). Interferon alpha is of benefit for carcinoid tumours that are somatostatin receptor negative (Oberg, 2000) but adding interferon to somatostatin analogues does not improve outcomes (Faiss et al., 2003). ^{131}I-met-iodobenzylguanidine has been used in patients with disabling symptoms in whom other therapeutic options have failed (Taal et al., 1996). Targeted agents including the mammalian target of rapamycin (mTOR) inhibitors such as everolimus (Yao et al., 2008a), and vascular endothelial growth factor receptor (VEGFR) inhibitors such as bevacizumab have been investigated (Yao et al., 2008b).

Symptom palliation in carcinoid syndrome includes therapy of diarrhoea (codeine phosphate, loperamide or diphenoxylate), β_2 adrenergic agonists for wheezing, and avoiding precipitating factors to reduce flushing (including alcohol and some foods).

Phaeochromocytoma

Catecholamine secreting tumours arise from the adrenal medulla (phaeochromocytomas) or other neural crest-derived tissues. Phaeochromocytomas derive from chromaffin cells of the sympathetic nervous system, usually in the adrenal medulla but occasionally in sympathetic ganglia (paragangliomas).

Table 14.2.3 Comparison of carcinoid tumours by site of origin

	Foregut (2–33% carcinoid tumours)	Midgut (75–87% carcinoid tumours)	Hindgut (1–8% carcinoid tumours)
Site	Respiratory tract, pancreas, stomach, proximal duodenum	Jejunum, ileum, appendix, Meckle's diverticulum, ascending colon	Transverse and descending colon, rectum
Tumour products	Low 5-HTP, multihormones[a]	High 5-HTP, multihormones[a]	Rarely 5-HTP, multihormones[a]
Blood	5-HTP, histamine, multihormones[a], occasionally ACTH	5-HT, multihormones[a], rarely ACTH	Rarely 5-HT or ACTH
Urine	5-HTP, 5-HT, 5-HIAA, histamine	5-HT, 5-HIAA	Negative
Carcinoid syndrome	Occurs but is atypical	Occurs frequently with metastases	Rarely occurs
Metastasises to bone	Common	Rare	Common

[a] Multihormones include tachykinins (substance P, substance K, neuropeptide K), neurotensin, PYY, enkephalin, insulin, glucagon, glicentin, VIP, somatostatin, pancreatic polypeptide, ACTH, α-subunit of human chorionic gonadotrophin.

5-HT, 5-hydroxytryptamine (serotonin); 5-HTP, 5-hydroxytryptophan; 5-HIAA, 5-hydroxyindole acetic acid.

Phaeochromocytomas commonly secrete norepinephrine and epinephrine but also occasionally significant quantities of dopamine. The catecholamines cause intermittent, episodic, or sustained hypertension and other manifestations including anxiety, tremor, palpitations, sweating, flushing, headaches, gastrointestinal disturbances, and polyuria. These symptoms are all attributable to excessive adrenergic stimulation, and when surgery and chemotherapy are unable to control the disease, palliative treatment is usually achieved by alpha and beta adrenergic receptor blockade. However, phaeochromocytomas rarely secrete other peptide hormones which cause symptoms refractory to adrenergic inhibition. Initial treatment should be alpha blockade to control hypertension (e.g. phenoxybenzamine 10 mg twice daily, gradually increasing the dosage until symptoms are palliated) followed by beta blockade to control tachycardia (e.g. propranolol 20–80 mg three times daily). This combination will control symptoms in most patients. If palliation is not achieved despite full adrenergic receptor blockade, α-methylparatyrosine (metirosine 250 mg twice daily increasing up to 4 g/day) may be used, but is only available on a named patient basis in the United Kingdom. Metirosine is a competitive inhibitor of tyrosine hydroxylase, the rate limiting enzyme in catecholamine synthesis, and reduces catecholamine production by up to 75%, but it is poorly tolerated due to sedation, extrapyramidal effects, and diarrhoea. The noradrenaline (norepinephrine) analogue metiodobenzylguanidine (MIBG) is taken up by catecholamine synthesizing tissues and ^{131}I-MIBG is useful for imaging phaeochromocytomas. At higher doses ^{131}I-MIBG may be used as therapy for phaeochromocytoma and neuroblastoma (Lenders et al., 2005).

Gonadotrophin secretion

Follicle-stimulating hormone, luteinizing hormone, and human chorionic gonadotrophin (hCG) may be secreted by pituitary, trophoblastic, or germ cell tumours and ectopically by tumours arising in other organs. All three gonadotrophins share the same β subunit with thyroid stimulating hormone but have a unique α subunit that confers biological activity. Excess gonadotrophins may result in precocious puberty in children, secondary amenorrhoea in women, gynaecomastia in men, and, rarely, hyperthyroidism.

Precocious puberty

Central precocious puberty occurs with central nervous system tumours secreting gonadotrophins. Incomplete or peripheral precocious puberty may result from hCG secretion by germinomas, teratomas, chorioepitheliomas, and hepatomas and oestrogen or testosterone production by adrenal, testicular (Leydig cell), and ovarian (granulosa thecal cell) tumours. The treatment of precocious puberty includes psychological counselling for boys with increased aggression and excessive masturbation. Medical therapy is required to control both the psychosocial aspects and sustained effects on skeletal maturation. Central precocious puberty is amenable to gonadorelin analogues which lead to pituitary gonadotrophin receptor desensitization resulting in suppressed luteinizing hormone and follicle-stimulating-hormone secretion. The management of incomplete precocious puberty is more difficult and requires the use of antiandrogens (e.g. flutamide, bicalutamide, cyproterone acetate and spironolactone) and

inhibitors of androgen synthesis (e.g. ketoconazole, dutasteride and finasteride).

Amenorrhoea

Secondary amenorrhoea occasionally may be a consequence of gonadotrophin, prolactin, oestrogen, or androgen-secreting tumours although iatrogenic causes are far more common. The vasomotor symptoms may be palliated by hormone replacement therapy and dyspareunia caused by vaginal atrophy may be alleviated by topical oestrogen preparations.

Gynaecomastia

Gynaecomastia results from elevation in the oestrogen:androgen ratio and is most often a consequence of drug therapy, either chemotherapy (alkylating agents, vinca alkaloids, nitrosoureas), antiemetics (metoclopramide and phenothiazines), antiandrogens (cyproterone acetate, flutamide, bicalutamide), or gonadorelin analogues (goserelin, leuprorelin, buserelin, and triptorelin). Occasionally, tumours secreting oestrogens or gonadotrophins may be responsible. Testicular Leydig cell tumours and feminizing adrenocortical tumours may secrete oestrogens, whilst peripheral aromatization of circulating androgens to oestrogens, is a feature of Sertoli cell tumours, trophoblastic germ cell tumours, sex cord tumours of the testes, and hepatocellular cancers. Elevated circulating oestrogen levels induce ductal, lobular, and alveolar growth of the breast. HCG-secreting tumours (including testicular tumours, non-small cell lung cancers, hepatoma, and pancreatic islet cell tumours) stimulate oestradiol production by interstitial and Sertoli cells of the testes resulting in gynaecomastia. Symptomatic therapy for gynaecomastia includes discontinuation of any incriminated drugs and treatment of the primary tumour. Tamoxifen, clomiphene, topical dihydrotestosterone, and danazol have all been used, as have liposuction, subcutaneous mastectomy, and low-dosage radiotherapy for palliation of painful gynaecomastia (Braunstein, 1993; Di Lorenzo et al., 2005).

Hyperthyroidism

On account of the structural similarities to thyroid stimulating hormone, hCG has intrinsic thyrotropic action via a thyroid stimulating hormone receptor spill-over effect (Fradkin et al., 1989) but clinically overt hyperthyroidism only occurs with tumours secreting very large quantities of hCG, usually trophoblastic tumours (Giralt et al., 1992). The hyperthyroidism resolves after successful tumour therapy, so palliation of the hyperthyroidism should be with drugs (e.g. carbimazole) rather than radioactive iodine or thyroidectomy.

Prolactin

Ectopic prolactin secretion from non-pituitary tumours is very rare and uncommonly causes galactorrhoea. Small cell lung cancer and renal cell cancer causing hyperprolactinaemia and galactorrhoea may be treated by the dopaminergic agonist bromocriptine.

Oxytocin

The molecular biology of oxytocin resembles that of AVP with similar genes, precursor proteins, and transport by axonal streaming. Furthermore, ectopic secretion of both oxytocin and its carrier protein neurophysin I have been demonstrated in small cell lung cancer, usually in conjunction with ectopic AVP production. Although water intoxication and hyponatraemia may follow oxytocin infusions in obstetrics, ectopic oxytocin secretion does not contribute to SIAD or any other clinical symptoms.

Pyrexia

Pyrexia is a common feature of advanced cancer and is usually attributable to infection or drugs. In one study of fever of unknown origin, 15% of cases were attributed to malignancy (Vanderschueren et al., 2003a), although amongst cancer patients, infection, chemotherapy, or other treatments account for most cases of pyrexia. Paraneoplastic pyrexia is a diagnosis of exclusion established after other causes of fever have been excluded. Lymphoma, leukaemia, renal cancer, hepatoma, myxoma, and osteogenic sarcoma account for most cases of paraneoplastic fever (Zell and Chang, 2005). Although neither C-reactive protein nor erythrocyte sedimentation rate differentiate paraneoplastic pyrexia from infection (Kallio et al., 2001), resolution of fever with naproxen 250 mg twice daily was diagnostic of paraneoplastic pyrexia in some (Chang, 1987), but not all, studies (Vanderschueren et al., 2003b).

Pathogenesis

Pyrogenic cytokines (including tumour necrosis factor, IL-1, IL-6, and interferons) stimulate the synthesis and release of prostaglandin E_2 from the hypothalamus which mediates thermal homeostasis. Tumour-related pyrexia is a consequence of pyrogenic cytokine production by neoplastic cells or normal cells in response to tumours.

Therapy

Definitive tumour therapy resolves paraneoplastic pyrexias in most cases of lymphoma. Sponging, ice-packs, and fans may relieve discomfort. Pharmacological agents such as paracetamol, aspirin, non-steroidal anti-inflammatory drugs, and steroids are effective antipyretics. Advances in the understanding of the pathogenesis of paraneoplastic pyrexia propose a role for cytokine antagonists in therapy.

Non-paraneoplastic complications

Hyperglycaemia

Aetiology

The prevalence of hyperglycaemia in cancer patients is higher than in the general population. Hyperglycaemia is both a risk factor for cancers and a consequence of their treatment. Diabetes mellitus increases the risk of cancers of the pancreas, liver by up to twofold, and to a lesser extent is a risk factor for other cancers (Vigneri et al., 2009; Gallagher and LeRoith, 2011). Several mechanisms may contribute to hyperglycaemia in advanced cancers, including increased gluconeogenesis and Cori cycle activity (conversion of muscle derived lactate to glucose), diminished glucose tolerance, and insulin resistance (Nelson et al., 1994; Poulson, 1997). These changes may arise as a consequence of hepatic dysfunction, altered glucose metabolism by tumour cells, and the secretion of insulin antagonists. Cancer treatments associated with glucocorticoid use, androgen receptor inhibition, or immunomodulation with cytokines, also predispose to the development of hyperglycaemia. Furthermore, the frequent use of corticosteroids in palliative medicine may contribute, since one in five patients on high-dose steroids will develop steroid-induced diabetes mellitus.

Treatment

The conventional treatment of diabetes advocates tight control of blood sugar to delay the onset of both macrovascular and microvascular complications. In contrast, the aims of therapy in palliative care of advanced cancer are to minimize symptoms associated with hypoglycaemia or marked hyperglycaemia. For this reason a higher range of blood sugar is usually advocated, although symptomatic hyperglycaemia (persistent blood sugar > 15 mmol/L) should be avoided (Poulson, 1997). As disease progresses, oral hypoglycaemic agents or insulin dose generally will need to be reduced with falling nutritional intake.

Steroid-induced diabetes, which occurs frequently in advanced cancer, is usually asymptomatic and requires no therapy; however, monitoring should be instituted for patients on moderate or high doses of exogenous glucocorticoids. If symptomatic hyperglycaemia develops, a short-acting sulphonylurea may be useful (e.g. gliclazide 40–80 mg once daily.)

Hypothalamic–pituitary–adrenal dysfunction

Dysfunction of the hypothalamic–pituitary–adrenal axis can occur as a direct result of cancer or as a consequence of treatment.

Growth hormone

Growth hormone deficiency occurs as a dose-dependent effect of cranial radiotherapy. It often presents years later with reduced bone and muscle mass, poor exercise tolerance, and diminished myocardial function (Sklar and Constine, 1995). Measurements of growth hormone, IGF-1, and gonadal function establish the diagnosis. Tumours of the pituitary or craniopharnyx can also cause growth hormone deficiency.

Sex hormones

Similarly, head and neck radiotherapy can affect sex hormone production, directly causing hyperprolactinaemia and gonadotrophin deficiency, or indirectly by disrupting growth hormone, thyroid, or adrenal function. Hyperprolactinaemia inhibits secretion of pituitary gonadatrophin causing secondary hypogonadism and occurs in 60% of brain tumour patients treated with cranial radiotherapy (Constine et al., 1993). Sex hormone deficiency may alter libido and affect metabolism of bones and lipids. Specialist assessment for sexual dysfunction is recommended, as there may be multifactorial causes.

Adrenocorticoid function

Adrenal function may be disrupted by bilateral metastases, infection in the immunocompromised, haemorrhage, surgery, chemotherapy, or other drugs which affect CYP enzymes (e.g. ketoconazole). Metastases to the adrenal glands are common, however clinically significant hypoadrenalism is rare, as over 80% of the adrenal tissue needs to be replaced to disrupt function (Cedermark and Sjoberg, 1981). Hypoadrenalism presents with profound weakness, gastrointestinal upset, hypotension, psychiatric manifestations, and, rarely Addisonian, crises. Standard replacement therapy is hydrocortisone 20 mg at 800 a.m. and 10 mg at 6 p.m. with fludrocortisone 0.05–0.15 mg daily.

Thyroid function

Thyroid function can be affected by surgery, radiotherapy, and systemic anticancer therapy. Radiotherapy is associated with hypothyroidism, transient hyperthyroidism related to an autoimmune thyroiditis, and thyroid cancer (Wasnich et al., 1973; Tami et al., 1992). Euthyroid sick syndrome, characterized by low serum triiodothyronine levels, occurs commonly with advanced malignancy but rarely causes clinical illness (McIver and Gorman, 1997).

Metabolic bone disease

Osteoporosis can be precipitated by glucocorticoids and chemotherapy (e.g. cisplatin) which cause renal loss of calcium, magnesium, and phosphate. In premenopausal women treated for breast or ovarian cancer and men with prostate cancer treated with androgen inhibition, osteoporosis is common (Gralow et al., 2009). Early assessment using bone mineral density measurement and treatment with oestrogens, if appropriate, or bisphosphonates should be considered to reduce the risk of skeletal events.

Renal failure

Renal failure is a common feature of advanced malignancy and many aetiological factors play a role in its pathogenesis (see Box 14.2.2) (Darmon et al., 2006). In the context of incurable malignant disease, reversible causes may be addressed but aggressive treatment, such as renal replacement therapy, is seldom appropriate. Conversely, there is increasing awareness of palliative measures and end-of-life care amongst nephrologists treating patients with end-stage renal failure (Poppel et al., 2003).

Potentially reversible metabolic causes of renal failure include urate nephropathy, hypercalcaemia, and tumour lysis syndrome

---

Box 14.2.2 Causes of renal failure in malignancy

- Infiltration by tumour
- Fluid depletion
- Electrolyte imbalance:
  - uric acid (tumour lysis syndrome)
  - hypercalcaemia
  - paraprotein (e.g. myeloma)
  - amyloid (e.g. myeloma)
  - lysozyme (e.g. acute myelomonocytic leukaemia)
  - mucoprotein (e.g. pancreatic adenocarcinoma)
  - nephrogenic diabetes insipidus (e.g. leiomyosarcoma)
- Urinary tract obstruction
- Iatrogenic
  - chemotherapy
  - radiotherapy
- Paraneoplastic:
  - membranous glomerulonephritis (e.g. carcinomas)
  - minimal change glomerulonephritis (e.g. Hodgkin's disease)
  - membranoproliferative glomerulonephritis (e.g. non-Hodgkin's lymphoma)
  - thrombotic microangiopathy
- Pre-existing chronic renal failure.

(Garnick and Mayer, 1978). Prerenal and obstructive renal failure may be reversible, although treatment may be inappropriate if the patient is very frail and antitumour options have been exhausted (Garnick and Mayer, 1978).

Nevertheless, symptomatic management of renal failure is important. Patients may experience nausea, vomiting, drowsiness, and confusion as the kidneys fail. Dry mouth and anorexia are frequent symptoms of advanced cancer and may be exacerbated by renal impairment. Appropriate and sensitive explanation to the patient and family should be accompanied by medication to relieve any unpleasant symptoms. In the context of renal failure, doses or dose frequency of some medications, including opioid analgesics, may need to be reduced or stopped to avoid drug accumulation or deterioration of renal function (see Chapter 15.6). Patients already receiving renal dialysis for pre-existing chronic renal failure may choose to continue, but should be supported to stop dialysis, if this is their wish (Smith et al., 2003).

Obstructive nephropathy may cause colicky pain in addition to the non-specific symptoms of renal failure. Although analgesics and antispasmodics may ameliorate the pain, longer lasting relief of symptoms can be achieved with percutaneous nephrostomy. This procedure, performed under sedation, can be followed by antegrade catheterization of the ureters. Nephrostomy tube insertion is an invasive procedure and is appropriate in selected cases where prognosis may be longer or antitumour treatment is planned (Harrington et al., 1995; Little et al., 2003).

Liver failure

Liver failure in cancer patients is usually a consequence of biliary obstruction, very extensive hepatic metastases, or drug therapy, although paraneoplastic hepatopathy has been described in Hodgkin's lymphoma (Dourakis et al., 1999) and renal cancer (Fang et al., 1992) (see Chapter 10.4). After excluding drug causes, it is important to differentiate obstructive and parenchymal causes, as the approach to palliation differs.

Biliary obstruction may be confirmed by ultrasonography and drainage may be undertaken to relieve jaundice and associated symptoms such as anorexia, nausea, and pruritus (see Chapter 10.4). The diagnosis is important since relief of obstruction can provide symptomatic relief and a prognosis of more than 6 months (Isayama et al., 2004), whereas hepatic failure from parenchymal replacement by malignant disease is likely to lead to death within weeks. Biliary drainage may be obtained temporarily by percutaneous transhepatic biliary drainage or directly by endoscopic retrograde biliary stenting.

Hepatic failure due to massive metastases may produce jaundice, pruritus, anorexia, liver capsule pain, ascites, disturbances of haemostasis, malabsorption, and electrolyte disturbances, culminating in hepatic encephalopathy. The palliative treatment of liver failure needs to be tailored to the particular symptoms of each patient. Liver capsule pain may be helped by non-steroidal anti-inflammatory drugs or corticosteroids together with conventional analgesics. Symptoms of functional gastric outlet obstruction may be relieved by metoclopramide before meals. Nausea secondary to liver failure may require centrally acting antiemetics such as haloperidol. Pruritus may be reduced by using emollients and night sedation. Naltrexone and stanozolol have also been found to be effective in pruritus from intrahepatic cholestasis and obstructive jaundice respectively (see Chapter 11.2).

Hepaticencephalopathyiscausedbyexcessgamma-aminobutyric acid (GABA) activity, ammonia, and other toxins in the central nervous system. Conventional therapies include restriction of dietary protein and sodium, bowel clearance with magnesium sulphate enemas and lactulose, as well as bowel sterilization with the non-absorbed antibiotic rifaximin (Bass et al., 2010). Since hepatic encephalopathy is a terminal event in advanced malignancy, these unpleasant treatments are rarely appropriate. The main symptom of encephalopathy is confusion, and after establishing the cause, familiar company, a light and quiet environment, and a regular routine should be provided, together with explanation, reassurance, and reorientation. Sedation may be necessary if the patient is agitated; haloperidol (1.5–5 mg) or levomepromazine (6.25–150 mg) may be given orally or subcutaneously, and also has antiemetic activity (see Chapter 18.2). Portal hypertension and abnormal coagulation predisposes to gastrointestinal haemorrhage. Major haemorrhage should usually be managed symptomatically (see Chapter 8.7).

Lactic acidosis

In cancer patients, lactic acidosis is most frequently type A, due to impaired tissue oxygenation secondary to hypoperfusion as a consequence of septicaemia shock. Less commonly, type B lactic acidosis occurs with large tumour burdens of haematological cancers. Increased lactate production by tumour cells owing to uncoupled oxidative phosphorylation and glycolysis, and reduced lactate clearance due to liver dysfunction, are implicated in the pathogenesis. Lactic acidosis presents with hyperventilation and hypotension and the diagnosis is established biochemically by the combination of wide anion gap acidosis and raised plasma lactate (> 2 mEq/L). High-volume haemofiltration and intravenous sodium bicarbonate may correct the metabolic acidosis, but should obviously only be used if effective anticancer therapy is available and appropriate (Fall and Szerlip, 2005).

Online materials

Complete references for this chapter are available online at <http://www.oxfordmedicine.com>.

References

Adrogue, H. and Madias, N. (2000). Hyponatremia. *The New England Journal of Medicine*, 342, 1581–1589.

Bass, N.M., Mullen, K.D., Sanyal, A., *et al.* (2010). Rifaximin treatment in hepatic encephalopathy. *The New England Journal of Medicine*, 362(12), 1071–1081.

Boscaro, M., Barzon, L., Fallo, F., and Sonino, N. (2001). Cushing's syndrome. *The Lancet*, 357(9258), 783–791.

Bouizar, Z., Spyratos, F., Deytieux, S., de Vernejoul, M.C., and Jullienne, A. (1993). Polymerase chain reaction analysis of parathyroid hormone-related protein gene expression in breast cancer patients and occurrence of bone metastases. *Cancer Research*, 53(21), 5076–5078.

Budayr, A.A., Nissenson, R.A., Klein, R.F., *et al.* (1989). Increased serum levels of a parathyroid hormone-like protein in malignancy-associated hypercalcaemia. *Annals of Internal Medicine*, 111, 807–812.

Carey, R.M., Varma, S.K., Drake, C.R., Jr, *et al.* (1984). Ectopic secretion of corticotropin-releasing factor as a cause of Cushing's syndrome. A clinical, morphologic, and biochemical study. *The New England Journal of Medicine*, 311(1), 13–20.

Decaux, G., Soupart, A., and Vassart, G. (2008). Non-peptide arginine-vasopressin antagonists: the vaptans. *The Lancet*, 371(9624), 1624–1632.

Di Lorenzo, G., Autorino, R., Perdonà, S., and De Placido, S. (2005). Management of gynaecomastia in patients with prostate cancer: a systematic review. *The Lancet Oncology*, 6(12), 972–979.

Ellison, D.H. and Berl, T. (2007). Clinical practice. The syndrome of inappropriate antidiuresis. *The New England Journal of Medicine*, 356(20), 2064–2072.

Feelders, R.A., de Bruin, C., Pereira, A.M., *et al.* (2010). Pasireotide alone or with cabergoline and ketoconazole in Cushing's disease. *The New England Journal of Medicine*, 362(19), 1846–1848.

Feldman, B.J., Rosenthal, S.M., Vargas, G.A., *et al.* (2005). Nephrogenic syndrome of inappropriate antidiuresis. *The New England Journal of Medicine*, 352(18), 1884–1890.

Fizazi, K., Lipton, A., Mariette, X., *et al.* (2009). Randomized phase II trial of denosumab in patients with bone metastases from prostate cancer, breast cancer, or other neoplasms after intravenous bisphosphonates. *Journal of Clinical Oncology*, 27(10), 1564–1571.

Gallagher, E.J. and LeRoith, D. (2011). Diabetes, cancer, and metformin: connections of metabolism and cell proliferation. *Annals of the New York Academy of Sciences*, 1243, 54–68.

Gorden, P., Hendricks, C.M., Kahn, C.R., Megyesi, K., and Roth, J. (1981). Hypoglycemia associated with non-islet-cell tumor and insulin-like growth factors. *The New England Journal of Medicine*, 305(24), 1452–1455.

Henry, D.H., Costa, L., Goldwasser, F., *et al.* (2011). Randomized, double-blind study of denosumab versus zoledronic acid in the treatment of bone metastases in patients with advanced cancer (excluding breast and prostate cancer) or multiple myeloma. *Journal of Clinical Oncology*, 29(9), 1125–1132.

Hillner, B.E., Ingle, J.N., Chlebowski, R.T., *et al.* (2003). American Society of Clinical Oncology 2003 update on the role of bisphosphonates and bone health issues in women with breast cancer. *Journal of Clinical Oncology*, 21(21), 4042–4057.

Kulke, M.H. and Mayer, R.J. (1999). Carcinoid tumors. *The New England Journal of Medicine*, 340(11), 858–868.

Lanske, B., Karaplis, A.C., Lee, K., *et al.* (1996). PTH/PTHrP receptor in early development and Indian hedgehog-regulated bone growth. *Science*, 273, 663–666.

Lenders, J.W., Eisenhofer, G., Mannelli, M., and Pacak, K. (2005). Phaeochromocytoma. *The Lancet*, 366(9486), 665–675.

Major, P., Lortholary, A., Hon, J., *et al.* (2001). Zoledronic acid is superior to pamidronate in the treatment of hypercalcemia of malignancy: a pooled analysis of two randomized, controlled clinical trials. *Journal of Clinical Oncology*, 19(2), 558–567.

Migliorati, C.A., Siegel, M.A., and Elting, L.S. (2006). Bisphosphonate-associated osteonecrosis: a long-term complication of bisphosphonate treatment. *The Lancet Oncology*, 7(6), 508–514.

Nieman, L.K., Biller, B.M., Findling, J.W., *et al.* (2008). The diagnosis of Cushing's syndrome: an Endocrine Society Clinical Practice Guideline. *Journal of Clinical Endocrinology and Metabolism*, 93(5), 1526–1540.

Orth, D. (1995). Cushing's syndrome. *The New England Journal of Medicine*, 332, 791–803.

Pollak, M. (2012). The insulin and insulin-like growth factor receptor family in neoplasia: an update. *Nature Reviews Cancer*, 12(3), 159–169.

Robertson, G.L. (2011). Vaptans for the treatment of hyponatremia. *Nature Reviews Endocrinology*, 7(3), 151–161.

Strewler, G.J. (2000). The physiology of parathyroid hormone-related protein. *The New England Journal of Medicine*, 342(3), 177–185.

Vigneri, P., Frasca, F., Sciacca, L., Pandini, G., and Vigneri, R. (2009). Diabetes and cancer. *Endocrine-Related Cancer*, 16(4), 1103–1123.

Vortkamp, A., Lee, K., Lanske, B., Segre, G.V., Kronenberg, H.M., and Tabin, C.J. (1996). Regulation of rate of cartilage differentiation by Indian hedgehog and PTH-related peptide. *Science*, 273, 613–622.

Warrell, R., Murphy, W.K., Schulman, P., O'Dwyer, P.J., and Heller, G. (1991). A randomised double-blind study of gallium nitrate compared to etidronate for acute control of cancer related hypercalcemia. *Journal of Clinical Oncology*, 9, 1467–1475.

Zell, J.A. and Chang, J.C. (2005). Neoplastic fever: a neglected paraneoplastic syndrome. *Supportive Care in Cancer*, 13(11), 870–877.

14.3

Bowel obstruction

Carla I. Ripamonti, Alexandra M. Easson, and Hans Gerdes

Introduction to bowel obstruction

In this chapter, malignant bowel obstruction (MBO) is defined as the clinical presentation of patients with symptoms, signs, and radiographic evidence of obstruction to the transit of gastrointestinal (GI) contents caused by cancer, or the consequences of anticancer therapy including surgery, chemotherapy or radiation therapy. Although some authors and investigators restrict the definition of MBO to the sites of obstruction in the small intestine alone, or any part of the bowel beyond the ligament of Treitz, for the purposes of this chapter, MBO will be considered as obstruction at any level from the stomach outlet to the anus. The signs and symptoms of MBO are not always pathognomonic, but when present in conjunction with the clinical history of abdominal and some extra-abdominal malignancies, should raise suspicion for the diagnosis. Similarly, radiographic testing may not always confirm the presence of obstruction in the presence of classical symptoms, while at times the radiographic changes may predate the onset of symptoms. Therefore, clinicians caring for cancer patients should always retain a high index of suspicion for this problem.

MBO is a well-recognized complication of advanced cancer in patients with abdominal and pelvic malignancies. Although it may develop at any time in the disease, it occurs most frequently at the advanced stage, with the highest incidence ranging from 5.5% to 42% in ovarian carcinoma and in 4.4–24% of patients with colorectal cancer depending on when it is measured in the disease trajectory (Castaldo et al., 1981; Krebs and Goplerud, 1983; Baines et al., 1985; Gallick et al., 1987; Fernandes et al., 1988, Beattie et al., 1989; Larson et all., 1989; Lund, 1989; Mercadante, 1997; Ripamonti et al., 2001). This chapter does not deal with bowel obstruction as the primary presentation of cancer, but rather MBO in the setting of advanced disease.

Mechanisms of bowel obstruction

The aetiology may be benign in 10–48% of cases at operation, caused by adhesions or radiation enteritis, or malignant with single-site, multiple-site, or diffuse disease.

The enlargement of the primary tumour or recurrence of abdominal masses, fibrosis, or adhesions may produce extrinsic occlusion of the lumen. Polypoidal lesions or annular narrowing due to disseminated disease may cause an intraluminal occlusion. Infiltration of the intestinal muscles or superimposed inflammation may produce intramural occlusion of the lumen. Intestinal motility disorders due to a deranged extrinsic neural control of viscera may produce delay in intestinal transit, resulting in a clinical picture similar to bowel obstruction, namely pseudo-obstruction. Concomitant disease, such as diabetes, para-neoplastic syndromes, or previous gastric surgery, may also contribute to dysmotility of this kind. Contributing factors include constipation, due to illness and/or to drugs such as those with anticholinergic side effects including opioids. Pain due to opioid-induced constipation, wrongly treated with increased doses of opioids, may result in faecal impaction producing signs consistent with bowel obstruction (Glare and Lickiss, 1992).

Pathogenesis

An occlusion of the lumen prevents or delays the propulsion of the intestinal contents from passing distally. The accumulation of non-absorbed secretions produces abdominal distension and colicky peristalsis to surmount the obstacle in the early stage, corresponding to a subobstructive state, possibly still reversible. Although there is little or no through-movement of intestinal contents, the bowel continues to contract with increased uncoordinated peristaltic activity. As a consequence, the bowel becomes distended, stimulating intestinal fluid secretion, thus creating a vicious cycle of distension–secretion, further stretching the bowel wall. Moreover, in bowel obstruction the abnormally increased flora may also produce gases in the small intestine, contributing to distension and pain (Mercadante, 1995a) (Fig. 14.3.1).

This will produce damage in the lumen with a consequent inflammatory response involving the activation of the cyclooxygenase pathway and the release of prostaglandins, potent secretagogues either by a direct effect on enterocytes or the enteric nervous reflex (Mercadante, 1995a). Vasoactive intestinal peptide (VIP) may be released into the portal and peripheral circulation and mediate local intestinal and systemic pathophysiological alterations as hyperaemia and oedema of the intestinal wall and an accumulation of fluid in the lumen (Nellgard and Cassuto, 1993; Nellgard et al., 1995).

Hypoxia, caused by the reduction in venous drainage from the obstructed segment interfering with oxygen consumption, is the primary stimulus for VIP release and for intraluminal bacterial overgrowth. High portal levels of VIP are known to cause hypersecretion and splanchnic vasodilatation (Basson et al., 1989). Experimental studies have shown that higher VIP content is

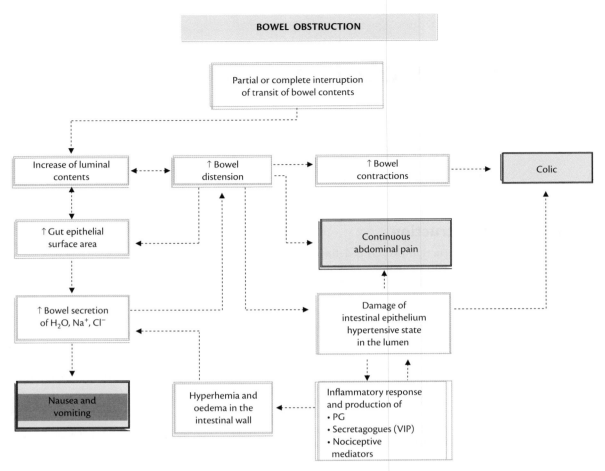

Fig. 14.3.1 Distension–secretion–motor activity causing gastrointestinal symptoms. PG, prostaglandins; VIP, vasoactive intestinal polypeptide. Reproduced courtesy of Carla Ripamonti.

present in the duodenal tissue when compared to colonic tissue content. This may also explain the finding of a redistribution of blood flow between the obstructed segment and the distal sites. Alterations of splanchnic flow are the basis of the appearance of multiple organ failure syndrome caused or worsened by systemic hypotension commonly observed in the late stage of bowel occlusion (Neville et al., 1991). Fluids and electrolytes are sequestered in the gut wall and in its lumen (third space) in the presence of vasodilatation.

Metabolic and septic consequences

The hypovolaemic state may induce functional renal failure due to a decrease in renal flow and, as a consequence, reduced glomerular filtration. Oliguria, azotaemia, and haemoconcentration may accompany dehydration. Metabolic disorders in intestinal obstruction depend on the site and duration of the obstruction and are caused by dehydration, electrolyte losses, and disorders of acid–base balance (Chan and Woodruff, 1992). The respiratory pattern will depend on the level of obstruction. Metabolic alkalosis, hypochloraemia, hyponatraemia, and hypokalaemia will be features of a high-level obstruction, in part due to intestinal stasis of biliary, pancreatic, intestinal, as well as gastric secretions (Mercadante, 1997). There will be acidosis due to ischaemic

lesions or septic complications (Scott Jones and Schirmer, 1989). The increased abdominal distension reduces the venous return and may impair pulmonary ventilation as a result of elevation of the diaphragm.

Sepsis may occur in the late stages of bowel obstruction. It consists of the passage of toxins from the intestinal contents through the intestinal wall into the lymphatic and systemic circulation, or bacterial translocation. This phenomenon results from the increase in endoluminal pressure, stasis, and intestinal ischaemia, together with intestinal gangrene and perforation, commonly observed in the late stages of persisting bowel obstruction. The time course of these events is variable, occurring over several days in malignant mechanical bowel obstruction.

Clinical and radiological diagnosis

In cancer patients, compression of the bowel lumen develops slowly and often remains partial. The level of obstruction determines the different patterns of symptoms (Table 14.3.1). The progression may be slow or fast, from partial obstruction to complete occlusion, each producing a different spectrum of symptoms, differing intensity of suffering, and ultimate outcome. Accumulation and increased production of secretions produce the principal symptoms, namely abdominal pain and distension,

Table 14.3.1 Common symptoms in cancer patients with MBO

Vomiting	Intermittent or continuous	It develops early and in great amounts in gastric, duodenum, and small bowel obstruction and develops later in large bowel obstruction	Biliary vomiting is almost odourless and indicates an obstruction in the upper part of the abdomen. The presence of bad smelling and faecaloid vomiting can be the first sign of a ileal or colic obstruction
Nausea	Intermittent or continuous		
Colicky pain	Variable intensity and localization due to distension proximal to the obstruction; secondary to gas and fluid accumulation most of which are produced by the gut	If it is intense, periumbelical and occurring at brief intervals, may be an indication of an obstruction at the jejunum–ileal level. In large bowel obstruction the pain is less intense, deeper, occurring at longer intervals and spreads toward the colon wall	An overall acute pain which begins intensely and becomes stronger, or a pain which is specifically localized, may be a symptom of a perforation or an ileal or colic strangulation. A pain which increases with palpation may be due to peritoneal irritation or the beginning of a perforation
Continuous pain	Variable intensity and localization	It is due to abdominal distension, tumour mass and/or hepatomegaly	
Dry mouth		it is due to severe dehydration, metabolic alterations but above all it is due to the use of drugs with anticholinergic properties and poor mouth care	
Constipation	Intermittent or complete	In case of complete obstruction there is no evacuation of faeces and no flatus	In case of partial obstruction the symptom is intermittent
Overflow diarrhoea		It is the result of bacterial liquefaction of the faecal material	

Reproduced courtesy of Carla Ripamonti.

vomiting, and constipation (Table 14.3.1). However, distension may be minimal in both jejunal involvement and fixed tumours extensively infiltrating the small bowel. In the presence of a high level of obstruction, such as in stomach, duodenum, or jejunum, vomiting develops early and in larger volumes. Nausea is persistent or occasionally subsides temporarily after an episode of vomiting. Continuous pain is due to a visceral mass growth compressing the intestine, intestinal distension, or hepatomegaly, while severe superimposed colic above the obstruction, in the small or large intestine, may worsen the distress. This activity is variable in intensity and site due to distension proximal to the obstruction. In large bowel obstruction, the pain is generally less intense.

The initial symptoms are frequently abdominal cramps, nausea, vomiting, and abdominal distension that usually present periodically and resolve spontaneously. These episodes are frequently followed by passage of gas or loose stools. GI symptoms caused by the sequence of distension–secretion–motor activity of the obstructed bowel occur in different combinations and intensity depending on the site of obstruction and tend to worsen. Dry mouth is associated with other symptoms, and is the consequence of severe dehydration and metabolic alterations, as well as pharmacological interventions such as anticholinergic drugs. No evacuation of faeces and no passing of flatus are typical features of complete obstruction. The eventual appearance of *paradoxical diarrhoea* results from leakage of faecal fluid from faecal impaction, generally in large bowel obstruction.

Vomiting can be assessed in terms of number of episodes, volume, and overall duration. Other symptoms such as nausea, pain (both colicky and continuous), somnolence, dyspnoea, and, at times even the sensation of hunger can be present and can be evaluated with visual analogue, numerical, or verbal scales.

The assessment of patients with suspected MBO should consider:

- other causes of nausea, vomiting, and constipation
- metabolic abnormalities
- type and dosages of drugs
- nutritional and hydration status
- bowel movements and the presence of overflow diarrhoea
- presence of abdominal faecal masses, distension of the whole abdomen or only above the obstacle, ascites, and painful sites
- presence of faeces in the rectal ampulla (rectal examination).

The diagnosis of intestinal obstruction is established or suspected on clinical grounds and confirmed with abdominal radiographs demonstrating air–fluid levels. Radiologic imaging in the evaluation of patients with the acute abdomen and the confirmation of the diagnosis of MBO has assumed a pivotal role. The preferred radiological procedure has evolved in recent years but it varies in different parts of the world according to the local expertise and the availability of each imaging modality. Table 14.3.2 reports the possible radiological investigations that might be performed in patients with symptoms and signs of bowel obstruction. These should only be used if they are going to directly inform clinical decisions.

Management of bowel obstruction: therapeutic approaches

The management of patients with MBO is one of the greatest challenges for physicians who care for cancer patients. Although MBO is usually associated with advanced-stage disease, when it occurs at the time of initial diagnosis, regardless of the primary site of malignancy, management generally proceeds with curative intent,

Table 14.3.2 Radiological investigations

Plain radiography	The usefulness of abdominal radiography taken is supine and standing position when small bowel obstruction is suspected in questionable; however, it remains an important step in the evaluation of most patients with acute and chronic abdominal symptoms. Plain X-ray can document the air-filled dilated loops of bowel, differential air–fluid levels, or both, but the accuracy for localizing the point and cause of obstruction is low. The sensitivity of plain films in making a decision of small bowel obstruction is 66%
Contrast GI series using barium suspension	Provide excellent radiological definition of the mucosal pattern and luminal patency, particularly in the assessment of the stomach and proximal small bowel but more distal points of small bowel obstruction may not be seen as clearly
	As it is not absorbed, the inability to eliminate it in the setting of obstruction can interfere with subsequent radiographic studies or cause severe impaction, overall in patients with a complete and inoperable bowel obstruction
	Barium small bowel series should be used selectively when acute obstruction has already been ruled out
	In large MBO, barium enema provides a quick, accurate, and inexpensive assessment of the location and cause of obstruction, but it should be used with caution to avoid the retention of the barium proximal to the obstruction leading to dehydration of the barium and potential impaction, especially in patients with incomplete and inoperable large bowel obstruction
	Gastrografin is useful in evaluating small and large bowel obstructions, but it usually only provides good visualization of proximal small bowel obstruction as the water soluble nature of the Gastrografin will result in it being diluted by the excess fluid retained in the distal small bowel
	Retrograde, transrectal contrast studies (enteroclysis) serve to insert the contrast under pressure resulting in full distension of the loops of small bowel, permitting better assessment of the mucosal pattern and patency, and improving the accuracy of diagnosis in small bowel obstruction
CT or MRI	CT provides superior results in the assessment of abdominal symptoms. MRI and CT are useful in evaluating the global extent of disease, to perform a staging and to assist in the choice of surgical, endoscopic, or simple pharmacological palliative intervention for relief of the obstruction

Reproduced courtesy of Carla Ripamonti.

and each patient should be managed according to appropriate principles/guidelines for the underlying malignancy. On the other hand, MBO as part of recurrent disease is often managed with palliative intent; in this context, different factors should be considered to determine the most appropriate treatment.

For patients with recurrent disease, MBO generally occurs in a chronic and slow fashion that results in narrowing of the diameter of the small or large bowel (or both simultaneously).

In the face of a clearly incurable situation, significant patient discomfort and suffering must be balanced with the short life expectancy. The goal in any decision we make needs to impact the quality of life (QOL) of the affected person in a positive way and each assessment and management needs to be tailored to the specific needs of the patients. Fig. 14.3.2 shows the algorithm for assessing and managing a patient with MBO. The physicians need to consider a series of questions when faced with terminal cancer patients (patients no longer responsive to specific oncological therapies) with bowel obstruction:

◆ Is the patient fit for surgery?

◆ Is there a place for stenting?

◆ Is it necessary to use a venting nasogastric tube (NGT) in inoperable patients?

◆ When should a venting gastrostomy be considered?

◆ What drugs are indicated for symptom control?

◆ What is the proper route for drug administration?

◆ What is the role of parenteral hydration and total parenteral nutrition?

Surgical procedures

An open or laparoscopic surgical procedure can successfully relieve obstruction in the appropriate patient (see also Chapter 12.4).

Endoscopic stent placement cannot be done beyond the length of the endoscope, cannot be done for long obstructions, and may not be possible due to previous surgical alterations of the anatomy. Because of a perforation rate of 7–14% and a long-term failure rate of 25–30%, stents are not always the best long-term solution and surgical palliation is likely to provide more durable palliation in patients where there is likely to be a longer survival, as demonstrated in a group of ovarian cancer patients (Abecasis et al., 2001; Dolan, 2011). The selection of patients who will benefit from these procedures is an ongoing challenge and can be done only by multidisciplinary teams working in close collaboration.

Surgical options include complete resection, operative bypass, lysis of adhesions, the creation of a diverting stoma, whether in the small or large bowel, or a combination of these. Complete resection of an obstructing lesion is only beneficial if all tumour in that area can be resected with negative margins, and therefore is most often possible for cancers originating within the digestive tract. In select cases of ovarian or colon cancer, such 'debulking' operation followed by chemotherapy may be of use. In a bypass procedure, if the tumour cannot be resected, but there is healthy non-obstructed bowel before and after the site of obstruction, the two healthy segments can be connected, allowing the bowel contents to go past the blockage. Diverting stomas bring the bowel out to the skin, allowing stool to empty into a bag, and effectively relieving distal obstruction. They can be made of either small or large bowel, and are created out of the most distal unaffected bowel segment. In small bowel stomas, it is necessary to have a minimum of 100 cm of small bowel before a stoma in order to maintain one's nutrition orally. Even so, high small bowel stomas may have high outputs and may cause significant fluid balance problems (Easson, 2007).

Patient selection for surgery

The decision to undergo a palliative procedure is facilitated if the goals and definition of success are clearly defined preoperatively.

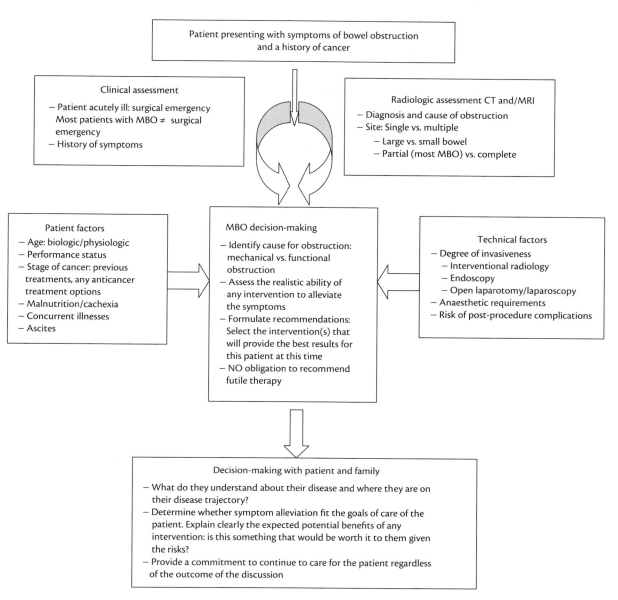

Fig. 14.3.2 Distension–secretion–motor activity causing gastrointestinal symptoms.

An accepted definition of palliative surgery is surgery used with the primary intent of improving patient QOL and symptoms (Krouse et al., 2002). In approaching these decisions, the patient must first have significant symptoms that, if they could be improved, will improve their QOL. The clinician then reviews which, if any, treatments are appropriate or feasible. The patient's understanding of the nature and prognosis of their underlying illness must be explored, as well as their expectations, goals and values. Their co-morbid medical conditions and expected prognosis are discussed. All treatment options including surgery, endoscopic procedures, interventional radiology, and aggressive medical management should be discussed, along with the complication rates and the expected success of each intervention. This discussion is an extraordinary opportunity to clarify goals of care, including suffering and QOL, adjust reasonable treatment plans,

and deepen the level of trust between the physician and surgeon. The surgeon should be prepared to make a recommendation rather than just providing information (Dunn et al., 2009). These discussions may take time as the patient comes to terms with their disease; fortunately MBO is rarely an emergency and thus the time should be available.

With careful preoperative planning it is possible to determine before the operation in most cases which operation is most likely to succeed; however, the final decision must be made in the operating room. The possibility that no surgical procedure may be possible should also be discussed preoperatively; the patient and family must be prepared for that option and consider advance directives or substitute decision-makers. Finally, there must be a commitment to ongoing care with a clear care plan whatever the outcome of the surgery.

Long-term outcomes from surgery

The likelihood of long-term relief of obstruction after surgery depends on the location of the bowel obstruction, with large bowel obstructions successfully relieved in 80% of cases, compared to 25% if both large and small bowel is involved (Bryan et al., 2004). The number of obstructed sites also affects the likelihood of success; a single site of obstruction has a high likelihood of success when compared to multiple sites of obstruction. It is worth emphasizing that MBO from generalized carcinomatosis is a distinct entity that responds poorly, or not at all, to surgical intervention and these patients are not surgical candidates (Abbas and Merrie, 2007; Helyer et al., 2007; Dolan, 2011).

The selection of patients who will benefit from these procedures is an ongoing challenge. The procedure that is the most likely to successfully relieve symptoms for the greatest length of time with reasonable morbidity is chosen (Krouse et al., 2002). Performance status remains one of the best predictors of lower complication rates and improved survival (Wright et al., 2010); patient factors associated with poor surgical outcomes include advanced age (both physiological and chronological), low albumin, psychological health and social support; and ascites, concurrent illness, and co-morbidities (Medina-Franco et al., 2008; Imai et al., 2010; Henry et al., 2012). Disease factors such as tumour type, grade and extent, time from primary presentation, and history of response to and availability of anti-cancer treatments also affects prognosis and likelihood of success (Henry et al., 2012). In patients with GI malignancy, relief of obstruction with surgery has been shown to increase the likelihood of receiving chemotherapy, with the potential that this may improve survival (Helyer et al., 2007). Several recent papers from large cancer centres have followed patients prospectively with MBO. Significant symptom relief can be obtained by selecting appropriate patients either for surgery or stenting with minimal procedural mortality (Imai et al., 2010; Wright et al., 2010; Chakraborty et al., 2011; Dalal et al., 2011). Henry et al. (2012) recently published two nomograms based on a retrospective analysis of 523 patients, providing a scoring system for 30-day mortality and likelihood of surgical success. Validation of these nomograms in a prospective fashion would be very useful.

Endoscopic procedures

Over the past two decades several endoscopic procedures have been developed in the management of MBO. Tumour ablative techniques were initially investigated including high-energy Nd:YAG (neodymium-doped yttrium aluminium garnet) laser therapy, alcohol injection, photodynamic therapy, and cryotherapy, but the insertion of a self-expandable metal stent (SEMS) and venting gastrostomy are more frequently non-surgical alternatives for relief of symptoms from MBO if intervention is indicated.

Multiple studies have demonstrated that these procedures can be performed both for palliation of symptoms from advanced disease. These treatments may not yet be available in all hospitals, but as the knowledge is disseminated and adopted more widely, they will allow clinicians to have more options to better tailor treatment for their patients according to their own clinical situation and individualized goals of therapy.

Endoscopic stenting for gastroduodenal and proximal jejunal obstruction

Malignant gastric-outlet and duodenal obstruction commonly occurs from neoplastic invasion or extrinsic compression by carcinoma of the stomach, head of the pancreas, gall bladder, and bile duct or from compression by metastatic lymphadenopathy in the porta hepatis from a number of abdominal and extra-abdominal primaries. Obstruction of the proximal jejunum is usually caused by primary jejunal tumours, but similarly can occur as a result of local extension from proximal GI tract cancers or metastases to the peritoneum from intra-and-extra abdominal malignancies.

Endoscopic placement of SEMSs has become the primary endoscopic approach to attempt luminal restoration in such patients. With the use of therapeutic gastroscopes with large operating channels, SEMSs can be inserted directly through the scope. Produced by several manufacturers, they come in several diameters and lengths, allowing clinicians to tailor treatment to the patient's needs. The procedure can be performed under conscious sedation, but because of the frequent presence of significant food retention in the stomach, the risk of aspiration is high, in which case general anaesthesia with airway intubation will help to minimize that risk. Combined endoscopic and fluoroscopic guidance permits accurate placement of stents resulting in quick and effective procedures, short hospital stays, or in selected cases with incomplete obstruction, outpatient procedures.

A number of small retrospective reviews have been published describing short-term results (Yim et al., 2001; Espinel et al., 2006; Chandrasegaram et al., 2012) and several prospective multi-institution series, and meta-analyses (Bryan et al., 2004, 2007; Dunn et al., 2009) report excellent technical and clinical success rates for stent placement for gastroduodenal obstruction as shown in Table 14.3.3 (Dormann et al., 2004; Telford et al., 2004; Kim et al., 2007). Very high technical and clinical success rates are associated with patient reports of improvement or resolution of their symptoms (nausea, vomiting and abdominal pain) while being able to consume at least semi-soft or pureed foods. One multicenter prospective study documented an improvement in ability to eat solid food by day 7 in 75% of patients and 80% by day 28 in a carefully selected cohort (Piesman et al., 2009).

Some comparative studies of treating malignant gastric outlet obstruction (GOO) with endoscopic stent placement versus surgery have shown stenting is associated with shorter hospital stay, lower periprocedural mortality (Lillemoe et al., 1999; Espinel et al., 2006), and more rapid food intake (Espinel et al., 2006; Jeurnink et al., 2007). Stent placement has even been shown to be effective in palliating symptoms from obstruction in the setting of limited degrees of peritoneal carcinomatosis (Mendelsohn et al., 2011).

A prospective study of 27 patients with malignant GOO, examining effects on QOL randomized patients to laparoscopic gastrojejunostomy or endoscopic stent placement and found that stent placement was associated with less pain and shorter hospital stay, with a greater improvement in physical health following stent placement relative to those managed surgically (Mehta et al., 2006). Other prospective non-randomized studies of patient administered questionnaires to quantify the effect of stents on symptoms and QOL noted that patients treated with stents reported significant improvements in nausea, vomiting, ability to eat, and several measures of QOL (Schmidt et al., 2009; Larssen et al., 2011).

Table 14.3.3 Summary of three studies of SEMS in palliation of malignant gastroduodenal obstruction

Reference	N	Outcome	Complications
Dormann et al. (2004) Pooled analysis	606	97% technical success 89% clinical success Med patency N/A	0% mortality 1.2% perforation/bleeding 18% re-obstruction 5% migration
Telford et al. (2004) US multicenter	176	98% technical success 84% clinical success Med patency 146 days	0% mortality 2% perforation/bleeding 6% migration 6% cholangitis
Kim et al. (2007) Radiologists	213	94% technical success 94% clinical success Med patency 270 days	0% mortality 1% bleeding (0% perforation) 17% re-obstruction 4% migration

Source: Data from Dormann A. et al., Self-expanding metal stents for gastroduodenal malignancies: systematic review of their clinical effectiveness, *Endoscopy*, Volume 36, Issue 6, pp.543–550, Copyright © Georg Thieme Verlag Stuttgart 2004; Telford, J.J. et al., Palliation of patients with malignant gastric outlet obstruction with the enteral Wallstent: outcomes from a multicenter study, *Gastrointestinal Endoscopy*, Volume 60, Issue 6, pp.916–920, Copyright © American Society for Gastrointestinal Endoscopy 2004; and Kim, J.H. et al., Metallic stent placement in the palliative treatment of malignant gastroduodenal obstructions: prospective evaluation of results and factors influencing outcome in 213 patients, *Gastrointestinal Endoscopy*, Volume 66, Issue 2, pp.256–264, Copyright © American Society for Gastrointestinal Endoscopy 2006.

Endoscopic stenting for obstruction beyond the third part of the duodenum is much more challenging because of the length of standard endoscopes and the more tortuous anatomy. Anecdotal and small series studies have reported success with the use of specialized overtubes designed for deep small bowel intubation, but such procedures are still in need of refinement and dissemination before distal small bowel stenting will become more widely available (Ross et al., 2006; Lennon et al., 2010).

Although endoscopic stenting has been demonstrated to be relatively safe, problems remain that reduce their long-term success rates. Delayed stent failure occurring in up to 18% of cases results in the potential need for reintervention, in some patients (Dormann et al., 2004). The most common causes of delayed stent failure are food impaction or re-obstruction caused by tumour ingrowth. Stent migration also occurs, sometimes in association with cancer treatment. In one study, the presence of ongoing anticancer therapy was reported to be associated with longer stent patency rates but a greater risk of stent migration (Kim et al., 2007). Re-obstruction due to tumour ingrowth can easily be managed with the placement of a second stent or tumour ablation by Nd:YAG laser or argon plasma coagulator (Holt et al., 2004). In comparative studies, those managed with stent did just as well initially as patients managed with surgical bypass, but they had a greater need for re-intervention because of delayed stent re-occlusion (Wong et al., 2002; Jeurnink et al., 2007). This should be considered when decisions on management are being made.

Patients who have slowly progressive disease with a relatively long life expectancy (> 60 days), few comorbidities, and a single site of obstruction near the gastric outlet are probably best managed with surgery. Those that are best suited for endoscopic stenting are patients with a short length of tumour, a single site of obstruction that is located near the pylorus or in the proximal two-thirds of the duodenum, with an intermediate to high performance status and a median life expectancy of greater than 30 days. Patients with a poor performance status, rapidly progressive disease, evidence of advanced carcinomatosis with moderate to severe ascites or multiple levels of obstruction on cross-sectional imaging, and a prognosis of less than 30 days are best served by managing their symptoms pharmacologically or by the insertion of a drainage percutaneous endoscopic gastrostomy (PEG) tube.

Endoscopic stenting for colorectal obstruction

Malignant colon and rectal obstruction occurs as a result of circumferential infiltration of the colonic wall by a primary colorectal cancer, extrinsic compression, or infiltration by nearby tumours, such as ovarian cancer, pancreas or gastric cancer, or from intra-peritoneal spread of tumours originating outside the abdomen, such as metastatic lung, or breast cancer. Regardless of the origin, the clinical manifestations vary depending on the location of obstruction in the colon and rectum. A common presentation is gradual development of constipation bloating and anorexia, eventually resulting in subacute or acute presentation with abdominal distension, abdominal pain, nausea, vomiting, and inability to pass faeces or even flatus. On occasion, patients present with acute obstruction without prior warning symptoms. The more severe cases are in danger of life-threatening bowel perforation and should be managed urgently.

Stent placement in the setting of malignant colorectal obstruction has been reported by investigators from several different countries and can be performed using colonoscopy or interventional radiology techniques using fluoroscopy, with catheters and guidewires (Mainar et al., 1999; Camunez et al., 2000; Law et al., 2000; Arya et al., 2011; Kim et al., 2011; Manes et al., 2011). The prior clearing of the bowel can often not be performed as customarily done for colonoscopy due to the obstruction and risk of perforation with vigorous oral laxatives, but should at the least involve clearing from below the obstruction with enemas.

In the case of the endoscopic approach, a sigmoidoscopy or colonoscopy is performed with the use of a therapeutic scope, which has a large operating channel that would permit the insertion of the constrained stent. In some cases the endoscope can be advanced through the area of obstruction, but in many cases with severe obstruction the 11–13 mm endoscopes are too large to pass the point of obstruction, but stent insertion can be facilitated with the use of guidewires or with concurrent fluoroscopic guidance to ensure accurate placement. Once properly aligned, the stent can be released from the insertion catheter, expanding spontaneously against the tumour stricture, gradually expanding the lumen. A successful stent deployment usually results in immediate passage of air and liquid faeces through the point of obstruction. This translates to rapid relief of symptoms for most patients, permitting resumption of oral intake. In some cases this procedure can be performed as an outpatient procedure, particularly for those with subacute obstruction.

Multiple retrospective studies and several pooled analyses of results have been published demonstrating the positive results of endoscopic and radiographically guided colorectal stent placement in treating malignant colon obstruction in selected patients

(Mainar et al., 1999; Camunez et al., 2000; Law et al., 2000; Khot et al., 2002; Sebastian et al., 2004; Arya et al., 2011; Kim et al., 2011; Manes et al., 2011; Meisner et al., 2011). On average, stent placement for palliative relief of malignant colorectal obstruction results in relief of symptoms in about 91% of patients with less than 4% risk of macroscopic perforation and 0.5% risk of death from complications caused by the procedure (Sebastian et al., 2004). In one retrospective study of long-term results from the Mayo Clinic, Rochester, Minnesota, mean stent patency was reported to be 145 days, and 88.5% of 122 patients treated with endoscopic stenting remained free of obstruction until death (Small et al., 2010). This group reported overall complications associated with palliative stenting of 24.4%, with 9% perforations, but most of the complications were not associated with the procedure, but rather at a delayed time; a mean of 27 days after stent for perforations and 143 days for reocclusion.

Although there have been few prospective studies comparing stenting with surgery in the palliation of malignant colorectal obstruction (Martinez-Santos et al., 2002; Carne et al., 2004; Xinopoulos et al., 2004), several retrospective studies have shown comparable results, with similar successes in relieving obstruction of about 94% for stent and close to 100% for surgery in selected patients, but with lower complications, shorter hospital stay, and lower hospital mortality with stenting (Nagula et al., 2010; Vemulapalli et al., 2010; Moore-Dalal et al., 2011). In addition to improving symptoms, stenting is also associated with an improvement in QOL (Nagula et al., 2010), even when the obstruction is caused by an extracolonic malignancy (Pothuri et al., 2004; Caceres et al., 2008; Shin et al., 2008; Nagula et al., 2010; Kim et al., 2011).

While most publications report excellent success with stenting there are some limitations to technical success which include a very proximal location which can be difficult to reach with the colonoscope, tortuous tumours which increase the difficulty of traversing the tumour with a guidewire or the stent, and tightly obstructing tumours which impair the ability of the stent to expand. Tumours that are very low in the rectum should not be treated with stenting as this will result in complete loss of continence, so such patients should be managed with surgical diverting colostomy. Stent migration can occur at times. Re-obstruction can occur as a result of tumour ingrowth, or stent occlusion from hard faecal material, but these problems can also be retreated with further endoscopic intervention, and treatment with mineral oil, stool softeners, and laxatives.

Endoscopic drainage gastrostomy and jejunostomy

Many patients with MBO cannot be successfully treated with endoluminal stenting. The presence of peritoneal carcinomatosis with multifocal bowel obstruction will often result in failure of both surgical and endoscopic attempts of luminal restoration. It may be reasonable to consider attempting stenting in the setting of two or three points of obstruction if radiographic evaluation clearly demonstrates functional patency of the rest of the gut; however, many patients who present with peritoneal carcinomatosis will have multiple sites of small bowel obstruction, or both small and large bowel obstruction. Such patients can often be successfully palliated with medicinal approaches, described in this chapter, to reduce gastric and bowel secretions and motility, in conjunction with analgesics. Some however

may experience intractable nausea and vomiting which is only relieved with the insertion of a NGT, or they may wish to continue to experience oral intake. For such people, the insertion of a drainage or venting tube in the stomach or jejunum can help relieve the nausea and vomiting, while allowing them to partake in the social experiences of eating and drinking for the rest of their shortened life (Campagnutta et al., 1996; Pothuri et al., 2005).

Although initial experiences used the same sized tubes that are used for feeding gastrostomies, Pothuri et al. showed that the use of a larger diameter PEG tube, 28 French, was feasible in 98% of patients with advanced recurrent ovarian cancer, even in patients with tumour encasing the stomach, diffuse carcinomatosis, and ascites (Pothuri et al., 2005). These larger tubes can also be used to temporarily palliate obstructive symptoms in patients with MBO still undergoing curative systemic therapy.

In some cases where the stomach has been partially or completely removed, as in Billroth II reconstruction, or where the position of the stomach impairs the insertion of a gastrostomy, a drainage PEJ (jejunostomy) tube can be inserted to serve the same purpose by draining the distended small bowel (Pothuri et al., 2005).

Pharmacological treatment of symptoms

The pharmacological management of MBO in inoperable patients focuses on the relief of nausea and vomiting, pain, and other possible distressing symptoms. It principally consists of a combination of antiemetics, antisecretory drugs, and analgesics whether the person is an inpatient or in the community. The drugs of choice vary widely, pending controlled studies which would give clearer therapeutic guidelines (Baines et al., 1985; Ripamonti et al., 2001).

Vomiting may be controlled either symptomatically, using antiemetic drugs with specific central effects, or with anticholinergic drugs able to reduce GI secretions. In the last years, steroids and somatostatin analogues have been successfully used as antisecretory–anti-inflammatory drugs. Clinical practice recommendations for the management of MBO in patients with end-stage cancer have recently been published by the Working Group of the European Association for Palliative Care (Ripamonti et al., 2001).

Route of administration

As oral administration is unreliable in most patients with nausea and/or vomiting, in the presence of bowel obstruction, an alternative route, mainly the parenteral one, is preferred. A continuous subcutaneous infusion or regular subcutaneous bolus administration allows a constant drug level to be maintained with similar pharmacokinetics demonstrated with either approach. In the presence of a pre-existing venous line, the intravenous route will be the route of choice. Morphine, haloperidol, cyclizine, and octreotide appear to be compatible in different combinations and can be mixed in the same syringe (Mercadante, 1995c; and Hutchings, 1997; Ripamonti et al., 2001). Rectal and sublingual administration can occasionally be used. Finally, some drugs, such as fentanyl and scopolamine, may be also administered by the transdermal route. Fig. 14.3.3 shows the drugs and their dosages used to control nausea and vomiting in bowel obstructed patients although formal dose ranging studies have not been done.

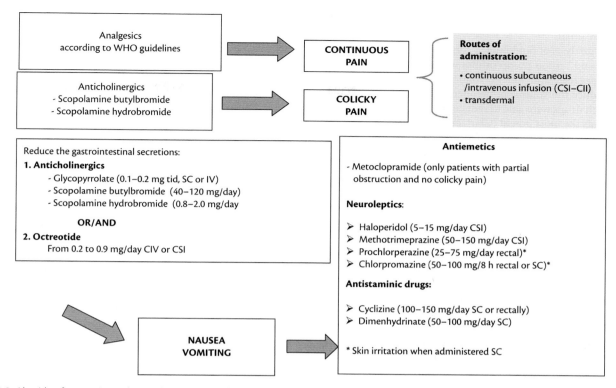

Fig. 14.3.3 Algorithm for assessing and managing a patient with malignant bowel obstruction. CII, continuous intravenous infusion; CSI, continuous subcutaneous infusion.
Reproduced courtesy of Carla Ripamonti.

The use of symptomatic pharmacological approach should be used in inoperable patients with the following aims:

◆ to relieve continuous abdominal pain and intestinal colic

◆ to reduce vomiting to an acceptable level for the patient without the use of a NGT

◆ to relieve nausea (Baines et al., 1985; Mercadante, 1997; Ripamonti et al., 2001; Ripamonti et al., 2008).

Pain

Opioid analgesics, administered according to the World Health Organization and European Society for Medical Oncology guidelines (World Health Organization, 1996; Ripamonti et al., 2012), are the most effective drugs for the management of abdominal continuous and colicky pain associated with bowel obstruction. The dose of opioids should be titrated against the effect, and most usually be administered parenterally.

Anticholinergic drugs such as scopolamine butylbromide, scopolamine hydrobromide, or glycopyrrolate can be associated to opioids in the presence of colicky pain if the opioids alone are not effective (Ventafridda et al., 1990; De Conno et al., 1991; Fainsinger et al., 1994; Mercadante, 1995b; Mercadante et al., 1997; Ripamonti et al., 2001) (Fig. 14.3.3).

Nausea and vomiting

Nausea and vomiting can be managed using two different pharmacological approaches (Fig. 14.3.3):

1. Administration of drugs that reduce GI secretions such as anticholinergics (hyoscine hydrobromide, hyoscine butylbromide, glycopyrrolate) and/or somatostatin analogues (octreotide) (Ventafridda et al., 1990; De Conno et al., 1991; Mercadante, 1995b; Mercadante et al., 2000; Ripamonti et al., 2000, 2001; Porzio et al., 2011).

2. Administration of antiemetics acting on the central nervous system, alone, or in association with drugs to reduce GI secretions. Metoclopramide is the drug of choice in functional intestinal obstruction, but it is not recommended in the presence of complete bowel obstruction because it may increase nausea, vomiting, and colicky pain. It is a prokinetic acting at the level of acetylcholine and dopamine receptors, thus stimulates the musculature of the GI tract. Other antiemetics are the butyrophenones, antihistaminic-antiemetic, and phenothiazines (prochlorperazine and chlorpromazine (Ripamonti et al., 2001) (Fig. 14.3.3). Haloperidol, a dopamine antagonist and a potent suppressor of the chemoreceptor trigger zone, is considered to be the antiemetic drug of first choice when the obstruction is complete. Haloperidol can be combined with scopolamine butylbromide and opioid analgesic in the same syringe.

There are no comparative studies on the efficacy of these different approaches. Generally, physicians are guided by drug availability, costs, and local practice.

Corticosteroids have been used as well because of their anti-inflammatory effect. There is no consensus regarding which is the most effective steroid in this condition, however dexamethasone and methyl-prednisolone are the most commonly used. A systematic review showed a tendency but no definite significant reduction in symptoms in the steroids group compared to the placebo. In terms of mortality, there was no difference between both groups (Feuer and Broadley, 1999), but the number of participants was relatively small.

In a meta-analysis of randomized controlled trials, histamine-2 antagonists and proton pump inhibitors (omeprazole, lansoprazole, pantoprazole, and rabeprazole) were compared for their ability to reduce the volume of preoperative gastric secretions in patients. Both drugs were able to reduce the gastric secretions, but ranitidine was the most potent (Clark et al., 2009).

Somatostatin and its analogues have been shown to inhibit the release and activity of GI hormones, modulate GI function by reducing gastric acid secretion, slow intestinal motility, decrease bile flow, increase mucous production, and reduce splanchnic blood flow. They reduce GI contents and increase absorption of water and electrolytes at intracellular level, via cyclic adenosine monophosphate and calcium regulation. The inhibitory effect of octreotide on both peristalsis and GI secretions reduces bowel distension and the secretion of water and sodium by the intestinal epithelium, thereby reducing vomiting. The drug may theoretically address hypersecretion and distension (Riley and Fallon, 1994).

Several uncontrolled studies have examined the use of octreotide in reducing GI secretions, nausea, and vomiting in patients with MBO (Ripamonti et al., 2001; Ripamonti and Mercadante, 2004; Shima et al., 2008; Hisanaga et al., 2010; Correa et al., 2011). In many cases NGT can be removed. Reported effective doses range from 100 to 600 micrograms per day either as a continuous infusion or as intermittent subcutaneous boluses. Octreotide has been co administered with numerous other agents including morphine, haloperidol and scopolamine butylbromide.

Controlled trials include two large studies of sustained release lanreotide, one large study of octreotide, and two smaller studies of octreotide (Mercadante et al., 2000; Ripamonti et al., 2000; Mystakidou et al., 2002; Laval et al., 2012; Mariani et al., 2012). Mystakidou and colleagues studied 68 people in a double blind, randomized controlled trial comparing octreotide to hyoscine butylbromide. Both arms received regular chlorpromazine. There was less nausea and vomiting at day 3, but not at day 6. Like the study by Hisanga et al., pain was not reduced in the octreotide arm (Mystakidou et al., 2002; Hisanaga et al., 2010).

More recently, studies have also looked at the use of long-acting octreotide in patients with advanced malignancies who developed MBO at some point during the course of the disease (Matulonis et al., 2005; Massacesi and Galeazzi, 2006). The efficacy and safety of octreotide long-acting release (LAR) at the dose of 30 mg on day 1 and ocreotide for 2 weeks was evaluated in a pilot study of 15 patients with advanced ovarian cancer. Of 13 evaluable patients, three patients had reductions in GI symptoms, two had minor response, four patients had no response, and four had progressive symptoms. No significant toxicities were due to LAR (Matulonis et al., 2005).

Recently Mariani et al. (2012) investigated the somatostatin analogue lanreotide as symptomatic treatment for inoperable bowel obstruction due to peritoneal carcinomatosis in 80 patients. The patients with inoperable MBO due to peritoneal carcinomatosis and two or more vomiting episodes daily or NGT who were previously treated with intravenous corticosteroids and proton pump inhibitors were randomly assigned to one 30 mg injection of lanreotide (43 patients) or placebo (37 patients) in a 10-day,

double-blind parallel-group phase. The primary end point was the proportion of patients responding on day 7: one or fewer episodes of vomiting per day or no vomiting recurrence after NGT removal. More patients receiving lanreotide than placebo were responders; this difference was not statistically significant for the intention-to-treat population.

These findings are reflected in another recent study combining regular monthly lanreotide with immediate-release octreotide for the first 6 days of the study in a placebo controlled, double-blind, randomized controlled trial (Laval et al., 2012). The study sought to measure vomiting on days 10–13 with success being defined as fewer than two episodes of vomiting per day for those four days. On an intention-to-treat basis, 37.5% (12/32) of patients on somatostatin analogue arm responded and 28.1% (9/32) in the placebo. This difference was not statistically significant.

Two of the three largest studies of a somatostatin analogue in the setting of MBO showed no additional benefit over and above a placebo (Mystakidou et al., 2002; Laval et al., 2012; Mariani et al., 2012).

Nutrition in the person with bowel obstruction

From the patient's view, the most important consequence of a bowel obstruction, no matter its cause, is the disruption of the ability to eat normally. This fundamental function is essential to maintain health and social ties, and when it is not possible, is a significant source of distress to the patient and more often, their caregivers. Patients with bowel obstruction mostly have little desire to eat, because it exacerbates their symptoms, and caregivers often do not understand that forcing nutrition on such a patient is of little benefit. Severe malnutrition is defined as at least one of the following risk factors: weight loss of 10–15% or more within 6 months; body mass index (BMI) of 18 kg/m^2 or lower, and serum albumin of 30 g/L or less (without evidence of renal and/or liver dysfunction) (Braga et al., 2009). The natural consequence of reduced intake is loss of weight and muscle mass, occurring over time, the cause is often multifactorial, whether from mechanical obstruction, anti-cancer treatments (chemotherapy/radiation), ascites, or cachexia. Cachexia is a catabolic metabolic state common in advanced illness, where intrinsic muscle, protein, and fat are metabolically breaking down (MacDonald et al., 2003). Associated with inflammation, hormonal changes, and the production of tumour factors, it can be difficult to diagnose. However, cachexia is not reversible by increasing nutritional intake, represents end-stage disease, and therefore interventions to improve oral intake will not be helpful. Unfortunately, in advanced cancer patients, cachexia and mechanical obstruction are often seen together and it can be difficult to identify if the weight loss can be reversed if the mechanical obstruction is relieved.

The use of parenteral nutrition in unrelieved MBO from advanced cancer is therefore generally not recommended. The exception may be for patients who are severely malnourished (BMI < 18.5–22 kg/m^2 depending on age), in whom a surgery is planned, and who cannot be enterally fed. Parenteral nutrition starting 7–10 days preoperatively may decrease the rate of postoperative infections, length of stay in hospital, and postoperative mortality. The postoperative duration of parenteral nutrition in such patients should be defined preoperatively and should be short (7–10 days). Short-term postoperative total parenteral nutrition (TPN) may be used for malnourished patients who required emergency surgery and therefore could not receive TPN preoperatively (Braga et al., 2009). For those patients with advanced cancer and poor nutritional status who will not have surgery, TPN is considered ineffective if there is no mechanical bowel obstruction. Also, TPN does not have a role as a supplement while patients are on either chemotherapy, radiation treatment or both therapies simultaneously and also are able to receive oral or enteral nutrition adequately (Bozzetti et al., 2009). Once the patient can eat, the value of oral nutritional support programmes for advanced cancer patients is unclear. In advanced head and neck cancer patients undergoing radiation, the group randomized to the nutritional support programme lost less weight but had an overall poorer outcome (Rabinovitch et al., 2006), and a review of nutritional support programme in lung cancer patients demonstrated no survival benefit (Rueda et al., 2011).

Conclusions

Bowel obstruction secondary to cancer or its treatments is encountered relatively frequently in supportive care as well as in hospice/palliative care practice, carries a poor prognosis, and is associated with significant symptoms. Careful clinical assessment and an understanding of the patient's disease trajectory are crucial in recommending the best way of providing palliation. In someone with a single-level obstruction and good functional status, surgery should be offered. Those with multilevel obstruction are almost never surgical candidates and should be managed with changes in oral intake and medications.

Online materials

Complete references for this chapter are available online at <http://www.oxfordmedicine.com>.

References

Ripamonti, C., Easson, A., and Gerders, H. (2008). Management of malignant bowel obstruction. *European Journal of Cancer* (Special Issue on Palliative Care), 44, 1105–1115.

Ripamonti, C. and Mercadante, S. (2004). How to use octreotide for malignant bowel obstruction. *Journal of Supportive Oncology*, 2(4), 357–364.

Ripamonti, C., Mercadante, S., Groff, L., Zecca, E., De Conno, F., and Casuccio, A. (2000). Role of octreotide, scopolamine butylbromide and hydration in symptom control of patients with inoperable bowel obstruction having a nasogastric tube. A prospective, randomized clinical trial. *Journal of Pain and Symptom Management*, 19, 23–34.

Ripamonti, C.I., Santini, D., Maranzano, E., Berti, M., and Roila, F. (2012). Management of cancer pain: ESMO Clinical Practice Guidelines for diagnosis, treatment and follow-up. *Annals of Oncology*, 23(Suppl. 7), vii139–vii154.

Ripamonti, C., Twycross, R., Baines, M., *et al.* (2001). Clinical-practice recommendations for the management of bowel obstruction in patients with end-stage cancer. *Supportive Care in Cancer*, 9, 223–233.

Skin problems in oncology

Sharon Merims and Michal Lotem

Introduction: skin in disease

Perception of reality is based on visual inputs, and part of living experience is a reflection of what meets the eye. The skin is the largest and most visible organ of the body. It can be a passive participant in states of disease or be directly involved by disease or by its treatment. The skin may manifest the disease or subtly hint at its existence. For the physician, the skin may be a diagnostic aid, though often enigmatic. For the patient, the skin is part of what his sense of illness derives from. In contrast to disease progression, which can be occult or more of an abstract notion, skin manifestations are easily perceived, measured, and followed. They focus attention and cause distress that often outsize their real risk, being a constant reminder of the harboured disease. In those with cancer particularly, the most alarming aspect of skin involvement may be the threat of disfigurement. When a distressing skin symptom is addressed and treated successfully, the patient may derive a renewed sense of hope that reflects on the motivation to participate actively in therapy.

Skin structure and function

The basic function of the skin is to serve as a barrier, separating the human body from the external environment. The skin is made up of three distinct layers:

Epidermis

The epidermis comprises mainly keratinocytes. Intercalated among them are the immigrant cells:

- melanocytes that produce melanin
- Langerhans cells, which serve as antigen presenting cells
- Merkel cells, which have neuroendocrine features and take part in mechano-reception.

Columnar keratinocytes at the base of the epidermis form the germinative layer of the skin, which is known as the basal layer. These keratinocytes undergo a process of differentiation while they move upwards towards the surface (Chu et al., 2008a). A small proportion of keratinocytes is constantly dividing to replace cells that are injured and removed. A pathological state associated with inflammation results in an increased turnover of keratinocytes.

Differentiating keratinocytes produce and contain keratin filaments arranged in bundles that anchor each keratinocyte to adjacent cells and produce adherent forces that resist external traction. Cellular adhesion is lost at the surface of the skin, where keratinocytes detach as flakes and scales, which are usually unnoticeable.

The regenerative potential of the skin is harboured in colony-forming cells that reside in the hair follicles (Oshima et al., 2001). In states of damage to the skin, it is these cells that generate a new epidermal covering.

The epidermis is anchored to the dermis through a basement membrane complex. This highly specialized basal lamina acts as a highly selective pathway for the migration of cells and transport of macromolecules. The basal cells are anchored to the basal lamina through an array of tonofilaments and hemidesmosomes. Epidermal integrity may be disrupted by any pathology that weakens keratinocyte adhesion or damages the basal lamina. Depositions of antibodies against proteins or collagen subtypes that build these structures can split the epidermis and lead to the formation of blisters. Excessive accumulation of fluids in the dermis can generate similar forces and damage skin integrity by distending the intercellular matrix, causing cells to detach from each other.

The skin appendages are specialized differentiated subunits with unique functions. They include the hair follicle, sebaceous gland, and the eccrine and apocrine sweat glands. The hair sebaceous unit in humans mainly serves a social function. The sweat glands are part of the thermoregulatory mechanism of the body.

Dermis

The dermis is a network of collagen and elastin fibres embedded in an amorphic extracellular matrix of mucopolysaccharides, which nests below the epidermis. The fibres and extracellular matrix of the dermis are synthesized by fibroblasts—cells that are dispersed throughout the dermis. The dermis also contains the blood supply for the non-vascularized epidermis tissue. Two webs of capillary blood vessels, deep and superficial, stretch along the dermis to oxygenate and nourish both layers. Parallel lymphatic vessels remove fluids from the skin back into the intravascular compartment. Trafficking immune cells traverse the lymphatic channels to and from regional lymph nodes as part of a screening and defence process against invasion. Inflammation of the skin—dermatitis—results in oedema of the dermis, vasodilatation, and accumulation of leucocytes and lymphocytes in the dermis.

Subcutaneous fat

This adipose tissue serves as a layer of padding and thermal isolation. In states of starvation and cachexia, the subcutaneous fat is severely depleted and the skin is exposed to pressure without the protective effect of fat.

Skin manifestations of neoplastic disease

The skin may be adversely affected by any serious medical illness, often as a secondary process related to infection, trauma, nutritional deficiencies, and other factors (see below). Disease-specific skin involvement occurs commonly in some conditions, and is best characterized in cancer.

Skin of the patient with advanced cancer is unique compared to other organs of the body. While the sequela of metastatic spread to internal organs often is replacement of normal tissue and resultant organ failure, widespread replacement of skin with a neoplasm is uncommon. Yet, even a local disruption of skin integrity can cause deterioration in the quality of life, debilitation, and even mortality. Other aspects of neoplastic disorders affecting the skin include accumulation of abnormally produced metabolites, adverse effects to treatment, and paraneoplastic syndromes.

Direct invasion of skin by tumour

Metastases to the skin are not an infrequent occurrence in cancer patients. In a retrospective series of 4020 metastatic cancer patients, 10% had skin involvement (Lookingbill et al., 1993). The skin may be involved with the primary tumour or may be the target of systemic metastatic spread (Brenner et al., 2001).

Direct invasion of the skin results from an uncontrolled local-regional disease, as in melanoma and breast cancer, where the tumour invades the superficial lymphatic vessels and infiltrates the skin. This commonly appears as discrete nodules, but can also form a diffuse pattern similar to oedema. An inflammatory plaque also may occur, which is often mistaken for erysipelas until diagnosed correctly. Any aggressive tumour that arises in an adjacent organ may directly extend to the overlying skin. The pressure of a tumour mass interferes with cutaneous blood supply and may lead to ulcerating wounds, which discharge foul smelling necrotic material and may require daily washing and the use of hydrocolloids or absorbent dressings. Metastatic cancer of the umbilicus, known as 'Sister Mary Joseph's nodule', has long been recognized as a clinical manifestation of intra-abdominal tumours that extend via the umbilical vessels into the peri-umbilical skin. Incisional metastases are also a common cause of abdominal skin involvement (Lookingbill et al., 1993).

Haematogenic spread to the skin may also occur with dermotropic distant metastases. Breast cancer, lung cancer, melanoma, and colon cancer are common neoplasms that tend to involve the skin (Brownstein and Helwig, 1972a). Common locations of skin metastases are the scalp, chest, and abdominal wall and less frequently to the limbs (Brownstein and Helwig, 1972b). Dermal metastases are more likely to cause pain and ulceration than metastases to the subcutaneous fat. Diagnosis of skin metastases is simple in the context of a patient already diagnosed with metastatic cancer.

Discoloration

The colour of the skin is based on the reflection of chromophores, which are normal constituents of skin that may form abnormal deposits as part of disease. Brown discoloration is intuitively attributed to melanin. Generalized melanosis—darkening of the skin because of a 'shower' of single melanoma cell dissemination—may occur with advanced melanin-producing metastatic malignant melanoma (Schuler et al., 1980). Dark urine often accompanies this condition.

Mild darkening of the skin may be seen with adrenal insufficiency, with adrenocorticotropic hormone-producing tumours such as primary tumours of the pituitary gland, or with other malignant tumours metastatic to the pituitary gland. Increased melanization of the basal layer, leading to hyperpigmentation, may be a side effect of chemotherapeutic agents (Alley et al., 2002). It may occur in skin overlying a vein used for chemotherapy, even if administered with no apparent extravasation injury; this is typical for 5-fluorouracil (5-FU). Bleomycin, busulphan, capecitabine and hydroxyurea can cause generalized persistent hyperpigmentation (Singal et al., 1991). Drug-induced hyperpigmentation may be limited to mucosae, nails, palms, and soles.

Brown discoloration may also result from haemosiderin sedimentation. Widespread inflammation of the skin from any cause results in post-inflammatory hyperpigmentation and persistent brown tint. Yellowish orange discoloration is associated with states of hyperbilirubinaemia.

Pruritus

One of the most distressing skin symptoms of advanced cancer is pruritus. In severe cases, it can lead to sleep deprivation and contribute to significant psychological distress. Biliary obstruction and cholestasis are the most common causes of pruritus in advanced disease, but many other factors may be important. The cancer itself can cause pruritus; the mechanism is unknown and possibly related to serotonin. Numerous other conditions, including common treatments such as systemic or intrathecal opioids (Ruan, 2007), also can cause or worsen the symptom.

Topical therapies for immediate itch relief include 1% menthol in cream base or lotion. Systemic therapy usually is required for better symptom relief, however, but unfortunately, first-line therapies, such as antihistamines, often have limited effectiveness and other types of therapies should be considered, if available.

The anticholestatic agent, cholestyramine, is effective for cholestatic pruritus but is of limited use in total biliary obstruction (Bosonnet, 2003). It chelates intestinal bile acids, thereby reducing the enterohepatic circulation of bile salts. Treatment consists of 4 g before meals, but some patients may find the preparation nauseating. Ursodeoxycholic acid (UDCA) exerts anticholestatic effects in various cholestatic disorders. Several potential mechanisms could explain its beneficial effects, including protection of injured cholangiocytes against the toxic effects of bile acids and stimulation of impaired hepatocellular secretion (Paumgartner, and Beuers, 2002).

Paroxetine, a selective serotonin reuptake inhibitor, may show some positive effect in cancer-related pruritus, and rifampicin, acting as a hepatic enzyme inducer, also has been reported to relieve itching (Tandon et al., 2007). Continuous infusion with granisetron, a 5-hydroxytryptamine type 3 receptor (5-HT$_3$) antagonist, also has been reported to relieve cancer-related pruritus (Porzio et al., 2004). Oral opioid mu-receptor antagonists (such as naltrexone and nalmefene) may be beneficial but cannot be used when an opioid analgesic is needed for pain. Topical application of naltrexone was recently reported as having anti-pruritic effects and the advantage of avoiding withdrawal (Bigliardi et al., 2007). For patients with good performance status, phototherapy using ultraviolet B spectrum is a good option (Seckin et al., 2007), but takes several weeks to exert its beneficial effect.

Dryness and erythroderma

General dryness, xerosis, is a common skin condition in cancer patients. Xerosis may follow chemotherapy administration, a period of decreased food intake, or hypoproteinaemia. Gentle flakes or larger scales generate an ichthyosiform appearance. Lack of elasticity of the drying skin creates cracking lines over the trunk and lower limbs, resulting in itching and soreness. Daily use of emollient may be helpful and should be encouraged.

The term 'erythroderma' refers to general redness of the skin. It often is associated with exfoliation and is, essentially, an end stage of many skin diseases, including psoriasis and papulo-squamous disorders. It also is a clinical hallmark of Sézary syndrome, which is a rare variant of cutaneous T-cell lymphoma. In the wider oncological context, erythroderma may accompany leukaemia and lymphoma (Robak and Robak, 2007), and, less commonly, solid tumours. The mechanism is unknown and it is sometimes managed with emollients and systemic steroids.

Radiation-induced toxicities

Radiation effects on the skin are usually divided into acute and chronic. Early effects occur during the course of radiation and the weeks thereafter, and late effects occur months and years later. The acute effects are thought to result from germinative cell failure to reproduce and replenish epidermal keratinocytes (Hopewell, 1990). Specifically, radiation destroys a section of the basal keratinocytes, stimulating non-cycling basal cells into a cycling phase; continued destruction of basal cells from ongoing radiation treatment overwhelms this process, however, and causes extensive injury. Radiation also damages dermal vasculature and leads to capillary disruption, extravasation, extracapillary cell damage, and inflammatory responses. The local release of histamine and serotonin induce vasodilation and hence erythema, oedema, and a burning sensation. Hair growth is interrupted as hair follicles revert to a resting phase and new hairs are shed. Complete hair loss depends on the total dose and fractionation of the radiation. Sweat and sebaceous glands can be permanently destroyed after approximately 30 Gy in fractions of 2 Gy per day.

Acute radiodermatitis

Clinically, the acute phase of radiation injury can present as an acute radiodermatitis. Erythema and oedema are the first to occur, appearing after 1–2 weeks of treatment and peaking around week 3–4. Dry desquamation and moist desquamation then ensue, and in severe cases erosions, and even ulcers, may develop and be associated with severe pain. Areas of skin folding are at particular risk of developing severe reactions.

Acute radiodermatitis varies in severity and is dependent on radiation energy, total dose and fractionation, the use of bolus material that reduces the skin-sparing effect of megavoltage units, and the individual's sensitivity (Denham et al., 1995). Co-morbidities, older age, and previous sun damage to the irradiated skin are aggravating factors (Porock, 2002). Addition of an electron beam boost to enhance the dose to the tumour is often associated with severe local skin reactions.

There is no effective prophylaxis for radiodermatitis. Daily washing with mild soaps, and avoiding the use of deodorants and electric razors, may help, and the basic care consists of ointments, creams, and lotions to moisten the skin, ease the burning sensation, restore elasticity, and prevent breakage and erosions. It is important to note that the vehicle of the beneficial preparation may be as influential in its effectiveness as the active component in it. Gels are soothing but increase drying. Fatty ointments protect well from moisture loss, but may increase itching. Corticosteroid creams and ointments may reduce vasodilation and inflammation, but have no preventative effect and their advantage over non-steroidal preparations is doubtful. Oil-in-water emulsions are a good option (such as Biafine® and aqueous creams), and calendula oil, sucralfate, and barrier films have been tried with favourable effects (McQuestion, 2006). Ulcers and erosions are treated with silver sulfadiazine (Silverol®) and hydrophilic dressings such as Tegaderm® and Vaseline® gauze.

Chronic radiodermatitis

Delayed damage to the skin is primarily a function of radiation effects on the vasculature. An initial wave of dermal atrophy is seen within 4–6 months. A second phase of dermal thinning tends to develop after more than 52 weeks, often accompanied by the appearance of telangiectasia (Hopewell, 1990). The skin is seen to appear thin and tight, hyperpigmented, and dry. Marked fibrosis may limit flexibility or movement. Radiation-induced skin necrosis and chronic ulcers may develop and persist indefinitely, especially over the scalp and leg. Trauma, chronic friction, and pressure contribute to the development of radiation ulcers. Keratoses and squamous cell carcinoma (SCC) may develop. Histopathology is often required to differentiate SCC from non-neoplastic radionecrosis.

For chronic radiodermatitis, the basic treatment for intact skin consists of oil-in-water emollients and prevention of trauma. Radiation ulcers are resistant to treatment and a realistic goal would be to prevent secondary infection, pain, and fetid smell. This can be achieved with the use of hydrocolloids, but the prospects of healing are limited.

Radiation recall

Radiation recall refers to inflammatory reactions triggered by the administration of cytotoxic chemotherapy, which develop in previously irradiated areas, mainly in the skin. The radiation could have been delivered days to years ago. Typically, chemotherapy is acutely followed by a well circumscribed erythema that perfectly fits the radiation field of the past treatment. The histopathology of this area reveals mixed non-specific inflammatory infiltrate. The most common chemotherapeutic agents implicated in radiation recall are anthracyclines and taxanes. Gemcitabine, a nucleotide analogue, was implicated recently in several cases (Friedlander et al., 2004).

Radiation recall may not require any special treatment. Withdrawal of the offending agent produces prompt improvement. If treatment is necessary, corticosteroids or the use of non-steroidal anti-inflammatory agents may help (Azria et al., 2005).

Paraneoplastic syndromes with skin manifestations

Paraneoplastic syndrome refers to a pathological state generated by cancer in an organ or system that is not directly affected by tumour. The syndromes may be due to the production, by the tumour or by the host, of substances that directly or indirectly cause disease, or by depletion of essential substances. There is a variety of paraneoplastic syndromes involving the skin and these skin manifestations can precede or follow the diagnosis of cancer, indicate a recurrence of disease, or have no correlation with the course of the neoplasm. In the patient with advanced illness, the discomfort caused by skin manifestations is often overshadowed by the neoplastic disease itself.

The most common paraneoplastic syndrome associated with skin pathology is dermatomyositis (DM). This is a systemic illness that primarily affects skeletal muscle and skin. It has been associated with almost every type of solid tumour, including ovarian, pancreatic, lung, stomach, or colorectal (Hill et al., 2001). Among adults older than 40 years who have melanoma or lymphoma, the disorder is especially common, affecting 15–50% of patients (Braverman, 2002).

In 1992, Sigurgeirsson et al. established the connection between DM and cancer. The relative risk of cancer in their series of 392 patients was 2.4 in males and 3.4 in females. In another series, the two independent predictive factors for malignancy ($p < 0.05$) in patients with DM were an older age at onset (> 45 years) and male sex (Chen et al., 2001). This connection with cancer distinguishes DM from polymyositis, which in the latter study had only a slight and statistically non-significant association with cancer.

The characteristic and possibly pathognomonic cutaneous features of DM are the heliotrope rash and Gottron's papules. The heliotrope is a violaceous rash with or without oedema involving periorbital skin. Gottron's papules are slightly elevated; violaceous papules and plaques are mainly found over the finger joints but also may be found overlying the elbows, knees, and feet. Other characteristic features include a slight scale and, on some occasions, a thick psoriasiform scale; telangiectasia; an erythematous eruption in a photosensitive distribution; and periungual changes.

The diagnosis of DM is based on the clinical presentation. Electrophysiological or laboratory evidence of myopathy, including elevations of creatine kinase, aldolase, lactic dehydrogenase, or alanine aminotransferase, are supportive. An evaluation of malignancy should be considered in all adult patients with a consistent syndrome (Callen, 1982).

Corticosteroids are the mainstay of DM therapy. In resistant cases, immunosuppressive agents, such as methotrexate, azathioprine, cyclophosphamide, mycophenolate mofetil, chlorambucil or ciclosporin, may be helpful in inducing remission. Skin lesions may persist even when positive systemic effects prevail. Skin pathology may be ameliorated by topical steroids or topical immunosuppressants, such as 0.1% tacrolimus ointment.

Skin toxicities of chemotherapeutic agents

The skin, hair, nails, and mucous membranes are composed of rapidly dividing cells and are therefore a natural target for toxicities and adverse effects of anti-cancer drugs. Cancer therapy has widened extensively during recent years. New molecular targeting therapies and monoclonal antibodies now comprise a larger part in the arsenal of anti-neoplastic drugs. Alongside new indications and combinations of these drugs, novel toxicities also appeared, including skin toxicity. Common skin toxicities of chemotherapy will be detailed first followed by those of the widely used epidermal growth factor receptor (EGFR) inhibitors.

Common adverse effects of chemotherapeutic agents

The potential effects of conventional chemotherapeutic agents are extremely diverse. Multiple syndromes have been defined and there is large inter-individual variation in presentation and severity.

Alopecia

The rapidly dividing and proliferating cells of hair follicles are targeted by many chemotherapies, and the resultant alopecia is one of the most common and distressing side effects of these drugs. Paclitaxel and doxorubicin are major causes of alopecia in the oncology clinic. Scalp hair is affected to a larger extent than the slowly growing eyelashes, eyebrows, and body hair.

Mucositis

Mucositis includes damage to mucous membranes, most frequently of the oral cavity, and is characterized by redness, swelling, white exudates, and in severe cases, ulceration. Difficulty in chewing, swallowing, and speech may arise. Patients avoid food intake and oral medications to avoid flares of pain. In severe cases, the patient may not be able to drink water due to distressing pain.

Almost all anti-neoplastic agents are associated with mucositis, but the severity is dependent on patient-related factors, the specific drugs employed in treatment, and varied comorbidities. Patient susceptibility to mucositis may be genetically determined, perhaps related to the expression levels of pro-apoptotic and anti-apoptotic genes (Sonis et al., 2004). Drugs that are administered continuously by slow-release mechanisms, such as continuous 5-FU, daily capecitabine, and liposomal doxorubicin, are relatively likely to produce mucositis. Other drugs with high rates of mucositis include methotrexate, cytarabine, and taxanes. Myeloablative conditioning prior to stem cell transplantation may cause severe stomatitis. The severity of mucositis may be greatly worsened by the occurrence of mucosal candidiasis secondary to reduced immunity. Superimposed herpes simplex infection also may severely complicate chemotherapy-induced stomatitis; extensive erosive components and circumscribed ulcers should raise the suspicion of herpes simplex virus infection. Damaged mucosal barriers give rise to a higher rate of septicaemia.

Prevention of chemotherapy-related oral complications is difficult. Good dental and oral hygiene are helpful. Daily chlorhexidine mouthwash is often recommended as a preventative, but its efficacy is doubtful. Povidone-iodine, NaCl 0.9%, water salt soda solution, and chamomile mouthwash also have been recommended and are not associated with dental staining typically produced by chlorhexidine (Potting et al., 2006). Topical non-steroidal anti-inflammatory agents and corticosteroids have been used with varying success, and mucosal protectants, such as sucralfate, have yielded inconsistent results (Pfeiffer et al., 1990; Nottage et al., 2003). Systemic administration of granulocyte macrophage colony-stimulating factor apparently reduces the development of radiation- and chemotherapy-related mucositis (Stokman et al., 2006). Palifermin (recombinant human keratinocyte growth factor) was recently shown to decrease the severity and duration of oral mucosal injury induced by intensive chemotherapy for haematological malignancies (Spielberger et al., 2004); data on the use of this drug in those with solid tumours are limited and its use is not advocated as there is a theoretical risk of stimulating tumour growth. In some cases pain may be so excruciating as to require opioid analgesics.

Nail changes and paronychia

Although less commonly encountered than alopecia and mucositis, nail changes can significantly interfere with manual activities and locomotion, due to their sensitive locations. Taxanes, especially docetaxel, are the major offenders, and cause nail abnormalities in 30–40% of patients (Hussain et al., 2000). Recently, paronychia was reported to occur with the new EGFR inhibitors (Hu et al., 2007). Discoloration, nail bed bleeding, and detachment of the corny material from the nail plate (onycholysis) may occur (Nicolopoulos and Howard 2002). The development of onycholysis seems to be unrelated to the drug dose or frequency of administration. In some cases, purulent exudates may accumulate beneath the nail and soft tissue swelling of the nail bed ensues.

There is a tendency for nail changes to resolve gradually over weeks, despite continued treatment (Flory et al., 1999). Nail changes may be partly reduced by soaking the tips of the fingers in ice water. Topical disinfectants like povidone iodine and 6% peroxide, and topical antibiotics can reduce secondary bacterial infection.

Hand–foot syndrome

Also known as toxic acral erythema and palmar–plantar erythrodysaesthesia syndrome, hand–foot syndrome is a common skin reaction among patients treated with conventional chemotherapy. The earliest sign is painful erythema of the palms, soles, and fingers that later becomes oedematous, changes colour to violet, then dries off and desquamates. In severe cases, blisters develop, later leaving erosive surfaces, with considerable impairment in function. Hand–foot syndrome is often a dose-limiting toxic effect, especially for liposomal doxorubicin. Pharmacologic agents that have been evaluated for hand–foot syndrome include pyridoxine or vitamin B_6, dexamethasone, amifostine, and COX-2 inhibitors. As of now, there are no established preventative strategies or treatments.

Chronic graft-versus-host disease

Allogeneic haematopoietic stem cell transplantation remains the major therapy that can consistently eradicate all evidence of chronic myeloid leukaemia, which is the most common indication of this treatment. The success of allogeneic stem cell transplantation depends on the degree of human leucocyte antigen (HLA) matching. The therapeutic success is offset by a large percentage of patients who develop clinical graft-versus-host disease (GVHD). GVHD is initiated when immunocompetent T cells from the graft react against the immunocompromised host via recognition of alloantigens displayed by host antigen-presenting cells. Th1

cytokines secreted by activated donor T cells are responsible in part for the acute phase changes, while Th2 cytokines, including interleukin (IL)-4 and IL-5 generate some of the chronic phase pathology (Okamoto et al., 2000; Hofmeister et al., 2004). Early withdrawal of post-transplant immunosuppression and use of donor lymphocyte infusions to incite a graft-versus-malignancy effect in patients with residual or progressive disease enhance acute and chronic GVHD. The majority of patients with chronic GVHD have had prior acute GVHD. In addition to the skin, the organs and systems that may be involved by GVHD include gastrointestinal tract, liver, respiratory tract, musculoskeletal system, and haematopoietic system. In HLA-matched marrow grafting with primarily methotrexate-based prophylaxis, skin (65–80%), mouth (48–72%), liver (40–73%), and eye (18–47%) involvement are most commonly reported (Sullivan et al., 1991).

The cutaneous hallmark of chronic GVHD is a lichenoid eruption, an erythematous, papular rash that resembles lichen planus and leaves hyperpigmented spots when resolved. In sclerodermatous GVHD the skin is thickened, tight, and fragile (Higman and Vogelsang, 2004). Atrophic patches of lichen sclerosus are often described. Poor wound-healing and ulcerations occur on areas subjected to tension or trauma. Hair loss and reduced sweating occur as a result of dermal fibrosis. Brittle hair, fingernails, and toenails develop and premature greying of hair may occur. Ocular GVHD presents with irritation, burning, dry eyes, or photophobia from irreversible destruction of the lacrimal glands (Higman and Vogelsang, 2004). Salivary gland dysfunction leads to xerostomia. Mucosal involvement by lichenoid eruption causes food sensitivity and in severe cases can develop to ulceration, especially at the biting line.

Basic skin lubrication to maintain flexibility, and eye and mouth wetting preparations are required in the management of GVHD. Antimicrobial agents against complicating herpes simplex infection also may be required. Extracorporeal photopheresis was reported to improve refractory GVHD, and effect that may be due to an increase in regulatory T cells that suppress autoreactivity (Biagi et al., 2007).

Skin toxicities of molecular targeted therapies

The newer molecular targeted therapies have greatly expanded treatment options for diverse types of cancer. Skin toxicity is a major problem associated with these drugs.

Epidermal growth factor receptor inhibitors

The EGFR inhibitors comprise monoclonal antibodies with varied modes of action. Some (e.g. cetuximab and panitumumab) target the extracellular ligand-binding domain of epidermal growth factor, thereby preventing binding of the ligand to the same receptor. Others (e.g. erlotinib and gefitinib) target the intracellular tyrosine kinase domain of the receptor. Yet others act by competing with adenosine triphosphate binding at the tyrosine kinase site.

Skin eruptions are the most common and sometimes distressing side effect of this category of drugs. Studies indicate that 45–100% of patients experience some type of cutaneous side effect (Perez-Soler and Saltz, 2005; Shepherd et al., 2005). The characteristic rash is composed of acneiform pustules on a background of seborrheic dermatitis-like erythematous plaques with oily scales. The typical distribution is on the face, upper chest and back, and less often the scalp. Unlike acne, closed and open comedones will not appear, and in contrast to steroid-induced acne, the EGFR inhibitors may induce oily scales and dried pus crusts with severe dermatitis rather than small pustular lesions which are prominent on normal skin. The rash begins during the first week of treatment and may vary in severity with repeated treatments, tending to increase initially and then partially decrease. A correlation between the clinical response to the drug and the presence of skin rash has been observed (Saltz et al., 2004).

Microscopically, the acneiform rash associated with the EGFR inhibitors is characterized by T-lymphocyte infiltration around the follicular infundibulum, which can be followed by superficial lymphocytic perifolliculitis. The latter condition can lead to follicular rupture and suppurative superficial folliculitis. Although secondary bacterial infection can occur, the pathology is directly related to the inhibition of the EGFRs on epidermal cells and is non-infectious.

Although most patients receiving EGFR inhibitors (EGFRIs) experience these toxicities, few controlled studies have been conducted to determine the best practices for their management. Instead, much of the literature contains prevention and treatment recommendations based on case reports or studies with small samples sizes and nonrandomized patient allocation. Nonetheless, comprehensive supportive care prevention and treatment recommendations for EGFRI-induced dermatological toxicities have been proposed (Lacouture et al., 2011). Hydrocortisone 1% combined with moisturizer, sunscreen, and doxycycline 100 mg twice daily recommended for the first 6 weeks of therapy, based on data from randomized clinical trials. Although prophylactic minocycline 100 mg daily is another effective agent in reducing the number of lesions during the first 8 weeks, doxycycline appears to have a more favourable safety profile, especially in patients with renal dysfunction; minocycline is less photosensitizing, however, and is preferable in geographic or seasonal locations with a high UV index. Oil-free moisturizing creams are used to relieve dryness and itching, and in severe cases, antihistamines can ameliorate pruritus. Dose reduction should be considered in non-remitting, severe skin symptoms (Lynch et al., 2007).

Non-specific tyrosine kinase inhibitors

Multikinase inhibitors have entered the clinic in the treatment of multiple systemic cancers. Two of these drugs, sorafenib and sunitinib, have become first-line agents for the treatment of advanced renal cell carcinoma and have brought hope to patients not responding to more traditional therapies. Dermatological side effects occur in more than 90% of patients treated with these drugs (Chu et al., 2008b) and the toxicities that appear overlap those observed with traditional chemotherapeutic agents, including mucositis, alopecia, and xerosis.

One of the most common reactions caused by the multikinase inhibitors is a hand–foot skin reaction (HFSR), which is distinct from the hand–foot syndrome caused by more traditional chemotherapy agents. Clinically, HFSR appears in the first 2–4 weeks of treatment as hyperkeratotic lesions with superficial blistering and callus formation usually affecting the flexural surfaces of the digits. The lesions typically have a peripheral halo of erythema. This is in contrast to the acute erythema, swelling, and desquamation seen in hand–foot syndrome. HFSR symptoms include paraesthesia, burning, pain, and decreased tolerance to contact with hot objects. The associated pain can have a large impact on health-related quality of life and impair the patient's activities of daily living. More severe involvement may require dose reduction,

temporary interruption in treatment, or even cessation of therapy (Porta et al., 2007).

There are no randomized controlled trials examining the treatment of HFSR. The goal of treatment should be focused on a balance between the patient's health-related quality of life and the continued administration of potentially life-prolonging therapy. Removal of pre-existing calluses and keratotic skin is recommended prior to initiation with sorafenib or sunitinib. Other preventive recommendations include orthotic devices to normalize weight-bearing and prevent friction, avoidance of friction and trauma to the hands and feet, especially during the first 2–4 weeks of treatment, and thick cotton socks and gloves to protect the hands and feet. For hyperkeratotic areas, agents that decrease keratinocyte proliferation can be used, including urea 20–40% cream, tazarotene 0.1% cream, and fluorouracil 5% cream. For erythematous areas, clobetasol propionate 0.05% ointment is recommended. Topical 2% lidocaine can help with pain, as can systemic medications, such as non-steroidal anti-inflammatory drugs, opioids, and perhaps pregabalin (Lacouture et al., 2008).

Imatinib mesylate

Imatinib mesylate selectively inhibits BCR/ABL-mediated oncogenic signalling and non-specific tyrosine kinases, such as c-kit and platelet-derived growth factor (PDGF) receptor. This drug has is well established as effective for Ph+ chronic myeloid leukaemia (CML); in the chronic phase of this disease, it induces complete haematological response in over 90% of patients and complete cytogenetic response in 50–80% of patients. Imatinib-related non-haematological side effects are reported in less than 10% of CML patients and include oedema, weight gain, nausea, vomiting, and muscle cramps. Cutaneous reactions are well-recognized events, occurring mostly in patients treated at doses of 600 mg/day and higher, either in stable or progressive disease.

A wide spectrum of dermatological toxicities has been associated with imatinib, among which a maculopapular rash is the most common event. In addition, a variety of pigmentary abnormalities of the skin and mucosal surfaces have been reported. Hypopigmentation is well recognized and paradoxical hyperpigmentation has only rarely been documented (Balagula et al., 2011). Inhibition of the PDGF receptor, which is expressed on blood vessels and negatively regulates transcapillary transport, may be responsible for an imatinib-mediated increase of dermal interstitial fluid pressure, capable of inducing oedema and subsequently erythema and desquamation. Generally, the majority of skin reactions are self-limiting or easily managed; occasionally, oral steroids are needed to continue therapy (Breccia et al., 2005) or therapy must be discontinued.

Selective BRAF inhibitors

BRAF is a human gene that makes a protein known as B-Raf and is associated with oncogenesis. Selective inhibitors, such as vemurafenib and dabrafenib, are approved for treatment of late-stage melanoma. These drugs generally are well tolerated and severe toxicities occur infrequently. Cutaneous side effects are common, however. In a recent multicenter, phase III study of vemurafenib in 336 patients, the most common grade 2 or 3 side effects induced by BRAF inhibition were arthralgia, exanthema (up to 18%), fatigue, photosensitivity (12%), cutaneous squamous cell carcinoma (12%), keratoacanthomas (8%), nausea, alopecia (8%),

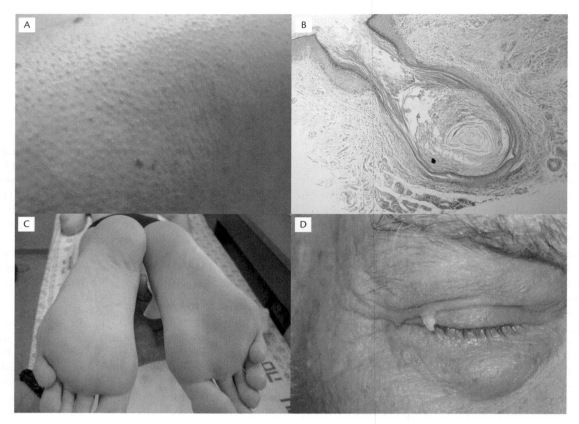

Fig. 14.4.1 Skin toxicities of B-RAF inhibitor vemurafenib. (A) Generalized keratosis pilaris; (B) histopathology of (A) showing lamellar hyperkeratosis and follicular plugging; (C) hyperkeratotic plaques on heels and metatarsal heads; (D) warty papule on upper eyelid.

pruritus (7%), and hyperkeratosis (6%) (Chapman et al., 2011). In a phase IIA trial, cutaneous squamous cell carcinoma occurred in eight of 92 patients (9%) with metastatic melanoma who received dabrafenib (Trefzer et al., 2011) (see Fig. 14.4.1).

In our experience the most common skin manifestation seen in patients treated with selected BRAF inhibitors is follicular accentuation clinically resembling generalized keratosis pilaris which was also observed by others (Wang et al., 2012). In a small number of patients, vitiligo was observed and rarely grade 3 vasculitis with pyrexia, leucocytosis, and elevated creatinine.

Immunotherapies

Targeted immunostimulatory drugs also have recently entered the therapeutic arena. They, too, are associated with cutaneous toxicities.

Ipilimumab

Ipilimumab is a novel, targeted, human immunostimulatory monoclonal antibody that blocks cytotoxic T-lymphocyte antigen4 (CTLA-4), an immune-inhibitory receptor expressed on activated T cells. Ipilimumab is well tolerated as an outpatient infusion therapy and multiple studies have confirmed significant activity against melanoma. A randomized trial has documented a survival benefit when ipilimumab was compared to a gp-100 vaccine-only arm (Hodi et al., 2010). Therapeutic responses peak between 12 and 24 weeks, with slow responses continuing up to and beyond 12 months. The major drug- related adverse effects (10–15% grade 3 or above) are immune related and consist most

commonly of rash, colitis, hypophysitis, thyroiditis, and hepatitis. Skin eruptions are mostly macula-erythematous (Di Giacomo et al., 2010). Pruritus often accompanies the eruption and may continue beyond clearing. In most patients, severity of the skin manifestations is mild and only rarely does skin toxicity necessitate treatment discontinuation (Weber et al., 2012). Vitiligo, an autoimmune-induced skin reaction, also has been observed in patients treated with ipilimumab. In contrast to the weak association between immune-related toxicities and tumour response in patients receiving IL-2 or interferon-alpha, this association appears to be much stronger for patients receiving ipilimumab (Bouwhuis et al., 2011).

Skin problems of bedridden patients

The patient with advanced illness who spends most of the day in bed is at risk for debilitating effects on many systems, including the skin. Immobilization, decreased body hygiene, urinary incontinence, and spilled body fluids expose the patient to the development of decubitus ulcers, hair follicle and sweat gland occlusion, irritant contact dermatitis, and skin infections caused by yeasts and dermatophytes.

Fungal skin infections

Tinea corporis and cruris

The typical presentation of tinea consists of large, confluent polycyclic or psoriasiform plaques extending over the buttocks, lower back, inguinal region, inner aspects of the thigh, pubic region, genitalia, and perianal skin. A common causative agent is the dermatophyte, *Trichophyton rubrum*. Although the clinical picture is useful for diagnosis, KOH skin scraping may reveal hyphae. Tinea corporis may resemble psoriasis, seborrheic dermatitis, and nummular eczema.

Topical agents such as the allylamines, imidazoles, tolnaftate, butenafine, or ciclopirox usually are effective in the treatment of tinea. In resistant cases, fluconazole 150 mg weekly for 4–6 weeks or terbinafine 250 mg daily for 2 weeks can be effective.

Mucocutaneous candidiasis

Candida albicans is an opportunistic human pathogen that produces skin infection. Debilitated and immune-compromised patients are at greatest risk. The non-albicans *Candida* species have been detected more frequently in clinical isolates in recent years, particularly from oropharyngeal cultures in patients who are HIV positive. White patches over buccal mucosa and a yellow velvety membrane over the tongue typically appear in oral candidiasis (also called 'oral thrush' and 'black hairy tongue') (Samaranayake and Yaacob, 1990). Once sloughing occurs, the tongue may appear red and atrophic. Angular cheilitis, or fissuring of the angles of the mouth, may accompany the oral infection.

Nystatin suspension, amphotericin B, and clotrimazole oral preparations are helpful (Hay, 1999). However, immune compromised hosts often do not respond to topical treatment. A short course of systemic fluconazole 100–200 mg daily for 5–10 days may expedite relief.

Other forms of skin infection with pathogenic *Candida* species include nail involvement and peri-ungual inflammation and intertriginous eczema. Treatment usually mirrors that used in mucocutaneous candidiasis.

Vaginal candidiasis

The clinical picture of candidal vulvovaginitis is quite similar to that of oral infection. The symptoms include irritation and discomfort associated with a creamy discharge (Sobel, 1984). Skin lesions may spread from the vulva to the groin area. Small 'satellite' pustules overlie intertriginous patches of the outer labial skin and groin region. The infection usually can be cleared using topically applied nystatin or miconazole. Alternatively, oral treatment with single-dose fluconazole or itraconazole for 3–5 days is effective.

Diaper dermatitis

Urinary incontinence leads to prolonged periods of wetness and soaking of the skin. Maceration of the skin and barrier damage enhances the irritant effect of urine and faeces. Inflamed patches evolve over affected regions, usually the buttocks and genitalia, and cause a burning sensation. Erosions may aggravate the pain. Preventive use of 5% dexpanthenol and zinc oxide ointments may restore the barrier and protect skin from the irritant effect of stool, urine and sweat (Wananukul et al., 2006). Topical corticosteroids are advocated when painful and disturbing dermatitis has already occurred, but should be combined with the barrier restoring agents and discontinued once improvement is detected.

Pressure ulcers

Immobilization puts the cancer patient at an immediate risk of developing pressure ulcers. Other factors, such as older age,

malnutrition, dehydration, immune suppression, cancer-related coagulopathy, hypoperfusion of skin, and increased susceptibility to skin infections, all can contribute to a significantly increased level of morbidity and deterioration (McDonald and Lesage, 2006). In the hospice population, 14%–28% develop ulcers, similar to the prevalence of this disorder in long-term care settings (2.3–28%) (Cuddigan et al., 2001).

Pressure ulcers often become a major source of distress for the patient, and for the caregiver, because of unsightliness, pain, odour, exudates, bleeding, and the potential of infection. Areas that are most affected are those subject to pressure. In the supine patient, for example, the most common ulcer affects the sacrum region.

The exact aetiology of pressure ulcers is unclear. Prolonged pressure obstructs capillaries, leading to dermal hypoxia and ischaemia. The ischaemia results in necrosis that progresses from superficial discoloration to full-thickness skin loss.

The key to good wound care is prevention, if possible. Frequent repositioning and weight support for better distribution of pressure on body parts is necessary. Alternating pressure mattresses and absorbing overlays aid in achieving this goal. Careful assessment for early evolving pressure wounds must be done on a daily basis.

When a pressure ulcer occurs, local wound care consists of absorbent dressing (activated charcoal, cellulose, or soft alginate), local and systemic infection control (metronidazole and antibiotics, respectively), and surgical debridement.

Conclusion

While there is much that cannot be changed during the course of a life-limiting illness, such as cancer, many dermatological aspects can be addressed successfully. It is important to give dermatological aspects of disease their appropriate attention, because these can be the ones that may be dealt with efficiently, using simple and effective treatments. The dermatologist is an important participant of the multidisciplinary team. An ambitious approach to seemingly minor aspects of disease can improve the patient's quality of life and provides a message of care, attention, and respect.

Online materials

Additional online materials for this chapter are available online at <http://www.oxfordmedicine.com>.

References

Alley, E., Green, R., and Schuchter, L. (2002). Cutaneous toxicities of cancer therapy. *Current Opinion in Oncology*, 14, 212–216.

Azria, D., Magne, N., Zouhair, A., *et al.* (2005). Radiation recall: a well recognized but neglected phenomenon. *Cancer Treatment Reviews*, 31, 555–570.

Balagula, Y., Pulitzer, M.P., Maki, R.G., and Myskowski, P.L. (2011). Pigmentary changes in a patient treated with imatinib. *Journal of Drugs in Dermatology*, 10, 1062–1066.

Biagi, E., Di Biaso, I., Leoni, V., *et al.* (2007). Extracorporeal photochemotherapy is accompanied by increasing levels of circulating CD4+CD25+GITR+Foxp3+CD62L+ functional regulatory T-cells in patients with graft-versus-host disease. *Transplantation*, 84, 31–39.

Bigliardi, P.L., Stammer, H., Jost, G., Rufli, T., Buchner, S., and Bigliardi-Qi, M. (2007). Treatment of pruritus with topically applied opiate receptor antagonist. *Journal of the American Academy of Dermatology*, 56, 979–988.

Bosonnet, L. (2003). Pruritus: scratching the surface. *European Journal of Cancer Care*, 12, 162–165.

Bouwhuis, M.G., Ten Hagen, T.L., Suciu, S., and Eggermont, A.M. (2011). Autoimmunity and treatment outcome in melanoma. *Current Opinion in Oncology*, 23, 170–176.

Braverman, I.M. (2002). Skin manifestations of internal malignancy. *Clinics in Geriatric Medicine*, 18, 1–19.

Breccia, M., Carmosino, I., Russo, E., Morano, S.G., Latagliata, R., and Alimena, G. (2005). Early and tardive skin adverse events in chronic myeloid leukaemia patients treated with imatinib. *European Journal of Haematology*, 74, 121–123.

Brenner, S., Tamir, E., Maharshak, N., and Shapira, J. (2001). Cutaneous manifestations of internal malignancies. *Clinics in Dermatology*, 19, 290–297.

Brownstein, M.H., and Helwig, E.B. (1972a). Metastatic tumors of the skin. *Cancer*, 29, 1298–1307.

Brownstein, M.H., and Helwig, E.B. (1972b). Patterns of cutaneous metastasis. *Archives of Dermatology*, 105, 862–868.

Callen, J.P. (1982). The value of malignancy evaluation in patients with dermatomyositis. *Journal of the American Academy of Dermatology*, 6, 253–259.

Chapman, P.B., Hauschild, A., Robert, C., *et al.* (2011). Improved survival with vemurafenib in melanoma with BRAF V600E mutation. *The New England Journal of Medicine*, 364, 2507–2516.

Chen, Y.J., Wu, C.Y., and Shen, J.L. (2001). Predicting factors of malignancy in dermatomyositis and polymyositis: a case-control study. *British Journal of Dermatology*, 144, 825–831.

Chu, D., Haake, A., Holbrook, K., and Loomis, C. (2008a). The structure and development of skin. In I. Freedberg (ed.) *Fitzpatrick's Dermatology in General Medicine* (6th ed.), pp. 58–88. New York: McGraw-Hill.

Chu, D., Lacouture, M.E., Fillos, T., and Wu, S. (2008b). Risk of hand-foot skin reaction with sorafenib: a systematic review and meta-analysis. *Acta Oncologica*, 47, 176–186.

Cuddigan, J., Berlowitz, D., and Ayello, E. (2001). Pressure ulcers in America: prevalence, incidence and implications for the future: an executive summary of the National Pressure Ulcer Advisory Panel Monograph. *Advances in Skin and Wound Care*, 14, 208–215.

Denham, J.W., Hamilton, C.S., Simpson, S.A., *et al.* (1995). Factors influencing the degree of erythematous skin reactions in humans. *Radiotherapy & Oncology*, 36, 107–120.

Di Giacomo, A.M., Biagioli, M., and Maio, M. (2010). The emerging toxicity profiles of anti-CTLA-4 antibodies across clinical indications. *Seminars in Oncology*, 37, 499–507.

Flory, S.M., Solimando, D.A., Jr., Webster, G.F., Dunton, C.J., Neufeld, J.M., and Haffey, M.B. (1999). Onycholysis associated with weekly administration of paclitaxel. *Annals of Pharmacotherapy*, 33, 584–586.

Friedlander, P.A., Bansal, R., Schwartz, L., Wagman, R. Posner, J., and Kemeny, N. (2004). Gemcitabine-related radiation recall preferentially involves internal tissue and organs. *Cancer*, 100, 1793–1799.

Hay, R.J. (1999). The management of superficial candidiasis. *Journal of the American Academy of Dermatology*, 40, S35–42.

Higman, M.A., and Vogelsang, G.B. (2004). Chronic graft versus host disease. *British Journal of Haematology*, 125, 435–454.

Hill, C.L., Zhang, Y., Sigurgeirsson, B., *et al.* (2001). Frequency of specific cancer types in dermatomyositis and polymyositis: a population-based study. *The Lancet*, 357, 96–100.

Hodi, F.S., O'Day, S.J., McDermott, D.F., *et al.* (2010). Improved survival with ipilimumab in patients with metastatic melanoma. *The New England Journal of Medicine*, 363, 711–723.

Hofmeister, C.C., Quinn, A., Cooke, K.R., Stiff, P., Nickoloff, B., and Ferrara, J.L. (2004). Graft-versus-host disease of the skin: life and death on the epidermal edge. *Biology of Blood and Marrow Transplantation*, 10, 366–372.

Hopewell, J.W. (1990). The skin: its structure and response to ionizing radiation. *International Journal of Radiation Biology*, 57, 751–773.

Hu, J.C., Sadeghi, P., Pinter-Brown, L.C., Yashar, S., and Chiu, M.W. (2007). Cutaneous side effects of epidermal growth factor receptor inhibitors: clinical presentation, pathogenesis, and management. *Journal of the American Academy of Dermatology*, 56(2), 317–26.

Hussain, S., Anderson, D.N., Salvatti, M.E., Adamson, B., McManus, M., and Braverman, A.S. (2000). Onycholysis as a complication of systemic chemotherapy: report of five cases associated with prolonged weekly paclitaxel therapy and review of the literature. *Cancer*, 88, 2367–2371.

Lacouture, M.E., Anadkat, M.J. Bensadoun, R.J., *et al.* (2011). Clinical practice guidelines for the prevention and treatment of EGFR inhibitor-associated dermatologic toxicities. *Supportive Care in Cancer*, 19, 1079–1095.

Lacouture, M.E., Wu, S., Robert, C., *et al.* (2008). Evolving strategies for the management of hand-foot skin reaction associated with the multitargeted kinase inhibitors sorafenib and sunitinib. *Oncologist*, 13, 1001–1011.

Lookingbill, D.P., Spangler, N., and Helm, K.F. (1993). Cutaneous metastases in patients with metastatic carcinoma: a retrospective study of 4020 patients. *Journal of the American Academy of Dermatology*, 29, 228–236.

Lynch, T.J., Jr., Kim, E.S., Eaby, B., Garey, J., West, D.P., and Lacouture, M.E. (2007). Epidermal growth factor receptor inhibitor-associated cutaneous toxicities: an evolving paradigm in clinical management. *Oncologist*, 12, 610–621.

McDonald, A., and Lesage, P. (2006). Palliative management of pressure ulcers and malignant wounds in patients with advanced illness. *Journal of Palliative Medicine*, 9, 285.

McQuestion, M. (2006). Evidence-based skin care management in radiation therapy. *Seminars in Oncology Nursing*, 22, 163–173.

Nicolopoulos, J., and A. Howard. (2002). Docetaxel-induced nail dystrophy. *Australasian Journal of Dermatology*, 43, 293–296.

Nottage, M., McLachlan, S.A., Brittain, M.A., *et al.* (2003). Sucralfate mouthwash for prevention and treatment of 5-fluorouracil-induced mucositis: a randomized, placebo-controlled trial. *Supportive Care in Cancer*, 11, 41–47.

Okamoto, I., Kohno, K., Tanimoto, T., *et al.* (2000). IL-18 prevents the development of chronic graft-versus-host disease in mice. *Journal of Immunology*, 164, 6067–6074.

Oshima, H., Rochat, A., Kedzia, C., Kobayashi, K., and Barrandon, Y. (2001). Morphogenesis and renewal of hair follicles from adult multipotent stem cells. *Cell*, 104, 233–245.

Paumgartner, G., and Beuers, U. (2002). Ursodeoxycholic acid in cholestatic liver disease: mechanisms of action and therapeutic use revisited. *Hepatology*, 36, 525–531.

Perez-Soler, R. and Saltz, L. (2005). Cutaneous adverse effects with HER1/EGFR-targeted agents: is there a silver lining? *Journal of Clinical Oncology*, 23, 5235–5246.

Pfeiffer, P., Madsen, E.L., Hansen, O., and May, O. (1990). Effect of prophylactic sucralfate suspension on stomatitis induced by cancer chemotherapy. A randomized, double-blind cross-over study. *Acta Oncologica*, 29, 171–173.

Porock, D. (2002). Factors influencing the severity of radiation skin and oral mucosal reactions: development of a conceptual framework. *European Journal of Cancer Care*, 11, 33–43.

Porta, C., Paglino, C., Imarisio, I., and Bonomi, L. (2007). Uncovering Pandora's vase: the growing problem of new toxicities from novel anticancer agents. The case of sorafenib and sunitinib. *Clinical and Experimental Medicine*, 7, 127–134.

Porzio, G., Aielli, F., Narducci, F., Cannita, K., Piccolo, D., and Marchetti, P. (2004). Pruritus in a patient with advanced cancer successfully treated with continuous infusion of granisetron. *Supportive Care in Cancer*, 12, 208–209.

Potting, C.M., Uitterhoeve, R., Op Reimer, W.S., and Van Achterberg, T. (2006). The effectiveness of commonly used mouthwashes for the prevention of chemotherapy-induced oral mucositis: a systematic review. *European Journal of Cancer Care*, 15, 431–439.

Robak, E. and Robak, T. (2007). Skin lesions in chronic lymphocytic leukemia. *Leukemia & Lymphoma*, 48, 855–865.

Ruan, X. (2007). Drug-related side effects of long-term intrathecal morphine therapy. *Pain Physician*, 10, 357–366.

Saltz, L.B., Meropol, N.J., Loehrer, P.J. Sr., Needle, M.N., Kopit, J., and Mayer, R.J. (2004). Phase II trial of cetuximab in patients with refractory colorectal cancer that expresses the epidermal growth factor receptor. *Journal of Clinical Oncology*, 22, 1201–1208.

Samaranayake, L. and Yaacob, H. (1990). Classification of oral candidiasis. In L.P. Samaranayake and T.W. MacFarlane (eds.) *Oral Candidiasis*, pp. 82–101. London: Wright.

Schuler, G., Honigsmann, H., and Wolff, K. (1980). Diffuse melanosis in metastatic melanoma. Further evidence for disseminated single cell metastases in the skin. *Journal of the American Academy of Dermatology*, 3, 363–369.

Seckin, D., Demircay, Z., and Akin, O. (2007). Generalized pruritus treated with narrowband UVB. *International Journal of Dermatology*, 46, 367–370.

Shepherd, F.A., Rodrigues Pereira, J., Ciuleanu, T., *et al.* (2005). Erlotinib in previously treated non-small-cell lung cancer. *The New England Journal of Medicine*, 353, 123–132.

Singal, R., Tunnessen, W.W. Jr., Wiley, J.M., and Hood, A.F. (1991). Discrete pigmentation after chemotherapy. *Pediatric Dermatology*, 8, 231–235.

Sobel, J.D. (1984). Vulvovaginal candidiasis—what we do and do not know. *Annals of Internal Medicine*, 101, 390–392.

Sonis, S.T., Elting, L.S., Keefe, D., *et al.* (2004). Perspectives on cancer therapy-induced mucosal injury: pathogenesis, measurement, epidemiology, and consequences for patients. *Cancer*, 100, 1995–2025.

Spielberger, R., Stiff, O., Bensinger, W. *et al.* (2004). Palifermin for oral mucositis after intensive therapy for hematologic cancers. *The New England Journal of Medicine*, 351, 2590–2598.

Stokman, M.A., Spijkervet, F.K., Boezen, H.M., *et al.* (2006). Preventive intervention possibilities in radiotherapy- and chemotherapy-induced oral mucositis: results of meta-analyses. *Journal of Dental Research*, 85, 690–700.

Sullivan, K.M., Agura, E., Anasetti, C., *et al.* (1991). Chronic graft-versus-host disease and other late complications of bone marrow transplantation. *Seminars in Hematology*, 28, 250–259.

Tandon, P., Rowe, B.H., Vandermeer, B., and Bain, V.G. (2007). The efficacy and safety of bile acid binding agents, opioid antagonists, or rifampin in the treatment of cholestasis-associated pruritus. *American Journal of Gastroenterology*, 102, 1528–1536.

Trefzer, U., Minor, D., Ribas, A., *et al.* (2011). BREAK-2: a phase IIA trial of the selective BRAF kinase inhibitor GSK2118436 in patients with BRAF mutation-positive (V600E/K) metastatic melanoma. *Pigment Cell & Melanoma Research*, 24, 990–1075.

Wananukul, S., Limpongsanuruk, W., Singalavanija, S., and Wisuthsarewong, W. (2006). Comparison of dexpanthenol and zinc oxide ointment with ointment base in the treatment of irritant diaper dermatitis from diarrhea: a multicenter study. *Journal of the Medical Association of Thailand*, 89, 1654–1658.

Wang, C.M., Fleming, K.F., and Hsu, S. (2012). A case of vemurafenib-induced keratosis pilaris-like eruption. *Dermatology Online Journal*, 18, 7.

Weber, J.S., Kahler, K.C., and Hauschild, A. (2012). Management of immune-related adverse events and kinetics of response with ipilimumab. *Journal of Clinical Oncology*, 30, 2691–2697.

14.5

Palliative issues in the care of patients with cancer of the head and neck

Barbara A. Murphy, Lauren A. Zatarain, Anthony J. Cmelak, Steven Bayles, Ellie Dowling, Cheryl R. Billante, Sheila Ridner, Kirsten Haman, Stewart Bond, Anne Marie Flores, Wisawatapnimit Panarut, and Bethany M. Andrews

Introduction to palliative issues in the care of patients with cancer of the head and neck

By convention, head and neck cancer (HNC) refers to tumours arising from the epithelial lining of the upper aerodigestive track. This includes patients with tumours of the oral cavity, larynx, pharynx, paranasal sinuses, and salivary glands. There are approximately 50 000 cases of HNC diagnosed annually within the United States. The vast majority of tumours (> 90%) are squamous cell carcinomas. Risk factors include use of tobacco, alcohol, and areca nuts; viral infection with human papilloma virus (HPV) or Epstein–Barr virus (EBV); and mucosal irritation by ill-fitting dentures or roughened dental edges (Blot, 1988). Due to higher rates of smoking and heavy drinking in males, HNC affects men disproportionately. Previously considered to be a disease of older adults, the epidemic of HPV-associated oropharyngeal cancers has led to a striking increase in HNC among middle-age adults.

Patients with HNC experience a wide array of palliative problems (Murphy et al., 2007a, 2007b). Symptoms may be related to the tumour, acute toxicities of treatment, or the long-term sequelae of therapy. Although some symptoms are common to all cancers, HNC patients experience a host of unique problems which require special consideration. In addition, palliation is a major issue throughout the disease trajectory. Symptoms are usually present at the time of diagnosis and remain problematic through the terminal phase. For those patients who are cured, long-term biopsychosocial sequelae may persist for years. Thus, assessment and treatment of palliative issues is an intrinsic and vital component of care for the HNC patient. This chapter will address the palliative issues unique to this cohort of patients. It has been divided into four sections: 'Presenting symptoms, evaluation, and treatment', 'Quality of life and psychosocial issues', 'Functional deficits' (speech and voice), and 'Specific symptom control issues'. The reader is referred to other chapters in this text to address general symptom control problems.

Presenting symptoms, evaluation, and treatment

Presenting symptoms

Presenting symptoms are often the result of encroachment of normal structures within the upper aerodigestive system and may be predictive of the primary tumour's location. Early in the disease process, symptoms may mimic routine complaints seen by a primary care physician, such as sore throat, nasal congestion, hoarseness, swollen glands, and ear ache. Symptoms, particularly in patients with risk factors of smoking and alcohol use, not resolving or improving spontaneously within 3 weeks of conservative measures warrant additional attention and specialty evaluation in order to limit diagnostic and treatment delays (Alho et al., 2006).

History and physical examination

Assessment begins with a comprehensive history and physical examination. Particular attention should be paid to identification of symptoms or functional deficits that require palliation or intervention. Patients with a known head and neck primary carcinoma carry an additional 5–15% risk of a synchronous primary elsewhere in the aerodigestive tract (Braakhuis and Leemans, 2005).

A thorough examination involves inspection and palpation of each region of the head and neck. A complete cranial nerve exam is necessary to assess signs of perineural spread or extension into the skull base. Otoscopy evaluates the possibility of serous effusion, which may herald a mass in the nasopharynx obstructing the Eustachian tube. Nasal exam begins with anterior rhinoscopy to assess the vestibule, turbinates, and septum. Bimanual palpation of the oral cavity and oropharynx may identify unvisualized submucosal masses and assesses for contiguous extension of visible primaries. Tumours of the base of tongue and tonsil are often missed because they are not immediately evident on simple visualization but are identifiable by palpation of a firm mass within the region. Larynx visualization is either accomplished with mirror examination or with a fibreoptic scope. The use of a fibreoptic scope through a transnasal route also allows for additional inspection of the nasopharynx, posterior soft palate, larynx, and hypopharyngeal inlet. Attention should be given to subsites of laryngeal involvement and the impact on vocal cord mobility, for this ultimately will impact overall tumour stage. Palpation of the neck with attention to nodal basins may suggest extracapsular extension if fixed to underlying carotid artery or deep neck musculature.

Radiographic and laboratory assessment

Computed tomography (CT) scans and magnetic resonance imaging (MRI) are routinely used in the assessment of head and neck carcinoma. MRI can be valuable in assessing skull base involvement and perineural spread of tumour, while CT scans are more useful for bone evaluation and nodal assessment. Work-up must include an evaluation for potential distant metastatic disease. Chest radiographs or CT of the chest are used to rule out metastatic disease or a second primary tumour. Increasingly, positron emission tomography (PET) scans are used as a part of the staging work-up and may be particularly useful in evaluating an unknown primary tumour (Rudmik et al., 2011). PET scans are used for follow-up where they may be helpful in distinguishing post-treatment scar tissue from recurrent disease (Nayak et al., 2007). Blood counts and complete metabolic profile screen for organ system dysfunction.

Endoscopy

Operative endoscopy is commonly performed to completely assess extension of tumour not easily viewed in the office setting. Additionally, due to the complexity and overlap of mucosal folds within the oral cavity, oropharynx, pharynx, and hypopharynx, standard images often fail to delineate the exact location of a tumour. Operative endoscopy offers the opportunity to manipulate the region and define the site of origin and extent of the tumour. Mapping of the tumour becomes critical in assessing resectability and defining the potential defect that would be created so a reconstructive effort may be planned. A panendoscopy procedure may be of value in high-risk patients to identify second primary tumours (Rodriguez-Bruno et al., 2011).

Treatment and outcome

The staging process must be carried out in a thorough and deliberate fashion since both treatment and outcome are heavily dependent on the extent of disease and the site of primary. Patients with early stage tumours ($T_{1-2}N_0M_0$) have a cure rate of between 70% and 90% with either radiation or surgery (Shah and Lydiatt, 1995). Unfortunately, the majority of patients present with locally advanced disease (T_{3-4} or N+). Patients with locally advanced disease or unresectable tumours are usually treated with combined modality therapy. Patients with resectable disease are treated with surgery followed by radiation therapy (with or without concurrent chemotherapy) in order to eliminate microscopic residual

disease. In some patients, surgical-based treatment may lead to severe functional compromise. Patients at particular risk for poor functional outcome with a surgical approach include those patients with laryngeal, hypopharyngeal, and base-of-tongue primaries. In this cohort of patients, a radiation-based treatment approach may be undertaken in order to avoid surgical morbidity (Forastiere et al., 2003). Depending on the stage, site of primary, smoking history, and HPV status, the 3-year survival for patients with resectable locally advanced disease varies from 30% to 90%. Historically the long-term survival for unresectable patients using aggressive chemoradiation is low, approximately 20–30% (Adelstein et al., 2000). In the subset of unresectable HPV positive patients who are non-smokers, the survival is higher (Ang et al., 2010). Combined modality therapy for locally advanced disease is associated with increases in both acute and long-term toxicities. The clinician is therefore challenged to provide sufficient symptom control to ensure completion of this aggressive therapy. In addition, attempts to minimize long-term sequelae of treatment through rehabilitation, nutritional counselling, and general support services are mandatory.

Quality of life and psychosocial issues

Quality of life and symptom burden

Quality of life (QOL) is a global construct that reflects a patient's general sense of well-being. It is influenced by numerous factors including beliefs, expectations, and personal experience (Osoba, 2000). There are four core domains included in health-related QOL: function, emotional, social, and physical well-being. It is important that QOL be distinguished from symptom assessment. Symptom assessment is directed at a specific problem or a related group of problems. Symptoms are a component of QOL assessment, but the emphasis of QOL assessment is on the overall sense of well-being, not specific contributing factors. The relationship between symptom burden and QOL is complex and may change over time as patients adapt to symptom control issues. Over the past decade, numerous tools have been developed to assess QOL and symptoms in patients with HNC (Murphy et al., 2007c): Functional Assessment of Cancer Therapy (FACT/FACIT) (Cella et al., 1993), European Organization for Research into the Treatment of Cancer Quality of Life Questionnaire (EORTC QLQ-30) (Sherman AC, 2000), Vanderbilt Head and Neck Symptom Survey (VHNSS) (Cooperstein et al., 2012), and the MD Anderson Symptom Survey—Head and Neck (Rosenthal et al., 2007).

Worth noting is the general trajectory of QOL in patients undergoing therapy for locally advanced disease. Regardless of the treatment approach used, patients with HNC experience an initial drop in QOL post-treatment. The QOL then rises slowly towards baseline levels as acute symptoms abate, function improves, and as patients adapt to new physical limitations (So et al., 2012).

Comorbid disease and ageing

Two of the primary risk factors for HNC include smoking and drinking, which may lead to comorbid disease (Blot et al., 1988). Between 30% and 90% of HNC patients have at least one comorbid disease at presentation with moderate to severe morbidities present in 8–55% of patients (Paleri et al., 2010). In the HNC population, comorbid disease is associated with decreased overall survival (Piccirillo et al., 2002) and holds true across the age spectrum (Singh et al., 1998; Reid et al., 2001). In addition, patients with comorbid disease experience increases in treatment-related toxicities and are more likely to die of competing causes such as co-morbid illness, second primary tumours, or treatment-related toxicity (Rose et al., 2011). Of interest, patients who have completed therapy for HNC have an increase in the number of post-treatment comorbidities indicating that treatment may contribute to the identification, development, or worsening of comorbidities (Yung and Piccirillo, 2008).

An extensive medical evaluation is mandatory for all patients prior to initiating therapy. In particular, clinicians should carefully assess those comorbidities that have been identified as 'prognostic for survival'. Patients with multiple comorbidities may be suitable for less aggressive therapy. Since ageing is associated with decrements in organ function that may predispose to the development of toxicity, elderly patients should be screened for function loss (Bond et al., 2012a).

Socioeconomic status

Family issue

HNC patients identify the family as their primary social support, followed by friends, health-care providers, and self-help groups (Hutton and Williams, 2001). Families play an important role in helping patients control the side effects of HNC and its treatment, as well as providing psychological support. HNC patients who do not have family support have worse adaptation and increased distress (de Leeuw et al., 2001). Social support is associated with improved health-related quality-of-life (Karnell et al., 2007).

From a family systems perspective, dysfunction or illness in one family member affects other family members, because a family unit functions as an interconnected whole (Firedman et al., 2003). Depression affects both patients and their caregivers (Wisawatapnimit et al., 2005). Caregiver burden is emerging as an important issue in the HNC population (Wisawatapnimit et al., 2006). HNC and side effects of treatment (in particular, facial disfigurement) negatively impact the QOL of patients and their partners (Vickery et al., 2003).

Both patients and their family reported similar concerns about fear of cancer recurrence (Watt-Watson and Graydon, 1995; Wisawatapnimit et al., 2006). However, there were some differences in concerns between HNC patients and their family members that highlight the importance of also assessing family members. Patients' concerns focused on their physical, functional, and social problems. On the other hand, family caregivers were concerned about their caregiver roles and about taking care of themselves (Watt-Watson and Graydon, 1995). Thus, individuals' concerns varied depending on their roles, and differences appear to increase with time after the surgery (Deschler et al., 2004).

Social issues

Disfigurement as a result of disease and treatment related is commonly experienced by HNC patients (Katz et al., 2000). Because of the highly visible nature of HNC-associated disfigurement, patients are particularly susceptible to experiencing body image disturbance. Body image concerns may exist before, during, or after treatment (He, 2008), with prevalence rates of 41–77% in the HNC population. Body image disturbance is characterized by dissatisfaction with appearance, anxiety, and depression (Katz et al., 2003).

Disfigurement leads to major social problems, most commonly altered social interaction and communication difficulties. HNC patients with visible scars and distorted features often feel stigmatized. There is a reluctance to participate in public activities such as speaking and eating, particularly in layngectomized patients. Moderate to severe effects on social activities occur in 60% of HNC patients (Epstein et al., 1999), with little improvement over time from treatment (de Graeff et al., 1999).

Financial issues, insurance, and work-related issues

In studies of HNC patients, over half of patients were unable to return to work after treatment (Taylor et al., 2004). Common causes for discontinuation of work include fatigue, eating issues, pain, and appearance (Buckwalter et al., 2007). Work-related issues result in a significant decrease in household income for 41.7% of patients (Vartanian et al., 2006), leading to financial consequences. Driving related to work is reduced, with approximately two-thirds of patients avoiding driving during therapy and less than one-third of patients driving less after therapy completion (Yuen et al., 2007).

Inadequate resources may impact both QOL and survival. Within the United States, HNC patients without insurance or those covered by Medicaid present with more advanced disease (Chen et al., 2007) and are at increased risk of death. Patients with a lower socioeconomic status have worse treatment outcomes than patients with a higher socioeconomic status (Boyd et al., 1999). Aggressive social work involvement is needed from the time of diagnosis and throughout treatment to aid the patient and the treatment team and optimize therapeutic outcome.

Functional deficits

HNC may profoundly affect two vital life functions: swallowing and vocalization. Abnormalities in swallowing and voice may be the result of either progressive tumour or treatment-related sequelae. For some patients, functional damage due to tumour may be irreparable; however, contemporary treatment regimens attempt to provide patients with a curative treatment that limits function loss. Access to appropriate rehabilitation services is critical for maximal functional outcomes; thus, the speech-language pathologist (SLP) should be considered an integral member of the multidisciplinary team.

Swallow dysfunction

Swallowing is a complex series of mechanical processes that allows for nutritional intake. A number of symptoms have been identified that herald swallow dysfunction. These 'trigger symptoms' include: (a) inability to control food, liquids or saliva in the oral cavity, (b) pocketing of food in the cheek, (c) excessive chewing, (d) drooling, (e) cough, choking or throat clearing with swallowing, (f) abnormal vocal quality after swallowing (wet or gurgled voice), (g) build-up or congestion after a meal, (h) complaint of difficulty swallowing, (i) nasal regurgitation, or (j) weight loss (Murphy and Gilbert, 2009). The presence of these trigger symptoms should initiate a swallow evaluation.

The two main instrumental assessments for swallowing evaluations include the modified barium swallow (MBS) and the fibreoptic endoscopic evaluation of swallowing (FEES). The MBS has been considered 'the gold standard' for swallowing assessment because it shows the entire oropharyngeal swallow as well as the aetiology of aspiration. FEES is an endoscopic procedure for the assessment of sensory and motor swallowing function. It may be used to evaluate airway protection as well as bolus transport. The MBS and the FEES provide information to the clinician regarding the effectiveness of diet modification and compensatory strategies that may be utilized to improve swallowing safety and function.

Studies on baseline swallowing abnormalities in patients with newly diagnosed HNC are mixed (Pauloski et al., 2000). The degree of impairment is site specific with hypopharyngeal and laryngeal patients experiencing the most impaired swallowing. Therefore, it is prudent to have a high index of suspicion for dysfunctional swallow at baseline and to refer patients for swallow assessment if any concerning signs or symptoms are present.

Patients who undergo surgery of an organ involved in deglutition should expect some alteration in function (Russi et al., 2012). The degree of functional deficit is largely dependent on site and extent of surgery, as well as reconstruction type (Logemann and Bytell, 1979). The only parameters prognostic for swallowing outcome are the percentage of oral and tongue base resected (McConnel et al., 1994). Abnormalities in oral and oropharyngeal swallow are noted by MBS and scintigraphy in more than half of patients at 6 months post treatment (Borggreven et al., 2007). Factors predictive for poor swallow outcome include comorbid condition, T3 or T4 tumours, and combined resection of the base of tongue and soft palate.

Dysphagia and odynophagia occur in patients who undergo primary or adjuvant radiation therapy. Common acute radiation induced toxicities contributing to dysphagia include mucositis, tissue oedema, xerostomia, and hyperviscous secretions. These side effects interfere with eating ability and overall swallow function. Most acute toxicities resolve slowly within 4–12 weeks of completing therapy; unfortunately, late effects may begin to appear simultaneous with the resolution of acute toxicities. The most commonly identified swallowing abnormalities include decreased tongue base retraction, decreased laryngeal elevation, decreased epiglottic inversion, decreased pharyngeal wall motion, and aspiration. Attempts have been made to limit radiation-induced dysphagia by avoiding or limiting the dose of radiation to critical structures involved in deglutition. These structures have become known as dysphagia-aspiration-related structures (DARS). Unfortunately, review of the literature fails to demonstrate conclusive evidence that conformal radiation decreases dysphagia (Roe et al., 2010).

One of the major complications of dysphagia is aspiration. Aspiration may lead to acute episodes of pneumonia or to chronic pneumonitis with associated decreased pulmonary function (Nguyen et al., 2007). Postoperative pneumonia is associated with increased morbidity, mortality, and hospital-related costs (Semenov et al., 2012). Aspiration is also a common late effect of therapy in up to 44% of patients (Campbell et al., 2004).

Patients with severe dysphagia may require a feeding tube for nutritional support during and immediately after completion of therapy. Early trials using primary chemoradiation therapy reported high rates of percutaneous endoscopic gastrostomy (PEG) feeding tubes 1–2 years post-treatment. It is now recognized that placement of a feeding tube for nutritional support may result in decreased use of muscles of deglutition, leading to disuse atrophy. In fact, periods of nil by mouth for as little as 2 weeks predict poorer swallowing outcomes (Gillespie et al., 2004). Patients are now encouraged to continue to swallow or to perform swallow exercises throughout the course of treatment and recovery in order to maintain pharyngeal function. Advancement to an oral diet is advocated as quickly as possible. In addition, SLPs should be actively involved in the care of HNC patients across the treatment trajectory.

Voice

The ability to communicate is a critical human function and vocalization is our most important communication method. Without an intact voice, patients experience a decrease in social interactions and ability to perform activities of daily living. Treatment of HNC often necessitates resection of structures critical to the production of normal speech, resonance, and voice. In general, greater extents of resection result in more severe communication disorders. Primary or adjuvant radiation may also affect vocalization.

Disordered speech may occur due to structural changes in lips, tongue, teeth, and hard palate. Altered articulation of bilabial sounds /b,p,m/, and labiodental sounds /f,v/ occur with reconstruction of labial structures and subsequent nerve paralysis. In the case of advanced disease, total glossectomy severely alters articulation. Loss of or extraction of teeth associated with tumour involvement or radiation therapy, or mandibular osteoradionecrosis, can negatively impact articulation and overall intelligibility. Hard palate defects resulting from maxillary involvement of tumour potentially affect the production of lingua-alveolar sounds /t,d,n,l/ and lingual-palatal sounds /sh,zh,ch,j/. Often a flap is used to close the defect.

Disordered resonance may occur due to tumour involvement or its treatment. Surgical resection of the soft palate creates velopharyngeal insufficiency. Similarly, when tumour involvement disrupts cranial nerves IX or X, the resulting unilateral palatal paralysis creates a velopharyngeal gap. There is inability of the soft palate to contact the posterior pharyngeal wall creating a constant air leak in the vocal tract. The abnormal leak of air through the nose during speech production results in hypernasal voice quality. Behavioural therapy or surgical correction of velopharyngeal gaps may facilitate articulation of speech sounds sufficient to reduce nasality and optimize intelligibility.

Voice disorders in HNC patients arise from neurologic abnormalities induced by tumour and surgical resection of the tumour. The voice disorder resulting from laryngeal paralysis is extremely debilitating. Most patients present with a very soft, breathy voice quality or even a whisper. Attempts to force enough vocal volume to be heard results in rapid fatigue of laryngeal and respiratory muscles, and patients may avoid communication because of the effort required. Phonosurgery attempts to reposition immobile vocal folds, restoring voice and preventing aspiration (Netterville et al., 1993). Operative procedures which spare some glottic structures and mobility yield varying voice results.

There are several options for communication rehabilitation in laryngectomized patients, including an artificial larynx (electrolarynx), oesophageal speech, or prosthetic speech. An electrolarynx is a device which provides an external sound source, producing a mechanical-sounding voice. The greatest advantage of the electrolarynx is that it provides immediacy of communication with minimal patient training. A second type of speech method is the use of oesophageal speech. This requires long commitments to therapy but allows for greatest communicative independence. In this method, air is pumped via swallow or inhaled into the cervical oesophagus and immediately exhaled. The pharyngo-oesophageal segment is vibrated by the expelled air and sound is produced, similar to a controlled belch. Prosthetic speech is achieved by creating a trachea-oesophageal tract to allow the insertion of a one-way valve. With the stoma occluded, air from the lungs is shunted through the prosthesis and into the oesophagus. The air vibrates tissue in the superior aspect of the oesophagus to produce sound.

Specific symptom control issues

Airway control

Airway compromise is one of the most distressing symptoms of progressive disease. Obstruction can occur anywhere along the airway but the symptoms and treatment differ depending on the level of obstruction. Initial assessment of the airway begins with an observation of breathing pattern. Sonorous mouth breathing without stridor would suggest obstruction at the level of base of tongue or oral cavity and is palliated with a nasal trumpet and upright patient positioning. Inspiratory or biphasic stridor is more indicative of a fixed laryngotracheal obstruction, often requiring bypass by tracheostomy. Anxiety, agitation, confusion, and claustrophobia are all signs of progressive hypercarbia and air hunger resulting from obstruction and immediate intervention is warranted. Laryngoscopy determines whether a patient may be amenable to intubation in the event of complete airway loss. Additional factors such as trismus and neck immobility complicate intubation. Ultimately for patients with known incurable disease, an honest discussion with the patient about the potential future need for tracheostomy and early placement may avoid emergent intervention under duress.

Auditory function

HNC patients may experience a decrease in hearing as a result of therapy. Sensorineural hearing loss may result from therapy with either radiation or systemic chemotherapy agents such as cisplatin (Bhandare et al., 2007), with 15–31% of patients demonstrating sensorineural hearing deficits 3 months post therapy. Hearing deficits improved over time in only 40% of patients. Predictive factors included age, pre-treatment hearing deficit, dose to cochlea, and concurrent chemotherapy. With the advent of intensity-modulated radiotherapy (IMRT), treatment plans may decrease radiation dose to the cochlea. Patients with a clinically significant sensorineural hearing loss should be referred for hearing aids.

Dermatitis

Patients receiving treatment with external beam radiation can develop severe dermal and soft tissue reactions (Hymes et al., 2006). Acute radiation dermatitis usually begins 2–3 weeks after therapy is initiated. Manifestations include erythema, oedema, blistering, ulceration, and sloughing. Dermal damage begins to heal within 2–4 weeks after radiation is completed. Late dermal effects of radiation occur weeks, months, or years after therapy. Late dermal effects commonly include atrophy, changes in pigmentation, development of telangiectasias, and hair loss. Grading systems are available for both acute and late dermal effects.

Several factors may increase the severity of acute radiation dermatitis. Patients with tracheostomy tubes in place may note increased irritation and ulceration in the peristomal region. Concurrent chemotherapy or epidermal growth factor receptor inhibitors may result in marked increase in radiation dermatitis (Lacouture et al., 2011).

Several guidelines have been developed for treatment for radiation dermatitis. Data supporting recommendations is scant (Bolderston et al., 2006). There is general consensus for cleaning the involved skin with mild soap but insufficient evidence exists for use of topical creams, enzymes, sucralfate or intravenous agents such as amifostine as preventive agents.

Laboratory abnormalities

Hypothyroidism

After primary surgery, neck dissection, or radiation, patients frequently develop hypothyroidism (Sinard et al., 2000). These effects are additive, with rates of hypothyroidism approaching 70% when both lobectomy and adjuvant radiation therapy are employed for laryngeal cancer. The risk for developing clinical or chemical hypothyroidism 3 years post treatment is 15% and 40% respectively, and may be higher with IMRT technologies, particularly if the thyroid gland is not spared. Routine follow-up should include a careful history and physical exam directed towards signs or symptoms of hypothyroidism. Periodic monitoring with a serum thyroid-stimulating hormone is appropriate for any patient who has received radiation to the low neck. For recommendations regarding treatment of hypothyroidism, please reference the American Thyroid Association Standards of Care Committee guidelines (Singer et al., 1995).

Anaemia

Anaemia is a common presenting haematological abnormality in patients with HNC and may worsen throughout the course of treatment. Compelling data demonstrate that anaemia is a strong predictor for outcome with radiation-based treatment regimens (Dische et al., 1986). It is hypothesized that low numbers of circulating red blood cells may increase the fraction of cancer cells that are hypoxic. Hypoxic tumour cells are resistant to radiation therapy and require two to three times higher radiation doses than those required to kill well-oxygenated cells (Gray et al., 1953). Thus anaemia may lead to increased radiation resistance. The absence of anaemia prior to treatment is associated with improvements in overall survival, local regional control, and radiation therapy complications (Cordella et al., 2011).

Studies evaluating erythropoietic agents for management of radiation-induced haematological toxicity raise concern about adverse treatment outcomes. Specifically, there are reductions in loco-regional control rates in HNC patients receiving radiation treated with epoetin beta when compared to placebo (Henke et al., 2003). Based on a re-review of the available data, it has been recommended that erythropoietic agents be used only as specified by regulatory agencies.

Lymphoedema

Lymphoedema is a condition in which excessive fluid and protein accumulate in the extravascular and interstitial space (see Chapter 11.3). This occurs when the lymphatic system can no longer transport the normal fluid and protein load from the blood capillary–interstitial interface into the lymphatic vessels or when there is increased lymph production. Lymphoedema incidence rates are up to 75% in HNC patients (Deng et al., 2011) and are due to alterations in the structures vital to fluid exchange at the blood capillary–interstitial–lymphatic interface and to the lymphatics related to surgery, radiation, and cancer itself. Lymphoedema may occur before or after surgery and/or radiation treatment.

Presenting symptoms vary depending on the site of involvement. Subtle or overt swelling of the soft tissues of the neck and face are often the first indicator of lymphoedema. HNC patients who develop lymphoedema may also experience other troubling symptoms such as feelings of heaviness, tightness, and stiffness in the swollen areas with the perception that something is stuck in the throat. Soft tissue swelling may progress rapidly over time resulting in fibrosis and impaired range of motion. Lymphoedema of the larynx may result in airway compromise or altered voice quality while pharyngeal oedema may impair swallowing. If swelling appears suddenly or if pre-existing lymphoedema worsens other medical conditions (renal failure, liver failure, cancer recurrence, etc.) should be considered. Thus, a thorough history coupled with a physical assessment is needed to ascertain causative factors and better plan treatment. The history should include onset of swelling, location of swelling, symptoms experienced, and exacerbation/remission patterns of symptoms. The physical assessment should include (a) laryngoscopic evaluation to assess oedema, and (b) careful examination of skin and soft tissues of the face, neck, and shoulders with attention to range of motion and signs of infection or inflammation.

Although controlled trials of lymphoedema therapy are lacking, clinical experience would indicate that appropriate treatment results in improved patient comfort, increased neck and shoulder range of motion, decreased respiratory compromise, improved swallowing function, and decreased risk of infection. Treatment of lymphoedema includes manual lymphatic drainage (MLD), the use of compression garments, and education. MLD should only be undertaken by lymphoedema therapists trained in head and neck drainage techniques. Education should include postural techniques to minimize symptoms, identification and prevention of infections, and exercises to maintain neck and shoulder mobility.

Mood and anxiety disorders

Clinical experience indicates that mental health issues are frequent in the HNC population (see Section 17). Many studies focus on 'psychological distress', which describes the psychological turmoil surrounding the cancer diagnosis and its treatment. However, distress is not synonymous with depressive or anxiety disorder. There are high rates of depressive disorder, alcohol use disorders, and anxiety disorders (Haman, 2008) in HNC patients. Over half of patients have an Axis 1 diagnosis: 27% depressive disorders, 14% anxiety disorders, and 11% with both a depressive and an anxiety disorder. The prevalence of new-onset depression and anxiety after treatment for cancer is 24% and 4%, respectively, with significant negative impacts on QOL.

In order to effectively address this issue, the aetiology of mood disorders in this patient population must be understood. For example, cancer treatment can result in the inability to communicate or impair the ability to eat, leading to social avoidance, depression, and anxiety. A close relationship exists between substance abuse and psychopathology with HNC patients having high rates of substance abuse (past and ongoing). These maladaptive coping strategies both result from and increase the likelihood of depression and anxiety.

Mood and anxiety disorders represent a significant problem in the HNC patient and can negatively impact QOL. They can undermine the ability of the patient to positively change modifiable risk factors (tobacco and alcohol), which can in turn affect disease-free survival. Males with HNC demonstrate some of the highest suicide rates of all cancer patients. In fact, characteristics common to the HNC population such as male gender, advanced disease, little social or cultural support, and limited treatment options all contribute to suicide risk (Kendel, 2007). Physicians who treat HNC must be sensitive to both the physical and psychological sequelae of the diagnosis and treatment.

Mucositis

Oral and pharyngeal mucositis is the most distressing acute complication of radiotherapy for HNC. Incidence rates for all grades of oral mucositis are reported as 60% in standard radiation, and up to 100% in hyperfractionation or accelerated hyperfractionation regimens (Montserrat et al., 2006), with grade 3–4 mucositis rates of 34–57% (Trotti et al., 2003). Oral mucositis clinically presents 10–14 days after radiation therapy is initiated. The initial observation is a transient patchy white discoloration of the mucosa followed by a confluent deep erythema and pseudomembrane formation. The most severe manifestation is frank ulceration of the mucosa.

Risk factors for the development of mucositis include: radiation with special attention to total dose, fraction size, volume irradiated, overall treatment time, fractionation regimen, and the use of concurrent chemotherapy (Murphy, 2007; Bensinger et al., 2008). Mucositis impairs eating, swallowing, and speech, often due to pain. When severe, mucositis may lead to hospitalization for malnutrition or dehydration in up to 15% of cases (Rodríguez-Caballero et al., 2012) and results in treatment interruptions or therapy modifications in 11% of patients (Murphy, 2007; Russo et al., 2008), thus leading to decreased local control and overall survival rates (Rosenthal, 2007). Once radiotherapy treatment has been completed, mucositis spontaneously subsides over a 2–6-week period.

A plethora of traditional treatments for oropharyngeal mucositis have been reported. The Multi-national Association for Supportive Care in Cancer (MASCC) and Cochrane systematic reviews routinely provide updates and generate guidelines on this rapidly expanding database in order to aid clinicians on prevention and treatment of oral mucositis (Keefe et al., 2007; Worthington et al., 2011). Good oral care is a standard component of mucositis management. The foundation of oral care should include regular assessments of oral cavity health and oral pain by dental professionals throughout treatment and follow-up. There is data to support a number of interventions; however, data is conflicting regarding the clinical significance and effectiveness. These interventions include palifermin, amifostine, low-level laser therapy, and multiple other agents for the prevention and treatment of oral mucositis. It is clear that new agents are needed for the prevention and treatment of this acute toxicity. Guidelines are available for review at <http://www.mascc.org>. For further information on treatment of mucositis and other oral cavity lesions, please see Chapter 8.5.

Neurocognitive impairment

HNC patients are at increased risk for neurocognitive impairment before, during, and after treatment. At the time of diagnosis, HNC patients may have baseline neurocognitive impairment due to alcohol abuse or comorbid medical and psychological conditions. Alcohol-dependent patients are at increased risk for greater preoperative neurocognitive impairment (McCaffrey et al., 2007). Almost half of patients have global neurocognitive impairment with the most commonly affected domains being verbal learning, executive function, verbal memory, and processing speed.

Acute neurocognitive impairment in HNC patients during treatment has been studied primarily in the context of delirium. The incidence of postoperative delirium in HNC patients ranges from 13% to 26% (Yamagata et al., 2005) and is attributable to many perioperative causes. HNC patients undergoing primary or adjuvant radiation-based therapies also experience delirium (Bond et al., 2012b), 9% with overt delirium and 45.3% exhibiting subsyndromal delirium (the presence of one or more delirium symptoms without meeting criteria for the full syndrome). Long-term neurocognitive effects of treatment result from incidental brain irradiation, despite improvements in treatment techniques. The pathogenesis of long-term neurocognitive impairment is multifactorial: radiation-induced vascular injury and inflammation, radionecrosis, radiation injury to subcortical white matter, pituitary and hypothalamic dysfunction, cerebral atrophy, and comorbid conditions (Abayomi, 2002).

The implications of neurocognitive deficits for the general management of HNC patients are considerable. Patients report difficulty learning new information and understanding the scope of their disease and treatment. It negatively affects treatment tolerance and compliance, follow-up, and rehabilitation, and leads to increased complications, decreased QOL, and increased psychological distress. Early identification and management of neurocognitive impairment in HNC patients is critical. Therefore, a thorough pre-treatment evaluation for HNC patients should include screening for neurocognitive impairment and associated factors such as alcoholism, depression, and comorbid medical conditions. Patients should be monitored for signs of delirium and ongoing neurocognitive impairment throughout and following treatment.

Nutrition

Nutritional deficits may be present in patients at the time of diagnosis and is prognostic for survival and ability to tolerate treatment (Pai et al., 2012) (see Chapters 4.8 and 10.4). Malnutrition is often multifactorial in nature. Decreased oral intake may be caused by oral pain, difficulty swallowing, or mechanical obstruction by tumour. If functional abnormalities are present, a swallowing evaluation and swallowing therapy may prove beneficial. In patients with mild to moderate swallowing deficits, soft, puréed foods and liquid supplements can stabilize weight loss. Patients with severe swallowing difficulty require more aggressive therapy such as placement of a feeding tube.

Weight loss secondary to treatment is almost universal in HNC patients, with average losses of 6–10% body weight while undergoing therapy. Patients who have extensive surgery resulting in dysphagia undergo PEG tube or nasogastric tube placement. Patients undergoing primary radiation therapy or combined chemoradiation develop severe mucositis resulting in profoundly diminished oral intake. Weight loss continues through the early recovery phase for most patients. The aggressive use of PEG feeding tubes may minimize weight loss during therapy and improve QOL (Brookes, 1985). However, as noted above, there is concern that prophylactic feeding tube placement may lead to increased rates of long-term feeding tube dependence due to disuse atrophy, loss of normal swallowing reflex, and psychological dependence (Oozeer et al., 2011; Langmore et al., 2012). Thus, patients with a feeding tube should be seen by a licensed SLP so that they may be given appropriate swallowing exercises to maintain swallow function. In addition, patients should be encouraged to transition to oral intake as soon as it is feasible. The placement of a feeding tube does not guarantee adequate caloric or fluid intake and requires considerable time and effort to manage. Elderly or debilitated patients who undergo feeding tube placement may require assistance from caregivers.

Post treatment, nutrition remains an issue of concern for many patients. There are numerous late effects that contribute to the dietary alterations noted in post-treatment HNC patients: (a) swallowing abnormalities due to tumour or treatment, (b) radiation-induced xerostomia inhibiting food bolus formation, (c) dental extractions altering ability to chew, (d) taste alterations causing food aversions, and (e) pain due to mucosal sensitivity. These factors lead to decreased food intake with or without restriction in the consistencies and type of foods ingested. Up to 1 year post treatment, 20% of patients require ongoing use of nutritional supplements and 72% report dietary modifications (Beecken and Calaman, 1994). Due to dietary alterations, a high percentage of patients are deficient in key micronutrients (Murphy et al., 2002), and have decreased energy and protein intake. Non-treatment-related factors which must be considered in the nutritional assessment include co-morbid diseases, the adequacy of socioeconomic support, and the presence of alcohol abuse. Periodic dietary assessment is critical to minimize late treatment effects on nutrition.

In addition to the functional causes of weight loss, patients with locally advanced, metastatic, or recurrent disease have cancer cachexia (Brookes, 1985). Cancers are able to profoundly affect the normal metabolic pathways resulting in weight loss, loss of lean muscle (Tisdale, 2000), and adipose tissue (Innui, 2002). These phenomena are at least partially mediated by cytokines and other pro-inflammatory mediators (Machon et al., 2012). Of note, patients undergoing aggressive therapy with chemoradiation may develop a similar clinical syndrome which is characterized by anorexia, rapid weight loss, loss of muscle mass, loss of subcutaneous fat, fatigue, and generalized weakness (Silver et al., 2007). It may be hypothesized that treatment results in local and systemic tissue damage. The body responds in a stereotypic fashion, activating biological pathways intended to aid in healing and repair. Unfortunately, when the biological response to tissue damage is over exuberant or protracted, repair mechanisms may actually adversely affect the host.

Osteoradionecrosis

Osteoradionecrosis (ORN) may be defined as ischaemic necrosis of bone in a previously radiated area with associated soft tissue necrosis. It presents as exposed bone with failure of mucosa to heal over 2–6 months. ORN most commonly affects the mandible and usually develops within 6–12 months of completing radiation therapy. Prevalence of ORN in HNC patients is 8.2% (Reuther et al., 2003), with lower reported rates with IMRT due to dose sparing of the mandible (Nguyen et al., 2012b). Rates vary depending upon total radiation dose, fractionation, volume irradiated, follow-up time, status of dentition, and reporting institution. It is more common in edentulous patients; however, ORN is often reported as occurring after dental extractions following irradiation.

Historically, the pathogenesis of ORN has been ascribed to the three 'Hs'—hypoxia, hypocellularity, and hypovascularity (Marx, 1983). More contemporary theories postulate a primary fibroatrophic process including endothelial damage, decreased cellularity, suppressed osteoblastic activity, disorganization of bone remodelling apparatus, avascularity, and fibrosis that leads to poor wound healing after dental trauma and an increased risk of secondary infection from bacterial flora (Chrcanovic et al., 2010).

Careful attention must be paid to the dentition and gingiva before, during, and after radiation treatment. Before initiation of treatment, patients receiving high dose (> 50 Gy) radiation require evaluation by a skilled dentist familiar with radiation side effects. Panoramic radiographs are integral for assessment of osteoradionecrosis (see Fig. 14.5.1). All grossly diseased maxillary and mandibular teeth should be extracted immediately. Antibiotic prophylaxis should be used, and a minimum of 14 days (preferably 21 days) should be allowed for healing prior to onset of radiation.

Prevention of ORN has naturally evolved around minimizing trauma or local irritants that have been shown to precipitate the process. A correlation between higher ORN and continued tobacco and alcohol use exists. Patients are encouraged to use fluoride before bedtime to minimize dental carries. Diseased teeth should be maintained through meticulous endodontic therapy. For periodontally involved or cariously unrestorable teeth, the retention of roots and the use of overdentures are preferable to extractions. ORN can resolve spontaneously with conservative management or may progress ultimately to fistula formation or pathological fracture. Treatment of ORN includes use of hyperbaric oxygen therapy (HBO), administering 100% oxygen under a pressure of greater than 1 atmosphere. Cochrane review found that HBO improved the probability of achieving mucosal coverage and restoration of bony continuity with ORN and prevented the development of ORN associated with dental extraction (Bennett et al., 2012).

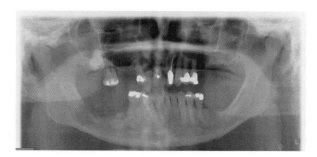

Fig. 14.5.1 Osteoradionecrosis of the right mandible after a dental extraction.

Pain

The reader is referred to Section 9 for general management strategies for cancer pain. There are, however, specific problems that confront HNC patients that merit special attention. Head and neck tumours are often deeply ulcerative causing severe somatic pain. Irritation of an ulcerative tumour via speech or swallowing movements makes pain control challenging. Tumour invasion into nerves can lead to refractory pain syndromes. Finally, maxillofacial pain thought to be due to benign processes such as sinusitis, temporomandibular joint dysfunction, or maxillofacial neuralgias can be the first manifestation of carcinomas. Determining the aetiology of pain in the head and neck patient requires familiarity with anatomy and often calls for consultation with the treating otolaryngologist and neuroradiologist.

Patients undergoing surgical resection will experience postoperative pain. Tracheostomy tube placement, loss of vocalization, or severe oral pain hinders effective communication, interfering with pain assessments. As patients recuperate, postoperative pain subsides. However, it is important to emphasize that chronic postoperative pain is common in the head and neck population. Two years following treatment, 26% of patients still experience pain (Chaplin and Morton, 1999), with moderate or severe pain in 14% of patients. Predictors for chronic pain included pain at 3 months post treatment and neck dissection. Patients may develop contractures and tissue scaring in the neck and shoulders, leading to severe and debilitating musculoskeletal pain. Physical therapy consultation can help guide patients in exercises to decrease contractures and preserve function and range of motion (Barrett et al., 1988).

Radiation doses used for the treatment of HNC is high (70 Gy for primary treatment and 50–60 Gy for adjuvant therapy) and are expected to result in significant damage to the mucous membranes, soft tissue, and skin. The severity of symptoms is usually related to the size of the radiation field and the area involved. Patients with large fields, and those receiving radiation to the oral cavity experience severe debilitating mucositis and radiation dermatitis. Mucositis-related pain is often severe and may dramatically impact function. Over the first 6 weeks of therapy, 76% patients experience severe mouth and throat pain, requiring opioid analgesics. The treatment of mucositis-induced pain requires close and frequent monitoring, with aggressive medication titration. Daily nursing assessment with aggressive treatment of mucositis results in decreased pain, improved sleep and eating, and better energy levels (Jannjan et al., 1992). Topical lidocaine solution and mixed opioid/non-opioid tablets are usually adequate during the initial weeks of radiation. By 4–5 weeks, oral and dermal pain begins to increase and swallowing decreases substantially. Fentanyl patches are a very convenient method for administering long-acting narcotics in this patient population. Short-acting liquid narcotics should be used for breakthrough pain. Pain due to radiation mucositis takes weeks to months to resolve.

Pain due to local recurrence is a major palliative issue in terminal HNC patients. More importantly, it may be the first symptom indicating recurrent disease. Pain is the first symptom indicating recurrence in 70% of patients, with a median lag time of 4 months between the onset of pain and the diagnosis of recurrent disease (Smit et al., 2001). Thus, new onset pain in a previously treated HNC patient should be carefully investigated.

Physical therapy examination and treatment

Surgical or radiation-based treatment approaches may result in head and neck specific and generalized alterations of physical performance. Examples of head and neck specific function loss include decreased range of motion in the jaw, neck, and shoulders. Generalized physical function abnormalities include weakness and deconditioning secondary to therapy. Prior to treatment, a baseline physical therapy evaluation will determine physical function and provide pre-treatment exercise programming and education to the patient and caregivers. An individualized home exercise programme targeting postural alignment, active and passive range of motion, muscle strengthening exercises, and balance/coordination activities are recommended.

During the immediate postoperative phase, the home exercise programme should be modified to account for postoperative movement and activity precautions. During this time, isometric exercises of the cervical and associated shoulder muscles help prevent muscle atrophy, excessive oedema, and decrease pain. Surgeries involving sternocleidomastoid resection will result in cervical rotation with the chin pointing toward the involved side. In severe cases, this may also result in cervical flexion, rotation and lateral flexion toward the uninvolved side mimicking torticollis. This dysfunctional movement pattern can be exacerbated with radiation induced tissue fibrosis. Left untreated, the cervical vertebrae lose mobility and abnormal biomechanics are translated up and down the involved vertebral segments. Similarly, a lack of preservation of the spinal accessory nerve will result in 'shoulder syndrome' in which both the sternocleidomastoid and trapezius are affected (Nahum et al., 1961; Cappiello et al., 2005). To compensate for the loss of the trapezius, the smaller scapular stabilizers are overused and can contribute to pain. The physical therapist will use therapeutic exercise, postural re-education, and manual therapy techniques to normalize altered cervical and shoulder biomechanics.

The goals of physical therapy after active cancer treatment are to maximize muscle strength, soft tissue length, postural alignment, endurance, balance/coordination, and scar and tissue mobility. Likewise, physical therapy aims to minimize pain, fatigue, lymphoedema, and improve overall physical function and return the patient to fitness. Trismus may be caused by a variety of mechanisms including the tumour occupying muscle tissue, radiation-induced tissue fibrosis, or muscle spasm of the masseters, pterygoids and/or temporalis muscles, leading to diminished mouth opening. Trismus directly affects nutritional intake and results in weight loss and energy imbalances. Trismus has been effectively treated with physical rehabilitation methods such as sustained stretch devices (e.g. Therabite®, Dynasplint®) and exercise (see Chapters 4.6, 4.9 and 4.10).

Taste alteration

Loss of taste is caused by chemotherapy drugs and radiation. Radiation therapy may result in severe and permanent alteration in taste sensation. Three models have been proposed to explain irradiation-triggered taste dysfunction: (1) disruption of contact between taste cells and nerves via radiation damage, (2) direct damage of taste cells, and/or (3) interruption of production of new taste cells (Nguyen et al., 2012a). Functional taste alteration reported by patients is congruent with taste bud cell degeneration, often beginning within the first week of radiation therapy (Mossman and Henkin, 1978), with more broad taste dysfunction reported by week 3 or 4 (Epstein and Barasch, 2010).

Loss of taste has profound effects on nutrition and QOL. Patients may describe an inability to take nutrition orally due to altered taste sensation. The taste of food may become noxious resulting in nausea and vomiting. Loss of umami taste appears to have the strongest correlation with QOL due to its role in triggering interest in eating via enjoyment and pleasure pathways (Shi et al., 2004). The impact of hyposalivation on taste loss is controversial (Epstein and Barasch, 2010).

The incidence of taste alteration in HNC patients undergoing radiation ranges from 75% to 100% (Comeau et al., 2001). Taste slowly returns over weeks to months after the completion of therapy for the majority of patients. However, some patients have a permanent alteration in taste sensation, especially with accumulated doses over 6000 cGy (Mossman, 1983). Late effects of taste alteration are more prominent than once realized, with 39% patients reporting moderate to severe taste alterations at greater than 6 months post treatment (Cooperstein et al., 2012). To date, there are no known preventative or treatment measures for taste alterations. Although small studies have reported that zinc improves taste alterations, randomized trials failed to demonstrate efficacy (Halyard et al., 2007).

Xerostomia

Xerostomia can be a severe and permanent complication of external beam radiation therapy (Chambers et al., 2007). The degree of xerostomia is related to the amount of salivary gland tissues within the radiation port and dose delivered. Salivary gland function drops rapidly to 5–30% of normal within the first 2–3 weeks of therapy and remains low following completion of radiation for a prolonged period of time (Frazen et al., 1992). The prevalence of xerostomia in HNC patients more than 6 months post radiation ranges from 73% to 93%, with 65% of patients reporting that symptoms are moderate to severe (Dirix et al., 2008). Xerostomia results in numerous symptoms and constitutes the most frequent patient complaint in those receiving radiation, resulting in a profound negative effect on QOL. Xerostomia impacts dietary choices, deglutition, and speech (Logemann et al., 2001; Roh et al., 2005; Brosky, 2007).

A number of palliative and therapeutic interventions can be attempted to improve symptoms of xerostomia. Patients swish and swallow liquids for soothing mucosal surfaces. Sodium bicarbonate rinses help maintain dental hygiene. Caphosol®, a concentrated calcium and phosphate solution, is approved by the Food and Drug Administration (FDA) in the United States for palliation of xerostomia. A number of commercial salivary gland substitutes are available. Although some patients find these products useful, the majority of patients fail to find significant benefit. For an extensive listing of palliative agents, please visit Oral Health in Cancer Therapy at <http://www.doep.org>.

A number of agents are used to increase salivary secretion in patients with established xerostomia. Pilocarpine is a parasympathomimetic that acts as a muscarinic agonist and demonstrates improvements in xerostomia-related symptoms, but not necessarily objective saliva production. Symptom relief is maximal at 4 months, but decreases once the sialagogue is discontinued (Vissink et al., 2010). Pilocarpine has been investigated as a prophylactic treatment during radiation therapy (Wong et al., 1994;

Scarantino et al., 2006). It should be noted that a frequent challenge to xerostomia study outcomes is the disconnect between subjective and objective data, in that patients' assessments of their dry mouth do not always correlate with salivary gland function (Fox et al, 1987).

Amifostine has been FDA approved for reduction in xerostomia in patients undergoing postoperative radiation treatment for HNC when the radiation port includes a large segment of salivary gland tissue (> 75% of both salivary glands included in the radiation port). The rate of acute xerostomia dropped from 78% to 51% and late xerostomia dropped from 57% to 35% (Brizel et al., 2000). A number of subsequent trials have been conducted to delineate more clearly the role of amifostine in the HNC population; however, the results were mixed. A meta-analysis suggests that amifostine decreased acute (odds ratio (OR), 0.24; confidence interval (CI) 0.15–0.36; $p < 0.00001$) and late xerostomia (OR 0.33; CI, 0.21–0.51; $p < 0.00001$) (Sasse et al., 2006). Long-term data suggest that amifostine did not compromise locoregional control rates, progression-free survival, or overall survival (Bourhis et al., 2011).

Wound care, fistulas, and carotid rupture

Despite newer reconstructive techniques, patients undergoing adjuvant radiation or combined chemoradiation therapy are at greater risk for wound breakdown as a result of the small vessel arteritis that reduces oxygen tissue exchange. Additionally, patients' preoperative nutritional status and smoking history complicate their wound healing capacity. Pharyngocutaneous fistulas result from wound breakdown if a watertight seal of the pharynx cannot be maintained. Patients who have had a breach of the pharynx during their resection are often maintained with nasogastric feedings to limit the contamination of the suture lines for 1–2 weeks. Fistula formation is usually heralded by erythema of the neck, tenderness, and low-grade fevers. The saliva in the neck must be drained and directed away from the carotid artery. Saliva, with its digestive enzymes, may necrose the great vessels resulting in life-threatening haemorrhage. Additionally, exposure of the vessels to the external environment leads to desiccation and potential carotid rupture. Exposure of the neck vessels or fistula formation represents a surgical emergency. The vessels should be covered with saline-soaked gauze until vascularized tissue can be placed over the vessels. Any continuous bleeding from an exposed area must be taken seriously for it may herald an early leak from the carotid artery and surgical exploration to repair the vessel may be necessary. If a fistula does form, and the great vessels are not exposed, the wound can often be managed conservatively until secondary healing occurs. The wound should be packed with wet to dry gauze dressings twice a day or more frequently if contamination is excessive.

In patients who have unresectable disease in the neck, ulceration of the tumour with necrotic debris may become problematic. Tumour hygiene can be achieved through gentle debridement with hydrogen peroxide. Desiccating powders may be applied if wound remains moist. Intermittent use of antibiotics to cover anaerobic floral contaminants will often assist with sterilizing the field and assist with odour control.

A carotid rupture is an uncommon but catastrophic complication of HNC and its therapy. Carotid rupture may occur in patients undergoing extensive resection, external beam radiation therapy,

brachytherapy, or those with recurrent/advanced cancers of the neck. Although initial retrospective reviews demonstrated carotid rupture rates as high as 14% (Marks et al., 1978), the numbers are much lower with contemporary treatment methods (Downey et al., 1999). When possible, patients with carotid rupture should undergo evaluation with angiography. In patients with controlled tumour, aggressive intervention with surgery or invasive radiologic procedures is indicated. Unfortunately data on the success of radiologic procedures (i.e. balloon occlusion and embolization) are scant (Citardi et al., 1995). In patients with terminal disease, palliative measures are usually undertaken (see Chapter 8.7).

Conclusions

Patients with HNC suffer a variety of cancer- and treatment-related symptom control problems. Some of the palliative issues are unique to the head and neck population. Optimal palliation requires a multimodality team of physicians, nurses, social workers, dentists, physical therapists, and speech/swallowing therapists in order to address the multitude of needs. Since many of these patients have poor social support systems, the treatment team may need to spend substantially more time with the patient to ensure adequate symptom palliation. The added effort and attention can result in improved cure rates, diminished long-term side effects, and decreased distress for the patient and family. For those patients who are destined to die of their disease, adequate medical support can mean the difference between an agonizing death and one that is both physically and emotionally comfortable.

References

Abayomi, O. (2002). Pathogenesis of cognitive decline following therapeutic irradiation for head and neck tumors. *Acta Oncologica*, 41, 346–351.

Adelstein, D., Adams, G., Wagner, H., *et al.* (2000). A phase III comparison of standard radiation therapy (RT) versus RT plus concurrent cisplatin (DDP) versus split-course RT plus CCP and F-fluorouracil (5FU) in patients with unresectable squamous cell head and neck cancer (SCHNC): an Intergroup study. *Proceedings of the American Society of Clinical Oncology*, 19, 411A Abstract#1624.

Alho, O.P., Teppo, H., Mäntyselkä, P., and Kantola, S. (2006). Head and neck cancer in primary care: presenting symptoms and the effect of delayed diagnosis of cancer cases. *Canadian Medical Association Journal*, 174, 779–784.

Ang, K.K., Harris, J., Wheeler, R., *et al.* (2010). Human papillomavirus and survival of patients with oropharyngeal cancer. *The New England Journal of Medicine*, 363, 24–35.

Barrett, N.V., Martin, J.W., Jacob, R F., and King, G.E. (1988). Physical therapy techniques in the treatment of the head and neck patient. *Journal of Prosthetic Dentistry*, 59, 343–346.

Beecken, L. and Calaman, F. (1994). A return to 'normal Eating' after curative treatment for oral cancer. *European Journal of Cancer Part B: Oral Oncology*, 30B, 387–392.

Bennett, M.H., Feldmeier, J., Hampson, N., Smee, R., Milross, C. (2012). Hyperbaric oxygen therapy for late radiation tissue injury. *Cochrane Database of Systematic Reviews*, 5, CD005005.

Bensinger, W., Schubert, M., Ang, K.K., *et al.* (2008). NCCN Task Force Report. prevention and management of mucositis in cancer care. *Journal of the National Comprehensive Cancer Network*, 6(Suppl. 1), S1–21.

Bhandare, N., Antonelli, P J., Morris, C.G., Malayapa, R.S., and Mendenhall, W. M. (2007). Ototoxity after radiotherapy for head and neck tumors. *International Journal of Radiation Oncology, Biology, Physics*, 67, 469–479.

Blot, W.J., McLaughlin, J.K., Winn, D.M., et al. (1988). Smoking and drinking in relation to oral and pharyngeal cancer. *Cancer Research*, 48, 3282–3287.

Bolderston, A., Lloyd, N.S., Wong, R.K., et al. (2006). The prevention and management of acute skin reactions related to radiation therapy: a systematic review and practice guideline. *Supportive Care in Cancer*, 14, 802–817.

Bond, S.M., Dietrich, M.S., and Murphy, B.A. (2012a). Neurocognitive function in head and neck cancer patients prior to treatment. *Supportive Care in Cancer*, 20(1), 149–157.

Bond, S.M., Dietrich, M.S., Shuster, J.L., and Murphy, B.A. (2012b). Delirium in patients with head and neck cancer in the outpatient treatment setting. *Supportive Care in Cancer*, 20, 1023–1030.

Borggreven, P.A., Leeuw, I.V., Rinkel, R.N., et al. (2007). Swallowing after major surgery of the oral cavity or oropharynx: a prospective and longitudinal assessment of patients treated by microvascular soft tissue reconstruction. *Head & Neck*, 29, 638–647.

Bourhis, J., Blanchard, P., Maillard, E., et al. (2011). Effect of amifostine on survival among patients treated with radiotherapy: a meta-analysis of individual patient data. *Journal of Clinical Oncology*, 29, 2590–2597.

Boyd, C., Zhang-Salomons, J.Y., Groome, P.A., and Mackillop, W.J. (1999). Associations between community income and cancer survival in Ontario, Canada and the United States. *Journal of Clinical Oncology*, 17, 2244–2255.

Braakhuis, B.J., Brakenhoff, R.H., and Leemans, C.R. (2005). Second field tumors: a new opportunity for cancer prevention? *Oncologist*, 10, 493–500.

Brizel, D.M., Wasserman, T.H., Henke, M., et al. (2000). Phase III randomized trial of amifostine as a radioprotector in head and neck cancer. *Journal of Clinical Oncology*, 18, 3339–3345.

Brookes, G.B. (1985). Nutritional status – a prognostic indicator in head and neck cancer. *Otolaryngology–Head and Neck Surgery*, 93, 69–74.

Brosky, M. (2007). The role of saliva in oral health: strategies for prevention and management of xerostomia. *Journal of Supportive Oncology*, 5, 215–225.

Buckwalter, A.E., Karnell, L.H., Smith, R.B., Christensen, A.J., and Funk, G.F. (2007). Patient-reported factors associated with discontinuing employment following head and neck cancer treatment. *Archives of Otolaryngology—Head & Neck Surgery*, 133, 464–470.

Campbell, B.H., Spinelli, K., Marbella, A.M., Myers, K.B., Kuhn, J.C., and Layde, P.M. (2004). Aspiration, weight loss, and quality of life in head and neck cancer survivors. *Archives of Otolaryngology—Head and Neck Surgery*, 130, 1100–1103.

Cappiello, J., Piazza, C., Giudice, M., De Maria, G., and Nicolai, P. (2005). Shoulder disability after different selective neck dissections (level II-IV versus levels II-V): a Comparative Study. *The Laryngoscope*, 115, 259–263.

Cella, D., Tulsky, D., Gray, G., Sarafian, B., Lium, E., and Bonnonni, A. (1993). The functional assessment of cancer therapy (FACT) scale: development and validation of a general measure. *Journal of Clinical Oncology*, 11, 570–579.

Chambers, M.S., Garden, A.S., Kies, M.S., and Martin, J.W. (2007). Radiation-induced xerostomia in patients with head and neck cancer: pathogenesis, impact on quality of life, and management. *Head & Neck*, 26, 796–2004.

Chaplin, J.M. and Morton, R.P. (1999). A prospective, longitudinal study of pain in head and neck cancer patients. *Head & Neck*, 21, 531–537.

Chen, A.Y., Schrag, N.M., Halpern, M.T., and Ward, E.M. (2007). The impact of health insurance status on stage at diagnosis of oropharyngeal cancer. *Cancer*, 110, 395–402.

Chrcanovic, B.R., Reher, P., Sousa, A.A., and Harris, M. (2010). Osteoradionecrosis of the jaws—a current overview—part 1: physiopathology and risk and predisposing factors. *Oral and Maxillofacial Surgery*, 14, 3–16.

Citardi, M.J., Chaloupka, J.C., Son, Y.H., Ariyan, S., and Sasaki, C.T. (1995). Management of carotid artery rupture by monitored endovascular therapeutic occlusion (1988–1994). *Laryngoscope*, 105, 1086–1092.

Comeau, T.B., Epstein, J.B., and Migas, C. (2001). Taste and smell dysfunction in patients receiving chemotherapy: a review of current knowledge. *Supportive Care in Cancer*, 9, 575–580.

Cooperstein, E., Gilbert, J., Epstein, J.B., et al. (2012). Vanderbilt head and neck symptom survey version 2.0: report of the development and initial testing of a subscale for assessment of oral health. *Head & Neck*, 34(6), 797–804.

Cordella, C., Luebbers, H.T., Rivelli, V., Grätz, K.W., and Kruse, A.L. (2011). An evaluation of the preoperative hemoglobin level as a prognostic factor for oral squamous cell carcinoma. *Head & Neck Oncology*, 3, 35.

De Graeff, A., de Leeuw, R.J., Ros, W.J.G., et al. (1999). A prospective study of quality of life of laryngeal cancer patients treated with radiotherapy. *Head & Neck*, 21, 291–296.

De Leeuw, J.R., de Graeff, A., Ros, W.J,. Blijham, G.H., Hordijk, G.J., and Winnubst, J.A. (2001). Prediction of depression 6 months to 3 years after treatment of head and neck cancer. *Head & Neck*, 23, 892–898.

Deng, J., Ridner, S.H., and Murphy, B.A. (2011). Lymphedema in patients with head and neck cancer. *Oncology Nursing Forum*, 38, E1–E10.

Deschler, D.G., Walsh, K., and Hayden, R.E. (2004). Follow-up quality of life assessment in patients after head and neck surgery as evaluated by lay caregivers. *ORL Head and Neck Nursing*, 22, 26–32.

Dirix, P., Nuyts, S., Vander Poorten, V., Delaere, P., and Van Den Bogaert, W. (2008). The influence of xerostomia after radiotherapy on quality of life: results of a questionnaire in head and neck cancer. *Supportive Care in Cancer*, 16, 171–179.

Dische, S., Suanders, M. I., and Warburton, M. (1986). Hemoglobin, radiation, morbidity and survival. *International Journal of Radiation Oncology, Biology, Physics*, 12, 1335–1337.

Downey, R.J., Friedlander, P., Groeger, J., et al. (1999). Critical care for the severely ill head and neck patient. *Critical Care Medicine*, 27, 95–97.

Epstein, J.B. and Barasch, A. (2010). Taste disorders in cancer patients: pathogenesis, and approach to assessment and management. *Oral Oncology*, 46, 77–81.

Epstein, J.B., Emerton, S., Kolbinson, D.A., et al. (1999). Quality of life and oral function following radiotherapy for head and neck cancer. *Head & Neck*, 21, 1–11.

Firedman, M.M., Bowden, V.R., and Jones, E.G. (2003). *Systems Theory*. Upper Saddle River, NJ: Prentice Hall.

Forastiere, A.A., Goepfert, H., Maor, M., et al. (2003). Concurrent chemotherapy and radiotherapy for organ preservation in advanced laryngeal cancer. *The New England Journal of Medicine*, 349, 2091–2098.

Fox, P.C., Busch K.A., and Baum, B.J. (1987). Subjective reports of xerostomia and objective measures of salivary gland performance. *Journal of the American Dental Association*, 115, 581–584.

Frazen, L., Funegard, U., Ericson, T., and Henriksson, R. (1992). Parotid gland function during and following radiotherapy of malignancies in the head and neck. *British Journal of Cancer*, 28, 457–462.

Gillespie, M.B., Brodsky, M.B., Day, T.A., Lee, F., and Martin-Harris, B. (2004). Swallowing-related quality of life after head and neck cancer treatment. *Laryngoscope*, 114, 1362–1367.

Gray L.H., Conger A.D., Ebert, M., Hornsey, S., and Scott, O.C. (1953). The concentration of oxygen dissolved in tissues at the time of irradiation as a factor in radiotherapy. *British Journal of Radiology*, 26, 638–648.

Halyard, M.Y., Jatoi, A., Sloan, J.A., et al. (2007). Does zinc sulfate prevent therapy-induced taste alterations in head and neck cancer patients? Results of phase III double-blind, placebo-controlled trial from the North Central Cancer Treatment Group (N01C4). *International Journal of Radiation Oncology, Biology, Physics*, 67, 1318–1322.

Haman, K. (2008). Psychologic distress and head and neck cancer: part 1—review of the literature. *Supportive Oncology*, 6, 155–163.

He, L. (2008). Changes of satisfaction with appearance and working status for head and neck tumour patients. *Journal of Clinical Nursing*, 17, 1930–1938.

Henke, M., Laszig, R., Rube, C., et al. (2003). Erythropoietin to treat head and neck cancer patients with anaemia undergoing radiotherapy: randomised, double-blind, placebo-controlled trial. *The Lancet*, 362, 1255–1260.

Hutton, J.M. and Williams, M. (2001). An investigation of psychological distress in patients who have been treated for head and neck cancer. *British Journal of Oral and Maxillofacial Surgery*, 39, 333–339.

Hymes, S.R., Strom, E.A., and Fife, C. (2006). Radiation dermatitis: clinical presentation, pathophysiology, and treatment 2006. *Journal of the American Academy of Dermatology*, 54, 28–46.

Innui, A. (2002). Cancer anorexia-cachexia syndrome: current issues in research and management. *CA: A Cancer Journal for Clinicians*, 52, 72–91.

Jannjan, N., Weissman, D., and Pahule, A. (1992). Improved pain management with daily nursing intervention during radiation therapy for head and neck carcinoma. *International Journal of Radiation Oncology, Biology, Physics*, 23, 647–652.

Karnell, L.H., Christensen, A.J., Rosenthal, E.L., Magnuson, J.S., Funk, G.F. (2007). Influence of social support on health-related quality of life outcomes in head and neck cancer. *Head & Neck*, 29, 143–146.

Katz, M.R., Irish J.C., Devins, G.M., Rodin, G.M., and Gullane, P.J. (2000). Reliability and validity of an observer-rated disfigurement scale for head and neck cancer patients. *Head & Neck*, 22, 132–141.

Katz, M.R., Irish J.C., Devins, G.M., Rodin, G.M., and Gullane, P.J. (2003). Psychosocial adjustment in head and neck cancer: the impact of disfigurement, gender and social support. *Head & Neck*, 25, 103–112.

Keefe, D.M., Schubert, M.M., Elting, L.S., et al. (2007). Updated clinical practice guidelines for the prevention and treatment of mucositis. *Cancer*, 109, 820–831.

Kendel, W. (2007). Suicide and cancer: a gender-comparative study. *Annals of Oncology*, 18, 381–387.

Lacouture, M.E., Anadkat, M.J., Bensadoun, R.J., et al. (2011). Clinical practice guidelines for the prevention and treatment of EGFR inhibitor-associated dermatologic toxicities. *Supportive Care in Cancer*, 19, 1079–1095.

Langmore, S., Krisciunas, G.P., Miloro, K.V., Evans, S.R., and Cheng, D.M. (2012). Does PEG use cause dysphagia in head and neck cancer patients? *Dysphagia*, 27, 251–259.

Logemann, J. and Bytell, D. (1979). Swallowing disorders in three types of head and neck surgical patients. *Cancer*, 44, 1095–1105.

Logemann, J., Smith, C., Pauloski, B., et al. (2001). Effects of xerostomia on perception and performance of swallow function. *Head & Neck*, 23, 317–321.

Machon, C., Thezenas, S., Dupuy, A.M., et al. (2012). Immunonutrition before and during radiochemotherapy: improvement of inflammatory parameters in head and neck cancer patients. *Supportive Care in Cancer*, 20(12), 3129–3135.

Marks, J.E., Freeman, R.B., Lee, F., Ogura, J.H. (1978). Pharyngeal wall cancer: an analysis of treatment results complications and patterns of failure. *International Journal of Radiation Oncology, Biology, Physics*, 4, 587–593.

Marx, R. (1983). A new concept in the treatment of osteoradionecrosis. *Journal of Oral and Maxillofacial Surgery*, 41, 351–357.

McCaffrey, J., Weitzner, M, Kamboukas, D., et al. (2007). Alcoholism, depression, and abnormal cognition in head and neck cancer: A pilot study. *Otolaryngology—Head and Neck Surgery* 136, 92–97.

McConnel, F., Logemann, J., and Rademaker, A. (1994). Surgical variables affecting postoperative swallowing efficiency in oral cancer patients: a pilot study. *Laryngoscope*, 104, 87–90.

Montserrat, V., Oster, G., Hagiwara, M., and Sonis, S. (2006). Oral mucositis in patients undergoing radiation treatment for head and neck carcinoma. *Cancer*, 106, 329–336.

Mossman, K. (1983). Quantitative radiation dose-response relationship for normal tissue in man. *Radiation Research*, 95, 392–398.

Mossman, K.L. and Henkin, R.I. (1978). Radiation-induced changes in taste acuity in cancer patients. *International Journal of Radiation Oncology, Biology, Physics*, 4, 663–670.

Murphy, B. (2007). Clinical and economic consequences of mucositis induced by chemotherapy and/or radiation therapy. *Supportive Oncology*, 5, 13–21.

Murphy, B.A., Friedman, J., Dowling, E., Cheatham, R., and Cmela, A. (2002). Dietary intake and adaptations in head and neck cancer patients treated with chemoradiation. *Proceedings of the American Society of Clinical Oncology*, 21, abstract # 932.

Murphy, B.A. and Gilbert, J. (2009). Dysphagia in head and neck cancer patients treated with radiation: assessment, sequelae, and rehabilitation. *Seminars in Radiation Oncology*, 19, 35–42.

Murphy, B.A., Gilbert, J., Cmelak, A., and Ridner, S.H. (2007a). Symptom control issues and supportive care of patients with head and neck cancers. *Clinical Advances in Hematology and Oncology*, 5, 807–822.

Murphy, B.A., Gilbert, J., and Ridner, S. H. (2007b). Systemic and global toxicities of head and neck treatment. *Expert Review of Anticancer Therapy*, 7, 1043–1053.

Murphy, B.A., Ridner, S., Wells, N., and Dietrich, M. (2007c). Quality of life research in head and neck cancer: a review of the current state of the science. *Critical Reviews in Oncology/Hematology*, 62, 251–267.

Nahum, A.M., Mullally, W., and Marmor, L. (1961). A syndrome resulting from radical neck dissection. *Archives of Otolaryngology*, 74, 424–428.

Nayak, J.V., Walvekar, R.R., Andrade, R.S., et al. (2007). Deferring planned neck dissection following chemoradiation for stage IV head and neck cancer: the utility of PET-CT. *Laryngoscope*, 117(12), 2129–2134.

Netterville, J., Stone, R., Luken, E., Civantos, F., and Ossoff, R. (1993). Silastic medializaton and arytenoid adduction: the Vanderbilt experience. A review of 116 phonosurgical procedures. *Annals of Otology, Rhinology, and Laryngology*, 102, 413–424.

Nguyen, H.M., Reyland M., and Barlow, L.A. (2012a). Mechanisms of taste bud cell loss after head and neck irradiation. *Journal of Neuroscience*, 32, 3474–3484.

Nguyen, N.P, Smith, H., Duttan, S., et al. (2007). Aspiration occurence during chemoradiation for head and neck cancer. *Anticancer Drugs*, 3B, 1669–1672.

Nguyen, N.P., Vock, J., Chi, A., et al. (2012b). Effectiveness of intensity-modulated and image-guided radiotherapy to spare the mandible from excessive radiation. *Oral Oncology*, 48, 653–657.

Oozeer, N.B., Corsar, K, Glore, R.J., Penney, S., Patterson, J., and Paleri, V. (2011). The impact of enteral feeding route on patient-reported long term swallowing outcome after chemoradiation for head and neck cancer. *Oral Oncology*, 47, 980–983.

Osoba, D. (2000). Guidelines for measuring health-related quality of life clinical trials. In M.J. Staquet, R.D. Hays, and P.M. Fayers (eds.) *Quality of Life Assessment in Clinical Trials, Methods and Practice*, pp. 19–35. Oxford: Oxford University Press.

Pai, P.C., Chuang, C.C., Tseng, C.K., et al. (2012). Impact of pretreatment body mass index on patients with head-and-neck cancer treated with radiation. *International Journal of Radiation Oncology, Biology, Physics*, 83, e93–e100.

Paleri, V., Wight, R.G., Silver, C.E., et al. (2010). Comorbidity in head and neck cancer: a critical appraisal and recommendations for practice. *Oral Oncology*, 46, 712–719.

Pauloski, B.R., Rademaker, A.W., Logemann, J.A., et al. (2000). Pretreatment swallowing function in patients with head and neck cancer. *Head & Neck*, 22, 474–482.

Piccirillo, J.F., Lacy, P.D., Basu, A., and Spitznagel, E.L. (2002). Development of a new head and neck cancer-specific comorbidity index. *Archives of Otolaryngology Head & Neck Surgery*, 128, 1172–1179.

Reid, B.C., Alberg, A.J., Klassen, A.C., et al. (2001). Comorbidity and survival of elderly head and neck carcinoma patients. *Cancer*, 92, 2109–2116.

Reuther, T., Schuster, T., Mende, U., and Kübler, A. (2003). Osteoradionecrosis of the jaws as a side effect of radiotherapy of head and neck tumour patients—a report of a thirty year retrospective review. *International Journal of Oral and Maxillofacial Surgery*, 32, 289–295.

Rodriguez-Bruno, K., Ali, M.J., and Wang, S.J. (2011). Role of panendoscopy to identify synchronous second primary malignancies in patients with oral cavity and oropharyngeal squamous cell carcinoma. *Head & Neck*, 33, 949–953.

Rodríguez-Caballero, A., Torres-Lagares, D., Robles-García, M., Pachón-Ibáñez, J., González-Padilla, D., Gutiérrez-Pérez, J.L. (2012). Cancer treatment-induced oral mucositis: a critical review. *International Journal of Oral and Maxillofacial Surgery*, 41, 225–238.

Roe, J.W., Carding, P.N., Dwivedi, R.C., *et al.* (2010). Swallowing outcomes following intensity modulated radiation therapy (IMRT) for head & neck cancer—a systematic review. *Oral Oncology*, 46, 727–733.

Roh, J.L., Kim, A.Y., and Cho, M.J (2005). Xerostomia following radiotherapy of the head and neck affects vocal function. *Journal of Clinical Oncology*, 13, 3016–3023.

Rose, B.S., Jeong, J.H., Nath, S.K., Lu, S.M., and Mell, L.K. (2011). Population-based study of competing mortality in head and neck cancer. *Journal of Clinical Oncology*, 29, 3503–3509.

Rosenthal, D. (2007). Consequences of mucositis-induced treatment breaks and dose reductions on head and neck cancer treatment outcomes. *Supportive Oncology*, 5, 23–31.

Rosenthal, D.I., Mendoza, T.R., Chambers, M.S., *et al.* (2007). Measuring head and neck cancer symptom burden: the development and validation of the M. D. Anderson symptom inventory, head and neck module. *Head & Neck*, 29, 923–931.

Rudmik, L., Lau, H.Y., Matthews, T.W., *et al.* (2011). Clinical utility of PET/CT in the evaluation of head and neck squamous cell carcinoma with an unknown primary: a prospective clinical trial. *Head & Neck*, 33, 935–940.

Russi, E.G., Corvò, R., Merlotti, A., *et al.* (2012). Swallowing dysfunction in head and neck cancer patients treated by radiotherapy: review and recommendations of the supportive task group of the Italian Association of Radiation Oncology. *Cancer Treatment Reviews*, 38(8), 1033–1049.

Russo, G., Haddad, R., Posner, M., and Machtay, M. (2008). Radiation treatment breaks and ulcerative mucositis in head and neck cancer. *Oncologist*, 13, 886–890.

Sasse, A.D., Clark, L.G., Sasse, E.C., and Clark, O.A. (2006). Amifostine reduces side effects and improves complete response rate during radiotherapy: results of a meta-analysis. *International Journal of Radiation Oncology, Biology, Physics*, 64, 784–791.

Scarantino, C., Leveque, F., Swann, R. S., *et al.* (2006). Effect of pilocarpine during radiation therapy: results of RTOG 97–09, a phase III randomized study in head and neck patients. *Journal of Supportive Oncology*, 4, 252–258.

Semenov, Y.R., Starmer, H.M., and Gourin, C.G. (2012). The effect of pneumonia on short-term outcomes and cost of care after head and neck cancer surgery. *Laryngoscope*, 122, 1994–2004.

Shah, J.P. and Lydiatt, W. (1995). Treatment of cancer of the head and neck. *CA: A Cancer Journal for Clinicians*, 45, 352–368.

Sherman, A.C., Simonton, S., Adams, D.C., Emre, V., Owens, B., and Hanna, E. (2000). Assessing quality of life in patients with head and neck cancer: cross-validation of the European organization for research and treatment of cancer (EORTC) Quality of Life Head and Neck Module (QLQ-H&N35). *Archives of Otolaryngology Head and Neck Surgery*, 126, 459–467.

Shi, H.B., Masuda, M., Umezaki, T., *et al.* (2004). Irradiation impairment of umami taste in patients with head and neck cancer. *Auris, Nasus, Larynx*, 31, 401–406.

Silver, H.J., Dietrich, M.S., and Murphy, B.A. (2007). Changes in body mass, energy balance, physical function, and inflammatory state in patients with locally advanced head and neck cancer treated with

concurrent chemoradiation after low-dose induction chemotherapy. *Head & Neck*, 29(10), 893–900.

Sinard, R.J., Tobin, E.J., Mazzaferri, E.L., *et al.* (2000). Hypothyroidism after treatment for nonthyroid head and neck cancer. *Archives of Otolaryngology–Head & Neck Surgery*, 126, 652–657.

Singer, P., Cooper, D., Levy, E., Ladenson, P., Braverman, L., and Daniels, G. (1995). Treatment guidelines for patients with hyperthyroidism and hypothyroidism. Standards of Care Committee. American Thyroid Association. *Journal of the American Medical Association*, 173, 80–812.

Singh, B., Bhaya, M., Zimbler, M., *et al.* (1998). Impact of comorbidity on outcome of young patients with head and neck squamous cell carcinoma. *Head & Neck*, 20, 1–7.

Smit, M., Balm, A., Hilgers, F., and Tan, I.B. (2001). Pain as sign of recurrent disease in head and neck squamous cell carcinoma. *Head & Neck*, 23, 372–375.

So, W.K., Chan, R.J., Chan, D.N., *et al.* (2012). Quality-of-life among head and neck cancer survivors at one year after treatment—a systematic review. *European Journal of Cancer*, 48(15), 2391–408.

Taylor, J.C., Terrell, J.E., Ronis, D.L., *et al.* (2004). Disability in patients with head and neck cancer. *Archives of Otolaryngology*, 130, 764–769.

Tisdale, M. (2000). Metabolic alterations in cachexia and anorexia. *Nutrition*, 16, 1013–1014.

Trotti, A., Bellm, L.A., Epstein, J.B., *et al.* (2003). Mucositis incidence, severity and associated outcomes in patients with head and neck cancer receiving radiotherapy with or without chemotherapy: a systemic review. *Radiotherapy and Oncology*, 66, 253–262.

Vartanian, J.G., Carvalho, A.L., Toyota, J., Kowalski, I.S., and Kowalski, L.P. (2006). Socioeconomic effects of and risk factors for disability in long-term survivors of head and neck cancer. *Archives of Otolaryngology—Head & Neck Surgery*, 132, 32–35.

Vickery, L.E., Latchford, G., Hewison, J., Bellew, M., and Feber, T. (2003). The impact of head and neck cancer and facial disfigurement on the quality of life of patients and their partners. *Head & Neck*, 25, 289–296.

Vissink, A., Mitchell, J.B., Baum, B.J., *et al.* (2010). Clinical management of salivary gland hypofunction and xerostomia in head-and-neck cancer patients: successes and barriers. *International Journal of Radiation Oncology, Biology, Physics*, 78, 983–991.

Watt-Watson, J. and Graydon, J. (1995). Impact of surgery on head and neck cancer patients and their caregivers. *Nursing Clinics of North America*, 30, 659–671.

Wisawatapnimit, P., Dwyer, K.A., and Murphy, B. (2005). *Predicting Depressed Mood in Head and Neck Cancer Patients*. Poster session presented at the 19th Annual Conference of the Southern Nursing Research Society, Atlanta, GA.

Wisawatapnimit, P., Dwyer, K.A., and Murphy, B. (2006). *Life Experience of Head and Neck Cancer Patients and their Caregivers after Treatment*. Poster session presented at the Southern Nursing Research Society Meeting, 2006 Memphis, TN.

Wong, W.W., Mick, R., Haraf, D., Weichselbaum, R.R., and Vokes, E. E. (1994). Time-dose relationship for local tumor control following alternate week concomitant radiation and chemotherapy of advanced head and neck cancer. *International Journal of Radiation Oncology, Biology, Physics*, 29, 153–162.

Worthington, H.V., Clarkson, J.E., Bryan, G., *et al.* 2011. Interventions for preventing oral mucositis for patients with cancer receiving treatment. *Cochrane Database of Systematic Reviews*, 4, CD000978.

Yamagata, K., Onizawa, K., Yusa, H., *et al.* 2005. Risk factors for postoperative delirium in patients undergoing head and neck surgery. *International Journal of Oral and Maxillofacial Surgery*, 34, 33–36.

Yuen, H.K., Gillespie, M.B., Day, T.A., Morgan, L., and Burik, J.K. (2007). Driving behaviors in patients with head and neck cancer during and after cancer treatment: a preliminary report. *Head & Neck*, 29, 675–681.

Yung, K.C. and Piccirillo, J.F. (2008). The incidence and impact of comorbidity diagnosed after the onset of head and neck cancer. *Archives of Otolaryngology–Head & Neck Surgery*, 134, 1045–1049.

Issues in populations with non-cancer illnesses

SECTION 15

Issues in populations with non-cancer illnesses

HIV/AIDS

Meera Pahuja, Jessica S. Merlin, and Peter A. Selwyn

Introduction to HIV/AIDS

In the current treatment era, human immunodeficiency virus (HIV) has become a complex chronic disease. This chapter will focus on contemporary palliative care issues in people living with HIV in developed countries, while also acknowledging key differences between developed and developing countries.

A changing epidemic: new needs for palliative care

Early in the epidemic, HIV infection was an inevitable and speedy death sentence. Managing opportunistic infections and end-of-life care was the main focus of HIV disease management. This was done mostly by primary care physicians who quickly learned to be good palliative care physicians, and many palliative care-trained clinicians were deeply involved in end-of-life care for patients with acquired immunodeficiency syndrome (AIDS). In 1996, the era of 'highly active antiretroviral therapy' (HAART) began, with the introduction of powerful protease inhibitor (PI) drugs active against HIV that for the first time significantly slowed the course of the disease. Since that time, increasingly tolerable regimens with smaller pill burdens have been developed; there are now over 35 drugs in five categories of antiretroviral agents, once-daily dosing is generally the norm, and there are two one-pill, once-daily combination drug formulations. In a startlingly short time, AIDS has been transformed in many settings from a rapidly progressive, uniformly fatal illness affecting young adults to a complex, chronic disease with a variable course affecting an ageing population over decades of time (Fig. 15.1.1).

As a result of these rapid changes, patients with HIV who know their diagnosis, are linked to care, and consistently take antiretroviral therapy (ART) can have a near-normal life expectancy. A study of US national HIV surveillance data indicated that life expectancy at diagnosis has increased from 10.5 to 22.5 years from 1996 to 2005 (Harrison et al., 2010). One study found that a 20-year-old individual starting ART could expect to live for another 43 years on average and a 35-year-old could expect 32 more years of life (Antiretroviral Therapy Cohort Collaboration, 2008). A study of a Danish cohort of people living with HIV found that median survival for patients on HAART was more than 35 years from HIV diagnosis (Lohse et al., 2007). Notably, however, this increase in life expectancy has also brought increased morbidity, including co-morbid chronic diseases and complications of ageing that occur earlier in HIV-infected individuals than in their uninfected counterparts (Gallant et al., 2011).

Increased life expectancy, combined with unchanged incidence rates of new HIV infections in the United States (approximately 40 000–50 000/year), also has led to a rise in the prevalence of persons living with HIV/AIDS. By 2009, the prevalence of HIV/AIDS in the United States had increased to an estimated 1.1 million people (Centers for Disease Control and Prevention, 2009a).

The changing nature of HIV disease has in turn expanded the palliative care needs of the population from more traditional end-of-life care into symptom management, co-morbidity disease management, and chronic care-coordination—all in addition to end-of-life care. HIV care in many developed countries now is delivered by infectious diseases specialists, or by primary care practitioners with additional training in HIV and large panels of HIV-infected patients. Because HIV-infected patients have increasingly complex primary care needs, new models of care have emerged, which often include access to an HIV specialist, a care coordinator, and subspecialty care for common comorbidities including liver disease, cardiopulmonary and renal disease, metabolic and bone disorders, malignancies, psychiatric illness, and substance abuse (Gallant et al., 2011). Ironically, as AIDS in the HAART era has become a more chronic, less rapidly fatal illness, palliative care needs have increased, and the need for expertise in palliative care is now expressed by a growing population of patients for longer periods of time. It is important for this palliative care expertise to be reintegrated in the ongoing care of patients with HIV.

In the pre-HAART era, the most common modes of HIV transmission in the United States and much of Europe included sexual contact in men who had sex with men (MSM), and injection drug use (IDU). In 2009, MSM still accounted for 55% of the new cases of HIV in the United States, but heterosexual sex accounted for 30% of the new cases, and IDU accounted for only 9% of the new cases (Centers for Disease Control and Prevention, 2009a). HIV infection disproportionately affects vulnerable populations. In the United States, for example, racial and ethnic minorities account for 71% of the new AIDS cases, 67% of the new HIV infections, and 70% of all AIDS deaths. Historically, poorer communities have higher rates of HIV/AIDS and patients with low socioeconomic status have lower survival rates (Gilman et al., 2012; Mills et al., 2012). Minorities also experience higher death rates even after starting ART (Levine et al., 2007). Though rates have declined in MSM, younger MSM and MSM of colour are still at especially high risk for infection. Women are also disproportionally affected—280 000 are living with HIV/AIDS in the United States (Centers for Disease Control and Prevention, 2009a) These disparities are due to increasing heterosexual transmission,

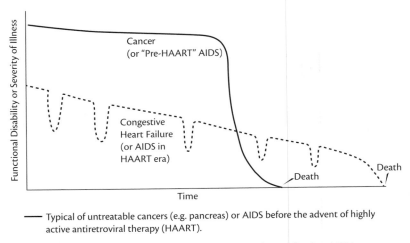

Fig. 15.1.1 Trajectories of illness over time in chronic, fatal diseases.
Reproduced from Joseph F. O'Neill et al., A Clinical Guide to Supportive and Palliative Care for HIV/AIDS, U. S. Department of Health and Human Services, Rockville, MD, USA, 2003, p.8, available from http://hab.hrsa.gov/deliverhivaidscare/files/palliativecare2003.pdf. Source: data from Joanne Lynn, Serving Patients Who May Die Soon and Their Families: The Role of Hospice and Other Services, Journal of American Medical Association, Volume 285, number 7, pp.925–32, Copyright © American Medical Association. All Rights Reserved.

delays in HIV diagnosis, and barriers in access/linkage to care (Gilman et al., 2012).

In developed countries, minorities, women, and older people (see below) also are more likely to present with more advanced disease than other populations, which raises important issues for health equity and palliative care. It is critical that these populations have access to HAART while making needed efforts to extend access to palliative care (Selwyn, 2008). Both in the developed and developing world, while advocating for better integration of palliative care with HIV care, it is important to be mindful not to implicitly endorse a double standard of 'HAART for the rich, and palliative care for the poor'.

The HIV-infected population is rapidly ageing. By 2015, half of the HIV-infected US population will be older than 50 (Centers for Disease Control and Prevention, 2009b; Mills et al., 2012). In 2009, more than 15% of both new HIV diagnoses and prevalent HIV infections, respectively, were in patients older than 50 (Centers for Disease Control and Prevention, 2009a). With ageing, HIV-infected patients accumulate comorbidities that were not historically associated with HIV, such as non-AIDS-defining malignancies, end-stage liver disease, atherosclerotic cardiovascular disease, chronic pulmonary disease, bone disorders, age-related neurocognitive decline, and frailty. These disorders appear at a faster rate than their non-HIV-infected counterparts (Onen and Overton, 2011). Frailty-prone HIV-infected patients experience fatigue and decreased mobility, and are at increased risk for bone pain and fractures (Womack et al., 2011).

Some have described a process of 'premature ageing' in HIV/AIDS, although the biological mechanism by which this occurs is not fully understood (Deeks and Phillips, 2009). As a result of this phenomenon, patients with HIV now encounter some of the same issues classically seen in geriatric patients. This accelerated ageing process further complicates the clinical management challenges for an already vulnerable population with multiple medical,

psychosocial, and environmental stressors: all of these issues further amplify the important role for palliative care interventions for HIV disease in the current era (Fig. 15.1.2).

Although advances in ART have increased life-expectancy, overall mortality for those living with HIV remains higher than the general population secondary to a myriad of factors, including delayed diagnosis, poor linkage and retention in care, and increasing co-morbid conditions. Although AIDS-related deaths have decreased, 1.8 million people died of AIDS in 2009 worldwide. In the United States, 15 000 die from AIDS-related causes annually, a number that has not decreased in recent years (UNAIDS, 2010). This underscores the importance of continued excellence in end-of-life care for this population.

Antiretroviral therapy

The two primary measures used to monitor patients with HIV are the CD4+ T-lymphocyte count, a measure of current immune function, and the HIV viral load, a measure of the current level of the virus in the patient's blood. The goal of ART is to achieve suppression of HIV replication such that the viral load is decreased to 'undetectable' levels (generally < 50 or 25 copies of viral RNA/mL, depending on the assay). This allows for immune reconstitution, which is represented by a rise in the CD4+ count and leads to reduced HIV-associated morbidity and mortality (Panel on Antiretroviral Guidelines for Adults and Adolescents, 2012).

In the developed world, guidelines currently advise considering ART in any patient infected with HIV, particularly those with a CD4 count lower than 500 cells/mm^3, and in all patients with certain conditions (e.g. pregnancy, hepatitis C, HIV nephropathy) (Panel on Antiretroviral Guidelines for Adults and Adolescents, 2012). This means that the majority of patients with HIV, if not all, ideally should be taking ART. This is a guideline, however, and clinicians often consider other factors to guide decisions about ART.

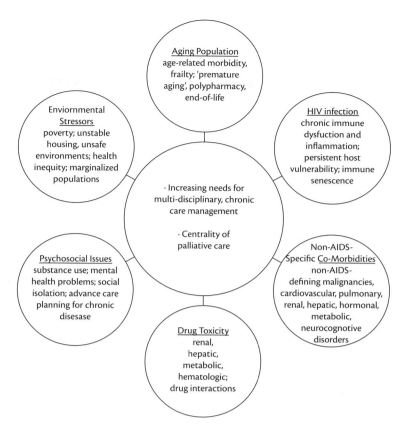

Fig. 15.1.2 Palliative care for HIV/AIDs as a complex, multifactorial chronic disease in an ageing population.

These include factors that influence treatment adherence, such as the patient's willingness to start treatment and the existence of a psychiatric disorder, such as substance abuse, or psychosocial issues.

Current ART guidelines for treatment-naïve patients recommend either: (1) a non-nucleoside reverse transcriptase inhibitor (NNRTI)-based regimen, (2) a ritonavir-boosted PI-based regimen, or (3) an integrase strand transfer inhibitor (INSTI)-based regimen. Each of these regimens includes two additional nucleoside reverse transcriptase inhibitors (NRTIs). Common first-line regimens in treatment-naïve patients include (1) a combination of emtricitabine plus tenofovir (two NRTIs) and efavirenz (NNRTI) in a one-pill once-daily formulation, (2) a two-NRTI combination pill plus a boosted PI (three to four pills once daily), or (3) two NNRTIs plus raltegravir, an INSTI (three pills daily in a twice-daily regimen). Though some of the newly developed medications have more favourable side-effect profiles (see Table 15.1.1), there are still many unknowns regarding their long-term side effects and influence on the development or evaluation of co-morbid conditions.

Adherence/retention

Key factors associated with increased life expectancy of HIV-infected patients include early diagnosis, linkage and retention in care, and adherence to ART regimens. Recent data from the United States suggest the need for improvement. Only 28% of persons with HIV achieved viral suppression (Centers for Disease Control and Prevention, 2011), and of patients who were aware of their HIV diagnosis, only 69% were linked to care and only 59%

were retained in care (Marks et al., 2010). Recent guidelines from the International Association of Physicians in AIDS Care focus on multidisciplinary interventions, such as adherence tools, education and counselling, health system and service delivery interventions, and special guidelines pertaining to vulnerable populations (such as pregnant women, homeless and marginally housed individuals, children and adolescents, and patients with substance use and mental health disorders) to improve entry into care, retention in care, and ART adherence (Thompson et al., 2012), As described below, palliative care interventions, particularly pain and symptom management, also may be especially important in achieving these aims through the provision of comprehensive HIV treatment services.

Co-morbid conditions

Co-morbid conditions which have not been historically associated with HIV, or which have become more common in long-surviving patients, such as cardiovascular, pulmonary, liver, and renal disease, non-AIDS-defining malignancies, frailty and bone disease, are now increasingly prevalent among HIV-infected patients. The accelerated nature of these disorders compared to non-infected patients is an area of active investigation. Multiple factors are suspected, including direct toxicity from the virus itself and/or related chronic inflammatory processes, chronic immunosuppression in patients living longer than in prior eras, toxicity secondary to ART, and increasing rates of smoking in this population. Each of these co-morbid conditions requires primary management, and together, they contribute to an increasing pain and symptom burden for HIV-infected patients.

Table 15.1.1 Classes of antiretrovirals, recommended first-line regimens, and common antiretroviral toxicities

Antiretroviral classes	Toxicities
Nucleoside reverse transcriptase inhibitors (NRTIs)	
Stavudine, (d4T)	Peripheral neuropathy, lipoatrophy, pancreatitis, lactic acidosis, hepatic steatosis
Didanosine (ddI)	Pancreatitis, peripheral neuropathy, nausea/vomiting
Zidovudine (AZT)	Anaemia, headache, nausea
Tenofovir (TDF)	Renal insufficiency, Fanconi syndrome, decreased bone mineralization, nausea, flatulence
Abacavir (ABC)	Hypersensitivity reaction[a], myocardial infarction (studies conflicted but should be used with caution in individuals at risk for myocardial infarction)
Lamivudine (3TC)	Minimal toxicity
Emtricitabine (FTC)	Minimal toxicity, hyperpigmentation/skin discoloration
Protease inhibitors (PIs)	
Lopinavir/ritonavir (LPV/RTV)	Diarrhoea, nausea, hyperlipidaemia, hyperglycaemia, pancreatitis
Atazanavir (ATV)	Indirect hyperbilirubinaemia, rare cardiac conduction abnormalities (PR prolongation), hyperlipidaemia, hyperglycaemia, fat maldistribution
Ritonavir (RTV)	Nausea, vomiting, diarrhoea, abdominal pain, fatigue, taste perversion, hepatotoxicity, headache, hyperlipidaemia, hyperglycaemia, fat maldistribution, circumoral paraesthesia
Darunavir (DRV)	Rash, hepatotoxicity, hyperlipidaemia, hyperglycaemia, diarrhoea nausea, fat maldistribution
Fosamprenavir (FAPV)	Rash, diarrhoea, nausea, headache, hyperlipidaemia, hyperglycaemia, fat maldistribution, transaminase elevation
Non-nucleoside reverse transcriptase inhibitors (NRRTIs)	
Entecavir (ETV)	Rash, nausea
Rilpivirine (RPV)	Rash, depression, insomnia, headache
Efavirenz (EFV)	Rash, neuropsychotic symptoms, transaminase elevation; teratogenic in non-human primates
Nevirapine (NVP)	Rash, hepatotoxicity (increased risk in women with CD4 counts > 250 cells/mm^3, and in men with CD4 counts > 400/mm^3)
Fusion inhibitors	
Enfuvirtide (INN)	Injection site pain and reactions
Integrase strand transfer inhibitors (INSTIs)	
Raltegravir (RAL)	Headache, nausea, diarrhoea
Elvitegravir (EVG)	Headache, nausea, diarrhoea, back pain

Recommended first-line treatment regimens

	Agents	Pills/day	Dosing schedule
NNRTI-based	TDF + FTC + EFV	1	Every day
PI-based	TDF + FTC + ATV/RTV	3	Every day
	TDF + FTC + DRV/RTV	4	Every day
INSTI-based	TDF + FTC + RAL	3	Twice a day

3TC, lamuvidine; ABC, abacavir; ATV, atazanavir; AZT, zidovudine; d4T = stavudine; DRV, darunavir; ddI, didanosine; EFV, efavirenz; EVG, elvitegravir; FTC, emtricitabine; ETV, entecavir; FAPV, fosamprenavir; INN, enfuvirtide; LPV, lopinavir; NPV, neviripine; RAL, raltegravir; RPV, rilpivirine; RTV, ritonavir; TDF, tenofovir.

[a] Hypersensitivity reaction seen primarily in patients who test positive for HLA-B*5701 allele; HLA screening recommended before initiation of this agent.

Reproduced from Panel on Antiretroviral Guidelines for Adults and Adolescents, *Guidelines for the use of antiretroviral agents in HIV-1-infected adults and adolescents*, US Department of Health and Human Services, available from http://aidsinfo.nih.gov/contentfiles/lvguidelines/adultandadolescentgl.pdf.

Cardiovascular disease

There is evidence that cardiovascular disease, in particular atherosclerosis and congestive heart failure, occurs earlier in HIV-infected population, and at higher rates, than in HIV-negative individuals (Glass et al., 2006). Some of this prevalence may be explained by a high prevalence of well-known and potentially modifiable risk factors. Smoking has been reported in 40–70% of HIV-infected patients, two- to threefold higher than the rate in the general population (Petoumenos et al., 2011), and HIV-infected patients are more likely to experience dyslipidaemias characterized by elevations in triglycerides, reduced high-density cholesterol, and variable increases in low-density and total cholesterol. In addition to these modifiable risk factors, HIV infection itself has been shown to increase the risk of atherosclerotic cardiovascular disease (El-Sadr et al., 2006); a combination of HIV viral load, immunological factors, and inflammation may be involved. PIs have also been associated with increased rates of myocardial infarction, which is thought to be secondary to increased rates of dyslipidaemia caused by this class of drugs, and abacavir (an NRTI) has been associated with cardiovascular disease risk as well (Kuritzkes and Currier, 2003; Friis-Moller et al., 2007). Accelerated atherosclerotic cardiovascular disease may be associated with painful or disabling symptoms, similar to patients not infected with HIV.

Pulmonary disease

HIV-infected patients developed numerous pulmonary complications. Some pulmonary opportunistic infections, such as *Pneumocystis jirovecii* pneumonia (PJP; previously *Pneumocystis carinii* pneumonia, PCP), are almost always seen only in HIV-infected patients with low CD4 counts (generally < 200 cells/mm^3); others, such as bacterial pneumonia, particularly pneumococcal pneumonia (Turett et al., 2001), and tuberculosis (Selwyn et al., 1989), are common in HIV-infected patients and may be seen at higher CD4 counts as well (generally < 400 cells/mm^3). There also is evidence in the current treatment era that certain pulmonary comorbidities, such as chronic obstructive pulmonary disease (Madeddu et al., 2013), pulmonary hypertension (Isasti et al., 2013), and lung cancer (Dubrow et al., 2012) may be relatively more common in HIV-infected patients. Whether this is due to higher rates of risk factors such as smoking, or due to the HIV infection itself, is still unknown. Respiratory symptoms experienced by patients with pulmonary comorbidities mirror those experienced by HIV-negative patients, and treatment strategies are similar. Dyspnoea, for example, may be treated with opioids, benzodiazepines, oxygen, and local environmental changes (e.g. open window, fan). Pulmonary comorbidities, like some of the other serious disorders experienced by HIV-infected patients, may cause more symptoms than the infection itself for those receiving successful ART regimens.

Liver disease

End-stage liver disease also is a significant cause of morbidity in HIV-infected patients. There are between 4 and 5 million people co-infected with HIV and hepatitis C virus (HCV) worldwide. Compared to non-HIV infected patients with hepatitis C, co-infected patients experience more rapid progression to fibrosis, increased HCV viral load, higher rates of viral persistence and higher rates end-stage liver disease and death (Operskalski and Kovacs, 2011). There also is evidence that HIV/HCV co-infected patients experience higher rates of neurocognitive impairment, peripheral neuropathy (Aronow et al., 2008), HIV-related kidney disease (Wyatt et al., 2008), and insulin resistance, glucose intolerance, and diabetes (Butt et al., 2009). Symptom burden also is relatively higher in co-infected patients, and studies show increased rates of abdominal pain, mental status change and bleeding risk, all of which may benefit from standard palliative care intervention in addition to disease modifying treatment (Braitstein et al., 2005).

Renal disease

In the pre-HAART era, common disorders of the kidney secondary to HIV disease included HIV-associated nephropathy, HIV-associated immune complex kidney disease, and thrombotic microangiopathy. These disorders remain an issue in those who are diagnosed late in infection or who are not receiving treatment. The risk of HIV-associated nephropathy may increase over time in chronically infected patients. HIV-associated kidney disease is itself an indication for initiation of ART.

Other aetiologies of kidney disease in the current treatment era have emerged. Drug-related nephrotoxicity has been associated with most classes of antiretrovirals, but in particular, with the NRTI tenofovir, and the PI indinavir (Izzedine and Deray, 2007). While indinavir has been replaced by other PIs with better safety profiles, tenofovir is in widespread use as a first-line NRTI (de Silva et al., 2007; Schmid et al., 2007). Serious renal events, such as renal failure and Fanconi syndrome, have been reported in 0.5% of patients taking tenofovir, and 2.2% of patients experience elevations in serum creatinine. There is evidence that older age, reduced renal function at baseline, lower body weight, low CD4 count and other nephrotoxic medications can increase rates of tenofovir-associated nephrotoxicity (Nelson et al., 2007). Tenofovir is thought to cause renal disease secondary to its action on the proximal tubular epithelial cells. This effect on the proximal tubule can also cause hypophosphatemia, which has important implications on bone mineralization and can lead to low bone mass and increased risk for osteoporosis and fractures (Cazanave et al., 2008).

Metabolic bone disease

Bone disease is becoming an increasingly burdensome issue for HIV-infected patients. The aetiology is multifactorial and includes hypogonadism, smoking/alcohol, direct inflammatory effects of HIV, ART (specifically tenofovir), vitamin D deficiency and low body weight. HIV-infected patients with osteoporosis are at increased risk for osteoporosis-related fractures. A recent study found that the prevalence of osteoporosis-related fractures was 60% higher in HIV-infected patients compared with HIV-uninfected patients (Triant et al., 2008).

Early detection of osteoporosis and treatment can reduce the burden of osteoporosis-associated fractures. Current screening guidelines recommend dual-energy X-ray absorptiometry scan for all HIV-infected postmenopausal women and men aged older than 50. Treatment for osteoporosis for HIV-infected patients is similar to HIV-uninfected individuals and includes weight-bearing exercise, muscle-strengthening exercises, smoking cessation, limitation of alcohol intake and adequate intake of calcium and vitamin D. Low vitamin D in particular has been associated with the aetiology of osteoporosis in HIV-infected patients (Walker Harris and Brown, 2012). A recent study found increased risk for vitamin D deficiency and insufficiency related to African American race, Hispanic ethnicity, and exposure to efavirenz and ritonavir (Dao et al., 2011). Despite the high prevalence of vitamin D deficiency, universal screening and treatment is controversial; however, in patients with known history of bone disease and certainly fractures, vitamin D levels should be tested, and if low, repleted (Walker Harris and Brown, 2012). Bisphosphonates have also been shown to improve bone mineral density in HIV-infected patients (Bolland et al., 2007).

Osteonecrosis

Osteonecrosis, or avascular necrosis, is also more common in HIV-infected patients than in the general population. Prevalence estimates are as high as 4.4% based on imaging studies, although many patients are asymptomatic (Miller et al., 2002). The pathogenesis is controversial; when the femoral head is involved, the pathogenesis may relate to interruption of blood supply, which can lead to instability and, most severely, collapse (Mankin, 1992; Mont and Hungerford, 1995). Risk factors in HIV-infected patients include any lifetime use of systemic corticosteroids, hyperlipidaemia, use of lipid-lowering agents, testosterone supplementation, weightlifting or bodybuilding, anticardiolipin antibodies, previous AIDS-defining illness, low CD4+ cell nadir, longer duration of exposure to ART, pancreatitis, and alcoholism (Scribner et al., 2000; Miller et al., 2002; Mary-Krause et al., 2006).

Osteonecrosis can involve any bone. The femoral head is most common, and the disease may be unilateral or bilateral (Yombi et al., 2009). Patients typically present with groin pain, although pain may also be in the buttock or thigh (Mankin, 1992; Steinberg, 1997; Allison et al., 2003). The recommended initial diagnostic strategy is to perform a plain radiograph of the affected joint. Magnetic resonance imaging is the diagnostic gold standard because of its high sensitivity (> 90%), however, and should be performed if the initial radiograph is negative (Mitchell et al., 1987; Chang et al., 1993; Guerra and Steinberg, 1995; Vande Berg et al., 1997; Sugano et al., 1999; Miller et al., 2002; Allison et al., 2003; Johnson and Decker, 2008).

Treatment depends upon the bone involved and the severity. Asymptomatic disease may be observed, and mild disease may be followed and treated with analgesics and medical management. Patients with more severe disease, efor example, disease involving more than 30% of the femoral head, as well as patients with symptomatic osteonecrosis, should be sent for orthopaedic evaluation. The type of procedure selected (joint-sparing procedures such as core decompression and osteotomy or hip replacement) depends on the severity of disease. In one study of patients with HIV and hip osteonecrosis, 59% underwent a total hip replacement by 10 months after diagnosis (Gutierrez et al., 2006).

Malignancies

Patients with HIV have increased rates of both HIV-related and non-HIV-related malignancies. AIDS-defining malignancies such as Kaposi's sarcoma, non-Hodgkin lymphomas (including Burkitt's lymphoma and primary central nervous system (CNS) lymphoma), and invasive cervical cancer still occur, but their rates have decreased substantially in the current treatment era. However, non-AIDS-defining malignancies, including Hodgkin's lymphoma, multiple myeloma, leukaemia, liver cancer, lung cancer, prostate cancer, invasive anal carcinoma and colon cancer, are increasingly prevalent in this population (Cheung et al., 2005; Palella et al., 2006; Simard and Engels, 2010). In fact, studies show twice the risk of non-HIV-related malignancies in HIV-infected patients compared with the general population (Bedimo et al., 2009). This enhanced risk corresponds to a two- to fivefold increase in risk for cancers such as melanoma, lung cancer, and hepatocellular carcinoma, and an even greater ten- to 30-fold increased risk for anal cancer and Hodgkin's lymphoma.

HIV-infected patients also have a higher prevalence of risk factors for cancer, such as smoking, alcohol consumption, and co-infection with HCV or human papilloma virus (HPV) infection (Silverberg et al., 2009a). Like cervical cancer, anal squamous cell carcinoma is associated with HPV; however, unlike cervical cancer, anal cancer is not considered an AIDS defining illness. Although HIV-infected MSM are at higher risk for anal cancer, there is evidence of an independent association of anal cancer with HIV infection in other patients as well (D'Souza et al., 2008; Piketty et al., 2008). Current guidelines for screening for anal cancer in HIV-infected patients have been borrowed from cervical cancer screening literature and include digital rectal exam and anal cytology testing (Sigel et al., 2011). Though the benefits of screening for anal cancer in HIV-infected patients have not been studied in randomized controlled trials, one observational cohort of HIV-infected MSM found that the median time of progression of high-grade anal intraepithelial neoplasia to cancer was 8.6 months, arguing the need for further study in this area (Kreuter et al., 2010).

The clinical challenge posed by the increasing prevalence of non-HIV related malignancies in HIV-infected patients has been compounded by the serious nature of these diseases. One study found that patients with non-AIDS-defining malignancies experienced a decreased 24-month survival compared to HIV-uninfected patients with equivalent malignancies (Biggar et al., 2005).

Neurocognitive disorders

Despite HAART, HIV-related cognitive disorders, variously described as HIV dementia, HIV encephalopathy and neurocognitive impairment, remain an important part of the disease burden in HIV-infected patients. HIV is a neuroinvasive virus and different HAART regimens have varying degrees of CNS penetration. The number of patients with HIV-related neurocognitive disorders, including HIV dementia and mild neurocognitive impairment, is expected to increase five- to tenfold by 2030 (Cysique et al., 2011). Although HAART can reduce the rates of some neurocognitive disorders, mild cognitive impairment is more difficult to treat, particularly in an ageing population characterized by comorbid disorders of brain function, including Alzheimer's disease. One study of HIV-associated neurocognitive disorders in the pre- and post-HAART eras found that increasing age was a risk factor for mild neurocognitive disorder (Heaton et al., 2011). Further research is needed to characterize the role of accelerated ageing in HIV-infected patients and its impact on HIV-related neurocognitive disorders.

Psychiatric comorbidities

Psychiatric disorders are relatively more common in the HIV-infected population. One study found that the prevalence of psychiatric disorders among HIV patients was more than twice that of non-infected patients (63% vs 30.5%) (Tegger et al., 2008). The most common psychiatric disorder in HIV-infected patients is major depressive disorder, with prevalence estimates as high as 36% (Bing et al., 2001), compared to 4.9% in the general population (Blazer et al., 1994). Generalized anxiety disorder also is common among HIV-infected patients, affecting about 16% (Repetto and Petitto, 2008). In some populations, other psychiatric illnesses, such as schizophrenia, also may be more prevalent. Epidemiologic research also has shown that psychiatric patients with chronic mental disorders such as schizophrenia are at higher risk for acquiring HIV infection (Kalichman et al., 1994).

Psychiatric illness, most significantly depression, has been associated with poor adherence to ART (Dalessandro et al., 2007; Mellins et al., 2009; Gonzalez et al., 2011). Further, a recent study of 198 HIV-infected patients initiated on HAART at a large academic medical centre in the United States found a higher predicted probability of any psychiatric disorder associated with a slower rate of virological suppression and a faster rate of overall virological failure (Pence et al., 2007). The authors suggest that there would be clinical benefit to screening and treating patients for psychiatric disorders prior to initiating HAART.

Access to mental health care is a vital part of HIV treatment and studies have shown that depressed patients who are started on antidepressants have higher levels of adherence than those that are untreated (Dalessandro et al., 2007). All of these themes suggest the central importance of psychosocial issues and mental health services in the care of patients with HIV/AIDS, and highlight the potential value of multi-disciplinary palliative care team intervention in routine care in this population.

Premature frailty

Frailty is a clinical syndrome that 'reflects biological rather than chronological age' (Onen and Overton, 2011). Frailty has been defined in numerous ways. The most widely accepted definition includes physical parameters only, that is, at least three of five criteria (unintentional weight loss of > 4.5 kg in the past year, exhaustion, low physical activity, weak grip strength, and slow walk time) (Fried et al., 2001). HIV researchers have suggested, however, that a more accurate representation of frailty in HIV-infected patients may include neuropsychiatric comorbidity as well (Onen and Overton, 2011).

The prevalence of premature frailty in HIV-infected individuals may be as high as 20%, even among populations of patients in their 40s and 50s, at least a decade younger than this occurs in non-HIV-infected patients. Premature frailty in HIV-infected patients is associated with having had AIDS and opportunistic infections in the past, lower CD4+ T-cell counts, uncontrolled viraemia, and medical comorbidity. The pathophysiology of this syndrome is not well understood, but may relate to immune dysregulation. Although evidence is limited, exercise seems to improve physical function (Onen and Overton, 2011).

Wasting

Wasting syndrome in HIV-infected patients is much less common in the current HIV treatment era, as fewer patients have advanced disease and active opportunistic infections. However, there is some evidence from more contemporary cohorts that wasting still occurs. To reflect syndromes seen more frequently in the current treatment era, and identify individuals with clinically meaningful weight loss, the Nutrition for Healthy Living Cohort defined wasting as (1) unintentional loss of greater than 10%, (2) a body mass index (BMI) of 20 or below, or (3) unintentional loss of more than 5% of body weight in 6 months that persisted for at least 1 year (Mangili et al., 2006). One study in the early post-HAART era found that the incidence of wasting per 1000 person-years was 7.5 in 1988–1990, 14.4 in 1991–1993, and 22.1 in 1994–1995, and decreased to 13.4 in 1996–1999 (Smit et al., 2002). Another study from the later post-HAART era found that the risk of a 5% weight loss over 6 months was greater in the years 1998–2003 than the years 1995–1997 (relative risk 1.52; 95% confidence interval 1.17–1.97) (Tang et al., 2005), and although seen at all CD4 counts, wasting was associated with lower CD4 count (Forrester et al., 2001) and increased mortality (Tang et al., 2002). The aetiology of wasting is often multifactorial, and can include inadequate nutrient intake secondary to oral and upper gastrointestinal problems, malabsorption, poor appetite, economic constraints, altered metabolism secondary to advanced HIV or opportunistic infections, and/or hormonal disorders such as hypogonadism or hyperthyroidism (Mangili et al., 2006).

In managing wasting, consideration should be given to consultation with an HIV specialist and initiation of ART in patients who are not receiving it. In addition to ART, other medical therapies have shown promise for the treatment of wasting. Moyle et al conducted a randomized, double-blind, placebo-controlled trial and found that 12 weeks of daily recombinant human growth hormone improved lean body mass, physical performance, and quality of life in patients with HIV-associated weight loss or wasting who were on ART (Moyle et al., 2004). Dronabinol, a synthetic delta-9-tetrahydrocannabinol is an approved treatment for HIV-associated weight loss and anorexia in the United States. Although studies have shown increased self-reported appetite and decreased nausea they have not shown significant increases in weight (Beal et al., 1995). Megestrol acetate, a synthetic progestational agent also has potent appetite stimulant properties and increases fat; compared to placebo, men taking 800 mg/day had increased caloric consumption and weight gains of up to 4 kg (Von Roenn et al., 1994).

Hypogonadism is highly prevalent in patients with HIV-associated wasting. Bhasin et al. demonstrated that testosterone replacement and resistance exercise increased lean body mass by 1.4 kg in HIV-infected, hypogonadal patients (Bhasin et al., 2000). Synthetic anabolic agents, such as oxandrolone, also have been shown to be effective in increasing lean body mass (Berger et al., 1996). Resistance exercise itself also has been shown to increase lean tissue in HIV-infected patients (Roubenoff et al., 1999).

Studies have shown that the combination of the above modalities have even further increases on weight gain and potential improvements in quality of life (Storer et al., 2005; Sardar et al., 2010). Effective treatment can be based on careful consideration of the aetiology of the weight loss and side effect profiles of the medical therapies.

Hypogonadism

As noted, low testosterone levels due to hypogonadism, specifically secondary hypogonadism, is a common problem among HIV-infected men in the current treatment era. Although prevalence rates are lower in the current treatment era, up to 6% of HIV-infected men have low testosterone levels (Dube et al., 2007). Hypogonadism increases with age. Relatively low testosterone also may exist in HIV-infected woman, but normative standards and guidelines for diagnosis and treatment are less clear for these patients.

With the ageing of the HIV-infected population, the consequences of male hypogonadism are becoming important primary care issues. Patients with low testosterone levels may report fatigue, depression, and decreased libido; decreased muscle mass and low bone mineral density may worsen (Bhasin et al., 2010). The clinical response to these problems starts with measurement of free and total testosterone levels. Measurement of free testosterone is important, especially since total levels may be normal as HIV-infected patients produce lower levels of sex hormone binding globulin (Martin et al., 1992; Bhasin et al., 2010). Treatment with testosterone replacement—available in topical, transdermal, and injectable preparations—is indicated in patients with poor libido, low bone mineral density, and low muscle mass. The benefits of testosterone replacement must be carefully weighed against potential risk of prostate cancer and cardiovascular disease (Bhasin et al., 2010).

Substance abuse

Substance use disorders are highly prevalent in the HIV-infected population. Studies report that 40–74% of patients have, or have had, comorbid substance use problems (McGowan et al., 2011). Substance abuse is related to the presence of other psychiatric illness, and recent estimates suggest that substance use and mental health disorders co-occur in at least one-quarter of all patients infected with HIV (Bing et al., 2001). Patients with substance abuse and concomitant psychiatric disorders have lower CD4 counts, and poorer HIV viral suppression and ART adherence (Lucas et al., 2001). While a recent review found that active substance abuse was related to poor adherence, the evidence also suggests that drug users can adhere effectively to medications if they receive structured care, including access to mental health treatment (Malta et al., 2008). All of these mental health and substance use issues pose special challenges and opportunities for palliative care interventions in patients with HIV/AIDS.

Pain and symptom burden

Earlier studies from the pre- and early HAART era documented high levels of pain in patients with AIDS (29–76%), as well as high levels of other non-pain symptoms (10–91% across many studies), with correspondingly high levels of under-diagnosis and under-treatment (Moss, 1990; O'Neill and Sherrard, 1993; Singer et al., 1993; Filbet et al., 1994; Foley, 1994; Larue et al., 1994; Breitbart et al., 1996, 1998; Fantoni et al., 1997; Kelleher et al., 1997; Larue et al., 1997; Wood et al., 1997; Fontaine et al., 1999; Vogl et al., 1999; Mathews et al., 2000). In the pre-HAART era, the aetiology of pain and other symptoms in HIV/AIDS was often due to opportunistic infections, AIDS-associated malignancies, and the systemic effects of progressive, untreated HIV infection. Although symptoms still may be due to these factors, patients in the HAART era also experience pain and other symptoms from numerous other sources, including chronic co-morbidities, frailty, bone disease, ageing-related processes, and the effects of chronic exposure to antiretroviral medications (Table 15.1.2). All of these factors highlight the importance of timely and effective palliative care interventions for the management of pain and other symptoms in patients with HIV/AIDS.

Recent studies have explored the prevalence of pain and other symptoms. A study of 156 ambulatory HIV-infected patients in the United States found that 48.7% reported pain, of whom 51.3% had moderate to severe pain intensity; 57.3% of participants felt that their pain caused moderate to severe interference with their lives (Merlin et al., 2012a). This high prevalence of pain has also been documented in numerous other studies in the current treatment era.

Since early in the epidemic, neuropathic pain has been reported in patients with HIV. HIV distal sensory polyneuropathy (DSP), which is the most common cause of neuropathic pain in HIV-infected patients, is a length-dependent degeneration of large and small peripheral nerve fibres (Cornblath and McArthur, 1988; Barohn et al., 1993; Griffen et al., 1998; Gonzalez-Duarte et al., 2008). Aetiologies include exposure to older ART regimens (e.g. stavudine (d4T), didanosine (ddI), and zalcitabine (DDC)), or more contemporary regimens such as PIs, and simply HIV infection (Gonzalez-Duarte et al., 2008). Although the prevalence estimates in the current treatment era are lower than in the pre-HAART era, DSP still affects many long-surviving HIV-infected patients, ranging from 4.3% to 21.8%, and the incidence of this disorder may increase in this population over time (Sacktor, 2002; Lichtenstein et al., 2005; Ellis et al., 2010; Evans et al., 2011).

Patients infected with HIV who develop DSP typically present with sensory signs in a stocking-glove distribution. The diagnosis is clinical, and initial workup should include testing for other common causes of neuropathy (e.g. diabetes, vitamin B_{12} deficiency, alcohol use). More invasive tests, such as nerve conduction studies, may be considered if the diagnosis is in question, but are often not needed (Gonzalez-Duarte et al., 2008). Treatment is symptomatic. Drugs with proven efficacy in HIV-infected patients include gabapentin (Hahn et al., 2004) and high-dose topical capsaicin (Estanislao et al., 2004). Although not specifically shown to be effective in HIV-infected patients, other drugs often are tried based on their efficacy in other types of peripheral neuropathy; these include various antidepressants, especially tricyclic antidepressants and duloxetine (a serotonin-norepinephrine (noradrenaline) reuptake inhibitor); opioids also are often employed effectively (Gonzalez-Duarte et al., 2008).

In addition to pain, overall symptom burden remains high for patients in the HAART era. Several recent studies have documented high prevalences of fatigue, weight loss, cough, memory loss, insomnia, depression and paraesthesias (Fontaine et al., 1999; Newshan et al., 2002; Harding et al., 2006, 2010a; Lee et al., 2009; Silverberg et al., 2009b; Cervia et al., 2010; Merlin et al., 2012b). A recent study that administered a 32-item symptom distress measure to patients in three separate outpatient HIV clinics in the United States found that, on average, patients reported 10.9–12.7 symptoms (Karus et al., 2005). The most common symptoms in this study were pain, lack of energy, shortness of breath, dry mouth, and nausea. In addition to physical symptoms, patients reported psychological symptoms, such as anxiety, depression, and difficulty sleeping. Half or more of the patients in this study described their symptoms as frequent, severe and distressing. The authors suggested that the prevalence of these symptoms is similar to those seen in a terminally ill cancer population (Karus et al., 2005). A recent systematic review looked at palliative care-related problems at HIV diagnosis and found physical and psychological symptoms were also highly prevalent at diagnosis (Simms et al., 2011).

Pain and non-pain symptom management in HIV-infected patients

Managing HIV-infected patients with frequent and severe symptoms is complex and special consideration needs to be given to frequent potential drug-drug interactions between antiretrovirals and common palliative care-related medications (Table 15.1.3). Notwithstanding these concerns, it is important to note that,

Table 15.1.2 Selected HIV-related symptoms, aetiologies, and management strategies in the pre-HAART and HAART eras

Symptom	Pre-HAART-era aetiologies	Management	HAART-era aetiologies	Management
Pulmonary				
Dyspnoea/cough	PJP	Antibiotics	COPD	Inhalers, steroids, oxygen
	Bacterial pneumonia	Antibiotics	Pulmonary hypertension	Pulmonary vasodilators, afterload reducers, HAART
	TB	Anti-mycobacterials	Congestive heart failure	Diuretics, afterload reducers, HAART
			Cardiomyopathy	Diuretics, afterload reducers, HAART
Gastrointestinal				
Nausea/vomiting	Oesophageal candidiasis	Antifungals	HAART	Change HAART regimen, antiemetics
	CMV	Antivirals	Anxiety	Selective serotonin reuptake inhibitors, cognitive behavioural therapy
	Disseminated MAC	Anti-mycobacterials	Gastroparesis	Prokinetic agents
			Oesophageal reflux/gastritis	H_2 blocker, proton pump inhibitors
Diarrhoea	Disseminated MAC	Anti-mycobacterials	HAART	Change HAART regimen, anti-diarrhoeals
	Cryptosporidiosis	Antifungals	Irritable bowel syndrome	Behavioural modification, dietary changes, fibre
	CMV	Antivirals		
Abdominal pain	Disseminated MAC	Anti-mycobacterials	Hepatic steatosis/hepatoma	Pain management
	CMV	Antivirals	Cirrhosis/ascites	Diuretics, pain management
			Chronic pancreatitis	Pancreatic enzyme replacement, pain management
			Hepatitis C	HCV specific therapy
Constitutional				
Fatigue, weight loss, anorexia, wasting	AIDS	Methylphenidate, dronabinol, testosterone, oxandrolone, megestrol acetate	Malignancy	Targeted chemotherapy, psychostimulants,
	Opportunistic infections	Treat opportunistic infections	Depression	Antidepressants, cognitive behavioural therapy
			Frailty, multimorbidity, ageing	Address comorbidities, exercise
Neuropsychiatric				
Dementia	AIDS-related dementia	Supportive care	AIDS-related dementia	HAART
Delirium	AIDS	Antipsychotics	Hepatic encephalopathy	Lactulose, rifaximin, HAART
Depression/anxiety		Antidepressants		Antidepressants
Pain				
Peripheral Neuropathy	HIV-related neuropathy	Anti-depressants, anti-convulsants, opioids	HAART-associated neuropathy	change HAART therapy
Musculoskeletal pain	Opportunistic infections	Treat opportunistic infections	Osteonecrosis (e.g. hip or other large joints)	NSAIDS, opioids, surgery
			Non-specific musculoskeletal pain syndromes (low back pain, other regional musculoskeletal pain)	Adjuvants, cognitive-behavioural therapy, opioids

Please note that this table is not meant to be an exhaustive list, but rather a list of examples of how symptoms may manifest in the current treatment era of highly active antiretroviral therapy (HAART), as compared to how they may have presented in the 'pre-HAART' era.

CMV—cytomegalovirus; MAC, *Mycobacterium avium* complex; PJP, *Pneumocystis jirovecii* pneumonia/formerly *Pneumocystis carinii* pneumonia (PCP).

Table 15.1.3 Potential cytochrome P450-related drug interactions between antiretrovirals, anti-infectives, and common palliative care medications

Cytochrome P450 inhibitors	
Antiretrovirals	Protease inhibitors (ritonavir, atazanavir, darunavir, fosamprenavir)
Antibiotics	Quinolones (ciprofloxacin), metronidazole, co-trimoxazole
Antifungals	Azoles (ketoconazole, fluconazole, itraconazole)
Antidepressants	Selective serotonin reuptake inhibitors (fluoxetine, paroxetine, sertraline)
Antipsychotics	Haloperidol, thioridazine[a]

Cytochrome P450 inducers	
Antiretrovirals	Non-nucleoside reverse transcriptase inhibitors (efavirenz, nevirapine)
Antimycobacterials	Rifampin, rifabutin
Anticonvulsants	Carbamazepine, phenytoin, phenobarbital

Cytochrome 3A4 substrates (levels decrease in the setting of an inducer, and increase in the setting of an inhibitor)	
Antiretrovirals	Protease inhibitors (ritonavir, atazanavir, darunavir, fosamprenavir), non-nucleoside reverse transcriptase inhibitors (efavirenz); CCR5 antagonists (maraviroc)
Antibiotics	Co-trimoxazole
Opioids	Methadone, oxycodone, codeine, fentanyl
Non-opioid analgesics	Naproxen, ibuprofen
Appetite stimulants	Dronabinol
Antidepressants	Tricyclic antidepressants (amitriptyline, nortriptyline), selective serotonin reuptake inhibitors (citalopram, paroxetine)
Benzodiazepines:	Clonazepam, diazepam, midazolam
Hypnotics	Zolpidem

[a] Withdrawn in some countries but used in the United States.

When initiating a new medication in a patient taking antiretroviral therapy, it is always best to use a drug–drug interaction programme to check for the presence of interactions. This list is not meant to be comprehensive, but rather introduce the reader to the high potential for drug–drug interactions between medications commonly prescribed to HIV-infected patients and to patients in palliative care settings.

Use drug interaction resources sites:

<http://www.ncbi.nlm.nih.gov/pmc/articles/PMC1312247/table/TU1/>
<http://www.hiv-druginteractions.org/>
<http://hivinsite.ucsf.edu/insite?page=ar-00-02>

Source: Data from *Guidelines for the Use of Antiretroviral Agents in HIV-1-Infected Adults and Adolescents*, AIDS *info*, U.S. Department of Health and Human Services (HHS), 2013, available from <http://aidsinfo.nih.gov/guidelines/html/1/adult-and-adolescent-arv-guidelines/32/drug-interactions>.

in general, the approach to managing many symptoms such as pain does not substantially differ from that in non-HIV-infected patients with similar symptoms.

However, pain management in the HIV population may pose some unique challenges related to the fact that both HIV and chronic pain are at the nexus of psychiatric illness and substance abuse. A complete discussion of this is beyond the scope of this chapter; interactive cases on HIV and pain that focus on these complex issues may be found on the International AIDS Society's website (https://www.iasusa.org/content/hiv-and-pain). The key concepts follow:

First, chronic pain is subjective, suggesting that a patient's self-report of pain must be taken seriously and worthy of investigation; moreover, the absence of an objective finding of physical pathology does not preclude trials of pain management interventions.

Second, patients with active psychiatric illness or substance abuse, many of whom may have comorbid personality disorders, may express pain or its consequences, and requests for pain management, in a manner that causes frustration and anger among staff. It is important to recognize one's own countertransference in such situations, and try not to let it interfere with the care of the patient. A history of substance use must not in itself become a disqualification for having pain assessed and treated in a patient reporting pain.

Third, aberrant opioid-related behaviours, such as frequent calls to the clinic requesting opioids, a focus on opioids during visits, a pattern of lost/stolen prescriptions, have a differential diagnosis. This differential diagnosis includes addiction, pseudoaddiction (problematic behaviours driven by uncontrolled pain), psychiatric disorders other than substance use disorders (including personality disorders, anxiety disorders and others), and even criminal intent (135). These potential diagnoses can coexist, further increasing the importance of a detailed assessment of problematic behaviours, should they occur.

Fourth, the complexity of chronic pain in the HIV population supports consideration of a multimodality (sometimes multidisciplinary) approach in every case. Pharmacologic therapies may include drugs in numerous classes, such as opioids, non-opioids, and analgesic antidepressants and anticonvulsants, as well as non-pharmacological therapies, such as rehabilitative approaches like physical therapy and exercise, and psychological approaches such as cognitive behavioural therapy. All of these modalities, and in some cases, others offered by pain specialists, should be investigated for patients with chronic pain (Chou et al., 2009). Although there is limited evidence to support the effectiveness of long-term opioid therapy in any population, clinical experience is very large and most clinicians agree that these drugs may be useful on a long-term basis for some carefully selected and monitored patients.

In every individual patient, the risk versus benefit of chronic opioid therapy must be weighed. For some patients, including those engaged in active alcohol or drug abuse, the risk may be too high to select this therapy, or to continue it (Chou et al., 2009).

Finally, the need to apply opioid risk mitigation strategies has become more accepted, but some, such as opioid treatment agreements ('contracts') are controversial, and even those that are widely accepted in the United States (e.g. urine drug screens), must be considered case by case. Other approaches that might be considered include limit-setting for the use of extra doses, general policies regarding non-replacement of reported lost or stolen prescriptions, avoidance of staff 'splitting', maintaining consistency of only one clinician providing ongoing prescriptions to the same patient, and others. Although there is a limited evidence base for all of these strategies, one or more are frequently used to try to monitor for aberrant opioid use and other illicit substance abuse (Starrels et al., 2010).

Symptoms and adherence

The increased symptom burden in patients with HIV/AIDS may have an effect on adherence with ART and other ongoing care, a key aspect of effective HIV disease management over time. High levels of long-term adherence with ART are critical for treatment success and even modest lapses in ART adherence below the 90% level for any period of time significantly increase the risk of the emergence of drug-resistant HIV. A study of symptom prevalence in an outpatient HIV setting which found that both physical and psychological symptoms were highly prevalent (including pain, lack of energy, worry, diarrhoea, and sexual dysfunction), also found on multivariate analysis that poorer ART treatment adherence was significantly and independently associated with psychological symptom burden (Harding et al., 2010a); lower educational achievement was also significantly associated with increased global symptom burden. Further studies are needed to evaluate the impact of appropriate and aggressive symptom management on adherence, but the evidence to date suggests another strategic role for palliative care intervention in the comprehensive management of patients with HIV/AIDS, where it may be of key importance in facilitating successful disease-modifying therapy.

End-of-life care

It is important to remember that many HIV-infected persons who die in developed countries at this time may not be dying of AIDS, but rather, of one of the comorbidities described earlier. A study of 230 patients with HIV in a palliative care programme in the United States found that, of the 120 deaths, 36% died of end-stage AIDS, 19% of non-AIDS defining cancers, 18% of bacterial pneumonia or sepsis, 13% of liver failure and/or cirrhosis, 8% of cardiac of pulmonary disease, 3% of end-stage renal disease, 2% of amyotrophic lateral sclerosis, and 2% of unknown causes (Shen et al., 2005). Mortality rates from some of these causes, for example, liver failure and other end-organ failure, may be increasing even further over time.

However, despite advances in treatment for HIV, people continue to die of AIDS-related causes in the United States and abroad. Although ART is widely available in the United States, only 25% of patients with HIV have an undetectable viral load. The reasons for this are multifactorial and include issues of adherence, retention and access to care for vulnerable populations (Giordano et al., 2005). From 1996 to 2007, HIV outpatient study (HOPS) investigators found that 331 of 3 754 patients who were on treatment for at least six months died. They further found that mortality was increased for patients with a CD4+ cell count less than 200, older age, and higher serum levels of HIV RNA. They also found that mortality was increased in patients who had public insurance compared to those that had private insurance when CD4+ cell counts were greater than 200 cells/mm^3. Since the publicly-insured patients had more frequent comorbidities, including cardiac disease, renal disease and chronic hepatitis, the investigators hypothesized that these treatable comorbidities contributed to the survival disparities seen between the publicly and privately-insured group (Palella et al., 2011).

In the current era, patients who actually die from AIDS per se typically fall into one of three categories: (1) those who were diagnosed late and have never been on ART or have only been on ART for a short time but are continuing to decline due to the severity of their illness at presentation (i.e. those for whom HAART is 'too little, too late'); (2) those who may have been diagnosed when their illness was at an early stage but due to a range of medical and/or psychosocial factors have never taken ART consistently and have progressed to irreversible and then to end-stage disease; and (3) those who have lived with HIV for many years, with multiple failed treatment regimens, who now have virus resistant to all current regimens.

Occasionally, an HIV-infected patient presenting with a late stage manifestation of AIDS, such as an opportunistic infection or malignancy, will be referred to hospice without a prior documented trial of ART. This can occur if the patient is newly diagnosed with HIV and first presents with end-stage AIDS. This may also occur in patients who have had persistent difficulties with retention in HIV primary care, poor adherence to ART, and/or struggles with psychiatric illness or substance abuse. While hospice referral may be appropriate based on the patient's illness severity, it is imperative that such patients be evaluated by an HIV specialist. Even in the sickest patients, a trial of ART and therapy directed at any other co-occurring life-threatening illnesses, is warranted. Many clinicians, even in hospice and palliative settings, have witnessed what has been described as the 'Lazarus syndrome', in which 'dying' patients with AIDS were placed, sometimes for the first time, on adequate ART, and soon experienced a dramatic return to their fully functional former lives (Brashers et al., 1999).

Advance care planning is an important consideration in caring for patients living with HIV. As with other chronic illnesses, goals of care should be addressed during the course of the disease and not only during times of exacerbation or crisis. A cross-sectional survey in the United States found that patients with AIDS are less likely to have discussed advance directives with their physicians compared with other chronically ill populations (Wenger et al., 2001). The investigators also found that practitioners discussed end-of-life care with black people and Latinos less often than with white people. In addition to racial disparities, they also found that patients infected with HIV via injection drug use and those with less education communicated the least about end-of-life issues. These end-of-life conversations may need to be addressed frequently and goals may change over the course of the disease given the non-linear progression of late-stage AIDS. There is some evidence to support the notion that physicians in HIV treatment settings may be uncomfortable addressing these issues with late-stage HIV infected patients and may themselves create unnecessary barriers to effective conversations about goals of care (Curtis and Patrick, 1997).

Prognostication has also been dramatically affected by ART in the current era, raising new challenges for both HIV specialists and palliative care clinicians. Prior to HAART, mortality rates for patients diagnosed with PJP admitted to an intensive care unit ranged from 53% to 62% (Morris et al., 2003). PJP mortality in the ICU has dropped to 29% and overall PJP mortality in the HAART era has declined to 11% (Radhi et al., 2008). Mortality secondary to opportunistic infections such as disseminated *Mycobacterium avium* complex (MAC), cytomegalovirus (CMV), *Mycobacterium tuberculosis* (TB), cryptococcus infection, progressive multifocal leucoencephalopathy (PML), and toxoplasmosis encephalitis have all decreased; however, all can still increase the risk of premature death or disability.

Since the advent of HAART, prognosis for those living with HIV is no longer simply a matter of viral load, CD4+ cell count, and history of specific opportunistic infections. A study looking at mortality of patients in an HIV palliative care programme at a large urban US medical centre found that for patients with late-stage AIDS, age and markers of functional status were more predictive of mortality than CD4+ count and viral load. This study also found that half of the deaths were attributed to non-AIDS specific causes such as cancer and end-organ failure (Shen et al., 2005). There is a vital need for more prognosis-related research in the current AIDS era, to further inform practitioners about when to refer for hospice and how to predict and anticipate the end of life in patients living with AIDS.

Hospice admission appropriateness

In the United States, hospice for most patients is a government-supported programme of comprehensive home-based services for end-of-life care. Eligibility for the programme requires that two physicians attest that the patient's life expectancy is 6 months or less if the disease runs its expected course. Prognostication is imprecise, of course, and physicians rely on predictive patient characteristics that have been endorsed based on limited data and experience. The most recent hospice admission criteria for patients with HIV/AIDS in the United States, along with those for other non-cancer diagnoses, were written by the National Hospice and Palliative Care Organization (NHPCO, formerly NHO) in 1996. These included: a CD4+ count of less than 25cells/mm^3 or viral load greater than 100 000 copies/mL, CNS lymphoma, untreated or refractory wasting, disseminated MAC, PML, systemic lymphoma, visceral Kaposi sarcoma, renal failure without dialysis, cryptosporidium infection, or refractory cerebral toxoplasmosis. In addition to meeting one more of the above criteria, patients must score less than 50% on the Palliative Performance Scale. With the advent of ART, some of these criteria are out of date, and most if not all of them could potentially be eliminated as predictors of early mortality in an individual patient by an adequate trial of appropriate ART. For this reason, patients with predictors of a short life expectancy typically are not considered eligible for hospice services unless there has been progressive disease despite ART, or the patient refuses a treatment trial.

Stopping ART and opportunistic infection prophylaxis

Despite the many guidelines in existence that address when to start ART in HIV-infected patients, there are no guidelines to inform clinicians and patients about when to stop ART or routine prophylaxis for opportunistic infections in patients with HIV at the end of life. As noted above, it is important to remember that most patients with HIV who die may not be dying of AIDS per se, but rather dying from a serious comorbid condition. This can make the decision about whether to stop ART and prophylaxis for opportunistic infections even more complex.

In general, the same decision-making process used for other medications—namely, a patient-by-patient burden versus benefit analysis—should apply to decisions about ART and prophylaxis. There are potential benefits of continuing HAART in late-stage disease, based on the assumption that continued viraemia could be associated with an increasing symptom burden. In one cohort study, more than one-third of patients who stopped ART experienced symptoms related to stopping the medication (Ahdieh

Grant et al., 2001). In late-stage disease, available regimens might only be partially active, but there is suggestion that treatment could possibly select for less fit virus even in the presence of elevated viral loads (Selwyn and Forstein, 2003). Maintaining CD4+ cell counts at higher levels also can be warranted, as it can provide protection against burdensome opportunistic infections. It is also known that peripheral viral load does not always correlate with CNS viral load (McArthur et al., 1997), and it is possible that continuing HAART may help sustain cognitive functioning and protect against HIV-associated encephalopathy or dementia (Frenkel and Mullins, 2001). Preserving mental status could have profound effects by allowing the patient with end-stage disease to remain clear about his/her goals and be a part of clinical decision-making. One could also argue in favour of the continuation of ART if there is a psychological benefit to the patient or family (e.g. the patient associates ART with a sense of well-being).

There are also reasons to consider discontinuing ART. If patient adherence was an issue prior to late-stage disease, then continuing ART might not have any therapeutic benefit and might actually contribute to patient anxiety over medication. Increased pill-burden has also been shown to be associated with decreased quality of life (Fincke et al., 1998). Continuing ART at the end of life could also contribute to drug-drug interactions between antiretroviral medication and common palliative care medications. Many ART medications need laboratory monitoring and dose adjustment which might not be consistent with end-of-life goals. Continuing ART while realizing its futility also could contribute to a type of therapeutic confusion, and therefore distract clinicians and/or patients from critical advanced care planning and end-of-life care. For patients entering into hospice or any other capitated system of care, the cost of ART may be an issue as well and might constitute a barrier to enrolling in hospice in some settings.

Terminal care

Much like any other end-stage chronic disease, the shift towards end-of-life palliation is a decision that requires much thought and collaboration between patients, families and caregivers. With HIV, there are disease-specific therapies and symptom-specific therapies that, when used together, can help manage patients' symptoms and significantly contribute to patient comfort (see Table 15.1.2). The disease-specific therapies are historically seen as justified by the effort to control the underlying disease and prolong life; however, they can contribute to patient comfort at the end of life. For instance, continuing treatment for PJP pneumonia might help treat dyspnoea, in addition to symptom–specific measures such as oxygen, opioids, and benzodiazepines. In some cases, the disease-modifying interventions may have no direct life-prolonging benefit but might help preserve quality of life in a dying patient (e.g. valganciclovir to suppress CMV and thus preserve sight in a patient with CMV retinitis); in others, they may both relieve immediate suffering, as well as prolong life (e.g. fluconazole or amphotericin B, in addition to adequate analgesics, for treatment of the odynophagia of oesophageal candidiasis, or the headache associated with cryptococcal meningitis).

Opportunities for integration

Given the complexity involved in the care of patients with HIV, whether treating symptoms when the virus is controlled or helping with advanced care planning at the end-of-life, palliative care teams can play an important role in supporting both patients and physicians throughout the disease process. For this reason, palliative care has been suggested as a useful adjunct for the treatment of patients with HIV (Greenberg et al., 2000; Selwyn, 2005). Recognizing the potential impact of integration of palliative care into routine care, the World Health Organization (WHO) has stated that 'palliative care should be incorporated as appropriate at every stage of HIV disease' (WHO, 2006). Similarly, UNAIDS guidelines state that all people living with HIV should be provided with effective palliative care throughout their treatment course (UNAIDS, 2009).

Existing programmes that incorporate palliative care into HIV care are heterogeneous, offering a variety of services, including hospital-based palliative care, outpatient palliative care clinics, home hospice services and inpatient hospice. Several have been described in the literature, including a multidisciplinary consultation team for HIV-infected patients at a large urban hospital in New York City, which helped to resolve patient symptoms (Selwyn et al., 2003), and hospital-based palliative care programmes in sub-Saharan Africa, which also improved patient-reported symptoms (Tapsfield and Jane Bates, 2011).

It is recognized that palliative care is not a substitute for provision of ART. It should be viewed as an adjunct, which when incorporated throughout the HIV disease process, can improve outcomes, as stated above. Early palliative care involvement not only improves quality of life (Davis, 2004), but also can favourably impact adherence to treatment (Ammassari et al., 2001). It is thus critical both for quality of life and potential disease outcomes and survival to prioritize palliative care integration into routine HIV care.

There are several approaches to changing the usual HIV clinical care paradigm that warrant further exploration. First, sound, rigorously designed clinical trials comparing integrated HIV palliative care to usual HIV clinical care must be tested to establish the impact of the integrated services on treatment outcomes, patient satisfaction, and cost. Second, approaches to ensuring early access to palliative care expertise in HIV care settings need to be examined. Finally, further research will be needed into the value of early palliative care involvement in discussion about advance directives and goals of care in HIV-infected populations.

Developing countries

As of 2009, 33 million people were living with HIV worldwide (UNAIDS, 2009). Availability of ART in resource-limited settings is increasing—over 4 million people are on ART in low- and middle-income countries—and as a result, the number of persons living with HIV in these areas is expected to grow (UNAIDS and WHO, 2009). Although ART is available, the choice of different regimens is limited by cost. The regimens available frequently have increased toxicity and side effect profiles, and are drugs that have already been phased out in developed country settings (e.g. stavudine and zidovudine). The ageing of the AIDS epidemic that has been seen in the developed world has begun to be reflected in developing countries as well. A recent modelling study found that, in South Africa, HIV infections in the elderly will increase by 50% in the next 15 years. With increasing access to HAART in developing countries, there are 20% fewer people dying of HIV-related

causes in 2009 than in 2004, suggesting that the same phenomena of a growing population of ageing long-term HIV survivors, with increasingly complex care needs over time, may emerge there as well (Hontelez et al., 2011).

It was estimated that 9.5 million people were still in need of HIV treatment in 2008 worldwide, and though this number is an improvement, it still highlights the overwhelming disparities in access to treatment between resource-poor and resource-rich countries. This delay in treatment leads to increased early mortality, increased rates of opportunistic illnesses, and increasing rates of tuberculosis (WHO et al., 2009). In efforts to promote starting treatment earlier, the 2009 WHO guidelines changed the threshold for starting HAART from 200 cells/mm^3 as stipulated in the 2006 guidelines, to 350 cells/mm^3 regardless of symptoms. Recognizing the significant toxicity of stavudine, especially with regards to lipodystrophy and peripheral neuropathy, the 2009 WHO guidelines also recommended phasing out stavudine and using alternatives such as zidovudine or tenofovir as the first-line NRTI of choice (WHO, 2009).

It also has been documented that patients have high symptom burdens in resource-limited settings. A study of HIV-infected patients in South Africa in both rural ($N = 125$) and urban ($N = 396$) areas found that 56–72% had pain and that this pain was moderate to severe in about 60% of patients in both areas. Increasing age was associated with increasing pain. In addition to these unacceptable rates of pain, much of this pain was untreated or severely undertreated. The authors note that no patients were receiving strong opioids and only 3% were receiving so-called weak opioids (Mphahlele et al., 2012). Other studies also have shown that a substantial proportion of patients' symptoms are either entirely untreated or substantially undertreated (Karus et al., 2005). In addition to practitioner hesitancy to prescribe opioids, lack of access to these drugs in countries or specific facilities contributes to this inadequacy of treatment (Harding et al., 2010b). Despite WHO guidelines, many patients in resource-limited settings also remain on stavudine. Peripheral neuropathy (distal sensory polyneuropathy) is a frequent symptom seen in resource-limited settings secondary to untreated HIV infection or the use of antiretrovirals, such as stavudine. A retrospective review in South Africa found that, in patients on at least 6 months of stavudine, the incidence of peripheral neuropathy was 90.4/100 person-years in patients taking the standard dose of 40 mg of stavudine twice daily, and although this decreased with a lower dose of 30 mg, the complication of neuropathy remained unacceptably high (Pahuja et al., 2012). As options for HAART are limited in many developing countries beyond first-line and second-line regimens, it is crucial that as governments improve access that they also provide adequate resources to support adherence and retention in care.

Summary

As patients survive longer in the current HAART era, HIV infection is now a chronic disease. Ironically, this new longevity has increased the risks of other co-occurring diseases and related complications. As co-morbid conditions such as cardiovascular, pulmonary, renal, and liver disease; malignancy; frailty; and neurocognitive disorders all increase in this population, they contribute significantly to patients' pain and symptom burden. Unlike in the 1980s and early 1990s when HIV infection was primarily a rapidly fatal, narrowly stereotypic illness, the current treatment era has changed and expanded the scope of palliative care needs for this population. Advance care planning also has become more complicated with longer and non-linear trajectories at the end of life. In addition to an ageing population, there are significant disparities still present in timely HIV diagnosis, treatment access, and outcomes. There is an overwhelming need to develop and study new models of care for chronic HIV disease that take into account these disparities and complicated co-morbidities. Integrating palliative care into routine HIV care not only improves patients' quality of life, but also has the potential to significantly impact mortality. In the early years of the AIDS epidemic, HIV care and palliative care were inseparable. Over a period of less than two decades, these two fields have both evolved rapidly, and in many ways diverged following the rapid advances in HIV treatment and the changing clinical manifestations of HIV disease. Once again, the rationale for integrating of HIV care and palliative care is strong and compelling. For effective disease management, improved symptom burden and quality of life, better care coordination, and facilitation of end-of-life care, palliative medicine has much to offer to the care of patients with HIV/AIDS in the HAART era. It is incumbent upon both HIV and palliative care providers to identify and help create opportunities for this re-integration.

Acknowledgement

The authors would like to thank Ms Tami Rivera for her expert assistance with manuscript preparation.

Online materials

Complete references for this chapter are available online at <http://www.oxfordmedicine.com>.

References

Ammassari, A., Murri, R., Pezzotti, P., et al. (2001). Self-reported symptoms and medication side effects influence adherence to highly active antiretroviral therapy in persons with HIV infection. *Journal of Acquired Immune Deficiency Syndromes*, 28, 445–449.

Ellis, R.J., Rosario, D., Clifford, D.B., et al. (2010). Continued high prevalence and adverse clinical impact of human immunodeficiency virus-associated sensory neuropathy in the era of combination antiretroviral therapy: the CHARTER Study. *Archives of Neurology*, 67, 552–558.

Karus, D., Raveis, V.H., Alexander, C., et al. (2005). Patient reports of symptoms and their treatment at three palliative care projects servicing individuals with HIV/AIDS. *Journal of Pain and Symptom Management*, 30, 408–417.

Mathews, W.C., McCutchan, J.A., Asch, S., et al. (2000). National estimates of HIV-related symptom prevalence from the HIV Cost and Services Utilization Study. *Medical Care*, 38, 750–762.

Merlin, J.S., Cen, L., Praestgaard, A., et al. (2012a). Pain and physical and psychological symptoms in ambulatory HIV patients in the current treatment era. *Journal of Pain and Symptom Management*, 43, 638–645.

Mills, E.J., Barnighausen, T., and Negin, J. (2012). HIV and aging—preparing for the challenges ahead. *The New England Journal of Medicine*, 366, 1270–1273.

Onen, N.F. and Overton, E.T. (2011). A review of premature frailty in HIV-infected persons; another manifestation of HIV-related accelerated aging. *Current Aging Science*, 4, 33–41.

Palella, F.J., Jr., Baker, R.K., Moorman, A.C., et al. (2006). Mortality in the highly active antiretroviral therapy era: changing causes of death and disease in the HIV outpatient study. *Journal of Acquired Immune Deficiency Syndromes*, 43, 27–34.

Panel on Antiretroviral Guidelines for Adults and Adolescents (2012). *Guidelines for the use of Antiretroviral Agents in HIV-1-Infected Adults and Adolescents*. [Online] Department of Health and Human Services. Available at <http://aidsinfo.nih.gov/contentfiles/lvguidelines/adultandadolescentgl.pdf>.

Piketty, C., Selinger-Leneman, H., Grabar, S., et al. (2008). Marked increase in the incidence of invasive anal cancer among HIV-infected patients despite treatment with combination antiretroviral therapy. *AIDS*, 22, 1203–1211.

Selwyn, P.A. (2005). Palliative care for patient with human immunodeficiency virus/acquired immune deficiency syndrome. *Journal of Palliative Medicine*, 8, 1248–1268.

Simms, V.M., Higginson, I.J., and Harding, R. (2011). What palliative care-related problems do patients experience at HIV diagnosis? A systematic review of the evidence. *Journal of Pain and Symptom Management*, 42, 734–753.

Womack, J.A., Goulet, J.L., Gibert, C., et al. (2011). Increased risk of fragility fractures among HIV infected compared to uninfected male veterans. *PLoS One*, 6, e17217.

World Health Organization (2006). *Palliative Care for People Living with HIV/AIDS: Clinical Protocol for the WHO European Region*. Geneva: World Health Organization.

Caring for the patient with advanced chronic obstructive pulmonary disease

Graeme M. Rocker, Joanne Michaud-Young, and Robert Horton

Introduction to caring for the patient with advanced chronic obstructive pulmonary disease

Chronic obstructive pulmonary disease (COPD) is an increasingly significant source of morbidity and mortality worldwide (Mannino and Buist, 2007). Despite under-diagnosis in early stages (the British Lung Foundation has referred to these patients as 'the hidden millions'), COPD is already the third leading cause of death in the United States and will be at this rank globally by 2020.

Historically, there has been an unjustified sense of nihilism towards treating the advanced stages of COPD. Although a phrase heard so often from physicians—'there is nothing more we can do for you'—may be seen as abandonment, it can imply a lack of knowledge and expertise in treating the myriad of distressing symptoms as the disease advances. Clinicians also experience frustration with the lack of accessible health system resources to ensure the provision of adequate care, and even helplessness when their prescribed biomedical treatments fail to alleviate symptoms in any appreciable way (Young et al., 2012a).

Given the considerable physical and psychosocial consequences of advanced COPD (Rocker et al., 2009), patients and families can be devastated by the message that there is nothing more to be done. To reduce the likelihood of this outcome, health professionals need a continual 're-thinking' of models of care and clinical interventions, and strong encouragement to provide the ongoing support needed by patients and families. This process can overcome the pervasive sense of professional nihilism that currently undermines efforts and worsens outcomes.

COPD is not 'just' a lung disease, but rather a complex systemic illness complicated by considerable psychosocial effects. As the illness advances, patients experience increasing symptom burden that also results in increasing stress for their family caregivers. Effective overall management requires complex, personalized interventions and proactive, collaborative models of care that address not only dyspnoea as the predominant symptom but also issues of hope, social isolation, strained relationships, and lack of responsive advance care planning. Our current health-care systems place a disproportionate focus on the provision of acute and facility-based services, which does little to address the complex needs of these patients and families who are for the most part housebound.

Primary care clinicians with whom patients and families have long-standing therapeutic relationships play a pivotal role throughout the trajectory of COPD (Young et al., 2012a). When patients' increasing symptom burden limits their ability to get out of their homes for non-emergent assessment, these crucial primary care services become less accessible and the care of patients with advanced and end-stage COPD becomes increasingly 'fragmented, episodic and reactive' (Crawford et al., 2013). Within this fragmented care framework, it is difficult to establish the extent of care provided by primary care physicians, specialist physicians, and hospice services (Horton et al., 2013). Patients are often caught in a cycle: without a better alternative, they may present repeatedly to the emergency room, to be admitted for aggressive care, and discharged back to a system that initially failed to meet their needs (Bailey, 2004). While the usual recorded admission diagnosis is acute exacerbation of COPD (AECOPD), the true precipitants of such presentations are often much more complex.

In this chapter, after briefly discussing conventional treatments, we highlight some newer understandings and approaches to care for advanced COPD. This includes a description of new information regarding the perception of dyspnoea that informs a rational approach to some innovative treatments, particularly for advanced disease. Subsequent sections focus on the use of individualized COPD 'action plans' (for AECOPD and for 'dyspnoea crises'), the value of engaging patients and their families in meaningful advance care planning dialogue, and the efficacy of newer models of care that employ the above interventions and aim to bridge the gap between chronic disease management and palliative care. In the final section, we review the use of opioids as a treatment for dyspnoea that is refractory to conventional COPD treatment.

Conventional COPD treatments

The goals of conventional management of COPD have changed little in recent years and professional society practice guidelines and consensus statements adequately outline standard approaches

(Marciniuk et al., 2011; Qaseem et al., 2011). Newer drug delivery devices and longer-acting agents have improved both patients' compliance and outcomes. While improvements in symptomatology may appear modest when assessed in clinical setting (especially in advanced disease), it is important that patients be encouraged to remain compliant with these treatments because they have been shown to significantly improve important clinical outcomes (Aaron et al., 2007; Calverley et al., 2007).

Inhaled therapy

Inhaled bronchodilator therapy should be optimized as per clinical practice guidelines (Marciniuk et al., 2011; Qaseem et al., 2011). Various formulations and delivery devices are available (metered-dose inhalers and spacers, dry powder inhalers, or wet nebulizers). Inhaler technique should be assessed to ensure that a patient is able to use a device effectively. In general, for patients with advanced disease, the combination of a long-acting anticholinergic, such as daily tiotropium, with an 'as needed' short-acting beta-agonist is a standard initial approach For the occasional patient who is unable to tolerate a long-acting anticholinergic, or when these agents are unavailable, a short-acting anticholinergic (ipratropium bromide) can be taken by metered dose inhaler and a spacer at a dose of up to 4–6 puffs four times daily. For many patients with advanced COPD, the addition of a combination inhaler containing a long-acting beta-agonist (LABA) and an inhaled corticosteroid (ICS) to a long-acting anticholinergic agent provides benefit in terms of symptom management and quality of life (Aaron et al., 2007; Calverley et al., 2007). As patients' symptoms become increasingly complex and beyond the range of inhaled therapy, other interventions will be required to optimize and preserve quality of life for as long as possible.

Systemic therapy

Theophyllines

Although theophylline-like medications have long been prescribed and are known for their effects on bronchodilation, the advent of newer and more selective inhaled LABA medications have provided clinicians with more effective alternatives. The effects of methylxanthines on bronchodilation are relatively weak and they are now considered a third-line treatment, notwithstanding some recent evidence that suggests new uses for this old drug. For example, theophylline has been shown to have beneficial anti-inflammatory effects and can reduce oxidative stresses that are increasingly recognized as a feature of COPD (Barnes, 2008). Nonetheless, side effects continue to be an issue and the adverse effects often outweigh benefits for many patients. Risks of toxicity through interactions with some antibiotics (e.g. clarithromycin) also pose potential limitations to their use and the need to monitor blood levels can be especially difficult for the many patients who are housebound as a result of their advanced disease.

Phosphodiesterase 4 (PDE$_4$) inhibitors

The emergence of PDE$_4$ inhibitors marks the first new COPD therapy in nearly 20 years. These drugs have been shown to reduce key inflammatory cells and mediators, but they do not have bronchodilator properties and their effect on patients' perception of dyspnoea is modest at best. Although they may be a viable option for those patients with moderate to severe COPD who have a chronic bronchitis phenotype, and who experience frequent exacerbations despite optimized therapies, their side effect profile continues to present challenges for many patients. The potential for side effects has tempered some clinicians' initial enthusiasm for their use. The most commonly reported adverse effects include diarrhoea, nausea, headache, and weight loss. The potential for gastrointestinal toxicity suggests that the PDE$_4$ inhibitors should be used with caution in cachectic patients.

Corticosteroids

Systemic steroids are not recommended for long-term use due to negative side effects and lack of compelling data demonstrating significant benefit (Pauwels et al., 2001). Nevertheless, despite this lack of data showing efficacy, some patients perceive symptomatic benefit and a trial of a long-acting steroid may be considered for the individual patient. Provided that continued assessment reveals benefits that outweigh risks, it is reasonable to ensure that patients, especially those with end-stage disease, are not denied a reasonable treatment approach that may provide them with an improvement in symptom control.

Oxygen therapy

During acute exacerbations of COPD

The use of oxygen in an AECOPD, especially for patients with known baseline hypercarbia, should be carefully controlled. A recent randomized trial demonstrated excess mortality in patients treated with uncontrolled oxygen en route to hospital (Austin et al., 2010) and the dangers of excess use of oxygen have been recognized since the 1960s (Campbell, 1960). It is critically important to choose the appropriate delivery device. The safest approach is to use a Venturi mask to supply an inspired oxygen concentration (FiO$_2$) of 24% or 28% to maintain a SpO$_2$ close to 89%. Inappropriately high FiO$_2$ (a risk with using nasal prongs in patients retaining CO$_2$) can cause a further increase in PaCO$_2$ by several mechanisms. The most significant effect is through worsening of V/Q mismatch via reversal of established pulmonary hypoxic vasoconstriction. Lesser effects are attributed to a lower minute ventilation through reduced hypoxic drive (for some patients), and reverse of the Haldane effect that causes displacement of CO$_2$ from more oxygenated haemoglobin into plasma.

Long-term oxygen therapy (LTOT)

For patients who are hypoxaemic, LTOT is prescribed for its benefits in reducing morbidity and mortality. Eligibility criteria vary between and within countries. While beneficial for many, LTOT can interfere with self-image and limit patients to their homes, and thus restrict activities that might otherwise contribute to a better quality of life (Eaton et al., 2002). While some patients will dislike the technical focus on machines, oxygen readings, or on unacceptable limitations, others adapt and endure, benefiting in some cases from improved health-related quality of life (Eaton et al., 2002).

Supplemental oxygen for the mildly hypoxaemic patient

Based on current evidence (Abernethy et al., 2010; Uronis et al., 2011), oxygen therapy for mild hypoxemia (i.e. PaO$_2$ > 55 mmHg without evidence of end-organ damage or PaO$_2$ > 60 mmHg with evidence of end-organ damage) cannot be recommended for routine use. Patients and caregivers often request oxygen in this setting and need to be helped to understand that their level of dyspnoea does not necessarily equate with 'oxygen starvation'. Nonetheless a therapeutic trial of oxygen may be indicated in the hospice setting for treatment of patients with persistent dyspnoea despite maximal therapy (see other treatments for refractory dyspnoea below).

Managing acute exacerbations

Exacerbations of COPD are defined as a sustained worsening of the patient's respiratory symptoms from his or her usual stable state, which is beyond normal day-to-day variations and is acute in onset (Anthonisen et al., 1987). Exacerbations of COPD are associated an accelerated decline in lung function, impaired quality of life, and increased mortality. The most commonly reported symptoms are worsening shortness of breath, increased cough (with or without increased sputum production), and a change in sputum colour. Other signs and symptoms include wheeze, chest tightness, fatigue, decreased appetite, and for some, change in mood. As COPD progresses to advanced stages, the frequency of acute exacerbations increases. The damage to lung tissue and subsequent effects on symptom burden make it important to act quickly when an AECOPD occurs. Those patients at high risk of frequent episodes should be provided with a written 'action plan' as per professional society guidelines to ensure that they can activate treatments at home when they observe or experience signs and symptoms consistent with an AECOPD. It is vitally important to provide focused education in terms of when to activate the plan. Access to a help line has also been beneficial in this regard (Rice et al., 2010). In addition to adjustment of medications, this action plan may involve the use of bi-level positive airway pressure (BiPAP). BiPAP has become a standard of care for patients presenting with hypercarbic respiratory failure and should be considered as an intervention that can also provide symptomatic relief, where this fits with overall goals of care.

COPD: symptom burden related to dyspnoea

Dyspnoea is nearly universal in patients with COPD and in those with advanced illness. The symptom often is refractory to conventional treatments (Elkington et al., 2005; Horton and Rocker, 2010). The significant physical, emotional, social, and/or spiritual/existential suffering associated with the context of 'total dyspnoea' has been acknowledged only recently (Abernethy and Wheeler, 2008; Parshall et al., 2012). Dyspnoea is defined as the subjective and usually unpleasant experience of discomfort with breathing (American Thoracic Society, 1999). For many patients, dyspnoea pervades all aspects of their lives and is a significant source of disability that can profoundly affect quality of life. As dyspnoea progresses, increasing disability can render patients housebound and at risk for profound social isolation (Elkington et al., 2005). The relative social isolation that comes with advanced disease may help explain COPD as an independent risk factor for development of depression (Schane et al., 2008). Effective treatment initiatives need to address not just the physical, but also the psychosocial and existential suffering that is so pervasive and damaging for both patients and their family caregivers (Gysels and Higginson, 2009; Simpson et al., 2010).

The recent appreciation of a neurobiological component to dyspnoea (von Leupoldt et al., 2008) also offers support for interventions that extend conventional therapies. Functional magnetic resonance imaging scanning has provided new insights into the central perception of dyspnoea. The amygdala and anterior insular cortex are activated (von Leupoldt et al., 2008; Parshall et al., 2012), particularly when dyspnoea and fear coexist. Fear, anxiety,

and panic are common in advanced COPD (Gore et al., 2000; Gudmundsson et al., 2005). Anxiolytics seem relatively unhelpful in the management of dyspnoea (Rose et al., 2002; Simon et al., 2010), but may be useful for treating a coexisting anxiety disorder that can worsen dyspnoea symptoms.

Fear, anxiety, and panic, when unrecognized, underestimated, and untreated, can cause overwhelming 'dyspnoea crises' the occurrence of which may augment fear of death when dyspnoea worsens (Bailey, 2001, 2004; Booth et al., 2003). These crises are defined in a recent American Thoracic Society (ATS) consensus statement (Mularski et al., 2013) as a 'sustained and severe resting breathing discomfort that occurs in patients with advanced, often life-limiting illness and overwhelms the patient and caregivers' ability to achieve symptom relief'. Understanding the components of these crises in individual patients is key to effective management. An example of a patient-specific 'action plan' that includes tips for managing 'dyspnoea crisis' is provided later in this chapter. Several professional societies have now recognized the need to provide adequate palliation for patients struggling with refractory dyspnoea (Mahler et al., 2010; Marciniuk et al., 2011; Mularski et al., 2013). The Canadian Thoracic Society (CTS) (Marciniuk et al., 2011) has provided suggestions for a 'start low go slow' titration schedule for opioids, an approach supported by recent clinical trial data (Rocker et al., 2013).

Current approaches to the management of dyspnoea in advanced COPD

The CTS has recently released a clinical practice guideline (Marciniuk et al., 2011) (available via <http://www.copdguidelines.ca>) that encapsulates an evidence-based approach to the management of dyspnoea (see Fig. 15.2.1). This guideline (Marciniuk et al., 2011) builds on the concept of the dyspnoea ladder described some years ago (Rocker et al., 2007) and emphasizes a stepwise approach to palliation of refractory dyspnoea using conventional therapies, non-pharmacological approaches, and carefully initiated and titrated opioids. In advanced COPD, conventional therapies should be maintained and optimized, however the symptomatic benefit realized by these biomedical approaches may wane and additional supportive initiatives may be required.

Neuromuscular electrical stimulation and chest wall vibration

Neuromuscular electrical stimulation and chest wall vibration techniques can be effective and data from some recent RCTs suggest that they may be promising adjuncts to conventional treatment. They are discussed in more detail in a recent clinical practice guideline (Marciniuk et al., 2011) but use in the context of specialist palliative care is likely to be limited.

Patient self-management education

Self-management programmes tend to include disease-specific education, promotion of healthy lifestyles, along with tips on how to conserve energy and to manage emotional symptoms. They may include the use of an 'action plan' that helps patients to decide when to initiate antibiotics and/or oral corticosteroids early in the course of an impending AECOPD (Trappenburg et al., 2009; Bischoff et al., 2010; Walters et al., 2010). The aims

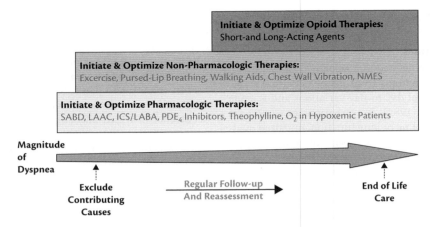

Fig. 15.2.1 Comprehensive approach to management of dyspnoea in patients with advanced COPD.
ICS, inhaled corticosteroids; LAAC, long-acting anticholinergics; LABA, long-acting beta-2 agonists; NMES, neuromuscular electrical stimulation; O_2, oxygen; PDE_4, phosphodiesterase 4; SABD, short-acting bronchodilators.
Reproduced with permission from Marciniuk, D. D. et al. for the Canadian Thoracic Society COPD Committee Dyspnea Expert Working Group, Managing dyspnea in patients with advanced chronic obstructive pulmonary disease: A Canadian Thoracic Society clinical practice guideline, *Canadian Respiratory Journal*, Volume 18, Issue 2, pp.1–10, Copyright © 2011 Pulsus Group Inc. All rights reserved. Source: data from O'Donnell DE et al. Canadian Thoracic Society recommendations for management of chronic obstructive pulmonary disease—2007 update, *Canadian Respiratory Journal*, Volume 14, Supplement B, pp.5B–32B, Copyright © 2007; O'Donnell DE et al. Canadian Thoracic Society recommendations for management of chronic obstructive pulmonary disease—2008 update—highlights for primary care, *Canadian Respiratory Journal*, Volume 15, Supplement A, pp.1A–8A, Copyright © 2008; and Rocker G et al., Advanced chronic obstructive pulmonary disease: Innovative approaches to palliation, *Journal of Palliative Medicine*, Volume 10, pp.783–97, Copyright © 2007.

of such programmes are to hasten recovery (Wilkinson et al., 2004), reduce morbidity, and health-care utilization (Bourbeau et al., 2004). Professional societies have espoused the use of 'action plans', but emphasize the need for *effective* education and reinforcement (Nici and ZuWallack, 2012). Recent randomized trials in Canada (Bourbeau et al., 2003), the United States (Rice et al., 2010), and Europe (Casas et al., 2006) have confirmed the efficacy of action plans within a broader model of self-management. Reductions (by approximately 40%) in emergency room visits and hospital readmission rates were similar in the three studies. A meta-analysis of self-management education (1066 patients, eight trials) has confirmed improvements in health status and reduction in hospital admissions (Effing et al., 2007). A recent trial of patient self-management was terminated early due to increased mortality in the intervention cohort (Fan et al., 2012). The reasons for increased mortality in this study are not clear and any potential for harm will need further study.

Pulmonary rehabilitation

The use of pulmonary rehabilitation to address dyspnoea and related symptoms in advanced COPD is supported by a substantial body of evidence including a Cochrane review (Lacasse et al., 2002). These programmes can ameliorate dyspnoea and enhance exercise tolerance, functional capacity and health-related quality of life. They also reduce health-care utilization (Bourbeau et al., 2003, 2004). Pulmonary rehabilitation 'is designed to reduce symptoms, optimize functional status, increase participation and reduce health-care costs through stabilizing or reversing systemic manifestations of the disease' (Nici et al., 2006). Exercise is central to pulmonary rehabilitation and may interrupt the 'spiral of disability' (Polkey and Moxham, 2006). Effects can wane over time (Soicher et al., 2011), however, for housebound patients, opportunities to improve symptoms and function inevitably fade. Patients should be referred for pulmonary rehabilitation well before this point.

The traditional approach to pulmonary rehabilitation has included 6–12 weeks of facility-based, individualized exercise training, self-management education, nutritional counselling, and psychosocial support when patients are stable and at their baseline. Some now advocate for initiating these programmes during an acute admission (Eaton et al., 2009). Social aspects of these programmes should not be underestimated and some improvements are associated with relief from ongoing anxiety and depression that occurs in the absence of changes in lung function (Nici et al., 2010; Harrison et al., 2011).

As an alternative to a facility-based approach to pulmonary rehabilitation, Maltais et al. (2008) have demonstrated equivalent benefit of home-based pulmonary rehabilitation. This concept will likely be explored further as a component of more community-based and integrated care.

The American Thoracic Society has defined integrated care as 'a continuum of patient-centred services organized as a care delivery value chain for patients with chronic conditions with the goal of achieving the optimal daily functioning and health status for the individual patient and to achieve and maintain the individual's independence and functioning in the community' (Nici and ZuWallack, 2012). Discussions of goals of care and advance care planning and provision of palliative care should be logical and complimentary components of this continuum (Reticker et al., 2012).

Addressing gaps in care through integrated care systems

Much has been written about the need for alternative models of care to address the needs of patients and caregivers who are living with advanced COPD (Simpson and Rocker, 2008; Booth et al., 2011a; Fromer, 2011; Ortiz and Fromer, 2011). Given that patients and family caregivers have repeatedly given voice to their unmet needs (Rocker et al., 2008; White et al., 2011; Crawford et al.,

2013), it is incumbent upon health professionals to build comprehensive, integrated programmes of care that can respond more appropriately to these needs. Implementation of disease specific self-management strategies has shown some efficacy at reducing emergency room utilization and hospital admissions (Bourbeau et al., 2003, Rice et al., 2010). However, augmentation of usual care by 'à la carte' addition of these programmes in the absence of a well thought out, comprehensive, integrated approach is likely to fall short of optimal effectiveness and efficiency. Important elements to consider include robust physician support, a detailed plan that is based on patient-driven goals of care and includes an individualized 'action plan' to deal with crisis symptoms in the home (Horton, 2013).

Fromer has stated that 'chronic care for COPD must reach beyond the primary care practice into patients' lives in the community on one hand, and into practices' linkages with specialty, ER and inpatient care on the other' (Fromer, 2011). One example of an innovative programme that embodies this philosophy is the INSPIRED programme in Halifax, NS, Canada. An acronym for 'Implementing a Novel and Supportive Program of Individualized Care for Patients and Families Living with Respiratory Disease', INSPIRED brings together a multidisciplinary team to address the needs of patients and families living with advanced COPD. Eligible patients are identified during hospital admission and upon discharge are enrolled in a structured programme that provides dedicated case management orchestrated by a skilled respiratory therapist (RT) educator who also acts as a care coordinator across care transitions. The care coordinator has robust support from fellow RTs, a pulmonary specialist with interest and expertise in community-based care in advanced COPD, and a spiritual care practitioner to address advance care planning issues. Patients are followed in their homes with bi-weekly visits spanning over a period of approximately 4 months. Emphasis is placed on providing proactive care through home-based education and support. Important elements of the programme include disease self-management education and advance care planning, help with navigating the local health-care system and gaining access to allied support services, improved communication with other health-care providers, and the provision of individualized action plans for both AECOPD and dyspnoea crisis.

INSPIRED has forged strong links with local primary care teams and palliative care programmes to improve the integration of care for patients living with advanced COPD in the community. Preliminary analysis of an initial cohort (Young et al., 2012b) continues and of 74 patients who completed the full programme revealed that participation in INSPIRED was associated with a 70% reduction in emergency room visits and length of hospital stay for those admitted (Graeme M. Rocker, personal communication, 31 January 2013).

Even with the best available home supports and detailed action plans, avoiding the emergency room may be impossible for some patients and families who are overwhelmed by panic and conditioned by years of reliance on the hospital when in crisis. A recent evaluation of home-based palliative care for patients with advanced COPD, found that despite access to comprehensive medical support that included after hours physician response, some patients continued to turn repeatedly to the emergency room when symptoms escalated rapidly (Horton et al., 2013).

Referrals to hospice/palliative care services may be seen by some as the most efficient way of addressing unmet needs in end-stage COPD. These services can be helpful in some cases. As they refine and adapt their programmes to address the needs of those with chronic non-cancer illness, however, it is important to recognize that the needs of the population with advanced COPD cannot be addressed by hospice/palliative care services in isolation from other elements of care that reflect best practices in COPD management (von Gunten, 2011).

The ideal care framework for advanced COPD combines the strongest elements of primary care and specialist expertise with implementation of an individualized and flexible multidisciplinary care approach. This approach should encompass education about disease progression and prognosis, emotional and practical support for caregivers, and treatments that integrate chronic disease management strategies with palliation of progressive symptoms. In addition, it is important to provide counselling about advance care planning and end-of-life decision-making, and assistance with practical interventions aimed meeting patient and family goals as illness progresses and death nears.

National support for such strategies are in their infancy in the United States and Canada, but are further advanced in the United Kingdom where there are clearly delineated standards and appointment of physician-leaders with responsibilities in both hospital and community settings.

Examples of an expanded approach used in the United Kingdom were recently described by Booth et al. (2011a). The 'Breathlessness Intervention Service' (BIS) has been established in Cambridge, United Kingdom, as a programme that focuses on patient-identified needs, regardless of diagnosis. BIS attends to symptoms and uses a flexible approach responsive to patient and carer(s), supplemented by education, and support. (Rocker et al., 2007; Booth et al., 2011a). The essence of the philosophy is to offer individualized evidence-based non-pharmacological interventions, along with conventional therapies (Bausewein et al., 2008). These include anxiety management (relaxation, visualization, and meditation techniques), positive psychological support, and attention to national guidelines standards, and COPD research objectives and best practices (Booth et al., 2006). In early assessments, participants indicated the importance they attached to having their concerns addressed (Booth et al., 2006), plus benefit to both patients and health-care systems as assessed through stages of the United Kingdom's Medical Research Council framework for complex interventions. Evaluation of the programme continues (Farquhar et al., 2009; Booth et al., 2011b; Farquhar et al., 2011) (Fig. 15.2.2).

Communication and advance care planning

Conventional systems of care often are characterized by a lack of timely and comprehensive care planning and communication that involves both patient and family, and key health professionals. As COPD becomes more advanced and numerous clinicians contribute to care, the responsibility to communicate with the patient and family about goals of care, including goals for end-of-life care, may become so diffused that no one ultimately takes on this role (Gott et al., 2009). Important discussions about advance care planning and end-of-life care may not occur because clinicians are unsure about who should initiate these conversations, as

---

Action Plan for Shorness of Breath (dyspnea)
Created for: [Patient Name +/− ID number]
Date: [Insert date plan was created]

A good morning routine to minimize shortness of breath first thing in the morning:

• Take 5 breaths from your incentive spirometer (slowly open airways). Use 4 time daily as needed
• Huffing/cough to clear your airway. Do your pursed-lip breathing if this helps
• Use your blue puffer, gray handihaler, and purple puffers as directed (don't forget to use your aerochamber and rinse after your purple puffer). Your blue puffer may be used as often as every four hours as needed
• Take your long-acting opioid medication [insert name, dose] as directed

---

When more short of breath than usual:

• With a slight increase in your shortness of breath at rest (not a result of infection or "crisis"), you can use an extra [insert dose] of your opioid syrup every 1–2 hours as needed for 'breakthrough' dyspnea between your regular doses
• For predictable shortness of breath with activity (i.e. getting up, dressed, bathed), time these activities ½ hour after your puffers and opioid dosing

---

For "crisis" shortness of breath (not due to infection) comes on suddenly, catches you by surprise:

• Use your hand-held fan and do pursed-lip breathing. Try recovery positions
• Use 2 puffs of your blue puffer (with aerochamber) or try your nebule instead
• Adjust oxygen flow from __ to __ litres/min for 10–15 mins only then re-adjust back to ___
• Take your anti-anxiety medication [insert name, dose], 1 tablet under the tongue
• If not setting, use Fentanyl, 12.5 ug from pre-prepared syringe. Let liquid dissolve under the tongue. Repeat in 10 mins if still not settling and call 911

For flare ups of COPD with increased sputum volume and mucky colour, use antibiotics and prednisone as per your COPD action plan.

Fig. 15.2.2 Sample of a personalized action plan for shortness of breath.
Reproduced with permission from Graeme M. Rocker and Deborah Cook, 'INSPIRED' Approaches to Better Care for Patients with Advanced COPD, *Clinical and Investigative Medicine*, Volume 36, Issue 3, e114–e120, Copyright © 2013 CIM.

well as where and when. Among the barriers to effective advanced care planning (Patel et al., 2012) identified by physicians are prognostic unpredictability/uncertainty, difficulty in identifying an 'end stage' in COPD, the potential to erode patients' hope, time constraints, inadequate communication skills (Knauft et al., 2005; Goodridge, 2006; Gott et al., 2009; Spence et al., 2009), and the possibility that the goals of such communication may conflict with those of chronic disease management (Gott et al., 2009). Two other factors include patients'/families' 'natural ageing' view of declining quality of life in advancing COPD (Pinnock et al., 2011) and clinicians' awareness of the lack of adequate palliative support for these patients no matter what is communicated. If these barriers are not recognized, the result may be that conversations either do not happen or are less than adequate. To help prevent this outcome the INSPIRED programme has incorporated an in-home 'advance care planning' component.

To realise the potential benefits of effective care planning, its intent must be understood. The *Respecting Choices* model (Gundersen Lutheran Medical Foundation, Inc., LaCrosse, WI), defines *advance care planning* as an organized ongoing process of communication to help an individual understand, reflect upon, and discuss goals, values, and beliefs for future his/her future care (Patel et al., 2012) (including health-care decisions). In contrast to

the 'ongoing process' orientation of this definition, more often than not, advanced care planning is reduced to a clinician-centred, one time 'code status' discussion that tends to occur during an illness crisis (Barnard, 2002) and in a suboptimal setting (e.g. emergency room or intensive care unit) (Patel et al., 2012). When patients have not previously considered or discussed their values and care preferences in terms of quality of life, dignity, respect, concerns about dying, perceptions of care, and who they might choose as a substitute decision-maker, being asked to do so in an already emotionally charged crisis atmosphere can add unnecessary suffering. It is hardly conducive to making an 'informed choice' and thus can heighten the potential for inadequate or erroneous representation of patients' care related values/preferences.

The ethical principles of informed choice and respect for individual autonomy in the context of COPD require clinicians to talk with patients, and those they choose to include, about their goals of care before major illness crises occur. The discussion should be revisited as the illness advances to ensure the care plan remains current. A skilled, self-reflective facilitator, relational communication, a focus on uncertainty/hope, attention to readiness and current care concerns, targeted information/education, inclusion of the substitute decision-maker, and contextual sensitivity are important elements for effective advanced care planning discussions. When patients are invited to reflect on their COPD experiences, hopes, and fears, clinicians are more likely to understand the personal values and perspectives that can help shape care plan relevant across the illness trajectory. In addition to their illness experiences, hopes, and fears, it is important to explore what provides patients' 'quality of life' and what they understand by terms such as personal dignity and respect. Patients may use phrases like 'no heroics', 'I don't want to be a vegetable', or 'I don't want to be kept alive on machines'. Clarifying exactly what prompts these comments and what the patient envisions in relation to them is also an important part of advanced care planning. Information about what is involved with various life-sustaining interventions as well as their potential burdens/benefits can help patients focus their preferences to better guide substitute decision-makers and clinicians. Taking time to ensure understanding and provide adequate emotional/existential support during and after these conversations is also an important aspect of effective advanced care planning.

Incapacitating dyspnoea, increasing dependency, isolation-induced social death, and profound uncertainty-related anxiety punctuate the experience of many of these patients and their informal caregivers/families. The burden of such symptoms demand advanced care planning that includes information (explanation plus burdens and benefits) on the range of potential life-sustaining treatment options as well as comfort measures including palliation of dyspnoea and anxiety through to the end of life. Topics to be covered should include cardiopulmonary resuscitation (including common complications and poor survival statistics), non-invasive ventilation (such as BiPAP), intubation and conventional mechanical ventilation, life-sustaining medications, intravenous hydration and/or nutrition, the role of feeding tubes and dialysis, and the meaning of comfort measures. Recent publications have addressed the role of non-invasive ventilation and how it may (or may not) fit with patients' overall goals of care (Curtis et al., 2007; Sinuff, 2011). Perhaps the most important element of every advanced care planning discussion is emphasizing the team's commitment to ongoing *care/non-abandonment* of the patient and family no matter what goals of care they set.

Ultimately the timing, setting, and manner in which advanced care planning occurs should be based on the needs of the patient and family or substitute decision-maker rather than those of health-care providers or institutions. Deciding 'when' to initiate such discussions is a matter of clinical judgement but should be informed by recognition of disease specific triggers that suggest the seriousness of the disease and might signal a time to engage the patient and family in advanced care planning:

◆ forced expiratory volume in 1 second less than 30%, oxygen dependence

◆ one or more AECOPD hospital admissions in the last year

◆ weight loss/cachexia

◆ decreased functional status

◆ increasing dependence on others

◆ age greater than 70

◆ lack of additional therapeutic options (Patel et al., 2012).

Health professionals also express confusion about the identity of the most appropriate person to initiate advance care planning

discussions with a patient and family. Competence and experience are key—professional discipline less so. Tasking other interested, skilled members of the health-care team to take on advance care planning responsibilities is a logical option, given the lack of time available to most physicians. Regardless of who facilitates the discussion, the final step in effective patient-centred advanced care planning includes collaborating with physicians and other members of the patient's health-care team so that care preferences ascertained through competent advanced care planning guide decision-making and impact outcomes. Patient preferences may change after hospitalization (Janssen et al., 2012), and advance care planning policies and strategies need to reflect and accommodate such possibilities.

The value of timely, effective advance care planning cannot be overstated. These discussions can help patients and loved ones begin to prepare themselves emotionally for illness progression. In terms of potential impact, sensitive, timely advance care planning may increase the likelihood that a patient's end-of-life care wishes will be known and followed. This can decrease the stress for family members and potential for complicated grief following the death: it also may decrease ethical distress and dilemmas for staff, and increase satisfaction with care for all concerned (Wright et al., 2008).

When patients with COPD more fully understand the range and implications of life-sustaining treatments available, they tend to choose fewer life-sustaining procedures or at most a time-limited trial of specific life-sustaining interventions. This lowers the rates of intensive care admissions and the costs associated with the final weeks of a patient's life (Au et al., 2006). For all these reasons, ethical care for these patients calls for ACP.

In summary, advance care planning as a patient-centred, ongoing process of adjusting goals of care is much more than a means to an end (Sudore and Fried, 2010). It is about improving care throughout the illness trajectory, not just at end of life.

Opioid therapy for dyspnoea in COPD

An increasing body of evidence supports the use (and safety) of opioids for refractory dyspnoea in patients with advanced COPD (see also Chapter 8.2). Nevertheless, long-held biases about the risk of opioid-induced respiratory depression continue to limit more widespread acceptance by physicians (Rocker et al., 2012) despite recommendations for their use in several recent professional society statements and/or clinical practice guidelines (Lanken et al., 2008; Mahler et al., 2010; Marciniuk et al., 2011) and despite qualitative studies indicate efficacy and acceptability from patient and caregiver perspectives (Rocker et al., 2012). Physicians in general practice, internal medicine, palliative care and chest medicine have suggested that lack of education and knowledge concerning opioids are among the greatest barriers to opioid use in advanced COPD (Rocker et al., 2012). They also worried about possible censure for prescribing opioids in this context. These physicians distinguished opioid prescribing for cancer for which clear guidelines endorse use and prescribing for dyspnoea in advanced COPD, for which many believed that opioids are not seen as 'standard of care' (Rocker et al., 2012).

Data from recently completed or ongoing clinical trials of opioid therapy for dyspnoea are encouraging with benefit outweighing side effects and patients finding them beneficial over the longer term

(Currow et al., 2011; Rocker et al., 2013). In a Canadian trial, the side effects were minimal for most patients, and outweighed by benefit. Patients made choices to continue with opioids based on improvements to quality of life, or to dyspnoea or both (Rocker et al., 2013).

In essence, both existing data and extensive clinical experience suggest these opioid drugs should be part of the treatment armamentarium for dyspnoea that is refractory to standard therapy. Our own clinical trial experience suggests that an initial 'start low, go slow' approach works well (Marciniuk et al., 2011; Rocker et al., 2013), and helps patients gain confidence with this medication. Often patients are reticent to try opioids, associating them with impending death or being fearful of side effects. Sensitive and careful explanations can usually diffuse concerns (Rocker et al., 2012, 2013). Once the daily requirements of an immediate-release preparation (e.g. morphine syrup 1 mg/mL) are established through a gentle titration schedule, patients can move on to a sustained-release preparation taken daily or twice daily with additional immediate-release opioid for 'breakthrough' dyspnoea.

Dyspnoea seems to respond to comparatively lower doses of opioids than pain. If one opioid preparation is not well tolerated, alternatives are available and can be tried. As newer formulations and modes of delivery of fast-acting lipophilic opioids become available, there will be new opportunities to incorporate these preparations into patient care plans (Horton and Rocker, 2010) that seek to provide patients and caregivers with the means to control episodic and frightening dyspnoea crises (Rocker, 2012). Clinicians should be aware that current product monographs continue to counsel explicitly against use in setting of lung disease, this despite the absence of any supporting evidence.

Conclusions

Health-care systems are faced with the need to care for an ageing population significantly burdened with chronic illnesses and frailty (Lynn, 2008; Murray and Sheikh, 2008). As the prevalence of COPD rises, more patients and families will live with the burdens of advanced or 'end-stage' COPD than ever before. Specific interventions can ease the illness burden associated with advanced COPD and models of care that employ interventions and holistic approaches to care can further improve patient and family outcomes. The move towards an integrated care approach to COPD will help patients and their families reach informed decisions about their care throughout the trajectory of COPD. Intensive medical treatment focused on increasing survival and holistic, supportive, and palliative approaches focused on quality of life are no longer mutually exclusive within the spectrum of care; the emphasis often simply changes over time. If we seek to provide care that is truly patient-centred, transitions within this spectrum should occur seamlessly and provide safe and effective care 'from beginning to end' (Partridge, 2003).

References

Aaron, S.D., Vandemheen, K.L., Fergusson, D., et al. (2007). Tiotropium in combination with placebo, salmeterol, or fluticasone-salmeterol for treatment of chronic obstructive pulmonary disease: a randomized trial. *Annals of Internal Medicine*, 146, 545–555.

Abernethy, A.P., McDonald, C.F., Frith, P.A., et al. (2010). Effect of palliative oxygen versus room air in relief of breathlessness in patients with refractory dyspnoea: a double-blind, randomised controlled trial. *The Lancet*, 376, 784–793.

Abernethy, A.P. and Wheeler, J.L. (2008). Total dyspnoea. *Current Opinion in Supportive and Palliative Care*, 2, 110–113.

American Thoracic Society (1999). Dyspnea. Mechanisms, assessment, and management: a consensus statement. *American Journal of Respiratory and Critical Care Medicine*, 159, 321–340.

Anthonisen, N.R., Manfreda, J., Warren, C.P., Hershfield, E.S., Harding, G.K., and Nelson, N.A. (1987). Antibiotic therapy in exacerbations of chronic obstructive pulmonary disease. *Annals of Internal Medicine*, 106, 196–204.

Au, D.H., Udris, E.M., Fihn, S.D., McDonell, M.B., and Curtis, J.R. (2006). Differences in health care utilization at the end of life among patients with chronic obstructive pulmonary disease and patients with lung cancer. *Archives of Internal Medicine*, 166, 326–331.

Austin, M.A., Wills, K.E., Blizzard, L., Walters, E.H., and Wood-Baker, R. (2010). Effect of high flow oxygen on mortality in chronic obstructive pulmonary disease patients in prehospital setting: randomised controlled trial. *BMJ*, 341, c5462.

Bailey, P.H. (2001). Death stories: acute exacerbations of chronic obstructive pulmonary disease. *Qualitative Health Research*, 11, 322–338.

Bailey, P.H. (2004). The dyspnea-anxiety-dyspnea cycle—COPD patients' stories of breathlessness: 'It's scary/when you can't breathe'. *Qualitative Health Research*, 14, 760–778.

Barnard, D. (2002). Advance care planning is not about 'getting it right'. *Journal of Palliative Medicine*, 5, 475–481.

Barnes, P.J. (2008). Frontrunners in novel pharmacotherapy of COPD. *Current Opinion in Pharmacology*, 8, 300–307.

Bausewein, C., Booth, S., Gysels, M., and Higginson, I. (2008). Non-pharmacological interventions for breathlessness in advanced stages of malignant and non-malignant diseases. *Cochrane Database of Systematic Reviews*, 11, CD005623.

Bischoff, E.W., Hamd, D.H., Sedeno, M., et al. (2010). Effects of written action plan adherence on COPD exacerbation recovery. *Thorax*, 66, 26–31.

Booth, S., Bausewein, C., and Rocker, G. (2011a). New models of care for advanced lung disease. *Progress in Palliative Care*, 19, 254–263.

Booth, S., Farquhar, M., Gysels, M., Bausewein, C., and Higginson, I. J. (2006). The impact of a breathlessness intervention service (BIS) on the lives of patients with intractable dyspnea: a qualitative phase 1 study. *Palliative Supportive Care*, 4, 287–293.

Booth, S., Moffat, C., Farquhar, M., Higginson, I.J., and Burkin, J. (2011b). Developing a breathlessness intervention service for patients with palliative and supportive care needs, irrespective of diagnosis. *Journal of Palliative Care*, 27, 28–36.

Booth, S., Silvester, S., and Todd, C. (2003). Breathlessness in cancer and chronic obstructive pulmonary disease: using a qualitative approach to describe the experience of patients and carers. *Palliative Supportive Care*, 1, 337–344.

Bourbeau, J., Julien, M., Maltais, F., et al. (2003). Reduction of hospital utilization in patients with chronic obstructive pulmonary disease: a disease-specific self-management intervention. *Archives of Internal Medicine*, 163, 585–591.

Bourbeau, J., Nault, D., and Dang-Tan, T. (2004). Self-management and behaviour modification in COPD. *Patient Education and Counseling*, 52, 271–277.

British Thoracic Society/The Primary Care Respiratory Society UK (n.d.). *Improving and Integrating Respiratory Services in the NHS*. Available at: http://www.networks.nhs.uk/nhs-networks/impress-improving-and-integrating-respiratory>.

Calverley, P.M., Anderson, J.A., Celli, B., et al. (2007). Salmeterol and fluticasone propionate and survival in chronic obstructive pulmonary disease. *The New England Journal of Medicine*, 356, 775–789.

Campbell, E.J. (1960). Respiratory failure: the relation between oxygen concentrations of inspired air and arterial blood. *The Lancet*, 2, 10–11.

Casas, A., Troosters, T., Garcia-Aymerich, J., et al. (2006). Integrated care prevents hospitalisations for exacerbations in COPD patients. *European Respiratory Journal*, 28, 123–130.

Crawford, G.B., Brooksbank, M.A., Brown, M., Burgess, T.A., and Young, M. (2012). The unmet needs of people with end-stage chronic obstructive pulmonary disease: recommendations for change in Australia. *Internal Medicine Journal*, 43(2), 183–190.

Currow, D.C., McDonald, C., Oaten, S., *et al.* (2011). Once-daily opioids for chronic dyspnea: a dose increment and pharmacovigilance study. *Journal of Pain and Symptom Management*, 42, 388–399.

Curtis, J.R., Cook, D.J., Sinuff, T., *et al.* (2007). Noninvasive positive pressure ventilation in critical and palliative care settings: understanding the goals of therapy. *Critical Care Medicine*, 35(3), 932–939.

Eaton, T., Garrett, J.E., Young, P., *et al.* (2002). Ambulatory oxygen improves quality of life of COPD patients: a randomised controlled study. *European Respiratory Journal*, 20, 306–312.

Eaton, T., Young, P., Fergusson, W., *et al.* (2009). Does early pulmonary rehabilitation reduce acute health-care utilization in COPD patients admitted with an exacerbation? A randomized controlled study. *Respirology*, 14, 230–238.

Effing, T., Monninkhof, E.M., van der Valk, P.D., *et al.* (2007). Self-management education for patients with chronic obstructive pulmonary disease. *Cochrane Database of Systematic Reviews*, 4 CD002990.

Elkington, H., White, P., Addington-Hall, J., Higgs, R., and Edmonds, P. (2005). The healthcare needs of chronic obstructive pulmonary disease patients in the last year of life. *Palliative Medicine*, 19, 485–491.

Fan, V.S., Gaziano, J.M., Lew, R., *et al.* (2012). A comprehensive care management program to prevent chronic obstructive pulmonary disease hospitalizations: a randomized, controlled trial. *Annals of Internal Medicine*, 156, 673–683.

Farquhar, M.C., Higginson, I.J., Fagan, P., and Booth, S. (2009). The feasibility of a single-blinded fast-track pragmatic randomised controlled trial of a complex intervention for breathlessness in advanced disease. *BMC Palliative Care*, 8, 9.

Farquhar, M.C., Prevost, A.T., McCrone, P., *et al.* (2011). Study protocol: Phase III single-blinded fast-track pragmatic randomised controlled trial of a complex intervention for breathlessness in advanced disease. *Trials*, 12, 130.

Fromer, L. (2011). Implementing chronic care for COPD: planned visits, care coordination, and patient empowerment for improved outcomes. *International Journal of Chronic Obstructive Pulmonary Disease*, 6, 605–614.

Global Initiative for Chronic Obstructive Pulmonary Disease (2010). *Global Strategy for the Diagnosis, Management, and Prevention of Chronic Obstructive Pulmonary Disease. Updated 2010.* [Online] Available at: <http://www.goldcopd.org>.

Goodridge, D. (2006). People with chronic obstructive pulmonary disease at the end of life: a review of the literature. *International Journal of Palliative Nursing*, 12, 390–396.

Gore, J.M., Brophy, C.J., and Greenstone, M.A. (2000). How well do we care for patients with end stage chronic obstructive pulmonary disease (COPD)? A comparison of palliative care and quality of life in COPD and lung cancer. *Thorax*, 55, 1000–1006.

Gott, M., Gardiner, C., Small, N., *et al.* (2009). Barriers to advance care planning in chronic obstructive pulmonary disease. *Palliative Medicine*, 23, 642–648.

Gudmundsson, G., Gislason, T., Janson, C., *et al.* (2005). Risk factors for rehospitalisation in COPD: role of health status, anxiety and depression. *European Respiratory Journal*, 26, 414–419.

Gysels, M.H. and Higginson, I. J. (2009). Caring for a person in advanced illness and suffering from breathlessness at home: threats and resources. *Palliative Supportive Care*, 7, 153–162.

Harrison, S.L., Greening, N.J., Williams, J.E., Morgan, M.D., Steiner, M.C., and Singh, S.J. (2011). Have we underestimated the efficacy of pulmonary rehabilitation in improving mood? *Respiratory Medicine*, 106, 838–844.

Horton, R. (2013). Reducing emergency room utilization in end-stage COPD—feasible or fantasy? *Chronic Respiratory Disease*, 10, 49–54.

Horton, R. and Rocker, G. (2010). Contemporary issues in refractory dyspnoea in advanced chronic obstructive pulmonary disease. *Current Opinion in Supportive and Palliative Care*, 4, 56–62.

Horton, R., Rocker, G., Dale, A., Young, J., Hernandez, P., and Sinuff, T. (2013). Implementing a palliative care trial in advanced COPD: a feasibility assessment (The COPD IMPACT Study). *Journal of Palliative Medicine*, 16, 67–73.

Janssen, D.J., Spruit, M.A., Schols, J.M., *et al.* (2012). Predicting changes in preferences for life-sustaining treatment among patients with advanced chronic organ failure. *Chest*, 141, 1251–1259.

Knauft, E., Nielsen, E.L., Engelberg, R.A., Patrick, D.L., and Curtis, J.R. (2005). Barriers and facilitators to end-of-life care communication for patients with COPD. *Chest*, 127, 2188–2196.

Lacasse, Y., Brosseau, L., Milne, S., *et al.* (2002). Pulmonary rehabilitation for chronic obstructive pulmonary disease. *Cochrane Database of Systematic Reviews*, 3, CD003793.

Lanken, P.N., Terry, P.B., Delisser, H.M., *et al.* (2008). An official American Thoracic Society clinical policy statement: palliative care for patients with respiratory diseases and critical illnesses. *American Journal of Respiratory and Critical Care Medicine*, 177, 912–927.

Lynn, J. (2008). Palliative care beyond cancer: reliable comfort and meaningfulness. *BMJ*, 336, 958–959.

Mahler, D.A., Selecky, P.A., Harrod, C.G., *et al.* (2010). American College of Chest Physicians consensus statement on the management of dyspnea in patients with advanced lung or heart disease. *Chest*, 137, 674–691.

Maltais, F., Bourbeau, J., Shapiro, S., *et al.* (2008). Effects of home-based pulmonary rehabilitation in patients with chronic obstructive pulmonary disease: a randomized trial. *Annals of Internal Medicine*, 149, 869–878.

Mannino, D.M. and Buist, A.S. (2007). Global burden of COPD: risk factors, prevalence, and future trends. *The Lancet*, 370, 765–773.

Marciniuk, D.D., Goodridge, D., Hernandez, P., *et al.* (2011). Managing dyspnea in patients with advanced chronic obstructive pulmonary disease: a Canadian Thoracic Society clinical practice guideline. *Canadian Respiratory Journal*, 18, 1–10.

Mularski, R.A., Reinke, L.F., Carrieri-Kohlman, V., *et al.* (2013). An Official American Thoracic Society Workshop Report: Assessment and Palliative Management of Dyspnea Crisis. *American Journal of Respiratory and Critical Care Medicine*, 10(5), S98–106.

Murray, S.A. and Sheikh, A. (2008). Palliative care beyond cancer: care for all at the end of life. *BMJ*, 336, 958–959.

Nici, L., Donner, C., Wouters, E., *et al.* (2006). American Thoracic Society/European Respiratory Society statement on pulmonary rehabilitation. *American Journal of Respiratory and Critical Care Medicine*, 173, 1390–1413.

Nici, L., Lareau, S., and Zuwallack, R. (2010). Pulmonary rehabilitation in the treatment of chronic obstructive pulmonary disease. *American Family Physician*, 82, 655–660.

Nici, L. and Zuwallack, R. (2012). An official American Thoracic Society workshop report: the integrated care of the COPD patient. *Proceedings of the American Thoracic Society*, 9, 9–18.

Ortiz, G. and Fromer, L. (2011). Patient-centered medical home in chronic obstructive pulmonary disease. *Journal of Multidisciplinary Healthcare*, 4, 357–365.

Parshall, M.B., Schwartzstein, R.M., Adams, L., *et al.* (2012). An official American Thoracic Society statement: update on the mechanisms, assessment, and management of dyspnea. *American Journal of Respiratory and Critical Care Medicine*, 185, 435–452.

Partridge, M.R. (2003). Patients with COPD: do we fail them from beginning to end? *Thorax*, 58, 373–375.

Patel, K., Janssen, D.J., and Curtis, J.R. (2012). Advance care planning in COPD. *Respirology*, 17, 72–78.

Pauwels, R.A., Buist, A.S., Calverley, P.M., Jenkins, C.R., and Hurd, S.S. (2001). Global strategy for the diagnosis, management, and prevention of chronic obstructive pulmonary disease. NHLBI/WHO Global Initiative for Chronic Obstructive Lung Disease (GOLD). Workshop summary. *American Journal of Respiratory and Critical Care Medicine*, 163, 1256–1276.

Pinnock, H., Kendall, M., Murray, S.A., *et al.* (2011). Living and dying with severe chronic obstructive pulmonary disease: multi-perspective longitudinal qualitative study. *BMJ*, 342, d142.

Polkey, M.I. and Moxham, J. (2006). Attacking the disease spiral in chronic obstructive pulmonary disease. *Clinical Medicine*, 6, 190–196.

Qaseem, A., Wilt, T.J., Weinberger, S.E., *et al.* (2011). Diagnosis and management of stable chronic obstructive pulmonary disease: a clinical practice guideline update from the American College of Physicians, American College of Chest Physicians, American Thoracic Society, and European Respiratory Society. *Annals of Internal Medicine*, 155, 179–191.

Reticker, A.L., Nici, L., and Zuwallack, R. (2012). Pulmonary rehabilitation and palliative care in COPD: two sides of the same coin? *Chronic Respiratory Disease*, 9, 107–116.

Rice, K.L., Dewan, N., Bloomfield, H.E., *et al.* (2010). Disease management program for chronic obstructive pulmonary disease: a randomized controlled trial. *American Journal of Respiratory and Critical Care Medicine*, 182, 890–896.

Rocker, G. (2012). Palliation of dyspnea. *Chronic Respiratory Disease*, 9, 49–50.

Rocker, G., Young, J., Donahue, M., Farquhar, M., and Simpson, C. (2012). Perspectives of patients, family caregivers and physicians about the use of opioids for refractory dyspnea in advanced chronic obstructive pulmonary disease. *Canadian Medical Association Journal*, 184, E497–504.

Rocker, G.M., Dodek, P.M., and Heyland, D.K. (2008). Toward optimal end-of-life care for patients with advanced chronic obstructive pulmonary disease: insights from a multicentre study. *Canadian Respiratory Journal*, 15, 249–254.

Rocker, G.M., Simpson, A.C., Young, J., *et al.* (2013). Opioid therapy for refractory dyspnea in patients with advanced chronic obstructive pulmonary disease: patients' experiences and outcomes. *Canadian Medical Association Open Access Journal*, 1, E27–E36.

Rocker, G.M., Sinuff, T., Horton, R., and Hernandez, P. (2007). Advanced chronic obstructive pulmonary disease: innovative approaches to palliation. *Journal of Palliative Medicine*, 10, 783–797.

Rocker, G.M., Young, J., and Simpson, A.C. (2009). Advanced chronic obstructive lung disease: more than a lung disease. *Progress in Palliative Care*, 17, 117–125.

Rose, C., Wallace, L., Dickson, R., *et al.* (2002). The most effective psychologically-based treatments to reduce anxiety and panic in patients with chronic obstructive pulmonary disease (COPD): a systematic review. *Patient Education and Counseling*, 47, 311–318.

Schane, R.E., Woodruff, P.G., Dinno, A., Covinsky, K.E., and Walter, L.C. (2008). Prevalence and risk factors for depressive symptoms in persons with chronic obstructive pulmonary disease. *Journal of General Internal Medicine*, 23, 1757–1762.

Simon, S.T., Higginson, I.J., Booth, S., Harding, R., and Bausewein, C. Benzodiazepines for the relief of breathlessness in advanced malignant and non-malignant diseases in adults. *Cochrane Database of Systematic Reviews*, 1, CD007354.

Simpson, A.C. and Rocker, G.M. (2008). Advanced chronic obstructive pulmonary disease: rethinking models of care. *Quarterly Journal of Medicine*, 101, 697–704.

Simpson, A.C., Young, J., Donahue, M., and Rocker, G. (2010). A day at a time: caregiving on the edge in advanced COPD. *International Journal of Chronic Obstructive Pulmonary Disease*, 5, 141–151.

Sinuff, T. (2011). Noninvasive positive pressure ventilation for acute respiratory failure: What role is there for patients declining intubation or choosing palliation?. *Progress in Palliative Care*, 19, 223–229.

Soicher, J.E., Mayo, N.E., Gauvin, L., *et al.* (2011). Trajectories of endurance activity following pulmonary rehabilitation in COPD patients. *European Respiratory Journal*, 39, 272–278.

Spence, A., Hasson, F., Waldron, M., *et al.* (2009). Professionals delivering palliative care to people with COPD: qualitative study. *Palliative Medicine*, 23, 126–131.

Sudore, R.L. and Fried, T.R. (2010). Redefining the 'planning' in advance care planning: preparing for end-of-life decision making. *Annals of Internal Medicine*, 153, 256–261.

Trappenburg, J.C., Koevoets, L., De Weert-Van Oene, G.H., *et al.* (2009). Action plan to enhance self-management and early detection of exacerbations in COPD patients; a multicenter RCT. *BMC Pulmonary Medicine*, 9, 52.

Uronis, H., Mccrory, D.C., Samsa, G., Currow, D., and Abernethy, A. (2011). Symptomatic oxygen for non-hypoxaemic chronic obstructive pulmonary disease. *Cochrane Database of Systematic Reviews*, 6, CD006429.

Von Gunten, C. (2011). Who should palliative care be asked to see? *Journal of Palliative Medicine*, 14, 2–3.

Von Leupoldt, A., Sommer, T., Kegat, S., *et al.* (2008). The unpleasantness of perceived dyspnea is processed in the anterior insula and amygdala. *American Journal of Respiratory and Critical Care Medicine*, 177, 1026–1032.

Walters, J.A., Turnock, A.C., Walters, E.H., and Wood-Baker, R. (2010). Action plans with limited patient education only for exacerbations of chronic obstructive pulmonary disease. *Cochrane Database of Systematic Reviews*, 5, CD005074.

White, P., White, S., Edmonds, P., *et al.* (2011). Palliative care or end-of-life care in advanced chronic obstructive pulmonary disease: a prospective community survey. *British Journal of General Practice*, 61, e362–370.

Wilkinson, T.M., Donaldson, G.C., Hurst, J.R., Seemungal, T.A., and Wedzicha, J.A. (2004). Early therapy improves outcomes of exacerbations of chronic obstructive pulmonary disease. *American Journal of Respiratory and Critical Care Medicine*, 169, 1298–1303.

Wright, A.A., Zhang, B., Ray, A., *et al.* (2008). Associations between end-of-life discussions, patient mental health, medical care near death, and caregiver bereavement adjustment. *Journal of the American Medical Association*, 300, 1665–1673.

Young, J., Donahue, M., Simpson, A.C., Farquhar, M., and Rocker, G. (2012a). Using opioids to treat dyspnea in advanced COPD: attitudes and experiences of family physicians and respiratory therapists. *Canadian Family Physician*, 58, e401–407.

Young, J., Simpson, A.C., Demmons, J., Conrad, W., and Rocker, G. (2012b). Evaluating the impacts of 'INSPIRED': a new outreach program for patients and families living with advanced chronic obstructive pulmonary disease (COPD). *American Journal of Respiratory and Critical Care Medicine*, 185, A3732.

Advanced heart disease

Steven Z. Pantilat, Anthony E. Steimle, and Patricia M. Davidson

Introduction to advanced heart disease

Heart disease is the leading cause of death in the developed world (Lindenfeld et al., 2010; Go et al., 2013). Heart failure (HF) is the final common pathway of many cardiac conditions, a major source of morbidity, and the most common reason that patients with advanced heart disease present to specialists in palliative care. More than 5 million Americans, 15 million Europeans (out of a population of 900 million), and 1.5–2% of Australians have HF (Dickstein et al., 2008b; Jessup et al., 2009; National Heart Foundation of Australia and the Cardiac Society of Australia and New Zealand, 2011).

HF has been defined as:

a complex clinical syndrome with typical symptoms [such as breathlessness, oedema, and fatigue] that can occur at rest or on effort, and is characterized by objective evidence of an underlying structural abnormality or cardiac dysfunction that impairs the ability of the ventricle to fill with or eject blood (particularly during physical activity). A diagnosis of HF may be further strengthened by improvement in symptoms in response to treatment. (National Heart Foundation of Australia and the Cardiac Society of Australia and New Zealand, 2011)

> Reproduced with permission from the *Guidelines for the prevention, detection and management of chronic heart failure in Australia.* Updated July 2011, Copyright © 2011 National Heart Foundation of Australia. Extract accurate at time of press, for update to information visit <HTTP://www.heartfoundation.org.au/>.

HF is divided into two types: *systolic*, which is also called HF with reduced ejection fraction (HFREF), and *diastolic*, or HF with preserved ejection fraction (HFPEF). The term HFPEF for the latter condition is preferred by some to emphasize the importance of contributing factors other than diastolic dysfunction. Systolic HF is characterized by the occurrence of the symptoms typical of this condition in association with a low ejection fraction; although somewhat arbitrary, this usually is taken as below 40%. In diastolic HF, the typical symptoms occur in association with a relatively normal ejection fraction, typically considered to be above 50%. Within the total population with HF, the prevalence of the systolic and diastolic types is roughly equal.

It is important for clinicians to know the underlying type of HF, as treatments differ based on type (Hunt et al., 2009). Additional categorization by class and stage also is relevant (Table 15.3.1) (Criteria Committee of the New York Heart Association, 1994; Hunt et al., 2009). The New York Heart Association (NYHA) class is a particularly helpful classification, as it provides some information about symptoms, functional status, and prognosis.

HF is a chronic illness characterized by periods of relative stability punctuated by exacerbations that may require hospitalization. It is the leading cause of hospitalization among Medicare beneficiaries in the United States and an increasing cause of hospital admission in Europe and Australia (Unroe et al., 2011). While most exacerbations can be managed effectively in hospital, each exacerbation is associated with a risk of death. Half of the patients diagnosed with HF die within 5 years of first hospital admission, a prognosis worse than many cancers (Stewart et al., 2001). Between one-third and one-half of patients die suddenly, irrespective of HF stage. This potential for sudden death creates an imperative for the discussion of preferences for care from the time of initial diagnosis.

Despite the high mortality, pharmacologic treatments for HF prolong survival and improve quality of life (Hunt, 2005; Heart Failure Society of America, 2006; Dickstein et al., 2008b; Jessup et al., 2009; McDonagh et al., 2011). Most patients respond to drug therapies, and some patients with advanced illness are eligible for specialized implanted therapies, such as cardiac resynchronization therapy (CRT) using a biventricular pacemaker, mechanical circulatory support with ventricular assist devices (VADs), and implantable cardioverter defibrillators (ICDs). A very small proportion of patients meet criteria for heart transplantation and have access to this surgery.

The availability of effective treatments, however, does not prevent illness-related suffering and burden. Even with optimal medical therapy, many patients with HF experience distressing symptoms, such as pain (41–78%), breathlessness (60–88%), fatigue (69–82%), and depression (9–56%) (McCarthy et al., 1996; Levenson et al., 2000; Bekelman et al., 2009; Pantilat et al., 2012). Some interventions, such as ICDs, may decrease the incidence of sudden death, and as a result, increase the proportion of patients who live with these debilitating symptoms (Stevenson and Stevenson, 2001; Heidenreich et al., 2002).

Many patients who receive an implanted technology experience the treatment itself as highly burdensome (Dickstein et al., 2008b; Tang et al., 2010). Approaches to care concerning these interventions are rapidly evolving and underscore the importance of consultation with HF specialists in treatment planning. This input is especially valuable for patients and their families as they make decisions about whether implanted therapies align with their values and goals. As in many areas of medical practice, the legal and ethical debates surrounding these decisions are still catching up with technological innovation (Sheehan et al., 2011).

Table 15.3.1 Definition of New York Heart Association (NYHA) heart failure class and American College of Cardiology/American Heart Association (ACC/AHA) stage (Criteria Committee of the New York Heart Association, 1964; Hunt et al., 2009)

NYHA class	Definition	ACC/AHA stage	Definition
None		Stage A	Presence of heart failure risk factors but no heart disease and no symptoms
Class I	No limitation of physical activity. Ordinary physical activity does not cause undue fatigue, palpitation, or breathlessness	Stage B	Heart disease is present but there are no symptoms (structural changes in heart before symptoms occur)
Class II	Slight limitation of physical activity. Comfortable at rest, but ordinary physical activity results in fatigue, palpitation, or breathlessness	Stage C	Structural heart disease is present AND symptoms have occurred
Class III	Marked limitation of physical activity. Comfortable at rest, but less than ordinary activity causes fatigue, palpitation, or breathlessness		
Class IV	Unable to carry out any physical activity without discomfort. Symptoms of cardiac insufficiency at rest. If any physical activity is undertaken, discomfort is increased	Stage D	Presence of advanced heart disease with continued heart failure symptoms requiring aggressive medical therapy

Source: data from Hunt, S.A. et al., Focused update incorporated into the ACC/AHA 2005 Guidelines for the Diagnosis and Management of Heart Failure in Adults A Report of the American College of Cardiology Foundation/American Heart Association Task Force on Practice Guidelines Developed in Collaboration With the International Society for Heart and Lung Transplantation, *Journal of the American College of Cardiology*, Volume 53, Issue 15, pp. e1–e90, Copyright © 2009 American College of Cardiology Foundation; and Criteria Committee of the American Heart Association NYCA 1964, *Diseases of the heart and blood vessels: Nomenclature and criteria for diagnosis*, Little, Brown and Co., Boston, USA, Copyright © 1964.

The high morbidity and mortality, the risk of sudden death at all stages of illness, the availability of interventions with significant burdens, and the chronic nature of the condition create an imperative for integrating palliative care into HF disease management (Goodlin et al., 2004; Pantilat and Steimle, 2004; Adler et al., 2009; Goodlin, 2009; Davidson et al., 2010; Janssen et al., 2011). Patients with HF, and their families, agree with guidelines developed by cardiology societies around the world and endorse an approach that provides palliative care alongside optimal medical management (Selman et al., 2007a, 2007b; Dickstein et al., 2008b; Hunt et al., 2009; Jaarsma et al., 2009; Bekelman et al., 2011; McDonagh et al., 2011; McKelvie et al., 2011; National Heart Foundation of Australia and the Cardiac Society of Australia and New Zealand, 2011). Broad agreement between cardiology and palliative care specialists support this integrated approach and should encourage palliative care clinicians to reach out to cardiologists and others who care for patients with HF (Low et al., 2011). While the involvement of palliative care specialists may be very limited for patients with class I HF, perhaps focusing on advance care planning, specialists may be required on a more regular basis for patients with class III and IV disease—to help manage persistent symptoms, discuss treatment preferences and goals of care, and provide support to the patient and family.

Despite agreement about the importance of palliative care in HF management, several barriers complicate the goal of simultaneous care (Selman et al., 2007b). First, prognosis in HF can be challenging and the severity of exacerbations can be difficult to gauge. Second, many cardiologists continue to misperceive palliative care as solely focused on the end of life. Combined with a reluctance to recognize the terminal nature of HF and a lack of training in symptom management and communication about advance care planning, this view can undermine optimal care and result in referral to specialized palliative care too late to realize the full benefits. Third, palliative care specialists may lack knowledge about medical management and interventions for HF, which may

have adverse consequences for patients and further reduce the willingness of cardiologists to refer. Fourth, patients with HF are medically complex and have comorbid conditions that may require the input of other specialists, complicating efforts to integrate best practices in cardiology and palliative care. This medical complexity also may impact on key decisions, such as the deactivation and withdrawal of devices, and thereby create added challenges for inter-professional cooperation. Finally, health-care systems typically lack palliative care services for people with HF and fail to adequately coordinate services to provide simultaneous care.

Palliative care specialists should work to overcome these barriers. Important strategies include continuing education about the trajectory and management of HF, ongoing efforts to develop good collaborations with cardiology colleagues, and participation in efforts to adapt the health-care system to serve the needs of patients with HF and their families.

Managing the disease of heart failure: optimal medical therapy and interventions

It is critical for palliative care specialists to understand the medications and interventions used to manage HF, as these treatments help patients live longer, avoid hospitalization, and achieve a better quality of life. In contrast to patients with advanced cancer, those with HF typically continue disease-modifying therapies until close to death. Although the benefits and burdens of individual drugs should be appraised regularly, the withdrawal of HF treatments places patients at increased risk of acute exacerbation, worsening symptoms and earlier death. Some treatments, however, may be less appropriate at the end of life because they do not directly affect cardiac function or relieve symptoms, and may require monitoring; for example, warfarin might be appropriately discontinued in the setting of advanced illness, particularly as the risk of over-anticoagulation increases with changes in drug metabolism associated with organ failure.

Palliative care clinicians also must recognize the many reversible cardiac lesions that can cause HF and be able to discuss these with patients and their families. For example, revascularization and valvular repairs using either percutaneous or surgical techniques may improve heart function and provide significant symptom benefits. Given the complexity of these treatments, it would be ideal if all patients with advanced heart failure were referred to a cardiologist who specializes in heart failure management; through consultation, this specialist may be able to maximize and fine tune medical therapy and determine whether procedural interventions would be beneficial.

The risks, benefits, and burdens must be considered in recommending invasive treatments for HF, and patients and their families must have accurate information in order to make informed decisions. Regardless of the setting in which patients receive palliative care, understanding the role of HF medications and interventions, and their potential side effects and risks, and knowing which medications to avoid, will make the palliative care specialist best able to help patients and collaborate effectively with other clinicians.

Drug therapies for systolic heart failure (HFREF)

For patients with systolic HF, one of the cornerstones of treatment is neurohormonal blockade with an angiotensin-converting enzyme inhibitor (ACEI), an angiotensin receptor blocker (ARB), a beta blocker, and a mineralocorticoid antagonist (MRA) (Table 15.3.2). These drugs slow the progression of cardiac dysfunction, reduce mortality, and prevent hospitalization (Lindenfeld et al., 2010; McMurray et al., 2012). Diuretics also are indispensable because of their ability to reduce fluid retention; these drugs are so accepted that a trial of their impact on mortality would be impracticable and has never been done (McMurray et al., 2012). Other medications, including digoxin and the vasodilator combination

hydralazine-isosorbide dinitrate, play a role in subgroups of HF patients.

Although neurohormonal blockers and diuretics are initiated for their life-prolonging effect, they also alleviate symptoms and improve functional status. They are, therefore, appropriate late in the course of illness, including when the focus shifts exclusively to palliative care. For this reason, HF medications are often continued until the end of life, as long as the burdens of therapy are acceptable.

As noted, the potential complexity of optimal medical management of advanced HF would be best addressed if all patients had access to cardiologists, particularly those who specialize in this condition. This type of care is not available throughout most of the world, and even in developed countries, most patients with HF are cared for by primary care providers, not cardiologists or HF specialists. Nonetheless, palliative care specialists should recognize the potential value of a referral to a HF specialist, if this is possible, particularly when patients have refractory symptoms.

Diuretics

HF may manifest with fluid retention or symptoms of low cardiac output, such as fatigue, breathlessness, and altered mentation, or both. Fluid retention is associated with oedema and breathlessness due to pulmonary congestion associated with volume overload. While there are other causes of breathlessness in patients with HF, diuretic treatment to remove excess fluid is essential in most cases for symptom relief (Hunt et al., 2009). These drugs usually are given orally, but when fluid retention is severe or acute, they may be given intravenously to ensure bioavailability and improve immediacy of effect; especially if gut oedema (suggested by abdominal bloating and nausea) has set in (Hunt et al., 2009). Occasionally, use of outpatient intravenous diuretics may help avoid hospitalization. Although diuretics have not been proven to increase survival, their ability to alleviate symptoms justifies continuation and active adjustment right up until the time of death.

Table 15.3.2 Appropriateness of drugs for systolic heart failure (LVEF < 40%) based on New York Heart Association (NYHA) class and impact on key outcomes

Drug	NYHA class I	NYHA class II	NYHA class III	NYHA class IV	Survival	Hospital admissions	Functional status
Diuretic	X	+	+	+	?	↓	↑
Angiotensin-converting enzyme inhibitor	+	+	+	+	↑	↓	↑
Beta blocker	+	+	+	+	↑	↓	↑
Mineralocorticoid antagonist	X	+	+	+	↑	↓	↑
Digoxin	X	X	+	+	↔	↓	↑

X: no evidence

+: evidence for benefit

↑: improves/increases

↓: worsens/decreases

↔: no impact.

Source: data from Lindenfeld, J. et al., HFSA 2010 Comprehensive Heart Failure Practice Guideline, *Journal of Cardiac Failure*, Volume 16, Issue 6, pp. e1–e2, Copyright © 2010 Published by Elsevier Inc. and McMurray, J. J., ESC guidelines for the diagnosis and treatment of acute and chronic heart failure 2012: The Task Force for the Diagnosis and Treatment of Acute and Chronic Heart Failure 2012 of the European Society of Cardiology. Developed in collaboration with the Heart Failure Association (HFA) of the ESC, *European Journal of Heart Failure*, Volume 14, Issue 8, pp.803–69, Copyright © 2010 The European Society of Cardiology 2012. All rights reserved.

Thiazide diuretics may be sufficient in mild cases of HF, but loop diuretics such as furosemide are more potent and typically are required as HF progresses, especially if renal insufficiency is present (Faris et al., 2002; McMurray et al., 2012). Fluid retention varies and diuretic dosing should be flexible to accommodate changing disease severity, weight, symptoms, and renal function; the dose required initially to remove excess fluid may be higher than that needed chronically to maintain 'dry weight'. At all times, the correct dose is the lowest dose sufficient to maintain euvolaemia. Often, patients can be taught to make dose changes based on daily self-monitoring. For example, patients can weigh themselves daily and when their weight increases by a certain amount over their baseline weight (typically by 2 lbs or 1 kg) they can take an extra dose of furosemide daily until they return to their baseline weight.

When diuresis is inadequate with furosemide, adherence to medications and sodium restriction should be reinforced. If this fails, the dose may be raised or, if the patient is already responding well to individual doses, the frequency of dosing can be increased. Alternatively, the loop diuretic can be changed to an alternative with better oral absorption, specifically bumetanide or torsemide, on the assumption that gut oedema is present and may be interfering with absorption.

Patients who are not responding adequately to appropriately dosed loop diuretics may respond to the addition of a thiazide diuretic, such as hydrochlorothiazide or metolazone, or a potassium-sparing diuretic, such as spironolactone or eplerenone. By blocking the nephron sequentially, the combination of loop and these distally acting diuretics work synergistically to remove fluid. However, potassium loss may be either potentiated or reduced by these combinations and must be monitored closely.

ACEIs, ARBs, and hydralazine-isosorbide dinitrate

ACEIs block the conversion of angiotensin I to angiotensin II in the pulmonary vasculature and thereby inhibit the renin–angiotensin–aldosterone system. This activity results in lower arteriolar resistance and increased venous capacity, increased cardiac output, lower renovascular resistance, and increased urinary sodium excretion. Multiple studies have confirmed that these drugs are essential in the management of systolic HF because they improve symptoms by enhancing forward blood flow and slowing ventricular remodelling, and reduce adverse outcomes, including hospitalization and mortality (Dickstein et al., 2008; Hunt et al., 2009; National Heart Foundation of Australia and the Cardiac Society of Australia and New Zealand, 2011) All patients with reduced ejection fraction should receive them in the absence of contraindications. They are typically begun along with diuretics as soon as HF or a HF exacerbation is diagnosed. They are continued until close to the end of life, as long as they are tolerated and there are no significant adverse effects on blood pressure or renal function. A common side effect of ACEIs is cough, and less common but more serious reactions include hyperkalaemia, renal insufficiency, allergy, and angio-oedema. Although they are not nephrotoxic, they can cause a rise in creatinine that usually is mild and should not discourage continued use.

Patients intolerant to ACEIs should be treated with ARBs, that have been shown to have similar effects on symptoms and mortality. Patients intolerant to both ACEIs and ARBs because of hyperkalaemia or progressive renal insufficiency should receive the combination of hydralazine and isosorbide dinitrate. The downside of this combination is that it requires two medications taken multiple times a day, whereas ACEIs and ARBs are typically given once daily. In African Americans with systolic HF, the combination of hydralazine and isosorbide dinitrate, and a beta blocker, significantly reduced death and hospitalization. Treatment with these drugs should be considered for this population; there is no evidence of effectiveness in other groups. Nonetheless, palliative care clinicians may encounter patients who are receiving hydralazine and isosorbide dinitrate in addition to standard HF therapy, especially those who require treatment for persistent hypertension or refractory symptoms.

Beta blockers

Beta blockers, which block the sympathetic nervous system, were once thought to be contraindicated in HF. Now it is known that sympathetic activation, like activation of the renin–angiotensin–aldosterone system, leads to progression of systolic dysfunction and worsening of HF. Clinical trials have found that three beta blockers, bisoprolol, carvedilol, and sustained-release metoprolol succinate, markedly reduce mortality and hospitalization in patients with systolic heart failure (Packer et al., 2001; Hunt et al., 2005, 2009; Dickstein et al., 2008; Jessup et al., 2009). However, beta blockers cause improvement gradually and when started acutely may worsen HF. Hence, they are begun only after patients are stabilized and euvolaemic. Therapy is initiated at a low dose, which is increased slowly.

Beta blockers should be continued during most HF exacerbations and have been shown to benefit even patients with severe HF and NYHA class IV symptoms (Packer et al., 2001). However, they may need to be reduced or stopped for severe exacerbations, symptomatic hypotension, bradycardia, or hypoperfusion leading to end-organ dysfunction. Some patients with low cardiac output may become intolerant of beta blockers at the end of life (Hunt, 2005).

Mineralocorticoid receptor antagonists

The MRAs, spironolactone and eplerenone, block aldosterone and have been found to reduce mortality, prevent hospitalization, and improve functional class for patients with an ejection fraction of 35–40% or lower, and persistent symptoms despite beta blockers and ACEIs (Hunt et al., 2005; Dickstein et al., 2008; Hunt et al., 2009; Jessup et al., 2009). Along with beta blockers and ACEIs/ARBs, they complete 'triple therapy', the trio of agents that improve survival in HF. It is important to monitor vigilantly for hyperkalaemia, which is a common side effect and can limit use in late stage HF when renal insufficiency is more common. Baseline hyperkalaemia and creatinine clearance less than 30 mL/min are contraindications to starting these medications. If gynecomastia from spironolactone is problematic, eplerenone may be used instead.

Digoxin

Digoxin may be added to standard therapy of ACEIs, diuretics, and beta blockers for systolic HF, to improve symptoms and reduce hospitalization. It does not prolong survival and hence should not be given when symptoms are mild or absent. However, digoxin can play a role when the goals of care are palliative, particularly since it does not lower blood pressure and can be given to patients with hypotension. Beta blockers, which also lower heart rate and have a much greater benefit, should be used preferentially when slow heart rate is limiting. Because higher serum levels have been associated with worse outcomes, digoxin should be used at a low dose and usually avoided with renal insufficiency.

Drug therapies for diastolic heart failure (HFPEF)

Nearly half of all patients with HF have preserved ejection fractions. Unfortunately, to date, no medication has been found to reduce mortality and morbidity in HFPEF. Hence, treatment is empiric and focused on treating concomitant conditions according to accepted guidelines: hypertension, rhythm abnormalities, ischaemia, and oedema. This approach often leads to the use of loop diuretics, beta blockers, and ACEIs in a fashion similar to systolic HF, though potentially with differences in rate and sequence of titration, dosing, or choices of agent.

Role of intravenous inotropes

Intravenous inotropes, such as milrinone or dobutamine, can improve cardiac function and relieve symptoms associated with HF. These drugs typically are used in hospitalized patients who develop hypotension during an exacerbation of HF, as an effort is being made to optimize medical management. Ideally, one of these drugs is given for a short period of time in a monitored environment, then tapered and discontinued as cardiac functioning improves with other treatments. Long-term use increases the risk of complications and sudden death, and should be avoided if possible. When weaning is accompanied by the reappearance of hypotension, however, and there are no options for advanced therapies such as mechanical circulatory support with a VAD or heart transplant, long-term therapy may be an option (Sherrod et al., 2009; Chua et al., 2011; Taitel et al., 2012). It should be recognized that inotrope dependence is a sign of very poor prognosis and the decision to proceed with this approach means acceptance of an increased risk of complications and death in order to palliate symptoms and potentially allow discharge from the hospital (Hauptman et al., 2006). Palliative care specialists may be called upon to assist with arranging outpatient inotrope infusions; in the United States, many home health, home infusion, and hospice agencies can provide these treatments.

Medications to avoid in people with HF

Medications of all types should be introduced cautiously in patients with advanced HF due to the potential metabolic disturbances associated with the disease. Some drugs used commonly in palliative care should be avoided all together, or used with extreme caution, due to their potential for worsening fluid retention or cardiac arrhythmia. For example, non-steroidal anti-inflammatory drugs (NSAIDs), including cyclooxygenase 2 selective inhibitors, can lead to fluid retention, volume overload, and HF exacerbation. Patients with advanced HF should be told to avoid NSAIDs in over-the-counter formulations. Thiazolidinediones used for management of diabetes also can cause fluid retention and should be avoided. Many drugs may affect the QTc interval and potentially predispose to arrhythmia, among which are methadone, tricyclic antidepressants, and venlafaxine; venlafaxine also can cause hypertension. All these drugs should be used with caution in patients with HF (Krantz et al., 2009). If goals of care are solely palliative, a patient could make an informed choice to use these medications and accept a small risk in exchange for better symptom control.

Non-pharmacologic disease management

Moderate restriction of sodium intake (< 2–3 g daily) is recommended for patients with more severe symptoms in the hope of relieving volume overload and potentially allowing lower diuretic doses (Dickstein et al., 2008b). Patients prone to hyponatraemia should also limit fluid intake to less than 1.5–2 L/day.

Exercise training probably improves survival in the population with HF (Piepoli et al., 2004) and has been found to lessen symptoms, increase stamina, reduce hospitalization, and improve depression (Belardinelli et al., 2012). Some exercise interventions may be too strenuous for patients with advanced HF, but all patients should be encouraged to be as active as possible to maintain maximal functional status.

Devices and interventions

The use of devices and interventions is a rapidly evolving area of HF disease management in developed countries. These therapies have risks and benefits, and the palliative care specialist should understand each intervention in order to help patients make informed decisions and manage these devices as the end of life approaches. The following information provides a background for the palliative care specialist, but does not offer definitive indications and protocols. The palliative care specialist should collaborate closely with HF specialists and those who insert these devices.

Implantable cardioverter defibrillators

ICDs are pacemaker-like devices implanted near the clavicle to sense ventricular arrhythmias or bradycardia and treat them with pacing or internal shock. More than 10 000 are being implanted each month in the United States alone (Hammill et al., 2010). They can reduce the risk of sudden death in patients with prior resuscitated arrest and selected patients with low ejection fractions (< 30–35%) despite optimal medical therapy.

While ICDs are highly effective when life-threatening dysrhythmias occur, it is difficult to identify patients at risk prior to a first episode. When used for primary prevention, follow-up data indicate that seven lives are saved over 5 years for every 100 devices implanted (Bardy et al., 2005). After considering the relative magnitude of this benefit, the potential exchange of a sudden death for a more prolonged death, and the fact that ICDs do not improve quality of life, some eligible patients choose not to undergo implantation. For some whose quality of life is poor, or who have comorbidities that shorten survival, the opportunity to avoid sudden cardiac death may not be a priority; for others, sudden death is preferable to one that occurs as the result of progressive HF with worsening symptoms.

When patients choose to have an ICD, they should be informed that the device can be turned off if their condition deteriorates and their goals of care change. Palliative care clinicians should have a clear plan for turning off an ICD if the patient prefers. To avoid painful shocks during the phase of active dying, events that may be very distressing to patients and families, there also should be a plan to discuss, and perhaps recommend, discontinuation of the device when the end of life is perceived to be soon (Goldstein et al., 2004; Russo, 2011). Although ICD firing is uncommon at the end of life, counselling about discontinuation is a marker of quality care (Clark et al., 2011; Bonow et al., 2012).

Specialists in palliative care should be able to discuss the technical aspects and the repercussions of ICD discontinuation. Turning off individual functions of ICDs and CRT pacemakers (see below) is simple and non-invasive and can be done in a few minutes with a programmer specific to the device by a technician or clinician trained in its use. Palliative care specialists should have clear procedures for how to manage ICD deactivation, including a collaboration with the treating cardiologist and device representative who can assist in deactivating the ICD (Lampert et al., 2010; Padeletti et al., 2010). The technician places the programmer's magnet over the device in order to deactivate therapies. In medical facilities lacking electrophysiological expertise, or when a patient is at home and too ill to come to clinic, a device company representative may be available to bring a programmer to the patient and provide technical assistance to on-site personnel (e.g. home-hospice nurse) under the direction of the treating physician (Lampert et al., 2010; Padeletti et al., 2010). If these options are unavailable, hospice nurses or other clinicians may carry a magnet which when left over the device will deactivate the shock therapy function.

While deactivating the shock function of an ICD is unlikely to have any immediate impact and thus does not typically require immediate management of symptoms, it can evoke anxiety in patients who viewed this function as potentially life-saving. Addressing such concerns in advance can alleviate this anxiety. Some patients may choose to withdraw some functions of an ICD and not others. Pacing for chronic bradycardia and anti-tachycardia pacing, which can prolong life but causes no symptoms, may continue, for instance, while therapies for tachyarrhythmias or shock therapy can be stopped. The choice of these options depends on a patient's goals for prolongation and quality of life. For pacemaker-dependent patients, death may occur immediately after the pacemaker is turned off or take longer if dependence is partial. Patients and their families should be prepared for these possibilities and appropriate symptom control readied if needed. Deactivation, especially when it could lead to immediate death, may make some practitioners uncomfortable and they should be reassured this intervention is ethically appropriate (Lampert et al., 2010; Grubb and Karabin, 2011). At the same time, no provider should be compelled to deactivate a device if this is against their personal beliefs, In such situations, another provider should be found.

Cardiac resynchronization therapy

In selected patients, CRT using a biventricular pacemaker can improve symptoms and extend life. CRT acts to synchronize the contraction of opposite sides of the left ventricle when impaired native electrical conduction results in less coordinated contraction and diminished cardiac output. CRT has been shown to improve ventricular function and slow HF progression. Because it offers both symptom relief and a greater mortality reduction than ICD, CRT is a very appealing option that should be considered in eligible patients. Initially, patients shown to benefit were those with low ejection fraction, NYHA class III/IV symptoms and electrocardiographic evidence of left ventricular dyssynchrony (i.e. left bundle branch block). More recently, patients with less severe symptoms have also been found to benefit (Heidenreich et al., 2002). CRT devices are usually but not always combined with an ICD, depending on a patient's interest in preventing sudden death versus relieving symptoms. As above, patients may choose to deactivate the ICD if their goals change, or less commonly, choose to deactivate both the ICD and CRT functions.

Mechanical circulatory support/ventricular assist devices

VADs are pumps that are implanted in the chest and connected to the heart to pump blood (Fig. 15.3.1). A cable (driveline) that connects the VAD to a control device and battery exits the body through the skin. The vast majority of VADs are connected to the left ventricle (left ventricular assist device or LVAD) and only a small number are connected to the right ventricle or to both ventricles. In the United States, since 2006, approximately 4500 VADs have been placed and currently about 1500 per year are implanted (Kirklin et al., 2012). Initially, LVADs were used exclusively in patients awaiting heart transplant. This approach to LVAD use was termed 'bridge to transplant' (BTT). During the past several years, however, there has been increasing evidence to support using LVADs in patients with advanced heart disease who are not candidates for transplant. This approach is called 'destination therapy' (DT), as the LVAD is not leading to another procedure. In 2006, in the United States, 44% of LVADs were for BTT and only 15% were for DT. By 2011, the percentages had flipped and only 24% were for BTT while 34% were for DT.

In some countries, palliative care specialists are increasingly likely to help care for patients with LVADs in both the DT and BTT scenarios. They must coordinate with cardiologists and support effective self-management and hope. Patients and their families should be amply prepared for potential adverse events, including bleeding, driveline infections, thrombosis and thromboembolism, device failure, and death. They should be reassured that the LVAD can be stopped if quality of life becomes too poor (Allen et al., 2012). They should also be informed about the survival with LVADs, which currently is 80% at 1 year and 70% at 2 years and considerably worse, however, in patients who are in acute cardiogenic shock at the time of implantation. Some patients, particularly those with advanced multisystem organ failure, may be too ill to benefit from mechanical circulatory support (Peura et al., 2012).

Palliative care specialists who are asked to help care for patients with LVADs may be called upon to assist in the treatment of symptoms should patients decide to turn off the machine, or help the primary team manage complications. It is valuable to have protocols in place to address specific complications and the need to consider device withdrawal (Wiegand and Kalowes, 2007). In a study of 20 patients with LVADs as DT who were able to participate in decision-making, 17 chose to turn off the device (Brush et al., 2010). The most common reason for the decision to turn off the LVAD was a new or worsened medical condition, such as sepsis, infection, cancer, and renal failure. For all 20 patients, the time from turning off the LVAD to death was less than 20 minutes and the majority of patients died at home. Understanding the process for stopping the LVAD and having plans to manage symptoms, such as breathlessness, alleviates anxiety and provides support to patients and caregivers. Developing a clear plan to manage symptoms in the event of device failure also is critical to ensure patient comfort and dignity (MacIver and Ross, 2005; Wiegand and Kalowes, 2007; MacIver and Ross, 2012). Although not specifically studied, it is appropriate to use opioids for breathlessness and benzodiazepines for anxiety, as would be used for these symptoms in other end-of-life situations.

Surgical approaches

Surgical approaches in HF include valve replacement, myocardial revascularization, and cardiac transplantation. Although cardiac

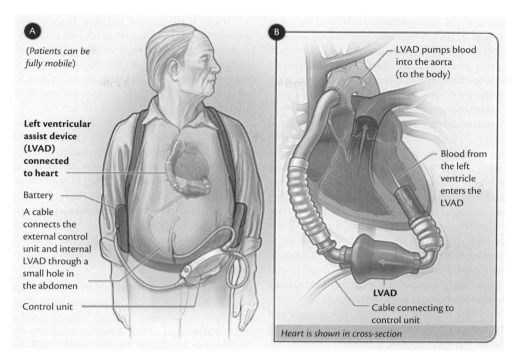

Fig. 15.3.1 Patient with a left ventricular assist device. The pump is implanted in the chest and the cable connecting it to the control unit exits the body.
Reproduced from *What Is a Ventricular Assist Device?*, National Heart, Lung and Blood Institute, U.S. Department of Health and Human Services, 2012, available from http://www.nhlbi.nih.gov/health/health-topics/topics/vad/.

transplantation is an effective option for HF, donor shortage and patient selection limit access (Mancini and Lietz, 2010; Glower, 2012). Patients who are candidates for surgery are best served by an approach that integrates palliative care, including symptom management.

Managing the symptoms of heart failure

Symptoms such as pain, dyspnoea, and fatigue are highly prevalent in patients with HF, as common as in patients with cancer, and diminish quality of life (McCarthy et al., 1996; Levenson et al., 2000; Bekelman et al., 2009; Pantilat et al., 2012). Symptoms are caused by HF itself, especially breathlessness and fatigue, but also relate to comorbid conditions common in patients with HF, such as osteoarthritis, low back pain, chronic pulmonary disease, and diabetes. A guideline jointly developed and published by the American College of Cardiology, American Heart Association, and American Medical Association includes symptom management as a key performance measure for patients with HF (Bonow et al., 2012). Because many cardiology specialists are not trained in symptom management, palliative care specialists play a key role in managing distressing symptoms for these patients.

Pain

Pain is present in up to 78% of patients with HF (Goebel et al., 2009; Pantilat et al., 2012). Pain can result from heart disease (e.g. angina), from comorbidities (e.g. peripheral neuropathy or back pain), or from interventions (e.g. implants and cardiac surgery). There are no randomized trials of treatments for pain in patients with HF. Given the prevalent aetiologies of pain and the commonalities between HF and other serious illnesses, an appropriate

general approach to pain would be modelled on other serious illnesses such as cancer. There are a few caveats to this perspective, however. As explained earlier, NSAIDs other than low-dose aspirin should be avoided in people with HF, as they cause fluid retention and can lead to HF exacerbations, and some drugs that can affect the QTc interval, such as methadone, venlafaxine and tricyclic antidepressants, should also be used with caution due to the risk of arrhythmia. Otherwise, the general approach to pain in those with advanced HF would emphasize pharmacotherapy as the mainstay therapies, and usually employ acetaminophen (paracetamol) for mild pain and opioids for moderate to severe pain. The use of these drug classes, and the so-called adjuvant analgesics, is guided by the widely published experience in the management of cancer pain.

Breathlessness

Breathlessness is a feared and distressing symptom for people with HF (see also Chapter 8.2). While breathlessness can be chronic for people with class III and IV, exacerbations of HF are typically associated with acute episodes of breathlessness that lead to emergency department visits and hospital admission. Establishing a plan with specific directions for patients and caregivers about how to respond to episodes of breathlessness is a critical role for the palliative care specialist. A practical plan and a well-educated patient and family can eliminate the use of the emergency department as the default for every episode. The complex interplay of breathlessness and anxiety mean that non-pharmacological strategies such as relaxation and breathing exercises may be of use.

Breathlessness associated with HF can result from a range of causes, including fluid congestion, leading to acute and chronic pulmonary oedema and pleural effusions, and skeletal muscle dysfunction. Optimal medical management, including titration of diuretics, is a key step in preventing and responding to both aetiologies of breathlessness. Non-pharmacological strategies such as exercise are also of importance. Large pleural effusions that persist despite best medical management can be drained with thoracentesis, if consistent with patient wishes and goals of care.

The acute onset of breathlessness from pulmonary oedema is typically managed in hospital with intravenous diuretics, supplemental oxygen, and oral nitrates. Opioids are also a useful strategy, and as with other indications, should be started at a low dose and increased slowly if needed. A similar approach can be applied to outpatient settings, including at home, although there are no data to confirm its effectiveness. Nonetheless, acute breathlessness in the home may be addressed with oral opioids, nitrates such as sublingual nitroglycerine, and oral diuretics such as furosemide. Providing the patient and caregiver with an algorithm of which medications to take, doses, and frequency, as well as clear instructions on when to call for help, may allow patients to avoid the emergency department.

Patients and caregivers should be alerted to signs of increasing pulmonary oedema, including weight gain, orthopnoea and worsening dyspnoea on exertion. If these signs gradually worsen and the patient is able to recognize them and has a plan for taking additional doses of diuretics in response, a more severe episode of breathlessness may be prevented. For chronic breathlessness, low dose opioids are effective and safe (Chua et al., 1997; Jennings et al., 2001). Supplemental oxygen plays a role in relieving breathlessness for patients who are hypoxic, but is not more effective than air for patients who are not hypoxaemic (Abernethy et al., 2010). Patients with refractory breathlessness despite optimal medical management of HF and treatment with opioids may be candidates for home intravenous inotropes, as described earlier, but the burden and risks of this approach should be carefully considered.

Oedema

Many patients with HF have chronic lower extremity oedema that can be painful and sometimes spontaneously weep. Explanation and reassurance to patients and their families is important. Limiting fluid and salt intake, and adjusting diuretics, to manage lower extremity oedema are key steps. Elevation of the legs, preferably above the level of the heart, may be helpful. Bandages and wraps for weeping lesions and blisters when oedema is severe can also provide symptomatic relief. In some instances, testicular oedema may be severe and appropriate support devices for patient comfort should be obtained.

Fatigue

Fatigue is a common symptom in patients with HF and is present in up to 82% of patients. Optimal medical management of the HF may ameliorate fatigue and other approaches can be used to target the symptom directly. The latter strategies have not been tested in the HF population, but are used in other illnesses. They include cognitive techniques to conserve energy (e.g. by pacing) and rehabilitative approaches such as special equipment (e.g. a shower chair) and therapeutic exercise. There are no studies of stimulant medications and the potential risks of these drugs in patients with severe HF limit their use. In one trial, however, caffeine at a dose equivalent to two cups of coffee improved exercise duration in patients with HF; this approach may have a role for HF patients with limited exercise tolerance (Notarius et al., 2006).

Fatigue also may be reduced if contributing factors can be safely and effectively managed. Fatigue may be related to anaemia, but routine correction of anaemia of chronic disease with blood transfusion or erythropoietin carries too much risk and is not recommended (Dickstein et al., 2008a). Similarly, obstructive sleep apnoea (OSA) can cause fatigue and may provide a target for therapy. While patients with HF are no more likely to have OSA than the age-matched general population (both have a prevalence of OSA of 2–10%), fatigue associated with obesity or refractory hypertension, should raise suspicion and prompt a work up for OSA (Sin et al., 1999, 2003). Treatment of OSA with continuous positive airway pressure (CPAP) in patients with HF can improve quality of life (McKelvie et al., 2011). Patients with advanced HF are more likely to have central sleep apnoea than the general population, but unfortunately, a trial of CPAP in these patients found no benefit of treatment (Bradley et al., 2005).

Depression

As many as half of patients with HF are depressed, and depression is associated with fatigue and poorer quality of life, as well as negative outcomes such as hospital readmission and mortality (Dracup et al., 1992; Albert et al., 2009; Bekelman et al., 2009; Johnson et al., 2012b; Pantilat et al., 2012; Rollman et al., 2012). Although a randomized trial showed that sertraline was not more effective than placebo for improving depression or cardiovascular outcomes in HF patients, depressed patients with HF would be expected to respond to treatment like other patients and should be treated with standard approaches (O'Connor et al., 2010). Based on clinical experience, selective serotonin reuptake inhibitors (SSRIs) are preferred for patients with HF; tricyclic antidepressants are associated with tachycardia and arrhythmia and should be avoided. Psychostimulants work quickly to treat depression in patients with cancer but studies are lacking in people with HF, and as noted, psychostimulants should be used with caution, if at all, due to the potential risk of arrhythmia and tachycardia. Exercise training and t'ai chi have been shown to reduce depressive symptoms in people with HF (Blumenthal et al., 2012; Redwine et al., 2012). Exercise training is especially recommended given its additional benefits of reducing fatigue.

Prognosis

Prognostication is challenging in HF. Although many cardiology specialists and patients may not consider HF a terminal illness, the prognosis is worse than for some cancers, with median survival from first admission of 5 years for both systolic HF and HFPEF (Stewart et al., 2001; Tribouilloy et al., 2008). At the same time, HF prognosis varies greatly depending on the presence of characteristics associated with worse prognosis. These markers of poor prognosis include higher NYHA class, weight loss/cachexia, advanced age, repeated hospital admissions, hyponatraemia, history of sudden death, hypotension, declining functional status, frailty, and comorbid conditions such as chronic obstructive pulmonary disease and end-stage renal disease (Harkness et al., 2012). Hence, younger patients responding well to medications who have NYHA class I/II symptoms, ICDs, and few comorbidities may have an annual mortality of 3% (Moss et al., 2009), while patients who are NYHA class IV despite optimal therapy may have an annual mortality greater than 70% (Rose et al., 2001).

There are many indices to aid in prognosis for people with HF but most are too complex to use easily at the bedside. The most commonly used and cited prognostic index in HF is the Seattle Heart Failure Model (SHF) (Levy et al., 2006; Mozaffarian et al., 2007; Kalogeropoulos et al., 2009). The SHF has five components, including demographic characteristics, medications, diuretics, devices, and laboratory values; an online calculator that is available on many portable device platforms simplifies its use, assuming the clinician has access to all the necessary data elements (<http://depts.washington.edu/shfm>). The Gold Standards Framework Prognostic Indicator Guide developed in the United Kingdom is simpler to use at the bedside and contains well established prognostic criteria, including NYHA class III or IV, a positive response to the so-called surprise question ('Would you be surprised if this patient died in the next 12 months?'), repeated hospital admissions with symptoms of HF, and difficult physical or psychological symptoms despite optimized tolerated therapy.

While either of these indices can help guide clinicians to identify patients with HF in need of specialist palliative care, neither index performed well in predicting 1-year mortality in a prospective trial (Haga et al., 2012). Nonetheless, the criteria in the Gold Standards Framework, some of which are familiar to palliative care specialists, combined with other factors associated with poor prognosis can provide guidance to patients, caregivers, and clinicians in planning for the future. The lack of sensitivity and specificity of these and other indices should not dissuade palliative care specialists from sharing with patients the best information they have about prognosis, including the fact that death can happen suddenly.

Advance care planning

A critical element of palliative care is effective communication and development of a clear plan for care (Pantilat and Steimle, 2004; Davidson, 2007). As a patient ages, the likelihood of dying from their cardiac condition or another terminal illness increases (Wiegand and Kalowes, 2007). Sadly, there are countless examples of the adverse consequences associated with inadequate communication, including needless distress and futile treatments (Quill and Holloway, 2012). To avoid these consequences, communication must be ongoing and address both present and future plans.

Advance care planning (ACP) is a patient-centred communication process allowing patients and their families to participate in discussions concerning their future care (Kirchhoff et al., 2012). The process allows patients to have their preferences known even if, at the time of crisis, they are too unwell to make decisions about their care. The term ACP is now commonly used, rather than 'advance directives'. The ACP process should involve a discussion of the patients' values and preferences regarding care, and a sharing of information that allows informed decision-making about life-sustaining and life-prolonging therapies.

Conversations about ACP can be challenging for health professionals and patients alike, and ideally, they should not take place during times of crisis (Davidson, 2007; Ahluwalia et al., 2012). It may be helpful to use models of shared decision-making, through which the individual is presented with options and collaborative decision-making is undertaken to elicit preferences (Allen et al., 2012). Religious and cultural factors should be part of the ACP process.

Because up to half of patients with HF die suddenly at any stage of illness, it is incumbent upon clinicians to discuss ACP early (Stevenson and Stevenson, 2001). Because exacerbations of HF are likely and sudden death is a real possibility, the discussion should cover patient preferences for hospitalization during exacerbations and for resuscitation in the event of cardiac arrest. When the issue is addressed openly, many patients will say that they prefer a sudden, quick and painless death from cardiac arrest and do not want to undergo resuscitation.

As discussed earlier, there are increasing numbers of individuals with implantable devices. These devices have important implications for future care and how a patient may die, and ACP is important for every patient considering an implant. ICDs are meant to prevent sudden death, and therefore, an implant may mean that a patient is more likely to die from progressive HF, with its associated symptoms of dyspnoea, fatigue, oedema, and functional decline. Among patients who have ACP conversations prior to implantation, two-thirds decide to have the device placed and one-third do not.

In those with implanted devices, ACP discussions also require consideration of device deactivation or LVAD withdrawal. The ethical and legal issues raised by deactivation of ICDs at the end of life are similar to those raised by withholding or withdrawing other life-sustaining medical interventions in other clinical settings. As discussed above, avoiding an arrhythmic death, with associated ICD activation, is often an important consideration, as device firings can cause distress to the patient and their family (Goldstein et al., 2004). To avoid this outcome, it may be appropriate for an ICD to be deactivated near the end of life, following discussion with the patient and family. There is a wide variation among individuals regarding their preferences, and this fact underscores the need to tailor and target approaches (Dev et al., 2012). The ACP process should employ open and sensitive communication with the patient and their family about prognosis and goals of care, and use reliable mechanisms for documenting patient preferences to ensure that the wishes of the patient are respected (Pantilat and Steimle, 2004).

ACP is an ongoing, iterative process and should not be considered as a single conversation or document (Davidson et al., 2007). Implicit in the process is providing psychosocial support to the family and caregivers, and ensuring communication across care settings to ensure that the patient's wishes are respected (Jaarsma et al., 2009). The conversations should focus on goals of care and not merely on specific interventions or devices. By first eliciting a patient's goals, the clinician can then help guide patients about the interventions and devices that may help achieve those goals and those that would be problematic. For example, optimizing medical management promotes better quality of life, being at home, and reduces symptoms. A patient that expresses these outcomes as goals may then be more willing and able to adhere to their medical regimen.

Psychosocial support

Patients with HF and their caregivers have the same needs for support—social, psychological, emotional, and spiritual—as those with other serious illnesses. Comprehensive palliative care should address all these issues. Many patients with HF worry about sudden death, and those with ICDs and LVADs may have concerns about the ICD firing or the LVAD failing. Patients may also worry about acute episodes of breathlessness and of suffocating. Anticipating these concerns, discussing them honestly and compassionately, eliciting and responding to questions and concerns, developing a clear plan for responding to urgent situations, and being available to the patient and caregiver may relieve anxiety and allay concerns.

Setting and approaches

The setting and approach to care will largely depend on available resources and funding models. In developed countries, the principles to be considered may include access to specialist expertise in both cardiology and palliative care; a multidimensional approach to care that considers physical, social, psychological, cultural, and existential issues, as well as concrete services for homebound patients; involvement of the family and support for caregivers; case management for complex patients; and coordination across care settings. Clear communication among providers and across settings, especially at times of transition, is critical to ensuring a consistent and coordinated approach to patient care. Ideally, the referral to specialist palliative care services should be on the basis of need, rather than clinical diagnosis or prognosis. All members of the health-care team, including the primary medical and nursing providers and cardiology specialists, are empowered and trained to address the complexity of HF care at the end of life. As a core principle, it is important to meet patients and their families where they are in terms of acceptance and acknowledgement of their situation. Open-ended questions such as, 'When you think about the future what do you hope for?' and 'When you look ahead what worries you the most?' can help establish what patients understand about their current situation and what values and goals are most important (Pantilat and Steimle, 2004; Pantilat, 2009).

Ideally, palliative care services for people with HF are available in all treatment settings, including hospital, home, outpatient/clinic, and nursing home. Because of the need for optimal medical management, most commonly the palliative care specialist serves in a consultative role. In all settings, collaboration among teams—primary, palliative care, cardiology, and others—and between disciplines—nurses, physicians, social workers, chaplains, pharmacists, and others—is most likely to promote the best care for the patient (Johnson et al., 2012a). Nurses often play a key role in managing patients in HF disease management programmes. These nurses that specialize in the care of people with HF should learn the core principles of palliative care and become adept at talking with patients about prognosis and ACP.

In HF, self-monitoring programmes can help patients manage their HF at home. Although there are conflicting data regarding the efficacy of these programmes (Chaudhry et al., 2010; Inglis et al., 2011) clinical experience is generally favourable. They typically include having patients weigh themselves daily and adjust diuretics in response to weight gain or symptoms of oedema. They may use telemonitoring of weight and symptoms by programme staff. Palliative care specialists can become engaged with self-monitoring programmes to assist in managing distressing symptoms and promoting ACP. Similarly, palliative care specialists can work with HF programmes in hospital and clinic settings to provide direct care to patients and to help teach their cardiology

colleagues about palliative care. Such close collaboration also serves to teach the palliative care specialist about managing HF.

In the United States, although heart disease is the leading cause of death, HF is the admitting diagnosis to hospice services in only 12% of cases (Teno et al., 2004). Similarly, palliative care and hospice are underutilized for patients with HF in other countries (Selman et al., 2007a, 2007b). Palliative care specialists can use data showing that hospice is associated with prolonged life in patients with HF to encourage their colleagues to refer more patients with HF to palliative care and hospice (Connor et al., 2007).

Conclusion

Heart disease is the leading cause of death in the developed world and causes significant morbidity and repeated hospitalization. With increasing use of optimal medical management and devices, including ICDs, CRT, and LVADs, survival and quality of life may improve. At the same time, greater access to such interventions introduces challenges, concerns, and expectations that must be managed. Palliative care specialists need to understand the important role of medical therapy and invasive interventions in maintaining quality of life and longevity for patients with HF. Ensuring that HF is managed optimally will address many symptoms and referral to HF specialists may be necessary in advanced illness. At the same time, palliative care treatments should be integrated at every stage of illness to promote the best possible quality of life. Palliative care should enhance the capacity for effective communication among clinicians, and the patient and family, and should provide more options in the management of symptoms. The key principles of palliative care should guide comprehensive care planning regardless of the setting or model of care. Integrating a palliative approach in HF care has the potential to increase quality of life, decrease suffering and health-care costs, and improve the quality of care.

Acknowledgements

Text extracts from National Heart Foundation of Australia and the Cardiac Society of Australia and New Zealand, *Guidelines for the prevention, detection and management of chronic heart failure in Australia, Updated October 2011*, National Heart Foundation of Australia, Copyright © 2011, reproduced with permission of National Heart Foundation of Australia. All rights reserved.

Online materials

Complete references for this chapter are available online at <http://www.oxfordmedicine.com>.

References

Adler, E.D., Goldfinger, J.Z., Kalman, J., Park, M.E., and Meier, D.E. (2009). Palliative care in the treatment of advanced heart failure. *Circulation*, 120, 2597–606.

Ahluwalia, S.C., Levin, J.R., Lorenz, K.A., and Gordon, H.S. (2012). Missed opportunities for advance care planning communication during outpatient clinic visits. *Journal of General Internal Medicine*, 27(4), 445–451.

Bekelman, D.B., Nowels, C.T., Retrum, J.H., *et al.* (2011). Giving voice to patients' and family caregivers' needs in chronic heart failure: implications for palliative care programs. *Journal of Palliative Medicine*, 14, 1317–1324.

Bradley, T.D., Logan, A.G., Kimoff, R.J., *et al.* (2005). Continuous positive airway pressure for central sleep apnea and heart failure. *The New England Journal of Medicine*, 353, 2025–2033.

Chaudhry, S.I., Mattera, J.A., Curtis, J.P., *et al.* (2010). Telemonitoring in patients with heart failure. *The New England Journal of Medicine*, 363, 2301–2309.

Chua, D., Buttar, A., Kaan, A., Andrews, H., Kealy, J., and Lam, S. (2011). Home inotrope program for patients with end-stage heart failure awaiting heart transplant. *Canadian Journal of Hospital Pharmacy*, 64, 292–293.

Chua, T.P., Harrington, D., Ponikowski, P., Webb-Peploe, K., Poole-Wilson, P.A., and Coats, A.J. (1997). Effects of dihydrocodeine on chemosensitivity and exercise tolerance in patients with chronic heart failure. *Journal of the American College of Cardiology*, 29, 147–152.

Criteria Committee of the New York Heart Association (1964). *Diseases of the Heart and Blood Vessels. Nomenclature and Criteria for Diagnosis*. Boston, MA: Little, Brown and Co.

Criteria Committee of the New York Heart Association (1994). *Nomenclature and Criteria for Diagnosis of Diseases of the Heat and Great Vessels* (9th ed.). Boston, MA: Little, Brown and Co.

Dev, S., Abernethy, A.P., Rogers, J.G., and O'Connor, C.M. (2012). Preferences of people with advanced heart failure—a structured narrative literature review to inform decision making in the palliative care setting. *American Heart Journal*, 164, 313–319.e5.

Faris, R., Flather, M., Purcell, H., Henein, M., Poole-Wilson, P., and Coats, A. (2002). Current evidence supporting the role of diuretics in heart failure: a meta analysis of randomised controlled trials. *International Journal of Cardiology*, 82, 149–158.

Glower, D.D. (2012). Surgical approaches to mitral regurgitation. *Journal of the American College of Cardiology*, 60, 1315–1322.

Goldstein, N.E., Lampert, R., Bradley, E., Lynn, J., and Krumholz, H.M. (2004). Management of implantable cardioverter defibrillators in end-of-life care. *Annals of Internal Medicine*, 141, 835–838.

Goodlin, S.J. (2009). Palliative care in congestive heart failure. *Journal of the American College of Cardiology*, 54, 386–396.

Harkness, K., Heckman, G.A., and McKelvie, R.S. (2012). The older patient with heart failure: high risk for frailty and cognitive impairment. *Expert Review of Cardiovascular Therapy*, 10, 779–795.

Janssen, D.J., Spruit, M.A., Schols, J.M., and Wouters, E.F. (2011). A call for high-quality advance care planning in outpatients with severe COPD or chronic heart failure. *Chest*, 139, 1081–1088.

Johnson, M., Nunn, A., Hawkes, T., Stockdale, S., and Daley, A. (2012a). Planning for end-of-life care in heart failure: experience of two integrated cardiology-palliative care teams. *British Journal of Cardiology*, 19, 71–75.

Kirchhoff, K.T., Hammes, B.J., Kehl, K.A., Briggs, L.A., and Brown, R.L. (2012). Effect of a disease-specific advance care planning intervention on end-of-life care. *Journal of the American Geriatrics Society*, 60(5), 946–950.

Low, J., Pattenden, J., Candy, B., Beattie, J.M., and Jones, L. (2011). Palliative care in advanced heart failure: an international review of the perspectives of recipients and health professionals on care provision. *Journal of Cardiac Failure*, 17, 231–252.

Mancini, D. and Lietz, K. (2010). Selection of cardiac transplantation candidates in 2010. *Circulation*, 122, 173–183.

McCarthy, M., Lay, M., and Addington-Hall, J. (1996). Dying from heart disease. *Journal of the Royal College of Physicians of London*, 30, 325–328.

McKelvie, R.S., Moe, G.W., Cheung, A., *et al.* (2011). The 2011 Canadian Cardiovascular Society heart failure management guidelines update: focus on sleep apnea, renal dysfunction, mechanical circulatory support, and palliative care. *Canadian Journal of Cardiology*, 27, 319–338.

Mozaffarian, D., Anker, S.D., Anand, I., *et al.* (2007). Prediction of mode of death in heart failure: the Seattle Heart Failure Model. *Circulation*, 116, 392–398.

Padeletti, L., Arnar, D.O., Bioncinelli, L., *et al.* (2010). EHRA Expert Consensus Statement on the management of cardiovascular implantable electronic devices in patients nearing end of life or requesting withdrawal of therapy. *Europace*, 12, 1480–1489.

Piepoli, M.F., Davos, C., Francis, D.P., and Coats, A.J. (2004). Exercise training meta-analysis of trials in patients with chronic heart failure (ExTraMATCH). *BMJ*, 328, 189.

Quill, T.E. and Holloway, R.G. (2012). Evidence, preferences, recommendations—finding the right balance in patient care. *The New England Journal of Medicine*, 366, 1653–1655.

Redwine, L.S., Tsuang, M., Rusiewicz, A., *et al.* (2012). A pilot study exploring the effects of a 12-week t'ai chi intervention on somatic symptoms of depression in patients with heart failure. *Journal of Alternative and Complementary Medicine*, 18, 744–748.

Sherrod, M.M., Graulty, R., Crawford, M., and Cheek, D.J. (2009). Intravenous heart failure medications: an update for home health clinicians. *Home Healthcare Nurse*, 27, 610–619.

Sin, D.D., Fitzgerald, F., Parker, J.D., *et al.* (2003). Relationship of systolic BP to obstructive sleep apnea in patients with heart failure. *Chest*, 123, 1536–1543.

Sin, D.D., Fitzgerald, F., Parker, J.D., Newton, G., Floras, J.S., and Bradley, T.D. (1999). Risk factors for central and obstructive sleep apnea in 450 men and women with congestive heart failure. *American Journal of Respiratory and Critical Care Medicine*, 160, 1101–1106.

Stevenson, W.G. and Stevenson, L.W. (2001). Prevention of sudden death in heart failure. *Journal of Cardiovascular Electrophysiology*, 12, 112–114.

Tribouilloy, C., Rusinaru, D., Mahjoub, H., *et al.* (2008). Prognosis of heart failure with preserved ejection fraction: a 5 year prospective population-based study. *European Heart Journal*, 29, 339–347.

Wiegand, D. L. and Kalowes, P. G. (2007). Withdrawal of cardiac medications and devices. *AACN Advanced Critical Care*, 18, 415–425.

15.4

Dementia

Eric Widera and Rachelle Bernacki

Introduction to dementia

Dementia is not a single disease, but rather a clinical syndrome characterized by the insidious onset and gradual progression of impairments in at least two of the following cognitive domains: (1) memory, (2) executive function (reasoning, planning, and judgement), (3) visuospatial ability, (4) language, (5) and personality or behaviour (McKhann et al., 2011). Importantly, the decline in cognitive abilities must be severe enough to interfere with social and/or occupational functioning, and cannot be accounted for by other psychiatric conditions such as depression or delirium.

An estimated 24 million individuals worldwide have dementia (Ballard et al., 2011). This number is expected to increase as more countries have ageing populations. The incidence increases with age, rising from 5% in those aged 71–79 years to over 30% in those aged 90 and older (Plassman et al., 2007). Alzheimer's disease represents the majority of these cases and is characterized by a progressive and irreversible cognitive and functional decline that ultimately leads to death. The advanced stages of dementia are associated with significant palliative care needs, including high symptom burden, frequent transitions in care, and the use of burdensome treatments at the end of life.

Screening for dementia

The clinical diagnosis of dementia often occurs well after the onset of cognitive impairment, making it important for palliative care providers to screen for dementia in older adults. Brief and effective screening tools are available that can aid in identifying dementia, including the Mini-Mental Sate Examination (MMSE), Montreal Cognitive Assessment (MoCA), and the Mini-Cog. Although long considered a standard, the MMSE lacks sensitivity to detect the early stages of cognitive impairment. The MoCA (<http://www.mocatest.org>) is a brief and validated screening tool that is available at no cost and has high sensitivity and specificity for detecting mild cognitive impairment (MCI) and dementia. The Mini-Cog, which can generally be done within 3 minutes, is an effective screening instrument that combines a three-item recall test with a clock-drawing test. The Mini-Cog is considered positive if a patient cannot recall all three items, or if the patient can recall one or two items and also has an abnormal clock draw.

Types of dementia

Alzheimer's disease

Alzheimer's disease is the most common type of dementia, accounting for 60–80% of all dementia cases. The clinical hallmark of Alzheimer's disease is a slowly progressive impairment in memory. Characteristic findings seen at autopsy include the accumulation of extracellular amyloid plaques, intracellular neurofibrillary tangles, and loss of neurons. These pathological findings are not specific, however, and can be found at autopsy in older adults who never had clinical evidence of dementia. Amyloid plaques are thought to be the result of abnormal metabolism of amyloid-β 40 and amyloid-β 42, which results in its accumulation in areas of the brain that are responsible for learning and memory, most notably the hippocampus and entorhinal cortex. Neurofibrillary tangles consist mainly of hyperphosphorylated tau protein, a microtubule assembly protein. It is still a matter of debate whether plaques and tangles are the mediators or the by-products of the pathogenesis of Alzheimer's disease and neuronal death (Querfurth and LaFerla, 2010).

Vascular dementia

Vascular dementia, the second most common type of dementia in the elderly, is the result of ischaemic or haemorrhagic cerebrovascular disease or ischaemic-hypoxic brain lesions. There are several subtypes of vascular dementia. Multiple lacunar infarcts or deep white matter changes related to chronic ischaemia may cause a subcortical dementia, which often has an insidious onset and a slowly progressive course. Multiple cortical infarcts usually occur in patients with multiple vascular risk factors and may progress in a 'stepwise' fashion characterized by the sudden onset of cognitive deficits followed by periods where deficits stabilize.

Dementia with Lewy bodies

Dementia with Lewy bodies (DLB) is another slowly progressive neurodegenerative disease that is associated with abnormal alpha-synuclein clumps (Lewy bodies). Patients with DLB experience a progressive cognitive decline, accompanied by vivid hallucinations, motor features of parkinsonism, and fluctuating cognition with pronounced variations in attention and alertness. Patients with DLB may be very sensitive to neuroleptic medications. If exposed to these medications, they may have a sudden exacerbation of parkinsonism, impaired consciousness, or a neuroleptic malignant syndrome. Parkinson's disease with dementia is a more appropriate diagnosis than DLB when the motor features of parkinsonism are present for longer than 12 months prior to onset of dementia.

Frontotemporal dementia

Frontotemporal dementia (FTD) is characterized by focal degeneration of the frontal and/or temporal lobes. Age of onset is typically younger than Alzheimer's disease, with most patients being diagnosed in their 50s and 60s. The most common presentation of FTD is that of progressive personality changes, including marked behavioural disinhibition or apathy, and loss of social awareness occurring early on in the disease. Patients with FTD have executive function deficits but their memory and visuospatial functions are mostly spared. However, over time FTD progresses to a more global dementia.

Natural history

There are significant differences in how different types of dementia present early in the course of the disease. In the advanced stages, however, patients with different disorders usually appear more similar in appearance.

Patients with the most common types of dementia may present with MCI, which refers to cognitive impairment that does not meet the criteria for dementia. In the amnestic subtype of MCI, which may represent a transitional stage from normal ageing to early Alzheimer's disease, individuals develop clinically observable memory impairment but no significant change in daily functioning. These patients often experience progression of memory impairment over time, and ultimately experience cognitive impairment that interferes with everyday function, which may fulfil the diagnostic criteria for dementia.

Over time, individuals with dementia require increased need for assistance and eventual complete dependence with more basic activities of daily living (ADLs), such as bathing, dressing, and feeding (Widera et al., 2011). In the most advanced forms of dementia, individuals lose the ability to ambulate independently, to communicate with others, to eat without assistance, and to maintain bowel and bladder continence. Persistently severe disability with complete dependence in basic ADLs is the predominant functional trajectory in the last year of life (Gill et al., 2010). Of note, rapid progression of cognitive and functional decline should be concerning for delirium and not be solely attributed to dementia (see Chapter 17.5).

The progression of dementia may be categorized into stages based on disease severity. Standardized cognitive assessment tools, such as the MoCA or the MMSE can be used to stage severity but they lack important functional measures. Global severity scales better rate severity as they include functional assessment. Three of the most commonly used global measures for staging include the Clinical Dementia Rating (CDR) scale, the Functional Assessment Stage (FAST) scale, and the Global Deterioration Scale (GDS). The CDR rates impairments in memory, orientation, judgement and problem-solving, community affairs, home and hobbies, and personal care. The CDR ranges from 0 to 3, with a score of 3 indicating advanced disease. The FAST scale consists of seven major stages split into 16 different substages (see Table 15.4.1), with stage 7 generally indicating advanced dementia. The GDS also divides the disease process into seven stages, assigning patients to a 1–7 scale, with the latter indicating very severe impairment.

Prognosis

The prolonged period of severe functional and cognitive impairment that occurs prior to death makes it difficult to determine short-term prognosis in advanced dementia (Brauner et al., 2000). However, longer-term prognosis is clear. The median survival after the diagnosis of Alzheimer's disease ranges from 4 to

Table 15.4.1 Summary of Functional Assessment Staging (FAST) (Anonymous, 1996)

Stage	Skill
1	No subjective or objective difficulties
2	Complaints of misplacing objects. Subjective word finding difficulties
3	Difficulties with job performance evident to co-workers. Difficulty with organization
4	Impairments in instrumental activities of daily living
5	Needs assistance with dressing to match weather or occasion
6 (a–e)	Difficulty dressing, bathing, toileting without assistance (stage 6a–c). Occasional or more frequent urinary incontinence (6d) and faecal incontinence (6e)
7 (a–f)	Speech limited to less than six intelligible words per day (7a) to one or less (7b). Inability to ambulate independently (7c), sit up without assistance (7d), smile (7e), and hold head up (7f)

Source: data from Reisberg B., Functional assessment staging (FAST), *Psychopharmacology Bulletin*, Volume 24, Issue 4, pp.653–9, Copyright © 1988.

6 years (Larson et al., 2004). For those with advanced disease, markers of poor short-term survival include aspiration, urinary tract infections, sepsis, pressure ulcers, fever, and weight loss (Luchins et al., 1997). One study observed that nursing home residents with advanced dementia and pneumonia had 6-month mortality rates of 47%; residents who had a febrile episode and those with an eating problem had mortality rates of 45% and 39%, respectively (Mitchell et al., 2009). Another study reported that advanced dementia patients hospitalized with either pneumonia or a hip fracture had a 6-month mortality rate exceeding 50% (Morrison and Siu, 2000b). These data suggest that, while patients with advanced dementia can survive for long periods of time with severe functional and cognitive decline, they are also at risk of sudden, life-threatening events such as respiratory and urinary tract infections.

Despite the poor prognosis, many patients and families, as well as some physicians, do not consider dementia a 'terminal illness' with a recognizable end-stage course. For instance, health-care providers have overly optimistic prognoses for individuals with advanced dementia. In one study of nursing home admissions, only 1% of residents were perceived to have life expectancy of less than 6 months, but 71% died within that period (Mitchell et al., 2004). Not perceiving dementia as a terminal illness can lead to poor quality outcomes at end of life. One study found that a family's perception of dementia as 'a disease you can die from' predicted higher patient comfort during the dying process (van der Steen et al., 2013). However, only 43% of family members in this study perceive dementia as a terminal illness (van der Steen et al., 2013).

In the United States, Medicare hospice eligibility criteria for dementia are based largely on whether a patient meets Stage 7 on the FAST and whether they have at least one complication from their dementia (aspiration, upper urinary tract infection, sepsis, multiple Stage 3–4 ulcers, persistent fever, or weight loss > 10% within 6 months) (Luchins et al., 1997). The FAST criteria are widely used, despite their limited reliability for prognostication and the observation that many patients do not follow FAST stages sequentially. While other validated models have been developed to predict survival in advanced dementia, their accuracy remains only moderate in predicting the risk of death within 6 months (Yaffe, 2010). The Advanced Dementia Prognostic Tool (ADEPT) (Mitchell et al., 2010) is one such tool, which is intended to identify nursing home residents with advanced dementia at high risk of death within 6 months and can be found online at <http://eprognosis.ucsf.edu/mitchell.php>.

Better tools for prognostication in dementia are needed. In their absence, at a minimum, clinicians can educate family members about the expected outcomes of advanced dementia and prepare families for the types of scenarios they might encounter. Such education, while time-consuming, is key to ensuring that high-quality care is provided to advanced dementia patients.

Place of death and multiple transitions

Most patients with advanced dementia require nursing home level of care at some point during their illness. Many of these patients die 'in place' at the nursing home. For example, a recent study reported that nearly half (49%) of Medicare patients with dementia died in a nursing home (Teno et al., 2013).

Simply knowing where someone dies may not say much about the care they received at the end of life. While patients with advanced dementia who received hospice at end of life in the United States increased dramatically from 19.5% in 2000 to 48% in 2009, the proportion of patients with very short hospice stays (< 3 days) doubled, from 5% to 10% (Teno et al., 2013). In addition, 65% of advanced dementia patients were hospitalized in the last 90 days of life (with 10% hospitalized more than three times) and 22% were hospitalized in the intensive care unit in the last 30 days of life (Teno et al., 2013). The median number of transitions per decedent increased from two in 2000 to three in 2009 (Teno et al., 2013). These transitions are costly and difficult for caregivers and reflect the chaos and 'churning' effect dementia patients may experience at end of life.

Costs of care

Dementia creates a substantial financial burden for patients, family members, and society. The total monetary cost of dementia in 2010 was estimated to be between $157 billion and $215 billion in the United States alone (Hurd et al., 2013). These costs are mainly attributable to the cost for providing institutional and home-based long-term care. This highlights an important point in dementia care across the globe. Despite the fact that many programmes, like Medicare in the United States, provide nearly universal health care coverage to the population aged 65 years or older, they do not cover the full financial cost associated with dementia. Data from the Health and Retirement Study, which measured out-of-pocket health-related expenditures, showed that the average total out-of-pocket costs in the 5 years prior to the death of a household head or spouse was $66 155 (Kelley et al., 2013). The average out-of-pocket spending for those with dementia was double that of the average spending of those dying from gastrointestinal disease or cancer.

Symptoms in dementia

There is a growing body of literature showing that individuals with dementia are at risk for the undertreatment of symptoms (Bernabei et al., 1998). Symptoms such as pain, dyspnoea, and agitation are common and increase in prevalence as patients approach the end of life (Mitchell et al., 2009). In one study of nursing home residents with advanced dementia, 46% had dyspnoea, 39% had pain more than 5 days per month, 39% had stage II–IV pressure ulcers, and 54% had agitation within the 18-month follow-up period (Mitchell et al., 2009).

Pain

Assessing and managing pain pose significant challenges in dementia, as evidenced by undertreatment of pain in this population independent of treatment setting. In a study of community-dwelling adults, individuals with dementia had a 20% decreased probability of receiving analgesics for daily pain relative to patients with normal cognition (Landi et al., 2001). In another study of residents living in long-term care, documentation of pain and analgesic use decreased as cognitive impairment increased (Reynolds et al., 2008). A hospital-based studied observed that patients with advanced dementia recovering from a hip fracture surgery received only one-third of the amount of opioid analgesia compared with comparable, but cognitively intact, adults (Morrison and Siu, 2000a).

One reason why individuals with dementia may be at risk for the undertreatment of pain is that they tend to report less pain to both their health-care providers and caregivers than cognitively intact adults. It is not a reduction in the actual experience of pain that leads to this underreporting, as numerous studies have shown that pain sensitivity and perceptual processing of pain remain largely intact even with advanced dementia (Widera and Smith, 2009). Rather, under-reporting is most likely due to poor patient recall and difficulty with the communication of painful symptoms.

Providers should include a combination of patient reports, caregiver reports, and direct observation of the patient when assessing pain in dementia. Patient report remains an important component of pain assessment, as even individuals with moderate to severe dementia may be able to communicate the presence and severity of pain. Verbal rating scales may be more difficult for individuals with dementia, and verbal descriptor scales, visual analogue scales, pain thermometers, and Faces Pain Scales should be considered as alternatives. Direct observations by health-care providers or caregivers should play a larger role in those with cognitive impairment than in cognitively intact older adults. Observational signs of distress may include changes in facial expressions, vocalizations, body movements, interpersonal interactions, activity patterns, and mental status. Agitation, irritability, and physical aggression may also occur, especially if there is exacerbation of pain during caregiver tasks.

Several pain scales based on non-verbal signs and symptoms have been developed and validated in older patients with cognitive impairment. The best validated tools include the Pain Assessment in Advanced Dementia (PAINAD), the Pain Assessment Checklist for Seniors with Limited Ability to Communicate (PACSLAC), and the Doloplus-2 scale (Pargeon and Hailey, 1999). After a tool is selected, it is best to continue to use the same tool for follow-up assessments.

The choice of analgesic for a patient with dementia should be based on several factors: the severity of pain, the previous responses to analgesic medications, the interaction of the analgesic with co-morbid conditions, and the care setting and support services. Acetaminophen (paracetamol) should be considered the first line of therapy for mild pain when caring for those with dementia. It can also be considered as a potential empiric treatment when the presence of pain is uncertain, as there is evidence that acetaminophen may lead to improved activity levels, social engagement, and behaviour symptoms in nursing home residents with moderate to severe dementia (Chibnall et al., 2005; Husebo et al., 2011). The use of non-steroidal anti-inflammatory drugs, including cyclooxygenase 2 selective inhibitors, should generally be used with great caution due to risks of gastroduodenopathy, renal failure, cardiovascular complications, and fluid retention.

An opioid may be appropriate for any patient with moderate or severe pain, or pain that does not respond to non-opioid therapy. Around-the-clock dosing and the use of a long-acting formulation should be considered, as individuals with dementia may not be able to readily request pain medications. Although the potential for precipitated delirium is an often-cited fear of using opioids in dementia, current evidence suggests that the undertreatment of pain is a greater risk factor for the development of delirium than the use of opioids in hospitalized adults with cognitive impairment (Morrison et al., 2003).

Neuropsychiatric symptoms

Nearly all patients with Alzheimer's disease develop neuropsychiatric symptoms, such as depression, psychosis, or agitation, at some stage in their illness (Ballard et al., 2009). The behavioural manifestations of these symptoms may take the form of repetitive mannerisms and vocalizations or physical aggressiveness. They may occur at any stage of illness, including in the severe and even terminal stages. In one study, 85% of hospice-eligible nursing home residents with advanced dementia exhibited one or more neuropsychiatric symptom (Kverno et al., 2008). These symptoms have been associated with decreased quality of life of both patients and their families, and an increased caregiver burden; they are associated with the caregiver's decisions for nursing home admission.

The management of neuropsychiatric symptoms should focus first on identifying a primary cause and creating a treatment plan to eliminate or mitigate this cause. Underlying physical or medical problems should be investigated, including that the development of a new illness, such as a urinary tract infection or delirium. New symptoms, such as pain and constipation, should be assessed for and treated. For instance, in one cluster randomized control study of nursing home patients with behavioural problems, an empiric stepwise protocol starting with a trial of scheduled acetaminophen resulted in a decrease in the number of symptoms, including agitation (Husebo et al., 2011). An evaluation of unmet needs, such as thirst, hunger, sleep difficulties, and sensory deprivation, also should be performed to identify possible causes of new behaviours. Documenting the antecedents of the behaviour, the behavioural disturbance, and the consequences of the behaviour (the ABCs) can help reveal unmet needs and triggers for a particular problem.

The treatment plan for neuropsychiatric symptoms includes management of the potential causes, various non-pharmacological interventions, and drug therapy. Among the non-pharmacological therapies with some evidence of efficacy are music therapy, massage, and physical activity (Hulme et al., 2010). Drug therapy is usually intended to reduce agitation. Antipsychotic medications are widely used, despite warnings to avoid them if possible, given their association with significant increases in stroke and death (Schneider et al., 2005; Sacchetti et al., 2010). There is limited evidence that these drugs help improve problematic behaviours in patients with advanced dementia with the exception of some modest efficacy for the treatment of aggression and psychosis over a short 6–12-week course (Ballard and Waite, 2006). There also is limited evidence of long-term benefit. For these reasons, antipsychotics should only be considered as additional therapies when non-pharmacologic approaches have failed or the behaviours are severe enough to become a safety issue.

There is little difference in effectiveness or side effects between first-generation antipsychotics (such as haloperidol) and second-generation drugs when used for short durations. Extreme caution is warranted when using these agents in patients who have DLB, as this illness is associated with severe and even life-threatening deterioration following exposure to this drug class.

Mood stabilizers, including valproic acid and divalproex, are also frequently prescribed to treat dementia-related behaviours. However, a Cochrane review revealed that these agents are ineffective to treat agitation and have an unacceptable rate of adverse effects, including somnolence, thrombocytopenia, infection (Lonergan and Luxenberg, 2009).

Depression

Depression occurs in up to 50% of individuals with Alzheimer's disease and is often chronic in nature (Steinberg et al., 2004). The diagnosis of depression is often difficult to make in a patient with dementia because cognitive impairment leads to poor recall and reporting of depressive symptoms. In addition, depression can present atypically in dementia, often manifesting as behavioural symptoms, such as physical aggression, vocalizations, or refusal to eat.

The evidence supporting the use of antidepressant drugs to treat depression in those with Alzheimer's disease is limited, with published controlled trials reporting equivocal results. The Depression in Alzheimer's disease study, phase 2 (DIADS-2) trial and the HTA-SADD study are the largest randomized controlled trials of an antidepressant to date in this population (Rosenberg et al., 2010; Banerjee et al., 2011). In DIADS-2, individuals with depression and mild-to-moderate Alzheimer's disease were randomly assigned to receive sertraline or placebo. No significant benefits were reported in mood, non-mood neuropsychiatric symptoms, function, quality of life, or global cognition at either 12 or 24 weeks. Adverse events were more frequent in patients randomized to receive sertraline than those who received placebo. Patients who received the drug experienced diarrhoea, dizziness, dry mouth, and pulmonary serious adverse events. The HCT-SADD trial compared both sertraline and mirtazapine against placebo and found no benefits at 13 and 39 weeks for both.

If the clinical decision is made to offer drug therapy to a patient with dementia and comorbid depression, the usual first-line treatment in patients with Alzheimer's disease should be a selective serotonin reuptake inhibitor (SSRI), serotonin and norepinephrine (noradrenaline) reuptake inhibitor (SNRI), or a norepinephrine reuptake inhibitor (NRI), as they have less risk for adverse effects than the tricyclic antidepressants and monoamine oxidase inhibitors. Choice of a specific agent should be based on past effectiveness, medical comorbidities, potential side effects, and pharmacologic interactions.

Cognitive decline

Individuals with Alzheimer's disease have decreased production of choline acetyl transferase, resulting in reduced acetylcholine synthesis and impaired cortical cholinergic function. Cholinesterase inhibitors, such as donepezil, galantamine, and rivastigmine, affect the clinical manifestations of Alzheimer's disease by increasing cholinergic transmission. Memantine, an N-methyl-D-aspartate (NMDA) antagonist, has a mechanism of action distinct from that of the acetylcholinesterase inhibitors.

Use of cholinesterase inhibitors or memantine in patients with moderate-to-severe Alzheimer's disease results in statistically significant improvements in cognitive, functional, and behavioural outcomes (Birks, 2006). However, the clinical significance of these outcomes is modest at best. The addition of memantine to acetylcholinesterase inhibitors also seems to be of little value (Howard et al., 2012). No significant benefits were observed from the combination of donepezil and memantine over donepezil alone in a trial of 295 patients with moderate to severe disease who were already taking donepezil (Howard et al., 2012).

Cholinesterase inhibitors also may improve outcomes in non-Alzheimer's dementia, including vascular dementia and DLB. In particular, patients with DLB may have significant improvements in behavioural symptoms and hallucinations, in addition to small improvements in cognition (McKeith et al., 2000).

Despite the lack of evidence that cholinesterase inhibitors and memantine are efficacious in individuals with very advanced dementia or those who are near the end of life, they are commonly used. For example, a study of hospice enrolees with dementia observed that 21.3% were prescribed at least one of these medications (Weschules et al., 2008). Nearly one-third of patients who receive cholinesterase inhibitors experience an adverse effect, with nausea, vomiting, and diarrhoea the most common (Birks, 2006), and in community-dwelling older adults, use of these drugs is associated with increased risks of syncope, bradycardia, permanent pacemaker insertion, and hip fracture (Gill et al., 2009). Given the lack of established benefit and risk of adverse events, both cholinesterase inhibitors and memantine generally should be discontinued or avoided in populations with far advanced dementia or short life expectancy.

Eating and swallowing problems

Eating and swallowing difficulties become nearly universal as dementia progresses to the advanced stages. In one prospective study, over 85% of 323 nursing home residents with advanced dementia developed eating problems during an 18-month study period. In those who died, over 90% developed eating problems in the last 3 months of life. When these difficulties arise, family members and health-care providers are likely to be confronted with the decision to administer food and fluids via a nasogastric tube or via a percutaneous endoscopic gastrostomy (PEG) tube. In the United States, placement of these tubes is common. Nearly one-third of nursing home residents with advanced dementia have feeding tubes placed, although there is great variation based on geography and nursing home characteristics (Ahronheim et al., 2001; Mitchell et al., 2003).

The frequency of feeding tube insertion is notable given the lack of evidence of benefit. Numerous observational studies have demonstrated that feeding tubes do not improve survival, prevent aspiration pneumonia, decrease the risk for pressure ulcers, or improve patient comfort (Finucane et al., 1999; Teno et al., 2012). Harms of feeding tube placement are well documented in the literature, although not often discussed by physicians prior to tube insertion (Teno et al., 2011). In one study, one in five tube-fed residents experienced a tube-related complication necessitating a hospital transfer in the year following insertion. Furthermore, over one-third of individuals required physical or pharmacologic restraints to prevent tube dislodgement (Teno et al., 2011).

It is important to consider potential modifiable factors when eating problems arise in individuals with dementia. Comorbid illnesses like depression, medication side effects, and oral health problems, such as xerostomia, are among the many conditions that may result in reduced oral intake, followed by weight loss. When no modifiable factors are identifiable, careful hand feeding and proper oral care should be recommended as better alternatives than PEG placement for individuals with advanced dementia (Yoneyama et al., 2002).

Palliative care interventions in dementia

In addition to symptom management, care for individuals with advanced dementia should involve a number of key palliative interventions, including advance care planning, avoidance of potentially inappropriate interventions, hospice referral, and caregiver support. There is now ample evidence showing improved outcomes for patients and caregivers when such interventions are performed (Engel et al., 2006).

Advanced care planning

Advance care planning is important for all patients with serious illness, but the types of decisions that have to be made are especially difficult when the patient suffers from advanced dementia and may not be able to communicate. Patient preferences are often not documented early despite the anticipated loss of capacity that occurs with dementia. A common reason for this is that family members often do not realize the importance of discussing advanced care plans with their love one until it is too late to have the discussion (Hirschman et al., 2008). Clinicians should routinely lead end-of-life planning conversations with dementia patients and families before moments of crisis, such as hospitalization for aspiration or fever. This is particularly important given the finding that nursing home residents whose health-care agents had an understanding of the poor prognosis and the clinical complications expected in advanced dementia were much less likely to have burdensome interventions in the last 3 months of life than were residents whose agents did not have this understanding (Mitchell et al., 2009).

Before clinicians discuss specifics, the planning conversations should explore overall patient values and goals, including whether comfort and quality of life are viewed as overriding priorities. Later, these views may be more helpful for surrogate decision-makers when asked to weigh the risks and benefits of the many interventions frequently performed on those with advanced dementia. Specific aspects of care, such as artificial nutrition and hydration, intubation, cardiopulmonary resuscitation, and other common medical interventions, should be discussed and this discussion should be documented in an advance directive.

A key element of this advance care planning is the selection by the patient of an agent, who would make decisions on behalf of the patient should he or she lack the capacity to do so. This agent is given written durable power of attorney to make health decisions when the patient loses capacity.

The discussion of prognosis is inextricably linked to the discussion of goals of care and advance care planning. Conveying information about prognosis is clinically challenging, and patients or families often misperceive or discount the information. This may result from a misunderstanding of medical terms, such as 'controlled' or 'terminal', or from a lack of consistency in the messages provided by different clinicians. Patients and families often ask several clinicians the same questions about prognosis, and all members of the clinical team should communicate the same information in a consistent fashion. Many physicians are concerned about destroying hope when discussing goals of care in the context of poor prognosis (Davison and Simpson, 2006). Clinicians should be able to provide direct information about the disease while supporting a wide spectrum of realistic hopes that patients and families may have depending on the situation. 'Hope for the best, prepare for the worst' acknowledges that hope can be sustained while also planning for the occurrence of clinical situations that may change quickly.

New tools are being used for helping patients and families understand the realities of their prognosis. Older adults who viewed a video depiction of a patient with advanced dementia after hearing a verbal description of the condition were more likely to opt for comfort as their goal of care compared with those who solely listen to a verbal description (Volandes et al., 2009). They also had more stable preferences over time (Volandes et al., 2007). In another study, the use of videos led to decision-making that was more patient focused, dealing with issues such as quality of life and effects on the family, and less conventionally treatment centric, with an intent to preserve life as long as possible (Deep et al., 2010).

Avoidance of potentially burdensome treatments

Hospitalization is often considered when individuals with advanced dementia develop infections such as pneumonia (Volicer et al., 2003). Hospitalization for an infection should be thought of as a significant event in the course of advanced dementia, as it heralds an increased short-term morbidity and mortality. Some data suggest that the hospital may not be the optimal setting for the treatment of pneumonia, at least for nursing home residents; mortality rates appear similar whether treatment is provided in a nursing home or hospital, with some evidence suggesting greater functional decline in hospitalized residents (Fried et al., 1995, 1997; Mylotte et al., 1998).

Pneumonia is the most commonly identified cause of death among individuals with advanced Alzheimer's disease and the treatment of pneumonia in this context may be challenging. In one recent prospective study of 323 nursing home residents with advanced dementia, antibiotic therapy for episodes of pneumonia improved survival compared with no antibiotic treatment, but also was associated with lower scores on the Symptom Management at End-of-Life in Dementia scale, indicating more discomfort compared to untreated residents (Givens et al., 2010). If antibiotics are not given, comfort can adequately maintained with aggressive use of antipyretics, analgesics, and oxygen if hypoxic.

Hospice

In the United States, hospice is a health-care system supported by the government and intended to provide specialist palliative care for patients approaching death and their families. Most patients are treated in the home, although care also can be provided in other settings, such as nursing homes. Other countries maintain other models of hospice, most focused on end-of-life care. Whatever the model, a specialized programme for end-of-life care, such as hospice, should be considered when patients with dementia progress into an advanced stage of the illness. In the United States, use of hospice in this population has been associated with improved patient and caregiver outcomes compared to usual care (Mitchell et al., 2007), including improved pain management, less aggressive care at the end of life (Miller et al., 2001), fewer unmet needs during the last 7 days of life (Kiely et al., 2010), and greater satisfaction among family members with end-of-life care (Shega et al., 2008). Individuals with advanced dementia who are enrolled in hospice are also more likely to die in their location of choice and less likely to die in the hospital (Shega et al., 2008).

Use of hospice services in the United States has been increasing over the last decade. For instance, Miller and colleagues found that hospice use for nursing home decedents with advanced dementia increased from 15% in 1999 to 43% in 2006 (Miller et al., 2010). The use of hospice benefits may be underutilized in part because prognostication is uncertain and restrictive hospice eligibility guidelines impact early referrals. In the same study by Miller and colleagues, a quarter of individuals were enrolled in hospice for 1 week or less prior to their death (Brickner et al., 2004; Miller et al., 2010).

Caregiver support

The majority of care provided to individuals with dementia is done at home and by family caregivers. This care is a physically, emotionally, and financially stressful experience that has been associated with a range of adverse health outcomes including high rates of anxiety and depression. There is now good evidence to suggest that interventions that combine caregiver education, counselling, and support can improve caregiver health. Callahan and colleagues developed a collaborative care model that involved advanced practice nurses integrated within a primary care clinic. In a randomized controlled trial of this intervention, the authors found significant improvements in caregiver distress and depression (Callahan et al., 2006). Another model, REACH II (Resources for Enhancing Alzheimer's Caregiver Health), focused on enhancing caregivers' coping skills and management of dementia-related behaviours by using a multicomponent home- and telephone-based intervention (Belle et al., 2006). REACH II significantly improved caregiver quality of life in terms of burden, depression, self-care and healthy behaviours, social support, and management of patient problem behaviours. Unfortunately, these proven multicomponent interventions are not available to most caregivers.

Conclusion

Although dementia is caused by a heterogeneous group of disorders, its relentless progression ultimately creates a common set of problems for the patients who are affected and their families. Meticulous assessment of unmet needs for palliative care will identify opportunities for interventions that can reduce suffering and illness burden, and ensure that clinical decisions in the setting of far advanced illness are medically appropriate and consistent with the values of the patient.

Online materials

Complete references for this chapter are available online at <http://www.oxfordmedicine.com>.

References

Brauner, D.J., Muir, J.C., and Sachs, G.A. (2000). Treating nondementia illnesses in patients with dementia. *Journal of the American Medical Association*, 283, 3230–3235.

Callahan, C.M., Boustani, M.A., Unverzagt, F.W., *et al.* (2006). Effectiveness of collaborative care for older adults with Alzheimer disease in primary care: a randomized controlled trial. *Journal of the American Medical Association*, 295, 2148–2157.

Gill, T.M., Gahbauer, E.A., Han, L., and Allore, H.G. (2010). Trajectories of disability in the last year of life. *The New England Journal of Medicine*, 362, 1173–1180.

Givens, J.L., Jones, R.N., Shaffer, M.L., Kiely, D.K., and Mitchell, S.L. (2010). Survival and comfort after treatment of pneumonia in advanced dementia. *Archives of Internal Medicine*, 170, 1102–1107.

Husebo, B.S., Ballard, C., Sandvik, R., Nilsen, O.B., and Aarsland, D. (2011). Efficacy of treating pain to reduce behavioural disturbances in residents of nursing homes with dementia: cluster randomised clinical trial. *BMJ*, 343, d4065.

Mitchell, S.L., Kiely, D.K., and Hamel, M.B. (2004). Dying with advanced dementia in the nursing home. *Archives of Internal Medicine*, 164, 321–326.

Mitchell, S.L., Miller, S.C., Teno, J.M., Kiely, D.K., Davis, R.B., and Shaffer, M.L. (2010). Prediction of 6-month survival of nursing home residents with advanced dementia using ADEPT vs hospice eligibility guidelines. *Journal of the American Medical Association*, 304, 1929–1935.

Mitchell, S.L., Teno, J.M., Kiely, D.K., *et al.* (2009). The clinical course of advanced dementia. *The New England Journal of Medicine*, 361, 1529–1538.

Morrison, R.S., Magaziner, J., Gilbert, M., *et al.* (2003). Relationship between pain and opioid analgesics on the development of delirium following hip fracture. *The Journals of Gerontology. Series A, Biological Sciences and Medical Sciences*, 58, 76–81.

Morrison, R.S. and Siu, A.L. (2000b). Survival in end-stage dementia following acute illness. *Journal of the American Medical Association*, 284, 47–52.

Schneider, L.S., Dagerman, K.S., and Insel, P. (2005). Risk of death with atypical antipsychotic drug treatment for dementia: meta-analysis of randomized placebo-controlled trials. *Journal of the American Medical Association*, 294, 1934–1943.

Teno, J.M., Gozalo, P.L., Mitchell, S.L., *et al.* (2012). Does feeding tube insertion and its timing improve survival? *Journal of the American Geriatrics Society*, 60, 1918–1921.

Teno, J.M., Mitchell, S.L., Kuo, S.K., *et al.* (2011). Decision-making and outcomes of feeding tube insertion: a five-state study. *Journal of the American Geriatrics Society*, 59, 881–886.

Volandes, A.E., Paasche-Orlow, M.K., Barry, M.J., *et al.* (2009). Video decision support tool for advance care planning in dementia: randomised controlled trial. *BMJ*, 338, b2159.

Widera, E., Steenpass, V., Marson, D., and Sudore, R. (2011). Finances in the older patient with cognitive impairment: 'He didn't want me to take over'. *Journal of the American Medical Association*, 305, 698–706.

15.5

Neurological disorders other than dementia

Raymond Voltz, Stefan Lorenzl, and Georg S. Nübling

Introduction to neurological disorders other than dementia

Whereas a palliative care approach is commonly accepted in the care of patients with glioblastoma or brain metastases, this is not yet so for many other neurological disorders. Having said that, it must be remembered that Dame Cicely Saunders, in her visionary concept, had included the care of patients with amyotrophic lateral sclerosis (ALS) or motor neuron disease. It has become clear in recent years that her 'total pain' concept, multiprofessional approach, early palliative care integration, and academic models all are very relevant to many patients suffering from neurological disorders.

Causes of death

What do patients with neurological disorders die of? How do they die? Very often this is not known to the specialist neurology services that typically stop caring for patients when they cannot attend clinics any more. These patients are then cared for at home or in nursing homes, often with little or no connection to palliative care or neurology.

Evidence is emerging that a palliative care approach would be very helpful for patients with many types of neurological diseases. One example is multiple sclerosis (MS). Although there is a common belief that patients do not die from MS (Voltz, 2010), the reality is that MS patients are threefold more likely to die prematurely in comparison to the general population (Hirst et al., 2008). Another common diagnosis classically not considered for palliative care services is ischaemic or haemorrhagic stroke. Although about 30% of patients die within the 'acute stroke' phase, defined as the first 30 days after the event (Roberts and Goldacre, 2003), and the event leaves another 30% permanently disabled with chronic deficits, this population is not recognized to have unmet palliative care needs. Experience with stroke patients is now emerging from palliative care services and it is apparent that specialist care can help with symptom control, psychosocial issues, and end-of-life decisions; the latter decisions often involve challenging scenarios such as withdrawal of mechanical ventilation, artificial nutrition, tracheostomy, and neurosurgical procedures (Burton et al., 2010; Holloway et al., 2010).

Palliative care may be very important even in more rare diagnoses, such as sporadic inclusion body myositis. Two recent, long-term observational studies demonstrated a high symptom burden of patients in end-stage disease; furthermore, 13% of patients died by euthanasia or terminal sedation, demonstrating the severe suffering of these patients near the end of their lives (Hohlfeld, 2011).

Although the proximate cause of death in neurological disorders often is an expected complication of a chronic illness, such as pneumonia (Hirst et al., 2008; Pennington et al., 2010), the downward trajectory of many of these illnesses means that decisions concerning withdrawal of life-sustaining therapy may be encountered before the acute terminal event occurs. In some settings that have legalized forms of physician-hastened death, the decisions are layered with even more complexity. In the Netherlands, for example, euthanasia seems to be even more an issue in neurological patients than in the cancer population. Whereas about 1% of the cancer population dies through euthanasia, it is about 20% in ALS, with the number being stable over recent years (Maessen et al., 2009). This potential for euthanasia increases the obligation to understand the nature of suffering associated with neurological conditions, and the varied means to address the contributing sources. In the example of ALS, both lay observers and professionals may believe that suffocation occurs at the end of life; this is not the case, however, and patients with ALS die a peaceful natural death, not only under hospice care but also in a neurology service (Neudert et al., 2001).

Neurological patients outside of the Netherland also seem to be at a high risk for developing a wish for hastening death or suicide. In MS, suicide is a frequent cause of death, and a long protracted course with severe neurological deficit in many leads to a wish for hastening death. In all these situations, the palliative care approach may identify the reasons behind this wish, assist and support, and may try to bring up the parallel existing will for life again (Voltz et al., 2011).

One of the obstacles in expanding access to palliative care for neurological patients is the relatively poor knowledge of palliative care approaches among the diverse professionals who care for these patients. Although palliative care is far broader than end-of-life care, the pivotal point that death is inevitable and likely to be soon may be a lever to improve palliative care skills in existing services, or to encourage referral to specialist palliative care. Teaching professionals about prognosis and the usual clinical course in advanced illness, such as by introducing 'death rounds' for physicians-in-training, is one way to underscore the life-limiting nature of neurological illnesses, teach about the role of palliative care throughout the course of the disease, and learn from a group while sharing the emotions around a death (Khot et al., 2011).

Amyotrophic lateral sclerosis

Motor neuron diseases are a group of syndromes affecting the primary and/or secondary motor neurons, with ALS being the most common and most severe manifestation. ALS is the most frequent neurological disease on palliative care wards. Thus, knowledge of the symptoms, course of disease, and treatment options is essential for palliative care specialists.

Amyotrophic lateral sclerosis: a brief summary

The incidence of ALS is estimated at approximately 2/100 000 per year, with a mildly elevated risk for male gender (Logroscino et al., 2010). The life expectancy of ALS patients averages at 2–4 years from symptom onset (Forsgren et al., 1983). Two manifestations of the disease are mainly recognized. The spinal variant is characterized by early, often asymmetric tetraparesis, and late onset of deficits in cranial nerve function. The bulbar variant occurs in approximately 20% of all cases and presents with a predominant affection of speech and swallowing, followed by progressive muscle weakness. Neurobehavioural dysfunction such as apathy, disinhibition, or dysexecutive behaviour occurs in a significant proportion of patients (Chio et al., 2012). In the course of the disease, patients suffer from decreased mobility, loss of speech and swallowing, and progressive dyspnoea. Additional symptoms frequently occur, including dysphagia, dysarthrophonia, dyspnoea, mucous congestion of airways, muscle cramps, and sleep disturbance.

Approaches to treatment

Since ALS is a fatal disorder invariably leading to progressive disability and death, treatment has to be adapted to the patient's preferences. While some patients may be willing to take any action to prolong survival, others refrain from invasive treatment options, given the severe disability and family burden accompanying late stages of the disease. Detailed discussions about the course of disease, benefits, and disadvantages of treatment options, as well as the patient's personal preferences are essential and should be addressed at an early stage of the disease, to help all personnel involved to best understand each patient's values and expectations. Advanced directives ensure the patient's autonomy and provide an important assurance for caregivers and clinicians. Importantly, the patient has to be aware that life-prolonging treatments do not have to be carried out indefinitely, and that symptom control is always an alternative.

Symptoms and treatment options

In ALS, symptoms occur at various time points and with various severities, rendering a stepwise treatment plan impossible. Early recognition and treatment are essential to preserve quality of life for patients and their caregivers. The diversity and rapid progression of symptoms often require a multidisciplinary approach. Treatment options are summarized in the section 'Medication at the end of life'.

Respiratory insufficiency

Respiratory insufficiency invariably occurs in the course of disease. The treatment strategy largely depends on the patient's preferences, and for this reason, prolonged artificial ventilation and tracheostomy should be discussed early. Pre-emptive measurements to prevent secondary causes of respiratory insufficiency, such as yearly influenza vaccinations or polyvalent pneumococcal vaccines, are recommended. Supplemental oxygen can lead to carbon dioxide retention and should not be used routinely.

Respiratory insufficiency is commonly treated with non-invasive positive pressure ventilation (NIPPV), which has been shown to prolong survival and improve quality of life (Bourke et al., 2006; Andersen et al., 2012). NIPPV is often started as a nocturnal measure in patients showing signs of nocturnal hypoventilation, such as morning headaches and increased daytime sleepiness. Objective measures that can be used to justify the start of NIPPV include percutaneous nocturnal oximetry and forced vital capacity (FVC). Although definite criteria for the initiation of NIPPV have not been established, there is some evidence suggesting a pronounced effect on survival if NIPPV is started at FVC values greater than 65% (Lechtzin et al., 2007). Furthermore, the indication for NIPPV treatment has to be appraised critically in patients with neurobehavioural impairment, where decreased efficiency was observed (Chio et al., 2012).

As the disease progresses, the use of NIPPV is often extended to daytime. The patient must be aware that NIPPV use cannot be extended indefinitely, and that termination of NIPPV in advanced respiratory failure without prior tracheostomy will result in rapid hypoventilation and death. Weaning off NIPPV in patients declining invasive ventilation must be carried out under morphine and benzodiazepine treatment to prevent dyspnoea and anxiety. Thus, advanced directives for the treatment strategy at this point are strongly recommended. It is an ongoing debate whether pre-emptive use of palliative sedation could be an option in this situation (Berger, 2012).

While tracheostomy extends life in ALS, its impact on patient and caregiver quality of life has to be considered carefully. Furthermore, patients with invasive ventilation are often denied access to palliative care wards. Dyspnoea, whether occurring during NIPPV treatment or spontaneously, is best controlled by opioids. Depending on concomitant symptoms, these can be administered orally, nasally, transdermally, or via continuous subcutaneous infusion using a syringe driver. Dyspnoea-related anxiety is best managed by addition of benzodiazepines, such as oral or sublingual lorazepam or midazolam.

Mucous congestion of the airways

Mucous congestion is difficult to manage in patients with impaired coughing. Treatment with mucolytics such as ambroxol or N-acetylcysteine may be attempted, but are of limited benefit. A combination of beta receptor antagonists, nebulized saline, and furosemide is recommended (Andersen et al., 2012). Guided respiratory exercise is mostly considered helpful by patients. The use of mechanical aids such as the CoughAssist*, high-frequency chest wall oscillation, or a home suction device can be applied.

Malnutrition

Malnutrition in ALS mainly results from dysphagia and hypermetabolism. Since malnutrition entails a poor prognosis, treatment of dysphagia plays an important role in ALS (Marin et al., 2011). Early swallowing deficits can be improved by speech and language therapy. At this time, referral to a dietician should also be discussed. Feeding tube placement should be discussed early, since many patients are reluctant to undergo this measure. Gastrostomy can be performed under endoscopic control, while radiologic guidance should be preferred in patients with respiratory insufficiency or severe mouth opening dystonia (Thornton et al., 2002; Desport et al., 2005). In patients with neurobehavioural dysfunction, gastrostomy showed poor outcome (Chio et al., 2012).

Sialorrhoea

Sialorrhoea and drooling are commonly associated with swallowing deficits. Non-pharmacological treatment options include sage tea and consultation with a speech and language therapist to improve swallowing. Pharmacological treatment should begin with low-dose amitriptyline or a hyoscine hydrobromide transdermal patch. Atropine sulphate can be used orally as a permanent medication. For the inpatient setting, subcutaneous atropine sulphate and glycopyrrolate are available. If pharmacological treatment fails, injections of botulinum toxin A or B in the salivary glands (Jackson et al., 2009; Guidubaldi et al., 2011) or salivary gland radiotherapy might be considered.

Spasticity and muscle cramps

Spasticity often occurs in patients with predominant affection of the primary motor neuron. Spasticity may lead to discomfort, pain, and decreased mobility. Physiotherapy should be applied to maintain a full range of motion and avoid contractures (Andersen et al., 2012). While pharmacological treatment with baclofen or tizanidine efficiently reliefs spasticity, patients often discontinue treatment due to side effects such as asthenia and general muscle weakness. Furthermore, treatment of lower limb spasticity can further decrease mobility in patients with preserved ambulatory function and should thus be considered carefully in these cases. Nabiximols, a synthetic cannabinoid, is approved for treatment of therapy-refractory spasticity in multiple sclerosis in several European countries and Canada, and may be considered as an off-label use to treat spasticity in ALS. Focal spasticity can be treated with repeated injections of botulinum toxin A, although literature concerning its use in ALS is sparse.

Muscle cramps often occur early, and can cause significant discomfort and sleep disturbance. The current guidelines from the European Federation of Neurological Societies (EFNS) recommend levetiracetam as first-line treatment (Andersen et al., 2012), but quinidine sulphate also offers effective relief and is the treatment of choice in our outpatient department. Alternatively, phenytoin or carbamazepine can be tried.

Insomnia and fatigue

Insomnia may occur due to various reasons such as muscle cramps, pain, respiratory distress, or depression. If treatment of these symptoms does not restore sufficient sleeping quality, antidepressants (amitriptyline, mirtazapine) or hypnotics (zolpidem) can be applied. For debilitating fatigue, modafinil or another psychostimulant such as methylphenidate may be tried (Andersen et al., 2012).

Pseudobulbar affect

Pseudobulbar affect results from corticobulbar degeneration and manifests in inappropriate laughter or crying incongruent to the patient's mood. It can largely affect social interactions and strain both patients and caregivers. It is of great importance to point out to relatives and caregivers that the patient is completely unable to control their emotional outbursts and that they do not reflect their actual mood, since these outbursts are often perceived to be offensive.

A combination of dextromethorphan and quinidine has been approved by the US Food and Drug Administration for use in pseudobulbar affect, but there also is evidence to suggest a positive treatment effect of antidepressants, mainly citalopram and amitriptyline (Pioro, 2011). Antidepressants might be attempted especially if concomitant depression is suspected.

Depression, suicidality, and death

The inevitable prognosis and continuous, rapid decline often lead to despair and depression in ALS patients. The widespread belief that death in ALS usually occurs through suffocation further increases many patient's wish for an early termination of their suffering through physician-hastened death. ALS patients must be monitored carefully and repeatedly for signs of depression. In particular, if continuous psychosocial support is insufficient or unavailable, antidepressants should be used (Andersen et al., 2012), with the choice of medication being partially directed by concomitant symptoms. For example, if drooling is present, a tricyclic antidepressant such as amitriptyline should be used.

Suicidality and the wish for physician-hastened death is an important issue in ALS. Up to 20% of ALS patients opt for physician-hastened death in countries where this is a legal option (Maessen et al., 2009). We repeatedly experience patients asking for physician-hastened death, both in our outpatient department and on our palliative care unit. The reasons for such requests are mainly the fear of an excruciating death, loss of personal autonomy, or fatigue (Maessen et al., 2009). However, in almost all cases patients can be convinced that appropriate symptom control and pre-emptive measurements to maintain a maximum of autonomy are sufficient to refrain from such measures. Most patients die a sudden, non-violent death, often while sleeping. This might be due to nocturnal hypoxia or autonomic failure may be due to constant hypoxia.

Patient management

ALS is a rapidly progressive disease requiring anticipatory planning and regular re-evaluation of the patient's condition. It is of great importance to inform patients and caregivers of the progressive nature of the disease, as well as of common symptoms such as tetraparesis, dyspnoea, and respiratory insufficiency. Advance directives should be issued early and updated regularly. Swift management of issues related to supportive care and assistive equipment is essential to avoid additional burden for both patients and relatives. Since caregivers are often over-challenged by the multitude of organizational tasks, bringing social workers or other organizational resources into care management can greatly alleviate caregiver burden. The symptoms occurring in the course of disease require a multiprofessional approach, which should best be organized by a single person or institution, for example, a nurse practitioner, a general practitioner, or a specialized ambulant palliative care team. The ALS Peer Workgroup recently suggested triggers for hospice referral for ALS patients (McCluskey and Houseman, 2004).

Given the often devastating course of disease in ALS, the psychosocial, spiritual, physical, and financial burden for the primary caregivers must always be considered. Caregivers are usually inexperienced in patient care. Furthermore, information on practical issues such as requesting therapeutic appliances is usually sparse.

Inpatient treatment of ALS patients offers the unique opportunity to address psychological, spiritual, as well as practical issues, with both patients and the caregivers.

Parkinsonian syndromes

Parkinson's disease and related conditions

Parkinson's disease (PD) and Parkinson-related conditions such as progressive supranuclear palsy (PSP), multiple system atrophy (MSA), and corticobasal degeneration (CBD), are more common than ALS and have a longer course of the disease. No disease-modifying or effective neuroprotective agents are currently available for PD. Disease trajectory is frequently divided into the supportive phase, the phase of transition, and the terminal phase (Bunting-Perry, 2006).

Distressing motor symptoms include bradykinesia, muscle rigidity, dystonia, instability of gait, and tremor. Physiotherapy is the mainstay of non-pharmacologic therapy to improve balance and self-confidence. Painful dyskinesias and dystonias are distressing for patients and carers and require aggressive management. More frequent and lower doses of carbidopa/levodopa might improve motor fluctuations. Controlled release preparations, adding a dopamine agonist, or amantadine are other considerations.

Autonomic dysfunction such as orthostatic hypotension is common in MSA but may occur in PD as well. Increased sweating, delayed gastric emptying, constipation, sialorrhoea, urinary urge incontinence, and erectile dysfunction are also part of the dysautonomic spectrum of Parkinson-related disorders.

Progressive dysphagia is due to rigidity and hypokinesis as well as the gradual involvement of the dorsal motor nucleus of the vagus nerve in the disease process. There is no evidence to suggest a survival or quality of life benefit by feeding tube placement in advanced parkinsonism (Yamazaki et al., 2011). This remains an individual decision following discussion with patient and caregivers.

Depression, panic attacks, and anxiety are frequent psychological features of parkinsonism. There are conflicting data on the effectiveness of selective serotonin reuptake inhibitors (SSRIs) versus tricyclic antidepressants in the management of depression associated with PD. SSRIs are frequently preferred because of their more favourable side effect profile. While a concern of many specialists, large studies have not demonstrated that SSRIs worsen motor symptoms in PD.

Psychosis, hallucinations, and delusions are common in Parkinson-related disorders. Dose reduction of antiparkinsonian medication often helps. If hallucinations are a source of distress, it is recommended that anticholinergic drugs should be withdrawn first, followed by amantadine, catechol-O-methyl transferase inhibitors, and dopamine agonists if necessary. Stopping levodopa treatment is not usually an option, but a dose reduction might be attempted. Low doses of atypical neuroleptics (e.g. quetiapine, 25 mg/day) can be beneficial without significantly worsening motor symptoms.

Day time sleepiness and complex sleep disorders are often associated with advanced PD. Restless legs syndrome responds well to low-dose dopamine agonists before bedtime. Valproic acid, gabapentin, and benzodiazepines are also useful in this situation. Rapid eye movement (REM) sleep behaviour disorder (RBD) is often an early symptom of PD, manifesting in complex active behaviour during REM sleep. Most dopaminergic drugs as well as anticholinergics worsen RBD.

Cognitive dysfunction is very common in this patient group and different from the neuropsychological features of Alzheimer's disease. Executive dysfunction and visuospatial impairment are usually present, while the initial memory impairment is less prominent. Cholinesterase inhibitors (CI) are used with moderate success (Rolinski et al., 2012). The potential benefit of CIs has to be weighed against worsening tremor and nausea.

Atypical parkinsonian disorders

The term 'atypical parkinsonian disorders' (APD) encompasses a group of conditions displaying Parkinson-like symptoms that do not or poorly respond to antiparkinsonian drugs. These syndromes frequently present with distinguishing symptoms that are seldom seen in PD. They are also referred to as Parkinson-plus disorders and have distinct neuropathological characteristics. The most common diseases of this group include PSP, CBD, dementia with Lewy bodies (DLB), and MSA. Despite these conditions being rapidly progressive, there is now evidence that quality of life can be preserved with high-quality palliative care. This is especially true in PSP and MSA.

In contrast to the normal life expectancy of patients suffering from PD, the median survival of APD is estimated at 6 years for PSP, 9.5 years for MSA, 7 years for CBD, and 9 years for DLB. Although these conditions do share similar features, their presentation and therapeutic challenges are very different. For example, increased sensitivity to neuroleptics is highly specific to DLB and presents with impaired consciousness and severe acute parkinsonism regardless of the dose administered. Anticholinergic agents and tricyclic antidepressant should be avoided if orthostatic hypotension is present, and benzodiazepines frequently cause paradoxical agitation in DLB.

Atypical Parkinsonian disorders are not traditionally managed by palliative care teams. However, since there are no disease-modifying agents available and the wide spectrum of symptoms have a significant impact on the quality of life of the patients and families, palliative care intervention has a lot to offer in the management of these conditions.

Symptomatic management of atypical parkinsonian disorders

Motor function

Motor symptoms are often the presenting symptoms in parkinsonian disorders, and dopaminergic agents may offer temporary relief. The most commonly used drugs are carbidopa/levodopa, amantadine, imipramine, and selegiline. Zolpidem has been reported to improve eye movements in PSP, but benefit is transient and sedation is likely (Cotter et al., 2010). As the antiparkinsonian medications become ineffective over time, they can be gradually reduced and even discontinued. As the patient becomes more and more disabled and persistent neuropsychiatric problems develop, the priority of care shifts to preservation of quality of life through effective symptom control.

Neck and back pain is very common in advanced atypical parkinsonian disorders. Similarly to PD, it arises from stiffness, rigidity, or dystonic spasms. Treatment with botulinum toxin can reduce dystonia and consequently dystonia-associated pain, but often fails to improve coordination and motor function. Alternatively, analgesics can be prescribed according to the World Health Organization analgesic ladder approach.

Falls occur frequently in PSP and MSA and can cause serious injuries. In PSP, amitriptyline might reduce the frequency of falls in the early stages of the disease. Occupational therapists often suggest helmets and other safety devices, such as transfer belts or grab bars to prevent or cushion falls. Despite these measures, insight and safety awareness becomes a problem as cognitive deficits develop.

Myoclonus might be present in PSP, CBD, and MSA, and treatment usually requires benzodiazepines (e.g. clonazepam) or levetiracetam. Blepharospasm or eyelid apraxia may be treated with botulinum toxin A injections, even in advanced stages of the diseases.

Dysautonomia

Dysautonomic symptoms are hallmark of MSA but occur across the whole spectrum of parkinsonian syndromes. Treatment options of orthostatic dysfunction include reduction of L-dopa, use of compression stockings, increased sodium intake, and improved hydration. If these measures prove to be ineffective, fludrocortisone (0.1–0.2 mg/day) and midodrine (2.5–10 mg three times a day) can be considered. Urgency and urinary incontinence are straining symptoms for patients with decreased mobility and occur frequently. If substances like oxybutinin or tolterodine show little effect, regular injections of botulinum toxin can be considered before suprapubic catheterization. Urinary tract infections should be identified early. Occasionally intermittent catheterization might be necessary. Erectile dysfunction might precede the onset of these conditions by years.

Dysarthria and dysphagia

Dysphagia and dysarthria are caused by extensive medullar neuronal loss and involvement of the corticobulbar pathways in the disease process. Oropharyngeal dystonia and impaired reflexes put patients at risk of choking and aspiration. However, feeding tube placement should be considered on a case-by-case basis, depending on the stage of the disease and respecting the patient's preferences. In dementia and parkinsonian syndromes, the decision between radiologically inserted gastrostomy versus percutaneous endoscopic gastrostomy depends on tolerance of sedation and local policies.

Psychiatric symptoms

Personality and mood changes are common in each of these disorders and a characteristic clinical feature of DLB. The cognitive domains affected initially in DLB are executive function, attention, and visuospatial function as opposed to the amnestic deficits of Alzheimer's disease. Cognitive changes in MSA are less likely and occur later in the course of the disease. In PSP and CBD, patients gradually develop subcortical dementia, characterized by mental slowing, language deficits, impaired memory, apathy, and irritability. A pronounced frontotemporal pattern was noted in a subset of patients with PSP. Cholinergic deficits are thought to underlie the cognitive impairment of PSP, but trials of cholinergic agonists and cholinesterase inhibitors have failed to show improvement. Impulsive behaviour might be treated with SSRIs, but amitriptyline can also be effective if the anticholinergic side effects are acceptable.

Sleep disorders

Sleep disorders such as insomnia, daytime somnolence, sleep apnoea, and restless leg syndrome are not uncommon in atypical parkinsonism and can be managed effectively. RBD is a prominent feature of DLB that describes complex motor manifestations of vivid dreams. Patients with RBD might harm themselves or their partners. Treatment options include bedtime clonazepam, and melatonin.

The last phase

In their last days of life, patients with parkinsonian syndromes often suffer from pneumonia. Bradykinesia increases dramatically, and often even spasticity is seen. Communication might not been possible due to severe generalized dystonia (including larynx and pharynx muscles as well as mouth opening dystonia). Eyes are often wide open, but apparently there is an inability to control eye movements. Seizures as well as myoclonic jerks occur frequently. Since extensive stiffness often is distressing for both patients and caregivers at this stage, transdermal dopamine agonists or subcutaneous apomorphine can be considered. Nausea and vomiting, a common complaint of apomorphine treatment, is usually not observed in late-stage patients. It is not rare for patients to exhibit profound cachexia, even if tube feeding has been placed earlier on. However, patients are often able to understand and make decisions. Therefore, decisions regarding life-limiting procedures should be discussed not only with the relatives but also with the patient. In our experience, most patients with parkinsonian syndromes refuse life-prolonging therapies.

Multiple sclerosis

MS is an inflammatory autoimmune disorder affecting about 2.5 million people worldwide and representing the most common cause of neurological disability among young adults in some countries. In recent years, novel immunomodulatory therapies have emerged and have been able to modify disease activity significantly (Miller and Rhoades, 2012). However, what this means in the long-term course of the disease remains to be seen, as MS remains incurable, and many patients who are severely affected today never had the chance to receive these modern treatments. Because of the complex clinical situation with a large range of physical symptoms and psychosocial issues, and a large proportion of patients with a wish for hastened death, care models are arising including palliative care services for severely affected patients.

What does it mean to be severely affected? The physical status is generally measured using the 'Expanded Disability Status Score' (EDSS). However, measuring only physical impairment, this alone is not sufficient to measure the full impact of the disease (Gruenewald et al., 2004). A purely subjective feeling of being 'severely affected' will identify MS patients with a longer disease duration, more likely to be of a progressive form, and having an EDSS of 6.5 (range 1–9.5) (Strupp et al., 2012).

In this patient group, there are many unmet needs. Starting with a mean of nine symptoms, mainly neurological symptoms, such as difficulty using legs or arms, fatigue, or spasticity, MS compares with other diagnoses that have conventionally been the targets for specialist palliative care, such as cancer, heart disease, or lung disease (Higginson et al., 2006). Patients, relatives, and

Table 15.5.1 Drug treatment options in symptoms in neurodegenerative disorders. Choice of therapy should be made considering optimal route of application and concomitant symptoms

Symptom control in neurodegenerative diseases	
Constipation	Ensure sufficient hydration
	Many options: (1) osmotic laxatives such as lactulose or polyethylene glycol, (2) stimulant laxatives such as senna, (3) 5-HT agonists such as prucaloprid, or (4) opioid antagonists such as methylnaltrexone
Dyspnoea	Opioids (e.g. in the opioid-naïve, oral morphine at a starting dose of 2 mg every 4 hours or transdermal fentanyl at 12 micrograms/hour)
Dyspnoea-related anxiety	Fast-acting anxiolytics (e.g. sublingual lorazepam 0.5–1.0 mg every 4 hours as needed) and/or continuous benzodiazepine therapy (e.g. lorazepam 1–2 mg every 6 hours or midazolam 10–30 mg/day)
Fatigue	SSRI (e.g. citalopram 20 mg/day) or a psychostimulant (e.g. modafinil starting at 100 mg daily or methylphenidate starting at 5 mg twice daily)
Muscle cramps	Quinidine sulphate 200 mg daily
Pain	Depending on severity and chronicity, trials of drugs such as tilidine, metamizole, tramadol, or tapentadol may be considered, or treatment with oral morphine or alternative pure mu agonist may be used; non-traditional analgesics, such as an analgesic antidepressant (e.g. a tricyclic or a serotonin-norepinephrine reuptake inhibitor), also are tried
Pseudobulbar affect	First choice: dextromethorphan/quinidine 20 mg/10 mg daily, increasing to twice daily after 1 week; an alternative choice would be a SSRI
Pseudohypersalivation	Sage tea
	Amitriptyline, 25 mg once a day
	Hyoscine hydrobromide transdermal patch, initially ¼ patch daily
	Botulinum toxin A, e.g. 50 IE injected in the salivary glands
	Salivary gland radiotherapy
Psychosis, agitation, irritability, dysphoria	Create a calm and stable environment
	Quetiapine (25–50 mg/day), clozapine
REM sleep behaviour disorder (RBD)	Clonazepam (0.25–1.5 mg), melatonin (3–12 mg)
Respiratory failure	NIPPV
	Tracheostomy
	Symptomatic treatment with opioids, e.g. morphine (see 'Dyspnoea')
Rigidity, brady-/akinesia Note: severe akinesia is rare	Amantadine IV, PO (600 mg/day)
	Rotigotine patch (2–8 mg/day)
	Apomorphine SC (6 mg/hour)
	Midazolam IV, SC (60 mg/day)
Sleeplessness	Zopiclone, zolpidem
	Amitriptyline (25 mg PO, especially if hypersalivation is present)
	Mirtazapine
	Quetiapine (25 mg PO)
Spasticity	Physiotherapy
	Baclofen (e.g. starting dose of 5 mg twice daily, titrated upwards as needed),
	Tizanidine (e.g. starting dose of 2 mg at night, titrated upwards as a twice-daily dose as necessary)
	Botulinum toxin A
Thick secretions	Ensure sufficient hydration
	Mucolytics, e.g. ambroxol, N-acetylcysteine
	Beta antagonists
	Supportive measures, such as nebulized saline, manually assisted coughing techniques, modified postural drainage, humidification, mechanical insufflation–insufflation devices, high-frequency chest wall oscillation

professionals all identify unmet needs in this population, and a full picture will only be achieved if all stakeholders' views are included (Golla et al., 2012).

One major aspect of care is the need for open communication about the disease status and fears arising from that. Patients constantly have to adapt to a new disease phase, sometimes a continuing process over years. The need for communication does not necessarily correlate with any 'objective' aspect of the disease, such as EDSS, duration of disease, age or the subjective feeling of being severely affected. Physicians just have to ask and find out how much patients want to know. Patients expect us to talk about serious issues in MS with themselves as well as their loved ones (Buecken et al., 2012).

So what does this mean for the management of these patients? First, all health professionals involved in the care of severely affected MS patients should implement the core aspects of palliative care as a best practice. Second, coordination of helping services in a given region must also focus on this patient group, and include palliative and hospice services. For example, encouraging results have been observed using a regional coordination palliative care MS hotline in Cologne, Germany, for severely affected patients. Beyond coordination, it is valuable for specialists in palliative care to provide advice and help to existing MS services, a model which has been tested very successfully in London. There, significant changes were seen in symptom control (e.g. identification and treatment of nausea, use of opioids for neuropathic pain), the burden of relatives was reduced, and there was a diminished need for inpatient admission (Edmonds et al., 2010).

Of course, the provision of palliative care services to patients with MS still seems counter-intuitive to some patients, relatives, and professionals. The future will show, however, that integration of this service will be of great benefit to MS patients. As the European Code of Good Practice states: 'Clinical experience and the results of recent studies lead us to conclude that patients severely affected by MS in Europe should have access to palliative care assessment and services.'

Medication at the end of life

To date, there is no cure for patients suffering from neurodegenerative diseases. Nonetheless, effective drug treatment can alter the individual's functional status, offer improved symptom control, and may even prolong life in many of these disorders, such as PD or MS. However, most of these drugs have their greatest effects when the disease is at a very early stage. They often fail to prove useful in advanced stages, when symptom burden is higher.

In these late stages, pharmaceutical options may be further limited, for example, by swallowing deficits, malabsorption, polypharmacy, or comorbidity. Especially in neurodegenerative diseases with deficits of swallowing, late-stage medication thus has to be applied via alternative routes, such as subcutaneous, transdermal, or rectal. Table 15.5.1 summarizes pharmaceutical options for symptom control in neurodegenerative diseases, with respect to alternative routes of administration. No distinction is made between different disorders, since comparable symptoms often occur in late-stage neurodegeneration irrespective of the underlying disease.

Online materials

Complete references for this chapter are available online at <http://www.oxfordmedicine.com>.

References

Andersen, P.M., Abrahams, S., Borasio, G.D., et al. (2012). EFNS guidelines on the clinical management of amyotrophic lateral sclerosis (MALS)—revised report of an EFNS task force. *European Journal of Neurology*, 19(3), 360–375.

Bourke, S.C., Tomlinson, M., Williams, T.L., Bullock, R.E., Shaw, P.J., and Gibson, G.J. (2006). Effects of non-invasive ventilation on survival and quality of life in patients with amyotrophic lateral sclerosis: a randomised controlled trial. *The Lancet Neurology*, 5(2), 140–147.

Buecken, R., Galushko, M., Golla, H., et al. (2012). Patients feeling severely affected by multiple sclerosis: how do patients want to communicate about end-of-life issues? *Patient Education and Counseling*, 88(2), 318–324.

Bunting-Perry, L.K. (2006). Palliative care in Parkinson's disease: implications for neuroscience nursing. *Journal of Neuroscience Nursing*, 38(2), 106–113.

Burton, C.R., Payne, S., Addington-Hall, J., and Jones, A. (2010). The palliative care needs of acute stroke patients: a prospective study of hospital admissions. *Age and Ageing*, 39(5), 554–559.

Desport, J.C., Mabrouk, T., Bouillet, P., Perna, A., Preux, P.M., and Couratier, P. (2005). Complications and survival following radiologically and endoscopically-guided gastrostomy in patients with amyotrophic lateral sclerosis. *Amyotrophic Lateral Sclerosis and Other Motor Neuron Disorders*, 6(2), 88–93.

Edmonds, P., Hart, S., Gao, W., Vivat, B., Burman, R., Silber, E., and Higginson, I.J. (2010). Palliative care for people severely affected by multiple sclerosis: evaluation of a novel palliative care service. *Multiple Sclerosis*, 16(5), 627–636.

Golla, H., Galushko, M., Pfaff, H., and Voltz, R. (2012). Unmet needs of severely affected multiple sclerosis patients: the health professionals' view. *Palliative Medicine*, 26(2), 139–151.

Higginson, I.J., Hart, S., Silber, E., Burman, R., and Edmonds, P. (2006). Symptom prevalence and severity in people severely affected by multiple sclerosis. *Journal of Palliative Care*, 22(3), 158–165.

Hohlfeld, R. (2011). Update on sporadic inclusion body myositis. *Brain*, 134(Pt 11), 3141–3145.

Khot, S., Billings, M., Owens, D., and Longstreth, W.T., Jr. (2011). Coping with death and dying on a neurology inpatient service: death rounds as an educational initiative for residents. *Archives of Neurology*, 68(11), 1395–1397.

Maessen, M., Veldink, J.H., Onwuteaka-Philipsen, B.D., et al. (2009). Trends and determinants of end-of-life practices in ALS in the Netherlands. *Neurology*, 73(12), 954–961.

Neudert, C., Oliver, D., Wasner, M., and Borasio, G.D. (2001). The course of the terminal phase in patients with amyotrophic lateral sclerosis. *Journal of Neurology*, 248(7), 612–616.

Pennington, S., Snell, K., Lee, M., and Walker, R. (2010). The cause of death in idiopathic Parkinson's disease. *Parkinsonism & Related Disorders*, 16(7), 434–437.

Rolinski, M., Fox, C., Maidment, I., and McShane, R. (2012). Cholinesterase inhibitors for dementia with Lewy bodies, Parkinson's disease dementia and cognitive impairment in Parkinson's disease. *Cochrane Database of Systematic Reviews*, 14(3), CD006504.

Strupp, J., Hartwig, A.J., Golla, H., Galushko, M., Pfaff, H., and Voltz, R. (2012). Feeling severely affected by multiple sclerosis: what does this mean? *Palliative Medicine*, 26(8), 1001–1010.

Voltz, R. (2010). Palliative care for multiple sclerosis: a counter-intuitive approach? *Multiple Sclerosis*, 16(5), 515–517.

15.6

End-stage kidney disease

Fliss E. M. Murtagh

Introduction to end-stage kidney disease

End-stage kidney disease (ESKD), like end-stage cardiac or respiratory disease, leads eventually to death. However, unlike cardiac or respiratory disease, life-sustaining treatment in the form of dialysis is available. Initially, dialysis was a short-term treatment for patients with acute renal failure, with no provision of longer-term maintenance dialysis for patients with chronic renal failure. But the first dialysis programmes started in the 1960s and have steadily expanded in subsequent decades. At first, older patients or those with multiple co-morbidities were excluded, but more recently, the criteria for dialysis have been relaxed, and many more patients have been accepted onto dialysis programmes. For example, the number of patients receiving dialysis in the United Kingdom rose fivefold, from 5000 in 1984 to 25 000 in 2006 (Ansell et al., 2007). This rise reflects several factors beyond increasing acceptance onto dialysis programmes, including an increase in the prevalence of renal disease, ethnic variations in renal disease, and an older population.

Despite technical advances and changes in the way dialysis is delivered, it still remains a challenging treatment for many patients. Dialysis usually requires invasive procedures and then protracted treatment sessions three times each week. While some uraemic symptoms are relieved by dialysis, the overall symptom burden of those receiving dialysis remains high (Murtagh et al., 2007c). For some patients with severe co-morbidity and short life expectancy, dialysis is either not feasible or is unlikely to improve quality or quantity of life. Other patients decide not to have dialysis, instead choosing conservative (non-dialytic) management of their renal disease. Their renal management then focuses on delaying progression of renal disease and controlling complications, alongside control of symptoms and psychosocial support as the disease progresses towards death.

There are, therefore, several groups of patients among those with ESKD who benefit from palliative care, whether that care is delivered by palliative care or nephrology clinicians, or by an integrated team which shares care across speciality boundaries. These patient groups are:

- those who choose or are advised not to embark on dialysis (conservative or non-dialytic management)
- those who are failing to thrive on dialysis, and who experience worsening quality of life and increasing symptom burden despite dialysis
- those who discontinue dialysis.

Epidemiology

It is estimated that the age-adjusted prevalence of stage 3–5 chronic kidney disease (CKD) in the United Kingdom is approximately 11% of women and 6% of men (Stevens et al., 2007). This is equivalent to 4 million people in the United Kingdom. A similar prevalence of CKD has been reported by studies from other countries (Chadban et al., 2003; Coresh et al., 2003). Only a small proportion of these will progress to ESKD, and to the time when a decision between conservative or dialysis treatment is required. Nevertheless, because the overall prevalence of CKD is relatively high, a large number of patients will reach ESKD.

Epidemiological studies also show that the prevalence of ESKD increases rapidly with advancing age. Stage 3–5 CKD is present in less than 1% of people under 35 years but is present in 40% of people over 75 years (Stevens et al., 2007). Initiation of dialysis is therefore much more frequent in the elderly, and the proportion increases sharply among those over 65 years, peaks between 75 and 85 years, and only drops off after 85 years. This strongly age-related nature of ESKD means that the numbers with ESKD will increase further as the overall population in developed countries ages. Certainly the number of patients on renal replacement therapy is increasing steadily and it is likely that this trend will continue for some years to come (Roderick et al., 2004). The United States Renal Data System (USRDS) reports 354 000 people on dialysis in 2006, with the prediction that this will increase to 533 000 by 2020 (USRDS, 2008). As the number of patients reaching ESKD increases, so will the number of patients choosing conservative treatment.

The exact number of patients who die of renal failure after conservative management (i.e. without receiving dialysis) is very difficult to ascertain, partly because of the lack of routinely collected data, but also because few population-based, rather than service-based, studies are conducted. Some patients with severe co-morbidity may never be referred to renal services. In reported series of patients known to renal services and managed in specialist low-clearance clinics, approximately 15–20% of those with declining renal function will follow a conservative pathway (Smith et al., 2003; Murtagh et al., 2007d). In reality, this figure is likely to vary considerably between units depending on the demographics of the catchment population, and on how services are structured. A national observational study in Australia indicates that about 14% (one in seven) of patients with ESKD referred to nephrologists plan not to dialyse (Morton et al., 2012b). Comprehensive service provision with integrated palliative care needs to be improved to meet the demands of the ageing population. There have always been some patients managed conservatively, without dialysis, but practice has varied over time and between countries (Lambie et al., 2006), and between individual nephrologists (Kee et al., 2000), and it is only recently that there has been greater recognition of the conservatively managed group of patients, with systematic study beginning to be undertaken in order to address some of these very relevant questions.

Survival

There is limited evidence about the duration of survival of conservatively managed patients. First, although there have always been patients managed without dialysis, only recently has this group been recognized as a distinct population needing study. Second, it has been difficult to identify when survival should be measured *from*—patients may not require dialysis until well into stage 5 CKD, as they begin to experience worsening uraemic symptoms. And even if dialysis is planned, some will die of co-morbid disease before dialysis can commence, and others experience only a very slow decline in renal function, such that dialysis is not actually needed for some time. Third, documented survival may well reflect the demographics, co-morbidity, and local practice at any one renal unit, rather than mortality data that is readily generalizable.

There have been no prospective randomized trials which assess the benefit of dialysis versus conservative management in this population. The ethical challenges that this would raise are such that a randomized trial is unlikely to occur, and only a small number of observational studies are currently available to inform practice. Smith et al. report survival of 38 patients who, after multidisciplinary assessment, were recommended palliative (conservative) treatment rather than dialysis (Smith et al., 2003). In this cohort, ten patients did not follow the recommendation and instead chose to have dialysis, while the remainder followed the conservative pathway as recommended. Statistically, survival was not significantly different between the two groups, although numbers were small. A second study considered all patients over 75 years with stage 5 CKD managed in specialist nephrology care (Murtagh et al., 2007d). Notably, this study excluded those referred into nephrology care late, after estimated glomerular filtration rate (eGFR) reached less than 15 mL/minute (late referrals are more likely to be managed conservatively (Joly et al., 2003), and are known to have worse survival). Seventy-seven patients (60%) were established on a conservative (non-dialytic) treatment pathway (Murtagh et al., 2007d). Patients managed without dialysis had a 1- and 2-year survival (measured from first reaching stage 5 CKD) of 68% and 47% respectively. Those managed conservatively had a significantly worse survival than those on a dialysis pathway, suggesting some benefit from dialysis for older patients, at least in terms of survival. However, it was impossible to exclude a selection bias, with fitter patients choosing dialysis, and factors other than dialysis were almost certainly contributing to the better survival in the dialysis group. If the patients with higher co-morbidity were considered in isolation, then the difference in survival between the two groups was much reduced. More recent evidence from a recent larger study shows that median survival from entry into stage 5 CKD was less in conservatively managed patients (21.2 months) than those on dialysis (67.1 months, p < 0.001), but similarly for patients over 75 years with high co-morbidity and diabetes, this survival advantage was lost (Chandna et al., 2011).

When there is no residual renal function, patients withdrawing from dialysis have a very short survival, with the evidence reporting a mean survival between 8 to 10 days (Murtagh et al., 2007a).

Most patients will have a shorter survival than this, living just a few days after dialysis is discontinued, but the range is 1–46 days. If there is residual renal function, for instance, after a brief trial of dialysis, then survival can be very much longer (sometimes months), according to the level of residual renal function and the underlying disease processes.

Symptoms

There has been little study into the symptoms of those managed conservatively, without dialysis, although this may change as this population grows and there is greater recognition of their specific needs. Most of the work to date has been undertaken in the United Kingdom (Murtagh et al., 2007b, 2011; Noble et al., 2007, 2008; Murtagh, 2009), but needs to be duplicated in other settings and countries. There is some work on the patient experience of conservative management (Noble et al., 2008), and the impact of it on families and carers (Ashby et al., 2005; Low et al., 2008).

The symptom work that has been done shows that patients with conservatively managed stage 5 CKD have a high prevalence of symptoms (Murtagh et al., 2007b), similar in terms of overall burden to patients with advanced cancer, although with differences in the patterns of symptoms and the level of distress caused. Patients with ESKD are among the most symptomatic of any chronic disease group (Solano et al., 2006). Identifying and controlling symptoms is a high priority for patients and families (Steinhauser et al., 2000), and notably improves their quality of life (Weisbord et al., 2003). For those with ESKD, excellent symptom management becomes an increasingly high priority as the duration of time they remain dependent on chronic renal replacement therapy increases (Singer et al., 1999; Steinhauser et al., 2000). It is also important to recognize that, while renal replacement therapy in the form of dialysis provides major benefit, including symptom relief, it will not always ameliorate or abolish symptoms and may sometimes contribute to them.

Prevalence of specific symptoms

Anxiety and depression

Anxiety is reported as occurring in 12–52% and depression in 5–71% of dialysis patients (Murtagh et al., 2007e). Much of this variation reflects variation in the populations assessed, the definitions of anxiety and depression used, and the instruments used to detect them. Screening tools, such as the Beck Depression Inventory, tend to identify a somewhat higher proportion (45–50%) of potential depression than diagnostic tools, depending on the level of cut-off used (Kimmel, 2001, Wuerth et al., 2005). Patients managed without dialysis probably have similar levels of anxiety and depression, although evidence remains limited, and the prevalence of anxiety and depression likely increases over time (Murtagh et al., 2007c). They have a high prevalence of the symptoms of feeling anxious or sad (63% and 50%, respectively), and 45% have depressive scores above the standard cut-off on the Geriatric Depression Scale (Murtagh et al., 2007c).

Pain

Pain is a common problem for patients with advanced renal disease. In a recent Canadian study, 50% of all haemodialysis patients reported chronic pain, and over half of these described their pain as severe (Davison, 2007). An Italian study reported a similar proportion (48%) of dialysis patients affected by pain (Mercadante et al., 2005), as did a US study which identified 50% of haemodialysis patients as reporting bone or joint pain (Weisbord et al., 2005). These studies demonstrate that pain is more common in dialysis patients than previously recognized. Pain prevalence in conservatively managed stage 5 CKD is similar, with baseline pain prevalence of 53% (Murtagh et al., 2007b), increasing markedly over time to affect 73% of patients by the month before death, with over half of these reporting severe pain (Murtagh et al., 2007c). For those withdrawing from dialysis, pain affects about 50% of patients (Cohen et al., 2000; Chater et al., 2006).

Pruritus

Numerous studies provide evidence on the prevalence of itch, suggesting that pruritus affects between 28% and 60% of patients on haemodialysis, and between 50% and 68% of those on peritoneal dialysis (Murtagh et al., 2007e). Four studies report higher prevalence still (between 70% and 74%) among haemodialysis patients (Merkus et al., 1999; Curtin et al., 2002; Subach and Marx, 2002; Dyachenko et al., 2006). Pruritus prevalence in those with stage 5 CKD managed without dialysis is also high (74%), suggesting it is similarly prevalent in those with ESKD not on dialysis (Murtagh et al., 2007b).

Restless legs

The reported prevalence of the symptom of restless legs among dialysis patients varies considerably, from 12% to 58% (Murtagh et al., 2007e). This compares with prevalence of at least 10–15% in the general population (Medcalf and Bhatia, 2006). For this symptom, perhaps more than any other, reported prevalence depends heavily on the definition used. Earlier studies have tended to use less well defined criteria, while more recent studies have used the specific criteria developed by the International Restless Legs Syndrome Study Group (IRLSSG) to define restless legs syndrome (RLS) (Allen et al., 2003). These latter studies indicate a somewhat lower prevalence of the syndrome of restless legs among patients receiving dialysis, between 12% and 22% (Manenti et al., 2009). Of those with stage 5 disease not receiving dialysis, 48% report the symptom of restless legs (Murtagh et al., 2007b), although this study did not formal IRLSSG criteria. As with pruritus, there is some indication that RLS is associated with poorer prognosis which may again be mediated partly through impaired quality of sleep (Hui et al., 2000).

Sleep disturbance

Sleep disturbance is a common problem in patients with ESKD but it is hard to determine the exact prevalence of this problem because of the challenges of definition. Insomnia affects at least 10–15% of the general population (Drake et al., 2003), but the prevalence of sleep disturbance in renal patients is notably higher. Several studies have described prevalence and findings range from 20% to 83% (Murtagh et al., 2007e). This wide range reflects varying definitions, but whatever definition is used, it is clear that this is a symptom which troubles many dialysis patients. Those stage 5 CKD patients who opt not to have dialysis and are managed conservatively also have a high prevalence of sleep disturbance, with 41% experiencing some difficulty with sleep, and 21% (of all conservatively managed patients) reporting severely distressing sleep disturbance (Murtagh et al., 2007b).

Fatigue

Tiredness or fatigue is also a symptom which is difficult to define, and therefore to quantify. Despite this, there is evidence that it is one of the most common symptoms experienced by renal patients; in most studies, between 70% and 97% of dialysis patients are affected by fatigue (Kutner et al., 1985; Chang et al., 2001; Kundhal and Lok, 2005; Jhamb et al., 2008). A very high proportion of conservatively managed stage 5 CKD patients are also affected by fatigue, with 90% of patients affected by fatigue, and 35% of all patients severely distressed by this (Murtagh et al., 2007c). Qualitative studies also suggest it is one of the most difficult symptoms for patients to cope with (Chang et al., 2001; Murtagh et al., 2007c).

Other symptoms

Other key symptoms have been shown to be important for patients with ESKD. These symptoms include nausea and vomiting, drowsiness, breathlessness, leg oedema, dry mouth, lack of appetite and altered taste, poor concentration, dry skin, and constipation. Some symptoms, for example, breathlessness, are frequently linked to co-morbidity, such as coexisting cardiac or respiratory disease, and their prevalence very much reflects the demographics of the population, with older populations and those conservatively managed (without dialysis)—who are almost always older patients—displaying a notably higher prevalence of these symptoms (Murtagh et al., 2007c).

Symptoms due to co-morbid conditions

In those with ESKD, it is not always clear whether uraemia, dialysis, or co-morbid conditions are the most dominant cause of each symptom, and for many patients a combination of causes and triggers contributes to their overall symptom burden. Co-morbid conditions do play a major part in causing symptoms, particularly for the older patient, who may have vascular disease, cardiac problems, diabetes mellitus, or other co-morbidities. Some of the commoner co-morbid conditions which contribute to symptom burden include diabetic gastroparesis, other diabetic neuropathies, other diabetic complications, cardiovascular disease, and peripheral vascular disease.

Diabetic patients with end-stage renal disease have often had their diabetes for many years, and may have other complications in addition to their renal impairment. Diabetic gastroparesis due to autonomic nerve damage is common in long-standing diabetes, and is characterized by anorexia, early satiety (feeling full), nausea, and sometimes vomiting. Advanced uraemia itself also leads to delayed gastric emptying, which can contribute to this problem. Delayed gastric emptying may itself cause gastric reflux and dyspepsia. Diabetic patients also suffer from other neuropathies, such as autonomic neuropathies affecting the mid and lower gut, and characterized by alternating diarrhoea and constipation. Non-autonomic diabetic neuropathies that affect the peripheral nerves may occur. The neuropathic pain associated with diabetic neuropathies can be severe, persistent, and difficult to control. Skin and soft tissue problems are also common in the diabetic patient; decubitus ulcers or diabetic foot may occur and amputation may sometimes be required. The severity of these skin and soft tissue problems may be such that these pains are sometimes difficult to control.

Assessment of symptoms

Global symptom measures

Several global symptom measures have been used to evaluate the whole range of symptoms in renal disease. These include instruments used in other advanced diseases, such as the Edmonton Symptom Assessment System (Parfrey et al., 1989; Davison et al., 2006a, 2006b), and the Memorial Symptom Assessment Scale short form (Weisbord et al., 2003; Murtagh et al., 2007b). Other measures have been validated specifically for use in those with renal disease. These include the Dialysis Symptom Index, developed from the Memorial Symptom Assessment Scale by Weisbord et al. (2004), and the renal version of the Patient Outcome Scale (symptom module) (Murphy et al., 2009), derived from the generic version of the Patient (or Palliative) Outcome Scale which is used across a wide number of conditions and countries.

Symptom-specific measures

Although the whole range of symptoms which patients experience needs to be assessed, there is a wider range of instruments which have been used to assess individual symptoms, such as pain, pruritus, or depression. These may provide a more detailed and accurate picture of each symptom, especially for research purposes. A range of measures are available for measurement of pain (Melzack, 1975; Daut et al., 1983), depression (Beck and Steer, 1984; Kutner et al., 1985; Martin and Thompson, 2000), pruritus (Majeski et al., 2007), or RLS (Allen et al., 2009). The Cambridge–Hopkins restless legs questionnaire is based on the IRLSSG criteria, but also distinguishes RLS from other conditions, with good sensitivity and specificity (Allen et al., 2009). A range of other measures for individual symptoms exist, and are useful for research purposes, but fairly brief validated measures which capture the whole range of symptoms may be most useful in the clinical setting.

Management of symptoms

Once symptoms have been identified and assessed, they need to be actively managed. Evidence shows that management of symptoms is often suboptimal for renal patients (Davison, 2003; Bailie et al., 2004). Renal impairment places a major constraint on use of medication, since many medicines are renally excreted, and may therefore accumulate substantially in renal impairment. For those on dialysis, careful consideration also needs to be given to the effect of dialysis on drug clearance.

Management of pain

As with any other disease group, the suspected causes of pain need to be carefully delineated, and management tailored to these causes. Removal or specific treatment of the underlying cause when feasible is always the best approach, and only when this cannot be achieved should palliation be the main focus. Non-opioid, opioid, and adjuvant analgesics can be used in the ESKD population, but careful consideration needs to be given to:

◆ potential risk of adverse effects, which may be exacerbated by uraemia

◆ whether there is risk of nephrotoxicity (it is critically important not to risk remaining renal function)

◆ elimination of the drugs used, and how this will be influenced by the renal impairment.

World Health Organization step 2 and step 3 opioids will be briefly considered here, but the reader is referred to extensive reviews of analgesic use for more details (Davies et al., 1996; Dean, 2004; Mercadante and Arcuri, 2004; Murtagh et al., 2007f).

Codeine and dihydrocodeine

There are reports of serious side effects following codeine use in patients with advanced renal failure, in particular profound hypotension (Parke et al., 1992), respiratory arrest (Talbott et al., 1997), and profound narcolepsy (Matzke et al., 1986). Dihydrocodeine is thought to have similar metabolism and elimination to codeine, and there are similar reports of prolonged narcosis (Barnes and Goodwin, 1983; Redfern, 1983). For these reasons, use of codeine and dihydrocodeine is not recommended in ESKD.

Tramadol

Ninety per cent of tramadol is excreted via the kidneys (Lee et al., 1993), and in renal impairment, there is about a twofold increase in the elimination half-life (Lee et al., 1993). Because of this increased elimination half-life, it is recommended that the dose interval be increased to 12-hourly, and the dose reduced. Uraemia also lowers the seizure threshold, and tramadol may be more epileptogenic in ESKD patients (Gardner et al., 2000). For these reasons, an alternative drug is preferred for ESKD patients, and if the use of tramadol is absolutely unavoidable, a dose of 50 mg 12-hourly should not be exceeded.

Morphine and diamorphine

Morphine and diamorphine are not recommended for use in ESKD, because of the problems with metabolite accumulation, and because at least some of these metabolites are clinically active.

Fentanyl

Less than 10% of fentanyl is excreted unchanged in the urine. In renal failure, no dose modification appears necessary when fentanyl is given as a bolus injection (Coral et al., 1980), but there is limited evidence on the pharmacokinetics when it is administered either in repeated doses or by continuous infusion. One study suggests that the parent compound may accumulate with sustained administration (Koehntop and Rodman, 1997), and a further study demonstrates reduced clearance of fentanyl in patients with renal failure (Scholz et al., 1996). Despite these concerns about accumulation, fentanyl is, on present limited evidence, one of the preferred opioids in ESKD, because the metabolites are inactive. Some authorities suggest dose reduction with declining renal function: 75% of normal dose if creatinine clearance is 10–50 mL/minute, and 50% normal dose if creatinine clearance is less than 10mL/min (Broadbent et al., 2003). Careful monitoring for any gradual development of accumulation and toxicity would certainly be wise in any case of sustained administration (beyond 1 or 2 days), and there may be some basis for gradual dose reduction if fentanyl is used over days or weeks. Transdermal patches can be used, but careful review, with vigilance for accumulation, is important. The very wide individual variations in its pharmacokinetics (Bentley et al., 1982; Labroo et al., 1997) would also support a cautious approach.

Alfentanil

Alfentanil is shorter acting than fentanyl, and is both less potent and less lipid soluble. Like fentanyl, it is highly protein bound and its protein binding is reduced by a high urea, but despite this the volume of distribution and elimination half-life appears unchanged in patients with renal failure (Chauvin et al., 1987). Alfentanil is therefore also one of the preferred opioids for use in ESKD, but is limited to end-of-life use, given that it is only available for parenteral use.

Buprenorphine

Buprenorphine is metabolized in the liver to norbuprenorphine, and buprenorphine-3-glucuronide, and these metabolites are principally excreted via the biliary system (Mercadante and Arcuri, 2004). Because of its high systemic clearance and largely hepatic metabolism, buprenorphine has the potential to be reasonably safe in patients with renal failure. Some evidence shows no change in the pharmacokinetics of buprenorphine in renal impairment (Summerfield et al., 1985), but other work shows some accumulation of metabolites (Hand et al., 1990). No adverse effects were reported, and specifically no sedation or respiratory depression. Buprenorphine also has the advantage of being available in sublingual, transdermal, and injectable preparations. Note that buprenorphine is omitted from some of the reviews of analgesia in renal impairment because it is not available in all countries.

Hydromorphone

A single-dose study indicates hydromorphone accumulation in renal impairment (Durnin et al., 2001) (with proportionately greater accumulation in severe renal impairment), and a further detailed pharmacokinetic case study over 14 days (Babul et al., 1995) demonstrated clear accumulation of H-3-G. Since H-3-G is known to be a more potent neuro-excitant, there has been considerable concern about the use of hydromorphone in severe renal impairment. However, a retrospective review by Lee and colleagues (Lee et al., 2001) suggests that hydromorphone may be reasonably better tolerated than morphine in patients with renal impairment, although levels of renal impairment were small. Overall, the evidence to support the safety of hydromorphone in renal impairment is extremely limited. It may be reasonable, given the available evidence, to use hydromorphone carefully in mild or even moderate renal impairment, provided doses are reduced and the dose interval increased, and with careful monitoring and titration. In severe renal impairment, its use cannot be recommended however, until there is more evidence available.

Methadone

Methadone is metabolized mostly in the liver, and excreted both renally and faecally (Davies et al., 1996). There is large inter-individual variation, but also considerable difference between acute and chronic phase dosing (Rostami-Hodjegan et al., 1999). Some evidence suggests that plasma concentrations are no higher than in those with normal renal function (Kreek et al., 1980), suggesting that faecal excretion might compensate in those with renal impairment. Because of this, and the limited possibilities for use of other opioids, methadone has been used reasonably often for patients with renal failure and no adverse effects have been reported. Caution should be exercised on two counts, however: firstly, because of a well-described risk of accumulation and toxicity, experienced specialist supervision of methadone use should be available, and secondly, because of the wide individual variation, doses and effects should be closely monitored. The titration and use of methadone is fully described elsewhere (Morley, 1998; Blackburn et al., 2002), but in severe renal impairment a dose reduction of 50–75% is recommended (Broadbent et al., 2003).

Oxycodone

A study by Kirvela et al. showed that the elimination of oxycodone in renal failure is significantly prolonged, and excretion of its metabolites is severely impaired (Kirvela et al., 1996), with wide inter-individual variation. Work by Kalso and colleagues also suggests that some of the effects of oxycodone may be mediated through its metabolites (Kalso et al., 1990). There are also reports of central nervous system toxicity and sedation with oxycodone in renal failure (Fitzgerald, 1991). This raises queries about the use of oxycodone in renal impairment, and there is insufficient evidence to determine whether or not it is safe to use in ESKD patients. Some clinicians use it with caution, reducing the dose and increasing the dose interval, while others avoid using it. Broadbent suggests the use of 75% of normal dose when creatinine clearance is 10–50 mL/minute, and 50% when creatinine clearance is less than 10 mL/minute (with unchanged dose intervals) (Broadbent et al., 2003).

Management of fatigue

Fatigue is multidimensional (Lee et al., 2007), with physical, cognitive, and emotional elements (O'Sullivan and McCarthy, 2007). There is a complex but poorly understood relationship between fatigue, sleep disturbance, physical functioning, and depression in those with renal disease (Brunier and Graydon, 1992; McCann and Boore, 2000). It is not clear, for instance, whether the reduced physical functioning which occurs with renal disease itself causes fatigue, or whether in fact the symptom of fatigue is a consequence of poor function. Fatigue is an important symptom because it is very common, highly distressing to patients, and there are a number of causes which are potentially treatable. These causes can be classified as related to the renal disease, to dialysis itself, or related to co-morbid conditions. The renal disease may cause anaemia, hyperparathyroidism, and uraemia, all of which may directly contribute to fatigue. Secondary to these direct effects are dietary and fluid restrictions, impaired nutrition, and the side effects of medications, all of which may contribute to fatigue, even if they are not the predominant causes of it. For those on dialysis, dialysis inadequacy, post dialysis fatigue, and the burden of dialysis itself may also play a part in instigating or perpetuating fatigue. Conditions unrelated to renal disease, such as hypothyroidism, should be considered and excluded. Non pharmacological managements of fatigue, such as exercise, cognitive and psychological approaches, and complementary treatments, are important, especially as pharmacological interventions become increasingly limited.

A systematic review of the use of erythropoietin-stimulating agents demonstrates that in renal patients there is a consistent relationship between haematocrit and energy/fatigue domains in quality of life (Ross et al., 2003); as haematocrit increases, so energy levels increase and fatigue reduces. When anaemia is due to kidney disease, which is likely if GFR is less than 30mL/min/1.73m^2 (less than 45 in diabetics) and no other cause (such as blood loss, folic acid or vitamin B_{12} deficiency) is identified, then active treatment with erythropoietin-stimulating agents is likely to improve fatigue. It is not clear, however, how long treatment should be maintained in those who are nearing the end of life; most clinicians continue treatment while the patient still continues to gain symptomatic benefit.

Management of nausea and vomiting

Nausea and vomiting are extremely unpleasant symptoms, and are often multifactorial. Assessment requires a thorough history including establishing the history and pattern of both nausea and vomiting separately. Profound nausea and/or repeated vomiting will prevent absorption of any medications taken orally, and alternative routes (such as sublingual, rectal, or subcutaneous routes) need to be considered, at least until nausea and vomiting is controlled.

The first step is to identify the specific cause of nausea and vomiting where possible, since cause-directed treatment is most likely to succeed. Uraemia and a variety of drugs (including opioids, anticonvulsants, antibiotics, and antidepressants) can cause this kind of persistent nausea. Gastroparesis or delayed gastric emptying, (which may be caused by drugs, such as opioids, or by primary diseases, such as diabetes mellitus), usually presents with a history of post-prandial nausea or vomiting of undigested food which relieves nausea. Bloating, epigastric fullness, flatulence, hiccough, or heartburn may accompany this. Nausea related to gastritis is often associated with heartburn, dyspepsia, or epigastric pain. Constipation may exacerbate nausea and vomiting.

For delayed gastric emptying or gastroparesis, metoclopramide can be use, although doses should be reduced by 50%, and there is an increased risk of dystonia. Haloperidol or levomepromazine is often used for nausea related to uraemia or drug-related nausea, although there is increased cerebral sensitivity, and both drugs need dose reduction. 5-hydroxytryptamine (serotonin) type 3 (5-HT$_3$) antagonists can also be used, although the side effect of constipation will need active management. Because gastritis is common among uraemic patients, there should also be a low threshold for treatment with a proton pump inhibitor if gastritis could be a contributory factor.

Management of pruritus

The aetiology and pathogenesis of pruritus in ESKD remain unclear, and treatment options are limited in their effectiveness. Pruritus is thought to arise in C fibres located in the skin, distinct from those which mediate pain (Schmelz et al., 1997). These C fibres transmit via the contralateral spinothalamic tract to the brain (thalamus and hypothalamus) via the reticular formation (Lugon, 2005). Connections to distinct cortical areas (the anterior cingulate process, supplementary motor area, and inferior parietal lobe) then mediate, via motor areas, the powerful, almost involuntary, desire to scratch. The difficulty is that pruritus could originate at any level in this pathway (in the skin at the level of the receptors, neuropathically in the afferent nerve pathway, neuropathically in central neural pathways, or centrally from psychogenic causes). In ESKD-related itch, complex interacting factors operate at more than one place in the pathway (Lugon, 2005), so that it is extremely difficult to elucidate any one discrete cause for itch. Current hypotheses postulate abnormal inflammatory/immune processes, dysfunction in the opioid receptor system, and/or neuropathic processes within the nervous system itself.

Immune modulators (such as ultraviolet (UV) B light, tacrolimus, and thalidomide) have been proposed to treat itch. These all act in various ways to decrease pro-inflammatory cytokines. Others have proposed disturbance in the endogenous opioids system as a cause of itch (Yosipovitch et al., 2003; Patel et al., 2007). Kappa (κ)-opioid receptor agonists have been shown to have anti-pruritic effects in animals, and κ-opioid receptor antagonists enhance itch in animal studies (Ikoma et al., 2006). It is for this reason that opioids such as butorphanol (which has mu

(μ)-opioid antagonist and κ-opioid agonist action) (Dawn and Yosipovitch, 2006), and opioids antagonists such as naloxone and naltrexone, have been proposed to treat itch. There is also some evidence that a relatively new κ-opioid agonist (nalfurafine) may be useful (Wikstrom et al., 2005). Evidence has emerged to support the link between itch and neuropathic processes. There are a number of features of itch which suggest a neuropathic process, and Akhyani and colleagues report association between clinical neuropathy and itch in haemodialysis patients (Akhyani et al., 2005). Neuropathic agents (lidocaine, gabapentin, and capsaicin) have been used to treat itch, with some success. However, the neuropathic component could be a secondary, rather than primary cause of ESKD-related pruritus. The role of histamine in acute itch is long established. Acute histamine-induced itch is well described, and histamine receptors appear to sensitize at least some of the C fibres which mediate itch. What is less clear is how this acute itch response relates to the chronic itch experienced by ESKD-related pruritus. Nevertheless, antihistamines are widely used in the management of ESKD-related pruritus, with varying results. A final important factor in ESKD-related itch is xerosis, or dry skin. Xerosis may be an important factor in older people with ESKD (Keithi-Reddy et al., 2007). And although uraemia is the most likely cause of pruritus, other common causes of pruritus need to be considered if the symptom is not resolving, such as skin disorders, skin infections such as scabies, and liver impairment.

The first step in management is to optimize renal management; high phosphate may contribute to pruritus (Lugon, 2005), and dietary advice and the use of phosphate binders should be considered to reduce phosphate levels. Hyperparathyroidism may also be a contributory factor and should be considered. Dry skin may both cause and contribute to pruritus, and so should be treated actively; liberal emollients should be used if dry skin is present. Older people living alone may find it hard to apply emollients easily; spray applications are often helpful in this instance. Preventive measures, such as nail care (keeping nails short) and keeping cool (light clothing, and tepid baths or showers), are useful concurrent measures.

The evidence as to which medications are effective is limited, often conflicting, and no one single preparation can be recommended above others. Choice of treatment should be influenced by the stage of disease—for instance, UV light may be practical for those who remain relatively well, while antihistamines may be more appropriate nearer end of life. Time should be taken to discuss with the patient the need to persist with any one medication, and to explain and minimize side effects where possible. A clear plan of management, and persistence in following treatment through, goes a long way to helping patients cope with the distress that this symptom can sometimes cause. The psychological and social dimensions of severe itch are considerable (Murtagh et al., 2007c), and psychological, family, and social support is an important component of management.

Management of restless legs

RLS is characterized by an urge to move the legs, uncomfortable sensations in the legs, and worsening of symptoms at rest, especially during the night. The formal IRLSSG criteria are (a) urge to move the legs, usually with unpleasant sensations in the legs, (b) worse during periods of rest or inactivity like resting or sitting, (c) partial or total relief by physical activity, and (d) worse symptoms in the evening or night rather than the day (Medcalf and Bhatia, 2006). The exact cause for restless legs is not well understood but the dopaminergic system in the central nervous system is somehow disrupted (Manenti et al., 2009). There is limited evidence in uraemic RLS that iron deficiency (O'Keeffe et al., 1993), low parathyroid hormone (Rijsman et al., 2004), hyperphosphataemia, and psychological factors (Takaki et al., 2003) may play a role. Treatment should involve correction of these factors, and reduction of potential exacerbating agents, such as caffeine, alcohol, nicotine, and certain drugs (sedative antihistamines, metoclopramide, tricyclic antidepressants, selective serotonin uptake inhibitors, lithium, and dopamine antagonists) (Manenti et al., 2009). Calcium antagonists may also exacerbate RLS (Telarovic et al., 2007).

There is very limited evidence about treatment of restless legs in CKD patients, and much of the evidence is extrapolated from patients with idiopathic restless legs (Silber et al., 2004). Gabapentin, dopamine agonists, co-careldopa, and clonazepam are the treatments most commonly used, with varying results. All need dose reduction, and gabapentin in particular accumulates rapidly if there is no dialysis; it can be given in low dose post dialysis sessions, and should be used with extreme caution in ESKD patients who are not receiving dialysis.

Management of sleep disturbance

A detailed history of any sleep disturbance is important, in order to identify sleep apnoea, RLS, and pruritus, which may be the underlying reason for the sleep disturbance; these each need treating in their own right initially to resolve any sleep problems. General sleep hygiene measures are important in addressing sleep disturbance; avoiding caffeine after lunch, reducing overall caffeine intake, avoiding alcohol (which is both depressant and stimulant), and avoiding daytime sleeping. If sleep apnoea is excluded, other exacerbating symptoms are treated optimally, and general measures are unsuccessful, then hypnotics may be necessary, ideally short term to attempt to re-establish sleep patterns. For those with a longer prognosis, hypnotics carry a risk of dependence, and this needs consideration in management. The shorter-acting hypnotics, such as zolpidem 5–10 mg or temazepam 7.5–10 mg, are preferable. These are generally safe in dialysis patients, although ESKD patients may be more sensitive to benzodiazepines in general, and lower doses are often required than in the general population.

Management of breathlessness towards end of life

The most common causes of breathlessness or dyspnoea in the renal patient are anaemia, pulmonary oedema (related to fluid overload or to coexisting cardiovascular disease), or co-morbidity (cardiac or respiratory disease). Anaemia produces significant symptoms including dyspnoea, and although anaemia is likely to be due to renal failure in the CKD patient, other causes should be considered and excluded. It is important to identify the underlying cause of breathlessness, since treating the underlying cause is almost always the most appropriate and effective first line of management. If volume overload is identified as a cause or contributor, more frequent or longer dialysis, with ultrafiltration, can be helpful. If treatment of the underlying cause has been exhausted, then symptomatic measures to relieve breathlessness will be required. These include general and non-pharmacological measures, psychological support, and pharmacological measures.

General measures in advanced disease include sitting upright rather than lying (which maximizes vital capacity), using a fan or stream of cool air which can provide effective symptom relief (Booth et al., 2004a), inhaled oxygen if hypoxia is confirmed or suspected (Booth et al., 2004b) and a calm, settled environment. For the patient whose mobility is limited by breathlessness, physiotherapy and occupational therapy can help to maximize mobility and provide appropriate aids to improve function constrained by breathlessness. Since breathlessness is a profoundly unpleasant symptom, assessment and management of the underlying psychological state is important. Breathlessness is very commonly associated with anxiety, often in an escalating cycle (anxiety causing worsening dyspnoea, which triggers worsening anxiety, and so on). Information, education, and support of patient and family are therefore critical.

As prognosis worsens, general and non-pharmacological measures will have less to offer, and pharmacological measures directed at the symptom of breathlessness itself may be more appropriate. Untreated moderate or severe dyspnoea at the end of life is very distressing, and should be treated as actively as pain or any other distressing symptom. Breathlessness is an increasingly important and dominant symptom in renal patients towards the end of life (Murtagh et al., 2007c), so it is important to try and anticipate and plan for future episodes. Not all patients will, for instance, choose to be admitted for maximal treatment with intravenous diuretics in the last days or weeks of life.

Pharmacological treatments directed specifically at breathlessness include opioids and benzodiazepines (especially if there is moderate or severe associated anxiety). Low-dose opioids are helpful in relieving breathlessness near the end of life in end-stage cardiac and respiratory disease (Jennings et al., 2001, 2002), and clinical experience suggests that this is true for renal patients too. However, there are considerable constraints on the use of opioids in renal patients; the guidance as for pain management should be followed, although dose of opioids for breathlessness is likely to be notably smaller (usually half or quarter the starting dose for pain) and titration upwards is undertaken to a lesser degree. If small doses are not at least partly effective, combining an opioid such as fentanyl with low dose midazolam towards the end of life (last few days or hours) may bring relief where either alone is only partially effective. This is often a better strategy than increasing the dose, since adverse effects quickly increase as doses rise.

Benzodiazepines are useful when there is coexisting anxiety (as there often is), but again need to be used with care and in reduced doses. Shorter-acting benzodiazepines are recommended, such as lorazepam 0.5–1 mg orally or sublingually four times a day (if used sublingually, it has a quicker onset of action and may more readily restore a sense of control to the frightened and anxious patient). If the patient is in the last days of life, midazolam (at 25% of normal dose if eGFR is less than 10) can be given subcutaneously and titrated according to effect. Midazolam can be given every 2–4 hours, although ESKD patients are sensitive to its effects and do not usually need frequent or large doses. A starting dose of 1.25 or 2.5 mg is common, and often sufficient. If more than one or two doses are required, a subcutaneous infusion over 24 hours is most practical.

Communication and advance care planning

There is growing evidence on the information provided to, and the communication needs of, patients with ESKD, as well as the kind of trade-offs that patients are willing to accept. In a recent study, patients were willing to forgo 23 months of life expectancy with home-based dialysis in order to decrease their travel restrictions, although there is inconsistency between patient and family preferences (Morton et al., 2012a). Communicating early and clearly about the options and possibilities is an important part of good quality care.

The evidence also provides wider pointers for clinicians. First, detailed discussions about the future and about preferences and priorities do not remove hope, as some professionals believe; rather, they sustain realistic hope and empower patients to work towards possibilities consistent with their own values (Davison and Simpson, 2006). They help patients and families to make the most of life, in the face of an advancing, life-threatening condition. Second, there are a variety of reasons why patients opt for conservative management (Noble et al., 2009). These will influence how patients and families view the future, after the decision is made; a patient who views conservative management as a 'logical and affirming choice' will respond differently to one who is 'angry and believed they were somehow giving up on life' (Noble et al., 2009). Subsequent advance care planning therefore needs to be responsive to the perspective patient and family bring to the process; it is about helping them towards greater empowerment, whatever the starting place, but some will have a very different psychological journey ahead, as compared with others. Third, advance care planning is not only about key medical decisions, such as decisions about dialysis, or agreement to 'not for resuscitation' order when in hospital. When done well, it also involves enhancement of the final days, weeks and months with positive decisions about family relationships, resolution of conflict, and living well until the end of life (Hines et al., 2001a); all priorities which patients themselves rate highly (Singer et al., 1998). This approach helps move away from isolated decisions about the utilization of medical supportive measures, which are sometimes influenced more by transient factors than by stable 'core' values (Fried et al., 2007), and builds on a more integrated person- and family-centred care.

There is some overlap between making dialysis decisions and planning ahead for subsequent care, because the former will inevitably involve some exploration of the patient's preferences and priorities. However, advance care planning becomes more far-reaching as the illness progresses. Patients and families often want advice and information, such as what to expect at different stages, when and why hospitalization might be appropriate, what other active management is right for them, who is available to care for them at home, and where do they prefer to be cared for and to die, if practicable. This is a dynamic and evolving process, not one or even a few fixed episodes, and there needs to be good liaison to ensure it is effective. Timing is critical; not all issues will be right to discuss at any one time, and there will need to be evolution in discussions as the disease itself advances. There is a fine balance between introducing issues for discussion too early, and leaving them too late, so that opportunities are missed, and 'default' care becomes inevitable (Holley, 2003). Family and other carers need to be actively involved in discussions whenever possible (Hines et al., 2001b) and according to patient preference, to enable consistent responses at times of crisis or decline. Communication among professionals is critical; there may be a number of professionals who also need to be aware of decisions, preferences, and priorities, including primary care professionals, who may have major responsibility if the patient is at home.

There has been some study of the experience of illness among conservatively managed stage 5 CKD patients (Murtagh, 2009), and this work suggests that loss of control and related uncertainty are a particular feature for these patients. Advance care planning can help reduce this sense of loss of control (Davison and Torgunrud, 2007). This is important, since for a number of these patients, the prospect of death was not their main concern; uncertainty about the path of their illness before death troubled them more. Above all, participants expressed a wish not to be a burden to their family and others (Murtagh, 2009); advance care planning helps to make explicit preferences and priorities about care, and identifies what can be provided to support families and reduce that burden (provided, of course, that appropriate services are available).

Conclusions

People with ESKD have extensive palliative care needs. They therefore need significant medical, nursing, psychological, and social care as their illness advances towards the end of life. This chapter has focused on the challenges of symptom recognition, assessment, and management, and the need for advance care planning, but has not addressed the considerable psychological, spiritual, and practical care that these patients need, or the high level of coordination between providers that is important for ensuring effective and accessible care.

Symptoms can arise directly from the renal disease itself, as a consequence of dialysis, or from co-morbid conditions (particularly in older patients). This diversity makes them harder to assess and address, and detailed assessments and interventions are needed. Pharmacological management of symptoms is one of the most challenging aspects of the care of those with ESKD. Although the emphasis in this chapter has been on pharmacological management, it should be stressed that psychological, social, and spiritual aspects of management are also important, especially towards the end of life. It is for this reason that care of renal patients is best managed with multiprofessional teams, including counsellors and psychologists, occupational therapists and physiotherapists, dieticians, and chaplains, and most importantly, professionals with both nephrology and palliative care skills.

Online materials

Complete references for this chapter are available online at <http://www.oxfordmedicine.com>.

References

Davison, S.N. (2007). The prevalence and management of chronic pain in end-stage renal disease. *Journal of Palliative Medicine*, 10, 1277–1287.

Dean, M. (2004). Opioids in renal failure and dialysis patients. *Journal of Pain and Symptom Management*, 28, 497–504.

Lugon, J.R. (2005). Uremic pruritus: a review. *Hemodialysis International*, 9, 180–188.

Booth, S., Farquar, M., Gysels, M., Bausewein, C., and Higginson, I.J. (2004a). The impact of a breathlessness intervention service (BIS) on the lives of patients with intractable dyspnea: a qualitative phase 1 study. *Palliative Supportive Care*, 4, 287–293.

Broadbent, A., Khor, K., and Heaney, A. (2003). Palliation and chronic renal failure: opioid and other palliative medications—dosage guidelines. *Progress in Palliative Care*, 11, 183–190.

Davies, G., Kingswood, C., and Street, M. (1996). Pharmacokinetics of opioids in renal dysfunction. *Clinical Pharmacokinetics*, 31, 410–422.

Davison, S.N., Jhangri, G.S., and Johnson, J.A. (2006b). Longitudinal validation of a modified Edmonton symptom assessment system (ESAS) in haemodialysis patients. *Nephrology Dialysis Transplantation*, 21, 3189–3195.

Davison, S.N. and Simpson, C. (2006). Hope and advance care planning in patients with end stage renal disease: qualitative interview study. *BMJ*, 333, 886.

Joly, D., Anglicheau, D., Alberti, C., *et al.* (2003). Octogenarians reaching end-stage renal disease: cohort study of decision-making and clinical outcomes. *Journal of the American Society of Nephrology*, 14, 1012–1021.

Low, J., Smith, G., Burns, A., and Jones, L. (2008). The impact of end-stage kidney disease (ESKD) on close persons: a literature review. *Nephrology Dialysis Transplantation*, 2, 67–79.

Mercadante, S. and Arcuri, E. (2004). Opioids and renal function. *Journal of Pain*, 5, 2–19.

Morton, R.L., Snelling, P., Webster, A.C., *et al.* (2012a). Dialysis modality preference of patients with CKD and family caregivers: a discrete-choice study. *American Journal of Kidney Diseases*, 60, 102–111.

Morton, R.L., Turner, R.M., Howard, K., Snelling, P., and Webster, A.C. (2012b). Patients who plan for conservative care rather than dialysis: a national observational study in Australia. *American Journal of Kidney Diseases*, 59, 419–427.

Murphy, E.L., Murtagh, F.E., Carey, I., and Sheerin, N.S. (2009). Understanding symptoms in patients with advanced chronic kidney disease managed without dialysis: use of a short patient-completed assessment tool. *Nephron Clinical Practice*, 111, c74–80.

Murtagh, F.E., Addington-Hall, J.M., Edmonds, P.M., *et al.* (2007b). Symptoms in advanced renal disease: a cross-sectional survey of symptom prevalence in stage 5 chronic kidney disease managed without dialysis. *Journal of Palliative Medicine*, 10, 1266–1276.

Murtagh, F.E., Addington-Hall, J., and Higginson, I.J. (2007c). The prevalence of symptoms in end-stage renal disease: a systematic review. *Advances in Chronic Kidney Disease*, 14, 82–99.

Murtagh, F.E., Chai, M.O., Donohoe, P., Edmonds, P.M., and Higginson, I.J. (2007f). The use of opioid analgesia in end-stage renal disease patients managed without dialysis: recommendations for practice. *Journal of Pain and Palliative Care Pharmacotherapy*, 21(2), 5–16.

Murtagh, F.E., Marsh, J.E., Donohoe, P., Ekbal, N.J., Sheerin, N.S., and Harris, F.E. (2007d). Dialysis or not? A comparative survival study of patients over 75 years with chronic kidney disease stage 5. *Nephrology Dialysis Transplantation*, 22, 1955–1962.

Murtagh, F.E., Sheerin, N.S., Addington-Hall, J., and Higginson, I.J. (2011). Trajectories of illness in stage 5 chronic kidney disease: a longitudinal study of patient symptoms and concerns in the last year of life. *Clinical Journal of the American Society of Nephrology*, 6, 1580–1590.

Roderick, P., Davies, R., Jones, C., Feest, T., Smith, S., and Farrington, K. (2004). Simulation model of renal replacement therapy: predicting future demand in England. *Nephrology Dialysis Transplantation*, 19, 692–701.

Singer, P.A., Martin, D.K., Lavery, J.V., Thiel, E.C., Kelner, M., and Mendelssohn, D.C. (1998). Reconceptualizing advance care planning from the patient's perspective. *Archives of Internal Medicine*, 158, 879–884.

Smith, C., Da Silva-Gane, M., Chandna, S., Warwicker, P., Greenwood, R., and Farrington, K. (2003). Choosing not to dialyse: evaluation of planned non-dialytic management in a cohort of patients with end-stage renal failure. *Nephron Clinical Practice*, 95, c40–46.

Weisbord, S.D., Carmody, S.S., Bruns, F.J., *et al.* (2003). Symptom burden, quality of life, advance care planning and the potential value of palliative care in severely ill haemodialysis patients. *Nephrology Dialysis Transplantation*, 18, 1345–1352.

Weisbord, S.D., Fried, L.F., Arnold, R.M., *et al.* (2004). Development of a symptom assessment instrument for chronic hemodialysis patients: the Dialysis Symptom Index. *Journal of Pain and Symptom Management*, 27, 226–240.

Palliative medicine in the intensive care unit

Nathan I. Cherny, Sharon Einav, and David Dahan

Introduction to palliative medicine in the intensive care unit

Approximately half of the patients admitted to an intensive care unit (ICU) are likely to die during ICU admission (Pronovost et al., 2002) and in some countries almost a fifth of the overall number of adult deaths occur in an ICU (Angus et al., 2004). Furthermore, the proportion of emergency ICU admissions has almost doubled within the last decade (Herring et al., 2013).

On admission to intensive care, both the severity and extent of pre-existing chronic diseases and the prognosis of the acute disease are often unknown, consequently it is difficult to predict the response to ICU treatment for an individual patient. In the ICU, the disease trajectory starts with a trial of major life-saving efforts. Often, however, these efforts fail to stabilize the patient and over time, it becomes increasingly apparent that the patient will either die or remain alive only with ongoing life support systems such as permanent ventilation (Truog et al., 2008).

Intensive care is not a homogenous concept or reality; ICU populations are varied in both case mix and age composition (Mosenthal et al., 2012). Thus, for example, surgical ICU decisions are often influenced by a 'covenantial'-like relationship between the surgeon and their patient characterized by a sense of obligation to protect the patient during the surgery and its aftermath and an exaggerated sense of accountability for the patient's outcome (Schwarze et al., 2010). Trauma ICUs are characterized by a disproportionately large number of relatively young patients, often without confounding pre-existing medical problems but with sudden onset of acute life-threatening catastrophic injuries (Deitch and Dayal, 2006). Neurological/neurosurgical ICUs are characterized by patients at risk of physiological survival despite vastly compromised neurological function (Patel et al., 2002; Bershad et al., 2008).

Irrespective, several factors characterize all of these settings: patients are fragile, their risk of mortality is high, and their immediate prognosis is often uncertain. Patients are often required to undergo unpleasant invasive procedures, they often suffer pain and discomfort, and are highly dependent. In addition, family members, who themselves are under duress are often required to be involved in decision-making processes. Under these circumstances, palliative care principles are critical in the relief of patient distress, communication with family members, and in the management of patients who are not responding to life-saving approaches (Curtis, 2008; Truog et al., 2008)

Why is delivery of palliative care different in the ICU?

Palliative and end-of-life care in ICU is characterized by a number of distinct factors that challenge the delivery of end-of-life care:

◆ *Professional culture*: the ICU physician and nurse training is primarily directed at life support and staff often have a professional culture regarding the primacy of saving lives, vital sign monitoring and stabilization, a low threshold for medical interventions, and, sometimes, a risk of 'depersonalizing' the individual.

◆ *Uncertainty*: almost every decision involved in ICU care is confounded by uncertainty and limited abilities to accurately predict outcomes for individuals. In particular, this relates to decisions to admit patients to ICU or not, and to decisions to continue or forego treatments. These decisions are influenced by both medical criteria (e.g. need for ventilatory and/or haemodynamic support, the likelihood of survival and morbidity) and non-medical criteria (e.g. patient wishes, values and goals, and cultural and religious beliefs), and how each should best factor into any decision-making.

◆ *Time course*: the typical course of an admission to ICU is acute, mostly within hours or days. This gives both patients and relatives little time to adjust to changes in expected life expectancy and often limits their ability to inform the ICU staff of their preferences.

◆ *Environment*: the patients are often in a room shared by other ICU patients, they are attached to multiple devices which create a noisy environment, and the room is often illuminated 24 hours a day. Families are often struck by the markedly changed appearance of the patient due to his/her medical condition, and often, fluid overload. Access to the bedside may be limited by stringent visiting hours and isolation measures and the patient is often attached to life-support devices such as ventilatory support, continuous dialysis, or infusions of vasoactive drugs, the discontinuation of which may result in rapid deterioration and death.

◆ *Patient communication*: most patients are not able to participate in discussions because of either their illness or sedation (Heyland et al., 2003).

◆ *Scarce and expensive resource*: due to its high demand on work force (often one nurse for two patients for all duty shifts) and its demand on high levels of medical technology, ICU is very costly. For the same reasons, ICU beds are a scarce resource (Zilberberg and Shorr, 2012) and both staff and family may be aware that the patient is consuming an expensive resource and there may be pressure to transfer the patient to a less intense environment for a more 'deserving' patient. The term 'inappropriate treatment' is often used by intensive care clinicians to describe care that involves the use of considerable resources without a reasonable hope that the patient will recover to a state of relative independence or ability to interact with their environment (Sibbald et al., 2007).

The scope of the issue

Palliative care in the ICU incorporates symptom control, goal setting, and communication which is essential for all patients, as well as the special issues related to the care of patients whose condition is not improving and who are approaching death. There is wide consensus regarding the need for palliative care competencies in the ICU; multiple authorities have published policy and guideline documents and standards on this subject. These standards were reviewed by Nelsen et al. (2010a) and are summarized into seven key points:

1. Patient care maintaining comfort, dignity, and personhood. Such care incorporates regular assessment and optimal management of pain and other distressing symptoms.

2. Timely, clear, and compassionate communication by clinicians with patients and families. Honest, complete, and repeated communication should be as dictated by the condition of the patient, with input from all pertinent members of the multiprofessional team.

3. Clinical decision-making processes which are led by patients' preferences, goals, and values.

4. Identification of, and respect for, patients' advanced medical directives and surrogate decision-makers.

5. Development of contingency plans for withdrawal of supportive interventions.

6. Interdisciplinary support of families during the critical illness and for families of patients who died in the ICU, in the bereavement period.

7. Emotional and organizational support for ICU clinicians. Support systems and resources for caregivers that address moral distress, burnout, and post-traumatic stress disorder. This should include a mechanism for staff members to request a debriefing or to voice concerns with the treatment plan, decompress, vent feelings, or grieve.

Practical issues

Among the key practice points for palliative care in the ICU are issues related to communication, assessment and management of symptoms, and end-of-life care transitioning and management

Communication with families

Family-centred care requires that patients be seen as embedded within a social structure and web of relationships (Truog et al., 2008; Jacobowski et al., 2010; Levin et al., 2010). Despite this, communication issues with clinicians are the most common source of complaints among families of deceased patients, with as many as 30% of family members feeling dissatisfied with communication in the ICU (Baker et al., 2000; Abbott et al., 2001) the major problems being inadequate dedicated time, inconsistent information, and provision of information by multiple health-care providers (Azoulay et al., 2000; Azoulay and Pochard, 2003). Suboptimal communication can also affect not only the psychological well-being of family members and satisfaction with care but also clinical decision-making (Jacobowski et al., 2010; Huang et al., 2012).

Family members need early and frequent interaction with the key clinical personal providing care and support to inform the family of the patient's condition and treatment, answer questions, and include the patient's surrogates in the decision-making process. Such meetings provide an important opportunity to clarify misunderstandings, talk about goals of care, prognosis, and contingency planning for worst case scenarios. Initial meetings should focus on a description of the patient's status, the measures undertaken to attempt to stabilize their condition, the level of risk and the likelihood of recovery, death, or permanent dependence on life support.

Good communication and regular family meetings not only improve the psychological well-being of family members (Lautrette et al., 2007; Wall et al., 2007; Gries et al., 2008) but may also be associated with a reduce length of ICU stay (Lilly et al., 2003; Norton et al., 2007).

Subsequent family meetings should be held when a change occurs in the medical status of the patient. This is particularly true if the treating clinicians believe that the goals of care should be reassessed and perhaps transitioned to palliation care and/or conflicts exist among family members, or between the family and treating clinicians regarding care issues.

Family members and relevant health-care providers, generally including physician, nurse, and social worker, should participate in the family meeting which should be led by a facilitator nominated from the clinical team. Since in most circumstances the family have no pre-existing relationship with the ICU staff, the participation of the patient's primary clinician is highly desirable. Additionally the nurse caring for the patient and a social worker should be included. To avoid presentation of conflicting information, it is prudent for the staff to corroborate their evaluations and understanding in preparation for the meeting. In situations where differences of opinion exist regarding management or prognosis, these should be explained to the family in a balanced manner that shows respect for all of the involved clinicians.

Additional factors that have been shown to improve satisfaction from family–clinician meetings include the ability of the clinician to listen, encourage questions, show empathy, provide emotional support, and be attentive to the patient's values and allowing family members sufficient opportunity to express themselves (Billings, 2011a, 2011b; Billings and Block, 2011).

Formal communication between providers and the family should be a continual process, and informal meetings with individual family members can occur in parallel even more frequently to provide updates and discuss pertinent issues and concerns.

Discussing prognosis

Meaningful participation in decision-making processes requires an understanding of prognosis (Bacchetta et al., 2006; Ford et al.,

2009; Aldawood, 2010; Billings, 2011a). Additionally, regular discussion of prognosis helps families prepare for the possibility of the patient's death. Discussion of prognosis should be framed in a context of probabilities. To this end, ICU physicians may use a range of prognostic tools including the SAPS (Metnitz et al., 2005; Moreno et al., 2005), Apache III (Knaus and Wagner, 1989; Knaus et al., 1991), and sepsis-related organ failure (SOFA) (Vincent et al., 1996). It is important to appreciate though that these scoring systems were developed to predict outcomes for *populations* and that they have limited accuracy in predicting survival for an individual patient (Rocker et al., 2004).

Additional methods to evaluate the extent and severity of the acute insult vary depending on the nature of the prevailing problem: for instance, in hypoxic brain damage clinical signs are supplemented by neurophysiological examinations (Wijdicks et al., 2006).

Uncertainty should always be openly acknowledged. However, this should be accompanied with an explanation of the factors that will help decrease the uncertainty and an estimate of when more accurate information will be available. The phrase 'hoping for the best and preparing for the worst' (Back et al., 2003) aligns with the family's hope that the patient will survive the hospitalization, while at the same time emphasizing the need to prepare for the contingency that the patient may not survive. Importantly, discussion of prognosis must be accompanied by an assessment of likely future functional outcome and mental state if the patient does survive.

End-of-life conversations

End-of-life conversations should be part of the natural progression of dialogue about the course of an illness. Such discussion should occur when considering the changing of goals of care, whether due to deterioration or due to failure to progress (Badger, 2005; Crighton et al., 2008). Transitioning to palliative care should be introduced as one of the potential contingencies if treatment does not go well (Glavan et al., 2008).

In the ICU, most patients are unable to express their preferences either because of their illness or because they are sedated. Unless the patient has a written advanced directive, decisions are made on their behalf by surrogates (usually family members) or a nominated healthcare proxy in coordination with the health-care team (Fried et al., 2002). If the patient's values and preferences are known they should be respected. This is called 'substituted judgement' or 'surrogate decision-making' (Fried et al., 2002).

Important questions in this process include (Ward et al., 2011):

◆ What are the essential clinical issues we are addressing?

◆ What are the clinically reasonable choices?

◆ What are the pros and cons of the treatment choices?

◆ What is the likelihood of success of treatment, and how confident are we in this estimate?

◆ Is the family now an 'informed participant,' with a working understanding of the decision?

◆ What role should the family play in making the decision?

◆ How will the decision impact the patient's life?

◆ What does the family think is the most appropriate decision for the patient?

The role of a surrogate is very challenging and should be addressed with extreme sensitivity and respect for the difficulty of the task at hand. While dealing with the complex emotions engendered by seeing their loved one in a state of profound illness they are also being asked to understand the illness, the life-sustaining interventions used, and the treatment options, and to be able to participate in decision-making with the health-care team not according to what they would want; rather, what the patient would want if still able to speak for him- or herself. This should be stressed and developed in part with substituted judgement. This approach is confounded by findings that patients rarely discuss specific treatment options with their family members, and surrogate decisions often do not correlate with what the patient would actually want done (Sulmasy et al., 1998; Shalowitz et al., 2006).

Situations in which the patient's preferences are unknown challenge both clinicians and family to find a mutual understanding of the patient's 'best interests'. Whenever possible, it is desirable to have a situation in which there is agreement between the involved clinicians and family members in a manner that is consistent with the patient's known wishes or values. In this shared process the family usually contributes their knowledge regarding the patient's values and treatment preferences while the physician contributes their knowledge regarding the patient's present medical condition and expected prognosis (Berger et al., 2008). The relative contribution towards the decision-making process from family members and physicians varies between countries due to differences in culture and legalities. Regardless, it should be clear that considerations regarding the forgoing of life support are a medical issue and the question to the family is to what extent such (in)action is consistent with the values of the patient. In this process the physician may offer a range of therapeutic strategies but also makes specific recommendations for their consideration and assent. It is never appropriate to make the patient and family feel solely responsible for the decision to forgo life-sustaining treatment and. indeed, some patients and families prefer to have physicians make these decisions without consultation (Searight and Gafford, 2005a, 2005a).

Legal guidelines regarding end-of-life decision-making are less clear when patients without capacity lack an appropriate surrogate and in practice, decisions are often made by the intensive care clinicians without judicial, peer, or institutional review (White et al., 2006).

Rarely, there may be times when sedatives and analgesics could be discontinued in the hope of engaging the patient in these decisions (Truog et al., 2008). More often than not, attempts may not result in a return to lucidity because the patient's illness is too severe. Furthermore, such attempts may be inappropriate when the patient's wishes are known, death is imminent, or discontinuing drugs would cause significant pain and suffering. In these situations, surrogates should be entrusted to make decisions for the patient as outlined above.

Organ and tissue donation is an integral part of end-of-life decisions and is grounded in respect for individuals and families, respectful communication and decision-making, and compassionate care (Williams et al., 2003). Patients and their families should be offered this opportunity as standard end-of-life care based on the presumption that organ donation may be consistent with the patient's values or recorded wishes. The request process for donation should focus on the benefit to the potential recipients and on the possibility of something good coming out of the tragedy of their loved one's death.

End-of-life decisions are stressful and monumental in the lives of those involved (Kesselring et al., 2007; Huang et al., 2012)., consequently the both patients and families must be given as much time as possible to reach their own decisions, and information should be delivered in ways that are sensitive to the patient's cultural, religious, and language needs.

Dealing with conflicts in intensive care

Conflicts regarding end-of-life decisions between families and health-care providers (Breen et al., 2001) or between members of the care team (Goold et al., 2000) are very common. The most common types of conflicts arise around decisions regarding whether to withdraw or withhold treatment (Studdert et al., 2003; Danjoux et al., 2009).

Such conflicts are often very damaging to trust and effective cooperation. From the clinician's perspective, polarization of views with efforts to persuade the family that they are wrong, may degenerate to questioning of the family's competence or intentions (Azoulay et al., 2009; Danjoux et al., 2009). From the family's perspective, this situation is associated with feelings of isolation, misunderstanding, abandonment, and doubt towards the integrity of the clinician's commitment to the patient's best interests (Azoulay et al., 2009; Danjoux et al., 2009).

Meetings to try to resolve conflicts should start by focusing on the common goals of caring for the patient and the family. Since the underlying issue is often distress over the patient's imminent demise, it is also important to acknowledge the emotions that underlie the conflict. Families may need time to come to grips with end-of-life decisions and sometimes simply allowing the family a day or two observe the ongoing deterioration in the patient's condition and to process the information that they received may be enough for them to acknowledge a patient's terminal condition. Often repeated discussions are needed since about half of the family members may not adequately understand the patient's diagnosis, prognosis, or treatment even after meeting with the physician (Azoulay et al., 2000). Many intensive care services work closely with bioethicists and social workers who may be invaluable in helping resolve conflicts (Schneiderman, 2006). It is often useful to have a 'trial of therapy' with agreed goals and timeframes that everyone can agree on (Lecuyer et al., 2007).

Conflicts between staff regarding issues of over treatment or premature forgoing of treatment are very common and are a major cause of moral distress and burnout among intensive care staff (Hamric and Blackhall, 2006; McAndrew et al., 2011; St Ledger et al., 2013). This underscores the importance of collegiality and interdisciplinary involvement in critical decision-making in which the opinions of all relevant staff members are respectfully considered (see Chapter 14.6).

Symptom management in intensive care

When patients are conscious, common symptoms can be evaluated using routinely available symptom assessment scales. However, among those patients who are delirious, sedated, or paralysed evaluations are notoriously difficult (Hawryluck et al., 2002).

There is very limited direct data on the prevalence and severity of symptoms in intensive care. What data are available highlight the prevalence of pain, dyspnoea, thirst, nausea, hunger, tiredness, anxiety, generalized discomfort, and depression (Nelson et al., 2001; Li and Puntillo, 2006; Puntillo et al., 2008, 2010). The high prevalence of post-traumatic stress disorder among survivors is indirect evidence of the severity of trauma involved for many patients (Davydow et al., 2013).

Evidence-based guidelines for the evaluation and management of pain, dyspnoea and delirium in the ICU have recently been updated by the American College of Critical Care Medicine in conjunction with Society of Critical Care Medicine and American Society of Health-System Pharmacists (Barr et al., 2013).

Pain

Pain in the ICU is often related to iatrogenic causes, procedures, and interventions. Moderately or severely uncomfortable procedures that are commonly performed in the ICU include suctioning, turning, catheter insertion, wound care, and the presence of endotracheal and nasogastric tubes (Puntillo et al., 2004). Despite this only a minority of patients receive adequate pain therapy for these procedures (Payen et al., 2007). Minimizing pain with pre-emptive analgesia or avoiding iatrogenic sources of pain should be part of the pain relief plan. Management of patient pain and discomfort with analgesia first, before resorting to sedative therapy, results in improved patient outcomes compared to standard sedative-hypnotic regimens (Devabhakthuni et al., 2012). ICU patients undergoing painful procedures often exhibit facial tension and expressions such as grimacing, frowning, and wincing. Additionally physical movement, immobility, and increased muscle tone may indicate the presence of pain. Tearing and diaphoresis in the sedated paralysed and ventilated patient represents autonomic responses to discomfort (Herr et al., 2006). Based on these observations, standardized pain scoring systems based on physiologic variables and behavioural observations have been developed. The Behavioural Pain Scale was developed and validated for use in the ICU with mechanically ventilated patients (Payen et al., 2001).

Agitation

Patients in intensive care commonly experience agitation and anxiety and the presence of these symptoms are associated with worse clinical outcomes (Atkins et al., 1997; Fraser et al., 2000). Agitation is an undifferentiated clinical symptom and it may be provoked by multiple mechanisms including pain, delirium, hypoxemia, hypoglycaemia, hypotension, or withdrawal from alcohol and other drugs.

Before resorting to sedative medications, steps to reduce anxiety and agitation should be undertaken including optimization of patient comfort, administration of adequate analgesia, frequent reorientation, and adjustment of the environment to maintain normal sleep patterns.

When necessary, sedation should be titrated to maintain a light rather than a deep level of sedation, unless clinically contraindicated. The Richmond Agitation-Sedation Scale (RASS) (Sessler et al., 2002) and Sedation-Agitation Scale (SAS) (Riker et al., 1999; Ryder-Lewis and Nelson, 2008) are the most valid and reliable sedation assessment tools for measuring quality and depth of sedation in adult ICU patients. Non-benzodiazepine medications, such propofol or dexmedetomidine, are associated with improved ICU patient outcomes, including a shortened duration of mechanical ventilation and intensive admission as well as a lower incidence of delirium and long-term cognitive dysfunction (Barr et al., 2013).

Dyspnoea

Dyspnoea and respiratory distress are common symptoms among patients admitted to an ICU (Nelson et al., 2001; Li and Puntillo, 2006; Puntillo et al., 2008, 2010). Evaluation of respiratory distress among non-verbal ventilated patients is challenging and is dependent on recognition of behavioural indicators of respiratory distress which include (in descending frequency) tachypnoea and tachycardia, a fearful facial expression, accessory muscle use, paradoxical breathing (diaphragmatic), and nasal flaring (Campbell, 2007). Patients undergoing mechanical ventilation generally need some degree of sedation in order to maintain a modicum of comfort. This is usually achieved with propofol or dexmedetomidine (Anger, 2013; Barr et al., 2013). Benzodiazepine medications such as midazolam, while commonly used, are not preferred since they are associated with, more prolonged duration of mechanical ventilation, and higher incidences of delirium and cognitive dysfunction (Barr et al., 2013).

Intravenous opioids and sedatives allow the assumption of greater control of respiratory function with mechanical ventilation, and to decrease the discomforts inherent in being on life support. Intermittent bolus doses of medications are used to supplement the infusions in anticipation of and in response to interventions that would be expected to increase pain and suffering. The use of continuous infusions results in better pain control and lower total doses of medication overall, yet many patients do require moderate to high doses of opioids and sedatives.

Patients who do not require ventilation will often require symptomatic therapy for dyspnoea including oxygen and systemic opioids (see Chapter 8.2).

Delirium

Delirium and agitated delirium are common among ICU patients as a consequence of their medical condition, substance intoxication or withdrawal, use of medication, lack of a day–night cycle, or a combination of these factors and others. Delirium is associated with increased ventilator dependency, an increased length of ICU admission, and higher short- and long-term mortality (Zhang et al., 2013). As with other symptoms, it is often overlooked or misdiagnosed because of the difficulty of assessing mental states in intubated patients.

The Confusion Assessment Method-Intensive Care Unit (CAM-ICU) Assessment Tool was specifically designed for use in non-verbal but rousable intensive care patients (Ely et al., 2001) and is the is the best documented method of diagnosing delirium in the ICU (Jacobi et al., 2002). With the CAM-ICU, delirium is diagnosed when patients demonstrate (a) an acute change in mental status or fluctuating changes in mental status, (b) inattention measured using either an auditory or visual test, and either (c) disorganized thinking, or (d) an altered level of consciousness. This very brief evaluation technique has a 93% sensitivity and 89% specificity for detecting delirium as compared to full DSM-IV assessment by a geriatric psychiatrist (Ely et al., 2001).

As an initial step, patients should be evaluated for distressing symptoms, such as pain or dyspnoea, which may contribute to delirium, and if identified these ought to be addressed. Non-pharmacological approaches include removing physical restraints, promoting sleep, reducing noise and lights, and providing a calming family or staff presence (Harvey, 1996). The use of haloperidol, while common, is contentious and is not well founded in evidence. There are limited data that atypical antipsychotics, such as quetiapine may reduce the duration of delirium in adult ICU patients. Neither of these should be used in patients at high risk for torsades de pointes (patients with baseline prolongation of QT interval, patients receiving concomitant medications known to prolong the QT interval, or patients with a history of this arrhythmia). Data suggests that dexmedetomidine may be the preferred option for delirium unrelated to drug or alcohol withdrawal (Anger, 2013; Barr et al., 2013).

Transitioning to palliative care and foregoing intensive care life-support

When intensive supportive measures are unlikely to achieve the patient's goals of care, or the duration or invasiveness of treatment required to achieve the patient's medical goals would be unacceptable to the patient, treatment goals change and the goals change from curing to a focus on palliative and end-of-life care. This almost always involves decisions regarding the withdrawal (discontinuation) of life support or not starting life support measures (see Chapter 5.8). Indeed, most patients who die in ICUs do so when life-supporting measures are withheld or withdrawn (Prendergast et al., 1998; Prendergast and Puntillo, 2002; Cook et al., 2003; Sprung et al., 2003). In most situations, the recognition that the patient will not survive occurs relatively quickly, most often in less than 4 days (Sprung et al., 2003). Both changing goals and making decisions to withhold/withdraw life-support are difficult for all involved, and implementing them requires planning skill and a high level of clinical vigilance and compassion.

Preparing the family members

Family preparation begins with discussions such as those described above (Truog et al., 2008). Clinicians must assist families through both the transition in goals and the dying process of the patient. Families need detailed explanations about the steps that will be taken to ensure patient comfort, and should also be prepared for the physical changes their loved one will likely undergo. The anticipated changes in respiratory pattern should be described as a normal part of the dying process. Clinicians should offer families the opportunity to spend more time with their loved one prior to withdrawal of life support and, if need be, to meet with a spiritual carer (e.g. chaplain) or a social worker.

Place of care

To the extent possible in the difficult environment of the ICU, the goal is to provide both patient and family a quiet, private space devoid of technology and alarms. This may be difficult in units where patient beds are separated by curtains. When the dying process is prolonged or when demands for an ICU bed cannot be met in other ways, transfer to another area in the hospital may be unavoidable. It is important to start communicating this possibility a day or two before it is necessary. This transfer should occur smoothly with deference to the needs of the patient and family. Some actively dying patients with difficult-to-treat symptoms may actually benefit from ongoing care in the ICU to ensure a comfortable death. Every effort should be taken to reassure family members that continuity of clinical and especially comfort care will be maintained.

Comfort measures

Ensure availability of analgesics and sedatives to rapidly treat distress. This should include infusions of opioids and sedatives, as well as bolus doses of rapidly acting agents to manage distress.

Discontinue interventions that are not consistent with the goals of care

All routine interventions that provide no comfort to the patient (e.g. routine vital signs, blood tests, and radiographs) should be discontinued. All therapies should be re-evaluated and those that do not contribute to patient comfort should be discontinued. An 'allow natural death' (AND) or 'do-not-resuscitate' (DNR) order should be documented (Truog et al., 2008). Unless there are specific objections by family members, electronic monitoring should generally be discontinued as it does not provide comfort and it may distract the family from care of the patient and of one another (Rubenfeld, 2004; Truog et al., 2008). Discontinuation of vasopressors, inotropes, and antibiotics results in no discomfort and they do not need to be weaned (Truog et al., 2008).

When a patient has specifically refused one form of life-sustaining treatment on the basis of personal values (e.g. when a patient refuses intubation while requesting other therapies) continuing limited sets of life-sustaining treatments is reasonable and appropriate. In general, these wishes should be followed as long as they are consistent with good quality care and they do not compromise the care of other patients.

Discontinuing medical ventilation

This is the most dramatic aspect of end-of-life care in the ICU. Discontinuing mechanical ventilation is often very difficult, and sometimes traumatic for clinicians and families alike. The goal is to discontinue ventilation in a manner compatible with staff and family sensitivities and at the same time to assure patient comfort during all phases of the procedure. Well-tested protocols have been developed and published to facilitate safe and effective approaches to withdrawing mechanical ventilation (Treece et al., 2004). Among the principal considerations are the following key elements:

Discontinue neuromuscular blockade

Neuromuscular blockade may mask patient distress and confound the physical assessment of stress (Brody et al., 1997). Neuromuscular blockade should be discontinued before withdrawal of life support either by allowing the paralytic agent to wear off or by pharmacologically reversing its effects. In the rare cases in which it is felt that waiting for the return of neuromuscular function would be excessively burdensome, deep sedation should be established before withdrawal of therapies (Truog et al., 2008).

Pre-emptive sedation

Many patients may need pre-emptive dosing of opioids and sedatives to prevent any sudden increase in dyspnoea which may occur even if the patient has been gradually weaned from ventilator support (Billings, 2012). The amount of opioids and sedatives required is variable and is influenced by the baseline dosing requirements prior to withdrawal and the patient's level of distress. There is wide interindividual variability for dosing requirements and, for some patients required doses may be high (Brody et al., 1997). Sedation should be administered continually with provision for bolus rescue doses as needed (Brody et al., 1997).

Whether discontinuation of ventilatory support should be accompanied by pre-emptive anaesthesia and deep sedation is controversial. While this is accepted practice in some places (Billings, 2012), it is not universal and some argue that this is a modified version of physician-assisted death (Rady and Verheijde, 2010; Carvalho et al., 2011).

Discontinuing ventilation support

Ventilator support is gradually withdrawn by decreasing the fraction of inspired oxygen and the amount of positive pressure ventilation over a period of 10–30 minutes in a way that allows the patient to comfortably transition to spontaneous breathing on room air through the endotracheal tube. The patient is assessed for signs of distress after each reduction in support and additional boluses of intravenous analgesics or sedatives should be administered as needed.

Extubation or not

Practices vary widely with regard to extubation (Brody et al., 1997). Extubation at the end of life is a complex decision that defies dogmatic approaches and agreement should be achieved between staff and the patients surrogate decision-makers regarding this issue. While some clinicians suggest extubating the patient to free the patient from unnecessary lines and tubes prior to death, and to facilitate a more natural appearance during the dying process this may not always be prudent. Patients who are extubated after receiving high levels of ventilator support, and those with difficulty clearing secretions or protecting their airway, often become distressed with struggling and gasping (Prendergast and Puntillo, 2002). Indeed, in many situations, especially when upper airway collapse is anticipated, it is acceptable to leave the endotracheal tube in place.

Continuing care

Patients should be cared for in a clinical setting that allows for monitoring of symptoms and the ability to treat them effectively. Some actively dying patients with difficult-to-treat symptoms may benefit from ongoing care in the ICU to ensure a comfortable death.

At the bedside of the imminently dying patient

Whenever possible, a member of the health-care provider team should offer to be available to be with the family as the patient is dying. Such a presence reinforces that the dying patient's welfare remains important, and provides support and guidance to the family at a time of extreme stress. In so doing, the health-care professional can defuse some of the strangeness of the situation for the family, and make it somehow more of a normal and natural process (as indeed it is).

When possible, encourage family participation in patient care (Prendergast and Puntillo, 2002). This promotes a sense of comfort, intimacy, and involvement when families are in an otherwise strange and tragic and, sometimes, impersonal situation. Family members can be encouraged to communicate with their loved one through speech, touch, song, prayer, or music. Caregiving activities can include assisting with face washing or hair combing, or gentle massage. For some family members, however, being present as the patient is dying is overwhelming and respect for emotional limits is itself a caring practice.

The role of the clinician at the bedside of the dying patient is to ensure adequate relief of patient distress and to provide support and guidance to the grieving family. The physician should evaluate the patient to ensure that the patient is comfortable. If present, pain, dyspnoea, agitation, or any other distressing symptoms that are remediable should be rapidly and effectively treated. Once adequate comfort is achieved, the physician should reassure the family that the patient is not in distress.

Families vary in the degree of professional support necessary at the bedside of the dying. Attentive and continual presence is often needed when family supports are limited or coping is frail. In other situations it may be more appropriate for the clinician to acknowledge the primacy of family and friends in this setting and to take a background position of availability if necessary.

If it is clear that breaths are agonal and the patient is about to die, it is often appropriate to indicate this to the family with the reassurance that the patient appears comfortable. The clinician should indicate that death has occurred when there are no signs of life and offer support and condolences. Families often talk and cry over the dead person, kiss them, and hug them. Adequate provision for time and privacy in this situation is strongly recommended.

After a patient death

The death of a patient stresses the physical and emotional resources of the professional health-care providers as well as the grieving family and friends. Members of the care team often require some degree of emotional recuperation. This process can be facilitated by expressions of mutual support and appreciation, and debriefing sessions in which the care of the patient is reviewed. The patient's family should be contacted personally to enquire about their well-being and to offer a meeting to address any outstanding issues regarding the patient's illness, treatment, and death.

Organizational issues for palliative care in the ICU

Models of care

A variety of models have been proposed to enhance palliative care involvement in the care of ICU patients. The Improving Palliative Care in the ICU (IPAL-ICU) project has identified two main models of palliative care involvement in ICUs (Strand and Billings, 2012).

A 'consultative model' seeks to increase the involvement of dedicated teams of palliative care clinicians in the care of ICU patients, especially for those patients at high risk for suffering and death. In this model, palliative care experts/teams are called in by the ICU team once the latter have recognized relevant problems with care. These tend to occur when the patient, family, and staff experience conflicts around goals and methods of care. Studies on the use of proactive palliative care consultations for patients at a high risk for dying, led to significant reductions in ICU length of stay, increased DNR ('do not resuscitate') orders, reduced non-beneficial resource utilization after a DNR order, and increased transition to goals focused on comfort, without affecting mortality rates (Campbell and Guzman, 2004; Norton et al., 2007). Proactive ethics consultations for patients at high risk of dying, have also demonstrated similar benefits, including reduced conflict among the staff members and between staff and family members (Schneiderman et al., 2000).

An 'integrative model' promotes integration of palliative care principles and education into the daily care of all ICU patients by ICU teams. This approach is less reliant on palliative care services or on the willingness of ICU staff to refer to palliative clinicians. This model focuses on interventions to increase staff awareness of patient/family palliative care needs, improve communication skills, and incorporate palliative care skills training in staff education. This model of care requires collaboration between ICU and palliative care leadership in the development of palliative care guidelines for use in ICU, and the training of ICU 'nurse experts' to promote palliative care principles in the ICU. Some departments combine the consultative and integrative approaches.

Education

Although there is a wide consensus that end-of-life care is a critical skill for intensive care clinicians, there are no uniform widely endorsed guidelines for the training of intensive care clinicians in palliative and end-of-life care and evidence suggests that the scope of actual training is variable (Kane et al., 1998; Nelson et al., 2006; Lofmark et al., 2008; Forte et al., 2012). The European COBATRICE core curriculum for ICU professionals includes palliative care competencies such as discussions of end-of-life care with patients and families, and the management of withholding and/or withdrawal of death deferring therapies but provides little detail on the scope or nature of the training and competencies to be achieved (Bion and Barrett, 2006).

Detailed curriculum guidance was developed by a multidisciplinary taskforce including intensive care specialists, palliative care specialists, ethicists, and consumer advocates (Danis et al., 1999). This very comprehensive document highlighted nine attitudes and skills critical for good palliative care performance by intensive care clinicians: appreciating the patient as a person; communicating effectively by listening well to patients and their families; being able to deal with prognostic uncertainty; being comfortable broaching the topic of death with patients and their families, and supporting them in facing this reality; negotiating the overall goals of care; switching from the simultaneous provision of life-supporting therapy and comfort care to comfort care only; providing excellent palliative care; giving explanations, ranging from small details to the large picture, in clear, understandable language; and working effectively in collaboration with a multidisciplinary health-care team. The American Association of Colleges of Nursing have developed a comprehensive modular training programme for end-of-life care specifically designed for nurses working in intensive care (Ferrell et al., 2007).

Improving palliative care practices in an established ICU

An international multidisciplinary working group has developed a practical guide for organizing initiatives to improve palliative care in an ICU (Nelson et al., 2010b). They advocate a phased mutistep process as outlined in the following sections:

Convene an interdisciplinary planning/implementation workgroup

Identify a core group of 'key stakeholders' who will collaborate to plan and lead implementation of the effort. These should include leaders from the ICU, the palliative care consultation service, and hospital administration. Representation of both physicians and nurses is essential, and involvement of staff educators and other disciplines such as social work, psychology, and chaplaincy is preferred.

Conduct a needs assessment

The needs assessment identifies opportunities and priorities for improvement, highlights the importance of the initiative, justifies the investment of resources including staff effort, helps to build support and collaboration within the ICU, and provides a baseline for evaluating results. This step should be completed before the development of strategies to improve care.

Define the problem

An ICU palliative care initiative is often prompted by concerns about one or more of the following: (1) high rates of death or other unfavourable outcomes in the ICU; (2) high utilization of ICU resources for patients who are unlikely to benefit, constricting availability for other patients in need; (3) distress or dissatisfaction reported by patients and/or families; (4) delayed and/or inconsistent performance of evidence-based palliative care processes such as identification of the patient's surrogate decision-maker, investigation of advance directive status, and proactive communication about prognosis and care goals between the interdisciplinary ICU team and the patient's family; (5) distress or burnout experienced by ICU staff; and (6) underutilization of palliative care specialists in care of ICU patients.

Evaluate resources for end-of-life care for ICU patients

This process should incorporate an inventory of available resources such as the availability of an adequately-staffed palliative care consultation service, social worker, mental health professional, chaplain, and ethics consultant. Educational resources are critical since clinicians may need to strengthen knowledge and skills in relevant areas of palliative care, such as management of multiple symptoms in the context of organ failure and adverse effects from first-line analgesic therapy; legal, regulatory, ethical, and empirical frameworks for surrogate decision-making and limitation of intensive care therapies; and approaches to prognostic uncertainty, strong emotions, and conflict in ICU family meetings.

This process should also seek alternative places of care for patients who no longer need or cannot benefit from continued ICU therapy. An increasing number of hospitals have created in-patient palliative care units that can accept ICU patients for whom comfort has become the paramount goal of care; some of these units will care for patients receiving mechanical ventilation. In other hospitals, ventilated patients whose care is focused on comfort can be transferred to a regular ward. Step-down units may also be available.

Develop an action plan

The report highlights five key steps in developing an action plan for a successful and sustainable ICU palliative care initiative: (1) establish overall goals that address unmet needs using available resources, and that are consistent with institutional priorities; (2) set initial targets that are clear and feasible within a specified time frame; (3) identify the changes in clinical practice and systems that are needed to achieve the targets; (4) address the need for new documentation processes to reflect clinical changes; and (5) plan for evaluation of progress toward specific targets and overall goals. For example, an ICU aiming to improve communication between the clinical team and families of critically ill patients may set a target that within 6 months at least half of families of patients in ICU for 5 or more days will have opportunity to meet with interdisciplinary ICU team for goal setting.

Conclusions

Intensive care patients have high degrees of morbidity and a relatively high risk of mortality. Under these circumstances, quality care demands a high level of skill in the core palliative care competencies, including communication, symptom control, goal setting, and end-of-life care. The particularities of the intensive care setting alter the context of discussions and decision-making and the particular issues relating to the foregoing of life-sustaining interventions as part of end-of-life care. The right of patients to adequate relief of unpleasant symptoms at the end of life and the right of family members to compassionate care imply duties incumbent upon individual clinicians working in this setting as well as on the organizational structures to ensure adequate levels of skill, compassion, and organization to meet the challenging needs of intensive care patients and their families.

Further research is required to optimize strategies for staff education, to reduce the incidence of conflict and moral distress surrounding these issues, which is common in this setting, and to optimize the delivery of palliative care in intensive care setting.

Online materials

Complete references for this chapter are available online at <http://www.oxfordmedicine.com>.

References

Abbott, K.H., Sago, J.G., Breen, C.M., Abernethy, A.P., and Tulsky, J.A. (2001). Families looking back: one year after discussion of withdrawal or withholding of life-sustaining support. *Critical Care Medicine*, 29, 197–201.

Anger, K.E. (2013). Dexmedetomidine: a review of its use for the management of pain, agitation, and delirium in the intensive care unit. *Current Pharmaceutical Design*, 19, 4003–4013.

Azoulay, E., Chevret, S., Leleu, G., *et al.* (2000). Half the families of intensive care unit patients experience inadequate communication with physicians. *Critical Care Medicine*, 28, 3044–3049.

Azoulay, E. and Pochard, F. (2003). Communication with family members of patients dying in the intensive care unit. *Current Opinion in Critical Care*, 9, 545–550.

Azoulay, E., Timsit, J.F., Sprung, C.L., *et al.* (2009). Prevalence and factors of intensive care unit conflicts: the Conflicus study. *American Journal of Respiratory and Critical Care Medicine*, 180, 853–860.

Bacchetta, M.D., Eachempati, S.R., Fins, J.J., Hydo, L., and Barie, P.S. (2006). Factors influencing DNR decision-making in a surgical ICU. *Journal of the American College of Surgeons*, 202, 995–1000.

Badger, J.M. (2005). Factors that enable or complicate end-of-life transitions in critical care. *American Journal of Critical Care*, 14, 513–521.

Barr, J., Fraser, G.L., Puntillo, K., *et al.* (2013). Clinical practice guidelines for the management of pain, agitation, and delirium in adult patients in the intensive care unit. *Critical Care Medicine*, 41, 263–306.

Billings, J.A. (2011a). The end-of-life family meeting in intensive care part i: indications, outcomes, and family needs. *Journal of Palliative Medicine*, 14, 1042–1050.

Billings, J.A. (2011b). The end-of-life family meeting in intensive care part II: family-centered decision making. *Journal of Palliative Medicine*, 14, 1051–1057.

Billings, J.A. and Block, S.D. (2011). The end-of-life family meeting in intensive care part III: a guide for structured discussions. *Journal of Palliative Medicine*, 14, 1058–1064.

Breen, C.M., Abernethy, A.P., Abbott, K.H., and Tulsky, J.A. (2001). Conflict associated with decisions to limit life-sustaining treatment in intensive care units. *Journal of General Internal Medicine*, 16, 283–289.

Brody, H., Campbell, M.L., Faberlangendoen, K., and Ogle, K.S. (1997). Withdrawing intensive life-sustaining treatment—recommendations for compassionate clinical management. *The New England Journal of Medicine*, 336, 652–657.

Cook, D., Rocker, G., Marshall, J., *et al.* (2003). Withdrawal of mechanical ventilation in anticipation of death in the intensive care unit. *The New England Journal of Medicine*, 349, 1123–1132.

Curtis, J.R. (2008). Caring for patients with critical illness and their families: the value of the integrated clinical team. *Respiratory Care*, 53, 480–487.

Danis, M., Federman, D., Fins, J.J., *et al.* (1999). Incorporating palliative care into critical care education: principles, challenges, and opportunities. *Critical Care Medicine*, 27, 2005–2013.

Ely, E.W., Margolin, R., Francis, J., *et al.* (2001). Evaluation of delirium in critically ill patients: validation of the Confusion Assessment Method for the Intensive Care Unit (CAM-ICU). *Critical Care Medicine*, 29, 1370–1379.

Forte, D.N., Vincent, J.L., Velasco, I.T., and Park, M. (2012). Association between education in EOL care and variability in EOL practice: a survey of ICU physicians. *Intensive Care Medicine*, 38, 404–412.

Fried, T.R., Bradley, E.H., Towle, V.R., and Allore, H. (2002). Understanding the treatment preferences of seriously ill patients. *The New England Journal of Medicine*, 346, 1061–1066.

Glavan, B.J., Engelberg, R.A., Downey, L., and Curtis, J.R. (2008). Using the medical record to evaluate the quality of end-of-life care in the intensive care unit. *Critical Care Medicine*, 36, 1138–1146.

Goold, S.D., Williams, B., and Arnold, R.M. (2000). Conflicts regarding decisions to limit treatment: a differential diagnosis. *Journal of the American Medical Association*, 283, 909–914.

Gries, C.J., Curtis, J.R., Wall, R.J., and Engelberg, R.A. (2008). Family member satisfaction with end-of-life decision making in the ICU. *Chest*, 133, 704–712.

Hawryluck, L.A., Harvey, W.R., Lemieux-Charles, L., and Singer, P.A. (2002). Consensus guidelines on analgesia and sedation in dying intensive care unit patients. *BMC Medical Ethics*, 3, E3.

Huang, H.L., Chiu, T.Y., Lee, L.T., Yao, C.A., Chen, C.Y., and Hu, W.Y. (2012). Family experience with difficult decisions in end-of-life care. *Psycho-Oncology*, 21, 785–791.

Kesselring, A., Kainz, M., and Kiss, A. (2007). Traumatic memories of relatives regarding brain death, request for organ donation and interactions with professionals in the ICU. *American Journal of Transplantation*, 7, 211–217.

Lautrette, A., Darmon, M., Megarbane, B., *et al.* (2007). A communication strategy and brochure for relatives of patients dying in the ICU. *The New England Journal of Medicine*, 356, 469–478.

Li, D.T. and Puntillo, K. (2006). A pilot study on coexisting symptoms in intensive care patients. *Applied Nursing Research*, 19, 216–219.

McAndrew, N.S., Leske, J.S., and Garcia, A. (2011). Influence of moral distress on the professional practice environment during prognostic conflict in critical care. *Journal of Trauma Nursing*, 18, 221–230.

Nelson, J.E., Angus, D.C., Weissfeld, L.A., *et al.* (2006). End-of-life care for the critically ill: a national intensive care unit survey. *Critical Care Medicine*, 34, 2547–2553.

Nelson, J.E., Campbell, M.L., Cortez, T.B., *et al.* (2010a). *Defining Standards for ICU Palliative Care: A Brief Review from The IPAL-ICU Project.* [Online] Available at: <http://ipal.capc.org/downloads/ipal-icu-defining-standards-for-icu-palliative-care.pdf>.

Nelson, J.E., Campbell, M.L., Cortez, T.B., *et al.* (2010b). *Organizing an ICU Palliative Care Initiative: A Technical Assistance Monograph from The IPAL-ICU Project.* [Online] Available at: <http://ipal.capc.org/downloads/ipal-icu-organizing-an-icu-palliative-care-initiative.pdf>.

Nelson, J.E., Meier, D.E., Oei, E.J., *et al.* (2001). Self-reported symptom experience of critically ill cancer patients receiving intensive care. *Critical Care Medicine*, 29, 277–282.

Payen, J.F., Chanques, G., Mantz, J., *et al.* (2007). Current practices in sedation and analgesia for mechanically ventilated critically ill patients: a prospective multicenter patient-based study. *Anesthesiology*, 106, 687–695.

Prendergast, T.J., Claessens, M.T., and Luce, J.M. (1998). A national survey of end-of-life care for critically ill patients. *American Journal of Respiratory and Critical Care Medicine*, 158, 1163–1167.

Prendergast, T.J. and Puntillo, K.A. (2002). Withdrawal of life support: intensive caring at the end of life. *Journal of the American Medical Association*, 288, 2732–2740.

Puntillo, K.A., Arai, S., Cohen, N.H., *et al.* (2010). Symptoms experienced by intensive care unit patients at high risk of dying. *Critical Care Medicine*, 38, 2155–2160.

Puntillo, K.A., Morris, A.B., Thompson, C.L., Stanik-Hutt, J., White, C.A., and Wild, L.R. (2004). Pain behaviors observed during six common procedures: results from Thunder Project II. *Critical Care Medicine*, 32, 421–427.

Rubenfeld, G.D. (2004). Principles and practice of withdrawing life-sustaining treatments. *Critical Care Clinics*, 20, 435–451, ix.

Schneiderman, L.J. (2006). Effect of ethics consultations in the intensive care unit. *Critical Care Medicine*, 34, S359–363.

Sprung, C.L., Cohen, S.L., Sjokvist, P., *et al.* (2003). End-of-life practices in European intensive care units: the Ethicus Study. *Journal of the American Medical Association*, 290, 790–797.

Strand, J.J. and Billings, J.A. (2012). Integrating palliative care in the intensive care unit. *Journal of Supportive Oncology*, 10, 180–187.

Truog, R.D., Campbell, M.L., Curtis, J.R., *et al.* (2008). Recommendations for end-of-life care in the intensive care unit: a consensus statement by the American College [corrected] of Critical Care Medicine. *Critical Care Medicine*, 36, 953–963.

SECTION 16

Issues of the very young and the very old

Talking with families and children about the death of a parent

Anna C. Muriel and Paula K. Rauch

Introduction to talking with families and children about the death of a parent

Anticipating the death of an adult who is the parent of young children is particularly distressing for families and medical providers. Concerns about the children's welfare, and impulses to protect children from the pain of parental loss, create challenges to honest communication. Nonetheless, attention to children's developmental stage and specific needs can guide clinicians in helping surviving family members to support children during the end-of-life period and into bereavement.

Clinicians and families alike may fear that parental loss during childhood will necessarily create mental health problems in the future, but studies show that the majority of bereaved children do not develop psychiatric disorders. While the loss of a parent during childhood will certainly affect a person's life, individuals usually go on to have meaningful lives and loving relationships. Studies of bereaved children from the time of a parent's death reveal that even though many children may develop non-specific, subclinical, and transient behavioural disturbances (Vida and Grizenko, 1989; Black, 1998) in the year following a parent's death, only one in five children develop a psychiatric disorder (Dowdney, 2000). Epidemiological studies highlight the importance of pre-existing psychosocial risk factors in families with an ill parent, and higher rates of subclinical psychiatric issues and decreased global function in children following the death of a parent (Kaplow et al., 2010). Rather than the simple fact of parental loss predicting future difficulties, studies also show that the quality of the surviving parent's care (Harris et al., 1986; Bifulco et al., 1987), or general home life (Breier et al., 1988) are better predictors of subsequent adult depression. Other factors that may mediate depression in adulthood are reports of warmth and empathy in surviving parents, and the opportunity to participate in the mourning process (Saler and Skolnick, 1992).

Research on normative childhood bereavement has found that children make active efforts to maintain a connection to their deceased parents, and construct a relationship that may shift with developmental stages in an effort to cope effectively with the loss (Silverman et al., 1992). The role of the surviving parent can be particularly important in providing the child with opportunities to remember and memorialize the dead parent, facilitating integration of the loss throughout different phases of growth and development (Nickman et al., 1998).

The terminal phase of parental illness may be a vulnerable time for children as they experience more anxiety and depression, lower self-esteem, fears, misconceptions, and behaviour changes (Christ et al., 1993, 1994; Siegel et al., 1996). The literature on children's coping with parental illness shows that children living with parental cancer have more anxiety associated with an inability to discuss the illness, decreased time spent in age-appropriate activities, and ongoing worries about the cancer (Nelson et al., 1994). These anxieties may be mediated by increased communication, as children given specific information about the illness have been shown to have lower rates of anxiety (Rosenheim and Reicher, 1985). However, these conversations between parents and children may not happen readily; even parents who are generally rated highly as communicators by their children are no more likely to disclose the probability of death than parents with low general communication ratings (Siegel et al., 1996).

Parental depression and family dysfunction in the context of parental illness are also important predictors of child emotional and behavioural problems (Thastum et al., 2009). Families coping with anticipated deaths may be additionally vulnerable to parent–child differences in coping due to the well parent's physical and emotional preoccupation with the dying spouse, as well as differences in cognitive understanding and therefore anticipation of the death (Saldinger et al., 2004). These differences may have implications for child coping and outcomes (Saldinger et al., 1999). There may also be a range of children's responses to the graphic experience of a parent's terminal illness with attendant changes in appearance, function, and dependence on medical equipment, which can sometimes, but not always, be mediated by overwhelmed adult caregivers (Saldinger et al., 2003).

Specific attention is needed for patients as parents, and targeted interventions may help mediate parental, family, and child distress. Some subsets of parents may have higher levels of concern about their children, including mothers, single parents, or those with metastatic or recurrent cancer, a subjective understanding of incurable disease, and current mental health treatment (Muriel et al., 2012). Parents of children under 18 years have higher rates of panic and anxiety than patients with advanced cancer who do not have dependent children. This population of parents has also been shown to prefer more aggressive treatment, and to be less likely to engage in advanced care planning. They were also judged by their caregivers to have worse quality of life in the last week of life (Nilsson et al., 2009). Palliative care clinicians are poised to address parenting issues directly and ease family suffering through open communication, planning, and support.

How children understand death at different ages

In thinking about how to talk with families and children anticipating parental death, it is essential to have a sense of how children at different ages understand death itself. This will be influenced by children's general level of cognitive and emotional development as well as by their exposure to death in their community. There will be individual variations in children's temperaments and development, and parents need to be respected in knowing their own children best. For clinicians, however, an understanding of basic needs at different ages provides a useful guide for recommendations for supporting children during the terminal phase of a parent's illness and death.

Infants and toddlers (0–2 years)

Infants and toddlers are working on the complex tasks of attachment, basic self-regulation, and trust in their environment and caregivers. These youngsters have no understanding of time, or of the finality of death. However, they are sensitive to separations, and will feel the absence of a familiar caregiver even with no comprehension of the permanence of death. They may be distressed by changes in regular routines, and will also probably be affected by the emotional distress of grieving adults around them.

While familiarity and structure are helpful for people of all ages during difficult times, it is even more essential for the youngest children. During the stressful months or weeks leading up to a parent's death, it is best if infants and toddlers can be cared for by a limited number of familiar caregivers who can get to know a child's routine and provide care in as consistent and predictable a way as possible. Feeding, nappy changing, bathing, and sleeping should have associated routines and things that help a child to feel secure: bottles and cups, stuffed animals and toys, blankets, and portable crib are examples of important items. The closest caregivers can provide schedules and instructions for other childcare helpers to ensure that important parts of the child's day proceed in a predictable manner even when they are not available.

Pre-schoolers (3–6 years)

Pre-school children have a wider range of social interactions, and particular ways of understanding the world around them. Egocentrism, associative logic, and magical thinking have strong bearings on how they understand parental illness and death. These self-referential ideas need to be mediated in order to prevent misunderstandings and guilt about what is happening in their family. For example, a 4-year-old may believe that something they did, like jump on a parent or misbehave, caused their parent's illness. A child who yells 'Bad Mummy' during a tantrum may think that saying this, or wishing her to 'go away', can actually make someone die and go away. Children of this age do not yet have an understanding of the irreversibility of death, and so they may also offer solutions to death, and expect the person to be 'all better'. They may also attribute the grief and distress of other adults to their own behaviour and need frequent reminders that they are not the cause of everyone's upset feelings.

Pre-schoolers, therefore, need regular conversations about how nothing a child says or does can make a parent ill or die. Adults need to enquire about how the child thinks their parent became ill or died, and dispel misconceptions repeatedly. In addition, caregivers may need to be patient with a natural disconnection of feelings and content, such that a child might talk about the death very matter-of-factly or make up a song about it, and yet might become cranky or have trouble with routine activities or changes in schedule. Parents of pre-schoolers can also expect some regression under stress, so that a fully toilet-trained child may have trouble using the potty, or a child may get upset being dropped off at a previously beloved nursery.

In discussing death with young children it is important to be concrete and use observable examples. Descriptions of death as 'going to sleep' can create worries about bedtime or not waking up. Heaven may be conceptualized as a place that one can visit or come back from. It is therefore helpful to talk about death as meaning that 'the body doesn't work anymore', that the person can't move or breathe, or think or feel, etc. Adult survivors are sometimes surprised and disturbed by how often young children need this explanation.

School-age children (7–12 years)

School-age children are immersed in mastering academic, physical, and social skills, and are working to understand cause and effect logic. They are often quite invested in fairness and are sensitive to things that set them apart from their peers. By 6 or 7 years of age children understand consistently the permanence of death. Their conceptions may still be very concrete, though, and they may have difficulty understanding more abstract or spiritual issues. In fact, they can be preoccupied with factual, medical, or physical aspects of death and dying that feel difficult for adults to discuss. The uncertainty about time that is inherent in terminal illness may be particularly hard for younger children to grasp, and so anticipating the death itself may become distorted. For example, a 10-year-old child hearing that a parent is very, very ill and 'coming home to die', may think that the parent will die that very night. School-age children are also vulnerable to worries about their own health or the health of their surviving family members, and need reassurances about this over time.

Because so much of these children's day is spent at school, it is important that the appropriate school personnel be informed about what is happening with an ill and dying parent. Children may not want to have teachers approach them to discuss the illness at school. However, they should know to whom they can go if they are having a difficult day. Teachers might adjust some expectations for schoolwork, but it is helpful for children to still have a certain level of responsibility and routines so that they understand that life will go on even in the context of a parent's illness and death. Children may also need additional help with school tasks and activities, and families may come to rely on other families in their community in order to support their children's participation in age-appropriate activities.

Adolescents (13 years and older)

Teenagers are in the process of identity formation and separation from parents. They have more adult capacities for abstract thinking, but their brains are not fully mature until into their twenties. Adolescents understand that death is final, irreversible, and

Box 16.1.1 How children understand death at different ages

Infants and toddlers (0–2 years)

Developmental context: establishing attachment and trust.

- Have no understanding of finality of separation, but feel absence of a familiar caregiver
- May be distressed by disruptions in routines
- Will be affected by the emotional distress/grief of surviving adult caregivers.

Pre-schoolers (3–6 years)

Developmental context: driven by egocentrism, magical thinking, associative logic.

- Are not able to understand that death is irreversible and permanent
- May attribute death or survivors' emotional distress to own actions or attributes
- Distress and behavioural changes may be fuelled by disruption in routine.

School-age children (7–12 years)

Developmental context: mastering skills, fairness, cause and effect logic, peer relationships.

- Understand that death is final and irreversible
- May have difficulty with abstract/spiritual issues
- May ask factual questions that can be painful or offensive to adults
- May struggle with unfairness of loss.

Adolescents (13 and above)

Developmental context: working on separation-individuation, identity formation.

- Understand that death is final, irreversible, and universal
- May struggle with existential issues
- May focus on personal effects of loss.

universal, and may think actively about existential and spiritual issues. They may also vacillate between abstract ideas about their parent's death, and being preoccupied with very specific and self-centred ways in which it affects their life. These young people are also likely to project forward into the future and worry about their life progressing without their parent, anticipating sadness about milestones that their parent will not be there to witness.

Surviving caregivers may need help to understand adolescent self-involvement as developmentally normal, and not attribute it to negative character flaws. In addition, adolescents will continue to need support and guidance, and be at risk of more independence than they are ready for in the context of a parental death. Families should be careful of teenagers who are taking on too many adult responsibilities, or are engaging in risky behaviours such as substance abuse or illegal activity. Older adolescents also need specific information about a parent's illness and probability of death as they make decisions about moving away from home for

employment or education. While parents may want to give them as much freedom as possible, these young adults need accurate information in order to make decisions that will be most comfortable for them, and minimize the possibility of regrets about being too close or too far away during the end of a parent's life (Box 16.1.1).

An approach to talking with families

With a basic understanding of where children are developmentally, clinicians can address parental concerns about helping their children through this difficult time. This task will also be influenced by the family culture around communication in general, the adults' capacities to integrate end-of-life care, and the expected progression of disease.

Clinicians can begin by assessing the adults' understanding and expectations of the illness and death. What do they understand about the expected time course? What do they know about the expected symptomatology? What do they hope for in terms of location and likely medical circumstances of the death?

The stage is then set to explore with the parents the children's understanding of the illness to date. What language has been used? What do they expect about the outcome of the illness? What prior experiences have the children had of major life changes, or death in their community or family? How have they managed these as a family? Do the parents have particular concerns about their children's coping with the illness so far? What are they worried about in terms of their coping with death? The answers to these questions will provide scaffolding for the discussion, and help parents to have honest conversations with their children while addressing worries and misconceptions along the way. Parents should be encouraged to use honest, straightforward, and age-appropriate language, checking frequently for the children's understanding, and welcoming questions as they arise. If the children have not yet been told the specific name of the illness, for example, 'leukaemia', 'glioblastoma', or 'cardiomyopathy', it is important to do so now, to minimize confusion and anxiety about illness in general.

With careful discussion with parents and adult caregivers, it may not be necessary for clinicians to meet directly with the children. In some clinical settings, it is not possible, and for most children information mediated by their parents is most easily integrated and discussed in varying iterations over time. However, when children are present during medical encounters by chance or by design, they should be welcomed into the discussion so that their questions can be addressed. Some older children may ask to participate in meetings with medical providers in order to feel included more fully in the family experience. Children may stump clinicians or parents with questions that are anxiety-provoking or out of the blue. Asking a child what got them thinking about that issue may help clarify exactly what the child is curious or worried about, and allow adults to provide specific answers without going into more detail than the child is interested in.

Timing of discussions with children

Families often wonder when to talk about the terminal nature of a parent's illness with the children. Sometimes it is hard for parents to talk openly, even when the children have already observed the parent's deteriorating status, or have overheard others talking about the likelihood of death. At other times, parents have trouble holding back the fact that there is a transition in care from curative to palliative treatment, even if there is no observable change in the parent's appearance or function, and death is probably many months away.

Generally, the worst way for a child to hear news is by overhearing it, and many children will experience well-intentioned protection as exclusion. A child left to their own conclusions about a parent's terminal illness may also be vulnerable to misconceptions about why the illness is progressing, or how their life will change after a parent dies. On the other hand, it is difficult for younger children to understand that a parent may live for some time even in the terminal phase, and it is confusing to be anticipating the death at every turn.

It is important to discuss the changes in a parent's appearance and functional status as they occur, and potentially use these markers to discuss the probability of death within weeks or days with children school-age or above. Many children will ask about death directly in the context of seeing a parent getting 'worse, or very, very sick'. For adults who feel worried about introducing the idea of death, asking, 'Do you know what could happen if Mum gets even more unwell? Or different parts of her body stop working?' will allow children to articulate that they are worried about death too. For the youngest children, acknowledging the functional changes as they pertain to their interactions with the parent may be enough: 'Dad used to be able to take walks with us and play with you, but now he can't because he is more unwell, so he stays in bed a lot.' Conversations with pre-school children about death may be most meaningful after the death has occurred.

Decisions about the setting for end-of-life care in a family context

One of the most important decisions for families facing an anticipated parental death is where they would like the death to occur. There is no one answer that will suit every family, and the ill adult may have prior experience or personal wishes that will dictate whether they die at home, in the hospital, or in an inpatient hospice setting. If families have choices, they should consider the needs of the children in addition to the medical or personal needs of the dying person.

Sometimes an inpatient hospice or hospital setting makes the most sense for families. In this case, the challenge may be that the well parent will have to divide their time between the inpatient setting with their spouse, and being at home with the children. Having thoughtful, familiar adults at home can ease this strain and allow the children to continue with their usual home and school activities. Visits with children should be facilitated whenever possible (see 'Visits between ill parents and children').

If families are interested in home hospice services, and expect a parent to die at home, attention to certain logistical details can make things more comfortable for children. Whenever possible, having the dying parent in a room with a door, as opposed to an open or family area, allows the children to titrate their own exposure to the ill parent and medical equipment. The advantage of having everyone at home is that the children can maintain their usual routines and probably have more access to their well parent. If there will be other adults staying in the home to help, they should also be aware of the children's needs for privacy and daily routines. A home death also makes it even more important to talk

about changes in medical status and check for questions or misconceptions about what is happening. Children may have particular fears about the death itself, and clinicians can help both adults and children who are curious by anticipating symptoms and treatments for pain, secretions, shortness of breath, etc., and explaining what the physical process of dying might look and sound like. This also allows older children to consider how much they want to be around during the final days and hours. When a parent dies at home, thought should be given to where the children will be when the undertaker arrives to remove the body.

Visits between ill parents and children

If a parent is expected to die in an inpatient or hospice setting, visits from children should be facilitated whenever possible. Children who express reluctance may have specific worries, for example, seeing blood, or having their parent die during the visit, and can usually be reassured with explanations and contingency plans. It is best to avoid an agitated or delirious parent who may be frightening, but a child can still visit a sedated parent. Older children and adolescents who are reluctant to visit need opportunities to discuss their concerns, and be able to make a decision for themselves that they can feel comfortable with over time.

Most importantly, children need to be prepared for the visit, with descriptions of the setting, medical equipment, roommates, as well as the physical and functional status of the parent. For younger children, these descriptions may need to be concrete comparisons to the last time they saw their parent. An additional supportive adult should accompany the child so that they can leave when the child is ready, even if the well parent would like to stay. Younger children may only be able to tolerate brief visits, or might need structured quiet play or drawing activities to do in the room. Touching a sick parent should never be forced, but can be modelled and supported if the child is willing. After the visit, adult caregivers should take some time to debrief and ask the child what was most interesting, fun, scary, or uncomfortable, in order to reassure the child and prepare better for the next visit. When personal visits are not possible, other kinds of contact between the ill parent and child should be encouraged. Children often enjoy making cards and notes that can be used to decorate a hospital room, and if able, parents can make recordings of themselves reading books or singing songs that can go home to young children (Box 16.1.2).

When death is imminent, last visits can be meaningful for children once they have an understanding of the finality of death. Older children may have the same wishes that adults do to have a few minutes alone with a dying parent, even if comatose, to say a last 'I love you', or share an important private moment. If possible, older school-age and teenage children should be asked about whether or not they want to be called to the bedside near the end of life or immediately after the death. For example, does a child want to be brought home from school, or woken in the middle of the night at the time of death, or not? Some children very much want to be included, while others may prefer to have healthier memories of their parent, or feel afraid and uncomfortable about seeing their parent very ill and dying. The guiding principle is to provide children with information so that they can make decisions that will help them feel that their needs and wishes are considered during this important time. It is important to remind families,

Box 16.1.2 Facilitating visits to an ill or dying parent

- ◆ Explore and alleviate worries or reluctance about visiting
- ◆ Prepare children for what they will see:
  - hospital or hospice setting
  - medical equipment
  - other patients
  - physical condition of parent
  - functional status of parent
- ◆ Bring an extra supportive adult who can leave when the child is ready
- ◆ Provide structure or activity for younger children
- ◆ Avoid an agitated or delirious parent
- ◆ Debrief after the visit
- ◆ Provide alternatives to a personal visit
- ◆ Remember that there are many opportunities to say goodbye.

however, that there are many opportunities to say goodbye before the death, immediately afterwards, during memorial services and funerals, as well as during private moments of reflection or prayer.

Legacy leaving

Parents who have come to terms with a diagnosis of a terminal illness often think about specific legacies or communications that they would like to leave for their children. Even the usual family photos and memorabilia become good foundations for telling stories about a parent after they have died. Parents may choose a variety of other more intentional communications, such as letters or audio recordings specifically for each child, or at particular milestones. There is little data on how these communications are received by children over time, but surviving children often look for indications from both the dead parent and surviving adults, about who the parent was as a person, their values and ideals, and what the parent saw in them, their child. Sometimes parents leave specific meaningful objects, or annotate books, music, or movies that have been important to them. Children may want to choose special objects to keep themselves either before or after the death. The wider community can also be engaged in legacy-leaving, as friends and relatives attending the memorial service can be asked to write down a memory or thought about the parent that can be compiled for the children and shared when they are curious later. Children spend a lifetime revisiting the loss of the parent, and may become interested in their parent as they themselves reach different phases in their own life.

Children's participation in funerals and memorial services

Children of any age may participate in different aspects of funerals and memorial services. Family tradition will dictate whether there is a wake, religious service, interment, or family gathering afterwards, and children may be included for all or part of these events. As with hospital visits, it is important to prepare children

for what the event will be like including the setting, who will be there, what the service will be like, what they will and will not be able to do, and that there may be a range of feelings expressed by people, from sadness to warmth and humour. Younger children will need a familiar adult to care for them throughout, and be responsive or leave when they are unable to sit still or remain quiet.

Older school-age and teenage children can be included in the planning or asked if they want to participate by reading, or playing music during the service. Many funeral homes will provide a private time for the family to have a special children's service or quiet visiting time. Children sometimes like to place a picture, note, or special object in or on top of the coffin. School-age children may have specific questions about the preparation of the body or cremation. Adult caregivers may want to learn about the process in advance, so that they can answer children's questions better. Alternatively, they should know whom to ask (funeral directors sometimes have age-appropriate information) about these issues during the difficult and chaotic days around the parent's death. Younger children, who do not yet fully understand death, may find the interment disturbing as they do not want to see their parent lowered into the cold, dark ground. Families may consider not having young children attend the burial itself, and be able to visit the gravesite at another time. For families who spread ashes or have non-traditional services that do not involve a burial site, it may still be important for the family to designate a special place to go to reflect or remember the parent.

Conclusion

The untimely death of a parent is one of the most challenging events for families and the clinicians who care for them. Attention to children's needs during this time is an important aspect of clinical care, and is much appreciated by adults in the family. A basic knowledge of child development and the ways that children understand illness and death can provide a template from which to engage families about how to help their children during this time and into bereavement. When clinicians support honest, child-centred communication, and help families anticipate common situations and questions, surviving adults are able to use their own best resources to provide thoughtful care for the children.

References

Bifulco, A.T., Brown, G.W., and Harris, T.O. (1987). Childhood loss of parent, lack of adequate parental care and adult depression: a replication. *Journal of Affective Disorders*, 12(2), 115–128.

Black, D. (1998). Coping with loss. Bereavement in childhood. *BMJ*, 316(7135), 931–933.

Breier, A., Kelsoe, J.R., Jr, Kirwin, P.D., *et al.* (1988). Early parental loss and development of adult psychopathology. *Archives of General Psychiatry*, 45(11), 987–993.

Christ, G.H., Siegel, K., Freund, B., *et al.* (1993). Impact of parental terminal cancer on latency-age children. *American Journal of Orthopsychiatry*, 63(3), 417–425.

Christ, G.H., Siegel, K., and Sperber, D. (1994). Impact of parental terminal cancer on adolescents. *American Journal of Orthopsychiatry*, 64(4), 604–613.

Dowdney, L. (2000). Childhood bereavement following parental death. *Journal of Child Psychology and Psychiatry*, 41(7), 819–830.

Harris, T., Brown, G.W., and Bifulco, A. (1986). Loss of parent in childhood and adult psychiatric disorder: the role of lack of adequate parental care. *Psychological Medicine*, 16(3), 641–659.

Kaplow, J.B., Saunders, J., Angold, A., and Costello, E.J. (2010). Psychiatric symptoms in bereaved versus nonbereaved youth and young adults: a longitudinal epidemiological study. *Journal of the American Academy of Child & Adolescent Psychiatry*, 49(11), 1145–1154.

Muriel, A.C., Moore, C.W., Baer, L., *et al.* (2012). Measuring psychosocial distress and parenting concerns among adults with cancer: The Parenting Concerns Questionnaire. *Cancer*, 118(22), 5671–5678.

Nelson, E., Sloper, P., Charlton, A., and While, D. (1994). Children who have a parent with cancer: a pilot study. *Journal of Cancer Education*, 9(1), 30–36.

Nickman, S.L., Silverman, P.R., and Normand, C. (1998). Children's construction of a deceased parent: the surviving parent's contribution. *American Journal of Orthopsychiatry*, 68(1), 126–134.

Nilsson, M.E., Maciejewski, P.K., Zhang, B., *et al.* (2009). Mental health, treatment preferences, advance care planning, location, and quality of death in advanced cancer patients with dependent children. *Cancer*, 115(2), 399–409.

Rosenheim, E. and Reicher, R. (1985). Informing children about a parent's terminal illness. *Journal of Child Psychology and Psychiatry*, 26(6), 995–998.

Saldinger, A., Cain, A., Kalter, N., and Lohnes, K. (1999). Anticipating parental death in families with young children. *American Journal of Orthopsychiatry*, 69(1), 39–48.

Saldinger, A., Cain, A., and Porterfield, K. (2003). Managing traumatic stress in children anticipating parental death. *Psychiatry*, 66(2), 168–181.

Saldinger, A., Porterfield, K., and Cain, A.C. (2004). Meeting the needs of parentally bereaved children: a framework for child-centered parenting. *Psychiatry*, 67(4), 331–352.

Saler, L. and Skolnick, N. (1992). Childhood parental death and depression in adulthood: roles of surviving parent and family environment. *American Journal of Orthopsychiatry*, 62(4), 504–516.

Siegel, K., Karus, D., and Raveis, V.H. (1996). Adjustment of children facing the death of a parent due to cancer. *Journal of the American Academy of Child & Adolescent Psychiatry*, 35(4), 442–450.

Silverman, P.R., Nickman, S., and Worden, J.W. (1992). Detachment revisited: the child's reconstruction of a dead parent. *American Journal of Orthopsychiatry*, 62(4), 494–503.

Thastum, M., Watson, M., Kienbacher, C., *et al.* (2009). Prevalence and predictors of emotional and behavioural functioning of children where a parent has cancer: a multinational study. *Cancer*, 115(17), 4030–4039.

Vida, S. and Grizenko, N. (1989). DSM-III-R and the phenomenology of childhood bereavement: a review. *Canadian Journal of Psychiatry*, 34(2), 148–155.

Care of children with advanced illness

John J. Collins, Kirsty Campbell,
Wendy Edmonds, Judith Frost, Martha
F. Mherekumombe, and Natasha Samy

Introduction to care of children with advanced illness

The World Health Organization (WHO) supports the global application of the principles of palliative care to every child with a life-limiting illness, irrespective of geographical location (WHO, 1998a) whilst acknowledging that treatment options are limited in some countries. The care of the child with advanced and progressive illness and their family requires a holistic approach to the often complex physical, social, psychological, and spiritual needs as well as support in bereavement. This inevitably requires a paediatric palliative care team with diverse skills and abilities to meet these needs.

This chapter will discuss the global perspective of paediatric palliative care and the role of the team, nursing, and volunteers in that care. The significant physical and psychosocial issues for the child with advanced illness will be discussed, as well as bereavement support of families. The necessity of quality improvement and strategies for setting up such a programme will be outlined. The reader is directed to Box 16.2.1 for additional resources and to Section 9 in this textbook regarding pain management for children needing palliative care.

Paediatric palliative care: a global perspective

Most of the world's children with advanced incurable illnesses die either in hospital or at home. Inpatient hospice units for children are an alternative for some children and are usually located in more affluent countries. While paediatric palliative care services are growing globally, approximately 70% of the world's children have no access to paediatric palliative care and only 6% have fully and multiple integrated services (Knapp et al., 2011). There is a greater disease burden in developing countries with more deaths, almost half of these occurring in Africa (Downing et al., 2012). Paediatric palliative care provision and delivery in developing countries can only happen through increased resources (Downing et al., 2012).

According to the World Bank, a developing country is one with a low- or middle-level economy per gross national product per capita and it also includes Hong Kong (China), Israel, Kuwait, Singapore, and the United Arab Emirates (World Bank, 2004). The funding required for palliative care services is often beyond the financial means of many developing countries. Palliative care service implementation is sometimes hindered by lack of economic and political government support. Funding sources in such circumstances are often from external resources and by non-governmental organizations (Callaway et al., 2007). Despite all the problems encountered in developing countries, there continues to be a growing awareness of the need for paediatric palliative care and the International Children's Palliative Care Network (ICPCN) is at the forefront of the global development of paediatric palliative care.

Africa

Just over 40% of African children are under the age of 15, with a mortality rate of 14.5%, mostly in sub-Saharan Africa (Downing et al., 2010). The under-5 child mortality rate in Sub-Saharan Africa is one in eight, more than 17 times the average for developed regions which is one in 143 (United Nations Children's Fund, 2011). Although most of the deaths are from communicable diseases and malnutrition, a large number of deaths are attributable to HIV/AIDS and cancer. HIV/AIDS has impacted on paediatric palliative care in Africa, resulting in an increased demand for services in already resource poor countries. Care is also complicated by late presentations, essential drug affordability, shortages especially of morphine, and lack of qualified health professionals (Amery, 2009; Downing et al., 2012).

Many African countries have made tremendous progress in paediatric palliative care provision and education. For example, Malawi has now integrated palliative care for children into all referral hospitals in all regions of the country. South Africa has pioneered paediatric palliative care in Africa (Marston et al., 2012). Education outreach has been mostly through Tanzania, Uganda, and South Africa to other regions in Africa. Integration has mostly been possible through organizations such as the Elizabeth Glaser Pediatric AIDS Foundation especially in Tanzania and Zambia, and the Paediatric AIDS Treatment in Africa (PATA) which works in 15 African countries. In addition, the Southern African Children's Palliative Care Network was launched in Cape Town in September 2012 in collaboration with and with support from the Hospice Palliative Care Association of South Africa, The Bigshoes Foundation, and the ICPCN (ehospice, 2012). The network arose to provide input and support for an integrated approach to improve palliative care for children across South Africa.

African services rely mostly on community volunteers and families for the identification of patients needing services. Palliative care models need to be adapted to the African setting and also take into consideration cultural variations and preferences. Home care is the most commonly used model of care in Africa because it is affordable. Unfortunately there are more patients than can be supported through such services, because of a shortage of skilled health workers (Harding et al., 2010).

Complex psychosocial issues impact on the care of children in Africa where there is a large number of children orphaned from AIDS. Stigmatization of children with HIV/AIDS, cultural beliefs, and rituals, mainly around death and dying also affect provision of effective palliative care services (Amery, 2009). These challenges require palliative care to be provided in a multidisciplinary team, which should include the family, nurses, doctors, social workers, community health workers, traditional healers, volunteers, and others as appropriate.

Asia

Of the 47 Asian countries, approximately 66% have no recognized paediatric hospice or palliative activity and only 2% of Asia has services integrated with mainstream services (Wright et al., 2008; Knapp et al., 2011). In Malaysia, through Hospis Malaysia, there are initiatives to set up a national paediatric care team to provide paediatric palliative care in hospitals and communities (Hamzah and Lan Kuan, 2012). Paediatric palliative care is provided mostly by adult physicians and various specialities. In Thailand, there are few paediatric palliative care programmes. Lack of palliative educational programmes, national palliative care guidelines, adequate finances, trained personnel, and a shortage of opioids are major challenges to effective delivery of services. Education is needed to change mind sets to focus on quality of life, improve symptom control, and address the misconceptions surrounding opioid use (Pairojkul, 2012).

India

India has palliative care services located mostly in the large cities and urban areas and 72% of the population living in rural areas have no access to these services (Mathews and Suresh Kumar, 2012). Services are provided by non-governmental organizations, public and private hospitals, and hospices. An estimated 200 000 children under the age of 15 live with HIV/AIDS, and only 4% of these have access to antiretroviral therapy. India has four established children's palliative care programmes with other programmes under development. Opioid use and availability in India has been affected greatly by current government legislature and fears surrounding its prescription. As a result, recent rulings should see opioid supply improve throughout the country (Pallium India, 2012).

Middle East

Paediatric palliative care in the Middle East is a new and developing concept driven mostly by non-governmental organizations. The Middle East has diverse cultures, political conflicts, various religions, and traditions which impact on the delivery of palliative services. There are also cultural taboos which impact on paediatric palliative care education. Palliative care providers need to be culturally sensitive to the different rituals and faiths but also sensitive and proactive to a family's needs to ensure a 'good death' and appropriate support in bereavement (Siblermann et al., 2012). Kuwait has taken a significant initiative with the development of Beyt Abdullah Children's Hospice.

Central America

Paediatric palliative care in Mexico has experienced similar challenges to other developing countries but has made substantial progress in the care of children with life-limiting diseases, with an increased awareness of paediatric palliative care (Okhuysen-Cawley et al., 2012). Mexico also has a shortage of trained paediatricians, medical specialists, and support services for terminally ill children. Difficult symptom management is, however, provided by the treating oncologists or anaesthesiologists with an interest in chronic pain management who are supported by paediatric palliative physicians in Costa Rica and Argentina and locally through the Associacion Mexicana de Cuidados Paliativos. In addition, the Instituto Nacional de Pediatria in Mexico City provides tertiary paediatric palliative care services (Okhuysen-Cawley et al., 2012). As with many developing countries, essential medications are available mostly in urban centres. Rural areas, where most indigenous people live, have limited access to contemporary medical care and rely on traditional remedies. Access to medical care is limited by poor accessibility, fear and distrust of health professionals, and strong traditional belief systems which emphasize life and death as a transcendental continuum (Okhuysen-Cawley et al., 2012).

Paediatric palliative care in Costa Rica is delivered mostly through the Paediatric Palliative Care and Pain Control Clinic (PPCPCC) which covers only an estimated third of the population of children with life-limiting illnesses (Quesada-Tristán and Masís-Quesada, 2012). This service is provided through the Children's National Hospital in collaboration with the Foundation for Palliative Care Unit a non-profit organization. There are number of barriers encountered by the PPCPCC which include identifying and mapping children who need to be referred to the programme. Comparable barriers include health professionals' misunderstanding of the concept of paediatric palliative care, limitation of resources, and finances. In Costa Rica, the paediatric palliative care programme is organized into four teams that operate in different areas of the country. The teams comprise a hospital-based team, day care centres, or home-based care and a team that is both day centre- and home-based, covering the entire country with a telephone support service for palliative patients (Quesada-Tristán and Masís-Quesada, 2012).

South America

Of the 23 South American countries about 67% have no demonstrable paediatric hospice-palliative care activity, whilst 8% of countries offer localized service (Knapp et al., 2011). In Brazil paediatric palliative care usually is offered when a child is dying and the Brazilian Pediatric Society is working towards improvement in collaboration with the Brazilian Intensive Care Association, local universities, and hospitals (Lago and Piva, 2012). Argentina has created Pediatric Palliative Care Units (PPCUs) distributed in the six provinces to provide medical care to children with life-limiting illnesses, palliative education, and research (Germ et al., 2012). Home care programmes have also been developed through the units. Challenges faced by the PPCU are similar to other countries. In Chile, paediatric palliative care is coordinated through paediatric hospitals, specifically in oncology units (Torres et al., 2012). Oncology children have access to pain and symptom management through the Pain Relief and Palliative Care programme (PR and PC) operating in National Child Antineoplastic Drugs Program (PINDA) cancer centres throughout Chile. Health reforms in Chile have incorporated PR and PC for care of children with advanced cancer (Torres, 2012). Palliative care services likewise operate in outpatient, hospital, or home settings with telephone follow-up. Despite palliative care services being limited to oncology patients with advanced disease, the Ministry of Health is creating committees to work in conjunction with paediatric palliative care units in hospitals, to extend services to other children with life-limiting illnesses.

The team in paediatric palliative care

Paediatric palliative care is delivered best by a team with a diverse skill set working together to enhance and deliver quality patient care. Care and support is coordinated and individualized to the patient and family (Baker et al., 2008). The team can include nurses, doctors, social workers, volunteers, chaplains, allied health practitioners, and other therapists (Crawford and Price, 2003). Excellent communication is vital to ensure good teamwork in the delivery of palliative care. This can be either formal, in the form of case conferences, or informal, via electronic means. It is important that clear lines of communication are established, particularly as to who the family should call should a change occur in the child's condition or if there is an exacerbation in pain or other debilitating symptoms. Case conferences are integral to the care planning, delivery of services, and help in the collaboration of care by defining and negotiating the roles of care as the patient's condition and psychosocial needs changes (Crawford and Price, 2003; Mitchell et al., 2008).

The role of nursing in the paediatric palliative care team

Palliative care nursing includes care planning and/or the provision of care to a child identified as needing palliative care, regardless of the projected duration of the child's illness and regardless of the location of care. The level and type of intervention provided will depend on the skill, expertise, or location of the nurse, as well as the needs of the child and their family. Paediatric palliative care nursing, whilst still relatively new as a specialty, has developed rapidly over the last 10–15 years.

Paediatric palliative care nursing is a mix of art and science that begins at diagnosis, or referral to palliative care, through to supporting the family in the bereavement process. These skills can support the family to adapt to the challenges of caring for a dying child and also empower the child to express needs, develop their goals of care, and work with his/her family to achieve them. Some children may require palliative care nursing for short periods while others require care over many months or years. 'Graduation' from palliative care needs can occur for a very few children as they either reach adulthood, obtain a treatment (e.g. liver transplant), or recover.

Aranda (2003) describes a framework for the role of nursing in palliative care. She describes three levels of nursing which are the palliative approach, specialist interventions, and specialist palliative care. The palliative approach is any care provided by any health professional with 'a core set of knowledge and skills' to a person with a life-threatening or terminal illness. This care is provided by a generalist nurse who may or may not have paediatric and/or palliative experience but is caring for a child receiving palliative care. Higher needs related to palliation are either carried out by the generalist nurse supported by a specialist palliative care nurse or, at times, provided by specialist palliative care nurse in collaboration with the generalist nurse. Aranda describes specialist interventions as those provided by specialists outside palliative care, such as wound care nurses and specialist palliative care by those with qualifications and advanced practice skills in palliative care whether these are in hospital, home, or hospice (Aranda, 2003).

Paediatric palliative care nursing at home is likely to fall under the auspices of community/domiciliary care of either generalist nurses or dedicated palliative care teams who are not necessarily familiar with paediatric needs. Direct care from a specialist tertiary paediatric palliative care service is less likely. More usually, care provided by domiciliary nurses will be overseen by a specialist paediatric palliative care service. Box 16.2.2 outlines the potential role of paediatric palliative care nursing in a child's home.

Family support volunteers in paediatric palliative care

A volunteer service within a paediatric palliative care team, if adequately supervised, is a flexible and cost-efficient way to alleviate a child's and family's distress. Volunteers can fill a support gap and not leave the family feeling indebted to friends and family. They can assist with practical help around the home, sibling support, craft and diversional activities for an unwell child, and social support for parents and family. They can undertake simple daily activities which are challenged by time and exhaustion in the family unit.

In Australia, there are two volunteer programmes supporting Paediatric Palliative Care families specifically at home. The Family Support Volunteer Program in Victoria is one of the services offered by Very Special Kids, a charity established for over 25 years, supporting families caring for children in palliative care

---

Box 16.2.2 The potential roles of paediatric palliative care nursing in the home

- Creating/implementing a care plan which includes assessment of symptoms and psychosocial needs in conjunction with the child's primary treating team and all other services involved

- Assessment of the home and relevant equipment needs

- Identifying the family unit and wider community support and ensuring relevant persons are present at family conferences

- Identifying and ensuring appropriate community clinicians are involved and planning of support such as contact details, details of home visiting, and so on.

- Providing appropriate information (at family's request) to community groups such as schools, cultural/religious support groups, volunteer services, interpreter services, and so on.

- Generating a plan for anticipated deterioration and/or emergency situations

- Generating a plan for end-of-life care which includes location of care and identifying family goals

- Accurate reporting systems for any interventions.

(Very Special Kids, n.d.). Part of a suite of services offered to families includes sibling support programmes, counselling, hospice respite, and end-of-life care. The volunteer programme provides practical and social support in the family home (Very Special Kids, n.d.).

The Family Support Volunteer Program at The Children's Hospital at Westmead (New South Wales) was established in 2009 and has been working as part of the palliative care team, providing both practical and social support for children, parents, and siblings. The service has a funded management position responsible for recruitment, training, and coordination of volunteers. The volunteers range in age from 21 to over 70 and come from a wide socioeconomic demographic and diverse cultural and ethnic backgrounds, widely reflecting the community they support.

Case study: volunteering and practical support

An 8-year-old girl with neurological disease was receiving palliative care. Both parents and a 13-year-old brother were living at home. The family were of Lebanese Australian background. Their oldest child died aged 2 of the same condition. Some extended family was available locally for support but the mother identified the length of her daughter's illness as a reason to not 'impose' on help offered. Due to the mother's caring responsibilities, the family were her main social contact. A 22-year-old female volunteer from an Australian/Asian background was placed with the family, initially to play with the unwell daughter and offer light practical help. As placement progressed, routines formed and as the home tasks were completed the mother, volunteer, and daughter started taking walks in their local area and visiting cafes. The mother commented, 'I really look forward to Fridays now, we get everything done and get out of the house. I wasn't able to do that previously.'

Case study: volunteering offering personal support and reducing impact on friendships

A single parent was caring for a 16-year-old boy profoundly disabled since birth, and a 15-year-old daughter. The family were supported by community organizations for respite care at home. A 55-year-old female volunteer was placed with family, initially to offer light practical support around the home and transport for the sibling to a local job after school. The placement lasted over 2 years with 6 months as a bereavement placement. The mother identified a valued difference in the support provided within the volunteer role which did not have the demands of reciprocity expected in friendship or the impersonality of paid service providers.

In current times of global migration, families may find themselves without family and community support, in a different country from their birth. These families face the added complexity of navigating health systems in second languages and in an alien culture, without wider family to provide support. Effective development of a volunteer programme could encompass education for palliative care volunteers, to provide tutoring in the local language and culture to support families in communicating with health and community services or to collaborate with other volunteer services which provide a home tutoring service.

Symptom management in children with advanced illness

Children with advanced illness are often highly symptomatic and their symptom burden may increase with time, especially when the terminal phase is reached (Drake et al., 2003). This symptom burden consists of physical, psychological, spiritual, and other factors and this entire matrix needs to be considered. Physical symptoms may be caused either by the underlying illness, side effects related to medical interventions and treatment, or causes unrelated to either the primary disease or its treatment. The assessment and diagnosis of symptoms is fundamental to the clinical care of the child with advanced illness. Palliative therapeutics generally should only be implemented once the underlying causative mechanisms have been established, since therapies directed at the primary cause may ultimately have a more effective outcome for symptom management. Clinical assessment of symptoms is complemented by symptom measurement. Measurement refers to the application of a metric to a specific dimension of symptom experience. The measurement of symptoms in children often utilizes formal scales that assess symptom intensity or frequency.

Symptoms, symptom burden, and quality of life in children

It is frequently assumed that a child's quality of life is directly related to their degree of symptom burden. This is not necessarily true as quality of life is a complex, multifactorial, and dynamic process. This complexity is compounded in paediatrics by quality of life (QOL) measurement. QOL measures frequently assess functional status rather than involve a comprehensive evaluation of the health-related quality of the child's physical, emotional, and social domains of life. Even with measures tailored appropriately to the child's capacity, a variety of barriers to the inclusion of QOL end points in clinical trials have been identified (Bradlyn et al., 1995). Attitudinal bias against self-reported health questionnaire data, lack of validated measures, and the absence of a QOL 'gold standard' are some of the difficulties faced when incorporating these measures into clinical research and practice (Bradlyn et al., 1995).

Symptom measurement and symptom management studies in children with life-threatening illness

The progress in symptom control for adults receiving palliative care does not have a parallel experience in children. This is due, in part, to the paucity of symptom control research in children and explains the reliance of best practice in paediatric palliative care on the best evidence in adult palliative care. In addition, most of the validated symptom assessment tools in paediatrics have focused on three common symptoms, pain, nausea (Zeltzer et al., 1983, 1984a, 1984; LeBaron and Zeltzer, 1984), and fatigue (Hockenberry-Eaton et al., 1998; Hockenberry et al., 2003). In contrast to instruments measuring nausea and vomiting, instruments measuring pain in children largely have been validated predominantly in the non-cancer setting. Systematic symptom assessment may be useful in assessing symptom burden as part of decision-making towards palliative care and in future epidemiological studies of symptoms in dying children.

One major difficulty in performing symptom management studies in dying children pertains to the heterogeneous nature of symptoms in this population. Children with cancer, for example, tend to receive therapies directed at control of their tumours until very late in the course of their illnesses and are frequently very ill and highly symptomatic. These epidemiological and treatment variables make it less likely that a subpopulation of children receiving palliative care exists who have a stable, chronic pattern of symptoms amenable to evaluation in a trial.

Multidimensional symptom assessment tools for children

The Memorial Symptom Assessment Scale (MSAS) 10–18 is a 30-item patient-rated instrument adapted from a previously validated adult version to provide multidimensional information about the symptoms experienced by children with cancer aged 10–18 (Collins et al., 2000). The analyses supported the reliability and validity of the MSAS 10–18 subscale scores as measures of physical, psychological, and global symptom distress, respectively.

A revised MSAS was created as an instrument for the assessment of symptoms in children with cancer aged 7–12 years (Collins et al., 2002). Validity was evaluated by comparison with the medical record, parental report, and concurrent assessment on visual analogue scales for selected symptoms. The data provide evidence of the reliability and validity of MSAS (7–12) and demonstrated that children with cancer as young as 7 years can report clinically relevant and consistent information about their symptom experience. The instrument appeared to be age appropriate and may be helpful to older children unable to independently complete MSAS 10–18.

Symptom management in children with advanced illness

The adequate, proficient, and timely management of symptoms in the dying child is of critical importance. Not only is it important from a humanitarian viewpoint, but also it is apparent that the memory of unrelieved symptoms in dying children may be retained by parents many years after their child has died (Wolfe et al., 2000). It will be impossible for children and their families to negotiate the domains of psychological and spiritual care if physical symptomatology has not been treated adequately. As few controlled studies of symptom management have been performed in childhood, many of the therapies used in children have been devised utilizing best practice for adults. The reader is referred to the adult section of this volume for the principles of management of unusual symptoms. An emphasis has been given in this chapter to the palliative care emergencies of childhood. Less urgent symptoms are discussed in alphabetical order in 'The palliation of other symptoms in childhood advanced illness'. Pain management for children is discussed in Chapter 9.13.

The palliative care emergencies of childhood

Seizure control

Seizures in paediatric palliative care patients may be either recent in onset or part of a long-standing, underlying seizure disorder. In the former situation, the onset will usually be frightening to patients and families and may be due to many possible causes (e.g. cerebral metastases, infection, metabolic disorder, hypoxia, etc.) which must be excluded, as treatment directed at the primary causes may be appropriate whilst anticonvulsant therapy is implemented. Worsening seizure control in a patient with an underlying seizure disorder may indicate either disease progression or factors related to anticonvulsant dose, class, or administration which should be reviewed.

Buccal midazolam has been shown to be at least as effective as rectal diazepam in the acute treatment of seizures (Scott et al., 2002). Administration via the mouth is more socially acceptable and convenient and may become the preferred treatment for long seizures that occur outside hospital. The buccal dose is the same as the oral dose of midazolam used for sedation (0.3 mg/kg per dose, maximum dose 15 mg) and should be used as a single dose only. Traditionally, refractory status epilepticus is treated with barbiturate-induced coma or general anaesthetics, both of which require invasive cardiorespiratory and haemodynamic monitoring and are associated with significant complications. Midazolam has been effective in terminating seizures refractory to diazepam, lorazepam, phenytoin, and phenobarbitone in paediatric patients (Scott et al., 2002).

Spinal cord compression

Spinal cord compression is an unusual complication of childhood cancer and occurs most often late in a child's illness. Back pain, more often than abnormal neurologic signs or symptoms, is the usual initial presenting sign of spinal cord compression in children (Lewis et al., 1986). Spinal cord compression is an emergency, since adult data show that if treated whilst a patient is ambulatory, the probability of retaining ambulant status is 89–94% (Loblaw and Laperriere, 1998). The mainstays of management are radiological diagnosis and treatment with radiotherapy for radio-sensitive tumour and corticosteroids (Abrahm, 1999).

Bleeding

Although the fear of external bleeding is paramount in the minds of families and caregivers of children dying of either haematological malignancy or liver failure, massive external bleeding as a mode of death in childhood is uncommon. While some children with malignancy receive blood products indefinitely, this is not always feasible or appropriate. Many families negotiate the use of blood products only if minor bleeding or anaemia becomes problematic. If the fear of external bleeding is overwhelming for families, this may influence their choice of location of the child's death and attitude towards blood product transfusion.

Terminal dyspnoea

Dyspnoea is an uncomfortable awareness of breathing (Bruera et al., 1993b). In the terminal phase it is often highly distressing to patients and for families to watch. Terminal dyspnoea may be due to a variety, and perhaps combination, of causes. These include pulmonary metastases, intrinsic lung disease or infection, cardiac failure, acidosis, muscle weakness, and so on. Diagnosis is important as this may influence choice of therapies. Non-invasive ventilation may be a viable choice for symptom management of dyspnoea related to muscle weakness, for example, and bronchospasm could be reversed easily with bronchodilators.

Most of the data on the management of terminal dyspnoea are from studies of adults with terminal malignancy. There are no data on the appropriate management of dyspnoea related to muscle weakness or complications of cystic fibrosis, for example. The goal of palliative therapies for terminal dyspnoea is to improve the patient's subjective sensation. The subjective sensation of dyspnoea is improved in patients receiving supplemental oxygen (Bruera et al., 1993a). In addition, systemic opioid therapy (Bruera et al., 1993b; Boyd and Kelly, 1997), cognitive behavioural strategies (Corner et al., 1996), and non-pharmacological strategies, such as using a handheld fan (Galbraith et al., 2010) benefit patients with dyspnoea related to terminal malignancy. As anxiety is often a component of terminal dyspnoea, judicious prescription of a benzodiazepine may be warranted.

Secretions

The management of noisy secretions in an unconscious patient is aimed at reducing the distress of the family, other patients, and staff. The sound of noisy secretions can be haunting to all concerned and should be given some priority by the attending clinician. Accepted management strategies include explanation to relatives, positioning, suction, and anticholinergics (e.g. hyoscine hydrobromide or glycopyrrolate) (Hughes et al., 1996).

Terminal delirium

Delirium during the final phase of dying is one of the most distressing symptoms for caregivers to watch, especially if the delirium is agitated. The interpretation of the latter may be that the delirium is a manifestation of an internal existential angst. This latter interpretation is unlikely, since the aetiology of delirium in the setting of an actively dying patient is usually multifactorial with a physical rather than psychological basis (e.g. hypoxia, metabolic derangement, central nervous system disease, infection, fever, etc.). Simple causes that can be corrected, hypoxia, for example, should be excluded. As terminal delirium cannot be predicted, a therapeutic plan for its management should be considered in every dying child. The usual therapies consist of haloperidol for delirium per se with consideration of adding a benzodiazepine if there is agitation as well.

The palliation of other symptoms in childhood advanced illness

Constipation

The aetiology of constipation is often multifactorial and may include reduced physical activity, mechanical obstruction, metabolic derangement, poor diet and low fluid intake, bowel atony due to opioids, and so on. Although unusual, bowel obstruction and faecal impaction must be excluded and treated urgently in any child presenting with constipation. Generally, dietary changes are recommended in the first instance (increased vegetables and fruity, bulk, prune juice, etc.). In addition, attention should be given to hydration, mobility, and other activities of daily living. Chronic opioid therapy necessitates the prescription of a regular laxative. There is little evidence to guide the prescription of laxatives in children. Whilst there are emerging adult data to suggest oral naloxone (Culpepper-Morgan et al., 1992) and subcutaneous methylnaltrexone (Portenoy et al., 2008; Thomas et al., 2008) may be appropriate for the management of opioid-induced constipation, a senna and lactulose combination is often prescribed in the adult population (Abu-Saad and Courtens, 2001). It is not clear if a senna/lactulose combination is appropriate for children. The osmotic laxative, Movicol-Half® is being used increasingly to treat constipation in children. There are, however, few data on its use in children.

Fatigue

Fatigue is a common symptom of children with cancer (Hockenberry-Eaton et al., 1998; Collins et al., 2000, 2002) and one that is often highly distressing. The aetiology of fatigue in children dying of cancer may be due to a combination of factors including anaemia, poor nutrition, insomnia, metabolic derangement, the increased effort of breathing in patients with dyspnoea, side effects of medication, and psychological factors. In the assessment of fatigue in a child, and the matrix of its potential causes, it is important to establish if this symptom is distressing to the child and/or their family. If so, the potential remediable causes should be considered. There are adult and limited paediatric data on the use of stimulant medication for the treatment of opioid-induced somnolence (Bruera et al., 1992a, 1992b; Yee and Berde, 1994). In children, it has become more common practice to switch opioids, for somnolence as a dose-limiting side effect of opioid therapy (Drake et al., 2004).

Insomnia

Sleep disturbance is common in children with advanced illness (Collins et al., 2000, 2002; Herbert et al., 2014). In the context of cancer, insomnia is both prevalent and distressing to children and, by inference, distressing to caregivers. The aetiology of insomnia is multifactorial and is often a combination of physical, psychological, and perhaps environmental factors. When depression is a factor, consideration should be given to psychotherapy and pharmacologic treatment. Fatigue often coexists with sleep disturbance. Lifestyle changes, including improved sleep hygiene, exposure to sunlight, and exercise may be helpful to improved sleep. Low-dose amitriptyline, if not contra-indicted, is often a helpful pharmacologic agent for the management of insomnia in terminally ill children, particularly if pain is a symptom management issue. An alternative consideration could be melatonin.

Mouth care and hydration

Routine mouth care promotes patient comfort and ability to eat and drink, prevents halitosis, and helps identify problems such as dry mouth, candidiasis, and ulceration (WHO, 1998b). Lip emollients and mouthwashes are important therapies for mouth care. The sensation of a dry mouth may be due to local (e.g. mouth breathing, candidiasis, radiotherapy to salivary glands, etc.) and systemic causes (e.g. dehydration, anticholinergic drugs uraemia, etc.) and is often distressing. The issue of hydration in dying patients is a contentious issue. Small but frequent volumes of fluid to maintain insensible losses may be appropriate via the oral route. However, this may be impossible in some instances unless other routes of administration are considered. As with all therapies, the benefits and deficits of any intervention must be discussed with the patient and family before any therapeutic intervention is implemented.

Nausea and vomiting

Nausea and vomiting are not uncommon in children receiving palliative care. Nausea and vomiting occur when the vomiting centre in the brain is activated by any of the following: cerebral cortex (e.g. anxiety), vestibular apparatus, chemoreceptor trigger zone (CTZ), vagus nerve, or by direct action on the vomiting centre. A clear diagnosis must be sought as to aetiology as the list of potential causes is great and therapies different, depending on the putative mechanism (WHO, 1998b).

Psychosocial issues in caring for a child with advanced illness

The emotional, psychological, and physical stress of caring for a child with a life-limiting illness impacts on the whole family unit. Issues such as social isolation and the impact of emotional and physical absence on relationships within the family can lead to high conflict and low support situations for parents and siblings (Mastroyannopolou et al., 1997). *The Hardest Thing We Have Ever Done* (Palliative Care Australia, 2004) is a social impact study of caring for terminally ill people in Australia and identifies that families with poor social support are at risk of experiencing coping and psychological distress. McGrath (2001a, 2001b) identifies the need of practical support by parents in the initial stages of a child's treatment, followed by emotional support to be able to cope with the challenges of caring for a palliative child.

The death of a child is uncommon in many societies. As a consequence, members of the community may be apprehensive and unsure of the approach to the child and family. In addition, staff working with dying children may be unaccustomed to providing palliative care and may be in a setting where specialist paediatric palliative care is unavailable. The death of a child challenges beliefs and assumptions about the world. Rosov (1994) suggests these include that parents will die before their children, that parents can protect their children from harm, and the sense of confidence, safety, and security as a parent. Psychosocial care can be defined as holistic care provided to address physical, social, psychological, and spiritual needs of children and their families (Davies et al., 2002). The following case studies illustrate some of the common psychosocial issues faced by children receiving palliative care and their families.

Case study: the impact on the family unit

Richard is an 8-year-old boy with a life-limiting congenital cardiac condition. He was referred to palliative care 8 months ago. Richard is one of two children of Paula and Adam.

Throughout his life, Richard has experienced many painful procedures, tests, and treatments. He was considered for heart transplant, and spent over a year living interstate with his parents in order to trial treatments. Richard's parents have coped with his illness by focusing on it to the detriment of other family relationships.

Upon Richard's referral to palliative care, his parents were told that he had 'weeks to months' to live. Paula and Adam spent time ensuring that Richard and his brother John were told about Richard's prognosis and had several broad discussions about death.

The family were able to use their faith as a guide to explain death and what happens when people die. It was important to Richard, who was aged 7 at the time of referral, and his family, to be baptised as soon as he turned 8. Richard's family believed that anyone who died aged younger than 8 would automatically go to Heaven because they were pure. Anyone aged 8 or older would need to be baptised. Given that Richard's health was up and down, it was unknown whether he would make it to his 8th birthday party, or to his baptism, which was scheduled for the following day.

He did, in fact, live to experience both his birthday and baptism, and continues to live with his family, almost a year after he was given weeks to months to live. Whilst he is still unlikely to live to adulthood, and there is still a risk that he will die suddenly at any moment, his parents have made him the focus of their lives. His sibling receives sporadic attention from their parents, and very little one-on-one time with them.

His brother, John, has begun to disassociate from his parents, preferring to spend time on his own. He does not argue or talk back the way other children his age would when refused something, such as a small snack or time on the computer. At school his confidence has dropped dramatically, and he is now fearful of activities that he cannot master. He is often cared for by his grandparents.

Whilst his parents are aware of the stress placed on the sibling, they do not allow themselves to be taken away from Richard and his needs. The family successfully engaged several celebrities to fulfil wishes, such as trips, toys, and visits to their home, and this appeared to be a primary focus for them.

The family unit is an invaluable resource in palliative care, in particular when the dying person is a child. The family unit is looked to for its ability to provide care, thus involving them intimately in the dying process (Kissane, 2000). Richard's parents have taken on much of his care at home; thereby isolating themselves from many respite services, and have also relied upon the extended family to fill in any gaps in care for the siblings.

In Richard's case, the assessment conducted indicated that religious rituals, such as his baptism, were important to him, as well as to his parents and grandparents. Richard also has taken an interest in his funeral, such as who will attend, who will give eulogies, and the kind of music that will be played. Whilst many adults may find this morbid and threatening, it is vital that dying children are given the emotional space to make their wishes known (Davies et al., 2002). A spiritual assessment conducted with the dying child is one method of beginning this discussion.

Kissane (2000) discusses the challenge in palliative care of balancing anticipatory grief and living life to the fullest. Richard and his entire family were caught in this very dilemma. His parents were trying to make the most of his life, given the unpredictability of his death, whilst his sibling coped with little time and attention from their parents. Additionally, his grandparents, who were reducing working hours and looking to retirement, took on the responsibility of caring for John and occasionally Richard. The involvement of grandparents as carers is growing, particularly as they often have more flexibility than working parents and are most often unpaid for the care they provide (Jenkins, 2012). Thus the changes to everyday life and the expectations placed on grandparents when a child is dying cannot be overestimated. Most of the palliative care—physical, emotional, spiritual, and psychological—was provided to Richard and his family in their home.

The parents' role as caregivers is usually redefined when their children become ill. Parents perceive themselves as 'decision-makers, nurturers, protectors, advocates, and caregivers' for their children (Bluebond-Langner et al., 2010). That said, adolescents involved in end-of-life decisions have been reported to understand the consequences of their decision and are also capable of participating in these complex decision processes (Hinds et al., 2005). In paediatric palliative care, psychosocial distress in a child or family is usually linked to illness-related factors. Appropriate interventions are often designed in response to these factors.

At times, good psychosocial care permits the child or family to not speak about issues with health professionals. The case of Chris, an 18-year-old boy with osteosarcoma, illustrates this. In keeping with family values and their cultural beliefs the family never discussed his impending death with him, despite giving him total control over his own symptom management including talking with palliative care services about his management. Discussions with his family were about updating them, addressing their own fears and questions, but never care planning. Three days before he died, Chris called a relative and gave them a detailed shopping list, including store names and specific gifts to buy for each of his family members. As the eldest child, he also called each of his two younger siblings to his bedside and gave them 'instructions about their future lives'. The value of the psychosocial support to this young teenager was to make time, to accept that he knew what was happening to him, and offer bereavement support in a request that we 'take care of his mum'.

Psychosocial issues are as diverse and individual as the families receiving care. The health professional who listens, who seeks to communicate openly with families by spending time just being 'present' with the family will increase awareness and understanding of the needs of the child and family. Integration of psychosocial care into paediatric palliative care includes establishing communication with the multidisciplinary team caring for the patient and a careful patient assessment. This includes assessing the family's ability to cope, their social and financial status, and linkage to appropriate social, community, and spiritual support (McSherry et al., 2007).

The clinician in bereavement support

The role of the clinician supporting a bereaved family can be multifaceted. As Bowlby (1961) indicated, the quality of the attachment to the deceased forms the basis of the grief reaction. The clinician will need to assess the quality of the relationship between the child, siblings, and parents. Additionally, it is beneficial to assess the attachment style of each member in the family to understand how they will grieve, and the most effective interventions for that particular attachment style (Bowlby, 1961).

Grieving rules describe the norms that are recognized in society as acceptable grief responses and they specify when, where, how long, and for whom people should grieve (Brabant, 2001). The clinician can ascertain some of the grieving rules that govern the bereaved person by inquiring what they think about grieving, and what they think others think about grieving (Brabant, 2001). This enables the clinician to address any grieving rules which may hamper the ability to manage grief.

Despite the acute pain associated with grief, the long-term impact of bereavement on siblings can be both positive and negative. As Oltjenbruns (2001) discusses, siblings who were not told about the serious nature of their brother's or sister's illness, may experience a number of difficulties. These can include an increased sense of isolation, a belief that others, such as parents, have minimized the significance of their loss, a diminished trust of those around them, and a misconception of what actually happened. With support from clinicians, bereaved siblings and parents should be able to work through these issues.

However, the impact of the death of a brother or sister is not always negative. Schaefer and Moos state that crises can be a catalyst for personal growth and that people can emerge from crises with enhanced social and personal resources, and new coping skills (Schaefer and Moos, 2001). The outcome of personal growth does not diminish the pain and devastation of the loss; however, once the individual has moved from the acute pain of grief, the search for meaning can lead to growth (Schaefer and Moos, 2001). In particular, children who experience bereavement are more likely to be less judgemental, more compassionate and tolerant, have a desire to help others who are grieving, and prioritize their family (Schaefer and Moos, 2001).

Considerations in bereavement work with families

The death of a child has been described as a 'loss like no other' (Rosov, 1994). Raphael (1983) describes that this is because the death of a child defies the natural order of life and societal expectations. A child represents the hopes and dreams for the future of his or her parents, grandparents, and extended family. The death of that child extinguishes those hopes and dreams and leaves the family with a devastating loss that can linger for years after death. Following the death of a child, the role of the counsellor is to support families to rebuild their lives whilst keeping the memory of their child alive.

Hope is a key element in bereavement work (Cutcliffe, 2004). The bereavement trajectory often reflects parents' lack of hope, the pursuit of hope, and the eventual regaining of hope. Hope represents a link to the future, and for many families, their children are representative of the hope they have for themselves and their family's future (Raphael, 1983). The following case history is illustrative:

Case history: the impact of past trauma

Rachel's family moved to Australia as refugees, after experiencing years of torture and persecution in their home country. They described moving to Australia as having a fresh start, and being an opportunity for their eight children to receive an education that would not have been possible in their home country. Their older children enrolled in practical courses which enabled them to work to contribute to the family's income. The family worked hard to establish themselves in Australia, facing the common struggles of refugee families—finding and maintaining work and accommodation, and adjusting to a new country, language, and culture. The children also faced the struggle of fitting in at school, making new friends, and integrating into a new education system.

Two years after moving to Australia, the second youngest child, Rachel, was diagnosed with a brain tumour. She received numerous trial treatments, before being referred to palliative care. Three months later, she died in hospital. Rachel's siblings were not told of her initial diagnosis, or of her poor prognosis. The parents explained that they did not want the children to worry, or to lose focus from their school work.

Rachel's sister, Mariam (17), was referred for bereavement counselling 6 months after Rachel's death. She explained that Rachel's death was a complete shock to her, and that she did not know that Rachel was so unwell. Mariam was in her final year at high school, and had her end of school exams approaching in 3 months. Prior to Rachel's death, Mariam was a bright student who was at the top of her class. Since Rachel's death, Mariam described being unable to concentrate on school work, that thoughts of Rachel intruded on her when she tried to study, and that she did not retain any information she read. Mariam was very worried that she would not receive the marks she needs to study at university.

Reflection on the case history

The move to Australia represented hope for Rachael's family. It was an opportunity to escape the persecution experienced in their home country and engendered hope for the parents that their children would receive a good education and be able to go on to develop worthwhile careers. However, Rachel's death has had an impact on all the members of her family. Not only were her parents mourning and less available to their children due to their own grief, but her sister Mariam's education was directly impacted upon. For Mariam, the impact of Rachel's death will linger for years, particularly as her final years of schooling were affected. This could have potential implications for further study or career path she had planned to pursue.

An important consideration in working with bereaved families is the impact of past trauma. It is not uncommon for children and adolescents who have experienced trauma to re-experience these symptoms following a secondary traumatic event (Cook et al., 2005). Given their past history of trauma, Rachel's parents and siblings were offered bereavement support in order to reduce the risk of complications during the grieving process.

The death of Rachel had a dual effect on her parents. Not only did they grieve the loss of their daughter but also one of the specific reasons that compelled them to leave their home country—securing a positive future for the children—was under threat as a result of their grief. Mariam's experience of grief not only left her unable to achieve her own goals but also the hopes and dreams of her parents for their children. Her parents were left questioning whether they made the right decision to leave their home country, now being bereaved in a country where they had limited social support.

Quality improvement and paediatric palliative care

Batalden and Davidoff (2007) define quality improvement as 'the combined and unceasing efforts of everyone—healthcare professionals, patients and their families, researchers, payers, planners and educators—to make the changes that will lead to better patient outcomes (health), better system performance (care) and better professional development (learning)'. These 'efforts' consist of processes to gather data about service provision, reviewing this information, identifying opportunities for improvement, trialling activities to improve the services, and re-evaluating the service.

All stakeholders receiving and delivering clinical care are interested in the quality and safety of care. Consumers wish to know that the services they are receiving care of a high standard. Clinicians wish to know that the services they provide are meeting defined standards. In addition, if clinicians aspire to attain standards of excellence in the services they deliver, a quality programme will be able to identify areas for improved performance in the quest for such a goal. Administrators and policymakers also have a vested interest in the quality and the outcomes of clinical services. At a governmental level, policymakers must ensure that health-care resources are being used well, that standards are being attained, and problematic clinical services identified quickly.

As paediatric palliative care has only become a specialty in its own right over the past 10–15 years and has been mainly focused on service development, it has had little opportunity to participate in quality improvement programmes. It is timely that quality improvement programmes are introduced into paediatric palliative care services as the status quo is never good enough and an honest appraisal of the quality of a clinical service will lead to improvement in the quest for excellence

The process of setting up a quality improvement programme in paediatric palliative care has been described previously (Collins et al., 2009) and is summarized in Box 16.2.3.

1. Identify a quality lead to create and implement a quality strategic plan

The appointment of a quality lead without a clinical load is important, given the specialized nature of the area, the lack of training in quality improvement included in clinical education, the lack of time on the part of the existing clinical personnel, and the need for a neutral person to be dealing with the sensitive areas of feedback and complaints should they arise.

Box 16.2.3 How to set up a quality improvement programme in paediatric palliative care

1. Identify a quality lead to create and implement a quality strategic plan
2. Identify defined standards and measure the clinical service against the standards
3. Develop measures of quality for palliative care
4. Collate and evaluate data from the quality programme and look for opportunities for improvement
5. Implement ongoing quality review as part of clinical care.

Source: Data from John J. Collins et al., Quality Improvement and Evolving Research in Pediatric Pain Management and Palliative Care, in José Castro-Lopes (Ed.), *Current Topics in Pain*, IASP Press, Seattle, Washington, USA, Copyright © 2009.

---

2. Identify defined standards and measure the clinical service against the standards

The document 'IMPaCCT: Standards for Paediatric Palliative Care in Europe' (Craig et al., 2008) outlines core standards for palliative care provision for children and their ethical and legal rights. In Australia, the *Standards for Providing Quality Palliative Care for All Australians* (Palliative Care Australia, 2005) guide care. This latter document influences the way care is delivered and planned. It moves away from the simplistic diagnostic basis for determining need, and focuses on establishing networks that allow patients to access the right care when needed. Palliative Care Australia developed a self-assessment review programme for services to use as a quality improvement tool—the National Self-Assessment Program (NSAP)—Paediatric (Palliative Care Australia, 2012). This enables paediatric services to review their clinical service against the standards to identify opportunities for improvement.

3. Develop measures of quality for palliative care

Consumer satisfaction as a measure of the quality of paediatric palliative care

There is controversy in the literature as to the meaning and value of consumer satisfaction surveys. The controversies relate to few alternatives to satisfaction being available, no widely held definition of satisfaction exists, methodological inconsistencies across studies (Aspinal et al., 2003), and a vulnerable population which may not feel free to express negative comments. It is essential that families are assured of the anonymity of survey responses, that the data are collated by a staff member who does not provide care to the survey population, and they are given contact details of a person outside of the department for support. Solely relying on consumer satisfaction surveys to determine clinical and policy change in paediatric palliative care may not be appropriate.

Measuring quality by identifying or creating outcome measures

Part of quality measurement involves the use of outcome measures. These may include clinical indicators (measures of clinical outcomes), process indicators (measures of clinical processes), and qualitative reflective review. Outcome measures are designed to identify the rate of occurrence (or non-occurrence) of an event which in turn reflects the care that was provided, or not. Data aggregated from all patients receiving the service can highlight areas that need improving, and can be used to measure the service against particular standards.

Process indicators for paediatric palliative care have been developed and implemented as a measure of care delivery for services in Australia and New Zealand. These indicators are linked closely to, and have been mapped against, the Australian Standards and are used in service evaluation. The indicators developed for use in Australia and New Zealand includes the following as key indicators of best care and are used to evaluate services:

◆ Equity of service provision (access to services, including respite care)

◆ Facilitating the right location of care (ensuring families have options for treatment at home)

◆ Child- and family-focused service delivery (including the family in decision-making)

◆ Access to the right place at the right time for end-of-life care

◆ Care planning and symptom management

◆ Family education and social support

◆ Holistic care

◆ Bereavement services.

4. Collate and evaluate data from the quality programme and look for opportunities for improvement

Data collection and collation should be an easy process with clear templates to collect the data and simple electronic or paper databases to collate it. Data can be compared with similar clinical services collecting the same indicators thus allowing benchmarking and peer review. Once an opportunity for improvement has been identified, work must begin to identify how the service can be improved.

5. Implement ongoing quality review as part of clinical care

A quality improvement programme needs to be designed in such a way as to be sustainable in the long term. This means the programme needs:

◆ input from all staff during development to share ownership of the programme

◆ a data collection system that is easy and not time-consuming

◆ timely distribution of results to maximize usefulness of data and support from clinical staff for ongoing collection

◆ to be dynamic, and change with changes in the delivery of care

◆ education for all clinical staff.

Some planning, including realistic time-frames and achievable goals, is necessary for a sustainable programme. Over time, the process becomes imbedded and normalized as part of the department's work. The available information can also be used showcase the department, particularly for external review or accreditation processes.

Conclusion

The care of the child with advanced and progressive illness and their family requires a holistic approach to the often complex physical, social, psychological, and spiritual needs including bereavement. This inevitably requires a paediatric palliative care team with diverse skills and abilities to meet these needs. Whilst the WHO supports the global application of the principles of palliative care to every child with a life-limiting illness, irrespective of geographical location (WHO, 1998a), the development of services for children will be contingent on the application of more resources.

Acknowledgement

Joan Marston, Chief Executive, International Children's Palliative Care Network kindly reviewed the section on 'Paediatric palliative care: a global perspective'. Her contribution is gratefully acknowledged.

References

Abrahm, J.L. (1999). Management of pain and spinal cord compression in patients with advanced cancer. *Annals of Internal Medicine*, 131, 37–46.

Abu-Saad, H.H. and Courtens, A. (2001). Pain and symptom management. In H.H. Abu-Saad, and A. Courtens (eds.) *Evidence-Based Palliative Care: Across the Lifespan*, pp. 63–87. Oxford: Blackwell Science.

Amery, J. (2009). *Children's Palliative Care in Africa*. Oxford: Oxford University Press.

Aranda, S. and O'Connor, M. (eds.) (2003). *Palliative Care Nursing: A Guide to Practice*. Melbourne: Ausmed Publications.

Aspinal, F., Addington-Hall, J., Hughes, R., and Higginson, I.J. (2003). Using satisfaction to measure the quality of palliative care: a review of the literature. *Journal of Advanced Nursing*, 42, 324–339.

Baker, J.N., Hinds, P.S., Spunt, S.L., *et al.* (2008). Integration of palliative care practices into the ongoing care of children with cancer: individualized care planning and coordination. *Pediatric Clinics of North America*, 55, 223–250, xii.

Batalden, P.B. and Davidoff, F. (2007). What is 'quality improvement' and how can it transform healthcare? *Quality & Safety in Health Care*, 16, 2–3.

Bluebond-Langner, M., Belasco, J. B., and Demesquita Wander, M. (2010). 'I want to live, until I don't want to live anymore': involving children with life-threatening and life-shortening illnesses in decision making about care and treatment. *Nursing Clinics of North America*, 45, 329–343.

Bowlby, J. (1961). Processes of mourning. *International Journal of Psychoanalysis*, 42, 317–340.

Boyd, K.J. and Kelly, M. (1997). Oral morphine as symptomatic treatment of dyspnoea in patients with advanced cancer. *Palliative Medicine*, 11, 277–281.

Brabant, S. (2001). A closer look at Doka's grieving rules. In K.J. Doka (ed.) *Disenfranchised Grief: New Directions, Challenges and Strategic Practice*, pp. 23–38. Champaign, IL: Research Press.

Bradlyn, A. S., Harris, C. V., and Speith, L. E. (1995). Quality of life assessment in pediatric oncology: a retrospective review of Phase III reports *Social Science & Medicine*, 41, 1463–1465.

Bruera, E., De Stoutz, N., Velasco-Leiva, A., *et al.* (1993a). Effects of oxygen on dyspnea in hypoxemic terminal cancer patients. *The Lancet*, 342, 13–14.

Bruera, E., Faisinger, R., Maceachern, T., and Hanson, J. (1992a). The use of methylphenidate in patients with incident pain receiving regular opiates: a preliminary report. *Pain*, 50, 75–77.

Bruera, E., Maceachern, T., Ripamonti, C., and Hanson, J. (1993b). Subcutaneous morphine for dyspnea in cancer patients. *Annals of Internal Medicine*, 119, 906–907.

Bruera, E., Miller, M. J., Macmillan, K., and Kuehn, N. (1992b). Neuropsychological effects of methylphenidate in patients receiving a continuous infusion of narcotics for cancer pain. *Pain*, 48, 163–166.

Callaway, M., Foley, K. M., De Lima, L., *et al.* (2007). Funding for palliative care programs in developing countries. *Journal of Pain and Symptom Management*, 33, 509–513.

Collins, J.J., Byrnes, M.E., Dunkel, I.J., *et al.* (2000). The measurement of symptoms in children with cancer. *Journal of Pain and Symptom Management*, 19, 363–377.

Collins, J.J., Devine, T.D., Dick, G.S., *et al.* (2002). The measurement of symptoms in young children with cancer: the validation of the Memorial Symptom Assessment Scale in children aged 7–12. *Journal of Pain and Symptom Management*, 23, 10–16.

Collins, J.J., Walker, S.M., and Campbell, K. (2009). Quality improvement and evolving research in paediatric pain management and palliative care. In J. Castro-Lopes (ed.) *Current Topics in Pain*, pp. 289–310. Seattle: IASP Press.

Cook, A., Spinazzola, J., Ford, J., *et al.* (2005). Complex trauma in children and adolescents. *Psychiatric Annals*, 35, 390–398.

Corner, J., Planth, H., Hern, R., and Bailey, C. (1996). Non-pharmacological interventions for breathlessness in lung cancer. *Palliative Medicine*, 10, 299–305.

Craig, F., Abu-Saad Huijer, H., Benini, F., *et al.* (2008). [IMPaCCT: Standards of Paediatric Palliative Care in Europe]. *Schmerz*, 22, 401–408.

Crawford, G.B. and Price, S.D. (2003). Team working: palliative care as a model of interdisciplinary practice. *Medical Journal of Australia*, 179, S32–34.

Culpepper-Morgan, J.A., Adelhardt, J., Foley, K.M., and Portenoy, R.K. (1992). Treatment of opioid-induced constipation with oral naloxone: a pilot study. *Clinical Pharmacological Therapy*, 52, 90–95.

Cutcliffe, J.R. (2004). The inspiration of hope in bereavement counseling. *Issues in Mental Health Nursing*, 25, 165–190.

Davies, B., Brenner, P., Orloff, S., Sumner, L., and Worden, W. (2002). Addressing spirituality in pediatric hospice and palliative care. *Journal of Palliative Care*, 18, 59–67.

Downing, J., Birtar, D., Chambers, L., Gelb, B., Drake, R., and Kiman, R. (2012). Children's palliative care: a global concern. *International Journal of Palliative Nursing*, 18, 109–114.

Downing, J., Powell, R.A., and Mwangi-Powell, F. (2010). Home-based palliative care in sub-Saharan Africa. *Home Healthcare Nurse*, 28, 298–307.

Drake, R., Frost, J., and Collins, J. J. (2003). The symptoms of dying children. *Journal of Pain and Symptom Management*, 26, 594–603.

Drake, R., Longworth, J., and Collins, J. J. (2004). Opioid rotation in children with cancer. *Journal of Palliative Medicine*, 7, 419–422.

ehospice (2012). *Launch of the South African Children's Palliative Care Network*. [Online] Available at: <http://www.ehospice.com/internationalchildrens/ArticleView/tabid/10670/ArticleId/853/language/en-GB/View.aspx>

Galbraith, S., Fagan, P., Perkins, P., Lynch, A., and Booth, S. (2010). Does the use of a handheld fan improve chronic dyspnea? A randomized, controlled, crossover trial. *Journal of Pain and Symptom Management*, 39, 831–838.

Germ, R., Marys Binelli, S., and Pose, M. (2012). Pediatric palliative care in Argentina. In C. Knapp, V. Madden, and S. Fowler-Kerry (eds.) *Pediatric Palliative Care: Global Perspectives*, pp. 405–416. London: Springer.

Hamzah, E. and Lan Kuan, G. (2012). Pediatric palliative care in Malaysia. In C. Knapp, V. Madden, and S. Fowler-Kerry (eds.) *Pediatric Palliative Care: Global Perspectives*, pp. 109–126. London: Springer.

Harding, R., Powell, R. A., Kiyange, F., Downing, J., and Mwangi-Powell, F. (2010). Provision of pain- and symptom-relieving drugs for HIV/AIDS in sub-Saharan Africa. *Journal of Pain and Symptom Management*, 40, 405–415.

Herbert, A.R., de Lima, J., Fitzgerald, D.A., Seton, C., Waters, K., and Collins J.J. (2014). An exploratory study of sleeping studies of children admitted to hospital. *Journal of Paediatrics and Child Health*, 50, 632–638.

Hinds, P.S., Drew, D., Oakes, L.L., *et al.* (2005). End-of-life care preferences of pediatric patients with cancer. *Journal of Clinical Oncology*, 23, 9146–9154.

Hockenberry-Eaton, M., Hinds, P. S., Alcosr, P., *et al.* (1998). Fatigue in children and adolescents with cancer. *Journal of Pediatric Oncology Nursing*, 15, 172–182.

Hockenberry, M. J., Hinds, P. S., Barrera, P., *et al.* (2003). Three instruments to assess fatigue in children with cancer: the child, parent and staff perspectives. *Journal of Pain & Symptom Management*, 25, 319–328.

Hughes, A. C., Wilcock, A., and Corcoran, R. (1996). Management of 'death rattle'. *The Lancet*, 12, 271–272.

Jenkins, B. (2012). *Grandparent Childcare in Australia: A Literature Review* [Online]. Available at: <http://www.uws.edu.au/data/assets/pdf_file/009/156339/Jenkins.pdf>.

Kissane, D.W. (2000). Death and the Australian family. In A. Kellehear (ed.) *Death and Dying in Australia*, pp. 52-67 Melbourne: Oxford University Press.

Knapp, C., Woodworth, L., Wright, M., *et al.* (2011). Pediatric palliative care provision around the world: a systematic review. *Pediatric Blood & Cancer*, 57, 361–368.

Lago, P. and Piva, J. (2012). Pediatric palliative care in Brazil. In C. Knapp, V. Madden, and S. Fowler-Kerry (eds.) *Pediatric Palliative Care: Global Perspectives*, pp. 417–430. London: Springer.

Lebaron, S. and Zeltzer, L. (1984). Behavioral intervention for reducing chemotherapy-related nausea and vomiting in adolescents with cancer. *Journal of Adolescent Health Care*, 5, 182.

Lewis, D.W., Packer, R.J., Raney, B., Rak, I.W., Belasco, J., and Lange, B. (1986). Incidence, presentation, and outcome of spinal cord disease in children with systemic cancer. *Pediatrics*, 78, 438–443.

Loblaw, D.A. and Laperriere, N.J. (1998). Emergency treatment of malignant extradural spinal cord compression: an evidence-based guideline. *Journal of Clinical Oncology*, 16, 1613–1624.

Marston, J.N., Nkosi, B., and Bothma, A. (2012). Pediatric palliative care in South Africa. In C. Knapp, V. Madden, and S. Fowler-Kerry (eds.) *Pediatric Palliative Care: Global Perspectives*, pp. 27–40. London: Springer.

Mastroyannopolou, K., Stallard, P., Lewis, M., and Lenton, S. (1997). The impact of childhood non-malignant life threatening illness on parents: gender differences and predictors of parental adjustment. *Journal of Child Psychology and Psychiatry*, 38, 823–829.

Mathews, L. and Suresh Kumar, K. (2012). Pediatric palliative care in India. In C. Knapp, V. Madden, and S. Fowler-Kerry (eds.) *Pediatric Palliative Care: Global Perspectives*, pp. 91–108. London: Springer.

McGrath, P. (2001a). Identifying support issues of parents of children with leukemia. *Cancer Practice*, 9, 198–205.

McGrath, P. (2001b). Trained volunteers for families coping with a child with a life-limiting condition. *Child and Family Social Work*, 6, 23–29.

McSherry, M., Kehoe, K., Carroll, J. M., Kang, T. I., and Rourke, M. T. (2007). Psychosocial and spiritual needs of children living with a life-limiting illness. *Pediatric Clinics of North America*, 54, 609–629, ix–x.

Mitchell, G. K., Tieman, J. J., and Shelby-James, T. M. (2008). Multidisciplinary care planning and teamwork in primary care. *Medical Journal of Australia*, 188, S61–64.

Okhuysen-Cawley, R., Garduno Espinosa, A., Paez Aguuirre, S., *et al.* (2012). Pediatric palliative care in Mexico. In C. Knapp, V. Madden, and S. Fowler-Kerry (eds.) *Pediatric Palliative Care: Global Perspectives*, pp. 345–358. London: Springer.

Oltjenbruns, K. (2001). *Handbook of Bereavement Research: Consequences, Coping and Care*. Washington, DC: American Psychological Association.

Pairojkul, S. (2012). Pediatric palliative care in Thailand. In C. Knapp, V. Madden, and S. Fowler-Kerry (eds.) *Pediatric Palliative Care: Global Perspectives*, pp. 185–207. London: Springer.

Palliative Care Australia (2004). *The Hardest Thing We Have Ever Done: The Social Impact of Caring for Terminally Ill People in Australia*. Deakin West: Palliative Care Australia. Available at: <http://www.palliativecare.org.au/portals/46/the%20hardest%20thing.pdf>.

Palliative Care Australia (2005). *Standards for Providing Quality Palliative Care for all Australians*. Deakin West: Palliative Care Australia. Available at: <http://www.palliativecare.org.au/portals/46/resources/StandardsPalliativeCare.pdf>.

Palliative Care Australia (2012). *National Standards Assessment Program*. [Online] Available at: <http://www.palliativecare.org.au/Ourwork/NationalStandardsAssessmentProgram.aspx>.

Pallium India (2012). *Supreme Court of India's Ultimatum Regarding Morphine*. [Online] Available at: <http://palliumindia.org/2012/08/supreme-court-of-indias-ultimatum-regarding-morphine-availability/>.

Portenoy, R.K., Thomas, J., Moehl Boatwright, M.L., *et al.* (2008). Subcutaneous methylnaltrexone for the treatment of opioid-induced constipation in patients with advanced illness: a double-blind, randomized, parallel group, dose-ranging study. *Journal of Pain and Symptom Management*, 35, 458–468.

Quesada-Tristán, L. and Masís-Quesada, D. (2012). Pediatric palliative care in Costa Rica. In C. Knapp, V. Madden, and S. Fowler-Kerry (eds.) *Pediatric Palliative Care: Global Perspectives*, pp. 323–344. London: Springer.

Raphael, B. (1983). *The Anatomy of Bereavement*. Lanham, MD: Rowman and Littlefield.

Rosov, B. (1994). *The Worst Loss: How Families Heal from the Death of a Child*. New York: Henry Holt and Company.

Schaefer, J.M. and Moos, R.H. (2001). *Bereavement Experiences and Personal Growth*. Washington, DC: American Psychological Association.

Scott, R.C., Besag, F.M., and Neville, B.G. (2002). Buccal midazolam and rectal diazepam for treatment of prolonged seizures in childhood and adolescence: a randomised trial. *The Lancet*, 353, 623–626.

Silbermann, M., Arnaout, A., Sayed, R.H.A., *et al.* (2012). Pediatric palliative care in the Middle East. In C. Knapp, V. Madden, and S. Fowler-Kerry (ed.) *Pediatric Palliative Care: Global Perspectives*, pp. 127–159. London: Springer

Thomas, J., Karver, S., Cooney, G.A., *et al.* (2008). Methylnaltrexone for opioid-induced constipation in advanced illness. *The New England Journal of Medicine*, 358, 2332–2343.

Torres, C.Z., Rodriguez Zamora, N., and Derio Palacios, L. (2012). Pediatric palliative care in Chile. In C. Knapp, V. Madden, and S. Fowler-Kerry (eds.) *Pediatric Palliative Care: Global Perspectives*, pp. 431–447. London: Springer.

United Nations Children's Fund (2011). *Child Mortality Report 2011*. New York: UNICEF.

Wolfe, J., Grier, H.E., Klar, N., *et al.* (2000). Symptoms and suffering at the end of life in children with cancer. *The New England Journal of Medicine*, 342, 326–333.

World Bank (2004). *World Bank Glossary of Terms* [Online]. Available at: <http://www.worldbank.org/depweb/english/beyond/global/glossary.html>.

World Health Organization (1998a). *Cancer Pain Relief and Palliative Care in Children*. Geneva: WHO.

World Health Organization (1998b). *Symptom Relief in Terminal Illness*. Geneva: WHO.

Wright, M., Wood, J., Lynch, T., and Clark, D. (2008). Mapping levels of palliative care development: a global view. *Journal of Pain and Symptom Management*, 35, 469–485.

Very Special Kids (n.d.). *Very Special Kids*. [Website] Available at: <http://www.vsk.org.au/>.

Yee, J.D. and Berde, C.B. (1994). Dextroamphetamine or methylphenidate as adjuvants to opioid analgesia for adolescents with cancer. *Journal of Pain and Symptom Management*, 9, 122–125.

Zeltzer, L., Kellerman, J., Ellenberg, L., and Dash, J. (1983). Hypnosis for reduction of vomiting associated with chemotherapy and disease in adolescents with cancer. *Journal of Adolescent Health Care*, 4, 84.

Zeltzer, L., Lebaron, S., and Zeltzer, P.M. (1984a). The effectiveness of behavioral intervention for reducing nausea and vomiting in children and adolescents receiving chemotherapy. *Journal of Clinical Oncology*, 2, 683–690.

Zeltzer, L., Lebaron, S., and Zeltzer, P.M. (1984b). A prospective assessment of chemotherapy related nausea and vomiting in children with cancer. *American Journal of Pediatric Hematology/Oncology*, 6, 5–16.

16.3

Palliative medicine and care of the elderly

Meera Agar and Jane L. Phillips

Introduction to palliative medicine and care of the elderly

Most deaths in the older patient occur in the context of chronic disease, often with multiple comorbidities and physiological change. Clinicians also need to be aware of particular geriatric syndromes that occur frequently, such as frailty, falls, and delirium. Managing symptoms and maintaining function are still important goals, however care may be delivered in residential care (nursing home) or community and hospital settings, with the older person particularly vulnerable during transitions in care. Advance care planning is also crucial to ensure care decisions are not made in crisis. Supporting caregivers is essential, with caregivers often either adult children who have their own family and work responsibilities to juggle or an older spouse who may have concurrent medical problems themselves. Although the fields of geriatric and palliative medicine have evolved separately, there is commonality of goals: maximizing quality of life by maintaining function and optimizing symptom control, continuity of care regardless of setting, and integrated care of the 'whole person'—in contrast to seeing the patient as a cluster of separate illness and organ systems (Geriatrics-Hospice and Palliative Medicine Work Group, 2012). This chapter will outline the principles of care for the older person, when one or several underlying illnesses continue to progress with death as the likely outcome.

Epidemiology of ageing

Epidemiological factors are crucial when considering the care of the older person and the role of palliative care. With the changing reasons for death as a result of modern medicine, most adults die when they are old, often from a non-malignant disease that they have had for some time and its associated multimorbidity (American Geriatrics Society Expert Panel on the Care of Older Adults with Multimorbidity, 2012), and after a significant period of disability (Lynn and Goldstein, 2003; Effiong and Effiong, 2012). In the United States, the life expectancy is 78.7 years (Minino et al., 2011; Minino and Murphy, 2012). The proportion of the world's population who are greater than 65 years will continue to rise (Mathers et al., 2009). By 2050 it is projected that 16% of the world's population will be over 65, totalling 1.5 billion people compared to 1950 where it was 5% (Mathers et al., 2009). At least half of people over 65 will have at least three coexisting chronic conditions, with one in five having five or more (Mangin et al.,

2012). This includes musculoskeletal, psychiatric, cognitive and chronic pain-related problems each often associated with substantive symptomatology and disability. The tendency for individuals to be treated in disease 'silos' and the risks associated with polypharmacy add to the burden of adverse outcomes (Mangin et al., 2012),

Death rates for 2010 in the United States showed decreased mortality in virtually all age groups, when compared to 2000 data; with the second largest decrease (13.3%) seen for those aged 65 and older (Minino et al., 2011; Minino and Murphy, 2012). Heart disease, cancer, chronic lower respiratory diseases, stroke, and accidents could account for 63% of deaths in 2010 in all age groups. In the group aged over 65 years, the leading five causes of death were heart disease, cancer, chronic lower respiratory diseases, stroke, and Alzheimer's disease (Minino et al., 2011; Minino and Murphy, 2012). Equally, ischaemic heart disease, cerebrovascular disease, cancer, and respiratory disease remain the predominant causes of death in Europe (Eurostat, 2011). In Australia, the top five causes of death are ischaemic heart disease, cerebrovascular disease, dementia, cancer, and chronic lower respiratory diseases (Australian Bureau of Statistics, 2010). Globally, utilizing World Health Organization statistics, ischaemic heart disease, cerebrovascular disease, and lower respiratory diseases similarly remain leading causes of death (Mathers et al., 2009).

Over 50% of the world's population over 65 live in low- and middle-income countries and this leads to the increasing trend of non-communicable diseases as leading causes of death (Mathers et al., 2009). In all regions, apart from Africa, in 50% or more of cases, non-communicable diseases were the cause of death (Mathers et al., 2009).

Assessing the needs of older people

Older people with progressive life-limiting illnesses are increasingly being managed in the community, often for longer periods and with significant levels of morbidity and associated disability. It is estimated that two-thirds of all older Americans who resided in the community require long-term care assistance with personal care and instrumental activities of daily living (Stone, 2000). A combination of age, co-morbidities, and psychosocial factors can complicate treatment for various chronic and complex conditions, and impact on an older person's capacity to adhere to treatment regimens. Community-dwelling older people are also at higher risk of developing a range of geriatric syndromes such as delirium, dementia, and depression, and are more likely to experience abuse, neglect, and social isolation (Moore et al., 2009). Medication use also tends to increases with age and even though many older people may benefit from taking fewer medications, clinicians are often reluctant to withdraw medication in the absence of robust evidence (Holmes et al., 2006). The effective management of the multiple co-morbidities associated with ageing are often clinically and managerially complex, time-consuming, and frequently challenging.

Within an aged population, there is a subset of older people who will not die of one specific terminal illness, but, rather, will experience progressive frailty (Carey et al., 2008). For these people, their slow and dwindling decline is characterized by multiple co-morbidities and progressive functional and cognitive impairment, resulting in a gradual loss of functional reserve, increased susceptibility to illness, and a reduced capacity to recover from such events (Carey et al., 2008). Many will require long-term care assistance at home until their care needs exceed available community resources, prompting an admission to a nursing home or an inpatient setting in crisis. It is important to distinguish older people with progressive life-limiting illnesses who may live for an extended period (even years), and who will benefit from screening, specific medical interventions, and advance care planning from those who are rapidly approaching the end of their lives and who may consequentl, benefit from appropriate palliative care services (Carey et al., 2008).

The ambiguity associated with determining the most appropriate time to initiate the transition from intensive medical treatment to palliative care for older people has promoted a range of international policy responses (Department of Health, 2008; Australian Government Department of Health and Ageing, 2011). The UK End of Life Care Strategy emphasizes the importance of improved recognition of an approaching death and advance care planning, with a view to increasing choice, particularly around the place of death (Department of Health, 2008). Clinicians are encouraged to consider whether the person they are caring for is at risk of dying with the next 12 months, before initiating the necessary end-of-life conversations and appropriate care and support required to meet the older person's palliative care needs (Department of Health, 2008). The rising burden of chronic conditions, population ageing, and increased demand on specialist palliative care services underpins policies advocating for a population-based approach to palliative care (Palliative Care Australia, 2005; Department of Health, 2008). This policy change has prompted specialist palliative care services to diversify to incorporate a wider range of populations, providers, and settings (Luckett et al., 2012). As part of the reorientation of health-care services, a 'palliative approach' has been identified as being essential to extending palliative care to underserved populations, such as older people. Such an approach is built around core competencies that every health professional should have for people who are dying, while specialist case is reserved for those who have more complex needs.

A palliative approach

A palliative approach is particularly relevant for older people with progressive life-limiting illnesses who need integrated and coordinated care well before they are dying (Wilhelmson et al., 2011). Integrating the elements of the World Health Organization's

(n.d.) vision of palliative care into the goals of care for older people living with progressive chronic conditions that cannot be cured is feasible with a palliative approach. A palliative approach allows for care to be targeted to the specific needs of the illness trajectory and the needs of the older person and their family. Whilst recognizing the inevitability of death, a palliative approach also focuses on optimizing older peoples' quality of life by maximizing comfort and function, and offering appropriate treatment and support for distressing symptoms (Australian Department of Health and Ageing and National Health and Medical Research Council, 2006). In addition to addressing the older person's psychological, spiritual, social, and cultural needs, a palliative approach acknowledges the needs of caregivers and actively encourages their input into care planning (Palliative Care Victoria, n.d.). Integrating a palliative approach into care for older people ensures that they are offered care in accordance with complexity and need, independent of their diagnosis or prognosis (Waller et al., 2008).

While models of cancer care are well defined and pathways to specialist palliative care evident, it is likely that the majority of the older people with chronic conditions, such as chronic heart failure and chronic respiratory disease, will continue to be cared for by their primary care team, with input from relevant medical specialists (Luckett et al., 2012). A palliative approach can be provided readily by the older person's usual care team; however, if the older person's needs or symptoms become more complex, specialist palliative care team input ought to be sought. As death nears, a palliative approach ensures that the care team is well prepared and able to support the older person to die in the preferred place of care (Palliative Care Victoria, n.d.).

Rethinking goal setting in the context of chronic illness in older adults: maximizing well-being and partnering with others

Initiating a palliative approach for an older person ought to be initiated long before the terminal phase of illness so that the impact of the co-morbidities are acknowledged, their comfort and dignity is optimized, and their caregivers' needs are adequately addressed. Older peoples' palliative care needs are frequently under-assessed and therefore under-treated, particularly in relationship to their pain, need for information to inform decision-making, access to support and care at home, specialist palliative care input, and palliative care in nursing homes assessment and care (Davies and Higginson, 2004). There are specific transitions when health professionals need to think about an older person's prognosis and need for a palliative approach to care, such as when:

- you answer 'yes' to the 'surprise question'
- the person has a newly diagnosed life-limiting condition
- there is a worsening prognostication markers for a specific disease
- there is a downward step in response to treatment
- the person has multiple hospital admissions
- there is admission to a nursing home
- if his/her spouse has recently died (Murray et al., 2005).

Palliative care needs assessment

Detecting the need for a palliative approach to care has been made simpler with the development of tailored assessment tools for both cancer and other chronic and complex illnesses (Waller et al., 2008). These palliative care specific needs assessment tools assist:

◆ to match the types and levels of need experienced by people with progressive illnesses and their caregivers with the most appropriate people or services to address those needs

◆ health professionals in general and in specialist practice, to determine which needs may be met in that setting and which needs are more complex and may be better managed by specialists

◆ to facilitate communication between primary and specialist care providers about patients and caregivers' needs and actions taken to address these (Waller et al., 2008).

Having identified the need for a palliative approach there are a number of innovations, particularly in the context of chronic illness, that ought to be considered in order to maximize function and well-being of older people with progressive life-limiting illnesses, including referrals where appropriate to:

◆ *Geriatric oncology:* despite cancer being essentially a disease of ageing, the routine assessment of performance status does not capture the full range of health and social problems that some older people experience, such as functional dependence, co-morbidity, polypharmacy, malnutrition, cognitive dysfunction, and depression (Hurria et al., 2007; Terret, 2008). To address this limitation, the National Comprehensive Cancer Network Guidelines (2009) recommends that a multidimensional comprehensive geriatric assessment be integrated into the treatment for all people aged over 70 years of age with cancer. Undertaking a comprehensive geriatric assessment helps to identify older people whose health and/or psychosocial problems may potentially interfere with proposed treatment (Hurria et al., 2007; Terret, 2008). Allowing additional support to be provided helps to identify remediable conditions influencing treatment decisions, establish treatment goals, and, if required, allows a modified treatment plan to be developed (National Comprehensive Cancer Network, 2009). Despite these benefits, the integration of a comprehensive geriatric assessment into routine oncology practice has been limited by cost and the lack of data to date of improved outcomes (Bellera et al., 2012). Regardless of local practices, assessing geriatric needs helps to ensure that the older person with cancer and their caregivers receive the most appropriate care and support to enable them to cope with the effects of cancer and its treatment.

◆ *Heart failure clinics:* referral to a heart failure clinic is highly relevant for many older people with this condition. Heart failure clinics aim to reduce mortality and rehospitalization rates and improve quality of life through individualized patient care (Hauptman et al., 2008). These positive outcomes are achieved through the consistent application of guidelines with a focus on:

• disease management

• functional assessment

• quality of life assessment

• optimizing medical therapy and drug evaluation

• device evaluation

• nutritional assessment

• follow-up

• advance care planning

• communication

• provider education

• quality assessment (Hauptman et al., 2008).

Attendance at these specialist clinics provides older patients and their caregivers with an opportunity to be involved in shared decision making and to have timely conversations about palliative and end-of-life care preferences (Waterworth and Gott, 2010).

◆ *Pulmonary rehabilitation:* chronic obstructive pulmonary disease (COPD) is a common disorder with a high prevalence among older people and an increasing mortality rate (Gelberg and McIvor, 2010). Older people affected by COPD are at an increased risk of cardiovascular events, osteoporosis, fractures, peripheral muscle wasting, depression, and anxiety. This array of problems makes a multidisciplinary approach optimal and such care should begin with stratification of disease severity and prognostic information for each patient (Gelberg and McIvor, 2010). However, if older people with COPD are well enough to participate in pulmonary rehabilitation, they are likely to derive a clinically significant benefit in terms of their dyspnoea, fatigue, and overall well-being (Lacasse et al., 2006). Advanced age on its own ought not be an exclusion criteria for referral to pulmonary rehabilitation given that no correlation between age and outcomes have been found (Gelberg and McIvor, 2010). Given this population's significant symptom burden, elevated risks of mortality and suboptimal access to pulmonary rehabilitation, a comprehensive assessment is an important element of a palliative approach for people with COPD (Reticker et al., 2012).

◆ *Breathlessness clinics:* for people with breathlessness any cause, there has been increased interest in the impact of nurse- or physiotherapist-led interventions, including breathlessness clinics. There is some evidence that a breathlessness clinic may improve management of dyspnoea in patients with advanced lung cancer (Scottish Intercollegiate Guidelines Network, 2005).

◆ *Rehabilitation:* the primary focus of rehabilitation is on restoring function, coping with disability, and decreasing the burden of chronic disease (Wu and Quill, 2011), making rehabilitation a highly appropriate consideration for older people with a range of chronic and complex illnesses, such as cancer, heart failure, renal failure, or stroke survivors with palliative care needs (Dy and Feldman, 2012). Integrating rehabilitation and palliative care helps maximize older people's function and autonomy, and minimize dependency, whilst balancing their quality of life and end-of-life preparation (Wu and Quill, 2011). The primary goal of palliative rehabilitation is to minimize dependence in domains such as mobility and self-care, while providing comfort and emotional support (Javier and Montagnini, 2011). This is achieved by focusing on:

• preventive strategies to minimize complications from the primary disease

- restorative strategies that help regain function and loss of strength due to treatment, disease or both
- supportive strategies to maintain function at the new baseline
- palliative strategies that reduce the burden of care and maximize quality of life (Dietz, 1980).

The input of multiple disciplines is required, with physiotherapists and occupation therapists playing a major role in helping to maintain older people's functional capacity. This is achieved through a range of targeted interventions, including use of various physical modalities to better manage pain, provision of adaptive and assistive equipment, environmental modification, exercise programmes and energy-conservation strategies (Javier and Montagnini, 2011). While benefits of palliative rehabilitation have been demonstrated in a series of smaller retrospective studies, there is a need for larger randomized controlled trials in this population (Javier and Montagnini, 2011)

Establishing care partnerships

The complexity of older people's care demands the formation of a collaborative partnership between primary care, geriatric and palliative care services, together with other health-care providers in accordance with need. While specialist palliative care services need to partner with primary care and geriatricians, there is also a need for geriatricians to access specialist palliative care teams for advice and support on management of older people's symptoms, communication, and psychological and spiritual support if necessary (British Geriatrics Society, 2010). Facilitating input from relevant disciplines to shape the treatment and care plan for older people in accordance with their priorities and needs may require the establishment of case management processes (Phillips et al., 2013). The sharing of information and honesty are integral aspects of all goals of care discussions, which need to be clearly documented.

Advance care planning

Advance care planning is an interactive process of ongoing communication between a competent patient, significant others, and their health-care team(s). The purpose of the advance care plan for older people is to record their wishes regarding treatment decisions and the values that underpin these decisions in order to extend their autonomy and to guide decision-making (Sudore et al., 2008). It plays an important role in clarifying treatment goals to inform care (Higginson and Sen-Gupta, 2000; Lorenz et al., 2006). Advance care planning is particularly relevant for frail older people who are at increased risk of loss of capacity as a result of dementia or a cerebrovascular accident (Dy and Feldman, 2012). However, the potential of advance care planning to improve care outcomes for older people is currently limited by the absence of systematic implementation and in many jurisdictions, no legislation that enshrines the wishes set out in such a plan. In non-cancer conditions and nursing homes where markers of prognosis can be less explicit, ensuring advance care plans are made in the context of patient and family wishes is important (Lynn and Goldstein, 2003). Promoting mechanisms of communicating these wishes across care settings has yet to be fully realized (Volandes et al., 2011). In the setting of dementia, caregivers are more likely than clinicians to want interventions to support (Sampson et al., 2005). Unless appropriate advance care plans are in place, health professionals in acute care may assume that aggressive treatments are in order for older people with dementia rather than care focusing on quality of life (Andrews, 2009; Hines, 2009).

Unfortunately, if the older person has already lost capacity, the opportunity to plan their care in advance or hold discussions with their families about their care preferences will be more limited. In this circumstance, the question that should be asked of families is 'What would I want under these circumstances?' and never simply what the caregiver would want for them. In this situation, there is a greater reliance on jurisdictional laws as to the required approach for managing their care needs and substitute decision making (Public Guardianship Office, 2005; NSW Guardianship Tribunal, 2011).

Managing older peoples' care transitions

Older people with complex care needs require models of care that facilitate smooth transitions across health-care interventions and settings. Transitional care describes a set of actions that involves the movement of a person from hospital, subacute and post-acute nursing facilities, home, primary, and specialty care offices or nursing home to another care setting or different levels of care within the same location (National Transitions of Care Coalition, 2008). Transitional care is based on a comprehensive plan of care and the availability of health-care practitioners who are well-trained in chronic care and have current information about the patient's goals, preferences, and clinical status. It includes logistical arrangements, education of the patient and family, and coordination among the health professionals involved in the transition and effective communication (National Transitions of Care Coalition, 2008). An integrated 'shared care' model of palliative care implemented by a Canadian specialist palliative care service reported a 7% reduction in the number of patients with cancer presenting to emergency departments (EDs) in the first 12 months (Lawson et al., 2009). A key feature of this model was the specialist service's capacity to cross all care settings from hospital, community, and palliative care unit. However, managing older populations with a non-malignant diagnosis poses tougher challenges, such as preventing avoidable hospital admissions by enhancing primary care and caregiver support (Jiwa et al., 2002; Shipman et al., 2008).

Palliative care in the home setting

Despite many older people preferring to die at home, it is not always feasible due to social or practical reasons. As older people near the end of their life, they frequently require significant assistance with transportation, homemaking services, nursing, and personal care, much of which is provided by informal and formal caregivers (Rolls et al., 2011). Enabling older people to be cared for at home until death is strongly linked to intensity of available home care support, living with relatives, and family support (Froggatt, 2005).

Contemporary health-care policy advocates case management, collaboration, and integrated teams to better support older people with complex and multiple needs through interprofessional practice (Trivedi et al., 2013). Although the effectiveness and cost-effectiveness evidence for interprofessional practice improving care outcomes for older people is weak, there is evidence that well-integrated and shared care models improve processes of care and have the potential to reduce hospital or nursing/care home use for older people (Trivedi et al., 2013). In the United States, a study exploring nurse practitioner models to better support the many older people with complex illnesses at home who would benefit from palliative care but who have elected not to accept hospice enrolment, found that additional funding is required to ensure the financial viability of such a role (Bookbinder et al., 2011).

Approximately half of all older people with advanced dementia will die at home (Mitchell et al., 2005). Achieving this outcome is dependent upon older people and their caregivers having access to a significant level of support over an extended period of time, as the average length of time from the onset of dementia symptoms to death is 4.5 years (Xie et al., 2008). Depending on the age at diagnosis and presence of co-morbidities, this illness trajectory can extent out to more than 10 years (Xie et al., 2008). This uncertainty reinforces the importance of implementing a palliative approach to care early in the older person's illness trajectory. There is widespread agreement that care for people in the advanced stages of dementia should be palliative (Alzheimers Australia, 2006). Bereaved family members of people with dementia in the United States who received hospice care reported higher ratings of the quality of care and quality of dying (Teno et al., 2011). Models are needed to support people with dementia over extended periods preceding the terminal phase of care and assist transitions when these are unavoidable (Luckett et al., 2012).

Living alone

Living alone influences both the place of care and place of death. Being older and living alone near the end of life is increasingly common as people, particularly women, live longer and families are smaller and frequently more dispersed (Grundy et al., 2004). The numbers of older people living in poverty is also increasing, whilst employment trends and other economic factors impact on the support older people living alone can expect to receive. These factors challenge the capacity for older people to age and die well in their preferred place of care (Rolls et al., 2011). Older people living alone near the end of life have practical, emotional, physical, and existential needs, underpinned by a desire to be independent and maintain a sense of dignity (Aoun et al., 2008). Those most vulnerable and least likely to be in a position to access palliative support include older people living in rural or inner city communities and people with fewer financial resources or smaller social networks (Rolls et al., 2011). Changes in living and social circumstances mean that, in times of crisis, older people no longer have such ready access to informal caregivers as in previous generations. The focus across the developed world on 'ageing in place' although well intended is largely dependent upon on the availability of a spouse, partner, or adult child who is prepared to take on the caregiver role, or a reliance on paid carers (Rolls et al., 2011). However, not all older people have continuous access to caregiver support making it difficult for them to be cared for at home as their care needs increase. This has implications for palliative care. Older people are more likely than younger people to request hospitalization as the end of life nears (Rigby et al., 2010), making confirming their place of care preferences important throughout their illness trajectory. When considering older people's preferences, two separate conversations are indicated to identify preference for current place of care as well as the preferred location for care immediately prior to death (Agar et al., 2008).

Palliative care in hospitals

Across the developed world, more than half of all deaths occur in hospitals, ranging from 56% in the United Kingdom (Department of Health, 2008), 65% in Australia, and 45% in the United States, with people aged 75–84 years having the highest death rate (Department of Health, 2008). In the United States, Canada, and recently in the United Kingdom, there is evidence that the number of people dying in hospitals is being averted with an increasing number of home deaths (Gomes et al., 2012). Despite this positive trend and the emphasis on remaining at home for end-of-life care, dying within the acute care setting will continue to be the reality for many older people.

The models of care largely adopted in the acute care sector are consultative models, inpatient palliative units/beds, and nurse practitioner models (Rabow et al., 2004; Sudore et al., 2008). Consultative acute care palliative care services tend to focus on (a) prognosis and goals of care conversations, (b) pursuing documentation of advance directives, (c) discussion about foregoing specific treatments and/or diagnostic interventions, (d) family and patient support, (e) discharge planning, and (f) symptom management (Manfredi et al., 2000). Hospital palliative care teams help to improve symptom control and quality of life, alleviate emotional burden, and improve caregiver and patient well-being (Hanks et al., 2002; Higginson et al., 2003), whilst also reducing hospital costs (Morrison et al., 2008). In the United States, palliative care provided to hospitalized patients with advanced disease has resulted in lower costs of care and less utilization of intensive care compared to similar patients receiving usual care (Penrod et al., 2010). The establishment of palliative care services within the acute care sector in the United States is more likely to occur in larger hospitals, academic medical centres, not-for-profit hospitals, and VA hospitals compared to other hospitals (Morrison et al., 2005). Meeting the end-of-life care needs of older people dying in the acute care sector demands greater attention and investment in a model of care that is responsive to the complex needs of this growing population.

Emergency departments

There is an increasing pressure on EDs, particularly by older people (Gruneir et al., 2011). A number of older people will die in the ED with few of these people being known to a specialist palliative care service (Beynon et al., 2011). ED presentations are frequently the end result of inadequate symptom control, absence of caregivers, or logistical (Agarwal et al., 2012). Many ED deaths may be prevented if a palliative approach is adopted and the older person's palliative care needs are identified earlier, appropriate referrals are made, and advance care planning is completed (Beynon et al., 2011). The capacity of coordinated models of care to decrease unnecessary ED usage has been demonstrated in heart failure (McAlister et al., 2004), and likely to be applicable to older people requiring palliative care. Previous ED attendance or admissions ought to be the trigger for initiating the necessary palliative supports to improve older people's quality of life, capacity to optimize their time at home or in their place of choice, whilst also reducing the pressure on busy EDs, which are not designed for delivering great palliative care (Beynon et al., 2011). Research exploring treatment uncertainty, quality of life, costs, ethical and social issues; optimizing timely and effective interactions between emergency and other health services; and strengthening community-based care are all required to inform end-of-life care delivery and policy in the ED (Forero et al., 2012). The importance of the ED as a setting for palliative care is explored further in Chapter 3.3.

Palliative care in nursing homes

The emphasis placed on supporting older people to live at home for as long as possible has resulted in nursing home residents becoming older and frailer. Nursing homes are increasingly the place of where many older people will live out their life for a relatively short period of time. The burden of disability and death that occurs in this care setting is significant, and the palliative care needs of nursing home residents and their caregivers is extensively detailed in Chapter 3.4.

Supporting caregivers

Informal caregivers play a major role in helping older people remain at home. The burden on informal caregivers is often profound, especially as the 'palliative phase' of an illness for both malignant and non-malignant conditions is often prolonged (Luckett et al., 2012). This is often also care that has no start date (with people slipping into the role and no time defined for an end date). Many caregivers of older people are themselves older and/ or ill, with this role impacting on their health (Mitchell et al., 2010a). Often older people are providing aspects of care for each other rather than one being sole caregiver for the other. While many caregivers may derive immense satisfaction from their role, for others there are often unintended adverse consequences, including (a) significant social, financial, and employment implications; (b) health implications; (c) increased risk of depression and anxiety which may increase as death approaches; (d) feelings of sadness, anger, resentment, isolation, and inadequacy; and (e) potential for increased risk of psychological morbidity and complicated grief, especially if the patient has unrelieved physical or psychological symptoms (Waller et al., 2008). Despite informal carers having high levels of need for support and psychological morbidity, a systematic review examining interventions to better support informal caregivers of people with palliative care needs found few well-designed studies generating high levels of evidence (Harding and Higginson, 2003). Caregivers of older people with dementia who are approaching the end of life have different but equally intense needs to carers of patients dying from other diseases (Schulz et al., 2003). Caregivers in this setting experience numerous losses associated with progressive dementia, as well as managing and coping with dementia-related behaviours (Goodman et al., 2010).

Elements of a palliative approach model of care for community dwelling older people

Despite the ambiguity in nomenclature describing palliative models of care and the scarcity of high-level evidence, a recent rapid review identified seven elements of care as being essential to addressing the needs of older people at the end of life and their caregivers:

1. Timely access to specialist palliative care knowledge and expertise, in accordance with needs

2. Case management, coordination, and promotion of communication across care settings

3. Support for home-based care including after-hours practitioner access

4. Tailoring and targeting services to the right population and setting, particularly when addressing cultural needs

5. Consideration of workforce issues across the care continuum

6. Collaboration across the health-care continuum including home, community, acute and residential aged care

7. Integrating health and social services to support palliative care in the community (Luckett et al., 2012).

Palliative care for specific diagnoses and geriatric syndromes

There are some specific diagnoses and syndromes that warrant special mention due to the prevalence in the older person and the specific clinical approaches needed to respond optimally. The term 'geriatric syndrome' is utilized in the context of a multimorbid process leading to specific phenomenology (Flacker, 2003). This concept focuses on common clinical conditions, which don't fall neatly into specific disease categories (Flacker, 2003; Inouye et al., 2007).

Dementia

Dementia is a progressive terminal illness for which there is no cure (Birch and Draper, 2008). Research advances in dementia treatments are unlikely to alter this picture significantly in the foreseeable future (Brodaty et al., 2011). From 1999 to 2008, 879 281 Alzheimer's disease-related deaths were identified in United States (Moschetti et al., 2012). The age-adjusted mortality rate for Alzheimer's disease increased from 45.3 per 100 000 population in 1999 to 50.0 per 100 000 in 2008. Dementia is now the third leading cause of death in Australia (Australian Bureau of Statistics, 2010). In the United States, between the years of 2000 and 2008, the proportion of deaths due to heart disease, stroke, and prostate cancer decreased by 13%, 20%, and 8%, respectively, whereas the proportion due to Alzheimer's disease increased by 66% (Alzheimer's Association, 2012). It is becoming the predominant reason for admission to residential aged care or nursing homes (Van Rensbergen and Nawrot, 2010). For example over half (53%) of all people living in residential aged care in Australia have a recorded diagnosis of dementia (Australian Institute of Health and Welfare, 2009).

There are several key challenges to delivering effective palliative care for the person with advanced dementia (Birch and Draper, 2008). Some areas which need special consideration include difficulties in identifying a well-defined terminal phase, a more protracted duration of end-stage illness over weeks to months (rather than hours to days), issues relating to communication and decision-making, assessment of pain in the cognitively impaired, and specific symptoms such as behavioural disturbance (Sachs et al., 2004).

Families of the person with dementia have many of the same needs as people caring for those with other life-limiting illnesses, including a need for information about:

◆ the patient's condition

◆ future changes

◆ the treatment plan.

There are also specific needs relating to dementia. Families often have limited knowledge about the dementia illness trajectory, resulting in expectations that differ from the health professionals providing their care (Hertogh, 2006). When these needs are unresolved, families are less prepared for end-of-life care and decision-making (Forbes et al., 2000). Having a relative with advanced dementia living in a residential aged care facility can be a significant burden and the role of a proxy decision-maker can be extremely stressful (Forbes et al., 2000; Caron et al., 2005). When the family members of residents with advanced dementia understand that prognosis is poor, there is a decreased likelihood of the resident having interventions in the last 90 days of their life that may be burdensome (Mitchell et al., 2009).

Communication issues with the patient, between services, between service and family, and the difficulties of advance care planning are major barriers to care provision. Decision-making and issues of consent surrounding treatment interventions are complex, particularly in relation to nutrition and hydration, treatment of pneumonia, and whether or not to send a resident to hospital, particularly when the wishes of the resident are unclear (Lamberg et al., 2005).

Predictors of mortality in residents with Alzheimer's disease living in aged care facilities include limitation of physical function, pressure sores, urinary incontinence, use of restraints, and indicators of delirium (Gambassi et al., 1999). Co-morbidities such as respiratory disease, cardiovascular disease, diabetes mellitus, and malnutrition are also strong predictors of mortality (Coventry et al., 2005). While they have limitations, there is mounting evidence to support criteria and tools that help with prognostication (Clelland, 2008).

The Functional Assessment Staging (FAST) tool is a seven-stage system to identify progressive functional decline and has been used to classify people with dementia (Coventry et al., 2005). There are concerns that FAST may not be valid for all types of dementia and that the Karnofsky Performance Status score may be more able to predict survival than FAST (Schonwetter et al., 2003). More recently Mitchell et al have assessed the validity of a mortality and risk score (Advanced Dementia Prognostic Tool (ADEPT) for residents with advanced dementia). The variables that best predicted survival were length of stay, age, gender, dyspnoea, pressure ulcers, total functional dependence, whether the person was bedfast, decreasing levels of oral intake, bowel incontinence, body mass index, weight loss, and congestive heart failure (Mitchell et al., 2010b). While it proved better than previous guidelines, the ADEPT tool was only moderately accurate at predicting survival (Mitchell et al., 2010b).

Nutrition and swallowing difficulties are common in the advanced stages of dementia (Palecek et al., 2010). Treatment decisions surrounding nutrition and hydration are often emotionally charged and raise ethical and moral issues for residents, families, the treating health professionals, as well as society (Wasson et al., 2001). This often results in staff as well as family members feeling compelled to 'do something' (Wasson et al., 2001). Studies have shown percutaneous endoscopic gastrostomy feeding for older people with end-stage dementia to result in adverse consequences including pain, gastrointestinal bleeding, use of restraints, faecal incontinence, and aspiration (Finucane et al., 1999). A higher incidence of pneumonia has been reported in tube fed patients (Bourdel-Marchasson et al., 1997). Further, a systematic review highlights that the use of feeding tubes has no survival benefit for this group of patients (Finucane et al., 1999).

Several studies highlight the poor recognition and treatment of pain in residential aged care facilities (McAuliffe et al., 2009; Corbett et al., 2012). Little is still known about the potential of dementia-related neuropathology contributing to the pain experience in dementia (Corbett et al., 2012). People with end-stage dementia appear to receive less medication for pain than patients without cognitive difficulties (The Australian Pain Society, 2005). Cognitive impairment and communication difficulties contribute to pain going unrecognized (Morrison and Siu, 2000). Not only are cognitively impaired residents prescribed less analgesia than other residents they also are administered less analgesia by the nurses caring for them (Chang et al., 2009).

Behavioural disturbances that impact on caregivers include a range of difficulties including wandering, agitation, aggression, sexual disinhibition, apathy, and shouting (O'Connor et al., 2008). Reducing behavioural disturbances and maintaining communication and personhood requires a range of approaches. A systematic review of psychosocial treatments for the management of behavioural and psychological symptoms of dementia (BPSD) (O'Connor et al., 2008) highlights the importance of clear communication, understanding triggers, social interaction, and environment (O'Connor et al., 2008). Moreover, non-pharmacological treatments worked best when they were adapted to the specific interests of the individual, and consistency and avoiding punishment are key (O'Connor et al., 2008). It is also important to rule out coexisting conditions such as constipation, depression and anxiety, and delirium. A comprehensive assessment undertaken by a professional with appropriate training in, for example, dementia care mapping can assist in devising individualized management plans for BPSD (O'Connor et al., 2008).

There are some aspects of end-of-life care that are particularly challenging or forgotten. For example, the spiritual care of persons with dementia is often overlooked. It is possible to nurture the spiritual well-being of people even when their dementia is advanced (Ryan et al., 2005). It is also important to consider the multiple losses experienced by caregivers prior to the death, such as loss of companionship and witnessing the loss of cognition of their loved one (Chan et al., 2012). Anticipatory grief may also be present at the time that decisions about the need for and transfer to institutional care are being made (Chan et al., 2012).

Delirium

Delirium is a medical illness characterized by change of level of consciousness and cognition, which develops rapidly and fluctuates, occurring in the context of an underlying medical condition (American Psychiatric Association, 2000.). Delirium is a common condition in the older person, and it is important to understand it is preventable and, if not prevented, then reversible in many cases. Increasingly, subsyndromal presentations are recognized, with less severe symptoms but all core domains of sleep–wake cycle, thought process, language, attention, orientation, and visuospatial ability present (Meagher et al., 2012; Trzepacz et al., 2012).

Delirium in older people is often under-recognized or misdiagnosed, yet is the most common complication of a hospital admission for older people (Young and Inouye, 2007). It develops in up to half of older adults postoperatively, and occurrence rates of delirium in medical inpatients vary between 11% and 42% (Siddiqi et al., 2006). Delirium in palliative care is covered in more detail in Chapter 17.5, and here we will highlight the pertinent issues when it occurs in the older adult. Increasing age, dementia and cognitive impairment, visual impairment, admission to hospital for fracture, and severe medical illness are important risk factors for delirium (National Institute for Health and Clinical Excellence (NICE), 2010). There are also multiple medications, which can precipitate or increase risk of delirium (Clegg and Young, 2011). Preventative strategies include orientating approaches, managing dehydration and constipation, avoiding unnecessary catheterization, optimizing oxygen saturation, encouraging mobility, and resolving reversible causes of sensory impairments by providing visual and hearing aids where needed (NICE, 2010). Caution should be exercised in prescribing antipsychotic medications to older people with delirium (Delirium Clinical Guidelines Expert Working Group, 2006). Non-pharmacological strategies (environmental, behavioural, social) are first-line strategies to manage the symptoms of delirium (Delirium Clinical Guidelines Expert Working Group, 2006). Delirium is a highly distressing experience and hence information about delirium should be made available to people who have experienced delirium after its presentation and their family/carers (Delirium Clinical Guidelines Expert Working Group, 2006).

Pain

The majority of older people with advanced illness will experience pain in some form, either as a result of diagnosed pathological processes or treatments trialled to manage their condition (Scottish Intercollegiate Guidelines Network, 2008). Many older people have more than one source of pain. Their pain is frequently underassessed and, as a consequence poorly managed. Age-related changes in pharmacokinetics and pharmacodynamics add to the challenges of effectively managing older people's pain (Dalacorte et al., 2011).

Constipation

Constipation is a prevalent problem in the older person (Gallegos-Orozco et al., 2012). On self-report, 26% of women and 16% of men over 65 years consider themselves constipated (Gallegos-Orozco et al., 2012). This rises to 34% and 26% respectively in the group aged 84 and older, and over half of the people in long-term care facilities. The symptomatology may not necessarily be reduced frequency of bowel movements, but straining and passage of hard stools may be reported (Gallegos-Orozco et al., 2012).

Constipation is associated with several medical conditions of high prevalence in the elderly population (including Parkinson's disease, diverticular disease, hypothyroidism, dementia, and stroke) and also medications (including iron and calcium tablets, calcium channel blockers, non-steroidal anti-inflammatory drugs, tricyclic antidepressants, and opioids). Intrinsic changes in colonic physiology including reduced number of neurons in myenteric plexus, increased collagen deposition, reduction in inhibitory nerve input, increased binding of plasma endorphins, and changes in anorectal function also occur and can predispose this population to develop constipation (Gallegos-Orozco et al., 2012).

Prevention of constipation is important as underlying illnesses progress and immobility and reduced oral fluid and fibre intake occurs. An elderly person with constipation requires a detailed history and examination, including a rectal examination.

Constipation management is discussed in more detail in Chapter 10.3.

Falls

Falls are often multifactorial in origin, and include motor problems (gait and balance, muscle weakness), sensory impairment (vestibular, vision, peripheral neuropathy), cognitive and mood impairments, postural hypotension, medication, and environmental hazards (Close and Lord, 2011). Fall risk is increased with medications for cardiovascular diseases (such as digoxin, type 1a antiarrhythmics and diuretics), benzodiazepines, antidepressants, antiepileptics, antipsychotics, anti-Parkinsonian drugs, opioids and urological spasmolytics and provide a modifiable risk factor (Huang et al., 2012). Once a person has fallen, it can lead to further immobility due to the fear of falling. Falls are associated with fractures, head injury, and further functional decline (Gates et al., 2008). It is important to regularly screen for falls risk, in particular when a change of environment, physical, or cognitive function has occurred (Close and Lord, 2011). A risk assessment also will allow individualized intervention, and to assess the patient's ability to understand and cooperate with falls risk reduction strategies, such as pushing the call bell to get assistance to go to toilet (Close and Lord, 2011).

Multifaceted interventions should be considered, addressing the factors specific to the individual include reducing environmental hazards, adjusting or ceasing psychoactive and hypotensive medications, gait retraining, use of assistive devices, and appropriate footwear (Gillespie et al., 2009; Close and Lord, 2011). The role of vitamin D supplementation is controversial (Verbrugge et al., 2012)

Frailty

Frailty has been variously defined as diminishing capacity to withstand stress or increased vulnerability to adverse outcomes (reduced ability to maintain or regain homeostasis), physical disability, impairment in activities of daily living, social withdrawal, slow motor processing, cognitive changes, weight loss, or negative energy balance (Boockvar and Meier, 2006; Sternberg et al., 2011). There is a point of contention as to whether disability and functional decline are components of frailty or its outcome (Sternberg et al., 2011). The definition developed by Fried and colleagues (Walston et al., 2006; Ko, 2011) is widely used for research purposes, and includes three or more of the following: unintentional weight loss, poor grip strength, self-reported exhaustion, low physical activity levels, and slow walking speed. It has been more difficult to develop an operationalized definition for use in clinical practice (Rodriguez-Manas et al., 2013). When caring for older adults, there is a spectrum of resilience ranging from the most frail and vulnerable to highly independent and robust (Walston et al., 2006). Though frailty is more common in older adults and those with multiple comorbidities, it can occur independent of age, disability, or illness (Ko, 2011).

Frailty is believed to be a complex interaction of several factors, including physiological alterations with ageing, comorbid disease, nutritional inadequacy, environmental impacts, and genetic and lifestyle factors (Heuberger, 2011). It is likely that the accumulation of factors has a synergistic effect (Heuberger, 2011). A key feature is weight loss and sarcopenia (Boockvar and Meier, 2006; Ko, 2011). Frailty can be present in the obese older adult, and the 'sarcopenic obese' is associated with significant health burden (Heuberger, 2011). Dysregulation of neuromuscular, endocrine, and immune systems seem key (Ko, 2011). Pro-inflammatory cytokines, activation of promoter genes relating to catabolism and catabolic cytokines, testosterone deficiency, hypovitaminosis D, low insulin-like growth factor, ghrelin, and growth hormone have been implicated in epidemiological studies (Heuberger, 2011; Ko, 2011; Shardell et al., 2012). Chronically high interleukin 6 is strongly associated with multiple disease states (diabetes, anaemia, atherosclerosis, heart failure, and dementia), and predicts increased disability, mortality, and sarcopenia in older adults (Ko, 2011).

Frailty has been associated with an increased risk of falling, hospitalization, reduced activities of daily living, disability, and death, after adjusting for health and socioeconomic status and disability (Ko, 2011). It has been estimated that 3–5% of deaths in older adults could be delayed if frailty was prevented (Shamliyan et al., 2012). Primary prevention of frailty includes addressing comorbid illness such as hypertension; chronic disease management, exercise, and nutrition are strategies for secondary prevention. The principles of good palliative care guide tertiary prevention, such as maintaining and improving function, control of symptoms, maintaining psychological well-being, and preventing hospital admissions where possible (Sternberg et al., 2011). Currently, the strategies, which have demonstrated benefits, are exercise and geriatric interdisciplinary assessment (Ko, 2011). Exercise strategies include progressive resistance exercise training, multicomponent training (resistance, endurance, balance, and flexibility), and t'ai chi, and have been demonstrated to improve performance of activities of daily living, reduce chronic elevation of inflammatory mediators, improve gait velocity, and decrease falls; whilst also improving quality of life and emotional health (Province et al., 1995; Chin et al., 2008; Ko, 2011). Exercise may have limited benefits in the severely frail.

To date there has been no definitive evidence demonstrating benefit of hormone replacement for improving muscle mass and strength in the treatment of frailty (Ko, 2011). Testosterone replacement can increase lean muscle strength but its effects on improved function have been mixed, and it has adverse effects that may be more problematic in the frail older person (Ko, 2011). Vitamin D replacement also can increase muscle strength, and decrease falls; however, its efficacy in frailty is yet to be determined (Ko, 2011). Medication may have a role in reducing incidence of frailty by inhibition of inflammatory pathways (statins, angiotensin-converting enzyme inhibitors), but the vast majority of medications are likely to have a net effect 'stressor' which could destabilize the frail person (Heuberger, 2011; Gnjidic and Hilmer, 2012).

Geriatric evaluation and management (GEM) and comprehensive geriatric assessment (CGA) are two models on interdisciplinary geriatric care, the first where the team directly delivers care, and the latter a consultative model (Ko, 2011). These assessments include a geriatrician, nurse, social worker, and occupational or physical therapist. The objectives of GEM and CGA are to improve physical and psychological function, reduce hospitalization and long-term care placement, and reduce early mortality (Ko, 2011). Similarly models in the outpatient or home setting such as the programme for all inclusive care of the elderly (PACE), and acute care setting (acute care for the elderly) have similar goals. More recently, longer time of enrolment in PACE is independently associated with: change of resuscitation status towards less aggressive care, reduced hospitalization, and death in a non-hospital setting (Pak et al., 2012).

Depression

Older age has been demonstrated as a risk factor for depression (Ellison et al., 2012; Zhao et al., 2012). Depression in the elderly is also associated with an increase by 50% in health-care costs, compared to the non-depressed with similar chronic medical illnesses (Ellison et al., 2012). Risk factors for later life depression include unmarried status, living alone, lack of social supports, negative life events such as bereavement, and lower socioeconomic status (Ellison et al., 2012). Depression often occurs in the context of comorbid psychiatric or medical illnesses. Specific medical disorders associated with a higher risk of depression include cardiovascular disease, Parkinson's disease, cancer, stroke, lung disease, arthritis, loss of hearing, and dementia (Ellison et al., 2012). It should be noted that 25–50% of family caregivers also experience depression (Ellison et al., 2012). Depressive symptoms such as anorexia, insomnia, fatigue, and weight loss may be non-specific, and reflect symptoms of concurrent comorbid medical illnesses. Older people may also have difficulty reporting symptoms due to cognitive impairment or due to fears of stigma associated with psychiatric illness. There are several scales validated for use in the older adult population, including the Geriatric Depression Scale, Cornell Scale for Depression in Dementia, Beck Depression Inventory, and Hamilton Depression Scale (Ellison et al., 2012). It is important to distinguish sadness and difficult coping with depression, and a common misperception is that depression is a part of normal ageing leading to its under-recognition and under-treatment.

Due to the frequency of concurrent cognitive impairment and depression, causal relationships have been explored but there is yet to be definitive evidence (Ellison et al., 2012). It has been demonstrated that older patients with depression demonstrate cognitive deficits in several neuropsychological domains, including processing speed, verbal and non-verbal memory, and executive functioning (Ellison et al., 2012). These cognitive symptoms sometimes do not fully respond to effective antidepressant treatment. Evolving evidence does support the concept that depression and the number of depressive episodes are independent risk factors for the future development of dementia (Ellison et al., 2012). Proposed mechanisms include hypothalamic–pituitary–adrenal axis dysregulation, cerebrovascular ischaemic white matter lesions, and inflammation in the central nervous system (Ellison et al., 2012).

Treatment of depression in the older patient with chronic illness requires a multifactorial approach, including psychological, cognitive, and behavioural interventions as well as medication (Ellison et al., 2012). Referral to specialist psychiatric services may be needed for those who have failed an adequate trial of depression treatments, those at risk of self-harm and suicide, those who abuse alcohol or other substances, those with comorbid psychiatric conditions or dementia, and those who need electroconvulsive therapy (Ellison et al., 2012). Time to onset of efficacy and the adverse event profile are important factors to inform therapeutic options in the older adult, especially if disease is progressive.

Managing multimorbidity

More than 50% of older adults have three or more chronic diseases (American Geriatrics Society Expert Panel on the Care of Older Adults with Multimorbidity, 2012). The best way to approach decision-making and clinical management in the older adult with multimorbidity remains challenging. It is important that the person is able to be adequately informed about the expected treatments benefits and harms (American Geriatrics Society Expert Panel on the Care of Older Adults with Multimorbidity, 2012). In particular when considering 'preference sensitive' decisions, based on values and preferences, the person will need to weigh up the potential therapies for each condition, the increased risk of adverse events, and the possibility of more limited benefits (American Geriatrics Society Expert Panel on the Care of Older Adults with Multimorbidity, 2012). It is also important to consider whether participants with multi-morbidity were included in the clinical trials evaluating the treatment options at hand (American Geriatrics Society Expert Panel on the Care of Older Adults with Multimorbidity, 2012).

Physiological changes with ageing

Hearing and vision changes

Age-related changes in hearing and vision are prevalent, and can impact on a wide range of issues relating to care. The person may not report symptoms due to embarrassment, and it may lead to difficulty in obtaining history and following management. Age-related hearing loss is known as presbycusis. Presbycusis is associated with progressive deterioration of auditory sensitivity, loss of the auditory sensory cells, and central processing functions, and is associated with the ageing process (Li-Korotky, 2012). Another common cause is cerumen impaction, which is more common due to decreased number of cerumen glands and activity.

Common causes of vision impairment in the older person include age-related macular degeneration, glaucoma, cataracts, and diabetic retinopathy, with one in three people over the age of 65 having some form of vision-reducing disorder (Quillen, 1999).

Sensory impairment increases risk of falls and delirium, as well as decreasing function and the ability to be self-caring.

Dry mouth, dysphagia, and tooth loss

Some studies have shown age-related changes in salivary constituents, but other contradict this, demonstrating age-stable production of salivary electrolytes and proteins in the absence of major medical problems and medication use (Turner and Ship, 2007). Hence complaints of xerostomia should not be only attributed to age. Salivary disorders in the ageing population usually are caused by systemic diseases and their treatments (e.g. anticholinergic medications or radiation therapy) (Turner and Ship, 2007). Several medical conditions (such as Sjögren's syndrome, diabetes, Alzheimer's disease, and dehydration), medications (e.g. anticholinergics), head and neck irradiation, and chemotherapy can cause or contribute to salivary gland dysfunction (Turner and Ship, 2007). Other medications which are implicated include antidepressants, sedatives, and tranquilizers; antihistamines; antihypertensives (alpha and beta blockers, diuretics, calcium channel blockers, angiotensin-converting enzyme inhibitors); cytotoxic agents; and medications to treat Parkinsonism and epilepsy (Turner and Ship, 2007). Xerostomia is associated with altered taste, difficulty chewing and swallowing food, mucosal breakdown, candidiasis, dental problems, and increased susceptibility to aspiration pneumonia (Turner and Ship, 2007).

Tooth loss prevalence varies between countries, and rates are generally reducing over time (Starr and Hall, 2010). Socioeconomic factors and related lifestyle and behavioural factors remain strong predictors (Starr and Hall, 2010). Ill-fitting dentures also can cause problems with chewing and swallowing. Dysphagia is also prevalent, in particular in those with dementia and stroke (Sura et al., 2012). Percutaneous endoscopic feeding only has a place in specific clinical scenarios, and is unlikely to offer benefit in the person with progressive and far advanced disease (Cullen, 2011).

Dermatological changes associated with ageing, pressure ulcers, and wound healing

The structure and the function of skin change with age (Yaar and Gilchrest, 2001). The epidermis becomes thinner and loses its undulating rete pattern, the stratum corneum loses its ability to retain water, and cell replacement, barrier function, and wound healing decrease (Yaar and Gilchrest, 2001). The dermis thins and loses elasticity, partly because of a decrease in the number of fibroblasts (Yaar and Gilchrest, 2001). Eccrine sweat glands shrink, reducing sweat production, and Langerhans cells decrease in number, affecting immune responsiveness (Yaar and Gilchrest, 2001). This has implications for pressure ulceration and may change absorption of transdermal medications (see Chapter 11.1). Other contributing factors may be corticosteroids, used in the context of COPD or for systemic indications.

Pharmacokinetics and pharmacodynamics and impacts on prescribing

There are pharmacokinetic and pharmacodynamic changes associated with ageing which are important. The effect of ageing on the small bowel transporter mechanism is not fully established, but absorption seems to be minimally effected with age (Cusack, 2004). Ageing is associated with some reduction in hepatic first-pass metabolism due to reduced liver mass and perfusion; hence the bioavailability of some medications can be increased (Klotz, 2009; Shi and Klotz, 2011). Changes in body composition also occur, with body fat and total body water increasing as lean body mass decrease. This leads to hydrophilic drugs having a smaller volume of distribution and lipophilic drugs have an increase, prolonging their half-life (Klotz, 2009; Shi and Klotz, 2011). Drugs with a high hepatic extraction ratio display some age-related decrease in systemic clearance, but for most drugs with a low hepatic extraction ratio, clearance is not reduced with advancing age (Klotz, 2009; Shi and Klotz, 2011). In general, cytochrome P450 enzyme activities are preserved in normal ageing. Drug transporters play an important role in pharmacokinetic processes, but their functional changes related to age are not fully understood. One-third of older people show no decrease in renal function. In the other two-thirds, the age-related decline of renal function is associated with coexisting cardiovascular diseases and other risk factors, rather than age alone (Klotz, 2009; Shi and Klotz, 2011). A progressive decline in homeostatic mechanisms leads to a reduced ability to mitigate many of the adverse effects of medications including hypotension and electrolyte disturbances (Turnheim, 2003). There is greater inhibition of synthesis of vitamin K-dependent clotting factors at similar plasma concentrations of warfarin in elderly compared with young patients (Mangoni and Jackson, 2004). Advancing age is associated with increased susceptibility to psychoactive medications (antidepressants, antipsychotics, lithium, and benzodiazepines) (Trifiro and Spina, 2011).

Conclusion

The older person presents unique clinical needs, where palliative care can make a substantial contribution. Understanding the epidemiology of the illnesses that cause death, multimorbidity, and the phenomenological manifestations of illness will allow the clinician to individualize care. Key principles include optimizing symptoms and function, supporting caregivers, and proactive monitoring for risks factors for common problems such as frailty, depression, and delirium. Continuity of care is required at points where the older person is most vulnerable: on presentation to hospital and transition to residential care. A multidisciplinary approach is paramount, as is an understanding of the values and beliefs of the individual to plan for future care.

Online materials

Complete references for this chapter are available online at <http://www.oxfordmedicine.com>.

References

Agar, M., Currow, D.C., Shelby-James, T.M., Plummer, J., Sanderson, C., and Abernethy, A.P. (2008). Preference for place of care and place of death in palliative care: are these different questions? *Palliative Medicine*, 22, 787–795.

Agarwal, S., Banerjee, J., Baker, R., *et al.* (2012). Potentially avoidable emergency department attendance: interview study of patients' reasons for attendance. *Emergency Medicine Journal*, 29(12), e3.

American Geriatrics Society Expert Panel on the Care of Older Adults with Multimorbidity (2012). Guiding principles for the care of older adults with multimorbidity: an approach for clinicians. *Journal of the American Geriatrics Society*, 60(10), E1–E25.

Australian Department of Health and Ageing and National Health and Medical Research Council (2006). *Guidelines for a Palliative Approach in Residential Aged Care—enhanced version.* Canberra: ACT.

Australian Government Department of Health and Ageing (2011). *Guidelines for a Palliative Approach for Aged Care in the Community Setting—Best Practice Guidelines for the Australian Context.* Canberra: Australian Government Department of Health and Ageing.

Bellera, C.A., Rainfray, M., Mathoulin-Pélissier, S., *et al.* 2012. Screening older cancer patients: first evaluation of the G-8 geriatric screening tool. *Annals of Oncology*, 23(8), 2166–2172.

Beynon, T., Gomes, B., Glucksman, E., *et al.* (2011). How common are palliative care needs among older people who die in the emergency department? *Emergency Medicine Journal*, 28, 491–495.

Birch, D. and Draper, J. (2008). A critical literature review exploring the challenges of delivering effective palliative care to older people with dementia. *Journal of Clinical Nursing*, 17, 1144–1163.

Boockvar, K.S. and Meier, D.E. (2006). Palliative care for frail older adults: 'there are things I can't do anymore that I wish I could. . . . *Journal of the American Medical Association*, 296, 2245–2253.

British Geriatrics Society (2010). *Palliative and End of Life Care for Older People.* [Online] Available at: <http://www.bgs.org.uk/index.

php?option=com_content&view=article&id=1301:palliativecare&catid=155:eolc&Itemid=784>.

Carey, E.C., Covinsky, K.E., Li-Yung, L., Eng, C., Sands, L.P., and Walter, L.C. (2008). Prediction of mortality in community-living frail elderly people with long-term care needs. *Journal of the American Geriatrics Society*, 56, 68–75.

Clegg, A. and Young, J.B. (2011). Which medications to avoid in people at risk of delirium: a systematic review. *Age and Ageing*, 40, 23–29.

Close, J.C. and Lord, S.R. (2011). Fall assessment in older people. *BMJ*, 343, d5153.

Corbett, A., Husebo, B., Malcangio, M., *et al.* (2012). Assessment and treatment of pain in people with dementia. *Nature Reviews Neurology*, 8, 264–274.

Coventry, P.A., Grande, G.E., Richards, D.A., and Todd, C.J. (2005). Prediction of appropriate timing of palliative care for older adults with non-malignant life threatening disease: a systematic review. *Age and Ageing*, 34, 218–227.

Cusack, B.J. (2004). Pharmacokinetics in older persons. *American Journal of Geriatric Pharmacotherapy*, 2, 274–302.

Dalacorte, R.R., Rigo, J.C., and Dalacorte, A. (2011). Pain management in the elderly at the end of life. *North American Journal of Medical Sciences*, 3, 348–354.

Ellison, J.M., Kyomen, H.H., and Harper, D.G. (2012). Depression in later life: an overview with treatment recommendations. *Psychiatric Clinics of North America*, 35, 203–229.

Forero, R., McDonnell, G., Gallego, B., *et al.* (2012). A literature review on care at the end-of-life in the emergency department. *Emergency Medicine International*, 2012, 486516.

Gallegos-Orozco, J.F., Foxx-Orenstein, A.E., Sterler, S.M., and Stoa, J.M. (2012). Chronic constipation in the elderly. *American Journal of Gastroenterology*, 107, 18–25.

Geriatrics-Hospice and Palliative Medicine Work Group (2012). Report of the Geriatrics-Hospice and Palliative Medicine Work Group: American Geriatrics Society and American Academy of Hospice and Palliative Medicine leadership collaboration. *Journal of the American Geriatrics Society*, 60, 583–587.

Hauptman, P.J., Rich, M.W., Heidenreich, P.A., *et al.* (2008). The heart failure clinic: a consensus statement of the Heart Failure Society of America. *Journal of Cardiac Failure*, 14, 801–815.

Heuberger, R.A. (2011). The frailty syndrome: a comprehensive review. *Journal of Nutrition in Gerontology and Geriatrics*, 30, 315–368.

Higginson, I., Finlay, I., and Goodwin, D. (2003). Is there evidence that palliative care teams alter end-of-life experiences of patients and their caregivers? *Journal of Pain and Symptom Management* 25, 150–168.

Hines, S.E.A. (2009). *Effectiveness and Appropriateness of a Palliative Approach to Care for People with Advanced Dementia: A Systematic Review.* Brisbane: Dementia Collaborative Research Centres. Available at: <http://www.dementia.unsw.edu.au/index. php?option=com_dcrc&view=dcrc&layout=project&Itemid=101&pid=125>.

Klotz, U. (2009). Pharmacokinetics and drug metabolism in the elderly. *Drug Metabolism Reviews*, 41, 67–76.

Mangin, D., Heath, I., and Jamoulle, M. (2012). Beyond diagnosis: rising to the multimorbidity challenge. *BMJ*, 344, e3526.

Mangoni, A.A. and Jackson, S.H. (2004). Age-related changes in pharmacokinetics and pharmacodynamics: basic principles and practical applications. *British Journal of Clinical Pharmacology*, 57, 6–14.

Mcauliffe, L., Nay, R., O'Donnell, M., and Featherstonehaugh, D. (2009). Pain assessment in older people with dementia: literature review. *Journal of Advanced Nursing*, 65, 2–10.

Meagher, D., Adamis, D., Trzepacz, P., and Leonard, M. (2012). Features of subsyndromal and persistent delirium. *British Journal of Psychiatry*, 200, 37–44.

Mitchell, S.L., Miller, S.C., Teno, J.M., Davis, R.B., and Shaffer, M.L. (2010b). The Advanced Dementia Prognostic Tool: a risk score to estimate survival in nursing home residents with advanced dementia. *Journal of Pain and Symptom Management*, 639–651.

National Institute for Health and Clinical Excellence (2010). *Delirium: Diagnosis, Prevention and Management*. [Online] Available at: <http://www.nice.org.uk/guidance/cg103>.

Rigby, J., Payne, S., and Froggatt, K. (2010). Review: what evidence is there about the specific environmental needs of older people who are near the end of life and are cared for in hospices or similar institutions? A literature review. *Palliative Medicine*, 24, 268–285.

Rodriguez-Manas, L., Feart, C., Mann, G., *et al.* (2013). Searching for an operational definition of frailty: a Delphi method based consensus statement. The Frailty Operative Definition-Consensus Conference Project. *The Journals of Gerontology: Series A*, 68(1), 62–67.

Sampson, E.L., Ritchie, C.W., Lai, R., Raven, P.W., and Blanchard, M.R. (2005). A systematic review of the scientific evidence for the efficacy of a palliative care approach in advanced dementia. *International Psychogeriatrics*, 17, 31–40.

Schulz, R., Mendelsohn, A.B., Haley, W E., *et al.* (2003). End-of-life care and the effects of bereavement on family caregivers of persons with dementia. *The New England Journal of Medicine*, 349(20), 1936–1942.

Siddiqi, N., House, A.O., and Holmes, J.D. (2006). Occurrence and outcome of delirium in medical in-patients: a systematic literature review. *Age & Ageing*, 35, 350–364.

Sternberg, S.A., Wershof Schwartz, A., Karunananthan, S., Bergman, H., and Mark Clarfield, A. (2011). The identification of frailty: a systematic literature review. *Journal of the American Geriatrics Society*, 59, 2129–2138.

Sura, L., Madhavan, A., Carnaby, G., and Crary, M.A. (2012). Dysphagia in the elderly: management and nutritional considerations. *Clinical Interventions in Aging*, 7, 287–298.

Terret, C. (2008). How and why to perform a geriatric assessment in clinical practice. *Annals of Oncology*, 19, vii300–vii303.

The Australian Pain Society (2005). *Pain in Residential Aged Care Facilities-Management Strategies*. Sydney: The Australian Pain Society. Available at: <http://www.apsoc.org.au/resources. php>.

Trifiro, G. and Spina, E. (2011). Age-related changes in pharmacodynamics: focus on drugs acting on central nervous and cardiovascular systems. *Current Drug Metabolism*, 12, 611–620.

Wu, J. and Quill, T. (2011). Geriatric rehabilitation and palliative care: opportunity for collaboration or oxymoron? *Topics in Geriatric Rehabilitation*, 27, 29–35.

Yaar, M. and Gilchrest, B. A. (2001). Skin aging: postulated mechanisms and consequent changes in structure and function. *Clinics in Geriatric Medicine*, 17, 617–630.

Young, J. and Inouye, S.K. (2007). Delirium in older people. *BMJ*, 334, 842–846.

Zhao, K. X., Huang, C. Q., Xiao, Q., *et al.* (2012). Age and risk for depression among the elderly: a meta-analysis of the published literature. *CNS Spectrums*, 17, 142–154.

SECTION 17

Psychosocial and spiritual issues in palliative medicine

Spiritual issues in palliative medicine

Susan E. McClement

Introduction to spiritual issues in palliative medicine

The focus of palliative care is the whole person, including biopsychosocial, cultural, and *spiritu*al dimensions of patient needs. That end-of-life care should incorporate some consideration of spiritual issues is consistent with both the vision of Dame Cicely Saunders, champion of the hospice movement (Saunders, 2001), and the World Health Organization's (WHO's) emphasis on integrating spiritual aspects of patient care as part of its definition of palliative care (WHO, n.d.). People confronted by serious illness often draw on religious or spiritual beliefs (Hamel and Lysaught, 1994; Matthew et al., 1998; Ehman et al., 1999), Taylor posits that, 'if left un-addressed spiritual distress may stifle the opportunity for growth at the end of life, lead to poorly controlled symptoms, and result in an "unquiet death"' (Taylor, 2001, p. 395). Clearly, such outcomes are inconsistent with the aims and goals of palliative medicine.

The burgeoning literature examining the topic of spirituality within health care in general, and within palliative care in particular, underscores the notion that attending to patients' spiritual care needs is a vital part of providing optimal palliative care (Chiu, 2004; Chochinov and Cann, 2005; Sinclair et al., 2006a). Competencies for spiritual care have been developed (Baldacchino, 2006); guidance on how to discuss religious and spiritual concerns with dying patients has been published; courses on spirituality are becoming more common in medical schools in the United States; and chapters devoted to spirituality are included within authoritative palliative medicine and nursing textbooks (Ferrell et al., 2001; Cassidy and Davies, 2003; Strang and Strang, 2006). Yet health-care providers frequently report that they feel ill equipped to provide spiritual care at the end of life and wrestle with many questions and uncertainties. What is spiritual care? What is spiritual suffering? Who should provide spiritual care? How is a spiritual assessment conducted? What are some spiritual interventions for end of life care? What are some future research directions in the area of spiritual care? Answers to these questions form the basis of this chapter (see Chapters 2.1, 4.4 and 7.4).

What is spirituality?

An ancient Chinese proverb reminds us that, 'the beginning of wisdom is to call things by their proper name' (Good Reads, 2014). Such wisdom presupposes conceptual clarity. To date, such clarity concerning spirituality remains elusive. Increased secularization of society has resulted in a shift from the traditional explicitly religious meaning given to spirituality (Cassidy and Davies, 2003; Strang and Strang, 2006). Numerous definitions of spirituality exist in the literature such that the concept of spirituality in relation to health research has been plagued by definitional ambiguity (Sinclair et al., 2006a). In an effort to address this issue, key stakeholders participated in a Consensus Conference aimed at improving the quality of spiritual care as a dimension of palliative care. The definition crafted at that conference defined spirituality within the health care context as 'the aspect of humanity that refers to the way individuals seek and express meaning and purpose, and the way they experience their connectedness to the moment, to self, to others, to nature, and to the significant or sacred' (Puchalski et al., 2009, p. 887).

The Consensus Conference definition of spirituality appears to reflect dying patients' perspectives of this concept. The empirical work in this area, though limited, is instructive. A qualitative study conducted by Chao and colleagues examining the essence of spirituality in a sample of terminally ill Buddhist and Christian patients ($N = 6$) identified four broad thematic areas: (1) communion with self (self-identity, wholeness, inner peace), (2) communion with others (love, reconciliation), (3) communion with nature (inspiration, creativity), and (4) communion with a higher being (faithfulness, hope, gratitude) (Chao et al., 2002).

Grant and colleagues identified spiritual issues and needs in a sample of patients with advanced cancer ($N = 13$) and advanced non-malignant disease ($N = 7$) from a variety of religious backgrounds. Content analysis of qualitative interviews revealed three main spiritual issues of concern to patients. These included (1) searching for meaning and identity within the illness experience; (2) searching for peace of mind, and freedom from a pervasive fear of dying; and (3) searching for a guide (e.g. nurse or physician) to help them make sense of what was happening as death drew near (Grant et al., 2004). Being treated as an individual and feeling valued and affirmed by their health-care provider were behaviours that helped address patients' spiritual care needs.

Smith-Stoner's qualitative survey examining end-of-life preferences for atheists ($N = 88$) evaluated the relevance of a threefold definition of spirituality that included domains related to the intrapersonal, interpersonal, and interconnectedness with the natural world (Smith-Stoner, 2007). The intrapersonal domain speaks to the importance these individuals place on finding meaning in their lives. Interpersonally, atheists identified the importance of maintaining connection with family and friends. Interconnectedness with the natural world concerns maintaining a connection with the natural world through spending time outdoors or with animals.

The notion of interconnectedness identified in studies conducted by Chao et al. (2002), Grant et al. (2004), and Smith-Stoner (2007) is consistent with Burkhardt and Jacobson's (2000) observation that, 'spirituality is known and experienced in relationships' (p. 95). The notions of communion and connectedness underscore the importance of 'relationship' in the spiritual well-being of patients, and the salience of spiritual care interventions that promote such connectedness.

Spirituality and religion

The term spirituality is sometimes used synonymously (and mistakenly) in place of the term religion (Schmidt and Mauk, 2004). Religion is typically equated with an organized system of beliefs, rituals, and practices an individual identifies with, which includes a relationship with a divine being. Religion may or may not be part of a person's spirituality (Smith, 2006), though spirituality is always part of a larger context, expressed within culture, religion, and/or society (Health Care Chaplaincy, 2012). A comparison of the characteristics associated with religion and spirituality identified by Robinson and colleagues (Robinson et al., 2003) is detailed in Table 17.1.1.

Some authors object that describing religion in terms of what it does is functionalist, reductionist, and implies negative attitudes towards religious belief (Clarke, 2006). Our purpose in seeking to distinguish between these two terms has no such nefarious purpose. Clinicians need to be aware of these related concepts because of the relative importance each may play in the lives of their patients. For example, research reviewed by Marler and Hadaway indicates that some patients see themselves as both spiritual and religious (Marler and Hadaway, 2002). Other patients who are religious may express their spirituality through identification and involvement within a particular religion. Other patients may claim to be highly spiritual, yet not religious. For these individuals, an important common denominator appears to be the notion of 'transcending the commonplace and searching their soul for deeper meaning' (Schmidt and Mauk, 2004, p. 3).

The concepts of spirituality and religion are also important because of their impact on health outcomes, though the exact mechanism through which this occurs remains unclear. Research suggests that religion and spirituality play a positive role in individuals coping with cancer and human immunodeficiency virus

(HIV) (Baider et al., 1999; Nelson et al., 2002). Studies among advanced cancer patients report that spiritual well-being and meaning are important buffers against hopelessness, depression, and desire for hastened death (Breitbart et al., 2000; Nelson et al., 2002; McClain et al., 2003). Ai and colleagues demonstrated that secular reverence—the ability for patients to experience deep respect, love, and the sublime in their relationships with others and nature—predicted shorter hospital stays following coronary bypass surgery after controlling for other key variables. Religious reverence showed no such impact on length of stay (Ai et al., 2011). These findings underscore the importance of understanding the various dimensions of spirituality and how interventions can address unmet needs in this area.

Spirituality and patient perspectives

Do terminally ill patients and those with life-threatening illnesses want health-care providers to be attuned to spiritual needs? Public opinion and empirical literature suggest that such attention would be welcomed by at least some patients. A Gallup survey (Gallup International Institute, 1997) examining spiritual beliefs and the dying process ($N = 1200$) indicated that in addition to turning to family (81%), close friends (61%), and clergy (36%) for companionship and support at the end of life, 30% of respondents would look to doctors for such support. Forty per cent of respondents indicated that it would be very important to have a physician who was spiritually attuned to them if they were dying.

King and Bushwick conducted a cross-sectional survey of family practice adult inpatients at two hospitals in the United States ($N = 203$). Though limitations of the study include patient homogeneity and variations in regional religiosity, the findings revealed that 77% of patients felt that physicians should consider patients' spiritual needs, and 37% of patients wanted their physicians to discuss religious beliefs with them more frequently. Of note is the finding that 68% of the patients in the study reported that their physician never discussed religious beliefs with them (King and Bushwick, 1994).

Ehman and colleagues explored the acceptability of physicians asking patients if they have spiritual or religious beliefs that would influence their medical decisions if they became gravely ill. Questionnaires were completed by a convenience sample of 177 ambulatory pulmonary outpatients, half of whom described themselves as religious, and 90% of whom believed that prayer may sometimes influence recovery from an illness. Forty-five per cent of respondents indicated that religious beliefs would influence their medical decisions in the context of grave illness. Ninety-four per cent of individuals with such beliefs agreed or strongly agreed that physicians should ask them whether they have these beliefs

Table 17.1.1 Concepts of religion and spirituality

Religion	Spirituality
Focused in institutions	Not institutionally bound
Concerned with defining orthodoxy and orthopraxy	
Meaning transmitted through doctrine and stories of the community	Concerned with discovery of meaning in the context of the level individual
May provide a motivational and disciplined framework for spiritual growth	Concerned with self-directed spiritual growth

Source: Data from Robinson, S., et al., *Spirituality and the practice of healthcare*, Palgrave McMillan, Basingstoke, UK, Copyright © 2003.

if they become gravely ill. Two-thirds of patients welcomed the idea of discussing these issues with their doctor, while nearly one-quarter of respondents found this prospect objectionable (Ehman et al., 1999).

Smith-Stoner's research examining end-of-life preferences for atheists identified that spiritual care that acknowledges the patients as caring and moral, focuses on issues of self-acceptance, the importance of family and friends, and connection to nature is welcome. Conversely, spiritual care that fails to respect an atheist's non-belief, or included proselytizing or praying was unacceptable to these individuals and was experienced as a violation of boundaries (Smith-Stoner, 2007).

Not all research regarding patients' attitudes towards spiritual dimensions of care is quite so definitive. A comparative qualitative study conducted by Murray and colleagues that explored the spiritual needs of people dying of lung cancer ($N = 20$) and heart failure ($N = 20$) found the extent to which patients wish to have spiritual care incorporated into their health care was unclear (Murray et al., 2004). Some patients, though in need of spiritual support, either did not see the provision of such support within the purview of the health professional or worried about burdening 'busy' professionals with this issue. That spiritual needs may not be readily expressed speaks to the importance of health-care providers creating a climate wherein patients feel comfortable to discuss spiritual care issues should they wish to do so.

Spiritual pain and existential suffering

The Tibetan Book of the Living and Dying (Rinpoche, 2002) notes that:

> Often we forget that the dying are losing their whole world: their house, their job, their relationships, their body, and their mind—they're losing everything. All the losses we could possibly experience in life are joined together in one overwhelming loss when we die. (p. 176)

Multiple spiritual issues arise in the wake of being diagnosed with a life-threatening illness. Patients, confronted with mortality, limitations, and loss, wrestle with questions about their life's purpose and meaning amidst suffering. But what is suffering? Cassell defined suffering as the state of distress brought about by an actual or perceived threat to the integrity or continued existence of the whole person. Suffering is 'an anguish that is experienced, not only as a pressure to change, but as a threat to our composure, our integrity, and the fulfillment of our intentions' (Cassell, 1991, p. 231).

The Concise Oxford Dictionary defines suffering as 'to undergo, experience, be subjected to (pain loss, grief, defeat, change, punishment wrong, etc.)' (Sykes, 1982, p. 1066). A central notion in this definition is that those who suffer submit (or are forced to submit) to a particular set of circumstances outside of their control. Such a situation has the potential to seriously erode one's autonomy (Younger, 1995), and foster hopelessness and loss of control.

Strang and Strang's study of hospital chaplains', palliative care physicians', and pain specialists' definitions of the term existential pain suggests that the term is used as a metaphor for suffering (Strang and Strang, 2002). This acknowledges that suffering can include physical pain and the reciprocal interaction between somatic pain and existential suffering. Suffering based on a perception of lost autonomy and control may express itself in patient requests for death hastening measures. McClain and colleagues demonstrated significant negative correlations between spiritual well-being and desire for hastened death ($r = -0.51$), hopelessness ($r = -0.68$), and suicidal ideation ($r = -0.41$) (McClain et al., 2003). These findings suggest that spiritual well-being may offer some protection against end-of-life despair based on the additional findings that depression was significantly correlated with desire for hastened death in patients will low spiritual well-being ($r = 0.40$) but not in those high in spiritual well-being ($r = 0.20$).

Research by Chochinov and colleagues also demonstrates the salience of existential issues as they affect the wish to go on living in the face of a progressing terminal illness. Examination of the concurrent influences on the will to live in a sample of 189 end-stage cancer patients revealed that physical issues played a secondary role to existential, psychiatric, and social variables, all of which were highly correlated with the will to live. Stepwise regression modelling was conducted to examine the relationship between will to live and patient characteristics. Hopelessness, burden to others, and dignity entered into the final model, demonstrating the profound influence of existential variables on patient outlook in the context of terminal illness (Chochinov et al., 2005b). Given their prominent influence on will to live amongst patients nearing death, health-care providers are well advised to more fully appreciate their importance.

Providing spiritual care: who, me?

Glass and colleagues note that 'responding to the spiritual needs of patients and families is not solely the domain of the chaplain, clergy, or other officially designated professionals. All members of the health care team share the responsibility of identifying and being sensitive to spiritual concerns' (Glass et al., 2001, p. 40). Numerous barriers to the provisions of spiritual care at the end of life have been identified in the literature. In their qualitative study with physicians ($N = 17$) at a university-based hospital, Chibnall and colleagues identified (a) the marginalization and devaluing of psychosocial and spiritual care during medical training, (b) lack of safe and supportive environment in which to discuss issues of loss and death, (c) time demands and busy clinical schedules, and (d) lack of training and skill regarding communication with patients about existential issues as significant barriers (Chibnall et al., 2004). Lack of training in spiritual assessment and care has also been identified by nurses as barriers to providing spiritual care to patients (Oldnall, 1996).

Research conducted by Sinclair and colleagues provides clinicians with a pragmatic yet empirically based framework for integrating spiritual care into routine bedside clinical care (Sinclair et al., 2012). A qualitative ethnographic study informed by the perspectives of palliative care leaders and front-line clinicians elicited five major categories of skills essential to the provision of spiritual care. These 'five senses' of spiritual care include (1) hearing: listening intuitively; (2) sight: seeing soulfully; (3) speech: taming the tongue; (4) touch: physical means of spiritual care; and (5) presence: the essence of spiritual care.

Health-care providers may assume that issues of spiritual care are best left to clergy or other types of spiritual leaders. Clearly if the results of a spiritual assessment indicate the need for further specialized care, or specific information related to religion, referrals to chaplains and clergy are warranted (Taylor, 2001). The literature, however, suggests that health-care providers should be able to respond to most of the questions posed to chaplains. In a Swedish national survey of hospital chaplains, religious questions accounted for only 8% of the questions regularly posed to them. Other questions concerned meaning, death and dying, pain and illness, and relationships.

McSherry and Ross caution that health-care providers cannot assume either that all patients have spiritual needs that require attention all of the time, or that they will look to health-care professionals to help meet these needs (McSherry and Ross, 2002). Thus the health-care team must make some determination regarding the extent to which the patient is desirous of their involvement regarding spiritual care issues. Inevitably, it is the clinician's own comfort level with providing spiritual care that will dictate their involvement in it. Palliative care clinicians may have palliative care expertise, but are not necessarily specialists in spiritual assessment and caregiving. It has been suggested that the provision of good spiritual care is dependent on the clinician's awareness of a spiritual dimension in his or her own life, honed communication skills (Tulsky, 2005), and the ability to establish a trusting relationship with patients, and drawing on one' own life experience and maturity (Pronk, 2005). Owing to differing spiritual or religious needs of both patient and caregiver, there will be individuals for whom one cannot provide spiritual care, but other members of the interdisciplinary team may be able to do so. Thus, an important part of spiritual care involves each member of the team recognizing their own limitations and that the needs of the terminally ill require multiple sets of skill and knowledge that may not be present in any one individual (Victoria Hospice Society, 1998; Walter, 2002).

In addition to being aware of the spirituality of their patients, the literature also suggests the importance of care providers being aware of their own spirituality. Kearney suggests that such awareness leads to healthier team functioning and ultimately better patient care (Kearney, 2000). There has been minimal research examining how health-care professionals experience spirituality personally or collectively in the work place. A notable exception is the ethnographic study conducted by Sinclair and colleagues that explored the collective spirituality of an interdisciplinary palliative care team (Sinclair et al., 2006b). The study involved face-to-face interviews and focus groups conducted with 20 participants to explore what members of the interdisciplinary team felt about their own spirituality, and how that related to the care they provided to patients. Content analysis of interview transcripts revealed that participants viewed spirituality as something inherently relational, consisting of wholeness, meaning, and personal journeying. The common goals, values, and belonging experienced by members of the palliative care team contributed to their experience of collective spirituality, which was then was manifest in clinical work through small daily acts of kindness and love, embedded within routine acts of caring. The kindness and respect or 'care tenor' (Chochinov et al., 2002b) that accompany these routine acts of caring are much more than mere niceties. Chochinov and colleagues' programmatic research examining dignity in end-of-life care demonstrates that health-care providers' attitudes and behaviours are integral in bolstering the dignity of dying patients (Chochinov et al., 2002a, 2005a, 2006; Hack et al., 2004; Chochinov, 2012).

Spiritual assessment

Naming and acknowledging spiritual distress allows for a greater awareness of what the patient is experiencing and thus increases possibilities for resolution. Such acknowledgment presupposes that clinicians be able to evaluate spiritual well-being in the patients for whom they are caring. Owing to the sensitive and personal nature of spirituality, prefacing the spiritual assessment with an acknowledgment of the sensitivity of the questions as well as the need for the assessment are important in setting the tone for the conversation to follow. Suggestions regarding how clinicians might preface the spiritual assessment with patients have been published (Maugens, 1996). To the extent that a patient's physiological status will permit it, base-line spiritual assessment data is typically collected from patients at the time of admission to hospital or hospice. Far from being a one-off assessment, continuous evaluation of spiritual care needs should occur.

A variety of models for spiritual assessment exist in the literature. Many of these involve the use of direct open-ended questioning. Maugens recommends the mnemonic SPIRIT as a way of structuring spiritual inquiry (Maugens, 1996). The S in SPIRIT stands for spiritual belief system that is the person's religious affiliation. P stands for personal spirituality and includes the person's spiritual views shaped by a person's unique life experiences. I stands for integration and involvement with a spiritual community and speaks to the importance of assessing the patient's involvement in spiritual communities and other supportive spiritual groups. R relates to ritualized practices and restrictions that individuals embrace as part of their lifestyle that may influence health. I refers to implications for medical care and is concerned with how spiritual beliefs and practices may shape the patient's participation in health care. T stands for terminal events planning and reminds the clinician about the importance of assessing patients' end-of-life concerns.

Puchalski and Romer offer the mnemonic 'FICA' for remembering four components to cover during a spiritual assessment (Puchalski and Romer, 2000). FICA stands for faith or beliefs (e.g. 'What is your faith or belief?'), importance and influence (e.g. 'What role do your beliefs play in regaining your health?'), community (e.g. 'Are you part of a spiritual or religious community?'), and address (e.g. 'How should this issues be addressed by health-care providers?'). Borneman and colleagues conducted a descriptive exploratory study to clinically evaluate the feasibility and usefulness of the FICA assessment tool in an ethnically diverse sample of 76 patients with a variety of cancer diagnoses drawn from an ambulatory medical oncology clinic. The authors found the FICA to be a feasible and effective measure of spirituality, tapping aspects of patients' lives related to spiritual support such as hope, meaning, and relationships (Borneman et al., 2010).

Ferszt and colleagues developed an approach to spiritual assessment that examines the areas of connection, meaning and joy, strength, and comfort. Questions asked within each of these areas of life are designed to serve as a springboard to conversation with the patient and uses language that is accessible and comfortable for clinicians and patients (Ferszt et al., 2001). These questions are summarized in Table 17.1.2.

Many of the approaches to conducting a spiritual assessment described in the literature use a qualitative approach to gathering information from the patient. Paper and pencil questionnaires

Table 17.1.2 Spiritual Assessment Tool

Area of assessment	Related questions
Connection	Who are the persons or communities you look to for support? What role do they have in your care
	Do you have an image of a power greater than yourself?
	Has your life situation now affected your feelings about yourself, your faith, or your relationships?
Meaning and joy	What has been most important in your life?
	What are you most thankful for?
	What makes or has made you happy?
	What do you feel the proudest of in your life?
Strength and comfort	Is there anything that is comforting to you now?
	What helped you get through difficult times in the past?
	Who or what is your source of strength now?
Hope and concerns	Is there anything that you hope for?
	Is there anything that feels unfinished?

Reproduced from McSherry, W. and Ross, L., Dilemmas of spiritual assessment: Considerations for nursing practice, *Journal of Advanced Nursing*, Volume 38, Issue 5, pp. 479–488, Copyright © 2002, with permission from John Wiley & Sons, Inc. All Rights Reserved.

to elicit information about spirituality also exist that may serve as a means of identifying and codifying patients' spiritual status, needs, and resources (Taylor, 2001). Such tools are not designed to replace interaction between patient and health-care provider, but rather to facilitate ongoing assessment and communication regarding spiritual care issues.

No single assessment approach, whether qualitative or quantitative, is likely to be ideal in all situations. An assessment method that works well with one client may be inappropriate with another. The ideal assessment tool for use in practice will be 'easy to use, flexible and take little time to assess the spiritual state of patients at different times and in different situations' (Catterall et al., 1998, p. 4).

Spiritual care interventions for end-of-life care

Both general and specific spiritual care interventions are identified in the literature (see Chapter 5.6). Arguably, palliative care in and of itself is a general intervention aimed at improving patients' quality of life, enhancing well-being, and reducing suffering. This finding was demonstrated in a study conducted by Cohen and colleagues of 88 patients admitted to five palliative care units in two distinct regions of Canada from whom scores on the McGill Quality of Life Scale were collected on admission and 1 week later. Qualitative data concerning patient changes in quality of life since admission to palliative care were also collected. The findings from this study indicated improved patient physical, psychological and existential well-being following admission to the palliative care unit, as well as a sense of deeper spiritual awareness (Cohen et al., 2001).

Kissane and associates assert that demoralization syndrome, with its attendant hopelessness and loss of meaning represents an important expression of existential distress in palliative care patients (Kissane et al., 2001). They advocate a broad range of approaches for the hopelessness, loss of meaning, and existential distress palliative patients may experience. These include (a) providing continuity of care and active symptom management, (b) exploring patients' attitudes toward hope and meaning in life, (c) balancing support for grief with promotion of hope, (d) fostering the search for a renewed purpose and role in life, (e) using cognitive therapy to reframe negative beliefs, f) involving pastoral care for spiritual support, (g) promoting supportive relationships and use of volunteers, (h) enhancing family functioning by conducting family meetings, and (i) reviewing the goals of care in multidisciplinary team settings. Preliminary reports regarding the validation of the Demoralization Scale have been published (Kissane, 2004); however, future research is needed to examine the feasibility and efficacy of the various interventions to manage demoralization syndrome.

Cole and Pargament developed a pilot psychotherapy programme of individuals with cancer that explored important existential issues identified to be important in those facing a life-threatening illness: control, identify, relationships, and meaning. Preliminary findings suggest that the majority of participants ($N = 10$) indicated they preferred to participate in this type of programme over others that did not contain a spiritual focus (Cole and Pargament, 1999).

Breitbart and associates have utilized meaning-centred group psychotherapy (MCGP) in ambulatory advanced cancer patients ($N = 90$). Using a combination of instruction, discussion, and experiential exercises, this eight-session group intervention aims to help patients sustain or enhance a sense of meaning and purpose in their lives and to optimize each group member's remaining life span. Patients with advanced solid tumour cancers were randomly assigned to either MCGP or supportive group psychotherapy (SGP). Measures of spiritual well-being, meaning, hopelessness, desire for death, optimism/pessimism, depression, anxiety, and overall quality of life were measured at baseline, upon completion of the 8-week intervention, and 2 months after completion. Compared to those in the SGP group, patients who participated in MCGP demonstrated significantly greater improvements on all outcome measures, suggesting that MCGP is a potentially beneficial intervention that can bolster advanced cancer patients' emotional and spiritual well-being (Breitbart et al., 2004).

Chochinov and colleagues' programmatic work (Chochinov et al., 2002a, 2002b, 2005a; Hack et al., 2004; Chochinov, 2012) examining dignity in the terminally ill has resulted in an empirically derived model of dignity towards the end of life, and the development of a therapeutic intervention called dignity therapy (Chochinov et al., 2005a; Chochinov, 2012) that targets depression and suffering along with enhancing palliative patients' sense of purpose, meaning, and will to live. A more extensive discussion of dignity therapy and the role of dignity in improving quality of life in terminal illness can be found Chapter 5.6.

Directions for future research

Although research from a variety of disciplines has enhanced our understanding about the connections between spirituality and health, many questions remain unanswered. Owing to its subjective, experiential, contextualized nature, some would argue that spirituality is not amenable to definition or measurement. This does not mean, however, that spirituality cannot be examined empirically. A methodological approach that honours the subjective meaning and experience of the individual within given historical, social, and cultural contexts can be realized through the use of qualitative research methods (Streubert and Carpenter, 1999). For researchers wishing to operationalize and measure spirituality, however, conceptual ambiguity is highly problematic, because approaches to measurement of a given construct follow conceptual decisions (Kristjanson, 1992). Incongruencies in conceptual and operational definitions threaten the validity of the research and pose significant challenges in the development of appropriate spiritual outcomes measures.

A recent survey of spiritual care needs of hospitalized children and their families found that quality of spiritual care was wanting, underscoring the need for ongoing research with this patient population (Feudtner et al., 2003). Future work in this area might include an explication of the spiritual care needs and preferences of hospitalized paediatric and adolescent patients and their parents.

Research points to health-care providers feeling inadequately prepared to address the spiritual concerns of patients, and in need of ongoing education in matters of spiritual care (McSherry and Ross, 2002). The optimal timing, nature, duration, and outcomes of such educational intervention need further examination. Walter asserts that the language or discourse of spirituality and spiritual care is largely restricted to the English-speaking world (Walter, 2002). Accordingly, the search for spirituality in health care has been cast in terms of primarily an Anglo-American debate (Pronk, 2005). Such an approach fails to encompass different notions of spirituality, as understood in many world religions (Markham, 1998). Given that we live and provide palliative care in a multicultural context, research is needed with diverse populations that will broaden our understanding of the relationships between spirituality and culture and the spiritual care concepts and issues that are salient to different constituencies (Chochinov and Cann, 2005).

The provision of spiritual care is a multidisciplinary endeavour (Victoria Hospice Society, 1998). This requires that clinicians and researchers come together to share their perspectives regarding spiritual care and jointly identify fruitful areas of collaborative investigation. There is increasing awareness of the need for palliation of individuals living with illnesses other than cancer (Addington-Hall et al., 2001). Expanding the focus of spiritual care research to include individuals with life-threatening illness apart from cancer is thus indicated.

Finally, a basic tenet of palliative care is that the patient and family constitute the unit of care (Ferrell et al., 2001). Yet, little is known regarding the role that spirituality plays in affecting bereavement outcomes for family members. Retrospective research and prospective cohort studies indicate that the outcome of bereavement is affected by religious belief (Lauer et al., 1989; Rosik, 1989; McIntosh et al., 1993), suggesting that the absence of such belief may be a risk factor for delayed or complicated grief. Ongoing research is needed to examine the extent to which strong beliefs may be a proxy for better adjustment and less psychological distress in the bereavement period. Such work may help to identify those family members who having difficulty in adjusting following the patient's death.

Conclusion

In defining palliative care, the WHO emphasizes that the control pain, of other symptoms, and of psychological social and spiritual problems is paramount (WHO, 2002). Patients experiencing life-threatening illnesses want and need meaning, perhaps more than at any other time in their lives. Thus spiritual care is an aspect of palliative care that must not be undervalued. Attending to the spiritual needs of palliative care patients may provide them with the opportunity 'to find meaning in the midst of suffering and to have the opportunity for love, compassion, and partnership in their final journey' (Puchalski et al., 2004, p. 711).

References

Addington-Hall, J. and Higginson, I.J. (eds.) (2001). *Palliative Care for Non-Cancer Patients*. Oxford: Oxford University Press.

Ai, A., Wink, P., and Shearer, M. (2011). Secular reverence predicts shorter hospital length of stay among middle-aged and older patients following open-heart surgery. *Journal of Behavioral Medicine*, 34, 532–541.

Baider, L., Russack, S., Perry, S., *et al.* (1999). The role of religious and spiritual beliefs in coping with malignant melanoma: an Israeli sample. *Psycho-Oncology*, 8, 27–35.

Baldacchino, D. (2006). Nursing competencies for spiritual care. *Journal of Clinical Nursing*, 15, 885–896.

Borneman, T., Ferrell, B., and Puchalski, C. M. (2010). Evaluation of the FICA tool for spiritual assessment. *Journal of Pain and Symptom Management*, 40, 163–173.

Breitbart, W., Gibson, C., Poppito, S., and Berg, A. (2004). Psychotherapeutic interventions at the end of life: a focus on meaning and spirituality. *Canadian Journal of Psychiatry*, 49, 366–372.

Breitbart, W., Rosenfeld, B., Pressin, H., *et al.* (2000). Depression, hopelessness, and desire for death in terminally ill patients with cancer. *Journal of the American Medical Association*, 284, 2907–2011.

Burkhardt, M. and Jacobson, M. (2000). Spirituality and health. In B. Dossey, L. Keegan, and G. Guzetaa (eds.) *Holistic Nursing: A Handbook for Practice* (3rd ed.), pp. 91–121. Gaithersburg, MD: Aspen.

Cassell, E. (1991). *The Nature of Suffering and the Goals of Medicine*. New York: Oxford University Press.

Cassidy, J. and Davies, D. (2003). Cultural and spiritual aspects of palliative medicine. In D. Doyle, G. Hanks, N. Cherny, and K. Calman (eds.) *Oxford Textbook of Palliative Medicine* (3rd ed.), pp. 955–957. Oxford: Oxford University Press.

Catterall, R., Cox, M., Greer, B., Sankey, J., and Griffiths, G. (1998). The assessment and audit of spiritual care. *International Journal of Palliative Nursing*, 4, 162–168.

Chao, C., Chen, C., and Yen, M. (2002). The essence of spirituality of terminally ill patients. *Journal of Nursing Research*, 10, 237–244.

Chibnall, J., Bennet, M., Videen, S., Duckro, P., and Miller, D. (2004). Identifying barriers to psychosocial spiritual care at the end of life: a physician group study. *American Journal of Hospice and Palliative Medicine*, 21, 419–426.

Chiu, L. (2004). An integrative review of the concepts of spirituality in the health sciences. *Western Journal of Nursing Research*, 26, 405–428.

Chochinov, H.M. (2012). *Dignity Therapy: Final Words for Final Days*. New York: Oxford University Press.

Chochinov, H.M. and Cann, B.J. (2005). Interventions to enhance the spiritual aspects of dying. *Journal of Palliative Medicine*, 88(Suppl. 1), S103–115.

Chochinov, H.M., Hack, T., Hassard, T., Kristjanson, L.J., McClement, S., and Harlos, M. (2002a). Dignity in the terminally ill: a cross-sectional, cohort study. *The Lancet*, 360, 2026–2030.

Chochinov, H.M., Hack, T., Hassard, T., Kristjanson, L.J., McClement, S., and Harlos, M. (2005a). Dignity therapy: a novel psychotherapeutic intervention for patients near the end of life. *Journal of Clinical Oncology*, 23, 5520–5525.

Chochinov, H. M., Hack, T., Hassard, T., Kristjanson, L. J., McClement, S., and Harlos, M. (2005b). Understanding the will to live in patients nearing death. *Psychosomatics*, 46, 7–10.

Chochinov, H.M., Hack, T., McClement, S., Kristjanson, L., and Harlos, M. (2002b). Dignity in the terminally ill: a developing empirical model. *Social Science & Medicine*, 54, 433–443.

Chochinov, H.M., Krisjanson, L.J., Hack, T.F., Hassard, T., McClement, S., and Harlos, M. (2006). Dignity in the terminally ill: revisited. *Journal of Palliative Medicine*, 9, 666–672.

Clarke, J. (2006). Religion and spirituality: a discussion paper about negativity, reductionism and differentiation in nursing texts. *International Journal of Nursing Studies*, 43, 775–785.

Cohen, S., Boston, P., Mount, B., and Porterfield, P. (2001). Changes in quality of life following admission to palliative care units. *Palliative Medicine*, 15, 363–371.

Cole, B. and Pargament, K. (1999). Re-creating your life: a spiritual/psychotherapeutic intervention for people diagnosed with cancer. *Psycho-Oncology*, 8, 395–407.

Ehman, J., Ott, B., Short, T., Ciampa, R., and Hansen-Flaschen, J. (1999). Do patients want physicians to inquire about their spiritual or religious beliefs if they become gravely ill? *Archives of Internal Medicine*, 159, 1803–1806.

Ferrell, B. and Coyle, N. (eds.) (2001). *Textbook of Palliative Nursing*. Oxford: Oxford University Press.

Ferszt, G., Teegan-Case, S., and Taylor, B. (2001). Spiritual assessment tool. In B. Poor and G. Poirrier (eds.) *End of Life Nursing Care*, pp. 175–187. London: Jones & Bartlett Publishers Inc.

Feudtner, C., Haney, J., and Dimmers, M. (2003). Spiritual care needs of hospitalized children and their families: a national survey of pastoral care providers' perceptions. *Pediatrics*, 111, e67–72.

Gallup International Institute (1997). *Spiritual Beliefs About the Dying Process*. Princeton, NJ: The George H. Gallup International Institute.

Glass, E., Cluxton, D., and Rancour, P. (2001). Principles of patient and family assessment. In B. Ferrell and N. Coyle (eds.) *Textbook of Palliative Nursing*, pp. 37–50. Oxford: Oxford University Press.

Good Reads (2014). *Confucius Quotes*. [Online]. Available at: <http://www.goodreads.com/quotes/106313>

Grant, E., Murray, S., Kendall, M., Boyd, K., Tilley, S., and Ryan, D. (2004). Spiritual issues and needs: perspectives from patients with advanced cancer and nonmalignant disease. A qualitative study. *Palliative & Supportive Care*, 2(4), 371–378.

Hack, T.F., Chochinov, H.M., Hassard, T., Kristjanson, L.J., McClement, S., and Harlos, M. (2004). Defining dignity in terminally ill cancer patients: a factor-analytic approach. *Psycho-Oncology*, 13, 700–708.

Hamel, H. and Lysaught, M. (1994). Choosing palliative care: do religious beliefs make a difference? *Journal of Palliative Care*, 10, 61–66.

Health Care Chaplaincy (2012). *Literature Review—Testing the Efficacy of Chaplaincy Care Executive Summary*. [Online] Available at: <http://www.healthcarechaplaincy.org/ userimages/doc/Templeton CFP/Testing_ the_Efficacy_of_Chaplaincy_Care-Literature_ Review_ and_References.pdf>.

Kearney, M. (2000). *A Place of Healing*. Oxford: Oxford University Press.

King, D. and Bushwick, B. (1994). Beliefs and attitudes of hospital inpatients about faith, healing and prayer. *Journal of Family Practice*, 39, 349–352.

Kissane, D.W. (2004). The demoralization scale: a report of its development and preliminary validation. *Journal of Palliative Care*, 20, 269–276.

Kissane, D.W., Clarke, D., and Street, A. (2001). Demoralization syndrome—a relevant psychiatric diagnosis for palliative care. *Journal of Palliative Care*, 17, 12–21.

Kristjanson, L.J. (1992). Conceptual issues related to measurement in family research. *Canadian Journal of Nursing Research*, 24, 37–52.

Lauer, M., Muilhern, R., Schell, M., and Camitta, B. (1989). Long term follow-up of parental adjustment following a child's death at home or hospital. *Cancer*, 63, 988–994.

Markham, I. (1998). Spirituality and the world faiths. In M. Cobb and V. Robshaw (eds.) *The Spiritual Challenge of Health Care*, pp. 73–87. Edinburgh: Churchill Livingstone.

Marler, P. and Hadaway, C. (2002). 'Being religious' or 'being spiritual' in America: a zero-sum proposition? *Journal for the Scientific Study of Religion*, 41, 289–300.

Matthew, D., McCullough, M., Larson, D., Koening, H., Sawyers, J., and Milano, M. (1998). Religious commitment and health status: a review of the research and implications for family medicine. *Archives of Internal Medicine*, 7, 118–124.

Maugens, T. (1996). The SPIRITual history. *Archives of Family Medicine*, 3, 129–137.

McClain, C., Rosenfeld, B., and Breitbart, W. (2003). Effect of spiritual well-being on end-of-life despair in terminally ill cancer patients. *The Lancet*, 361, 1603–1607.

McIntosh, D., Silver, R., and Wortman, C. (1993). Religion's role in adjustment to a negative life event: coping with the loss of a child. *Journal of Personality and Social Psychology*, 65, 812–821.

McSherry, W. and Ross, L. (2002). Dilemmas of spiritual assessment: considerations for nursing practice. *Journal of Advanced Nursing*, 38, 479–488.

Murray, S., Kendall, M., Boyd, K., Worth, A., and Benton, T. (2004). Exploring the spiritual needs of people dying of lung cancer or heart failure: a prospective qualitative interview study of patients and their carers. *Palliative Medicine*, 18, 39–45.

Nelson, C., Rosenfeld, B., Breitbart, W., and Balietta, M. (2002). Spirituality, religion and depression in the terminally ill. *Psychosomatics*, 43, 213–220.

Oldnall, A. (1996). A critical analysis of nursing: meeting spiritual needs of patients. *Journal of Advanced Nursing*, 23, 138–144.

Pronk, K. (2005). Role of the doctor in relieving spiritual distress at the end of life. *American Journal of Hospice and Palliative Care*, 22, 419–425.

Puchalski, C., Ferrell, B., Virani, R., *et al.* (2009). Improving the quality of spiritual care as a dimension of palliative care: the report of the Consensus Conference. *Journal of Palliative Medicine*, 12, 885–904.

Puchalski, C.M., Dorff, E., and Hendi, I. (2004). Spirituality, religion, and healing in palliative care. *Clinics in Geriatric Medicine*, 20, 689–714.

Puchalski, C.M. and Romer, A. (2000). Taking a spiritual history allows clinicians to understand patients more fully. *Journal of Palliative Medicine*, 3, 129–137.

Rinpoche, S. (2002). *The Tibetan Book of Living and Dying*. San Francisco, CA: Harper.

Robinson, S., Kendrick, K., and Brown, A. (2003). *Spirituality and the Practice of Healthcare*. Basingstoke: Palgrave McMillan.

Rosik, C. (1989). The impact of religious orientation in conjugal bereavement among older adults. *International Journal of Aging and Human Development*, 28, 251–260.

Saunders, C. (2001). The evolution of palliative care. *Journal of the Royal Society of Medicine*, 94, 430–432.

Schmidt, N. and Mauk, K. (2004). Spirituality as a life journey. In Mauk, K., and Schmidt, N. (eds.) *Spiritual Care in Nursing Practice*, pp. 2–19. Philadelphia, PA: Lippincott Williams & Wilkins.

Sinclair, S., Pereira, J., and Raffin, S. (2006a). A thematic review of the spirituality literature within palliative care. *Journal of Palliative Medicine*, 9, 464–478.

Sinclair, S., Raffin, S., Chochinov, H., Hagen, N.A., and McClement, S. (2012). Spiritual care: how to do it. *BMJ Supportive & Palliative Care*, 2(4) 319–327

Sinclair, S., Raffin, S., Pereira, J., and Guebert, N. (2006b). Collective soul: the spirituality of an interdisciplinary palliative care team. *Palliative & Supportive Care*, 4, 13–24.

Smith, A. (2006). Using the synergy model to provide spiritual nursing care in critical care settings. *Critical Care Nursing*, 26, 41–47.

Smith-Stoner, M. (2007). End-of-life preferences for atheists. *Journal of Palliative Medicine*, 10, 923–928.

Strang, S. and Strang, P. (2002). Questions posed to hospital chaplains by palliative care patients. *Journal of Palliative Medicine*, 5, 857–864.

Strang, S. and Strang, P. (2006). Spiritual care. In E. Bruera, I.J. Higginson, C. Ripamonti, and C. Von Gunten (eds.) *Textbook of Palliative Medicine*, pp. 1019–1028. London: Hodder Arnold.

Streubert, H. and Carpenter, D. (1999). *Qualitative Research in Nursing: Advancing the Humanistic Imperative*. Philadelphia, PA: Lippincott.

Sykes, J. (1982). *The Oxford Concise Dictionary*. Oxford: Clarendon Press.

Taylor, E.J. (2001). Spiritual assessment. In B. Ferrell and N. Coyle (eds.) *Textbook of Palliative Nursing*, pp. 379–406. Oxford: Oxford University Press.

Tulsky, J. (2005). Interventions to enhance communication among patients, providers, and families. *Journal of Palliative Medicine*, 8, S95–102.

Victoria Hospice Society (1998). Spiritual care. In *Medical Care of the Dying* (3rd ed.), pp. 534–537. Victoria, BC: Victoria Hospice Society.

Walter, T. (2002). Spirituality in palliative care: opportunity or burden? *Palliative Medicine*, 16, 133–139.

World Health Organization (2002). *National Cancer Control Programmes: Policies and Managerial Guidelines* (2nd ed.). Geneva: World Health Organization.

World Health Organization (n.d.). *WHO Definition of Palliative Care*. [Online]. Available at: <http://www.who.int/cancer/palliative/definition/en/>.

Younger, J. (1995). The alienation of the sufferer. *Advances in Nursing Science*, 17, 53–72.

Coping in palliative medicine

Simon Wein and Lea Baider

Introduction to coping in palliative medicine

Coping is a universal experience which ranges from coping with a rude clerk at the bank to all of the consequences of serious illness. The psychological literature has theorized extensively about coping in an attempt to conceptualize this common human trait. Although most coping is a day-to-day experience, researchers have developed theories and therapies to assist psychologists and palliative medicine health-care workers in managing their patients. The literature on coping comes from various disciplines hence there are many different ways to cope.

Coping in palliative medicine mitigates against anxiety, existential distress, physical discomfort, depression, anger, and the wish to die. Initially the literature looked at coping as simply overcoming stress, maintaining the status quo, and surviving. The literature also addressed failed coping, specifically coping styles that are not beneficial, such as anger. However in recent years, especially as applied to palliative medicine, researchers have emphasized and encouraged 'psychological growth' as a response to the stress.

Many research questions remain: what allows some people to cope better than others? Can coping be measured? What should be the goals of coping? Is coping the same in different areas of palliative medicine? How do different cultures cope differently?

This chapter will present various coping models in palliative medicine and show how eclectic, flexible, and highly individual coping can be and it will also address approaches to augment coping.

Definitions

Wai Man in an article about coping with death defined it as: 'a process by which a person deals with stress, solves problems or makes decisions'. And: 'stress is a particular relationship between a person and the environment that is appraised by the person as taxing or exceeding his or her resources and endangering his or her well-being' (Man, 2009).

Folkman and Moskowitz described coping as 'the thoughts and behaviours used to manage the internal and external demands of situations that are appraised as stressful' (2004). The situation is stressful because personally important goals and values are threatened, harmed, or lost. These assessments often elicit distressing and negative emotions. Carver and Connor-Smith describe coping as 'efforts to prevent or diminish threat, harm, and loss, or to reduce associated distress' (Carver and Connor-Smith, 2010).

It is important to note that often it is not just one stressor that precipitates a crisis but several that have accumulated, often in a short time, and exceeded the usual coping strategies.

Successful coping will see a reduction in the negative emotional response by either a change in self or in the stressor itself. Initially coping can be understood as a cognitive response—'How am I going to manage this problem?'—in order to regulate distressing emotions. Folkman et al. divided coping into two categories: (1) problem-focused coping (which is directed at removing, evading, or diminishing the impact of the stressor itself) and (2) emotion-focused coping (which aims to minimize the distress caused by the stressors, including meditation, crying, yelling, or avoidance). Often these two coping behaviours complement each other (Folkman et al., 1986).

The literature notes that coping is dynamic and fluctuating and each person may use a range of coping strategies and these strategies may change over time (Folkman and Moskowitz, 2004). Coping is an interactive, fluid, and dynamic process especially with friends and family.

Liao and Arnold emphasize that we should be sensitive to the question of what constitutes normal coping. 'Normal' is determined by both the individual and the culture. Conversely our own culture, psychology, and beliefs influence our judgements about 'normal' coping by the patient. They point out that successful coping reflects the balance between how important we think a particular life event is, and how we respond to the stressors (Liao and Arnold, 2006).

A major problem with coping is there is no gold standard of how to measure or assess it. Coyne and Gottlieb emphasize the limitations of standardized checklists or questionnaires currently used to assess coping. They observe that these screening or diagnostic tools often produce 'an incomplete and distorted picture of coping' because they are unable to measure the 'interactional dynamic' of stress and coping. Most of the tools have a lot of recall bias and give inconsistent results. They claim it is better to use semi-structured interviews, specific checklists for testing hypotheses, and diaries (Coyne and Gottlieb, 1996).

Concepts and theories

Specific theories have been developed to explain coping and make it operational for research and treatment. However, other psychological theories not specifically related to coping literature will be presented as they also help us to help our patients cope (Box 17.2.1).

Coping theory

Folkman et al. described two steps in the coping process. They observed that appraisal and coping are iterative processes in response to a stress. First an appraisal or assessment of the stressful situation is made, second a coping response is made—and then a re-appraisal, followed by a response and so forth. Thus the appraisal influences the coping and vice versa (Folkman et al., 1986). Along with Greer, Folkman subsequently expanded on this model by noting numerous factors needed to sustain psychological well-being during serious illness. These include personality (optimism, personal control), cognitive appraisal, goal-directed planning, and hope—all involve positive and negative feedback loops which are interactional (Folkman and Greer, 2009). Greer studied these concepts and looked at 62 women with non-metastatic breast cancer in terms of denial (avoidance), fatalism (stoic acceptance), and helplessness/hopelessness. They found that women who coped best, viewed the stresses not as threats but as challenges (Folkman and Greer, 1987).

In subsequent studies, Folkman and Moskowitz confirmed improved psychological coping by applying a three-stage intervention: (1) change the conditions from threat to challenge (by establishing meaning, aims and person control), (2) encourage productive behaviour to achieve goals (address loss of confidence, despair; start with small and concrete goals); and (3) maintain background positive mood (including control of physical symptoms; psychotherapy) (Folkman and Moskowitz, 2010).

Symbolic immortality

Lifton coined the expression 'symbolic immortality' through research on coping mechanisms of survivors of the Hiroshima atom bomb. He viewed 'symbol formation as a fundamental process of man's psychic life . . . a compelling universal urge'. Clearly it is through symbols that we communicate—be they words, music, images. Lifton, however, was not referring to the fixed symbols of society—flags and anthems. Rather he observed the ongoing process of creating new symbols for ourselves as we cope with the challenges of meaning-making. These symbols help us to cope with our mortality, though not as denial. A symbol of immortality helps us to cope with our personal death.

Lifton observed five activities of life which create symbols of immortality: (1) biological: having children ensures our continuity after death; (2) theological belief of life after death via the immortality of the soul or its resurrection; (3) creativity: in a real way Mozart and Rembrandt are alive today through their creations; (4) feeing part of eternal universe, most commonly through nature; (5) experiential transcendence where sense of time is lost: this symbol enables us to connect to a higher power or spirit and escape our earthly fate. All these activities provide tools with which to cope (Lifton, 1976).

Sense of coherence

Antonovsky developed the 'sense of coherence model' which is 'a global orientation that expresses the extent to which one has a

pervasive, enduring though dynamic feeling of confidence that one's internal and external environments are predictable and that there is a high probability that things will work out' (Antonovsky, 1979). This concept also underpins coping. He understood from his research that for certain individuals, no matter what terrible circumstances they had experienced (he had researched Holocaust survivors from the Second World War), they coped with life and thrived. His research indicated that the main variable was 'the way of looking at the world'.

A strong sense of coherence means that one responds to stressors with a conviction that life will continue to be meaningful and function in a predictable way—that it 'makes sense' and that tomorrow will be the same as today. One sees the future as reasonably predictable and this security helps one to cope with variables and unbidden stressors. Through his research, three components emerged: the ability for people to understand what happens around them, to what extent they were able to manage the situation on their own or through their social network, and the ability to find meaning in a given situation. These three elements, comprehensibility (cognitive), manageability (instrumental/behavioural), and meaningfulness (motivational), provide a sense of coherence (Eriksson and Lindstrom, 2005).

Personality

Personality is an essential part of our ability to cope. However, defining personality and making generalizations about personalities is problematic. Carver and Connor-Smith suggested that personality 'is the dynamic organization within the persons of the psychological and physical systems that underlie that person's patterns of actions, thoughts, and feelings' (Carver and Connor-Smith, 2010).

There are aspects of personality that are generalizable (part of the biology of human nature). Other aspects emphasize individual differences which have been describes in a five-factor personality model: extraversion (assertiveness, spontaneity, confidence, sociability), neuroticism (moodiness, anxiety, depression, vulnerability), agreeableness (friendly, helpful, empathic, inhibit negative feelings, maintenance of relationships), conscientiousness (planning, goal-making, persistence, reliability, impulse control, optimism), and openness-to-experience (curiosity, flexibility, imaginativeness, intellect) (Digman, 1990).

Challenges (such as threat to life or goals) become a stress when one's resources to manage are stretched or threatened. In terms of personality style extraversion, conscientiousness and openness respond to stressors as challenges and not threats. High neuroticism plus low conscientiousness predicts high stress levels and readily perceiving a stress as a threat (Digman, 1990).

Chochinov and colleagues studied neuroticism (which they defined as a trait with the tendency to experience psychological distress) as a variable in coping. They examined 211 patients towards the end of life and found a significant correlation between neuroticism and increased psychological and existential distress. Identifying the neurotic personality as a marker of poor coping, could help direct resources and be realistic about management goals, given that it is a life-long trait (Chochinov et al., 2006).

Resources and therapies

Applying these theories and concepts to augment coping requires practical items including patients' and carers' internal and external resources and therapeutic interventions by the staff.

Internal resources

Weisman writes with wisdom about coping (Box 17.2.2). In the chapter 'Hoping is Coping' (Weisman, 1979) he notes that most patients cope with anxiety and uncertainty using common-sense interpersonal and intrapersonal resources. He asks how do we judge 'good' coping? 'Good coping regardless of the medical outcome is clearly an extension of how well a patient coped in their healthier days' (Weisman, 1979). Resourceful people cope better because they do not restrict themselves in range of coping strategies whereas more rigid people are confined to a narrow range of tools, are less flexible, and find coping more difficult (Weisman, 1979).

Courage and fighting spirit

Courage is critical to coping. Courage is defined as being aware of the fear but facing the challenge anyway, whether one succeeds or not. If one is unaware of the fear it is uncertain whether that virtue was courage. Many factors contribute to a courageous response to a challenge—character, self-esteem, sense of purpose, culture, hope, love, faith, emotional support, past successes, and dignity (Wein, 2007).

Greer coined the phrase 'fighting spirit' as a coping strategy (Greer and Moorley, 1997). He characterized this as a determination not to give in, an optimism, having a knowledge of the illness, being active in treatment, and living as 'normal a life' as possible in the face of adversity. The utility of courage is to boost a 'fighting-spirit', to resuscitate morale and to enable one to cope.

Clinicians can help to augment courage with prudent inspiration, such as other patients' success stories, and by exploring with the patient previous challenges they have successfully overcome. It is often effective to say to the patient: 'I think you have been very courageous' for some small fear they overcame. The bottom line is to improve their self-esteem and belief in themselves.

Reminiscences

Reminiscences are memories that 'recall past events, feelings, and thoughts in order to facilitate pleasure, quality of life, or adaptation to present circumstances' (Parker, 1995). These memories may be long-forgotten experiences or events frequently recalled. Reminiscing may be dreams, reflections, meditations, art-therapy, talking-therapy, and psycho-analysis.

Reminiscing serves two functions: the first is as a pleasurable way of recalling significant life events, and by placing a perspective on and summing up one's life. The other function is to re-evaluate life with the intention of resolving and integrating past conflicts and finding new significance. The process of recounting the scene and recollected thought and memory helps to put it into a context

---

Box 17.2.2 Internal mechanisms of coping

- ◆ Hope
- ◆ Dignity
- ◆ Meaning
- ◆ Reminiscence
- ◆ Courage
- ◆ Fighting spirit
- ◆ Resilience.

---

to enable 'psychological growth'. Reminiscences can process the memory in a psychological-emotional (or spiritual) way (Butler, 1963, 1974; Parker, 1995). Reminiscences can be something one goes over and over, like an artist repainting the same scene again and again until he understands it.

However, not everyone chooses to reminisce, since for some people it is too painful. For others, however, reminiscence have been shown to help families bond or reconcile, even if temporarily, at difficult times by using common 'good' memories to help overcome differences (Butler, 1974).

Reminiscent-based theory and therapy has been described and studied (Haight, 1992; Wholihan, 1992; Haight et al., 2000). It is a cognitive therapy and has similarities to dignity therapy (Chochinov et al., 2011) and life narrative therapy (Viederman, 1983; Pickrel, 1989) which, by expressing and integrating experiences, has been shown to provide meaning, reduce depression, and reverse emotional withdrawal (Haight et al., 2000). Bohlmeijer and colleagues performed a meta-analysis of 25 controlled studies and concluded that reminiscence therapy enhance psychological well-being in older adults (Bohmeijer et al., 2007).

Hope

Dufault and Martocchio describe hope as 'a multidimensional dynamic life force characterized by a confident yet uncertain expectation of achieving a future good which, to the hoping person, is realistically possible and personally significant' (Dufault and Martocchio, 1985).

Using semi-structured interviews, Sachs et al. studied 22 terminally ill cancer patients with the aim of examining the relationship between hope and hopelessness. Positive interpersonal relationships enhanced hope, and uncontrolled physical pain increased hopelessness. They concluded that hope is associated with 'greater psychological and spiritual well-being' and 'more effective coping strategies' (Sachs et al., 2013).

Chochinov (2003) and McLement and Chochinov (2008) reviewed the literature and found 'hope in advanced cancer is a coping mechanism protecting patients from the experience of distress and suffering'. Several studies indicated that positive relationships, living in the moment, cognitive reframing of negative thoughts, and ritual exercises improve hope and thereby aid coping.

Chi noted a positive relationship between a higher level of hope and effective coping style. Hope, they concluded, was essential for coping with chronic stress of serious illness since it enables patients to accept death whilst still engaging in day-to-day living. Hopelessness was a stronger predictor of poor coping in the terminally ill as evidenced by suicidal ideation and desire for hastened death. They noted in their study that uncontrolled pain, disability, depression, and other symptoms caused a sense of hopelessness and poorer ability to cope with illnesses stressors (Chi, 2008).

Eclectic

An interesting qualitative study from Sand et al. analysed 20 non-religious people in Sweden and how they cope despite the threat of impending death. The findings showed that they coped using 'every means available' including cognitive, emotional, other people, animals, nature, a transcendental power, imagination, and magical thinking. The focus of the coping was to keep death at a respectable distance whilst seeking togetherness, involvement, hope, and continuance, as palliatives to the 'hurtful feelings' of dying (Sand et al., 2009).

Maybe this finding best describes the real-life way people cope—as best as they can, and with whatever tools work for them.

External resources and therapies

Many resources and therapies are available to help patients and their families cope (Boxes 17.2.3 and 17.2.4). Typically in a supportive and palliative care service this would include psychotherapy, psychopharmacology, spiritual, religious, social work, physiotherapy, occupational therapy, physical symptom control, and the various supportive and complementary therapies. These all assist coping and should be used in combination as suitable.

Therapeutic relationship

Weisman notes that, in order to maintain morale and facilitate coping, the treating clinicians must develop the trust and confidence of the patient and their family. Coping, he notes, at its most basic is getting from one problem to the next. He calls it 'the enduing and incessant process of coping' (Weisman, 1979). He advocates that the clinician invest in relationship building and that, in the context of a caring relationship, the clinician should enquire about how the patient copes: what problems has the illness created? How do you plan to deal with them? What do you do when faced with a problem? What usually happens? To whom do you turn when you need help? What has happened in the past when you asked for help? What kind of problems make you upset? (Weisman, 1979). Murray-Parkes contends that an important way we have of helping patients cope with cancer and other life-threatening illnesses is to offer frightened or grieving people a 'secure base', a relationship of respect and trust—with a person who has the time, knowledge, and willingness to remain involved—that will last them through the bad times; to explore the situation they face, share the feelings that arise, and review the implications of loss (Murray-Parkes, 1998).

Weisman also advises of the importance of honesty in coping with stress: 'More problems are solved by awareness and acceptance than by disavowal, avoidance and denial' (Weisman, 1979).

Weisman emphasizes that one cannot cope with the psychological, social, and spiritual stressors of a life-threatening illness if physical symptoms are not properly controlled. Meticulous care of physical suffering is critical to coping. This responsibility lies with the palliative medicine clinicians.

Meaning and dignity-based approaches

An important aspect of coping with stressors is the search for meaning. Greenstein and Breitbart (2000) describe a psychotherapy programme using meaning as a way of coping. Sessions focus on responsibility to self (reappraising the meaning of the problem) and others (survivors, family, legacy), creativity (artistic, work), transcendence, ascertaining one values, and understanding the role of goals—all as means of coping with terminal illness. The power of their programme is its didactic interactions together with experiential exercises.

Chochinov has taken the common concept of dignity, defined and studied it, and developed dignity therapy, a form of cognitive behavioural treatment (Chochinov et al., 2011). His research has shown 'the importance of self-perception and the way in which patients experience themselves to be seen or appreciated, as a powerful mediator of preservation of one's sense of dignity' (Chochinov et al., 2011). The principle is to help patients with a limited life-expectancy to identify values that are important to them. Transcripts of the interviews are prepared and returned to the patients who may then choose to pass on to family and loved ones. This has been shown to help patients cope by improving dignity, self-esteem, meaning, and reinforcing the will to live (see Chapter 5.6).

Information to enhance coping

McPherson et al. made a systematic review of the literature and found ten randomized controlled studies showed that information interventions (over and above usual care) such as audiotapes, pamphlets, and educational programmes improved factual recall, symptoms control, satisfaction, and use of health-care facilities (McPherson et al., 2001). However, the majority of studies showed no benefit on psychological measures. Nevertheless this is a useful activity to encourage coping (Johnson, 1986).

Spiritual care and religious coping and chaplaincy

Hanson studied 103 recipients (seriously ill patients and family carers) of spiritual care in a tertiary medical institution. The 237 spiritual care providers (clergy, family, health-care) provided 21 different types of spiritual care. They found that 87% of the recipients identified 'helped coping with the illness' as the key activity (Hanson et al., 2008).

Religious coping, as an item separate from spiritual coping, has been extensively studied and reviewed in the literature. Pargament et al. (2000) called religion 'a search for significance related to the sacred'. Religious coping responds to the triggering event by creating meaning and purpose, and by reappraising the values and goals of life. Religious strategies have been grouped as follows: spiritual, congregational, moral reframing, orientation to agency and control, and rituals. In a summary of the literature

---

Box 17.2.3 External resources

- Supportive and complementary therapies
- Magic and alternative therapies
- Psychopharmacology
- Psychotherapy
- Caregivers
- Volunteers
- Palliative care
- Religion.

Box 17.2.4 Therapies that assist coping in palliative medicine

- Meaning-based therapies
- Dignity therapy
- Cognitive behavioural therapy
- Psychopharmacology
- Supportive and complementary therapies: art, relaxation, music.

of the clinical use of religious coping, studies have shown up to 70–80% of patients use religion as a coping strategy, especially in cancer, HIV, and psychotic inpatients (Dull and Skokan, 1995; McClain et al., 2003).

Whilst it is not the role of the clinician to prescribe prayer or other religious practices to the patient, the clinician may refer them to a chaplain or faith-person to assist in coping. Pargament et al. developed a validated measure (RCOPE) for religious coping and showed that in hospitalized, elderly patients, better adjustment (stress-related growth, physical health, emotional health) was found in those who coped by using benevolent religious reappraisal and religious forgiveness/purification. Religious coping offered sense of meaning, comfort, control, and personal growth in face of life-threatening illnesses (Pargament et al., 2000).

Whilst most studies show benefit, some have revealed negative outcome of religious coping because of discontent with god, punishment, guilt, and disappointment with their congregations (Dull and Slokan, 1995; McClain et al., 2003). This together with the move away from formal religious adherence by young people in recent years, especially in Europe, in part explains the greater interest in spirituality, unaligned to formal religion (Pargament et al. 2000; Block, 2006). Tarashekwar et al. studied 170 patients using a structured interview and after controlling for sociodemographic and lifetime history of depression, found that greater use of positive religious coping was associated with better quality of life scores including existential well-being. Rarely, negative religious coping (anger at god, feelings of guilt, or a sense of community abandonment) actually lead to worse quality of life (Tarashekwar et al., 2006). Phelps et al. noted in a study of 345 patients with advanced cancer, that positive religious coping is more likely to be associated with receipt of intensive and more aggressive life-prolonging medical care near the end of life. The study was not designed to analyse the reasons (Phelps et al., 2009).

Positive psychology

Positive psychology prescribes the role of hope, wisdom, spirituality, courage, and responsibility in adapting to stress (Carver et al., 1994). However, Coyne and Tennen vigorously dispute the positive psychologists in cancer care whose claims go beyond achieving coping. Their paper examines and rejects the scientific basis for the claims that a fighting spirit prolongs life, that it influences immune function and cancer progression, and can be shown to contribute post-traumatic growth following serious illness. They carefully reject the scientific basis and therefore reject therapies which advocate these claims (Park et al., 1996; Coyne and Tennen, 2010).

Folkman and Moskowitz argue for the positive outcome of coping—that is, therapists should aim for more than holding (or returning to) the status quo. New life skills, perception of improved self-esteem, spiritual or religious transformation, deeper understanding of life, and improved social relationships are justifiable aims (Folkman and Moskowitz, 2000). They advocate research on how to better understand how people build and maintain positive 'coping' in face of stress. That is, how good can come out of bad (Lazarus, 1968).

However, Parker challenged the ultimate goal of happiness as 'mindless or tyrannical optimism' and 'unthinking positive psychology'. Coping does not necessarily mean happiness, and coping is not the equivalent of a positive psychological outcome. It is distinct, he claims. Coping, he suggests, is used in a narrow sense of 'returning to the mean', that is, to the pre-stress state (Parker, 2011).

Integrative medicine approaches

Many patients use complementary, supportive, and alternative therapies to help cope with their illnesses, so much so that many of the major cancer centres have incorporated these therapeutic options into their institutions in order to provide patients with this care and to supervise the types of therapies they are receiving. Studies have repeatedly shown that patients find therapies that include unproven, alternative, and magic help them cope better by providing a sense of control, better bedside manners, more trusting practitioners, and that the therapies fit in with their world-view and therefore provide meaning (Wein, 2000).

Burstein and colleagues looked at how psychological and physical factors influenced use of unproven therapies in early-stage breast cancer (Burstein et al., 1999). They found that initiation of unproven therapies after surgery was associated with a worse quality of life characterized by depression, fear of recurrence, lower sexual satisfaction, and more physical symptoms. Therefore, Holland editorialized that when a patient reveals use of unproven therapies the follow-up question should be how she or he is coping with the illness especially in terms of anxiety and depression (Holland, 1999). Referral to a psycho-oncology service might be considered next.

Evaluating coping effectiveness

There is no agreed-upon method of measuring coping effectiveness. The effectiveness of a given coping strategy depends on the individual using it, the culture, and the particular circumstance. Thus a strategy may be useful in one situation but not tomorrow. Furthermore, the event causing the stress is variable. Generalizations about what constitutes successful coping should be issued cautiously. Nevertheless, there are some coping strategies that in general are not helpful and should be identified and managed by staff. These include anger, aggression, illicit drug use, and abuse of prescription medications. Weisman listed a number of mechanisms that we use to cope with cancer. The mechanisms he described were both helpful and harmful. General strategies included: seeking information; laugh it off; submit to the inevitable, be fatalistic, do something however impractical; use alcohol, drugs and danger; blame someone or something, and blame yourself. Strategies Weisman considered that good copers used are: 'avoid avoidance: do not deny'; 'confront realities and take appropriate action'; create solutions; consider alternatives; don't stop talking to loved ones; accept support even if against the grain; self-esteem is vital to good health, and 'hope is self-pride, not self-deception' (Weisman, 1979).

Health professionals and coping

Effective coping is important to health-care professionals. Whilst our stressors might be different, failed coping such as in burnout, drug and alcohol abuse, and emotional fatigue are real problems. These topics are dealt with elsewhere in the textbook, however it should be noted that the principles of coping as outlined earlier, including therapies such as meaning, and talking, and issues such as courage, heroism, and religious identity, are also relevant (Khot et al., 2011).

Coping by family and carers

Hudson used a semi-structured interview to study 45 family caregivers of patients with advanced cancer 2 months after the patient died. Only 7% of caregivers met the criteria for traumatic grief and the vast majority identified 'positive aspects associated with the experience'. The repeated message of the caregivers was the importance and value of a 'multidisciplinary specialist care services' and of 'comprehensive information to prepare them for the future' (Hudson, 2006). Notwithstanding the vast literature on coping, its styles, problems, and therapies, most patients, families, and carers seem to cope well.

Conclusion

Although much of the literature on coping appears obvious, it is important to objectively classify and describe our common-sense impression in order to understand the factors that allow some people to thrive under stress and adapt, and to know which therapy works best, with whom, and when (Billings and Moos, 1981).

After reviewing many observations and theories we should take a step back and ask what happens to the individual when s/he says 'I can't cope'. The inability to control the stress in turn threatens the self-esteem of the person. They might start berating themselves and a vicious cycle ensues causing them to be more distressed, more unable to focus on a task, and to feel helpless and hopeless. Conversely when the individual feels 'I can cope', the daily tasks once again fall into place, seem manageable, and one feels in control.

Coping, in its general meaning, implies restoring equilibrium. The equilibrium does not necessarily refer to returning to what was—since often circumstances have changed, such as advancing cancer or indeed personal growth. More precisely it refers to regaining the equilibrium of self-esteem.

A good rule of thumb is, if the mechanism of coping is not causing harm then leave well alone. The patient's choice of coping might not lead to personal growth or deep self-insights—this is not for us to judge—but if it enables survival in the face of threat to life and limb then it is beneficial.

Coping mechanisms can evolve, change, and adapt over a lifespan. Coping is complex because it stands as a sentinel in the ever-changing interaction between the whole person and his/her environment. It demands that we strive to change the stressor if we can, but also change ourselves to fit in to a new reality. Changing ourselves implies acceptance. This process of acceptance in its fullest development demands that as we cope with change, we grow and become more fully aware of ourselves.

References

Antonovsky, A. (1979). *Health, Stress and Coping*. San Francisco, CA: Jossey-Bass.

Billings, A.G. and Moos, R.H. (1981). The role of coping responses and social resources in attenuating the stress of life events. *Journal of Behavioral Medicine*, 4, 139–157.

Block, S.D. (2006). Psychological issues in the end-of-life care. *Journal of Palliative Medicine*, 9(3), 751–772.

Bohmeijer, E., Roemer, M., Cuijpers, P., and Smit, F. (2007). The effect of reminiscence on psychological well-being in adults: a meta-analysis. *Aging and Mental Health*, 11(3), 291–300.

Burnside, I. and Haight, B.K. (1992). Reminiscence and life review: analyzing each concept. *Journal of Advanced Nursing*, 17, 855–862.

Burstein, H.J., Gelber, S., Guadagnoli, E., and Weeks, J.C. (1999). Use of alternative medicine by women with early-stage breast cancer. *The New England Journal of Medicine*, 340, 1733–1739.

Butler, R.N. (1963). The life review: an interpretation of reminiscence in the aged. *Psychiatry*, 26, 65–76.

Butler, R.N. (1974). Successful aging and the role of the life review. *Journal of the American Geriatrics Society*, 22, 529–535.

Carver, C.S. and Connor-Smith, J. (2010). Personality and coping. *Annual Review of Psychology*, 61, 679–704.

Carver, C.S., Pozo-Kaderman, C., Harris, S.D., et al. (1994). Optimism versus pessimism predicts the quality of women's adjustment to early stage breast cancer. *Cancer*, 73(4), 1213e1220.

Chi, G.C. (2007). The role of hope in patients with cancer. *Oncology Nursing Forum*, 34(2), 415–424.

Chochinov, H.M. (2003). Thinking outside the box: depression, hope, and meaning at the end of life. *Journal of Palliative Medicine*, 6(6), 973–977.

Chochinov, H.M., Kristjanson, L.J., Breitbart, W., et al. (2011). Effect of dignity therapy on distress and end-of-life experience in terminally ill patients: a randomised controlled trial. *The Lancet Oncology*, 12(8), 753–762.

Chochinov, H.M., Kristjanson, L.J., Hack, T.F., et al. (2006). Personality, neuroticism, and coping towards the end of life. *Journal of Pain and Symptom Management*, 32, 332–341.

Coyne, J.C. and Gottlieb, B.H. (1996). The mismeasure of coping by checklist. *Journal of Personality*, 64(4), 959–991.

Coyne, J.C. and Tennen, H. (2010). Positive psychology in cancer care: bad science, exaggerated claims, and unproven medicine. *Annals of Behavioral Medicine*, 39(1), 16–26.

Digman, J.M. (1990). Personality structure: the emergence of the five-factor model. *Annual Review of Psychology*, 41, 417–440.

Dufault, K. and Martocchio, B.C. (1985). Hope: its spheres and dimensions. *Nursing Clinics of North America*, 20(2), 379–391.

Dull, V.T. and Skokan, L.A. (1995). A cognitive model of religion's influence on health. *Journal of Social Issues*, 51, 49–64.

Eriksson, M. and Lindstrom, B. (2005). Validity of Antonovsky's sense of coherence scale: a systematic review. *Journal of Epidemiology and Community Health*, 59, 460–466.

Folkman, S. and Greer, S. (2009). Promoting psychological well-being in the face of serious illness: when theory, research and practice inform each other. *Psycho-Oncology*, 9, 11–19.

Folkman, S., Lazarus, R.S., Dunkel-Schetter, C., et al. (1986). Dynamics of a stressful encounter: cognitive appraisal, coping, and encounter outcomes. *Journal of Personality and Social Psychology*, 50(5), 992–1003.

Folkman, S. and Moskowitz, J.T. (2000). Positive affect and the other side of coping. *American Psychologist*, 55(4), 647–654.

Folkman, S. and Moskowitz, J.T. (2004). Coping: pitfalls and promise. *Annual Review of Psychology*, 55, 745–774.

Greenstein, M. and Breitbart, W. (2000). Cancer and the experience of meaning. *American Journal of Psychotherapy*, 54(4), 486–500.

Greer, S. and Moorley, S. (1997). Adjuvant psychological therapy for cancer patients. *Palliative Medicine*, 11, 240–244.

Greer, S. and Watson, M. (1987). Mental adjustment to cancer: its measurement and prognostic significance. *Cancer Surveys*, 6, 439–453.

Haight, B., Michel, Y., and Hendrix, S. (2000). The extended effects of the life review in nursing home residents. *International Journal of Aging and Human Development*, 50, 151–168.

Hanson, L.C., Dobbs, D., Usher, B.M., et al. (2008). Providers and types of spiritual care during serious illness. *Journal of Palliative Medicine*, 11(6), 907–914.

Harrison, M.O., Koenig, H.G., Hays, J.C., Eme-Akwari, A.G., and Pargament, K.I. (2001). The epidemiology of religious coping: a review of recent literature. *International Review of Psychiatry*, 13, 86–93.

Holland, J.C. (1999). Use of alternative medicine—a marker for distress? *The New England Journal of Medicine*, 340, 1758–1759.

Hudson, P.L. (2006). How well do family caregivers cope after caring for a relative with advanced disease and how can health professionals enhance their support? *Journal of Palliative Medicine*, 9(3), 694–703.

Johnson, J. (1982). The effects of a patient education course on persons with a chronic illness. *Cancer Nursing*, April, 117–123.

Khot, S., Billings, M., Owens, D., and Longstreth, W.T. Jr. (2011). Coping with death and dying on a neurology inpatient service: death rounds as an educational initiative for residents. *Archives of Neurology*, 68(11), 1395–1397.

Lazarus, R. (1968). *Psychological Stress and the Coping Process*. New York: McGraw-Hill.

Liao, S. and Arnold, R.M. (2006). The importance of addressing psychological issues in palliative medicine—editorial. *Journal of Palliative Medicine*, 9(6), 749–750.

Lifton, R.J. (1976). *The Life of the Self*. New York: Simon and Schuster.

Man, W.L. (2009). Coping strategies in the face of death. *Hong Kong Society of Palliative Medicine Newsletter*, 2, 28–32.

McClain, C.S., Rosenfled, B., and Breitbart, W. (2003). Effect of spiritual well-being on end-of-life despair in terminally ill cancer patients. *The Lancet*, 361, 1603–1607.

McClement, S.E. and Chochinov, H.M. (2008). Hope in advanced cancer patients. *European Journal of Cancer*, 44(8), 1169–1174.

McPherson, J.C., Higginson, I.J., and Hearn, J. (2001). Effective methods of giving information in cancer: a systematic literature review of randomized controlled trials. *Journal of Public Health*, 23(3), 227–234.

Murray-Parkes, C. (1998). Facing loss. *BMJ*, 316(7143), 1521–1524.

Pargament, K.I., Koenig, H.G., and Perez, L.M. (2000). The many methods of religious coping: development and initial validation of the RCOPE. *Journal of Clinical Psychology*, 56, 519–543.

Park, C.L., Cohen, L.H., and Murch, R.L. (1996). Assessment and prediction of stress-related growth. *Journal of Personality*, 64(1), 71–105.

Parker, M. (2011). Not so great expectations: why we should accept and respect hopelessness and futility. *Journal of Law and Medicine*, 19, 36–42.

Parker, R.G. (1995). Reminiscence: a continuity theory framework. *Gerontologist*, 35(4), 515–525.

Phelps, A.C., Maciejewski, P.K., Nilsson, M., *et al.* (2009). Religious coping and use of intensive life-prolonging care near death in patients with advanced cancer. *Journal of the American Medical Association*, 301(11), 1140–1147.

Pickrel, J. (1989). Tell me your story: using life review in counseling the terminally ill. *Death Studies*, 13, 127–135.

Sachs, E., Kolva, E., Pessin, H., Rosenfeld, B., andBreitbart, W. (2013). On sinking and swimming: the dialectic of hope, hopelessness, and acceptance in terminal cancer. *American Journal of Hospice Palliative Care*, 30, 121–127.

Sand, L., Olsson, M., and Strang, P. (2009). Coping strategies in the presence of one's own impending death from cancer. *Journal of Pain and Symptom Management*, 37(1), 13–22.

Tarakeshwar, N., Vanderwerker, L.C., Paulk, E., *et al.* (2006). Religious coping is associated with the quality of life of patients with advanced cancer. *Journal of Palliative Medicine*, 9(3), 646–657.

Viederman, M. (1983). The psychodynamic life narrative: a psychotherapeutic intervention useful in crisis situations. *Psychiatry: Journal for the Study of Interpersonal Processes*, 46(3), 236–246.

Wein, S. (2000). Cancer, unproven therapies, and magic. *Oncology*, 14(9), 1345–1350.

Wein, S. (2007). Is courage the counterpoint of demoralization? *Journal of Palliative Care*, 23(1), 40–43.

Weisman, A.D. (1979). *Coping with Cancer*. New York: McGraw-Hill.

Wholihan, D. (1992). The value of reminiscence in hospice care. *The Journal of Hospice and Palliative Care*, 9, 33–35.

Depression, demoralization, and suicidality

David W. Kissane and Matthew Doolittle

Introduction to depression, demoralization, and suicidality

Any loss of happiness, morale, or hope will have a substantial impact on a patient's journey through palliative care. Although under-recognized, depression can generally be well managed with evidence-based strategies and medications familiar to the competent clinician. Restoring threads of coherence to a life torn by illness, pain, and loss may require different skills and greater wisdom. Demoralization may lead to a desire for hastened death, which is one of the greatest challenges a clinician may face, yet successful treatment can help the patient to live life to the fullest extent permitted by sickness and frailty. The worth, dignity, value, and meaning of each person's life are central concerns for palliative care. In this chapter, we examine and compare the nature, diagnosis, and management of depression, demoralization, and suicidality in the settings of advanced and terminal diseases.

Depression

Depression in the medically ill is not only associated with reduced quality of life, but also with decreased adherence to treatments, increased inpatient stays, thoughts of suicide, and poorer survival (Grassi et al., 2005). The profound sadness or pervasive guilt associated with depression can interfere with the integration of information, reduce tolerance for the symptoms or humiliations of serious disease, and contribute to social withdrawal and disengagement from things previously cherished, spoiling what remains of a patient's life.

The nature of depression

Psychiatrists define depression as the loss of interest or pleasure, an anhedonic state, which may be associated with a lowered or sad mood, generally present for most of the day and on most days, and accompanied by a number of additional symptoms, including several somatic symptoms (Dimatteo et al., 1994). Clinical depression is present when this specified combination of symptoms persists for at least 2 weeks but, for most sufferers, depression represents a continuum of unhappiness. The word 'depressed' is used broadly in the community to describe both deep desperation and sad moods, however brief, and this complicates the use of the term and blurs the boundary between 'depression' and appropriate responses to loss or grief.

Diagnosis of depression in palliative medicine

Serious disease and its treatment may cause somatic symptoms that are readily attributed to depression, including changes in appetite, weight, concentration, sleep, energy, and fatigue. Debate exists about including or excluding such symptoms from criteria when diagnosing depression in the medically ill, but somatic symptoms correlate highly with other symptoms and add a worthwhile contribution to diagnostic accuracy (Akechi et al., 2003; Grabsch et al., 2006; Guo et al., 2006). Endicott takes another approach, suggesting alternatives for somatic symptoms in the medically ill: depressed demeanour or appearance; social withdrawal or reduced talkativeness; brooding, self-pity, or pessimism; and loss of responsiveness (Endicott, 1984). Whatever the approach, pervasive anhedonia or sustained low mood are central to the diagnosis of a Major Depressive Episode. Regression-tree analysis has shown *Diagnostic and Statistical Manual of Mental Disorders*, fourth edition (DSM-IV) Major Depression to be highly associated with combinations of either (a) pessimism and worthlessness, or (b) pessimism, loss of interest and thoughts of death (McKenzie et al., 2010), and these factors can often be readily identified or excluded in patients with physical illnesses.

Depressive Disorder Due to Another Medical Condition (DSM-5) is a related diagnosis that is understood as a direct physiological result of such conditions as hypothyroidism, chronic uraemia, presence of cancer-induced cytokines, or medication effects of steroids, interferon-alpha, or chemotherapy agents (Miller and Massie 2010). DSM-5 retains a category of Depressive Disorder Not Elsewhere Classified for brief depressive episodes or those with mixed anxiety-depressive symptoms. DSM-5 also allows a diagnosis of Major Depressive Episode even if symptoms result from bereavement (American Psychiatric Association, 2013).

Prevalence of depressive disorders

Prevalence rates for major depression in oncology may be as high as 38%, while the prevalence of depression spectrum disorders has been found to be as high as 58%—compared with 6.6% 12-month prevalence and 16.6% lifetime prevalence in the general community (Hotopf et al., 2002; Massie, 2004). Rates are similarly high in palliative medicine (Massie et al., 2012). A meta-analysis of 94 oncology and palliative care studies suggested that the prevalence of depression spectrum disorders may be 38%, which is comparable to rates found in a general palliative care setting (Mitchell et al., 2011). Depression is associated with greater physical, social, and existential distress, and with measurable reductions in the quality of life (Wilson et al., 2007).

A diagnosis of cancer may precipitate or enhance risk for depression both directly through the use of treatment agents that have psychiatric side effects and indirectly by posing emotional and logistical challenges that exhaust patients' material and psychological resources. In the classic PSYCOG study, only 11% of cases of depression had evidence of past psychiatric disorder, and most depression seemed to develop in the setting of the cancer (Derogatis et al., 1983; Wilson et al., 2007; Mitchell et al., 2011).

Depression as a cause of cancer

The role, if any, that depression may play in causing cancer is less intuitive and less direct. Depression is not directly associated with an increased rate of cancer in the general community (Sihvo et al., 2010). Moreover, life events such as bereavement do not cause cancer (Ewertz, 1986) and stress is no longer considered a cause of cancer (Li et al., 2002). However, in the third National Health and Nutrition Examination Survey, depression seems to increase the risk of obesity in women (odds ratio 1.82; 95% confidence interval 1.01–3.3) (Onyike et al., 2003). Obesity, in turn, increases endometrial and breast cancer through oestrogenic mechanisms (Kulie et al., 2011). The relationship between depression, obesity, and cancer is less consistent in men. Depression is also associated with smoking and alcoholism (Graham et al., 2007; Azevedo et al., 2010), both of which increase incidence of cancer (Murphy et al., 2010). Co-morbidities associated with depression including obesity, smoking, physical inactivity, and alcohol use do increase risk for malignancies (Chwastiak et al., 2011).

The consequences of depression in cancer or advanced disease

Untreated depression has been associated with worsened medical outcomes. Patients who are helpless, hopeless, depressed (Temoshok et al., 1985; Watson et al., 1999, 2005), socially alienated (Goodkin et al., 1986), and socially deprived (Boesen et al., 2007) have had shorter survival times. Fatalistic and stoical attitudes may also handicap survival (Pettingale et al., 1985; Temoshok et al., 1985). Psycho-oncology has a role in promoting coping, treating depression, and helping patients be connected to supports. Whether group therapy can improve survival remains contentious, but in the advanced cancer setting, it did prevent the development of depression (Kissane et al., 2007).

Untreated depression affects treatment adherence (DiMatteo et al., 2000). One meta-analysis finds that depressed patients are three times more likely than non-depressed patients to be non-adherent (DiMatteo and Hanskard-Zolnierek, 2011). Depression interferes with adherence via cognitive, motivational, and resource-related pathways (see Box 17.3.1). The goal of psycho-oncology interventions is to treat depression and promote coping and social support that may improve both the quality of life and outcomes.

Contributors to depression in palliative patients

Oestrogen receptors have a significant role in the mood-regulating limbic circuits of the brain and gender is one of the most important risk factors for depression (Cutter et al., 2003; Kendler et al., 2006). In one study of women with breast cancer, patients were found to have double the rate of depression of women in the general community (Kissane et al., 2004). On the other hand, male cancers such as prostate cancer are associated with rates of depression quite close to those seen in the general population (Couper et al., 2006). Rates of depression among wives of men with prostate cancer can approach twice the rates of the general female population (Couper et al., 2006). Research on the husbands of cancer patients is more limited, but seems to show that rates among husbands are either not elevated (Hagedoorn et al., 2000; Hinnen et al., 2008), or that they are elevated to a lesser degree than that found in studies of patients' wives (Langer et al., 2003). Women seem to bear the burden of emotional distress.

Other contributory factors (see Box 17.3.2) include younger age, advanced disease with pain and poor symptom control, co-morbid neurological disorders, and a range of other metabolic and endocrine disorders (Wilson et al., 2009). Many medications have a direct effect on depression or its treatment, including interferon, interleukin 2 (IL-2), steroids, certain chemotherapy agents (vincristine, vinblastine, procarbazine, L-asparaginase, vinorelbine, paclitaxel, docetaxel), hormonal agents (tamoxifen, cyproterone, leuprolide), as well as antihypertensives (propranolol, reserpine, methyldopa) and antibiotics (amphotericin). Specific cancers that have been linked to depression include pancreas cancers, which like lymphomas and lung cancers may increase pro-inflammatory cytokines (IL-1, IL-6, tumour necrosis factor-alpha) (Musselman et al., 2001; Ebrahimi et al., 2004), and many other cancers can be associated with paraneoplastic syndromes that can also cause mood disturbance. Neurodegenerative disorders including Parkinson's disease, endocrine disorders including Cushing's disease and hypothyroidism, metabolic disorders including hypercalcaemia, and such nutritional deficits as pellagra may all cause Depressive Disorder Due to Another Medical Condition (DSM-5).

Barriers to recognition of depression

The potentially confounding effect of medical symptoms is only one of several barriers to the recognition of depression in palliative medicine (Greenberg, 2004). The stigma attached to mental illness may cause the patient to withhold data. For family and medical staff, acknowledging depression may appear to deny the reality of the patient's distress, or seem a criticism of the sufferer's coping. 'Isn't this normal?' or 'Wouldn't you be depressed?' are statements that both reflect suffering and express indignation that it should be observed. In fact, responding to such complicated emotions, or acting in accord with cultural beliefs, family

---

Box 17.3.1 Associations between depression and treatment adherence

1. Reduced understanding
2. Ambivalent decision-making about palliative treatments
3. Decreased motivation for care and healthy behaviours
4. Pessimism about the outcome and benefit
5. Poorer tolerance of side effects
6. Poorer family support and greater isolation
7. Reduced use of community resources.

Box 17.3.2 Risk factors for depression in palliative medicine
1. Female gender
2. Younger age
3. Past history and family history of depression
4. Poor social support, including family dysfunction
5. Pain and poor symptom control
6. Illness and treatment-related factors
7. Declining functional status
8. Unaddressed existential concerns.

members may deliberately or inadvertently conceal their relative's distress. The most basic barrier to recognizing depression, though, may be the limited time of clinicians. Physicians may be trained to focus on physical symptoms and may avoid opening what is feared to be a Pandora's box of unsolvable problems (Wilson et al., 2007).

Screening for depression

To assist clinicians in recognizing depression, the National Comprehensive Cancer Network Distress Management Panel recommends periodic screening of all patients (National Comprehensive Cancer Network, 2003). Brief self-report instruments are most practical, though they will return more false positives than structured psychiatric interviews (Passik and Lowery, 2011). A systematic review of screening scales suggests that the Beck Depression Inventory (BDI), the General Health Questionnaire-28 (GHQ-28), and Center for Epidemiological Studies—Depression Scale (CES-D) are reliable and valid (Vodermaier et al., 2009). The Patient Health Questionnaire-9 (PHQ-9) is briefer than any of these measures, freely available, highly reliable, and widely used (Passik and Lowery, 2011). The Distress Thermometer is a single unitary measure with less reliability, but is rapid and straightforward (Roth et al., 1998). Even asking the single question, 'Are you depressed?' can identify the majority of patients who should have further evaluation (Miller et al., 2006).

Demoralization

Kissane and colleagues recognized a group of patients who sought hastened death because of their conviction that their lives were pointless and meaningless, even when they were not thought to be clinically depressed (Kissane et al., 1998). Kissane followed others in proposing that 'demoralization syndrome' captures this phenomenon (Kissane et al., 2001). Constructs such as acedia (the tedious meaninglessness of life), spiritual torpor, Engel's 'giving up-given up' complex (Engel, 1967), Gruenberg's social breakdown syndrome (Gruenberg, 1967) in the chronically institutionalized, and Seligman's 'learned helplessness' (Miller et al., 1975) had all identified aspects of demoralization, and some version of the concept has long been recognized clinically. An empirical study identified demoralization as a non-specific form of distress in the community (Dohrenwend et al., 1980). Frank saw its correction as the vital therapeutic component of all successful psychotherapy (Frank, 1974). De Figueiredo suggested with Frank that the development of a state of subjective incompetence was the hallmark of demoralization (de Figueiredo and Frank, 1982).

Nature of demoralization

Folkman's studies of the coping among caregivers of men dying from AIDS in San Francisco in the early 1990s recognized 'meaning-based coping', which had been omitted from her earlier descriptions of 'emotion-based' and 'problem-based' coping strategies (Folkman, 1997). New impetus was given to recognition of the loss of meaning and hope, especially in the medically ill. Clarke and Kissane have described the process whereby sufferers begin to feel they cannot cope with stressful situations, feeling helpless, hopeless, and even ashamed, until the pointlessness of their situation invokes disheartenment and despair (Clarke and Kissane, 2002). Ordinarily a strong generalized hope about the value and worth of life will preserve meaning when illness appears to destroy immediate hopes. Similarly, robust self-esteem will sustain self-worth against the infirmity of illness. Demoralization seems to ensue when these mechanisms break down.

Loss of morale spans a spectrum of mental states, ranging from disheartenment (a mild loss of confidence), through despondency (starting to lose hope and sense of purpose), to despair (where all hope is lost), and demoralization (where meaning and purpose are lost). Psychiatric involvement is indicated in the more severe end of this spectrum, where meaninglessness, pointlessness, and hopelessness can all lead to suicidal thinking. Indeed, suicidality may not follow directly from anhedonia, the inability to take pleasure in the moment, but rather may develop from reflection about worthlessness, hopelessness, or the meaninglessness of life—a conviction that there will be no satisfaction in the future. Indeed, Klein and colleagues thought that a distinguishing feature of demoralization was its loss of anticipatory pleasure (through loss of meaning and hope), although consummatory pleasure remained possible (Klein et al., 1980). In contrast, depression involves loss of available and expected pleasure in the here and now.

Diagnosis of demoralization syndrome

The DSM defines adjustment disorders as impairments and symptoms not meeting criteria for other major psychiatric diagnoses, and which arise in response to an identified stressor. The judgement of the clinician in determining whether an anxious or depressed affect or behavioural change reaches a threshold for disordered 'adjustment' has made this a difficult diagnostic category to apply in the medically ill.

In contrast, a focus on the phenomenology of meaninglessness, hopelessness, and loss of purpose that brings existential dimensions to the fore may enable palliative care clinicians to recognize the lived experience of patients (Fava et al., 1995). More directly reflecting the language actually used by patients experiencing existential distress, the development of a diagnostic category for a demoralization syndrome might facilitate recognition of a significant form of suffering without requiring the complex judgement about adaptiveness currently necessary to identify adjustment disorder (Box 17.3.3).

Prevalence of demoralization

The introduction of methodical instruments including the Demoralization Scale has begun to allow estimates of the extent of the phenomenon (Kissane et al., 2004). The frequency of high demoralization among cancer patients has been estimated at 16% (Mehnert et al., 2011). Among methadone patients in a Dutch sample, rates of demoralization were twice that in the

Box 17.3.3 Diagnostic criteria for demoralization syndrome

1. Loss of meaning or purpose in life
2. Loss of hope for a worthwhile future
3. Sense of being trapped or pessimistic
4. Feel like giving up
5. Unable to cope with the predicament
6. Socially isolated or alienated
7. Potential for desire to die
8. Phenomena persist for more than 2 weeks; may be co-morbid or distinct from depressive disorders.

community (Jong et al., 2008). The Bologna group developed diagnostic criteria for psychosomatic disorders and identified demoralization in medical illnesses, reporting for instance a rate of 31% after cardiac transplantation (Grandi et al., 2001) and 29% among breast cancer patients (Grassi et al., 2004). Loss of meaning and hope has been found in 37% of terminally ill patients in Japanese studies (Morita et al., 2000). More elevated rates of demoralization and suicidality have been described in patients with amyotrophic lateral sclerosis, while more elevated rates of anhedonia were found among patients with advanced cancer (Clarke et al., 2005a).

Demoralization has been associated with younger age, female sex, living alone, family dysfunction, high physical symptom burden, use of resignation and avoidant coping, and emotional, spiritual, and practical problems (Kissane et al., 2004; Clarke et al., 2005a; Mehnert et al., 2011). Conversely, lower levels of demoralization have been measured in people with high spiritual meaning and sense of coherence to their life (Lethborg et al., 2006; Boscaglia and Clarke, 2007; Lethborg et al., 2007; Mullane et al., 2009).

Correlation between demoralization, anxiety, and depression

Trait anxiety predicts the development of both demoralization and depression (Clarke et al., 2005b), with anxiety having a higher correlation with demoralization ($r = 0.71$) than depression ($r = 0.61$) (Mehnert et al., 2011). Feelings of helplessness and a sense of existential uncertainty help to explain this association between anxiety and demoralization.

A high correlation has also been shown in several studies between demoralization and clinical depression. Patients can develop major depression with or without demoralization, and some studies have shown cases of demoralization without depression (Kissane et al., 2004; Mehnert et al., 2011), while others have not (Mullane et al., 2009). Mehnert and colleagues found that 60% of subjects with moderate demoralization had no clinical depression, whereas only 5% of patients with severe demoralization (more than one standard deviation above the mean) were without depression. As clinical status worsened, co-morbid states of depression, anxiety, and demoralization all became more likely.

Empirical studies of demoralization

Beck first recognized that hopelessness predicted suicide independently of depression (Beck et al., 1975), and this finding has been replicated among psychiatric inpatients and suicidal adolescents (Wetzel et al., 1980; Dori and Overholser, 1999), and in the settings of cancer (Owen et al., 1994), HIV (Breitbart et al., 1996), and primary care (Gutkovich et al., 1999). Latent trait analyses of psychopathology in the medically ill have shown that demoralization, anhedonia, anxiety, grief, and somatization are distinct, suggesting the existence of an identifiable and measurable phenomenon requiring further study (Clarke et al., 2000). Field trials are needed to examine more comprehensively a typology of existential distress and to identify empirical diagnostic criteria for demoralization.

Suicidality

Nature of desire for hastened death

An intense and abiding desire to die develops from a sense that life is worthless, pointless or hopeless. This loss of the meaning and value of life can lead to thoughts that one might be better dead, and if the process continues, to the development of plans to hasten death. The more abject the sense of loss of purpose, the more agitation and desperation that develops, the more active and consuming these plans may become. When lethal means are available, the danger can be grave. Admission, close observation, and active treatment of depression, hopelessness, and demoralization are needed for actively suicidal patients.

Psychiatrists often receive consultations for 'suicidality' in cases of patients who have no desire to die, but who have instead accepted their own death. Such acceptance is based on awareness of disease progression, frailty, and the inevitability of death. Some patients close to death develop an adaptive conservation-withdrawal syndrome (Ironside, 1980), in which they retreat as they accept the pending closure of their life. Conservation-withdrawal needs to be differentiated from depression. Other patients develop fleeting, passive thoughts of suicide, in contrast to those who develop active plans with intent (Chochinov et al., 1995).

Another variation of the desire for hastened death in palliative care is the request for physician-assisted suicide or euthanasia. Much clinical discernment is needed to differentiate when such a request is based on a philosophical conviction about controlling the dying process and when it has developed from demoralized and depressed themes about the worthlessness, hopelessness, and pointlessness of life, even in the setting of potential for months of further living. Many patients use a question about hastened death as a 'cry for help' to cope with and manage a challenging illness experience. When such a request represents more than a need for better support or for improved control of symptoms, the care paradigms of legally supported physician-assisted suicide and psychiatric care for the suicidal patient appear contradictory and competing (Hamilton and Hamilton, 2005). Optimal psychotherapeutic support for such patients can be handicapped by a physician's willingness to hasten their death (Kelly et al., 2004).

Prevalence of suicidality and suicide

Suicide and suicidality are generally believed to be higher among the medically ill, and the phenomenon seems more significant in the cancer population. Transient wishes to die are frequent in the general palliative care setting. One Canadian study identified a fleeting desire for death in 44.5% of palliative patients, whereas 8.5% developed a more persistent wish (Chochinov et al., 1995).

One study in the United States reported that 25% of cancer patients had seriously thought about euthanasia and 12% had discussed this with their physicians (Emanuel et al., 1996), while another study, also in the United States, found that 17% of hospice patients identified a high desire for hastened death (Breitbart et al., 2000). In the Netherlands, euthanasia and physician-assisted suicide comprise between 1% and 5% of all deaths and 7.4% of cancer-related deaths (Onwuteaka-Philipsen et al., 2003). By 2006, cancer patients comprised 87% of some 292 patients who had used assisted suicide in the US state of Oregon since it was first legalized in 1994 (Oregon Department of Health Services, 2006). Studies have generally suggested an increased rate of completed suicide in the cancer setting, especially for older men (Louhivuori and Hakama, 1979; Fox et al., 1982; Allebeck and Bolund, 1991; Hem et al., 2004). These rates, in the range of 1–2%, are higher than the community prevalence of suicide; for instance, from 1960 to 1999, males in Norway's Cancer Registry were 55% more likely to die by suicide than the general population; female suicides were 35% more likely (Hem et al., 2004).

Risk factors for suicidality

Some of the complex factors contributing to a desire for hastened death are summarized in Fig. 17.3.1. In general, risks for suicidality include depression, demoralization, pain, and poor symptom control, though other important factors include debility, social isolation, delirium, alcohol or other substance abuse, and past history of psychiatric disorder. Such cancers as lung and head and neck cancers are associated with greater physical morbidity and therefore increased suicide rates.

Dutch studies have shown that depressed patients are four times more likely to request euthanasia than are the non-depressed (van der Lee et al., 2005). A series of studies has explored the change that can be seen in patients' interest in life-sustaining treatment when depression is actively treated (Ganzini et al., 1994; Breitbart et al., 1996; Hooper et al., 1996). In these studies, depressed people tended to select only six out of 14 potential medical therapies

(e.g. the use of oxygen, blood transfusion, or being treated with antibiotics), whereas when depression was successfully treated, they selected on average ten out of 14 therapies. A study of seven people seeking legal euthanasia in Darwin, Australia highlighted the contribution of inadequately treated depression, unrecognized demoralization and poor symptom control to these patients' desire for death (Kissane et al., 1998; Kissane 2002). Zylicz found that 25% of patients in a palliative care programme in the Netherlands wanted to discuss euthanasia. The most important reasons for their requests included fear of the process of dying, 'burnout' (equivalent to demoralization), need for control, depression, and poor symptom management (Zylicz, 2002). Moreover, Chochinov has described a wide fluctuation in the will to live among the terminally ill, with anxiety, depression, and dyspnoea predicting this variation (Chochinov et al., 1999).

Assessment of the suicidal patient

Whenever patients express a desire to die, clinicians need to evaluate whether this is a readiness to accept death when it arrives or active suicidal thinking. Evaluation for the presence of depression or demoralization is paramount, assessing for meaninglessness, pointlessness, hopeless-helpless thinking, or worthlessness as pathways to suicidal thinking (see Fig. 17.3.1). Ask for thoughts about the mode of suicide—gun, hanging, jumping, car accident, or medications—and enquire about definite plans to act. If a patient appears desperate, agitated, and strongly resolved to act, the danger is grave and warrants urgent management as described later in this chapter.

Treatment of depression, demoralization, and suicidality

Pharmacological and psychotherapeutic treatments are combined in treating depression. Less empirical guidance is available for demoralization, although newer meaning-centred and dignity-conserving therapies are relevant. Creating a safe environment is crucial for those actively suicidal.

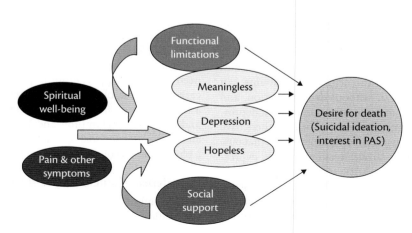

Fig. 17.3.1 Factors associated with desire for hastened death, including physician-assisted suicide (PAS).

Pharmacological treatment of depression

Only modest or negligible differences in efficacy have been found among common antidepressants, and as in the general psychiatry setting, the choice of antidepressant medication in palliative care is governed largely by the potential side effect profile, which can be harnessed advantageously (Cipriani et al., 2010; Omori et al., 2010). However, medically ill patients do require additional care to avoid drug interactions and reduced quality of life (see Table 17.3.1).

Selective serotonin reuptake inhibitor (SSRI) medication is the first-line treatment for depression. SSRIs and selective noradrenaline (norepinephrine) reuptake inhibitor (SNRI) medications have been demonstrated to be effective for depression in the settings of cancer, coronary artery disease, and medical illnesses generally (Lloyd-Williams, 2004; Price and Hotopf, 2009; Dowlati et al., 2010; Rayner et al., 2010). Some case reports or smaller studies do support specific palliative care indications of standard medications (e.g. paroxetine and sertraline to prevent and treat depressive

Table 17.3.1 Use of antidepressants in palliative medicine

Class	Action	Advantageous effects or side effects	Harmful side effects	Use in palliative care	Daily dose ranges (may have ER forms)
Tricyclics, e.g. amitriptyline	Inhibits 5-HT and NA uptake, antimuscarinic, antihistaminic, anti-alpha 1	Co-analgesic Sedative	Constipation Dry mouth Urinary retention Hypotension Syncope	Pain Insomnia Depression	Amitriptyline 25–150 mg
Selective serotonin reuptake inhibitors (SSRI), e.g. citalopram, fluoxetine, paroxetine, sertraline, escitalopram	Inhibition of 5-HT reuptake	Citalopram safe with tamoxifen	Sexual dysfunction ($5-HT_{2A}$); GI—nausea, vomiting, diarrhoea ($5-HT_3$); QTc prolongation at higher doses	Depression Anxiety Obsessive–compulsive PTSD	Citalopram 10–60 mg; fluoxetine 10–80 mg; paroxetine 10–60 mg; sertraline 25–200 mg; escitalopram 5–20 mg.
Selective serotonin and noradrenaline reuptake inhibition (SSNRI), e.g. venlafaxine, desvenlafaxine, duloxetine, milnacipran	Inhibition of 5-HT and NA reuptake	Co-analgesic	Hypertension in higher doses Nausea, GI tract	Severe depression Anxiety	Venlafaxine 37.5–450 mg; desvenlafaxine 50–200 mg (care with hepatorenal insufficiency); duloxetine 15–60mg; milnacipran 50–200mg
Selective dopamine and noradrenaline reuptake inhibitors, e.g. bupropion	Inhibition of dopamine and noradrenaline reuptake	Improve attention and concentration; reduce fatigue; lowest impact on sexual function	Anxiety Seizures Agitation	Depression Fatigue	Bupropion 150–450mg
Noradrenergic and specific serotonergic antidepressants, e.g. mirtazapine	Increases 5-HT and NA activity, antihistaminic	Stimulates appetite Helps sleep	Dry mouth Drowsiness Neutropenia rare	Depression Anxiety Appetite and weight gain Insomnia	Mirtazapine 15–60 mg
Serotonin antagonists and reuptake inhibitors, e.g. trazodone	Increases 5-HT activity, anticholinergic	Helps sleep	Dry mouth Constipation Urinary retention Drowsiness	Sleep Depression	Trazodone 50–300 mg
Psychostimulants, e.g. methylphenidate, modafinil, dextroamphetamine	Increase dopamine activity	Counter opioid sedation Alertness Counter fatigue Rapid effect	Agitation Insomnia Anorexia Seizures Hallucinations Psychosis Arrhythmia Nightmares	Depression Opioid sedation	Methylphenidate 5–60 mg; modafinil 100–400 mg; dextroamphetamine 5–60 mg

5-HT, 5-hydroxytryptamine (serotonin); GI, gastrointestinal; NA, noradrenaline.

effects of interferon) (Musselman et al., 2001; Reddy et al., 2008), or indications for non-standard treatments in the medically ill, including, for example, ketamine (Irwin and Iglewicz, 2010) or scopolamine (Furey and Drevets, 2006). Electroconvulsive therapy has also been effective in some medically ill patients (Rasmussen and Richardson, 2011).

Monoamine oxidase inhibitors (MAOIs) should be avoided because of a risk of drug interactions, especially with opiates or other serotonergic medications. Tricyclics, mirtazapine, trazodone, and SSRIs including fluoxetine and sertraline can rarely exacerbate neutropenia (Albertini and Penders, 1978; Kasper et al., 1997; Duggal and Singh, 2005). Anticholinergic side effects of antidepressants can worsen the constipating effect of opiates or complicate painful mucositis, or exacerbate delirium. Constipating effects may be particularly risky in patients with pelvic or abdominal masses.

In patients with brain lesions or other reasons for risk of seizures, bupropion and psychostimulants should be avoided and mirtazapine may also pose a risk; therapeutic doses of citalopram have been associated in most general population studies with no increased risk of seizure, or even with a decreased risk, though studies in the cancer population are lacking (Favale et al., 2003; Waring et al., 2008).

Methylphenidate or other stimulants may be beneficial both for adjunct treatment of depression and for fatigue in the terminally ill (Minton et al., 2008; Hardy 2009). Modafinil is a newer agent that may be better tolerated, but its use may be limited by cost (Breitbart and Alici, 2010). All stimulants may precipitate or exacerbate a delirium. Bupropion may also reduce fatigue (Cullum et al., 2004; Moss et al., 2006).

Mirtazapine or tricyclics may help with sleeplessness, with the added benefit of improving appetite (mirtazapine) or treating pain (tricyclics). Venlafaxine and duloxetine may also be helpful for adjunct treatment of pain along with opiates. The literature supports the use of venlafaxine and mirtazapine for hot flashes in both men and women undergoing hormonal treatments, but other antidepressants may also be helpful if these are not tolerated (Biglia et al., 2007; Loibl et al., 2007; Buijs et al., 2009). Haloperidol and olanzapine have been used for nausea, and atypical antipsychotics may also be effective for anxiety or sleep in medically ill patients (Critchley et al., 2001; Tan et al., 2009). Pruritus from various causes may respond to paroxetine or mirtazapine when standard treatments have been ineffective or are contraindicated (Zylicz et al., 1998; Demierre and Taverna, 2006).

Finally, a trial of steroids to elevate mood and overall well-being may be used in patients with a very short life expectancy. Methyl prednisolone 30 mg per day or dexamethasone 4 mg per day are used, with due care in watching for side effects, as steroids may cause dysphoric mood in some patients. Dexamethasone is metabolized by cytochrome P450 (CPY) 3A4, potentially interacting with venlafaxine, and dexamethasone is less bound to plasma proteins, therefore reaching higher concentrations in the CSF.

Tamoxifen and cytochrome P450 cytochrome interactions

Tamoxifen is a selective oestrogen receptor modulator used to reduce recurrence or treat metastatic disease in oestrogen receptor-positive breast cancers. Most common antidepressants are believed to induce some degree of inhibition of CYP2D6, the enzyme catalysing the conversion of tamoxifen to its active form, and use of the more potent CYP2D6 inhibitors fluoxetine, paroxetine, and sertraline has been associated with increased recurrence and mortality (Aubert et al., 2009; Kelly et al., 2010). Citalopram and escitalopram are less potent CYP2D6 inhibitors, and in retrospective studies they do not seem to be associated with increased cancer risk (Cronin-Fenton et al., 2010). Venlafaxine and mirtazapine are believed to be weak CYP2D6 inhibitors and are generally believed to be safe (Aubert et al., 2009).

Irinotecan and SSRIs

Irinotecan is a colon cancer agent that also requires conversion to its active form by the CYP system. SSRI medications and tricyclics may increase levels of the active drug through CYP interaction, and the combination can also rarely cause rhabdomyolysis by an unclear mechanism. Antidepressants should be used cautiously in the setting of Irinotecan (Richards et al., 2003).

Serotonin syndrome

Serotonin syndrome is a rare but potentially fatal autonomic dysregulation caused by excessive serotonin. Manifestations are usually mild but may become severe, progressing from shivering, sweating, and nausea to tachycardia, mydriasis, myoclonus, and hyper-reflexia, and finally to psychomotor agitation and disorientation, hyperthermia, hypertension, metabolic acidosis, and renal failure leading to possible seizure, disseminated intravascular coagulation, coma, and even death (Kim and Fisch, 2006). Treatment involves withdrawal of the offending agents and supportive management. Linezolid is an oxazolidinone antibiotic with MAOI-like properties that could precipitate a serotonin syndrome when combined with antidepressants; administration within 2 weeks of antidepressant use should be avoided if possible. Antidepressants are generally contraindicated in patients receiving the chemotherapy agent procarbazine, which has well-documented MAOI action. In rare cases, many common medications including opiates (especially meperidine), ondansetron, and granisetron may precipitate serotonin toxicity when given with antidepressants (Lee et al., 2009; Takeshita and Litzinger, 2009).

Psychological treatment for depression

Meta-analyses of psychotherapies in cancer patients document clear benefits (Meyer and Mark, 1995), with communication of specific knowledge through psychoeducation most easily demonstrated (Devine and Westlake, 1995). Both individual and group psychotherapeutic interventions seem to have benefit in proportion to the experience and skill of the therapist and the length of intervention (Sheard and Maguire, 1999). In eight of 13 studies of interpersonal psychotherapy focusing on grief, life transitions, social isolation, and interpersonal conflicts, de Mello et al. showed that the intervention was superior to control at improving depression (de Mello et al., 2005).

Behavioural activation strategies

Depression is readily maintained by social withdrawal and avoidance behaviours. Strategies such as scheduling, self-monitoring, rating daily levels of pleasure and accomplishment, and exploring alternative roles with rehearsal during therapy have been found to help alleviate depression (Dimidjian et al., 2006; Dobson et al., 2008).

Couple therapy

A randomized controlled trial of active coping for couples compared with usual care in the breast cancer setting showed a reduction in women's depressive symptoms up to 6 months after active treatment (Manne et al., 2005). Couple therapy assists adaptation when body image changes (e.g. mastectomy, colostomy, ileal conduit, and limb amputation), when sexuality is affected (e.g. erectile dysfunction after prostate cancer and dyspareunia after gynaecological cancers), or when issues of shame, guilt, doubt, despair, or depression arise, and the partner is a prime source of support (Zaider and Kissane, 2011).

In working with couples to promote effective mutual support, it is important to maintain awareness of patterns of demand-withdrawal that can represent a protest at the burden of illness and lead to disengagement and diminished safety. Couple therapy that identifies existential fears and supports intimacy in the face of death has been shown beneficial in reinforcing resilience and protecting against demoralization and depression (Dobson et al., 2008).

Group therapy

In cognitive-existential group therapy, the goals are to promote a supportive environment, facilitate grief for multiple losses, alter maladaptive cognitive patterns, enhance problem-solving and coping skills, foster a sense of mastery, and encourage review of lifestyle priorities (Kissane et al., 1997). In supportive-expressive group therapy (SEGT), the goals are to build bonds, express emotions, detoxify death, redefine life's priorities, fortify families and friends, enhance doctor–patient relationships, and improve coping (Classen et al., 2001). Through an emphasis on transforming existential ambivalence into creative living and promoting adherence to anti-cancer treatment (Kissane et al., 2004), SEGT has been shown to prevent depression (Kissane et al., 2007).

Family therapy

In a randomized controlled trial targeting 'at-risk' palliative care families, family-focused grief therapy (FFGT) has been shown to reduce depression and support mourning (Kissane et al., 2006). The goals of FFGT are to optimize family relational functioning through promotion of effective communication, enhanced cohesion and adaptive resolution of conflict. The more pronounced the relational dysfunction, the greater the number of family sessions needed during the bereavement phase. In general, families with mild communication breakdown can be aided by four to six sessions, whereas ten to 12 sessions are preferred for severe family dysfunction. Openness to discussion of death and dying and early containment of conflict prove beneficial until improved communication and closeness help family members tolerate differences of opinion (Kissane and Zaider, 2011). Therapists make use of circular questions to reveal family dynamics and offer regular summaries to help families integrate understanding of their patterns of relating and coping with loss and change (Dumont and Kissane, 2009). Commencing therapy while the cancer patient is still alive and present to contribute establishes a model of family care that is preventive, cost-effective, and enables continuity of support to be carried into bereavement.

Pharmacological treatment for demoralization

Where co-morbid major depression and demoralization exist, medications for the treatment of depression are indicated. When demoralization exists without co-morbid depression, the mainstay of treatment is psychotherapeutic, without current research evidence to guide the use of antidepressants or other medications (Angelino and Treisman, 2001).

Psychological treatment for demoralization

New models of treatment including dignity and meaning-centred therapies allow more focus on demoralization and other states of existential or spiritual distress (Griffith and Gaby 2005).

Dignity therapy

Dignity therapy (DT) is a brief focused intervention near the end of life that is designed to address psychosocial and existential distress (Chochinov et al., 2005). Its goals are to sustain generativity and continuity of self, to maintain pride and hope, to preserve the patient's cherished roles, to alleviate concerns about being a burden to others, and, if desired, to leave a legacy document that summarizes the sufferer's accomplishments and values in life. DT seeks to celebrate life and affirm the worth of each person, addressing critical aspects of demoralization and enriching the life lived.

Meaning-centred therapies

Based on Frankl's model of logotherapy, meaning-centred therapy (MCT) has been used with groups and individuals (Breitbart et al., 2004). Its goals are to review concepts and sources of psychological meaning and value, together with the impact of palliative care, and to acknowledge the finiteness of life and therefore highlight its value and worth. The therapy often includes creativity and good deeds, appreciation of nature, art and humour, and a focus on taking stock of the depth of meaning that sustains worthwhile living. MCP is anticipated to be effective in alleviating demoralization and promoting dignity of the person.

The psychodynamic life review is a narrative approach that identifies key accomplishments and personal strengths alongside vulnerabilities, in order to frame the crisis of illness as an opportunity for growth in the setting of an ongoing life story (Viederman 1983). The containing frame of support generated actively by the therapist is intended to maintain adaptive defences and draw attention to the value and meaning of continued life. Meaning and purpose therapy is another brief, individual model that focuses on the patient's intention and ability to derive meaning (Lethborg et al., 2012).

Treatment of suicidality

Many who complete suicide have recently denied the presence of suicidal ideation and have not made prior attempts (Busch et al., 2003). The warning signs of an imminently impending suicide attempt differ from demoralization, depression, and other risk factors discussed above, and include agitation and increasing anxiety, desperation, and easy access to a mode of dying. This is a medical emergency. Immediate admission to hospital, use of one-to-one observation, careful assessment, and active treatment of depression and demoralization are crucial to protect such patients from self-harm (Olden et al., 2009). When patients express a desire for hastened death in the setting of hospice or palliative care, therapeutic communication is central, with empathic responsiveness, active listening, management of realistic expectations, permission to discuss psychological distress, and psychiatric referral as needed (Hudson et al., 2006).

Conclusion

Depression and demoralization are interrelated experiences that have a measurable effect on the lives of cancer patients and their course of illness. Desire for hastened death or even suicidality can develop from severe demoralization or depression. Treatments including medications and psychotherapies with patients and their families have been shown to be both promising and effective in alleviating suffering and improving the quality of cancer treatment and medical care.

Online materials

Complete references for this chapter are available online at <http://www.oxfordmedicine.com>.

References

American Psychiatric Association (2013). *Diagnostic and Statistical Manual of Mental Disorders* (5th ed.). Arlington, VA: American Psychiatric Publishing.

Aubert, R.E., Stanek, E.J., Yao, J., et al. (2009). Risk of breast cancer recurrence in women initiating tamoxifen with CYP2D6 inhibitors. *Journal of Clinical Oncology*, 27(18S), CRA508.

Boesen, E.H., Boesen, S.H., Frederiksen, K., et al. (2007). Survival after a psychoeducational intervention for patients with cutaneous malignant melanoma: a replication study. *Journal of Clinical Oncology*, 25(36), 5698–5703.

Breitbart, W., Gibson, C., Poppito, S.R., and Berg, A. (2004). Psychotherapeutic interventions at the end of life: a focus on meaning and spirituality. *Canadian Journal of Psychiatry*, 49(6), 366–372.

Buijs, C., Mom, C.H., Willemse, P.H., et al. (2009). Venlafaxine versus clonidine for the treatment of hot flashes in breast cancer patients: a double-blind, randomized cross-over study. *Breast Cancer Research and Treatment*, 115(3), 573–580.

Busch, K.A., Fawcett, J., and Jacobs, D.G. (2003). Clinical correlates of inpatient suicide. *Journal of Clinical Psychiatry*, 64(1), 14–19.

Chochinov, H.M., Hack, T., Hassard, T., Kristjanson, L.J., McClement, S., and Harlos, M. (2005). Dignity therapy: a novel psychotherapeutic intervention for patients near the end of life. *Journal of Clinical Oncology*, 23(24), 5520–5525.

Chochinov, H.M., Wilson, K.G., Enns, M., et al. (1995). Desire for death in the terminally ill. *American Journal of Psychiatry*, 152(8), 1185–1191.

Chwastiak, L.A., Rosenheck, R.A., and Kazis, L.E. (2011). Association of psychiatric illness and obesity, physical inactivity, and smoking among a national sample of veterans. *Psychosomatics*, 52(3), 230–236.

Clarke, D., Kissane, D., Trauer, T., and Smith, G. (2005a). Demoralization, anhedonia and grief in patients with severe physical illness. *World Psychiatry*, 4(2), 96–105.

Clarke, D., Mackinnon, A., Smith, G., McKenzie, D., and Herrman, H. (2000). Dimensions of psychopathology in the medically ill. A latent trait analysis. *Psychosomatics*, 41(5), 418–425.

Clarke, D., McLeod, J., Smith, G., Trauer, T., and Kissane, D. (2005b). A comparison of psychosocial and physical functioning in patients with motor neurone disease and metastatic cancer. *Journal of Palliative Care*, 21(3), 173–179.

Clarke, D.M. and Kissane, D.W. (2002). Demoralization: its phenomenology and importance. *Australian & New Zealand Journal of Psychiatry*, 36(6), 733–742.

Couper, J.W., Bloch, S., Love, A., Duchesne, G., Macvean, M., and Kissane, D.W. (2006). The psychosocial impact of prostate cancer on patients and their partners. *Medical Journal of Australia*, 185(8), 428–432.

Critchley, P., Plach, N., Grantham, M., et al. (2001). Efficacy of haloperidol in the treatment of nausea and vomiting in the palliative patient: a systematic review. *Journal of Pain and Symptom Management*, 22(2), 631–634.

Cronin-Fenton, D., Lash, T.L., and Sorensen, H.T. (2010). Selective serotonin reuptake inhibitors and adjuvant tamoxifen therapy: risk of breast cancer recurrence and mortality. *Future Oncology*, 6(6), 877–880.

De Figueiredo, J. and Frank, J. (1982). Subjective incompetence, the clinical hallmark of demoralization. *Comprehensive Psychiatry*, 23(4), 353–363.

De Mello, M.F., de Jesus Mari, J., Bacaltchuk, J., Verdeli, H., and Neugebauer, R. (2005). A systematic review of research findings on the efficacy of interpersonal therapy for depressive disorders. *European Archives of Psychiatry and Clinical Neuroscience*, 255(2), 75–82.

Demierre, M.F. and Taverna, J. (2006). Mirtazapine and gabapentin for reducing pruritus in cutaneous T-cell lymphoma. *Journal of the American Academy of Dermatology*, 55(3), 543–544.

Derogatis, L.R., Morrow, G.R., Fetting, J., et al. (1983). The prevalence of psychiatric disorders among cancer patients. *Journal of the American Medical Association*, 249(6), 751–757.

DiMatteo, M.R. and Hanskard-Zolnierek, K.B. (2011). Impact of depression on treatment adherence and survival from cancer. In D.W. Kissane, M. Maj, and N. Sartorius (eds.) *Depression and Cancer*, pp. 101–124. Oxford: Wiley-Blackwell.

Dimidjian, S., Hollon, S.D., Dobson, K.S., et al. (2006). Randomized trial of behavioral activation, cognitive therapy, and antidepressant medication in the acute treatment of adults with major depression. *Journal of Consulting and Clinical Psychology*, 74(4), 658–670.

Dohrenwend, B., Shrout, P., Egri, G., and Mendelsohn, F. (1980). Nonspecific psychological distress and other dimensions of psychopathology. Measures for use in the general population. *Archives of General Psychiatry*, 37(11), 1229–1236.

Duggal, H.S. and Singh, I. (2005). Psychotropic drug-induced neutropenia. *Drugs of Today*, 41(8), 517–526.

Dumont, I. and Kissane, D. (2009). Techniques for framing questions in conducting family meetings in palliative care. *Palliative & Supportive Care*, 7(2), 163–170.

Ebrahimi, B., Tucker, S.L., Li, D., Abbruzzese, J.L., and Kurzrock, R. (2004). Cytokines in pancreatic carcinoma: correlation with phenotypic characteristics and prognosis. *Cancer*, 101(12), 2727–2736.

Emanuel, E.J., Fairclough, D.L., Daniels, E.R., and Clarridge, B.R. (1996). Euthanasia and physician-assisted suicide: attitudes and experiences of oncology patients, oncologists, and the public. *The Lancet*, 347(9018), 1805–1810.

Endicott, J. (1984). Measurement of depression in patients with cancer. *Cancer*, 53(10 Suppl.), 2243–2249.

Ewertz, M. (1986). Bereavement and breast cancer. *British Journal of Cancer*, 53(5), 701–703.

Folkman, S. (1997). Positive psychological states and coping with severe stress. *Social Science & Medicine*, 45(8), 1207–1221.

Frank, J. (1974). Psychotherapy: the restoration of morale. *American Journal of Psychiatry*, 131(3), 271–274.

Furey, M.L. and Drevets, W.C. (2006). Antidepressant efficacy of the antimuscarinic drug scopolamine: a randomized, placebo-controlled clinical trial. *Archives of General Psychiatry*, 63(10), 1121–1129.

Grassi, L., Holland, J.C., Johansen, C., Koch, U., and Fawzy, F. (2005). Psychiatric concomitants of cancer, screening procedures, and training of health care professionals in oncology: the paradigms of psycho-oncology in the psychiatry field. In G.N. Christodolou (ed.) *Advances in Psychiatry*, pp. 59–66. Athens: Beta Publishing.

Grassi, L., Rossi, E., Sabato, S., Cruciani, G., and Zambelli, M. (2004). Diagnostic criteria for psychosomatic research and psychosocial variables in breast cancer patients. *Psychosomatics*, 45(6), 483–491.

Griffith, J.L. and Gaby, L. (2005). Brief psychotherapy at the bedside: countering demoralization from medical illness. *Psychosomatics*, 46(2), 109–116.

Guo, Y., Musselman, D.L., Manatunga, A.K., *et al.* (2006). The diagnosis of major depression in patients with cancer: a comparative approach. *Psychosomatics*, 47(5), 376–384.

Hamilton, N.G. and Hamilton, C.A. (2005). Competing paradigms of response to assisted suicide requests in Oregon. *American Journal of Psychiatry*, 162(6), 1060–1065.

Hem, E., Loge, J.H., Haldorsen, T., and Ekeberg, O. (2004). Suicide risk in cancer patients from 1960 to 1999. *Journal of Clinical Oncology*, 22(20), 4209–4216.

Hinnen C, Ranchor RV, Sanderman R, Snijders TAB, Hagedoorn M, Coyne JC. (2008). Course of distress in breast cancer patients, their partners, and matched control couples. *Annals of Behavioral Medicine*, 36(2), 141–148.

Hooper, S.C., Vaughan, K.J., Tennant, C.C., and Perz, J.M. (1996). Major depression and refusal of life-sustaining medical treatment in the elderly. *Medical Journal of Australia*, 165(8), 416–419.

Irwin, S.A. and Iglewicz, A. (2010). Oral ketamine for the rapid treatment of depression and anxiety in patients receiving hospice care. *Journal of Palliative Care*, 13(7), 903–908.

Jong, C.d., Kissane, D., Geessink, R., and Velden, D.v.d. (2008). Demoralization in opioid dependent patients: a comparative study with cancer patients and community subjects. *Open Addiction Journal*, 1, 7–9.

Kelly, B.J., Burnett, P.C., Pelusi, D., Badger, S.J., Varghese, F.T., and Robertson, M.M. (2004). Association between clinician factors and a patient's wish to hasten death: terminally ill cancer patients and their doctors. *Psychosomatics*, 45(4), 311–318.

Kendler, K.S., Gatz, M., Gardner, C.O., and Pedersen, N.L. (2006). A Swedish national twin study of lifetime major depression. *American Journal of Psychiatry*, 163(1), 109–114.

Kim, H.F. and Fisch, M.J. (2006). Antidepressant use in ambulatory cancer patients. *Current Oncology Reports*, 8(4), 275–281.

Kissane, D., Clarke, D., and Street, A. (2001). Demoralization syndrome—a relevant psychiatric diagnosis for palliative care. *Journal of Palliative Care*, 17(1), 12–21.

Kissane, D.W., Bloch, S., Miach, P., Smith, G.C., Seddon, A., and Keks, N. (1997). Cognitive-existential group therapy for patients with primary breast cancer—techniques and themes. *Psycho-Oncology*, 6(1), 25–33.

Kissane, D.W., Grabsch, B., Clarke, D.M., *et al.* (2004). Supportive-expressive group therapy: the transformation of existential ambivalence into creative living while enhancing adherence to anti-cancer therapies. *Psycho-Oncology*, 13(11), 755–768.

Kissane, D.W., Grabsch, B., Clarke, D.M., *et al.* (2007). Supportive-expressive group therapy for women with metastatic breast cancer: survival and psychosocial outcome from a randomized controlled trial. *Psycho-Oncology*, 16(4), 277–286.

Kissane, D.W., McKenzie, M., Bloch, S., Moskowitz, C., McKenzie, D.P., and O'Neill, I. (2006). Family focused grief therapy: a randomized, controlled trial in palliative care and bereavement. *American Journal of Psychiatry*, 163(7), 1208–1218.

Kissane, D.W., Street, A., and Nitschke, P. (1998). Seven deaths in Darwin: case studies under the Rights of the Terminally Ill Act, Northern Territory, Australia. *The Lancet*, 352(9134), 1097–1102.

Kissane, D., Wein, S., Love, A., Lee, X., Kee, P., and Clarke, D. (2004). The Demoralization Scale: a preliminary report of its development and validation. *Journal of Palliative Care*, 20(4), 269–276.

Kulie, T., Slattengren, A., Redmer, J., Counts, H., Eglash, A., and Schrager, S. (2011). Obesity and women's health: an evidence-based review. *Journal of the American Board of Family Medicine*, 24(1), 75–85.

Lethborg, C., Aranda, S., Bloch, S., and Kissane, D. (2006). The role of meaning in advanced cancer-integrating the constructs of assumptive world, sense of coherence and meaning-based coping. *Journal of Psychosocial Oncology*, 24(1), 27–42.

Lethborg, C., Schofield, P., and Kissane, D. (2012). The advanced cancer patient experience of undertaking meaning and purpose (MaP) therapy. *Palliative & Supportive Care*, 10(3), 177–188.

Li, J., Johansen, C., Hansen, D., and Olsen, J. (2002). Cancer incidence in parents who lost a child: a nationwide study in Denmark. *Cancer*, 95(10), 2237–2242.

Manne, S.L., Ostroff, J.S., Winkel, G., *et al.* (2005). Couple-focused group intervention for women with early stage breast cancer. *Journal of Consulting and Clinical Psychology*, 73(4), 634–646.

McKenzie, D., Clarke, D., Forbes, A., and Sim, M. (2010). Pessimism, worthlessness, anhedonia, and thoughts of death identify DSM-IV major depression in hospitalized, medically ill patients. *Psychosomatics*, 51(4), 302–311.

Mehnert, A., Vehling, S., Höcker, A., Lehmann, C., and Koch, U. (2011). Demoralization and depression in patients with advanced cancer: validation of the German version of the Demoralization Scale. *Journal of Pain and Symptom Management*, 42(5), 768–776.

Meyer, T.J. and Mark, M.M. (1995). Effects of psychosocial interventions with adult cancer patients: a meta-analysis of randomized experiments. *Health Psychology*, 14(2), 101–108.

Miller, K. and Massie, M.J. (2010). Depressive disorders. In J.C. Holland, W.S. Breitbart, P.B. Jacobsen, M.S. Lederberg, M.J. Loscalzo, and R. McCorkle (eds.) *Psycho-Oncology*, pp. 177–186. New York: Oxford University Press.

Minton, O., Richardson, A., Sharpe, M., Hotopf, M., and Stone, P. (2008). A systematic review and meta-analysis of the pharmacological treatment of cancer-related fatigue. *Journal of the National Cancer Institute*, 100(16), 1155–1166.

Mitchell, A.J., Chan, M., Bhatti, H., *et al.* (2011). Prevalence of depression, anxiety, and adjustment disorder in oncological, haematological, and palliative-care settings: a meta-analysis of 94 interview-based studies. *The Lancet Oncology*, 12(2), 160–174.

Morita, T., Tsunoda, J., Inoue, S., and Chihara, S. (2000). An exploratory factor analysis of existential suffering in Japanese terminally ill cancer patients. *Psycho-Oncology*, 9(2), 164–168.

Murphy, J.M., Gilman, S.E., Lesage, A., *et al.* (2010). Time trends in mortality associated with depression: findings from the Stirling County study. *Canadian Journal of Psychiatry*, 55(12), 776–783.

Onwuteaka-Philipsen, B.D., van der Heide, A., Koper, D., *et al.* (2003). Euthanasia and other end-of-life decisions in the Netherlands in 1990, 1995, and 2001. *The Lancet*, 362(9381), 395–399.

Onyike, C.U., Crum, R.M., Lee, H.B., Lyketsos, C.G., and Eaton, W.W. (2003). Is obesity associated with major depression? Results from the Third National Health and Nutrition Examination Survey. *American Journal of Epidemiology*, 158(12), 1139–1147.

Passik, S.D. and Lowery, A.E. (2011). Recognition of depression and methods of depression screening in people with cancer. In D.W. Kissane, M. Maj, and N. Sartorius (ed.) *Depression and Cancer*, pp. 81–100. Oxford: Wiley-Blackwell.

Pettingale, K.W., Morris, T., Greer, S., and Haybittle, J.L. (1985). Mental attitudes to cancer: an additional prognostic factor. *The Lancet*, 1(8431), 750.

Price, A. and Hotopf, M. (2009). The treatment of depression in patients with advanced cancer undergoing palliative care. *Current Opinion in Supportive and Palliative Care*, 3(1), 61–66.

Rayner, L., Price, A., Evans, A., Valsraj, K., Higginson, I.J., and Hotopf, M. (2010). Antidepressants for depression in physically ill people. *Cochrane Database of Systematic Reviews*, (3), CD007503.

Richards, S., Umbreit, J.N., Fanucchi, M.P., Giblin, J., and Khuri, F. (2003). Selective serotonin reuptake inhibitor-induced rhabdomyolysis associated with irinotecan. *Southern Medical Journal*, 96(10), 1031–1033.

Sheard, T. and Maguire, P. (1999). The effect of psychological interventions on anxiety and depression in cancer patients: results of two meta-analyses. *British Journal of Cancer*, 80(11), 1770–1780.

van der Lee, M.L., van der Bom, J.G., Swarte, N.B., Heintz, A.P., de Graeff, A., and van den Bout, J. (2005). Euthanasia and depression: a prospective cohort study among terminally ill cancer patients. *Journal of Clinical Oncology*, 23(27), 6607–6612.

Vodermaier, A., Linden, W., and Siu, C. (2009). Screening for emotional distress in cancer patients: a systematic review of assessment instruments. *Journal of the National Cancer Institute*, 101(21), 1464–1488.

Waring, W.S., Gray, J.A., and Graham, A. (2008). Predictive factors for generalized seizures after deliberate citalopram overdose. *British Journal of Clinical Pharmacology*, 66(6), 861–865.

Watson, M., Homewood, J., Haviland, J., and Bliss, J.M. (2005). Influence of psychological response on breast cancer survival: 10-year follow-up of a population-based cohort. *European Journal of Cancer*, 41(12), 1710–1714.

Wilson, K.G., Chochinov, H.M., Skirko, M.G., *et al.* (2007). Depression and anxiety disorders in palliative cancer care. *Journal of Pain and Symptom Management*, 33(2), 118–129.

Zaider, T.I., and Kissane, D.W. (2011). Couples therapy in advanced cancer: using intimacy and meaning to reduce existential distress. In M. Watson and D.W. Kissane (eds.) *Handbook of Psychotherapy in Cancer Care*, pp. 163–171. Chichester: Wiley-Blackwell.

Zylicz, Z. (2002). Palliative care and euthanasia in the Netherlands. In K. Foley and H. Hendin (eds.) *The Case Against Assisted Suicide—For the Right to End-of-Life Care*, pp. 122–143. Baltimore, MD: Johns Hopkins University Press.

17.4

Adjustment disorders and anxiety

Simon Wein and Limor Amit

Introduction to adjustment disorders and anxiety

The American Psychiatric Association's *Diagnostic and Statistical Manual of Mental Disorders* (DSM) has a category called Adjustment Disorders (ADs) (American Psychiatric Association, 2000). This category is problematic because it is not grounded in a body of reproducible research or a clear and agreed-upon definition (Strain 1998; Gur et al., 2005; Laugharne et al., 2009). Being unable to adjust to a stressor may result in the patient developing pathological and distressing symptoms. It is a common clinical observation to see patients who initially cope, but then with another and added stressor are unable to adjust. The category of AD has a practical and intuitive appeal that makes it useful at the bedside.

Anxiety, like the ADs, is a common response to the stressors caused by physical illnesses, especially those that are life-threatening (Noyes et al., 1998; Stark et al., 2002; Lederberg, 2003; Kangas et al., 2007; Teunissen et al., 2007; Roy-Byrne et al., 2008). Anxiety may or may not be pathological. It can be a stimulus to adaptation, or occur along a spectrum of clinical syndromes and diagnoses. Too little anxiety can kill through neglect, whereas too much can lead to decompensation, and psychiatric or even physical illness (Stevens and Price, 2000).

ADs and anxiety, therefore, occupy a grey zone between an individual's healthy adaptation to stressors and pathological decompensation. Given the importance and variability in the stressors encountered by those with serious illness, they are highly relevant phenomena in the practice of palliative care.

Stressors

The precipitating event for an AD or anxiety is a stressor, which is a stimulus that disturbs the normal physiologic or psychological equilibrium (Gur et al., 2005), but may not be objectively quantifiable. Stressors can be internal or external, inherited or acquired, and physical or non-physical. In the medically ill, stressors can be numerous and extremely complex. The specific nature of the stressors may guide therapy.

A case is illustrative: a young, single mother treated for locally advanced cervical cancer presents on the anniversary of her diagnosis with extreme anxiety and severe back pain, requiring intravenous morphine. The morphine lessens the pain, but the patient's distress remains very high. Magnetic resonance imaging shows a ruptured intervertebral disc. After being told, the patient quickly reports symptomatic improvement and a desire to return home.

The stressors in this scenario probably included both physical pain and fear of cancer recurrence. Other stressors may have been prominent but would remain hidden unless elicited through the clinical interview. The complexity of the factors driving this patient's anxiety exemplify the biopsychosocial model of ill health and underscore the potential value of careful assessment and a varied therapeutic response. When enmeshment of different response systems occurs, such as the response to pain and the response to fear of recurrence, no one type of treatment, such as medication alone, should be viewed as the best management (Engel, 1977). Indeed, the complexity of treatment decisions in populations with advanced illness is reflected by the need to understand and address the broad range of emotional reactions, such as anxiety, depression, grief and anger, as well as coping and adaptation, as highly varied stressors wax and wane (Murray-Parkes, 1998; Lederberg, 2003; Jordan and Okifuji, 2011).

In populations with advanced illness, some stressors appear to be relatively common. They include knowledge that death is imminent, family feuds, inability to work, financial crisis, the perception of becoming a burden or losing control due to illness, physical pain or other symptoms, and being unable to complete life's tasks, Other stressors relate to premorbid physical or psychiatric problems, such as obsessive–compulsive neurosis. Yet others occur as system issues, such as the threat of non-coverage by a health insurance company.

In assessing the possibility of an AD, clinicians should seek evidence of the diverse events, situations, conditions and cognitions that can become stressors in the context of medical illness. At the same time, however, this assessment must be informed by the reality that overt connections between stressors and distress may not be found. There is no direct correlation between patients' responses and either the severity or type of stressor, and up to 30% of ADs are diagnosed without an obvious recent (within 3 months) identified external stressor (Gur et al., 2005).

When is adjustment or anxiety psychopathology?

Patients living with progressive incurable illness must continually adjust to new situations, realities, and losses. The psychological processes underpinning coping and adaptation are repeatedly challenged, and the degree of distress and dysfunction that occur may vary with the severity and type of stressor, individual resilience, premorbid psychological health, education, and preparation, support from family and health professionals, and other factors. Distress associated with adjustment is common, and to some extent, entirely normal.

How can a health professional judge that a patient's response is abnormal, that in fact an AD is occurring? The DSM suggests that the distinction can be made by considering (1) the severity of symptoms and (2) the extent of disruption of normal functioning or of homeostatic adaptation (American Psychiatric Association, 2000).

Ideally, the assessment parameters that would distinguish normal from pathological would be defined empirically through research. Unfortunately, it is difficult to conduct quality research in palliative care because of the practical and ethical challenge in recruiting sick patients, short and unpredictable follow-up, difficulty in controlling multiple variables, high attrition rate, and the overlap between psychological and physical symptoms (Grande and Ingleton, 2008). Indeed, a large systematic review of psychological distress and psychiatric morbidity in advanced cancer confirmed the difficulty in recruiting 'large and representative samples' due to patient ill health or refusal, and emphasized the need for greater flexibility in research design and different ethical guidelines (Ryan et al., 2012). Given the limitations in the extant literature, many of the principles for assessment of the ADs and their treatment are extrapolated from the general psychiatric literature and rely on empirical 'N-of-1' studies, and expert opinion.

The type of assessment needed to determine whether a patient's distress in association with a stressor is best labelled an AD is exemplified by grief.

'Uncomplicated grief . . . is an entirely normal emotional response to loss. The medical profession should normalize, not medicalize, grief' (Friedman, 2012). Grieving patients may evince profound sadness, rumination about the loss, and difficulty functioning. Categorizing this phenomenology as a psychiatric syndrome carries the risk of medicalizing emotions and relying on medical therapies, particularly drugs, to address the distress. The symptoms associated with grief can, however, reach a clinical threshold defined by character, severity, or duration that appropriately leads to a diagnosis of pathological grief. The diagnosis, in turn, impels consideration of treatment.

Even in the latter situation, however, treatment should not be taken to mean common medical interventions, like drugs, along. Grieving, like coping with the stress of illness, and indeed dying itself, are life tasks. Health professionals should not presume that the goal is to abort the type of psychological or spiritual work that may be needed by the patient to process, cope, and recover. In a sense, the clinician risks infantilizing the patient by 'doing' the psychological work for them. Recognizing this complexity provides a strong rationale for the use of traditional talking therapy in addressing ADs or uncomfortable emotions like anxiety. Through psychotherapy, uncomfortable emotions can be tools to allow insight (Stevens and Price, 2000).

The clinical assessment of the severity of response is a key to distinguishing an AD from normal adjustment, or identifying times that anxiety calls for clinical intervention. Anxiety, for example, can help or cripple. The clinician must decide whether this particular person in the context of the particular stressor is expressing a degree of anxiety that is pathological, and if so, how best to manage it (McHugh and Slavney, 2012). The assessment may require corroborative evidence from family, friends, or the family doctor (with the patient's consent), so that the presenting symptoms can be contrasted with premorbid behaviour

Adjustment disorder

In DSM-IV, the ADs are divided into subcategories: Depressed Mood, Anxiety, Disturbance of Conduct, Mixed Anxiety and Depressed Mood, and Mixed Disturbance of Emotions and Conduct (American Psychiatric Association, 2000). The literature does not offer a precise definition of AD, but the concept overall, and these phenomenological distinctions, are clinically easy to use by applying DSM criteria (Baumeister and Kufner, 2009). As noted, the assessment should seek to define the stressors associated with a potential AD. Symptoms that suggest an AD can develop up to 3 months after a stressor; the symptoms typically remit by 6 months after the stressor resolves. Identifying a key stressor may warrant a targeted intervention, even if research has not established with any predictive accuracy which stressors are beneficial or destructive (Casey et al., 2001), and the relationship between individual stressors and ADs is indeterminate. For example, marital problems, financial difficulties, and moving place of residence are common stressors in the general population (Maercker et al., 2007), and the specific impact of a disease, such as a cancer or other chronic illness, is a common stressor in hospitalized patients, but neither the development nor the severity of AD is directly related to the existence or severity of these problems (Strain et al., 1998; Gur et al., 2005). Nonetheless, once identified by the patient as a source of distress, clinical efforts to ameliorate a stressor can be beneficial.

The resilience of the individual, which is one determinant of ability to adjust, is influenced by character, 'ego strength', social support, culture, belief system, and past ability to deal with stressors. While overall resilience does not usually change late in life, stressors associated with a fatal illness may precipitate unexpected reactions (Greer and Watson, 1987; Lederberg, 2003). To the extent that efforts to support resilience are possible, they may be worthy to explore if an AD occurs.

To diagnose an AD, the distressing symptoms may not be explicable by another disorder and cannot be due to bereavement. This is problematic, since up to 60% of medically ill patients have another Axis 1 psychiatric disorder, such as Major Depression. Diagnosis is further complicated by the clear potential for overlap between ADs and post-traumatic stress disorder, and later on, with bereavement. It remains unclear whether any particular AD is part of a spectrum of disorders, or is a distinct entity, and as noted, the criteria that define a transition between normal adjustment and psychopathology are ill defined (Strain et al., 1998; Casey et al., 2001; Maercker et al., 2007; Baumeister and Kufner, 2009; Laugharne et al., 2009). Nonetheless, some authors claim that ADs have distinct profiles and represent a category between no mental disorder and affective disorders, specifically depression and anxiety disorders (Fernández et al., 2012). Consistent with the latter view, AD has been labelled a subthreshold disorder (American Psychiatric Association, 2000).

Depending on the specific symptoms, other elements in the differential diagnosis of the ADs may include other types of depression, somatization, personality disorder, suicidality, anger, generalized anxiety disorder, and insomnia. As noted, the information needed for diagnosis must first come from the patient, but also may originate from multiple other sources. If the patient is receiving care from a palliative care team, valuable information may be forthcoming from any member of the team, particularly social workers.

A high index of clinical suspicion is needed to diagnose, anticipate, and prevent psychiatric problems, including ADs. These disorders may be misdiagnosed as physical complaints or dismissed as 'normal' responses. If one or more of the stressors common in advanced illness, such as progressive disease, physical limitations, dependency, financial stress, anticipatory loss, failed goals, or a family in crisis, has occurred or worsened, this may assist in the diagnosis of an AD or present an opportunity for prevention.

If suspicion is high and assessment is performed competently, the diagnosis of AD can be distinguished from normal adjustment and other psychiatric disorders. The diagnosis of ADs can be made in as many as 13% of inpatients in a general hospital situation, 10% in outpatients, and 13% in emergency rooms, In the general population, AD is associated with suicidal thoughts (30%); 58% of suicide attempters and 9–19% of suicide completers may be diagnosed with an AD. A study of 209 terminally ill cancer patients found that AD was present in 11–17%, compared to a depression prevalence of 7–12%; lower performance status, inadequate social support, and concern about being a burden were significantly associated with the diagnosis (Akechi et al., 2004).

Anxiety

Anxiety, fear, or nervousness is almost universal at some point in life, especially when life is threatened by illness. 'We may take for granted that the fear of death is always present in our mental functioning. . . . It must be properly repressed to keep us living with any modicum of comfort' (Zilboorg, 1943). Anxiety can be adaptive or maladaptive. Too little fear is dangerous, whereas too much (as in a crippling neurosis) can paralyse (Stevens and Price, 2000). DSM-IV subdivides anxiety into generalized, adjustment, panic, phobias, post-traumatic, and due to general medical condition (American Psychiatric Association, 2000).

In the context of advanced illness, anxiety may be linked to a set of thoughts and concerns. Murray-Parkes documented these common fears in a hospice: separation from loved ones, becoming a burden to others, losing control, knowing that dependents will suffer, having pain or other symptoms, being unable to complete life tasks, dying or being dead, and the fears of others (reflected) (Murray-Parkes, 1998).

Although the expression of anxiety varies from person to person, severe anxiety is associated with common symptoms and signs, some of which are related to hyperactivity of the sympathetic nervous system. These include restlessness and irritability, difficulty concentrating, increased muscle tension, somatization, acute stress with nightmares, sleep disturbance, worries that cannot be rationally allayed, and panic-like attacks. The differential diagnosis of anxiety also can include specific phobias, obsessive–compulsive disease, post-traumatic stress disorder, and delirium (American Psychiatric Association, 2000).

Most studies indicate that between 10% and 30% of cancer patients have an identifiable anxiety disorder, as opposed to a prevalence of general anxiety disorder of 5% in the community (Stiefel and Razavi, 1994; Rasic et al., 2008; Wein et al., 2010; Traeger et al., 2012). The prevalence may be underestimated because diagnosis can be difficult if the patient does not have the vocabulary to express an unaccustomed frightening inner feeling. Some part

of the prevalence is a related to an exacerbation of a previous or underlying psychiatric disorder by the stresses of an intercurrent illness, or by the use of medications that can produce anxiety as a side effect (Wein et al., 2010) (Box 17.4.1). The prevalence of anxiety disorder does not include common situational anxiety that may come and go in response to a specific threat such as waiting for results, receiving bad news, experiencing a new symptom, or starting a treatment (Palmer et al., 2004).

Diagnosis

Failure to diagnose anxiety increases the likelihood of anxiety-related problems. These can include trouble making decisions about treatment or adhering to treatment, and more visits to the physician's office and emergency rooms for symptoms such as dizziness, palpitations, breathlessness, insomnia, or pain (Greer and Watson, 1987; Roy-Byrne et al., 2008). In terminally ill cancer patients, depression and anxiety appeared to increase the desire

---

Box 17.4.1 Classification and aetiology of anxiety

- Situational
- Existential
- Psychiatric
- Organic
- Central nervous system neoplasm
- Carcinoid syndrome
- Pulmonary: emboli, bronchospasm, hypoxia, oedema, lymphangitis
- Endocrine: thyrotoxicosis, phaeochromocytoma
- Hyponatremia, hypoglycaemia
- Cardiac: tachyarrhythmias, pericardial disease
- Pain
- Delirium
- Medications
- Antipsychotics
- Metoclopramide
- Flumazenil
- Antibiotics: cephalosporins, isoniazid, ciprofloxacin
- Thyroxine
- Baclofen
- Corticosteroids
- Interferon
- Serotonergic syndrome: SSRI, SNRI
- Withdrawal states: benzodiazepines, opioids, alcohol, tobacco, caffeine
- Theophylline.

Source: Data from Rasic DT, et al., Cancer, mental disorders, suicidal ideation and attempts in a large community sample, *Psycho-Oncology*, Volume 17, Issue 7, p.660–7, Copyright © 2008.

for hastened death, in contrast to pain alone, which does not (Kolva et al., 2011).

To prevent these problems and directly address a symptom that commonly undermines quality of life, it is essential to diagnose and manage anxiety. Although the prevalence of psychiatric disorders in chronic diseases can be as high as 40% in some studies (Palmer et al., 2004; Kangas et al., 2007; Rasic et al., 2008; Mitchell et al., 2011), the diagnosis can be missed if an assessment focuses on somatic symptoms and comments about the patient's emotional state are narrow ('Wouldn't you be anxious if you were sick?'). There are many physical illnesses with symptoms of anxiety that mimic existential or psychological distress, and these, too, must be evaluated to understand the anxiety. Examples include dyspnoea and uncontrolled pain (Teunissen et al., 2007; Roy-Byrne et al., 2008). In the same way, both premorbid and comorbid psychiatric illnesses must be assessed because many, including depression, demoralization, personality disorder and delirium, are associated with anxiety.

In particular, it is difficult to establish a diagnosis of either anxiety or an AD in patients who are suffering with uncontrolled pain or other physical symptoms. Symptom distress should be promptly relieved if possible, before the psychiatric assessment of an AD or pathological anxiety is done.

The diagnosis of anxiety relies on both verbal and non-verbal cues, and the importance of non-verbal cues may explain the observation that physicians miss the diagnosis in as many as one-third of patients (Stiefel and Razavi, 1994; Kangas et al., 2007). Some authors have found that men are less able to verbally express their emotions and the clinician must rely on collateral information more often when assessing male patients (Wein et al., 2010). Although the Hospital Anxiety Depression Scale (Zigmond and Snaith, 1983) and the Edmonton Symptom Assessment Scale (Jacobsen et al., 1991) are commonly used and validated tools that measure anxiety, the gold standard remains the clinical interview and observation of the non-verbal cues (Mitchell et al., 2011).

As noted, diagnosis of an anxiety disorder in the medically ill patient is predicated on an assessment of premorbid and comorbid psychiatric disorders. This need for a careful psychiatric assessment mirrors the approach taken to diagnose an AD. It should have a high index of suspicion for illnesses such as depression, insomnia and somatization, phenomena like anger and sadness, and altered body image. Common psychological defences are denial and hope. One needs to know the patient's social milieu and to ask leading questions about psychological state, just as one would when taking a history of a physical illness. In assessing anxiety, it is important to know what sort of a person the patient was before the illness began and this may be clarified by interviews with family members or the family doctor, if the patient consents.

In the cancer population, screening for anxiety has not been shown to result in better mental health and lower distress than results obtained by patient self-referral or clinician referral (Jacobsen, 2007). There are many potential reasons for this finding: a person identified with significant psychological symptoms may not want to be referred for treatment, or there may be inadequate resources to cope with the referrals (which raises ethical questions). Screening also may be problematic because the cut-off points in the screening tool for what constitutes psychopathology have not been fixed by research (Jacobsen, 2007; Meijer et al., 2011). These data suggest that the diagnosis of an anxiety disorder in

medically ill populations is most efficiently accomplished through astute assessment during routine clinical care.

Management of adjustment disorders and anxiety

Comprehensive palliative care is multidisciplinary care and is structured in varied ways. In all situations, however, the physician who is primarily responsible for the patient should know the principles of diagnosis and management of ADs and anxiety, and help organize and monitor care, even if through collaboration with a mental health specialist (Wein et al., 2010).

Treatment should aim to relieve unpleasant feelings or distress, and improve functioning and adherence to medical care. The goal usually is not to eliminate negative feelings or entirely prevent distress. If anxiety is the target symptom, effective treatment also may improve sleep and enable the patient to communicate more openly with their families and significant others. Given the association between anxiety and an increased desire to die, symptom relief also may reduce the risk of suicidal ideation (Kolva et al., 2011).

Evolutionary psychiatry asks whether there is value in psychological distress. Can it lead to deeper understanding? If anxiety is chemically 'removed,' does this mean the patient will not do the psychological work needed to grow? On the other hand, too much stress can make it difficult to think and function (Stevens and Price, 2000).

The treatment of both ADs and anxiety begins with consideration of primary therapies for those factors identified as stressors, triggers, or aetiologies of the symptoms. It is important not to presume what is causing the anxiety. Asking intimate questions directly with empathy and caring will neither frighten nor offend a patient. If anxiety or distress is related to the perception of imminent death, it may be helpful to describe in detail the process leading to death. Many have not seen death before and Rodin and colleagues showed that discussing life expectancy and prognosis can lead to a reduction in anxiety (Rodin et al., 2009). Yalom (2002) noted that death anxiety is inversely proportional to life satisfaction. Building a trusting relationship with honesty and empathy is important for later on when difficult decisions need to be made. Very attentive control of physical symptoms, especially nausea, pain and dyspnoea, also goes a long way to relieving anxiety.

Symptomatic therapies should be considered even if a treatable source of distress is identified and managed. Therapy is both psychological and pharmacological, with judicious use of alternative therapies (Jackson and Lipman, 2004; Davidson et al., 2012). Effective management may include medications, talking therapy, hypnosis, relaxation, and supportive therapy (McQuellon et al., 1998; Roth and Massie, 2007; Arch and Craske, 2009; Otte et al., 2011; Reinhold et al., 2011). Many patients find other complementary therapies helpful, which may include the entire gamut from meditation and reflexology, to Chinese herbs and spices (Wein, 2000; Anderson and Taylor, 2012).

Talking therapies

Psychoeducational interventions provide information about the nature of the disease, the treatments, side effects, and outcomes. These interventions can facilitate initial adjustment to the new situation and help the patient regain a sense of control (Jacobs et al., 1983). Discussing with the patient the causes of anxiety and ways people adjust to stress, and providing anonymous examples is extremely helpful. Explaining to the patient that fear of the disease or its treatment, and fear of dying, are common to everyone can often help them feel less isolated and more in control. Every patient (just as every person) has a thought or fear about death. Talking about it will not cause permanent damage. Most patients (as with most people) will activate psychological defence mechanisms according to their needs. Today, much information is available via the Internet and patients should be encouraged to explore this, and discuss it. Some studies have shown that up to 50% make use of these sources, although others show that fewer patients do so (Helft et al., 2005; Hesse et al., 2005). Many of the larger health centres have resources specifically available for patients and families.

Cognitive behavioural therapy (CBT) is a short-term (up to 20 sessions), goal-oriented intervention aimed at changing the patterns of thinking and behaviour that lead to anxiety and distress (Otte, 2011). The cognitive interventions aim to modify maladaptive cognitions, self-statements, or beliefs. Cognitive techniques include thought stopping, prioritizing worries, distraction, disruption of thought patterns, labelling distortions, and development of replacement imagery. Behavioural techniques include scheduling activities, relaxation training, learning social skills, assertiveness training, rehearsing stressful situations, and *in vivo* exposure (Leichsenring et al., 2009). A recent study assessing the efficacy of CBT in the various anxiety disorders showed that it was an effective treatment (Leichsenring et al., 2009). Encouraging physical exercise has also been shown to improve psychological well-being (Helft et al., 2005).

Chochinov and colleagues developed dignity therapy, a form of CBT, for patients with advanced cancer (Chochinov et al., 2005). The principle is to help patients with a limited life expectancy to identify values in their lives that are important to them. Transcripts of interviews are prepared and returned to the patients, who may then chose to pass them on to family and loved ones. This has been shown to improve dignity, self-esteem, meaning, reduce distress, and reinforce the will to live (Chochinov et al., 2011) (see Chapter 5.6).

Group psychotherapy is a well-established method of treating anxiety and ADs (Yalom and Leszcz, 2005). There is some evidence that it can prolong survival, but this is controversial (Yalom and Leszcz, 2005; Stefanek et al., 2009). Group psychotherapy manages a number of patients at a time, uses patient interactions therapeutically, provides social support, offers an opportunity to express oneself in a peer group, and facilitates learning about the disease process from other patients. The limitations include mixing different diseases (e.g. breast and colon cancers), as well as the problem of patients dying and leaving the group. Many people find publically expressing their feelings socially prohibitive.

Breitbart and colleagues developed a group therapy programme for cancer patients based on meaning and spirituality, and the ideas of Frankl (one can achieve meaning and a sense of control in life even in the most dire and extreme situations) (Frankl, 1959/1988; Breitbart, 2002; Breitbart et al., 2012). The programme is a mixture of didactic, psychoeducational, and cognitive therapies. It has been manualized for group psychotherapy over 8 weeks. A recent pilot study showed that, compared with a standard supportive group therapy, meaning-centred group therapy participants had less anxiety, distress and hopelessness, and a greater wish to live

(Breitbart et al., 2010).The therapy may enable a re-evaluation of life's priorities by facing existential concerns, talking specifically about fears, and ultimately detoxifying the fear of death (Lee et al., 2006).

Family meetings with the staff are critical to any therapeutic intervention, including discharge planning. Family is important, for better or worse, and for emotional support and psychological well-being (Gueguena et al., 2009; Hudson et al., 2009).

Regardless of the talking therapy selected, an effective therapist should be flexible in direction, content, and methodology. Therapy should not be theory driven, but rather, relationship driven. Thus the choice of therapy is eclectic. It is the therapist that plays the central role, not the technique (Yalom, 2002).

Psychopharmacology

The pharmacological choices to address the symptoms of an AD, or anxiety specifically, comprise several classes, including the anxiolytics, antidepressants, and antipsychotics (Schwartz et al., 1989; Lederberg, 2003; Breitbart et al., 2010; Davidson et al., 2010; Koen and Stein, 2011; Traeger et al., 2012). All medications should be prescribed initially for a limited time, with regular review to assess effectiveness and side effects. In physically sick patients, delirium, biochemical disturbances, and drug–drug interactions require specific attention. In the elderly, there is no better adage than 'start-low and go-slow', especially if they are also physically ill.

The medications used to manage acute anxiety disorder in populations with advanced illness are those used for general anxiety disorder. There are few studies of psychopharmacology in palliative care populations (Breitbart et al., 2010), and most clinical decisions are extrapolated from studies in the general population. This is based on reasonable assumptions, as long as caution is exercised about specific drug interactions. For example, certain selective serotonin reuptake inhibitors (SSRIs) are strong inhibitors of the isoenzyme cytochrome P450 2D6 (including fluoxetine, fluvoxetime, and paroxetine) and may lower levels of tamoxifen (Kelly et al., 2010; Lash et al., 2010). For this reason, other SSRIs (including sertraline, citalopram, and escitalopram), or venlafaxine should be considered as alternatives.

There is a theoretical concern that SSRIs used together with tramadol may cause a serotonergic syndrome. However, clinical experience shows that if the medications are combined at low doses and carefully titrated and monitored, they can be safely used together (Sansone and Sansone, 2009).

When only a partial response to a specific drug occurs, or intolerable side effects develop, combination therapy may be helpful. It often is prudent to ask for psychiatrist input when considering combinations of psychotropics (Adson et al., 2005; Brawman-Mintzeret al., 2005). For example, an antipsychotic with sedating characteristics, such as promethazine or methotrimeprazine, may be indicated at a low dose if delirium or other cognitive disturbance accompanies anxiety.

Most placebo-controlled studies in general anxiety have shown benzodiazepines and antidepressants are effective for short-term (up to 12 weeks) anxiolytic therapy (Stocchi et al., 2003; Breitbart et al., 2010; Kolva et al., 2011). They often are used for longer periods based on clinical observation.

Benzodiazepines presumably exert their therapeutic benefit by promoting gamma aminobutyric acid (GABA) activity. In addition to managing anxiety, they can treat insomnia, and in certain circumstances can be antiemetic (e.g. lorazepam). Clonazepam and diazepam have long half-lives and are effective in suppressing symptoms, whilst alprazolam and lorazepam act rapidly, can be given sublingually, and are useful for acute anxiety or panic attack. Benzodiazepines have a particular role in controlling acute anxiety and can be used to manage symptoms until a SSRI or serotonin noradrenaline reuptake inhibitor (SNRI), such as venlafaxine or duloxetine, take effect. After this, they may be used intermittently or as an adjuvant. The main side effect associated with benzodiazepine therapy is sedation. Central nervous system depression is additive to other drugs, including the opioids and anticonvulsants, and this may exacerbate their risks. Tolerance may develop to the sedative effects.

SSRIs and SNRIs have been shown in controlled studies to improve anxiety, especially where there are depressive symptoms (Stocchi et al., 2003; Davidson et al., 2005). These drugs are generally well tolerated, but a significant subgroup of patients (up to 20%) are unable to tolerate them due to nausea, insomnia, agitation, somnolence, or weight gain (Stocchi et al., 2003). Trazodone is useful as second-line antidepressant/anxiolytic, especially if the anxiety is associated with insomnia, sleep disturbance, or hot flashes. Although tricyclic antidepressants (TCAs) are used less often, they too retain a role, especially when there is associated neuropathic pain or when their side effects (such as somnolence) can be used beneficially. Schwartz et al. found support for the use of TCAs to manage ADs in the medically ill (Schwartz et al., 1989).

Antipsychotics are also effective anxiolytics, although the evidence is mainly as augmentation for antidepressants. The atypical antipsychotics, such as risperidone and olanzapine, are generally preferred in the palliative care setting. When patients have comorbid cachexia, the side effect of weight gain can be an advantage (Breitbart et al., 2010).

There is evidence that pregabalin is efficacious in generalized anxiety disorder (Rickels et al., 2005). It is a first-line agent for neuropathic pain. Like gabapentin, this drug is a ligand of the alpha-2-delta protein of specific presynaptic calcium channels. Its mode of action involves inhibition of release of glutamate and other neurotransmitters. The side effects of somnolence and dizziness may be dose-limiting.

Since the 1980s, in part driven by the success of DSM in providing 'diagnostic criteria for all mental disorders' and in part by the pharmaceutical industry's success in promoting drugs for psychiatric disorders, psychiatrists have self-identified increasingly as psychopharmacologists (Angell, 2011). As a consequence, they have less focus on exploring the life stories of their patients and may be less attuned to the human complexities inherent in suffering. The problem of course is that suffering, existential distress, meaning, divorce, death, financial ruin, and losses are not subserved by any specific brain neurotransmitters. Labelling patients as having an anxiety disorder or an AD should not be used as a shortcut to a medication or as a replacement for understanding the person. There is an extensive literature about loss, anger, control, dignity, humiliation, and so forth, which can help guide clinicians in learning how to best communicate with the patient. Psychological techniques, such as Viederman's 'life narrative' (Viederman, 1980; Viederman and Perry, 1983), should be integrated into the management strategy even as drugs are administered to improve symptom distress.

Other therapies

In some countries, medical marijuana (cannabis) is available. In Israel, for example, almost 8000 people have a licence to use it (Y. Baruch, pers. comm.). The main indications are spasticity of multiple sclerosis, chronic non-malignant pain, AIDS-related anorexia, and cancer-related symptoms. In the cancer population, it is used in the management of nausea related to chemotherapy, pain (especially neuropathic pain), anorexia, anxiety, distress, and insomnia (Gray, 1998; Carter et al., 2011; Twycross and Wilcock, 2011). Research in populations with cancer or other serious illness is limited and there are no randomized controlled studies. Unfortunately, commercial interests and widespread acceptance in society make the possibility of randomized studies less likely (Gray, 1998; Tikum Olam, n.d.). Nonetheless, one review found support for cannabis in the treatment of anxiety and insomnia (Robson, 2001), and based on clinical observations, it is likely that cannabis also can be helpful for some patients with insomnia. It is essential that research, preferably blinded studies, be undertaken to document cannabis's role in palliative care.

Complementary therapies play a role in managing anxiety and ADs. Many patients have faith that these therapies help (Burstein, 1999; Holland, 1999; Wein, 2000); that in itself may reduce anxiety and distress. It is important to distinguish between complementary therapies that are provided with the idea of reversing the disease and those that are provided to help cope with the disease. The former, if lacking evidence, have no place in palliative care. Those that may reduce distress or improve quality of life may play a role, as long as they cause no harm, even if they have not been proven in randomized studies. Some complementary therapies, such as art therapy (Oster et al., 2006) and music therapy have been shown in randomized studies to relieve suffering and anxiety.

Rarely, the anxiety and existential distress at the end of life causes severe and intractable suffering, despite medications and talking therapy. In this situation, some specialists in palliative care will consider the use of palliative sedation, as long as the patient consents and the family and colleagues agree (Cherny and Radbruch, 2009). The depth of the sedation is usually just enough to provide sleep, and thus relief, and by agreement may be temporary. Other specialists do not endorse this approach and limit the use of palliative sedation to patients with intractable suffering related to physical problems such as pain, dyspnoea, or delirium.

Anxiety and adjustment of staff

Anxiety, guilt, ADs, personal problems, burn-out, compassion fatigue, and depression are not uncommon in health-care professionals. This is important as regards the health of the professionals, but it can also impact on care of the patients and communication with other staff members. There is a clear role for colleagues to identify staff at risk and departments should have measures and procedures in place to help and assist. Doctors in particular tend to adopt a heroic and a 'never-give-up approach', which can also be their undoing (see Chapter 14.6).

Conclusion

Identifying ADs and anxiety is important in populations with advanced illness because they are common and there are many stressors, both physical and existential, that may precipitate them.

Clinicians must be prepared to diagnose appropriately and treat wisely.

Suffering includes physical and psychosocial components. Physical symptoms, such as dyspnoea and pain, are generally treated with medications or other physical interventions. To manage psychological suffering, both pharmacotherapy and talking therapy should be considered. For patients with advanced illness, for whom many stressors are existential in nature and not due to long-standing pre-morbid psychiatric disorders, it is important to combine the two arms of therapy and not just to rely on psychotropic medications. A family meeting is critical to the understanding of the patient and for developing plans for ongoing care and discharge.

Clinicians need to 'clinically screen' patients by proactively asking about psychological symptoms. There is, however, no strong evidence that formally screening all patients improves outcome.

The clinical significance of ADs and anxiety is based on the assessment of symptoms and the degree of impairment of social or occupational functioning. It is neither a realistic nor appropriate goal to eliminate all symptoms. A sufficient aim is to control the symptoms enough to reduce distress and improve the ability to function. The goal of the palliative medicine clinician is to help the patient move from an AD to adjustment, and from anxiety to acceptance.

Online materials

Complete references for this chapter are available online at <http://www.oxfordmedicine.com>.

References

Breitbart, W., Rosenfeld, B., Gibson, C., *et al.* (2010). Meaning-centered group psychotherapy for patients with advanced cancer: a pilot randomized controlled trial. *Psycho-Oncology*, 19(1), 21–28.

Casey, P., Dowrick, C., and Wilkinson, G. (2001). Adjustment disorders: fault line in psychiatric glossary. *British Journal of Psychiatry*, 179, 479–481.

Greer, S. and Watson, M. (1987). Mental adjustment to cancer: its measurement and prognostic significance. *Cancer Surveys*, 6, 439–453.

Holland, J.C. (1999). Use of alternative medicine—a marker for distress. *The New England Journal of Medicine*, 340, 1758–1759.

Jackson, K.C. and Lipman, A.G. (2004). Drug therapy for anxiety in palliative care. *Cochrane Database of Systematic Reviews*, 1, CD004596.

Koen, N. and Stein, D.J. (2011). Pharmacotherapy of anxiety disorders: a critical review. *Dialogues in Clinical NeuroSciences*, 13, 423–437.

Kolva, E., Rosenfeld, B., Pessin, H., Breitbart, W., and Brescia, R. (2011). Anxiety in terminally ill cancer patients. *Journal of Pain and Symptom Management*, 42(5), 691–701.

Lederberg, M.S. (2003). Psycho-oncology. In B.J. Sadock and V.A. Sadock (eds.) *Kaplan and Sadock's Synopsis of Psychiatry* (9th ed.), pp. 1351–1365. Philadelphia, PA: Lippincott Williams and Wilkins Press.

Murray-Parkes, C. (1998). Coping with loss: the dying adult. *BMJ*, 316, 1313–1315.

Stark, D., Kiely, M., Smith, A., Velikova, G., House, A., and Selby, P. (2002). Anxiety disorders in cancer patients: their nature, associations, and relation to quality of life. *Journal of Clinical Oncology*, 20, 3137–3148.

Viederman, M. (1983). The psychodynamic life narrative: a psychotherapeutic intervention useful in crisis situations. *Psychiatry*, 46(3), 236–246.

Wein, S., Sulkes, A., and Stemmer, S. (2010). The oncologists' role in managing depression, anxiety and demoralization in advanced cancer. *Cancer Journal*, 16(5), 493–499.

Zilboorg, G. (1943). Fear of death. *Psychoanalytic Quarterly*, 12, 465–475.

17.5

Delirium

Meera Agar, Yesne Alici, and William S. Breitbart

Introduction to delirium

Delirium is the most common neuropsychiatric disorder experienced by patients with advanced illness. It is characterized by disturbances in level of alertness, attention, thinking, perception, cognition, psychomotor behaviour, mood, and sleep–wake cycle. Acute onset and fluctuation of symptoms are critical features. Although conceptualized as a reversible process, it may not be reversible in the context of advanced illness, and indeed, may be a harbinger of imminent death (Breitbart and Alici, 2008).

The occurrence of delirium indicates significant physiological disturbance, usually involving multiple aetiologies. It may be associated with significant immediate morbidity, increased costs due to prolonged hospitalization, and long-term cognitive decline (Breitbart and Alici, 2008). It often distresses both families and staff (Breitbart et al., 2002) and can interfere with the recognition and control of other physical symptoms, such as pain.

Unfortunately, delirium often is under-recognized and under-treated. The heterogeneity of neuropsychiatric signs and symptoms, and the fluctuating course, may delay diagnosis and treatment. Specialists in palliative care must be able to screen for delirium, diagnose it accurately, undertake appropriate assessment of aetiologies, and be familiar with risks and benefits of pharmacological and non-pharmacological treatment options.

Definition

Delirium is a complex syndrome with a multifactorial aetiology, characterized by disturbance of cognition, arousal, and attention (Lipowski, 1990a; Caraceni and Grassi, 2011). The term 'delirium' is derived from the Latin word *delirare*, which means to 'go out of the furrow' (Lipowski, 1990b).

Epidemiology of delirium in advanced illnesses

Based on data from five studies, delirium prevalence on admission to palliative care units or hospices ranges from 13.3% to 42.3% and the incidence after admission ranges between 3% and 45% (Hosie et al., 2013). Two studies that explored delirium rates during the period prior to death observed a prevalence of 58.8–88% (Lawlor et al., 2000a; Hosie et al., 2013).

Pathophysiology

Recent studies indicate that delirium has a multifaceted pathophysiology. In addition to perturbations in dopamine-containing and cholinergic pathways, other neurotransmitters and neurobiological pathways have been implicated (Flacker and Lipsitz, 1999; Trzepacz, 2000; van der Mast and Fekkes, 2000; Wilson et al., 2005; MacLullich et al., 2008), Disturbances in serotonin, gamma-aminobutyric acid (GABA), cortisol, cytokines, and oxygen free radicals may be involved (Flacker and Lipsitz, 1999; Trzepacz, 2000; van der Mast and Fekkes, 2000; Wilson et al., 2005; MacLullich et al., 2008). Drug-induced delirium may be related to transient thalamic dysfunction caused by medication-induced interference with central glutamatergic, GABAergic, dopaminergic, and cholinergic pathways at critical sites of action (Gaudreau and Gagnon, 2005).

A recent model classifies the proposed aetiologies of delirium into (a) direct brain insults and (b) aberrant stress responses (MacLullich et al., 2008). Direct brain insults include general and regional energy deprivation (e.g. hypoxia, hypoglycaemia, and stroke), medication effects, and metabolic abnormalities (e.g. hyponatraemia, hypercalcaemia) (MacLullich et al., 2008). Aberrant stress responses may involve systemic inflammation, the sickness behaviour response, and activity of the limbic–hypothalamic–pituitary–adrenal axis (MacLullich et al., 2008).

Delirium assessment: clinical features and phenomenology

The gold standard for clinical diagnosis is a clinician assessment utilizing standard diagnostic criteria, most commonly the *Diagnostic and Statistical Manual of Mental Disorders* (DSM), fourth edition—text revised (DSM IV-TR), or alternatively, the International Classification of Disease, version 10 (ICD-10) of the World Health Organization (WHO) (American Psychiatric Association, 2000; WHO, 2010). The major components of the DSM IV-TR classification are disturbance of consciousness, a change in cognition, short and fluctuating chronology, and presence of an underlying medical condition. The fifth edition of the DSM (DSM-5) was released in May 2013 (American Psychiatric Association, 2013).The term consciousness has been removed from the delirium diagnostic criteria in DSM-5 to avoid diagnostic confusion between delirium and coma states. There has been much controversy and currently no data to inform implications of the DSM-5 for clinical care and research. The ICD-10 classification has the main components of impairment of consciousness and attention, global disturbance of cognition, psychomotor disturbance, disturbance of sleep–wake cycle, and emotional disturbance.

Delirium includes both cognitive and non-cognitive neuropsychiatric symptoms, including changes in motor behaviour, sleep–wake cycle, affective expression, perception, and thinking (Box 17.5.1) (Gupta et al., 2008). Both the frequency and specificity

Box 17.5.1 Delirium clinical features

Disturbance in consciousness

Cognitive deficits

- Attention
- Orientation to time, place, and person
- Short-term, verbal, visual, and long-term memory
- Executive functions.

Perceptual disturbance

- Illusions
- Hallucinations, in particular visual
- Metamorphoses.

Delusions

- Paranoid delusions, poorly formed.

Thought disorder

- Tangentiality
- Circumstantiality
- Loose associations.

Sleep–wake disturbance

- Fragmented sleep
- Reversal of normal sleep–wake cycle
- Sleeplessness.

Language disturbance

- Word finding difficulty
- Paraphasia
- Dysnomia
- Dysgraphia
- Severe delirium can mimic receptive/expressive aphasia.

Altered affect

- Incongruent mood to context
- Anger
- Increased irritability
- Hypoactivity misdiagnosed as depression
- Lability
- Fear.

Motor behaviours

- Increased or decreased activity
- Increased or decreased speed of actions
- Loss of control of activity
- Wandering
- Restlessness

- Combativeness
- Apathy/listlessness.

Source: Data from Trzepacz, P. T. & Meagher, D. J., Neuropsychiatric aspects of delirium, in Yudofsky, S. C. & Hales, R. E. (Eds.), *The American Psychiatric Publishing Textbook of Neuropsychiatry and Behavioural Neurosciences*, American Psychiatric Publishing, Washington DC, USA, Copyright © 2002; and Meagher, D., Motor subtypes of delirium: past, present and future, *International Review of Psychiatry*, Volume 21, Number 1, pp. 59–73, Copyright © 2009 Informa Plc. All rights reserved.

of these symptoms have been part of the debate in developing a definition of delirium, and approaches to classify and measure it. The frequency of core symptoms varies: attentional deficits 97–100%, thought process abnormalities 54–79%, disorientation 76–96%, memory deficits 88–96%, sleep–wake disturbance 92–97%, motoric alterations 24–94%, language disturbance 57–67%; and the non-core symptoms such as perceptual disturbance 50–63%, delusions 21–31%, and affective changes 43–86% (Webster and Holroyd, 2000; Meagher et al., 2007; Gupta et al., 2008).

Delirium screening instruments can be helpful to characterize clinical symptoms and potentially improve delirium detection rates. Commonly used screening instruments include the Confusion Assessment Method (Ryan et al., 2009) and the Nursing Delirium Assessment Scale (Gaudreau et al., 2005a).

The most studied delirium assessment tools for populations with cancer or advanced illness are the Memorial Delirium Assessment Scale (Breitbart, 1997) and the Delirium Rating Scale—Revised 98 (Trzepacz et al., 2001; Leonard et al., 2008b). These instruments assist clinicians in operationalizing DSM-IV criteria and monitoring severity.

In particular, patients who have predisposing risk factors, such as visual and hearing impairment, age greater than 65, pre-existing cognitive impairment, dehydration, immobility, multiple medications, and comorbid illness, should be monitored closely for delirium symptoms (National Institute for Health and Clinical Excellence (NICE), 2010). The studies exploring risk factors in cancer patients have been small, but implicate psychoactive medication, low albumin, and bone, liver, and intracranial metastases as additional risk factors (Fann et al., 2002; Ljubisavljevic and Kelly, 2003; Gaudreau et al., 2005b).

Delirium subtypes

Three clinical subtypes of delirium have been identified based on psychomotor features and arousal levels (Meagher, 2009). Patients with the hypoactive subtype appear lethargic and drowsy, respond slowly to questions, do not initiate movement, and have reduced awareness of surroundings (Breitbart and Alici, 2012). The hypoactive presentation often leads to misdiagnosis (fatigue or depression) (Meagher and Trzepacz, 2000.). Patients with the hyperactive subtype have restlessness, agitation, and psychomotor overactivity (Camus et al., 2000.). Perceptual disturbance and delusions are more common in this subtype than in hypoactive delirium (Boettger and Breitbart,

2011). More recently, longitudinal studies have demonstrated a group of delirious patients—the so-called no subtype—who have minimal motor activity change (Meagher et al., 2012b). Once established, the type of delirium seems to remain stable over time (Meagher et al., 2012b).

The DSM IV-TR criteria for delirium do not include categories to define psychomotor subtype (Meagher and Trzepacz, 1998, 2000). Methods that have been used include the presence or absence of particular psychomotor behaviours, quantitative measurement of psychomotor activity, validated scales to rate agitated behaviours (not specific for delirium), and most recently, the development of the delirium motor subtype scale (O'Keeffe, 1999; Meagher et al., 2008a, 2008b). There is poor concordance between these different methods of subtyping (Meagher et al., 2008b). It has been suggested that focusing on purely motoric features (Meagher et al., 2008a), and using independent quantitative methods such as electronic motion analysis (accelerometry), may assist in determining the true relationships between clinical subtypes, aetiologies, and outcomes (Leonard et al., 2007; Godfrey et al., 2010).

Increasing subsyndromal presentations also are recognized. For example, some patients with delirium present with symptoms in all core domains of sleep–wake cycle, thought process, language, attention, orientation, and visuospatial ability, but less severe symptoms overall (Meagher et al., 2012a; Trzepacz et al., 2012). This presentation can be particularly difficult to diagnose.

Several studies have explored delirium subtypes in varied populations, including those receiving specialist palliative care, those with advanced cancer, and those with haematological malignancies. These studies suggest that 40–78% of patients with delirium have the hypoactive subtype (Lawlor et al., 2000b; Morita et al., 2001; Lam, 2003; Fann et al., 2005; Gaudreau et al., 2005c; Spiller and Keen, 2006).

There has been much effort to determine if the delirium subtype has implications for differential diagnosis, aetiology, treatment, or prognosis (Meagher and Trzepacz, 1998; O'Keeffe, 1999; Gupta et al., 2008). This work has led to some tentative conclusions.

Differential diagnosis should consider that hyperactive delirium may mimic psychosis or anxiety disorders, whereas hypoactive delirium may be confused with depression or uncooperative behaviour (O'Keeffe, 1999).

It has been postulated that different neurotransmitter abnormalities may associate with delirium subtype (O'Keeffe, 1999.). For example increased GABA and reduced glutamate activity have been demonstrated in hepatic encephalopathy, and this may relate to the high prevalence of hyperactive delirium with this condition (O'Keeffe, 1999.). Some neurotransmitter abnormalities can cause varied phenomenology, for example, anticholinergic medication is typically associated with the hyperactive subtype but also can cause hypoactive and mixed presentations (Itil and Fink, 1966). The concentration of the melatonin metabolite, urinary 6-sulphatoxymelatonin, is highest in hypoactive delirium, lower in delirium with mixed presentation, and lowest in hyperactive delirium (Balan et al., 2003). Interleukin 6 has been associated with the hyperactive and mixed subtypes (van Munster et al., 2008).

Localized neuroanatomical lesions are also associated with particular presentations. For example, hyperactivity has been linked with middle temporal gyrus damage and frontostriatal injury has been associated with hypoactive presentations (Gupta et al., 2008).

In the main, the evidence seems to point to the hypoactive subtype having poorer outcomes (Meagher et al., 2011). Differences in morbidity include more pressure sores and hospital-acquired infection in hypoactive delirium and more falls in hyperactive presentations (O'Keeffe and Lavan).

Diagnostic workup

The presence of delirium implies the existence of an underlying medical disorder and a detailed history and examination should be undertaken to identify the aetiologies and determine whether they are reversible. Most episodes of delirium have an average of three precipitants (Leonard et al., 2008a). Common aetiologies include infection, substance withdrawal (alcohol and nicotine), metabolic abnormalities (e.g. hypercalcaemia), hypoxia, and psychoactive medications (corticosteroids, opioids, anticholinergics, and benzodiazepines) (Lawlor et al., 2000a; Breitbart et al., 2008; Leonard et al., 2008b). Predisposing delirium risk factors should be reviewed including older age, physical frailty, multiple medical comorbidities, dementia, admission to the hospital with infection or dehydration, visual impairment, deafness, polypharmacy, renal impairment, and malnutrition (Inouye, 2006).

The evaluation of delirium may require laboratory test, imaging, or an electroencephalogram. Laboratory tests can identify metabolic abnormalities (e.g. hypercalcaemia, hyponatraemia, and hypoglycaemia), hypoxia, or disseminated intravascular coagulation. Imaging can detect brain metastases or leptomeningeal disease, intracranial bleeding, or ischaemia. An electroencephalogram may rule out seizures. Occasionally, a lumbar puncture is needed to assess the possibility of leptomeningeal carcinomatosis or infectious meningitis (Breitbart and Alici, 2008).

When confronted with delirium in the terminally ill or dying patient, a differential diagnosis should always be formulated as to the likely aetiology or aetiologies. However, consideration of individual goals of care, and prior function and disease trajectory, is needed to determine the extent to which these aetiologies are investigated (Leonard et al., 2008a).

Differential diagnosis of delirium

Many of the clinical features of delirium can be associated with other psychiatric disorders such as depression, mania, psychosis, and dementia (Breitbart and Alici, 2008). Delirium, particularly the hypoactive subtype, is often initially misdiagnosed as depression. In distinguishing delirium from depression, particularly in the context of advanced disease, an evaluation of the onset and temporal sequencing of depressive and cognitive symptoms is particularly helpful. Importantly, the degree of cognitive impairment in delirium is much more severe than in depression, and usually has a more abrupt onset. Additionally, disturbance in level of alertness, which is characteristic of delirium, is not a feature of depression (Breitbart and Alici, 2008).

A manic episode may share some features of a hyperactive or mixed subtype of delirium. The temporal onset and course of symptoms, the presence of a disturbance in level of alertness, as well as of cognition, and the identification of a presumed medical aetiology for delirium are helpful in diagnosis. A past psychiatric history or family history of mood disorders is usually evident in patients with depression or a manic episode (Breitbart and Alici, 2008).

Delirium that is characterized by vivid hallucinations and delusions must be distinguished from a variety of psychotic disorders. In delirium, such psychotic symptoms occur in the context of advanced medical illness with features of disturbance in level of alertness and impaired attention span, as well as memory impairment and disorientation, which is not the case in other psychotic disorders (Breitbart and Alici, 2008).

The most challenging differential diagnostic issue is whether the patient has delirium, or dementia, or a delirium superimposed upon a pre-existing dementia. Both delirium and dementia are cognitive impairment disorders and share such common clinical features as impaired memory, thinking, judgement, aphasia, apraxia, agnosia, executive dysfunction, and disorientation. Delusions and hallucinations can occur in both disorders. To distinguish delirium from dementia, specific differences should be sought. In a study of 100 cancer patients that compared patients with delirium superimposed on dementia to those with delirium in the absence of dementia, the former presentation was characterized by more severe cognitive symptoms, poorer response to treatment, and a lower rate of resolution (Boettger et al., 2011). Clinically, the patient with dementia is alert and does not have the disturbance of level of alertness that is characteristic of delirium. The temporal onset of symptoms in dementia is more subacute and chronically progressive. Delirium is an acute change from the patient's baseline cognitive functioning, even if the patient has dementia or other cognitive disturbances at baseline (Breitbart and Alici, 2008). Treatment may lead to reversal of the symptoms and signs of delirium, even in the patient with advanced illness; this also distinguishes the syndrome from dementia. However, as noted previously, delirium may not be reversible in the last 24–48 hours of life. A number of instruments can aid clinicians in the diagnosis of delirium, dementia, or delirium superimposed on dementia (Wong et al., 2010).

Management of delirium

The management of delirium should include both correction of underlying causes, if possible, and treatment of the symptoms and signs of the disorder (Breitbart and Alici, 2012). To minimize distress to patients, staff, and family members, treatment of the symptoms and signs should be initiated before, or in concert with, a diagnostic assessment of the aetiologies. In the terminally ill patient who develops delirium in the last days of life ('terminal' delirium), management may present a number of dilemmas, and the desired clinical outcome may be significantly altered by the dying process. The desired and often achievable outcome is a patient who is awake, alert, calm, comfortable, cognitively intact, not psychotic, not in pain, and communicating coherently with family and staff (Breitbart and Alici, 2008).

Non-pharmacological interventions

In addition to seeking out and potentially correcting underlying causes of delirium, non-pharmacological and supportive therapies are important (Box 17.5.2). Fluid and electrolyte balance, nutrition, measures to help reduce anxiety and disorientation; interactions with and education of family members may be useful. A quiet, well-lit room with familiar objects, a visible clock or calendar, and the presence of family may help reduce anxiety and disorientation. In non-palliative care settings, there is evidence that these non-pharmacological interventions result in faster

> **Box 17.5.2** Summary of non-pharmacological interventions used in the prevention and treatment of delirium
>
> - Reducing polypharmacy
> - Control of pain
> - Sleep hygiene
> - Monitor for fluid/electrolyte disturbances
> - Monitor nutrition
> - Monitor for sensory deficits
> - Encourage early mobilization (minimize the use of immobilizing catheters, intravenous lines, and physical restraints)
> - Monitor bowel and bladder functioning
> - Reorient the patient frequently
> - Place an orientation board, clock, or familiar objects in the patient's room
> - Encourage cognitively stimulating activities.
>
> Source: Data from Breitbart W. and Alici Y., Agitation and delirium at the end of life: 'We couldn't manage him', *Journal of the American Medical Association*, Volume 300, Number 24, pp. 2898–2910, Copyright © 2008 American Medical Association. All Rights Reserved.

improvement in delirium and slower deterioration in cognition. However, they were not found to have any beneficial effects on mortality or health-related quality of life when compared with usual care (Milisen et al., 2005; Pitkälä et al., 2006, 2008; Flaherty et al., 2010).

Physical restraints should be avoided in patients who are at risk for developing delirium and for those with delirium (Breitbart and Alici, 2008). Recent evidence suggests that restraint-free management of patients should be the standard of care for prevention and treatment of delirium (Flaherty and Little, 2011). One-to-one observation may be necessary while maintaining safety of the patient without use of any restraints.

Pharmacological interventions

There have been an increasing number of delirium prevention and treatment studies published within the last decade. Although there are no drugs specifically approved by the US Food and Drug Administration (FDA) for the treatment of delirium, antipsychotic or sedative medications often are required to control the symptoms or signs (Breitbart and Alici, 2012). Antipsychotics, cholinesterase inhibitors, and alpha-2 agonists are the three groups of medications studied in randomized controlled trials in different patient populations. In palliative care settings, the evidence is supportive of short-term, low-dose use of antipsychotics in the control of symptoms of delirium with close monitoring for possible side effects especially in older patients with multiple medical comorbidities (Breitbart and Alici, 2012).

Antipsychotics

There have been a number of case reports, case series, retrospective chart reviews, open-label trials, randomized controlled comparison trials, and most recently placebo-controlled trials with antipsychotics in the treatment of delirium (Breitbart et al., 1996; Han and

Kim, 2004; Hu et al., 2004; Jackson and Lipman, 2004; Lonergan et al., 2007; Devlin et al., 2010; Girard et al., 2010; Tahir et al., 2010; Grover et al., 2011; Breitbart and Alici, 2012). Study populations mostly include medically ill patients, postoperative patients, and patients in intensive care unit settings. Only a few studies focus specifically on patients with delirium in palliative care settings.

The American Psychiatric Association practice guidelines published in 1999 recommended the use of antipsychotics as the first-line pharmacological option in the treatment of symptoms of delirium (American Psychiatric Association, 1999).The guidelines recommend low-dose haloperidol (i.e. 1–2 mg orally (PO) every 4 hours as required or 0.25–0.5 mg PO every 4 hours for the elderly) as the treatment of choice when medication is necessary (American Psychiatric Association, 1999).

A 2004 Cochrane review concluded that haloperidol was the most suitable medication for the treatment of patients with delirium near the end of life, with chlorpromazine being an acceptable alternative based on one randomized controlled trial with haloperidol, chlorpromazine, and lorazepam (Jackson and Lipman, 2004).

A 2007 Cochrane review that compared the efficacy and adverse effects of haloperidol and atypical antipsychotics concluded that, like haloperidol, selected atypical antipsychotics (risperidone, olanzapine) were effective in managing delirium (Lonergan et al., 2007). Haloperidol doses greater than 4.5 mg/day resulted in increased rates of extrapyramidal symptoms compared with the atypical antipsychotics, but low-dose haloperidol (i.e. < 3.5 mg/day) was not shown to result in a greater frequency of extrapyramidal adverse effects (Lonergan et al., 2007).

Based on these published data, low-dose haloperidol continues to be the first-line agent for treatment of symptoms of delirium (Breitbart and Alici, 2012). In those with advanced illness, haloperidol is preferred due to its efficacy, tolerability (due in part to few anticholinergic effects), and its lack of active metabolites (Breitbart and Alici, 2008). It also may be given by various routes of administration. When used intravenously, however, the US FDA has warned about the risk of QTc prolongation and torsades de pointes; therefore, monitoring QTc intervals closely during intravenous haloperidol has become standard clinical practice. If haloperidol is not tolerated, the atypical antipsychotics are effective alternatives (Lonergan et al., 2007; Breitbart and Alici, 2012).

Based on clinical experience, lorazepam often is added to haloperidol to manage an acute delirium, particularly when hyperactive. Lorazepam (0.5–1.0 mg every 1–2 hours PO or intravenously (IV)) may be more effective in rapidly sedating the agitated delirious patient and may minimize extrapyramidal side effects associated with haloperidol. An alternative strategy is to switch from haloperidol to a more sedating antipsychotic, such as chlorpromazine. The latter approach is most acceptable when the patient is in a monitored setting and blood pressure can be checked frequently. It is important to monitor for anticholinergic and hypotensive adverse effects of chlorpromazine, particularly in elderly patients (Breitbart and Alici, 2012).

The potential risks associated with antipsychotic drug treatment should be considered before the first dose is given. These risks include the possibility of extrapyramidal effects, sedation, anticholinergic side effects, cardiac arrhythmias, and possible drug–drug interactions. These concerns are particularly salient in older patients with dementia. The US FDA has issued a warning about the increased risk of mortality associated with the use of antipsychotics in elderly patients with dementia-related behavioural disturbances. This warning was based on a meta-analysis by Schneider et al of 17 placebo-controlled trials involving patients with dementia (Schneider et al., 2005). The risk of death in patients treated with atypical antipsychotic agents was 1.6–1.7 times greater than in those who received placebo. Most deaths were associated with cardiovascular disease or infection. A second, retrospective study of nearly 23 000 older patients found that mortality rates were higher with typical than with atypical antipsychotics—whether or not they had dementia (Wang et al., 2005). This finding led to an extension of the FDA warning to typical antipsychotics, including haloperidol.

Other studies that have evaluated the risk of excess mortality during antipsychotic drug treatment have yielded mixed results. A retrospective cohort study of Medicaid enrolees in Tennessee demonstrated an increased risk of serious ventricular arrhythmias and sudden cardiac death among users of both typical and atypical antipsychotics (Ray et al., 2009). In contrast, a retrospective, case–control analysis of 326 elderly hospitalized patients with delirium at an acute care community hospital included 111 patients who received an antipsychotic and found non-significant odds ratios of dying during treatment of 1.53 (95% confidence interval (CI) 0.83–2.80) in univariate and 1.61 (95% CI 0.88–2.96) in multivariate analyses (Elie et al., 2009). Additional prospective studies with larger sample sizes will be needed to clarify this association further.

In palliative care settings, the evidence is most clearly supportive of short-term, low-dose use of antipsychotics for the control of symptoms of delirium. Close monitoring for possible side effects is essential, especially in older patients with multiple medical comorbidities (Table 17.5.1) (Breitbart and Alici, 2012).

Psychostimulants

The use of psychostimulants in the treatment of hypoactive subtype of delirium has been suggested by case reports and one open-label study (Keen and Brown, 2004; Gagnon et al., 2005). These drugs can precipitate agitation and exacerbate psychotic symptoms, however, should be used very cautiously in palliative care settings.

Cholinesterase inhibitors

Impaired cholinergic function has been implicated as one of the final common pathways in the pathogenesis of delirium (MacLullich et al., 2008). Despite case reports of beneficial effects of donepezil and rivastigmine, a 2008 Cochrane review concluded that there is currently no evidence from controlled trials supporting the use of cholinesterase inhibitors in the treatment of delirium (Overshott et al., 2008). On the basis of the existing evidence from general hospital and critical care settings, and the lack of studies in palliative care settings, cholinesterase inhibitors cannot be recommended in the treatment of delirium.

Dexmedetomidine

Dexmedetomidine is a selective alpha-2 adrenergic receptor agonist indicated in the United States for the sedation of mechanically ventilated adult patients in intensive care settings and in non-intubated adult patients prior to and/or during surgical and other procedures. It has analgesic effects and has been considered for the prevention and treatment of delirium (Riker et al.,

Table 17.5.1 Antipsychotic medications used in the treatment of delirium

Medication	Dose range	Routes of administration	Side effects	Comments
Typical antipsychotics				
Haloperidol[a]	0.5-2 mg every 2–12 hours	PO, IV, IM, SC	Extrapyramidal adverse effects can occur at higher doses. Monitor QT interval on electrocardiogram	Remains the gold-standard therapy for delirium. May add lorazepam (0.5–1 mg every 2–4 hours) for agitated patients. Double-blind controlled trials support efficacy in treatment of delirium. A pilot placebo-controlled trial suggests lack of efficacy when compared to placebo
Chlorpromazine[a]	12.5–50 mg every 4–6 hours	PO, IV, IM, SC, PR	More sedating and anticholinergic compared with haloperidol. Monitor blood pressure for hypotension. More suitable for use in intensive care unit settings for closer blood pressure monitoring	May be preferred in agitated patients due to its sedative effect. Double-blind controlled trials support efficacy in treatment of delirium. No placebo-controlled trials
Atypical antipsychotics				
Olanzapine[a]	2.5–5 mg every 12–24 hours	PO[b], IM	Sedation is the main dose-limiting adverse effect in short-term use	Older age, pre-existing dementia, and hypoactive subtype of delirium have been associated with poor response. Double-blind comparison trials with haloperidol and risperidone support efficacy in the treatment of delirium. A pilot placebo-controlled prevention trial suggested worsening in delirium severity. A placebo-controlled study is supportive of efficacy in reducing delirium severity and duration
Risperidone[a]	0.25–1 mg every 12–24 hours	PO[b]	Extrapyramidal adverse effects can occur with doses > 6 mg/day. Orthostatic hypotension	Double-blind comparison trials support efficacy in the treatment of delirium. No placebo control trials
Quetiapine[a]	12.5–100 mg every 12–24 hours	PO	Sedation, orthostatic hypotension	Sedating effects may be helpful in patients with sleep–wake cycle disturbance. Pilot placebo-controlled trials suggest efficacy in treatment of delirium. However, studies allowed for concomitant use of haloperidol which makes the results difficult to interpret
Ziprasidone	10–40 mg every 12–24 hours	PO, IM	Monitor QT interval on electrocardiogram	Placebo-controlled, double blind trial suggests lack of efficacy in the treatment of delirium
Aripiprazole[c]	5–30 mg every 24 hours	PO[b], IM	Monitor for akathisia	Evidence is limited. A prospective open label trial suggests comparable efficacy to haloperidol. No placebo-controlled trials

[a] Despite shortcomings of the studies described in the text there is US Preventive Services Task Force (USPSTF) level I evidence for the use of haloperidol, risperidone, olanzapine, and quetiapine in the treatment of delirium.

[b] Risperidone, olanzapine, and aripiprazole are available in orally disintegrating tablets. There have been no intervention or prevention trials with the use of recently released antipsychotics including paliperidone, iloperidone, asenapine, or lurasidone in the treatment or prevention of delirium.

[c] There is USPSTF level II-2 evidence for the use of aripiprazole in the treatment of delirium.

Originally published by the American Society of Clinical Oncology. Breitbart W. and Alici Y, Evidence-Based Treatment of Delirium in Patients with Cancer, Volume 30, Number 11, pp. 1206–1214, Copyright © 2012 by American Society of Clinical Oncology. Source: data from Breitbart W. and Alici Y., Agitation and delirium at the end of life: 'We couldn't manage him', *Journal of the American Medical Association*, Volume 300, Number 24, pp. 2898–2910, Copyright © 2008 American Medical Association. All Rights Reserved.

2009; Pandharipande et al., 2010; Prommer, 2011). Clinical trials in the intensive care unit have shown mixed results for the prevention and treatment of delirium (Riker et al., 2009; Pandharipande et al., 2010) and there have been no studies in palliative care settings.

Prevention of delirium

The development of effective strategies to prevent delirium should be a high priority in palliative care settings. Promising results in the elderly hospitalized population have been observed with various non-pharmacological interventions (Inouye et al., 1999; Siddiqi et al., 2007; NICE, 2011). In the latter population, the study effect sizes suggest that the incidence of delirium may be reduced by as much as one-third with multicomponent interventions (Siddiqi et al., 2007; NICE, 2012). In contrast, a simple multicomponent preventive intervention was found to be ineffective in reducing delirium incidence or severity among cancer patients ($N = 1516$) receiving end-of-life care; no difference was observed between the intervention and the usual-care groups in delirium incidence (odds ratio 0.94, p = 0.66), delirium severity (1.83 vs 1.92, p = 0.07), total days in delirium (4.57 vs 3.57 days, p = 0.63), or duration of first delirium episode (2.9 vs 2.1 days, p = 0.96) (Gagnon et al., 2010).

A variety of pharmacological interventions have also been considered for the prevention of delirium. Antipsychotics, cholinesterase inhibitors, melatonin, and dexmedetomidine have been evaluated in randomized controlled studies conducted in different settings (Kalisvaart et al., 2005; Liptzin et al., 2005; Sampson et al., 2007; Gamberini et al., 2009; Riker et al., 2009; Larsen et al., 2010; Pandharipande et al., 2010; Prommer 2011; NICE, 2012). A 2007 Cochrane review concluded that the evidence for the effectiveness of interventions to prevent delirium was sparse and no recommendations could be made regarding the use of drug therapy for delirium prevention (Siddiqi et al., 2007). Studies published since 2007 have shown mixed results with cholinesterase inhibitors, antipsychotics, melatonin, and dexmedetomidine (Breitbart and Alici, 2012), and there continues to be no established treatment to prevent delirium in palliative care settings.

Controversies in the management of terminal delirium

Delirium that evolves to active dying is terminal delirium. The management of this syndrome is controversial. One study showed that physicians from different disciplines manage terminal delirium differently (Agar et al., 2012); medical oncologists were found to be more likely to manage terminal delirium with benzodiazepines or benzodiazepine and antipsychotic combinations, whereas palliative care physicians were more likely to use antipsychotics to manage delirium symptoms, including the hypoactive subtype of delirium.

Some have argued from a philosophical perspective that pharmacological interventions with antipsychotics or benzodiazepines are inappropriate in the dying patient because delirium is a natural part of the dying process and should not be altered. Clinical experience, however, indicates that the development of delirium can be highly distressing to the patient and family and that the use of antipsychotics to manage agitation, paranoia, hallucinations or altered sensorium is safe, effective and often quite appropriate (Breitbart and Alici, 2008). The use of drug therapy in those believed to be approaching death is best managed on a case-by-case basis, balancing a 'wait and see' approach without the use of pharmacological interventions against the level of overt distress and the knowledge that patients with hypoactive delirium—who may not appear distressed—may quickly and unexpectedly become agitated. It is important to remember that, by their nature, the symptoms of delirium are unstable and fluctuate over time.

Perhaps the most challenging clinical problem is the management of the dying patient with a 'terminal' delirium that is unresponsive to standard antipsychotic interventions, whose symptoms can only be controlled by sedation to the point of a significantly decreased level of consciousness. While antipsychotics are most effective in diminishing agitation, clearing the sensorium and improving cognition is not always possible in delirium which complicates the last days of life. Approximately 30% of dying patients with delirium do not have their symptoms adequately controlled with antipsychotic medications (Fainsinger et al., 2000; Rietjens et al., 2008). Processes causing delirium may be ongoing and irreversible during the active dying phase. In such cases, a reasonable choice is the use of sedative agents such as benzodiazepines (e.g. midazolam, lorazepam) or propofol (and sometimes an opioid, if the drug has proved to be demonstrably sedative) to achieve a state of quiet sedation (Fainsinger et al., 2000; Rietjens et al., 2008). Indeed, delirium has been identified as the main indication for the use of palliative sedation (Fainsinger et al., 2000; Sykes and Thorns, 2003; Lo and Rubenfeld, 2005; Rietjens et al., 2008). Clinicians who are concerned that the use of sedating medications can hasten death via respiratory depression, hypotension, or even starvation, should note that studies in hospice and palliative care settings have not confirmed this association (Bercovitch and Adunsky, 2004; Vitetta et al., 2005).

Before administering a sedative to achieve a calm and comfortable but sedated and unresponsive patient, the clinician must first take several steps. The clinician must have a discussion with the family (and the patient, if there are lucid moments when the patient appears to have capacity), eliciting their concerns and wishes for the type of care that can best honour their desire to provide comfort and symptom control during the dying process. The clinician should describe the optimal achievable goals of therapy as they currently exist. Family members should be informed that the goal of sedation is to provide comfort and symptom control, not to hasten death. Sedation in such patients is not always complete or irreversible; some patients have periods of wakefulness despite sedation, and many clinicians will periodically lighten sedation to reassess the patient's condition. Ultimately, the clinician must always keep the goals of care in mind and communicate these goals to the staff, patient, and family members. The clinician must weigh each of the issues outlined above in making decisions on how to best manage the dying patient who presents with delirium that preserves and respects the dignity and values of that individual and family (Breitbart and Alici, 2008).

Prognostic implications of delirium in the terminally ill

It is important to emphasize the prognostic value of delirium in terminally ill patients. Delirium is a relatively reliable predictor of approaching death in the coming days to weeks (Casarett and Inouye, 2001). In the palliative care setting, several studies provide support that delirium reliably predicts impending death in patients with advanced cancer (Morita et al., 2011). Given the prognostic significance of delirium, recognizing an episode of delirium in the late phases of an illness is critically important in treatment planning and in advising family members.

Conclusion

Palliative care clinicians commonly encounter delirium as a major neuropsychiatric complication of terminal illness. Screening, assessment, diagnosis, and management of delirium are essential in improving quality of life and minimizing morbidity in palliative care settings for patients, families, and health-care professionals.

Online materials

Complete references for this chapter are available online at <http://www.oxfordmedicine.com>.

References

Agar, M., Draper, B., Phillips, P.A., *et al.* (2012). Making decisions about delirium: a qualitative comparison of decision making between nurses working in palliative care, aged care, aged care psychiatry, and oncology. *Palliative Medicine*, 26(7), 887–896.

American Psychiatric Association (1999). Practice guidelines for the treatment of patients with delirium. *American Journal of Psychiatry*, 156(5 Suppl), 1–20.

American Psychiatric Association (2000). *Diagnostic and Statistical Manual of Mental Disorders* (4th ed., text revision). Washington, DC: American Psychiatric Association.

American Psychiatric Association (2013). *Diagnostic and Statistical Manual of Mental Disorders* (5th ed.). Arlington, VA: American Psychiatric Publishing.

Bercovitch, M. and Adunsky, A. (2004). Patterns of high-dose morphine use in a home- care hospice service: should we be afraid of it? *Cancer*, 101(6), 1473–1477.

Boettger, S., Passik, S., Breitbart, W. (2011). Treatment characteristics of delirium superimposed on dementia. *International Psychogeriatrics*, 23(10), 1671–1676.

Breitbart, W. (1997). The memorial delirium assessment scale. *Journal of Pain & Symptom Management*, 13, 128–137.

Breitbart, W. and Alici, Y. (2008). Agitation and delirium at the end of life: 'We couldn't manage him'. *Journal of the American Medical Association*, 300, 2898–2910.

Breitbart, W. and Alici, Y. (2012). Evidence-based treatment of delirium in patients with cancer. *Journal of Clinical Oncology*, 30, 1206–1214.

Casarett, D.J. and Inouye, S.K. (2001). American College of Physicians-American Society of Internal Medicine End-of-Life Care Consensus Panel. Diagnosis and management of delirium near the end of life. *Annals of Internal Medicine*, 135(1), 32–40.

Devlin, J.W., Roberts, R.J., Fong, J.J., *et al.* (2010). Efficacy and safety of quetiapine in critically ill patients with delirium: A prospective, multicenter, randomized, double-blind, placebo-controlled pilot study. *Critical Care Medicine*, 38, 419–427.

Elie, M., Boss, K., Cole, M.G., *et al.* (2009). A retrospective, exploratory, secondary analysis of the association between antipsychotic use and mortality in elderly patients with delirium. *International Psychogeriatrics*, 21, 588–592.

Fainsinger, R.L., Waller, A., Bercovici, M., *et al.* (2000). A multicentre international study of sedation for uncontrolled symptoms in terminally ill patients. *Palliative Medicine*, 14(4), 257–265.

Fann, J.R., Alfano, C.M., Burington, B.E., *et al.* (2005). Clinical presentation of delirium in patients undergoing hematopoietic stem cell transplantation. *Cancer*, 103, 810–820.

Flacker, J.M. and Lipsitz, L.A. (1999). Neural mechanisms of delirium: current hypotheses and evolving concepts. *Journals of Gerontology Series A – Biological Sciences & Medical Sciences.* 54(6), B239–246.

Flaherty, J.H., Steele, D.K., Chibnall, J.T., *et al.* (2010). An ACE unit with a delirium room may improve function and equalize length of stay among older delirious medical inpatients. *Journals of Gerontology Series A – Biological Sciences & Medical Sciences*, 65, 1387–1392.

Flaherty, J.H. and Little, M.O. (2011). Matching the environment to patients with delirium: lessons learned from the delirium room, a restraint-free environment for older hospitalized adults with delirium. *Journal of the American Geriatrics Society*, 59(Suppl. 2), S295–300.

Gagnon, B., Low, G., and Schreier, G. (2005). Methylphenidate hydrochloride improves cognitive function in patients with advanced cancer and hypoactive delirium: a prospective clinical study. *Journal of Psychiatry & Neuroscience*, 30, 100–107.

Gagnon, P., Allard, P., Gagnon, B., *et al.* (2012). Delirium prevention in terminal cancer: Assessment of a multicomponent intervention. *Psycho-Oncology*, 21, 187–194.

Gamberini, M., Bolliger, D., Lurati Buse, G.A., *et al.* (2009). Rivastigmine for the prevention of postoperative delirium in elderly patients undergoing elective cardiac surgery: a randomized controlled trial. *Critical Care Medicine*, 37, 1762–1768.

Girard, T.D., Pandharipande, P.P., Carson, S.S., *et al.* (2010). Feasibility, efficacy, and safety of antipsychotics for intensive care unit delirium: the MIND randomized, placebo-controlled trial. *Critical Care Medicine*, 38, 428–437.

Grover, S., Kumar, V., and Chakrabarti, S. (2011). Comparative efficacy study of haloperidol, olanzapine and risperidone in delirium. *Journal of Psychosomatic Research*, 71, 277–281.

Han, C.S. and Kim, Y.K. (2004). A double-blind trial of risperidone and haloperidol for the treatment of delirium. *Psychosomatics*, 45, 297–301.

Hu, H., Deng, W., and Yang, H. (2004). A prospective random control study: Comparison of olanzapine and haloperidol in senile delirium. *Chongqing Medical Journal*, 8, 1234–1237.

Inouye, S.K., Bogardus, S.T., Jr., Charpentier, P.A., *et al.* (1999). A multicomponent intervention to prevent delirium in hospitalized older patients. *The New England Journal of Medicine*, 340, 669–766.

Jackson, K.C. and Lipman, A.G. (2004). Drug therapy for delirium in terminally ill patients. *Cochrane Database of Systematic Reviews*, 2, CD004770.

Kalisvaart, K.J., de Jonghe, J.F., Bogaards, M.J., *et al.* (2005). Haloperidol prophylaxis for elderly hip-surgery patients at risk for delirium: a randomized placebo-controlled study. *Journal of the American Geriatrics Society*, 53, 1658–1666.

Keen, J.C. and Brown, D. (2004). Psychostimulants and delirium in patients receiving palliative care. *Palliative and Supportive Care*, 2, 199–202.

Larsen, K.A., Kelly, S.E., Stern, T.A., *et al.* (2010). Administration of olanzapine to prevent postoperative delirium in elderly joint-replacement patients: a randomized, controlled trial. *Psychosomatics*, 51, 409–418.

Lawlor, P.G., Gagnon, B., Mancini, I.L., *et al.* (2000a). Occurrence, causes, and outcome of delirium in patients with advanced cancer: a prospective study. *Archives of Internal Medicine*, 160, 786–794.

Leonard, M., Raju, B., Conroy, M., *et al.* (2008b). Reversibility of delirium in terminally ill patients and predictors of mortality. *Palliative Medicine*, 22(7), 848–854.

Liptzin, B., Laki, A., Garb, J.L., et al. (2005). Donepezil in the prevention and treatment of post-surgical delirium. *American Journal of Geriatrics and Psychiatry*, 13, 1100–1106.

Lo, B. and Rubenfeld, G. (2005). Palliative sedation in dying patients: "we turn to it when everything else hasn't worked." *Journal of the American Medical Association*, 294(14), 1810–1816.

Lonergan, E., Britton, A.M., Luxenberg, J., *et al.* (2007). Antipsychotics for delirium. *Cochrane Database of Systematic Reviews*, 2, CD005594.

MacLullich, A.M.J., Ferguson, K.J., Miller, T., De Rooij, S.E.J.A., and Cunningham, C. (2008). Unravelling the pathophysiology of delirium: a focus on the role of aberrant stress responses. *Journal of Psychosomatic Research*, 65, 229–238.

Meagher, D. (2009). Motor subtypes of delirium: past, present and future. *International Review of Psychiatry*, 21, 59–73.

Meagher, D., Adamis, D., Trzepacz, P., and Leonard, M. (2012a). Features of subsyndromal and persistent delirium. *British Journal of Psychiatry*, 200, 37–44.

Milisen, K., Lemiengre, J., Braes, T., *et al.* (2005). Multicomponent intervention strategies for managing delirium in hospitalized older people: systematic review. *Journal of Advanced Nursing*, 52, 79–90.

Morita, T., Tsunoda, J., Inoue, S., and Chihara, S. (1999). Survival prediction of terminally ill cancer patients by clinical symptoms: development of a simple indicator. *Japanese Journal of Clinical Oncology*, 29(3), 156–159.

National Institute for Health and Clinical Excellence (2010). *Delirium: Diagnosis, Prevention and Management*. Clinical Guideline 103. London: NICE. Available at: <http://www.nice.org.uk/nicemedia/live/13060/49908/49908.pdf>.

Overshott, R., Karim, S., and Burns, A. (2008). Cholinesterase inhibitors for delirium. *Cochrane Database of Systematic Reviews*, 1, CD005317.

Pandharipande, P.P., Sanders, R.D., Girard, T.D., *et al.* (2010). Effect of dexmedetomidine versus lorazepam on outcome in patients with sepsis: an a priori-designed analysis of the MENDS randomized controlled trial. *Critical Care*, 14, R38.

Pitkälä, K.H., Laurila, J.V., Strandberg, T.E., *et al.* (2006). Multicomponent geriatric intervention for elderly inpatients with delirium: a randomized, controlled trial. *The Journals of Gerontology Series A: Biological Sciences and Medical Sciences*, 61, 176–181.

Pitkälä, K.H., Laurila, J.V., Strandberg, T.E., et al. (2008). Multicomponent geriatric intervention for elderly inpatients with delirium: effects on costs and health-related quality of life. *The Journals of Gerontology Series A: Biological Sciences and Medical Sciences*, 63, 56–61.

Prakanrattana, U. and Prapaitrakool, S. (2007). Efficacy of risperidone for prevention of postoperative delirium in cardiac surgery. *Anaesthesia and Intensive Care*, 35, 714–719.

Prommer, E. (2011). Review article. Dexmedetomidine: does it have potential in palliative medicine? *American Journal of Hospice and Palliative Medicine*, 28, 276–283.

Ray, W.A., Chung, C.P., Murray, K.T., Hall, K., and Stein, C.M. (2009). Atypical antipsychotic drugs and the risk of sudden cardiac death. *The New England Journal of Medicine*, 360(3), 225–235.

Rietjens, J.A., van Zuylen, L., van Veluw, H., van der Wijk, L., van der Heide, A., and van der Rijt, C.C. (2008). Palliative sedation in a specialized unit for acute palliative care in a cancer hospital: comparing patients dying with and without palliative sedation. *Journal of Pain and Symptom Management*, 36(3), 228–234.

Riker, R.R., Shehabi, Y., Bokesch, P.M., et al. (2009). Dexmedetomidine vs midazolam for sedation of critically ill patients: a randomized trial. *Journal of the American Medical Association*, 301, 489–499.

Ryan, K., Leonard, M., Guerin, S., Donnelly, S., Conroy, M., and Meagher, D. (2009). Validation of the confusion assessment method in the palliative care setting. *Palliative Medicine*, 23, 40–45.

Sampson, E.L., Raven, P.R., Ndhlovu, P.N., et al. (2007). A randomized, double-blind, placebo-controlled trial of donepezil hydrochloride (Aricept) for reducing the incidence of postoperative delirium after elective total hip replacement. *International Journal of Geriatric Psychiatry*, 22, 343–349.

Schneider, L.S., Dagerman, K.S., and Insel, P. (2005). Risk of death with atypical antipsychotic drug treatment for dementia: meta-analysis of randomized placebo-controlled trials. *Journal of the American Medical Association*, 294, 1934–1943.

Siddiqi, N., Stockdale, R., Britton, A.M., et al. (2007). Interventions for preventing delirium in hospitalised patients. *Cochrane Database of Systematic Reviews*, 2, CD005563.

Sykes, N. and Thorns, A. (2003). Sedative use in the last week of life and the implications for end-of-life decision making. *Archives of Internal Medicine*, 163(3), 341–344.

Tahir, T.A., Eeles, E., Karapareddy, V., et al. (2010). A randomized controlled trial of quetiapine versus placebo in the treatment of delirium. Journal of Psychosomatic Research, 69, 485–490.

Trzepacz, P.T. (2000). Is there a final common neural pathway in delirium? Focus on acetylcholine and dopamine. *Seminars in Clinical Neuropsychiatry*, 5(2), 132–148.

Trzepacz, P.T., Mittal, D., Torres, R., Kanary, K., Norton, J., and Jimerson, N. (2001). Validation of the Delirium Rating Scale-revised-98: comparison with the delirium rating scale and the cognitive test for delirium. [Erratum appears in *Journal of Neuropsychiatry & Clinical Neurosciences* 2001, 13(3), 433]. *Journal of Neuropsychiatry & Clinical Neurosciences*, 13, 229–242.

Van Der Mast, R.C. and Fekkes, D. (2000). Serotonin and amino acids: partners in delirium pathophysiology? *Seminars in Clinical Neuropsychiatry*, 5(2), 125–131.

Vitetta, L., Kenner, D., and Sali, A. (2005). Sedation and analgesia-prescribing patterns in terminally ill patients at the end of life. *American Journal of Hospice and Palliative Care*, 22(6), 465–473.

Wang, P.S., Schneeweiss, S., Avorn, J., et al. (2005). Risk of death in elderly users of conventional vs atypical antipsychotic medications. *The New England Journal of Medicine*, 353, 2335–2341.

Wilson, K., Broadhurst, C., Diver, M., Jackson, M., and Mottram, P. (2005). Plasma insulin growth factor-1 and incident delirium in older people. *International Journal of Geriatric Psychiatry*, 20(2), 154–159.

Wong, C.L., Holroyd-Leduc, J., Simel, D.L., and Straus, S.E. (2010). Does this patient have delirium?: value of bedside instruments. *Journal of the American Medical Association*, 304(7), 779–786.

17.6

The family perspective

Carrie Lethborg and David W. Kissane

The family, not just the patient, deals with and attempts to understand the meaning of cancer, and it is the meaning of cancer to the family that sets the context within which dynamic processes occur. (Lewis 1990, p. 759)

Reproduced from Lewis, F. M., Strengthening family supports—cancer and the family, Cancer, Volume 65, Supplement 3, pp. 752–759, Copyright © 1990, with permission from John Wiley & Sons, Inc.

Introduction to the family perspective

More often than not, a person's family background, over and above any other factor, influences the meaning they ascribe to a serious illness. Each person is shaped by, and in turn shapes, their world view. A major component of any person's world view is their family, defined here simply as 'those individuals considered as family by that person' (Ferrell, 1998). The family provides the individual with their history, a strong pattern of beliefs (including those about serious illness and its treatment), traditions, and an identity. Each individual is inextricably linked to and affected by the life of their family, which in turn, responds to changes in the individual. In order to fully understand the impact of an illness on a patient then, we do a disservice to them unless the impact on and of the family as a whole is also considered.

If the health-care professional is serious about providing whole-patient care, it is imperative that the context in which patients *live with* their illness is understood. A family-centred approach to palliative care then, is crucial to any comprehensive service (Northouse, 1984; Quinn and Herndon, 1986; Pederson and Valanis, 1988; Zabora and Smith, 1991).

In addition to understanding the patient within their family context, it is also important to understand the impact of serious illness *on* the wider family. According to systems theory, family members are reciprocally affected by illness in each other. Thus, Northouse and (1993) described serious illness as an assault on the entire family. Indeed, throughout the illness trajectory, a family's emotional, physical, and financial resources can be sequentially challenged by a series of medical crises (Jacobs et al., 1998). Failure to understand this impact leads to inadequate support for the complete range of people affected (Hacialioglu et al., 2010).

Moreover, families should be considered an important *resource* to the health-care team. Often providing the majority of home-based care for palliative patients, they form a crucial component of any programme. If patients are viewed in isolation, both the care provided to them and the resources that could be mobilized are limited. Consistently, the literature has strongly argued

that in palliative care, treatment of the whole family is the optimal approach (Cassileth and Hamilton, 1979; Rait and Lederberg, 1989; Bluglass, 1991; Baider et al., 1996; Lederberg, 1998).

This chapter will explore the concept of the patient in context, the impact of serious illness on the family, and the family as caregiver. It will also consider the assessment of families and their needs and some of the interventions that clinicians can utilize to better assist the family in the setting of palliative care. Families who are well supported will, in turn, be better able to care for their loved ones.

The impact of serious illness on the family

The key to understanding the way illness impacts on the family as a whole is to make sense of two important characteristics of its overall system: (a) the sharing of suffering and (b) the homeostatic force within the family to maintain its usual patterns of relating and living.

The interchange of suffering within the family

Life with a beloved suffering from serious illness may be more difficult than having such an illness oneself (Hilton, 1993; Marshall et al., 2011). Firstly, there is what the Sutherland group (1956) described as *the intimate reciprocity of suffering*. Levels of despair or optimism in patients and family carers are interrelated and are a significant predictor of each other's mental health (Given and Given, 1992; Kurtz et al., 1995; Wittenberg-Lyles et al., 2011). Relatives of the seriously ill thus have higher levels of depression and anxiety than the general population (Stuber et al., 1991). Rates of psychological distress for spouses of cancer patients, for example, have ranged between 18% and 35% (Buckley, 1977; Plumb and Holland, 1977; Maguire, 1981; Gotay, 1984; Ell et al., 1988; Northouse, 1989; Kissane et al., 1994a). In one Australian study, one-quarter of adult offspring of cancer patients exhibited significant distress (Kissane et al., 1994a).

The suffering of the palliative patient, especially in the face of poorly controlled physical symptoms, is a particular trigger for increased anxiety and physical concerns for family members themselves (Ferrell, 1998, Lewis, 1986; Northouse, 1988; Sales, 1991; Hilton, 1993, Kristjanson and Aoun, 2004). In fact, the anguish involved in caring for someone who is living with advanced disease promotes such a level of stress that one should think of close family members as 'second-order patients' (Rait and Lederberg, 1989). Hudson et al. (2011) reported that in a cohort of 302 family caregivers of patients with advanced, life-threatening disease, 44% had anxiety and/or depressive disorders.

While family members can provide a type of 'buffering' to protect and sustain patients (Wilson and Morse, 1991; Sabo et al., 1986), this support is not necessarily mutual in that the patient may have a diminished ability to reciprocate. Their carers may thus find they are responsible for the majority of the emotional support in the relationship. Conflict and greater family disharmony can grow from dissatisfaction with these relationships.

The tendency towards sustaining stability

The second important characteristic to understand in relation to the family system in the setting of illness is that in most cases families gravitate towards maintaining equilibrium in its structure. This homeostatic pull promotes the maintenance of a structure of predictability, security, and cohesiveness (including both positive and negative traits), and will often struggle when faced with uncertainty (Lederberg, 1998). The family affected by serious illness must maintain itself through many changes. These include adoption of the role of the ill member (breadwinner, mother, or patriarch), adjustment to loss, meeting the emotional needs of members in crisis, and continuing to perform standard family functions.

The structure that the family strives to maintain is informed by its unique culture, values, attitudes, norms, roles, and the beliefs peculiar to each family. There are unspoken, yet powerful, regulating actions and relationships, based on a power structure whereby decisions are made and consequences enforced. The family's attitudes towards autonomy, desired medical communication, explanatory models of illness, and the roles of its members all influence its harmony and well-being (Gotay, 2000, pp. 99–101).

Family traditions are translated into a 'script' (Byng Hall, 1988), a subtle yet definitive influence on each member, in varying degrees, throughout their lives. These manifest like a tape recording that is played in each individual's mind to guide their choices. An example is the patient who still hears their father's voice saying, 'Don't trust doctors'. Clinicians need to consider that there are specific traditions for each patient and family when providing information and discussing decision-making. The following vignette illustrates how the family's culture can impact on the medical consultation process:

> Joseph Ramirez was a 68-year-old man, newly diagnosed with end-stage prostate cancer. He had been married to Maria for 49 years and they had three sons: Michael (aged 48), Marko (45), and Frederik (40). Since Joseph had retired, his health had deteriorated and, as weakness increased, he had begun to hand over his position of 'head' of the family to Michael—asking him to make financial and lifestyle decisions. Maria had always been quite passive in her marriage and she was comfortable with whatever her son decided.
>
> When Joseph was diagnosed, Michael felt quite anxious about the additional burden placed on him—especially given his own responsibilities as a husband, father, and with work. When he and his father attended the first consultation with his specialist, Dr Sinclair, Joseph constantly turned to Michael for advice, causing Michael to take a

lead role in the meeting, pre-empting questions and pressing for definitive answers about treatment and prognosis.

> Dr Sinclair found this consultation disconcerting and was worried that Joseph was being held back from directing his own care. He tried to redirect questions back to Joseph asking 'Well what do *you* think, Mr. Ramirez?'
>
> At the end of the consultation, all parties left feeling frustrated. Joseph felt confused and pressured; his son Michael felt offended, stressed, and was contemplating getting a second opinion for his father. Dr Sinclair felt annoyed that Michael was interfering with his care of his father.

If Dr Sinclair had taken some additional time to understand the family's dynamics, he may have found it easier to work with them. Recognizing the potential relevancy of the son's attendance, he could have started by asking Joseph about his family and his feelings regarding his illness and then enquired of Michael, asking him about *his* concerns prior to launching into the medical issues of the consultation. Often a short time taken to get to know the family background will save time in the future and avoid both confusion and anger. Clinicians ought not impose their own value systems but be curious about those of the family. Although Dr Sinclair presumed that patients would make their decisions autonomously, he may have foreseen how consultation within the Ramirez family could also work.

This vignette raises a common dilemma in the palliative setting which is worth special mention. Truth telling, or relaying bad news to a patient, one of the most challenging and complex areas of patient/doctor communication, can be further complicated by the request from a relative to not tell the patient specific information such as diagnosis, prognosis, and/or treatment plans. In Western countries, it is generally accepted that it is the patient's right to be told the truth about their diagnosis and prognosis in a manner in which they can fully grasp its consequences and be a full participant in decision-making. Indeed, breaking bad news is a growing aspect of training in both undergraduate and postgraduate medical education. Yet, the idea that full disclosure is 'best' for the patient is not necessarily shared in all cultures or all families (O'Kelly et al., 2011).

Some families believe that full disclosure of a poor prognosis to patients places an unacceptable burden on them, reducing hope and the will to fight their disease. In some cases, the family perceives that the patient will 'give up' and die because of the words of the physician. The family expects to be told the diagnosis and prognosis and make decisions for the patient to 'shield' them (Hook, 2000). These situations raise difficulties for the health-care team and families alike and it is important to develop guidelines to manage this sensitively. The following broad principles can be helpful:

◆ There are legal and ethical standards, which necessitate that the patient is informed about their medical condition and that they understand this information sufficiently to be competent to the extent that they are able to give informed consent about treatment-related issues. In addition, there are privacy laws that govern what information about a patient can and can't be shared with others.

◆ Refusing to take into account the genuine wishes of the family about how they chose to manage a crisis such as serious illness can result in communication breakdown between the patient/family and treatment team. Such tension only adds to the trauma for the family and the level of difference for the treatment team.

◆ Though it should never be assumed, it is important to remember that in many cases, patients who say they don't want to know their diagnosis are in fact aware of it at some level, but chose to manage their illness through avoidance and or denial.

◆ The wishes of families and patients about how information is communicated require compassion on the part of the treating team to understand the issues for each member. Being able to discuss fear surrounding the breaking of bad news or poor prognosis can often dispel myths and enable collaboration about how the family and the team *can* work together.

Keeping these concepts in mind, it is clearly prudent to aim to prevent the situation where the family is at the patient's door asking the physician to not enter and reveal the results of diagnostic and/or prognostic tests. There is benefit, whenever possible, in talking to all patients about *how* they would like to be told the outcomes of various tests *prior* to undertaking them—this would include where and when they would like to be told, the complexity of the information they would like revealed and who they would like to be present (Clayton and Kissane, 2010). When present with the patient, it is always pertinent to start with what the patient already understands and to again ask what they want to know about specific aspects, before launching into giving any information (Kissane, 2010). Families who have raised concerns about truth-telling should be advised that this will be the manner in which the information will be shared, proportional to what the patient requests and with sensitive delivery.

The family as caregiver

At the same time that family members are adjusting to the impact of serious illness and its uncertainty, many are also expected to take on the complex role of primary caregiver (Given and Given, 1992) and, indeed, many see this role as their duty (McLaughlin et al., 2011). Moreover, the medical system is often funded on the premise that patient care will occur as much as possible in the home to reduce the cost of inpatient services.

Increasingly sophisticated treatments such as chemotherapy are now being offered in the home and the philosophy of hospice care emphasizes patient support in this setting. Given the complexity involved, one could argue that never in history has as much been demanded of family members as carers.

In this context, direct care tasks for the family include dispensation of medications, assistance with nausea, vomiting, and pain relief, washing and other personal care tasks, meal preparation as well as tending to laundry, visitors, and answering phone calls from concerned friends. These tasks would require in the inpatient setting a range of staff, but they are provided by the family on a 24-hour basis, often including support during the night.

While the toll from these tasks could be overwhelming even without complications, there are certain activities that are especially complex: (a) provision of medication for pain, (b) maintenance of nutrition, (c) provision of emotional support for the patient, and (d) the practical nursing and care-provision tasks. For example, the introduction of morphine could be wrongly viewed as the beginning of the dying process and the development of cachexia can cause conflict as the caregiver pushes food as a means towards increasing strength (Reid et al., 2009). In addition, regular roles, such as being husband or wife, mother or daughter are easily lost, when intimacy is crucial. However, families generally make a valiant effort and, in the process, often display great courage.

The longer the caregiving role, the more difficult it is to sustain energy to provide both physical as well as psychological care. Psychological symptoms may increase proportional to the length of illness (Lederberg, 1998). In the article titled, 'Sleeping with one eye open', Hearson and associates (2011) described the extent of the impact of sleep deprivation on family caregivers in palliative care, illustrating that almost 40% experienced excessive daytime sleepiness. The sustained effort, compounded by anxiety, adds to the exhaustion that comes with the burden of care in the palliative setting, and the reluctance of many to ask for help for themselves (Richards et al., 2011).

Yet, though the role of carer is clearly stressful in many ways, it is important to remember the positives involved for both patient and caregiver. There is consistent evidence linking successful family-based support with increased psychosocial adaptation for all concerned (Bloom, 1978; Woods and Earp, 1978; Northouse and Swain, 1987; Northouse, 1988; Mishel and Braden, 1989). Families serve as the primary referent and emotional support base for their members who become medically ill (Litman, 1974). Families also provide essential, instrumental functions that enable patients to adhere to arduous treatment protocols and manage the debilitating side effects associated with modern cancer treatment. The effectiveness of symptom control in palliative care is greatly enhanced by the presence of the family as caregiver (Schachter and Coyle, 1998). Families, in turn, also report a number of positives in their own lives and relationships as a result of their experience (Folkman, 1997).

The needs of the family-based caregiver

Much of the suffering of families in the palliative setting results from being ill prepared and struggling with uncertainty and helplessness (Cherny et al., 1994). Family carers often state that they wish they had been taught some of the skills required for their caring role by health-care providers rather than having to work them out for themselves through 'trial and error'. There are a number of unmet needs among caregivers. Some of the most commonly reported needs include:

◆ information about diagnosis and expected prognosis (Wright and Dyck, 1984; Tringali, 1986; Schofield et al., 1998; Finney Rutten et al., 2005)

◆ assistance in dealing with the patients' physical symptoms (Tringali, 1986; Hileman and Lackey, 1992; Kristjanson and Ashcroft, 1994; Watson, 1994; Harrington et al., 1996; Schofield et al., 1998)

◆ assistance in dealing with feelings such as inadequacy, guilt, anxiety, fear, and grief (Northouse, 1984; Stetz, 1987; Woods et al., 1989; Wingate and Lackey, 1989; Hileman and Lackey, 1990; Nolan et al., 1990; Schofield et al., 1998)

◆ managing the personal impact of caring such as sleep disturbance, weight loss, maintaining family stability, and recognition of altered roles and choices (Northouse and Peters-Golden, 1993; Schofield et al., 1998)

◆ guidance about coping strategies (Klagsburn, 1994; Given and Given, 1996; Schofield et al., 1998, Meyers et al., 2011).

In addition to these psychological and physical needs of the family, there are considerable costs involved with caring for a loved one with serious illness. These can be both direct and indirect, with at least 25% of family carers being unable to continue employment, thus suffering substantial losses of income (Schofield et al., 1998). Many carers also find they lose friends (though others are surprised by those who *are* supportive), and are unable to continue prior levels of involvement with sport or other interests. Given the wide ranging effects of the caregiving role, comprehensive assessment is required when considering supportive care of these families.

Assessing the family for intervention

While the impact of serious illness can be considered to be catastrophic enough to argue for an evaluation of *each* family, this is clearly not a practical option (Zaider and Kissane, 2009). It is more common for staff to develop concerns for family members when they are not providing expected practical or emotional support (Jacobs et al., 1998). This is also not an effective basis for decisions about resource allocation. What *is* necessary is the ability to screen for those families who are at greater risk of maladaptive outcome, so that scarce resources can be allocated to those in greater need (Kissane et al., 2007–2008).

An interesting approach to the identification of those families in most need of supportive intervention grew out of empirical observations about the significant association between family functioning and psychosocial outcome during palliative care and bereavement (Kissane et al., 1994). Dysfunctional families carried significantly more psychosocial morbidity among their members, such that screening for family functioning provided a method of recognition of those in greater need. Indeed, the 12-item Family Relationships Index (FRI) (derived from the Family Environment Scale; Moos and Moos, 1981) provides information on the family's cohesiveness, shared expression of thoughts and feelings, and conflict, and thus serves as a simple pencil-and-paper screening test. Well-functioning families are cohesive and score more than 9 out of 12 on an FRI. Families at risk of poorer outcome have been termed *hostile*, *sullen*, or *intermediate*, reflecting varying levels of conflict, poor communication and lack of any sense of togetherness (Kissane et al., 1998, 2003). A model of intervention that targets enhancing these dimensions of family functioning has been described as family-focused grief therapy (FFGT) (Kissane et al., 2006). It is initiated during the stage of advanced disease, as the family becomes more involved with care, and is continued into bereavement to maintain continuity of care. Such an approach to screening families, with preventive intervention for those at risk, will become the necessary working model for the future.

Family assessments should be aimed at leading the health professional to an increased understanding of the medical and psychosocial situation of the family system (Schachter and Coyle, 1998). Developing an understanding of the major concerns of individual members and the family as a whole empowers planning of appropriately focused interventions. We find a checklist as portrayed in Box 17.6.1 helpful to ensure that family assessments are thorough in their detail.

Understanding the impact of practical issues on the family is also important for effective functioning. Practical issues include the financial impact of serious illness on the family, the impact on work and home life, division of labour in the family, availability

Box 17.6.1 Themes warranting evaluation during family assessment
◆ Family understanding of the illness, key symptoms, and treatment
◆ Major concerns at this moment: prognosis, death and dying, caregiving needs
◆ Liaison with medical team, when to seek help
◆ Family functioning: cohesion, communication, and conflict
◆ Developmental and past history: prior experience of loss and relational strains
◆ Useful coping strategies: problem-solving, team work, emotional support
◆ Social issues: employment, finances, living arrangements
◆ Community resources: meals, cleaning, volunteers, respite
◆ Presence of children at home and their needs
◆ Spiritual needs
◆ Expectations and future concerns, what to expect as death approaches, how to talk with the patient about dying, how to say goodbye and how to manage a death in the home
◆ How to help each other in bereavement.

of family members to provide the care needs required, and the appropriateness of the physical surroundings to care for someone.

In addition to the specific concerns of the family, the clinician needs to consider each family's ability to adjust to change that is inevitable during palliative care. While a normal grief response is expected following each change in disease status, the level of intervention required will depend on the ability of family members to comfort and support each other.

Family-centred principles for intervention

In general, interventions for families in the setting of advanced disease are provided in two broad areas: (1) those that are preventive, supportive, and focus on enhancing coping; and (2) those that deal with actual dysfunction in the family. However there are a number of general principles of family-centred therapy that apply to all interventions (Kovacsa et al., 2006). Box 17.6.2 outlines the key goals and principles in conducting family meetings.

Open communication and information provision

Open communication from the health-care team is crucial in attempting to include the family in the treatment plan. To begin with, the provision of information is empowering to the family. Knowledge relieves family anxiety, improves problem-solving, and enhances both emotional and physical well-being (Stewart, 1996). Yet in response to encouraging open discussion of the family's experience, the practitioner must go on to provide emotional comfort and legitimization of their feelings and concerns.

All information about palliative care and advanced disease is value-laden for those living with the disease. Specific discussion about deterioration and dying can be difficult to process. Clinicians need to proceed sensitively, respectfully, and also model

Box 17.6.2 Key goals and principles in conducting family meetings

- Open communication and willing provision of medical information
- Identification of issues or concerns held by family members
- Recognition of current and past patterns of relating
- Problem-solving around the provision of instrumental care
- Encouragement of acceptance of community support
- Affirmation of strengths and courage of the family as a whole
- Comfort for the inherent suffering yet optimism about their capacity to cope.

Box 17.6.3 A clinical roadmap to run a family meeting in palliative care

1. Planning and prior set-up to arrange the family meeting—who to invite?
2. Welcome and orientation of the family to the goals of the family meeting
3. Check each family member's understanding of the illness and its prognosis
4. Check for consensus about the current goals of care
5. Identify family concerns about the management of key symptoms and care needs
6. Clarify the family's view of what the future holds
7. Clarify how family members are coping and feeling emotionally
8. Identify family strengths and affirm their level of commitment and mutual support for each other
9. Close the family meeting by final review of agreed goals of care and consensus about future care plans.

the openness that is possible. Some families grow closer as a result of this challenge (Bloom, 1982; Neuling and Winefield, 1988), but others get stuck in awkwardness and avoidance (Reiss et al., 1993). Prior patterns of intimacy, comfort, and support can be fostered during this time if information is shared in a sensitive way to promote understanding and teamwork (Griffith and Griffith, 1994).

Recognition of past patterns of relating

Families develop patterns of relating and coping that influence the way they subsequently handle the impact of serious illness (Sales et al., 1992). Past stress and loss affect the attitude and resources a family brings to this experience (Bloch et al., 1994). Recognition and acknowledgment of transgenerational patterns of relating can empower adoption of new choices for mutual support (Kissane and Bloch, 2002).

Encouragement of acceptance of outside support

The emotional cost to the caregiving family is seldom raised by members themselves, whose focus is so clearly on the patient, their relative. It is not surprising, therefore, that families underutilize support programmes and assistance from health providers (Davis-Ali et al., 1993). In one Australian study, Schofield and colleagues (1998) found that 38% of carers reported problems with coping, one-third health concerns, and over half, unmet needs. However, a meagre 12% received counselling! An important challenge may be to get these families to accept outside help.

Struggling to manage the caregiving role without support can bring about a sense of burden, which family members may feel guilty about, but unable to articulate (Given et al., 1993). A comprehensive appraisal of carer needs can ameliorate the fatigue experienced by family members (Jensen and Given, 1991). Community support in the form of respite provided by volunteers, home nursing, or cleaning services are examples of support that may make the difference between families coping with home-based care or not. Careful matching of services to needs and encouragement of their acceptance is critical.

Discussions with the family as a whole

Use of a family meeting is crucial to family-centred care and should be considered a routine component of care today. Box 17.6.3 outlines a useful schema for clinicians to follow in running this meeting (Guergen et al., 2009; Coyle and Kissane, 2010). The presence of all important members of the patient's family (including the patient)

in one room allows the clinician to see how the family relates and provides a multitude of data about who influences decision-making, how open the family as a group is to discuss difficult issues, what their view of treatment is, and so on. This type of information can only be gained by experiencing the family in action.

Many clinicians avoid family meetings as they consider them to be too time-consuming and likely to open up difficult issues with which the team must deal. In reality, a family meeting can be time-saving and allow for many issues to be considered in a short time. Often the clinician finds that the family meeting prevents them from having to answer phone calls from numerous family members repeating the same questions over and over. Such meetings deal with what information can be shared with whom, as the patient is present to provide permission for each topic to be covered. Many issues are resolved in a family meeting more swiftly than when pursued individually. Summarized agreements of these meetings can be included, with the family's permission, in the patient's records to enhance communication throughout the team (Hudson et al., 2008). In addition, a family genogram (Barker, 1986) can be completed and added to records for a succinct visual overview of the family structure. For example, Fig. 17.6.1 illustrates a genogram of the previously mentioned Ramirez family.

Such a family meeting empowers allocation of tasks among family members and the clinician can understand the impact this will have on each. When roles can be shared among members, so that the family becomes a team, there is reduced burden (Given and Given, 1994). Many of the everyday tasks, exemplified by housework, shopping, and transport, can be sorted out through problem-solving during the session, while the family grows in mutual understanding. On the other hand, when decisions about task allocation are made individually and without full consultation within the family, plans can be unconsciously sabotaged by those who do not feel they were included in the decision-making.

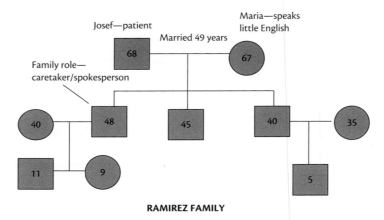

Fig. 17.6.1 Genogram of the Ramirez family described as a clinical vignette, where the eldest son takes up a culturally-consistent decision-making role in the family, a dynamic that the treatment team must recognize.

Box 17.6.4 Specific facilitation techniques used in family meetings

◆ *Circular questions*: ask each family member to comment in turn on the concerns and coping of others to promote curiosity and reflection by the group as a whole. For example, 'How are your parents and sisters coping with Dad's illness? Who is most upset in your view?'

◆ *Reflexive questions*: invite the family to reflect on possibilities, hypotheses, and a range of outcomes to stimulate their internal efforts to improve family life. For example, 'What benefits might come from caring for Dad at home? In what ways might this be hard for you as a family group?'

◆ *Strategic questions*: here a solution might be incorporated into the wording of the question to more directly guide the family toward an outcome that is considered preferable. For example, 'What change in Dad's symptoms (e.g. level of agitation) would need to occur for you to realize that admission to an inpatient hospice bed is necessary?'

◆ *Integrative summary of the family's concerns*: the family's views are reflected back to highlight levels of tension or discordance in different member's opinions, while maintaining professional neutrality, yet inviting further problem-solving by the family. For example, 'As a family, you recognize your father's desire to die at home, your mother's commitment to meet his wishes, and yet your concern that his confusion is becoming unmanageable and a burden to your mother. There is no easy answer here, as whichever solution you adopt will appear to demand more of each of you for a time.'

The family meeting also provides opportunity for the expression of genuine feelings individual members may have, both positively and negatively. For example, the chance is created for adult offspring to reassure their parents about the gratification they derive when reciprocating some of the love and attention they received during childhood (Hinton, 1994). Disagreement about plans or task allocation can be safely raised in this setting and appropriately problem solved. Box 17.6.4 outlines some key skills that clinicians need to facilitate routine family meetings (Dumont and Kissane, 2009). A more detailed coverage of

these skills is found in a series of useful articles by Karl Tomm (Tomm, 1988).

Family meetings may need to be arranged at each juncture of the treatment programme. As the goals of treatment change, or new information is ascertained, the family should be reconvened to review the situation.

Support during unpreventable emotional suffering

There is much distress and suffering that arises from caring for a seriously ill family member, which cannot be prevented or relieved. Though there appears to be an expectation or belief that modern medicine can prevent all suffering, this is an often unrecognized myth (Callahan, 1995). Support throughout the illness that includes frank discussion of side effects and tempering of unrealistic expectations can lessen any consequent emotional impact, but sometimes suffering can only be assuaged (Ferrell et al., 1991a, 1991b, 1991c; Kissane, 1998).

Specific interventions

Preventive and supportive interventions

Most well-functioning families who have become carers benefit from a single family meeting that mobilizes their inherent strengths and resources. Such consultative interventions aim to assist families expand and adapt their own successful problem-solving methods (Jacobs et al., 1998). They would begin where the family is at and provide additional encouragement to enhance coping.

Interventions that challenge dysfunction

Serious illness often provides a timely opportunity to intervene with a dysfunctional family. Indeed, such transition points in the life cycle are fertile occasions to effect change. Hence families that oncology services find challenging because of their long term dysfunction may become amenable to help at exactly this point in their lives—the threat of death of a loved one.

Challenging families include those that are rigid in their structure and processes, and find it difficult to accept change, or where their relationships are chaotic and unstable, with distress generating psychiatric disorder such as major depressive episode. Concern for these families develops when (a) their conflict and behaviours prevent members from providing effective care-provision, or (b), when the negative impact on the family becomes disruptive and unbearable, producing mental illness. Such difficult families warrant referral to psycho-oncology services for ongoing family therapy. For example:

> Wartime separation had led the parents of this family to be raised in an orphanage during their childhood, challenging their ability to later cope with stress in life. The subsequent illness with advanced breast cancer of the mother brought great worry to the family. Her children teamed reasonably but the father's aloof and retreating manner created a gulf that interfered with effective communication. In family sessions, the construction of a transgenerational genogram and sharing of narrative about the deprivations of war helped this family to better understand and tolerate their father's solitariness. Thereafter, his children made renewed endeavours to include him in family activities and provided improved support for him during his bereavement.

Interventions with the family of a dying patient

Supporting a family through the chronic phase of advanced disease is largely a matter of maintenance and different to the kind of support required when the patient is dying. Yet a common mistake made by the treatment team is in not being clear about the shift from cure or maintenance to palliative care. While the presence of hope is crucial to all families, and, indeed, many hold onto this hope in the face of extreme deterioration, it is important that it is balanced with some sense of realism, which often needs to come from the health care team (Parkes, 1972). There can be hesitancy in giving an honest appraisal about prognosis because of the emotional response involved with anticipatory grief. Yet there are two important reasons for clinicians to be brave and open in this setting.

To begin with, the time that the family spends together when a member is dying can be one of extreme intimacy and poignancy. This period involves finishing-up for the patient and those around them (Lethborg, 1994). As Hinton (1981) suggested, saying goodbye, while often perceived to be a final act, in practice evolves gradually as a temporal process. Finishing-up can include a period of life review, of completing projects, and of saying farewell. Equally, for the family, there can be review of relationships with the ill member, affirmation of the contribution of each person, completion of unfinished business, and expression of gratitude for the good times shared (Meares, 1981).

This period can also be one of great stress and emotional pain, especially when excessive anticipatory grief occurs. With skilled guidance, this existential pain can be processed through reminiscence and externalization, eventually leading to increased acceptance (Yalom, 1980; Kissane, 1998; Breitbart, et al., 2010; Chochinov, 2011; Lethborg, et al., 2012). The tasks involved in saying goodbye can easily be postponed by well-intentioned families, motivated to protect their dying member from distress. Guidance is distinctly helpful so that families do not misjudge the time remaining for this farewell.

Secondly, successful management of this palliative phase is a form of preventive therapy in relation to the mental health of the family during bereavement. Care provided to families during the course of a terminal illness has a profound influence on bereavement following the death (Ferrell, 1998). The experience of a family member dying at home thereafter becomes part of the narrative of the whole family (Coyle, 1996).

By screening palliative care families to identify those 'at some risk' for maladaptive outcomes, randomized trials of family intervention starting during palliative care and continued into bereavement have shown the ability to prevent complicated grief and depressive illness in the bereaved (Kissane et al., 2006, 2012). Palliative medicine presents a unique opportunity to establish a therapeutic alliance with families in need, in a manner that does effectively support their transition through this stressful experience (Kissane et al., 1998). Through a focus on enhancing family functioning, families are helped to support one another, communicate more effectively, tolerate differences and deal with conflict adaptively. This approach is a preventive model that offers therapy through a brief and empirically driven technique, and sustains continuity of care to the family across a period of major change in their lives. While very chaotic families decline to meet, accepting distance and separation as the practical solution to their differences, many other families with more mild to moderate disturbance in their relationships welcome the help delivered through this family-centred model of care. Through this FFGT approach, bereavement care actually begins during palliative care.

Conclusion

Serious illness should be viewed as 'a bio-psychosocial and spiritual problem that occurs in the context of an intense interpersonal relationship that affects, and is affected by, the disease process in reciprocal circularity' (Northouse, 1993, p. 70). Never is this truer than for the family of a patient with advanced disease. The serious progression of this disease towards terminal events inevitably involves the family in key relationships with the health team and their dying relative. These relationships are pivotal in determining the ultimate outcome of the experience for all. Families are second-order patients in their own right, and the bearers of the burdens and joys of loving relationships. Family-centred care is challenging as a paradigm but a useful harness to improved quality of life, one that warrants the effort involved to ease the suffering of all.

Online materials

Complete references for this chapter are available online at <http://www.oxfordmedicine.com>.

References

Baider, L. and Kaplan De-Nour, K. (2000). Cancer and couples—its impact on the healthy partner: methodological considerations. In L. Baider, C.L. Cooper, and A. Kaplan De-Nour (eds.) *Cancer and the Family*, pp. 41–51. Chichester: Wiley.

Breitbart, W., Rosenfeld, B., Gibson, C., *et al.* (2010) Meaning-centered group psychotherapy for patients with advanced cancer: a pilot randomized controlled trial. *Psycho-Oncology*, 19, 21–28.

Cherny, N.I., Coyle, N., and Foley, K.M. (1994). Suffering in the advanced cancer patient: a definition and taxonomy. *Journal of Palliative Care*, 10, 57–70.

Chochinov, H.M. (2011). *Dignity Therapy, Final Words for Final Days*. New York: Oxford University Press.

Clayton, J. and Kissane, D.W. (2010). Communication about transitioning patients to palliative care. In D.W. Kissane, B.D. Bultz, P.N. Butow, and I. Finlay (eds.) *Handbook of Communication in Oncology and Palliative Care*, pp. 203–214. Oxford: Oxford University Press.

Coyle, N. and Kissane, D.W. (2010). Conducting a family meeting. In D.W. Kissane, B.D. Bultz, P.N. Butow, and I. Finlay (eds.) *Handbook of Communication in Oncology and Palliative Care*, pp. 165–176. Oxford: Oxford University Press.

Dumont, I. and Kissane, D.W. (2009). Techniques for framing questions in conducting family meetings in palliative care. *Palliative & Supportive Care*, 7, 163–170.

Finney Rutten, L.J., Arora, N.K., Bakos, A.D., Aziz, N., and Rowland, J. (2005). Information needs and sources of information among cancer patients: a systematic review of research (1980–2003). *Patient Education and Counseling*, 57, 250–261.

Folkman, S. (1997). Positive psychological states and coping with severe stress. *Social Science & Medicine*, 45, 1207–1221.

Given, B.A. and Given, C.W. (1994). Family home care for individuals with cancer. *Oncology*, 8, 77–88.

Gotay, C.C. (2000). Culture, cancer, and the family. In L. Baider, C.L. Cooper, and A. Kaplan De-Nour (ed.), *Cancer and the Family*, pp. 95–110. Chichester: Wiley.

Gueguen, J., Bylund, C.L., Brown, R., Levin, T.T., and and Kissane, D.W. (2009). Conducting family meetings in palliative care: themes, techniques and preliminary evaluation of a communication skills module. *Palliative & Supportive Care*, 7, 171–179.

Hacialioglu, N., Ozer, N., Yilmaz Karabulutlu, E., Erdem, N., and Erci, B. (2010). The quality of life of family caregivers of cancer patients in the east of Turkey. *European Journal of Oncology Nursing*, 14(3), 211–217.

Hearson, B., McClement, S., McMillan, D.E., and Harlos, M. (2011), Sleeping with one eye open: the sleep experience of family members providing palliative care at home. *Journal of Palliative Care*, 27(2), 69–78.

Hileman, J.W., Lackey, N.R., and Hassanein, R.S. (1992). Identifying the needs of home caregivers of patients with cancer. *Oncology Nursing Forum*, 19, 771–777.

Hilton, B.A. (1993). Issues, problems and challenges for families coping with breast cancer. *Seminars in Oncology Nursing*, 9, 88–100.

Hinton, J. (1994). Can home care maintain an acceptable quality of life for patients with terminal cancer and their relatives? *Palliative Medicine*, 8, 183–186.

Hook, C.C. (2000). Cancer, medical ethics, and the family. In L. Baider, C.L. Cooper, and A. Kaplan De-Nour (eds.) *Cancer and the Family*, pp. 497–512. Chichester: Wiley.

Hudson, P., Quinn, K., O'Hanlon, B., and Aranda, S. (2008). Family meetings in palliative care. *Multidisciplinary Clinical Practice Guidelines*, 19, 7–12.

Jacobs, J., Ostroff, J., and Steinglass, P. (1998). Family therapy: a systems approach to cancer care. In J. Holland (ed.) *Psycho-Oncology*, pp. 994–1003. New York: Oxford University Press.

Kissane, D.W. (1994). Grief and the family. In S. Bloch, J. Hafner, E. Harari, and G.I. Szmukler (eds.) *The Family in Clinical Psychiatry*, pp. 71–91. Oxford: Oxford University Press.

Kissane, D.W. (2010). Communication training to achieve shared decision making. In D.W. Kissane, B.D. Bultz, P.N. Butow, and I. Finlay (eds.) *Handbook of Communication in Oncology and Palliative Care*, pp. 127–134. Oxford: Oxford University Press.

Kissane, D.W. and Bloch, S. (2002). *Family Focused Grief Therapy: A Model of Family-centred Care during Palliative Care and Bereavement*. Buckingham and Philadelphia: Open University Press.

Kissane, D.W., Lichtenthal. W.G., and Zaider, T.I. (2007–2008). Family care before and after bereavement. *Omega*, 56, 21–32.

Kissane, D.W., McKenzie, M., Bloch, S., Moskowitz, C., McKenzie, D.P., and O'Neill, I. (2006). Family focused grief therapy: a randomized controlled trial in palliative care and bereavement. *American Journal of Psychiatry*, 163, 1208–1218.

Kissane, D.W., McKenzie, M., McKenzie, D.P., Forbes, A., O'Neill, I., and Bloch, S. (2003). Psychosocial morbidity associated with patterns of family functioning in palliative care—baseline data from the Family

Focused Grief Therapy controlled trial. *Palliative Medicine*, 17, 527–537.

Kissane, D.W., Zaider, T.I., Li, Y., and Del Gaudio, F. (2012). Family therapy for complicated grief. In M. Stroebe, H. Schut, and J. Van Den Bout (eds.) *Complicated Grief: Scientific Foundations for Health Care Professionals*, pp. 248–262. New York: Routledge.

Kovacsa, P., Hayden Bellinb, M., and Fauria, D. (2006). Family-centered care. *Journal of Social Work in End-Of-Life & Palliative Care*, 2(1), 13–27.

Kristjanson, L. and Aoun, S. (2004). Palliative care for families: remembering the hidden patients. *Canadian Journal of Psychiatry*, 49(6), 359–365.

Lethborg, C., Schofield, P., and Kissane, D. (2012). The patient experience of undertaking meaning and purpose (MaP) therapy. *Palliative and Supportive Care*, 10(3), 177–188.

Lewis, F.M. (1990). Strengthening family supports—cancer and the family. *Cancer*, 65, 752–759.

Marshall, C., Larkey, L., Curran, M., *et al.* (2011). Considerations of culture and social class for families facing cancer: the need for a new model for health promotion and psychosocial intervention. *Families, Systems and Health*, 29(2), 81–94.

McLaughlin, D., Hasson, F., Kernohan, W.G., *et al.* (2010). Living and coping with Parkinson's disease: perceptions of informal carers. *Palliative Medicine*, 25(2), 177–182.

Meyers, F.J., Carducci, M., Loscalzo, M.J., Linder, J., Greasby, T., and Beckett, L.A. (2011). Effects of a problem-solving intervention (COPE) on quality of life for patients with advanced cancer on clinical trials and their caregivers: simultaneous care educational intervention (SCEI): linking palliation and clinical trials. *Journal of Palliative Medicine*, 14(4), 465–473.

Mishel, M.H. and Braden, C.J. (1989). Finding meaning: antecedents of uncertainty in Illness. *Nursing Research*, 37, 98–103.

Moos, R.H. and Moos, B.S. (1981). *Family Environment Scale—Manual*. Palo Alto, CA: Consulting Psychologists Press.

Nolan, M.R., Grant, G., and Ellis, N.C. (1990). Stress is in the eye of the beholder: reconceptualizing the measurement of cancer burden. *Journal of Advanced Nursing*, 15, 544–555.

Northouse, L. (1984). The impact of cancer on the family. *International Journal of Psychiatry in Medicine*, 14, 215–242.

Northouse, L.L. (1993). Cancer and the family: strategies to assist spouses. *Seminars in Oncology Nursing*, 9, 74–82.

O'Kelly, C., Urch, C., and Brown, E. (2011). The impact of culture and religion on truth telling at the end of life. *Nephrology Dialysis Transplantation*, 26(12), 3838–3842.

Rait, D. and Lederberg, M.S. (1989). The family of the cancer patient. In J.C. Holland and J.H. Rowland (eds.) *Handbook of Psycho-Oncology*, pp. 585–597. New York: Oxford University Press.

Reiss, D., Steinglass, P., and Howe, G. (1993). The family's organization around the illness. In R.E. Cole and D. Reiss (eds.) *How Do Families Cope with Chronic Illness?*, pp. 173–214. Hillsdale, NJ: Erlbaum.

Reid, J., Fitzsimons, H., Fitzsimons, D., and McCance, T. (2009). Fighting over food: patient and family understanding of cancer cachexia. *Oncology Nursing Forum*, 36(4), 439–445.

Richards, S.H., Winder, R., Seamark, C., *et al.* (2011). The experiences and needs of people seeking palliative health care out-of-hours: a qualitative study. *Primary Health Care Research Development*, 12(2), 165–178.

Schofield, H., Bloch, S., Herrman, H., Murphy, B., Nankervis, J., and Singh, B. (1998). *Family Caregiver's Disability, Illness and Ageing*. Melbourne: Allen and Unwin.

Stuber, M.L., Nader, K., and Yasuda, P. (1991). Stress responses following pediatric bone marrow transplantation: preliminary results of a prospective, longitudinal study. *Journal of the American Academy of Child and Adolescent Psychiatry*, 30, 952–957.

Tomm, K. (1988). Interventive interviewing: part III. Intending to ask lineal, circular, strategic or reflective questions? *Family Process*, 27, 1–15.

Watson, M. (1994). Psychological care for cancer patients and their families. *Journal of Mental Health*, 3, 453–461.

Wittenberg-Lyles, E., Demiris, G., Oliver, D.P., and Burt, S. (2011). Reciprocal suffering: caregiver concerns during hospice care. *Journal of Pain Symptom Management*, 41(2), 383–393.

Zabora, J. and Smith, E.D. (1991). Family dysfunction and the cancer patient: early recognition and intervention. *Oncology*, 5(12), 31–35.

Zaider, T.I. and Kissane, D.W. (2009). The assessment and management of family distress during palliative care. *Current Opinion in Oncology*, 3, 67–71.

17.7

Bereavement

David W. Kissane and Talia I. Zaider

Introduction to bereavement

Mourning is an essential adaptive response to the inevitable experience of loss. In many ways it is the debt that has to be repaid for investment in the joys of life. Familiarity with and confidence in responding to grief is a sine qua non for all clinicians working in palliative medicine, including the capacity to differentiate healthy from maladaptive adjustment. Many losses are experienced as patients and their families move through the phases of progressive illness towards death. Related grief is thus current as well as anticipatory of future loss. Support for the grieving process in both the patients and their carers clearly begins during palliative care and places the clinician in an ideal position to sustain continuity of this care into bereavement.

Family-centred care is integral to this supportive process as the family's understanding of the illness and its treatment influences their later adjustment (Kissane et al., 2007–2008). Every word uttered by the treating team, the related tone, and sensitivity shown contributes to the experience for the bereaved, who generally need to understand the process of death and discuss any features of concern. Palliative care teams are ideally placed to recognize those at greater risk of poor outcome and provide care prophylactically to prevent bereavement morbidity (Williams and McCorkle, 2011).

Although words such as grief, mourning, and bereavement are commonly used interchangeably, the following definitions indicate their use in this chapter:

◆ Bereavement is the state of loss resulting from death (Parkes, 1998).

◆ Grief is the emotional response associated with loss (Stroebe et al., 1993).

◆ Mourning is the process of adaptation, including the cultural and social rituals prescribed as accompaniments (Raphael, 1983).

◆ Anticipatory grief precedes the death and results from the expectation of that event (Raphael, 1983).

◆ Pathological grief represents an abnormal outcome involving psychological, social, or physical morbidity (Rando, 1993). Complicated grief and chronic or prolonged grief are variants.

◆ Disenfranchised grief represents the hidden sorrow of the marginalized where there is less social permission to express many dimensions of loss (Doka, 1989).

In this chapter, the theoretical models that have been developed to explain bereavement phenomena and the process of mourning are considered with a view to generating an understanding of the clinical features of grief. Recognition of those at risk of complicated outcome is mandatory to offer preventative interventions (Guldin et al., 2011). Models of follow-up and management of complicated grief are fully explored, as is variation across the life cycle and the impact of stigmatized deaths. Spiritual aspects of bereavement highlight the contributions of the world's major religions in supporting the bereaved. Bereavement research in the future will be aided by use of validated measures, which are summarized towards the chapter's end as a handy resource. Finally, to conclude, the recognition that personal growth is a common outcome despite the sadness of loss reminds us that creativity often emerges as a result of resolution of the mourning process.

Theoretical models of bereavement phenomena

Dating from Darwin's observation of monkeys 'weeping' from grief, ethology has pointed out that social birds and mammals do grieve (Darwin, 1872). Indeed, mourning appears to be the price paid for the evolutionary adaptiveness of social relationships. This universality of grief suggests it is imprinted into the biological processes of the species, consistent with the experience that death seems to be difficult for people everywhere. Yet, social constructionists remind us that the shape and content of grief is culturally determined. It varies markedly across places, times, and social groups, with noteworthy differences in the expression of anger, emotionality, self-mutilation, rituals, and public versus private grief (Rosenblatt, 2001).

A conceptual framework that illuminates what underpins the phenomena of bereavement aids our clinical understanding of the experience of the bereaved (see Table 17.7.1). Explanatory models favoured by bereavement researchers were ranked in the following order of importance: attachment, psychodynamic, sociological, cognitive behavioural, and ethology (Middleton et al., 1993). Although limited by the available list of potential theories (for instance, continuing bonds, interpersonal, systemic, and traumatic were not offered), these models help practitioners work flexibly with pertinent issues.

Attachment theory posits that the development of close affectionate bonds to particular others generates security and survival potential (Bowlby, 1997). From a secure base, the capacity for curiosity emerges to generate creativity in autonomous adult life. Parents, especially the mother, constitute the usual subject of primary attachments, but these behaviours become enduring throughout adult life and the spouse eventually replaces the parents as the recipient of the strongest bonds. The family thus

Table 17.7.1 Theoretical models explaining bereavement phenomena

Name of model	Key contributors	Main features
Attachment theory	Bowlby, Ainsworth, Parkes, Weiss	The bonds of close relationships are severed by loss
Psychodynamic theory	Freud, Klein, Horowitz, Kohut	Early relationships lay down a template that guide future relationships
Interpersonal model	Sullivan, Bonnano, Horowitz, Benjamin	Relational influences are dominant in grief outcome
Psychosocial transition	Parkes, Janoff-Bulman	Changed assumptive world view
Sociological model	Rosenblatt, Klass, Walter	Cultural influences shape the form and content of grief
Family systems theory	Walsh, McGoldrick, Kissane, Shapiro	Family are the main source of support; family functioning determines outcome
Cognitive stress coping theory	Stroebe, Kavanagh	Conditioned or learnt patterns become entrenched
Traumatic model	Horowitz, Pynoos, Prigerson, Jacobs	Intrusive aspects of trauma dominate
Ethology	Darwin, Lorenz	Biological and physiological processes underpin the phenomena across species
Meaning-centred model	Neimeyer, Lichtenthal	Narrative methods guide the reconstruction of meaning after the loss

forms the setting for the major constellation of bonds. Through studying parent–child relationships, Mary Ainsworth differentiated secure from insecure attachments, the latter appearing as either anxious, avoidant, or disorganized/hostile (Ainsworth et al., 1978). A transgenerational influence is evident between the parental style of attachment and that found in children, such that families can transmit insecure patterns of relating through the generations. The nature of attachments in a person's life influences the impact of loss when these bonds are changed, determining the work of mourning as this separation is dealt with (Parkes, 1985; Jacobs et al., 1987/1988).

While related to attachment theory, the psychodynamic model places greater emphasis on the development of the person, with all of their childhood and earlier life influences, including their sense of self, confidence, and resilience that comes with a robust self-esteem, and their learnt capacity to mourn. Schematic representations of early relationships construct a template (technically termed object relations) that lays down the operating principles guiding the emotional experience of relationships. Once the infant has developed feelings of concern for its mother, Klein described the early pining evident when the mother was absent (Klein, 1940). Mourning was thus recognized as a life-long mechanism of adaptation to cope with the inevitable traumas of life.

Interpersonal theories have emerged recently to throw further light on bereavement (Shapiro, 2001) and complement the psychodynamic model. Cyclical relational patterns are understood to result from current relational selections based on their resonance with the past, often confirming previous expectations. Schemas of the 'who the self is' are constructed through relational interactions to establish a role for the person pertaining to these relationships (Young et al., 2003). Horowitz has made particular use of these schemas using a stress–response model for grief (Horowitz, 1989). For instance, ambivalence towards the deceased is associated with greater distress, but restructuring the 'ambivalent' schema is possible through its observation in current relational patterns and the introduction of strategic variations to alter this habitually dysfunctional pattern. Horowitz and colleagues have tested a model of therapy based on these premises (Horowitz et al., 1993).

Transition theorists highlight the adaptation to change that is inherent in any resolution of grief. Parkes suggested that alteration to an individual's set of ideas and beliefs about their environment—their assumptive world—was central to adaptation (Parkes, 1975b). Development of acceptance of change is implicit in such a view. Meaning-making and the reconstruction of a continuing bond help reconfigure the assumptive world (Neimeyer, 2011).

In their contribution to a sociological model of bereavement, post-modern writers emphasize the various discourses that indicate a multiplicity of perspectives. The notion of the 'breaking of the bonds' of relationship, first hinted at by Freud (1912), is thus socially determined. Klass and colleagues highlighted the process of continuing bonds through reverence for the dead as both ancestors and moral guides (Klass et al., 1996). Walter noted that conversations about and with the deceased served as one means of sustaining a relationship (Walter, 1996). It becomes a personal choice whether the bereaved moves on to a new relationship or sustains the attitude of a 'broken heart'.

The sociological view also recognizes the loneliness of the bereaved and the value of groups or networks, including the family, to counter the social isolation that otherwise might prevail. Patterns of socialization of the bereaved vary with cultures, but networks of support have a vital influence on adjustment. The manner in which a family grieves and how its members continue to relate to each other is crucial to outcome. Families wreaked by conflict, reduced cohesion, and poor communication struggle to support each other—high rates of psychosocial morbidity are found in dysfunctional families (Kissane et al., 1996). Family systems theory makes particular use of intergenerational and family life-cycle perspectives (Walsh and McGoldrick, 1991).

Mourning can be triggered by unexpected life events, natural disasters, and traumas that violate the person and introduce an unwelcome element to the experience that is described as 'shocking'. Traumatic grief captures something that is unique to the trauma and challenges the bereaved with the intrusion of any resultant distressing memories. Prigerson and Jacobs have argued for recognition of the specifically traumatic nature of some deaths and their impact on grief (Prigerson and Jacobs, 2001).

Finally, behavioural models offer their contribution to bereavement theory through the challenge of chronic grief, in which the bereaved become stuck in an entrenched state of distress (Kavanagh et al., 1990). Patterns such as social withdrawal, 'memorialization' of the deceased through preserving their bedroom, clothes, and possessions intact as if a shrine, or chronic weeping upon mention of the deceased's name illustrate these behaviours. Cognitive behavioural approaches such as activity scheduling generate clinical improvement and point to an element of conditioned response in chronic grief.

The number of overlapping dimensions to these conceptual models is noteworthy, yet none by itself is a sufficient and complete explanation of bereavement phenomena. However, the intrapsychic, interpersonal, systemic, and sociological features of these models deliver an intersecting and overall coherence, which aids our eventual understanding of the complex phenomena observed in grief.

Stroebe and Schut have pointed out that while these general theories of grief explain the broad range of phenomena observed, they do not inform fully about the specific coping pathways that grieving individuals go down (Stroebe and Schut, 2001). They have suggested a dual-process model of bereavement-specific coping, in which oscillation occurs between loss-orientation, in which there is a focus on the loss itself, and restoration-orientation, in which the focus shifts to attending to ongoing life. Active 'grief work' occurs when the bereaved are loss-oriented, but excessive negative emotion could lead to a deterioration in coping, and so active confrontation of grief sits in a dynamic equilibrium with some degree of avoidance of grief. The individual needs at times to pull back and take 'time out' from the distress of the loss. They may do so through use of the restorative track in which the negative emotions are countered by some degree of positive reappraisal and of construction of meaning about the event. This promotes positive affects and eventually opens up new goals and plans for the future. Complex regulation exists in getting this balance right between grieving and restoring, with both interpersonal and cultural influences guiding this balance. Dissonance between bereaved members of a family, for instance, will challenge the balance and lead systemically to some readjustment by some or more members.

The bereaved cope therefore through adjusting the balance between expression of negative and positive emotions in emotion-based coping, and incorporating appropriate degrees of problem-solving and meaning-generation to guide their sense of purpose and control. They need to sustain the normal operation and functioning in their lives while also grieving the loss that has occurred irrevocably.

The nature of normal grief

The expression of normal grief is evident through its emotional, cognitive, physical, and behavioural features (Parkes, 1998). Eric Lindemann provided the first systematic study of these through his observations of people who lost a relative in Boston's Cocoanut Grove Nightclub fire (Lindemann, 1944). Somatic distress with numbness, preoccupation with sad memories of the deceased, guilt, anger, loss of the regular patterns of conduct, and identification with symptoms of the deceased formed the key dimensions that Lindemann observed.

Emotional distress occurs in waves that last for minutes at a time and involves unavoidable crying, loss of concentration and purpose while preoccupied with thoughts about the deceased, and a range of associated affects including sadness, anger, despair, anxiety, and guilt. Cognitive processes become dominated by memories, reflected in storytelling, reminiscences, and conversations about the deceased. Physical responses include numbness, restlessness, tension, tremors, sleep disturbance, anorexia, weight loss, fatigue, and a variety of aches and pains. Finally, behavioural aspects are variously reflected in social withdrawal, wandering, searching, and seeking company and consolation.

A number of physiological changes have been identified in neuroendocrine functioning (Jacobs et al., 1997) (e.g. challenge studies like the dexamethasone suppression test), immune indices (Esterling et al., 1996) (e.g. natural killer cell functioning), and sleep efficiency (Hall et al., 1998). Exploration of these physiological changes not only suggests that grief and depression lie on a biological continuum but also provides understanding for the morbidity, both somatic and psychosocial, that is associated with bereavement.

The clinical presentations of grief

As the family journey through palliative care, the clinical phases progress from anticipatory grief through to the immediate news of the death, to the stages of acute grief and, potentially for some, the complications of bereavement.

Anticipatory grief

When news of cancer recurrence or disease progression reaches the patient and family, grief is initiated as they anticipate eventual death. However, not all of this grief is about the final loss, as many changes unfold with the illness and its treatment. Loss of health can be accompanied by loss of work, leisure activities, financial security, independence, sense of certainty about life and further physical impairments, body image change, and altered perception of well-being. The clinician is challenged to understand the meaning of the loss to each person and evaluate therein their grief response.

Anticipatory grief generally draws the supportive family into a configuration of mutual comfort and greater closeness as the news of the illness and its proposed management is grappled with. For a time this perturbation advantages the care of the sick, until the pressures of daily life draw the family back towards their prior constellation. Movement back and forth is evident thereafter as news of illness progression unfolds. Periods of grief become interspersed with phases of contentment and happiness. When the family is engaged in the domiciliary care of their ill member, their cohesion potentially increases as they share their fears, hopes, joy, and distress.

In contrast, difficulties emerge for some families as they express their anticipatory grief. Impaired coping is exhibited through protective avoidance, denial of the seriousness of the threat, anger, or withdrawal from involvement. Sometimes family dysfunction is so glaring that clinicians are rapidly drawn into its snares. More commonly, however, subthreshold or mild depressive or anxiety disorders develop gradually as individuals struggle to adapt to unwelcome changes. While anticipatory grief was historically suggested to reduce post-mortem grief (Parkes, 1975a), intense distress is now well recognized as a marker of risk for complicated grief.

During this phase of anticipatory grief, clinicians can usefully help the family that is capable of effective communication by encouraging them to openly share their feelings as they pay attention to the material needs of their dying family member or friend. Saying goodbye needs to be recognized as a process that evolves over time, with opportunities for reminiscence, celebration of the life and contribution of the dying person, expressions of gratitude and completion of any unfinished business (Meares, 1981). These tasks have the potential to generate meaningful and positive emotional aspects of what is otherwise a sad time for all.

Grief of family and friends gathered around the death bed

When relatives or close friends gather to keep watch by the bed of a dying person, not only do they support the sick, but they also help their own subsequent adjustment. The solidarity shared through this experience cements these carers into mutually supportive relationships. As staff go about nursing the ill patient, they need to comfortably relate to the family, whether in the home, hospice, or hospital. For years to come, these poignant moments will be recalled in immense detail—the sensitivity and courteous respect of health professionals is crucial (Maguire, 1985). Clinicians can helpfully comment on the process of dying, explaining the breathing patterns, and commenting on any noises, secretions, patient reactions, and comfort (Kissane et al., 2012a). The experience needs to be normalized empathically and the family reassured whenever concern develops. Discussion about pain, reasons for medications, and skilled prediction of events will assuage worry and build a collaborative approach to the care of the dying.

Religious rituals warrant active facilitation, including appropriate notification of a religious minister or pastoral care worker. Respect for the body remains paramount once death has occurred and the expression of sympathy from clinicians is greatly appreciated. The family will be invariably grateful for time spent alone with the deceased, while regard for cultural approaches to the laying out of the body is essential (Parkes et al., 1997) (discussed in the section on cross-cultural bereavement practices in the online Appendix). The bereaved are commonly bewildered and benefit from guidance about what to do next—making contact with the undertaker is an obvious example.

When relatives have not been present at the moment of death, informing them by telephone of the fact is generally undesirable. The invitation for them to attend in person is often based on a stated deterioration in the patient's condition. On arrival, the news can be sensitively shared in an appropriate setting before accompanying them to see the deceased. To help the family to integrate an understanding of all that has occurred, clinicians should explain the sequence of medical events culminating in the death. Questions need to be sensitively answered and time taken to comfort the bereaved in their distress.

From time to time, the cause of death will remain uncertain and an autopsy may be indicated. A senior clinician should outline the pertinent issues, emphasizing the positive aspects of the information that will be gleaned and indicating that it will be subsequently shared with the family in a follow-up meeting. Unless there is a legal requirement for a coroner's post-mortem, the family's views on autopsy need to be fully respected.

Sometimes staff will have concerns about the emotional response of the bereaved. If there is uncertainty about its cultural appropriateness, consultation with an informed cultural intermediary may prove helpful. The prescription of short-acting benzodiazepines will help some, while others will prefer to manage without medication. A follow-up telephone call on the next day is worthwhile to check on coping and identify the need for continued support.

Caution is needed in settings where grief could be marginalized, well exemplified by ageism (Doka, 1989). If a death is normalized because it appears in step with the life cycle, family members can be given less support and reduced permission to express many aspects of their loss. In the process, the disenfranchised can be ignored in their sorrow.

Acute grief and time course of bereavement

The sequence or phases through which the bereaved move over time are never rigidly demarcated but merge gradually one into the other (Raphael. 1983; Parkes, 1998). They assist the clinician to recognize aberration from the normal evolution. From the (1) initial numbness and sense of unreality, (2) waves of distress begin to occur as the bereaved suffer intense pining and yearning for their lost one. Memories of the deceased trigger these acute pangs of grief. Then as the pain of separation grows, (3) a phase of disorganization emerges as loneliness resulting from the loss sets in. Hofer described this phase aptly as a constant background disturbance of restlessness, inattention, sadness, and despair with social withdrawal that can last for several months (Hofer, 1984). Eventually (4) a phase of reorganization and recovery develops as nostalgia replaces sadness, morale improves, and an altered world view is constructed. Personal growth can be recognized at this stage and new creativity is expressed (Polloch, 1989).

The time course of mourning is proportional to the strength of attachment to the lost person and also varies with cultural expression, there being no sharply defined end point to grief. Just as a mother's grief following sudden infant death syndrome lasts longer than grief following a neonatal death, so to with adult loss, the mourning that follows many years of marriage is generally longer than brief relationships. Older widows and widowers may continue to display their grief for several years (Zisook and Schuchter, 1985). This can correspond with a continuing relationship with the deceased, which for some is their choice and leads to chronic grief. The clinical task is then to differentiate those who remain within the spectrum of normality from those who cross the threshold of complicated grief

Pathological grief

Normal and abnormal responses to bereavement span a spectrum in which intensity of reaction, presence of a range of related grief behaviours, and time course determine the differentiation. Psychiatric conditions that commonly accompany grief include clinical depression, anxiety disorders, alcohol abuse or other substance abuse and dependence, psychotic disorders, and post-traumatic stress disorder (PTSD). When frank psychiatric disorders complicate bereavement, their recognition and management is straightforward; subthreshold states present the greater clinical challenge as studies of the bereaved indicate groups in which clusters of intense grief symptoms are distinct from the normal trajectory of grief (Parkes and Weiss, 1983; Prigerson et al., 1995a, 1995b). The *Diagnostic and Statistical Manual of Mental Disorders*, fifth edition (DSM-5) of the American Psychiatric Association proposes further study on its proposed criteria for what has been called 'Persistent Complex Bereavement Disorder' (American Psychiatric Association, 2013). For at least 12 months following the death, intense longing or yearning for the deceased will be accompanied by intense sorrow and significant social impairment. Recognition of pathological grief calls for an experienced clinical judgement that does not normalize the distress as necessarily understandable. In practice, a set of criteria by which these patients can be identified as high risk and the application of preventive models of bereavement care eliminate some of the academic debate about their characteristics.

Inhibited or delayed grief

While use of avoidance may serve some as a temporary coping mechanism, its persistence is sometimes associated with relationship difficulties or the emergence of a hypomanic state in individuals with bipolar disorder. There are scenarios, however, in which the absence of significant distress and impairment immediately following loss may be understandable, perhaps indicative of resilience. Bonnano cogently argues that the prevailing model of grief that has become popularized in our culture (e.g. the need for 'grief work') is based on poorly supported assumptions, and does not allow for the full range of grief responses that may prove adaptive among the bereaved (Bonnano, 2004). In keeping with this view, Bonnano identifies a subgroup of individuals who show little distress or disruption to normal functioning following a loss, with relatively stable, healthy functioning up to 2 years following the event. Rather than consider them delayed or avoidant in their grief, Bonnano instead refers to this group as resilient, noting that research to date has failed to find any evidence for the phenomenon of delayed grief. On this basis, he challenges the assumption that the absence of grief is necessarily pathological, that it indicates a superficial bond with the deceased or that it necessarily warrants clinical intervention. Still, it is important to highlight that cultural variation influences grief expression. Additionally, among those who present with symptoms of complicated grief (see following section), avoidance of activities or situations reminiscent of the loss is common and may indeed require targeted intervention.

Complicated grief

An impressive body of empirical work supports the validity of complicated grief as a clinical entity, distinct from normal grief responses and related pathological states (e.g. major depression). After an extended debate about whether complicated grief constitutes a bona fide psychiatric disorder (Stroebe et al., 2000; Prigersonet al., 2007), DSM-5 (American Psychiatric Association, 2013) includes a chronic grief syndrome as Persistent Complex Bereavement Disorder (PCBD). For at least 12 months following the death of a close relative or friend, the individual experiences intense yearning or longing for the deceased, intense sorrow and preoccupation with the deceased on more days than not. This reaction must be out of proportion to the bereaved's culture and cause significant impairment in social, occupational, or other important areas of functioning. More significant mental disorders (e.g. major depression, PTSD) take precedence as diagnoses over PCBD (Hogan et al., 2003–2004). A variety of other phenomena may accompany this, including non-acceptance of the death, intense anger, a diminished sense of self, a feeling that life is empty, and indecisiveness

about the future, whether with activities or relationships (Prigerson et al., 1995c, 1996, 2009). Such prolonged grief has been independently associated with risk for a range of health problems, including cardiac distress, hypertension, increased alcohol and cigarette consumption and suicidal ideation (Prigerson et al., 1999).

Using the Inventory of Complicated Grief (Prigerson et al., 1995c), cases of complicated grief were identified with high sensitivity and specificity (Prigerson et al., 1999). Moreover, a substantial and growing number of cross-validation studies have successfully replicated the unique clustering of the proposed criteria as a coherent and distinct syndrome (Prigerson and Maciejewski, 2005–2006). Results from a DSM-5 field trial conducted with a community sample of 317 bereaved persons indicated that the presence of complicated grief at 6–12 months post loss predicted much higher risk for morbidity than its presence within the first 6 months following loss (Prigerson et al., 2007). The diagnostic criteria adopted by the DSM-5 committee stayed with the conservative time frame of longer than 12 months, while opting to further study the predictive nature of intense distress persisting across 6–12 months.

Who is most likely to develop complicated grief in response to the death of a loved one? Attachment processes are believed to play a central role in predicting the grief response, with separation distress most strongly activated following the loss of a 'security-enhancing attachment bond' (Neimeyer, 2005–2006). The loss of a close and stabilizing attachment figure may be especially harrowing to those with a history of childhood neglect or abuse. Indeed, evidence suggests that these subgroups are especially prone to develop complicated grief (Silverman et al., 2001). Bereaved individuals who suffered a traumatic or unexpected loss, had an intimate relationship with the deceased, and experienced little support following the death are also at heightened risk for complicated grief (Silverman et al., 2001; Prigerson et al., 2007).

Chronic grief is particularly associated with overly dependent relationships in which a sense of abandonment is avoided by perpetuation of the relationship through memorialization of the deceased and maintenance of continuing bonds. A stuck situation emerges in which the tearfulness is induced by any reminder of the deceased without any cognitive transition being achieved in the world view of the bereaved. Social withdrawal and depression are common. A fantasy of reunion with the deceased can cause suicide to be an increasingly attractive option. Active treatment using pharmacology for depression and cognitive behavioural therapy to reality test the loss and promote socialization (via activity scheduling) is appropriate for chronic grief. Treatment of complicated grief employs multimodal therapy incorporating retelling the story of loss, written and imaginal exposure exercises and behavioural activation exercises to resocialize (Shear et al., 2005; Boelen et al., 2007).

Traumatic grief

When death has been unexpected or its nature in some way shocking—traumatic, violent, stigmatized, or perceived as undignified—its integration and acceptance may be interfered with by the arousal and increased distress that memories can trigger. Intensive recollections including flashbacks, nightmares, and recurrent intrusive memories cause hyperarousal, disbelief, insomnia, irritability, and disturbed concentration, which distorts normal grieving (Prigerson and Jacobs, 2001). The shock of the death can precipitate mistrust, anger, detachment, and an unwillingness to accept its reality. These reactions at a subthreshold level merge with the full features of PTSD, but the subthreshold state has been observed to persist for years and contribute substantial morbidity.

Depressive disorders

Rates of major depression in the bereaved have varied between 16% and 50%, peaking over the first 2 months (Stroebe et al., 2000; Bonnano, 2004), and gradually decreasing to 15% across the next 2 years (Hogan et al., 2003–2004; Prigerson et al., 2007). The features of any major depressive episode post bereavement resemble major depression at other points of the life cycle (Prigerson et al., 1995c). There is a tendency to chronicity, considerable social morbidity, and risk of inadequate treatment.

Anxiety disorders

These take the form of adjustment disorders, generalized anxiety disorder, and phobic states and occur in up to 30% of the bereaved (Prigerson et al., 1996). Patients present commonly to general practitioners with a range of somatic concerns. Separation anxiety of a heightened nature can be distinguished from anxiety symptoms of a general kind.

Alcohol and substance abuse/dependence

Typically an exacerbation of pre-existing psychiatric states, individuals predisposed to alcohol abuse or dependence on other substances such as benzodiazepines relapse during bereavement (Prigerson et al., 1996). Other family members often raise the alarm.

Post-traumatic stress disorder

While clearly related to unnatural deaths, deaths involving profound breakdown of bodily surfaces (Rudge and Holmes, 2010), gross disfigurement due to head and neck cancers, or other causes of relatives perceiving the illness to cause loss of dignity may generate traumatic memories in the bereaved. Prigerson and colleagues found that PTSD was often correlated with the perceived inadequacy of the goodbye, and suggested that rituals to complete this be incorporated into related grief therapies (Prigerson et al., 1999).

Psychotic disorders

Bereavement is a common precipitant of relapse of psychotic illnesses such as bipolar disorder or schizophrenia in individuals so predisposed; occasionally, mania presents for the first time in such a setting.

Family grief

The family is one of the primary contexts in which grief is recognized and expressed. As survival time has increased for those with terminal illness, a new grief has emerged for families, reflecting the cumulative losses that families anticipate and cope with across a longer period of time. Indeed, death from illness is less often a sudden and unexpected event. The opportunity to prepare for the dying process enables families to strive for a 'good death', and thus changes the conditions under which subsequent grief unfolds. The extended nature of grief as it occurs across a family's journey with illness underscores the importance of family-centred care from diagnosis to death.

It has long been recognized that the family, when functioning optimally, empowers mutual support, either through direct and open expression of sadness, shared performance of rituals, or informal opportunities for remembrance before and after loss (Kissane et al., 2007–2008). In addition to supporting the adaptation of its individual members, the grieving family faces the task of reconstituting its key roles and functions without the lost member (e.g. parenting and sustaining important traditions). In some cases, grief that is shared brings opportunities to forge or strengthen new relationships among surviving members, and can prompt tremendous growth and resilience (Zaider and Kissane, 2007).

Therapists have long recognized the salience of family processes to mourning and their systemic influence on outcome (Prigerson and Maciejewski, 2005–2006). Exploration of the interplay between family functioning and individual members' bereavement morbidity has highlighted the manner in which dysfunctional relationship patterns predict increased rates of psychosocial morbidity in the bereaved (Kissane et al., 1996). A typology of family functioning during both palliative care and bereavement was created using cluster analysis in the Melbourne-based family grief studies (Kissane et al., 1994, 1996). Dimensions of cohesiveness, expressiveness, and conflict from the Family Environment Scale (Moos and Moos, 1981) determined five classes of families illustrated in Table 17.7.2. While over half the families met in a palliative care setting demonstrate resilience through their family functioning, and do not need particular psychological assistance to achieve an adaptive outcome from bereavement, the remainder have identifiable characteristics predictive of a higher risk of morbid outcome and can be specifically targeted through a preventive model of family care (Kissane and Bloch, 2002).

During early bereavement, families at risk have been shown to decompensate through deterioration in their functioning with loss of cohesiveness, communication breakdown, and increased conflict. A proportion of families with intermediate characteristics of functioning changes to become 'Sullen' or 'Hostile' in type. Importantly, these dysfunctional families carry the bulk of the psychosocial morbidity observed to occur during bereavement, thus highlighting the potential benefits of a family form of intervention. Screening of families on their admission to palliative care through the use of a well-validated measure such as the Family Relationships Index (Moos and Moos, 1981) provides an ideal means to recognize those families at greater risk of morbid outcome during bereavement.

Recognizing those at risk of complicated bereavement outcome

Palliative care teams are ideally placed to recognize those at increased risk of complicated grief and plan preventive interventions in an endeavour to circumvent morbidity. To accomplish this, bereavement care planning does not begin post death but at the point of entry into the palliative care service. The continuity of supportive care that flows from this builds a strong therapeutic alliance, which will be more likely to survive ambivalence about the death than if a bereavement counsellor attempts to begin post death. Avoidance hinders many attempts to engage the bereaved after the death.

In times of resource scarceness and economic rationalism, services are under pressure to direct their clinical staff to appropriate areas of need. When relatives appear resilient and well supported,

Table 17.7.2 Typology of palliative care and bereaved families (Kissane et al., 1994; 1996)

Category: family type	Rate of occurrence (%)	Features
Well-functioning types		
Supportive	32	Strongly cohesive families who grieve adaptively
Conflict resolving	20	Cohesion and effective communication empowers tolerance of difference of opinions
Dysfunctional types		
Hostile	6–12	Poorly cohesive with high conflict, ineffective communication, and fractured relationships; families resist help
Sullen	9–18	Muted anger generates highest levels of depression; families seek help
Intermediate	20–33	Mid-range levels of communication, cohesion, and conflict place these families at risk of deterioration when stressed by life events

clinicians can wisely respect their capacity to cope with loss adaptively. The best predictors of an adaptive outcome include a gradually resolving trajectory of emotional distress that began from a moderate rather than excessive initial level, open communication with others, good supports, robust self-esteem, and evidence of personal competency in the daily tasks that are ordinarily pursued (Lund et al., 1993). Moreover, empirical evidence confirms that when preventive interventions are targeted to those at risk, benefits ensue (Raphael, 1977), whereas when they are broadly offered to a bereaved population regardless of risk, no such benefit is discernible (Parkes, 1981). In the latter type of study, the well functioning dilute any evidence of benefit to those at risk. In contrast with a broadly supportive bereavement follow-up programme that utilizes condolence cards and invitations to memorial services, seriously intended preventive interventions should be directed towards those at increased risk.

Pathological grief can be recognized by the presence of greater degrees of separation distress, emotional numbing and dissociation, mood symptoms, impaired social functioning, and maladaptive coping styles. The coping styles contributing to this include elements of avoidance or denial, distortion through excessive anger, despair, guilt, idealization or somatization, and prolongation that culminates in chronicity of distress.

Risk factors to aid recognition of those at greater risk of complicated grief are summarized in Table 17.7.3. These should be assessed at entry to the service and upgraded during the phase of palliative care, including revision shortly after the death. Completion of the family genogram presents an ideal time for such assessment as relationships, prior losses, and coping are considered. Some palliative care services have developed checklists based on such risk factors to generate a numerical measure of risk. There has been insufficient validation of such scales at this stage, but the presence of any single factor in Table 17.7.3 signifies greater risk. Continued observation of the pattern of grief evolution over time is appropriate whenever such concern exists.

Health consequences of bereavement

Over 15 studies of mortality following bereavement provide evidence for an increased rate of deaths in the 45–75 age range,

Table 17.7.3 Risk factors for pathological grief outcomes

Category	Range of circumstances
Nature of the death	Untimely within the life cycle (e.g. death of child)
	Sudden and unexpected (e.g. death from septic neutropenia during chemotherapy)
	Traumatic (e.g. gross cachexia and debility)
	Stigmatized (e.g. AIDS or suicide)
Strengths and vulnerabilities of the carer/bereaved	Past history of psychiatric disorder (e.g. depression)
	Personality and coping style (e.g. intense worrier, low self-esteem)
	Cumulative experience of losses
Nature of the relationship with the deceased	Overly dependent (e.g. clinging, symbiotic)
	Ambivalent (e.g. angry and insecure with alcohol abuse, infidelity, gambling)
Family and support network	Dysfunctional family (e.g. poor cohesiveness and communication, high conflict)
	Isolated (e.g. new migrant, new residential move)
	Alienated (e.g. perception of poor support)

with these occurring over the first year post loss, particularly the first 6 months from acute cardiovascular causes (Stroebe and Stroebe, 1993). While some studies have only identified increased mortality in men, a well-controlled study of 12,522 spouse pairs in a prepaid health-care plan showed increased mortality for both women and men, adjusting for age, education, and other mortality predictors (Schaefer et al., 1995). Other noteworthy causes of death in addition to cardiovascular events include accidents, suicide, alcohol and substance abuse, and cirrhosis while the association evident in large epidemiological studies of increased mortality with social isolation and alienation is also relevant (House et al., 1988).

Early studies by Saunders (1999) and Parkes (1984) identified the increased use of health services—both greater consultations and hospitalizations—by the recently bereaved, with increased psychological distress, somatic health complaints, more days of disability, and greater reliance on medications. Some 20–25% were noted to develop depressive disorders (Clayton, 1990; Harlow et al., 1991; Zisook and Schuchter 1991; Karam, 1994; Zisooket al., 1994), but increased rates of anxiety disorders, including PTSD in settings of traumatic loss, also occur (Hofer et al., 1972). Some of the explanations for these health consequences lie in the development of complicated grief, others in altered behaviours and lifestyle including diet, smoking, and alcohol consumption. Studies have also highlighted effects on the cardiovascular, neuroendocrine, and immunological systems: several studies have shown increased rates of myocardial infarction post bereavement (Stroebe and Stroebe, 1993); altered cortisol levels were seen in parents following death of their children from leukaemia (Hofer et al., 1972); altered lymphocyte response to mitogens and lowered natural killer cell activity were also seen in bereaved spouses (Hofer et al., 1977; Schleifer et al., 1983; Irwin et al., 1987). Immunosuppressed patients, either chemically induced or as a result of AIDS, develop specific malignancies such as lymphomas or Kaposi's sarcomas. However, the clinical relevance of the immunological changes described in bereavement is uncertain in the light of a series of large epidemiological studies that fail to show increased rates of cancer in the bereaved (Helsing et al., 1982; Jones and Goldblatt, 1986; Kaprio et al., 1987).

Bereavement follow-up by the treatment team

Once the patient has died, the palliative care team should routinely review the death and the bereavement-related risk factors in the next available multidisciplinary team meeting. Was the death perceived to impact significantly on key family members? What level of bereavement follow-up should be adopted?

Two broad levels of follow-up are possible. The first involves the expression of condolences via the telephone, sympathy card, visit by the nurse or general practitioner, staff attendance at the funeral, and subsequent family invitation to a periodic commemorative service arranged by the palliative care team. This model provides both encouragement and support while normalizing the grief that relatives express and respecting their mourning process without undue intrusion. Where greater concern does emerge, an opportunity presents to intervene appropriately. The staff who have developed the closest relationships with the family are wisely selected by the team to take up this observing model of follow-up as it provides them with a means of gradual farewell. Their formal identification and documentation is nonetheless important to ensure completion of the process over time. Final contact is often shortly after the first anniversary.

The second model of follow-up is for those individuals or families judged to be at greater risk and thought likely to benefit from a preventive intervention. Studies have shown that such prevention effectively reduces morbidity when delivered to those 20% likely otherwise to develop complicated grief (Schut et al., 1997). Teams vary in their pursuit of this depending on staff availability; in other instances, general practitioners provide active

individual support. Individual, group, or family approaches are valid and selected on the basis of personal needs. Where continuity of involvement of the counsellor from palliative care into bereavement is possible, direct knowledge of the deceased is advantageous, as is the continuing relationship with the bereaved. Attempts to establish bereavement counselling only after the death meet high rates of defensive avoidance blocking this form of support. Where social isolation is noteworthy, the additional support derived from a group approach maximizes connectedness (Yalom and Vinogradov, 1988; Lieberman and Yalom, 1992). Others will seek the personal support of individual therapy.

For many, a family approach is cost-effective in reaching several at risk when the nature of the family's functioning has been shown by screening to be dysfunctional. family-focused grief therapy (FFGT) offers continuity from palliative care through to bereavement and, in promoting family functioning, it fosters the role of the family as a natural and sustainable source of ongoing support (Kissane, 2000). Engaging the distressed family in supportive meetings can prove challenging, particularly for the protective family whose members wish to avoid distressing topics, or for the conflictual family in which the lack of emotional safety is barrier to open communication (Kissane, 1999). A flexible, yet focused model of family support that is guided by a collaboratively formed agenda helps the clinician to establish realistic parameters of care and protects against efforts to resolve more complex, longstanding issues (e.g. prior marital affairs). FFGT is also easily adapted to families of Hispanic and Asian origin, for whom culturally based values that promote family closeness and prioritize the caregiving role are well suited to a model of care that engages the family as a whole (Mondias et al., 2012; Del Gaudio et al., 2013).

The diverse range of clinicians in palliative care teams, including chaplains or pastoral care workers, nurses, social workers, psychologists or psychiatrists, general practitioners, volunteers, and generic bereavement counsellors ensure that there is no shortage of staff to support the bereaved. Nevertheless, staff caught up with the business of acute patient care will neglect the bereaved despite their best of intentions. Team leadership needs to actively monitor programmes of bereavement follow-up to ensure its adherence to an intended protocol and to initiate appropriate cross-referral of those at greater risk.

Grief therapies

Indications

For the majority, although bereavement is painful, their personal resilience will ensure their normal adaptation. There can, therefore, be no justification for routine intervention as grief is not a disease. Those considered at risk of maladaptive outcome are the ones that should be treated preventatively and those who later develop complicated bereavement need active treatments.

General considerations

The spectrum of interventions spans individual-, group-, and family-oriented therapies, and encompasses all schools of psychotherapy as well as appropriately indicated pharmacotherapies. Adoption of any model is predicated on the clinical issues and associated predicaments that arise. Thus, variation will be influenced by age, perception of support, the nature of the death, the personal health of the bereaved, and the presence of co-morbid states. Clinicians generally plan for an intervention to proceed as six to eight sessions over several months and do well to map this out at the beginning. In this sense, grief therapy is focused and time limited, but multimodal therapies are commonplace. Thus, group as well as individual therapies better support the lonely so that socialization complements interpersonally any intrapersonal change. As loss is so ubiquitous within palliative care, all clinicians need skill in the application of grief therapies.

General supportive aids

Basic aids to any form of grief counselling include the use of evocative rather than sensitive language to assist the expression of feelings, the sharing of photo albums and special letters from the loved person, writing about any unfinished business to draw it to a close, and optimizing attendance at cultural or religious rituals to support the process of mourning. Children can be encouraged to make up a 'scrap' or memory book about a deceased parent as an aide to their adaptive mourning. Complementary forms of therapy such as art (Simon, 1982) and music (Bright, 1986) therapy can also make a valuable contribution to any programme for the bereaved. Any individual differences in the intensity and progress of mourning need to be normalized as appropriate. For instance, research has repeatedly confirmed that mothers express grief more intensely than fathers do (Kissane and Bloch, 1994). Time must be allowed to permit the process to unfold naturally and the length of mourning is helpfully appraised as proportional to the strength of attachment to the deceased.

Supportive–expressive therapy

The most basic model is a supportive–expressive intervention in which the person is invited to share their feelings about the loss to a health professional, who will listen and seek to understand the other's distress in a comforting manner. The key therapeutic aspects of this encounter are the sharing of distress and, through the relational understanding that is acknowledged, some shift in cognitive appraisal of the reality that has been forever altered. In supportive therapy, guided mourning is an approach to 'grief work' that promotes narrative review of the story, with repetitive recollections of the deceased being actively encouraged to relive and eventually revise the relationship experienced, ultimately redefining the reality of self and situation (Melges and Demaso, 1980; Mawson et al., 1981). In the process, Worden emphasized the accomplishment of four basic tasks of mourning: accepting the reality of loss, working through the pain of grief, adjusting to a new environment without the loved person, and establishing a collection of positive and useful memories of the deceased for future reference (Worden, 1991).

Reality testing and adaptation to the separation leads to what Parkes termed an altered assumptive world in which the ideas, attitudes, and beliefs about the self and the world are fundamentally altered (Parkes, 1975b; Janoff-Bulman, 1989, 1992). The inherent cognitive change is vital to future equanimity. Even when culture prescribes some level of continuing bonds with one's ancestors, creativity and generativity emerge from resolution of the mourning process (Parkes et al., 1997). Raphael has tended to understand much of this guided grief therapy within the rubric of 'crisis' intervention, placing additional emphasis on the mobilization of support to assist and comfort the bereaved (Raphael, 1983).

Interpersonal psychotherapy

This places emphasis on the nature of relationships and how the bereaved functions within these (Klerman et al., 1984). Any psychodynamic understanding of the patterns of relationship from childhood that repeat in adult life will inform these interpersonal approaches (Horowitz et al., 1984). The mixed feelings underpinning ambivalent relationships warrant expression and understanding, while the past influences on insecure and overly dependent patterns of relating help to consider future needs. The nature of the continuing relationship with the deceased is explored alongside any desire to replace the lost person. The urge for reunion with the deceased merits active discussion as suicidal desire easily grows out of persistence of such ideas. Gersie highlighted the dangerous pull that reunion fantasies can have when the dependent bereaved lament their loss and search to re-establish connection (Gersie, 1991). Increased suicide risk also occurs among socially isolated, elderly widowers, those who abuse alcohol, and those with a current or past history of depressive disorder.

Cognitive behavioural therapy

This offers a special contribution to chronic grief (Kavanagh, 1990; Shear et al., 2005; Boelen et al., 2007). Here, continued connectivity with the deceased may be valued, promoting some memorialization as 'stuckness' that prevents other progress in life. Repeated exposure to cues that induce sadness may deepen depressive illness in these circumstances. Behavioural approaches regulate exposure to these cues, optimize socialization through activity scheduling, moderate inappropriate drug and alcohol use, and promote graduated involvement in new roles and experiences. Related cognitive reframing of negative ideas such as unfairness and hopelessness steers towards a constructive adaptation.

Complicated grief treatment

This form of therapy was recently developed and evaluated by Shear and colleagues (Shear et al., 2005), and integrates techniques from interpersonal and cognitive behavioural therapies in order to specifically target symptoms of complicated grief. It draws upon the dual-process model of adaptive coping (Stroebe and Schut, 2001), thus focusing simultaneously on discussion of the loss and restoration of adaptive functioning. Attention to the loss and associated affect is alternated with pragmatic facilitation of identified life goals. In order to address the trauma-like symptoms presented in complicated grief (e.g. intrusive thoughts of death, avoidance of reminders of death), exposure-based exercises are adapted from cognitive behavioural therapies for PTSD. To address loss-related symptoms (e.g. yearning and longing for deceased) and encourage a revised connection to the deceased, the bereaved is invited to engage in an imaginal conversation with the deceased and to generate a list of positive memories. A randomized controlled trial compared standard interpersonal psychotherapy (IPT) with complicated grief treatment (CGT) among men and women who met criteria for complicated grief (Shear et al., 2005). Treatment response was evident in 51% of participants who received CGT, compared to only 28% of those treated with IPT. Furthermore, CGT was associated with significantly better outcome than IPT on self-report measures of complicated grief symptoms, depression, work and social functioning. Interestingly, among participants who had experienced a violent or traumatic loss, response rates were higher for CGT than for

IPT. Furthermore, response to CGT varied by type of loss, with loss of a spouse, friend or relative associated with higher response to CGT than loss of a child. In their trial, Boelen and colleagues found that exposure was more potent than cognitive restructuring; exposure is importantly located early in the therapy (Boelen et al., 2007).

When an overly dependent relationship has formed the basis of a complicated grief reaction, the bereaved's self-image changes from 'being valued and cared for' to being now 'alone and useless'. Patterns of perceived abandonment may re-emerge from earlier relationships. Therapy needs to target boosting self-esteem, confidence, and sense of security. The combination of both group and individual therapy has special merit since the group process promotes socialization in an individual otherwise at risk of isolation (Vachon et al., 1980). Brief group psychotherapy (Lieberman and Yalom, 1992) can be offered as a complementary programme of support for the more needy, and both variety and creativity can enhance such programmes, exemplified by one programme that combined group behaviour therapy with art therapy (Vachon et al., 1996).

Family-focused grief therapy

This family approach to grief intervention is a brief, manualized model of therapy (Kissane and Bloch, 2002). It aims to improve family functioning while also supporting the expression of grief and, as mentioned, can be applied preventatively to those families judged through screening to be at high risk of such morbid outcome (Kissane, 2000). Evidence from two randomized controlled trials of FFGT suggests that this model of care can benefit highly distressed families, is easily applied by clinicians of various disciplines and training backgrounds, and can be delivered in the outpatient setting, at the hospital bedside, or in the home (Kissane et al., 2006; Del Gaudio et al., 2012). Working with distressed families in the context of grief presents multiple challenges, such as how to sustain a systemic view, remain neutral to family conflicts, formulate realistic goals and be mindful of boundaries, particularly when working in the home. Peer support for clinicians in the form of supervision groups is an invaluable resource when conducting FFGT (Del Gaudio et al., 2012).

Commencing thus during palliative care and including the ill member in the family work, FFGT continues through the early phases of bereavement until there is confidence that morbidity has been prevented or appropriately treated. This approach invites the family to identify and agree to work on aspects of family life that they recognize as a cause of concern. Through enhancing cohesion, promoting open communication of thoughts and feelings, and teaching effective problem-solving to reduce conflict and optimize tolerance of different opinions, the improved functioning of the family as a unit becomes the means to accomplish adaptive mourning. The continuity of care and the personal knowledge that the therapist achieves of the dying family member empowers considerable maturation in the family unit not only as carers but also as comforters of the bereaved. Parentally bereaved children can also be greatly helped by family therapy (Sandler et al., 2010).

Pharmacotherapy accompanying grief therapies

Pharmacotherapies are widely used to support the bereaved—judicious prescribing is nonetheless important. Benzodiazepines allay anxiety and assist sleep, but words of caution should be offered about intermittent use to avoid tachyphylaxis and dependence. Antidepressants are indicated whenever bereavement is complicated by the development of depressive disorder, panic attacks, and moderate to severe adjustment disorders (Jacobs et al., 1987; Pasternak et al., 1991). If insomnia is prominent, tricyclics (e.g. dothiepin, nortriptyline, desipramine) or tetracyclics (e.g. mianserin) are beneficial; otherwise, selective serotonergic reuptake inhibitors (e.g. sertraline, paroxetine, citalopram, fluvoxamine, or fluoxetine) or combined noradrenergic and serotonergic reuptake inhibitors (e.g. venlafaxine, duloxetine, or mirtazapine) are indicated. Occasionally, antipsychotics are needed for hypomania or other forms of psychosis.

An integrated approach to the treatment of complicated grief incorporates balanced combinations of pharmacology (e.g. antidepressants or antianxiety agents), individual psychotherapy, and socialization through family or group work (Jacobs, 1993). Where the experience of death has been in some manner 'shocking', incomplete assimilation of the event can develop, leading to intrusive recollections and numbing. Here, the bereaved need to make clear sense of the loss, understanding the mechanisms involved in the death, and attributing responsibility to appropriate factors (Rynearson, 1987). Benzodiazepines have a particular role in reducing autonomic arousal, lessening intrusive symptoms, and allaying anxiety so that avoidant responses are minimized (Jacobs, 1993). The treatment team helps further by bringing the bereaved back in the weeks after the death to review overall understanding of events and report on findings from any autopsy. Whenever a coroner's inquiry follows a death, the bereaved are to be encouraged to attend to increase their integration of understanding of such events.

The notion of recovery is important and recognized by the return of equanimity in discussion of the deceased. A process of social transition has been accomplished (Silverman, 1986). New interests or roles are adopted, with new friendships emerging. Eventually, the bereaved see their future with reprioritized and altered world views. As ultimate evidence of completed mourning, new generativity and creativity emerges in the activities and lives of the bereaved (Polloch, 1989).

Special types of loss

Particular needs arise for bereaved children, the very elderly, and when loss is especially stigmatized, for instance, death from AIDS. The timing of such deaths within the life cycle explains some of the special considerations that arise.

Children and bereavement

The general principle of open communication with children about cancer or serious illness, its nature and meaning, treatment, and prospect of death is important (Adams-Greenly, 1984; Eiser and Havermans, 1992) (see also Chapter 16.1). Concepts need to be presented in an age-appropriate manner, recognizing that the finality of death only becomes more completely understood around the age of 9–10 years (Rowland, 1989). Younger children believe that death is reversible; after age 5, the understanding is more in terms of separation with a gradual recognition of its irreversibility. Families can teach children a healthy understanding of the life cycle and support the child through identification of and reassurance by available, surviving adults who commit to remaining involved with the child in the future. Such processes may help a child to mature more rapidly and grow in their appreciation of death as cessation of life. Children display a variety of bereavement symptoms including sadness, fear, guilt, insecurity, and behavioural problems (Webb, 1993). A programme that guides parents in what to say and do to assist their children was found to be helpful (Adams-Greenly and Moynihan, 1983; Moore and Rauch, 2010).

The death of either a parent or sibling is a significant and distressing occurrence that prompts many children to ask questions such as: 'Why? Did I cause it? Who will care for me?' Careful discussion of death causation is worthwhile to avoid prophylactically any misinterpretation by the child. In the setting of advanced cancer, when death can be anticipated, preparation of the child through involvement in care activities and open discussion of realities facilitates acceptance and adjustment. Subsequent involvement of children in funeral and anniversary rituals (Silverman and Worden, 1992) normalizes the experience of loss and promotes the family as the continuing, supportive environment (Wells, 1988).

The long-term effects of childhood bereavement are not completely clear, as studies have been hampered by being retrospective, but they have suggested that the loss of a mother prior to age 12 predicts an increased risk of adult depression. However, the quality of the relationship to subsequent care providers may be more significant in determining outcome than the parental loss (Tennant et al., 1980). Nonetheless, should such children develop cancer themselves in adult life, their memories of their dying parent and related identifications are powerful influences on their overall adjustment.

After accidents, cancer is the second leading cause of death in childhood. The family typically focuses on the dying child with the risk of relative neglect of other children. They in turn may try to replace the dead child and experience survivor guilt. Openness of family communication about all aspects of the illness and death is the best formula to promote normal grieving and family meetings can especially model this. The grief of the parents needs support alongside the grief of the children, empowering the parents to attend to their children's grief, rather than the children being parentified as a support for their parents. Parents may become hypervigilant about their surviving children's health, unwittingly promoting hypochondriasis in later life if too much attention is placed on somatic symptoms and fear of cancer. Attention to the functioning of the family provides the most useful model for recognition of those at greater risk of poorer outcome (Davies et al., 1986). Families that block discussion, suppress sharing of feelings, and concentrate rigidly on concrete events fare more poorly than families that comfort one another with empathy and teamwork.

The elderly and bereavement

When couples have been married for many years, the length and depth of their attachment may predispose them to profound grief, further complicated by the acute loneliness they can experience if many of their friends and sources of support have already died. Elderly bereaved men can have particular needs in these circumstances (Byrne and Raphael, 1994). Moreover, despite apparent support from within the family, the bereaved spouse may carry an especially painful level of loneliness (Large, 1989). The social support of the elderly bereaved warrants special consideration, including use of volunteer programmes (Lopata, 1986).

Bereavement during adulthood

Although the loss of a spouse has received most attention in research, loss of a parent or sibling during adult life is a common event and will generate distress proportional to the degree of emotional closeness to the deceased. Increased maturity is one potential outcome of such losses (Malinak et al., 1979). Where there is a high familial incidence of cancer raising questions of genetic risk, as in familial polyposis, breast, or colon cancer, the death of a sibling increases the sense of vulnerability of family members and highlights the importance of genetic testing and counselling when relevant.

When comparisons have been made between the death of a spouse, parent, or child, the most intense bereavement reactions are found following the death of a child, an event clearly out of step with life-cycle expectations (Saunders, 1979; Saunders et al., 1998). Parents have a strong and powerful investment in their children such that their premature death shakes the adult personality to its very roots (Rubin, 1993). Its impact is life-long—although the distress slowly declines with the passage of time, it plateaus eventually to a steady state of continued influence, although the meaning of this continues to change throughout the life cycle (Neimeyer et al., 2000). For many it is a disruptive and life-shattering experience, necessitating a continuing life-long accommodation, but this is affected to some degree by the quality of the relationship before the child's death and the relationship that exists with other surviving children (Dyregrov and Dyregrov, 2008).

Aware of such inherent challenges, palliative care teams do well to involve parents in the care of terminally ill children (including adult offspring), foster open communication of feelings about the death, and seek views on their philosophy of life. Where parents can find some meaning and sense of purpose in their child's life, their acceptance of the death, despite its inherent unfairness, is likely to be greater (Spinetta et al., 1981). The incorporation of parents into the model of family-centred care remains important when a middle-aged adult is dying and predeceasing elderly parents; often the focus of the palliative care team is on the nuclear family, supporting the spouse and children to the neglect of parental grief.

Hospices for dying children allow particular care to be taken of the family, including continuity of this care into bereavement. Active discussion of the choice between death at home or in the hospice is important and a family-centred model of care will consider the potential impact on usually three generations of family membership. Well-functioning families are perceived to cope better with death in the home, while respite admissions can bring relief to those families more stressed by the emotional demands of caring for the dying child. Irrespective of whether death is affecting a young child, an adolescent or young adult, grief is intense and potentially protracted; sustained support of family members is especially important when the functioning of the family has been stressed or is clearly dysfunctional.

Bereavement and AIDS

The stigma associated with human immunodeficiency virus (HIV) infection handicaps the adjustment of both patients and their families and adds a risk factor for complicated grief. Caregiving partners of men with AIDS experience several stressors that induce role conflict and burden (Folkman et al., 1994). Mean scores for depressive symptoms were found in one longitudinal study to remain at one standard deviation above the general community norm 3 years after the death (Moskowitz et al., 1988). The families also display complex dynamics related to their degree of acceptance of a homosexual relationship, any ambivalence about which potentially complicates the mourning process (Wolfe, 1993).

Spirituality and bereavement

The existential quest to understand the meaning of life creates an endeavour to understand the uniqueness and special contribution of each and every person. This spiritual orientation influences adaptation both to dying and to bereavement. Clinicians do well to inquire about the spiritual dimensions and philosophy of life of both their patients and families (Doka, 1993). For some, this will be expressed in the language of their religious beliefs; for others, cultural custom and traditions will inform their set of values and the philosophy by which they have lived. Using these values to understand the life of the deceased helps in appraising their accomplishments, the sort of person they were, and the meaning their life had. When consensus about this can be achieved with the bereaved, it assists their acceptance of the death. Moreover, when the latter has been peaceful, this will console the bereaved, but when the death was difficult, disappointing, or in some manner horrifying, there is considerable work to do in helping the bereaved to understand and come to terms with this final outcome. A spiritual understanding of the person's life may help in accepting the limitations of palliative care or coming to terms with any unfinished business that remained in the deceased's life. Philosophically this may be akin to letting go of the ideal and accepting a life lived with a goodness that is sufficient (Kissane et al., 2012b).

Ritual is an important component of religious and cultural tradition as it creates a proven pathway down which the bereaved tread (Faschingbauer, 1981). The wisdom of centuries is often woven into such rituals as a means of assisting the bereaved to mourn. Respect for such ritual is important and clinicians help the bereaved by endorsing its value. Familiarity with different ethnic traditions is worthwhile in palliative care. Nonetheless, should a clinician meet an unfamiliar ethnic group, they should seek from the relatives an understanding of their tradition and strive to cooperate with them in a culturally sensitive manner.

Positive outcome and personal growth

The adaptation that follows the wrenching loss of bereavement is associated with personal growth for a sizeable proportion. Although this personal growth manifests itself most clearly after the acute pain of grief, it is actually identifiable across all phases of the bereavement process (Hogan et al., 1996). Renewed sense of meaning, self-awareness, increased empathy, appreciation of family and relationships, independence, reprioritized goals and values, deepened spirituality, and increased altruism can all result from positive reappraisal, seeking for help and enhanced social resources.

Clinicians can helpfully reassure bereaved people about these beneficial outcomes, especially at times when the going is hard. Providing information about the longitudinal course of the mourning process including the prospect of such personal growth creates a feedback loop that nurtures adaptive recovery through cognitive appraisal and active coping.

Conclusion

Bereavement care is an integral dimension of palliative medicine as clinicians sustain continuity of care in assisting the family or carers of their deceased patient. Knowledge of and competence in assessing grief is essential to enable recognition of the 20% of the bereaved who get into difficulties and need additional assistance. Routine assessment of the bereaved for risk factors for complicated grief provides a responsible method through which treatment teams can intervene preventatively or early to reduce unnecessary morbidity. Effective therapies are available to assist in the management of complicated grief and palliative care practitioners should be skilled in their application or understand the circumstances when referral for further specialist help is appropriately made. Grief is an inevitable dimension of our humanity, an adaptive adjustment process, and one that with support can be approached with courage. Grief that is shared is grief that is healed.

Online materials

Additional online materials and complete references for this chapter are available online at <http://www.oxfordmedicine.com>.

References

Ainsworth, M., Blehar, M., Waters, E., and Wall, S. (1978). *Patterns of Attachment: A Psychological Study of the Strange Situation*. Hillsdale, NJ: Erlbaum.

Doka, K. (1989). Disenfranchised grief. In K. Doka (ed.) *Disenfranchised Grief: Recognizing Hidden Sorrow*, pp. 3–11. Lexington, MA: Lexington Books.

Doka, K. (1993). The spiritual crisis of bereavement. In K. Doka and J. Morgan (eds.) *Death and Spirituality*, pp. 185–193. New York: Baywood.

Faschingbauer, T. (1981). *Texas Revised Inventory of Grief Manual*. Houston, TX: Honeycomb.

Folkman, S. (2001). Revised coping theory and the process of bereavement. In M. Stroebe, R. Hansson, W. Stroebe, and H. Schut (eds.) *Handbook of Bereavement Research: Consequences, Coping, and Care*, pp. 563–584. Washington, DC: American Psychological Association.

Freud, S. (1912). *Totem and Taboo*. London: Hogarth Press.

Gersie, A. (1991). *Storymaking in Bereavement: Dragons Fight in the Meadow*. London: Jessica Kingsley Publishers.

Hogan, N., Morse, J., and Tason, M. (1996). Toward an experiential theory of bereavement. *Omega*, 33, 43–65.

Jacobs, S. (1993). *Pathological Grief*. Washington, DC: American Psychiatric Association Press.

Janoff-Bulman, R. (1992). *Shattered Assumptions. Towards a New Psychology of Trauma*. New York: Free Press.

Kissane, D. (2000). Family grief therapy: a new model of family-centered care during palliative care and bereavement. In L. Baider, G. Cooper, and A. Kaplan De Nour (eds.) *Cancer and the Family* (2nd ed.), pp. 175–197. Chichester: Wiley.

Kissane, D. and Bloch, S. (2002). *Family Focused Grief Therapy: A Model of Family-Centered Care during Palliative Care and Bereavement*. Buckingham: Open University Press.

Klass, D., Silverman, P., and Nickman, S. (eds.) (1996). *Continuing Bonds: New Understandings of Grief*. Washington, DC: Taylor & Francis.

Klerman, G., Weissman, M., and Rounsaville, B. (1984). *Interpersonal Psychotherapy of Depression*. New York: Basic Books.

Lund, D., Caserta, M., and Dimond, M. (1993). The course of spousal bereavement. In M. Stroebe, W. Stroebe, and R. Hansson (eds.) *Handbook of Bereavement: Theory, Research and Intervention*, pp. 240–254. Cambridge: Cambridge University Press.

Moos, R. and Moos, B. (1981). *Family Environment Scale Manual*. Palo Alto, CA: Consulting Psychologists' Press.

Moskowitz, J., Acree, M., and Folkman, S. (1998). *Depression and AIDS-related Bereavement: A 3-Year Follow-Up. New Perspectives on Depression in AIDS-Related Caregiving and Bereavement.* Presentation at the Annual Meeting of the American Psychological Association, San Francisco, CA.

Neimeyer, R. and Hogan, N. (2001). Quantitative or qualitative? Measurement issues in the study of grief. In M. Stroebe, R. Hansson, W. Stroebe, and H. Schut (eds.) *Handbook of Bereavement Research: Consequences, Coping, and Care*, pp. 89–118. Washington, DC: American Psychological Association.

Neimeyer, R., Keese, B., and Fortner, M. (2000). Loss and meaning reconstruction: propositions and procedures. In R. Malkinson, S. Rubin, and E. Witztum (eds.) *Traumatic and Non-traumatic Loss and Bereavement: Clinical Theory and Practice*, pp. 197–230. Madison, CT: Psychosocial Press/International Universities Press.

Parkes, C. (1998). *Bereavement: Studies of Grief in Adult Life* (3rd ed.) Madison, CT: International Universities Press.

Parkes, C., Laungani, P., and Young, B. (eds.) (1997). *Death and Bereavement Across Cultures.* London: Routledge.

Parkes, C. and Weiss, R. (1983). *Recovery from Bereavement.* New York: Basic Books.

Polloch, G. (1989). *The Mourning-Liberation Process.* New Haven, CT: International University Press.

Prigerson, H. and Jacobs, S. (2001). Traumatic grief as a distinct disorder: a rationale, consensus criteria, and a preliminary empirical test. In M. Stroebe, R. Hansson, W. Stroebe, and H. Schut (eds.) *Handbook of Bereavement Research: Consequences, Coping, and Care*, pp. 613–637. Washington, DC: American Psychological Association.

Rando, T. (1993). *Treatment of Complicated Mourning.* Champaign, IL: Research Press.

Raphael, B. (1983). *The Anatomy of Bereavement.* London: Hutchinson.

Rowland, J. (1989). Developmental stage and adaptation: child and adolescent model. In J. Holland and J. Rowland (eds.) *Handbook of Psycho-Oncology*, pp. 519–543. Oxford: Oxford University Press.

Rubin, S. (1993). The death of a child is forever: the life course impact of child loss. In M. Stroebe, W. Stroebe, and R. Hansson (eds.) *Handbook of Bereavement Research: Theory, Research, and Intervention*, pp. 285–299. Cambridge: Cambridge University Press.

Saunders, C. (1999). *Grief: The Mourning After: Dealing with Adult Bereavement* (2nd ed.). New York: Wiley.

Saunders, C., Mauger, P., and Strong, P. (1985). *A Manual for the Grief Experience Inventory.* Blowing Rock, NC: Center for the Study of Separation and Loss.

Shapiro, E. (2001). Grief in interpersonal perspective: theories and their implications. In M. Stroebe, R. Hansson, W. Stroebe, and H. Schut (eds.) *Handbook of Bereavement Research: Consequences, Coping, and Care*, pp. 301–327. Washington, DC: American Psychological Association.

Silverman, P. (1986). *Widow to Widow.* New York: Springer.

Stroebe, M. and Schut, H. (2001). Models of coping with bereavement: a review. In M. Stroebe, R. Hansson, W. Stroebe, and H. Schut (eds.) *Handbook of Bereavement Research: Consequences, Coping, and Care*, pp. 375–403. Washington, DC: American Psychological Association.

Stroebe, M. and Stroebe, W. (1993). The mortality of bereavement: a review. In M. Stroebe, W. Stroebe, and R. Hansson (eds.) *Handbook of Bereavement Research: Theory, Research, and Intervention*, pp. 175–195. Cambridge: Cambridge University Press.

Stroebe, M., Stroebe, W., and Hansson, R. (eds.) (1993). *Handbook of Bereavement Research: Theory, Research, and Intervention.* Cambridge: Cambridge University Press.

Walsh, F. and McGoldrick, M. (eds.) (1991). *Living Beyond Loss.* New York: Norton.

Webb, N. (ed.) (1993). *Helping Bereaved Children.* London: Guilford.

Wells, R. (1988). *Helping Children Cope with Grief.* London: Sheldon.

Wolfe, B. (1993). AIDS and bereavement. In K. Doka and J. Morgan (eds.) *Death and Spirituality*, pp. 257–278. New York: Baywood.

Worden, J. (1991). *Grief Counseling and Grief Therapy: A Handbook for the Mental Health Practitioner* (2nd ed.). New York: Springer.

SECTION 18

The terminal phase

Management of the actively dying patient

Judith Lacey

Introduction to management of the actively dying patient

Just as each phase of the illness journey has its unique challenges, so too does the care of the actively dying patient. The period leading to death is characterized by increasing prevalence and intensity of physical, psychological, existential, and social concerns, and it is often a challenging time for patients, their families, and health-care providers.

Addressing the whole-person needs of the patient at this time with excellent clinical skills, compassion, and understanding can greatly reduce the suffering experienced as well as support and maintain patients' dignity and autonomy (Cassem, 1991; Thompson and Chochinov, 2010). The goal of care during this phase is to minimize distress for patients and their families by meticulous symptom control and supportive care, while maintaining the well-being and moral integrity of all.

Ethical and relationship issues in the transition to end-of-life care

The premises that underlie end-of-life care are:

◆ the ethical imperative to provide adequate relief of suffering

◆ that dying patients should not be subjected to ineffectual treatments which cause further distress

◆ that all patients have a right to adequate relief of physical and psychological symptoms, and social support

◆ that all patients have the right to care that enables them to have the best possible life given the constraints of their prevailing circumstances (Cherny et al., 1996).

The idea of a 'good death' is a concept that medicine is trying to identify and quantify, although the construct is itself also controversial (see Chapter 2.4) (Miyashita et al., 2007; Hughes et al., 2008). Whilst ensuring that goals of care shift to allow for those priorities that contribute to a 'good death'—this transition must also be characterized by non-abandonment.

Specific skills and knowledge to ensure high-quality end-of-life care

Assessment and prognostication

Recognizing that a patient is imminently dying is the prerequisite for providing appropriate end-of-life care. Indeed one of the common problems in the care of the dying is failure to appreciate that the patient is indeed close to death. Prognostication and recognizing that death is near is, therefore, a cardinal clinical skill (Glare and Sinclair, 2008).

Establishing a short-term prognosis is part of the therapeutic alliance and yet is one of the most challenging aspects of care for many. Using and communicating this knowledge requires an individualized, patient-centred, and culturally appropriate approach (see Chapter 2.3).

Defining and recognizing the terminal phase

The terminal phase is defined *as a period of irreversible decline in functional status prior to death.* The terminal phase can last from a few hours to days and very occasionally to weeks. Worsening of certain symptoms is indicative of entering the terminal phase (Pitorak, 2003):

◆ weight loss

◆ profound weakness and fatigue

◆ social withdrawal

◆ disinterest in food and drink

◆ dysphagia and difficulty in swallowing medication

◆ refractory delirium

◆ changes in breathing

◆ drowsy for extended periods

◆ reduced urine output

◆ skin that is cool to touch

◆ a waxy look to the skin.

Recognizing this phase allows for the pre-emptive planning of care for the patient, preparation of family, patient, and staff, and may involve discussions around preferences for end-of-life care, place of death, and anticipated symptom control.

Whilst there are situations where it is possible to identify the terminal phase with some accuracy, many diseases have a natural history of progression and exacerbations that make the terminal phase difficult to identify (Lunney et al., 2003).

Communication with patients and families about end-of-life care

End-of-life care discussions make a difference. Well-conducted discussions about end-of-life care foster trust and non-abandonment for patients and carers and improve end-of-life outcomes for both the patient and the bereaved (Steinhauser et al., 2000; Detering et al., 2010). Discussing the approaching terminal phase and end of life with patients and families reduced the number of aggressive medical interventions near death, and, compared to those who had not had these conversations, reduced distress and improved quality of life of both patient and family/caregiver. Importantly, recent studies have demonstrated that end-of-life discussions were not associated with increased patient emotional distress or psychiatric disorders (Emanuel et al., 2004; Wright et al., 2008; Mack et al., 2010) and Mack and colleagues found a reduction in family/caregiver bereavement morbidity when the dying patient had the benefit of end-of-life discussions (Mack et al., 2010).

When the terminal phase is recognized, this needs to be communicated to the family and patient with empathy and equanimity. This is a task requiring sensitivity and skill, which can be improved with specific training. It is important for health-care professionals to be aware of their own feelings of grief, fear, anxiety, and guilt, and to acknowledge the impact this can have on the way they approach this conversation and ongoing communication (Curtis et al., 2004; Hancock et al., 2007).

Cultural awareness is extremely important and influences how and what information is communicated. Using interpreters can be vital (Crawley, 2005; Searight and Gafford, 2005; Volker, 2005). Frequently patients and families fear uncontrolled pain and other distressing symptoms, and should be confidently reassured about the management of these. When discussing future care planning and possible symptoms to anticipate, the family and the patient may have different information needs. Ideally the aim is to maintain a balance between supporting the patient's and family's sense of control and dignity, reducing their fear of suffering, and maintaining the hope for good quality of living, whilst preparing for death (Steinhauser et al., 2001).

Preparing the family and family well-being

Care of the family is integral to caring for a dying patient. Surveys of families of patients dying from advanced cancer have identified a series of critical needs (Table 18.1.1). These can be used as a checklist for assessing family needs, preparing for terminal care at home, and promoting family well-being. Families with dependent children have complex needs and make choices around end of life that have been found to differ from others (Nilsson et al., 2009).

Discussing advanced care planning and resuscitation

Among patients with chronic disease, life-threatening events and death occur in two distinct situations:

Anticipated dying

In patients with terminal illness, cardiopulmonary resuscitation (CPR) may prolong, but cannot reverse, the dying process; however, the patient, family, and indeed some health-care professionals may not fully comprehend the ineffectiveness of this intervention for the patient. It is important to discuss with patients, family, and team members the role of CPR and not for resuscitation/do not resuscitate orders as failure to discuss these may result in patients receiving unwanted interventions

Table 18.1.1 Families' support and information needs during the terminal phase

Patient comfort	Prompt and effective relief of patient symptoms is essential to support the family as a whole
Information and communication	Communication needs to be honest, direct, and compassionate, and must allow for the concerns and opinions of the family to be heard and appreciated. Family members need information about the likely course of the patient's illness. Potential symptoms and plans for their monitoring and management should be explained
Evaluation of family needs and resources	The degree with which the family is able and willing to participate in care is a major determinate in formulating a care plan. If the family are considering caring for a patient at home, family members need information regarding the daily care needs of the patient, likely clinical problems, available resources for routine care, and availability of emergency care
Care education	Irrespective as to whether the patient is at home or in hospital, family members require guidance regarding ways in which they can contribute to the comfort care of the patient
Emergency provisions	If the family are considering caring for a patient at home, the family need to know what to do and who to call in case of uncontrolled symptoms and when the patient dies Link to a 24-hour phone support service is important in this situation
Review of family coping	Family coping should be regularly assessed to enable early intervention to address unmet emotional or supportive needs of the family or previously unappreciated patient problems
Care of the family when the patient is unconscious	Continued vigilance and reassurance that comfort is being achieved are essential for the well-being of the family
Preparing the family for the dying process	When death is imminent, the family should be forewarned of the process that they are likely to witness

Adapted from Hematology/Oncology Clinics of North America, Volume 10, Issue 1, Cherny, N. I et al., Guidelines in the care of the dying cancer patient, pp. 261-86, Copyright © 1996, with permission from Elsevier, http://www.sciencedirect.com/science/journal/08898588.

(Hofmann et al., 1997; Loggers et al., 2009). This conversation is particularly difficult because it highlights the reality that the person's death is imminent. Such discussions are frequently avoided until the days just before death. However, these discussions have not been found to change patient or surrogate satisfaction with the clinician (Anderson et al., 2011). Despite being extremely unwell and aware of their disease process, dying patients differ in their capacity to acknowledge prognosis, with the majority only partially aware of the proximity of death (Chochinov et al., 2000; Mack, 2010).

The conversation should focus on the positives of what can and will be done for the person at the end of their life (Harlos, 2009)—with the emphasis on their dignity, comfort, and the prevention of distress. This should be done with sensitivity and empathy, allowing time to deal with the questions, concerns, and sometimes strong emotions associated with this issue (Lacey and Sanderson, 2010).

Advanced care planning for patients with unanticipated threatening events

The effect of the illness on the body and, sometimes, its treatment can cause sudden life-threatening medical crises for patients with advanced chronic illness. Some of these events may be reversible, some may have a very small chance of being reversed, and some may not be reversible at all.

Given their state of chronic ill health and ultimate incurability, patients vary in their approach as to how they would want to be treated in this situation. Opinions are often influenced by any one of many factors, such as religious or cultural beliefs, fear of suffering, fear of death, unfinished life plans, or the advanced stage of the disease:

- Some patients would want every possible treatment tried.
- Some would want to try some treatments but not others. For example, some patients give advanced directives that they would want to have artificial feeding, but would not want to be dependent on a machine to help them breathe.
- Some say that they would want aggressive treatments to be tried but, if they were not responding, they would want these stopped and replaced with comfort measures only.
- Some patients indicate that they would not want aggressive therapies, rather comfort measures only, allowing them either to recover with simple measures or to die in comfort.

The issues regarding advance care planning for patients with anticipated dying from vital organ failure as a consequence of their disease are different from the issues of those patients with unanticipated, acute life-threatening events. It is inappropriate to conflate these two issues in ascertaining patient preferences for end-of-life care.

It is important that this discussion and any subsequent decision is clearly documented in the patient's medical records and communicated to other health-care providers.

Identifying substitute decision-makers and advance care planning

As a person approaches death, their ability to make decisions may become impaired. Encouraging advance care planning, directives, or discussions with the patient prior to the terminal phase greatly reduces the burden on the substitute decision-maker and ensures the patient's choices are respected (Detering et al., 2010; Keating et al., 2010).

Symptoms management in the final days of life

Addressing psychosocial and existential concerns at the end of life

At the end of life, studies clearly suggest that existential and psychosocial issues greatly concern dying patients (Boudreau and Cassell, 2010). Through understanding and addressing factors that may potentially overwhelm the patient, family, and/or health-care providers, the necessary preconditions for coping can be established (Chochinov et al., 2008; Cherny, 2009; Cassell, 2010; Cassell and Rich, 2010). This is a vital and integral part of the care of the actively dying person and is discussed in detail in Section 17 of this textbook.

General principles for management of physical symptoms in end-of-life care

Problems of weakness, fatigue, and loss of appetite become more evident as death approaches. In the terminal phase, these problems usually start to assume relatively less significance for patients—although not necessarily for families. Comfort-related symptoms become increasingly important—particularly pain, dyspnoea, delirium, fear/anxiety, and respiratory secretions. Active assessment and pre-emptive management of these problems is crucial, especially as the patient becomes less able to communicate. Whilst the overall approach to managing these problems is presented elsewhere, the following discussion relates to the end-of-life setting, which creates some specific challenges.

Discontinuing non-essential medications

Only essential medications should be given and they should be administered by the least invasive route that can provide adequate relief. An appropriate rule is to identify and cease any drug which does not contribute to the patient's immediate comfort. Likewise observations and investigations that do not contribute to comfort should be ceased. Families will need reassurance that meticulous care continues with comfort being the goal of care (Abrahm, 2005). If persistent reservations about the withdrawal of a medication that is not causing the patient harm (such as an antibiotic) are expressed by the patient and/or family, the medication may be continued. It is often helpful to set a time limit on such treatment, whilst identifying specific improvements that would justify further treatment beyond that point.

Medications for pain and symptom control should be continued and the route converted from oral to transdermal and/or parenteral (the subcutaneous route is preferred wherever possible as it is less traumatic for the patient). Loss of the ability to swallow in the terminal phase should be anticipated and planned for by provision of as-needed (PRN) medications so that patients are not left without adequate symptom control, especially for a crisis (e.g. seizure, airway obstruction, bleeding, and so on). As a person's physical condition changes so too can their renal function and metabolism of medications. Careful monitoring and adjustment of medications is frequently required (see Table 18.1.2).

Table 18.1.2 Essential medications for management of symptoms in the actively dying patient

Symptom/indication	Medication	Application route	Dosage	Over 24 hours via syringe driver (SD)
Pain				
	Morphine or opioid equivalent	SC /IV injection or transdermal fentanyl	Convert oral medication to parenteral equivalent	Morphine compatible in SD with most medications
Neuropathic pain	Lignocaine/ketamine	SC/IV	Continue as previously or initiate if required for neuropathic pain	Yes
Breathlessness				
	Morphine or equivalent opioid	SC/IV injection	1–2.5 mg q4 h SC for breathlessness in the opioid naïve	24 h total dose in SD
With anxiety	Lorazepam	Tablet for SL	0.25–1 mg tds	
Refractory breathlessness	Midazolam	IV or SC	1–5mg q4 h	Estimate 24 h total dose and add to SD
Nausea				
Useful if prokinetic required	Metoclopramide	SC or IV	10–20mg tds–qid or via SD over 24 h	30–80 mg/24 h via SD
Primarily central	Haloperidol	SC or IV	0.5–1.5 mg bd–tds	1–15 mg over 24 h via SD. Usually up to 5 mg
Primarily central	Levomepromazine	SC	6.25–12.5 mg qid	25–100 mg/24 h
Primarily central	Cyclizine	SC	25–50mg	300 mg/24 h via SD. Compatibility issues
Gastrointestinal obstruction				
With colicky abdominal pain	Buscopan (hyoscine butylbromide)	IV or SC	20–40 mg qid	Up to 240 mg/day
With refractory vomiting	Octreotide	IV or SC	100–300 micrograms tds	Up to 1200 mg/24 h
Terminal restlessness/agitation/refractory hyperactive delirium				
Antipsychotic required	Haloperidol	SC or IV	1.5–5 mg tds SC	3–15 mg/day
	Levomepromazine	SC	25–50 mg qid	Up to 200 mg/day
	Olanzapine wafers	PO	2.5–10 mg bd	
	Chlorpromazine HCL	PR	50–100 mg bd	
Benzodiazepine required	Midazolam	SC/IV	2.5–5 mg q4 h	Up to 60 mg/day
	Clonazepam	SL/SC	0.5–1 mg bd	SC via SD. Compatibility issues
Other sedation required	See section on terminal sedation			
Respiratory secretions				
When unconscious	Hyoscine	SC	0.4 mg q2–q4 h	2.4 mg/24 h
When conscious	Glycopyrrolate	SC	0.2–0.4 mg q2–4 h	2.4 mg/24 h
Acute crisis episode				
Sedation required (also see other sedatives)	Midazolam	SC or IV	2.5–10 mg stat and q2 h PRN	Consider continuous dose
Acute pain syndrome	Morphine or parenteral opioid equivalent	SC or IV	10 mg in opioid naïve or 1/6 total opioid dose	Consider increasing baseline 24 h dose

(continued)

Table 18.1.2. (Continued)

Symptom/indication	Medication	Application route	Dosage	Over 24 hours via syringe driver (SD)
Seizure				
Acute and maintenance	Midazolam	SC, IV, buccal	2.5–10 mg stat or continuous	10–20 mg maintenance for seizure prevention
	Clonazepam	SL drops, or SC amps	0.5–1 mg stat, bd	1–2 mg continuous for seizure prevention
Anxiety/distress	Midazolam/clonazepam/lorazepam	IV/SC or SL	See 'Breathlessness' and 'Agitation'	Continuous if sedation required

bd, twice a day; h, hour; IV, intravenous; mg, micrograms; PO, orally; PR, rectally; q, every; qid, four times a day; SD, syringe driver (e.g. Grasby); SC, subcutaneous; SL, sublingual; tds, three times a day.

Pain

Pain management continues to be crucial. Based on a precautionary principle, it is important not to discontinue analgesics in the dying patient. Ensure availability of medications to be given by a non-oral route (preferably subcutaneous) and review the clinical need for any medications for which there is no parenteral form available, for example, some of the adjuvant analgesics. Whilst decreased levels of physical activity may mean that pain control is adequate despite ceasing oral adjuvants, if this is not the case, opioids may need to be increased to cover additional requirements. Alternative adjuvant medications, for example, anti-inflammatory or antineuropathic agents that can be delivered subcutaneously may be required (see Section 9 of this textbook for details of pain management).

Dyspnoea

Up to 70% of patients experience dyspnoea in the last 6 weeks of life, and its prevalence, severity, and associated distress increase as death approaches (Ben-Aharon et al., 2008; Kamal et al., 2012) (see also Chapter 8.2). It is usually multifactorial. Though it may be clinically appropriate to manage reversible causes of dyspnoea, in the final days of life dyspnoea can be more refractory to interventions, as the dominant causes become less amenable to modification (e.g. obstructing tumour; general weakness and frailty; restrictive conditions, including chest wall disease; lymphangitis carcinomatosis; pleural infiltrate or refractory effusions; diffuse extensive lung pathology or infection.) In this setting, pharmacological management with oral or parenteral opioids to reduce the distress of dyspnoea has been shown to be of benefit (Allard et al., 1999; Ben-Aharon et al., 2008) (see Box 18.1.1). Benzodiazepines may be useful for reducing panic and anxiety frequently associated with dyspnoea but have not been shown to improve dyspnoea itself. Oxygen therapy has been found to improve dyspnoea in the hypoxic patient (Booth and Wade, 2004; Gallagher and Roberts, 2004; Cranston et al., 2008; Uronis et al., 2008). Whilst non-pharmacological measures such as a fan and positioning are simple techniques that can improve the patient's comfort, in contrast, relaxation and breathing techniques take considerable concentration and are difficult to initiate late in the terminal phase (Zhao and Yates, 2008). For the patient with refractory dyspnoea and severe distress in the terminal phase, sedation is an option to consider for maintaining adequate symptom control and reducing suffering (see Chapter 8.2).

Delirium and agitation

In the terminal phase, delirium has been found to be present in up to 88% of patients when carefully screened for (Lawlor et al.,

2000a, 2000b) (see also Chapter 17.5). Delirium may be hypoactive or hyperactive (de Rooij et al., 2005). Although witnessing agitated delirium is upsetting for family, caregivers, and health-care professionals alike, the degree of patient distress associated with the thought-disordered states of hypoactive delirium should also not be underestimated (Leonard et al., 2008; Chochinov and Breitbart, 2009). Refractory delirium is a poor prognostic factor and often heralds the terminal phase (Maltoni et al., 2012).

In a patient with hours to days to live, the key issue is deciding whether to symptomatically manage delirium rather than burdening the patient and family with a search for causes or

---

Box 18.1.1 Pharmacological options for management of dyspnoea at the end of life

For the opioid naive patient

Starting dose of 2.5–5 mg morphine PO every 4 hours regularly or PRN may be sufficient. Alternative opioids at an equivalent dose can be tried if there is intolerance to morphine; however, most studies on dyspnoea have used morphine and evidence for other agents is lacking. Titrate upwards as tolerated.

For the patient already on opioids

Increase the usual morphine (or alternative opioid) dose by 25% (and up to 50%)—shown to be effective and tolerated, although evidence as to what dose increment is most effective is limited. Therefore starting lower and titrating up or adding a 25% of total dose PRN initially is acceptable, safe practice.

Addition of benzodiazepines

Used as second-line management of refractory dyspnoea associated with distress. Midazolam 2.5 mg four times a day is a reasonable starting dose. Lorazepam can also be used 0.5–1 mg three times a day sublingually.

Refractory dyspnoea

A combination of opioids and benzodiazepines/sedatives can be used to manage distress (see Chapter 18.2).

Reproduced from Judith Lacey and Christine Sanderson, The Oncologist's Role in Care of the Dying Cancer Patient, Cancer Journal (ISSN: 1528-9117), Volume 16, Issue 5, pp. 532-541, Copyright © 2010, with permission from Lippincott Williams & Wilkins, Inc. Source: data from Hematology/Oncology Clinics of North America, Volume 10, Issue 1, Cherny, N. I et al., Guidelines in the care of the dying cancer patient, pp. 261-86, Copyright © 1996.

trial of management for reversibility. The aim is to maintain the patient's dignity, reduce any agitation and associated risks to the patient and caregivers, and to ease distressing hallucinations, delusions, and restlessness (Caraceni and Simonetti, 2009). The symptoms of delirium at the end of life need to be palliated confidently, with compassion, reassurance, and clear explanation of the impact of pharmacological and non-pharmacological strategies to improve symptom control (Breitbart and Alici, 2008). Medications for treating agitation and delirium in the terminal phase include antipsychotics able to be given parenterally—such as haloperidol, levomepromazine, risperidone, or olanzapine (by sublingual wafers) and chlorpromazine (which can be given rectally). Benzodiazepines may be required for more rapid control of agitation and anxiety, but can potentially worsen delirium if used alone. The doses used should be the lowest dose that is effective for the symptoms of concern (see Chapter 17.5).

The condition identified as 'terminal restlessness' is a frequently described though little-studied state of agitation and reduced conscious level which appears to be closely associated with the onset of the terminal phase (Brajtman, 2005). Diagnostically it is most consistent with a refractory agitated delirium in an actively dying patient, possibly triggered by the onset of the terminal phase itself. However, before making this diagnosis it is worthwhile to consider, and exclude if clinically appropriate, other physical, medication-related, or medical causes of agitation. The latter includes status epilepticus, akathisia, serotonergic syndrome, myoclonus, hypoxia, physical pain or discomfort in an obtunded patient (e.g. from itch, urinary retention, or faecal impaction), medication toxicity, or paradoxical reaction (White et al., 2007). If no other cause is found and the clinical context is consistent with the onset of the terminal phase, palliation should be prompt and effective using sedating antipsychotics with or without benzodiazepines to reduce patient awareness and motor agitation.

Terminal secretions (death rattle)

During the last hours to days of life, terminal secretions (the 'death rattle') may become evident. They have been found to occur in around 44% of dying patients (Morita and Hyodo, 2004). The mechanism remains uncertain, but it may be due to pooling of saliva and secretions in the upper airways along with reduced swallowing reflexes, dysphagia, and inability to expectorate. This has been called type I death rattle or 'true' death rattle (Bennett et al., 2002; Wildiers and Menten, 2002) in contrast to type II rattle, which is due to pooling of bronchial secretions. Type II or 'pseudo' death rattle can appear over days and may not respond as well to antimuscarinic/anticholinergic medications. Included in type II are other causes of retained secretions, such as bronchorrhoea from primary lung tumour, infection, dysphagia, bleeding, airway obstruction, pulmonary oedema, or tracheo-oesophageal fistula (Bennett et al., 2002; Mercadante et al., 2011). No significant association has been found between hydration status and the development of death rattle (Ellershaw et al., 1995; Morita and Hyodo, 2004). The true death rattle is a strong predictor of approaching death—in one study 76% of patients died within 48 hours of its onset (Wildiers and Menten, 2002).

Antimuscarinic agents can be used to reduce the salivary secretions. Although most studies of the efficacy of antimuscarinic agents on reducing salivary secretions are mostly based on single-dose studies, a randomized trial of three anticholinergic agents in 333 patients (Wildiers et al., 2009) showed beneficial responses in up to 76% of patients by salivary secretion reduction. This was less marked in secretions thought to be of bronchial origin or 'pseudo death rattle'. The evidence supporting this practice is not robust but therapeutic trial is reasonable, paying attention to the adverse effects profiles (Wee and Hillier, 2008; Mercadante et al., 2011,). It is important to reassure families that terminal secretions are rarely distressing for the patient, although they may be distressing for the family.

Addressing functional decline and increased need for assistance

With progression of illness and reduced overall function there is an associated reduced ability to carry out independent activities of daily living. Transferring may require assistance and the environment of care may often require modification to improve access, safety, and comfort. If available, the input of an occupational therapist and physiotherapist is very useful preferably prior to the onset of the terminal phase.

Mobility, skin, and mouth care

Meticulous nursing and active monitoring for symptom distress is essential in the care of dying patients. Common problems include immobility, pressure area care, care of bladder and bowel, secretions, xerostomia, and odours. For the imminently dying patient, measuring and recording patient data not directly related to comfort (such as pulse and blood pressure) is superfluous and can be discontinued unless there are religious, cultural, or other concerns (Cherny et al., 1996).

Bowel and bladder function

Incontinence of urine, reduced mobility impacting on toileting options, and urinary retention are all potential problems. These can impact on a person's sense of dignity and should be dealt with sensitively. Catheterization or, if no retention, incontinence pads, are often required. Ultrasound bladder scanning is a valuable investigation to minimize inappropriate catheterization. Judicious rectal intervention may be appropriate to maintain regular bowel motions if the patient is uncomfortable. Faecal impaction and urinary retention can cause severe distress and should always be excluded as a cause of agitation in the obtunded patient.

Refractory symptoms and suffering: approach to care

Uncontrolled suffering in a dying patient is considered a medical emergency (Cherny, 2009), but suffering cannot be treated unless it is recognized and diagnosed (Cassell, 1999) (see also Chapter 18.2). Occasionally in the terminal phase, symptoms and suffering are refractory to all standard palliative interventions. Suffering is considered refractory if, despite use of aggressive and concerted efforts to determine and treat the cause, suffering persists. Refractory suffering can relate to intractable symptoms including complex pain, severe dyspnoea, nausea and vomiting, neuropsychiatric symptoms including agitated delirium, fitting, and very occasionally severe anxiety or depression, or other irreversible crises. All available and appropriate diagnostic, therapeutic, and consultative processes need to be exhausted (including

---

Box 18.1.2 Criteria for determination of refractoriness of a severe symptom

Diagnosis

Aggressive efforts to diagnose the severe symptom are either successful or are exhaustive but unsuccessful within a reasonable time frame

Treatment

Aggressive efforts to relieve the severe symptom using all available resources are unsuccessful within a reasonable time frame

Consultation

All available colleagues who might assist in diagnosing or treating the symptom or in providing psychosocial support to the patient or family within a reasonable time frame have been consulted

Transfer

Transfer to another location where more potentially helpful resources are available is either not feasible or has been refused by the patient

Persistent suffering

The patient continues to report intolerable suffering despite all above interventions, or a patient lacking the ability to communicate verbally appears to the surrogate decision-maker, the responsible physician, and at least one other clinician to be in severe distress despite all above interventions

Reproduced from Judith Lacey and Christine Sanderson, The Oncologist's Role in Care of the Dying Cancer Patient, Cancer Journal (ISSN: 1528–9117), Volume 16, Issue 5, pp. 532–541, Copyright © 2010, with permission from Lippincott Williams & Wilkins, Inc. Originally adapted from Eric L. Krakauer and Quinn E. Thomas, Sedation in palliative medicine, Table 19.2.1, pp.1560–1588, in Cherny et al. (Eds.), Oxford Textbook of Palliative Medicine, Fourth Edition, Oxford University Press, Oxford, UK, Copyright © 2010, by permission of Oxford University Press.

---

consultation with pain, palliative care, psychiatry, and other relevant experts if available) before classifying suffering as refractory (Krakauer and Quinn, 2009) (Box 18.1.2).

The role of sedation in the care of dying patients

Palliative sedation is an option in the terminal phase if refractory suffering is present. The importance of using the minimum level of sedation required to adequately manage refractory symptoms and suffering is stressed. Existential distress and suffering can be viewed as intrinsically linked to the impact of terminal illness on the whole (Cassell and Rich, 2010) (see Chapter 18.2 for further discussion on sedation).

Symptom crisis at the end of life and contingency planning

Identification of patients at high risk for uncontrolled pain, dyspnoea, nausea and vomiting, agitated delirium, acute airway obstruction, or massive haemorrhage is crucial. It allows contingency planning for a crisis, and occasionally prophylactic

management. This usually enables a family to often care for their dying relative at home or in the desired setting with minimal angst and distress.

The specific drugs, doses, and routes of administration ordered as part of a crisis plan should be appropriate to the clinical situation. If severe symptoms requiring rapid relief are anticipated, maintenance of parenteral access is recommended. This might include a subcutaneous butterfly. In the home care situation, whenever possible, family members/carers must be instructed in preparation and administering medications for an emergency (see Table 18.1.2).

Discussing specific issues in end-of-life care—nutrition and hydration

In the last days to weeks of life, anorexia, weight loss, and swallowing difficulties are common. In patients with disease-related dysphagia or bowel obstruction, the ability to maintain adequate nutritional intake is reduced. Weakness, cognitive deterioration, or other factors increase aspiration risk and further compromise a person's ability to eat.

Reduced oral intake is often distressing for the family. Requests for artificial nutrition via enteral or parenteral routes are common. As the patient's conscious level deteriorates, aspiration risk is greater and the risk versus benefit of oral intake with regard to aspiration needs to be explored with the family. Often compromises are reached at this stage. However, concerns about cessation or non-initiation of enteral or parenteral feeding often poignantly relate to the expectations and hopes that patient and family still hold (McClement et al., 2003, 2004).

The discussion needs to be centred on the ineffectiveness and burden of artificial nutrition versus any likely benefit. If there are religious or culturally based reservations about discontinuing nutritional support, it may be maintained, unless there is evidence of patient harm from the intervention (Cherny et al., 1996).

In the actively dying patient who is comatose or poorly responsive, the decision to provide artificial hydration is based on clinical judgement, and assessment of the burden of the intervention. Where families are concerned about the need for fluids, provision of gentle hydration is reasonable. Excessive hydration, particularly in the hypoalbuminaemic patient, may exacerbate oedema and discomfort, and if a trial of therapy is offered, the family should be warned that worsening oedema or other signs of fluid overload would be a reason to cease the treatment (Hanks et al., 2009). Reassurance can be given, particularly in the last days, that maintaining good mouth hygiene alleviates much of the sensation of thirst and discomfort. The majority of trials conducted at the very end of life show no significant burden nor benefit from hydration. If it is decided to administer fluids in the last days or weeks of life, the subcutaneous route is a well-tolerated and minimally invasive option. 1–1.5 L over 24 hours of normal saline can be delivered in this manner (Dalal et al., 2009).

At the bedside of the dying patient

The clinician at the bedside of the dying patient should ensure adequate relief of patient distress, and provide support and guidance to the grieving family. This often includes responding to family members who ask what to expect, and how to recognize the dying process. The physician and nurse's role is to evaluate and treat the patient for pain, dyspnoea, agitation, or any other distressing symptoms. Once adequate comfort is achieved, the clinician can reassure the family that the patient is not distressed.

Families vary in the degree of professional support necessary at this time. Increased involvement is valuable when family supports are limited or coping is frail. In other situations, it may be enough for the clinician to acknowledge the primacy of family and friends in this moment, taking a background role, but available if necessary.

At and after death

If it is clear that breaths are agonal and the patient is about to die, explain this to the family with the reassurance, again, that the patient appears comfortable. Adequate provision for family privacy and time with the patient is crucial. Awareness and respect for cultural and/or religious practices related to death is important. If the death occurs in an institution, provision for necessary cultural practices should be made and the family should be reassured of this. At the time of death, families often talk and cry over the dead person, and kiss and hug them. An offer of condolences from clinicians may be very comforting for a distressed family.

Most palliative care services provide bereavement support, and can refer those affected by the patient's illness and death to an associated bereavement service after the patient has died. Adults need to recognize when a dependent, grieving child needs help. When a parent of dependent children is dying, offering their children age-appropriate grief and bereavement counselling and education may be very reassuring for the dying parent (Auman, 2007; Sandler et al., 2010).

Difficult end-of-life scenarios

It is important to prepare for some of the more difficult and unusual end-of-life care scenarios. These include unanticipated sudden events, such as trauma, postoperative overwhelming sepsis, or failure of treatment for acute potentially reversible disease as well as other treatment-related deaths. Young parents and other young people (adolescents), children, the isolated, incarcerated, or mentally ill, those in care isolation wards, and those in an intensive care unit are other unique groups whose end-of-life care may require a unique and thoughtful, planned approach. The unanticipated sudden event requires action to be taken with care to alleviate suffering and provide appropriate support to the family and carers. For those with advanced care plans, communication and respect for the plans is key to provision of care. 'Crisis medications' should be available on the hospital wards and in the home for adequate symptom control for those at risk of an acute event. Preparing a patient, family, and team may not always be possible and the grief and bereavement support become a very important part of care.

Young people and young children and their families may request more active management even at the end of life. Here, care for the family and early psychosocial support is vital with many wishing to return home (or remain at home) for end-of-life care in the final days. The isolated or incarcerated person may have little access to adequate multidisciplinary care and modifying limited resources and mobilizing adequate support may prove the greatest

challenge. Provision of the minimal essential drugs is imperative and may require thoughtful proactive intervention.

Professional aspects of end-of-life care

Communication between colleagues

It is the role of the treating team to ensure that all of their colleagues are 'on the same page', and that at this advanced stage of illness the patient and their family are receiving the same message regarding stage of disease, prognosis, and goals of care. The nursing and allied health professionals involved in the care of the patient should also have a clear understanding of goals of care and approach to the patient entering the terminal stage.

Despite sounding straightforward, much conflict and angst between staff members stems from lack of such communication. Furthermore, for staff faced with a dying patient on their ward, particularly nursing staff who do not often care for dying patients, the entire process may be distressing and confronting. It can be worthwhile to acknowledge the impact the patient's dying and the family's distress could be having on the team. For many treating team members, there are long associations with their patients and close relationships formed. Grieving needs to be recognized and space provided for this to occur.

Support for junior staff and distressed staff members

As a member of a team caring for patients at the end of life, the anticipated and non-anticipated death can have a significant impact on staff and team members. Junior staff are often more vulnerable. It is important to recognize this and for appropriate support to be offered in the form of structured professional supervision, a time and space for debriefing, discussions, and willingness of senior team members to be available to respond to the distressed staff member. Many resources are available that may assist and these should be chosen based on suitability to staff and service needs.

Conclusion

Care of patients in the final stages of a life-limiting illness requires a high level of clinical vigilance and skill in order to ensure that the passage from life to death is as free from suffering as possible. Patients who are dying have a right to adequate relief of physical and psychological symptoms, and they and their families have a right to adequate support. The care of patients and their families requires (a) interdisciplinary cooperation of a health-care team incorporating physicians, nurses, social workers, and other allied health staff, and (b) a high level of clinical flexibility to address the evolving needs of the patient and family. Contingency planning and communicating expected symptoms and signs to family and carers, coupled with provision of adequate access to medications and non-pharmacological resources, can allow a person to die peacefully at home or in the desired setting with minimal distress. Participation in this process challenges the clinician's emotional resources and medical skills. There is, however, much professional satisfaction in helping to ensure a 'good death' since relief of suffering is at the very heart of medicine. Familiarity with guidelines in the care of the dying can reduce the potential for distress in this important clinical endeavour.

Acknowledgements

Chapter adapted from Judith Lacey and Christine Sanderson, The Oncologist's Role in Care of the Dying Cancer Patient, Cancer Journal (ISSN: 1528–9117), Volume 16, Issue 5, pp. 532–541, Copyright © 2010, with permission from Lippincott Williams & Wilkins, Inc.

Thank you to Dr Joanne Doran and Dr Jan Maree Davis for review and comments.

Online materials

Complete references for this chapter are available online at <http://www.oxfordmedicine.com>.

References

Anderson, W.G., Pantilat, S.Z., Meltzer, D., *et al.* (2011). Code status discussions at hospital admission are not associated with patient and surrogate satisfaction with hospital care: results from the multicenter hospitalist study. *American Journal of Hospice and Palliative Care*, 28, 102–108.

Ben-Aharon, I., Gafter-Gvili, A., Paul, M., Leibovici, L., and Stemmer, S. M. (2008). Interventions for alleviating cancer-related dyspnea: a systematic review. *Journal of Clinical Oncology*, 26, 2396–2404.

Booth, S., Wade, R., Johnson, M., *et al.* (2004). The use of oxygen in the palliative of breathlessness. A report of the Expert Working Group of the Scientific Committee of the Association of Palliative Medicine. *Respiratory Medicine*, 98, 66–77.

Boudreau, J.D. and Cassell, E.J. (2010). Abraham Flexner's 'mooted question' and the story of integration. *Academic Medicine*, 85, 378–383.

Brajtman, S. (2005). Terminal restlessness: perspectives of an interdisciplinary palliative care team. *International Journal of Palliative Nursing*, 11, 170, 172–178.

Caraceni, A. and Simonetti, F. (2009). Palliating delirium in patients with cancer. *The Lancet Oncology*, 10, 164–172.

Cassell, E.J. (1999). Diagnosing suffering: a perspective. *Annals of Internal Medicine*, 131, 531–534.

Cassem, N. (1991). *The dying patient*. In T.P. Hackett and N.H. Cassem (eds.) *Massachusetts General Hospital Handbook of General Hospital Psychiatry*, pp. 332–352. St. Louis, MO: Mosby Year Book.

Cherny, N.I., Coyle, N., and Foley, K.M. (1996). Guidelines in the care of the dying cancer patient. *Hematology/Oncology Clinics of North America*, 10, 261–286.

Chochinov, H.M., Hassard, T., McClement, S., *et al.* (2008). The patient dignity inventory: a novel way of measuring dignity-related distress in palliative care. *Journal of Pain and Symptom Management*, 36, 559–571.

Chochinov, H.M., Tataryn, D.J., Wilson, K.G., Ennis, M., and Lander, S. (2000). Prognostic awareness and the terminally ill. *Psychosomatics*, 41, 500–504.

Dalal, S., Del Fabbro, E., and Bruera, E. (2009). Is there a role for hydration at the end of life? *Current Opinion in Supportive and Palliative Care*, 3, 72–78.

Detering, K.M., Hancock, A.D., Reade, M.C., and Silvester, W. (2010). The impact of advance care planning on end of life care in elderly patients: randomised controlled trial. *BMJ*, 340, c1345.

Ellershaw, J., Sutcliffe, J., and Sauders, C. (1995). Dehydration and the dying patient. *Journal of Pain and Symptom Management*, 10, 192–195.

Glare, P. and Sinclair, C. (2008). Palliative medicine review: prognostication. *Journal of Palliative Medicine*, 11, 84–103.

Hancock, K., Clayton, J.M., Parker, S.M., *et al.* (2007). Truth-telling in discussing prognosis in advanced life-limiting illnesses: a systematic review. *Palliative Medicine*, 21, 507–517.

Harlos, M. (2009). The terminal phase. In G. Hanks, N.I. Cherny, N.A. Christakis, M. Fallon, S. Kaasa, and R.K. Portenoy (eds.) *Oxford Textbook of Palliative Medicine* (4th ed.), pp. 1549–1459. Oxford: Oxford University Press.

Kamal, A.H., Maguire, J.M., Wheeler, J.L., Currow, D.C., and Abernethy, A.P. (2012). Dyspnea review for the palliative care professional: treatment goals and therapeutic options. *Journal of Palliative Medicine*, 15, 106–114.

Keating, N.L., Landrum, M.B., Rogers, S.O. Jr., *et al.* (2010). Physician factors associated with discussions about end-of-life care. *Cancer*, 116, 998–1006.

Lacey, J. and Sanderson, C. (2010). The oncologist's role in care of the dying cancer patient. *Cancer Journal*, 16, 532–541.

Lawlor, P., Fainsinger, R., and Bruera, E. (2000a). Delirium at the end of life: critical issues in clinical practice and research. *Journal of the American Medical Association*, 284, 2427–2429.

Loggers, E.T., Maciejewski, P.K., Paulk, E., *et al.* (2009). Racial differences in predictors of intensive end-of-life care in patients with advanced cancer. *Journal of Clinical Oncology*, 27, 5559–5564.

Mack, J.W., Weeks, J.C., Wright, A.A., Block, S.D., and Prigerson, H.G. (2010). End-of-life discussions, goal attainment, and distress at the end of life: predictors and outcomes of receipt of care consistent with preferences. *Journal of Clinical Oncology*, 28, 1203–1208.

Maltoni, M., Scarpi, E., Pittureri, C., *et al.* (2012). Prospective comparison of prognostic scores in palliative care cancer populations. *Oncologist*, 17, 446–454.

Mcclement, S.E., Degner, L.F., and Harlos, M. (2004). Family responses to declining intake and weight loss in a terminally ill relative. Part 1: fighting back. *Journal of Palliative Care*, 20, 93–100.

Mcclement, S.E., Degner, L.F., and Harlos, M.S. (2003). Family beliefs regarding the nutritional care of a terminally ill relative: a qualitative study. *Journal of Palliative Medicine*, 6, 737–748.

Mercadante, S., Villari, P., and Ferrera, P. (2011). Refractory death rattle: deep aspiration facilitates the effects of antisecretory agents. *Journal of Pain and Symptom Management*, 41, 637–639.

Miyashita, M., Sanjo, M., Morita, T., Hirai, K., and Uchitomi, Y. (2007). Good death in cancer care: a nationwide quantitative study. *Annals of Oncology*, 18, 1090–1097.

Morita, T. and Hyodo, I.Y.T., Ikenaga, M., *et al.* (2004). Incidence and underlying etiologies of bronchial secretion in terminally ill cancer patients: a multicenter, prospective, observational study. *Journal of Pain and Symptom Management*, 27, 533–539.

Nilsson, M.E., Maciejewski, P.K., Zhang, B., *et al.* (2009). Mental health, treatment preferences, advance care planning, location, and quality of death in advanced cancer patients with dependent children. *Cancer*, 115, 399–409.

Sandler, I.N., Ma, Y., Tein, J.Y., *et al.* (2010). Long-term effects of the family bereavement program on multiple indicators of grief in parentally bereaved children and adolescents. *Journal of Consulting and Clinical Psychology*, 78, 131–143.

Searight, H.R. and Gafford, J. (2005). Cultural diversity at the end of life: issues and guidelines for family physicians. *American Family Physician*, 71, 515–522.

Steinhauser, K., Christakis, N., Clipp, E., McNeilly, M., McIntyre, L., and Tulsky, J. (2000). Factors considered important at the end of life by patients, family, physicians, and other care providers. *Journal of the American Medical Association*, 284, 2476–2482.

Thompson, G.N. and Chochinov, H.M. (2010). Reducing the potential for suffering in older adults with advanced cancer. *Palliative and Supportive Care*, 8, 83–93.

Wee, B. and Hillier, R. (2008). Interventions for noisy breathing in patients near to death. *Cochrane Database of Systematic Reviews*, 1, CD 005177.

Wildiers, H., Dhaenekint, C., Demeulenaere, P., *et al.* (2009). Atropine, hyoscine butylbromide, or scopolamine are equally effective for the treatment of death rattle in terminal care. *Journal of Pain and Symptom Management*, 38, 124–133.

Wright, A.A., Zhang, B., Ray, A., *et al.* (2008). Associations between end-of-life discussions, patient mental health, medical care near death, and caregiver bereavement adjustment. *Journal of the American Medical Association*, 300, 1665–1673.

18.2

Sedation at the end of life

Eric L. Krakauer

Introduction to sedation at the end of life

The need for palliative sedation at the end of life

The most fundamental task of palliative medicine, and indeed of medicine in general, is to relieve suffering (Cassell, 1982). Among terminally ill patients whose primary goal is comfort, severe suffering occurs occasionally that is refractory to standard palliative interventions. Controlled sedation, sometimes to unconsciousness, may be the only effective means of relieving suffering in these unusual situations.

Patients and their families fearful of severe, refractory terminal suffering may feel quite relieved when informed that palliative sedation is available as an option should all standard interventions fail. Thus, clinicians who are fully prepared to provide sedation for refractory terminal suffering often will be able to comfort fearful patients simply by discussing it with them (Cherny, 2006).

While there is consensus in the literature about the need for and permissibility of sedation for refractory suffering of a terminally ill patient, there remains debate about nomenclature, about the definition of palliative sedation, and about the ethics of specific practices (Quill et al., 2009). This chapter will provide guidance for palliative sedation based upon a synthesis of current debates.

Definitions

Palliative sedation may be defined as controlled induction of sedation, sometimes to the point of unconsciousness, to relieve severe refractory suffering of a terminally ill patient.

Severe, refractory suffering may be a result of severe, refractory physical symptoms such as pain, dyspnoea, or vomiting or severe, refractory neuropsychiatric problems such as seizure, agitated delirium, anxiety, or depression. While severe social problems such as discrimination or rejection, and 'existential' distress due to loss of dignity or of a sense of meaning in life, also may cause severe suffering in a terminally ill patient, they may respond to intensive interventions including 'dignity therapy', psychological counselling, spiritual guidance, and social interventions such as emotional, legal, and financial support (Chochinov, 2007; Schuman-Olivier et al., 2008; Cassell and Rich, 2010). Thus, palliative sedation should be considered as a response to social or 'existential' problems only in the most extraordinary circumstances.

Suffering is refractory when it cannot be adequately relieved despite aggressive and concerted efforts both to determine its causes and to treat them using standard palliative interventions without inducing sedation. Adequate relief is reduction of the patient's suffering to a tolerable level. Because pain, many other physical and neuropsychiatric symptoms, social suffering, and 'existential' distress are subjective and not amenable to easy measurement, both 'tolerability' and 'adequate relief' can be defined only by each individual patient. Aggressive and concerted efforts are those that make use of the best available diagnostic techniques, palliative medications, and other interventions and have enlisted the help of the best available experts (see Box 18.1.2 in Chapter 18.1).

Nomenclature

Various names have been used for sedation for refractory suffering of dying patients (Claessens et al., 2008). It is important to distinguish between ordinary palliative sedation and palliative sedation to unconsciousness. Ordinary sedation is sedation that occurs commonly in the standard practice of palliative care for a variety of reasons. Palliative sedation to unconsciousness designates deep sedation for severe suffering that is refractory to all reasonable and aggressive interventions including ordinary sedation (American Academy of Hospice and Palliative Medicine, 2006). The key point is that the level of sedation should be proportional to an individual patient's suffering in that it should be just deep enough to provide the desired relief. By definition, death is never intended by palliative sedation. Thus, the term 'terminal sedation', that inevitably connotes sedation intended to terminate or euthanasia, should not be used in palliative care (Krakauer, 2000).

Experience with palliative sedation

The frequency and success of palliative sedation is impossible to determine accurately because of lack of consensus and clarity in the literature about the definition of palliative sedation and about indications, goals, and appropriate medication regimens. Reports of the frequency of palliative sedation in palliative care programmes range from 1% to 88% (Sykes and Thorns, 2003). Practice patterns vary widely in part due to differing cultural beliefs and values (Fainsinger et al., 2000a; Moyano et al., 2008). In some studies, it is unclear whether patients received light or deep sedation or were sedated to varying degrees. The frequency of palliative sedation also may be changing in settings where palliative care is becoming more available, where physicians of more specialties are providing palliative sedation, and where guidelines for palliative sedation have been established (Fainsinger et al., 2000a; Rietjens et al., 2008a; Seale, 2010; van Deijck et al., 2010).

There is some consistency in the literature about some aspects of palliative sedation. Multiple studies list some or all of the same refractory symptoms as the most common indications for palliative sedation: pain, dyspnoea, agitated delirium, or vomiting (Fainsinger et al., 2000b; Rousseau, 2001; Van Deijck et al., 2010). Studies of physicians from multiple countries and cultures reveal a widespread opinion that palliative sedation for refractory suffering is sometimes needed and is ethically acceptable (Chater et al., 1998; Morita et al., 2002; de Graeff and Dean, 2007; Claessens et al., 2008). In addition, there is some concurring evidence that palliative sedation may not hasten death (Sykes and Thorns, 2003; Rietjens et al., 2008b; Mercadante et al. 2009; Maltoni et al., 2012).

Ethical issues

Moral imperative

There is broad agreement that physicians have a moral imperative to respond to the suffering of terminally ill patients, particularly when the suffering is extreme (Wanzer et al., 1989; Hasselaar et al., 2009; Russell et al., 2010). While severe refractory suffering is uncommon, it demands that physicians be prepared to provide palliative sedation as 'the end of the continuum of symptom management' (Quill and Byock, 2000).

Informed consent

The physician should determine the goal or goals of care for any patient with a terminal illness in consultation with the patient or surrogate. When a terminally ill patient is experiencing severe, refractory suffering, palliative sedation should be considered only if the overriding goal of care is comfort and the patient or surrogate has decided to forego life-sustaining treatment (Cherny and Portenoy, 1994).

Even when these conditions obtain and palliative sedation is being considered, it may not be initiated without informed consent (Quill et al., 1997b). The patient or surrogate should be informed of and capable of understanding both the clinical predicament that makes palliative sedation a legitimate treatment option and any alternative options. Religious or ethical concerns of the patient should be explored and religious counselling from a chaplain should be offered if appropriate. Because a decision about palliative sedation may have a lasting emotional impact on the patient's family and loved ones, efforts should be made to achieve consensus (Cherny, 2006). However, the clear request of a competent patient or a legal surrogate decision-maker should be honoured even over objections of other family members or friends.

In the rarest of cases, there may be a terminally ill patient with severe, refractory suffering who lacks both decision-making capacity and any surrogate decision-maker. If palliative sedation is being considered in such a case, consensus should be sought from at least one other senior physician—a palliative care specialist if possible—and from the hospital ethics committee.

Principle of double effect

The principle of double effect provides guidance for decisions when all possible actions risk bad consequences. Its applicability to decisions about treatments to relieve suffering in dying patients is widely accepted. The principle states that an action with two or more possible effects, including at least one possible good and one possible bad effect, is morally permissible if four provisos are met (Quill et al., 1997a; Sulmasy and Pellegrino, 1999):

- The action must not be immoral in itself.
- The action must be undertaken with the *intention* of achieving only the good effect or effects. Possible bad effects may be *foreseen* but must not be *intended*.
- The action must not achieve the good effect by means of a bad effect.
- The action must be undertaken for a proportionally grave reason (the rule of proportionality).

When palliative sedation is considered in cases of severe refractory suffering of terminally ill patients, sedation as a means to relieve suffering would be the intended good effect. Possible side effects of the sedative such as respiratory depression, hypotension, and hastening death may be foreseeable but not intended. The act of giving medication to relieve suffering is not immoral as long as the patient or surrogate requests relief and accepts the risk of side effects, and there are no safer means to achieve an acceptable degree of relief. Such serious side effects must be risked only for a proportionally grave reason such as the relief of severe refractory suffering of a terminally ill patient who does not wish to suffer (Krakauer et al., 2000).

Some have criticized the principle of double effect or questioned its applicability to palliative sedation in part because the principle relies on the distinction between the intended and the merely foreseen (Quill et al., 1997a). It is argued that clinical intentions may be ambiguous and difficult to discern. Because of the complexity and potential ambiguity of clinical intentions, physicians working to relieve the suffering of frail terminally ill patients should think through their intentions carefully, document them in the medical record, and demonstrate them with their actions (Hallenbeck, 2000). The least toxic medications should be used at the minimum doses that achieve the desired effect. The patient's response to the medication and level of comfort should be assessed and documented frequently and changes in the dose or type of medication should be made and documented based on these assessments. In this way, clinical intentions are made as clear as possible, the benefits of the intervention maximized, and the risk of bad effects minimized (Cherny et al., 2009).

Distinction from voluntary active euthanasia and physician-assisted suicide

Application of the principle of double effect to palliative sedation also has been criticized because of the assumption associated with the principle that intentionally hastening death is always wrong. It is argued that some patients wish for death and that intentionally helping a patient to shorten an intolerable existence may not be wrong (Quill et al., 1997a). However, it is widely accepted that palliative sedation can and should be clearly distinguished in theory and in practice from both voluntary active euthanasia and physician-assisted suicide (see Chapter 5.7) (Cowan and Palmer, 2002; De Graeff and Dean, 2007; Russell et al., 2010).

In palliative sedation, the physician's intention or goal is only to relieve severe refractory suffering using sedation as a last resort. The goal is not to end the patient's life as in euthanasia and physician-assisted suicide (Cherny, 2006). In practice, palliative sedation entails titration of medications to achieve the goal of comfort. The physician administers just enough medication to induce adequate sedation and thereby assure comfort. Once comfort is achieved, the lowest doses that maintain comfort are used. Euthanasia and physician-assisted suicide entail no titration, no calculation or maintenance of minimum doses needed for comfort, because the goal is death (Hallenbeck, 2000).

Withholding and withdrawal of artificial nutrition and hydration

The decision whether or not to use any medical intervention, including artificial nutrition and hydration, should be based on the patient's values and medical condition and on agreed-upon goals of care. Frequently, patients who have a terminal illness and are unable to eat decline artificial nutrition and hydration. To provide these interventions against patients' wishes would not only infringe on their right to autonomy. Because these interventions also may cause harm by prolonging the dying process or by exacerbating pulmonary oedema, pleural effusions, respiratory secretions, ascites, or anasarca with resultant dyspnoea or pain, providing them also risks violating the principle of non-maleficence.

The situation is morally no different when a patient is receiving palliative sedation for severe refractory suffering. For patients still able to eat prior to sedation, it is the patient's terminal illness that makes the sedation necessary and thereby precludes further eating. When the overriding goal is comfort and the patient or surrogate does not request artificial nutrition or hydration, there should be no presumption that an unwanted and potentially noxious intervention should be provided. When artificial nutrition and hydration are withheld or withdrawn in this situation, the patient dies of the terminal illness, not at the hand of the physician by euthanasia, nor by physician-assisted suicide (De Graeff and Dean, 2007; Cherny et al., 2009; Kirk and Mahon, 2010). When palliative sedation is being considered, the physician should suggest to the patient or surrogate that artificial nutrition and hydration be withheld or withdrawn if palliative sedation is implemented.

There may be patients or surrogates who believe that artificial hydration and/or nutrition should not be withheld or withdrawn during palliative sedation based on religious beliefs, cultural norms, or personal history. There should be no absolute prohibition of artificial nutrition and hydration in patients receiving palliative sedation as long as the harms of these medical interventions do not grossly outweigh the potential benefits by the patient's values (Cherny, 2006). The patient's personal beliefs should be explored as carefully as possible and every effort made to assure that palliative sedation or any proposed treatment is compatible with cherished beliefs and values.

Misuse of palliative sedation

Studies from several countries have revealed that physicians occasionally intend to hasten death even where euthanasia and physician-assisted suicide are illegal (Meier et al., 1998; Rietjens et al., 2004; Seale, 2010). These data raise the concern that palliative sedation may be used to intentionally hasten death and that physicians may try to hide their intention by invoking the principle of double effect. Therefore, it is extremely important for physicians who provide palliative sedation to demonstrate their intentions as clearly as possible by documenting carefully in the medical record the regimen used and the patient's response.

Informing other clinicians

It is often helpful to involve key members of the patient's care team such as the primary nurse and social worker in the process of decision-making about palliative sedation. Before initiating palliative sedation, the physician always should inform all members of the patient's care team of the plan, the indication for palliative sedation, and the receipt of informed consent (Cherny, 2006). No clinician should be required to participate in non-emergent palliative sedation—or in withdrawal of life-sustaining treatment—if they conscientiously object (Quill and Byock, 2000).

Legal issues

Laws in most rich Western countries recognize the right of a competent patient to refuse any medical treatment including life-sustaining treatment. In the same countries, interventions to relieve the severe, refractory suffering of terminally ill patients generally are permitted even if they might unintentionally hasten death (Van der Heide et al., 2004). In criminal law in the United States, for example, actions that might put another's life at risk are justifiable if the potential benefits of the action are likely and important enough. This precept reflects the rule of proportionality that is part of the principle of double effect (Quill et al., 1997a).

Practical guidelines for palliative sedation

Indications and prerequisites

Palliative sedation should be considered only under the following circumstances:

1. The patient must have a *severe, chronic, life-threatening illness* such as, but not limited to:

   a. advanced incurable cancer

   b. end-stage major organ failure, and organ transplantation and organ replacement therapy either are not feasible or have been declined by the patient

   c. advanced AIDS, and antiretroviral therapy either is no longer effective, causes intolerable side effects, or has been declined by the patient

   d. advanced neuromuscular disease

   e. advanced dementia, unable to take adequate oral nutrition.

2. The patient must be suffering from one or more *severe physical or neuro-psychiatric symptoms* such as, but not limited to pain, dyspnoea, vomiting, seizures, agitated delirium, anxiety, or depression.

3. The distressing symptom or symptoms must be *refractory to standard palliative interventions* such as, but not limited to:

   a. medications such as opioids, neuroleptics, anticonvulsants, anxiolytics, and antidepressants

   b. neuromodulatory procedures for pain such as nerve block and intrathecal analgesia

   c. palliative radiation therapy

   d. palliative endoscopic or surgical procedures

   e. consultation by the best available medical specialists from disciplines relevant to the patient's disease or symptoms such as palliative care, pain medicine, or psychiatry and by those who can provide psychosocial support such as social workers and chaplains.

4. *Comfort must be the overriding goal* of the patient's care as determined by the responsible physician in dialogue with the patient or, if the patient does not have capacity to make medical decisions, with the legal surrogate decision-maker.

   a. If there is doubt about a patient's capacity to understand her diagnosis and prognosis, to explain her values, or to make a specific decision, psychiatric consultation is recommended (Cherny et al., 2009).

   b. If a patient does not have capacity and there is no legal surrogate decision-maker, the goals of care should be determined by the responsible physician in discussion with a non-legal surrogate who is the most knowledgeable person available about the patient's values regarding healthcare and suffering.

   c. If no surrogate decision-maker is available, consensus on the goals of care should be sought from at least one other senior physician—a palliative care specialist if possible—and from the hospital ethics committee if one exists.

   d. In any case, both the goal of comfort and the discussion in which this goal was decided upon must be documented in the medical record.

5. Where possible, *an active order must exist to withhold life-sustaining treatments* including at least the following:

   a. chest compressions

   b. defibrillation

   c. endotracheal intubation

   d. mechanical ventilation

   e. non-invasive ventilatory support.

6. *Informed consent* for palliative sedation that may unintentionally hasten death must be obtained in advance from the patient or from an appropriate surrogate decision-maker identified following the procedure outlined in item 4 (a–d) above. The informed consent or decision-making process must be documented in the medical record.

7. If possible, all *staff members involved in caring for the patient should be informed* in advance of the plan to initiate palliative sedation. In particular, the patient's nurse, respiratory therapist, and pharmacist should be informed.

   a. Once palliative sedation has been initiated, clinical staff who will be assigned to the case should be informed in advance of the plan of care.

   b. In non-emergent situations, staff members who conscientiously object to the care plan should be given the opportunity to excuse themselves from participation in the patient's care once a replacement is found. Every effort should be made in keeping with any institutional policies on conscientious objection to find a replacement for any essential staff member.

Special circumstances

Severe, refractory social or 'existential' suffering

Very rarely, a patient's severe social or 'existential' problems such as social isolation, loss of dignity, or loss of a sense of meaning in life may cause severe suffering that is refractory to intensive and sustained intervention by the best available clinicians and supporters. In these very rare cases, respite sedation to unconsciousness may be considered (see following section). Only after respite sedation has been tried at least once in addition to all other intensive palliative interventions without an acceptable reduction in the patient's suffering should permanent palliative sedation be considered (Cherny, 1998; Rousseau, 2001).

Respite sedation

Time-limited sedation to unconsciousness or respite sedation may be used for terminally ill patients with severe refractory suffering in a variety of situations:

◆ *Incident pain*: some patients may experience particularly severe pain or other symptoms due to therapeutic or diagnostic procedures or to necessary movement for other clinical care (Del Rosario et al., 2001).

◆ *Severe refractory social or 'existential' suffering*: one or more trials of respite sedation may 'break a cycle of anxiety and distress' that has evoked a request for palliative sedation (Cherny, 1998; Rousseau, 2001).

◆ *Patient requests trial of temporary sedation to unconsciousness*: some patients with severe refractory physical or neuropsychiatric symptoms who are not imminently dying may benefit from a temporary respite from their discomfort. The respite may relieve severe fatigue that could influence the patient's perception that the symptoms or the attempts to alleviate them are intolerable (Cherny 2006). The patient may then decline further palliative sedation.

The mandatory informed consent discussion for respite sedation to unconsciousness should include the possibility that the patient may not reawaken and that death may be unintentionally hastened. Respite sedation may be provided for as little as a few minutes or as long as a few days. In general, artificial hydration should be provided if respite sedation is expected to last longer than a few hours. A decision on monitoring of heart rate and rhythm, blood pressure, and oxygen saturation should be based on the patient's values, the agreed-upon goals of care, and the clinical situation.

Terminal discontinuation of mechanical ventilation

In terminally ill patients receiving mechanical ventilation for respiratory failure, terminal extubation of the trachea or discontinuation of mechanical ventilation without extubation is likely to cause dyspnoea unless the patient is well pre-medicated, unconscious, or in a persistent vegetative state (see also Chapter 15.7). Some patients may wish to receive only enough medication to reduce to a tolerable level the feeling of air hunger in the hope that they can remain awake during the process. However, it is reasonable to consider palliative sedation to unconsciousness when a patient or the surrogate of a patient not in a persistent vegetative state decides to terminally discontinue mechanical ventilation (Billings, 2012; Truog et al., 2012).

Palliative sedation for terminal discontinuation of mechanical ventilation is medically and ethically slightly different from palliative sedation for severe refractory symptoms:

◆ Sedation may be intended not to relieve existing severe refractory symptoms but rather to assure that the patient does not experience severe dyspnoea in the time between removal of the ventilator and death. The other prerequisites for palliative sedation apply in this situation as well: terminal illness, a decision that the overriding goal of care is comfort, an order to withhold or withdraw life-sustaining treatment, informed consent, an informed and prepared staff.

♦ If the patient already is receiving sedation to treat or prevent discomfort from mechanical ventilation, this sedation should continue and adjustments should be made to assure comfort during and after the removal of the ventilator.

♦ Because most agents used for palliative sedation have no analgesic effect and some do not specifically relieve dyspnoea, opioid therapy usually should be continued or added to the sedative regimen. In the absence of pain or other indications for opioid therapy, the opioid dose should be titrated to a normal respiratory rate and the absence of laboured breathing while the sedative is titrated to the appropriate depth.

♦ Sedation and opioid therapy should be initiated before the ventilator is removed. The adequacy of the treatment should be checked with a trial of reduced ventilatory support. This can be done by setting the fraction of inspired oxygen at room air and changing the ventilation mode to pressure support at a setting adequate only to overcome the resistant of the endotracheal tube (approximately 5 cmH_2O for a tube 7.5 mm in internal diameter). Patients should be observed for 10–15 minutes on this ventilator setting (to allow their arterial partial pressure of oxygen to decrease and the partial pressure of carbon dioxide to increase).

  • If the patient develops tachypnoea, agitation, grimacing, or other evidence of discomfort, the previous level of ventilatory support should be reinstituted, the doses of sedative and/or opioid should be increased and the assessment repeated.

  • If the patient is apnoeic and is not thought to have pain, the opioid dose and/or sedative dose should be reduced and the trial repeated once the effects of the higher opioid and/or sedative doses have worn off. However, the sedative should not be reduced to the point of allowing the patient to awaken if the goal is unconsciousness.

  • If the minimum opioid and/or sedative doses necessary to control the patient's pain and/or maintain comfort also cause both unconsciousness and apnoea, and there are no other reversible causes of apnoea, the removal of the ventilator may proceed.

♦ Any neuromuscular blocking agents should be stopped and the effects allowed to wear off before initiating palliative sedation so that the patient's respirations are not unnecessarily depressed and the effects of the sedation can be assessed.

  • If the effects of a neuromuscular blocking agent persist longer than 24 hours after the last dose and there is a compelling reason to withdraw the ventilator quickly, the withdrawal may proceed but care must be taken to assure that the patient is sedated to unconsciousness since the patient will be paralysed and unable to show any signs of discomfort (Truog et al., 2000).

Medications

Ideal medications for palliative sedation have a rapid onset of action and a short duration of action that facilitate titration to the desired effect. They should reliably induce sedation and, if necessary, unconsciousness, and cause minimal side effects. Agents mentioned in the literature include opioids, benzodiazepines, neuroleptics, barbiturates, and other general anaesthetic induction agents (Krakauer et al., 2000). In general, medications for palliative sedation should be given via continuous and/or intermittent intravenous or subcutaneous infusion. Intramuscular injections generally should be avoided as the injections themselves may be painful. Administration of sedatives transdermally, rectally, or via tube gastrostomy or jejunostomy generally is not suitable for palliative sedation to unconsciousness because of the delayed onset of action and the greater difficulty in titrating the dose to the desired effect.

Opioids

Strong opioids such as morphine, hydromorphone, or fentanyl are the best available agents to relieve dyspnoea and many types of pain, but they are not reliable sleep-inducing agents by themselves. While opioids often cause drowsiness and may occasionally induce unconsciousness, especially in patients obtunded by other medications or by their medical conditions, increasing the opioid dose beyond that needed for relief of pain or dyspnoea puts the patient at increased risk of counter-productive and uncomfortable side effects such as myoclonus, hyperalgesia, and agitated delirium. Thus, opioids should not be used alone for palliative sedation. When pain or dyspnoea are present or expected, opioid therapy should be continued or added in combination with a sedative.

Benzodiazepines

Several benzodiazepines are cited in the literature on palliative sedation, lorazepam and midazolam most frequently. Midazolam has the most rapid onset of action and is the easiest to titrate and is widely used. However, benzodiazepines sometimes fail to provide adequate sedation (Krakauer et al., 2000; Cheng et al., 2002). They also may cause paradoxical agitation and psychotic reactions particularly in elderly patients and those with impaired liver function (Breitbart et al., 1996; Shafer, 1998). Therefore, benzodiazepines should be used with caution for palliative sedation and are not ideal agents for palliative sedation to unconsciousness.

Neuroleptics

Antipsychotic drugs available in parenteral forms such as haloperidol, chlorpromazine and levomepromazine (formerly called methotrimeprazine) are cited in the literature on palliative sedation. Levomepromazine also has analgesic properties while haloperidol and chlorpromazine are good treatments for agitated delirium. However, none of these drugs alone reliably induce unconsciousness.

Barbiturates

Barbiturates including pentobarbital, thiopental, and phenobarbital reliably induce unconsciousness. All are available in parenteral form. Pentobarbital and especially thiopental have rapid onset and short duration of action for ease of titration. Pentobarbital also has beneficial antiemetic and anticonvulsant properties. Either thiopental or pentobarbital are excellent agents for palliative sedation to any degree including unconsciousness (Truog et al., 1992). Pentobarbital may be easier to obtain outside of an intensive care unit.

Anaesthetic induction agents

Anaesthetic induction agents that have been used for palliative sedation include propofol and ketamine. While ketamine has both sedative and analgesic properties and is less likely to cause

Table 18.2.1 Protocol for palliative sedation to unconsciousness using continuous intravenous infusion of midazolam, pentobarbital or propofol

Physician responsibilities

1. Confirm that:
   a. the patient's overriding goal of care is comfort
   b. the patient has an advanced terminal illness
   c. the patient is suffering from severe refractory physical or neuropsychiatric symptoms or psychosocial problems
   d. there is an order to withhold life-sustaining treatment
   e. informed consent for palliative sedation to unconsciousness has been obtained
2. Document all of the above in the medical record
3. Inform the patient's clinical team of the plan
4. Specify in the orders:
   a. the loading dose, if any
   b. the initial infusion rate
   c. the amount of drug in mg/hour and time interval for infusion rate increases
   d. the dose and time interval for any bolus doses
5. Ensure that the medication is titrated optimally by frequent assessment of the patient and/or by reading the documentation by nurses of all dose adjustments and of comfort levels before and after dose adjustments
6. Document in the medical record the efficacy of this therapy at least daily

Nurse responsibilities

1. Administer the medication as a continuous infusion by an infusion pump that is clearly labelled with the name of the medication
2. Once the desired level of sedation is achieved, reduce the infusion to the lowest rate that maintains the desired level
3. Should the patient exhibit any evidence of pain or other distress, increase the infusion rate as ordered
4. Once an initial steady dose rate is found that maintains the desired level of sedation, document the reason (intention) for any dose adjustment and the level of comfort before and after the adjustment
5. Do not reduce the infusion rate for low blood pressure, low respiratory rate, or other abnormal vital signs if the patient exhibits any evidence of pain or other distressing symptoms
6. When the medication is running out, call for additional medication well in advance so that there is no interruption in the infusion

Midazoam administration	Pentobarbital administration	Propofol administration
1. Inspect midazolam solution prior to administration. If precipitation is present, do not use	1. Inspect pentobarbital solution prior to administration. If precipitation is present, do not use	1. Use strict aseptic technique when administering propofol. Change infusion tubing every 12 hours. Discard vial and any unused drug if not fully infused after 12 hours
2. Loading dose for benzodiazepine-naïve patient: 0.03–0.05 mg/kg slow intravenous push (over 2–5 minutes)	2. Loading dose: 2–3 mg/kg slow intravenous push (no faster than 50 mg/minute)	2. Infuse only through central venous catheter.
3. Loading dose may be repeated every 5 minutes to achieve desired effect	3. A physician should give loading dose and remain at bedside for 15 minutes to observe the effect	3. Start infusion at 2.5–5 micrograms/kg/min (for adults approximately 10–20 mg/hour) and titrate to desired level of sedation every 10 minutes by increments of 10–20 mg/hour
4. A physician should give each loading dose and remain at bedside for 10 minutes to observe the effect	4. At time of loading dose, start infusion at 1–2 mg/kg. Titrate to desired level of sedation	4. Use bolus doses of 10–20 mg every 10 minutes only for rapid control of extreme symptoms
5. At time of loading dose, start infusion at 0.02–0.1 mg/kg/hour depending on patient's prior exposure to and tolerance for benzodiazepines. Titrate to desired level of sedation	5. Because tolerance may develop rapidly, assess the patient's comfort level frequently and adjust infusion rate as needed	5. During initiation of therapy, a physician should be present and remain at the bedside for 5 minutes to observe the effects. Any initial bolus doses should be given by a physician
6. Additional bolus doses equal to the hourly infusion dose may be given as often as every 15 minutes. A physician or nurse should remain at the bedside for 10 minutes to observe the effects of each bolus dose		6. During subsequent dose titration and bolus dosing, a physician or nurse should remain at the bedside for 5 minutes to observe the effects
		7. The infusion should not be interrupted longer than 60 seconds when changing vials or tubing

hypotension and respiratory depression than propofol or barbiturates, it commonly causes unpleasant dissociative or dysphoric reactions. It is not recommended as a single agent for palliative sedation. Propofol has an onset of action, duration of action, and half-life shorter than midazolam and any of the barbiturates. This greatly facilitates titration to the desired effect. Liver disease and renal disease do not appear to significantly affect its pharmacokinetics (Mirenda and Broyles, 1995). It also has anxiolytic, antiemetic, antipruritic, anticonvulsant, antimyoclonic, and muscle relaxant effects. Propofol therefore appears to be an excellent agent for palliative sedation to any degree including unconsciousness (Krakauer et al., 2000; Lundström et al., 2005).

Combinations of sedatives

Many patients who require palliative sedation already will be receiving standard palliative medications such as an opioid and/or a benzodiazepine and/or a neuroleptic. Opioid therapy for pain should be continued despite the risk of hypotension and respiratory depression when a barbiturate or propofol is added because these latter agents have no analgesic effect. A benzodiazepine generally may be tapered once adequate sedation is achieved with another agent. However, if the sedative does not have strong anticonvulsant properties, the taper should proceed slowly to minimize the risk of seizure. Neuroleptic therapy may be reduced or discontinued provided adequate sedation can be maintained easily without it. Ketamine should be used only in combination with a benzodiazepine.

Recommended protocols

Recommended protocols for palliative sedation with midazolam, pentobarbital, and propofol are provided in Table 18.2.1.

Conclusions

Palliative sedation is a well-accepted therapy that should be considered in the rare situations when a terminally ill patient whose overriding goal is comfort experiences severe suffering that is refractory to all available standard palliative interventions. Its availability alone may be very comforting to patients fearful of terminal suffering. Informed consent must be obtained and strict medical and ethical guidelines for providing, monitoring, and documenting palliative sedation should be followed.

References

American Academy of Hospice and Palliative Care (2006). *Statement on Palliative Sedation*. [Online] Available at: <http://www.aahpm.org/positions/sedation.html>.

Billings, J.A. (2012). Humane terminal extubation reconsidered: the role for preemptive analgesia and sedation. *Critical Care Medicine*, 40, 625–630.

Breitbart, W., Marotta, R., Platt, M.M., *et al.* (1996). A double-blind trial of haloperidol, chlorpromazine, and lorazepam in the treatment of delirium in hospitalized AIDS patients. *The American Journal of Psychiatry*, 153, 231–237.

Cassell, E.J. (1982). The nature of suffering and the goals of medicine. *The New England Journal of Medicine*, 306, 639–645.

Cassell, E.J. and Rich, B.A. (2010). Intractable end-of-life suffering and the ethics of palliative sedation. *Pain Medicine*, 11, 435–438.

Chater, S., Viola, R., Paterson, J., and Jarvis, V. (1998). Sedation for intractable distress in the dying—a survey of experts. *Palliative Medicine*, 12, 255–269.

Cheng, C., Roemer-Becuwe, C., and Pereira, J. (2002). When midazolam fails. *Journal of Pain and Symptom Management*, 23, 256–265.

Cherny, N.I. (1998). Sedation in response to refractory existential distress: walking the fine line. *Journal of Pain and Symptom Management*, 16, 404–406.

Cherny, N.I. (2006). Sedation for the care of patients with advanced cancer. *Nature Clinical Practice Oncology*, 3, 492–500.

Cherny, N.I. and Portenoy, R.K. (1994). Sedation in the management of refractory symptoms: guidelines for evaluation and treatment. *Journal of Palliative Care*, 10, 31–38.

Cherny, N.I. and Radbruch, L., and the Board of the European Association of Palliative Care (2009). European Association of Palliative Care recommended framework for the use of sedation in palliative care. *Palliative Medicine*, 23, 581–593.

Chochinov, H.M. (2007). Dignity and the essence of medicine: the A, B, C, and D of dignity conserving care. *BMJ (Clinical Research Ed.)*, 335, 184–187.

Claessens, P., Menten, J., Schotsmans, P., and Broeckaert, B. (2008). Palliative sedation: a review of the research literature. *Journal of Pain and Symptom Management*, 36, 310–333.

Cowan, J.D. and Palmer, T.W. (2002). Practical guide to palliative sedation. *Current Oncology Reports*, 4, 242–249.

De Graeff, A. and Dean, M. (2007). Palliative sedation therapy in the last weeks of life: a literature review and recommendations for standards. *Journal of Palliative Medicine*, 10, 67–85.

Del Rosario, M.A., Martín, A.S., Ortega, J.J., and Feria, M. (2001). Temporary sedation with midazolem for control of severe incident pain. *Journal of Pain and Symptom Management*, 21, 439–442.

Fainsinger, R.L., de Moissac, D., Mancini, I., and Oneschuk, D. (2000a). Sedation for delirium and other symptoms in terminally ill patients in Edmonton. *Journal of Palliative Care*, 16, 5–10.

Fainsinger, R.L., Waller, A., Bercovici, M., *et al.* (2000b). A multicentre international study of sedation for uncontrolled symptoms in terminally ill patients. *Palliative Medicine*, 14, 257–265.

Hallenbeck, J.L. (2000). Terminal sedation: ethical implications in different situations. *Journal of Palliative Medicine*, 3, 313–320.

Hasselaar, J., Verhagen, S., Reuzel, R., van Leeuwen, E., and Vissers, K. (2009). Palliative sedation is not controversial. *The Lancet Oncology*, 10, 747–748.

Kirk, T.W. and Mahon, M.M. (2010). Palliative Sedation Task Force of the National Hospice and Palliative Care Organization Ethics Committee. National Hospice and Palliative Care Organization position statement and commentary on the use of palliative sedation in imminently dying terminally ill patients. *Journal of Pain and Symptom Management*, 39, 914–923.

Krakauer, E.L (2000). Responding to intractable terminal suffering. *Annals of Internal Medicine*, 133, 560.

Krakauer, E.L, Penson, R.T., Truog, R.D., King, L.A., Chabner, B.A., and Lynch, T.J. (2000). Sedation for intractable distress of a dying patient: acute palliative care and the principle of double effect. *The Oncologist*, 5, 53–62.

Lundström, S., Zachrisson, U., and Fürst, C.J. (2005). When nothing helps: propofol as sedative and antiemetic in palliative cancer care. *Journal of Pain and Symptom Management*, 30, 570–577.

Maltoni, M., Scarpi, E., Rosati, M., *et al.* (2012). Palliative sedation in end-of-life care and survival: a systematic review. *Journal of Clinical Oncology*, 30, 1378–1383.

Meier, D.E., Emmons, C.A., Wallenstein, S., Quill, T., Morrison. R.S., and Cassel, C.K. (1998). A national survey of physician-assisted suicide and euthanasia in the United States. *The New England Journal of Medicine*, 338, 1193–1201.

Mercadante, S., Intravaia, G., Villari, P., Ferrera, P., David, F. and Casuccio, A. (2009). Controlled sedation for refractory symptoms in dying patients. *Journal of Pain and Symptom Management*, 37, 771–779.

Mirenda, J. and Broyles, G. (1995). Propofol as used for sedation in the ICU. *Chest*, 108, 539–548.

Morita,T., Akechi, T., Sugawara, Y., Chihara, S., and Uchitomi, Y. (2002). Practices and attitudes of Japanese oncologists and palliative care physicians concerning terminal sedation: a nationwide survey. *Journal of Clinical Oncology*, 20, 758–764.

Moyano, J., Zambrano, S., Ceballos, C., Santacruz, C.M., and Guerrero, C. (2008). Palliative sedation in Latin America: survey on practices and attitudes. *Supportive Care in Cancer*, 16, 431–435.

Quill, T.E. and Byock, I.R. (2000). Responding to intractable terminal suffering: the role of terminal sedation and voluntary refusal of food and fluids. *Annals of Internal Medicine*, 132, 408–414.

Quill, T.E., Dresser, R., and Brock, D.W. (1997a). The rule of double effect—a critique of its role in end-of-life decision making. *The New England Journal of Medicine*, 337, 1768–1771.

Quill, T.E., Lo, B., and Brock, D.W. (1997b). Palliative options of last resort: a comparison of voluntary stopping of eating and drinking, terminal sedation, physician-assisted suicide, and voluntary active euthanasia. *Journal of the American Medical Association*, 278, 2099–2104.

Quill, T.E., Lo, B., Brock, D.W., and Meisel, A. (2009). Last-resort options for palliative sedation. *Annals of Internal Medicine*, 151, 421–424.

Rietjens, J., van Delden, J., Onwuteaka-Philipsen, B., Buiting, H., van der Maas P., and van der Heide, A. (2008a). Continuous deep sedation for patients nearing death in the Netherlands: descriptive study. *BMJ (Clinical Research Ed.)*, 336, 810–813.

Rietjens, J.A.C., van der Heide, A., Vrakking, A.M., Onwuteaka-Philipsen, B.D., van der Maas, P.J., and van der Wal, G. (2004). Physician reports of terminal sedation without hydration or nutrition for patients nearing death in the Netherlands. *Annals of Internal Medicine*, 141, 178–185.

Rietjens, J.A.C., van Zuylen, L., van Veluw, H., van der Wijk, L., van der Heide, A., and van der Rijt, C.C. (2008b). Palliative sedation in a specialized unit for acute palliative care in a cancer hospital: comparing patients dying with and without palliative sedation. *Journal of Pain and Symptom Management*, 36, 228–234.

Rousseau, P. (2001). Existential suffering and palliative sedation: a brief commentary with a proposal for clinical guidelines. *The American Journal of Hospice & Palliative Care*, 18, 151–153.

Russell, J.A., Williams, M.A., and Drogan, O. (2010). Sedation for the imminently dying: survey results from the AAN Ethics Section. *Neurology*, 74, 1303–1309.

Schuman-Olivier, Z., Brendel, D.H., Forstein, M., and Price, B.H. (2008). The use of palliative sedation for existential distress: a psychiatric perspective. *Harvard Review of Psychiatry*, 16, 339–351.

Seale, C. (2010). Continuous deep sedation in medical practice: a descriptive study. *Journal of Pain and Symptom Management*, 39, 44–53.

Shafer, A. (1998). Complications of sedation with midazolam in the intensive care unit and a comparison with other sedative regimens. *Critical Care Medicine*, 26, 947–956.

Sulmasy, D.P. and Pellegrino, E.D. (1999). The rule of double effect: clearing up the double talk. *Archives of Internal Medicine*, 159, 545–550.

Sykes, N. and Thorns, A. (2003). The use of opioids and sedatives at the end of life. *The Lancet Oncology*, 4, 312–318.

Truog, R.D., Berde, C.B., Mitchell, C., and Grier, H.E. (1992). Barbiturates in the care of the terminally ill. *The New England Journal of Medicine*, 327, 1678–1682.

Truog, R.D., Burns, J.P., Mitchell, C., Johnson, J., and Robinson, W. (2000). Pharmacologic paralysis and withdrawal of mechanical ventilation at the end of life. *The New England Journal of Medicine*, 342, 508–511.

Truog, R.D, Brock, D.W., and White, D.B. (2012). Should patients receive general anesthesia prior to extubation at the end of life? *Critical Care Medicine*, 40, 631–633.

Van Deijck, R.H.P.D., Krijnsen, P.J.C., Hasselaar, J.G.J., Verhagen, S.C.A.H.H.V.M, Vissers, K.C.P., and Koopmans, R.T.C.M. (2010). The practice of continuous palliative sedation in elderly patients: a nationwide explorative study among Dutch nursing home physicians. *Journal of the American Geriatrics Society*, 58, 1671–1678.

Van der Heide, A., van Delden, J.J.M., and van der Wal, G. (2004). Doctor assisted dying: what difference does legalization make? *The Lancet*, 364(Suppl. 1), s24–25.

Wanzer, S.H., Federman, D.D., Adelstein, J., *et al.* (1989). The physician's responsibility toward hopelessly ill patients: a second look. *The New England Journal of Medicine*, 320, 844–849.

SECTION 19

Research in palliative medicine

Research in palliative care

Stein Kaasa and Karen Forbes

Ignorance has risks, but they are largely unseen and unnoticed. Gaining knowledge has risks which are noticed, but largely unpredictable, and it is very costly (though less so than prolonged ignorance). It focuses blame, whereas ignorance dispels it. So, maintaining ignorance often seems more attractive than gaining knowledge. (Vere, 1981)

Vere, D., Controlled clinical trials: the current ethical debate, *Journal of the Royal Society of Medicine*, Volume 74, Number 2, pp. 85–8, Copyright © 1981 by The Royal Society of Medicine. Reprinted by Permission of SAGE.

Introduction to research in palliative care

Duncan Vere was Professor of Clinical Pharmacology and Therapeutics at the London Hospital and one of the key advisors to Cicely Saunders when she founded St Christopher's Hospice in 1967. Vere is an expert in clinical trials and analgesic clinical pharmacology and was one of the first people to undertake and supervise research in a hospice setting. The quotation is taken from a paper he presented at the Royal Society of Medicine in London in 1981 in a debate about the ethical aspects of randomized controlled trials (RCTs). He was not talking specifically about research in palliative care but making a general point that it was easy to be deterred from undertaking rigorous scientific research in a clinical setting. He went on to highlight that such research is crucial to the advancement of reliable knowledge.

We have used Vere's quotation to open this chapter on research in palliative care in all four of the previous editions of this textbook because it is an apposite comment on the relatively slow progress of research in palliative care. The initial enthusiasm and urgency to gain a basic understanding of the physiology and pharmacology of the dying or severely ill patient and to evaluate the care provided and the treatment that was given did not grow and mature as Cicely Saunders had wished. Research in palliative care has remained in the doldrums until relatively recently, in spite of wide recognition of its importance amongst palliative care practitioners. In contrast, the continued development of new clinical services has continued apace around the world.

The provision of new services has not been driven by research findings. We do not have data which demonstrate the most cost-effective model of service delivery of palliative care (Grande, 2009), nor can we answer the more fundamental question of what models are effective. There remain large areas of clinical practice in palliative care that are founded on clinical experience and anecdote rather than high-quality evidence, and this has applied even to core activities such as the control of pain.

Recently a debate about whether the Liverpool Care Pathway (LCP) is relevant for routine use in palliative care has been ongoing (Fainsinger, 2008). One element in the debate is the lack of scientific evidence supporting the content of the pathway, and there has been a lack of scientific evidence in the effect of implementation of the pathway into clinical practice until recently (Costantini et al., 2014).

This frustrating state of affairs has changed and is changing (Fainsinger, 2008). During the last decade there have been major developments in palliative care research in terms of funding, and the development of infrastructure and support for academic teaching and research. Substantial investment in departments that have the critical mass and facilities to allow high-quality research to be undertaken would take research in palliative care a quantum leap forward. During the last decade, in different parts of the world, new funding streams for palliative care research have become available.

Obstacles to research in palliative care

It has taken much time for research to become embedded within the culture of palliative care. The issues of the primacy of the individual and whole-person care versus the 'greatest happiness of the greatest number' are brought sharply into focus in palliative care. The physician's obligation to privilege the patient's best interests is a fundamental precept of medical practice which is given great emphasis in palliative care. However, the physician also has an obligation to promote the acquisition of scientific knowledge. These obligations constitute a real conflict and raise difficult ethical dilemmas; in time-pressured, daily clinical practice, patient care will always take precedence over research.

There have been problems in attracting high-quality researchers into palliative care. This is partly a consequence of the uncertain career structures and a relative lack of training opportunities (which reflects the lack of funding and investment). The need for academic palliative care researchers affiliated to formalized research groups within the main academic hospitals, made up of a sufficient number of scientists representing a variety of disciplines working together has been highlighted in a topical review (Kaasa et al., 2006). Research groups need to have core funding to enable them to apply for further project grants. Symptom control research is always likely to be less attractive to grant awarding bodies than molecular genetics, however, it is increasingly apparent that molecular biology may be a fertile area for exploring research questions of direct relevance to palliative care clinical practice. For example, a recent review summarizes the available evidence for the influence of human gene polymorphisms on variability in response to opioid analgesics in terms of both analgesia and side effects (Skorpen et al., 2008). There is some evidence in palliative care patients that mu opioid receptor polymorphisms may be related to the need for higher doses of morphine (Klepstad et al., 2004) and a catechol-o-methyl transferase (COMT) polymorphism may influence morphine requirements in cancer pain patients (Rakvåg et al., 2005). Translational research is thus one of the priority areas for palliative care: academic departments of palliative care may need to broaden their base to include laboratory scientists as well as social anthropologists, ethicists, and clinicians.

National and international organizations have a key role to play in palliative care research. The European Association for Palliative Care Research Network (EAPC RN) was established in 1996, implicitly recognizing that networks are essential for palliative care research (Blumhuber et al., 2002). The number of patients available for clinical research in any one centre is always relatively small which means that collaborative studies are necessary to recruit sufficient patients in a reasonable period of time. It became clear in the mid 1990s that palliative care research activity and expertise in different countries in Europe varied considerably, and it was not feasible to launch large multi-centre clinical trials at the outset of the EAPC RN because only a handful of centres were in a position to participate in them; this had been one of the initial ideas behind the setting up of the Research Network.

The EAPC RN therefore adopted a different strategy in its early years. Expert working groups were set up to review areas of clinical controversy or areas that were particularly topical, and to draw up clinical guidelines based on the available evidence. These guidelines have generally proved to be highly influential (1996) and, for the researchers, were useful in identifying gaps in the evidence base and prioritizing areas for research. Latterly the EAPC RN, supported by the European Palliative Care Research Centre (PRC) (2009), has conducted one large cross-sectional study (CSA study) (Hjermstad et al., 2012), and the first large international prospective study on multiple symptoms in advanced cancer patients is about to be finalized. A multicentre randomized feasibility study of the management of cachexia (Clinicaltrials.gov, 2011) is to be followed by a larger ($N = 300$) prospective randomized study with participating institutions from Europe and Canada. These, among other clinical studies, show that palliative care research can be undertaken through collaboration and international networking. The future for palliative care research lies with networks, be they local, regional, national, or international.

Consolidating for future developments in palliative care research

Reports from the United Kingdom and Canada have identified a number of needs: the need to establish multidisciplinary research groups of sufficient strength and size, the need for long-term planning, and the need for international as well as national collaboration reflected by the membership of the groups. Some groups individually, or in collaboration with others, are working for international consensus on patient-centred outcomes (e.g. health-related quality of life and subjective symptoms) and patient cohort classification. The long-term goal for clinical palliative care research should be to move from descriptive to interventional studies. New research initiatives as well as the establishment of new academic chairs of palliative medicine and palliative care nursing will enable researchers to address complex research questions in the field of palliative care.

The most urgent needs for the future, which should be partly realized through the output of the new collaboratives/collaboration are that:

◆ groups of sufficient size and sufficient output need to take the responsibility for further development of research

◆ national and international funding needs to continue, and successful collaboratives need to achieve further funding without unnecessary gaps

◆ it is vital to train a sufficient number of clinicians and scientists in palliative care research.

Research governance

In recent years there has been a trend towards increasingly explicit guidelines and regulations relating to research involving patients. In the United Kingdom, these guidelines are described under the heading of 'research governance'. Research can involve an element of risk regarding both the safety and well-being of participants and the return on investment. Research governance guidelines are designed to minimize risk and improve research performance and they provide a useful framework, particularly for those new to research, which has general applicability and is also relevant outside the United Kingdom.

Research governance is the means by which we ensure high scientific, ethical, and financial standards for the conduct of research and involves transparent decision-making processes, clear allocation of responsibilities, and robust monitoring arrangements. The research governance framework for health and social care in the United Kingdom encompasses five domains. These are ethics (the dignity, rights, safety, and well-being of participants); science (the quality and appropriateness of research); information (the requirements for free access to research information); health, safety, and employment (of participants and research and other staff); and finance and intellectual property.

In the United Kingdom the introduction of these regulations and procedures added considerable time to the process of having an application to do research approved by the various bodies involved. The changes have not been universally welcomed (Jones and Bamford, 2004; Reid, 2004) because of their potential negative effects, not merely on the research process but also on researchers, particularly junior staff first embarking on a research career. It is crucial that some balance is maintained in striving to make the process as safe and as user-friendly as possible for patients, remembering that researchers too need to be supported and not deterred from doing research because of the bureaucracy and inevitable delays that are involved.

Controlled clinical trials and informed consent in palliative medicine

Austin Bradford Hill set out the ethical precepts for RCTs in his Marc Daniels Lecture at the Royal College of Physicians in London in 1963 (Hill, 1963). In the United States, Henry Beecher had a similar influence on the development of ethical guidelines for clinical research (Sackett et al., 1996) and the subject has been debated in many places since. It is not appropriate to discuss this subject in detail here, but the reader is referred to these reviews, which make two important points. The first is that the prospective RCT is the most efficient, scientific way of evaluating a new treatment or of comparing alternative treatments, and the second is that it is not the only way of ensuring the advance of reliable knowledge.

Controlled clinical trials are necessary in palliative medicine, and the usual guidelines and ethical principles apply. Some points need particular emphasis in the palliative care setting. Patients are invariably unwell and many are elderly and frail; most have a multitude of physical and emotional as well as social and spiritual problems. When they come to the palliative care unit or team, many of these problems will be dealt with, and some, particularly the psychosocial issues, may receive attention for the first time. The supportive environment in palliative care may make patients particularly keen to give something back to their carers, to show their gratitude for the care they are receiving. All of these factors make patients particularly vulnerable when they are asked to participate in any sort of research project; many will feel almost obliged to accede to such a request. Researchers in palliative care must be on their guard not to take advantage of this situation.

In palliative care, cognitive impairment and often frank confusion are encountered in many patients; when this is obvious, they will be excluded from consideration for entry to a study. However, the impairment may be mild or variable. Such patients need careful assessment, and, wherever there is any doubt that the patient is able to understand what is being asked of them, he or she should not be considered for inclusion.

There is a fine balance that needs to be achieved. The special vulnerability of patients receiving palliative care dictates the need for great care in obtaining consent to participate in research but at the same time the researcher must enable those patients able and wishing to take part to do so.

Evidence-based palliative care

The principles of evidence-based medicine underpin our day-to-day clinical practice. Evidence-based medicine 'is the conscientious, explicit, and judicious use of current best evidence in making decisions about the care of individual patients. The practice of evidence-based medicine means integrating individual clinical expertise with the best available external clinical evidence from systematic research' (Beecher, 1966).

Evidence-based medicine is not new. The evolution of current thinking about evidence-based medicine is described in Chapter 19.2.

Evidence-based medicine is about finding ways in which to bridge the gap between the huge amount of published data and its application to clinical practice, and encompasses a number of strategies. One of these has been the development of scientific methods (systematic reviews and meta-analyses) to combine data from a number of different randomized studies of the same or similar treatments in any particular condition. Systematic reviews differ from other types of review in that they adhere to a strict scientific design in order to make them more comprehensive, to minimize the chance of bias, and so ensure their reliability.

Taken at face value, it seems reasonable to assume that the data from several studies, which have been combined according to agreed scientific methodology, should be more meaningful than the evidence from single studies. This is increasingly accepted; however, there is no doubt that the methodology and application of these techniques must continue to be looked at critically. Systematic reviews and meta-analyses are, however, powerful tools in aggregating and evaluating large amounts of data and have become an important area of research activity in palliative medicine. One function they serve is to highlight research questions and thus contribute to the research agenda by careful and comprehensive review of the available evidence.

Evidence-based medicine and the future of palliative care

Evidence-based medicine has already had a major impact on the development of health care in a time of ever-increasing demands and limited resource. It is likely that resource allocation will increasingly be based on evidence, not just of efficacy, but also of cost effectiveness. Where proof of efficacy is lacking, funds will not be provided by government or other health-care agencies. This has particular implications for palliative care because where such research-based evidence is sparse. There are many activities within palliative care which are not amenable to investigation by randomized controlled studies; however, as noted earlier, the RCT is not the only valid method of ensuring knowledge advances. The focus on evidence-based medicine makes investment in high-quality palliative care research all the more urgent.

The scope of research in palliative care

One of the challenges in palliative care research is setting boundaries around the field. Because death and dying are at the centre of practitioners' concerns, it can be tempting to include all dimensions of scholarship related to 'death' within the field of interest. Death, as a major rite of passage for individuals, families, and societies, attracts research on its many ramifications, manifestations, and meanings in everyday life. The cultural context in which people present themselves as patients, come to approach death, and are cared for through their dying, is open to wide and varied interpretations drawn from historical, sociological, anthropological, theological, philosophical, and psychological perspectives; each with its own research traditions. Understanding the significance of death as a rite of passage as well as a biological or medical event is important for the practitioner when faced with the challenges raised by dying patients and their families, and so it could be argued that the field of palliative care research is in fact immense. Practically, however, the field is generally focused on a narrower range of interests of immediate concern and relevance to practitioners and planners.

The principal questions that face palliative care professionals are those of clinical effectiveness and acceptability, service efficiency and organization, and meeting the changing needs of the population. These are basic questions concerned with what palliative care practitioners do, and how they do it. The research skills to answer these questions are commonly drawn from the traditions of clinical research (medical, nursing, and allied health professional), health services research, and also epidemiology.

Epidemiological research

Descriptive epidemiology seeks to describe the prevalence and incidence of conditions within defined populations. Assessing the need for palliative care in different sectors of the population is clearly important for informing the process of service development and planning. In relation to palliative care, epidemiological research has been hampered by an absence of clearly defined population indicators linked to levels of clinical need, as well as changing perceptions within the profession of palliative care as to the appropriate 'catchment population'. The extended application of palliative care from its original main constituency of cancer patients at the end of life, to patients with any life-limiting illness, from point of diagnosis onwards, poses problems of classification. The majority of health service utilization data and measures of morbidity and mortality are based on disease categories. These do not give an indication of symptom burden or dependency levels, and thus little indication of the need for different forms of palliative care.

Clinical research

Clinical research traditionally tends to focus on biochemical, microbiological, and physiological processes and the effect of pharmacological and other therapeutic agents. In palliative care, this focus is much broader because of the complexity of advanced disease and the high prevalence of psychological and existential distress. Clinical trials are based on an experimental approach and will often use outcomes from the laboratory derived from body samples (blood, tissue) or images (X-rays or scans) as well as patient responses recorded by questionnaire or structured interview. It is at the level of clinical research that trial based research methodologies are most effective and applicable. The need for access to skilled technicians and laboratory facilities may limit research capacity for researchers working in non-academic or community settings.

Health services research

Health services research is primarily focused on the evaluation of the organization and delivery of health care. Frequently, the research is applied to particular problems faced by policymakers, managers, practitioners, and patients, and can range from questions of cost and effectiveness, policy formulation and implementation, the evaluation of new technologies, through to patient and public preferences and perceptions. Research approaches include those that underpin the social sciences as well as the more experimentally based approaches of the natural sciences. Much of the multidisciplinary research carried out in palliative care is focused on questions of innovation and organization in services, and assessing the need for and access to different types of intervention.

Humanistic research

The contribution of other disciplines and research traditions to the body of research in palliative care is well recognized and valued.

Concern with the ethical, moral, spiritual, and philosophical dimensions of care for the dying and bereaved from all perspectives informs a body of scholarship, which broadens out the focus of research that can be relevant to palliative care practitioners. However, lack of familiarity with disciplinary roots and epistemological theory can make the contributions from the social sciences and humanities more difficult to assimilate for practitioners schooled in the natural sciences.

Defining the patient population

A particularly complex issue is the definition of a palliative care patient population. The lack of strict criteria for defining the patient population is a threat to both the internal and external validity of research in palliative care. In this context, internal validity can be understood as the ability to define the cohort of patients included in a given study. For example, if the true patient population is more heterogeneous than the one defined, the heterogeneity might obscure, or even obliterate the positive effect of a particular intervention. External validity is about the representativeness of the sample. Research data might be inappropriately applied in clinical practice if the precise characteristics of the population included in a particular research project are not accurately described. Research methods are generally predicated on the comparison of one population with another; studies of effectiveness are only meaningful when one treatment is set against another within similar or homogeneous populations. Palliative care populations are difficult to standardize however, since referral to a palliative care team is made for a wide variety of reasons, most of which will be patient-generated, but will also include reasons that involve the patient's family and professional carers, and the facilities available to the patient. Prognosis on referral is one way of categorizing patients, however this is generally a matter of clinical judgement and use of dependency scores, while time from referral to death is another way; but this is only possible retrospectively. Another possibility is symptom burden—which is in most cohorts closely related to expected survival (Kaasa et al., 1989; Maltoni et al., 1995; Vigano et al., 2000).

Methodology

In a recent European study, a basic set of core variables were identified as necessary and sufficient to describe a palliative care patient population (Sigurdardottir et al., 2014). This EAPC basic dataset consists of 31 core variables divided into patient and health-care professional forms.

The evaluation of the effectiveness of treatments in palliative care has either not been undertaken or has been conducted using poor or inadequate research methodologies. This was also the case in clinical medicine generally until the late 1960s and early 1970s. Only in recent years has it become evident that properly designed and well-conducted clinical trials are needed in palliative care as much as in any other area of medicine. Most of the published studies of the effectiveness of treatments in palliative care have been related to pain and often the patients included have been at an early stage of their disease. Whether the results of these studies can be extrapolated to palliative care patients is open to question.

A clinical trial is any investigation that follows the principles of a scientific experiment, allowing for the evaluation of the clinical effect of an intervention in a valid and reliable way. The term 'clinical trial' is not synonymous with 'randomized controlled trial' (RCT). A clinical trial in the broadest sense of the term may mean any kind of planned experiment in patients, ranging from open descriptive studies to RCTs. The trial design will, and should be, determined by the research question.

The choice of an appropriate study design will depend on what is already known about the particular question to be investigated. With the recent emphasis on evidence-based medicine, there has been much discussion about the need for RCTs with reference to the RCT as the 'gold standard' and the most robust method for evaluating new treatments. However, many research questions do not need to be answered by an RCT. Furthermore, when attempting to design a randomized study, a lack of sufficient descriptive data may make it difficult to decide upon a study design and appropriate outcomes, or to perform a valid sample size calculation. This is commonly the case in palliative care research. The choice of trial design is crucial and, in this process, collaboration between experts is essential. This is the stage at which a project group should be established, at the very beginning of the planning process of a study.

In palliative care, a pilot study or simply a non-systematic observation of a particular intervention is not a rigorous research experiment but is the first step in the research plan. A step-by-step approach is necessary and highlights the fact that clinical research is a time-consuming process. Researchers and clinicians should not expect too many answers from each study.

Guidelines and books (Pocock, 1984; Karlberg and Tsang, 1998) on clinical trial methodology are widely available. The objectives and design of a study will be driven by the research questions and the resources available. This is not just about funding but also about academic and clinical resources and the availability of sufficient patients. A common problem in clinical research (not unique to palliative care) is that investigators invariably and substantially overestimate the number of patients they are likely to see who would be suitable for a particular study. Changes in treatment policies might influence the availability of patients for a particular study even more if the entry criteria are based on previous policy.

A general criticism of palliative care research is that too many small studies are performed with an open non-comparative design, and thus the impact of the results in terms of changing practice will be limited. For example, in a recent systematic review of ketamine in cancer-related pain, the reviewers found 32 case series, but only two RCTs of good quality (and these involved a total of only 20 patients). This makes it impossible to draw firm conclusions about the efficacy of ketamine (Bell et al., 2003).

How to plan a clinical trial

The planning process of any clinical study often starts with new encouraging data from the laboratory or, probably more often in palliative care, from chance or non-systematic observations in the clinic. Aside from the need to collect together background information, the planning process involves a series of basic steps, which will need to be considered to provide the framework for the study (Box 19.1.1).

Usually one will start with a literature review to see what is known about an intervention and the target condition or symptom. If the review indicates that a formal study is necessary or worthwhile, a research question or hypothesis should be formulated and this will determine the aim of the study.

Box 19.1.1 The evolution of a research project in palliative care

1. Describe clearly the clinical problem or observations which prompted the idea for a study.
2. Discuss the relevance and validity of the observations with clinical colleagues.
3. Carry out a comprehensive review of the literature to find out what is already known about the topic.
4. Formulate the research question(s). These will define the aim of the study.
5. Define the patient population.
6. Decide on the appropriate study design.
7. Decide on the outcomes to be measured.
8. With these decisions made, write the protocol.

A common mistake in clinical research is to bring too many ideas together and try to answer too many questions at the same time. Many studies are too complex, with many research questions, which cannot be answered with a limited number of patients.

Explicit definition of the aim of the study is crucial. Many clinical research projects are undertaken without a clear and concise aim, and the consequence is a lack of precision in the subsequent planning process, and ultimately a poor study or one that is impossible to complete. The aim should be written in clear and understandable language and, ideally, it should be easily understood by a lay person. It should be possible to formulate it briefly in one or two sentences. It is often expressed as a general question and this is broken down into specific research questions or hypotheses.

The research questions will determine the patient population to be studied. There are several factors to take into consideration such as 'Which group of patients will best give an answer to these questions?' For example, if a study was designed to examine patients' attitudes toward euthanasia and physician-assisted suicide in palliative care, the researchers would need to decide whether to ask the patient directly. In similar studies, patients themselves have not been asked, but the questions have been put to proxies or the general public. If the researchers decide to ask patients, they must then decide how to select patients, (in this example perhaps 'not too ill, but not too far away from being confronted with death and dying'). The patient sample must also be representative of the population of patients to whom the results will be applied. In other words, if a selected sub-group of the general population is recruited to a study, the usefulness and applicability of the results (the external validity or generalizability) will be compromised.

In studies evaluating the effect of adjuvant chemotherapy in breast cancer or combination therapy for HIV, the primary outcomes are easy to select, for example, tumour response or survival time (Early Breast Cancer Trialists' Collaborative Group, 1998). However, more recently, in oncology trials, criticisms have been made about limiting the outcomes to survival or cure and not taking account of late side effects of the treatment. During the last decade, for example, several studies have described the high prevalence of subjective side effects, such as fatigue, in Hodgkin's disease survivors (Loge et al., 1999). These experiences emphasize that the selection of outcomes, even in curative treatment studies, might be less straightforward than it at first appears. In palliative care, the patient population is complex and studies have been reported with ten to 20 and even more outcome measures. This multiplicity of outcomes is further driven by the multidimensionality of the concept of health-related quality of life and the range of scales and single items found in these measures (Aaronson et al., 1993; Cohen et al., 1995). It is important not to fall into this trap. In general, one or two primary outcomes and perhaps two to three secondary outcomes are the most that should be included.

All of these issues should be thoroughly discussed by the researchers and the involved clinicians, together with the larger study group, before the research protocol can be finalized.

Randomization and blinding

The concept of random allocation of patients when comparing different treatments (or any other intervention) is important in the design of a clinical experiment. The purpose of randomization is to reduce selection bias. Non-randomized trials have a tendency to overestimate the effect of treatment. Randomization also provides a basis for the use of standard methods of statistical analysis. When a new treatment is introduced, enthusiastic clinicians and researchers tend to overestimate its beneficial effects. For example, in the early open studies of cisplatin in the treatment of non-small-cell lung cancer, the response rate was double what was found in later randomized studies (Kaasa et al., 1988). The same tendency is also seen when using historical controls as a comparison group or when using other quasi-experimental designs.

In palliative care, randomized studies are particularly difficult to undertake and complete. Therefore, other types of study must be considered and might be preferable. Caution needs to be exercised in the analysis and interpretation of data from non-randomized studies. Other designs may be appropriate and may represent a slightly less robust option than an RCT but still produce persuasive data. For example, in the evaluation of palliative care programmes, cluster randomized designs have been used (Jordhøy et al., 2000; Costantini et al., 2014).

Unblinded trials also overestimate the effect of treatment. Blinding may be difficult to achieve and needs to be thought about early in the planning process, particularly if it involves the manufacture of placebo formulations or other manufacturing processes to conceal the identity of treatments. Palliative care researchers should consult with statisticians and clinical trial methodologists early in the planning process of the study, and preferably include these advisors in the project group. There are useful texts on clinical trial methodology (Pocock, 1984), study design (Rothman and Greenland, 1998), introduction to statistics (Rosner, 2000), and more comprehensive textbooks on medical statistics (Altman, 1991). Such texts provide useful basic background reading for researchers.

Statistical considerations

The project group will need to consult with a statistician, or preferably include a statistician. Medical statisticians have skills and expertise in several areas of clinical research, that is, study design, sample size estimation, and in the analysis of the data. A statistician should be consulted early in the process of designing the study and should have continuing input throughout the project.

One essential step in the planning process of any clinical study is to decide how many patients will be needed to get a valid result.

The purpose of this 'sample size' calculation is to ensure that the study is large enough to detect a clinically important difference should one exist, or exclude the possibility of such a difference should none be detected. In order to estimate the sample size, the statistician will want to know how small a difference it is important to be able to detect in the main outcome measures in terms of clinical significance. For example, the number of patients treated with a new opioid, reaching a numerical rating scale (NRS) score below three within 2 weeks of the initiation of treatment. In comparative studies of pain relief, the mean value of the NRS is often used as a primary outcome. The clinicians need to specify how small a difference between groups will be considered to be of clinical significance (e.g. 2 on a 0–11 NRS scale). It would also be helpful to have information about what could be expected to happen in the control group (mean and standard deviation) and this information may be derived from a pilot study or from published literature. The required number of patients is calculated according to how confident one wants to be about detecting a difference between interventions if one exists (the power of the study).

The protocol

The process of developing a rough draft of a study protocol through to a stage where all aspects of the study have been considered and piloted is a major research effort on its own. In theory, it means that short of actually carrying out the study, everything that could be done has been done. In practice, researchers who skimp on the protocol and associated development work will often find themselves faced with untenable or impractical research studies.

Access to patients

A major challenge in palliative care research needing to involve relatively large numbers of patients is in identifying the patient population and gaining access to them. When research involves selected patients in a clinic, or on a ward, identifying those appropriate for research may not be problematic, especially if the clinician involved is carrying out the research. However, for non-clinical researchers, or for clinical researchers wanting to recruit patients from settings other than their own, identification and access are crucial aspects of patient recruitment. In these situations, cooperation will be needed from other health-care professionals caring for the patients. To gain access to patients may require lengthy negotiation, involving presentations at clinical meetings, permission from professional bodies, as well as a strategy for communication and keeping the research project uppermost in clinicians' minds.

It can be useful to develop information sheets, specific for each professional concerned, early on in the stages of introducing a project to those who are affected. Thinking through likely questions and their answers can help to take the project off the drawing board and ground it in the reality of clinical life. Colleagues and peers will be concerned that the research is well designed and addresses a clinically important question. Justifying the purpose and value of a research project to one's peers is particularly critical in relation to palliative care research where non-palliative care colleagues may question the probity of carrying out research with this patient group. There are probably few palliative care researchers who have not, at some time, had their research intentions questioned. In addition, it will be important to listen to colleagues' concerns and offer flexibility in carrying out the research. Colleagues will be particularly resistant to participating in anything that involves more paperwork or disruption to routines. The effort and time involved in securing access from professional colleagues should not be underestimated.

It is also important to feed back to practitioners who have been involved in the research through facilitating access to patients, or providing information, at the end of the research. Knowing what the findings are, and what importance they hold for future service configurations, helps make the research a collaborative experience, and can be an element in service development and change where that is indicated. This affirms the stakeholder role, which professional carers hold in the research process.

Significant others to the patient—non-professional carers

Care at the end of life embraces not only the patient, but also those close to him or her. Supporting family carers in their caring role is important in relieving some of the practical difficulties and burdens that are encountered during protracted periods of high-dependency care in the home, as well as addressing the psychological distress which is associated with the loss of a close relative. Research similarly may involve not only the patient but also those close to the patient in a primary caring role. Research interest may take several forms; it may focus on the long-term health of those who survive the patient (bereavement studies), but it may also focus on how patients and their home carers cope with the illness together, or the perceptions of the home carers of the professional care received by the patient. Even when research is solely concerned with patient-based indicators, those close to the patient are important in the research process by acting as intermediaries. Home or family carers can take on a number of roles in relation to patients' involvement in research and each role needs to be appreciated by the research team.

Gatekeepers/protectors

Family members adopting a primary caring role act as 'gatekeepers' to patient. This is likely to be increasingly critical as the patient declines, when dependency increases, and when the patient him/herself may have delegated certain aspects of decision-making to a trusted family carer. When patients are approached for recruitment into a research study, it is generally advisable, therefore, to approach also whoever appears to be most in contact with the patient (in hospital or at home), with the patient's consent. Research can appear threatening to those who are striving to care for the patient; primarily they may worry about the research tiring the patient, or about questions upsetting the patient—either by providing too much information or opening up areas of contemplation that may further disturb the patient. When time is perceived to be short, carers may well resent the patient's attention being taken by people outside of the family. How family carers weigh up the benefits of participating in a research study (short-term benefits of additional monitoring and attention versus the long-term benefits to society) against the costs to the patient (and themselves) of time commitments and possibly extra upset will be pivotal in the recruitment process.

The family carer's role as gatekeeper is often regarded negatively by researchers, as one of the barriers to achieving adequate sample sizes. While researchers should regard adult patients as autonomous, self-determining individuals who can decide for themselves whether they want to participate in research, the vulnerability of some palliative care patients can make this problematic. The tensions between dealing with a patient as a family member rather than as simply an individual are all too apparent. Participation in research is an intervention in itself (patients are not 'passive subjects') with consequences that cannot be wholly predicted, however meticulously procedures are followed. Being involved in research can involve the wider family context, and so the extended boundaries of the palliative care patient need to be appreciated by researchers, with procedures in place to inform and include family members.

Interpreters, substitutes, and advocates

When patients have difficulty communicating their thoughts and feelings, family members may take on the role of interpreter and substitute (proxy). Interpretation can be needed for both speech and language difficulties. In the face of cognitive impairment, the views of family carers may be used as a substitute for the patient's views. A number of studies have investigated the validity of proxy ratings, concluding that proxies tend to underestimate the severity of certain symptoms (pain and depression) but that in the absence of patient derived data, proxy data is valuable.

A role that sits between gatekeeper and interpreter is that of advocate. The extent to which family carers take on this role varies with their own confidence and the situations within which they find themselves. Researchers should be aware that advocacy can work in different ways; at times making sure that the patient's best interests are promoted, at others, following an agenda that is not the patient's but that of the family member. This is another reason for extreme sensitivity to be exercised by the research team.

Significant others to the patient—professional carers

Professional carers can also act as gate-keepers, interpreters, substitutes, and advocates, with all the cautions outlined above. Similarly, they are also a subject of great interest in their own right from the point of view of service/practitioner efficiency and effectiveness, and understanding the process of delivering high-quality palliative care. There is a growing body of research on the training and educational needs of practitioners, the dynamics of inter-professional and multidisciplinary team working, and management processes to preserve and enhance occupational health.

Finance and management

There are many sources of funding that are relevant to palliative care, but securing funds for research in this area is a competitive exercise, as it is in any area of health care. As indicated at the beginning of this chapter, palliative care research is a relatively neglected area as far as the major funders of cancer research are concerned. The great majority of patients currently being treated by palliative care services are patients with cancer and funding for studies in non-cancer patients is in even shorter supply. However, the climate is changing, and this is happening in many different parts of the world. It is not possible here to give detailed information about funding sources since these will vary from country to country. This sort of information is obviously of considerable relevance to future researchers and it is one area where the scientific journals available in palliative care could play a useful role.

Finance for individual projects: the length of time between securing financial support for a project and actually starting data collection is always underestimated. This period can be divided into two main phases: the time before project funds are actually drawn upon, when research staff are being recruited and when a considerable amount of planning and groundwork is being carried out; and phase two, when the funds are being disbursed and piloting work is being undertaken. It is crucial that as much work as possible is carried out in the first phase, even though the work is essentially not funded. Efficient management of time and resources from the very start of a project are obviously key factors in its successful running.

Project group

All research projects benefit from being exposed to a group of people who have experience in the subject under research and who are interested in the project. This is particularly important for large studies. The role of a project group can vary from being highly involved in the administration and day-to-day concerns of the project, to being relatively distant, and receiving information about the project on a regular though infrequent basis.

Depending on the size of the project, it can sometimes be helpful to institute a steering group of key stakeholders who are sympathetic to the research but who do not have much time to devote to it, and a management group of people who are accessible regularly and become close to project and data collection, and who report back to the steering group.

Piloting the study and study procedures

Research studies do not start as fully formed projects. Indeed, it is impossible to anticipate all the challenges that a study will face at the planning stage. The word 'pilot' derives from the job of steering a boat on its course and the metaphor of guiding a ship through uncertain and troubled waters is an apt one. Without preliminary studies, it is difficult to steer the course of a large project. Pilot work is important for testing all aspects of research design, from the face validity and acceptability of data collection procedures, to the workability of allocation schedules and administration tasks. Dealing with the questions and issues raised by pilot studies can be demanding at a stage when there is impatience to start the main study, not least due to the pressure of obtaining funds for research and the need to work to deadlines. However, learning the lessons from pilot work can be critical to the success of the project. For researchers working alone, the use of a research journal can encourage a reflective attitude to pilot work, and help to refine the research design. For researchers in a team, frequent meetings at this stage, with records made of the discussions and decisions will help to re-define and re-model the research into a workable proposition. Re-writing the protocol with the findings of the pilot work is important for the auditing of the research project.

Administration and paperwork

It will be readily appreciated that a research study will quickly develop different strands of paperwork, reflecting the different administrative tasks:

- Background work relating to the development of the study, reviews of the scientific literature, and any position papers and early proposals.

- Paperwork relating to the funding and approval of the study (sponsors, ethics committees, other professional and regulatory bodies).

- Correspondence and paperwork relating to the formation of the steering and project groups, together with the minutes and agendas of each formally convened meeting.

- A record of the protocol as it develops through successive drafts with careful version control.

- Sources of information targeted at specific sectors of the study population: information sheets for patients and their professional and non-professional carers, information posters for hospital or hospice wards or other settings, information in local media about the study.

- Paperwork used for collecting data, ranging from consent forms and case record forms, to questionnaires and data abstraction forms. This might also include letters or cards sent by the research team to patients and carers after data collection, to thank them for their participation, as well as any correspondence from the study population regarding the research, including letters of complaint or inquiry. Restricting access to this kind of documentation is central to preserving patient confidentiality (lockable rooms or filing cabinets).

- A developing account of the way the study is progressing. Most projects benefit from regular review, although this will depend on size and timescale. Even in the absence of interim analysis, it can be important to monitor recruitment rates, protocol deviations, and any other problems with the management of the project. This can also be an opportunity for informal reflections on the study, particularly from the point of view of the day-to-day researchers.

- Paperwork relating to data preparation and data analysis, including any conventions used in coding data, and where the data are held and in what form. This aspect of project administration is most important for the understanding and interpretation of data in analysis.

- Finally, the project will be written up as a report in various formats for various audiences, and it is important to keep records of the drafts as they develop and become finalized.

Efficient administration is essential for two main reasons. One is where a project is required to audit its activities and give an account of the funds that have been used and the procedures that have been followed. This can happen as a result of a rolling programme of research audit within an institution or sector, or can happen as a result of a special investigation, triggered by a number of different concerns (perhaps unrelated to the study). Another more common scenario is where researchers move away from the project before its conclusion; this may seriously affect the smooth running of a study, but the effect can be minimized by comprehensive paperwork. Again, the role of a project group is critical to the orientation of a new researcher, mid-study, with the dangers of keeping decision-making and discussion to too small a group all too evident.

Monitoring of study

Supporting researchers and the clinical team (keeping it going)

The initial rush of enthusiasm for a project is difficult to sustain over time without conscious management of the research team.

Box 19.1.2 Submitting a paper for publication
1. Decide which journal to go for. Are the data relevant to a general journal (*The New England Journal of Medicine, The Lancet, BMJ*) or a specialist journal (*Cancer, Journal of Clinical Oncology, Palliative Medicine*)? It is more difficult to achieve publication in the general journals.
2. Aim high (but appropriately so) because sometimes you will catch an editor's interest. With the leading journals you will usually get a very rapid response if the paper is rejected.
3. Try to learn from rejection. Usually authors will get some feedback explaining why the paper has been rejected. This should enable them to improve the paper before submitting it to another journal.
4. Before submission to any journal, study the 'Instructions to Authors' and abide by them strictly, particularly in terms of length, style, and references.
5. In general, it is not worth arguing with editors if they have made it clear that they do not wish to publish your paper. However, if you believe the comments of referees or editors are unreasonable or erroneous it is perfectly legitimate to challenge them. Occasionally an editor may change their mind!
6. If your paper is accepted but the referees or editors suggest changes which you are not happy with, respond and explain why you feel the changes are not justified.
7. After publication, make sure you read the journal (even if it is not one you regularly take) so that you can respond to any correspondence about your paper.

Studies can get into difficulty quite quickly when unexpected problems start to shake the confidence of the supporting clinical teams or the front-line researchers. Encountering slow patient recruitment or high dropout rates, for example, can be disillusioning and demotivating. However, a project that is conceived as a collaborative venture, where support from others is openly valued, and where there is a commitment to teamwork, is likely to develop mechanisms for keeping the study going. Attention needs to be focused on the individual needs and group dynamics of the research team, as well as the wider group of staff who are involved in facilitating the study. Morale and support for the study can be promoted in a number of ways:

◆ For clinical staff, provision of regular feedback and direct contact with the study team to answer queries and address any concerns is desirable. This is also important considering the high turnover of clinical staff; new staff will need to be identified and inducted especially during a long-running study. Busy clinical staff will tend to forget about studies, and an important aspect of regular contact is to remind them that the study is still running.

◆ Within the research team, time should be set aside for team-building activities (e.g. away days and social events), and to help prevent 'burn-out', the provision of mentoring, co-counselling, or debriefing should be considered.

Submitting a paper for publication

Much research is undertaken and completed, and even presented at scientific meetings, but is never published in a peer-reviewed journal. There may be many reasons for this and it is not possible briefly to discuss them all here. However, Box 19.1.2 gives some advice about submitting papers for publication.

Conclusions

Research in palliative care is essential for maintaining standards and advancing knowledge and improving practice. It is challenging, sometimes daunting, often frustrating, but always exciting and rewarding when a study is successfully completed, whether the outcome is positive or negative. We hope that this chapter will help those who are new to research to get started, to proceed and complete it, and contribute to improving outcomes for patients with advanced disease, which is ultimately the aim of this endeavour.

References

Aaronson, N.K., Ahmedzai, S., Bergman, B., *et al.* (1993). The European Organization for Research and Treatment of Cancer QLQ-C30: a quality-of-life instrument for use in international clinical trials in oncology. *Journal of the National Cancer Institute*, 85, 365–376.

Altman, D. (1991). *Practical Statistics for Medical Research*. London: Chapman and Hall.

Beecher, H.K. (1966). Ethics and clinical research. *The New England Journal of Medicine*, 274, 1354–1360.

Bell, R., Eccleston, C., and Kalso, E. (2003). Ketamine as an adjuvant to opioids for cancer pain. *Cochrane Database of Systematic Reviews*, 1, CD003351.

Blumhuber, H., Kaasa, S., and De Conno, F. (2002). The European Association for Palliative Care. *Journal of Pain and Symptom Management*, 24, 124–127.

ClinicalTrials.gov (2011). *A Feasibility Study of Multimodal Exercise/ Nutrition/Anti-inflammatory Treatment for Cachexia—the Pre-MENAC Study*. [Online] Available at: <http://ClinicalTrials.gov>.

Cohen, S.R., Mount, B.M., Strobel, M.G., and Bui, F. (1995). The McGill Quality of Life Questionnaire: a measure of quality of life appropriate for people with advanced disease. A preliminary study of validity and acceptability. *Palliative Medicine*, 9, 207–219.

Costantini, M., Romoli, V., Leo, S.D., *et al.* (2014). Liverpool Care Pathway for patients with cancer in hospital: a cluster randomised trial. *The Lancet*, 383, 226–237.

Early Breast Cancer Trialists' Collaborative Group. (1998). Tamoxifen for early breast cancer: an overview of the randomised trials. *The Lancet*, 351, 1451–1467.

European Palliative Care Research Centre (2009). *European Palliative Care Research Centre (PRC)* [Online]. Available at: <http://www.ntnu.no/prc>.

Expert Working Group of The European Association For Palliative Care (1996). Morphine in cancer pain: modes of administration. *BMJ*, 312, 823–826.

Fainsinger, R. (2008). Global warming in the palliative care research environment: adapting to change. *Palliative Medicine*, 22, 328–335.

Grande, G. (2009). Palliative care in hospice and hospital: time to put the spotlight on neglected areas of research. *Palliative Medicine*, 23, 187–189.

Hill, A.B. (1963). Medical ethics and controlled trials. *British Medical Journal*, 1, 1043–1049.

Hjermstad, M.J., Lie, H.C., Caraceni, A., *et al.* (2012). Computer-based symptom assessment is feasible in patients with advanced cancer: results from an international multicenter study, the EPCRC-CSA. *Journal of Pain and Symptom Management*, 44(5), 639–654.

Jones, A.M. and Bamford, B. (2004). The other face of research governance. *BMJ*, 329, 280–281.

Jordhøy, M.S., Fayers, P., Saltnes, T., Ahlner-Elmqvist, M., Jannert, M., and Kaasa, S. (2000). A palliative-care intervention and death at home: a cluster randomised trial. *The Lancet*, 356, 888–893.

Kaasa, S., Hjermstad, M.J., and Loge, J.H. (2006). Methodological and structural challenges in palliative care research: how have we fared in the last decades? *Palliative Medicine*, 20, 727–734.

Kaasa, S., Mastekaasa, A., and Lund, E. (1989). Prognostic factors for patients with inoperable non-small cell lung cancer, limited disease. The importance of patients' subjective experience of disease and psychosocial well-being. *Radiotherapy and Oncology*, 15, 235–242.

Kaasa, S., Thorud, E., Høst, H., Lien, H.H., Lund, E., and Sjolie, I. (1988). A randomized study evaluating radiotherapy versus chemotherapy in patients with inoperable non-small cell lung cancer. *Radiotherapy and Oncology*, 11, 7–13.

Karlberg, J. and Tsang, K. (1998). *Introduction to Clinical Trials*. Hong Kong: University of Hong Kong.

Klepstad, P., Rakvåg, T.T., Kaasa, S., *et al.* (2004). The 118 A > G polymorphism in the human mu-opioid receptor gene may increase morphine requirements in patients with pain caused by malignant disease. *Acta Anaesthesiologica Scandinavica*, 48, 1232–1239.

Loge, J.H., Abrahamsen, A.F., Ekeberg, O., and Kaasa, S. (1999). Hodgkin's disease survivors more fatigued than the general population. *Journal of Clinical Oncology*, 17, 253–261.

Maltoni, M., Pirovano, M., Scarpi, E., *et al.* (1995). Prediction of survival of patients terminally ill with cancer. Results of an Italian prospective multicentric study. *Cancer*, 75, 2613–2622.

Pocock, S. (1984). *Clinical Trials: A Practical Approach*. New York: Wiley.

Rakvåg, T.T., Klepstad, P., Baar, C., *et al.* (2005). The Val158Met polymorphism of the human catechol-O-methyltransferase (COMT) gene may influence morphine requirements in cancer pain patients. *Pain*, 116, 73–78.

Reid, C.M. (2004). Research bureaucracy in the United Kingdom: ask for help. *BMJ*, 329, 624.

Rosner, B. (2000). *Fundamentals of Biostatistics* (5th ed.). Pacific Grove, CA: Duxbury.

Rothman, K. and Greenland, S. (1998). *Modern Epidemiology*. Philadelphia, PA; Lippincott.

Sackett, D.L., Rosenberg, W.M., Gray, J.A., Haynes, R.B., and Richardson, W.S. (1996). Evidence based medicine: what it is and what it isn't. *BMJ*, 312, 71–72.

Sigurdardottir, K.R., Kaasa, S., Rosland, J.H., Bausewein, C., Radbruch, L., and Haugen, D.F. (2014). The European Association for Palliative Care basic dataset to describe a palliative care cancer population: results from an international Delphi process. *Palliative Medicine*, 28(6), 463–473.

Skorpen, F., Laugsand, E.A., Klepstad, P., and Kaasa, S. (2008). Variable response to opioid treatment: any genetic predictors within sight? *Palliative Medicine*, 22, 310–327.

Vere, D. (1981). Controlled clinical trials: the current ethical debate. *Journal of the Royal Society of Medicine*, 74, 85–88.

Vigano, A., Bruera, E., Jhangri, G.S., Newman, S.C., Fields, A.L., and Suarez-Almazor, M.E.(2000). Clinical survival predictors in patients with advanced cancer. *Archives of Internal Medicine*, 160, 861–868.

The principles of evidence-based medicine

Amy P. Abernethy

Introduction to the principles of evidence-based medicine

Originally introduced by Thomas Kuhn in the 1960s, the term 'paradigm' refers to a frame of reference in the sciences. In the vernacular sense, it has come to mean a global framework for organizing current information and understanding reality (Kuhn, 1962). A paradigm shift occurs when a new global framework, and its corresponding way of thinking, supplants an old one. In this process, inadequacies, defects, and errors in the prevailing paradigm make it no longer tenable. The new paradigm emerges not as incremental change but as a discontinuity.

In medicine, the emergence of evidence-based medicine (EBM) can be viewed as a paradigm shift encompassing philosophical, cultural, and logistical changes that are transforming medical practice.

As defined by Kuhn, a paradigm shift is irreversible. Once a new paradigm permeates a field's consciousness, individuals are no longer able to revert to their prior way of thinking. For example, germ theory completely and irrevocably replaced the previous view of disease as caused by spontaneous generation, a hypothesis that had held sway since Aristotle's time. Likewise, the basic concept of EBM, described below, is here to stay. Embracing this paradigm will be essential if palliative care is to establish itself as a peer to other medical disciplines, communicate and collaborate with them, and progress as a field in the contemporary biomedical research and health-care environment. Arguably, as well, adoption of EBM in palliative care represents the current best approach to improving quality of care and patient outcomes in this, as in other, disciplines.

What is evidence-based medicine?

EBM was first defined, and described as a global approach to medical practice, in the 1990s. In a seminal manuscript published by the *British Medical Journal* in 1996, David Sackett and colleagues provided the most commonly cited definition of EBM: 'Evidence-based medicine is the conscientious, explicit, and judicious use of current best evidence in making decisions about the care of individual patients' (Sackett et al., 1996). Here Sackett set down the central parameters of EBM: it is a personalized approach to patient care, in which the physician determines the best treatment plan for each patient, based on best research data, and tempered by clinical experience and wisdom.

A more general term than EBM is evidence-based practice (EBP), defined by Muir Gray in 2001 as follows: 'Evidence-based clinical practice is an approach to decision making in which the clinician uses the best evidence available, in consultation with the patient, to decide upon the option that suits that patient best' (Muir Gray, 2001) (Fig. 19.2.1). The terms EBM and EBP are often used interchangeably, acknowledging the distinction between them. For simplicity's sake this chapter will use the term EBM throughout.

Sackett's now-classic definition of EBM clearly specified the aim, but did not spell out the processes by which to attain it. Meanwhile, between 1993 and 2000, Gordon Guyatt and colleagues in the Evidence-based Medicine Working Group published, in the *Journal of the American Medical Association* (*JAMA*), a seminal series of 31 articles designed to provide educational content, tools, and strategies that could enable clinicians to interpret evidence from published research and integrate it into their care of patients. These 'User's Guide to the Medical Literature' articles, now compiled and published as a text (Guyatt et al., 2008) by the American Medical Association Press, rapidly attained the status of a classic in medicine.

What is evidence?

The practice of EBM requires, first, a clear understanding of what constitutes 'evidence'. In the history of medicine, the conviction that clinical care should be based on data from research studies is quite new. The modern clinical trial, characterized by the use of eligibility criteria, concurrent comparison, placebo or control conditions, randomization, and blinding, emerged in the late nineteenth and early twentieth century. Prior to that time, medical knowledge accrued through, and medical decisions were largely based on, observation and anecdote often painstakingly assembled. Though these forms of information served as 'evidence' in earlier times, today they are generally considered to be of lesser value than information derived from more quantitative or standard scientific methods.

The boundaries circumscribing what will be included in the evidence considered, and what will be excluded, vary. Some authors narrow Sackett's definition to only include evidence from clinical trials, randomized controlled trials (RCTs), or secondary clinical research based on RCTs (Hampton, 2002). These requirements narrow the definition of evidence and exclude much non-trial evidence such as observational, epidemiological, and qualitative studies (Giacomini, 2001; Hampton, 2002). Other authors seek to expand the definition of evidence so as to include the basic sciences

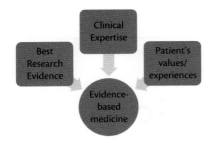

Fig. 19.2.1 Core inputs to evidence-based medicine.
Source: data from Muir Gray, J. A., *Evidence-Based Healthcare: How to Make Health Policy and Management Decisions*, Second Edition, Churchill Livingstone Edinburgh, UK, Copyright © 2001.

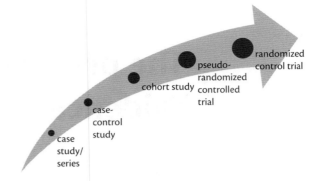

Fig. 19.2.2 Evidence hierarchy for primary clinical research into new interventions.

and clinical knowledge (Sackett et al., 1996; Guyatt et al., 2000; Youngblut and Brooten, 2001). With the advent of medical informatics and administrative databases, the definition of evidence is being expanded further to include aggregated data from multiple patient encounters with a clinician or across a health system or of multiple experiences of an individual patient accumulated over time (Bakken, 2001). The N-of-1 trial may be the ultimate evidence source for an individual patient (Guyatt et al., 2000). Qualitative studies that explore social phenomena and enlighten clinicians about why, when, and how treatments take effect are increasingly recognized as important sources of supportive information (Giacomini and Cook, 2000a). In the future, 'evidence' may even encompass information appearing on bulletin boards, global chat-rooms, and personal electronic databases (Abbasi et al., 2002). Today, a massive volume of evidence is available and pertinent to virtually every discipline, specialty, and subspecialty. In palliative care, it is often not the availability of evidence, but rather the availability of reliable evidence and the clinician's ability to differentiate between high- and low-quality evidence and apply this knowledge into practice for the individual patient, that is critical to EBM.

Quality of evidence

General consensus holds that not all evidence is of equal strength or quality. As methods of generating evidence have developed and evolved, an evidence hierarchy has taken shape to assign relative merit to different sorts of evidence (Fig. 19.2.2). In general, experimental studies are believed to generate higher-level evidence than comparative (observational and non-randomized) studies. Among the latter, study designs are ranked in quality (low to high) as follows: case series, historical controls, case–control, cohort study. The RCT remains the 'gold standard' of study design, considered to generate the highest-quality and most reliable evidence for evaluating interventions.

Generally, the quality of evidence reported in a clinical trial is defined by its 'internal validity', a term referring to the extent to which the investigators have minimized bias in study design and execution (Juni et al., 2001). Various types of bias can threaten the internal validity of a study. *Selection bias* results when participants in a sample do not truly represent the baseline population, population of interest, or population to which results should pertain. *Performance bias* occurs when participants receive unequal care, apart from the treatment under evaluation. Potential

for procedure selection bias is present when the intervention is chosen in a non-random way for or by the participant. For example, healthier patients may preferentially select or be selected for a particular treatment, and study results may be correspondingly skewed. In post-entry exclusion, certain patients are omitted from the final analyses often due to missing data points or deviation from protocol by introducing significant bias making the study's results no longer legitimately generalizable to the target population. *Attrition bias*, in which certain participants are lost to follow up, causes similar effects. In *assessment bias*, participants, investigators, or both are aware of intervention assignments and this awareness can affect outcome assessments.

Biases lower the quality and reliability of evidence by decreasing the confidence that the observed effect is the true effect (Sackett et al., 1991). Non-randomized studies are prone to selection and assessment bias. Compared to RCTs, non-randomized studies can dramatically under- or overestimate the treatment effect; they most commonly show that the treatment is far better than it really is (Kunz and Oxman, 1998). Chalmers et al. documented this trend as early as 1983, in their review of 145 clinical trials of treatment for acute myocardial infarction. Outcome differences between treatment and control groups were identified in 9% of studies that were blinded and randomized, 24% of unblinded but randomized studies, and 58% of non-randomized studies (Chalmers et al., 1983). A review of RCTs versus historical control trials from the same time period reported that most of the positive findings of historical control trials were later repudiated by RCTs (Sacks et al., 1982, 1983). These findings were corroborated in 1995, with estimations of treatment effect exaggerated by 41% in inadequately concealed trials (Schulz et al., 1995).

There is also the potential for bias after the study is completed. The most relevant example in EBM is *publication bias* in which the results of only a portion of trials relevant to a clinical question are available in the published medical literature (Dickersin et al., 1994; Piantadosi, 1997). In general, positive results are more likely to be published than negative results (Song et al., 2009).

Specific skills required for evidence-based medicine

The 'information paradox', another term that has joined the lexicon associated with present-day medicine, refers to the current situation in which clinicians face an exploding volume of information but, despite a wealth of information, they have trouble

Table 19.2.1 JAMA's 'users' guides to the medical literature' from the evidence-based medicine working group

Article	Lead author	Title
I	Oxman, AD (Oxman et al., 1993)	How to get started
II-A	Guyatt, GH (Guyatt et al., 1993)	How to use an article about therapy or prevention. A. Are the results of the study valid?
II-B	Guyatt, GH (Guyatt et al., 1994)	How to use and article about therapy or prevention. B. What were the results and will they help me in caring for my patients?
III-A	Jaeschke, R (Jaeschke et al., 1994a)	How to use an article about a diagnostic test. A. Are the results of the study valid?
III-B	Jaeschke, R (Jaeschke et al., 1994b)	How to use an article about a diagnostic test. B. What are the results and will they help me in caring for my patients?
IV	Levine, M (Levine et al., 1994)	How to use an article about harm
V	Laupacis, A (Laupacis et al., 1994)	How to use an article about prognosis
VI	Haynes, RB (Haynes et al., 1986)	How to store and retrieve articles worth keeping
VII-A	Richardson, WS (Richardson and Detsky, 1995a)	Are the results of the study valid?
VII-B	Richardson, WS (Richardson and Detsky, 1995b)	What are the results and will they help me in caring for my patients?
VIII-A	Hayward, RS (Hayward et al., 1995)	Are the recommendations valid?
VIII-B	Wilson, MC (Wilson et al., 1995)	What are the recommendations and will they help you in caring for your patients?
IX	Guyatt, GH (Guyatt et al., 1995)	A method for grading health care recommendations
X	Naylor, CD (Naylor and Guyatt, 1996a)	How to use an article reporting variations in the outcomes of health services
XI	Naylor, CD (Naylor and Guyatt, 1996b)	How to use an article about a clinical utilization review
XII	Guyatt, GH (Guyatt et al., 1997)	How to use articles about health-related quality of life
XIII-A	Drummond, MF (Drummond et al., 1997)	How to use an article on economic analysis of clinical practice. A. Are the results of the study valid?
XIII-B	O'Brien BJ (O'Brien et al., 1997)	How to use an article on economic analysis of clinical practice. B. What are the results and will they help me in caring for my patients?
XIV	Dans AL (Dans et al., 1998)	How to decide on the applicability of clinical trial results to your patient
XV	Richardson, WS (Richardson et al., 1999)	How to use an article about disease probability for differential diagnosis
XVI	Guyatt, GH (Guyatt et al., 1999)	How to use a treatment recommendation
XVII	Barratt, A (Barratt et al., 1999)	How to use guidelines and recommendations about screening
XVIII	Randolph, AG (Randolph et al., 1999)	How to use an article evaluating the clinical impact of a computer-based clinical decision support system
XIX-A	Bucher, HC (Bucher et al., 1999)	Applying clinical trial results. A. How to use an article measuring the effect of an intervention on surrogate end points
XIX-B	McAlister, FA (McAlister et al., 1999)	Applying clinical trial results B. Guidelines for determining whether a drug is exerting (more than) a class effect
XX	McAlister, FA (McAlister et al., 2000)	Integrating research evidence with the care of the individual patient
XXI	Hunt, DL (Hunt et al., 2000)	Using electronic health information resources in evidence-based practice
XXII	McGinn, TG (McGinn et al., 2000)	How to use articles about clinical decision rules
XXIII-A	Giacomini, MK (Giacomini and Cook, 2000a)	Qualitative research in health care A. Are the results of the study valid?
XXIII-B	Giacomini, MK (Giacomini and Cook, 2000b)	Qualitative research in health care B. What are the results and how do they help me care for my patients?
XXIV	Richardson, WS (Richardson et al., 2000)	How to use an article on the clinical manifestations of disease

finding and understanding pertinent information both at the time when it is needed and especially at point-of-care (Muir Gray and de Lusignan, 1999). Information access, apprehension, and application are key challenges to clinicians seeking to implement EBM. To overcome the information paradox—a plethora of evidence, but an inability to use it—clinicians need a new set of competencies

that enable them to ask explicit questions, access relevant evidence, evaluate its quality, critique it in light of what is currently known, and assess its applicability to the patient at hand.

Basic steps in practising EBM have been defined beginning with *The Users' Guide to the Medical Literature* series (Table 19.2.1) and in books by Sackett, Guyatt, and colleagues: *Evidence-Based*

Table 19.2.2 Critical appraisal skills

ASSESS the patient	The process begins with the patient who has a clinical problem or question arising from their care
ASK the question	A well-constructed clinical question is derived
ACQUIRE the evidence	Conduct a search and choose the most appropriate resources
APPRAISE the evidence	Appraise the evidence: valid and applicable?
APPLY: talk with the patient	Integrate: evidence and clinical expertise with patient's preferences and apply
EVALUATE: review outcomes and process	Evaluate the patient's outcomes and performance

Source: Data from Sackett, D. L., et al., *Evidence-based Medicine: How to Practice and Teach EBM*, Second Edition, Churchill Livingstone Edinburgh, UK, Copyright © 2000.

Medicine: How to Practice and Teach EBM (Sackett et al., 1997, Sackett et al., 2000), *Clinical Epidemiology: A Basic Science for Clinical Medicine* (Sackett et al., 1991), and *Users' Guides to the Medical Literature: Essentials of Evidence-Based Clinical Practice* (Guyatt et al., 2008). Subsequently, the core approach and skill set, commonly termed 'critical appraisal skills' have been well described (Table 19.2.2).

1. Assess

The starting point of EBM is genuine clinical equipoise: what is the best course of treatment for the patient at hand, or a class of patients? Methods of patient assessment, and thus of defining the clinical scenario and pinpointing the clinical need or question, are addressed in other chapters. In the practice of EBM, the use of robust, validated assessment instruments to fully describe the patient's condition will yield information vital to tailoring the course of care to the individual, in light of best available evidence.

2. Ask

Once the patient's situation has been assessed, clear articulation of the clinical question is a next step essential to EBM. A well-built clinical question includes four elements, usually collapsed into the acronym 'PICO': (1) the specific clinical *Patient, Problem Population*; (2) the *Intervention* in question, including aetiology of the illness in question, prognostic factors, and treatments; (3) a *Comparison* intervention when relevant; and, (4) the clinical *Outcome* or outcomes of interest (Sackett et al., 1997). A helpful framework for categorizing questions about managing specific clinical scenarios appears in Table 19.2.3 (Sackett et al., 2000). Clarification of the question at hand, with respect to a particular patient, focuses the practitioner on the most appropriate intervention, alternative actions (i.e. comparison interventions), and outcome(s) of interest. This, in turn, helps determine the best study design, that is, the study type most likely to generate evidence that will help answer the question (Sackett et al., 1997). Once the question has been formulated, the practitioner is ready for the next step, searching for relevant and appropriate evidence.

3. Acquire

Successful practice of EBM requires the identification of appropriate, high-quality evidence. Pragmatically, for EBM to become the modus operandi of palliative care, clinicians must have convenient access to the evidence (Rubin et al., 2000). The quantity of current evidence may seem to make the task of accessing relevant evidence highly burdensome, time-consuming, and even frustrating. Information technology (IT), however, has dramatically simplified the 'Acquire' step of EBM. Given the volume of evidence that may or may not be relevant to any given clinical question, mastery of this third critical appraisal skill in today's health-care environment requires the ability to use computerized evidence resources and to apply a stratified approach to these resources (Guyatt et al., 2000).

A '4S Model' has been suggested as a hierarchical approach to evidence acquisition. In this model, evidence sources are prioritized in the following order (lowest to highest priority): *Studies* (published reports of clinical trials and other original research), *Syntheses* (meta-analyses and systematic reviews), *Synopses* (evidence-based abstracts printed in journals and other credible sources), and *Systems* (computerized search and decision support systems) (Haynes, 2001).

The clinician seeking evidence begins at the Systems level. Several computerized decision support systems are currently available, such as *Up-to-Date*. The practitioner should note, however, that these sites can lack explicit detail as to how studies were selected for inclusion (Haynes, 2001; Up-to-Date, 2003; WebMD Professional Publishing, 2003). Evidence-based clinical practice guidelines are also at this level of the 4S ladder, especially when IT-enabled, however, such guidelines have varying levels of reliability depending upon approach to development and updates.

At the second level of evidence acquisition, the practitioner accesses synopses of individual studies and reviews, provided in secondary publications such as *ACP Journal Club* (Sackett et al., 1997; Haynes, 2001; Up-to-Date, 2003). The *ACP Journal Club* reviews over 6000 original internal and general medicine articles published each year and from these, culls approximately 300 highest-quality studies (Davidoff et al., 1995). A virtue of these resources is that the publisher has performed an initial review of each study for quality and validity.

Syntheses such as the *Cochrane Database of Systematic Reviews*, exemplifying the third level in the 4S model, incorporate specific methods of review and assembly of data (Haynes, 2001; The Cochrane Collaboration, 2003). Addressing a great number of common clinical concerns, these evidence-based reviews provide an efficient and invaluable resource to busy practitioners. They are however limited to the studies available, and still have a process of selecting the studies to be included.

Finally, in seeking evidence to support EBM, practitioners often go directly to the ever-expanding volume of original studies. Various search tools, such as MEDLINE, Google Scholar, and other electronic bibliographies, are available to facilitate this task. Many universities have proprietary search engines that assist institutionally affiliated clinicians in performing targeted searches of the literature. Subscription services and search tools offered to members by professional associations are also available.

In using the 4S approach to seek evidence, the practitioner looks for the highest-level evidence available for the clinical question at hand (Haynes, 2001; Hunt et al., 2000), considering first what is the highest and likely most accessible level on which to find the answer to the problem, searching for evidence at that level, and if there is no answer there, moving to the next-highest level.

Table 19.2.3 Categories of common clinical questions

Category	Possible questions
Clinical findings	How should findings from the history and physical be interpreted?
Aetiology	Can any causes for the disease be identified?
Clinical manifestations of disease	When, and how often, are clinical manifestations of disease present?
	Can this information help classify the patient's illness?
Differential diagnosis	What other diseases might manifest similarly?
	How do we select those that are likely serious and responsive to treatment?
Diagnostic tests	How are diagnostic tests selected and interpreted?
	How are selected tests used to confirm or exclude a diagnosis?
	What is the precision, accuracy, acceptability, expense, safety, etc. of selected tests?
Prognosis	Can the clinical course of a patient's disease be estimated?
	How likely are complications to occur?
Therapy	How are treatments selected?
	How likely are selected treatments to do good or harm?
	What is the cost/benefit relationship?
	Is the treatment worth the effort?
Prevention	What are the risk factors of the disease?
	Can the risk of the disease be reduced by modifying the risk factors?
	Can the disease be diagnosed early with screening and if so, what screening tests are best?
Experience and meaning	How can we as caregivers empathize with our patient's situation?
	How can we appreciate the meaning that our patients find in their experience?
	Can we improve our understanding of how this meaning influences healing?
Self-improvement	What is the best way for we caregivers to keep up-to-date?
	How can we improve our clinical and personal skills to run a better and more efficient practice?

Adapted from Sackett, D. L., et al., *Evidence-based Medicine: How to Practice and Teach EBM*, Second Edition, Table 1.2, p.19, Churchill Livingstone Edinburgh, UK, Copyright © 2000, with permission from Elsevier.

Evidence can be sought at more than one level to confirm conclusions, and/or to provide depth and nuance to findings.

However, clinicians should beware of the frustration of 'no evidence is available'. The concept of 'best available evidence' implies that the EBM-practitioner uses the best information that is available—which may be a trial, a summary in *Up-to-Date*, or anecdote relayed by a close colleague. The tenets of EBM risk 'lack-of-evidence paralysis' unless the EBM practitioner can confidently adapt the evidence hierarchy to the realities of day-to-day care, and acknowledge that there is not a study to guide every scenario.

4. Appraise

Once evidence has been identified, it must be evaluated before it is applied to a patient in clinical practice. Evaluation of evidence from a study involves assessment of both (a) the appropriateness of the study's methodology to the problem at hand, and (b) the study's methodological quality. Consideration of the former requires an understanding of study type and the outcome(s) being studied. For example, a cross-sectional survey design is an appropriate gold standard design to answer clinical questions related to disease burden, symptom prevalence, or an intervention's acceptability, whereas an RCT is the best design to answer questions related to treatment effectiveness or assess any intervention in the most rigorous way (National Health and Medical Research Council, 2000; Muir Gray, 2001). If the study's methodology appears appropriate to the clinical question, then the EBM practitioner proceeds to consider the validity of its results that depends, fundamentally, on the study's methodological quality.

Assessment of methodological quality demands a systematic approach to reading an article, with a focus on the methods section. Initial review should take note of the study's design, recruitment procedures, eligibility criteria, intervention and comparator, outcomes, measures to assess them, methods to reduce bias (e.g. randomization, blinding), calculation of sample size, duration, and completeness of follow-up (Greenhalgh, 1997). If these aspects appear rigorously described and reasonable, a more in-depth examination begins. Main questions to answer (sometimes referred to as 'primary guides') include:

Were patients randomly assigned to treatments under study?

Was randomization concealed from patients and investigators?

Were all patients enrolled in the trial included in analyses, in the groups to which they were randomized?

A valid study will yield a 'yes' answer to each of these questions. If any of these questions is answered in the negative, the study design is fatally flawed. A finer level of questions to be asked ('secondary guides') include:

Were patients and investigators kept 'blind' to the treatment being received?

Other than the intervention under study, were patients in each group treated equally?

Were groups similar at the outset of the study?

These questions represent important but non-essential elements that may or may not invalidate a study. If a study fails to meet these criteria, the practitioner should critically consider whether or not to use the study in decision-making for a patient (Guyatt et al., 1993, 1994; Guyatt et al., 2008).

What happens when a practitioner encounters a 'no' answer to one or more of the validity questions? Perhaps the study chosen is not a RCT, but no RCT is available and the study being evaluated is the only one published about the clinical question at hand. How does the practitioner resolve this dilemma? Guyatt et al's 'Users' Guides' help the practitioner work through the implications of a negative result (Guyatt et al., 2008). The Users' Guide focused on studies of harm offering instruction for critical evaluation of cohort studies, case-control studies, case series, and case reports (Levine et al., 1994). The practitioner examines studies with an eye to potential sources of bias and discounts studies early if they are not valid. When only lower-quality evidence is available, the practitioner must ask whether or not reliance on best clinical judgement can value add to the decision-making process.

5. Apply

Application of evidence, and in particular the results of a specific study, to an individual patient entails consideration of the generalizability and applicability of the results. Generalizability, also termed external validity, refers to the extent to which a study's findings can be extrapolated beyond the study setting and study population (National Health and Medical Research Council, 2000). Applicability refers to the extent to which a study can be applied to an individual or to a specified group of patients (National Health and Medical Research Council, 2000)

A study's inclusion criteria are the usual starting place for determining whether results are applicable to a patient or clinical population. However, rather than dismissing a high-quality study simply because its eligibility criteria and setting were not consistent with characteristics of the individual patient in question, the practitioner should consider, based on the study's external validity, whether there is a compelling reason that it should not be applied to this individual (Guyatt et al., 1994). In order to be relevant to the individual, the study must consider potential outcomes, harms, and costs that would be important to this individual (Guyatt et al., 1994). Key factors to consider include the individual's risk of a target disorder, likelihood that the biology of the treatment effect will be similar in this individual, risk to this individual of adverse effects, and local availability of the intervention (Dans et al., 1998).

Questions to guide the practitioner's evaluation of applicability include:

Can the intervention be reproduced in this setting?

Can the results be applied to this setting?

Can the results be applied to this individual?

If these questions can be answered affirmatively, then the clinical option should be discussed with the patient (and loved ones, where appropriate) in the context of the patient's preferences and values (National Health and Medical Research Council, 2000; Sackett et al., 2000). Together, the clinician and patient should consider the full range of outcomes that the patient values, and whether, in the case of the clinical option being discussed, the potential benefits outweigh the potential harms and costs (Guyatt et al., 1994).

Both the founders of EBM and its current advocates have underscored the point that EBM is not 'cook book' or 'one size fits all' medicine. The individualized nature of this clinical paradigm is most apparent at the 'Apply' stage, where evidence deemed to be relevant, appropriate, and valid is considered in the process of making clinical decisions, with a specific focus on the patient's unique circumstances, goals of care, values, and preferences.

In EBM, the practitioner integrates valid and meaningful results with knowledge of the individual patient. Chris Silagy, a leading international expert in EBM, noted several important points to be heeded when applying the evidence in patient care. Good doctors and nurses listen and listen and listen to their patients.

◆ Trust is essential to a good doctor–patient relationship.

◆ Honesty is important but so is some hope . . .

◆ Treatment choices need to take account of a patient's values and preferences.

◆ Survival statistics are just that—probabilities of what may happen not what will happen . . .

◆ One can learn to live with uncertainty (Silagy, 2001).

These poignant statements based, in part, on Silagy's experience as a cancer patient are especially salient to the practice of EMB in palliative care.

Practitioners, and palliative care clinicians in particular, must be sensitive to patients and their emotional needs. Even the early publications about EBM remind us that, 'Understanding patient's suffering and how that suffering can be ameliorated by the caring and compassionate physician are fundamental requirements [of evidence-based practice]' (Evidence Based Medicine Working Group, 1992). EBM in practice is about explicitly integrating the findings from systematic acquisition and appraisal of the literature or other evidence resources with patients' needs, fears, desires, and preferences.

Recognizing the paramount importance of the patient's unique characteristics, the initial step in individualizing care in an EBM approach, is to determine the extent to which the individual wants to be involved in decision-making (McAlister et al., 2000). Shared decision-making entails three principal components: (1) disclosure of information, (2) exploration of values about the therapy and potential health outcomes, and (3) actual decision-making (Elwyn et al., 1999; McAlister et al., 2000). Each of these steps requires excellent communication skills as the practitioner must translate concepts and results described in the evidence base into meaningful information that the patient (and his or her loved ones, as appropriate) can understand. Formal decision aids and other forms of evidence-based patient education are available to help the practitioner communicate choices to patients and families (O'Connor et al., 1999; McNutt, 2000; O'Connor, 2001).

In palliative care, the evidence often contains uncertainty about prognosis; 'difficult conversations' are a standard aspect of clinical practice. EBM is well aligned with the principles and practice of palliative care in stressing the need for partnership with patients and/or family members, sensitive communication of relevant information even when it is uncomfortable or entails uncertainty, truthfulness, and respect for the patient's communication preferences. Thus the art encompassed in EBM resides in the integration of science with compassion to guide sensitive communication and optimal, individualized decision-making.

6. Evaluate

Evaluation is an iterative, ongoing process in EBM. With respect to patient outcomes, the practitioner should systematically collect data that can be analysed to evaluate the benefit, and relative harm, of applied interventions. Electronic health records (EHRs) are making this process more efficient, enabling more ready access to data, and facilitating real-time review of the results of intervention. In the future, interoperability of EHR datasets will add power to retrospective analyses of intervention results. Once the practitioner has applied evidence in practice, routine evaluation of the effects of the clinical choice can inform future practice. This continuous feedback guides and improves clinical practice and is the essence of 'learning health care'.

A model advanced by the Institute of Medicine and other agencies, learning health care describes a system in which (1) processes of care are standardized, based on the latest research evidence;

(2) each patient's care is routinely documented in an electronic health record; (3) patients' data are secure, standardized, and interoperable; (4) clinicians have ready access to real-time data and other information relevant to the each patient's care; (5) outcomes of care are regularly assessed to evaluate effectiveness and to identify opportunities for improvement; and, (6) the system 'learns' by refining its activities and functions based on results (Abernethy et al., 2010b; Abernethy, 2011). Although currently most health-care systems fall short of this ideal, the concept of learning health care is gaining traction and will likely provide a powerful framework to house the practice of EBM in years to come.

Self-evaluation, on the part of the practitioner, should take place at each step in practising EBM. The most important evaluations are likely those that the practitioner designs and carries out in his or her own clinical practice, to assess both process and outcomes. Formal audit processes and feedback systems can support self-evaluation, and these methods should constitute the backbone of the practitioner's regular self-evaluation. However, a process for ongoing informal self-evaluation can also provide a framework in which to consider a current situation, a mode of continuous review of care process and results, and insights to guide the development of strategies to improve care.

Principal categories of questions for self-evaluation include:

How well did the EBM process go?

How well was the information applied to the patient?

How well does the practitioner perform in this area for all patients? (Sackett et al., 2000)

The importance of IT to evidence-based medicine

The nature, locus, and quantity of evidence available to support twenty-first century medical care makes IT an indispensable tool for EBM, and IT fluency a necessary skillset for the EBM practitioner. Without an adequate IT infrastructure, clinicians will remain mired in the 'information paradox', unable to implement critical appraisal skills well and in a timely way (Rosenberg and Donald, 1995; Muir Gray and de Lusignan, 1999; Rubin et al., 2000; Bakken, 2001).

Medical informatics, a new and rapidly growing discipline, is the science of information and communication in health care. Recent advances in medical informatics relevant to EBM include a surge in resources available via the internet, computer-based reminder systems for clinicians, secondary databases of summarized evidence that is ready for clinical application, secondary publications, and a host of applications for mobile devices and new software solutions (Haynes et al., 1997). Due to differences in their organizations and clinical environments, palliative care clinicians will vary in the extent to which their practice of EBM is supported by IT infrastructure. Best IT-supported EBM will rest upon five building blocks of an informatics infrastructure: (1) standardized technologies, (2) electronic data, (3) data exchange standards, (4) informatics processes, and (5) informatics competencies (Bakken, 2001).These elements facilitate both the execution of EBM and the generation of evidence to support it. The creation of this infrastructure within any institution requires both considerable investment in terms of resources, education, and leadership, while simultaneously considering critical issues such as the quality of electronic data, methods for synthesizing and presenting evidence, debugging and maintaining IT systems,

and the requirements of multi-disciplinary teams (Haynes et al., 1995). IT systems should be designed with close attention to the information needs of all relevant health-care professionals, rather than unquestioningly choosing the latest technology available (Smith, 1996).

Regardless of their institution's IT infrastructure, all clinicians can avail themselves of the Internet and administrative databases. Web browsing and hypertext links provide convenient portals to an ever-increasing amount of information, though identifying appropriate and reliable content quickly is difficult for the unskilled searcher and busy clinician (Muir Gray and de Lusignan, 1999). Synthesized access points such as the Health Information Resources (formerly National Library for Health) maintained through the National Health Service in the United Kingdom, (National Health Service Information Authority, 2003). PubMed Clinical Queries (National Center for Biotechnology Information, 2003) and the National Guideline Clearinghouse (National Guideline Clearinghouse, 2003) can provide busy practitioners with quick access to high-quality clinical information. For-profit sites such as *Up-to-Date* (<http://www.UpToDate.com>) may provide more extensively synthesized information, although the requirement to join and log on may create a barrier to use (MDConsult, 2003).

The digitalization of health-care data, made possible through IT, has created phenomenal new opportunities for examining various types of evidence. Administrative databases house demographic, organizational, financial, and basic clinical data elements such as deaths, in-hospital complications, hospital length of stay, and readmissions. Insurers and hospitals maintain these databases for administrative tasks like billing, patient flow, and strategic planning. While these databases provide valuable opportunities to review and compare outcomes for large populations, issues related to data quality must first be addressed, including the following (Naylor and Guyatt, 1996b):

- Important patient outcomes such as disability, performance status, distress, and satisfaction are generally not entered

- Coded outcomes may not be measured or entered consistently across the population, inhibiting comparisons

- Interventions may be administered differently, but the variability of administration is often not recorded

- Inaccurate recording and poor data quality ('dirty data') are rampant.

The rationale for EBM in palliative care

Several compelling arguments underlie the effort to promote EBM in palliative care. First in importance is the argument for quality of care. As defined by the Institute of Medicine, 'quality of care is the degree to which health services for individuals and populations increase the likelihood of desired health outcomes and are consistent with current professional knowledge' (Chassin and Galvin, 1998). Embedded in this definition are the concepts of effectiveness and standards of care, both of which are commonly understood to be closely related to evidence. One could make the claim that, indeed, this definition of quality care comes close to restating the original definition of EBM. EBM, and in particular a reliance upon highest-quality available evidence, clinical practice guidelines, and evidence-based decision aids, has been proposed as one method to improve and uphold quality of care. The assumption is that provision of best evidence and convincing information will lead to optimal decision making and thus optimal care (Grol, 2001). Evidence-based secondary research methodologies are critical to quality-focused tasks such as highlighting the most effective interventions, critiquing inferior ones, and identifying areas in which the evidence is inconclusive and which warrant further research.

A second rationale for advancing EBM in palliative care is the argument that increased demand will lead health-care systems to offer more palliative care services and that health-care systems should do so in a rational manner. Demand for palliative care is increasing worldwide, fuelled by ageing of national populations, longer lifespans, and a shift in disease burden from primarily acute illnesses and events to predominantly chronic conditions. Growing public awareness, and expectations on the part of both patients and providers, are also cited as factors helping to increase demand (Muir Gray, 2001), as are trends in disease management, earlier detection of cancers and initiation of palliative care throughout the duration of curative treatment for these patients, and increased referral of non-cancer patients to palliative care. As demand increases, health-care providers will seek to offer services that meet it—to the extent that those services effectively, demonstratively, meet population needs. EBM offers a system for intelligently and intentionally selecting the services that will be made available.

The increasing need and demand for palliative care, leading to provision of more services, will result in greater overall costs of care. In this context, the presence of an evidence base supporting palliative care services and interventions will be critical for sustaining funding and government support. Naturally, health systems of the twenty-first century are striving to restrain potential increases in costs through rational approaches to service delivery, including the practice of palliative care. They are looking for 'best value' health care, wherein an intervention is provided to an individual based upon the physician's advice, evidence that benefits outweighs adverse effects, and 'value for the money' in relation to other interventions (Muir Gray, 2001). In short, in an effort to enhance the value of medical care attained for the expenditure made, they are beginning to require EBM.

As health-care funders begin to mandate an evidence-based approach to care, palliative care will not be immune. The EBM framework synthesizes efficiency, quality, and effectiveness into a systematic process for medical decision-making. For this reason, private and public health-care funders increasingly look to EBM as an effector of health-care reform (Muir Gray, 2001). The practice of EBM provides a mechanism for optimizing value in health care, one physician at a time. When each physician evaluates the effectiveness of interventions using explicit criteria and matches interventions to appropriate clinical patients and settings, aggregate medical care will achieve best results cost-efficiently (i.e. with minimal waste).

EBM offers a viable mechanism for palliative care to meet new performance and reporting requirements. Organizational expectations and policies are changing in ways that emphasize evidence-based practice, with accountability distributed across all levels and types of medical practice. Health care today, a highly competitive and market-driven system, faces increasing directives from financiers to control escalating costs (DeBourgh, 2001). It is no longer sufficient to provide safe and individualized patient care. While managing complex acute and chronic caseloads, practitioners must also demonstrate that the desired patient outcomes are attained in a cost-effective manner, and they must show improvement in the quality of care—all to the satisfaction of regulatory agencies and increasingly informed health-care consumers. EBM can help palliative care practitioners, and palliative care as a discipline, meet these emerging expectation.

Next, to evolve further as a medical discipline and on a par with numerous other specialties and subspecialties, palliative care will need to join its peers in the current paradigm shift. EBM is now commonly recognized throughout medicine as a new paradigm, replacing the long-standing perception of medicine as a healing art with its blended scientific/systematized/personalized basis. Palliative care has been slower to adopt EBM due to the lack of high-quality evidence, numerous barriers to scientifically conducted research, cultural barriers, and difficulty implementing new knowledge into practice (Lunder et al., 2004; Abernethy et al., 2007). As the new paradigm undeniably takes hold, health-care systems, regulatory agencies, and patients will insist upon evidence-based practice in all realms of care and by all practitioners. Credibility of the field of palliative medicine is at stake. Unless palliative care embraces the movement toward EBM, it stands to be relegated to second-class status, marginalized as 'unscientific' at a time when the need for its services is growing exponentially. A similar challenge has been described in the field of nursing: 'Important areas of nursing practice are blighted by the stigma of poor evidence and subtly devalued' (Forbes and Griffiths, 2002). Without EBM, palliative care risks a similar fate.

A final rationale for the adoption of EBM in palliative care is that EBM provides a structured framework to constantly improve the care provided. As new data supporting (or refuting) inventions become available, the explicit EBM approach provides a mechanism to update response to a clinical question with contemporary information. Research advances palliative care interventions and knowledge, while EBM provides the mechanism to advance palliative care practice and policy.

Barriers to evidence-based medicine in palliative care

Estimates claim that only half of palliative care decisions are evidence based, at best. As Irene Higginson highlighted at the end of the past century, part of the problem is a paucity of convincing research evidence in palliative care (Higginson, 1999). The evidence base in this discipline has been expanding over recent years, but even when evidence exists, palliative care practitioners do not consistently apply a systematic, evidence-based approach to the care of patients with advanced and/or life-limiting illness (Lunder et al., 2004). The overall prevalence of palliative care practitioners who possess EBM skills and who routinely implement an EBM approach would be difficult to quantify, but likely remains low.

A variety of philosophical, organizational, and practical reasons have hindered the incorporation of EBM into palliative care. The most important of these barriers have been the lack of a high-quality body of evidence upon which to base clinical practice, barriers to the conduct of rigorous scientific research, and challenges to translation of new evidence into meaningful changes in clinical practice (Lunder et al., 2004; Abernethy et al., 2007). A major task of the palliative care community is to demand research that brings evidence to practice. International clinical trials groups such as the Palliative Care Clinical Studies Collaborative (PCCSC) in Australia (Shelby-James et al., 2012), the Palliative Care Research Cooperative Group (PCRC) in the United States (Abernethy et al., 2010a), and the European Association for Palliative Care Research Network (<http://www.eapcnet.eu/Home.aspx>) are starting to generate the large-scale evidence needed to answer commonly encountered questions.

Traditional critical appraisal skills have seemed ill-suited to the palliative care literature. The perception is that these skills need to be adapted to accommodate the heterogeneity of palliative care scenarios and the nuances of palliative care practice (Lunder et al., 2004; Abernethy et al., 2007; Currow et al., 2009). Rather than denounce EBM critical appraisal skills as irrelevant, the palliative care community must develop tailored solutions fit requirements for working with this population. For example, Currow, Abernethy, and colleagues are developing a templated framework for reporting clinical studies in palliative care so that users of new research data can efficiently generalize and apply findings within their local practice (Currow et al., 2009, 2012; Wheeler et al., 2012). Similarly, the team with (<http://www.caresearch.com.au>) is developing, validating, and curating a portfolio of pre-defined search strategies to support efficient searching of the medical literature for topics pertinent to palliative medicine (Tieman et al., 2005, 2010; Sladek et al., 2006). Suppose a user is looking for palliative care relevant clinical trials about anorexia; a click on the 'anorexia' link will provide a real-time search of PubMed using a validated search string that will identifies trials, sorted by strength of evidence and toggled by timeframe.

Medical disciplines face common challenges as they move toward more evidenced-based approaches, including: unmotivated clinicians, deficiencies of research and critical appraisal skills, unsupportive organizational cultures, inconsistent approaches to evidence, and inadequate IT. EBM cannot be implemented equally well in any practice setting. Prerequisites to the success of EBM, according to Muir Gray, are motivation, competency, and overcoming of the barriers to the EBM approach (Muir Gray, 2001). Evidence-based decision-making requires that clinicians be not only motivated but also equipped with key skills such as critical appraisal, astute clinical judgement, and ability to elicit and incorporate patient preferences (Sackett et al., 1996; Sackett et al., 2000). Muir Gray also emphasized the role of barriers in impeding, or facilitating (if they are overcome), EBM and good clinical decision-making.

Barriers to EBM must be tackled for the clinician to perform well in this new paradigm. The lack of a body of evidence and easy access to the evidence—key requirements of evidence-based practice—represent current and formidable barriers to EBM in many palliative care settings (Rubin and Thomas, 1996). Clinician-level barriers such as inadequate skills, over-reliance on authority, or disinterest (Sackett et al., 1997) also serve to slow the adoption of EBM in this field. The organization within which the palliative care practitioner works can be either a motivator and facilitator, or a barrier, to EBM. Ideally, the organizational culture will support EBM, offer institutional endorsement and incentives, and provide resources and mechanisms, such as IT infrastructure, to facilitate its uptake.

Limitations of evidence-based medicine

As EBM becomes the dominant paradigm across medical disciplines including palliative care, it is important to recognize its inherent limitations. No approach to patient care, old or new, will be without limitations, and conscious attention to these can improve the integrity and quality of care.

In 1999, Straus and McAlister prepared a structured review of published criticisms to evidence-based practice (Straus and McAlister, 2000). Abernethy recapitulated the Straus and McAlister literature search in 2007, focusing on papers written after 1999 (Greenhalgh and Meadows, 1999; McAlister et al., 1999; Woolf, 1999; Trinder and Reynolds, 2000; Scott et al., 2000; Bakken, 2001; Kerigan, 2001; Caplan, 2001; Forbes and Griffiths, 2002; Ford et al., 2002; Hampton, 2002; Temple, 2002; Guyatt et al., 2008; Montori et al., 2008) Principal limitations included the following:

◆ Shortage of coherent, consistent, scientific evidence to inform clinical practice in a variety of areas.

◆ Difficulties in applying evidence to the care of individual patients. There is, as yet, no rubric that provides definitive guidance on how to extrapolate from data presented in studies to its application in the individual patient and variation from individual to individual will continue to make this step challenging. Some interventions supported by the evidence may be unavailable or impractical.

◆ Dependence on physician factors, including willingness to develop new skills and to change modes of practice.

◆ Time and resource constraints. EBM requires time and resources that the busy clinician may not have. IT infrastructure may be insufficient while access to digital libraries and librarians may be unavailable.

◆ Weaknesses of currnet EBM tools. Secondary research methodologies are still crude. Secondary studies quickly become out-dated, and their design poorly accommodates subjective outcomes or a variety of primary outcome measures—which are critical in palliative care. Clinical practice guidelines are relatively new, and are frequently consensus-based rather than evidence-based (with varying levels of embedded conflicts of interest).

◆ Potential for distortion of purpose and principles. Health-care systems can use the banner of EBM as justification for cost-cutting measures. Expansion of for-profit research, and its inclusion as 'evidence' in EBM, could threaten the quality and integrity of the evidence base. A focus on IT, quantitative research, and critical appraisal skills could overshadow other elements of EBM that are also vital, such as traditional skills of performing a physical exam and interviewing patients and families for an adequate and detailed history.

Palliative care practitioners intending to adopt EBM as their mode of practice should be advised that there is a paucity of evidence that EBM works. Because it is hard to conceive of a high-quality RCT of EBM versus usual care, this evidence may not be forthcoming. Moreover, use of an evidence-based approach does not always ensure good decisions (Kerridge et al., 1998). In the delivery of high-quality palliative care, the practitioner's wisdom, human perceptiveness, and judicious and thoughtful consideration of the individual patient must help shape the path indicated by robust evidence.

Concluding remarks

Evidence-based medicine has become the norm across medical disciplines. Its principles are becoming inextricably interwoven into clinicians' expectations of approach to decision-making, organizations' expectations of providers' performance, and patients' and families' expectations of the care they will receive. The many potential advantages of EBM over the previous paradigm include greater effectiveness of the treatment(s) selected for the individual patient, greater consistency in the application of interventions, with interventions being applied in appropriate patients and populations, a studied and conscientious blend of science and compassion, and ultimately, better outcomes for patients, populations, and health-care systems.

The adoption of EBM in palliative care will benefit the field since wide adoption of EBM principles will help establish the position of palliative care among other medical disciplines in which EBM is now the dominant paradigm. Practitioners will benefit from their integration of EBM into their clinical care because its framework will provide them with a systematic and manageable approach to the overwhelming and increasing quantity of available evidence. Patients will benefit when their palliative care providers employ evidence-based best practices by receiving care that is most likely to be effective for them specifically, and that is tailored to their personal needs, characteristics, and preferences.

References

Abbasi, K., Butterfield, M., Connor, J., et al. (2002). Four futures for scientific and medical publishing. *BMJ*, 325, 1472–1475.

Abernethy, A.P. (2011). 'Learning health care' for patients and populations. *Medical Journal of Australia*, 194, 564.

Abernethy, A.P., Ahmad, A., Zafar, S.Y., Wheeler, J.L., Reese, J.B., and Lyerly, H.K. (2010a). Electronic patient-reported data capture as a foundation of rapid learning cancer care. *Medical Care*, 48, S32–38.

Abernethy, A.P., Etheredge, L.M., Ganz, P.A., et al. (2010b). Rapid-learning system for cancer care. *Journal of Clinical Oncology*, 28, 4268–4274.

Abernethy, A.P., Hanson, L.C., Main, D.S., and Kutner, J.S. (2007). Palliative care clinical research networks, a requirement for evidence-based palliative care: time for coordinated action. *Journal of Palliative Medicine*, 10, 845–850.

Bakken, S. (2001). An informatics infrastructure is essential for evidence-based practice. *Journal of the American Medical Informatics Association*, 8, 199–201.

Barratt, A., Irwig, L., Glasziou, P., et al. (1999). Users' guides to the medical literature: XVII. How to use guidelines and recommendations about screening. Evidence-Based Medicine Working Group. *Journal of the American Medical Association*, 281, 2029–2034.

Bucher, H.C., Guyatt, G.H., Cook, D.J., Holbrook, A., and McAlister, F.A. (1999). Users' guides to the medical literature: XIX. Applying clinical trial results. A. How to use an article measuring the effect of an intervention on surrogate end points. Evidence-Based Medicine Working Group. *Journal of the American Medical Association*, 282, 771–778.

Caplan, L.R. (2001). Evidence based medicine: concerns of a clinical neurologist. *Journal of Neurology, Neurosurgery and Psychiatry*, 71, 569–574.

Chalmers, T.C., Celano, P., Sacks, H.S., and Smith, H., Jr. (1983). Bias in treatment assignment in controlled clinical trials. *The New England Journal of Medicine*, 309, 1358–1361.

Chassin, M.R. and Galvin, R.W. (1998). The urgent need to improve health care quality. Institute of Medicine National Roundtable on Health Care Quality. *Journal of the American Medical Association*, 280, 1000–1005.

Currow, D.C., Tieman, J.J., Greene, A., Zafar, S.Y., Wheeler, J.L., and Abernethy, A.P. (2012). Refining a checklist for reporting patient populations and service characteristics in hospice and palliative care research. *Journal of Pain and Symptom Management*, 43(5), 902–910.

Currow, D.C., Wheeler, J.L., Glare, P.A., Kaasa, S., and Abernethy, A.P. (2009). A framework for generalizability in palliative care. *Journal of Pain and Symptom Management*, 37, 373–386.

Dans, A.L., Dans, L.F., Guyatt, G.H., and Richardson, S. (1998). Users' guides to the medical literature: XIV. How to decide on the applicability of clinical trial results to your patient. Evidence-Based Medicine Working Group. *Journal of the American Medical Association*, 279, 545–549.

Davidoff, F., Haynes, B., Sackett, D., and Smith, R. (1995). Evidence based medicine. *BMJ*, 310, 1085–1086.

Debourgh, G.A. (2001). Evidence-based practice: fad or functional paradigm? *AACN Clinical Issues*, 12, 463–467.

Dickersin, K., Scherer, R., and Lefebvre, C. (1994). Identifying relevant studies for systematic reviews. *BMJ*, 309, 1286–1291.

Drummond, M.F., Richardson, W.S., O'Brien, B.J., Levine, M., and Heyland, D. (1997). Users' guides to the medical literature. XIII. How to use an article on economic analysis of clinical practice. A. Are the results of the study valid? Evidence-Based Medicine Working Group. *Journal of the American Medical Association*, 277, 1552–1557.

Elwyn, G., Edwards, A., Gwyn, R., and Grol, R. (1999). Towards a feasible model for shared decision making: focus group study with general practice registrars. *BMJ*, 319, 753–756.

European Association for Palliative Care Research Network (n.d.). *European Association for Palliative Care Research Network*. [Online] Available at: <http://www.eapcnet.eu/Themes/Research/AbouttheEAPCResearchNetwork.aspx>.

Evidence-Based Medicine Working Group (1992). Evidence-based medicine. A new approach to teaching the practice of medicine. *Journal of the American Medical Association*, 268, 2420–2425.

Forbes, A. and Griffiths, P. (2002). Methodological strategies for the identification and synthesis of 'evidence' to support decision-making in relation to complex healthcare systems and practices. *Nursing Inquiry*, 9, 141–155.

Ford, S., Schofield, T., and Hope, T. (2002). Barriers to the evidence-based patient choice (EBPC) consultation. *Patient Education and Counseling*, 47, 179–185.

Giacomini, M.K. (2001). The rocky road: qualitative research as evidence. *ACP Journal Club*, 134, A11–A13.

Giacomini, M.K., and Cook, D.J. (2000a). Users' guides to the medical literature: XXIII. Qualitative research in health care A. Are the results of the study valid? Evidence-Based Medicine Working Group. *Journal of the American Medical Association*, 284, 357–362.

Giacomini, M.K., and Cook, D.J. (2000b). Users' guides to the medical literature: XXIII. Qualitative research in health care B. What are the results and how do they help me care for my patients? Evidence-Based Medicine Working Group. *Journal of the American Medical Association*, 284, 478–482.

Greenhalgh, J. and Meadows, K. (1999). The effectiveness of the use of patient-based measures of health in routine practice in improving the process and outcomes of patient care: a literature review. *Journal of Evaluation in Clinical Practice*, 5, 401–416.

Greenhalgh, T. (1997). How to read a paper. Assessing the methodological quality of published papers. *BMJ*, 315, 305–308.

Grol, R. (2001). Improving the quality of medical care: building bridges among professional pride, payer profit, and patient satisfaction. *Journal of the American Medical Association*, 286, 2578–2585.

Guyatt, G., Rennie, D., Meade, M.O., and Cook, D.J. (eds.) (2008). *Users' Guides to the Medical Literature: Essentials of Evidence-Based Clinical Practice* (2nd ed.). New York: The McGraw-Hill Companies.

Guyatt, G.H., Haynes, R.B., Jaeschke, R.Z., et al. (2000). Users' guides to the medical literature: XXV. Evidence-based medicine: principles for applying the Users' Guides to patient care. Evidence-Based Medicine

Working Group. *Journal of the American Medical Association*, 284, 1290–1296.

Guyatt, G.H., Naylor, C.D., Juniper, E., Heyland, D.K., Jaeschke, R., and Cook, D.J. (1997). Users' guides to the medical literature. XII. How to use articles about health-related quality of life. Evidence-Based Medicine Working Group. *Journal of the American Medical Association*, 277, 1232–1237.

Guyatt, G.H., Sackett, D.L., and Cook, D.J. (1993). Users' guides to the medical literature. II. How to use an article about therapy or prevention. A. Are the results of the study valid? Evidence-Based Medicine Working Group. *Journal of the American Medical Association*, 270, 2598–2601.

Guyatt, G.H., Sackett, D.L., and Cook, D.J. (1994). Users' guides to the medical literature. II. How to use an article about therapy or prevention. B. What were the results and will they help me in caring for my patients? Evidence-Based Medicine Working Group. *Journal of the American Medical Association*, 271, 59–63.

Guyatt, G.H., Sackett, D.L., Sinclair, J.C., Hayward, R., Cook, D.J., and Cook, R.J. (1995). Users' guides to the medical literature. IX. A method for grading health care recommendations. Evidence-Based Medicine Working Group. *Journal of the American Medical Association*, 274, 1800–1804.

Guyatt, G.H., Sinclair, J., Cook, D. J., and Glasziou, P. (1999). Users' guides to the medical literature: XVI. How to use a treatment recommendation. Evidence-Based Medicine Working Group and the Cochrane Applicability Methods Working Group. *Journal of the American Medical Association*, 281, 1836–1843.

Hampton, J.R. (2002). Evidence-based medicine, opinion-based medicine, and real-world medicine. *Perspectives in Biology and Medicine*, 45, 549–568.

Haynes, R.B. (2001). Of studies, syntheses, synopses, and systems: the '4S' evolution of services for finding current best evidence. *ACP Journal Club*, 134, A11–A13.

Haynes, R.B., Hayward, R.S., and Lomas, J. (1995). Bridges between health care research evidence and clinical practice. *Journal of the American Medical Informatics Association*, 2, 342–350.

Haynes, R.B., Jadad, A.R., and Hunt, D. L. (1997). What's up in medical informatics? *Canadian Medical Association Journal*, 157, 1718–1719.

Haynes, R.B., McKibbon, K.A., Fitzgerald, D., Guyatt, G.H., Walker, C.J., and Sackett, D.L. (1986). How to keep up with the medical literature: VI. How to store and retrieve articles worth keeping. *Annals of Internal Medicine*, 105, 978–984.

Hayward, R.S., Wilson, M.C., Tunis, S.R., Bass, E.B., and Guyatt, G. (1995). Users' guides to the medical literature. VIII. How to use clinical practice guidelines. A. Are the recommendations valid? The Evidence-Based Medicine Working Group. *Journal of the American Medical Association*, 274, 570–574.

Higginson, I.J. (1999). Evidence based palliative care. There is some evidence—and there needs to be more. *BMJ*, 319, 462–463.

Hunt, D.L., Jaeschke, R., and Mckibbon, K.A. (2000). Users' guides to the medical literature: XXI. Using electronic health information resources in evidence-based practice. Evidence-Based Medicine Working Group. *Journal of the American Medical Association*, 283, 1875–1879.

Jaeschke, R., Guyatt, G., and Sackett, D.L. (1994a). Users' guides to the medical literature. III. How to use an article about a diagnostic test. A. Are the results of the study valid? Evidence-Based Medicine Working Group. *Journal of the American Medical Association*, 271, 389–391.

Jaeschke, R., Guyatt, G.H., and Sackett, D.L. (1994b). Users' guides to the medical literature. III. How to use an article about a diagnostic test. B. What are the results and will they help me in caring for my patients? The Evidence-Based Medicine Working Group. *Journal of the American Medical Association*, 271, 703–707.

Juni, P., Altman, D.G., and Egger, M. (2001). Systematic reviews in healthcare: assessing the quality of controlled clinical trials. *BMJ*, 323, 42–46.

Kerigan, A. (2001). Modern doctoring. *Clinical Medicine*, 1, 154.

Kerridge, I., Lowe, M., and Henry, D. (1998). Ethics and evidence based medicine. *BMJ*, 316, 1151–1153.

Kuhn, T.S. (1962). *The Structure of Scientific Revolutions*, Chicago, IL: University of Chicago Press.

Kunz, R. and Oxman, A.D. (1998). The unpredictability paradox: review of empirical comparisons of randomised and non-randomised clinical trials. *BMJ*, 317, 1185–1190.

Laupacis, A., Wells, G., Richardson, W. S., and Tugwell, P. (1994). Users' guides to the medical literature. V. How to use an article about prognosis. Evidence-Based Medicine Working Group. *Journal of the American Medical Association*, 272, 234–237.

Levine, M., Walter, S., Lee, H., Haines, T., Holbrook, A., and Moyer, V. (1994). Users' guides to the medical literature. IV. How to use an article about harm. Evidence-Based Medicine Working Group. *Journal of the American Medical Association*, 271, 1615–1619.

Lunder, U., Sauter, S., and Furst, C. J. (2004). Evidence-based palliative care: beliefs and evidence for changing practice. *Palliative Medicine.*, 18, 265–266.

McAlister, F.A., Laupacis, A., Wells, G.A., and Sackett, D.L. (1999). Users' guides to the medical literature: XIX. Applying clinical trial results B. Guidelines for determining whether a drug is exerting (more than) a class effect. *Journal of the American Medical Association*, 282, 1371–1377.

McAlister, F.A., Straus, S.E., Guyatt, G.H., and Haynes, R.B. (2000). Users' guides to the medical literature: XX. Integrating research evidence with the care of the individual patient. Evidence-Based Medicine Working Group. *Journal of the American Medical Association*, 283, 2829–2836.

McGinn, T.G., Guyatt, G.H., Wyer, P.C., Naylor, C.D., Stiell, I.G., and Richardson, W.S. (2000). Users' guides to the medical literature: XXII: how to use articles about clinical decision rules. Evidence-Based Medicine Working Group. *Journal of the American Medical Association*, 284, 79–84.

McNutt, R. (2000). Review: health care decision aids to improve knowledge, decrease decisional conflict, and increase active participation. *ACP Journal Club*, 132, 66.

MD Consult. (2003). *MD Consult member log on page* [Online]. Elsevier. Available at: <http://home.mdconsult.com/bin/login?Tag=/&URI=/>.

Montori, V.M., Guyatt, G.H., Montori, V.M., and Guyatt, G.H. (2008). Progress in evidence-based medicine. *Journal of the American Medical Association*, 300, 1814–1816.

Muir Gray, J.A. (2001). *Evidence-Based Healthcare: How to Make Health Policy and Management Decisions*. Edinburgh: Churchill Livingstone.

Muir Gray, J.A. and De Lusignan, S. (1999). National electronic Library for Health (NeLH). *BMJ*, 319, 1476–1479.

National Center for Biotechnology Information (2003). *PubMed Clinical Queries*. [Online] National Library of Medicine. Available at: <http://www.ncbi.nlm.nih.gov/entrez/query/static/clinical.html>.

National Guideline Clearinghouse (2003). *National Guideline Clearinghouse* [Online]. United States Agency for Healthcare Qualtiy and Research, Department of Human Services. Available at: <http://www.guideline.gov>.

National Health and Medical Research Council (2000). *How to use the Evidence: Assessment and Application of Scientific Evidence*. Canberra: Commonwealth of Australia, NHMRC.

National Health Service Information Authority (2003). *National Electronic Library for Health (pilot site)*. [Online] National Health Service. Available at: <http://www.nelh.nhs.uk/>

Naylor, C.D. and Guyatt, G.H. (1996a). Users' guides to the medical literature. X. How to use an article reporting variations in the outcomes of health services. The Evidence-Based Medicine Working Group. *Journal of the American Medical Association*, 275, 554–558.

Naylor, C.D. and Guyatt, G.H. (1996b). Users' guides to the medical literature. XI. How to use an article about a clinical utilization review. Evidence-Based Medicine Working Group. *Journal of the American Medical Association*, 275, 1435–1439.

O'Brien, B.J., Heyland, D., Richardson, W.S., Levine, M., and Drummond, M.F. (1997). Users' guides to the medical literature. XIII. How to use an article on economic analysis of clinical practice. B. What are the results and will they help me in caring for my patients? Evidence-Based Medicine Working Group. *Journal of the American Medical Association*, 277, 1802–1806.

O'Connor, A. (2001). Using patient decision aids to promote evidence-based decision making. *ACP Journal Club*, 135, A11–A12.

O'Connor, A.M., Rostom, A., Fiset, V., *et al.* (1999). Decision aids for patients facing health treatment or screening decisions: systematic review. *BMJ*, 319, 731–734.

Oxman, A.D., Sackett, D.L., and Guyatt, G.H. (1993). Users' guides to the medical literature. I. How to get started. The Evidence-Based Medicine Working Group. *Journal of the American Medical Association*, 270, 2093–2095.

Piantadosi, S. (1997). *Clinical Trials: A Methodologic Perspective*. New York: John Wiley & Sons, Inc.

Randolph, A.G., Haynes, R.B., Wyatt, J.C., Cook, D.J., and Guyatt, G.H. (1999). Users' Guides to the Medical Literature: XVIII. How to use an article evaluating the clinical impact of a computer-based clinical decision support system. *Journal of the American Medical Association*, 282, 67–74.

Richardson, W.S. and Detsky, A.S. (1995a). Users' guides to the medical literature. VII. How to use a clinical decision analysis. A. Are the results of the study valid? Evidence-Based Medicine Working Group. *Journal of the American Medical Association*, 273, 1292–1295.

Richardson, W.S. and Detsky, A.S. (1995b). Users' guides to the medical literature. VII. How to use a clinical decision analysis. B. What are the results and will they help me in caring for my patients? Evidence Based Medicine Working Group. *Journal of the American Medical Association*, 273, 1610–1613.

Richardson, W.S., Wilson, M.C., Guyatt, G.H., Cook, D.J., and Nishikawa, J. (1999). Users' guides to the medical literature: XV. How to use an article about disease probability for differential diagnosis. Evidence-Based Medicine Working Group. *Journal of the American Medical Association*, 281, 1214–1219.

Richardson, W.S., Wilson, M.C., Williams, J.W., Jr., Moyer, V.A., and Naylor, C.D. (2000). Users' guides to the medical literature: XXIV. How to use an article on the clinical manifestations of disease. Evidence-Based Medicine Working Group. *Journal of the American Medical Association*, 284, 869–875.

Rosenberg, W. and Donald, A. (1995). Evidence based medicine: an approach to clinical problem-solving. *BMJ*, 310, 1122–1126.

Rubin, D.B. and Thomas, N. (1996). Matching using estimated propensity scores: relating theory to practice. *Biometrics*, 52, 249–264.

Rubin, G.L., Frommer, M.S., Vincent, N.C., Phillips, P.A., and Leeder, S. (2000). Getting new evidence into medicine. *Medical Journal of Australia*, 172, 180–183.

Sackett, D.L., Haynes, R.B., Guyatt, G.H., and Tugwell, P. (1991). *Clinical Epidemiology: A Basic Science for Clinical Medicine*. Boston, MA: Little, Brown and Company.

Sackett, D.L., Richardson, W.S., Rosenberg, W., and Haynes, R.B. (1997). *Evidence-based Medicine: How to Practice and Teach EBM*. Edinburgh: Churchill Livingstone.

Sackett, D.L., Rosenberg, W.M., Gray, J.A., Haynes, R.B., and Richardson, W.S. (1996). Evidence based medicine: what it is and what it isn't. *BMJ*, 312, 71–72.

Sackett, D.L., Straus, S.E., Richardson, W.S., Rosenberg, W., and Haynes, R.B. (2000). *Evidence-based Medicine: How to Practice and Teach EBM*. Edinburgh: Churchill Livingstone.

Sacks, H., Chalmers, T.C., and Smith, H., JR. (1982). Randomized versus historical controls for clinical trials. *American Journal of Medicine*, 72, 233–240.

Sacks, H.S., Chalmers, T.C., and Smith, H., Jr. (1983). Sensitivity and specificity of clinical trials. Randomized v historical controls. *Archives of Internal Medicine*, 143, 753–755.

Schulz, K.F., Chalmers, I., Hayes, R.J., and Altman, D.G. (1995). Empirical evidence of bias. Dimensions of methodological quality associated with estimates of treatment effects in controlled trials. *Journal of the American Medical Association*, 273, 408–412.

Scott, I., Heyworth, R., and Fairweather, P. (2000). The use of evidence-based medicine in the practice of consultant physicians. Results of a questionnaire survey. *Australian and New Zealand Journal of Medicine*, 30, 319–326.

Shelby-James, T.M., Hardy, J., Agar, M., *et al.* (2012). Designing and conducting randomized controlled trials in palliative care: a summary of discussions from the 2010 clinical research forum of the Australian Palliative Care Clinical Studies Collaborative. *Palliative Medicine*, 26(8), 1042–1047.

Silagy, C. (2001). A view from the other side: a doctor's experience of having lymphoma. *Australian Family Physician*, 30, 547–549.

Smith, R. (1996). What clinical information do doctors need? *BMJ*, 313, 1062–1068.

Song, F., Parech-Bhurke, S., Hooper, L., *et al.* (2009). Extent of publication bias in different categories of research cohorts: a meta-analysis of empirical studies. *BMC Medical Research Methodology*, 9, 79.

Straus, S.E. and McAlister, F.A. (2000). Evidence-based medicine: a commentary on common criticisms. *Canadian Medical Association Journal*, 163, 837–841.

Temple, J. (2002). Why general practitioners do not implement evidence. Evidence seems to change frequently. *BMJ*, 324, 674.

Tieman, J.J., Abernethy, A.P., Fazekas, B.S., and Currow, D.C. (2005). CareSearch: finding and evaluating Australia's missing palliative care literature. *BMC Palliative Care*, 4, 4.

Tieman, J.J., Abernethy, A.P., and Currow, D.C. (2010). Not published, not indexed: issues in generating and finding hospice and palliative care literature. *Journal of Palliative Medicine*, 13, 669–675.

Sladek, R., Tieman, J.J., Fazekas, B.S., Abernethy, A.P., and Currow, D.C. (2006). Development of a subject search filter to find information relevant to palliative care in the general medical literature. *Journal of the Medical Library Association*, 94, 394–401.

The Cochrane Collaboration (2003). *The Cochrane Library*. [Online] The Cochrane Collaboration. Available at: <http://gateway1.ovid.com/ovidweb.cgi>.

Trinder, L. and Reynolds, S. (eds.) 2000. *Evidence-Based Practice: A Critical Appraisal*. Oxford: Blackwell Science.

Up-To-Date (2003). *Up-to-Date*. [Online] Available at: <http://www.uptodate.com>.

WEBMD Professional Publishing (2003). *Scientific American Medicine*. [Online] WebMD Professional Publishing. Available at: <http://www.samed.com>.

Wheeler, J.L., Greene, A., Tieman, J.J., Abernethy, A.P., and Currow, D.C. (2012). Key characteristics of palliative care studies reported in the specialized literature. *Journal of Pain and Symptom Management*, 43, 987–992.

Wilson, M.C., Hayward, R.S., Tunis, S.R., Bass, E.B., and Guyatt, G. (1995). Users' guides to the Medical Literature. VIII. How to use clinical practice guidelines. B. what are the recommendations and will they help you in caring for your patients? The Evidence-Based Medicine Working Group. *Journal of the American Medical Association*, 274, 1630–1632.

Woolf, S.H. (1999). The need for perspective in evidence-based medicine. *Journal of the American Medical Association*, 282, 2358–2365.

Youngblut, J.M. and Brooten, D. (2001). Evidence-based nursing practice: why is it important? *AACN Clinical Issues*, 12, 468–476.

Understanding clinical trials in palliative care research

John T. Farrar

Introduction to understanding clinical trials in palliative care research

Components of the randomized, controlled trial (RCT) have been part of clinical research for several centuries but the modern concept of the importance of the random selection of a control group can be traced to one of the first studies of streptomycin for pulmonary tuberculosis conducted by the British Medical Research Council and published in 1948 (Anonymous, 1948, 1998). Prior to that time, the evaluation of health care relied on what today would be considered anecdotal evidence. The RCT represents the gold standard for the evaluation of the efficacy of new medical therapies. Despite their status, several potential scientific and ethical difficulties continue to limit the use of RCTs in some clinical contexts such as palliative care, and hinder the generalizability of their results in others. Understanding these limitations and how to apply the results of such studies to clinical care is important.

By presenting the various strengths and limitations that are common to all RCTs and how they apply to trials of palliative care interventions, we will be considering how decisions made regarding trial design, conduct, and analysis can influence the trial's results. Basic issues in the analysis of clinical trial data as they apply to the interpretation of RCT results will also be considered. This chapter will provide palliative care clinicians with a proper understanding of the structure and inherent problems with clinical trials. No research experiment can ever be perfect, but the information provided by RCTs is extremely useful as a basis for evidence-based approaches to clinical care. With this knowledge, the reader of science should be able to ascertain whether the results of published trials are (1) likely to be valid and (2) likely to apply to their patients.

The anatomy of a trial

To maximize the usefulness of clinical trials, study design issues must be considered from conceptualization, through implementation, and ending with the interpretation of results. Decisions made regarding every component of an RCT can dramatically influence the quality of the data and the outcome of a trial. Subtle flaws at any stage may lead to inappropriate conclusions.

Even when a clinical trial is perfectly designed, there is no guarantee of finding the right answer to a specific research question. Because of random variation from a sample of the whole population of interest, there is always a probability of reaching a false positive or a false negative conclusion simply by chance. Statistical analyses are necessary to define the extent of this probability.

A statistical analysis is conducted primarily to (1) summarize the data by estimating the size of the effect being observed that can be attributed to the treatment being tested and (2) to estimate the probability that the results obtained occurred simply by chance. The conventional selection of a p-value cut-off point of 0.05 means that we are willing to accept a 1/20 probability of getting a false positive answer by chance alone. The selection of the power for the study to detect a true change if one exists (often set at 90%) accepts a 10% chance of a false negative. As a result, replication of a trial's results is always preferable before clinicians can confidently make decisions about patient care, since no single trial should ever be considered definitive proof of the presence or absence of efficacy.

The question

The initial step in designing any trial or understanding the results is to define what research question is being asked. This can seem like a relatively simple process, but it is often a tremendous challenge to replicate a clinical reality in the research setting. To properly design a clinical trial requires reducing an important clinical question into a testable hypothesis. Many clinically relevant questions cannot be studied because the appropriate population is not available, the number required may be prohibitively large, or for ethical issues.

In such situations it is often necessary to modify the research question to one that is more readily answerable or to choose a different clinical study design, such as an observational cohort study. It is important to understand that getting an answer to a different question, may or may not allow its application to the original clinical scenario. Attempting to answer the right question may result in compromises in the study design, sacrificing either precision or protection from bias. In some cases, alteration of the design may reduce the value of the knowledge, and hence alter the risk–benefit calculation used to justify the research (Freedman, 1987; Emanuel et al., 2000). From the outset, an alternative design should be considered if the investigators are not clear about the clinical importance of answering the proposed question.

The choice of an appropriate outcome and choice of the measure to be used to collect the data are important steps. To ensure that the research question can be answered a clinically relevant primary outcome must be selected that can be appropriately measured, analysed, and the results interpreted. This must be done a priori, that is, before the data are collected or analysed. In order to maintain acceptable limits on the probability of arriving at an incorrect result by chance both the clinical importance of the effect of an intervention and the characteristics of the data to be collected must be defined. Although multiple secondary outcomes are often also tested within a single trial, each should be identified at the outset, and none should subsequently be designated as the primary outcome after the data have been collected and analysed (a posteriori).

Choosing outcomes is often dependent on the disease area to be studied. A recently published summary of outcomes created in conjunction with the Agency for Healthcare Research and Quality (AHRQ) have specified areas, including symptom management, quality of life (QOL), function and satisfaction, family burden, and quality-of-death measures. There are a number of evaluative tools that have been used over time or recommended by various groups, but they are beyond the scope of this chapter and well described elsewhere (Mularski et al., 2007). Almost all of the measures used for palliative care studies are patient-reported outcomes, which require a thoughtful approach to collection, analysis, and interpretation.

Types of trials

Part of the process of answering the appropriate clinical question is choosing the correct design of the trial. While there are many different variations on an RCT, the two basic formats are to design a trial to demonstrate an effect (either beneficial or harmful) of an exposure (or treatment) over no exposure; or to design a trial to demonstrate equivalence between two different treatments. In both cases, the goal is to demonstrate a difference in outcome between the treatment groups that usually has a less than 5% probability of occurring by chance (i.e. a p-value < 0.05) and with an appropriate probability of detecting a difference, if one truly exists (i.e. a power of > 80% or 90%). While the statistical issues need to be determined appropriately, the more difficult concerns usually involve other issues in clinical trial design. The majority of this chapter will focus on the other issues involved in the design and interpretation of clinical trials.

Efficacy trials

An efficacy trial is designed to demonstrate that the two groups are not the same (i.e. also described as rejecting the null hypothesis). This trial benefits from the fact that demonstrating two things are different is substantially easier than proving that two things are the same. The determination of an appropriate sample size is based on established probability calculations that take into consideration the underlying variability of the measurement and the size of the effect to be evaluated, in addition to the appropriate p-value and power.

Non-inferiority and equivalence trials

When there are significant concerns about the difficulties in conducting a placebo-controlled trials, investigators may design a clinical trial to show that a new drug is 'no worse than' a treatment that is commonly accepted as effective (i.e. a non-inferiority or equivalency trial). In evaluating therapeutics for conditions in which the risks of placebo assignment are widely regarded as too great, such as thrombolytic agents for acute myocardial infarction

or stroke, active-controlled, non-inferiority trials are the standard (Anonymous, 1997a, 1997b).

These trials are presently not considered standard for problems such as hypertension, hyperlipidaemia, and pain, because there are several potential problems with interpreting such studies (Jones et al., 1996; Temple, 1996, 1997; Van De Werf et al., 1999; Fleming, 2000). The first problem is that equivalence trials essentially aim to confirm the conventional null hypothesis of no treatment difference. Since a lack of difference in the outcomes detected between treatment groups can be the result of an inappropriate study design, problems with the study conduct, or other unexpected difficulties with the clinical trial, questions frequently remain about the validity of the results of such trials. This may create inappropriate incentives for conducting 'sloppy' research (Ellenberg and Temple, 2000). Secondly, such trials generally require larger numbers of participants, because equivalence or non-inferiority must be documented within relatively narrow margins to be clinically relevant. Thirdly, demonstrating that two treatments have the same outcome does not show that either of them work. This problem is related to 'assay sensitivity', because such trials require the assumption that the standard therapy would have proven superior to placebo had a placebo arm been included in the study design used (Temple, 1996). Because of these concerns, current regulatory guidelines still call for placebo-controlled trials to evaluate treatments for problems such as pain and other symptoms (Food and Drug Administration, 2001) where no established gold standard therapy exists.

Randomization

The most important feature of an experimental clinical trial is the equivalence of the comparison groups at baseline such that any differences measured at the end can be attributed only to the differences between the treatments administered. Random selection of subjects from a sufficiently large single population equally distributes known and unknown factors that might otherwise influence the outcome, such as age, sex, race, and disease severity.

This is in contrast to observational studies (e.g. case–control, cohort, or cross-sectional studies) which depend on nature to set up the experiment. In these types of studies, there is a substantial possibility that known or unknown factors may create differences between the comparison groups at baseline, limiting our ability to attribute any subsequent changes to the treatment. By using statistical methods to adjust for potentially important confounders, some of these factors can be taken into consideration; however, unmeasured confounding or bias can potentially lead to the wrong conclusion from the study. In experimental studies, randomization is the primary mechanism used to create equivalence between the comparison groups. By minimizing the possibility of differences at baseline, an RCT enables investigators to more confidently attribute observed changes over time to the assigned treatments.

True randomization is accomplished by generating a set of random numbers, and distributing them via a mechanism that protects the integrity of the random assignment. A centrally managed randomization scheme may help to ensure consistent application of the procedure across sites and staff. Central control of the randomization will also prevent members of the study team, from knowingly or unknowingly influencing the assignment, especially if they are not be blinded to a patient's treatment allocation.

Randomization works correctly only when sufficient numbers of patients are enrolled to ensure an equal distribution of all important factors. In smaller trials, or in large, multicentre trials with few participants from a given centre, chance alone may cause significant differences in the distributions of important demographic or disease-related characteristics between groups. In order to reduce the likelihood of such occurrences, investigators can use a block randomization scheme to ensure that selected participant characteristics will be equally distributed. For example, if investigators wished to guarantee an equal sex distribution among two treatment arms at multiple sites, they may randomize in blocks of six participants each, within each of which three participants would be male and three would be female. To assess the success of the randomization process, the analysis of all clinical trials should include a careful comparison of the baseline characteristics of the treatment groups to assure that they are approximately equivalent.

Control group

The purpose of the control group is to provide an appropriate comparison for the treatment group, in order to be able to attribute causality to the treatment if a difference is found. The treatment can be as specific as an individual medication such as an opioid (Abernethy et al., 2003), a physical treatment modality such as massage therapy (Kutner et al., 2008), or as complex as a whole-system approach such as inpatient hospice care (Gade et al., 2008). Assuming that the treatment groups are equivalent at baseline (through randomization), then the differences seen in outcome of the groups can be attributed to differences in the treatment. The degree to which blinding is applied to each group is important in defining what aspect of care is being studied and for the ability to interpret the resulting data (see following paragraphs).

There are three primary types of control groups that have a role in clinical trials: (1) a no-treatment control, (2) a placebo control, and (3) an active control. Each type provides different information in comparison to the active treatment group, and the usefulness will depend on the research question that is being explored by the study. The unblinded no-treatment control group can provide information about changes that happen based on the (1) natural history of the disease (i.e. normal variation in the status of any disease state) and (2) regression to the mean (i.e. patients with severe symptoms tend to get better), but does not control for the effect of patient's knowing their treatment group (i.e. a mind–body interaction). The placebo treated control group, when properly blinded, also controls for the mind–body interaction that occurs either from participating in a clinical trial or because of the subject's belief in the therapy. The mind–body response is an especially important part of many symptomatic therapy trials. An active control group is best thought of as a standard to test if the design and conduct of the clinical trial was to detect a difference if the study treatment has a real effect. By administering a drug known to be active in the disease being tested, a positive result provides evidence that the study has been properly designed and conducted. If the experimental agent then does not demonstrate an effect, the negative result is more convincing. Conversely, if the active agent does not produce an effect, the design and conduct of the trial are called into question. In this situation, a negative result with the experimental agent is as likely to be due to the problems in the design as a true lack of efficacy.

No-treatment-controlled trials

An unblinded no-treatment or standard of care control group, where participants receive no intervention or a delayed intervention, is applicable in two primary situations. The first situation arises when there are practical and/or ethical problems with using a placebo or sham control. For example, it is often difficult to construct an appropriate sham intervention for many trials of surgical interventions. Even if adequate shams could be constructed, some feel that assigning patients to receive an invasive, but non-active, intervention is unethical (Hrobjartsson and Gotzsche, 2001). A randomly assigned control group is still a major advantage over not having a control group, but the results must be viewed cautiously since there are many factors that can affect a subject's response to a treatment, when both the subject and the investigator know the group assignment. As discussed in the following paragraphs, it is important that the study staff that collect and record the outcome measures are blinded to the subject's group.

The second situation occurs when one of the goals of the trial is to determine the magnitude of the mind–body placebo effect. The placebo treated group will have a response that is a mix of the natural history of disease and regression to the mean, along with the mind–body placebo effect. By having a no-treatment-control group, the mind–body placebo effect can be estimated. In a meta-analysis of 114 trials employing both placebo- and no-treatment-controls, the placebo effect was less than might be expected, but in symptomatic relief the effect can be large (Hardy et al., 2012). In pain research, the placebo-control group patients typically have a more favourable outcome than those in no-treatment-control groups (Chaput de Saintonge and Herxheimer, 1994).

Blinded placebo-controlled trials

A blinded placebo control group is the best known and most widely used of the possible control groups. A placebo is defined as an inactive treatment designed to mimic as closely as possible, the characteristics of the active treatment. The purpose is to have the control group treated exactly the same as the treatment group except for the specific component being tested. The usefulness of a placebo assumes that at least the study subject and data collector will be blinded to the type of therapy being administered. Creating a placebo for a drug trial is relatively straightforward. An inactive substance is formulated to have similar appearance, route of administration, and, if appropriate, taste as the active treatment. Procedure-oriented therapies are much harder to mimic and therefore, it is significantly harder to obtain true blinding (see following paragraphs). In the absence of blinding, the placebo group is equivalent to the no-treatment group.

The primary benefit of using a blinded placebo control group, rather than a no-treatment control group, is that it enables the specific efficacy of the new intervention to be distinguished from the many non-specific effects that occur with most therapies, including the well-known mind–body interaction (also called the placebo effect) (Freedman et al., 1996a, 1996b). The placebo control group is a group of patients who are treated with a placebo. The response measured in this group results from all three separate processes, namely (1) natural history of the disease, (2) regression to the mean, and (3) the mind–body interaction. The mind–body interaction is a change in brain function that, at least temporarily, leads to improvement in the bodily signs or symptoms. The mind–body interaction is also sometimes known as a non-specific action of treatment, while the direct effect of the therapy on the disease is known as a specific action of the therapy.

Assuming a simple additive model of treatment effects, the magnitude of the placebo effect in a given study can be estimated by the mean (or median) response in the placebo group and subtract the response in the no-treatment group. In addition, the placebo group response can be subtracted from the mean response in the active treatment group to estimate the specific efficacy of the new intervention. Though the existence of true placebo effects across a broad range of clinical interventions can vary depending on the disease being treated, the treatment modality, and the outcome expectation of the patients, the effect is generally larger in studies of the treatment of symptoms and in the management of pain (Hrobjartsson and Gotzsche, 2001). In such therapy trials, it is unclear if this additive model applies, complicating the assessment of the specific effect (Enck et al., 2011).

A placebo control group assumes the study will be conducted in a double-blind fashion. This helps to avoid the biases that may ensue if patients, investigators, or both, knew who would be receiving which treatment. But there are also costs to using a placebo control. The first, and most obvious, is that placebo-controlled trials require that some patients be given an inactive treatment. This is ethically questionable if there are effective interventions in existence, especially in palliative care trials, and remains a hotly debated topic (Rothman and Michels, 1994; Freedman et al., 1996a, 1996b; Temple and Ellenberg, 2000), and is considered further elsewhere in this book. The second cost to conducting placebo-controlled trials is that, while they remain the gold standard for documenting absolute efficacy, they do not always answer a clinically relevant question. For practising clinicians, who have several symptomatic therapies at their disposal, knowing whether another medication works better than nothing is not as important as knowing how the new therapy compares to the existing standard of care (Halpern and Karlawish, 2000).

Participant selection

Another critical decision for investigators designing trials, and for clinicians who use the data, regards the selection of study participants. There are two conflicting priorities: (1) ensuring similarities between participants in the experimental and control groups and (2) testing a new treatment in a sample of patients likely to reflect all those who could benefit from using the intervention. To meet the first goal, investigators would attempt to enrol patients who are relatively homogenous so there are fewer differences to equalize with randomization. Strict inclusion and exclusion criteria allow greater confidence that the observed differences in outcomes are attributable to the treatments being compared, rather than to undetected confounding variables related to the compositions of participants in each group.

By contrast, meeting the second goal requires enrolling participants from a more heterogeneous population. Because of the large interpersonal variability inherent in such a population, this approach can substantially increase the number of participants required to assure that the trial has adequate statistical power to document a treatment difference, if one exists. If a large enough sample size is available, a heterogeneous sample allows subgroup analyses to be conducted, and so potential variations in a

treatment's efficacy among higher- and lower-risk patients may be identified. As a result, early investigations of efficacy are commonly conducted using a select group of participants, whereas later, more definitive trials attempt to enrol more broadly representative patient samples often termed effectiveness studies. Physicians should, therefore, consider the composition of a given trial's sample in order to determine the extent to which the results are applicable to their own patients.

In palliative care populations, there is the additional issue of the frailty of the population and the potential lack of stability in their disease state over time. Finding patients who will remain relatively stable for the duration of the trial can be a difficult challenge. In addition, vulnerable populations may make choices that are not always consistent with the goals of a trial, either to participate out of desperation or to not participate because they do not want to be part of an experiment. There is frequently the additional problem of the ability of some patients to understand enough about their disease to be able to give an informed consent. When patients are cognitively challenged in addition, the process of recruitment can become a seemingly overwhelming task. The ethical issues surrounding these problems are considered elsewhere in this book (White and Hardy, 2010).

Blinding

Over the last century, a growing understanding of the ability of the mind to influence functions of the body, along with the desire to enhance the experimental rigor of clinical trials has increased appreciation of the need for blinding. Recall that the primary goal of a clinical trial is to ensure that any changes between groups seen at the end of the trial may be attributed to a specific treatment being studied. To accomplish this, not only must all comparison groups be similar at the start, but participants in all groups should feel that they have the same probability of getting the real treatment. Thus, the blinding of the study participants is of substantial importance, and investigators must design the study to prevent the participants from unblinding themselves. In particular, if a medication has a specific taste, common side effects, or other distinctive traits, it is important that the placebo treatment mimic these characteristics as closely as possible. Although the evaluation of more invasive interventions for some medical conditions have occasionally used sham procedures (Cobb et al., 1959; Macklin, 1999) this has no place in palliative care research.

In addition to creating a suitable placebo, investigators should plan to determine whether the blinding was maintained by asking participants what treatment they think they received and why. Such questions should be posed to participants occasionally during the trial, and at the trial's completion (Morin et al., 1995). If the blinding is successful, the participants' guesses should be no more accurate than chance (e.g. 50% in a typical two-arm trial). Blinding can be difficult to maintain (Karlowski et al., 1975; Brownell and Stunkard, 1982; Howard et al., 1982; Byington et al., 1985; Rabkin et al., 1986; Moscucci et al., 1987; Fisher and Greenberg, 1993; Basoglu et al., 1997). Study participants can often predict their receipt of placebo due to the absence of side effects, or their receipt of the real treatment by noting adverse effects of the intervention. However, common side effects often occur in the placebo group by chance helping to blind the patients (Sanderson et al., 2013).

When only participants are blinded to the treatment received, the study is labelled as a single-blind trial. The standard use of the term double-blind applies when both the participants and investigators are blinded, assuming that the investigator is collecting the outcome data. If the investigator is not collecting the data, it is critical to blind the person who is, so as to minimize the chance that evaluators will more favourably rate those receiving the innovative treatment, thereby biasing the trial toward finding a benefit of that treatment. Even in studies where the subject fills out their own forms, blinding of the investigator remains important to minimize the possibilities that they would impart different levels of enthusiasm, or prescribe different co-interventions, to patients in the different treatment groups.

Sample size

The statistical power of an RCT to show a difference between treatments is determined by:

1. The size of the effect—treatment effect (i.e. difference in the response among groups) that is deemed to be clinically important to be able to detect.

2. The variance—variability of the outcomes in each treatment group.

3. The p-value (α or type I error rate)—probability of *finding* a difference in the treatment effect of the size detected in the study or larger by chance alone when *there is not* a true effect. This is usually chosen to connote statistical significance and typically set at 0.05.

4. The power (1 − β or 1 − type II error rate)—β is the probability of *not finding* a difference in the treatment effect of the size detected in the study or smaller by chance alone when *there is* a true effect. Power is 1 − β and adequate power is usually set to be 80–90% (i.e. β is set to 10–20%)

In general, the size of the sample to be tested (i.e. sample size) is the variable investigators most commonly adjust to obtain adequate power to detect a meaningful treatment difference when one truly exists and the p-value is outcome of the statistical test conducted upon completion of the clinical trial. It is a truism that with a sufficiently large sample size, any real difference between groups, no matter how small or clinically irrelevant, can be shown to be statistically significant. The converse is also true: a large, clinically important difference (CID) between treatments can fail to reach statistical significance when inadequate numbers of participants are enrolled.

The most common method of calculating the sample size required to achieve 80% power (or greater) is to first determine (1) the size of the effect that would be considered clinically important, (2) the anticipated response in the control group, and (3) the expected variability of the outcomes among the groups. This last determination may be particularly difficult to estimate, and should, when possible, be based on evidence from prior studies of similar diseases and/or treatments. An alternate method used when the sample size is fixed is to calculate the size of the effect that would need to be present to produce a statistically significant outcome. This approach is rarely preferable to setting the sample size to detect a specified difference but is commonly used when the available population is fixed.

Outcome measurement

Another critical decision to be made in planning an RCT involves how to measure the chosen outcome of interest. For example, if investigators are interested in studying the effects of a new antihypertensive agent on systolic and diastolic blood pressure, should they measure these values with a mercury sphygmomanometer or via an arterial line? In addition to how the outcome will be measured, investigators must further consider when and how often to measure the outcome. Are single readings once each week adequate, or should participants be equipped with ambulatory blood pressure monitors to obtain multiple readings throughout the day? Finally, investigators must consider how to account for other variables that could alter the measurement, such as body position, when the blood pressure is assessed. In palliative care, a frequent concern about the outcome is whether to measure a specific symptom (e.g. pain) or sign (e.g. physical function) or the more general outcome of quality of life. Similar to the hypertension model, the question of which measure to use and time period to consider is an important decision to consider in the design of a trial. Ultimately this decision is best made based on the clinical or scientific question that is primary reason for conducting the clinical trial.

Regardless of what measurement technique is chosen, it should be characterized by three features. Firstly, the measurement should be reliable—if the same measure is used repetitively in the same person under identical conditions without this person's condition changing, then the measure should produce the same results each time. Secondly, the measure should be valid—it should measure exactly what it is intended to measure. Thirdly, the measure should be responsive—it should change over time if the condition being measured has truly changed. Though a full discussion of these concepts is beyond the scope of this chapter, the topics are well covered in many textbooks (Streiner and Norman, 2003). If the outcome measure has been not routinely used in other similar research, its reliability, validity, and responsiveness should be formally tested and documented in the intended population.

The criteria of reliability, validity, and responsiveness also depend on what form the outcome takes. For example, in pain management, the primary goal is to improve the patient's subjective sense of comfort. For this purpose, investigators might ask a simple question, such as, 'Do you feel better, yes or no?' Because such a measure has only two possible responses, it may not provide an adequately responsive measure of pain relief.

To help differentiate the level of response, investigators might ask, 'What percentage of pain relief do you get from the treatment?' However, such questions require patients to remember their previous conditions in order to report the change over time. Alternatively, investigators could use a 0–10 numerical rating scale at both the beginning and end of the study to calculate the change in pain over time. Deciding which measurement is most appropriate for a given situation should be informed by considerations of how much change in the measure would be important to the patient, and the ability of the chosen scale to detect such a change.

Another measurement concern in palliative care trials relates to the fact that a change in pain or nausea may only provide one component of an overall change in quality of life. Thus, symptomatic reports may be incomplete surrogate markers for changes in the more complete outcome, the overall quality of life. The use of surrogate markers is a widespread practice in clinical trials. For example, investigators routinely monitor changes in serum cholesterol as a surrogate measure for one of the risk factors for myocardial infarction. However, using this surrogate measure requires making the assumption that a reduction in cholesterol will lead to a reduced risk of myocardial infarction. Similarly, if the use of an experimental analgesic agent relieves pain but produces substantial side effects, the patient may not consider its use as an improvement in quality of life. Therefore, if investigators wish to know an intervention's effects on both the level of pain and the overall quality of life, then they must employ tools to measure both. Since there is no single measurement strategy that is universally applicable, it is important to carefully consider whether the measured outcome is appropriate to answer the research question being posed in the clinical trial. The systematic reporting of the benefits and harms of an intervention allows a net effect to be calculated.

Analysis

Like other aspects of a clinical trial, the specific analytic strategy should be defined before commencing the study. Many different analytic approaches are possible and each will produce an answer to a slightly different research question. It is important that the chosen strategy be appropriate to evaluate the primary research question, and be compatible with the numerical distribution of the data collected. The primary role of the analysis is to summarize the data (size of the effect) and to provide an estimate of the likelihood that the result was obtained by chance alone (i.e. statistical significance).

Effect size

The first, and most important, result of any analysis is a summary value of the size of the effect resulting from the experimental therapy. In RCTs, the size of the effect is estimated by determining a summary value for the primary outcome in each treatment groups, and then calculating the difference between these values to reveal the difference in the treatment effect. There are only two primary forms for the summary value for a set of trial data: (1) the central tendency (e.g. mean, median, or mode) of the response among participants, or (2) the proportion of participants who achieve a defined level of response.

For example, in a hypertension trial, investigators can report the mean change in diastolic blood pressure (central tendency), or the proportion of patients who achieve a diastolic blood pressures below 90 mmHg (proportion of responders). If one were interested in the effect of a hospice intervention on hospital length of stay, it might be acceptable to report either the median time spent in the hospital for each group (central tendency), or the proportion of patients in each group who die before discharge or some other predefined time period. Finally, in trials of pain management, in which the outcome of reported pain symptoms is provided on a numeric scale, investigators might either report the mean response in each group, or the percentage of patients in each group reporting pain reductions of 33% (or 50%) or greater in pain intensity. In each case, the units of these summary values should correspond to the units of the outcome measure.

Choices regarding how to best present the summary measures should reflect the type of information that is most relevant for the scientific or clinical question. In addition, ultimately results will need to have applicability to practising clinicians. For most health-care providers, the question of interest is whether a given treatment will work for a given patient rather than the average change that is likely in a population. The average change does not provide a unique answer to the question of the number of people who are likely to improve. For example, suppose investigators reported that the mean response in the active treatment group was an improvement of 10% on a standard pain scale. This same result could apply to data indicating that (1) every patient in the active treatment group improved by 10% (a unimodal distribution), (2) half of the patients in the treatment group improved by 20% and half had no improvement (a bimodal distribution), or (3) half of the patients in the active treatment group improved by 40%, and half deteriorated by 20% (a bimodal distribution in which some patients improve and other deteriorate). Because these three descriptions of the underlying data could yield strikingly different clinical decisions, it is important to present an analysis of the proportions of patients in each group who improve or deteriorate by a clinically important amount.

What is a clinically important difference?

A common concern about presenting the proportion of 'responders' in each group is the need to define a level of response to be considered clinically important. Thus, the determination of a CID in a patient's symptoms plays a key role in the interpretation of symptomatic studies. Two methods for determining the CID are 'expert opinion', and an assessment of how changes in symptom scales correspond to responses to global questions (Jaeschke et al., 1989, 1991; Todd, 1996). Regardless of the method used, however, each requires that a somewhat arbitrary decision be made in defining the scale to be considered the standard.

Recent studies of pain have adopted an alternative method of displaying response data, but graphing the proportion of responders at each possible outcome level for all the groups in a clinical trial (Farrar et al., 2006). This display is a form of a cumulative distribution and allows the readers of the published report to select the level of improvement that they feel is clinically important and then determine the difference between the various groups at that level.

Statistical considerations

Statistical significance (p-values and confidence intervals)

A p-value of 0.05 or higher is the most commonly accepted statistical test of the probability that a given result occurred by chance. However, this value is strictly arbitrary and is an indication that we are willing to accept a 1/20 chance of getting the wrong answer. This traditional method of hypothesis testing, in which p-values are reported to quantify the significance of a result, is gradually being replaced by methods used to gauge the range of plausible results that are compatible with the data. The most common method for presenting this range is to report a point estimate of the effect size, along with a 95% confidence interval around this estimate. A 95% confidence interval will include the true population value of the effect 19 times out of 20 (95%). Thus, it can help readers determine the uncertainty inherent in any result—the narrower the interval, the more precise the estimate of the true effect, and thus, the more confident readers can be that the reported result is 'correct'.

Multiple comparisons

It is also important to realize that when investigators choose a p-value of 0.05 as an acceptable type I (false positive) error rate, this value only applies to a single comparison between groups. In most clinical trials, however, performing multiple comparisons can be informative. However, the greater the number of comparisons, the more likely it is that at least one of them will be spuriously positive by chance alone. If an a priori decision is made to perform multiple comparisons, the p-value must be adjusted. Of the several available methods for adjusting this value, the simplest is to divide the p-value for one comparison by the number of comparisons to be performed, and to then use this new p-value as the cut-off for statistical significance across all analyses, called the Bonferroni adjustment (Hilsenbeck and Clark, 1996). While valid, this is a very conservative estimate, and alternative methods have been developed to deal with multiple comparisons (Liu et al., 1997).

A related issue regards the distinction between comparisons chosen a priori, and those which investigators choose to conduct post hoc, or after the data have been collected. There are times when post hoc comparisons can be informative, but the results of such analyses should never be considered conclusive because they were not explicitly planned at the outset. Rather, results of post hoc analyses may be considered exploratory, intended to guide future investigations by defining or refining new hypotheses. Authors can help highlight this distinction by reporting which comparisons were chosen a priori, and which were not.

Evidence from secondary measures

In addition to the reported effect size and statistical significance of the primary outcome results, corroborative evidence from secondary outcome analyses should be used to support a study's hypothesis. If multiple related measures are obtained, and the analyses of each show similar results, then it is less likely that any one of the positive results arose by chance. While there is no specific statistical test to document this phenomenon, showing that multiple related measures, all producing similar types of effects, lends support to the conclusions drawn from the primary outcome.

Evaluating side effects

Evaluating side effects of interventions tested in clinical trials is subject to the same considerations as those used to evaluate measures of efficacy. It is important to compare the relative incidence in the active treatment and control groups. Differing rates of side effect must be evaluated with caution, since clinical trials are rarely powered to detect such differences, and the large number of different side effects that are possible make it likely that one or more of the differences observed, will be due to chance. Such differences should not be ignored; but observing similar results in multiple trials can increase one's confidence that the findings may be specifically attributed to the treatment received.

Publication

Thorough presentation of methods and results

Given that many components of a trial are central to interpreting the results, it is vital that trial reports be accurate, complete, and objective in their presentation of all important aspects of the trial. In particular, the a priori hypothesis should be clearly stated,

and the discovery of other findings properly identified. All randomized participants must be accounted for in the publication, and an intention-to-treat analysis of all participants is typically appropriate. Subsequent subgroup analyses can focus on those who complete the trial, but these should not be considered as the primary result. A careful description of the randomization and blinding procedures is also important to assure readers that the trial was properly conducted. Finally, brief descriptions of the rationale behind the choice of measurement tools and analytic strategies can be helpful.

Negative studies are as important as positive ones

There is now good evidence for a publication bias against negative studies, since authors prefer to write up positive ones and editors prefer to publish them (Begg and Berlin, 1988; Reidenberg, 1998). This can lead to difficulties for clinicians who want a true picture of the nature of the evidence for a particular treatment.

Potential limitations of RCTs

There are several issues inherent in the design and conduct of RCTs that may threaten the internal validity of the results—that is, the likelihood that the treatment comparison is free from bias. Furthermore, even when the comparison is internally valid, the external validity, or generalizability of the results, can be limited. Finally, because the conditions in which trials are conducted only weakly approximate clinical reality, physicians must be cautious in using the results as the only guide in clinical decision-making. We will briefly discuss each of these potential problems in the following paragraphs. More detailed discussions of these issues are provided by Feinstein (1983) and by Kramer and Shapiro (1984).

Under-enrolment

Under-enrolment occurs when too few research participants are enrolled to provide adequate statistical power to answer the study's primary research questions. The inability to recruit sufficient numbers of eligible patients is the most common cause of insufficient statistical power in RCTs (Freiman et al., 1978; Altman, 1980; Collins et al., 1980; Meinert, 1986; Hunninghake et al., 1987; Nathan, 1999). Such under-enrolment has been attributed to characteristics of (1) clinicians who refer their patients (Taylor et al., 1984, 1994; Taylor, 1992), (2) patients who choose to be screened (Greenlick et al., 1979) or enrolled (Barofky and Sugarbaker, 1979), (3) investigators who design the trials (Collins et al., 1984), and (4) institutions at which the trials are conducted (Begg et al., 1982; Shea et al., 1992).

Among the challenges to adequate participant recruitment, potential participants' reluctance to enrol in RCTs is likely to be the most formidable, especially in palliative care populations. Ways of addressing these issues specifically in palliative care studies have been carefully codified (LeBlanc et al., 2013). It has been observed that patients are generally less willing to participate in RCTs than in non-randomized, observational studies (Kramer and Shapiro, 1984). In addition to yielding unacceptably high probabilities for type II errors, the resulting under-enrolment substantially reduces the trial's precision in quantifying the treatment effect.

Selective enrolment

Even when properly designed and carefully conducted, clinical trials can only provide information specific to the population from which the study participants were drawn. Selective enrolment occurs when particular subgroups within the target population enrol in proportions greater or lesser than their representation in that population (Mant, 1999; Halpern et al., 2001). If this population does not include, for example, elderly patients, or children, then applying the results to these clinical populations requires extrapolation. While extrapolating results may sometimes be reasonable, it must always be done cautiously because both the beneficial and adverse effects of an intervention can vary across populations.

The level of response detected by a single trial will depend on the patient population enrolled. For example, when first studying a novel treatment for a condition for which there is no adequately effective treatment, all patients with the condition are more likely to be willing to volunteer. By including people with relatively early or mild symptoms, the response rate may be higher than expected, although the response in the placebo group may also be larger. In contrast, when a treatment is tested in a population where an effective treatment already exists, only people who do not obtain a response to the available treatments are likely to enrol. This more recalcitrant group may have a lower response rate than expected in the total population, thereby underestimating the treatment's potential usefulness.

Poor participant adherence

In RCTs, participants may not adhere completely to their prescribed treatment regimens (Kramer and Shapiro, 1984). Especially if participants believe they are receiving a non-preferred treatment, their enthusiasm for the trial, and subsequent adherence to their assigned treatment, may wane. This is further complicated if the participants have access to and decide to take either the experimental therapy or a concomitant additional therapy outside of the trial. This occurs more frequently in trials where participants are able to overcome the blinding. There is accumulating evidence that a significant number of study participants make concerted efforts to unblind themselves, and that participants who become aware of their treatment assignment maybe more likely to drop out of the study. For example, many participants assigned to the placebo groups in both the initial phase II trial of AZT (azidothymidine/zidovudine) for patients with AIDS (Fischl et al., 1987), and in a randomized trial of vitamin E for patients with Alzheimer's disease (Sano et al., 1997), appear to have become unblinded, and even to have obtained the active agents outside the trial (Kodish et al., 1990; Epstein, 1996; Karlawish and Whitehouse, 1998). Even more problematically, widespread unblinding in one AIDS Clinical Trial Group study (Volberding et al., 1990) not only allowed approximately 9% of those assigned to the placebo to receive AZT, but contributed to the drop-out rate in the placebo group being one-third higher than it was in the active treatment group (Merigan, 1990).

Participant non-adherence and drop-out can substantially bias the results of a trial (Peto et al., 1995). Though intention-to-treat analyses may mitigate this bias, if non-adherence or drop-out rates are higher in one group than in the other, such analyses may also prevent a true effect of treatment from being detected. Thus, investigators should make concerted efforts to monitor participant adherence and drop-outs. When such problems exist, the results of the trial must be interpreted cautiously.

Ethical issues in palliative care research

As with all clinical research, palliative care studies require informed consent of the participants and, when cognitive impairment is an issue, from the appropriate family member or medical surrogate. Especially in situations where curative therapies are not likely to be effective, there are a number of important issues to consider and detailed discussions of this topic are covered in Section 5 of this book. The most important issue is to consider the balance between the ethical issues of right of the individual to receive compassionate care and the needs of the population for information on the efficacy and safety of specific therapies. When conducting clinical trials, the investigator must carefully protect the rights and well-being of the subjects in the study. One possible alternative is the use of innovative approaches for the conduct of clinical trials (Streiner, 2007). Although beyond the scope of this chapter, trials designs such as response-adaptive randomization procedures (e.g. 'play-the-winner' or 'drop-the-loser') may be more ethically appropriate for the testing of therapies in conditions that may have significant consequences on the quantity and/or quality of life that may result in the palliative care population. Such designs focus on minimizing the expected treatment failures while maintaining the power and randomization benefits (Rosenberger and Huc, 2004). 'Add-on' trials, where a new treatment is added to the current treatments the patient is receiving, may reduce the consequences to the individual patients from being randomized to a placebo treatment. Building in rescue strategies to the trial design can also reduce the potential risk to study participants (Boers, 2003). Crossover trial designs may also be useful in studies of diseases but are only applicable when symptoms are relatively stable. Using patients as their own control markedly increases the power of the study, but concerns about carryover effects between treatment periods are a serious risk to the validity of the study (Garcia et al., 2004; Simon and Chinchilli, 2007).

Conclusions

This chapter has outlined several fundamental considerations for investigators planning clinical trials, and for clinicians attempting to discern the applicability of such trials to their practices. There has been special consideration to the nuances of clinical trials for palliative care interventions. In summary, randomized, controlled trials remain the best available means of evaluating novel palliative care interventions, and for determining how these interventions may be optimally used. Despite the strengths of the design, readers of trial reports should be mindful of the many difficulties inherent in extrapolating from the results obtained in a trial setting to the use of these same interventions in clinical practice. Further advances in our understanding of how best to apply clinical trials in the evaluation of pain and palliative care will depend on improved understanding of the underlying pathophysiology and the anatomy of clinical trials (Farrar, 2010).

Online materials

Complete references for this chapter are available online at <http://www.oxfordmedicine.com>.

References

Anonymous (1948). Streptomycin treatment of pulmonary tuberculosis. *British Medical Journal*, 2, 769–782.

Chaput De Saintonge, D. M. and Herxheimer, A. (1994). Harnessing placebo effects in health care. *The Lancet*, 344, 995–998.

Farrar, J.T. (2010). Advances in clinical research methodology for pain clinical trials. *Nature Medicine*, 16, 1284–1293.

Freiman, J.A., Chalmers, T.C., Smith, H., Jr., and Kuebler, R.R. (1978). The importance of beta, the type II error and sample size in the design and interpretation of the randomized control trial. Survey of 71 'negative' trials. *The New England Journal of Medicine*, 299, 690–694.

Hardy, J., Quinn, S., Fazekas, B., *et al.* (2012). Randomized, double-blind, placebo-controlled study to assess the efficacy and toxicity of subcutaneous ketamine in the management of cancer pain. *Journal of Clinical Oncology*, 30, 3611–3617.

Jaeschke, R., Singer, J., and Guyatt, G. H. (1989). Measurement of health status. Ascertaining the minimal clinically important difference. *Controlled Clinical Trials*, 10, 407–415.

Leblanc, T.W., Lodato, J.E., Currow, D.C., and Abernethy, A.P. (2013). Overcoming recruitment challenges in palliative care clinical trials. *Journal of Oncology Practice*, 9, 277–282.

Mularski, R.A., Rosenfeld, K., Coons, S.J., *et al.* (2007). Measuring outcomes in randomized prospective trials in palliative care. *Journal of Pain and Symptom Management*, 34, S7–S19.

Sanderson, C., Hardy, J., Spruyt, O., and Currow, D.C. (2013). Placebo and nocebo effects in randomized controlled trials: the implications for research and practice. *Journal of Pain and Symptom Management*, 46, 722–730.

Streiner, D.L. (2007). Alternatives to placebo-controlled trials. *Canadian Journal of Neurological Sciences*, 34(Suppl. 1), S37–41.

Taylor, K.M., Feldstein, M.L., Skeel, R.T., Pandya, K.J., Ng, P., and Carbone, P.P. (1994). Fundamental dilemmas of the randomized clinical trial process: results of a survey of the 1,737 Eastern Cooperative Oncology Group investigators. *Journal of Clinical Oncology*, 12, 1796–1805.

Temple, R. and Ellenberg, S.S. (2000). Placebo-controlled trials and active-control trials in the evaluation of new treatments. Part 1: ethical and scientific issues. *Annals of Internal Medicine*, 133, 455–463.

White, C. and Hardy, J. (2010). What do palliative care patients and their relatives think about research in palliative care? A systematic review. *Supportive Care in Cancer*, 18, 905–911.

Qualitative research

Kate Flemming

Introduction to qualitative research

This chapter will seek to explore the role for qualitative research within palliative care. It is not a chapter about how to 'do' qualitative research, as there are numerous texts that provide detailed information on the design and conduct of qualitative research to answer questions for practice and policy. More, it is a chapter that seeks to outline the role and purpose of qualitative research for palliative care by looking at the kind of questions qualitative research can answer; exploring qualitative research and its relationship to evidence based practice; the role of qualitative research within mixed methods research; the synthesis of qualitative research; and perhaps most practically how to go about finding qualitative research and undertaking an appraisal of its quality.

What kind of questions can qualitative research answer?

Qualitative research is a form of naturalistic enquiry, which seeks to study people in social settings and to collect data on the meanings people attach to their social world. Qualitative research relies on the power of words to describe social phenomena, rather than numbers.

Traditionally there has been seen to be a division between qualitative and quantitative research methods. Each has been identified by a distinct paradigm (Flemming, 2007). Research has been conducted within the constraints of these paradigms with the differences apparent at a number of levels, from epistemology and theoretical framework, to methods and data collection techniques (Brannen, 1992). Whilst the distinction between qualitative and quantitative research should be informed by epistemology and theory, it most commonly occurs at the level of method. There have been ongoing debates as to the role and purpose of each approach since the mid-nineteenth century (Flemming, 2007). Historically, quantitative methods dominated enquiry at this time and developed further during the early part of the twentieth century, as more complex statistical methods developed. This continued until the mid 1960s, when qualitative research underwent resurgence, though predominantly at this point in the disciplines of anthropology, sociology, and psychology (Brannen, 1992; Hammersley, 1992). By the 1970s, researchers in social work, nursing, community services, and health promotion were embracing qualitative methods. By the late 1980s, a substantial body of methodological writing on qualitative research was in evidence (Clark, 1997).

As the modern hospice movement developed in the United Kingdom, so research in palliative medicine developed. In the early 1970s, randomized controlled trials (RCTs) in palliative medicine

were undertaken by Dr Robert Twycross at St Christopher's Hospice, London (Twycross, 1972, 1976). Alongside this, narrative methods of research were also developing. Kübler-Ross's seminal work *On Death and Dying*, published in 1969, was developed through interviews with people who were dying talking about their experiences. In 1974, John Hinton published work in which he explored dying patients' perceptions of their conversations with doctors and nurses. These early examples of qualitative research in palliative medicine, demonstrate its potential to answer many of the questions fundamental to the care of people receiving palliative care.

How research is carried out should be determined by the nature of the research question being posed, rather than it being driven by a particular theoretical or methodological assumption (Hammersley, 1992). Research questions which are best informed by qualitative methods are those which seek to explore processes and/or meanings: the 'why' type questions (Payne, 2007). These questions can then be answered through a number of different qualitative approaches.

Qualitative research is an umbrella term representing a range of epistemologies (theories of knowledge), which subsequently inform methodologies, which themselves dictate the types of methods used to collect qualitative data. There are a core set of methodological approaches to conducting qualitative research which commonly feature in health research and that have relevance to palliative medicine (Table 19.4.1). Once the methodology is established, this justifies the data collection techniques used by the researchers. Some methodologies are more prescriptive than others about method, but all should 'provide researchers with an overall strategy for formulating, articulating, analysing, and evaluating their methods' (Carter and Little 2007, p. 1318). The practicalities of research in health care, however, often mean that the supposed linear relationship from epistemology to method often becomes interrupted or distorted as different influences such as funding sources, social organization, political orientations of research teams, and clinical speciality, exert forces over the research process (Bryman, 1988).

Qualitative research and its relationship to evidence-based practice

The aim of evidence-based practice (EBP) is to reduce uncertainty in clinical decision-making by incorporating appropriate, current research evidence in decision-making processes (Flemming, 2008). What constitutes 'best evidence' is dependent on the question being asked. Whilst qualitative research did not feature prominently in the early development of EBP, since the late 1990s

Table 19.4.1 Methods of data collection used in qualitative research (Clark, 1997; Bowling, 2002; Carter and Little, 2007)

Methodology and aim	Data collection method	Examples
Phenomenology: aims to understand the lived experiences of individuals or groups	Interviews: *unstructured, structured, individual, conjoint, group* Focus groups	A phenomenological study to understand patient and family experiences of health care services in the palliative stages of Parkinson's disease (Giles and Miyasaki, 2009)
Grounded theory approaches: aim to generate analytical categories and dimensions and the relationships between them in order to understand social processes	Observation and Participant observation Focus groups Interviews (see above)	A grounded theory study to explore attitudes and beliefs among emergency care providers regarding the provision of palliative care services in the emergency department (Grudzen et al., 2012)
Ethnography: aims to understand the social world of people from a cultural perspective	Observation Interviews Documentary analysis Case studies	An ethnographic study tracing the changing notions of a good death held by hospice and palliative care practitioners (McNamara, 2004)

Source: Data from Bowling 2002; Carter and Little 2007; Clark 1997; Giles and Miyasaki 2009; Grudzen et al. 2012; and McNamara 2004.

it has started to contribute in a number of traditional and more novel ways (Murphy et al., 1998).

EBP began with the development of evidence-based medicine (EBM) in the early 1990s. At this time, medicine was seeking to ensure continuing medical education was effective and that new types of research evidence were being translated into clinical practice (Sackett et al., 1997). Positivist research methods evaluating the effectiveness of health-care interventions through RCTs and systematic reviews emerged as the core of EBM. Critics of EBP have focused on this perceived over-emphasis on RCTs and systematic reviews, citing a privileging of 'science' over other forms of knowledge in clinical decision-making (Freshwater, 2004). RCTs are, however, the most appropriate research design for evaluating the effectiveness of interventions and provide an evidence base appropriate to the kinds of questions for which clinicians need answers. A common problem with RCTS, particularly in trials of palliative care interventions, is inadequate sample sizes leading to different or discrepant findings between seemingly similar studies (Ciliska et al., 2008). Systematic reviews of primary research can overcome some of the limitations associated with single studies, by using rigorous methods for searching, research retrieval, appraisal of quality and validity, data extraction, and synthesis. Systematic reviews provide summaries of research-based knowledge on a topic, and their usefulness to clinicians has led to their privileged position in the hierarchy of evidence in EBP.

Qualitative research has not traditionally fitted into the evidence hierarchy proposed by EBP. Whilst qualitative research will never be able to answer effectiveness questions, its focus of obtaining insightful and rich data on complex issues (Bowling, 2002) ensures it has a role in contributing to the evidence base for practice, answering clinical questions quite different to addressed by RCTs.

The role of qualitative research within mixed methods research for palliative care

There is a growing appreciation that health care needs to be evaluated and informed through a variety of research methods and that it is clinical uncertainty or policy requirements that need to drive evaluation, rather than an allegiance to a particular research methodology. Clinicians can face a multitude of decision challenges within a single consultation (Thompson et al., 2004) and need an evidence base which supports this complexity.

The best available evidence should be used to inform and provide insight into decision-making processes. The Medical Research Council (2000, 2008) produced guidance on evaluating complex interventions recommending that researchers recognized and adopted appropriate methods for evaluation. Using multiple methods to evaluate health-care is now part of mainstream research funding and practice.

Circumstances of research, rather than methodological or epistemological positions, are beginning to drive research agenda. By removing some of the distinctions between qualitative and quantitative research, a greater range of options for evaluating the complex nature of health care have become available. Quantitative and qualitative research methods are gaining an independence from their original epistemological positions. Each approach has its own strengths and weaknesses for conducting health-care research and this is behind the rationale for their integration (Bryman, 1988). The conventional distinction of two opposing standpoints is being replaced by the idea of a range of positions which are located in more than one dimension, particularly as all research assumes there is a social reality which is amenable to observation (Hammersley, 1992).

Qualitative research is gaining increased prominence as mixed-method approaches to research have become more popular. The traditional gulf between qualitative and quantitative methods has narrowed, as the consensus of two methodological paradigms has been challenged (Hammersley, 1992). The previously mentioned difficulty in maintaining the linear relationship between epistemology, theory and method, is another factor that has led to an increased interest in mixed-method research to evaluate health care.

Evaluation of the effectiveness of palliative treatments has been central to the speciality since its inception in the late 1960s, but has been beset with difficulties. Conducting research with dying patients and their families is difficult. Broad ethical dilemmas and methodological issues need to be overcome, for example, poor recruitment leads to under-powered trials and unreliable results. Employing qualitative methodologies in the planning and execution in trials of palliative care interventions may overcome many methodological and ethical issues. The process of a clinical trial begins with its inception and ends with its dissemination and implementation. Incorporating qualitative research into study planning, recruitment, conduct and implementation has the potential to enhance the final outcomes of the research and ensure it has meaning beyond its initial conduct (Flemming et al., 2008). An example is the recognition that few palliative care patients participate in trials for which they are eligible (Grande and Todd, 2000).

The ability to answer complex questions is crucial in the evaluation of palliative care. It is essential to understand not only which treatments are effective in palliative care, but also how the context of delivery can influence implementation. Improving the quality and relevance of research by ensuring that the methods employed answer clinical questions in their totality, can help ease the ongoing and dynamic tension surrounding the role of research in palliative care, the maintenance of an ethical stance and developing an evidence base for practice. Good quality evidence is needed on which to base future interventions, but at the same time researchers need to remain sensitive about involving people (and their families) in research when they are facing the end of their lives (Flemming et al., 2008). Using qualitative research to enhance the utility, effectiveness, and applicability of findings from RCTs and other methods, may start to ease some of the tensions arising from patient participation.

There are some very practical challenges to conducting qualitative research alongside other research methods. These include ensuring research teams have relevant expertise to conduct the research; persuading research commissioners to fund longer, more expensive projects; difficulties in publishing mixed-methods research in its entirety; and mixed-methods research being used inappropriately in favour of more traditional approaches, to the detriment of outcomes.

While combining qualitative and quantitative research will not eradicate all methodological problems associated with palliative care research, there is definite potential to enhance the utility of RCTs. Doing this may assuage some of the ethical concerns regarding participation in research, and reduce the ongoing tension which exists between providing care for the individual now, and improving care for the patients of the future.

Synthesis of qualitative research

Earlier in the chapter it was discussed about the role of systematic reviews of effectiveness have played within EBP. More recently, methodological developments have occurred that enable the synthesis of qualitative research.

Interest in the development of methods to synthesize qualitative research developed for a number of reasons. Some mirrored the drive behind the synthesis of RCTs, that is, the need to overcome problems associated with isolated, single, primary studies that individually have little impact in practice. Another driving factor is the recognition that a range of evidence is required for health care, beyond those established for the systematic reviewing of RCTs. The synthesis of qualitative research complements the 'rationalist' model of synthesis provided by traditional systematic review methods (Flemming, 2007).

A number of different methods have been developed for the synthesis of qualitative research, each of which produces a

different type of review. How the synthesis of qualitative research is approached is driven by the research question (Dixon-Woods et al., 2005). Approaches to research synthesis can be viewed as a continuum, with aggregative reviews at one end, and interpretative reviews at the other (Noblit and Hare, 1988). Aggregative reviews are those which assemble and pool data and use techniques such as meta-analysis to summarize data. Interpretive reviews seek to develop concepts and theories that integrate those concepts. The end point of an interpretive synthesis is the development of theory grounded in the studies included in the review (Dixon-Woods et al., 2006). The synthesis of qualitative research naturally sits at the interpretive end of the continuum. In reality, however, many syntheses include elements of both interpretation and aggregation, seen as a principle of good synthesis (Flemming, 2007).

Many aspects of the methods associated with systematic reviewing of RCTs such as question formulation, literature searching, appraisal of studies, and methods of synthesis are in the early stages of development in the synthesis of qualitative research. It is unlikely that a standardized set of procedures will ever be developed in quite the way that has been achieved with systematic reviews of RCTs. More probably, a 'methodological palette' will be developed from which reviewers can draw methods most relevant to the focus of their review (Flemming, 2007).

Interest in the use of multiple and mixed-methods in primary research to develop the evidence base for practice has also manifested itself at the level of synthesizing research (Pope and Mays, 2006). Methods for synthesizing RCTs are well established, with organizations such as the Cochrane Collaboration producing and disseminating systematic reviews of effectiveness (Khan et al., 2003). As previously mentioned, this 'rationalist' model of synthesis may not provide answers to the complex, multifactorial decisions posed by health care. Therefore interest has developed in producing techniques for the synthesis of wider research methods to address such limitations.

Methods for synthesizing qualitative research have been developed over the last decade. In 1998, the Cochrane Qualitative Methods Group was formed to advance the synthesis of qualitative research and to develop methods for including qualitative syntheses into effectiveness reviews. Others, including the Joanna Briggs Institute in Australia and specific research groups in the United Kingdom, have developed a variety of methods for synthesizing qualitative research. Many of these syntheses have contributed to the evidence base for palliative care, for example:

- Do hospital-based palliative teams improve care for patients or families at the end of life? (Higginson et al., 2002)

- Health professionals' knowledge of, attitudes towards, and ability to deliver educational interventions for symptom and disease management (Flemming et al., 2012)

- Patients' experiences of breathlessness (Gysels et al., 2007)

- Preferences for place of care and death among advanced cancer patients (Higginson and Sen-Gupta, 2000)

- Knowledge and information needs of informal caregivers in palliative care (Docherty et al., 2008)

- The use of morphine to treat cancer related pain (Flemming, 2010).

Synthesizing qualitative research is not universally accepted. For qualitative researchers who consider that each piece of qualitative research is a unique representation of multiple truths or realities, synthesis is an anathema (Pope and Mays, 2006). Those that do accept synthesis of qualitative research as a feasible methodological option acknowledge that all research studies try to capture an underlying social reality, albeit in different ways (Pope and Mays, 2006). Adopting this pragmatic position of 'subtle realism' (Hammersley, 1992) ensures that the synthesis of qualitative research may be seen as acceptable in contributing to the evidence base for practice, which is in keeping with the interpretive approach advocated by qualitative research.

It is recognized that considerable work is needed to create mutually agreed upon approaches to the synthesis of qualitative research. Any resolution of debates will be driven by the pragmatism required for successful health services research. Despite the current lack of consensus, the potential for syntheses of qualitative research to influence clinical practice and policy in health care is beginning to be realized.

Finding qualitative research

One of the key aspects of using qualitative research to inform practice is to be able to identify the research in the first place. Whilst it is increasingly acknowledged that qualitative research has an important role of play in developing the evidence base for practice, there is consensus that searching for and identifying relevant qualitative research can be both frustrating and difficult (Campbell et al., 2011).

One of the commonest approaches to identifying research literature of any sort is by searching electronic databases. As the EBP movement began to grow, so did work by information specialists on how best to retrieve research evidence from databases. It was increasingly apparent that there were potentially detrimental effects of missing key research articles through using poorly constructed searches (Grant, 2004). In keeping with the development of EBP, initial work focused on developing strategies for identifying quantitative research. More recently, and alongside developments for synthesizing qualitative research, work has been undertaken to optimize ways of searching for qualitative research. Some of this work has highlighted the following challenges (Evans, 2002; Campbell et al., 2011; Saini and Shlonsky, 2012):

Non-specific titles

While many reports of randomized controlled trials include the research method in the title for example, 'The imPaCT study: A randomised controlled trial to evaluate a hospital palliative care team' (Hanks et al., 2002), this is not the case for many qualitative research publications. Such reports often use quite descriptive titles, reflecting the focus of the research undertaken, but not identifying the methodology used (Evans 2002). Some examples include: 'Negotiating leave-taking events in the palliative medicine unit' (Hadders, 2011); 'Striving for emotional survival in palliative cancer nursing' (Sandgren et al., 2006); 'Relieving existential suffering through palliative sedation: discussion of an uneasy practice' (Bruce and Boston, 2011). Such titles make the selection of papers by key terms quite difficult, leading to potentially relevant studies being missed (Evans, 2002).

Abstracts

The content of abstracts within qualitative research can also vary greatly. As electronic databases include abstracts as part of the information retrieved about publications, these also form part of the search. If the abstract contains no mention of the research method, then there is increased difficulty in locating these studies (Evans, 2002). In contrast, searches that are too broad to capture the variety of ways that concepts are defined by authors, may result in the retrieval of many thousands of irrelevant papers (Saini and Shlonsky, 2012).

Indexing within electronic databases

The quality of indexing of qualitative research is another well-documented problem that besets those searching for qualitative research (Dixon-Woods et al. 2001; Evans 2002). Index terms are those that identify both the subject and method of research publications (Evans 2002). Databases vary in the way that use methodological indexing terms to describe qualitative research designs (Campbell et al., 2011) with some databases using many more index terms for qualitative research than others. For example when the index terms for the same piece of qualitative research were compared, it was found that the Cumulative Index for Nursing and Allied Health Literature (CINAHL) used twice as many terms as MEDLINE, including many methodological terms (Evans, 2002). Indexers are, however, reliant on authors providing enough detail of their methods to enable accurate indexing, and this can be problematic if insufficient detail is provided (Flemming and Briggs, 2007). Given the range of methodologies that sit under the umbrella term 'qualitative research' and the variety of ways these are enacted and reported, the complexity of indexing of qualitative research becomes apparent.

Strategies for searching for qualitative research

Searching for research takes place for a number of different reasons. Those wanting information to find an answer a question arising from clinical practice will need a different approach to searching than someone undertaking a systematic review of qualitative research. Some good texts are available to guide readers in more detailed and complex searching (e.g. McKibbon and Marks, 2008a, 2008b; Finfgeld-Connett and Johnson, 2012; Saini and Shlonsky, 2012). There are however some core principles that are relevant to both and it is worth focusing on an answerable question when thinking about developing an efficient search strategy. For example, it is worth establishing:

- Who are the population I am interested in?
- What aspect(s) of their health care experience am I interested in finding out about?

An example of a searchable question is: 'What are health professionals' attitudes towards delivering educational interventions for symptom management to patients with advanced cancer?'
In this there are two *populations*:

1. The group whose experiences you are interested in establishing, that is, health professionals

2. The 'clinical' focus of the type of patients, that is, those with advanced cancer.

The focus of the *aspect of health-care experience* is health professionals' attitudes towards delivering education.

A focused question becomes the basis for literature searching in order to identify relevant evidence from research. Framing the question in a way which lends itself to searching while still reflecting the specific patient or service focus is an important stage to get right. That way, when searching for evidence on a chosen topic, the volume of research will be more manageable than if non-focused searching had been undertaken (Flemming, 2008).

The individual parts of the question are vital aspects to remember when it comes to searching for evidence. Sometimes reading some background research papers can help to focus the question and to identify the search terms required, which arise from the clinical question. Question formulation is fundamental to searching, as it converts situations and problems from practice into the focus of searching. The keywords of the question become the key terms for a search; time spent developing a focused question can save a great deal of searching time. In addition, consulting a health information specialist can help develop a search strategy and to identify and target the best places to search (Flemming, 2008).

When searching electronic databases, search strategies are best constructed using a combination of the relevant 'clinical' terms identified through focussing an answerable question and 'qualitative' terms in the form of a filter (Shaw et al., 2004; Flemming and Briggs, 2007). Both research and personal experience of the author has shown that a simple three-line search strategy using broad-based terms can identify most qualitative research for both clinical and systematic review purposes (Flemming and Briggs, 2007; Flemming, 2010; Flemming et al., 2012). These terms are:

◆ qualitative

◆ findings

◆ interviews.

More detailed filters are also available. Shaw et al. (2004), when evaluating qualitative filters to identify research on breastfeeding, found three separate search strategies were required to optimize searching for qualitative research: thesaurus terms, free text terms, and broad-based terms. It was concluded that relying on any one strategy risked missing relevant records. As with many methodological developments in qualitative research, there is a lack of consensus as to the best way forward, and it is down to individuals to decide the optimum way of searching that matches the purpose of their search.

Other forms of searching exist such as footnote chasing, hand searching, use of personal knowledge, reference chaining, and consultation with experts. These additional methods of searching may be needed when undertaking a detailed systematic search in order to locate studies that may have been missed by electronic searching (Saini and Shlonsky, 2012). It can be important also to identify grey literature, that is, those studies more difficult to retrieve through conventional searching methods. Grey literature consists of conference proceedings, research reports, government reports, book chapters, policy documents etc. and can be found through grey literature websites. Up-to-date information about such websites can be accessed through locally based information specialists.

Appraising the quality of qualitative research

Once qualitative research has been identified, it is helpful to be able to appraise its quality, in order to determine its usefulness in practice. It has to be noted that appraisal of the quality of qualitative research remains a contentious issue, reflecting some of the tensions apparent in qualitative research itself (Dixon-Woods

et al., 2007). A pragmatic approach is, however, often taken, in that there is utility in establishing a set of appraisal criteria that are unique to qualitative research (Saini and Shlonsky, 2012).

The most common approach to appraisal has been in the form of structured checklists. As with methods of searching for qualitative research however, there is lack of consensus on an actual tool to guide decision-making when trying to establish quality, with over 100 quality appraisal lists available (Saini and Shlonsky, 2012). Given that 'qualitative research' is an umbrella term for a range of methodologies, it is perhaps not surprising that there is a lack of consensus as to which single quality appraisal checklist is deemed suitable against all methodologies, nor that so many exist. Certainly there is no analogous 'quantitative research' appraisal checklist; different checklists are available for RCTs, cohort studies, surveys, etc.

Having said this, qualitative appraisal checklists do exist, and they are deemed important for ascertaining the merits and limitations of qualitative studies on their own terms (Drisko, 1997). Due to space constraints within journals affecting the potential to adequately address qualitative standards of reporting, it is recognized that quality appraisal may become an exercise of judging the quality of the published report, rather than being an evaluation of the research process itself (Sandelowski and Barroso, 2002; Atkins et al. 2008).

For a clinician trying to ascertain the quality of an identified piece of qualitative research in order to inform practice, these academic debates may seem a distraction from getting the job done. There are well established appraisal tools, which have been developed to enable EBP and qualitative research is included in these. One of the longer standing and more commonly used has been developed by the Critical Appraisal Skills Programme (CASP). The programme aims to enable individuals to develop the skills to find and make sense of research evidence, helping them to put knowledge into practice.

The checklist begins with two screening questions which enable the reader to quickly determine whether it is worth reading the paper in more depth:

1. Was there a clear statement of the aims of the research?

2. Is a qualitative methodology appropriate?

These are followed by more detailed questions:

3. Was the research design appropriate to address the aims of the research?

4. Was the recruitment strategy appropriate to the aims of the research?

5. Were the data collected in a way that addressed the research issue?

6. Has the relationship between researcher and participants been adequately considered?

7. Have ethical issues been taken into consideration?

8. Was the data analysis sufficiently rigorous?

9. Is there a clear statement of findings?

10. How valuable is the research?

Reproduced with permission from Critical Appraisal Skills Programme (CASP), 10 questions to help you make sense of qualitative research, Copyright © CASP, – www.casp-uk.net, available from http:// media.wix.com/ugd/dded87_951541699e9edc71ce66c9bac4734c69.pdf.

The checklist is particularly helpful for those less experienced in appraising research. Within each question prompts are provided as to what to look for in the paper to help ascertain its quality, enabling clinicians to establish whether the paper is worthy of informing practice.

Conclusion

This chapter on qualitative research has outlined its importance as a research methodology that can provide answers to clinical questions arising in palliative medicine. The roles of qualitative research as a primary research method, within systematic reviews and also alongside quantitative methodologies have been discussed, and the place for qualitative research within EBP has been established.

The chapter has also addressed some of the more practical aspects of searching for qualitative research and undertaking an appraisal of its quality, whilst acknowledging that these are contested areas undergoing methodological development.

Online materials

Complete references for this chapter are available online at <http://www.oxfordmedicine.com>.

References

Atkins, S., Lewin, S., Smith, H., Engel, M., Fretheim, A., and Vomink, J. (2008). Conducting a meta-ethnography of qualitative literature: lessons learnt. *BMC Medical Research Methodology*, 8, 21.

Brannen, J. (1992). Combining qualitative and quantitative approaches: an overview. In J. Brannen (ed.) *Mixing Methods: Qualitative and Quantitative Research*, pp. 3–38. Aldershot: Ashgate Publishing Company.

Bowling A. (2002). Qualitative and combined research methods, and their analysis. In *Research Methods in Health: Investigating Health and Health Services*, pp. 351–401. Buckingham: Open University Press.

Campbell, R., Pound, P., Morgan, M., *et al.* (2011). Evaluating meta-ethnography: systematic analysis and synthesis of qualitative research. *Health Technology Assessment*, 15, 43.

Dixon-Woods, M., Fitzpatrick, R., and Roberts, K. (2001). Including qualitative research in systematic reviews: opportunities and problems. *Journal of Evaluation in Clinical Practice*, 7(2), 125–133.

Flemming, K., Adamson, J., and Atkin, K. (2008). Improving the effectiveness of interventions in palliative care: the potential role of qualitative research in enhancing evidence from randomized controlled trials. *Palliative Medicine*, 22, 12–131.

Flemming, K. and Briggs, M. (2007). Electronic searching to locate qualitative research. *Journal of Advanced Nursing*, 57(1), 95–100.

Hammersley, M. (1992). Deconstructing the qualitative–quantitative divide. In J. Brannen (ed.) *Mixing Methods: Qualitative and Quantitative Research*, pp. 39–55. Aldershot: Ashgate Publishing Company.

Murphy, E., Dingwall, R., Greatbach, D., Parker, S., and Watson P. (1998). Qualitative research methods in health technology assessment: a review of the literature. *Health Technology Assessment*, 2, 16.

Pope, C. and Mays, N. (2006). Synthesising qualitative research. In C. Pope and N. Mays (eds.) *Qualitative Research in Health-Care* (3rd ed.), pp. 142–152. Oxford: Blackwell Publishing.

Saini, M. and Shlonsky, A. (2012). *Systematic Synthesis of Qualitative Research*. Oxford: Oxford University Press.

Research into psychosocial issues

David W. Kissane, Annette F. Street,
Erin E. Schweers, and Thomas M. Atkinson

Introduction to research into psychosocial issues

Psychosocial research examines issues and concerns in the psychological, social, spiritual, and existential domains of human experience, including quality of life studies and interventions that seek to optimize outcomes. Psychosocial research needs to be conducted in accordance with the core values and principles of palliative care. Patient- and family-centred care acknowledges the unique experience of each person and their family members. Key values include respect for the dignity of all, advocacy on behalf of their expressed wishes, and equity in access to services. In response, psychosocial researchers seek not only the most effective interventions, but are also concerned with the meaning such treatments have for patient and family. To do so, psychosocial researchers increasingly create multidisciplinary teams and draw on a variety of methods.

In this chapter, we want to highlight the scope of psychosocial questions and interests by drawing on a number of different methods that have formed the basis of psychosocial research. In doing so, we have made choices. Detailed explanations of relevant methods are covered in detail in other chapters in this section on research. We highlight formative and current research, delineate the problems involved in conducting research with dying people, and make some suggestions about where future psychosocial research should be directed. A feature of the chapter is a section analysing the various instruments in use in psychosocial research. Sometimes, researchers are unaware of the potential range of validated questionnaires that can aid psychosocial research. Similarly, we have analysed a range of computer-assisted qualitative analysis programmes

The scope of psychosocial research in palliative medicine

Research activity can be grouped into broad domains or themes of inquiry. Many interesting questions and controversies arise in each domain. These are listed in Box 19.5.1.

The choice of research issue is commonly determined by awareness of unmet needs, concern about the standard of care, or a desire to improve the outcomes of treatment. We illustrate pertinent issues about a number of these domains and useful methods for addressing them and return to the challenges for the future at the end of this chapter.

Literature review and meta-analysis

A comprehensive literature review is a *sine qua non* as many ideas have been considered before. Exploring the boundaries of knowledge necessitates firstly identifying what is known, what aspects remain unclear, and thinking through where the benefits of further study will lie. A formal literature search is thus crucial before the hypothesis is generated or aims and objectives of the study are delineated.

While the history of any construct and its application is of interest, the recent emphasis on a clinical approach that is evidence-based (see Chapter 19.2) requires a systematic approach to any literature review. Recently, more systematic reviews of psychosocial palliative care topics have been conducted. Systematic reviews have explored the effects of multidisciplinary palliative care teams (Hearn and Higginson, 1998; Higginson et al., 2003), the level of need for palliative care (Franks et al., 2000), and effective methods of information giving to cancer patients (McPherson et al., 2001). Meta-synthesis of qualitative studies can also inform understanding of patient experiences (Seymour et al., 2003).

Concept and construct development

The building up of a theory provides a conceptual framework on which further observations can be based and ultimately delivers an empirical basis for the development of interventions. The qualitative approach to concept development begins in grounded theory, while quantitative methodology creates instruments to measure constructs, which in turn need to be carefully validated and demonstrated to have reliability for recurrent use.

Instrument development

The commonly used rating scales used in psychosocial research in palliative medicine have been summarized in Tables 19.5.1, 19.5.2, 19.5.3, 19.5.4, 19.5.6, 19.5.7, 19.5.8, 19.5.9, 19.5.10, 19.5.11, 19.5.12, 19.5.13, 19.5.14 and 19.5.15. Instruments that measure distress, mood states, coping, quality of life, support, and family functioning tend to be well validated, while measures of spirituality, dignity, and existential domains warrant further work.

Rating scales can be used for screening, diagnosis, measurement of severity, and change—attention needs to be paid to the purpose for which any instrument was designed and its reliability and validity in that role. In choosing an instrument, the researcher needs to consider what they seek to measure and for what purpose. For instance, sensitivity of scales to detect small changes will vary, sometimes at the expense of specificity, and the scales' practicality

- Communication studies: breaking bad news, discussing prognosis and dying
- Coping and adaptation to change
- Cultural issues including those of indigenous peoples
- Dying process
- Ethics of end-of-life care
- Family studies: carers, family support
- Grief and bereavement
- Interventions: psychotherapy, pharmacological, and physical
- Lived experience of illness: impact on self, the body, dignity, and burden on others
- Paediatric aspects of adaptation, coping, and care
- Psychiatric disorders: anxiety, depression, delirium, etc.
- Quality of life
- Sexuality and intimacy
- Social issues: relationships, recreation, work, and living arrangements
- Suffering, existential and spiritual distress.

and brevity will often be important when considered for use with palliative patients. It is also important to evaluate the content/face validity in detail for each study by asking the question: 'What is the real content of this instrument and will it apply to my study?' Such an examination needs to be in detail and each question should be evaluated by the researcher in order to have insight into the content validity of any assessment scale.

Grounded theory studies (see Chapter 19.4) have provided understanding of psychosocial concerns such as 'enduring', 'uncertainty', 'suffering', and 'hope', and then examining their interrelationships (Morse and Penrod, 1999) or exploring how decision-making occurs at the end of life for family caregivers and health-care providers in long-term-care settings (Caron et al., 2005).

Cohort and longitudinal studies

Observational studies may be either retrospective or prospective. In the former, past events are studied through case notes or by interview. They may be limited by incomplete recording or biased recall, but are inexpensive and serve as a useful beginning. Such studies should probably be regarded as hypothesis-generating and be carefully applied when one wants to change practice, for example, in the development of evidence-based guidelines. In contrast, prospective studies eliminate the bias of memory and permit examination of a number of associations, but may be limited by the availability of suitable subjects for recruitment within a reasonable time frame. In many studies, due to low recruitment rates, one needs to consider collaboration between centres, that is, by conducting national, or international, multicenter studies. In addition, subjects may be lost to follow-up.

Cross-sectional studies

Cross-sectional studies are both observational and descriptive, typically being used to measure the prevalence of a symptom or illness. They can be further used to identify clinical associations, well exemplified by the study of the 'desire for death' by Chochinov and colleagues in 200 Canadian hospice inpatients, which was found to be genuine and persistent in 8.5% and significantly associated with depressive disorder, isolation from family, and pain (Chochinov et al., 1995).

Table 19.5.1 Instruments measuring *anxiety* and *fear*

Instrument name	Item number (response style)	Factor structure	Reliability	Validity	Comments on utility
Beck Anxiety Inventory (BAI) (Beck et al., 1988)	21 items (4-point scale)	1. somatic 2. panic symptoms	$\alpha = 0.92$; test–retest = 0.75	r = 0.51 (HAM-A)	Designed to assess anxiety in a clinical population
Death Anxiety Scale (DAS) (Templer, 1970)	15 items (true/false)	1 factor	$\alpha = 0.76$; test–retest = 0.83	Well validated	Designed to assess preoccupation with and anxiety about death
Generalized Anxiety Disorder-7 (GAD-7) (Spitzer et al., 2006)	7 items (4-point scale)		$\alpha = 0.92$	r = 0.72 (BAI)	Designed as a self-assessment of anxiety
Hamilton Anxiety Rating Scale (HAM-A) (Hamilton, 1959)	14 items (5-point scale)	1. psychic anxiety 2. somatic anxiety	$\alpha = 0.79–0.86$	r = 0.56 (BAI)	Clinician-administered measure designed to assess global anxiety
Hospital Anxiety and Depression Scale (HADS) (Zigmond and Snaith, 1983)	14 items (4-point scale)	1. anxiety 2. depression	$\alpha = 0.89$; test–retest r = 0.74	Well validated	Designed as a rapid assessment tool in a non-psychiatric setting
State Trait Anxiety Inventory (STAI) (Spielberger et al., 1970)	40 items (4-point scale)	1. state 2. trait	$\alpha = 0.83–0.92$ on subscales	Well validated	Designed to assess how subjects respond to psychological stress. STAI-Y (revised) available.

Table 19.5.2 Instruments measuring *depression*

Instrument name	Item number (response style)	Factor structure	Reliability	Validity	Comments on utility
Beck Depression Inventory (BDI) (Beck et al., 1961)	21 items (4-point scale)	1. cognitions 2. somatic symptoms	$\alpha = 0.81$	$r = 0.62{-}0.66$ with clinician ratings	Designed to assess depressive symptoms. BDI-II and BDI-SF available
Brief Case Find for Depression (Jefford et al., 2004)	4 items		Sensitivity = 67%; Specificity = 75%	Satisfactory	Designed to screen for depression in medical patients
Geriatric Depression Scale (GDS) (Yesavage et al., 1982)	30 items (yes/no)		$\alpha = 0.94$	$r = 0.84$ (Zung SDS) and 0.83 (HAM-D)	Designed to assess depression in a geriatric population. GDS-15 and GDS-5 available
Patient Health Questionnaire (PHQ-9) (Kroenke et al., 2001)	9 items (4-point scale)		$\alpha = 0.86$	$r = 0.73$ (BDI); $r = 0.59$ (GHQ12)	Designed to assess depression. Self-report subscale of PRIME-MD
Brief Zung Self Rating Scale for Depression (Dugan et al., 1998)	11 items (4-point scale)	1 factor	$\alpha = 0.84$	$r = 0.92$ (SRS-D)	Designed to assess depression in the medically ill (eliminates somatic symptoms)

Table 19.5.3 Instruments measuring *distress*

Instrument name	Item number (response style)	Factor structure	Reliability	Validity	Comments on utility
Brief Symptom Inventory (Zabora et al., 2001)	18 items (5-point scale)	1. anxiety 2. depression 3. somatization	$\alpha = 0.89$	$r = 0.84$ (GSI of BSI)	Designed to assess symptoms of distress. 53-item BSI available.
Distress Thermometer (DT) (Roth et al., 1998)	1 VAS (+34) (yes/no)	Domains related to distress can be endorsed	Sensitivity = 84%; Specificity = 61%	Well validated in cancer studies	Designed for rapid assessment of patient distress. New variation uses an additional impact thermometer (Akizuki et al., 2005)
General Health Questionnaire (GHQ 12) (Johnstone and Goldberg, 1976)	12 items (4-point scale)	1 factor	Split-half = 0.95	Well validated	Designed as a distress screening measure. GHQ28 and GHQ60 available
Impact of Events Scale Revised (IES-R) (Creamer et al., 2003)	22 items (5-point scale)	1. intrusion 2. avoidance 3. hyperarousal	$\alpha = 0.79{-}0.90$	$r = 0.84$ (PCL-C)	Designed to assess subjective distress and intrusive thoughts. IES available

Table 19.5.4 Instruments measuring *pain* and *symptom management*

Instrument name	Item number (response style)	Factor structure	Reliability	Validity	Comments on utility
Brief Pain Inventory (Cleeland and Ryan, 1994)	23 items (11-point scale)	1. severity 2. interference	$\alpha = 0.95$	$r = 0.71$ (VAS)	Brief measure of pain. Short form available
Brief Pain Inventory for Ambulatory Care (Maunsell et al., 2000)	5 items (4-point scale)		$\alpha = 0.87{-}0.92$	$r = 0.65$ (EORTC pain)	Designed to assess pain intensity, impact, and medication doses
Edmonton Symptom Assessment System (ESAS) (Bruera et al., 1991)	9 items (11-point scale)		Satisfactory	Well validated	Designed to assess symptoms in palliative care patients
Memorial Symptom Assessment Scale (MSAS) (Portenoy et al., 1994)	32 items (4-point and 5-point scales)	1. psychological 2. physical	$\alpha = 0.58{-}0.88$	Well validated	Designed to assess cancer related symptoms. MSAS-SF available

Table 19.5.5 Instruments measuring *suffering*, *existential*, and *spiritual issues*

Instrument name	Item number (response style)	Factor structure	Reliability	Validity	Comments on utility
Demoralization Scale (DS) (Kissane et al., 2004)	24 items (5-point scale)	1. loss of meaning 2. dysphoria 3. disheartenment 4. helplessness 5. sense of failure	$\alpha = 0.94$; 0.71–0.89 on subscales	Good concurrent validity	Designed to assess existential distress in palliative care patients
Functional Assessment of Chronic Illness Therapy-Spiritual (FACIT-Sp) (Peterman et al., 2002)	12 items (5-point scale)	1. meaning 2. faith	$\alpha = 0.81$–0.88	$r = -0.54$ (POMS)	Designed to assess spiritual well-being in the general population. Expanded version available
Meaning in Life Scale (Warner and Williams, 1987)	15 items (5-point scale)		$\alpha = 0.78$	$r = 0.53$ (PIL)	Designed to assess sense of purpose and beliefs of hospice patients
Posttraumatic Growth Inventory (PTGI) (Tedeschi and Calhoun, 1996)	21 items (6-point scale)	1. relating 2. new possibility 3. strength 4. spiritual 5. appreciation	$\alpha = 0.90$	$r = 0.23$ (LOT) and $r = 0.50$ (religious participation)	Designed to assess perceived positive outcomes from traumatic events
Sense of Coherence/Orientation to Life (Antonovsky, 1993)	29 items (7-point scale)	1 factor	$\alpha = 0.84$–0.93	$r = 0.39$ (Rotter's I-E)	Designed to assess sense of coherence/meaningfulness
Shame and Stigma Scale (SSS) (Kissane et al., 2013)	20 items (5-point scale)	1. shame with appearance 2. sense of stigma 3. regret 4. speech/social concerns	$\alpha = 0.94$	$r = 0.60$ (DS)	Designed to assess adaptation after treatment of patients with head and neck cancer
Spiritual Involvement and Beliefs Scale (Hatch et al., 1998)	26 items (5-point scale)	1. ritual 2. fluid 3. existential 4. humility	$\alpha = 0.92$	$r = 0.80$ (SWB)	Designed to assess spiritual beliefs across religions
System of Beliefs Inventory (SBI-15) (Holland et al., 1998)	15 items (4-point scale)	1. beliefs/practice 2. social support	$\alpha = 0.93$	Well validated	Designed to assess spiritual beliefs in medically ill patients

Table 19.5.6 Instruments measuring *coping* and *adaptation*

Instrument name	Item number (response style)	Factor structure	Reliability	Validity	Comments on utility
Brief COPE (Carver, 1997)	28 items (4-point scale)	1. substance use 2. religion 3. humour 4. disengagement 5. support 6. coping 7. venting 8. denial 9. acceptance	$\alpha = 0.50$–0.90 on subscales	Well validated	Designed to assess coping strategies of individuals. Original version available
Life Orientation Test Revised (LOT-R) (Scheier et al., 1994)	10 items (5-point scale)	1 factor	$\alpha = 0.78$; test–retest = 0.79 at 28 months	Well validated	Designed to assess optimism
Mini Mental Adjustment to Cancer (Mini-MAC) (Watson et al., 1988, Watson et al., 1994)	29 items (4-point scale)	1. fighting spirit 2. preoccupation 3. fatalism 4. help/hopeless 5. avoidance	$\alpha = 0.62$–0.88 on subscales	Well validated	Designed as to assess responses to a cancer diagnosis

Table 19.5.7 Instruments measuring *delirium*

Instrument name	Item number (response style)	Factor structure	Reliability	Validity	Comments on utility
Confusion Assessment Method (CAM) (Inouye et al., 1990)	9 items		Sensitivity = 94–100%; Specificity = 90–95%	r = 0.82 (VAS)	Designed to assess delirium
Delirium Rating Scale (DRS) (Trzepacz et al., 1988)	10 items	1 factor	α = 0.90	r = 0.66 (Trailmaking)	Designed to clinically assess delirium
Memorial Delirium Assessment Scale (MDAS) (Breitbart et al., 1997)	10 items (4-point scale)	1 factor	α = 0.91	r = 0.88 (DRS)	Designed to assess medically ill patients for symptoms of delirium
Mini Mental State Exam (MMSE) (Folstein et al., 1983)	Interviewer administered		α = 0.82–0.84	Well validated	Designed as a quick standardized assessment of mental status

Table 19.5.8 Instruments measuring *social issues*

Instrument name	Item number (response style)	Factor structure	Reliability	Validity	Comments on utility
Bottomley Social Support Scale (Bottomley, 1995)	9 items (5-point scale)		α = 0.78; test–retest = 0.73–0.79	r = 0.38 (DHD)	Designed to assess social support in cancer patients
Duke-UNC Functional Social Support Scale (Broadhead et al., 1988)	8 items (5-point scale)	1. confident 2. affective	Test–retest = 0.66	Well validated	Designed to assess perceived social support
MOS Social Support Scale (Sherbourne and Stewart, 1991)	19 items (5-point scale)	1. emotion/information 2. tangible 3. affectionate 4. positive social interaction	α = 0.97	r = 0.67 (loneliness)	Designed to assess the perceived availability of social support
Multidimensional Scale of Perceived Social Support (Zimet et al., 1988)	12 items (7-point scale)	1. family 2. friends 3. significant others	α = 0.88	Well validated	Designed to assess the perceived availability of social support
Short Saranson Social Support Questionnaire (SSSSQ) (Sarason et al., 1983; Sarason et al., 1987)	6 items (6-point scale)	1. number 2. satisfaction	α = 0.94–0.97	r = −0.52 (loneliness)	Designed to assess the perceived availability of social support. Original version available

Table 19.5.9 Instruments measuring *caregiving issues*

Instrument name	Item number (response style)	Factor structure	Reliability	Validity	Comments on utility
Caregiver QOL Scale-Cancer (Weitzner et al., 1999)	35 items (5-point scale)	1. burden 2. disruptiveness 3. positive adaptation 4. financial concerns	α = 0.73–0.90	r = 0.49–0.65 (SF36)	Designed to assess QOL of caregivers
Caregiver Reaction Assessment (CRA) (Given et al., 1992)	24 items (5-point scale)	1. caregiver esteem 2. family support 3. finances 4. schedule 5. personal health	α = 0.80–0.90 on subscales	Good construct validity (CESD, ADL)	Designed to assess reactions to caring for ill elderly patients
Family Appraisal of Caregiving Questionnaire -Palliative Care (FACQ-PC) (Cooper et al., 2006)	25 items (5-point scale)	1. strain 2. positive appraisals 3. distress 4. family well-being	α = 0.73–0.86 on subscales	Well validated (FRI)	Designed to assess caregivers' appraisal of the caregiving process

Table 19.5.10 Instruments measuring *family issues*

Instrument name	Item number (response style)	Factor structure	Reliability	Validity	Comments on utility
FAMCARE Scale (Kristjanson, 1993)	20 items (5-point scale)	1. information giving 2. care availability 3. psychosocial care 4. physical care	$\alpha = 0.93$; test–retest = 0.91	r = 0.77–0.80 (McCusker Scale)	Designed to assess family satisfaction with advanced cancer care
Family Crisis Oriented Personal Evaluation Scales (F-COPES) (McCubbin et al., 1996)	30 items (5-point scale)	1. social support 2. reframing 3. spiritual support 4. mobilizing family 5. passive appraisal	$\alpha = 0.87$; 0.62–0.87 on subscales	Well validated	Designed to assess family coping strategies in difficult situations
Family Relationships Index (Edwards and Clarke, 2005)	12 items (true/false)	1. cohesion 2. expressiveness 3. conflict	$\alpha = 0.56$–0.70 on subscales	Well validated	Designed to assess family dysfunction. Subscale of the Family Environment Scale

Table 19.5.11 Instruments measuring *pediatric aspects* of advanced illness

Instrument name	Item number (response style)	Factor structure	Reliability	Validity	Comments on utility
Childhood Cancer Stressors Inventory (Hockenberry-Eaton et al., 1997)	18 items (true/false and 4-point scale)		$\alpha = 0.82$	r = −0.63 (CACI)	Designed to assess stressors in children with cancer
Miami Pediatric Quality of Life Scale (Armstrong et al., 1999)	56 items (5-point scale)	1. social competence 2. emotional stability 3. self-competence	$\alpha = 0.89$	Good discriminant validity	Designed to assess QOL in children with cancer
Multidimensional Anxiety Scale for Children (MASC) (March et al., 1997)	39 items (4-point scale)	1. physical symptoms 2. harm avoidance 3. social anxiety 4. separation anxiety	$\alpha = 0.90$; 0.74–0.85 on subscales	r = 0.63 (RCMAS)	Designed to assess paediatric anxiety
Pediatric Cancer QOL Inventory (PCQL) (Varni et al., 1998)	32 items (4-point scale)	1. disease 2. physical 3. psychological 4. social 5. cognitive	$\alpha = 0.91$ patient and 0.92 parent	Good convergent and discriminant validity	Designed to assess global QOL in paediatric cancer patients
Pediatric Inventory for Parents (PIP) (Streisand et al., 2001)	42 items (5-point scale)	1. communication 2. emotional functioning 3. medical care 4. role function	$\alpha = 0.80$–0.96	Good construct validity	Designed to assess parenting related stress in caring for an ill child

Case–control studies

The case–control study is used generally to test an aetiological hypothesis, by comparing a group with a disease or specific treatment, matched with controls. The methodological challenge is in the selection criteria for the cases to ensure that they are a representative sample and similarly the variables on which matching is achieved, and whether this is by random community selection or paired match. For instance, studies of men with prostate cancer have shown global quality of life to be equivalent to community samples of similarly aged men, but urinary incontinence,

impotence, and bowel symptoms to be causally related to the treatments these men have received (Litwin et al., 1995).

Cohort studies

Cohort studies are both observational and analytical in prospectively following groups of patients with key differences to assess outcome. They provide valuable information on the nature of a relationship and whether there is a causal association. Thus, the King's College cohort of women with breast cancer was followed across 15 years of illness to determine the influence of coping style

Table 19.5.12 Instruments measuring *communication* and *satisfaction with care*

Instrument name	Item number (response style)	Factor structure	Reliability	Validity	Comments on utility
Decisional Conflict Scale (O'Connor, 1995)	16 items (5-point scale)	1. uncertainty about alternatives 2. factors of uncertainty 3. decision effectiveness	$\alpha = 0.78–0.92$; test–retest $= 0.81$	Well validated	Designed to assess decisional uncertainty in patients facing a medical decision
Decision Regret Scale (Brehaut et al., 2003)	5 items (5-point scale)	1 factor	$\alpha = 0.81–0.92$	Well validated	Designed to assess decisional regret after making a medical decision
Patient Satisfaction Index (Guyatt et al., 1995)	23 items (7-point scale)	1 factor	$\alpha = 0.94$; test–retest $= 0.86$	Well validated	Designed to assess patient satisfaction with treatment
Satisfaction with Decision Scale (SWDS) (Wills and Holmes-Rovner, 2003)	6 items (5-point scale)	1 factor	$\alpha = 0.85$	$r = -0.26$ (SF20)	Designed to assess patient satisfaction with medical decisions

Table 19.5.13 Instruments measuring *sexuality* and *intimacy*

Instrument name	Item number (response style)	Factor structure	Reliability	Validity	Comments on utility
Abbreviated Dyadic Adjustment Scale (ADAS) (Spanier, 1976)	32 items (6-point scale)		$\alpha = 0.73–0.96$	Well validated	Designed to assess the quality of marital relationships
Changes in Sexual Function Questionnaire (CSFQ-14) (Keller et al., 2006)	14 items (5-point scale)	1. pleasure 2. frequency 3. interest 4. arousal 5. orgasm	$\alpha = 0.89–0.90$	Good concurrent validity	Designed to assess change in sexual activity and satisfaction due to illness
Female Sexual Function Index (FSFI) (Rosen et al., 2000)	19 items (5-point and 6-point scales)	1. desire 2. lubrication 3. orgasm 4. satisfaction 5. pain/discomfort	Test–retest $= 0.79–0.80$	Well validated	Designed to assess sexual function in women
International Index of Erectile Function (IIEF) (Rosen et al., 1997)	15 items (5-point and 6-point scales)	1. erectile function 2. orgasmic function 3. desire 4. intercourse satisfaction 5. overall satisfaction	$\alpha = 0.91$	Well validated	Designed to assess erectile function in men with various medical conditions. IIEF-5 available
Relationship Assessment Scale (RAS) (Hendrick, 1988)	7 items (5-point scale)		$\alpha = 0.86$	$r = 0.80$ (DAS)	Designed to assess relationship satisfaction in couples

on survival (Greer et al., 1990). Women who were fatalistic, overly anxious, or hopeless/helpless in their cognitions died earlier than those using positive avoidance or fighting spirit. Time available for follow-up is an obvious limitation in palliative medicine.

Clinical case reports

Clinical reports of individual patients have always served an important function in highlighting relevant issues of presentation, diagnosis, or management. One example was a series of patients who sought euthanasia under the Northern Territory of Australia's Rights of the Terminally Ill legislation, which operated for 9 months in 1996 (Kissane et al., 1998). These cases exemplified

non-recognition of depression, a poor standard of medical care, and disagreement over the terminal status of patients, highlighting the defective gate-keeper roles set up by the legislation. Building up collections of case reports points to the need for cohort and longitudinal studies as observational evidence is mounted. The corresponding narrative inquiry of the qualitative approach brings an equally worthwhile persepective.

Ethnographic case studies

Longitudinal ethnographic case studies draw on many of the techniques of ethnography to develop an in-depth and detailed case account to explore issues for a cultural or ethnic group.

Table 19.5.14 Instruments measuring *quality of life* and *functional status*

Instrument name	Item number (response style)	Factor structure	Reliability	Validity	Comments on utility
Assessment of Quality of Life at End of Life (Axelsson and Sjoden, 1999)	22 items (10-point scale)	1. physical 2. psychological 3. social 4. existential	Test–retest = 0.52–0.90	Strong correlations with CIPS	Designed to assess QOL in palliative patients.
EORTC-QLQ-C15 Palliative (Groenvold et al., 2006)	15 items (4-point scale)		Based on EORTC-QLQ-C30	C30 well validated; C15 in development	Designed to assess QOL in palliative patients. EORTC-QLQ-C30 available
Hospice Quality of Life Index Revised (McMillan and Weitzner, 1998)	25 items (100 mm VAS)		α = 0.83–0.87	Good content validity; further work needed	Designed to assess QOL in hospice patients
McGill Quality of Life Questionnaire (MQOLQ) (Cohen et al., 1995)	16 items (11-point scale)	1. physical 2. psychological 3. existential 4. support	α = 0.83	Well validated	Designed to assess QOL in palliative patients
McMaster Quality of Life Scale (Sterkenburg et al., 1996)	32 items (7-point scale)		α = 0.80	r = 0.70 (Spitzer QLI)	Designed to assess QOL in palliative patients
Palliative Care Outcomes Scale (Hearn and Higginson, 1999)	12 items (4-point scale)		α = 0.70	r = 0.43–0.51 (EORTC-C30)	Designed to assess outcomes in palliative patients and their families
Palliative Care Quality of Life Inventory (Mystakidou et al., 2004)	28 items (3-point and 5-point scales)	1. activity 2. self-care 3. health 4. treatment choice 5. support 6. communication 7. psychological affect	α = 0.79	r = 0.44–0.94 (AQEL)	Designed to assess QOL in palliative patients
Quality of End of Life Care and Satisfaction (QUEST) (Sulmasy et al., 2002)	30 items (5-point scale)		α = 0.88–0.93	r = 0.38–0.47 (PSI)	Designed to assess QOL and satisfaction with care in palliative patients
Quality of Life at End of Life (Steinhauser et al., 2003)	31 items (5-point scale)	1. life completion 2. provider relationship 3. symptom management 4. preparation 5. social support	α = 0.68–0.87	r = 0.62 (FACIT-Sp)	Designed to assess QOL in palliative patients

A study that identified unmet support needs of family caregivers caring for people with AIDS in Southern Thailand (Nilmanat and Street) led to a World Health Organization-funded study to develop policy and models of care to improve the situation. An innovative study exploring the experiences of men with prostate cancer used the technique of photo-novella where the men were asked to provide photos to express their experiences along with the interview texts. Some men chose to photograph themselves, others contributed photos of places or symbols that helped them make meaning from their experiences.

Narrative inquiry

Narratives constructed from research interviews mirror the social life of the person, with language forming the major cultural resource that participants draw on jointly to create meaning (Charmaz, 1999). The seminal work of Kleinman (1988) on illness narratives and Frank's (1995) writings on the wounded storyteller have shaped a narrative tradition designed to offer explanatory models of the world of people experiencing life-limiting illnesses. Recent nursing work has developed individual and group narratives to explore close nurse–patient relationships in palliative care (Aranda and Street, 2001).

Textual and electronic studies

Increasingly researchers are examining ways of researching palliative care practice in ways that are less intrusive to patients and allow them to write or respond at their own convenience in terms

Table 19.5.15 Instrument measuring the *dying process*

Instrument name	Item number (response style)	Factor structure	Reliability	Validity	Comments on utility
Beck Hopelessness Scale (BHS) (Beck et al., 1974)	20 items (true/false)	1. future feelings 2. loss motivation 3. future expectations	$\alpha = 0.85-0.93$	$r = 0.62-0.74$ with clinical ratings	Designed to assess suicidality
Life Closure Scale (Dobratz, 2004)	20 items (5-point scale)	1. self-reconciled 2. self-restructuring	$\alpha = 0.87$	Correlation with ABS	Designed to assess psychological adaptation at the end of life
Needs at End of Life Screening Tool (NEST) (Emanuel et al., 2001)	13 items (11-point scale)	1. financial burden 2. access to care 3. closeness 4. caregiving needs 5. psychological distress 6. spirituality 7. settledness 8. sense of purpose 9. patient clinician relations 10. information	$\alpha = 0.63-0.85$	Well validated	Designed to assess needs at the end of life
Schedule of Attitudes Towards Hastened Death (SAHD) (Rosenfeld et al., 2000)	20 items (true/false)	1 factor	$\alpha = 0.83$	$r = 0.67$ (DDRS)	Designed to assess a patient's interest in a hastened death

of time and place. These include the analysis of public domain texts such as published stories, media texts, and diaries or stories from the Internet. Other electronic sources include the use of online support groups (Høybye et al., 2004). Interviews and supportive therapy interventions conducted by telephone (Sandgren et al., 2000) and web interface are a new direction.

Controlled clinical trials

Preventive or therapeutic interventions are generally tested through controlled studies such as the randomized controlled trial (RCT), which could be double-blinded, placebo-controlled, or cross-over in design.

The place of controlled trials has been much debated in palliative medicine, yet they are vital when outcome is examined as the end point. The study of family-focused grief therapy during palliative care and bereavement delivered to 'high-risk' families selected by screening and thereafter randomized to intervention or control is another example of a carefully designed and methodologically sound study, this time a psychotherapeutic intervention (Kissane et al., 2006).

Methodological difficulties experienced in controlled trials include patient refusers and withdrawals, undeclared confounding treatments, dose variations and fidelity of the treatment applied, defaults in interim assessments, and deaths prior to outcome measurements. Despite such inherent challenges, the quality of evidence achieved necessitates greater utilization of these designs in future research in palliative medicine.

Mixed methods

Increasingly, psychosocial research is being designed utilizing a combined methods approach. Mixed methods can be conducted sequentially where one method leads to another to further explore a construct or phenomena. Triangulation of different data sets can confirm and explain findings more comprehensively. Similarly a study can be designed so that two or more methods complement and inform each other. An excellent recent example of this is found in a study of coping during illness with HIV (Folkman, 2001). Seeking to identify the predictors of coping outcome, Folkman and colleagues began a longitudinal study in 1990 with a cohort of 253 carers of gay men dying from AIDS during the era before triple therapies became available. Bimonthly assessment occurred over 2 years, during which two-thirds became bereaved. The researchers expected to focus on negative affects, but were struck by the interviewees' desire to share positive experiences. Further analysis of 106 narratives revealed that meaning-centred coping increased self-worth, sense of resilience, wisdom, and a perspective that no longer feared death. The importance of meaning-based coping emerged to expand the earlier theory of coping (problem- or emotion-focused processes that regulate distress).

A problem with many mixed method approaches is that one or more methods may not be developed with sufficient rigor to do justice to the method or topic. Development of expertise is equally important for both qualitative and quantitative research and collaboration between such researchers generates a powerful armamentarium.

Characterization of psychological outcome can be through both form and content. Quantitative studies mostly emphasize the content through measurement of specific dimensions, which can be compared to controls over time, but usually at specific points. Qualitative studies add insight into form, with recognition of the pattern of change in outcome over time. Then, repeated measures analysis, with attention to the slope and variability of change using qualitative techniques, enriches understanding of the evaluation process.

Computer-assisted qualitative data analysis software

Computers have become an integral part of the repertoire of tools for qualitative analysis (Fielding, 2001). There are a number of packages available from the relative simple text retrievers that are useful to sort and manage data into categories of information, to the highly sophisticated new-generation multimedia capacities of interpretive theory building and mapping packages. Some products are free and may be all that is needed for small, straightforward projects. Complex project usually need the facilities of commercial software, preferably with user assistance provided as part of the package. It is important to understand what capabilities are needed for the research process before deciding on a software package (see Table 19.5.16).

Table 19.5.16 Comparing features of computer-assisted qualitative data analysis packages

FUNCTIONS	ATLAS.ti V7	HyperRESEARCH 3.0.3	MaxQDA 10	nVivo 10	QDA Miner 4	Dedoose 4.2
File placement	External files	External files	Imported files	Imported files	Imported files	External files
File types	Text and multimedia Survey data Geo data PDF	Text and multimedia	Text and multimedia Geo data PDF	Text and multimedia Datasets Social network and web page media Geo data PDF Bibliographic data Evernote	Text and multimedia PDF Spreadsheets Databases Geo data Social network media	Text and multimedia Survey data PDF Survey Monkey NVivo projects
Coding	Non-hierarchical Drag and drop Codes Margin coding PDF coding	Hierarchical Drag and drop Case based Code frequencies Code statistics	Hierarchical Drag and drop Codes Weights Frequencies	Hierarchical Drag and drop Coding stripes Aggregate coding Cases Relationships Matrices PDF coding Social media coding	Hierarchical Drag and drop Cases Variables Code margin Geo and time tagging	Hierarchical—vertical and horizontal Drag and drop Time variables Weights Frequencies
Project management	Document families Network visualizations	Cases Code group sets	Variables Document sets Visualization tools Colour coding	Classifications Attributes Sets Report and Extracts Visualization tools Colour coding	Cases Socio-demographic Report manager Visualization tools	Excerpts Descriptors Reports Interactive visualizations Colorization
Interrogating database	Query tool Boolean, semantic and proximity based operators	Case selection Hypothesis tool	Matrix Frequency table	Text Search Word Frequency Coding query Matrix coding Compound query Coding comparison Group coding Relationships	Case selection Hypothesis tool Statistical functions Text retrieval Frequency Co-occurrence Coding agreement Query By Example Filtering	Filters Database query tool
Writing tools	Memo Comments	Annotations Memos	Memos Tables	Memos Annotation	Annotations Memos	Memos
Teamwork	Shared documents Individual and Team Libraries	Merge	Merge Import Team member protocol creation	Merge Import NVivo Server option	Multiple long-on Merge Duplicate Coding agreement	Web-based Online Chat

(continued)

Table 19.5.16 Continued

FUNCTIONS	ATLAS.ti V7	HyperRESEARCH 3.0.3	MaxQDA 10	nVivo 10	QDA Miner 4	Dedoose 4.2
Interface Language	English	English	English German Spanish French Japanese Italian Chinese Portuguese Turkish Polish Thai	English French German Spanish Portuguese Japanese Chinese	English French Spanish	English Picture-based
Operating System	Windows Mac (+ Windows emulator)	Cross platform: Windows Mac	Windows Mac (+ Windows emulator)	Windows Mac Tablets Smartphones	Windows Mac (+ Windows emulator)	Web-based AND Desktop app Platform independent Tablets (with Photon app)
Additional features	Hyperlink and mapping	Hyperlink and mapping Code Mapping	Mapping Additional dictionary Qualitative and quantitative data analysis	MS Outlook interface See also links Hyperlink Static or dynamic mapping Spellcheck	Thesaurus searching Numerical and textual content analysis Optional Statistical analysis module	Integrates qualitative and quantitative data analysis Data downloadable

Methodological difficulties in psychosocial research in palliative medicine

Psychosocial researchers encounter significant specific difficulties in conducting research with dying people (Glare, 1999; Field et al., 2001). The recruitment of patients, attainment of an adequate sample size (Jordhoy et al., 1999), attrition rates, and the variability of the patient's condition (Kirkham and Abel, 1997) create problems for researchers internationally (Bakitas et al., 2006). Employment of trained data managers, adoption of several recruitment methods, and use of well-thought out inclusion criteria does assist sampling problems (Jordhoy et al., 1999). Moreover, ethical debates exist regarding the impact of research on patients at the end of their lives (de Raeve, 1994), the withholding of treatment in controlled trials (Corner, 1996), and the informed consent process when delirium is present (Karim, 2000). Extensive interviews and use of batteries of questionnaires can be stressful and intrusive at a vulnerable and potentially poignant time in the life cycle (Atkinson and Silverman, 1997). Despite the challenges involved in such psychosocial research, its value is beyond question and critical to our endeavours to improve the care of the dying.

Outcomes in psychosocial research and future directions

The clinical significance or utility of each study merits careful reflection so that standards of care are steadily improved. Quality assurance programmes have highlighted the importance of the feedback loop, which leads to altered practice, innovation, and change (Lawton, 1971). This should be a cyclical activity.

For palliative medicine to grow as a discipline, its research activity must be scholarly and generate the needed evidence that informs purposeful clinical activity. Psychosocial research is a cardinal component of such endeavours. It needs to grow through well thought out national and international collaborations, utilizing integrated methodologies of the highest standards. For too long, clinicians have defensively avoided good science through flawed claims about the unsuitability of palliative patients for research. Fortunately, the specialty is maturing and recognizes the imperative for its future of excellence in research studies.

Psychosocial research in the future needs to embrace RCTs to establish a sound evidence base for its practice. Further, RCTs are needed of pharmacotherapies and particularly meaning-centred therapies to treat existential and spiritual distress. Interpersonal psychotherapy is one manualized and standardized intervention waiting to be applied in palliative care—its emphasis on grief, transitions, roles, and relationships makes it particularly suitable with this population. Interventions need to be both patient- and family-centred.

Suffering remains a cardinal domain for future research activity. Observational studies using mixed methodologies are needed to explore demoralization, dignity, shame, and unworthy dying, incorporating the experience of patients, families and carers, doctors and nurses, and all related support staff to build a complete gestalt of the many intersecting influences on outcome. Over the next decade, such a body of work should guide future intervention studies aimed at further improving the standard of psychosocial care.

Communication studies have developed in oncology over the past decade but remain a vital research domain for palliative medicine. Discussion of prognosis and preparation for death are some of the most challenging conversations, yet there is a corresponding dearth of systematic research to guide the approach that clinicians take. Promotion of adaptive coping and maintenance of hope alongside acceptance of the reality of impending death constitute a fundamental feature of the effective communication needed in palliative medicine.

More systematic research into decision-making and informed consent in end-of-life care is also needed that provides patient- and family-centred outcomes in terms of quality of care and satisfaction with the process, whilst outcomes that evaluate staff compliance with advance care planning and other decisions are required to provide empirical evidence to inform the otherwise theoretical ethical debate that abounds globally.

Finally, an urgent requirement in many countries of the world is the training of dedicated researchers who can then address many of these problems. Without solid education and experience, the pitfalls appear formidable; skill development in research methodology is crucial to respond to the many challenges emerging in this young discipline.

Online materials

Complete references for this chapter are available online at <http://www.oxfordmedicine.com>.

References

Bakitas, M.A., Lyons, K.D., Dixon, J., and Ahles, T.A. (2006). Palliative care program effectiveness research: developing rigor in sampling design, conduct, and reporting. *Journal of Pain and Symptom Management*, 31, 270–284.

Bruera, E., Kuehn, N., Miller, M.J., Selmser, P., and Macmillan, K. (1991). The Edmonton Symptom Assessment System (ESAS): a simple method for the assessment of palliative care patients. *Journal of Palliative Care*, 7, 6–9.

Cohen, S.R., Mount, B.M., Strobel, M.G., and Bui, F. (1995). The McGill Quality of Life Questionnaire: a measure of quality of life appropriate for people with advanced disease. A preliminary study of validity and acceptability. *Palliative Medicine*, 9, 207–219.

Edwards, B. and Clarke, V. (2005). The validity of the family relationships index as a screening tool for psychological risk in families of cancer patients. *Psycho-Oncology*, 14, 546–554.

Folstein, M.F., Robins, L.N., and Helzer, J.E. (1983). The Mini-Mental State Examination. *Archives of General Psychiatry*, 40, 812.

Higginson, I.J., Finlay, I.G., Goodwin, D.M., et al. (2003). Is there evidence that palliative care teams alter end-of-life experiences of patients and their caregivers? *Journal of Pain and Symptom Management*, 25, 150–168.

Kissane, D.W., Wein, S., Love, A., Lee, X.Q., Kee, P.L., and Clarke, D.M. (2004). The Demoralization Scale: a report of its development and preliminary validation. *Journal of Palliative Care*, 20, 269–276.

Kroenke, K., Spitzer, R.L., and Williams, J.B. (2001). The PHQ-9: validity of a brief depression severity measure. *Journal of General Internal Medicine*, 16, 606–613.

Peterman, A.H., Fitchett, G., Brady, M.J., Hernandez, L., and Cella, D. (2002). Measuring spiritual well-being in people with cancer: the functional assessment of chronic illness therapy—Spiritual Well-being Scale (FACIT-Sp). *Annals of Behavioral Medicine*, 24, 49–58.

Steinhauser, K., Clipp, E., Bosworth, H., et al. (2003). Measuring quality of life at the end of life: validation of the QUAL-E. *Gerontologist*, 43, 200–200.

Zigmond, A.S. and Snaith, R.P. (1983). The hospital anxiety and depression scale. *Acta Psychiatrica Scandinavica*, 67, 361–370.

Ethical issues in palliative care research

David Casarett

Introduction to ethical issues in palliative care research

Recent growth in palliative care research has created a heterogeneous field that encompasses both qualitative and quantitative techniques, and descriptive as well as interventional study designs. Despite the valuable knowledge that has been produced by this research, and the promise of future important advances, its progress has been impeded by a persistent uncertainty about the ethics of these studies (Casarett et al., 2003). For instance, there have been concerns raised about whether patients near the end of life should ever be asked to participate in research (de Raeve, 1994; Annas, 1998) although others have objected to this extreme position (Mount et al., 1995; Casarett and Karlawish, 2000). Nevertheless, the combination of ethical and practical issues can create substantial barriers to palliative care research (Aktas and Walsh, 2011).

This chapter discusses five ethical aspects of palliative care research that investigators and clinicians should consider in designing and conducting palliative care research. These include (1) the study's potential benefits to future patients, (2) the study's potential benefits to subjects, (3) the study's risks to subjects, (4) subjects' decision-making capacity, and (5) the voluntariness of subjects' choices about research participation. Although none of these aspects is unique to palliative care research, palliative care investigators can use these overarching principles to enhance the ethics of palliative care research.

Benefits to future patients: a study's validity and value

Palliative care research should eventually improve care for future patients. These benefits to future patients can be described in terms of validity and value.

Validity

To ensure the ethical foundation of palliative care research, investigators should use valid techniques of design and data analysis, and intend to produce knowledge that is generalizable. Indeed, generalizability is the cornerstone of one definition of research used in the United States: 'a systematic investigation, including research development, testing and evaluation, designed to develop or contribute to generalizable knowledge' (Department of Health

and Human Services, 1991, §46.102(d)). These requirements collectively describe a study's validity (Freedman, 1987). Indeed, it is unethical to expose human subjects to risks in studies that peer reviewers agree cannot adequately answer a research question (Rutstein, 1970).

Value

Above this threshold of validity, palliative care studies may offer more or less importance, or 'value'. Broadly, value can be defined as the likelihood that a study's results will improve the health and well-being of future patients (Casarett et al., 2003). Like validity, value is an important measure of a study design's scientific quality. It is also a measure of its ethical quality, however, because a central goal of research is to produce knowledge that will ultimately be 'important' (Department of Health and Human Services, 1991), 'fruitful' (Brody, 1998, p. 213), or 'valuable' (Freedman, 1990). In fact, one reason that subjects participate in clinical research is to produce knowledge that will benefit others (Advisory Committee on Human Radiation Experiments, 1995; Casarett et al., 2001). Because subjects are willing to accept risks and burdens of research at least in part in order to benefit others, investigators have an ethical responsibility to maximize the probability that a study will be able to do so.

Maximizing validity and value in palliative care research

There are several ways in which investigators can enhance the validity and value of palliative care research. First, a study's sample size should be adequate to answer the research question that is posed. Problems of underpowered studies, and particularly clinical trials, are both widespread and well described (Meinert, 1986). But they are particularly relevant to palliative care research, in which random variation can be quite large (Moore et al., 1998) and recruitment can be difficult (Aktas and Walsh, 2011). To minimize these problems, it can be useful to establish consortia or collaborative groups that can participate in multicentre studies (Kutner et al., 2008). Efforts to integrate data collection into usual care have been promising (Abernethy, 2010), and use of electronic medical record data has allowed large-scale studies at minimal cost (Casarett et al., 2012).

Second, palliative care investigators can increase the generalizability of its results. These steps might include sample size calculations that permit analysis of groups of patients that have typically not been the focus of investigation, such as patients with non-cancer diagnoses, ethnic minorities, or elderly patients. The generalizability of a study's results might also be enhanced by recruiting subjects outside the usual academic medical settings through outreach to community clinics and hospices.

Benefits to subjects

Palliative care investigators can also enhance the ethical rigor of a study by maximizing the benefits that it will offer to subjects, either during the study or after the study ends. During interventional studies, for example, a treatment could offer the possibility of a meaningful improvement. These potential benefits can be enhanced by choosing an active control design, rather than a placebo. Even if a placebo is used, a study's potential benefits can also be improved by altering the standard 1:1 randomization scheme in a placebo-controlled trial in a way that increases subjects' chances of receiving an active agent (Farrar et al., 1998) or by using a crossover design, if possible. Of course, the potential benefits of study interventions are never certain and a trial is only ethically acceptable only if there is legitimate uncertainty, or equipoise (Freedman, 1987), regarding the relative benefits of an intervention. Therefore, although investigators have an obligation to consider the benefits that a study offers to prospective subjects, this should not be interpreted as a requirement that all interventional studies should offer potential benefits.

Descriptive studies can also offer benefits to subjects who participate. For instance, data gathered during a descriptive study may identify pain that is inadequately treated, dissatisfaction with pain management, or related clinical problems like depression. In anticipation of instances like these, investigators can design standard operating procedures that help to ensure that these problems are identified and triaged appropriately, including communication with the patient's health-care provider if appropriate (Casarett and Karlawish, 2000).

An interventional or descriptive study also might benefit a subject after it is over. Subjects may benefit from learning about a study's aggregate results. For example, if a study comparing two pain medications found that one resulted in fewer side effects, this knowledge may help a subject make a more informed choice among available medications. Others may benefit if the study permits continued access to an intervention after the study ends, often through reduced rate programmes or open-label extension phases. This benefit may be particularly important in palliative care research, if subjects are unlikely to live long enough to see a study medication's approval for clinical use, or to see a study's results published and translated into improved care.

Minimizing risks and burdens

Investigators can also enhance a study's ethical rigor by taking steps to minimize a study's risks (e.g. medication side effects) and burdens (e.g. additional clinic visits or time required for surveys). The criteria by which study risks and burdens are identified and evaluated apply the concept of incremental or 'demarcated' risks imposed by participation in a study (Freedman et al., 1992). For instance, a study that compares two commonly used sustained-release opioids for pain may not present a significantly increased ('demarcated') risk to the patient because treatment with one of the drugs would have occurred off protocol. In contrast, a study that evaluates a sustained-release opioid in a condition for which it is not typically used (e.g. pruritus) poses risks that must be justified in the study's design. In either case, however, the risks of any medication in a clinical trial should be disclosed in the informed consent process.

Minimizing risks in an interventional trial: the choice of control

Perhaps one of the most contentious and emotional questions in palliative care research (Hardy, 1997; Kirkham and Abel, 1997), and indeed in research generally (Rothman and Michels, 1994; Macklin, 1999; Temple and Ellenberg, 2000), is whether a placebo or sham control arm is ethically appropriate. Broadly, placebos can be defined as interventions that are 'ineffective or not specifically effective' for the symptom or disorder in question (Shapiro and Shapiro, 1998, p. 12). The consensus that all subjects in a clinical trial should have access to the best available standard of care (World Medical Association, 2000) highlights the potential for unethical use of placebo. For example, all subjects with meningitis must have access to an antimicrobial agent that has proven effective; a placebo control in a trial of a new antibiotic would be unethical. In some types of research, however, such as symptom research, the placebo response can be substantial and mimics an active intervention. Moreover, the symptom under study may be transient, such as incident pain. In these situations, a placebo control may be ethically acceptable, particularly if one or more of several other conditions are met. First, placebos are acceptable if subjects receive a placebo in addition to the standard of care, such as a design that randomly assigns patient to receive an opioid plus an adjuvant agent for pain or an opioid plus a placebo. Second, a placebo arm is justified if the symptom under study has no effective treatment. Third, a placebo control is justified if subjects have adequate access to breakthrough, or 'rescue' treatment. This may in turn alter a trial's end points, and may require the inclusion of these doses as a study endpoint (Dhaliwal et al., 1995; Silverman et al., 1993; Broomhead et al., 1997).

Although sham procedures are difficult to define, the term generally is applied to a procedure that is administered in a way that makes it ineffective (Polati et al., 1998). These create ethical concerns because some subjects are exposed to the risks of the procedure without any hope of its benefits (Macklin, 1999). Like placebo controls, though, the use of a sham procedure may be ethical in some studies if the risks to subjects are minimized, some subjects are likely to benefit from non-specific effects, and the research question has high value. For instance, Leonard Cobb's research in the 1950s effectively debunked a widely used cardiac procedure that, if it had been widely disseminated, would eventually have put thousands of patients at risk. Designing a sham-controlled study so that the procedure itself (whether sham or real) poses few if any additional or 'incremental' risks above and beyond usual care also can reduce concerns about ethical acceptability. For example, investigators might insert a sham epidural catheter that would then be used for postoperative analgesia (Haak van der Lely et al., 1994) or a crossover design can be used to ensure that all subjects who bear the risks of the sham procedure also have access to the real procedure's potential benefits. This crossover sham design has been used in other settings (Hahn et al., 1996), and might be appropriate for pain research when the risks or discomforts of the sham procedure are substantial.

Minimizing burdens

For the most part, opportunities to minimize burdens are readily apparent. For instance, it seems reasonable wherever possible to minimize surveys, interviews, and additional study visits (Bruera, 1994). The importance of these actions may be accentuated when study subjects are very ill and an additional appointment or the requirement to complete another measure may increase distressing symptoms, such as fatigue, Investigators who conduct palliative care research should be particularly attuned to strategies that minimize these burdens, such as telephonic data collection.

Palliative care investigators may also need to consider the burdens that a study creates for friends and family members who often take on substantial burdens as caregivers (Steele and Fitch, 1996; Emanuel et al., 1999). By building flexibility into a study design (e.g. use of brief telephone interviews, multiple options for timing of clinic visits), investigators may be able to reduce the burdens of research participation on others.

Ensuring decision-making capacity

Patients who consent to participate in research should have adequate decision-making capacity, which refers to subjects' ability to understand relevant information, appreciate the significance of that information, and reason through to a conclusion that makes sense for them (Grisso and Appelbaum, 1998). Concerns have been raised about capacity in research involving patients with dementia (Marson et al., 1994) and psychiatric illness (Elliott, 1997), and patients in the intensive care setting (Lemaire et al., 1997), among others.

Concerns about the potential for impaired decision-making capacity are reasonable when research involves a population with advanced illness. The prevalence of cognitive impairment is high in this setting (Breitbart et al., 1995; Pereira et al., 1997), occurring in 10–40% of patients in the final months of life and in up to 85% of patients in the last days of life. Cognitive impairment may be difficult to identify because decision-making capacity varies over time (Bruera et al., 1995) and because impairment may result from the experimental or therapeutic medications themselves, such as opioids, benzodiazepines, or corticosteroids (Bruera et al., 1989; Stiefel et al., 1989). Investigators who conduct trials of medications will encounter these challenges even more frequently if trials are designed to evaluate treatments for delirium, for which impairment is an inclusion criterion (Breitbart, 1996).

Concern about impaired capacity also is increased by the potential comorbidity of clinical depression, which occurs in between 5% and 25% of patients near the end of life (Derogatis et al., 1983; Brown, 1986; Kathol et al., 1990; Massie and Holland, 1990). Clinically significant adjustment disorders may be even more common (Derogatis et al., 1983), and it is possible that these disorders may impair either comprehension or decision-making, or both (Elliott, 1997).

Decision-making capacity also can be undermined by severe symptoms, the experience of which may impair comprehension if patients are unable to concentrate on the information offered in the informed consent process (Kristjanson et al., 1994). This concern is particularly relevant in clinical trials that require the presence of one or more poorly-controlled symptom as an inclusion criterion.

The challenges encountered in ensuring decision-making capacity among research subjects may be magnified in longitudinal studies. Even if patients have the capacity to consent at the time of enrolment, they may not retain that capacity throughout the study. Days or weeks after patients give consent to participate, they may be unable to understand changes in their condition clearly enough to withdraw. The result can be a 'Ulysses contract', in which research subjects find it easier to enrol than they do to withdraw (Dresser, 1984).

None of these challenges is easily remedied. Indeed, it is obstacles like these that lead some authors to argue that patients near the end of life should not be allowed to enrol in research (de Raeve, 1994; Annas, 1998). To address the concern and enhance the ethical rigor of palliative care research when decision-making capacity is uncertain, it is important to briefly assess understanding in either open-ended or multiple choice format whenever studies involve subjects who may be near the end of life (Penman et al., 1984; Miller et al., 1996). In some situations, investigators may wish to assess decision-making capacity more formally using validated instruments (Grisso and Appelbaum, 1995). This need not be employed in all studies, but rather considered whenever the prevalence of cognitive impairment is likely to be high and the study design includes risks that must be balanced against benefits (Casarett et al., 2001). For instance, when palliative care research involves only interviews or behavioural interventions that pose minimal risks, informal capacity assessments are generally sufficient. When research poses greater than minimal risks, but offers potential benefits, a structured assessment of understanding may be appropriate. Finally, when a study poses greater than minimal risks but does not offer potential benefits, a formal evaluation of capacity should be considered.

If a patient does not have the capacity to give consent, a legally authorized representative may be able to give consent for research. This approach is justified by the argument that surrogate decision-makers should be allowed to consent to research just as they are allowed to consent to medical therapy, using either a substituted judgement of the patient's preferences or an assessment of what would be in the patient's best interests. If a patient does not have the capacity to consent, but is still able to participate in decisions, investigators should obtain assent from the patient and informed consent from the patient's surrogate (High, 1993; High et al., 1994). This 'dual consent' ensures that patients are as involved in the decision as possible, yet provides the additional protection of a surrogate's consent.

If a patient has decision-making capacity intermittently, or is expected to lose capacity, investigators may obtain advance consent. This innovative approach has been used in a study of treatment for delirium, in which informed consent was obtained from patients while they had decision-making capacity (Breitbart, 1996). Advance consent should be obtained only for specific studies, and should be obtained close to the planned start of research (e.g. at the time of hospitalization or enrolment in a hospice or palliative care programme).

Protecting voluntariness

Another way that investigators can enhance the ethical soundness of a study's design is to examine ways in which subjects' voluntary participation can be protected. In general terms, a choice is voluntary if it is made without significant controlling influences (Faden and Beauchamp, 1986, pp. 241–268; Beauchamp and Childress,

2001, p. 123). Voluntariness can be protected by ensuring that a subject's choice to enrol is made with full knowledge of available alternatives and with the understanding that he or she can withdraw at any time.

Recruitment of subjects from an environment with excellent standards of palliative care enhances the likelihood that decisions about research participation will be voluntary. If patients receive excellent care, they will be best able to make a free and uncoerced choice about research participation. Patients without access to excellent care may view research participation more favourably out of desperation, or may be less willing to withdraw from research because of the perception that effective palliative interventions (e.g. opioids) are not readily available off protocol.

Conclusion

The field of palliative care, and the standard of care that it represents, depends upon rigorous research to provide data that will guide clinical care. Although this research raises ethical questions, these questions need not curtail what promises to be a valuable and highly productive area of research. Ethical questions can be addressed through careful attention to the study's consent process and scientific design. With proper attention to strategies that ensure the ethical conduct of studies, missteps that have produced scandals in other fields will be avoided.

Online materials

Complete references for this chapter are available online at <http://www.oxfordmedicine.com>.

References

Breitbart, W., Marotta, R., Platt, M.M., *et al.* (1996). A double-blind trial of haloperidol, chlorpromazine, and lorazepam in the treatment of delirium in hospitalized AIDS patients. *American Journal of Psychiatry*, 153(2), 231–237.

Brody, B. (1998). *The Ethics of Biomedical Research. An International Perspective.* New York: Oxford University Press.

Casarett, D. and Karlawish, J. (2000). Are special ethical guidelines needed for palliative care research? *Journal of Pain and Symptom Management*, 20, 130–139.

Dresser, R. (1984). Bound to treatment: the Ulysses contract. *Hastings Centre Reports*, 14, 13–16.

Freedman, B. (1987). Equipoise and the ethics of clinical research. *The New England Journal of Medicine*, 317, 141–145.

Freedman, B. (1990). Placebo-controlled trials and the logic of clinical purpose. *IRB*, 12, 1–6.

Freedman B. (1987). Scientific value and validity as ethical requirements for research: a proposed explication. *IRB*, 9, 7–10.

Macklin, R. (1999). The ethical problems with sham surgery in clinical research. *The New England Journal of Medicine*, 341, 992–996.

Marson, D.C., Schmitt, F.A., Ingram, K.K., and Harrell, L.E. (1994). Determining the competency of Alzheimer patients to consent to treatment and research. *Alzheimer Disease & Associated Disorders*, 8(Suppl. 4), 5–18.

Quality of life in palliative care: principles and practice

Stein Kaasa and Jon Håvard Loge

Introduction to quality of life in palliative care

Quality of life (QOL) is the main goal of palliative care. This is not a new idea; one of the main goals of the health-care system in ancient Greece was to improve what we might now interpret as the patients' quality of life (Aristotle, 1975). Such improvement has therefore been, and will continue to be, an overall goal for palliative care specifically as it is for health care in general.

In a sociological context, QOL is described in theories of human welfare (defined as level of education, and economic and industrial growth). Studies from the 1950s found that economic improvement did not necessarily result in greater levels of happiness, lower levels of worries, or a better outlook (Bradburn, 1969). It was recognized that there was a need for alternative indicators of welfare in addition to the economic and material indicators used at that time. On this background, indicators of human welfare, based upon subjects' perceptions, were developed. Different terminologies have been used by different groups to describe this phenomenon of subjective well-being; subjective indicators, general well-being, or QOL (Andrews and Withey, 1976; Campbell et al., 1976). The common denominators were that the respondents' perceptions were asked for and that the information was collected by means of interviews or questionnaires.

Despite the widespread use of the term QOL as a theoretical concept, in politics and in empirical studies, no precise agreed-upon definition exists. However, in order to simplify the discussion on the content of the term, one may target two general approaches in the understanding of its meanings. Firstly, QOL may be regarded as a broad concept that encompasses 'how is your life, everything taken in consideration' and secondly QOL may be regarded as a more distinct health-oriented concept focusing on specific aspects of health or health care, including symptom levels and functioning. These are not mutually exclusive concepts, but rather a continuum of issues between two extremes allowing an intuitive flexibility in defining quality of life in terms of an overall general phenomenon or as a single sign or symptom, as illustrated in Fig. 19.7.1.

Overall quality of life

In sociological, psychological, and medical contexts, QOL has been used as a broad concept. One major distinction is between QOL as a social phenomenon in which access to health care, education, etc. are seen as indicators of QOL, and QOL as a subjective phenomenon in which the individual's subjective perception is the indicator of QOL. The different definitions of QOL in the latter meaning, all connect psychological, mental, and spiritual domains of a person's life. In the process of finding indicators of these phenomena, satisfaction, happiness, morale, positive and negative affects have been put forward as important components of the quality of life concept. In some of the literature there is an emphasis on normality, viewing QOL as fulfilment of life and the possibilities to live a normal life, while others focus more on mental capacity, to think clearly, to feel well, to love and be loved, to make decisions for oneself, to maintain contact with family and friends, to live at home and/or to be physically active. The ability to make individual decisions has also been emphasized as an important aspect of QOL, including capacity of the individual to realize his life, which includes a perception of personal meaning.

According to these conceptualizations, QOL is strongly linked to normality, including normal function or that a minimum of human needs are met. Such a minimum of needs were also described by Maslow (1970), which is often referred to as 'Maslow's hierarchy of needs', consisting of biological needs, needs for close relationships, needs for meaningful occupation, and need for change. This concept has further been elaborated in a QOL context, viewing quality of life as the level of a person's activity, the ability to relate to others, self-esteem, and a basic mood of happiness (Moum et al., 1988).

Inclusion of normality and biological fulfilment into the global QOL concept is strongly challenged by empirical findings of many patients with major physical and/or psychological limitations reporting a high degree of global QOL (Hjermstad et al., 1999). These empirical findings fit well with another theory, the so-called gap theory of Calman (1984). He described QOL as an inverse relationship of the difference between an individual's expectations and its perception of the given situation: 'the smaller the gap the better quality of life'. According to this gap theory, as illustrated in Fig. 19.7.2, a change in QOL from T0 to T1 can be caused by changes in both expectations and experience, case A and B report the same QOL at T0 and T1, however the underlying causes of the change from T0 to T1 are different in the two individuals.

The gap theory may be used to explain unexpected findings between groups and within groups over time in intervention studies. In other words, one needs to explore the magnitude of all

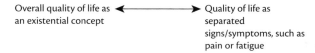

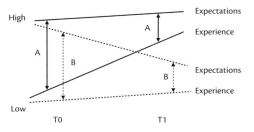

Fig. 19.7.1 Quality of life as a continuum from existentiality to single symptoms.

Fig. 19.7.2 Quality of life as the gap between expectations and experience.

relevant factors that may contribute to changes. This is especially important to consider in non-controlled intervention studies that use patient-reported outcomes.

Quality of life in medicine

In health-care research, QOL encompasses a range of components that are measurable and related to health, disease, illness, and medical interventions. In health care as well as in other contexts, QOL might have different meanings for different actors and take different meanings according to illness, experience, support, etc. A professional focus may also influence the perception of QOL. For example, a medical oncologist may rate tumour response after delivering combination chemotherapy to a patient with a non-Hodgkin's lymphoma as the most important achievement to improve QOL, while a nurse may focus on patients' ability to deal with daily activities. For a physician in palliative medicine, improvement of QOL for one patient may mean pain control, and for another the establishment of necessary social support. In the context of clinical trials one is rarely interested in QOL as a global concept, but rather as a specific outcome related to the intervention in question, such as improved pain control during night-time by delivery of slow-release morphine at bedtime, or reduced dyspnoea after chest irradiation for a patient with lung cancer. Despite the unresolved issue about how to define QOL, most researchers and clinicians agree that QOL in palliative medicine is related to symptom control, physical function, social functioning, psychological well-being and meaning and fulfilment (existential and spiritual issues). This multidimensional health-oriented concept has been named by many clinicians and researchers as health-related quality of life (HRQOL) (Priestman and Baum, 1976; Bergner et al., 1981; Coates et al., 1983; Goldberg and Williams, 1988; Wade and Collin, 1988). During the last decade, the terms QOL and HRQOL have been challenged by another terminology—'patient-reported outcomes' (PROs). In essence it is a more neutral term which includes all types of measure completed or reported by the patients.

As early as 1947, the World Health Organization (WHO), in its definition of health, described it as multidimensional: 'Health is not only the absence of infirmity and disease, but also a state of complete physical, mental and social well-being' (WHO, 1958). This definition has been identified by several researchers as the beginning of a new era in relation to health and health care. In spite of being highly disputed, the definition includes three dimensions of health that later have been included in the HRQOL concept: physical health, mental health, and social functioning.

Another event that subsequently influenced the development of the QOL concept in health care was proposed by Karnofsky in 1948. He evaluated the palliative effects of nitrogen mustard on various malignant tumours by means of subjective improvement, objective improvement, and performance status (Karnofsky et al., 1948). Performance status was defined according to specific criteria, which have become widely used and known as the Karnofsky Performance Status scale. This simple scale has been shown to be a significant predictor of survival in patients with metastatic disease, as have measurers of HRQOL (Kaasa et al, 1989; Maltoni, 1995; Coates et al., 1997). In a topical review, it was advocated for the use of complementary prognostic factors such as indicators of cachexia, dyspnoea, delirium, and some biological factors (Maltoni, 2005).

During the 1970s, standardized questionnaires were developed in cooperative groups and in academic settings. 'Linear analogue self-assessment scales' (LASAs) were used to capture the QOL of specific cancer groups, such as breast cancer patients. These measures included a variety of subjective domains, such as general well-being, mood, anxiety, activity, pain, and social activity (Priestman and Baum, 1976; Coates et al., 1983). Others developed measures of health status in order to capture patients' general perceptions of health, some examples are the Sickness Impact Profile (Bergner et al., 1981), Nottingham Health Profile (Hunt and McEwen, 1980), Short Form 36 (SF-36) (Ware and Sherbourne, 1992; Ware, 1995), and more physically oriented scales such as the Barthel index (Wade and Collin, 1988). Other measures, which are also classified as QOL measures focus primarily on psychological domains, such as the General Health Questionnaire (GHQ) (Goldberg and Williams, 1988) and Profile of Mood States (McNair et al., 1971).

At the same time a similar development of measures were seen within the area of pain assessment based upon the definition of pain launched by The International Association for the Study of Pain (IASP). IASP defined pain as 'an unpleasant sensory and emotional experience associated with actual or potential tissue damage, or described in terms of such damage' (IASP Task Force on Taxonomy, 1994). These definitions are conceptually very similar to most definitions of QOL and the WHO definition of health in that the subjective perception of the individual is recognized as the key component of health, pain, and QOL respectively. By looking into the content of the so-called broad measures of QOL, health, and pain, they contain to a large degree the same domains. Recently it is also shown that sleep and psychological distress correlate significantly with pain intensity (Knudsen et al., 2012). Previously pain measurement had involved standardized external stimulants, such as radiant heat, which were used to obtain a psycho-physiological standard to measure clinical pain. A 'language of pain' was developed, which is well illustrated by the McGill Pain Questionnaire (MPQ) (Melzack and Torgerson, 1971). During this development the concept of pain was broadened from previously focusing on pain as a neurobiological entity to a multidimensional concept like QOL. More simple tools were also used to assess pain intensity in order to simplify the assessment in clinical practice, such as Verbal Rating Scales (VRS), Numerical Rating Scales (NRS), and Visual Analogue Scales (VAS) (Jensen, 1986). A work group in the European Association for Palliative Care (EAPC) has recommended to measure pain intensity on an 11-point NRS using the following anchoring points: 'no pain' and 'pain as bad as you can imagine' (Kaasa et al., 2011).

Assessment methodology

Most of the measurement tools for HRQOL, pain, and other aspects of subjective health are built upon the questionnaire concept, where a standardized paper-based questionnaire is to be completed by the patients. This approach is more or less well suited for palliative care patients. For severely ill patients assessment by means of interviews or standardized observations may be more appropriate. Interviews are flexible and provide detailed information, but are expensive and time-consuming to perform. Further, their usefulness might be limited in multicentre trials where HRQOL is often assessed at several time points (Kaasa, 1992).

Standardized observations of behaviours or functions are alternatives to self-report questionnaires for assessment in specific groups of palliative patients such as pain assessment in cognitively impaired or assessment of functioning such as activities of daily living (ADLs). On a theoretical level one may dispute whether these are assessments of QOL since the observer's and not the patient's perceptions are registered. In cognitively impaired patients, for example, pain is recommended to be measured by observation, which is probably the only valid methodology as of today. On a practical level we do not know the optimal assessment method for a given situation. For example, is physical functioning best assessed by asking the patient or by observing him/her? At what level of cognitive impairment is pain best assessed by standardized observations of behaviour and not by asking the patient? In spite of these and other unresolved issues, assessment of QOL by use of questionnaires has become the far most commonly used approach. The questionnaires have until now mostly existed in paper format, but administration in an electronic format seems to become increasingly popular, especially in research (Velikova et al., 1999).

Patient-reported outcomes and QOL

Another term, PROs, has been launched in order to improve the terminology with regards to measurement of patients' subjective health status. A PRO has been defined as a measurement of any aspect of a patient's health status that comes directly from the patient, without the interpretation of the patient's responses by a physician or anyone else. This implies that the term PRO is an umbrella that covers a wide range of measurements but is used specifically about questionnaires in paper or electronic format that are completed by the patient. QOL is in this context considered a broad concept referring to *all* aspects of a person's well-being. PRO can measure QOL in this broad meaning of the term, but can also focus more narrowly on a single symptom such as pain, or on a function such as physical functioning (Bren, 2006; US Food and Drug Administration, 2009).

The introduction of the term PRO must be understood in the context of manufacturers' claims of treatments' positive effects on patients' QOL. Such claims should be documented by an evaluation of the impact of a given treatment on *all* aspects of a person's well-being since QOL in its broad meaning includes assessment of the physical aspects of disease (i.e. symptoms and function), the person's emotional state, feelings, coping behaviours, self-identity (psychological functioning), and the person's ability to interact with others (social functioning) (US Food and Drug Administration, 2009). In most cases, however, claims by a manufacturer on a treatment's positive effect on QOL have not been based on such a broad assessment. In most cases the claims are based on improvement within specific domains such as reduced levels of pain or less fatigue. A 'Guidance for Industry' on these issues published by the US Food and Drug Administration is a strong support for the relevance of outcomes based on patients' reports but also restricts the use of the term QOL to a more clearly specified situation than has been practised by most until now (US Food and Drug Administration, 2009).

Barriers to the use of patient-reported outcomes in the clinic

Reports indicate that doctors' and health professionals' recognition of subjective symptoms both in general oncology and in palliative care are suboptimal (Cull et al., 1995; Passik et al., 1998; Shuster et al., 1999), and measurement of HRQOL has not become an integral part of clinical practice. These shortcomings have been on the agenda for decades. Recently it was well documented in a study that subjective toxicity, which is a key parameter in the evaluation of cancer treatment and is not consistent across various symptoms, is underestimated by physicians (Gravis et al., 2014). The clinical interpretation is that physicians fail to report symptoms and consequently do not address them in a treatment plan. There are probably several explanations for these shortcomings, such as the content of the measures, that is, many of the scales may not have enough clinical relevance, clinicians do not believe in the importance of assessing subjective experience and/or the impracticalities of using comprehensive measures in daily clinical practice (Chang, 2007). Further, physical functioning is of great importance for palliative patients and thus of high relevance for clinical decisions and clinical studies. Still, it has been demonstrated that adequate measures for use in palliative care is lacking (Jordhøy et al., 2007).

The complexity of HRQOL measures makes them difficult to interpret and they are not easily accessible in the clinical decision-making process. For research purposes there are also needs for improvement of HRQOL measurements: clinical trials often use different measures to assess the same concepts, many measures are unresponsive to changes, many represent a burden on research participants and personnel, many measures have not been validated specifically in the clinical population during the study, and some/many lack sufficient evidence for validity (Garcia et al., 2007).

Computer-based assessment

The progress in information technology has expanded the use of computer systems in the clinic. Presently there is a major shift from paper-based medical records to electronic medical records (EMRs). These can also integrate other clinical electronic information systems such as digital imaging in radiology and laboratory data. The EMR may in the near future be complemented by clinical computerized support systems. As of today, the configuration and methods of data collection and the data entry varies. Systematic reviews have provided evidence on the effect of computer-based decision systems (Jaspers et al., 2011; Roshanov et al., 2013).

Various research groups in cancer care are in the process of developing computer-based assessment systems for general cancer care (Cella et al., 2010; Petersen et al., 2013). In palliative care, a computer-based tool for assessment of PRO, communication support, and decision support is under development (NTNU Technology Transfer AS, 2014).

Computer systems can also make the communication between patients and health-care providers dynamic as opposed to the static paper-based questionnaire. Furthermore, the computerized form will allow for more flexible ways of administering the tool, including downloading it from the Internet, administration by proxies, and the employment of handheld devices. Scores will be computed immediately and in digital forms. In total, such a development can make integration with other clinical parameters easier, support clinical decision-making, and finally be stored in the EMR.

Plethora of publications and instruments

The enormous increase in publications indexed under the subject heading QOL in MEDLINE reflects the increased focus on patients' QOL during the last 35–40 years. Seven papers were published in the period of 1966–1970 while nearly 40 000 papers were published in 2006–2011. A textbook published in 1996 included more than 200 different measures of quality of life in the broad sense (Spilker, 1996). A database on PRO and QOL instruments established in 2002 (the PROQOLID) now includes 886 instruments (PROQOLID, 2008). The rapidly increasing number of papers and newly developed questionnaires represents a challenge for the researcher and the clinician when they shall select the most appropriate assessment tool for their purpose

This increase in papers and questionnaires also points to a need for collaboration on development of a common nomenclature, as well as standardized and agreed-upon assessment tools. These suggestions have been put forward by several research groups for at least a decade both in HRQOL-assessment in general (Anderson et al., 1993) and in palliative care specifically (Kaasa et al., 2007; Kaasa and Radbruch, 2008). Despite these suggestions it was recently found in the area of pain assessment that new instruments are still being developed and published (Hjermstad et al., 2008). Most of these instruments are rarely used in later empirical studies.

HRQOL in palliative care

The goals of palliative care are acknowledged to include HRQOL as well as spirituality, loss/grief, family involvement, and coping. Many of the most common HRQOL tools have been thought inadequate by researchers for use in palliative care. The instruments have been criticized for being too narrow by only including physical, psychological, and social aspects of a patient's life. Outcome measures require questions that reflect the specific goals of palliative care (Hearn and Higginson, 1997), such as improving the QOL before death, controlling symptoms, and supporting the

---

Box 19.7.1 HRQOL measurement in palliative care

Content of measures—dimensions:

- Symptoms
- Physical function
- Emotional function
- Existential issues (spirituality).

Proxy ratings:

- Health-care providers
- Family members.

Quality of life:

- Patient and family assessment.

---

family (Box 19.7.1). It has been proposed that also meaning should be included, as well as purpose, spirituality, and grief (Cohen and Mount, 1992; Byock and Merriman, 1998; Waldron et al., 1999).

During end-stage disease, patients will often not be able to complete HRQOL instruments and proxies will be the only possible source of collection of information, either by means of interviews (open, semi-structured, or structured) or questionnaires. One possible strategy is to let the health-care provider or a family member complete the HRQOL instrument. However, many studies have shown that assessments by health-care providers or family members differ from the responses obtained from the patients. In some conditions, observers overestimate the psychological burden of disease, while pain and other symptoms are often underestimated.

In summary, HRQOL is the patient's perceptions of their health that are collected directly from the patient without interpretation of others. It is a dynamic phenomenon and different dimensions might be focused on, depending on individual factors, disease factors, symptomatology, coping ability, closeness to death, etc. The content is influenced by the setting, that is, the severity of physical symptoms, general health, spirituality, coping, existentially, etc. Still there is a general agreement to at least include relevant symptoms, physical, psychological, and social domains into the measures, and in many circumstances existential and spiritual domains also seem appropriate to include.

Patient population in palliative care and compliance with QOL assessment tools

There are several issues one must take into account when assessing HRQOL in palliative care. The patients are often sick and frail. Valid and reliable data may therefore be difficult to collect, particularly in the latest stages of life. Patients often have multiple symptoms at the same time and physical symptoms may give raise to psychological problems (and vice versa). These relationships in palliative care in general and specifically in end-of-life care have been discussed and addressed empirically.

What is a palliative care population?

A palliative care population is not a well-defined group of patients. In some programmes most patients are dying while in others the majority of the patients have a longer life expectancy.

Table 19.7.1 Patient population in palliative care—a proposal for classification

	Expected survival	**Karnofsky**
Combined oncology and palliative care	>12 months	>70
Primary palliation	>6–9 months	60–70
Early palliation	2–3 months	50–60
Late palliation	<1 month	30–40
Imminently dying	<1–2 weeks	<10

Source: Data from David A. Karnofsky et al., The use of the nitrogen mustrads in the palliative treatment of carcinoma—with particular reference to bronchogenic carcinoma, *Cancer*, Volume 1, Issue 4, pp. 34–56, Copyright © 1948 American Cancer Society.

In discussing the use of methodology to collect HRQOL data, the patient population in question should be specified as well as all research questions that are to be answered. Several indicators might be used to describe the population, such as expected survival, type of tumour-directed treatment, do not resuscitate (DNR) status, symptom burden, type of oncological treatment, etc. Recently a research group based on a collaboration within the EAPC has proposed a minimum dataset to use in the description of a palliative care cohort in clinical work as well as in quality assurance and research (Sigurdardottir et al., 2014).

Most patients in trials on palliative chemotherapy have a Karnofsky Performance Status above 60–70 and consequently an expected survival time of more than 6 months with large variations depending on the primary diagnosis. Newer types of chemotherapy, however, such as protein kinase inhibitors and growth factors inhibitors have improved survival substantially in many cancer patients with metastatic disease. Therefore it is argued that palliative care needs to be presented earlier in the disease trajectory (Kaasa, 2013). A second category of patients are those admitted to a palliative care programme, either as inpatients or as outpatients, with an average survival of 1–3 months. A third category may be the imminently dying patients with a Karnofsky Performance Status of 30–40 and lower. This latter category can be further divided into cognitively intact and cognitively impaired patients (Table 19.7.1).

The content of the assessment tools, the number of items in the instrument, and the use of proxy raters are some of the important issues to consider in relation to the patient population being investigated.

Compliance and patient population

Missing data can be defined as data that are anticipated but not returned. There are two main types of missing data: missing items (item non-response) and missing forms (unit non-response). The first relates to uncompleted question(s) within a QOL instrument and the second to a whole QOL assessment missing. Missing data is a potential source of selection bias in cancer research, quality assurance programmes, and in research in palliative medicine (Bernhard et al., 1998). Randomly missing data are not a problem except for some possible loss of power. Usually 1–2% of the responses to a given item within a questionnaire will be missing. However, in most cases missing data are due to a mixture of randomly missing data and data missing not at random (Fielding

et al., 2006). When data are missing for some patients, basic questions arise as to whether these patients differ from those with complete data sets. The patients in poorest health and with the shortest life expectancy are at the highest risk for both types of missing data (Anderson et al., 2000). In order to evaluate a scientific report and to compare cohorts between studies, a standard reporting system of compliance including all available information, should be required. Compliance is often defined as the number of questionnaires completed as a proportion of the number expected. The issue of compliance is described in more detail in textbooks (Fayers and Machin, 2007) and statistical literature (Colton et al., 1998). In this chapter some issues relating to compliance in palliative care will be discussed.

When patients become increasingly ill with progressive disease, they will find it difficult to complete questionnaires. Acceptable compliance can be achieved with HRQOL questionnaires in palliative care, though several patients will need assistance to complete the measures. During end-of-life care, the last 1–2 months of the patient's life, more patients will need help to complete the assessment tools due to physical deterioration, cognitive impairment, severe symptom distress, and/or emotional burdens. Compliance will decrease substantially if help is not provided (Jordhøy et al., 1999) (Fig. 19.7.3). Patients who are immediately dying will experience many distressing symptoms, but if they are excluded from not just research, but quality assurance and in evaluating clinical practice, there is a great risk for lack of empirical knowledge needed for development of systematic treatment procedures for this fragile population (Sneeuw et al., 1997). As of today, HRQOL questionnaires are in a paper-and-pencil format. All patients need to answer all questions in often extensive questionnaires. By using modern information technology systems and developing appropriate software, a custom-made approach can be applied by using systems where patients are only answering relevant questions according to symptoms and conditions in general. (See paragraph on computer-based assessment earlier in this chapter.)

Based on these facts, there are two main strategies in relation to missing data. The first is to reduce the risk of missing data to a minimum. This will include careful consideration of the length of the questionnaire, collection of data by use of optimal procedures for the population at stake, standardized procedures for

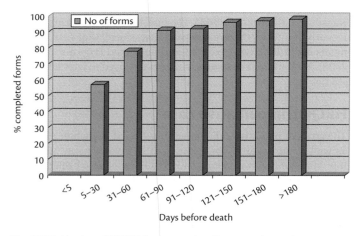

Fig. 19.7.3 Number of HRQOL forms completed in proportion to those distributed within various time frames prior to patients' death.

data collection, and careful observation of the data collection, especially towards 'gate-keeping', which implies that the data collector for some reason wants to shield the patient from participation. The ethics are clear on this point, it is the eligible patient's right to choose to participate or not. The second strategy is to carefully analyse for systematic patterns of missing data (both missing forms and missing items) in order to discover a biased data set.

Proxy ratings

Proxies may be considered as an alternative or complementary source of information, especially during end-of-life care (Brunelli et al., 1998). However, there has been a generally negative attitude towards the use of proxy ratings in the HRQOL literature because it has been repetitively demonstrated that assessment directly from the patient is the most valid way of collecting data on subjective health.

Review articles (Sprangers and Aaronson, 1992; Higginson et al., 1994), commentaries (Lampic and Sjoden, 2000; Sprangers and Sneeuw, 2000), and recent studies (To et al., 2012) have addressed the topic of caregivers and significant others as raters. Most of the published articles that address this issue, relate to general cancer populations or those in 'early palliation'. The studies have been criticized because of small sample sizes, major limitations in methodology, and use of unstandardized ad hoc instruments. The findings of the published studies are not totally consistent but can be summarized as follows:

◆ Health-care providers tend to overestimate patients' anxiety, depression, and general psychological distress.

◆ Agreement between health-care providers and patients' ratings was better in the absence of distress, than in the presence of distress.

◆ Pain and other symptoms seem to be underestimated by proxies.

◆ Proxy rating seems to be more accurate when the domains are concrete and observable.

There are several unanswered questions related to the use of proxy raters (Box 19.7.2): the limitation of proxy data, the content of proxy rating instruments, and the development of a common measure.

Even with these limitations caregivers or health-care providers can be used as proxy raters and it is probably best to use one of the short validated tools in order to compare data between studies and to optimize the clinicians' understanding of the content of the measures. The COOP/WONCA chart (Van Weel, 1993), Edmonton Symptom Assessment Schedule (ESAS) (Bruera et al.,

1991), and EORTC QLQ C-30 (Aaronson et al., 1993) are examples of such instruments. Another alternative is the SF-8 (Ware et al., 2001). However, the SF-8 has not been validated in palliative care populations. The SF-8 is an 8-item version of the SF-36. It yields a comparable 8-dimension health profile and comparable estimates of the physical and mental summary score as the SF-36 (Ware and Sherbourne, 1992).

However, before proxy ratings can be recommended outside a methodological research setting in palliative care, measurement tools and report systems need to be further developed into a user-friendly format and the strengths and limitations of proxy ratings need to be further addressed in research settings.

Choice of questionnaires

In the following, a comprehensive presentation of instruments for use in palliative medicine will not be given; instead some principles with concrete recommendations will be outlined.

The first step of the selection procedure is to specify the overall aim of the project. The overall aim then needs to be followed by an outline of the specific research questions or hypotheses. For each research question a clinical outcome should be decided upon. This will subsequently guide the selection of an assessment tool or even specific scales or items within a tool (Box 19.7.3).

It is generally recommended to assess HRQOL with multidimensional instruments because such measures are more comprehensive than uni-dimensional scales (Osoba, 1994). The HRQOL-measures are commonly divided into *generic, disease-specific*, and *domain-specific*. The *generic* measures are not specific to any population or disease. They are therefore applicable for subjects with more than one condition, and they make comparisons across populations and conditions possible. The *disease-specific* measures are developed for specific groups of patients, for example, such as the EORTC-QLQ-C30 and the FACT-G (Aaronson et al., 1993; Cella et al., 1993) developed for cancer patients or instruments specifically developed for palliative care. Most of the instruments include various aspects of functioning such as physical, role and social functioning and subjective appraisal of symptoms and well-being (Muldoon et al., 1998). Most recent generic and disease-specific instruments also assess positive health; that is, good health and well-being and not merely the absence of problems (Ware, 1995). The *domain-specific* instruments assess specific domains within the overall concept of HRQOL, such as fatigue, pain, or psychological distress.

Assessments of HRQOL will often include combinations of generic, disease-specific, and domain-specific instruments based on the specific purpose of the study. For example, if one wants

---

Box 19.7.2 Limitations of proxy ratings
◆ Lack of understanding of when and why proxies' ratings and patients' ratings differ
◆ Lack of short and intuitively understandable assessment tools
◆ Uncertainty about the instruments' psychometric properties when used by proxies
◆ Uncertainty about the comparability between patients' and proxies' ratings.

Box 19.7.3 A generic guide for selection of outcomes
◆ Step 1. Define the overall aim(s) of the project
◆ Step 2. Define the research question(s) or hypotheses
◆ Step 3. Agree upon the (clinical) outcome(s) for each recommended question
◆ Step 4. Select the assessment tool or scales within a tool, guided by the clinical outcome.

to compare the effects of single-fraction irradiation with multiple fractions in a population with painful bone metastasis, a multidimensional disease-specific questionnaire such as the EORTC-QLQ-C30 in combination with a domain-specific questionnaire on pain might be relevant. The number of questionnaires must fit the purpose for the assessment, but must also be balanced against the burden on the respondents and the costs of the data collection. The increased amount of information gained by including domain-specific measures is not always obvious and is clearly dependent on the content, the psychometric properties and the sensitivity of the instruments. For example, if a domain-specific instrument on fatigue does not have better measurement qualities than the fatigue scale within a generic or disease-specific instrument, it is not recommended to include it because of the increased burden to the patient.

Comparative data on different instruments measuring the same constructs are relatively scarce. The cancer-specific instrument EORTC QLQ-C30 and the generic instrument SF-36 were compared in patients with chronic non-malignant pain (Fredheim et al., 2007). Scales assumed to measure the same constructs were highly correlated, and for these scales the SF-36 scales tended to have better internal consistencies. On the other hand, the EORTC QLQ-C30 includes several symptoms that are not assessed by the SF-36.

The researcher might be best off by choosing instruments that are commonly used and found relevant within similar populations and settings. By choosing commonly used instruments, one's findings can more easily be evaluated by other researchers and put in a broader context. The psychometric properties of an instrument might vary across populations, therefore applying a questionnaire for the first time within a 'new population' requires a minimum of testing of some basic psychometric properties of the instrument in that particular population. The downside of this approach is that instruments with sub-optimal measurement qualities are used repetitively due to the costs associated with development and introduction of new and possibly better instruments.

In the following some commonly used instruments are briefly discussed. This does not imply that these instruments are superior to other available instruments.

Generic instruments

The first instruments were published in the 1970s and 1980s, such as the Sickness Impact Profile (SIP) (Bergner et al., 1976) and the Nottingham Health Profile (Hunt and McEwen, 1980). For a more detailed description we refer to other reviews (Bowling, 1995; Ware, 1995; Spilker, 1996). The first generation of instruments was generally lengthy and time-consuming to fill in.

The SF-36 is a second-generation instrument, developed from a larger questionnaire (Ware and Sherbourne, 1992). Eight concepts that were not specific to any disease, age, population, or treatment group were chosen to measure health conceptualized in two main dimensions: physical and mental health. The psychometric properties of the eight scales are generally very good with Cronbach's alphas in the range 0.80–0.93 (Ware, 1996). A revised version (version 2) was published in 2000 (QualityMetric, n.d.). The SF-36 version 2 is licensed and usage is depending upon a signed licence agreement and a fee. SF-36 Version 1 is available for usage without any costs as Rand SF-36 or Rand-36.

The SF-36 physical and mental component summary scales capture about 85% of the reliable variance in the instrument (McHorney et al., 1993). On this background, a shortened questionnaire was constructed. Twelve items from the SF-36 were selected and the instrument labelled SF-12 (Ware and Keller, 1996; QualityMetric, n.d.), and later the even shorter SF-8 (Ware et al., 2001; QualityMetric, n.d.). The SF-12 reproduces the eight-scale profile of the SF-36 but yields less precise scores. A revised version of the SF-12 (version 2) was published in 2002 (QualityMetric, n.d.). The revision followed the same principles as used for the revision of SF-36.

WHOQOL

The World Health Organization has developed the WHO Quality of Life Assessment Instrument (WHOQOL) (1993). The instrument was developed, according to a standardized protocol, simultaneously in several languages and cultures at 15 international centres (Szabo, 1996). The original instrument encompasses five domains measured by 100 items; physical health, psychological health, level of independence, social relationship, spirituality and environment. Each domain includes several facets, in total 24. Each facet contains four items, and the last four items measure overall quality of life and general health. Because of the limitations posed upon the use of the instrument's length, a 26 item abbreviated scale has been published, primarily for use in epidemiological studies (1998).

Disease-specific measures
EORTC QLQ-C30

The development of the cancer-specific questionnaires, the EORTC QLQ-C30 (European Organization for Research and Treatment of Cancer) was finalized in 1993 (Aaronson et al., 1993). Modified versions have been published and the group recommends version 3.0 of the questionnaire (EORTC). The questionnaire covers five functional scales (physical, role, cognitive, emotional and social), general QOL, three symptom scales (fatigue, pain and nausea and vomiting) and six single items. The single items assess common symptoms in cancer patients such as dyspnoea, loss of appetite, insomnia, constipation and diarrhoea.

The timeframe for the assessment is 1 week, which may be of particular relevance in clinical trials. The instrument has good psychometric properties including test/retest reliability (Bjordal and Kaasa, 1992; Hjermstad et al., 1995).

The so-called modular approach adopted by the EORTC Quality of Life Group infers that the core questionnaire can be supplemented with additional questionnaires designed for specific cancer sites (Aaronson et al., 1994). Updates on the latest development of the EORTC questionnaires are found on the website (EORTC, n.d.).

A shortened version containing 15 items intended for use in the palliative care setting, the EORTC QLQ-C15-PAL, was published in 2006 (Groenvold et al., 2006). Pain, physical function, emotional function, fatigue, global health status/QOL, nausea/vomiting, appetite, dyspnoea, constipation, and sleep were retained in the questionnaire. The EORTC QLQ-C15-PAL is a 'core questionnaire' for palliative care. Depending on the research questions or the purpose for use, it may be supplemented by additional items, modules, or questionnaires (Groenvold et al., 2006).

FACT-G

The Functional Assessment of Cancer—General Version (the FACT-G) was first published in 1993. In 1997 it was included as a core questionnaire in a measurement system called Functional Assessment of Chronic Illness Therapy (FACIT) intended for use in chronic diseases. Thus, FACIT is a broader, more encompassing system that includes the FACT questionnaires under its umbrella.

The FACT-G includes 27 items arranged in subscales covering four dimensions: physical well-being, social/family well-being, emotional well-being and functional well-being (Cella et al., 1993). It is considered appropriate for use in patients with any type of cancer. The time frame is 1 week, and the psychometric properties are reported as comparable to the EORTC QLQ C30 (Cella et al., 1993). There seems to be a tendency of the FACT-G being used more frequently in the United States than in Europe, while the EORTC QLQ-C30 is used primarily in Europe.

The FACIT measurement system has also adopted a modular approach with cancer-specific, symptom-specific and treatment-specific subscales. An update on the complete FACIT measurement system is found at the group's website (FACIT, n.d.).

Domain-specific measures

Generic or disease-specific instruments might not be sensitive enough for detection of differences in HRQOL. Questionnaires, also called domain-specific instruments, have been designed to assess specific symptoms, such as pain, fatigue, and anxiety. In some instances these types of instruments might be preferable. For example, in a study of patients with advanced prostate cancer, the EORTC QLQ-C30 fatigue scale did not detect variations in fatigue over time whereas two fatigue-specific instruments captured group differences (Stone et al., 2000). This finding is probably related to the so-called floor- and ceiling-effects. Numerous instruments are available and for a more comprehensive description we refer to relevant textbooks and websites (Bowling, 1995; Spilker, 1996; PROQOLID, 2008; FACIT, n.d.; QualityMetricQualityMetric, n.d.).

Anxiety, depression, and psychological distress

Many frequently used domain-specific instruments for measurement of anxiety and depression are old and can be characterized as first-generation instruments. For example, the Hospital Anxiety and Depression Scale (the HADS) was constructed in 1983 (Zigmond and Snaith, 1983). Other commonly used instruments for measurement of depression such as the Beck Depression Inventory (BDI) and Hamilton Depression Scale (HDS) were first published as early as the 1960s (Hamilton, 1960; Beck et al., 1961). At the time the psychiatric disorders (anxiety and depression) were defined differently than they are in 2014 (American Psychiatric Association, 2013).

When measuring anxiety and depression in palliative care it is important to examine whether the instrument includes somatic items (fatigue, weight loss, loss of appetite, etc.). Such symptoms are valid symptoms of anxiety and depression disorders in psychiatric and healthy populations, and the symptoms are included in the present diagnostic criteria for these disorders (American Psychiatric Association, 2013). However, these symptoms are not valid symptoms of anxiety and depression in palliative care patients because they are strongly affected by the underlying somatic disease.

A review on assessment of depression in palliative care identified 198 papers in which 105 different assessment methods had been used (Wasteson et al., 2009). Just a few studies had used structured interviews which are the 'gold standard' for diagnosing *depression disorders*. Sixty instruments had been used only once, and usage was not based on definition of depression and rather seemed to reflect local traditions. Regional differences were also detected as HADS was most commonly used in Europe but seldom in the United States or Canada.

HADS is one of the most frequently used instruments for measuring anxiety (seven items) and depressive symptoms (seven items) in oncology and palliative medicine. Four of the items constituting the depression subscale are about anhedonia, two items are about mood and one is about retardation. It has been demonstrated that a total score, including both the anxiety and depression subscales is a better predictor of major depression disorder in palliative care patients than the depression subscale (Le Fevre et al., 1999).

In order to bring the PRO on depression more in line with the diagnostic criteria for depression disorder as formulated in the DSM-IV, the Patient Health Questionnaire 9 (PHQ-9) was launched in 1999 (Spitzer et al., 1999). The instrument assesses all the nine depression diagnostic criteria including duration and functional consequences for major depression disorder and has good psychometric properties. A two-item version including the two major diagnostic criteria for depression disorder (lowered mood and anhedonia) has also demonstrated good screening properties (Mitchell, 2008). However, depression screening in cancer patients is debated, and we presently lack documentation that such screening improves depression outcomes compared to routine clinical examinations (Meijer et al., 2011).

Anxiety is more prevalent in palliative care patients than in the general population but has received less attention in the literature than depression. As for depression the term is used both for symptoms and disorders; generalized anxiety disorder (GAD), panic disorder or post-traumatic stress disorder (PTSD) (Roth and Massie, 2007). In a clinical perspective the common co-existence of anxiety symptoms and depression symptoms is of high relevance (Brenne et al., 2013). Assessing both anxiety and depression symptoms is therefore often recommendable. Still, the choice of instruments should reflect what shall be measured (i.e. symptoms or disorders) and the purpose for the assessment. Several PROs on anxiety are available. The HADS is probably the most commonly used instrument in a palliative care setting (Zigmond and Snaith, 1983). The anxiety subscale consists of six items on general anxiety (such as tension and worrying) and one item on panic.

An expert group introduced an alternative term, *distress*, for political reasons in 1997 (National Comprehensive Cancer Network, n.d.). The term was first introduced by one of the pioneers in stress research, H. Selye, who in 1975 defined it as 'persistent stress that is not resolved through coping or adaptation, deemed distress, may lead to anxiety or withdrawal (depression) behavior'. Thus distress implies that the stressor exceeds the individual's coping abilities which effectively handle the so-called good stress (eustress).

The term distress was chosen because it was assumed to be more acceptable/less stigmatizing than psychiatric, emotional or psychosocial, it sounded normal and less embarrassing and it could be measured by self-report (National Comprehensive Cancer Network, n.d.). Distress was conceptualized as a continuum from normal reactions to depression, anxiety and delirium thus mirroring the whole spectre of psychiatric/psychological aspects of palliative care without distinguishing between them.

The introduction of the term distress was rapidly followed by the introduction of an assessment method; the distress thermometer (Roth et al., 1998). The thermometer was a single item with a zero to ten response alternative designed as a thermometer. The instrument has later been supplemented by other items on related phenomena and with the original thermometer as the response alternative.

Instruments for assessing distress are defined differently. One review identified 33 instruments including the HADS (Vodermaier et al., 2009). Another review identified other instruments also assessing psychiatric disorders such as delirium and subscales from HRQOL instruments (Kelly et al., 2006).

Fatigue

Fatigue can be defined as a subjective feeling of tiredness, weakness, or lack of energy (Radbruch et al., 2008). Fatigue is the most frequent symptom in palliative care and is experienced by nearly all patients with advanced disease (Coyle et al., 1990; Stone et al., 1999). In palliative care, as opposed to healthy populations, fatigue relatively weakly correlates with psychological distress and in many cases reflects the subjective experience of being seriously ill (Stone et al., 1999).

Instruments specifically designed for measuring fatigue were first published in the late 1980s. At present several instruments are available (Loge and Kaasa, 1998; Stone et al., 1998; Stone and Minton, 2008), and most of these should be classified as first-generation instruments. A single item with an 11-point NRS for the responses has been proposed for screening purposes (National Comprehensive Cancer Network, n.d.). The Functional Assessment of Cancer Therapy- Fatigue scale is a 13-item free-standing part of the FACT-Anaemia Scale within the FACIT measurement system (Cella et al., 1993). The 13 fatigue items are available as a separate instrument (the FACIT-Fatigue) which is a uni-dimensional measure of physical fatigue (FACIT). However, most researchers agree that fatigue is a multidimensional phenomenon, but the number and types of dimensions is debated. All present fatigue measures include physical fatigue, which corresponds to the subjective feeling of being exhausted and lacking energy. A short (11 items) fatigue-instrument (Fatigue Questionnaire (FQ)) measures fatigue in two dimensions—physical and mental fatigue (Chalder et al., 1993)—and is commonly used in studies of cancer-related fatigue (Stone and Minton, 2008; Minton and Stone, 2009).

A review on instruments to be used in patients with advanced cancer identified more than 40 instruments published between 1985 and 2008 (Seyidova-Khoshknabi et al., 2011). The authors concluded that most instruments were too burdensome for those with advanced cancer. They proposed shorter unidimensional instruments such as the the Brief Fatigue Inventory or the 3-item scale on fatigue in the European Organization for Research and Treatment Quality of Life Questionnaire Fatigue Scale (EORTC QLQ-C30) (Seyidova-Khoshknabi et al., 2011). By this they point to an important aspect in choosing instruments for severely diseased populations. Still, the number of items must be evaluated in a broader context including the purpose of the data collection and the total number of items in the questionnaire package. A short instrument might be feasible if data on fatigue is collected as part of a broad symptom assessment or as a secondary endpoint. On the other hand, a short three-item uni-dimensional scale might lack sensitivity in for example intervention studies.

Pain

Pain is the second most prevalent symptom in palliative care, and for the majority of patients it is the most distressing symptom. It is well documented that pain is underdiagnosed and undertreated (Grond et al., 1996). Pain is the aim for different interventions both clinical and for research purposes in palliative care. In most situations, pain intensity will be the main target for assessments of pain. Additional aspects such as variation of pain over time, pain triggered by physical activity, or breakthrough pain might be of relevance in many situations. In such cases, available instruments must be evaluated for their properties in measuring these aspects of the pain experience.

In general, pain is included as single items or as separate subscales in all existing generic and disease-specific instruments. In these, pain is measured as a uni-dimensional construct (Hølen et al., 2006). However, it is important to underline that pain is a complex and also a controversial area for assessment, although some of the problems are reflecting challenges for HRQOL assessments in general (Hølen et al., 2006). Some major unresolved issues in relation to pain assessments in palliative care are: to what extent shall a pain assessment include assessment of physical and emotional distress caused by pain (Stenseth et al., 2007) (= pain interference)? How should pain be measured in patients receiving analgesics? How to deal with pain thresholds which vary between individuals and with individual access to support? What about differentiating between specific types of pain? How to measure specific cancer pains such as breakthrough pain? How is pain best measured in patients with cognitive impairment who are not able to respond to self-report questionnaires?

Domain-specific tools for measurement of pain such as the McGill Pain Questionnaire measure pain as a multidimensional phenomenon, but it is rather extensive and therefore difficult to apply in debilitated palliative care patients (Melzack, 1975). A shorter version of this instrument has been developed and validated (Melzack, 1987). Others, for example, the BPI (Daut et al., 1983), measure the impact of pain on physical functioning in addition to measuring pain intensity. There is reason to question whether consequences of pain can be validly separated from functional limitations due to other factors (Radbruch et al., 1999). This is of particular concern in palliative care patients due to the complexity of their diseases, the functional limitations they present and their experience of several symptoms at the same time.

An expert working group of the EAPC recommended that selection of tools for pain assessment should be based on the study population and the specific study design (Caraceni et al., 2002). The recommendations of the expert group apply to adults without cognitive impairment. For assessment of changes in pain intensity, single items with NRS were recommended while the Brief Pain Inventory short form (BPI-sf) were recommended for broader assessments (National Palliative Care Research Center, n.d.). The recommendations were recently updated with a simple algorithm for pain in assessment (Kaasa et al., 2011). The Short Form McGill Pain Questionnaire (SF-MPQ) (Melzack and Katz, 2001) was recommended for studies of pain qualities, such as studies focusing on diagnoses and characterization of pain syndromes. For assessments in cognitively impaired, several instruments are available but not sufficiently tested for explicit recommendations (Zwakhalen et al., 2006).

Use of single items

The use of single items either as self-constructed items or as items borrowed from a complete instrument is generally not recommended. An exception to this is simple questions about facts such as sick leave status where the items assess concretes and not underlying constructs. The validity of self-constructed items is generally uncertain and moving an item from its context might affect the responses.

Cognitive impairment

Cognitive impairment as part of dementia, amnestic disorder or delirium is prevalent in palliative care (Robinson, 1999; Casarett and Inouye, 2001). Among patients with terminal cancers, 20–40% develop delirium or other neuropsychiatric conditions (Pereira et al., 1997). We are not aware of HRQOL studies in cancer patients which have discussed their results in relation to possible cognitive impairment among the subjects. Cognitive impairment might affect completion rates, data quality, and the validity of HRQOL studies in palliative care.

Interviews conducted by health-care providers by means of specific interview guides and observation of behaviour are the appropriate methods for the detection of cognitive impairment (Hjermstad et al., 2004). The subjective experience of cognitive impairment is weakly correlated to neuropsychiatric disturbances but much stronger to psychological distress (Cull et al., 1996). Consequently, cognitive functioning scales within HRQOL questionnaires probably measure mental fatigue rather than cognitive functioning.

The most commonly used interview-based instruments in assessments of cognitive impairment are the Mini Mental State Examination (MMSE) and the Memorial Delirium Assessment Scale (MDAS) (Folstein et al., 1975; Breitbart et al., 1997). Physicians or other health professionals can use these measures without specific preparation, although it is wise to compare first time performances with more experienced personnel as part of the introduction routines into a research project or clinical practice. The MDAS is a brief, reliable tool for assessing delirium severity, while the MMSE is designed for detection of cognitive impairment irrespective of the cause or neuropsychiatric diagnosis. For the MMSE it has been demonstrated that the scores of selected items are equally effective as the sum-score of all the 20 items in identifying cognitive impairment in elderly patients and delirium (Braekhus et al., 1992; Fayers et al., 2005). However, more research is needed before such an abbreviated version can be recommended for general use. The present documentation on the usage of shortened instruments indicates that the standard clinical evaluation of consciousness and orientation are good screeners for detecting cognitive impairment.

Palliative care specific instruments

Several instruments have been developed and validated within palliative care. Most of these instruments are not used extensively in clinical research or in clinical practice today. Clinicians and researchers seem to use either generic instruments such as the SF-36 or disease-specific instruments, the EORTC QLQ- C30, this instrument's shortened version (the EORTC QLQ-C15-PAL) or the FACT-G. These instruments are described earlier in this chapter. The generic instruments may be supplemented by domain-specific measures. Examples are instruments which measure pain, anxiety, depression, fatigue, and aspects at end of life.

HRQOL in the dying

Research on QOL for the dying patient is sparse—probably related to several factors, such as a lack of focus on dying patients and the dying process in general ('the battle is lost—why bother with it'). Furthermore, the dying patient is vulnerable and the ethics related to the research is debated.

There are several methodological challenges related to HRQOL assessment in the dying, including the rapid change in most biological processes and loss of cognition, which is highly relevant for the ability to collect subjective data. As previously pointed out, there are major problems with compliance in this sub-population when using traditional HRQOL questionnaires. In most palliative care programmes the aim is to support the family to care for the dying at home as well as providing specialist professional care. Consequently the team is caring for the patient in a family network. In end-of-life care 12 important aspects of care have been identified; acceptability and continuity, team co-ordination and communication, communication with patients, patient education, inclusion and recognition of family, competence, pain and symptom management, emotional control, personalization, attention to patient values, respect and humanity, and support for patient decision-making (Curtis et al., 2001). Another group involved in the development of assessment tools for patients with life-limiting illness, reached similar conclusions: the outcomes should be patient-focused and family-centred, clinically meaningful, administratively manageable, and psychometrically sound (Teno et al., 1999).

Quality of life assessment is by definition subjective in nature. In the dying patient, who is cognitively impaired, 'subjective data' needs to be collected by observers. There is a lack of validated instruments specifically designed for dying patients; however, there is an increase in literature addressing measurement issues for this patient population, focusing on the development of a conceptual framework (Singer et al., 1999; Stewart et al., 1999). Several attempts have been made to develop observation-based instruments to measure pain in the cognitively impaired (Zwakhalen et al., 2006).

In summary one may say that the patient-focused assessment recommended is very similar to the strategy developed earlier in life, focusing on symptom control and how to relieve the patient burden. However, during end-of-life care, spiritual and existential

---

Box 19.7.4 Quality at the end of life

Important domains

- Symptom management
- Avoiding inappropriate prolongation of dying
- Achieving sense of control
- Reliving burden
- Strengthening of relationship between loved ones.

Box 19.7.5 Challenges related to interpretation of HRQOL outcomes

- Multidimensionality: generic
- Content of the measure: generic
- No common metric: generic
- Heterogenic intervention: palliative care specific
- Multiple problems (symptoms): palliative care specific
- Progressive disease: palliative care specific.

---

issues need to be addressed in more detail in addition to family members' perception of quality of care (Box 19.7.4).

Family satisfaction, HRQOL, grief, and other domains may be used as outcomes of quality of death. A variety of instruments have been used in the published studies to examine different aspects and models of care (Rinck et al., 1997; Hearn and Higginson, 1998; Smeenk et al., 1998; Salisbury et al., 1999), and no consensus on content nor on type of instruments seem to be agreed upon. In several studies a general high level of satisfaction with care has been observed and only minor differences between various palliative care programmes, which may indicate a poor ability of the existing instruments to discriminate between groups when measuring satisfaction with care and HRQOL (Kane et al., 1984; Zimmer et al., 1985; Addington-Hall et al., 1992; Hughes et al., 1992; Jordhøy et al., 2000, 2001).

Practical measurement of HRQOL during end-of-life care

The complexity, length, and content of the existing HRQOL instruments seem inappropriate for use during the dying process. Shorter and simpler instruments are needed here. To our knowledge there is no single instrument widely used for this purpose, but simple NRS have been developed. The Edmonton Symptom Assessment Schedule (ESAS) is a short ten-item instrument (Bruera et al., 1991) that has been extensively used in several scientific reports by the group. Other symptom assessment schedules are also used, such as the Memorial Symptom Assessment Scale Short Form (MSAS-SF), which is one of the several alternatives for symptom assessment (Chang et al., 2000). Still there is a lack of consensus on how to measure HRQOL in the dying patient. New, shorter, and more comprehensive instruments are therefore needed, which ideally could be completed both by the patient and proxy raters in sequence.

Interpretation of data

What is the clinical relevance of a summary score on a single item when comparing groups of patients or individuals? This is one basic question to ask both in daily clinical practice, in interpreting clinical research, and in sample size calculation in the planning process of a clinical trial. The clinical significance is related to the importance of the symptoms or the signs.

In pain assessments a single item on pain intensity rated on a NRS ranging from 0 to 10 is often used as the outcome. When discussing the clinical significance of a pain score, two important questions need to be answered. What is a relevant cut-off point in order to classify the score of those in need of intervention? What is the minimum difference on a pain score, say on a 0–10 scale, in a randomized trial comparing two different pain medications that is of clinical importance? Some major challenges related to interpretation of HRQOL outcomes are presented in Box 19.7.5.

Change in any clinical variable, independent of the nature of the variable, that is, physiological (blood pressure), psychological (anxiety), and performance (physical function) needs to be interpreted in a clinical framework. It is not a methodological or statistical question whether a change of 20 on a scale from 0 to 100 is of clinical significance. In order to be able to make a valid judgement on the magnitude of a measure in order to regard it as 'clinically significant', the clinician needs at least to understand the nature of the measure, including insight into the content of the composite score, the clinical meaning of the measure, and how it relates to individual patients. The discussion about clinical significance is not unique to QOL assessment. Similar discussions arise, for example, in interpreting the clinical significance of blood pressure medication, interpreting the reduction of tumour size caused by chemotherapy, and the importance of change in median survival in patients with non-small cell lung cancer admitted to a randomized chemotherapy trial.

These are some of the general problems. A more specific problem related to palliative care is the interpretation of change in several QOL estimates in the same study. QOL estimates are by nature multidimensional and each estimate is often based on a summary of responses to several questions. A common metric does not apply between scales and domains (i.e. is 40 on a pain measure similar to 40 on a nausea measure in symptom burden?). In palliative care, where most patients are living with a progressive disease, improvement in overall condition cannot be expected, thus the 'improvement' may actually be nearly 'slowing down' or stabilization of symptom burden. The complexity of human biology may cause an increase in intensity in one symptom when another symptom is relieved. Furthermore, most patients have a mosaic of symptoms, which often needs broad interventions, and consequently one specific outcome may be difficult to identify.

Conclusion

QOL is a term with quite differing meanings, and new terms have been suggested in order to improve the terminology. Presently the term is preferably used in the broad meaning of overall QOL.

The term QOL instruments should not be used unless in the context of overall quality of life. PROs is the common term for all instruments assessing the patient's perspectives.

Multidimensional measures of HRQOL cover physical, psychological, and social aspects of life. In palliative care these measures have been criticized for not covering the existential and spiritual issues sufficiently. A series of measures for use in health care in general (generic instruments) and for use in specific diagnostic groups, such as cancer (cancer specific) and palliative care (palliative care specific), have been developed. A third category of instruments is the domain specific measures. The latter is developed for assessing specific symptoms or signs, such as pain, fatigue, depression, anxiety, physical function, spirituality, etc. The plethora of instruments is a challenge for the users of the instruments, the readers of scientific reports, and for the performance of meta-analyses.

Most instruments have been developed for use in research and may not be suited for use in daily clinical practice. Many instruments for measurement of the same constructs are available and validation has often been insufficient both in relation to the palliative population and on a more general level. However, ongoing efforts include multinational research collaborations in order to develop instruments that are based upon experts' evaluations and input from patients, that are computer based with better measurement capabilities, and that are well suited for use in clinics and research. In the meantime a reasonable strategy is to choose one of the most commonly used HRQOL instruments. Still, the content of a questionnaire always needs to be cautionary investigated to assure that it fits the purpose for the assessment in clinical research, in quality assurance, or in clinical practice.

Online materials

Complete references for this chapter are available online at <http://www.oxfordmedicine.com>.

References

Aaronson, N., Cull, A., Kaasa, S., and Sprangers, M.A.G. (1994). The European Organization for Research and Treatment of Cancer (EORTC) modular approach to quality of life assessment in oncology. *International Journal of Mental Health*, 23, 7–96.

Cella, D.F., Tulsky, D.S., Gray, G., *et al.* (1993). The Functional Assessment of Cancer Therapy scale: development and validation of the general measure. *Journal of Clinical Oncology*, 11, 570–579.

FACIT (n.d.). *The Functional Assessment of Chronic Illness Therapy (FACIT) Measurement System Overview*. [Online] Available at: <http://www.facit.org/FACITOrg/Overview>.

Fielding, S., Fayers, P.M., Loge, J.H., Jordhøy, M.S., and Kaasa, S. (2006). Methods for handling missing data in palliative care research. *Palliative Medicine*, 20, 791–798.

Groenvold, M., Petersen, M.A., Aaronson, N.K., *et al.* (2006). The development of the EORTC QLQ-C15-PAL: a shortened questionnaire for cancer patients in palliative care. *European Journal of Cancer*, 42, 55–64.

Hearn, J. and Higginson, I. (1997). Outcome measures in palliative care for advanced cancer patients: a review. *Journal of Public Health Medicine*, 19, 193–199.

Jordhøy, M.S., Fayers, P., Loge, J.H., Ahlner-Elmqvist, M., and Kaasa, S. (2001). Quality of life in palliative cancer care: results from a cluster randomized trial. *Journal of Clinical Oncology*, 19, 3884–3894.

Kaasa, S., Loge, J.H., Fayers, P., *et al.* (2007). Symptom assessment in palliative care: a need for international collaboration. *Journal of Clinical Oncology*, 26, 2367–2373.

Maltoni, M. (2005). Prognostic factors in advanced cancer patients: evidence-based clinical recommendations – a study by the Steering Committee of the European Association for Palliative Care. *Journal of Clinical Oncology*, 23, 6240–6248.

NTNU Technology Transfer AS (2014). *Eir Health*. [Online] Available at: <http://www.eirhealth.com>.

Rinck, G.C., Van Den Bos, G.A., Kleijnen, J., De Haes, H.J., Schade, E., and Veenhof, C.H. (1997). Methodologic issues in effectiveness research on palliative cancer care: a systematic review. *Journal of Clinical Oncology*, 15, 1697–1707.

19.8

Health services research in palliative care and end-of-life care

Tinne Smets and Luc Deliens

What is health services research?

In 1979, the Institute of Medicine of the United States stated that the aim of health services research is 'to produce knowledge about the structure, processes, and effects of personal health services' (Institute of Medicine, 1979). A broader definition was offered in 2002 by the American Academy for Health Services Research and Health Policy:

> Health services research is the multidisciplinary field of scientific investigation that studies how social factors, financing systems, organisational structures and processes, health technologies, and personal behaviors affect access to health care, the quality and cost of health care, and ultimately our health and well-being. Its research domains are individuals, families, organizations, institutions, communities, and populations. (Lohr and Steinwachs, 2002)

These definitions emphasize that health services research analyses many aspects of care and is a multidisciplinary field drawing on many disciplines, including biostatistics, epidemiology, health economics, medicine, nursing, psychology, and sociology (Ginzberg, 1991; Institute of Medicine, 1991; Scott and Campbell, 2002). It involves the systematic search for knowledge that will lead to improvements in the delivery of health care (Crombie and Davies, 1996).

Health services research in palliative care and end-of-life care

During the last century, achievements in public health and improved living conditions in developed countries have led to an increase in life expectancy and a significant rise in the proportion of the elderly in the population (Seale, 2000). Death usually occurs from chronic and degenerative diseases, and typically is preceded by a prolonged terminal illness (United Nations Population Division, 2002; Lunney et al., 2003). High illness burden prior to death may be ameliorated by interventions identified as palliative care or delivered by services that provide specialist palliative care. Palliative care could potentially benefit between 50% and 89% of the 50 million people worldwide who die annually (McNamara et al., 2006).

Ensuring equal and adequate access to quality palliative care presents a major public health challenge (Davies and Higginson, 2004). Public health policy is ideally informed by an up-to-date and unbiased evidence base, which can be provided only by health services research. Investigating and interpreting the use of palliative care, including its costs, quality, accessibility, delivery, organization, and outcomes, is important in determining the most effective public health strategies.

During the past two decades, clinical research relevant to the domains of palliative care has increased rapidly. The development of evidence-based guidelines, such as the European Association for Palliative Care (EAPC) recommendations on opioid therapy for cancer pain (Caraceni et al., 2012), exemplifies this trend. At the same time, rapid developments in health services research have generated complementary knowledge about the organizational aspects of palliative care and the experiences of patients and professionals involved in the services. Health services studies have evaluated the caregiving process and the feasibility and effectiveness of one or more particular service or intervention (Steinwachs and Hughes, 2008). Researchers in palliative and end-of-life care have examined topics such as need, access, and quality, and the feasibility, effectiveness and cost of palliative and end-of-life care services and interventions.

Studies of access to palliative care may expose possible disparities. The principle of equitable distribution of health care and the commitment to ensuring equitable access is widely acknowledged (European Union, 2000; Van Doorslaer et al., 2006). Equitable access is often defined as horizontal equity, which means that people with equal needs are treated equally (Wagstaff et al., 1991). Health services research has attempted to identify situations in which patients with specific palliative care needs are denied care on the basis of ethnicity, gender, age, socioeconomic status, educational level, or geographical isolation, or because of inadequate service levels (Scott and Campbell, 2000). For example, a retrospective cohort study in Belgium acquired data from a nationwide sentinel network of general practitioners to analyse end-of-life care in a nationwide representative sample of people who died non-suddenly in 2005–2007, and demonstrated that the less well-educated are disadvantaged in terms of access to specialist palliative care services and contacts with a general practitioner at the end of life compared with the better educated (Bossuyt et al., 2011); while they were no less likely to have a palliative treatment goal, they used multidisciplinary palliative care services less often, moved between care settings less frequently, and had fewer contacts with their general practitioner in the last 3 months of life. These type of data can be used to redress disparities in care through system-level changes.

Evaluation of palliative and end-of-life care services and interventions raises the question of whether the service or intervention is feasible, achieves its stated goals and objectives, and is cost-effective. Although the development of palliative care services and interventions should be based on evidence that they will increase the likelihood of desired outcomes, clear information on feasibility and effectiveness is often lacking (Kaasa et al., 2006; Costantini and Beccaro, 2009).

Research designs for service evaluation of complex interventions

Palliative care services and interventions are complex and health services research must deal with their complexities (Costantini and Higginson, 2008). Most interventions are not single-component interventions, such as a drug therapy, but rather have several interacting components, such as care by different professionals or coordination in different health-care settings. Patient and family needs also change over time, further complicating the assessment of a range of possible outcomes in the target population (Campbell et al., 2000; Medical Research Council, 2008; Craig et al., 2008).

Practical guidance for developing, evaluating and implementing complex interventions comes from the Medical Research Council (MRC) in the United Kingdom. In 2000, the MRC published a *Framework for the Development and Evaluation of RCTs for Complex Interventions to Improve Health* (MRC, 2000) which was updated in 2008 as *Developing and Evaluating Complex Interventions: New Guidance* (MRC, 2008). According to the MRC framework, interventions should be developed and tested systematically using a phased approach (Campbell et al., 2000). In a preclinical phase, a researcher must identify evidence that the intervention might have the desired effect (Campbell et al., 2000); a review of relevant theory and empirical evidence may provide this. In phase I, the relevant components of the intervention are defined, often through qualitative research such as focus groups or case studies. Qualitative studies can also give insight into the barriers and facilitators to the eventual implementation of the intervention and help explain how it works. In phase II, the exploratory phase, the intervention and study design of the main trial are developed and the feasibility of delivering the intervention, and its acceptability to health-care providers and patients, can be tested. During this phase, the content of the control group also is decided and the outcome measures are piloted. Phase III is the main trial. Experimental designs such as randomized controlled trials (RCTs), cluster RCTs, or stepped wedge designs often are preferred for the evaluation of complex palliative care interventions (MRC, 2008). Phase IV involves examination of its implementation in practice and can explore the rate of uptake of the intervention, its stability, and the possible existence of adverse effects (Campbell et al., 2000). The four phases may not always follow a linear sequence (Craig et al., 2008).

Randomized controlled trials

RCTs are often considered as the gold standard for clinical trials (Cochrane, 1979; Elley et al., 2004; Davis and Mitchell, 2012) and informed consent by an individual patient aware of the random allocation is essential. The elements of this design may be difficult to implement in groups of patients with advanced illness who are receiving palliative care interventions. It may be difficult to obtain informed consent from people who are dying (Hardy, 2000) and random allocation of individuals to a study

intervention or a 'usual care' or control group may not be possible when patients are receiving care on the same ward or by the same team. Contamination, that is, the risk that the demonstrated effect of the intervention will be weakened because control group patients unintentionally receive some or all of the intervention, is a significant concern when the intervention is complex (Elley et al., 2004). For example, if the intervention is the introduction of a palliative care service in a hospital or in a specific ward, all patients in the hospital or ward will potentially have contact with the intervention. Contamination can also occur during the delivery of the intervention, especially when it is related to the health-care provider's behaviour or a service's way of working (Elley et al., 2004), for example, when the intervention is aimed at improving patient/health-care provider communication. When random allocation of individuals is not possible or there is substantial concern about contamination, a cluster RCT design may be preferable (MRC, 2002).

In some situations, a conventional RCT is possible. For example, Temel et al. (2010) examined the effect of introducing palliative care soon after diagnosis on patient-reported outcomes and end-of-life care among ambulatory patients with newly diagnosed metastatic non-small cell lung cancer. Newly diagnosed patients were randomly assigned to receive either early palliative care integrated into standard oncological care or standard oncological care alone. The study found that those receiving early palliative care had a longer median survival, better quality of life, and fewer depressive symptoms than those receiving standard care. The study concluded that introducing early palliative care for this patient population led to important improvements in quality of life and mood.

Cluster randomized controlled trials

Cluster RCTs are a type of RCT in which clusters or groups of subjects rather than individuals are randomized (MRC, 2002). When randomization occurs at group or cluster level, all participants from the same cluster—for example, hospital ward, hospice, or family practice—are allocated either to the intervention or to the control group. Cluster RCTs are mainly used when delivery of an intervention is at the group level and outcomes are measured at the patient level (Elley et al., 2004).

The main advantage of the cluster RCT design is that randomizing a whole group of individuals reduces the risk of contamination; individuals from the intervention and control groups are less likely to have contact with each other (Elley et al., 2004). Another is that informed consent may be obtained not from the individual patient but for an entire cluster of patients from their 'cluster guardian' who decides whether the cluster as a whole should participate in the trial (MRC, 2002; Fowell et al., 2004, 2006). A 'cluster gatekeeper' takes responsibility for individual patients and can withdraw them from the trial if deemed necessary (Elley et al., 2004). A disadvantage of cluster RCTs is that individuals within the cluster are not independent from each other; for example, patients of the same family practitioner are more likely to share some characteristics and thus to respond to an intervention in a similar way than those who do not share those characteristics. The variation in outcomes between clusters is thus greater than would be expected in RCTs. The resulting loss of power can be avoided by using a larger sample than would be required in an RCT (Campbell et al., 1998; Elley et al., 2004).

One example of the use of a cluster RCT in palliative care is the phase III trial to assess the effectiveness of the Liverpool Care Pathway for the Dying Patient (LCP) performed by Costantini et al. (2011, 2014) in Italy. The LCP was developed in the United Kingdom to improve the quality of care in the last days of life and provides a comprehensive template of evidence-based multidisciplinary care. In this study, pairs of eligible medical wards from different hospitals were randomized to receive the LCP programme or no intervention. The main outcome measure was the difference in the overall quality of end-of-life care provided on the wards that received or did not receive the LCP. The cluster RCT showed that after implementation of the Italian LCP programme, no significant difference was found in the distribution of the overall quality of care toolkit scores between the wards in which the LCP programme was implemented and the control wards (Costantini et al., 2014).

Stepped wedge design

In a stepped wedge design, an intervention is rolled out sequentially to the individuals participating in the trial—as individuals or as clusters of individuals—at different time points (Brown and Lilford, 2006). The order in which the individuals or clusters receive the intervention is determined at random. By the end of the random allocation, all individuals or clusters will have received the intervention. Data are collected at each point when a new group, or step, receives the intervention (Brown and Lilford, 2006). To determine the effectiveness of an intervention, the data points in the control section of the wedge are compared with those in the intervention section (Brown and Lilford, 2006). This design is especially interesting when it is expected that the intervention or service will do more good than harm and denial of the service or intervention to the control group is deemed unethical, which is often the case in palliative care interventions for the dying.

One example of a study using a stepped wedge design is the multicentre, stepped wedge cluster RCT performed by Leontjevas et al. (2013) in the Netherlands. The objective of that study was to estimate the effectiveness of a structural approach to the management of depression in nursing home residents. This structural approach entailed the implementation of a multidisciplinary care programme called Act in Case of Depression (AiD). A network of nursing homes in the Netherlands was asked to enrol one dementia and one somatic ward per nursing home. In the wards, the nursing staff recruited eligible residents. The enrolled nursing home wards were randomly allocated to one of five groups and the intervention was implemented at different time points in each group. The primary outcome measure was the prevalence of depression in the wards using the Cornell scale for depression in dementia. The study found that in the somatic wards the intervention reduced the prevalence of depression but the effect was not significant in the dementia wards.

Observational designs

If an experimental approach is unnecessary, inappropriate, impossible, or inadequate, non-experimental designs, such as observational or before-and-after designs, can be considered (MRC, 2008).

In observational designs the researcher only observes and does not carry out any intervention. Observational designs include cohort studies, prospective as well as retrospective, cross-sectional studies, and case–control studies (Mann, 2003). Cohort studies are used to study incidence, cause, and prognosis. Because they measure events in chronological order, they can be helpful in clarifying cause and effect. Cross-sectional studies are used to determine prevalence. Case–control studies compare groups retrospectively to identify possible predictors of an outcome (Mann, 2003).

An example of an observational study is the phase II study performed by Follwell et al. in Canada, which evaluated the impact of an Oncology Palliative Care Clinic on symptom distress and satisfaction (Follwell et al., 2009). Patients with metastatic cancer who were newly referred to an Oncology Palliative Care Clinic received a consultation by a palliative care team and provided baseline data on the Edmonton Symptom Assessment Scale (ESAS) and the patient-adapted Family Satisfaction with Advanced Cancer Care (FAMCARE) scale. These measures were repeated after 1 week and after 1 month, and comparison of the latter scores to baseline demonstrated improvements in both symptom control and patient satisfaction.

Before-and-after designs can be controlled or uncontrolled. Uncontrolled before-and-after studies measure outcomes before and after some planned event or introduction of an intervention. Observed changes are assumed to be due to the intervention (Eccles et al., 2003). One of the main disadvantages of this design is that trends or changes in practice or in the law governing end-of-life care make it difficult to attribute observed changes to the intervention (Eccles et al., 2003).

In controlled before-and-after designs, a control group with characteristics similar to the group undergoing the planned event or intervention is identified and data are collected from both groups before and after the change. Analysis compares post-intervention performance in the intervention and control groups and observed differences are assumed to be due to the intervention (Eccles et al., 2003).

An example of a study which used an uncontrolled before-and-after design is Veerbeek et al.'s (2008) study of the effect produced by the LCP on the documentation of care, symptom burden, and communication in three health care settings in the Netherlands. During the baseline period, care in the dying phase was provided as usual. During the intervention period, the LCP was used for all patients for whom the multidisciplinary team had evaluated that the dying phase had started. The study demonstrated that the use of the LCP was followed by significantly more comprehensive documentation and lower average total symptom burden.

Challenges in the evaluation of palliative care interventions and services

Trials that enrol patients with advanced illness present unique challenges, both ethical and methodological (Grande and Todd, 2000). Studies that have attempted to do so have revealed problems, including failure to define the intervention, failure to determine appropriate outcome measures, problems with randomization of patients to intervention or control group, problems with achieving recruitment and minimizing attrition, failure to consider the heterogeneity of the patient group, and difficulties with obtaining informed consent (Rinck et al., 1997; Goodwin et al., 2002; Harding and Higginson, 2002; Higginson et al., 2003; Harding et al., 2005; El-Jawahri et al., 2011). Care must be taken to minimize these problems.

Defining the intervention

An intervention refers to 'a set of actions with a coherent objective to bring about change or identifiable outcomes' (Costantini et al., 2008). The experimental intervention and its alternative need to be clearly and precisely defined. This may be difficult with palliative care interventions, as palliative care is by nature holistic, multidisciplinary, and tailored to an individual patient's needs (Grande and Todd, 2000). It is possible that, alongside the intervention, other services with similar characteristics may be delivered to patients from both the intervention and the control group, and these confounding treatments may be difficult or unethical to eliminate or control (Grande and Todd, 2000). Patients who receive home palliative care services as the intervention may, for instance, also receive supportive care from their family physician, making it difficult to define the effect of the intervention. It is advised that clearly defining the intervention and control conditions in trials, and documenting additional care, may improve the quality of trials in palliative care and facilitate the interpretation of results (Rinck et al., 1997).

Determining outcome measures

The outcomes chosen for assessment must be relevant to the intervention or an effect cannot be demonstrated. Additionally, the timing of measures must be such that they pick up the effects of the intervention (Grande and Todd, 2000). It is suggested that the first assessment after baseline should be consistent with the shortest period likely to give a clinically significant effect (Jordhoy et al., 1999). Bad timing may lead to under-recording of the effects of the intervention. In one study (McWhinney et al., 1994), for example, pain was measured at baseline and 1 month later, but the possibility could not be excluded that a patient with no pain at baseline and at 1 month might have had a pain crisis in between that was successfully managed by the palliative care home support team (McWhinney et al., 1994).

The measurement of the outcomes can be difficult in palliative care research. Patients and caregivers may have difficulty completing questionnaires, which can result in a loss of data. For this reason, researchers may rely on proxy measures and retrospective accounts, but the validity of these assessments may be questioned (Jordhoy et al., 1999). Trained interviewers can also be used to collect data (McWhinney et al., 1994) by helping patients and caregivers to interpret the questions and by taking account of cognitive impairment, exhaustion and distress (McWhinney et al., 1994). For palliative care research, it is essential that means are explored to obtain valid outcome measurements; feasibility studies and extensive piloting are necessary.

Randomization

Randomization should always be considered as it is the most robust method of preventing selection bias (Eccles et al., 2003), but trials of palliative care pose particular ethical challenges in terms of randomization of patients. Denial of a service or treatment to the control group may be unethical, and a waiting list control does not solve the problem as palliative care patients are a vulnerable patient group for whom there is often no second opportunity to improve care. For patients who are aware that they are dying, even a short waiting list may be too long (Grande and Todd, 2000). As noted, the use of a cluster RCT design or a stepped wedge design may reduce these concerns by randomizing at a group level before

the patient is identified. In a cluster RCT, access to the service or intervention may be less related to study procedures than to other factors, such as the geographical location of the hospital or general practice, and in the stepped wedge design, all patients eventually receive the intervention.

Achieving recruitment and minimizing attrition

A large enough sample is needed to ensure that differences between the intervention group and the control group can be detected. However, screening and enrolling patients into palliative care trials can be difficult. Many patients understandably choose not to participate and physicians may be reluctant to enrol patients because they may find it hard to accept that cure is no longer possible (Grande and Todd, 2000). As a result, many patients who would otherwise be eligible to be included in a trial are left out. Patients may also die before they can enter the trial or before data can be collected (McWhinney et al., 1994). Furthermore, patients may be lost from the trial due to early death or withdraw due to progressive illness (Jordhoy et al., 1999). Problems with recruitment and attrition may lead to inadequate statistical power. These possible problems should be taken into consideration when calculating sample size.

Heterogeneity of the patient group

Patients requiring or receiving palliative care are a diverse group with different illnesses and different illness courses (Grande and Todd, 2000). In RCTs, it is assumed that the different characteristics of the study population are evenly distributed among the intervention and control group, and outcome differences between the groups result from the intervention. When variation within the study population is very large, however, there is a concern that randomization may not be successful in ensuring equal distribution of important variables among study groups. A possible solution is stratified randomization according to important variables. Particular key variables for stratification are those that the intervention seeks to address such as symptom burden (Grande and Todd, 2000).

Obtaining informed consent

Obtaining informed consent from patients for participation in palliative care trials can be challenging for several reasons (Hardy, 2000; Agar et al., 2013). First, patients may have impaired or fluctuating decision-making capacity. Second, palliative care trials may focus on times in the illness trajectory when consent is impossible to obtain due to concerns about an unethical imposition of requests unrelated to the provision of care; this may occur, for example, when a study focuses on patients perceived to be in the last hours of life. Third, patients may not always have full knowledge of their illness or prognosis, in which case seeking informed consent is a very sensitive issue. Finally, in the advance stages of illness, patients fatigue easily and may find it difficult to concentrate on processes like consent (Hardy, 2000; Agar et al., 2013).

There are several ways in which informed consent for trials in palliative care can be sought (Hardy, 2000; Agar et al., 2013). The gold standard is to ask the patient's informed consent at the time of enrolment in the study. If this is not possible, proxy consent can offer a solution when the patient is unable to give informed consent him or herself. Proxy consent, which has often been used in dementia research (Karlawish, 2003; National Health and Medical Research Council, 2007), means that another person must be authorized to consent on behalf of the patient to the patient's participation in the research (Agar et al., 2013). When the trial focuses on times in the illness when the patient is unlikely be unable to give informed consent, informed consent can be obtained from the patient in advance, for instance, if the study focuses on symptoms in the last days or hours of life (Hardy, 2000; Agar et al., 2013).

Conclusion

Clear information about the effectiveness of services and interventions is often lacking in palliative care service planning. In order to stimulate growth and quality in palliative care research, good quality studies in health services research are needed. Health services research in palliative care covers topics such as palliative care needs, access to palliative care, quality of care and feasibility, effectiveness, and cost of palliative care services and interventions. Patients needing palliative care often have complex needs and require complex services and interventions; most interventions in palliative care are indeed complex interventions. The MRC framework for developing and evaluating complex interventions offers useful guidance for researchers.

To evaluate complex services and interventions, a wide ranch of study designs, both experimental and non-experimental, can be used. In planning a study of palliative care, researchers should also keep in mind possible difficulties with choosing and measuring appropriate outcomes, with the ethical problems raised by randomization of dying patients, with attrition due to early death or withdrawal of patients due to progressive illness, with obtaining informed consent from dying patients, and with the ethical aspects of imposing on people at the end of their lives.

Online materials

Complete references for this chapter are available online at <http://www.oxfordmedicine.com>.

References

Costantini, M. and Higginson, I.J. (2008). Health services research. In D. Walsh, A. Caraceni, R. Fainsinger, et al. (eds.) *Palliative Medicine*, pp. 165–170. Philadelphia, PA: Saunders Elsevier.

Costantini, M., Romoli, V., Leo, S.D., *et al.* (2014). Liverpool Care Pathway for patients with cancer in hospital: a cluster randomised trial. *The Lancet*, 383(9913), 226–237.

Craig, P., Dieppe, P., Macintyre, S., Michie, S., Nazareth, I., and Petticrew, M. (2008). Medical Research Council Guidance. Developing and evaluating complex interventions: the new Medical Research Council guidance. *BMJ*, 337, a1655.

Eccles, M., Grimshaw, J., Campbell, M., Ramsay, C. (2003). Research designs for studies evaluating the effectiveness of change and improvement strategies. *Quality & Safety in Health Care*, 12, 47–52.

Elley, C.R., Chondros, P., and Kerse, N.M. (2004). Primary Care Alliance for Clinical Trials (PACT) network. Randomised trials—cluster versus individual randomization. *Australian Family Physician*, 33(9), 759–763.

Fowell, A., Johnstone, R., Finlay, I.G., Russell, D., and Russell, I.T. (2006). Design of trials with dying patients: a feasibility study of cluster randomization versus randomized consent. *Palliative Medicine*, 20, 799–804.

Grande, G.E. and Todd, C.J. (2000). Why are trials in palliative care so difficult? *Palliative Medicine*, 14, 69–74.

Jordhoy, M.S., Kaasa, S., Fayers, P., *et al.* (1999). Challenges in palliative care research; recruitment, attrition and compliance: experience from a randomized controlled trial. *Palliative Medicine*, 13, 299–310.

McWhinney, I.R., Bass, M.J., and Donner, A. (1994). Evaluation of a palliative care service: problems and pitfalls. *BMJ*, 309, 1340.

Medical Research Council (2002). *Cluster Randomized Trials: Methodological and Ethical Considerations*. London: Medical Research Council.

Medical Research Council (2008). *Developing and Evaluating Complex Interventions: New Guidance*. London: Medical Research Council.

Clinical audit in palliative medicine

Irene J. Higginson

Quality of care: a worldwide concern?

Quality and value for money in health care is now centre stage in many countries. Whatever the funding system, most developed countries place a high priority on 'consumer' choice and accountability. Scandals related to poor care continue in many countries, higher public expectations, increased health-care spending, and the move towards quality service in many public and private companies have all heightened the desire to introduce quality assurance, clinical audit and evaluation into clinical care (Shaw, 1980a–1980e; Selman and Harding, 2010; Eastman and Martin, 2012) The move from palliative and hospice care from being a concern of primarily the voluntary and charitable sector, to the greater involvement of public and, increasingly, private sector services bring with it a growing need to continuously monitor quality through clinical audits. Audits allow clinicians, managers, and governments to standardize practice and support 'best' possible practice (Shaw, 1988, 1989, 1990). Audit data also can be the foundation for future research—testing methods, identifying potential recruits, or better understanding the focus of research (Currow et al., 2010; Evans et al., 2013; Higginson et al., 2013).

Although many terms in the quality dictionary are new, many of the ideas, such as clinical review, are not. The history of quality improvement and audit can be traced back as far as 1700 BC in Egypt when King Hammurabi (the King who proposed the code of 'eye for an eye') introduced penalties for different degrees of 'surgical incompetence' (Rosser, 1985). This included a proposal that: 'if a doctor operates on a patient and the patient dies, the doctor's hand will be cut off' (Rosser, 1985). In 1518, the Charter of the Royal College of Physicians included: 'to uphold the standards of medicine both for their own honour and public benefit'. The General Nursing Council (GNC) was established in 1919 to 'monitor nurses' practice and conduct'. Florence Nightingale was one of the first clinicians to insist on measuring the outcome of care for her patients, to evaluate treatment. Grand rounds, postgraduate lectures, and clinical presentations all contributed to the review of medical and nursing performance.

References in the medical and nursing literature to quality assurance and clinical audit began in the late 1970s. They continue to rise, although the terms have changed over time (Fig. 19.9.1), including terms such as continuous quality improvement, clinical governance, standards, and preferred practices (Shaw, 1980a, 1988, 1991; Higginson, 1994). The new emphasis on clinical audit, quality improvement, and governance has brought four main differences:

◆ Explicit criteria for good practice should be applied by all clinicians rather than those in exemplary centres

◆ All patients in care and all centres should be included in quality monitoring rather than a few 'interesting' cases

◆ Patients and their families should be able to seek empowerment

◆ Funding or accreditation may be withheld from those units which do not comply with quality standards or which are found to be ineffective or inefficient (Shaw, 1980a; Higginson, 1994; Higginson and Bruera, 2002).

Why perform clinical audit in palliative medicine?

Palliative care arose out of a desire to improve the quality of care for patients with advancing disease and their families. This was based on evidence that care for people with progressive illness, and care for the imminently dying, was lacking (Higginson and Evans, 2010). Many of the early evaluations of palliative services compared hospice, home, and hospital care (Higginson et al., 2003) and some sought to influence those working in oncology and other professions (Buckingham et al., 1976; Higginson, 1993, 1994; Ling, 2000; Lee et al., 2001). Later, palliative care often led the way in developing ways to examine the quality of care generally and its core precepts were seen to align with public preferences. A recent survey of 9344 citizens across Europe found that respondents highlighted (a) a need for improved quality of end-of-life and palliative care, and access to this care for patients and families and (b) the recognition of the importance of death and dying and holistic care including comfort and support (Daveson et al., 2014).

Palliative and hospice care have grown rapidly such that there are services in all countries of the globe. This growth has been accompanied by the development of many tools and measures to assess and audit the quality of palliative care. The use of these tools is becoming more common and national and international guides for quality are now available (Dudgeon, 2007; Ferrell, 2007). There is now evidence demonstrating the effectiveness of palliative care and hospice services, based on empirical studies in different sites and systematic literature reviews (Higginson et al., 2003; Higginson and Evans, 2010; Gomes et al., 2013a). Although the importance of this

Audit by any other name: combine terms from the table below

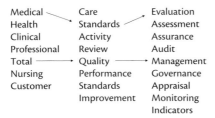

Fig. 19.9.1 Different approaches.

work is undeniable, the lack of comparison of different models of care has been criticized (Higginson and Evans, 2010). Practice still varies from one country to another, from one part of a country to another, and from one service to another, even in simple aspects such as staffing levels and mix within a hospice or home care team, the catchment populations, the operational policies and the throughput (Higginson and Evans, 2010). Even today, we need to know which models of care work best and for which types of problems palliative care is most effective. Those providing and those who resource palliative services need to know which interventions and in what combination work best, for what kinds of patients and families, and in which type of localities. Research is important in discovering some of these aspects, but equally audit or quality assessment, is important to identify what works best, for whom and when.

Hospices and palliative services bring new therapies, such as new treatments for symptoms, support and counselling services, or complementary and alternative medicine therapies. These new therapies must be evaluated and audited to determine if and in whom these are useful. Otherwise hospices' resources and the patient's time will be wasted. There is a great danger on concentrating on only current concerns without reviewing previous failings and using those findings to plan improved care in the future.

Clinical audits have been slow to materialize in some settings. Antipathy to the approach is based on various arguments, such as:

◆ There is no problem, since the high quality of palliative care is evident, as shown by thank you letters

◆ Palliative care is self-auditing, because staff spend time with patients and families

◆ The outcomes of palliative care cannot be measured—they are too complicated or intangible

◆ Measuring more simple outcomes of palliative care, such as pain or symptom control, is not enough, and until we can measure everything, audit should not be attempted

◆ Resources, information, and time are not available

◆ Audit looks back at practice which has gone, not the problems which lie ahead.

None of these arguments can be supported by evidence. Numerous audits and quality assessments of palliative care have helped to improve care (Charlton et al., 2002; Cooper and Hewison, 2002; Galvin, 2002; Higginson and Bruera, 2002; Ackroyd, 2003; Burt et al., 2004; Galbraith and Booth, 2004; Hunt et al., 2004; Newbury and Hatherell, 2004; Bausewein et al., 2005; Brandt et al., 2005; Currow and Abernethy, 2005; Harding and Leam, 2005; Morita

et al., 2005; Veerbeek et al., 2006; Godfrey and Poole, 2007; Kaasa et al., 2007; Le and Ashby, 2007; Payne, 2007; Amigo et al., 2008; Currow et al., 2008a, 2008b; Deane et al., 2008; Eisenchlas et al., 2008; Miller and Hopkinson, 2008; Morita et al., 2008; Tsai et al., 2008; Eagar et al., 2010; Harding et al., 2010; Nadimi and Currow, 2011; Benitez-Rosario et al., 2012).

Audit has been recommended in national strategies (Kaasa et al., 2007) and has had major impact in the development of hospice and palliative care in much of Europe, Canada and Australia. The results have been used in the following ways:

◆ Assisting the development of local and regional palliative care programmes.

◆ Providing outcomes information that have allowed the programme leaders to advocate for increased funding.

◆ Demonstrating the effectiveness of different interventions and allowed for increased patient referrals

◆ Reviewing the quality of work and identification of ways to improve it so that services are planned to ensure future patients and families will not suffer the same failings.

◆ Identifying areas where care is effective and where it is not; this allows services to be better targeted and will mean that patients and families receive the most up-to-date care.

◆ Developing procedures for the systematic assessment of patients and families to ensure that key aspects of care are less likely to be overlooked, communication between patients and families and professionals is not overlooked and problems identified by patients and families are brought to the attention of staff, there is a more holistic approach to care, and new staff have a clearer understanding of what should be assessed and how appropriate assessments are done.

◆ Assisting in the development of predictive models that promote early referral of patients or families who may experience problems.

Audit or clinical governance can help most patients and families receiving palliative care, because it looks at routine practice, rather than at a few 'special' cases. Quite apart from mistakes, suboptimal care may be due to professional or administrative problems which tend to escape anecdotal case reviews. Audit also is important for education and training, because the structured review allows analysis, comparison, and evaluation of individual performance; it promotes adherence to local clinical policies and offers opportunity for publication of results. Educational programmes can be constructed to meet the demonstrated needs of individuals or groups. Increasingly, audit, clinical governance, or quality review are required for the recognition of training posts and for the revalidation of doctors. Royal Colleges and Faculties increasingly seek evidence of formally organized review and could withdraw recognition from departments that do not provide this.

Audit is important for those who resource palliative care, such as commissioners, primary care trusts, and health-care insurance agencies, because it provides tangible evidence that the service is seeking the most effective use of existing clinical resources and aims to improve the quality of care. This is increasingly important when competing for health-care contracts (Clark et al., 1995). Requirements for audit and the implementation of research findings may well be included in such contracts (Clark et al., 1995).

The costs of not auditing are as important as the benefits of auditing (Shaw, 1980a–1980e; Higginson, 1994). In the absence of review, there is a risk that inappropriate treatment may be undertaken, uncontrolled symptoms may cause admission to hospice or hospital, or delay discharge, or unnecessary services may be delivered. All this activity wastes the patients' and families' time and resources, as well as staff time and resources.

Clinical audit takes time and resources (Shaw, 1980a–1980e; Higginson, 1994). These should not be underestimated. Indeed, it may be impossible to undertake audit if a service is struggling, with insufficient numbers of staff to give even basic care such as washing and administering drugs. Perhaps the audit here is to show simply that the service cannot even measure and assess a patient's needs properly. Indeed, simple assessments, such as whether follow-up occurs, can be useful in assessing practice (Selman and Harding, 2010). The resources needed for audit and quality assessment can include:

◆ Time from all staff to prepare for audit, to agree the standards or topic and to review the findings

◆ Time from some staff to carry out the audit and to analyse its results and document the findings and any recommendations

◆ Commitment from *all* staff, managers, nurses, doctors, etc. to consider the results and act upon them

◆ Resources to pay for the staff time involved, plus any other analytical or computing support needed.

Computers are not necessary for audit, but they are increasingly becoming part of routine health care. A number of computer programmes are available for palliative care and other services, many from commercial companies. The audit measures can be included within these programmes, and increasingly application in clinical practice is aided by staff or patients using mobile computing devices. However, if the audit is small or in its early stages, too rigid use of computers by inexperienced staff can be a hindrance, because the need to update the computer delays the evolution of the audit.

The costs of audit mean that it is important to ensure that the audit itself is as effective as possible. What is the purpose of collected audit data if the changes are not acted on? Mechanisms to review the audit and to ensure it is effective are discussed in a later section.

What do we mean by quality?

Quality, as defined in many dictionaries, pertains to 'degree of excellence' or 'general excellence'. But what constitutes excellence in the context of a service, who defines it, and what components should be addressed? For example, should 'excellence' be limited to clinical skills, or should it encompass broader aspects, such as whether the service reaches all those in need? Surely, when measuring quality of a service all the features and characteristics that bear on its ability to satisfy the stated or implied needs of the users of that service should be assessed. Quality in health care is a multidimensional concept, and as such, a multidimensional approach to measurement and assessment of that quality is required (Donabedian, 1966, 1976, 1981a, 1997, 2005).

Numerous authors have identified some of the dimensions that should be included when assessing the quality of a service. For example, Maxwell identifies the following as dimensions of care that need to be measured when monitoring quality (Maxwell, 1984, 1986, 1992):

◆ Effectiveness

◆ Acceptability

◆ Efficiency

◆ Access

◆ Equity

◆ Relevance.

Black agreed with all these, but added a further dimension: humanity, a dimension which would be particularly important for palliative care services (Black, 1990).

So how do we determine whether we are offering a good quality service if we have to consider all these dimensions? One method is to conduct a programme of review and improvement of the service, a process that incorporates clinical audit, quality assurance and quality improvement.

How do we assess the quality of palliative care?

Donabedian and others have translated the assessment of the quality of health care into:

1. Structure/or inputs: resources in terms of manpower, equipment and money

2. Process: how the resources are used (such as domiciliary visits, beds, clinics, drugs or treatments given)

3. Output: productivity or throughput (such as rates of clinic attendance or discharge, throughput—rate that patients are seen)

4. Outcome: change in health status or quality of life that can be attributed to health care (Donabedian, 1978, 1980, 1981b, 1997, 2005).

This model is built on manufacturing industry and, despite limitations discussed below, it has value in that it defines the steps in which health and social care are delivered.

Structural aspects influence the process of care so that its quality can be either diminished or enhanced. Similarly, changes in the process of care, including variations in its quality, will influence the output, and in turn, the effect of care on health status and outcomes. Thus, there are functional relationships (Fig. 19.9.2).

Structure is easiest to measure because its elements are the most stable and identifiable. However, it is an indirect measure of the quality of care and its value depends on the nature of its influence on care. Structure is relevant to quality in that it increases or decreases the probability of a good performance. Process and output are closer to changes in the health status of individuals and their measurement reflects the most immediately discernible attributes of care activities. However, they are only valuable as a measure once the elements of process are known to have a clear relationship

structure → process → output → outcome.

Fig. 19.9.2 Functional relationship.

with the desired changes in health status. Outcome reflects the true change in health status, and thus is the most relevant for patients and society. However, it is difficult to eliminate other causes for change, such as prior care or external events. A useful approach is to focus on the difference between the desired outcome and the actual outcome. Services can then identify whether or not their goals are being achieved and investigate any failings.

Organizational audits usually assess the structure and process of care, whereas clinical audits often measure the process and outcome of care. Although structure is easiest to measure it is furthest from influencing change in the patient and family. Outcome is most difficult to measure but is of direct relevance to the patient and family. Standards of structure or process are most useful when these are of proven effectiveness, or if there is an overwhelming consensus that these are desirable. Structure, process, and outcome measures which have been either used or advocated to assess palliative care are shown in Table 19.9.1.

Stewart et al. have extended the model, subdividing the 'structure' elements into (1) personal and social environment of the patient and family and (2) the structure aspects of care (Stewart et al., 1999). They also subdivided the outcomes into (a) satisfaction and (b) quality and length of life. These subdivisions are consistent with the earlier model of Donabedian, and those proposed for palliative care audit in the United Kingdom. However, Stewart et al.'s differentiation of the personal and social environment is a useful demonstration of how audit results may be different because of different settings, or with a different 'case mix' where patients and families have differing conditions or problems. Casarett et al. have built further on this model, proposing a minimum data set (Casarett et al., 2006).

A rose by any other name would smell as sweet: the evolving terms—audit, quality improvement, governance?

Over the last 30 years, it has been interesting to observe how different terms have come in and out of vogue to describe the evolving approaches to assessing and ensuring the quality of health care. There are also differences among countries. Somewhat disappointingly, the literature in one country tends to ignore audit and quality improvement initiatives in another, thereby reducing the chance to learn. In the United Kingdom and many other European countries, clinical audit (as opposed to financial audit, concerned only with financial matters), became the initial term of choice. Later this was accompanied by quality assurance (which tended to include a programme of several audits, all working together). Such a programme was similar to the development of total (or continuous) quality improvement in the United States and many other countries, which incorporated a cycle called Plan, Do, Study, Act. Some of the widely accepted definitions are shown in Table 19.9.2.

There are elements common to all types of clinical audit or quality review. These include systematic assessment in a cycle that includes the monitoring of care, review of results, and change to improve practice (Fig. 19.9.3). The cycle is repeated and the process should become part of the organization's culture. Practice changes usually are made to be consistent with standards of care that are set locally or nationally, but it is possible to enter the audit cycle at any point; standards can be developed after practices are observed and change is made based on the results.

Table 19.9.1 Aspects of care that could be measured to assess structure, process, output or outcome in palliative care

Type of measure	Examples
Structure	Values or aims of the service
	Financial resources
	Home care/hospital/hospice services
	Day hospice places
	Number of staff or services per cancer patient in the population
	Staffing mix, grades
	Number of staff per patient
	Drugs and equipment available
	Building design
	Physical environment—e.g. safety, pleasantness of surroundings
Process	Number of visits
	Number of admissions
	Procedures followed
	Documentation
	Time taken in a visit
	Policies and procedures for staff training and working
	Mechanism for handling complaints and the documentation of this
	Adherence ethical and legal codes
	Staff support given
Output	Rate of discharge
	Number of completed consultant episodes
	Throughput
	Rate of equipment given out
	Drugs given
	Well-coordinated care—telephone communication etc.
	Supply of medicines after discharge
	Completed patient management plans
	Early arrival of discharge information to GP
	Satisfaction of professionals referring to the service
Outcome	Reduction in distressing symptoms
	Improved mental health of patient and carer
	Patient and carer satisfaction
	Satisfied with place of care
	Open and honest communication as the patient wishes.
	Resolved communication, fears, grief, anger
	Resolved need to plan future events—e.g. funeral or meetings
	Good use of remaining time
	Any spiritual problems resolved or fulfilment
	Reduced carer strain
	Improved carer health
	Resolved grief after death (if appropriate)

Table 19.9.2 Common definitions: audit and quality assurance

Term	Definition
Medical audit	The systematic critical analysis of the quality of medical care including the procedures used for diagnosis and treatment, the use of resources, and the resulting outcome and quality of life of the patient (Higginson, 1994)
Clinical audit	The systematic critical analysis of the quality of clinical care including the procedures used for diagnosis and treatment, the use of resources, and the resulting outcome and quality of life of the patient
	Clinical audit is like medical audit but involves all professionals and volunteers rather than only doctors
Nursing audit	The methods by nurses compare their actual practice against pre-agreed guidelines and identify areas for improving their care
Prospective audit	The standards and measures are recorded on patients and their families during their care
Retrospective audit	This looks back at the care of patients who have been discharged or have died, and the standards are applied to the information available from case notes or by asking families about the care after the patient has died
Quality assurance	The definition of standards, the measurement of their achievement and the mechanisms to improve performance
	The quality assurance cycle is as for medical audit or clinical audit. However, quality assurance implies a planned programme involving the whole unit or health services. Clinical or medical audit is usually described as one part of a quality assurance programme

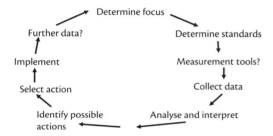

Fig. 19.9.3 Cycles of clinical audit, quality improvement, and performance measurement.

Some common distinctions

Clinical audit

Clinical audit is the systematic critical analysis of the quality of clinical care (Higginson, 1994). It may focus on the procedures used for diagnosis and treatment, the use of resources, or the resulting outcome and quality of life for the patient. It can be prospective, where the standards and measures are agreed at the start and are recorded on patients and families during their care, or retrospective, which looks back at the care of patients using either the clinical notes and extracting the information or by asking families. Although early forms of audit involved only single professions—for example, medical or nursing audit (Table 19.9.2)— it is now widely accepted that audit in palliative care should be multiprofessional, to reflect the multiprofessional nature of care.

Organizational audit

The Kings Fund Centre in London originally described organizational audit as the developmental and voluntary stage towards accreditation (Higginson, 1994). Accreditation schemes exist in many countries and usually operate nationally. The audit focuses on the organization and compares specific aspects against agreed standards. These standards usually consider only the structure and process of care, and may try to identify administrative delays, uncoordinated care, poor environment or sign-posting, poor staff training, etc. Organizational standards need to be straightforward enough to be monitored by an external surveyor.

Quality assurance and total quality management programmes

Although there are various definitions for quality assurance, a widely accepted one is the 'definition of standards, the measurement of their achievement and the mechanisms to improve performance'. Clinical audit lies within the frame of quality assurance. Audits may involve the review of the quality of a local clinical practice on a regular basis, for example, through internal 'peer review' by practising clinicians.

Total quality management is a recent term, which has been defined as a strategy to get an organization working to its maximum effectiveness and efficiency. It has been facilitated by closer working relationships between clinicians and managers (Higginson, 1994), builds on the other definitions, and switches the focus from quality practised within professionals to quality within the whole organization. Thus, clinical audit would lie within a total quality management programme. It also introduces the concept of managing the quality process, such as cataloguing reports of local quality initiatives (Higginson, 1994) and using managers to ensure that improvements in quality occur.

Clinical governance

Clinical governance has developed recently because of concerns about variations in clinical practice, particularly assessment, diagnosis, and prescribing. This is of increasing concern in modern medicine because of the rapid development of diagnostic investigations and treatments that may have potentially dangerous effects if not carried out properly. Clinical governance programmes assess what doctors (and most recently nurses) do, and examines both their training and continuing professional development, and all components of their practice. It aims to ensure and develop the practice of all clinicians. Participation in clinical governance is already required of many health-care services, and will soon be required to ensure the revalidation of doctors in many countries (Ferrell et al., 2007).

Who carries out clinical audit and what is measured?

The different approaches to audit and the assessment of quality can be categorized according to two axes. The first is defined by the identity of the auditor. This could be clinicians, managers, or an organization. The second is defined by the object of the audit,

INTERNAL   EXTERNAL

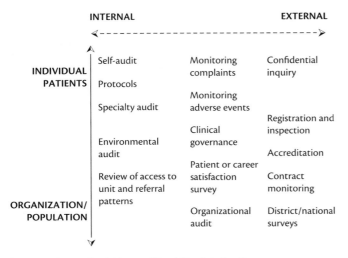

Fig. 19.9.4 Range of activities possible within clinical audit.

INTERNAL   EXTERNAL

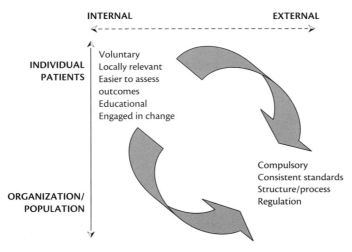

Fig. 19.9.5 Effect of activities within clinical audit.

whether it focuses on the care of an individual or a few patients, or on the whole organization or population. Common forms of audit according to these two axes–internal versus external and individual versus organization/population—are shown in Fig. 19.9.4. The type of audit should be determined by the setting and goals. Those focused on improving specific practices often are more oriented towards internal and individual assessment. They are more likely to be educational and voluntary. Those that are external and focused on the overall clinical quality of care are more likely to rely on organizational or environmental standards, determine whether professionals are employing proven high quality treatments, examine structural elements such as staff mix, and note whether quality activities such as a clinical audit programme is in place. These types of audits are more likely to be mandatory and to provide funding or accreditation (see Fig. 19.9.5).

Applying clinical audit to palliative medicine

Clinical audits and other quality activities should be actively embraced by those working in palliative care. Specific steps should be taken to implement the audit processes:

1. Know what we are trying to achieve: goals, standards, and desired outcomes

The definitions of palliative care and palliative medicine provide good guidance on the goals of palliative care, and the appropriate outcomes that might be measured in clinical audit. These include aspects of pain and symptom control, improving the quality of life for the patient, relieving fears and anxiety, and caring for the family members or carers. Therefore, in analysing the goals or standards of care, many have audited their effectiveness in improving outcomes such as control of symptoms, their effect on a patient's quality of life or psychological well-being, or the patient's or family members' satisfaction with care. A European-wide survey of public attitudes recently found that pain, breathlessness, and burden to others were top concerns that needed to be addressed near the end of life (Bausewein et al., 2013).

Specialists in palliative care often focus on end-of-life care and those undertaking clinical audits may choose to evaluate specific concerns encountered in the care of the dying. Kellehear described the features of a modern 'good death' as 'awareness of dying, social adjustments and personal preparations, public preparations (legal, financial, religious, funeral, medical), work or activities reduced, and farewells' (Kellehear, 2000, 2001, 2009) Singer et al. identified five domains of quality end-of-life care: receiving adequate pain and symptom management, avoiding inappropriate prolongation of dying, achieving a sense of control, relieving burden, and strengthening relationships with loved ones (Singer et al., 1999, 2000). Payne et al. identified similar concerns from family members (Payne et al., 1999). These definitions might suggest audit of aspects of patient and family awareness of the illness or their planning of personal and public preparations, and such aspects have been included in some measures, such as the Support Team Assessment Schedule (Higginson et al., 1992; Bausewein et al., 2011a).

In many countries, the role of palliative care in supporting, advising and educating other professions is stressed. For example, family practitioners and hospital clinicians may identify educational needs for symptom control and patient and family support. Therefore, another form of audit could examine the educational and supportive role of palliative care services.

Poor communication is a frequent cause of stress for patients and families. Doctors and nurses need to communicate well with patients and their families rather than withdrawing or appearing hurried or abrupt in their manner. Communication also is needed among professional staff caring for the patient and family member, to ensure liaison and to prevent duplication or delay. Usually patients and family members want to be involved in decision making, and patients want their family members to make decisions when they are not able to, although this wish is not universal (Daveson et al., 2013, 2014). These aspects are also goals suitable for audit.

Total pain has been described as including physical, emotional, social, and spiritual components. Although the earlier discussions have covered the emotional and physical aspects of palliative care, it is also important to consider audit of the social and spiritual aspects. Social aspects might include whether the patient and family have sufficient practical and financial support to remain at home, or whether they have been cared for in their place of choice, usually home (Gomes et al., 2013b). Spiritual audit might consider whether patients are able to raise aspects of spiritual concern to them and find a mechanism to relieve problems, or whether patients are in any form of spiritual crisis. Guidelines for spiritual practice have been developed, and several of the more recent measures that can be used for audit include spiritual aspects, measuring items such as peace and feeling good about self (Selman et al., 2010, 2011).

There are also simple goals, such as place of death, or meeting other patient or family preferences, or access to services by certain patient groups (such as those from ethnic minorities, or non-cancer conditions) that might be suitable for audit. In auditing the processes and outcomes associated with these goals, clinicians must recognize and accommodate variation. For example, although around 70% of patients would prefer to die at home, increasingly patients choose hospice as a second choice, wishes are very individual, are little understood in some sections of society and are altered by experience (Gomes et al., 2013b). Thus this indicator, like other process indicators, needs to be reviewed cautiously.

How can these goals be turned into standards? Any goal or standard which is set must be measurable, sufficiently challenging but achievable. It would be unrealistic to set a goal or standard that all patients would be free from pain, but it would be reasonable to set a goal of what proportion of patients' pains might be controlled and in what circumstances pain might be uncontrolled. A baseline could be established from current practice. Standards of action when pain is uncontrolled could be audited. Such an approach has been used in developing audit programmes in many countries, including Africa (Harding et al., 2010; Selman and Harding, 2010).

When standards are ill-defined, achievement of goals can be compared across services. This approach has been used successfully by the Australian Palliative Care Outcomes Collaborative, which has compared data on the assessment of symptoms and concerns using the Palliative care Outcome Scale (Eagar et al., 2010).

2. Have a way of assessing and re-assessing the quality of care

For all of the above aspects, measurement tools or indicators are needed. There are now a number of these available in palliative care which have been validated to different degrees. The Association for Palliative Medicine of the United Kingdom established a working party to review these and subsequently published a 'which tool' guide (Clinical Effectiveness Working Group et al., 2002). The group carried out a MEDLINE search to identify potential measures and to check whether they had been used in more than one centre. Then the group provided a preliminary guide as to whether they would recommend the tools in research or clinical audit palliative care.

More recently, a Europe-wide project PRISMA surveyed clinicians internationally on outcome measures used in clinical audit, clinical practice and research, and examined the barriers to using outcomes in routine clinical practice and for audit (Bausewein et al., 2011b; Harding et al., 2011). Key findings were that:

◆ There was disharmony in the tools used. Of the 311 participants who completed a survey, 99 tools in clinical care and audit, and 94 in research, were cited by fewer than ten participants (Harding et al., 2011).

◆ Time constraints, burden, and lack of training and guidance were the main reasons for not using outcome measures in practice. Participants expressed the need for more guidance and

training in the use of outcome measures in clinical practice and audit (Bausewein et al., 2011b).

◆ In clinical care and audit, assessment of the patient's situation, monitoring changes, and evaluation of services were the main reasons for use of outcome measures (Bausewein et al., 2011b).

◆ The most common outcome measures used in clinical practice were, in order of frequency of use:

• the Karnofsky Performance Status or Palliative Performance Scale (both measures of functional activity/consciousness)

• the Edmonton Symptom Assessment System (ESAS)

• the Palliative care Outcome Scale (POS)

• the Symptom Distress Scale (SDS)

• the Support Team Assessment Schedule (a precursor to POS).

Some measures used in clinical audit have been validated in many languages and settings. Table 19.9.3 shows examples of these. The two most common multidimensional measures used in clinical audit, the ESAS (Bruera et al., 1991; Amigo et al., 2008; Richardson and Jones, 2009; Bergh et al., 2011; Carvajal et al., 2011; Selby et al., 2011; Watanabe et al., 2012a; Hui and Bruera, 2013) and the POS (see Box 19.9.1 for an example of one item in this measure, pain) (Hearn and Higginson, 1999; Bausewein et al., 2005; Brandt et al., 2005; Stevens et al., 2005; Siegert et al., 2010; Higginson et al., 2012) (see also <http://www.pos-pal.org>) have both had extensive research into their validity, reliability, and factor structures, as well as translations and cultural adaptations in many languages. This includes determining factor structures, clinically important differences, and use for screening for depression and other symptoms (Siegert et al., 2010; Bergh et al., 2011; Selby et al., 2011; Zimmermann et al., 2011; Harding et al., 2013; Watanabe et al., 2012b; Hui and Bruera, 2013; Saleem et al., 2013). POS builds on an earlier widely used measure, the Support Team Assessment Schedule (STAS) (Box 19.9.2) but was designed for use by patients as well as staff and families.

An alternative to multidimensional assessment is audit of single symptoms or other problems, for example, constipation, communication, or access to care. This is called topic review. Other approaches are also possible, although seldom used. Box 19.9.3 reviews these.

In contrast to the use of these measures to perform internal audits of individual patient care issues, other strategies often are used for organizational audits or peer review systems. These have tended to employ indicators that can be used in inspections of services, and concentrate on the structure and process of care, such as:

◆ Service values—a statement of service values and objectives related to the palliative care service guides the organization and delivery of high-quality care

◆ Organization and management—the palliative care service or Organization is managed efficiently to ensure patients and families receive suitable and effective multidisciplinary care

◆ Organizational and operational policy—Organizational and operational policies reflect current knowledge and principles and are consistent with the requirements of statutory bodies, purchasing authorities and service objectives

◆ Physical environment for care—the physical environment is safe and accommodates individual and shared needs

Table 19.9.3 Common outcome measures used in clinical audit

Measure, scale or tool	Used in . . .	Strengths	Limitations	Useful for: Clinical—☆ Research—▲
Karnofsky Performance Status (KPS) Scale	All settings	Quick and widely used	Assesses only function	☆▲
Edmonton Symptom Assessment Scale (Aaronson et al., 1993)	All settings	Simple and short, can be used either by patient or with nurse assistance, widely used and validated	Potential bias introduced by change in the person recording the answers as care continues. Patient may have wider concerns than those included	☆▲
POS—Palliative care Outcome Scale (POS) (Higginson et al. 1999; Hughes et al. 2001)	All settings	Simple and short—has patient completion, family completion and staff completion versions; tested for validity and reliability, has items for individual patient generation	Patient may have wider concerns than those included	☆▲
Support Team Assessment Schedule (STAS) (Cartwright 1990; McGee et al., 1991; Finlay and Dunlop 1994; Hearn and Higginson 1999)	Used by community palliative care teams, hospital teams, day care, inpatient units and hospital at home services	A wide ranging checklist looking at clinical and communication issues; available in other languages and has been modified with additional specific items	Teams need to actively use this questioning each section, not just ticking boxes; professional completion. Now often replaced by shorter POS, although not all aspects included in POS	☆▲
PACA—Palliative Care Assessment (Hearn and Higginson 1999)	Hospital palliative care team and outpatient	Short and relatively simple to use	Professional completion. Not so widely used	☆
EORTC—European Organisation for Research into Treatment of Cancer—QLQ C30 (Cella, and Tulsky 1990; Cella 2004)	Developed for chemotherapeutic cancer trials—lung cancer patients; work of palliative module underway	Reliable and valid in research settings, broad ranging	Functional questions may cause distress if asked repeatedly	▲
FACT, Functional Assessment of Cancer Therapies	General cancer settings in United States, especially research studies—has a palliative module	Major validation programme	Use in palliative care not yet widely reported	▲
McGill Quality of Life Questionnaire (Cohen et al. 1995, 1997; Ellershaw et al. 1995)	Advanced cancer and HIV patients at home or in-patient palliative care unit	Includes an existential domain, as well as symptoms and psychological issues	Not been widely tested in UK settings	▲
Symptom Distress Scale	Life-threatening cancer and heart disease	Some validation; looks at symptoms and mood in relation to quality of life	Patient completion in presence of interviewer	▲
Other possible audit measures—usually more orientated to process of care				
Proportion who die at home	Used by health authorities to monitor overall care	Quick and easy to measure and aggregate. Easy to make comparisons	Home death may not have been patient choice. May be distorted by lack of appropriate inpatient provision	
Proportion who die in their place of choice	Used by some palliative home care and primary care teams.	Reflects patient choice and individual wishes	Difficult to get information in some circumstances, choice may change over time	
Proportion of final weeks spent at home	A proxy measure that can give some indication of the availability of community support services	Quick and easy to measure and aggregate. Clear operational definitions allow valid comparisons between districts	May be distorted by lack of appropriate inpatient provision	

- Self-determination and climate for care—the caring environment for patients and families is conducive to independence, self-esteem and participation in daily life

- Direct patient and family care—professional staff manage to ensure that patient and family needs are assessed, planned, implemented and evaluated on an individual basis

- Multidisciplinary working and team work—a range of skills is available to meet service goals, and specific contributions are identified and integrated

- Staffing and skill mix—good employment practices are in place and staffing levels are systematically determined in order to meet service needs

Box 19.9.3 Types of audit: an appraisal of their uses in palliative care

Key indicators

These can be based on the structure or process of care, as in organizational audit or can be based on clinical indicators, such as in clinical audit. In organizational audit the indicators are reviewed by inspection, in clinical audit they are reviewed by the clinical team (see Fig. 19.9.3 and Fig. 19.9.4).

Routinely collected data, such as throughput, visits, or re-admission rates can be used in some areas of health care, but in palliative care these may not be appropriate and the clinical record may have to be amended to include relevant items. In clinical audit, a few key indicators are chosen and recorded prospectively and examined after a period of care. In organizational audit or peer review the survey team ask for information about the indicators and then seek evidence of these. In clinical audit, measures such as those shown in Table 19.9.3 are used.

Topic review

A topic is chosen and reviewed prospectively or retrospectively. Although the latter often revels inadequacies in the clinical records it is often valuable in providing a baseline for later comparison. Examples of topics are medical records and letters, referral or admission procedures, control of a particular symptom, prescribing practice, or the diagnostic procedures used.

Random case review

Here notes are selected at random and critically reviewed by doctors not involved in that person's care. This method may lose direction if the aims and criteria for quality are not clear. One way to focus the audit is to develop a previously agreed checklist for use in the critical review. The method can be linked with key indicators—a random sample of notes are examined for the key indicators.

Patient or family satisfaction

The simplest method is to analyse patient and family complaints. However, in palliative care patients may die before they are able to complain. Surveys of patients' or families' views may be included in the overall quality improvement plan of a hospice or hospital, see Table 19.9.3 for examples of how this may be used.

Adverse patient events

This systematically identifies events during a patient's treatment which may indicate some lapse in the quality of care. Patients' clinical records are reviewed retrospectively by a health professional or a ward clerk for examples of agreed adverse events. This method is of value in specialities such as surgery, where adverse events (e.g. death or postoperative infection) are usually recorded in the patient's records. However, in palliative care the method is awkward, because adverse palliative events are more difficult to identify routinely and may not be included in the patient's records unless these are standardized.

◆ Education, training, and staff development—staff have access to education and training programmes, which reflect the different levels of activity and practice necessary to meet service goals, provide appropriate care and respond to change

◆ Staff support—staff support systems are in place as an integral part of the Organization and a healthy working environment is promoted, which recognizes the possible physical and emotional effects of work on staff

◆ Ethics and law—there is guidance and support for staff to comply with statutory requirements and use a systematic approach to decision-making where ethical and legal status issues are involved.

3. Change practice to improve care and/or ensure that any deficiencies are corrected

Ideally, the audit cycle should include a period to implement change to improve quality based on the findings of the audit. Data should be discussed with the whole team to determine what changes might be appropriate. Decisions also may involve a review of the literature or consulting with other individuals to determine whether they have solutions to particular problems. For example, in London we identified that our control of breathlessness in the last weeks of life was not reaching our targets: this was the most severe symptom in patients (Higginson and McCarthy, 1989). To decide what change was needed we had to consult chest physicians, physiotherapists, and other colleagues about what treatment might be appropriate in the home, review the literature on effective treatment, and examine the possible causes of breathlessness. This led us to substantially change our practice and it also has probably led to further research into the management of breathlessness.

In larger specialist palliative care services, difficulties in implementing the change have been described (Higginson et al., 1996). These include the following:

◆ Inadequate cascading of the information from those present at the audit meetings to other staff

◆ Difficulties in ensuring that those with hands-on patient contact but at the end of the cascade, such as auxiliary nurses, feel ownership of any changes and therefore are willing to take part in them

◆ Difficulties if the main communicator is a resistor to change. Many healthcare professionals have inane conservatism to resist the change of long cherished views. This may be partly from fear of their deficits being revealed.

The change management process is a vital component of clinical audit but is often neglected. Continuing education is important and can be targeted to ensure that those to be educated feel part of the teaching or learning process. A systematic review by Antunes et al. shows how the process of introducing routine outcome measurement into practice requires leadership, facilitation, education, and ongoing support, including attitude change in staff (Antunes et al., 2014).

Audit in developing countries

It is appropriate to ask whether audit is yet relevant in developing as well as developed countries? Palliative care programmes in these countries have relatively few health-care professionals, and these have varied levels of training. In addition, some patients and families have high levels of illiteracy, making self-completion of assessment forms impossible. The burden of illness and symptom distress in patients dying of AIDS, tuberculosis, malaria, and even cancer-related syndromes may be different, just as belief systems vary, and therefore assessment tools may need to be adjusted in these populations (Higginson and Bruera, 2002).

Nonetheless, the professionals who deliver health care in the developing world document the results of interventions and use them to guide future direction in a manner not different than professionals in developed countries. Symptom control, information needs, and physical, emotional, spiritual, and social support for patients and families are important, just as in Europe, Australia, and North America (Selman et al., 2009). It can be argued that the limited resources make it even more imperative to ensure that, as the programmes evolve, they are capable of serving the largest possible number of patients and families in the most effective possible way. Audit is one way to minimize the risk of failure, and to learn, at an early stage, about potential problems and to identify success. A good example of a successful adaptation are the programmes of clinical audit now well established in Africa, with culturally adapted and validated forms of existing measures, in particular the African APCA POS (see Fig. 19.9.6). The tool is used to aid assessment, conduct clinical audit and in research (Harding et al., 2010). Considerable progress has now been made in Africa with audits using this measure to identify successes and shortcomings and ways to improve care (Harding et al., 2013).

Conclusion

Audit approaches and methods are now well advanced in palliative care, especially in clinical audit. We have a choice of possible and already tried methods and measures which we can adapt for our own needs, rather than having to undertake much of the development ourselves. Practical tools for clinical audit may use multidimensional measures, such as the Support Team Assessment Schedule, the new shorter Palliative care Outcome Scale, or the Edmonton Symptom Assessment Scale, or specific measures for topic audits. Clinical audits which use satisfaction surveys or surveys after bereavement are probably more costly, but are still possible. Apart from completing the audit cycle, clinical audit can look to developing clinical protocols for treatment, or algorithms to predict patient problems and the need for specialized care. Organizational audit and peer review is also now well established, and different systems are available.

Audit, or the various alternative terms that describe this assessment of the quality of care, is here to stay, and is now widely accepted. But it requires resources, and so it must be sure to benefit patients and families, be kept as simple and efficient as possible, and have a strong educational component. Further work is needed to evaluate the impact of different audit approaches and methods on improving care, so that we know which approach is most cost-effective. In addition, there is a need to develop and test methods of audit in developing countries. If palliative approaches extend backwards to include patients earlier in care, rather than those just near to death, then the audit could become a means for clinical dialogue and education between specialties. Palliative medicine could take the lead in encouraging this, promoting

APCA AFRICAN POS

PATIENT ID _____   **Staff name** _____

Date _____   **POS no** 1st ☐ 2nd ☐ 3rd ☐ 4th ☐ 5th ☐ 6th ☐

ASK THE PATIENT	POSSIBLE RESPONSES
Q1. Please rate your pain (from 0 = no pain to 5 = worst/overwhelming pain) during the last 3 days	**0 (no pain)- 5 (worst/overwhelming pain)** 0 ☐ 1 ☐ 2 ☐ 3 ☐ 4 ☐ 5 ☐
Q2. Have any other symptoms (e.g. nausea, coughing or constipation) been affecting how you feel in the last 3 days?	**0 (not at all)- 5 (overwhelmingly)** 0 ☐ 1 ☐ 2 ☐ 3 ☐ 4 ☐ 5 ☐
Q3. Have you been feeling worried about your illness in the past 3 days?	**0 (not at all)- 5 (overwhelming worry)** 0 ☐ 1 ☐ 2 ☐ 3 ☐ 4 ☐ 5 ☐
Q4. Over the past 3 days, have you been able to share how you are feeling with your family or friends?	**0 (not at all)- 5 (yes, I've talked freely)** 0 ☐ 1 ☐ 2 ☐ 3 ☐ 4 ☐ 5 ☐
Q5. Over the past 3 days have you felt that life was worthwhile?	**0 (no, not at all)- 5 (yes, all the time)** 0 ☐ 1 ☐ 2 ☐ 3 ☐ 4 ☐ 5 ☐
Q6. Over the past 3 days, have you felt at peace?	**0 (no, not at all)- 5 (yes, all the time)** 0 ☐ 1 ☐ 2 ☐ 3 ☐ 4 ☐ 5 ☐
Q7. Have you had enough help and advice for your family to plan for the future?	**0 (not at all)- 5 (as much as wanted)** 0 ☐ 1 ☐ 2 ☐ 3 ☐ 4 ☐ 5 ☐

ASK THE FAMILY CARER	
Q8. How much information have you and your family been given?	**0 (none)- 5 (as much as wanted)** **N/A ☐** 0 ☐ 1 ☐ 2 ☐ 3 ☐ 4 ☐ 5 ☐
Q9. How confident does the family feel caring for _____?	**0 (not at all)- 5 (very confident)** **N/A ☐** 0 ☐ 1 ☐ 2 ☐ 3 ☐ 4 ☐ 5 ☐
Q10. Has the family been feeling worried about the Client over the last 3 days?	**0 (not at all)- 5 (severe worry)** **N/A ☐** 0 ☐ 1 ☐ 2 ☐ 3 ☐ 4 ☐ 5 ☐

Fig. 19.9.6 APCA African POS.

Reproduced with permission from Palliative Care Outcome Scale (POS): A Resource for Palliative Care, Copyright © 2012 Cicely Saunders Institute, available from http://pos-pal.org/maix/

methods among their medical and surgical colleagues and presenting their own results.

References

Ackroyd, R. (2003). Audit of referrals to a hospital palliative care team: role of the bilingual health-care worker. *International Journal of Palliative Nursing*, 9, 352–357.

Amigo, P., Fainsinger, R.L., Nekolaichuk, C., and Quan, H. (2008). Audit of resource utilization in a regional palliative care program using the Edmonton Classification System for Cancer Pain (ECS-CP). *Journal of Palliative Medicine*, 11, 816–818.

Antunes, B., Harding, R., and Higginson, I.J. (2014). Implementing patient-reported outcome measures in palliative care clinical practice: a systematic review of facilitators and barriers. *Palliative Medicine*, 28(2), 158–175.

Aaronson, N.K., Ahmedzai, S., Bergman, B., *et al.* (1993). The European Organization for Research and Treatment of Cancer QLQ-C30: a quality-of-life instrument for use in international clinical trials in oncology. *Journal of the National Cancer Institute*, 85, 365–376.

Bausewein, C., Calanzani, N., Daveson, B.A., *et al.* (2013). 'Burden to others' as a public concern in advanced cancer: a comparative survey in seven European countries. *BMC Cancer*, 13, 105.

Bausewein, C., Fegg, M., Radbruch, L., *et al.* (2005). Validation and clinical application of the German version of the palliative care outcome scale. *Journal of Pain and Symptom Management*, 30, 51–62.

Bausewein, C., Le Grice, C., Simon, S., and Higginson, I. (2011a). The use of two common palliative outcome measures in clinical care and research: a systematic review of POS and STAS. *Palliative Medicine*, 25, 304–313.

Bausewein, C., Simon, S.T., Benalia, H., *et al.* (2011b). Implementing patient reported outcome measures (PROMs) in palliative care—users' cry for help. *Health and Quality of Life Outcomes*, 9, 27.

Benitez-Rosario, M.A., Castillo-Padros, M., Garrido-Bernet, B., and Ascanio-Leon, B. (2012). Quality of care in palliative sedation: audit and compliance monitoring of a clinical protocol. *Journal of Pain and Symptom Management*, 44, 532–541.

Bergh, I., Kvalem, I.L., Aass, N., and Hjermstad, M.J. (2011). What does the answer mean? A qualitative study of how palliative cancer patients interpret and respond to the Edmonton Symptom Assessment System. *Palliative Medicine*, 25, 716–724.

Black, N. (1990). Quality assurance of medical care. *Journal of Public Health Medicine*, 12, 97–104.

Brandt, H.E., Deliens, L., Van Der Steen, J.T., Ooms, M.E., Ribbe, M.W., and Van Der Wal, G. (2005). The last days of life of nursing home patients with and without dementia assessed with the palliative care outcome scale. *Palliative Medicine*, 19, 334–342.

Bruera, E., Kuehn, N., Miller, M.J., Selmser, P., and MacMillan, K. (1991). The Edmonton Symptom Assessment System (ESAS): a simple method for the assessment of palliative care patients. *Journal of Palliative Care*, 7, 6–9.

Buckingham, R.W., 3rd, Lack, S.A., Mount, B.M., Maclean, L.D., and Collins, J.T. (1976). Living with the dying: use of the technique of participant observation. *Canadian Medical Association journal*, 115, 1211–1215.

Burt, J., Barclay, S., Marshall, N., Shipman, C., Stimson, A., and Young, J. (2004). Continuity within primary palliative care: an audit of general practice out-of-hours co-operatives. *Journal of Public Health*, 26, 275–276.

Cartwright, A. (1990). *The Role of the General Practitioners in Caring for People in the Last Year of Their Lives*. London: King Edward's Hospital Fund for London

Carvajal, A., Centeno, C., Watson, R., and Bruera, E. (2011). A comprehensive study of psychometric properties of the Edmonton Symptom Assessment System (ESAS) in Spanish advanced cancer patients. *European Journal of Cancer*, 47, 1863–1872.

Casarett, D.J., Teno, J., and Higginson, I. (2006). How should nations measure the quality of end-of-life care for older adults? Recommendations for an international minimum data set. *Journal of the American Geriatrics Society*, 54, 1765–1771.

Cella, D.F. and Tulsky, D.S. (1990). Measuring quality of life today: methodological aspects. *Oncology*, 4, 29–37

Cella, D. (2004). The Functional Assessment of Cancer Therapy-Lung and lung cancer subscale assess quality of life and meaningful symptom improvement in lung cancer. *Seminars in Oncology*, 31, 11–15

Charlton, R., Smith, G., White, D., Austin, C., and Pitts, M. (2002). Audit tools for palliative care services: identification of neglected aspects of care. *The American Journal of Hospice & Palliative Care*, 19, 397–402.

Clark, D., Neale, B., and Heather, P. (1995). Contracting for palliative care. *Social Science & Medicine*, 40, 1193–1202.

Clinical Effectiveness Working Group, Higginson, I.J., Campion-Smith, C., Miller, M., Thomas, K., and Wee, B. (2002). *The 'Which Tool' Guide*. Southampton: Association for Palliative Medicine.

Cohen, S.R., Mount, B.M., Strobel, M.G., *et al.* (1995). The McGill Quality of Life Questionnaire: a measure of quality of life appropriate for people with advanced disease. A preliminary study of validity and acceptability. *Palliative Medicine*, 9, 207–219

Cohen, S.R., Mount, B.M., Bruera, E., *et al.* (1997). Validity of the McGill Quality of Life Questionnaire in the palliative care setting: A multi-centre Canadian study demonstrating the importance of the existential domain. *Palliative Medicine*, 11, 3–20

Cooper, J. and Hewison, A. (2002). Implementing audit in palliative care: an action research approach. *Journal of Advanced Nursing*, 39, 360–369.

Currow, D.C. and Abernethy, A.P. (2005). Quality palliative care: practitioners' needs for dynamic lifelong learning. *Journal of Pain and Symptom Management*, 29, 332–334.

Currow, D.C., Christou, T., Smith, J., *et al.* (2008a). Do terminally ill people who live alone miss out on home oxygen treatment? An hypothesis generating study. *Journal of Palliative Medicine*, 11, 1015–1022.

Currow, D.C., Shelby-James, T.M., Agar, M., *et al.* (2010). Planning phase III multi-site clinical trials in palliative care: the role of consecutive cohort audits to identify potential participant populations. *Supportive Care in Cancer*, 18, 1571–1579.

Currow, D.C., Ward, A.M., Plummer, J.L., Bruera, E., and Abernethy, A.P. (2008b). Comfort in the last 2 weeks of life: relationship to accessing palliative care services. *Supportive Care in Cancer*, 16, 1255–1263.

Daveson, B.A., Alonso, J.P., Calanzani, N., *et al.* (2014). Learning from the public: citizens describe the need to improve end-of-life care access, provision and recognition across Europe. *European Journal of Public Health*, 24(3), 521–527.

Daveson, B.A., Bausewein, C., Murtagh, F.E., et al. (2013). To be involved or not to be involved: a survey of public preferences for self-involvement in decision-making involving mental capacity (competency) within Europe. *Palliative Medicine*, 27, 418–427.

Deane, A., Young, R., Chapman, M., and Fraser, R. (2008). A clinical audit of the efficacy of tegaserod as a prokinetic agent in the intensive care unit. *Critical Care and Resuscitation*, 10, 71.

Donabedian, A. (1966). Evaluating the quality of medical care. *The Milbank Memorial Fund Quarterly*, 44(Suppl.), 166–206.

Donabedian, A. (1976). Some basic issues in evaluating the quality of health care. *American Nurses Association Publications*, 3–28.

Donabedian, A. (1978). The quality of medical care. *Science*, 200, 856–864.

Donabedian, A. (1980). Methods for deriving criteria for assessing the quality of medical care. *Medical Care Review*, 37, 653–698.

Donabedian, A. (1981a). Advantages and limitations of explicit criteria for assessing the quality of health care. *The Milbank Memorial Fund Quarterly*, 59, 99–106.

Donabedian, A. (1981b). Criteria, norms and standards of quality: what do they mean? *American Journal of Public Health*, 71, 409–412.

Donabedian, A. (1997). The quality of care. How can it be assessed? 1988. *Archives of Pathology & Laboratory Medicine*, 121, 1145–1150.

Donabedian, A. (2005). Evaluating the quality of medical care. 1966. *The Milbank Quarterly*, 83, 691–729.

Dudgeon, D. (2007). Ontario, Canada: using networks to integrate palliative care province-wide. *Journal of Pain and Symptom Management*, 33, 640–644.

Eagar, K., Watters, P., Currow, D. C., Aoun, S. M., and Yates, P. (2010). The Australian Palliative Care Outcomes Collaboration (PCOC)—measuring the quality and outcomes of palliative care on a routine basis. *Australian Health Review*, 34, 186–192.

Eastman, P. and Martin, P. (2012). Factors influencing survival after discharge from an Australian palliative care unit to residential aged care facilities: a retrospective audit. *Journal of Palliative Medicine*, 15, 327–333.

Eisenchlas, J.H., Harding, R., Daud, M.L., Perez, M., De Simone, G.G., and Higginson, I.J. (2008). Use of the palliative outcome scale in Argentina: a cross-cultural adaptation and validation study. *Journal of Pain and Symptom Management*, 35, 188–202.

Ellershaw, J.E., Peat, S.J., and Boys, L.C. (1995). Assessing the effectiveness of a hospital palliative care team. *Palliative Medicine*, 9, 145–152.

Evans, C. J., Harding, R., and Higginson, I.J. (2013) 'Best practice' in developing and evaluating palliative and end-of-life care services: a meta-synthesis of research methods for the MORECare project. *Palliative Medicine*, 27(10), 885–898.

Ferrell, B.J., Connor, S.R., Cordes, A., *et al.* (2007). The National Agenda for Quality Palliative Care: The National Consensus Project and the National Quality Forum. *Journal of Pain and Symptom Management*, 33, 737–744.

Finlay, I.G. and Dunlop, R. (1994). Quality of life assessment in palliative care. *Annals of Oncology*, 5, 13–18

Galbraith, P.S. and Booth, S. (2004). Audit of the use of a formatted postcard to communicate between a hospital palliative care team and general practitioners. *Palliative Medicine*, 18, 666–667.

Galvin, J. (2002). An audit of pressure ulcer incidence in a palliative care setting. *International Journal of Palliative Nursing*, 8, 214–221.

Godfrey, J. and Poole, L. (2007). An audit of the use of the Barthel Index in palliative care. *International Journal of Palliative Nursing*, 13, 543–548.

Gomes, B., Calanzani, N., Curiale, V., McCrone, P., and Higginson, I. J. (2013a). Effectiveness and cost-effectiveness of home palliative care services for adults with advanced illness and their caregivers. *The Cochrane Database of Systematic Reviews*, 6, CD007760.

Gomes, B., Calanzani, N., Gysels, M., Hall, S., and Higginson, I. J. (2013b). Heterogeneity and changes in preferences for dying at home: a systematic review. *BMC Palliative Care*, 12, 7.

Harding, R. and Leam, C. (2005). Clinical notes for informal carers in palliative care: recommendations from a random patient file audit. *Palliative Medicine*, 19, 639–642.

Harding, R., Selman, L., Agupio, G., *et al.* (2010). Validation of a core outcome measure for palliative care in Africa: the APCA African Palliative Outcome Scale. *Health and Quality of Life Outcomes*, 8, 10.

Harding, R., Selman, L., Simms, V. M., et al. (2013). How to analyze palliative care outcome data for patients in Sub-Saharan Africa: an international, multicenter, factor analytic examination of the APCA African POS. *Journal of Pain and Symptom Management*, 45, 746–752.

Harding, R., Simon, S.T., Benalia, H., *et al.* (2011). The PRISMA Symposium 1: outcome tool use. Disharmony in European outcomes research for palliative and advanced disease care: too many tools in practice. *Journal of Pain and Symptom Management*, 42, 493–500.

Hearn, J. and Higginson, I.J. (1999). Development and validation of a core outcome measure for palliative care: the palliative care outcome scale. Palliative Care Core Audit Project Advisory Group. *Quality in Health Care: QHC*, 8, 219–227.

Higginson, I. (1993). Palliative care: a review of past changes and future trends. *Journal of Public Health Medicine*, 15, 3–8.

Higginson, I. (1994). Clinical audit and organizational audit in palliative care. *Cancer Surveys*, 21, 233–245.

Higginson, I. and McCarthy, M. (1989). Measuring symptoms in terminal cancer: are pain and dyspnoea controlled? *Journal of the Royal Society of Medicine*, 82, 264–267.

Higginson, I.J. and Bruera, E. (2002). Do we need palliative care audit in developing countries? *Palliative Medicine*, 16, 546–547.

Higginson, I.J. and Evans, C.J. (2010). What is the evidence that palliative care teams improve outcomes for cancer patients and their families? *Cancer Journal*, 16, 423–435.

Higginson, I.J., Evans, C.J., Grande, G., *et al.* (2013). Evaluating complex interventions in end of life care: the MORECare statement on good practice generated by a synthesis of transparent expert consultations and systematic reviews. *BMC Medicine*, 11, 111.

Higginson, I.J., Finlay, I.G., Goodwin, D.M., *et al.* (2003). Is there evidence that palliative care teams alter end-of-life experiences of patients and their caregivers? *Journal of Pain and Symptom Management*, 25, 150–168.

Higginson, I.J., Hearn, J., and Webb, D. (1996). Audit in palliative care: does practice change? *European Journal of Cancer Care*, 5, 233–236.

Higginson, I.J., Jarman, B., Astin, P., *et al.* (1999). Do social factors affect where patients die: an analysis of 10 years of cancer deaths in England. *Journal of Public Health Medicine*, 21, 22–28

Higginson, I.J., Simon, S.T., Benalia, H., *et al.* (2012). Republished: which questions of two commonly used multidimensional palliative care patient reported outcome measures are most useful? Results from the European and African PRISMA survey. *Postgraduate Medical Journal*, 88, 451–457.

Higginson, I.J., Wade, A.M., and Mccarthy, M. (1992). Effectiveness of two palliative support teams. *Journal of Public Health Medicine*, 14, 50–56.

Hui, D. and Bruera, E. (2013). Minimal clinically important differences in the Edmonton symptom assessment system: the anchor is key. *Journal of Pain and Symptom Management*, 45, e4–5.

Hughes, R., Higginson, I.J., Addington-Hall, J., *et al.* (2001). Project to impROve Management Of TErminal illness (PROMOTE). *Journal of Interprofessional Care*, 15, 398–399.

Hunt, J., Keeley, V. L., Cobb, M., and Ahmedzai, S. H. (2004). A new quality assurance package for hospital palliative care teams: the Trent Hospice Audit Group model. *British Journal of Cancer*, 91, 248–253.

Kaasa, S., Jordhoy, M. S., and Haugen, D. F. (2007). Palliative care in Norway: a national public health model. *Journal of Pain and Symptom Management*, 33, 599–604.

Kellehear, A. (2000). Spirituality and palliative care: a model of needs. *Palliative Medicine*, 14, 149–155.

Kellehear, A. (2001). The changing face of dying in Australia. *The Medical journal of Australia*, 175, 508–510.

Kellehear, A. (2009). On dying and human suffering. *Palliative Medicine*, 23, 388–397.

Le, B.H. and Ashby, M.A. (2007). Audit of deaths and palliative care referrals in a large Australian teaching hospital. *Journal of Palliative Medicine*, 10, 835–836.

Lee, L., White, V., Ball, J., *et al.* (2001). An audit of oral care practice and staff knowledge in hospital palliative care. *International Journal of Palliative Nursing*, 7, 395–400.

Ling, J. (2000). Audit in practice: the referral of dying patients to palliative care. *International Journal of Palliative Nursing*, 6, 375–379.

McGee, H.M., O'Boyle, C.A., Hickey, A., *et al.* (1991). Assessing the quality of life of the individual: the SEIQoL with a healthy and a gastroenterology unit population. *Psychological Medicine*, 21, 749–759

Maxwell, I. (1986). Quality assurance: simple, rational and desirable. *Dimensions in Health Service*, 63, 36–37.

Maxwell, R.J. (1984). Quality assessment in health. *British Medical Journal*, 288, 1470–1472.

Maxwell, R.J. (1992). Dimensions of quality revisited: from thought to action. *Quality in Health Care: QHC*, 1, 171–177.

Miller, J. and Hopkinson, C. (2008). A retrospective audit exploring the use of relaxation as an intervention in oncology and palliative care. *European Journal of Cancer Care*, 17, 488–491.

Morita, T., Fujimoto, K., Namba, M., *et al.* (2008). Palliative care needs of cancer outpatients receiving chemotherapy: an audit of a clinical screening project. *Supportive Care in Cancer*, 16, 101–107.

Morita, T., Fujimoto, K., and Tei, Y. (2005). Palliative care team: the first year audit in Japan. *Journal of Pain and Symptom Management*, 29, 458–465.

Nadimi, F. and Currow, D. C. (2011). As death approaches: a retrospective survey of the care of adults dying in Alice Springs Hospital. *The Australian Journal of Rural Health*, 19, 4–8.

Newbury, J. and Hatherell, C. A. (2004). Audit on discharging patients from community specialist palliative care nursing services. *International Journal of Palliative Nursing*, 10, 24–31.

Payne, M. (2007). Safeguarding adults at end of life: audit and case analysis in a palliative care setting. *Journal of Social Work in End-Of-Life & Palliative Care*, 3, 31–46.

Payne, S., Smith, P., and Dean, S. (1999). Identifying the concerns of informal carers in palliative care. *Palliative Medicine*, 13, 37–44.

Richardson, L.A. and Jones, G.W. (2009). A review of the reliability and validity of the Edmonton Symptom Assessment System. *Current Oncology*, 16, 55.

Rosser, R. (1985). A history of the development of health indices. In G.T. Smith (ed.) *Measuring the Social Benefits of Medicine*, pp. 31–49. London: Office of Health Economics.

Saleem, T. Z., Higginson, I. J., Chaudhuri, K. R., Martin, A., Burman, R., and Leigh, P. N. (2013). Symptom prevalence, severity and palliative care needs assessment using the Palliative Outcome Scale: a cross-sectional study of patients with Parkinson's disease and related neurological conditions. *Palliative Medicine*, 27(8), 722–731.

Selby, D., Chakraborty, A., Myers, J., Saskin, R., Mazzotta, P., and Gill, A. (2011). High scores on the Edmonton Symptom Assessment Scale identify patients with self-defined high symptom burden. *Journal of Palliative Medicine*, 14, 1309–1316.

Selman, L. and Harding, R. (2010). How can we improve outcomes for patients and families under palliative care? Implementing clinical audit for quality improvement in resource limited settings. *Indian Journal of Palliative Care*, 16, 8–15.

Selman, L., Harding, R., Gysels, M., Speck, P., and Higginson, I. J. (2011). The measurement of spirituality in palliative care and the content of tools validated cross-culturally: a systematic review. *Journal of Pain and Symptom Management*, 41, 728–753.

Selman, L., Harding, R., Speck, P., *et al.* (2010). *Spiritual Care Recommendations for People from Black and Minority Ethnic (BME) Groups Receiving Palliative Care in the UK*. London: Cicely Saunders Institute.

Selman, L., Higginson, I. J., Agupio, G., et al. (2009). Meeting information needs of patients with incurable progressive disease and their families in South Africa and Uganda: multicentre qualitative study. *BMJ*, 338, b1326.

Shaw, C.D. (1980a). Aspects of audit. 1. The background. *British Medical Journal*, 280, 1256–1258.

Shaw, C.D. (1980b). Aspects of audit. 2. Audit in British hospitals. *British Medical Journal*, 280, 1314–1316.

Shaw, C.D. (1980c). Aspects of audit. 3: Audit in British general practice. *British Medical Journal*, 280, 1361–1363.

Shaw, C.D. (1980d). Aspects of audit. 4: Acceptability of audit. *British Medical Journal*, 280, 1443–1446.

Shaw, C.D. (1980e). Aspects of audit. 5: Looking forward to audit. *British Medical Journal*, 280, 1509–1511.

Shaw, C.D. (1988). Management and medical audit. *Australian Clinical Review/Australian Medical Association [and] the Australian Council on Hospital Standards*, 8, 185–187.

Shaw, C.D. (1989). Audit in internal medicine. *British Journal of Hospital Medicine*, 42, 19.

Shaw, C.D. (1990). Criterion based audit. *BMJ*, 300, 649–651.

Shaw, C. (1991). Specifications for hospital medical audit. *Health Services Management*, 87, 124–125.

Siegert, R.J., Gao, W., Walkey, F.H., and Higginson, I. (2010). Psychological well-being and quality of care: a factor-analytic examination of the palliative care outcome scale. *Journal of Pain and Symptom Management*, 40, 67–74.

Singer, P.A., Martin, D.K., and Bowman, K. (2000). Quality end-of-life care: where do we go from here? *Journal of Palliative Medicine*, 3, 403–405.

Singer, P.A., Martin, D.K., and Kelner, M. (1999). Quality end-of-life care: patients' perspectives. *Journal of the American Medical Association*, 281, 163–168.

Stevens, A.M., Gwilliam, B., A'hern, R., Broadley, K., and Hardy, J. (2005). Experience in the use of the palliative care outcome scale. *Supportive Care in Cancer*, 13, 1027–1034.

Stewart, A.L., Teno, J., Patrick, D.L., and Lynn, J. (1999). The concept of quality of life of dying persons in the context of health care. *Journal of Pain and Symptom Management*, 17, 93–108.

Tsai, L.Y., Li, I.F., Liu, C.P., Su, W.H., and Change, T.Y. (2008). Application of quality audit tools to evaluate care quality received by terminal cancer patients admitted to a palliative care unit. *Supportive Care in Cancer*, 16, 1067–1074.

Veerbeek, L., Van Zuylen, L., Gambles, M., *et al.* (2006). Audit of the Liverpool Care Pathway for the Dying Patient in a Dutch cancer hospital. *Journal of Palliative Care*, 22, 305–308.

Watanabe, S.M., Nekolaichuk, C.L., and Beaumont, C. (2012a). The Edmonton Symptom Assessment System, a proposed tool for distress screening in cancer patients: development and refinement. *Psycho-Oncology*, 21, 977–985.

Watanabe, S.M., Nekolaichuk, C.L., and Beaumont, C. (2012b). Palliative care providers' opinions of the Edmonton symptom assessment system revised (ESAS-r) in clinical practice. *Journal of Pain and Symptom Management*, 44, e2–3.

Zimmermann, C., Cheung, W.Y., Lo, C., and Rodin, G. (2011). Edmonton Symptom Assessment System screening and depression at the end of life. *Journal of Clinical Oncology*, 29, 3107–3108.

Index

Note: Page numbers in **bold** indicate major coverage of a topic. Those in *italics* refer to figures, tables, and boxes.